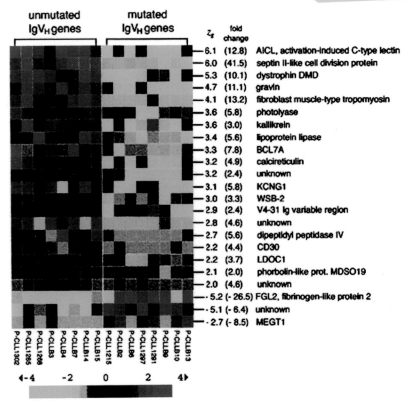

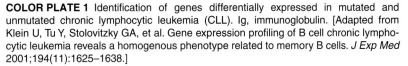

COLOR PLATE 1 Identification of genes differentially expressed in mutated and unmutated chronic lymphocytic leukemia (CLL). Ig, immunoglobulin. [Adapted from Klein U, Tu Y, Stolovitzky GA, et al. Gene expression profiling of B cell chronic lymphocytic leukemia reveals a homogenous phenotype related to memory B cells. *J Exp Med* 2001;194(11):1625–1638.]

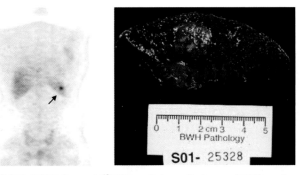

COLOR PLATE 2 Coronal [^{18}F]-fluoro-2-deoxy-D-glucose (FDG)–positron emission tomography (PET) section through the spleen showing focal abnormal uptake (*arrow*) and correlative pathologic splenic sample confirming focal recurrence as suggested by the FDG-PET scan.

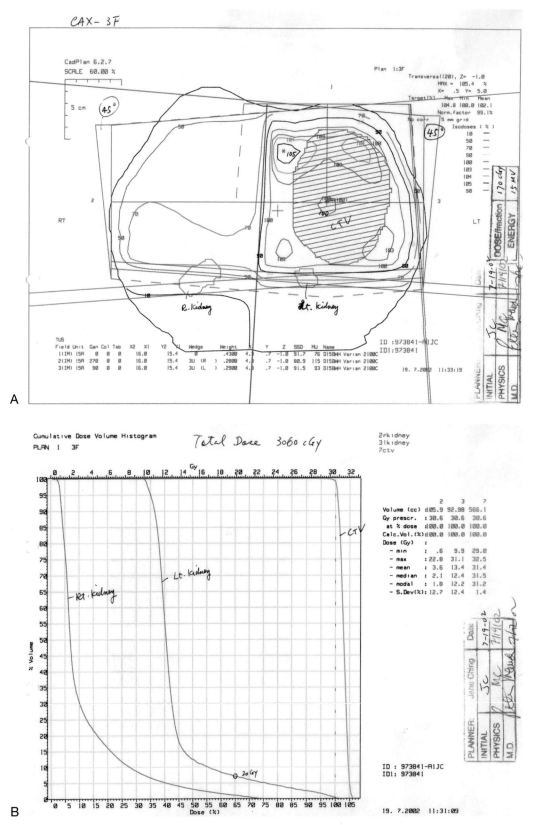

COLOR PLATE 3 Three-field radiation treatment for a gastric lymphoma. **A:** Graphic plan for the three-field technique, showing isodose distribution to the clinical target volume (CTV) and the kidneys. **B:** Dose-volume histograms of the CTV and the kidneys, showing the sparing of most of the right kidney with the three-field technique. Lt., left; Rt., right.

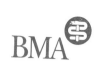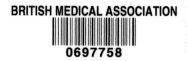

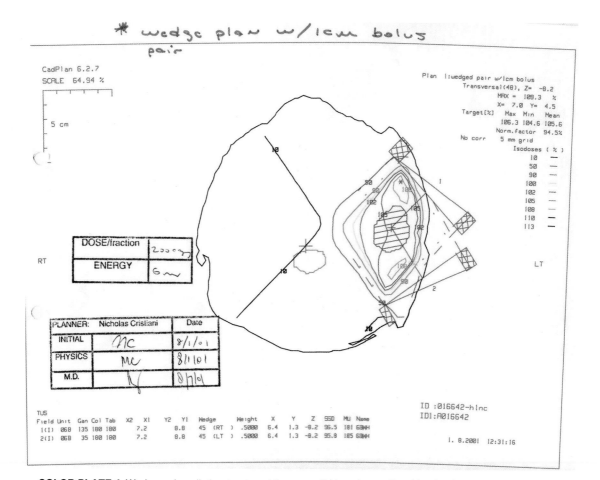

COLOR PLATE 4 Wedge pair radiation treatment for a parotid lymphoma. Graphic plan for the wedge pair technique, showing isodose distribution to the clinical target volume and the spinal cord, with sparing of the contralateral parotid.

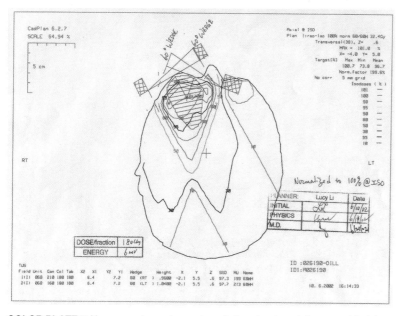

COLOR PLATE 5 Narrow-angle wedge pair radiation treatment for an orbital lymphoma. Graphic plan for the narrow-angle wedge pair technique, showing isodose distribution to the involved right orbit and the contralateral, uninvolved orbit.

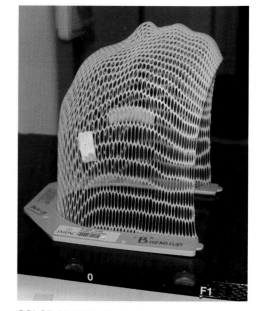

COLOR PLATE 6 Customized Aquaplast mask for patient immobilization when receiving radiation therapy to the head and neck region.

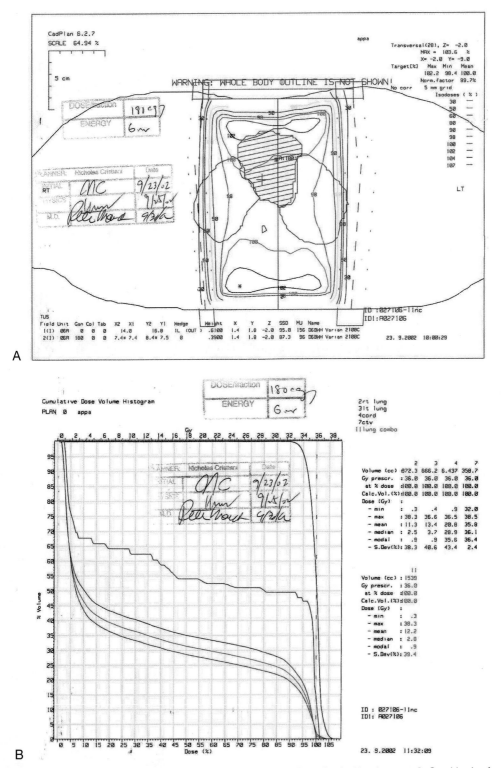

COLOR PLATE 7 A modified mantle field in a lymphoma patient with mediastinal involvement. **A:** Graphic plan for modified mantle field, showing isodose distribution to the clinical target volume and the surrounding normal lungs. **B:** Dose-volume histograms of the clinical target volume, lungs, and spinal cord. Approximately 30% of the lungs were receiving 20 Gy in this case. LT, left; RT, right.

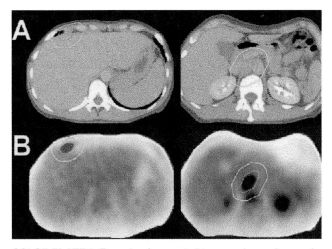

COLOR PLATE 8 Example of computed tomography–positron emission tomography (CT-PET) image fusion. Simultaneous contouring of the target volumes on the treatment-planning CT **(A)** and PET **(B)** scans improve anatomic accuracy. The yellow contour depicts the planning target volume, whereas the aqua color depicts the gross tumor volume.

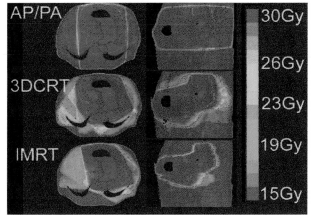

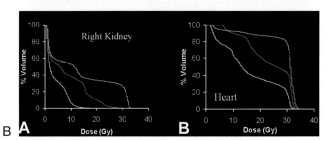

COLOR PLATE 9 Definitive external beam radiation therapy for gastric mucosa–associated lymphoid tissue lymphoma. **A:** The representative axial and sagittal color-wash displays compare the dose distributions using an anterior/posterior (AP/PA) technique, three-dimensional conformal radiotherapy (3DCRT), and intensity-modulated radiation therapy (IMRT). Computed tomography (CT)–based treatment planning and IMRT improve dose conformality and homogeneity. **B:** Dose-volume histograms are shown for an AP/PA technique, 3DCRT, and IMRT. The green curve represents the IMRT plan, the violet curve the 3DCRT, and the yellow curve the AP/PA. The IMRT plan is superior in minimizing the dose to the right kidney and the heart, thereby reducing the risk of treatment-related toxicity.

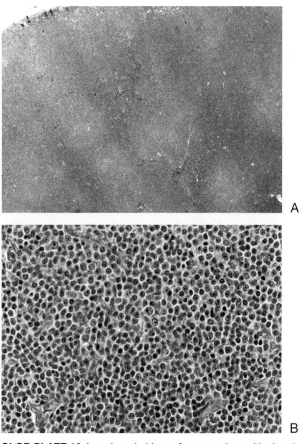

COLOR PLATE 10 Lymph node biopsy from a patient with chronic lymphocytic leukemia. At low magnification **(A)**, there is a vaguely nodular (pseudofollicular) pattern. **B:** Higher magnification shows a predominance of small lymphocytes with scattered larger cells known as *prolymphocytes* and *paraimmunoblasts*.

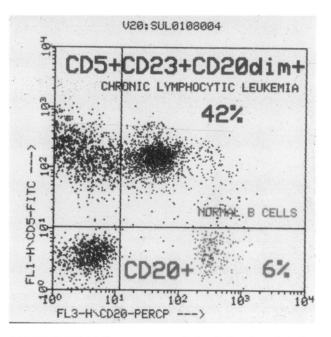

COLOR PLATE 11 Flow cytometry of chronic lymphocytic leukemia. The cells express dim CD20, dim CD5, and CD23. (Courtesy of Dr. Frederick I. Preffer, Department of Pathology, Massachusetts General Hospital, Boston, MA.)

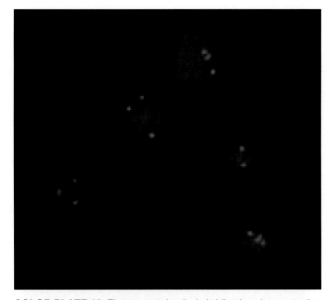

COLOR PLATE 12 Fluorescent *in situ* hybridization demonstrating trisomy 12 in chronic lymphocytic leukemia.

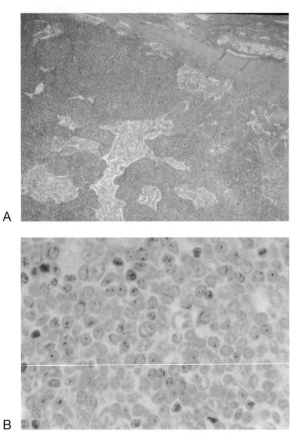

A

B

COLOR PLATE 13 Lymph node from a patient with Waldenström's macroglobulinemia. **A:** At low magnification, there are open sinuses with a histiocytic reaction to secreted immunoglobulin. **B:** At high magnification, there is a mixture of lymphocytes, plasma cells, and intermediate cells with lymphocyte-like nuclei and plasma cell–like cytoplasm, known as *plasmacytoid lymphocytes.*

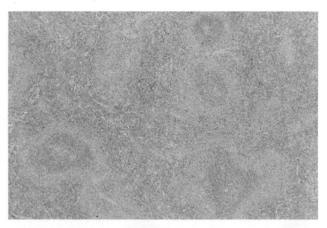

COLOR PLATE 14 Histologic image of a typical splenic marginal zone lymphoma case, showing micronodular infiltrate, biphasic cytology, and marginal zone differentiation.

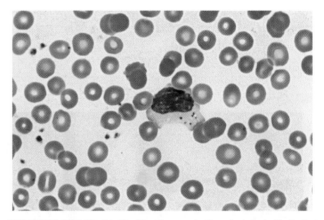

COLOR PLATE 15 A typical large granular lymphocyte is illustrated in this peripheral blood film. Note sparse, yet prominent, cytoplasmic granules in this mature-appearing lymphoid cell. (Wright's stain.)

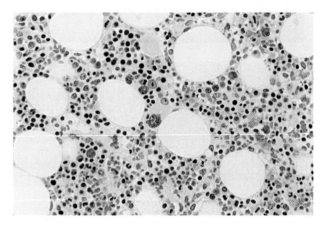

COLOR PLATE 16 Although inconspicuous on hematoxylin and eosin sections of this hypocellular bone marrow specimen, significant infiltration by T-cell large granular lymphocytic leukemia was documented by specialized techniques. (See Color Plates 17 and 18.)

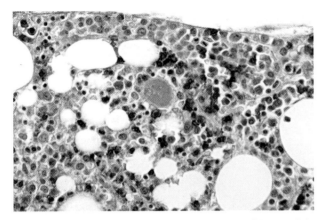

COLOR PLATE 17 Immunoperoxidase staining for CD3 highlights significant numbers of both clustered and individually dispersed T cells, in this case with subtle bone marrow involvement by T-cell large granular lymphocytic leukemia. (Immunoperoxidase staining for CD3.)

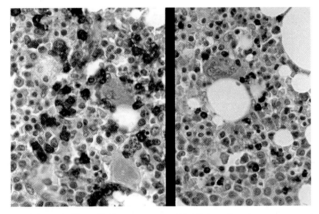

COLOR PLATE 18 This composite highlights the immunoperoxidase staining for CD8 (*left*) and TIA-1 (*right*) in this bone marrow biopsy section exhibiting subtle involvement by T-cell large granular lymphocytic leukemia. Note sinusoidal involvement on CD8 stain. (Immunoperoxidase staining for CD8 and TIA-1.)

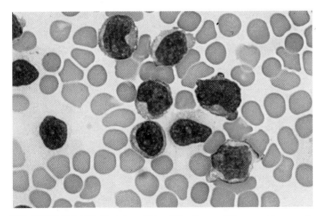

COLOR PLATE 19 Peripheral blood film from a 65-year-old man who presented with a white blood cell count of 280×10^9/L showing lymphocytes with distinct nucleoli and cytoplasmic blebbing. (Wright's stain.)

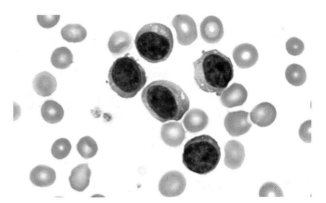

COLOR PLATE 20 Peripheral blood film from a 69-year-old man with a white blood cell count of 112×10^9/L, hemoglobin of 8 g/dL, and a platelet count of 50×10^9/L showing mature lymphocytes with condensed chromatin and inconspicuous nucleoli mimicking chronic lymphocytic leukemia. (Wright's stain.) This case represents an example of the small-cell variant of T-cell prolymphocytic leukemia.

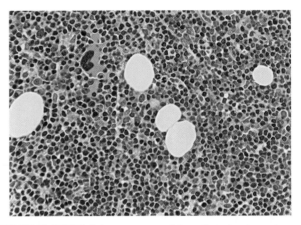

COLOR PLATE 21 A bone marrow clot section showing a hypercellular bone marrow in a 65-year-old man with T-cell prolymphocytic leukemia. Note extensive diffuse interstitial infiltration. (Hematoxylin and eosin stain.)

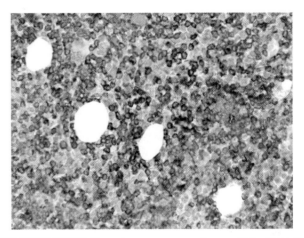

COLOR PLATE 22 Same bone marrow section as Color Plate 20 showing extensive CD3 positivity by the immunoperoxidase technique.

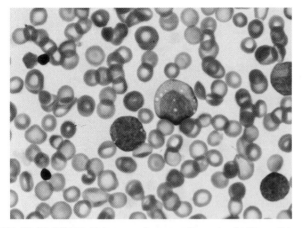

COLOR PLATE 23 This case of aggressive natural killer–cell leukemia/lymphoma in a native American patient is characterized by immature, blastic nuclear features. Note cytoplasmic granules. (Wright-Giemsa stain.)

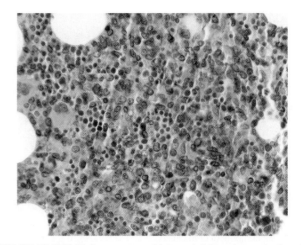

COLOR PLATE 26 Immunoperoxidase staining for cytoplasmic CD3ε in a case of aggressive natural killer–cell leukemia/lymphoma.

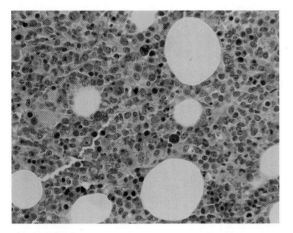

COLOR PLATE 24 Bone marrow clot section showing an extensive interstitial infiltrate of blastic large cells confirmed to be natural killer cells by immunophenotypic assessment (see Color Plates 26–28). (Hematoxylin and eosin stain.)

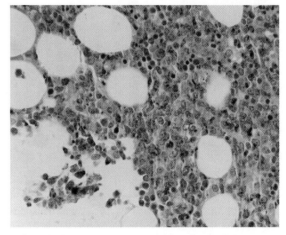

COLOR PLATE 27 Immunoperoxidase staining for TIA-1 cytoplasmic staining in a case of aggressive natural killer cell leukemia/lymphoma.

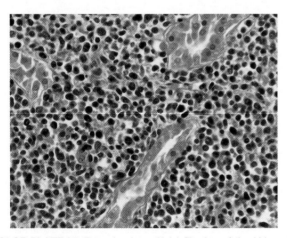

COLOR PLATE 25 Extensive interstitial infiltration of the kidney by aggressive natural killer–cell leukemia/lymphoma is evident. Note pleomorphism of leukemia/lymphoma cells. (Hematoxylin and eosin stain.)

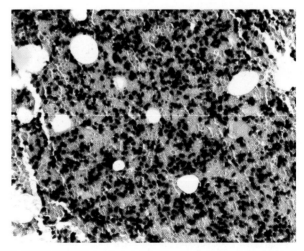

COLOR PLATE 28 *In situ* hybridization for EBER (Epstein-Barr virus RNA) in a case of aggressive natural killer–cell leukemia/lymphoma.

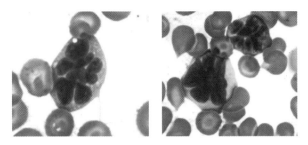

COLOR PLATE 29 The markedly polylobated neoplastic cells of adult T-cell leukemia-lymphoma in the peripheral blood. They have been termed *flower cells* based on the petal-like appearance of the nuclear lobes.

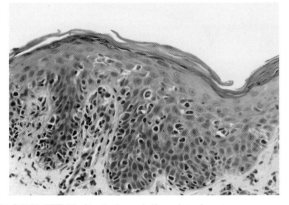

COLOR PLATE 30 Atypical cerebriform lymphocytes are arranged in a linear pattern along the dermoepidermal junction. Similar atypical lymphocytes are scattered within the upper epidermal layers, without accompanying spongiosis.

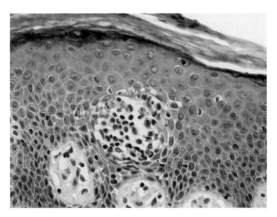

COLOR PLATE 31 Pautrier collections of atypical lymphocytes are characteristic of mycosis fungoides but are seen in only a minority of early-stage lesions.

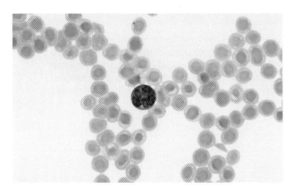

COLOR PLATE 32 Sézary cell within peripheral blood. Note the cerebriform nuclear convolution.

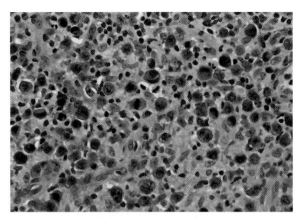

COLOR PLATE 33 In cases of large-cell transformation, the dermis demonstrates many large, cytologically atypical lymphocytes with prominent nucleoli and easily appreciated mitotic activity.

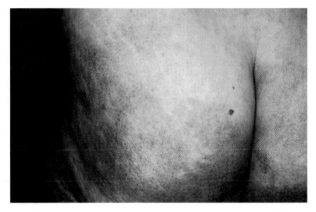

COLOR PLATE 34 Typical erythematous patch disease in the bathing trunk distribution.

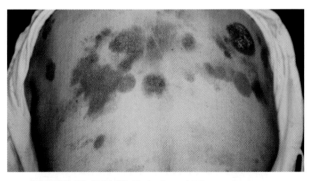

COLOR PLATE 35 Typical patch/plaque disease.

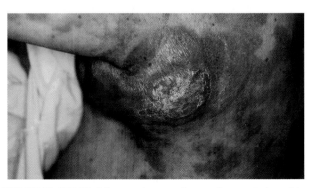

COLOR PLATE 36 A large cutaneous tumor of mycosis fungoides in a background of patch/plaque disease.

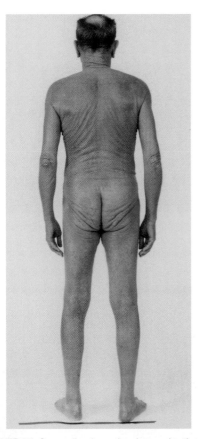

COLOR PLATE 37 Generalized erythroderma in the context of Sézary syndrome.

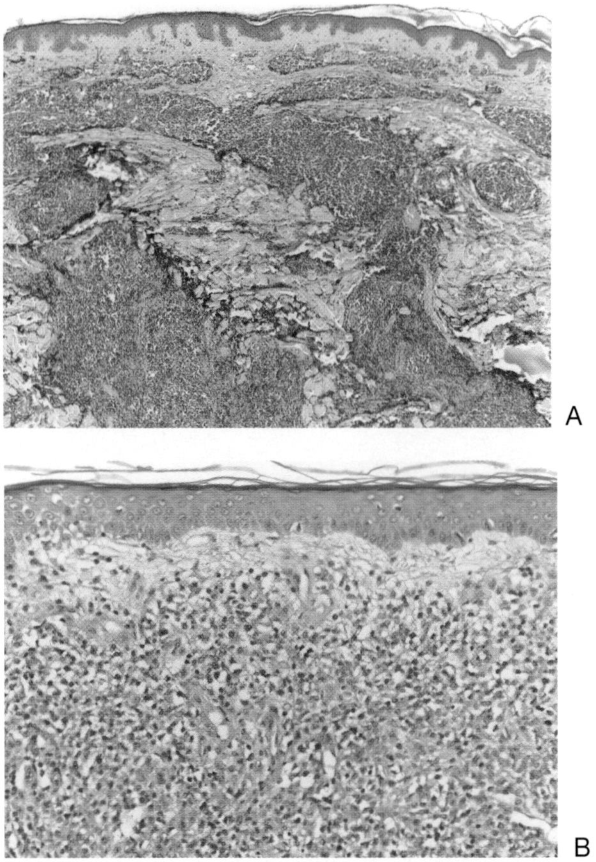

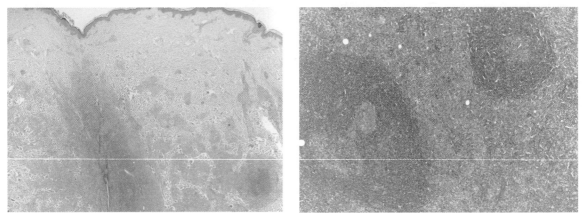

A

B

COLOR PLATE 38 Cutaneous follicular lymphoma. **A:** This dense lymphoid infiltrate occupies the superficial and deep dermis and is separated from the epidermis by a grenz zone of uninvolved dermis. No significant epidermal changes are present. Lymphoid follicles are present but may be inconspicuous. **B:** This B-cell lymphoma is composed of centrocytes and centroblasts with a surrounding infiltrate of nonneoplastic T cells.

A

B

COLOR PLATE 39 Cutaneous marginal zone B-cell lymphoma (low grade B-cell lymphoma of mucosa-associated lymphoid tissue-type). **A:** This dense lymphoid infiltrate occupies the superficial and deep dermis and is separated from the epidermis by a grenz zone of uninvolved dermis. No significant epidermal changes are present. Lymphoid follicles are present and surrounded by an infiltrate of neoplastic B cells. **B:** Neoplastic plasma cells and marginal zone B cells with small cleaved nuclei and variably abundant amphophilic cytoplasm are present in the dermis between two reactive lymphoid follicles.

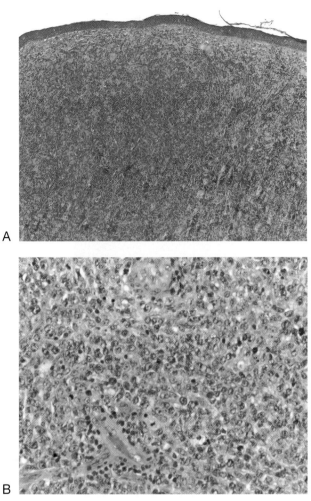

A

B

COLOR PLATE 40 Diffuse large B-cell lymphoma. **A:** This diffuse infiltrate of lymphocytes occupies the dermis with atrophy of the overlying epidermis. **B:** The tumor is composed of large neoplastic B cells, predominantly centroblasts and immunoblasts, with scattered centrocytes.

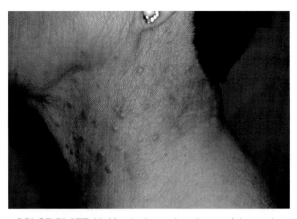

COLOR PLATE 42 Marginal zone lymphoma of the trunk.

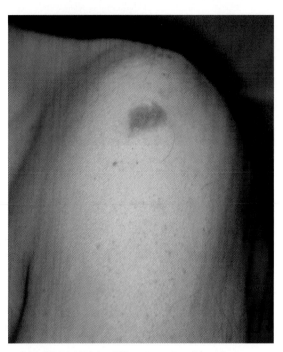

COLOR PLATE 43 Diffuse large B-cell lymphoma.

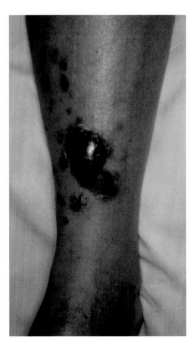

COLOR PLATE 41 Diffuse large B-cell lymphoma of the leg.

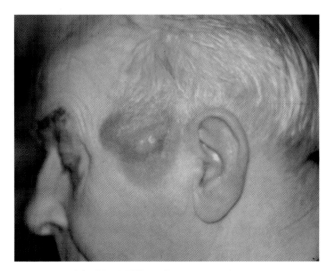

COLOR PLATE 44 Follicular lymphoma.

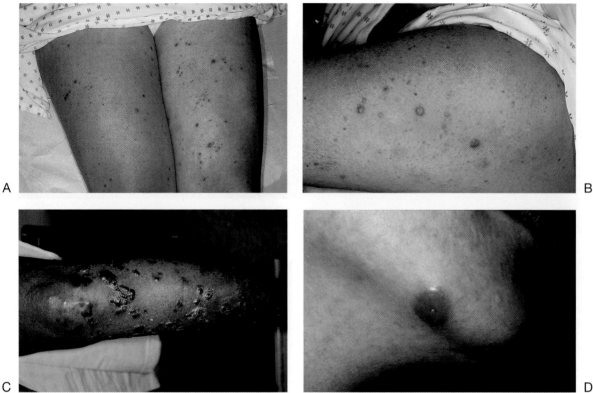

COLOR PLATE 45 Clinical appearance of CD30⁺ cutaneous lesions. **A,B:** Multiple lesions of lymphomatoid papulosis in various stages of regression on the leg of a female patient. **C:** Multiple nonregressing tumors of CD30⁺ cutaneous anaplastic large-cell lymphoma on the leg of a male patient. **D:** Borderline lesion on the mandible of young female patient.

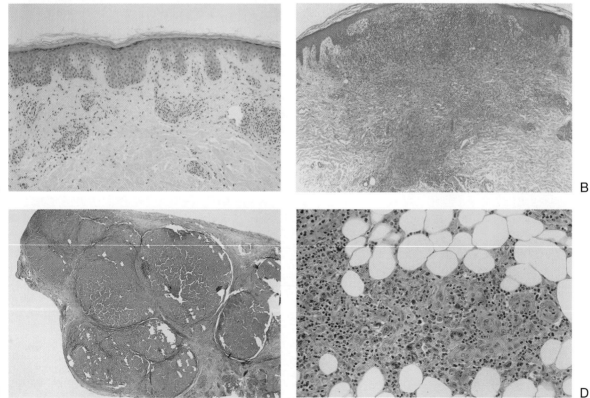

COLOR PLATE 46 Distribution of lymphoid infiltrate in CD30⁺ cutaneous lesions. **A:** Early lesion of lymphomatoid papulosis showing perivascular accumulation of atypical lymphocytes. **B:** Fully developed wedge-shaped lesion of lymphomatoid papulosis. **C:** Extensive multinodular lesion of CD30⁺ cutaneous anaplastic large-cell lymphoma. **D:** Extension of anaplastic large-cell lymphoma into subcutis.

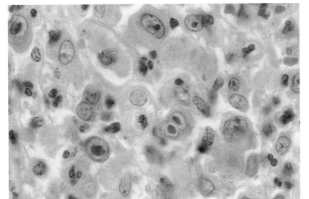

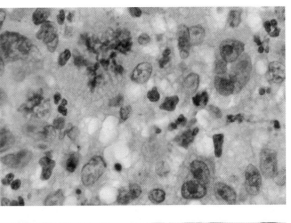

A

B

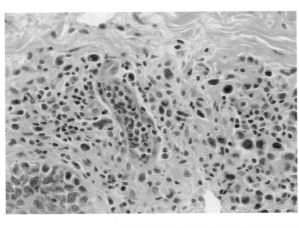

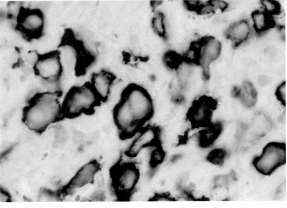

C

D

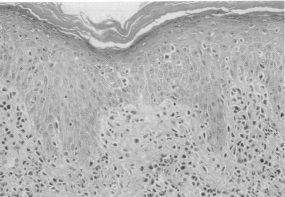

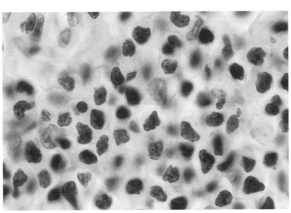

E

F

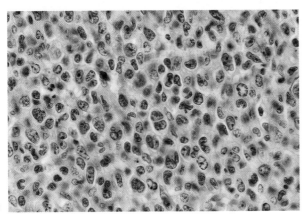

COLOR PLATE 47 Histopathology of lymphomatoid papulosis.
A: Type A lesion of lymphomatoid papulosis with Reed-Sternberg–like cells. B: Type A lesion with abnormal mitosis and
Reed-Sternberg–like cells surrounded by neutrophils and eosinophils. C: Type A lesion with neutrophils within a blood vessel.
D: Type A lesion with an immunoperoxidase stain showing many
atypical cells staining for CD30. E: Type B lesion showing atypical lymphocytes in superficial papillary dermis with migration into
the epidermis. F: Convoluted cerebriform lymphocytes in a type
B lesion of lymphomatoid papulosis. G: Type C lesion with the
monotonous appearance of atypical lymphocytes.

G

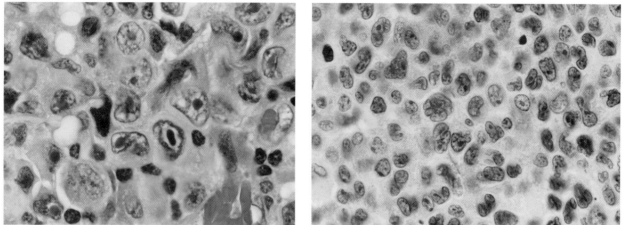

COLOR PLATE 48 Histopathology of two CD30$^+$ cutaneous large-cell lymphomas. **A:** Anaplastic lymphocytes with prominent eosinophilic nucleoli. **B:** Pleomorphic lymphocytes with irregular nuclei and small nucleoli.

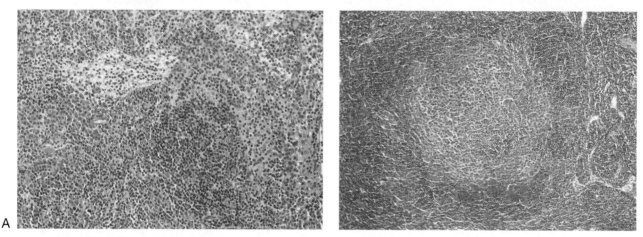

COLOR PLATE 49 Histopathology of nodal marginal zone B-cell lymphoma. **A:** An atrophic follicle is surrounded by an infiltrate of small plasmacytoid cells (interfollicular and perisinusoidal pattern). **B:** A reactive follicle is colonized by large transformed cells, simulating follicular lymphoma (grade 3). The low-grade component can be recognized in the interfollicular area.

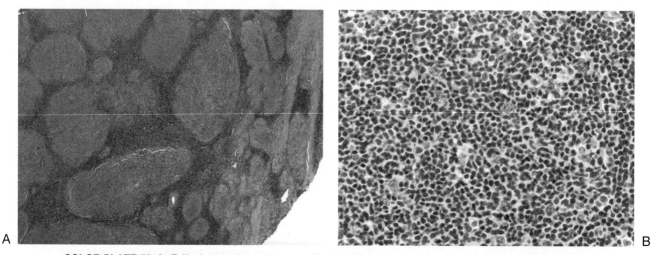

COLOR PLATE 50 A: Follicular lymphoma, low magnification. There are closely packed follicles of varying sizes, extending beyond the lymph node capsule into the fat, associated with sclerosis. **B:** Follicular lymphoma, grade 1/3, high magnification. The majority of the cells are small centrocytes with cleaved nuclei; there are rare large non-cleaved centroblasts with small nucleoli.

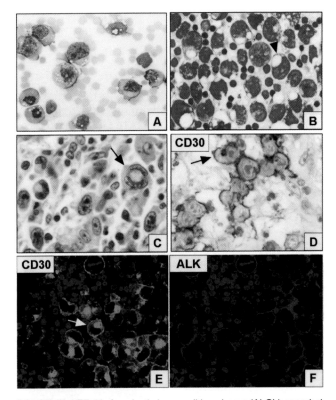

COLOR PLATE 51 Anaplastic large-cell lymphoma (ALCL): morphology and phenotype. **A:** ALCL, common type. Large tumor cells showing vacuolized cytoplasm (ascitic fluid; May-Grunwald-Giemsa; ×800). **B:** ALCL with "signet-ring" appearance (*arrowhead*) (lymph node imprint; May-Grunwald-Giemsa; ×800). **C:** ALCL, common type (lymph node paraffin section). The arrow points to a large tumor cell with a bizzarre nucleus (hematoxylin and eosin; ×800). **D:** ALCL cells show strong CD30 positivity at the surface and in the Golgi area (*arrow*) (APAAP technique; ×800). **E,F:** Double immunofluorescence labeling (rhodamin/fluorescein) of tumor cells for CD30 (E) and anaplastic lymphoma kinase (F) in lymph node paraffin sections from ALCL, common type. The arrow in (E) points to a neoplastic cell showing positivity on the cell surface and Golgi area. (E amd F from Falini B, Mason DY. Proteins encoded by genes involved in chromosomal alterations in lymphoma and leukemia: clinical value of their detection by immunocytochemistry. *Blood* 2002;99:409–426, with permission.)

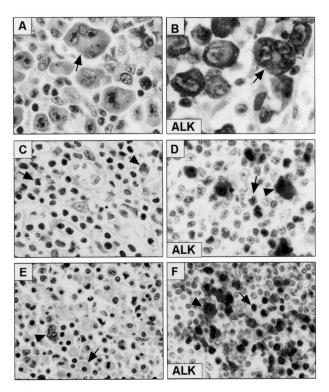

COLOR PLATE 52 Anaplastic large-cell lymphoma (ALCL): morphologic variants and anaplastic lympoma kinase (ALK) expression. **A,B:** ALCL, common type (lymph node paraffin sections). **A:** The arrow points to a "hallmark cell" (hematoxylin and eosin; ×800). **B:** Tumor cells from the same case show cytoplasmic-restricted labeling for the ALK protein (*arrow*) (monoclonal antibody ALKc; APAAP technique; ×800). **C,D:** ALCL, small-cell variant (lymph node paraffin sections). **C:** Small (*arrow*) to medium-sized (*arrowhead*) tumor cells showing a clear cytoplasm and irregular nuclei (hematoxylin and eosin; ×800). **D:** Large anaplastic tumor cells show ALK expression both in the cytoplasm and the nucleus (*arrowhead*). In the smaller cells with irregular nuclei, ALK labeling is restricted to the nucleus (*arrow*) (monoclonal antibody ALKc; APAAP technique; ×800). **E,F:** ALCL, lymphohistiocytic variant (lymph node paraffin sections). **E:** Small- and large-sized (*arrowhead*) tumor cells are admixed with a high number of reactive histiocytes (*arrow*) (hematoxylin and eosin; ×800). **F:** The small tumor cells show a nucleus-restricted positivity for the ALK protein (*arrow*), whereas the large neoplastic elements are ALK$^+$ both in the cytoplasm and the nucleus (*arrowhead*) (monoclonal antibody ALKc; APAAP technique; ×800). (**C,D,E,** and **F** from Falini B. Anaplastic large cell lymphoma: pathological, molecular and clinical features. *Br J Haematol* 2001;114: 741–760, with permission.)

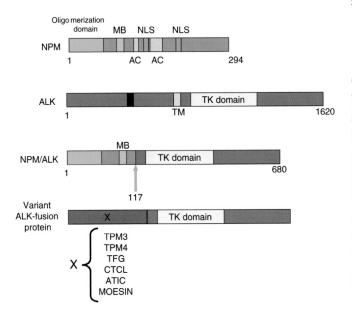

COLOR PLATE 53 Molecular structure of nucleophosmin (NPM), anaplastic lymphoma kinase (ALK), and ALK chimeric proteins. The NPM molecule consists of an oligomerization domain (residues 1–83), a metal binding domain (MB; residues 104–115), two acidic aminoacid clusters (AC; residues 120–132 and 161–188) functioning as acceptor regions for nucleolar targeting signals, and two nuclear localization signals (NLS). The ALK protein is a transmembrane tyrosine kinase (TK) receptor that contains an extracellular portion, a transmembrane domain (TM), and a TK domain in the N-terminal part of the intracytoplasmic tail. Approximately 85% of ALK$^+$ ALCL bear the NPM-ALK-fusion protein in which the extracellular and TM domains of ALK are replaced by the oligomerization domain and the metal-binding region of NPM. Approximately 15% of ALK$^+$ ALCL bear ALK-variant fusion proteins in which the extracellular and TM domains of ALK are replaced by the oligomerization domains of proteins (X) other than NPM. In all ALK fusion proteins, with the exception of moesin-ALK (see Chapter 25), the fusion point is at codon 117.

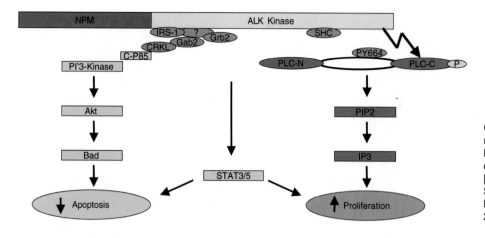

COLOR PLATE 54 Alterations of signaling pathways in anaplastic lymphoma kinase–positive (ALK+) anaplastic large-cell lymphoma. NPM, nucleophosmin. [Modified from Duyster J, Bai RY, Morris SW. Translocations involving anaplastic lymphoma kinase (ALK). *Oncogene* 2001;20:5623–5634, with permission.]

ANAPLASTIC LARGE-CELL LYMPHOMA EXPRESSING NPM-ALK

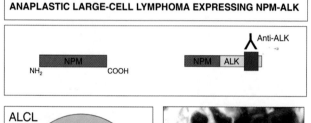

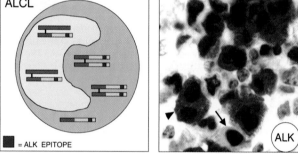

COLOR PLATE 55 Patterns of oligomerization and subcellular distribution of the nucleophosmin–anaplastic lymphoma kinase (NPM-ALK) fusion protein in ALK+ anaplastic large-cell lymphoma (ALCL) with t(2;5). ALK expression is localized only in the nucleus (*arrow*) or nucleus and cytoplasm (*arrowhead*) of tumor cells. Normal residual lymphoid cells are ALK− (lymph node paraffin section; monoclonal antibody ALKc; APAAP technique; ×800).

ANAPLASTIC LARGE-CELL LYMPHOMA EXPRESSING VARIANT ANAPLASTIC LYMPHOMA KINASE FUSION PROTEIN

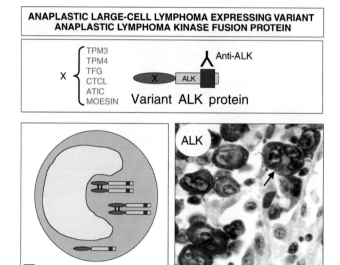

COLOR PLATE 56 Patterns of oligomerization and subcellular distribution of the anaplastic lymphoma kinase (ALK)-variant fusion proteins in ALK+ anaplastic large-cell lymphoma without t(2;5). ALK expression is localized only in the cytoplasm of tumor cells (*arrow*). Normal residual lymphoid cells are ALK− (lymph node paraffin section; monoclonal antibody ALKc; APAAP technique; ×800).

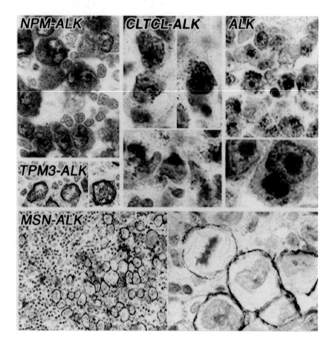

COLOR PLATE 57 Different patterns of anaplastic lymphoma kinase (ALK) immunostaining in lymphomas. All tumors contain a hybrid ALK protein, except for that marked ALK, an example of the rare subtype of large B-cell lymphoma in which full-length wild-type ALK protein is expressed. Notice the typical granular cytoplasmic positivity for ALK in tumor cells bearing the chlatrin (CLTCL)-ALK and the surface expression for ALK in anaplastic large-cell lymphoma cells containing moesin (MSN)-ALK (immunoperoxidase technique in paraffin sections; ×800 to 1,000). (From Falini B, Mason DY. Proteins encoded by genes involved in chromosomal alterations in lymphoma and leukemia: clinical value of their detection by immunocytochemistry. *Blood* 2002;99:409–426, with permission.)

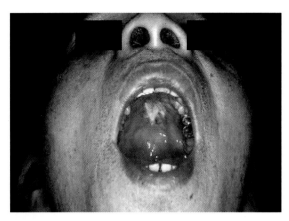

COLOR PLATE 58 Clinical photograph of a patient with nasal natural killer–cell lymphoma involving the hard palate.

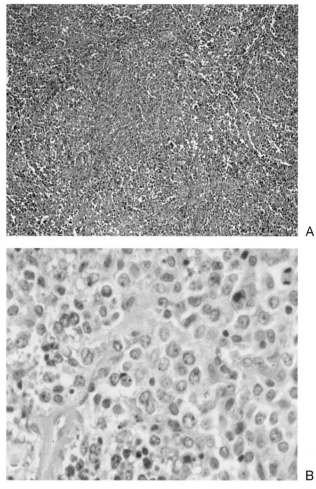

COLOR PLATE 60 Morphologic features of primary mediastinal large B-cell lymphoma. **A:** Low magnification showing compartmentalizing sclerosis. **B:** High magnification showing large cells with pale to clear cytoplasm.

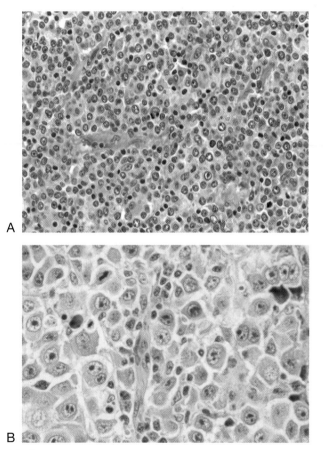

COLOR PLATE 59 Diffuse large B-cell lymphoma. **A:** The majority of cases contain a mixture of large cells that resemble centroblasts with peripheral nucleoli and a minority of large cells that resemble immunoblasts with central nucleoli. **B:** Occasional cases have a predominance of large cells with prominent central nucleoli and abundant cytoplasm, resembling immunoblasts.

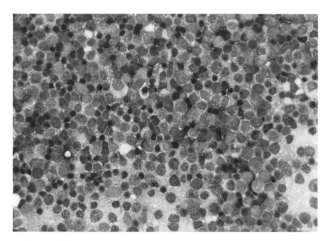

COLOR PLATE 61 Imprint preparation of classic Burkitt's lymphoma stained with Wright-Giemsa. Note the numerous Burkitt's lymphoma cells with basophilic cytoplasm and vacuoles.

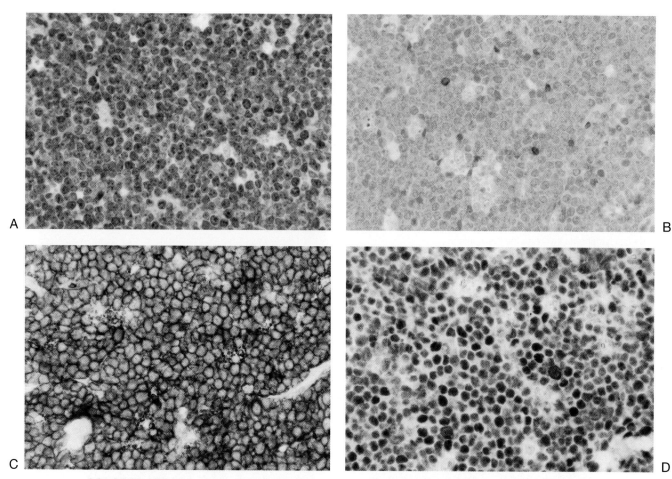

COLOR PLATE 62 Immunostains of MIB-1 **(A)**, Bcl-2 **(B)**, CD10 **(C)**, and Bcl-6 **(D)** in a case of classic Burkitt's lymphoma. Note that all cells are proliferating as defined by positive MIB-1 staining, except the phagocytic histiocytes in the section. CD10 is strongly expressed by the malignant cells, and Bcl-2 is negative. Note several small, reactive lymphocytes in the section staining positively for Bcl-2 that serve as an internal control. Bcl-6 staining **(D)** shows strong nuclear expression.

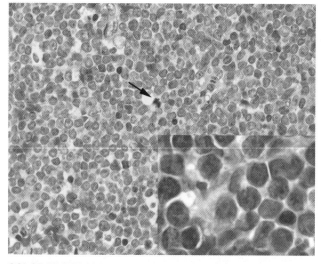

COLOR PLATE 63 Histologic section of lymphoblastic lymphoma, showing the characteristic uniform population of medium-sized cells, with mitotic figures (*arrow*). At high power (*inset*), the chromatin is finely dispersed, and nucleoli are inconspicuous.

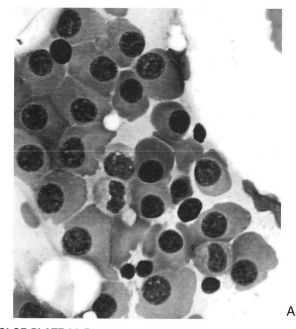

COLOR PLATE 64 Bone marrow examination in myeloma. **A:** Wright-Giemsa–stained aspirate smear of a plasma cell aggregate composed of mature plasma cells with eccentric nuclei and paranuclear halo admixed with more immature plasma cells with central nuclei and more dispersed chromatin. (*continued*)

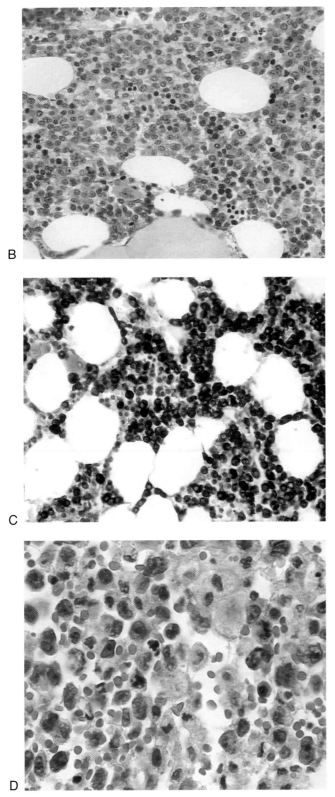

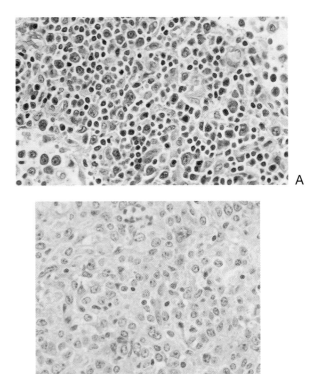

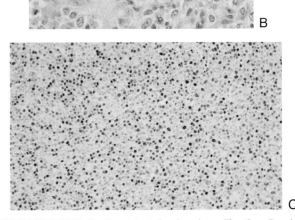

COLOR PLATE 64 Continued B: Bone marrow core biopsy with a diffuse infiltrate of mature and immature plasma cells present in clusters and solid sheets comprising most of the cellularity. Scattered maturing hematopoietic elements are admixed. C: Immunohistochemical study demonstrating monoclonal staining of plasma cells for κ light chain immunoglobulins. D: Anaplastic myeloma composed of large cells with vesicular nuclei, prominent nucleoli, and abundant cytoplasm.

COLOR PLATE 65 Posttransplantation lymphoproliferative disorder (PTLD) with distinct infectious mononucleosis–like and monomorphic diffuse large B-cell PTLD (see Fig. 40.1 for low-magnification images). A: At higher magnification, the abdominal lymph node shows a polymorphic population of variably sized lymphocytes, including a moderate number of transformed cells or immunoblasts, seen both in the nodal parenchyma and in the sinus. These findings would suggest the diagnosis of an infectious mononucleosis–like PTLD because of the polymorphic cell population and architectural preservation. B: The presence of numerous large transformed lymphoid cells that are marked as B cells present in the colonic lesion indicates that this is a monomorphic diffuse large B-cell lymphoma–type PTLD. This case, therefore, illustrates the principle that regional lymph nodes or other adjacent tissues may demonstrate what appears to be an early-type PTLD in the face of a coexisting monomorphic PTLD. C: The Epstein-Barr early region in situ hybridization stain for the Epstein-Barr virus shows numerous positive cells.

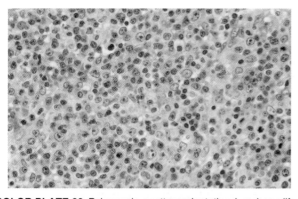

COLOR PLATE 66 Polymorpic posttransplantation lymphoproliferative disorder (Epstein-Barr virus postive) (see Fig. 40.2 for low magnification). The proliferation is composed of variably sized and shaped lymphoid cells, including both many small lymphocytes and a moderate number of scattered transformed cells/immunoblasts. A Reed-Sternberg–like cell is seen in the upper right. A clonal B-cell population was documented by Southern blot analysis.

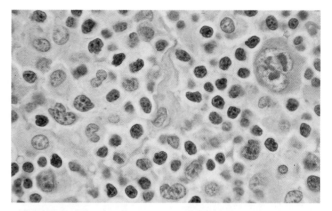

COLOR PLATE 68 Monomorphic peripheral T-cell lymphoma–type posttransplantation lymphoproliferative disorder (see Fig 40.3 for low magnification). At higher magnification, the variably sized lymphoid cells, some of which have irregular nuclear contours and many of which have abundant pale cytoplasm, can be seen. Occasional, much larger, transformed and Reed-Sternberg–like cells are also present.

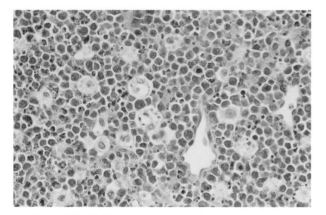

COLOR PLATE 67 Monomorphic Burkitt's lymphoma–type posttransplantation lymphoproliferative disorder (Epstein-Barr virus negative) in an abdominal mass from 46-year-old man status post–liver transplant. Note the very uniform population of relatively small transformed B cells with a starry sky appearance caused by the admixed tingible body macrophages.

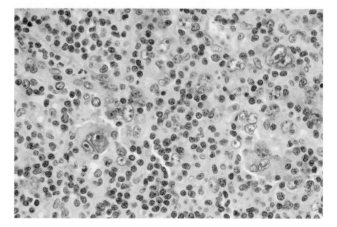

COLOR PLATE 69 Hodgkin's lymphoma–like posttransplantation lymphoproliferative disorder (Epstein-Barr virus positive) in a lymph node from a 57-year-old woman 12 years status post–renal transplant. There are Reed-Sternberg cells surrounded by many small lymphocytes and occasional histiocytes.

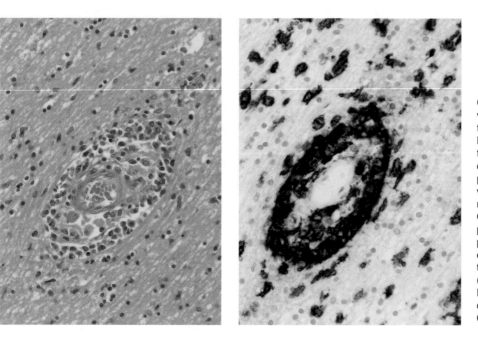

COLOR PLATE 70 A: This blood vessel in the cerebral white matter is cuffed by large, atypical lymphoid cells—a growth pattern characteristic of primary cerebral non-Hodgkin's lymphoma (×100). **B:** The same vessel is shown with an immunohistochemical preparation for CD20. Note labeling of nearly all perivascular cells for this B-lymphocyte antigen and the presence of lymphoma cells infiltrating the neural parenchyma (×100). (Photomicrographs from Dr. Marc Rosenblum, Department of Pathology, Memorial Sloan-Kettering Cancer Center, New York, NY.)

A,B

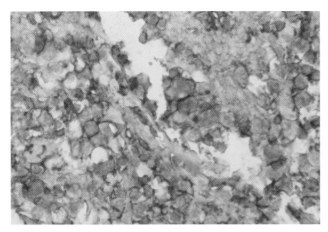

COLOR PLATE 71 Extranodal natural killer/T-cell lymphoma, nasal cavity. Neoplastic cells are positive for the T-cell associated antigen CD45RO (immunoperoxidase technique on paraffin section).

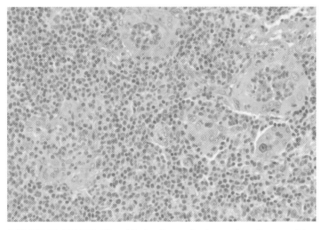

COLOR PLATE 72 Thyroid gland, marginal zone lymphoma arising in association with Hashimoto's thyroiditis. Marginal zone lymphoma, with more extensive obliteration of thyroid parenchyma and prominent lymphoepithelial lesions.

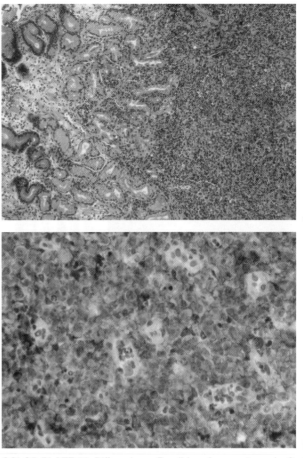

A

B

COLOR PLATE 73 Diffuse large B-cell lymphoma, stomach. **A:** A dense diffuse cellular infiltrate occupies much of the tissue and infiltrates overlying mucosa. **B:** Neoplastic cells are CD20⁺, helping to confirm the diagnosis of lymphoma (immunoperoxidase technique on paraffin sections).

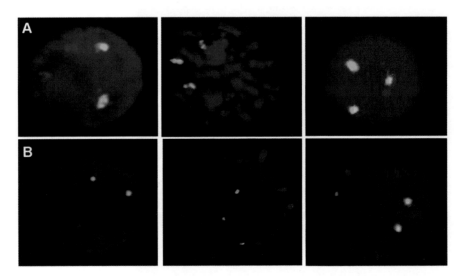

COLOR PLATE 74 Florescent *in situ* hybridization analysis of t(11;14)(q13;q32) **(A)** and t(14;18)(q32;q13) **(B)** translocations. **A:** Left, a normal interphase nucleus showing two green (chromosome 11) and two red (chromosome 14) signals. In the middle and right, respectively, are a metaphase and an interphase of an mantle cell lymphoma showing one green, one red, and two fusion signals identifying the translocation. **B:** Left, a normal interphase nucleus showing two green (chromosome 18) and two red (chromosome 14) signals. In the middle and right, respectively, are a metaphase and an interphase of a follicular lymphoma, showing one green, one red, and two fusion signals identifying the translocation. (Images courtesy of Nallasivam Palanisamy and Cancer Genetics, Inc., Cambridge, MA.)

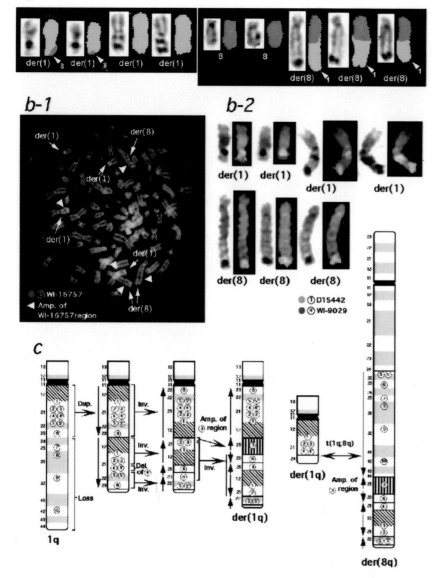

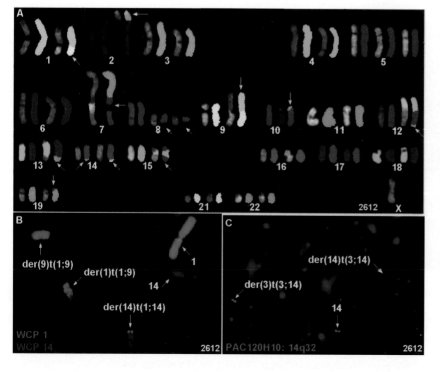

COLOR PLATE 75 Analysis of complex abnormalities involving chromosome 1q by florescent *in situ* hybridization. **A:** Spectral karyotyping analysis (inverted G-banding patterns by 46'-diamidino-2-phenylindole-2 HCl on the left) of chromosome 1 in two cases. **B2:** Florescent *in situ* hybridization (inverted G-banding patterns by 46'-diamidino-2-phenylindole-2 HCl on the left) of chromosome 1 in the same two cases. D1S442 (*green*) and WI-9029 (*red*) are the probes used. **C:** Schematic representation of the possible origin of the 1q aberrations analyzed. Numbers in circles on the schema are the positions of signals studied. The near-tetraploid abnormal karyotype showed seven rearrangements involving chromosomes 1 and 8: der(1)t(1;1)(q21;q?), der(1)t(1;8)(q21;q24), and der(8)t(1;8)(q?;q24). Florescent *in situ* hybridization analysis indicated at least six rearranged regions in 1q12–22. Rearrangements included translocation, inversion, and duplication. The case also showed high-level amplification of the *WI-16757* locus **(B1)**. (From Itoyama T, Nanjungud G, Chen W, et al. Molecular cytogenetic analysis of genomic instability at the 1q12-22 chromosomal site in B-cell non-Hodgkin lymphoma. *Genes Chromosomes Cancer* 2002;35:318–328, with permission.)

COLOR PLATE 76 Multiple chromosome rearrangements identified by spectral karyotyping in a case of primary effusion lymphoma. **A:** Spectral karyotype of a metaphase cell. For each chromosome, on the left is the so-called display color as detected by the spectral system, and on the right is the so-called classification color resulting from an assigned pseudocolor. Note multiple rearrangements, many of which cannot be detected by conventional banding techniques. **B,C:** Further refinement of rearrangements is achieved by whole chromosome painting (WCP) and florescent *in situ* hybridization (FISH). **B:** A metaphase spread hybridized with WCP probes for chromosomes 1 (*green*) and 14 (*red*) show a green signal on chromosome 14 identifying a der(14)t(1;14)(?;32). **C:** FISH analysis using a chromosome 14q32 probe (PAC120H10) identifies a t(3;14)(q27;q32) translocation and establishes the nonreciprocal nature of the der(14)t (1;14)(?;q32) identified by whole chromosome painting. (From Nanjangud G, Rao PH, Hegde A, et al. Spectral karyotyping identifies new rearrangements, translocations, and clinical associations in diffuse large B-cell lymphoma. *Blood* 2002;99:2554–2561, with permission.)

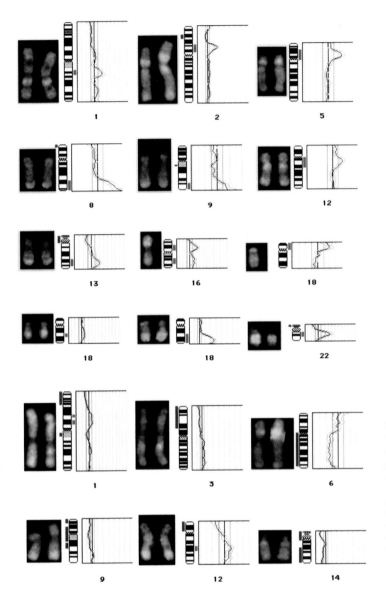

COLOR PLATE 77 Chromosome-based genomic hybridization images (left) and corresponding ratio profiles (right) of several chromosomes in diffuse large B-cell lymphoma illustrating gain, amplification, and loss of chromosomal regions. The averaged green to red fluorescence–signal ratio along the length of the chromosome is shown. The blue line in the ratio profile represents the mean of eight to ten chromosomes, and the yellow line represents the standard deviation. The vertical thin red and green bars on the right of the ideogram indicate threshold values of 0.8 and 1.2 for loss and gain, respectively. The thick red bars (right) represent loss and the green bar (right) gain/high level amplification. (From the laboratory of R. S. K. Chaganti and Gouri Nanjangud.)

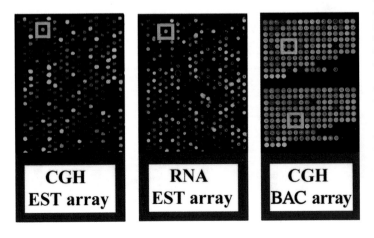

COLOR PLATE 78 Identification of amplicons by array-based comparative genomic hybridization (A-CGH). **Left and middle panels:** A-CGH and expression analysis using an endodermal sinus tumor array. In the case of a germ cell tumor with a 12p amplification, genomic DNA (control, placental DNA) (*left panel*) and complementary DNA (control, normal testis complementary DNA) (*middle panel*) are hybridized to identical arrays. The green color of the same clone on both arrays identifies an amplified and over-expressed target. (From Bourdon V, Naef F, Rao PH, et al. Genomic and expression analysis of the 12p11-p12 amplicon using expressed sequence tag arrays identifies two novel amplified and overexpressed genes. *Cancer Res* 2002;62:6218–6223, with permission). **Right panel:** A-CGH using a bacterial artificial chromosome array. Genomic DNA (control, placental DNA) from a diffuse large B-cell lymphoma is hybridized to a 2- to 4-Mbp–resolution bacterial artificial chromosome array, printed in duplicate. Replicated green hybridization of a clone mapped to 2p12-16 identifies amplification of the REL region. (From the laboratory of R. S. K. Chaganti and Gouri Nanjangud.)

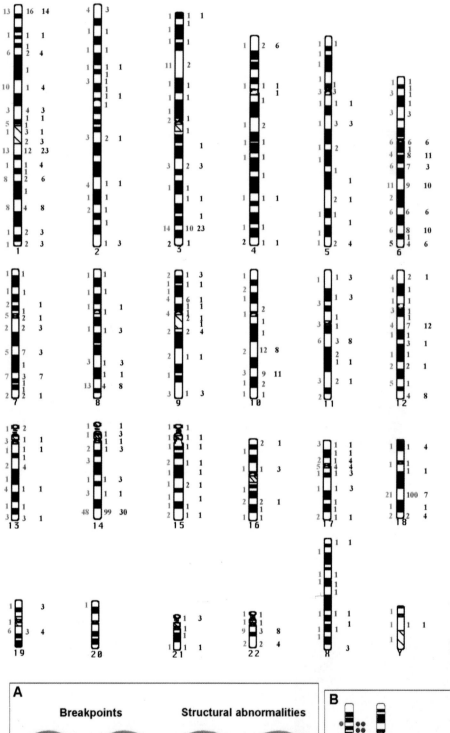

COLOR PLATE 79 Idiogram showing the distribution of breakpoints identified by G-banding in follicular lymphoma and diffuse large B-cell lymphoma. On the right are breakpoints noted in the t(14;18)(q32;q21)-positive (*red*) and -negative subsets (*black*) of follicular lymphoma, and on the left are breakpoints noted in diffuse large B-cell lymphoma. Numbers indicate percentages. (From the laboratory of R. S. K. Chaganti and Gouri Nanjangud.)

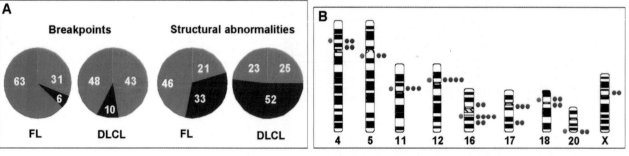

COLOR PLATE 80 A: Refinement of breakpoints and structural abnormalities by spectral karyotype (SKY) in follicular lymphoma and diffuse large B-cell lymphoma. Green indicates the percentage of new breakpoints and structural abnormalities identified by SKY. Blue and red indicate the percentage of G-banded breakpoints and structural abnormalities that were confirmed and revised by SKY, respectively. B: Idiogram showing new recurring breakpoints identified by SKY in diffuse large B-cell lymphoma. Breakpoints identified by SKY are shown on the right and breakpoints identified by G-banding on the left. Each dot represents a single breakpoint. (From the laboratory of R. S. K. Chaganti and Gouri Nanjangud.)

Non-Hodgkin's Lymphomas

Non-Hodgkin's Lymphomas

Editors

Peter M. Mauch, M.D.
Professor of Radiation Oncology
Harvard Medical School
Department of Radiation Oncology
Brigham and Women's Hospital
Dana-Farber Cancer Institute
Boston, Massachusetts

James O. Armitage, M.D.
Joe Shapiro Professor of Medicine
Department of Internal Medicine
University of Nebraska Medical Center
Omaha, Nebraska

Bertrand Coiffier, M.D., Ph.D.
Professor of Medicine
Department of Hematology
Hospices Civils de Lyon
Université Claude Bernard
Lyon, France

Riccardo Dalla-Favera, M.D.
Uris Professor of Pathology and Professor of Genetics and Development
Institute for Cancer Genetics
Columbia University College of Physicians and Surgeons
New York, New York

Nancy Lee Harris, M.D.
Professor of Pathology
Department of Pathology
Harvard Medical School
Massachusetts General Hospital
Boston, Massachusetts

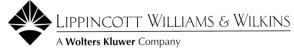

LIPPINCOTT WILLIAMS & WILKINS
A **Wolters Kluwer** Company
Philadelphia · Baltimore · New York · London
Buenos Aires · Hong Kong · Sydney · Tokyo

Acquisitions Editor: Jonathan Pine
Developmental Editor: Stacey L. Baze
Supervising Editor: Mary Ann McLaughlin
Production Editor: Erica Broennle Nelson, Silverchair Science + Communications
Manufacturing Manager: Colin Warnock
Cover Designer: Christine Jenny
Compositor: Silverchair Science + Communications
Printer: Maple Press

© 2004 by LIPPINCOTT WILLIAMS & WILKINS
530 Walnut Street
Philadelphia, PA 19106 USA
LWW.com

Printed in the USA

Library of Congress Cataloging-in-Publication Data

Non-Hodgkin's lymphomas / editors, Peter M. Mauch ... [et al.].
   p. ; cm.
  Includes bibliographical references and index.
  ISBN 0-7817-3526-2
  1. Lymphomas. I. Mauch, Peter M.
  [DNLM: 1. Lymphomas, Non-Hodgkin. WH 525 N81191 2003]
  RC280.L9N6592 2003
  616.99' 446--dc22

                       2003058867

10 9 8 7 6 5 4 3 2 1

Contents

SECTION I: HISTORICAL ASPECTS

SECTION II: DIAGNOSIS, STAGING, AND INITIAL EVALUATION

SECTION III: TREATMENT PRINCIPLES AND TECHNIQUES

SECTION VII: ETIOLOGY, EPIDEMIOLOGY, AND BIOLOGY

CONTRIBUTING AUTHORS

Richard Frederick Ambinder, M.D., Ph.D.
James B. Murphy Professor
Department of Oncology, Pharmacology,
  and Pathology
Director, Division of Hematologic Malignancies
Johns Hopkins University School of Medicine
Baltimore, Maryland

Hesham M. Amin, M.D.
Assistant Professor
Department of Hematopathology
University of Texas Medical School at Houston
M.D. Anderson Cancer Center
Houston, Texas

Kenneth C. Anderson, M.D.
Kraft Family Professor of Medicine
Department of Medical Oncology
Harvard Medical School
Dana-Farber Cancer Institute
Boston, Massachusetts

Marc P. E. André, M.D.
Department of Hematology and Oncology
Center Hospitalier Notre Dame et Reine Fabiola
Charleroi, Belgium

Patricia Aoun, M.D., M.P.H.
Assistant Professor
Department of Pathology and Microbiology
Medical Director
Flow Cytometry Laboratory
University of Nebraska Medical Center
Omaha, Nebraska

James O. Armitage, M.D.
Joe Shapiro Professor of Medicine
Department of Internal Medicine
University of Nebraska Medical Center
Omaha, Nebraska

Ramsey D. Badawi, Ph.D.
Assistant Professor of Radiology
Department of Nuclear Medicine
Harvard Medical School
Dana-Farber Cancer Institute
Boston, Massachusetts

Frederick G. Behm, M.D.
Vice Chair
Department of Pathology

St. Jude Children's Research Hospital
Memphis, Tennessee

Costan A. Berard, M.D.
Former Chief
Hematopathology Section
National Cancer Institute
National Institutes of Health
Bethesda, Maryland

Françoise Berger, M.D., Ph.D.
Professor of Pathology
Department of Hematopathology
Centre Hospitalier Lyon Sud
Pierre Bénite Cedex, France

Joseph R. Bertino, M.D.
Professor
Departments of Medicine and Pharmacology
University of Medicine and Dentistry of
  New Jersey—Robert Wood Johnson
  Medical School
Associate Director
Cancer Institute of New Jersey
New Brunswick, New Jersey

Philip J. Bierman, M.D.
Associate Professor of Medicine
Department of Internal Medicine
Section of Oncology and Hematology
University of Nebraska Medical Center
Omaha, Nebraska

Michael J. Borowitz, M.D., Ph.D.
Professor of Pathology and Oncology
Department of Pathology
Johns Hopkins University School of Medicine
Baltimore, Maryland

Günter Brittinger, M.D.
Professor (Emeritus) of Medicine
Department of Hematology
University of Essen
Essen, Germany

Alan K. Burnett, M.D., F.R.C.P., F.R.C.Path.,
  F.Med.Sci.
Professor of Haematology
Head, Department of Haematology
University of Wales College of Medicine
Cardiff, United Kingdom

Fernando Cabanillas, M.D.
Professor
Department of Lymphoma/Myeloma
University of Texas Medical School at Houston
M.D. Anderson Cancer Center
Houston, Texas

Francisca I. Camacho, M.D.
Molecular Pathology Program
Lymphoma and Lung Cancer Group
Centro Nacional de Investigaciones Oncológicas
Madrid, Spain

Daniel Catovsky, M.D., D.Sc.
Professor of Haematology
Department of Academic Haematology
The Institute of Cancer Research
London, United Kingdom

Franco Cavalli, M.D., F.R.C.P.
Professor of Medicine
Oncology Institute of Southern Switzerland
Ospedale San Giovanni
Bellinzona, Switzerland

Ignacio Chacón
Medical Oncology Service
Department of Pathologic Anatomy
Hospital Virgen de la Salud
Toledo, Spain

R. S. K. Chaganti, Ph.D., F.A.C.M.G.
Member and Professor
William E. Snee Chair
Department of Medicine and Cell Biology Program
Memorial Sloan-Kettering Cancer Center
New York, New York

Bertrand Coiffier, M.D., Ph.D.
Professor of Medicine
Department of Hematology
Hospices Civils de Lyon
Université Claude Bernard
Lyon, France

Joseph M. Connors, M.D.
Clinical Professor of Medicine
Department of Medicine
Division of Medical Oncology
University of British Columbia Faculty of Medicine
British Columbia Cancer Agency
Vancouver, British Columbia
Canada

Miguel A. Cruz
Department of Oncology

Hospital Virgen de la Salud
Toledo, Spain

Riccardo Dalla-Favera, M.D.
Uris Professor of Pathology and Professor of
  Genetics and Development
Institute for Cancer Genetics
Columbia University College of Physicians
  and Surgeons
New York, New York

Lisa M. DeAngelis, M.D.
Professor and Chairman
Department of Neurology
Cornell University Joan and Sanford I. Weill Medical
  College and Graduate School of Medical Sciences
Memorial Sloan-Kettering Cancer Center
New York, New York

Volker Diehl, M.D.
Prof. Dr. med. Dr. h.c.
Klinik I für Innere Medicine
University of Cologne
Cologne, Germany

Ronald F. Dorfman, M.D.
Professor of Pathology Emeritus
Stanford University School of Medicine
Stanford, California

Martin H. Dreyling, M.D.
PD (Lecturer of Medicine)
Department of Medicine
Ludwig-Maximilians University
University Hospital Grosshadern
Munich, Germany

Lyn M. Duncan, M.D.
Associate Professor of Pathology
Department of Pathology
Harvard Medical School
Massachusetts General Hospital
Boston, Massachusetts

Brunangelo Falini, M.D.
Professor of Hematology
Institute of Hematology
University of Perugia
Perugia, Italy

Judith A. Ferry, M.D.
Associate Professor of Pathology
Department of Pathology
Massachusetts General Hospital
Boston, Massachusetts

Kenneth A. Foon, M.D.
Professor of Medicine
Department of Internal Medicine
University of Pittsburgh Cancer Institute
Pittsburgh, Pennsylvania

Kathryn Foucar, M.D.
Professor of Pathology
Department of Pathology
University of New Mexico Health Sciences Center
Albuquerque, New Mexico

Arnold S. Freedman, M.D.
Associate Professor of Medicine
Department of Medical Oncology
Harvard Medical School
Dana-Farber Cancer Institute
Boston, Massachusetts

Jonathan W. Friedberg, M.D.
Assistant Professor of Medicine
James P. Wilmot Cancer Center
University of Rochester School of Medicine and Dentistry
Rochester, New York

Juan F. García, M.D., Ph.D.
Staff Scientist
Molecular Pathology Program
Lymphoma and Lung Cancer Group
Centro Nacional de Investigaciones Oncológicas
Madrid, Spain

Randy D. Gascoyne, M.D., F.R.C.P.C.
Clinical Professor of Pathology
Department of Pathology and Laboratory Medicine
University of British Columbia Faculty of Medicine
British Columbia Cancer Agency
Vancouver, British Columbia
Canada

Christian Gisselbrecht, M.D.
Professor of Hematology
Institut d'Hématologie
Hôpital Saint Louis
Paris, France

Mary K. Gospodarowicz, M.D., F.R.C.P.C., F.R.C.R. (Hon.)
Professor, Faculty of Medicine
Department of Radiation Oncology
University of Toronto Faculty of Medicine
Princess Margaret Hospital
Toronto, Ontario
Canada

Andre H. Goy, M.D.
Assistant Professor
Department of Lymphoma/Myeloma
University of Texas Medical School at Houston
M.D. Anderson Cancer Center
Houston, Texas

Timothy C. Greiner, M.D.
Associate Professor
Departments of Pathology and Microbiology
University of Nebraska Medical Center
Omaha, Nebraska

John G. Gribben, M.D., D.Sc.
Associate Professor of Medicine
Department of Medical Oncology
Harvard Medical School
Dana-Farber Cancer Institute
Boston, Massachusetts

Thomas M. Habermann, M.D.
Department of Medicine
Division of Hematology
Mayo Clinic
Rochester, Minnesota

Jorgen L. Hansen, M.S.
Instructor in Radiation Therapy
Harvard Medical School
Staff Physicist
Department of Radiation Oncology
Brigham and Women's Hospital
Dana-Farber Cancer Institute
Boston, Massachusetts

Nancy Lee Harris, M.D.
Professor of Pathology
Department of Pathology
Harvard Medical School
Massachusetts General Hospital
Boston, Massachusetts

Patricia Hartge, Sc.D., M.A.
Deputy Director
Epidemiology and Biostatistics Program
Division of Cancer Epidemiology and Genetics
National Cancer Institute
National Institutes of Health
Bethesda, Maryland

Jeff D. Harvell, M.D.
Department of Pathology
Stanford University
Stanford, California

Michel Henry-Amar, M.D., Ph.D.
Université de Caen-Basse Normandie
Centre François Baclesse
Caen, France

Wolfgang Hiddemann, M.D., Ph.D.
Professor of Medicine
Department of Internal Medicine III
Ludwig-Maximilians University
University Hospital Grosshadern
Munich, Germany

Richard T. Hoppe, M.D.
Henry S. Kaplan-Harry Lebeson Professor of
  Cancer Biology
Department of Radiation Oncology
Stanford University School of Medicine
Stanford, California

Steven M. Horwitz, M.D.
Clinical Assistant Attending Physician
Department of Medicine
Lymphoma Service
Memorial Sloan-Kettering Cancer Center
New York, New York

Liangge Hsu, M.D.
Assistant Professor of Radiology
Department of Neuroradiology
Harvard Medical School
Brigham and Women's Hospital
Boston, Massachusetts

Peter G. Isaacson, D.M., D.Sc., F.R.C.Path.
Professor
Department of Histopathology
University College London
London, United Kingdom

Andrew S. Jack, B.Sc., M.D., Ch.B., Ph.D.,
F.R.C.Path.
Consultant Haematopathologist
Haematological Malignancy Diagnostic Service
Leeds Teaching Hospitals
Leeds, United Kingdom

Elaine S. Jaffe, M.D.
Chief
Hematopathology Section
Deputy Chief
Laboratory of Pathology
National Cancer Institute
National Institutes of Health
Bethesda, Maryland

Marshall E. Kadin, M.D.
Associate Professor of Pathology
Department of Pathology
Harvard Medical School
Beth Israel Deaconess Medical Center
Boston, Massachusetts

Youn H. Kim, M.D.
Department of Dermatology
Stanford University
Stanford, California

Ralf Küppers, Ph.D.
Department of Internal Medicine I
University of Cologne
Cologne, Germany

Anton W. Langerak, Ph.D.
Immunologist, Consultant Medical Immunology
Department of Immunology
Erasmus MC, University Medical Center Rotterdam
Rotterdam, The Netherlands

Stanislav Lechpammer, M.D., Ph.D.
Research Associate
Department of Nuclear Medicine
Harvard Medical School
Dana-Farber Cancer Institute
Boston, Massachusetts

Karl Lennert, M.D.
Professor of Pathology Emeritus
Former Director, Institute of Pathology
Christian Albrecht University
Kiel, Germany

Georg Lenz, M.D.
Department of Internal Medicine III
Ludwig-Maximilians University
University Hospital Grosshadern
Munich, Germany

Alexandra M. Levine, M.D.
Distinguished Professor of Medicine
Department of Medicine
Keck School of Medicine of the University of
  Southern California
Los Angeles, California

Raymond H. S. Liang, M.D., F.R.C.P., F.R.A.C.P.
Professor of Haematology and Oncology
Department of Medicine
University of Hong Kong
Queen Mary Hospital
Hong Kong, China

T. Andrew Lister, M.D.
Department of Medical Oncology
St. Bartholomew's Hospital
London, United Kingdom

Howard L. Liu, M.D.
Resident, Former Fellow of Cutaneous Lymphoma

Department of Dermatology
Stanford University School of Medicine
Stanford, California

Ian T. Magrath, D.Sc.(Med.), F.R.C.P., F.R.C.Path.
Professor of Pediatrics (USUHS)
International Network for Cancer Treatment and Research
Brussels, Belgium

Karen J. Marcus, M.D.
Assistant Professor of Radiation Oncology (Pediatrics)
Harvard Medical School
Children's Hospital
Dana-Farber Cancer Institute
Boston, Massachusetts

Estella Matutes, M.D., Ph.D., F.R.C.Path.
Reader in Haemopoietic Malignancies
Academic Department of Haematology
Institute of Cancer Research
Royal Marsden Hospital
London, United Kingdom

Peter M. Mauch, M.D.
Professor of Radiation Oncology
Harvard Medical School
Department of Radiation Oncology
Brigham and Women's Hospital
Dana-Farber Cancer Institute
Boston, Massachusetts

L. Jeffrey Medeiros, M.D.
Professor
Department of Hematopathology
University of Texas Medical School at Houston
M.D. Anderson Cancer Center
Houston, Texas

Manuela Mollejo
Department of Pathology
Hospital Virgen de la Salud
Toledo, Spain

Gouri Nanjangud, Ph.D.
Research Fellow
Cell Biology Program
Memorial Sloan-Kettering Cancer Center
New York, New York

Andrea K. Ng, M.D., M.P.H.
Assistant Professor of Radiation Oncology
Department of Radiation Oncology
Harvard Medical School
Brigham and Women's Hospital
Dana-Farber Cancer Institute
Boston, Massachusetts

Carl J. O'Hara, M.D.
Associate Professor of Pathology
Department of Pathology
Boston University School of Medicine
Boston, Massachusetts

Laura Pasqualucci, M.D.
Assistant Professor of Clinical Pathology
Institute for Cancer Genetics
Columbia University College of Physicians
*   and Surgeons*
New York, New York

Miguel A. Piris, M.D.
Director Molecular Pathology Program
Department of Molecular Pathology
Centro Nacional de Investigaciones
*   Oncológicas*
Madrid, Spain

Mark Raffeld, M.D.
National Cancer Institute
National Institutes of Health
Bethesda, Maryland

Noopur Raje, M.D.
Clinical Fellow
Department of Adult Oncology
Dana-Farber Cancer Institute
Boston, Massachusetts

Klaus Rajewsky, M.D.
Professor of Pathology
Department of Pathology
Harvard Medical School
Senior Investigator
Center for Blood Research
Boston, Massachusetts

Sumul N. Raval, M.D.
Clinical Instructor
Department of Neurology
Memorial Sloan-Kettering Cancer Center
New York, New York

Félix Reyes, M.D.
Professor of Clinical Hematology
Service d'Hématologie Clinique
Centre Hospitalo-universitair Henri Mondor
Créteil, France

Ama Z. S. Rohatiner, M.D., F.R.C.P.
Professor of Haemato-Oncology
Department of Medical Oncology
St. Bartholomew's Hospital
London, United Kingdom

Malek M. Safa, M.D.
Assistant Professor of Medicine
Department of Hematology and Oncology
University of Cincinnati College of
*   Medicine*
Barrett Cancer Center
Cincinnati, Ohio

Jonathan W. Said, M.D.
Professor of Pathology
Department of Pathology and Laboratory Medicine
University of California, Los Angeles, David Geffen School
*   of Medicine at UCLA*
UCLA Center for Health Sciences
Los Angeles, California

Gilles A. Salles, M.D., Ph.D.
Professor of Medicine
Department of Hematology
Université Claude Bernard
Hospices Civils de Lyon
Pierre Bénite Cedex, France

John T. Sandlund, M.D.
Associate Professor of Pediatrics
Department of Hematology-Oncology
St. Jude Children's Research Hospital
Memphis, Tennessee

Kerry J. Savage, M.D., F.R.C.P.C.
Instructor in Medicine
Department of Medical Oncology
Harvard Medical School
Dana-Farber Cancer Institute
Boston, Massachusetts

David T. Scadden, M.D.
Associate Professor of Medicine
MGH Cancer Center and AIDS Research
*   Center*
Massachusetts General Hospital
Boston, Massachusetts

Kitt Shaffer, M.D., Ph.D.
Associate Professor of Radiology and Assistant Chief
Department of Radiology
Dana-Farber Cancer Institute
Boston, Massachusetts

Margaret A. Shipp, M.D.
Associate Professor of Medicine
Department of Medical Oncology
Harvard Medical School
Director, Lymphoma Program
Dana-Farber Cancer Institute
Boston, Massachusetts

Lena Specht, M.D., Ph.D.
Chief Oncologist and Associate Professor
*   of Oncology*
Department of Oncology
The Finsen Centre
Rigshospitalet, Copenhagen University Hospital
Copenhagen, Denmark

Frank J. T. Staal, M.D.
Department of Immunology
Erasmus MC, University Medical Center Rotterdam
Rotterdam, The Netherlands

John W. Sweetenham, D.M., F.R.C.P.
Professor of Medicine
Department of Medical Oncology
University of Colorado School of Medicine
University of Colorado Health Sciences Center
Denver, Colorado

Steven H. Swerdlow, M.D.
Professor of Pathology
Department of Pathology
Division of Hematopathology
University of Pittsburgh School of Medicine
UPMC-Presbyterian Hospital
Pittsburgh, Pennsylvania

Lode J. Swinnen, M.D., Ch.B.
Professor of Medicine
Department of Oncology
Division of Hematologic Malignancies
Johns Hopkins University School of Medicine
Baltimore, Maryland

Richard J. Tetrault, B.S., C.N.M.T., R.T.N.
Department of Nuclear Medicine
Dana-Farber Cancer Institute
Boston, Massachusetts

Kensei Tobinai, M.D., Ph.D.
Chief, Hematology Division
National Cancer Center Hospital
Tokyo, Japan

Alexandra Traverse-Glehen, M.D.
Service d'Anatomie Pathologique
Centre Hospitalier Lyon-Sud
Pierre Bénite Cedex, France

Lois B. Travis, M.D., Sc.D.
Senior Investigator
Division of Cancer Epidemiology and Genetics
National Cancer Institute
National Institutes of Health
Bethesda, Maryland

Lorenz H. Trümper, M.D.
Professor of Medicine
Department of Hematology and Oncology
Georg August University
Göttingen, Germany

Richard W. Tsang, M.D., F.R.C.P.C.
Associate Professor
Department of Radiation Oncology
University of Toronto Faculty of Medicine
Princess Margaret Hospital
University Health Network
Toronto, Ontario
Canada

Annick D. Van den Abbeele, M.D.
Associate Professor of Radiology
Department of Radiology/Nuclear Medicine
Harvard Medical School
Director of Nuclear Medicine/Positron-Emission Tomography
Dana-Farber Cancer Institute
Boston, Massachusetts

Jacques J. M. van Dongen, M.D., Ph.D.
Professor of Immunology
Department of Immunology
Erasmus MC, University Medical Center Rotterdam
Rotterdam, The Netherlands

Flora E. van Leeuwen
Department of Epidemiology
The Netherlands Cancer Institute
Amsterdam, The Netherlands

Hemachandra Venkatesh, M.D.
Oncologist/Hematologist
Department of Medical Oncology and Hematology
Central Indiana Cancer Centers, US Oncology
Indianapolis, Indiana

Sophia S. Wang, Ph.D.
Investigator
Division of Cancer Epidemiology and Genetics
National Cancer Institute
National Institutes of Health
Bethesda, Maryland

Toshiki Watanabe, M.D., Ph.D.
Associate Professor
Department of Cancer Biology
Division of Pathology
University of Tokyo
The Institute of Medical Science
Tokyo, Japan

Dennis D. Weisenburger, M.D.
Professor of Pathology and Director of Hematopathology
Department of Pathology and Microbiology
University of Nebraska Medical Center
Omaha, Nebraska

J. Patrick Whelan, M.D., Ph.D.
Instructor in Pediatrics
AIDS Research Center
Massachusetts General Hospital
Boston, Massachusetts

Wyndham H. Wilson, M.D., Ph.D.
Senior Investigator
Experimental Transplantation and Immunology Branch
National Cancer Institute
National Institutes of Health
Bethesda, Maryland

Thomas E. Witzig, M.D.
Department of Medicine
Division of Hematology
Mayo Clinic
Rochester, Minnesota

Elisa J. Wu, M.D.
Clinical Assistant Attending Radiation Oncologist
Department of Radiation Oncology
Memorial Sloan-Kettering Cancer Center at Mercy Medical Center
Rockville Centre, New York

Joachim Yahalom, M.D.
Professor of Radiation Oncology in Medicine
Department of Radiation Oncology
Cornell University Joan and Sanford I. Weill Medical College and Graduate School of Medical Sciences
Memorial Sloan-Kettering Cancer Center
New York, New York

Pier Luigi Zinzani, M.D., Ph.D.
Professor of Hematology
Institute of Hematology "Seràgnoli"
University of Bologna
Bologna, Italy

Emanuele Zucca, M.D.
Head, Lymphoma Unit
Division of Medical Oncology
Oncology Institute of Southern Switzerland
Ospedale San Giovanni
Bellinzona, Switzerland

PREFACE

Hodgkin's disease, non-Hodgkin's lymphomas, and leukemias were uniformly fatal diseases before 1960. Hodgkin's disease and childhood leukemia were the first cancers discovered to be highly curable with the development of multiagent chemotherapy and modern radiation therapy. Many of the strategies used to cure these two diseases have been successfully applied in improving the survival and cure rates of patients with non-Hodgkin's lymphomas and adult leukemias. The outgrowth of the successful treatment of these diseases also has provided a prototype for strategies for the curative treatment of other cancers over the past 30 years.

This is the first definitive text by Lippincott Williams & Wilkins on non-Hodgkin's lymphomas. The current title, *Non-Hodgkin's Lymphomas,* was chosen to complement the text *Hodgkin's Disease*, published by Lippincott Williams & Wilkins in 1999.

In designing the current text, we chose to be as inclusive as possible. We wanted a broad representation of the knowledge and treatment of the non-Hodgkin's lymphomas, and we wished to credit those who have made important contributions to our understanding of these diseases. As a result, the editors represent the disciplines of radiation oncology, medical oncology, molecular biology, and pathology. There are more than 100 contributors from all parts of the world.

Advances in molecular biology, immunology, and cytogenetics have greatly improved our understanding of the pathogenesis of lymphoma. As a result, lymphoma and leukemia have been reclassified over the last decade, first through the Revised European-American Lymphoma Classification, and, more recently, through the World Health Organization Classification. *Non-Hodgkin's Lymphomas* is organized using these new reclassification systems for lymphoma and leukemia.

Non-Hodgkin's Lymphomas is divided into seven sections to represent the many advances in the treatment of these diseases that have occurred over the last decade. Each chapter has been designed to stand alone and to comprehensively cover a topic. By intent, portions of a topic may be addressed in more than one chapter.

Early contributions to the understanding and treatment of the non-Hodgkin's lymphomas are covered in Section I. Section II, composed of seven chapters on diagnosis, staging, and initial evaluation, highlights the many new technical advances in radiologic staging and in the development of prognostic factors that help guide treatment. Treatment principles and techniques are presented in Section III and help provide a general understanding of the specific treatment approaches for patients.

Section IV contains 19 chapters that portray what is known of the pathogenesis, current treatment options, and ongoing trials of the major types of lymphoma. These chapters should prove to be a valuable resource to physicians, nurses, medical students, and patients.

The late effects of treatment are covered in Section V. This is an area of increasing importance as the treatments for non-Hodgkin's lymphomas become more effective. Special topics are covered in the eight chapters in Section VI. Because of the varied pathogenesis of the different types of lymphoma, this section should help guide management of the patient in the clinic.

Perhaps the greatest changes in our knowledge of non-Hodgkin's lymphomas have been advances in biology, which have allowed for the development of new strategies for diagnosis and treatment, and are highlighted in each of the specific disease chapters (Section IV) and in Section VII.

We had several goals in designing this book. We wanted to provide a reference text for training programs and researchers. We wanted to provide information and guidance for practicing physicians. Finally, we hoped to provide a foundation for new ideas in laboratory and clinical investigation. We look forward to advances that will enable us to better understand the pathophysiology and etiology of the non-Hodgkin's lymphomas. These advances should aid in prevention and in the development of safer and more effective treatment approaches.

P.M.M.
J.O.A.
B.C.
R.D-F.
N.L.H.

ACKNOWLEDGMENTS

We are deeply indebted to all of the authors whose expertise and promptness have eased the preparation of this text. We would like to thank our families, who endured our efforts in the preparation of this work, and our colleagues, who provided support and made numerous valuable suggestions.

We also want to thank Jonathan Pine, Editor, Oncology Program at Lippincott Williams & Wilkins, whose guidance helped shape the book; Stacey L. Baze of Lippincott Williams & Wilkins and Erica Nelson of Silverchair Science + Communications, whose pleasant but firm manner helped keep us on schedule; and Elaine Ryan (Omaha, Nebraska) and Barbara Silver (Boston, Massachusetts), who assisted in preparation of materials for the book.

SECTION I

Historical Aspects

CHAPTER 1

Non-Hodgkin's Lymphoma: A History of Classification and Clinical Observations

Lorenz H. Trümper, Günter Brittinger, Volker Diehl, and Nancy Lee Harris,

with contributions from Ronald F. Dorfman, Karl Lennert, and Costan A. Berard

In many aspects, lymphomas are a model for the progress that has been achieved in the diagnosis, classification, and treatment of malignant diseases. This is illustrated by the historical developments in the classification and treatment of lymphomas that are summarized in this chapter.

EARLY DESCRIPTIONS OF LYMPHOMAS

The first century of lymphoma classification consisted of the sequential recognition by a variety of observers of different disease entities that were characterized by distinctive morphology and clinical behavior (Table 1.1) [reviewed in (1–3)]. To determine with certainty the time at which lymphomas were recognized as a separate disease entity is all but impossible. The starting point of the history of malignant lymphomas is generally thought to be the identification of Hodgkin's disease by Thomas Hodgkin in 1832 in a paper that is entitled "On some morbid appearances of the absorbent glands and spleen" (4). Even though his observation was lost for more than a generation, Hodgkin is to be credited with distinguishing a condition that was separate from the then more common causes of lymphadenopathy—namely, infectious diseases, such as tuberculosis; amyloidosis; and carcinomas (5). Among the malignant disorders of the lymph nodes that Thomas Hodgkin described in his first paper, three or four (out of seven) fulfilled the criteria of the entity that we now refer to as Hodgkin's disease (6,6a,7). However, even the original small series of lymphomas that was presented by the author included malignant tumors of the lymphatic tissue that differed in their morphology from Hodgkin's disease. It later became evident that the tumors belonged to a large and heterogenous group of lymphomas that is now called *non-Hodgkin's lymphomas* to distinguish them from the original lymphoma, Hodgkin's disease (5).

In the nineteenth century and the first six decades of the twentieth century, when the functions of the lymphatic tissues were still largely unknown, lymphomas could only be classified by their macro- and microscopic appearance. As summarized by Lennert and colleagues (3) and Dorfman (2), the first use of the terms *lymphoma* and *lymphosarcoma* is attributed to Rudolf Virchow, who, in 1863 (7a), distinguished lymphosarcoma from leukemia, which he had described in 1845 (7b). In 1865, the term *pseudoleukemia* was created by Cohnheim, a student of Virchow, based on a case with enlarged lymph nodes, spleen, liver, and kidney without leukemia, which replaced Virchow's aleukemic leukemia (7c). The term *malignant lymphoma* is attributed to the famous surgeon Theodor Billroth, who coined this term in 1871 (7d). At the end of the nineteenth century, Dreschfeld (7e) and Kundrat (8) separated pseudoleukemia (including some forms of Hodgkin's disease) from lymphosarcoma; the first clear description of the pathology of lymphosarcoma is attributed to Kundrat (8). In 1898 and 1902, Carl Sternberg (9) and Dorothy Reed (10) independently described the characteristic binucleate giant cell that came to be called the *Reed-Sternberg* or *Sternberg-Reed cell* and gave a more precise histologic definition of Hodgkin's disease. In 1908, Sternberg described an aggressive mediastinal tumor in a young male (11); initially known as *Sternberg sarcoma*, this was later recognized as *lymphoblastic lymphoma* (12).

Jackson and Parker (13a) credit Ewing with proposing in 1914 that tumors of lymphoid tissues could arise from reticulum cells (14). In 1928, Oberling coined the term *reticulosarcoma* for a tumor of the bone or bone marrow and suggested the existence of a similar neoplasm in the lymph nodes (14a). Comparable tumors that were called *retothelsarcoma* were described by Roulet, who defined the immature, mature, and combined (with leukemia or Hodgkin's disease) types of retothelsarcoma as independent tumors of the lymph nodes that differ from lymphosarcoma (15). In their paper discussing most of the malignant lymphomas that were distinguished at the time (1916), Ghon and Roman (16) also described cases of lymphosarcoma in which

TABLE 1.1. *Time line of lymphoma descriptions and classification (partial listing)*

Diseases defined

   Hodgkin's disease: Hodgkin (1832*)*, Wilks (1856, 1865), Sternberg (1898), Reed (1902)

   Leukemia: Virchow (1845)

   Lymphosarcoma: Virchow (1863), Billroth (1871–malignant lymphoma), Kundrat (1893) (Dreschfeld, 1892, and Kundrat, 1893–distinction of lymphosarcoma from pseudoleukemia, including some forms of Hodgkin's disease)

   Multiple myeloma: Bence Jones, MacIntyre, Watson, and Dalrymple (1845), von Rustizky (1873), Wright (1900)

   Reticulum cell sarcoma: Ewing (1914), Oberling (1928), Roulet (1930)

   Follicular lymphoma: Brill, Baehr, Rosenthal (1925), Symmers (1927,1938), Gall, Morrison, Scott (1941)

   Burkitt's lymphoma: Burkitt (1957), O'Conor (1961)

Lymphoma classifications

   American Registry of Pathology (1934)

   Robb-Smith (1938)

   Rössle (1939)

   Gall and Mallory (1942)

   Jackson and Parker (1937, 1947)

   Rappaport (1956, 1966)

   Lennert (1967)

   Lukes and Collins (1974)

   Kiel (1974)

   British National Lymphoma Investigation (1974)

   Dorfman (1974)

   World Health Organization (1976)

reticulum cells apparently took part in the proliferative process. Others adopted the term *reticulum cell sarcoma* (17).

The term *reticulum cell* had been applied to a large cell that is found within the supporting fibrous reticulum of lymphoid tissues (it was not generally believed to produce the reticulum) (13a,18). Some observers considered it to be related to an endothelial cell, some believed it to be an immature lymphoid cell, and some believed it to be a pluripotent stem cell, whereas others believed it was identical to the histiocyte or macrophage, also known as the *clasmatocyte*. The term *reticulum cell sarcoma* was generally applied to large-cell neoplasms (13a,18)—this uncertainty about the lineage of large-cell neoplasms of lymphoid tissues persisted well into the latter half of the twentieth century—whereas the term *lymphosarcoma* was applied to those neoplasms that are composed of smaller cells recognized as lymphocytes. Because the cell type of reticulum cell sarcoma was unclear, Edward Gall and Tracy Mallory commented that "when such variation of opinion exists it seems probable that the individual authors…cannot be describing the same tumor" (18).

In 1925, Brill et al. (19) described an enlargement of lymph nodes that was characterized by a proliferation of lymphoid follicles; additional cases were reported by Symmers (20,21). As with Hodgkin's disease, there was initial confusion about

whether this represented a neoplasm or a progressive reactive process, and it is likely that initial reports contained, in addition to examples of what we would now call *follicular lymphoma*, cases of florid reactive follicular hyperplasia. By 1941, however, follicular lymphoma, or *giant follicle lymphoma*, was recognized and confirmed by Gall et al. (22) to be a distinctive form of lymphoid neoplasm, with frequent disseminated disease and a long natural history.

The essential features of multiple myeloma were described in three steps. In 1845, Henry Bence Jones, together with William MacIntyre and Thomas Watson, observed a new protein with a peculiar reaction to heat, now referred to as *Bence Jones protein*, in the urine of a patient with "Mollities Ossium." Based on the clinical picture, rapid lethal course, and postmortem histologic examination performed by John Dalrymple, the authors considered this hitherto undescribed disease "essentially malignant in nature" affecting the "osseous system" (23,23a). J. von Rustizky (23b) in 1873 recognized that the multiple tumors he had found in the bones of a patient originated from the bone marrow and, therefore, he introduced the term *multiple myeloma*. Finally, in 1900, James Homer Wright was able to identify multiple myeloma as a neoplasm of plasma cells with the application of the Wright's stain (24). Mycosis fungoides was described as a clinical syndrome as far back as 1806 (24a), whereas Sézary syndrome (24b) and Waldenström's macroglobulinemia (24c) were recognized as distinct entities by the mid-1940s.

In 1958, Burkitt described a tumor of African children, which was rapidly recognized as a new and distinctive type of lymphoma (25–27) that also occurred in western countries (28). The discovery of this *African lymphoma*, which represents the endemic variant of Burkitt's lymphoma, warrants further description, because it highlights the unique steps that led from Burkitt's clinical description of a rare jaw tumor in African children to the discovery of a unique, now well-understood, sequence of events in the pathogenesis of a lymphoma.

Denis Burkitt and the Discovery of African Lymphoma

Denis Burkitt's astute clinical observation in 1957, which led to the recognition of Burkitt's lymphoma as a distinct clinical entity (29–31) and, ultimately, to the discovery of Epstein-Barr virus (EBV) (32), is an excellent example of how clinical observations can lead to unexpected discoveries and promote the development of novel research areas—in this example, cancer epidemiology and research into the viral etiology of cancer. During his time as a surgeon in the East African country of Uganda, Burkitt noted the occurrence of bizarre jaw tumors in children that lead to "massively swollen faces with bizarre lesions involving both sides of upper and lower jaws. The teeth were loose and features grossly distorted" (31). In most of the fast-growing tumors, biopsy results "suggested some form of sarcoma." Burkitt was baffled by the observation that many of the children who were affected by this disorder also had large abdominal masses and involvement of other organs, which suggested a systemic, and probably malignant, process. Together with his colleagues from the Department of Pathology, O'Conor and Davies, Burkitt discovered that these tumors, which were identified previously as Ewing's sarcoma or neuroblastoma, represented a form of a particularly fast-growing lymphoma that had been observed in this area of Africa for several decades.

Intrigued by the observation that these tumors did not seem to occur in areas of southern Africa, Burkitt started (with a minimum funding of £25!) epidemiologic research that, after a famous journey into West Africa that is known as the *long safari*, yielded the important observation that this tumor only occurred in regions of Africa with a minimum mean temperature of 15°C and a minimum rainfall of 20 in. per year—the definition of the so-called *lymphoma belt* in Africa. The climatic dependence of the incidence of tumors made Burkitt believe that this novel tumor (which has borne his name since the 1963 Paris meeting of the Union Internationale Contre le Cancer) might be caused by a vector-borne virus. Even though—as we know now—endemic Burkitt's lymphoma is not caused by the vector-borne disease with which it is associated (i.e., malaria), nor is the virus that causes its malignant transformation (i.e., EBV) vector-borne, Burkitt's early hypothesis laid the foundation for several seminal discoveries.

After a talk he gave at the Middlesex Hospital in London, England, Burkitt was approached by a young experimental pathologist named M. A. Epstein who, said Burkitt, "had realized that what I was talking about was just what he had been looking for for years" (31). In one of the African lymphoma biopsies that was provided by Denis Burkitt, Epstein, Achong, and Barr subsequently found the DNA virus that is now referred to as *EBV* (32). The initial hypothesis that EBV could be the tumor virus that Burkitt had been seeking did not prove true, because it was ultimately found that EBV is prevalent even in areas in which Burkitt's lymphoma is uncommon.

Another geographically distributed disease provided the clue that led to the discovery of the now well-known sequence of events in the development of Burkitt's lymphoma. Kafuko and Burkitt (33) demonstrated that the incidences of Burkitt's lymphoma and malaria were directly related in different districts of Uganda. The proposed causal relationship was further supported by the finding that children with sickle cell hemoglobin, which is known to protect against malaria, developed Burkitt's lymphoma less frequently than age- and sex-matched controls. It is now established that the specific suppression of T-cell clones that control the proliferation of EBV-infected B cells in patients with malaria supports the uncontrolled proliferation of B cells that carry activated c-*myc* oncogenes [reviewed in (34)]. The current hypothesis is that EBV infection in early childhood, followed by chronic malaria infection that induces suppression of cytotoxic T cells, forms the substrate for the development of Burkitt's lymphoma. The fact that immunosuppression, by drugs or human immunodeficiency virus, can also cause the development of EBV-positive B-cell lymphomas further supports this hypothesis. When the last step that characterizes this lymphoma, a chromosomal translocation t(8;14) that activates the c-*myc* oncogene, which, in turn, induces uncontrolled B-cell proliferation, was discovered, one of the first multistep carcinogenesis models in humans was completed (34). Burkitt's clinical observations in 1957 thus led to the delineation of one of the first complete pathways of development of a neoplasm.

Being a physician driven to "serve the less privileged" (30) in his chosen country of work, Burkitt also made significant contributions to our knowledge of the clinical course and treatment of Burkitt's lymphoma. This includes the observation of spontaneous regressions (35), as well as the excellent response of this fast-growing lymphoma to vincristine (36) and other cytotoxic drugs. The evolution from drug monotherapy to the principles of multiagent and multicycle chemotherapy, as later defined by DeVita and others, also starts with the observation that a fast-growing lymphoma, such as Burkitt's lymphoma, responds well to cytotoxic drugs but develops resistance early to this therapy, if drug monotherapy is used. Burkitt's lymphoma thus rightly serves as a model lymphoma entity in many aspects; initiated by the curiosity of a surgeon serving in East Africa, this lymphoma deservedly carries Burkitt's name.

CLASSIFICATIONS OF LYMPHOMAS

Although the list of malignant diseases of the lymphatic tissues that were outlined previously already comprised a form of lymphoma classification, reproducibility of the histologic diagnoses was poor, largely because of a lack of agreed-on morphologic criteria for classification. In the first half of the twentieth century, the existing terms *lymphoma*, *lymphosarcoma*, *giant follicle* or *follicular lymphoma*, *lymphocytoma*, *lymphoblastoma*, *reticulum cell sarcoma*, and even *Hodgkin's disease* were used heterogeneously by different pathologists and understood variably by clinicians. Nevertheless, important observations as to the natural history and the course of these disorders could be made. Because most patients were diagnosed in an advanced stage of their disease for which no effective therapy was available at that time, clinicians could only describe the natural history of the disorders. Reflecting the heterogeneity of the non-Hodgkin's lymphomas, this course differed from case to case and varied between a rapid exacerbation of the disease with early death and a rather slow progression over many years, particularly in patients with follicular lymphoma (18,37,38). Even in these early days, some of the patients with localized lymphoma could be cured by surgery or local radiotherapy (18,38,39).

Early Classifications

In the 1930s and 1940s, several attempts were made to develop a comprehensive list of the lymphomas that had been recognized into what might be called a classification, and these attempts were published in the United States and Europe. Although those nostalgic for what they believe to have been a simpler past are fond of suggesting that early classifications contained only three diseases—lymphosarcoma, reticulum cell sarcoma, and Hodgkin's disease—review of these early classifications actually reveals a far different picture. In fact, as early as 1948, Willis complained that "nowhere in pathology has a chaos of names so clouded clear concepts than in the subject of lymphoid tumors" (40). One of the earliest American attempts at a lymphoma classification came in 1934 from the American

TABLE 1.2. *The American Registry of Pathology Classification of lymphatic and reticular tumors (1934)*

Lymphocyte
  Leukemic lymphocytoma
    Chronic
    Acute
  Aleukemic lymphocytoma
    Diffuse
    Nodular
  Lymphosarcoma (lymphatic leucosarcoma)
    Aleukemic
    Leukemic
Reticulum cell
  Reticulocyte monocyte
    Leukemic reticulocytoma (monocytic leukemia)
    Aleukemic reticulocytoma
    Reticulum cell sarcoma
  Hodgkin's disease
    Localized (sclerosing)
    Generalized (cellular)
    Sarcomatous

From Callender GR. Tumors and tumor-like conditions of the lymphocyte, the myelocyte, the erythrocyte and the reticulum cell. *Am J Pathol* 1934;10:443–465.

TABLE 1.3. *The Robb-Smith Classification of reticulosis and reticulosarcoma (1938)*

Reticuloses
  A. Follicular reticuloses
    i. Lymphoid (follicular lymphoblastoma of American writers)
    ii. Myeloid (experimental only)
    iii. Lymphoid and histiocytic (Flemming's centres: reactive hyperplasia)
    iv. Giant cell and fibrillary
  B. Sinus reticuloses
    i. Histiocytic (sinus catarrh)
    ii. Giant-cell histiocytic (Stengel-Wolbach sclerosis)
    iii. Histiosyncytial
  C. Medullary reticuloses
    i. Lymphoid (lymphoid leukosis)
    ii. Myeloid (myeloid leucosis and myeloid transformations)
    iii. Monocytic (monocytic leukosis)
    iv. Reticulum-celled (Letterer-Siwe syndrome)
    v. Storage reticulum-celled (lipoidosis)
    vi. Histiocytic
    vii. Pro-histiocytic-fibrillary
    viii. Fibro-myeloid (Hodgkin's disease)
Reticulosarcoma
  A. Undifferentiated reticulosarcoma (syncytial)
    1. Diffuse
    2. Trabecular (stroma reaction)
  B. Differentiation to histioid cells
    1. Dictyosyncytial (fibrillo-syncytial) reticulosarcoma
    2. Dictyocytic (fibrillary) reticulosarcoma
  C. Differentiation to haemic cells
    1. Lymphocytoma
      i. Lymphoblastic sarcoma
        a. Medullary
        b. Follicular
      ii. Lymphosarcoma
    2. "Plasmocytoma"
    3. Monocytoma
    4. Myeloblastoma
    5. Erythroblastoma
  D. Mixed type (polymorphic reticulosarcoma)
  E. Differentiation of sinus-lining cells
    a. Undifferentiated cell type (reticulo-endothelio-sarcoma)
    b. Differentiated cell type (histiocytoma)

From Robb-Smith AH. Reticulosis and reticulosarcoma: a histological classification. *J Pathol* 1938;47:457–480.

Registry of Pathology, the predecessor to the Armed Forces Institute of Pathology (AFIP) (41) (Table 1.2). This classification incorporated morphologic and clinical information into a scheme that included multiple categories for each morphologic type, depending on its clinical presentation and extent of disease. A reading of this paper is instructive, in that it illustrates the complexity that can come from attempts to categorize with insufficient data. In 1938, Robb-Smith published a classification of benign and malignant disorders of lymph nodes, which was based on the concept of the reticuloendothelial system and the relationship of neoplasms to these normal counterparts, and escalated the complexity even further (Table 1.3) (42). At roughly the same time (1939), Rössle (42a) proposed a classification of lymphatic diseases that included multiple myeloma, based on the distinction between myeloblasts, lymphoblasts, and reticulum cells (Table 1.4).

Gall and Mallory

Several years later, Edward Gall and Tracy B. Mallory, pathologists at Massachusetts General Hospital (18), reviewed their own extensive material—618 cases—and concluded that the American Registry of Pathology proposal was not a practical approach; they proposed a classification that was based predominantly on morphology but showed that the different categories that were described did indeed have distinctive clinical behavior (Table 1.5). In addition, the morphologic features of the different subtypes were care-

fully described and illustrated, so that pathologists could learn and use the classification. The terminology reflected that in use in other publications but provided further subdivisions based on morphology: they suggested that the term

TABLE 1.4. *The Rössle Classification of hemoblastoses (1939)*

Mother cell	Undifferentiated mesenchymal cell			
	Erythroblast	Myeloblast	Lymphoblast	Reticulum cell
Type of neoplasia				
Benign	Erythroblastoma?	Myeloma?	Lymphoma?	Retothelioma?
Systemic	Erythroblastosis	Multiple myeloma	Lymphadenosis	Reticulosis (retotheliosis)
Locally malignant	Erythroblastic sarcoma (liver)	Myelosarcoma	Lymphosarcoma	Retothelsarcoma
Systemically malignant	?	Myelosarcomatosis	Lymphosarcomatosis	Reticulosarcomatosis
Leukemic	Polycythemia	Myeloid leukemia	Lymphatic leukemia	Monocytic leukemia

From Rössle R. Das Retothelsarkom der Lymphdrüsen. Seine Formen und Verwandtschaften. *Beitr Path Anatomie* 1939;103: 385–415, with permission.

lymphosarcoma should be discarded and divided into *lymphocytic lymphoma* and *lymphoblastic lymphoma*, *reticulum cell sarcoma* was divided into *clasmatocytic* (a term for a tissue histiocyte) and *stem cell lymphomas*, and *follicular lymphoma* was recognized as a distinctive morphologic and clinical entity. The classification included what have come to be known as *non-Hodgkin's lymphomas* and *Hodgkin's disease*; the classification of the non-Hodgkin's lymphomas appears to have been the first generally accepted classification of these disorders in the United States. In 1937 and 1947, Jackson and Parker, at Boston University Hospital, also published a comprehensive lymphoma classification; however, their primary focus was on Hodgkin's disease and the classification of the other lymphomas did not achieve widespread use (Table 1.6) (13,13a).

Modern Lymphoma Classifications

In the second half of the twentieth century, a large number of new lymphoma classifications were proposed, several of which achieved widespread use and greatly influenced the biologic understanding and clinical management of these diseases. The authors of some of these lymphoma classifications were invited to comment on the process and thinking that underlies their classifications. Contributions were received from Ronald Dorfman, Karl Lennert, and Costan Berard and are included in the Working Classification of Non-Hodgkin's Lymphoma (Dorfman), Kiel Classification (Lennert), and International Working Formulation (Berard) sections of this chapter.

Rappaport Classification

In 1957, Edward Gall and Henry Rappaport co-moderated a workshop on lymphoma at the American Society of Clinical Pathology (43); out of this collaboration, Rappaport developed a new classification proposal, which was based on the principles of the Gall and Mallory Classification (Table 1.5). The Rappaport Classification, which was published initially in 1956 in a report that was focused primarily on follicular lymphoma and fully developed in the AFIP fascicle of 1966 (44,45), took as its primary stratification the pattern of the lymphoma and considered that all lymphomas—including Hodgkin's disease—could be nodular

TABLE 1.5. *The Gall and Mallory Classification (1942)*

Stem cell lymphoma	
Clasmatocytic lymphoma	
Lymphoblastic lymphoma	⎫ "Reticulum cell sarcoma"
Lymphocytic lymphoma	
Hodgkin's lymphoma	
Hodgkin's sarcoma	
Follicular lymphoma	

From Gall EA, Mallory TB. Malignant lymphoma. A clinicopathologic survey of 618 cases. *Am J Pathol* 1942;18:381–429, with permission.

TABLE 1.6. *The Jackson and Parker Classification (1937, 1947)*

Reticulum cell sarcoma
Lymphocytoma
Lymphoblastoma
Lymphosarcoma
Giant follicle lymphoma
Plasmocytoma
Hodgkin's disease
    Early Hodgkin's disease, Paragranuloma
    Granuloma (Classical Hodgkin's disease)
    Sarcoma

From Jackson H Jr. The classification and prognosis of Hodgkin's disease and allied disorders. *Surg Gynec & Obst* 1937;64:465–467 and Jackson H Jr, Parker F Jr. *Hodgkin's disease and allied disorders.* New York: Oxford University Press, 1947, with permission.

TABLE 1.7. *The Rappaport Classification (1956, 1966)*

Nodular lymphomas	Diffuse lymphomas
Well-differentiated lympho-cytic	Well-differentiated lympho-cytic
Poorly differentiated lympho-cytic	Poorly differentiated lympho-cytic
Mixed lymphocytic and histi-ocytic	Mixed lymphocytic and histio-cytic
Histiocytic	Histiocytic
Undifferentiated	Undifferentiated
Hodgkin's disease	Hodgkin's disease

From Rappaport H. Tumors of the hematopoietic system. In: *Atlas of tumor pathology*, 3rd section, fasc 8. Washington: Armed Forces Institute of Pathology, 1966; and Rappaport H, Winter WJ, Hicks EB. Follicular lymphoma. A re-evaluation of its position in the scheme of malignant lymphoma, based on a survey of 253 cases. *Cancer* 1956;9:792–821, with permission.

or diffuse (Table 1.7). Within each tumor type, those with a nodular pattern had a better prognosis in general than those with a diffuse pattern. Rappaport modified the terminology of the Gall and Mallory Classification but continued to believe, as did others at the time, that neoplasms of large cells were derived from nonlymphoid stromal or other cells—the term *histiocytic* replaced the *reticulum cell* and *undifferentiated* replaced the *stem cell* of Gall and Mallory (the newly recognized Burkitt's lymphoma was considered *undifferentiated*).

Rappaport was concerned by the tendency of the day for pathologists and clinicians to believe that follicular hyperplasia was a precursor lesion or that it formed a continuum with follicular lymphoma. He recognized, as is generally accepted today, that there was no evidence that reactive follicles actually progressed to neoplastic ones. He further questioned whether the nodules of follicular lymphoma were in any way related to normal lymphoid follicles. To avoid this confusion, he proposed the term *nodular* to replace *follicular*, when it describes the pattern of the lymphoma (45). He further observed that most cytologic types of lymphoma could have a nodular or diffuse pattern, including Hodgkin's lymphoma. Thus, the previously well-defined *follicular lymphoma* of Gall and Mallory became lost among the four categories of *nodular lymphoma*: well-differentiated lymphocytic, poorly-differentiated lymphocytic, mixed lymphocytic and histiocytic, and histiocytic.

Although now there is general agreement that follicular lymphomas do not derive from follicular hyperplasia, we do recognize—as did many observers in the early twentieth century—that, in fact, the nodules of follicular lymphoma are neoplastic follicles, which are analogous to the neoplastic glands of an adenocarcinoma. By 1966, when the Rappaport Classification was published in full, the phenomenon of lymphocyte transformation had been described (46), and it was known that large cells could be lymphoid in origin; despite this knowledge, the erroneous designation of *histiocytic* was

retained for large-cell neoplasms. Finally, the entity of lymphoblastic lymphoma, which had been recognized in the Gall and Mallory Classification as a separate entity, was subsumed under diffuse poorly-differentiated lymphocytic lymphoma, thus mingling the distinctive *Sternberg sarcoma* and nodal infiltrates of acute lymphoblastic leukemia with diffuse variants of follicle center lymphomas.

Thus, the Rappaport Classification was somewhat of a paradox. It was concise but comprehensive, describing most of the entities known at the time, with clear morphologic criteria that were well illustrated in the 1966 AFIP fascicle, thus making it possible for pathologists to learn and use the classification. However, it ignored much of what was currently known about lymphocyte biology—the morphologically obvious relationship of neoplastic follicles to germinal centers and the understanding that lymphoid cells could be large.

Clinical Relevance of the Rappaport Classification

When physicians started to use the Rappaport Classification, they quickly learned to appreciate its clinical and prognostic relevance. In 1973, a large-scale study of patients from Stanford (47) confirmed the clinical predictive value of the Rappaport Classification for adult patients in the United States and ensured its adoption as the American standard (48). Thus, except for some disorders, such as nodular "histiocytic" and diffuse well-differentiated lymphocytic lymphoma (the latter corresponds to the lymphocytic lymphomas of the Kiel Classification), the most favorable natural history was observed in patients with entities that were characterized by lymphocytes and nodular architectural features, whereas patients with untreated diffuse "histiocytic" lymphomas showed an aggressive course and an unfavorable prognosis. Most patients with advanced lymphocytic and nodular lymphomas had good, even repeated, responses to irradiation or conventional cytotoxic chemotherapy, or both, with high rates of remission, but cures could not be achieved.

In their early pioneer work that was published in 1975, DeVita et al. (49) were able to demonstrate that, in a considerable proportion of patients with advanced diffuse "histiocytic" lymphoma, combination chemotherapy with mechlorethamine, vincristine, procarbazine, and prednisone (MOPP) induced durable complete remissions, thus indicating that patients with lymphomas of unfavorable histology can be cured by conventional chemotherapy (see Chapter 12).

The question arises, if the Rappaport Classification was biologically incorrect, why was it so successful in predicting patient outcome? The reason lies in the epidemiology of lymphomas in the United States and western Europe. Follicular lymphoma, which accounts for the vast majority of lymphomas with a nodular pattern, comprises almost 40% of adult non-Hodgkin's lymphomas in the United States (47,50). Because the vast majority of these behave in an indolent manner, the recognition of a nodular or follicular pattern alone would identify a large number of patients with indolent disease. Diffuse large B-cell lymphoma, which comprises approximately 70%

of diffuse lymphomas, is roughly equal in frequency to follicular lymphoma; because this is an aggressive disease, solely the recognition of a diffuse pattern would identify an aggressive lymphoma in the majority of the cases. Because pattern recognition has been shown to be the only truly reproducible feature of this classification, and because pattern alone identifies the two most common types of lymphoma, which have different clinical behavior, this simple approach to classification proved to have clinical relevance, even though it was biologically incorrect. It was not, however, useful for childhood lymphomas, because follicular lymphoma is rare in children, and the category of lymphoblastic lymphoma was not recognized as a distinct entity (51). It was also less useful in parts of the world in which follicular lymphoma is less common.

Immunologic Advances of the 1960s and 1970s

In the 1960s, two discoveries revolutionized the understanding of the immune system and its neoplasms. These discoveries were (a) the potential of lymphocytes, which had been thought to be end-stage, terminally differentiated cells, to transform into large, proliferating cells in response to mitogens or antigens (46) and (b) the existence of several distinct lymphocyte lineages (T, B, and natural killer) that could not be reliably predicted by morphology but that had different functions and physiology (52,53,56). In the early 1970s, lymphoid cells were found to have surface antigens or receptors that could be exploited to identify the lineage of normal and neoplastic cells (55). These observations led to the recognition that lymphomas were tumors of the immune system (54). In response to the new information, pathologists quite appropriately began to try to apply this knowledge to the classification of lymphomas.

Working Classification of Non-Hodgkin's Lymphomas

Ronald F. Dorfman has provided us with the following account of the development of his Working Classification.*

When I was a young pathologist working at the South African Institute for Medical Research in Johannesburg, in 1955, I was required by my professor to memorize and to use a complex classification of the progressive hyperplasias and neoplasias of lympho-reticular tissues, proposed in 1938 by A. H. T. Robb-Smith of the Pathology Department, St. Bartholomew's Hospital, London [42] (Table 1.3). By his own admission, Robb-Smith described his classification "as avoiding the fallacy of oversimplification!"

It was with some relief, therefore, that I encountered a new classification that was proffered in 1956 by Henry Rappaport in collaboration with Winter and Hicks of the AFIP [45]. It was clearly more utilitarian than that of Robb-Smith, and I was determined to use it from then on in my studies of malignant lymphomas that were occurring in South Africa. I had

also been impressed by the reported concepts of Gall et al. [22] in regard to the "follicular type of malignant lymphoma." They concluded that follicular lymphoma *was* a form of malignant disease of lymphoid tissues and that it had a distinct identity, with many characteristic clinical and structural features. On the other hand, Rappaport et al. [45] held that "there was no conclusive evidence that the so-called follicles of follicular lymphomas arose in, originated from, or were related to reactive secondary nodules." For this reason, Rappaport favored the term *nodular lymphoma*.

In 1961 [57], I concurred that lymphomas with a follicular pattern should be fitted into the general classification of malignant lymphomas; however, contrary to the view held by Rappaport et al. [45], I concluded that the clinical behavior of these follicular lymphomas, particularly with regard to race and sex incidence and their more favorable prognosis, warranted their separation from the diffuse lymphomas. For these reasons, I also felt that they should be regarded as distinct clinicopathologic entities.

After emigrating to the United States in 1963, I successfully persuaded the pathologists and the medical and radiation oncologists at Washington University School of Medicine in St. Louis, Missouri, to adopt the Rappaport Classification. In 1968, I was equally successful in convincing the pathologists and clinicians at Stanford University Medical Center of the inadequacy of the outdated terms *reticulum cell sarcoma*, *lymphosarcoma*, and *giant follicular lymphosarcoma* to characterize the malignant lymphomas. My membership in Rappaport's National Lymphoma Panel for Clinical Trials, which was instituted at the behest of Vincent DeVita [58], proved helpful in gaining adoption of the Rappaport terminology at Stanford. For the next decade, many important national clinical trials were successfully conducted and completed, using this uniform terminology, which had also been adopted at the National Cancer Institute by Costan Berard and Louis B. Thomas.

The recognition that malignant lymphomas represent neoplasms of the immune system resulted in attempts by Lukes and Collins and by Lennert to correlate morphology with function. The elegant studies of Jaffe and colleagues [59] illustrated the role of new immunologic techniques in the identification of cellular elements that comprised the so-called "nodular lymphomas" and provided evidence that supported their origin from follicular B lymphocytes. Thus, the validity of Rappaport's terminology and his concepts came under fire. This applied particularly to the concept of "differentiation" of lymphocytes, to the existence of mixed lymphocytic and histiocytic or predominantly histiocytic types of nodular lymphoma, and to the precise origin of cells in many lymphomas that were designated heretofore as *histiocytic* or *reticulum cell*. There was increasing evidence that these large cells were derived from small lymphocytes that had undergone transformation to "large lymphoid cells." Like those of Jaffe et al. [59], my own immunologic studies [60] provided further evidence of the origin of nodular lymphomas from follicular B lymphocytes, thus substantiating the term *follicular lymphoma*.

In 1973, at a Workshop on Classification of Non-Hodgkin's Lymphomas that was held at the University of Chicago, Farrer-Brown, Bennett, and Henry presented their own system, which had been accepted as the Working Classification for the British National Lymphoma Investigation (BNLI) of Non-Hodgkin's Lymphomas.

In an attempt to reach a compromise among the concepts of Rappaport, which had been so usefully applied to collaborative studies, those propounded by Lukes and Collins, and those of Farrer-Brown, Bennett, and Henry in England, I presented my own Working Classification of Non-Hodgkin's Lymphomas at the 1974 meeting of the International Acad-

*Ronald F. Dorfman, M.D., Professor of Pathology Emeritus, Stanford University School of Medicine, Stanford, California.

TABLE 1.8. *Working Classification of non-Hodgkin's lymphomas (Dorfman 1974, 1976)*

Follicular lymphomas

  (Follicular or follicular and diffuse)

  Small lymphoid

  Mixed small and large lymphoid

  Large lymphoid

Diffuse lymphomas

  Small lymphocytic

  Atypical small lymphoid

  Lymphoblastic

    Convoluted

    Non-convoluted

  Large lymphoid

  Mixed small and large lymphoid

  Histiocytic

  Burkitt's lymphoma

  Mycosis fungoides

  Undefined

(Composite lymphomas, sclerosis, plasmacytoid differentiation, and presence of epithelioid cells noted when present)

From Dorfman RF. Classification of non-Hodgkin's lymphomas [Letter]. *Lancet* 1974;1:1295–1296 and Dorfman RF. Pathology of the non-Hodgkin's lymphomas: new classifications. *Cancer Treat Rep* 1977;61:945–951, with permission.

TABLE 1.9. *The Kiel Classification (1974, 1988)*

B-Cell	T-Cell
Low Grade Malignancy	Low Grade Malignancy
Lymphocytic:	Lymphocytic:
CLL	CLL
Prolymphocytic leukemia	Prolymphocytic leukemia
Hairy-cell leukemia	Small, cerebriform cell - mycosis fungoides, Sézary's syndrome
Lymphoplasmacytic/cytoid (immunocytoma)	Lymphoepithelioid (Lennert's lymphoma)
Plasmacytic	Angioimmunoblastic (AILD, LgX)
Centroblastic/centrocytic	T zone
- follicular ± diffuse	
- diffuse	
Centrocytic	Pleomorphic, small cell (HTLV-1±)
High Grade Malignancy	High Grade Malignancy
Centroblastic	Pleomorphic, medium and large cell (HTLV-1 ±)
Immunoblastic	Immunoblastic (HTLV-1±)
Large cell anaplastic (Ki-1 +)	Large cell anaplastic (Ki-1 +)
Burkitt lymphoma	
Lymphoblastic	Lymphoblastic
Rare Types	Rare Types

AILD, angioimmunoblastic lymphadenopathy with dysproteinemia; CLL, chronic lymphocytic leukemia; HTLV-1, human T-cell leukemia virus type I; LgX, lymphogranulomatosis X.

From Gérard-Marchant R, Hamlin I, Lennert K, et al. Classification of non-Hodgkin's lymphomas [Letter]. *Lancet* 1974;2:406–408 and Stansfeld AG, Diebold J, Kapanci Y, et al. Updated Kiel classification for lymphomas [Letter]. *Lancet* 1988;1:292–293;603, with permission.

---

emy of Pathology in San Francisco [Table 1.8]. My hope was that this classification would eliminate controversial terminology, introduce new designations that were based, to some extent, on the functional capacity of the component cells, and yet use terms that would be acceptable to the pathologist in his or her everyday diagnostic work and to the hematologist and oncologist who were burdened with the choice of therapy for patients who were affected by the non-Hodgkin's lymphomas. Subsequently, I submitted this classification in the form of a letter to *The Lancet* (June 22, 1974) [61]. In 1976, I modified this slightly to include lymphoblastic lymphoma, convoluted and non-convoluted types, and added footnotes in regard to composite lymphomas, those lymphomas that show plasmacytoid differentiation, and those diffuse lymphomas that are associated with epithelioid cells [62].

The response to my letter in *The Lancet* was a little like opening Pandora's box! In short order, *The Lancet* published letters that were received from Bennett, Farrer-Brown, and Henry in support of the BNLI Classification [63] and from a European consortium in support of the Kiel Classification [64], which was largely based on the concepts of Karl Lennert and of Robert Lukes, whose classification was also published in 1974 [65] [Tables 1.9, 1.10, 1.11].

I was not entirely surprised when *The Lancet* published H. E. M. Kay's hilarious "Classification of non-Hodgkin's lymphomas" [66] [Table 1.12]. I was then given the opportunity to respond to all these letters, including that of Kay [61a]. I indicated that my colleagues and I had derived great amusement from Kay's letter and that, by all means, we should retain our sense of humor about this controversy; however, in the interest of amicable transatlantic relations, I hoped that we could reach a compromise, because there was no doubt about

the similarities in the proposed systems, even though there were differences of opinion, which needed clarification. In my letter, and in a subsequent review [62], I emphasized that my clinical colleagues viewed this controversy with dismay, because they had come to rely on the Rappaport Classification as being most useful in correlating response to therapy with morphologic designations. I concluded by indicating that, if a conference were to be arranged in the Caribbean, I fully intended to propose Dr. Kay as the moderator!

Kiel Classification

Professor Karl Lennert has provided us with the following account of the development of the Kiel Classification.*

The Kiel Classification is based on relating the proliferating cell types to their normal counterparts in lymphoid tissues.

---

*Karl Lennert, M.D., Professor of Pathology Emeritus; former Director, Institute of Pathology, Christian Albrecht University, Kiel, Germany.

TABLE 1.10. *The Lukes-Collins Classification (1974)*

I. U cell (undefined cell) type

II. T cell types

Mycosis fungoides and Sézary's syndrome

Convoluted lymphocyte

? Immunoblastic sarcoma (of T cells)

? Hodgkin's disease

III. B cell types

Small lymphocyte (chronic lymphocytic leukemia)

Plasmacytoid lymphocyte

Follicular center cell (FCC) types (follicular, diffuse, follicular and diffuse, and sclerotic)

Small cleaved

Large cleaved

Small noncleaved

Large noncleaved

Immunoblastic sarcoma of B cells

IV. Histiocytic type

V. Unclassifiable

From Lukes RJ, Collins RD. Immunologic characterization of human malignant lymphomas. *Cancer* 1974;34:1488–1503, with permission.

TABLE 1.12. *"Classification of classifications" (1974)*

Well-defined, high-grade, oligosyllabic

Poorly differentiated, polysyllabic

Diffuse

Circumlocutory

With dyslexogenesis

Unicentric

Derivative

Neologistic

Multicentric, cycnophilic (Greek κυκνος = swan)[a]

Cleaved and convoluted types

Rappaport (non-Lukes)

Lukes (non-Rappaport)

Note: This system makes no claim to be comprehensive or even comprehensible, so there may well be scope for other classifications of classifications and, ultimately, one hopes, a classification of classifications of classifications. At that point, we shall need a conference in the Caribbean.

[a]A former colleague of Dr. Kay's commented that this term was derived from the tendency of pathologists who had proposed lymphoma classifications to be found "swanning about" from one conference on classification to another.

From Kay HEM. Classification of non-Hodgkin's lymphomas [Letter]. *Lancet* 1974;2:586, with permission.

Identification of the cell type is based essentially on a combination of two elements: (a) subtle cytomorphology, which is studied in imprints and sections by using the same hematologic stains (Giemsa) for both, and (b) data and techniques from the field of modern immunology. By comparative

TABLE 1.11. *The British National Lymphoma Investigation classification (1974)[a]*

Grade 1

Follicular lymphomas

Follicle cell, predominantly small

Follicle cell, mixed small and large

Follicle cell, predominantly large

Diffuse lymphomas

Lymphocytic, well differentiated (small round lymphocyte)

Lymphocytic, intermediate differentiation (small follicle cell)

Grade 2

Lymphocytic, poorly differentiated

Mixed, small lymphoid and undifferentiated large cell

Undifferentiated large cell

Plasma cell

True histiocyte

Unclassified

[a]Plasmacytoid differentiation in lymphocytic tumors and banded or fine sclerosis are recorded.

From Bennett MH, Farrer-Brown G, Henry K, et al. Classification of non-Hodgkin's lymphomas [Letter]. *Lancet* 1974;2:405–406, with permission.

analysis of imprints and Giemsa-stained sections, it was possible as early as the 1960s to identify various previously unrecognized cell types in normal and reactive lymph nodes: centroblasts, centrocytes, immunoblasts, two types of plasma cells, and later plasmacytoid T-zone cells and monocytoid B cells [67].

Because the Kiel Classification is based on the proliferating cell types, not on purely histologic features, it was necessary to identify the cells that constitute the various types of lymphoma. For many lymphomas, this could be done with morphologic examination of Giemsa-stained sections; in this way, several lymphomas of germinal center cells were identified [68]. In other types, this was more difficult. The biggest problem concerned the type of lymphoma that was composed of large cells (at the time designated as *histiocytic* or *reticulum cell*). With Giemsa staining, it could be seen that these cells had basophilic cytoplasm, similar to some large cells in the lymph node (centroblasts and immunoblasts). A chance opportunity to investigate a case by means of electron microscopy provided the first clues. The cytoplasm was found to contain large amounts of rough endoplasmic reticulum, similar to plasma cells. Therefore, the tumor was interpreted as "immunoblastic sarcoma" [69]. Unfortunately, the next cases of large-cell lymphoma contained only very little endoplasmic reticulum but instead contained many polyribosomes (corresponding to the cytoplasmic basophilia).

We then turned to the technique of gel electrophoresis to study a case of highly basophilic large-cell lymphoma from which fresh, unfixed tissue homogenates could be investigated. The tumor contained large amounts of immunoglobulin M (IgM). Three further cases of large-cell lymphoma also revealed increased IgM. Other lymphomas showed increased amounts of IgM, immunoglobulin G, or even immunoglobulin A. These findings stimulated us to begin a preliminary study on fresh lymphoma cases.

The results, which were presented by Stein and Lennert in Vienna in 1972, served as the impetus for a cooperative study that involved a number of German and Austrian hospitals. Led by A. Stacher and G. Brittinger, this group was known as the Kiel Lymphoma Study Group (KLSG). The immunochemical data were correlated with entities that were distinguished on the basis of morphologic differences. Because, in most types of lymphoma, increased amounts of immunoglobulin were found in tissues, it became clear that most of the lymphomas must be of the B-cell type. Histiocytic types were not found. The first summary of the data was presented at a meeting organized by H. Rappaport in Chicago in June, 1973.

Subsequently, the participating European lymphoma pathologists met in Kiel for a three-day symposium in May, 1974 to study the details of the new approach to lymphoma classification. This symposium began with an extensive demonstration of bone marrow and lymph node cells in imprints and Giemsa-stained sections. After this demonstration, slides that demonstrated all of the various types of lymphoma were distributed to the participants and jointly studied. Agreement was reached that two groups should be distinguished. In accordance with the rules of general pathology, lymphomas that consisted of small cells (*cytes*), with or without some interspersed large cells (*blasts*), were to be referred to as *low-grade* (instead of *well-differentiated*), whereas lymphomas composed only of large cells (*blasts*) were to be called *high-grade* (instead of *undifferentiated*). The low-grade lymphomas included chronic lymphocytic leukemia, immunocytomas, and centrocytic and centroblastic-centrocytic lymphomas. The high-grade lymphomas consisted of centroblastic, lymphoblastic, and immunoblastic lymphomas. Additionally, an unclassified group was included. At the beginning of the meeting, the terms *germinoblastic* and *germinocytic* were used, but these were replaced by *centroblastic* and *centrocytic*, because Lukes feared confusion with germ-cell tumors. No distinction was made between leukemias and solid tumors of the same cell types. The classification was given the name *Kiel Classification* by analogy to the Rye Classification of Hodgkin's lymphomas.

At that meeting, the pathologists who were present decided to form a group, which was called the European Lymphoma Club. The members were R. Gérard-Marchant, I. Hamlin, K. Lennert, F. Rilke, A. G. Stansfeld, and J. A. M. van Unnik. The members of the club returned to their laboratories and studied their current cases to see whether the classification could be used in practice. After a one-day discussion on July 6, 1974, Stansfeld presented a paper, which had been read and edited by Lennert during the night. A brief discussion followed, and, at Amsterdam Airport, all club members signed a letter to the editor to be sent to *The Lancet* [64] [Table 1.9]. The morphologic details of the Kiel Classification were presented by Lennert, N. Mohri, E. Kaiserling, and H. Stein at the Congress of the International Society of Haematology in London in August, 1975 [70].

Over the following years, the club met two to three times a year to study difficult cases that were presented by the various members. Additionally, more immunologic data became available. The clinicians of the KLSG also met two to three times a year to exchange their experiences with the various types of lymphoma, and it became clear that we were dealing with real entities [71,78,79]. On the basis of the large amounts of new immunologic data, it became possible to classify lymphomas not only according to the categories low- and high-grade, but also as B- and T-cell lymphomas of low and high grade. The updated Kiel Classification, which was published in 1988, was the result of these studies [72]. It was described in detail in a book that was published by Lennert together with A. C. Feller [73].

Centrocytic lymphoma, which, thanks to new immunologic techniques, was later recognized as mantle cell lymphoma, was included as an entity from the beginning and not merely considered the equivalent of Lukes' cleaved cell lymphoma [3]. Clinically, it was also recognized as an entity [71,74,78,79]. In the category of high-grade lymphomas, *lymphoblastic* lymphomas (or precursor cell lymphomas) were distinguished from Burkitt's lymphomas and large-cell anaplastic (Ki–1+) lymphomas, and a group of rare types was added.

Subsequent cytogenetic and molecular genetic studies [75] and molecular genetic techniques [76] supported our definitions of distinct entities related to the B- and T-cell lineage. The clinicians became more and more convinced that they were applying a clinically relevant, and by no means esoteric, classification. At the "Non-Hodgkin's Lymphoma Classification Project Meeting" (September 8–10, 1997; Omaha, Nebraska) the results of a clinical evaluation (77) were discussed which demonstrated that the International Lymphoma Study Group (REAL) classification (97) identifies clinically distinctive types of non-Hodgkin's lymphomas and has prognostic relevance. As pointed out by Dr. Saul Rosenberg at the conference, these data were equivalent to those obtained with patients diagnosed according to the updated Kiel Classification whereas the Working Formulation had to be considered outdated and should be abandoned.

Clinical Relevance of the Kiel Classification

In Europe, where the Rappaport Classification had been used only occasionally, the Kiel Classification gained widespread endorsement by pathologists and clinicians. In the late 1970s, a retrospective analysis of the clinical and prognostic features of 405 patients who had lymphomas that were classified according to the Kiel Classification was carried out by the KLSG and published in German (78,79). Subsequently, a prospective observation study was performed in which 1,127 patients were followed for as many as 10 years by the KLSG (71). Several histopathologic entities appeared as distinct entities from both a clinical and a prognostic point of view, as evidenced by a fan-like arrangement of the survival curves. In general, patients who had low-grade malignant lymphomas had a more favorable prognosis than patients who had high-grade malignant entities. However, the survival curves of patients who had advanced low-grade lymphomas had an almost linear decline without any evidence of a plateau, thus suggesting that treatment was not curative. This observation was validated by all subsequent studies that used different classification systems and remained true, even when more intensive therapeutic regimens were used.

The early investigations by the KLSG also showed that patients with advanced lymphomas of high-grade malignancy had a different shape of their survival curves, which were characterized by an early steep decline and a subsequent plateau, thus suggesting the possibility of cure in a proportion of patients by chemotherapy alone. These findings agreed with the earlier observations by DeVita et al. (49) of patients with diffuse "histiocytic" lymphomas, as classified according to the Rappaport Classification (and corresponding to high-grade lymphomas of the Kiel Classification).

Evaluation of survival data of patients with advanced centrocytic lymphoma by the KLSG (71,78,79) showed that patients with this newly defined entity differed in their prognosis from those with any other lymphoma. Although the shape of the survival curve was similar to that of patients with low-grade lymphomas, the decline was much steeper, with a median survival of only approximately 2.5 years (71). In a later randomized treatment trial (74), it was demonstrated that even an anthracycline-containing combination chemotherapy, such as cyclophosphamide, doxorubicin, vincristine, and prednisone (CHOP), was not able to induce long-lasting complete remissions as the prerequisite for cure.

The category of immunocytoma included two subtypes: lymphoplasmacytic, which is equivalent to the tissue counterpart of Waldenström's macroglobulinemia, and lymphoplasmacytoid, which is now believed to be a variant of chronic lymphocytic leukemia, with plasmacytoid differentiation. The investigations of the KLSG (71,74a) showed that patients with this lymphoplasmacytoid variant of chronic lymphocytic leukemia had a significantly less favorable prognosis than patients with typical chronic lymphocytic leukemia.

Important Features of the Kiel Classification

The original Kiel Classification recognized that most lymphomas resembled cells of the germinal center and were therefore of B-cell lineage (centrocytic, centroblastic-centrocytic, and centroblastic), with a smaller number composed of B cells of nonfollicular type (chronic lymphocytic leukemia, immunocytoma, immunoblastic lymphoma, Burkitt's lymphoma, plasmacytoma), and a minority of types showing evidence of T-cell derivation (mycosis fungoides, mediastinal lymphoblastic lymphoma, an immunoblastic sarcoma of T-cell lineage, and rare cases of nodal lymphomas that are called *T-zone lymphoma*). However, rather than sorting lymphomas primarily as T-cell and B-cell types, it focused on carefully defining disease entities by a combination of morphology, available immunophenotyping studies, and clinical features (3). It was thus a practical classification that could be applied by pathologists in daily practice, and it achieved widespread use in Europe.

The Kiel Classification never achieved general acceptance in the United States. Possible reasons include the terminology, which included new names for most cell types and disease categories; the lack of inclusion of pattern as a major defining feature; and the lack of subclassification (grading) of nodular (follicular) lymphoma, which was perceived as having prognostic importance in the United States. Interestingly, follicular lymphoma was reported at the time to be less common in Europe than in North America (3), a fact that probably influenced the attention that was paid to this disease by the two classifications.

In fact, these problems were more a matter of perception than reality. The terminology was not particularly difficult and reflected usage that was adopted by immunologists (such as the term *immunoblast*); newly described cell types had to be named, and the convention of hematologists was used—small resting cells were named with the suffix *-cytes* and large, transformed, or proliferating cells were named with the suffix *-blasts*. Follicular lymphoma was indeed recognized as an entity: it was given the cumbersome name *centroblastic-centrocytic* lymphoma and subclassified as follicular, follicular and diffuse, or diffuse. It was also graded, in the sense that this category included only the low-grade categories of "poorly differentiated lymphocytic" and "mixed lymphocytic and histiocytic" in the Rappaport scheme; cases composed of predominantly large cells (Rappaport's "nodular histiocytic") were classified as centroblastic, follicular—a category of high-grade lymphoma. Thus, although cell type, rather than pattern, was the primary method of classification, the importance of pattern within this category was indeed recognized.

In retrospect, there is no question that the Kiel Classification represented the first major conceptual advance in classification since Gall and Mallory; it recognized and defined important disease entities and correctly predicted their relationships to normal cellular counterparts. It also incorporated important features of the Rappaport Classification: careful morphologic descriptions of entities and clear illustrations that permitted pathologists to learn and use the classification (3). Finally, it represented the first attempt at a consensus among pathologists on a lymphoma classification; although Karl Lennert was the primary force behind the classification, the involvement of a large group of pathologists, who studied cases together and had input into the terminology and organization of the classification, represented yet another conceptual advance.

The Lukes-Collins Classification

In the late 1960s and early 1970s, R. Lukes and J. Parker studied the morphology of lymphocyte transformation by mitogens (80,81,83). Similar to the work of Lennert and his colleagues, they emphasized the importance of special stains to demonstrate nuclear and cytoplasmic features of lymphoid cells at various stages of differentiation, by using the methyl green pyronin and Giemsa stains (82,84). Lukes attended the meetings in Europe and Asia that were described by Lennert in the Kiel Classification section earlier in this chapter, and the two groups shared concepts and ideas about an immunologic approach to the understanding and classification of lymphomas. In 1974, Lukes and Robert Collins published an immunologically based classification of lymphomas (Table 1.10) (65). It was based on essentially the same observations and immunologic data as the Kiel Classification, but the approach to the definition of diseases was somewhat different. The authors made use of *camera lucida* drawings to delineate cell types in lymph nodes based on their nuclear contours. The major disease categories were then based on the resemblance of the cells to those found in lymph node germinal centers and extrafollicular areas. Diseases were categorized as T- or B-cell lineage derived, based on morphologic features. Pattern (follicular or diffuse) was not considered an important feature for classification, because the authors anticipated that cell type would be the most important predictor of clinical behavior.

The Lukes-Collins Classification predicted, similar to the Kiel Classification, that the vast majority of lymphoid neoplasms were derived from follicular center cells, including what we now know as follicular lymphoma (small cleaved follicular center cell, large cleaved follicular center cell), most cases of diffuse large B-cell lymphoma (large cleaved follicular center cell, large noncleaved follicular center cell), and Burkitt's lymphoma (small noncleaved follicular center cell). B- and T-immunoblastic lymphomas were also recognized, as were small lymphocytic lymphomas of B- and T-cell types and the T-cell lymphomas, mycosis fungoides and lymphoblastic lymphoma. This classification did not distinguish between the two types of "small cleaved cell lymphomas" of the Kiel Classification (centrocytic and centroblastic-centrocytic).

In several subsequent studies, the morphologic and clinical features of some of the disorders that were defined in the Lukes-Collins Classification were delineated (85–90). However, similar to the Kiel Classification, this classification did not achieve widespread acceptance in the United States. The requirement for assigning lineage based on morphology and the difficulty in relating the disease categories to the familiar categories of the Rappaport scheme resulted in resistance to this classification on the part of pathologists and oncologists. An additional problem was that in neither its original description nor in subsequent publications were clear criteria for diagnosis presented and illustrated; thus, it was difficult for pathologists to learn and apply the classification.

Other Classifications of the 1970s: British National Lymphoma Investigation and World Health Organization

Shortly after the publication of the Dorfman, Kiel, and Lukes-Collins classifications, other proposals appeared in the literature, including the proposal of Bennett et al. (63), which became the BNLI classification (Table 1.11), and the World Health Organization (WHO) classification of Mathé et al. (Table 1.13) (91). To varying extents, these classifications attempted to apply terminology that reflected immunologic advances—that is, the recognition that large-cell lymphomas were lymphoid, rather than histiocytic—to the basic framework of the Rappaport Classification (Table 1.7). The BNLI classification was used for many years in Britain.

International Working Formulation for Clinical Usage

By the mid 1970s, at least five new proposals for lymphoma classification had been made, in addition to the standard Rappaport Classification. This situation was the subject of much humor, as previously described by Ronald Dorfman (Table 1.12) (66), but also a cause for consternation among oncologists, who were concerned that the results of clinical trials from different institutions would be impossible to interpret. Several meetings were organized by oncologists in the United States and Europe in the mid 1970s, in an attempt to produce a consensus among the expert pathologists on a unified approach to lymphoma classification; unfortunately, these attempts were unsuccessful.

Dr. Costan Berard contributed the following recollections of the events that led up to the development of the Working Formulation for non-Hodgkin's lymphomas.*

TABLE 1.13. *World Health Organization (WHO) Classification (1976)*

A. Lymphosarcomas
  1. Nodular lymphosarcoma
  2. Diffuse lymphosarcoma
    (a) Lymphocytic
    (b) Lymphoplasmacytic
    (c) Prolymphocytic
    (d) Lymphoblastic
    (e) Immunoblastic
    (f) Burkitt's tumour
B. Mycosis fungoides
C. Plasmacytoma
D. Reticulosarcoma
E. Unclassified malignant lymphomas
F. Hodgkin's disease
  1. With lymphocyte predominance
  2. With nodular sclerosis
  3. With mixed cellularity
  4. With lymphocyte depletion
G. Others
  1. Eosinophilic granuloma
  2. Mastocytoma

From Mathé G, Rappaport H, O'Conor GT, et al. *Histological and cytological typing of neoplastic diseases of haematopoietic and lymphoid tissues (International Histological Classification of Tumors No. 14).* Geneva: World Health Organization, 1976, with permission.

Vincent DeVita and Henry Kaplan were the driving force behind the project, because of the chaos of nomenclature that became apparent at the 1974 Cancer Congress in Florence, Italy. "Not only couldn't the clinicians understand what the pathologists were saying, the pathologists couldn't even understand each other!" DeVita and Kaplan arranged a meeting of clinicians and the hematopathologists who had proposed classifications at Airlie House, Warrenton, Virginia, in September of 1975. Ronald Dorfman and I were appointed co-chairs. We hoped that the proponents of the major proposals could reach a consensus through rational discussion. It was a disaster! The meeting ended with one clear conclusion: only a study to generate data had any chance of breaking the stalemate. I was invited, as the only expert who was not the author of a classification, to devise a study plan to put forward for funding a project to move ahead. I designed the study, with the collaboration of Eli Glatstein and a Stanford statistician named Byron Brown and input from a few others. Each of the experts approved the study design and agreed to participate. DeVita funded the project through a National Cancer Institute contract. The plan called for six control pathologists, and I agreed to serve as one of those, in addition to my major role as National Cancer Institute Project Officer.

Histologic slides and clinical data from more than 1,000 patients who had been treated on prospective clinical trials in four institutions around the world (Milan Tumor Institute, University

---

*Costan A. Berard, M.D., former Chief, Hematopathology Section, National Cancer Institute, National Institutes of Health, Bethesda, Maryland.

of Minnesota, Stanford University, and Tufts University) were reviewed, in an attempt to develop data that could be used to determine which of the classifications was most effective in predicting the clinical behavior of lymphomas. Authors of each of the six classifications (the experts) traveled to the different sites and reviewed histologic sections, each classifying them according to his or her own scheme. In addition, six other pathologists (control pathologists) attempted to classify each case according to all six schemes. Several endpoints were used as markers of the validity of each classification; the most important was the overall actuarial survival of patients whose slides were reviewed, but inter- and intra-observer reproducibility were also evaluated.

Three years later, at the conclusion of this investigation, it became clear that each of the systems had merit, as applied by the expert pathologists or the control group. All classifications were found to be able to attribute the lymphomas to different groups of low, intermediate, and high clinical grade, as shown by the corresponding survival data. The reproducibility by individual pathologists (second review of the same slide) and the concordance of various examiners in reproducing a diagnosis within a given scheme were not satisfactory, possibly due, in part, to technical problems. In the end, none of the classifications could be agreed on as the standard. At a series of meetings at Stanford in 1979 and 1980, the *Working Formulation for Clinical Usage* was developed to translate between the various classifications [Table 1.14] [50]. In its original concept, this scheme was not designed to be a free-standing lymphoma classification but rather was meant to be superimposed on whatever classification was in use at a particular center, to permit the results of clinical trials to be generalized across different centers that used different classifications. However, it rapidly became the primary classification that was used in the United States.

Important Features of the Working Formulation

The WF essentially used categories of lymphomas that were recognized in the Rappaport Classification but substituted terminology—primarily from the Lukes-Collins Classification—that was believed to be biologically more correct: for example, *small lymphocytic* was used instead of *well-differentiated lymphocytic*, *small cleaved cell* instead of *poorly differentiated lymphocytic*, *large cleaved* or *noncleaved cell* or *immunoblast* instead of *histiocytic*, and *follicular* rather than *nodular*. It also recognized that not all lymphomas could have a truly follicular pattern. Unfortunately, in adapting the Lukes-Collins terminology, important modifying terms were left out, which led to a lack of specificity and clarity in the WF terminology. In the Lukes-Collins scheme, a *small cleaved follicular center cell* was a distinctive cell of the germinal center; this term did not apply to any cell with nuclear irregularity. Similarly, a *small noncleaved follicular center cell* was a distinctive blastic cell (corresponding to Burkitt's lymphoma cells), which was small only in comparison to *large noncleaved follicular center cells*. The term *small noncleaved cell*, however, could be confusing, because a small lymphocyte is also *small* and *noncleaved*.

The WF categories were deliberately defined broadly, so that (a) all lymphomas could be classified, and (b) all categories of all existing classifications could be accommodated, thus fulfilling its function as a sort of pathologic *lingua franca* or Esperanto. Thus, the category of *diffuse mixed small and large cell* included diffuse follicle center lymphomas and peripheral T-cell

TABLE 1.14. *The Working Formulation for Clinical Usage (1982)*

Low grade
  A. Malignant lymphoma, small lymphocytic
      Consistent with chronic lymphocytic leukemia
      Plasmacytoid
  B. Malignant lymphoma, follicular, predominantly small cleaved cell
      Diffuse areas
      Sclerosis
  C. Malignant lymphoma, follicular, mixed, small cleaved and large cell
      Diffuse areas
      Sclerosis
Intermediate grade
  D. Malignant lymphoma, follicular, predominantly large cell
      Diffuse areas
      Sclerosis
  E. Malignant lymphoma, diffuse, small cleaved cell
      Sclerosis
  F. Malignant lymphoma, diffuse, mixed, small and large cell
      Sclerosis
      Epithelioid cell component
  G. Malignant lymphoma, diffuse, large cell
      Cleaved cell
      Non-cleaved cell
      Sclerosis
High grade
  H. Malignant lymphoma, large cell, immunoblastic
      Plasmacytoid
      Clear cell
      Polymorphous
      Epithelioid cell component
  I. Malignant lymphoma, lymphoblastic
      Convoluted cell
      Nonconvoluted cell
  J. Malignant lymphoma, small noncleaved cell
      Burkitt's
      Follicular areas
Miscellaneous
  Composite
  Mycosis fungoides
  Histiocytic
  Extramedullary plasmacytoma
  Unclassifiable
  Other

From National Cancer Institute sponsored study of classifications of non-Hodgkin's lymphomas. Summary and description of a working formulation for clinical usage. The Non-Hodgkin's Lymphoma Pathologic Classification Project. *Cancer* 1982;49:2112–2135, with permission.

lymphomas, and the category of *large cell immunoblastic* included B- and T-cell cases. To further deemphasize the idea of disease entities, each category was given a letter designation (A through J), which could be used instead of the category name.

An important and novel feature of the WF was the separation of the lymphomas into clinical prognostic groups, or *clinical grades*, as they came to be called. These groupings differed from the *histologic grades* of the Kiel Classification in that they were based on the actuarial survival curves of the patients in the international study and not on morphologic features, such as cell size, nuclear immaturity, or proliferative activity. The oncologists who were involved in the study believed that these groupings were necessary to help clinicians to deal with the large number of morphologic categories by combining them into groups that could be used to suggest appropriate treatment. Thus, *low-grade* lymphomas were treated palliatively, with an expectation of long survival that was unaffected by treatment; *intermediate-grade* lymphomas were treated aggressively, with an expectation of cure; and *high-grade* lymphomas were treated intensively, often with central nervous system prophylaxis.

In the mid 1970s, clinical studies had begun to show that some aggressive lymphomas (diffuse "histiocytic") could be cured with combination chemotherapy (49,92). At least one study appeared to show that histologic subclassification of these lymphomas could predict which cases could be cured with this treatment (93). Thus, there was considerable optimism that morphologic features could be used to predict the outcome of patients with large-cell lymphomas. This hypothesis was tested in the National Cancer Institute study; unfortunately, the pathologists were unable to agree on subclassification of many of the cases. Nonetheless, in a subset of the cases that could be classified as immunoblastic, there was a small but statistically significant decrease in survival compared to the large cleaved and noncleaved types (50).

The WF thus divided large-cell lymphomas into two categories: large-cell (cleaved or noncleaved) and immunoblastic. The immunoblastic category was placed in the *high-grade* clinical group, with Burkitt's and lymphoblastic lymphomas, whereas the large-cell category was considered *intermediate* grade. Unfortunately, clear and reproducible criteria for the separation of large-cell and large-cell immunoblastic lymphomas were not given in the paper, and pathologists found this distinction difficult to make. Thus, although the distinction could theoretically lead to important differences in treatment, it proved impossible for pathologists to make it reliably (94).

The WF did not represent a true consensus, because Lukes, Collins, and Lennert disagreed with it in a commentary accompanying its publication and in later publications (95). The major criticisms were the lumping of distinct entities into broad categories that clouded biologic entities and the lack of incorporation of even the somewhat limited immunophenotyping studies that were available at the time. The three main groups of low-, intermediate-, and high-grade lymphomas had been solely defined by prognostic criteria (survival curves) and were based only in part on individual biologic entities, as determined by cytologic and immunologic parameters. As a consequence of this prognosis-oriented approach, lymphomas that were considered entities by the Kiel Classification, such as centroblastic-centrocytic lymphoma, were present in several categories of the low- and intermediate-grade lymphomas of the WF, whereas centrocytic lymphoma did not appear at all.

Berard comments:

> We all knew that, but the driving force was the stalemate to *clinical* research, and there were no good data regarding important clinical or therapeutic implications of the proposed B-cell versus T-cell neoplasms, whether lymphoblastic, mixed cell, or large cell. The driving force in the WF's distinctions were survival curves, and they formed the backbone of clinical trials for almost 20 years. During that time, the biologic entities that we all knew existed were greatly clarified, with the introduction and use of immunologic, cytogenetic, and molecular biologic tools that were not available at the time of the WF study (1976–1980).

However, for these reasons, the WF was not universally accepted, and, in several parts of the world, especially in Europe, the Kiel Classification continued to be applied. In addition, many centers in the United States used the Lukes-Collins Classification, alone or with the WF. Nonetheless, the WF served the purpose of standardizing terminology for clinical trials. Because the most common lymphoma types—follicular lymphoma and diffuse large B-cell lymphoma—were in fact recognized, this classification, similar to the Rappaport Classification, had clinical utility, despite its lack of an immunologic basis. In addition, this experience impressed on pathologists and clinicians the need for consensus among pathologists and clinical data to support any pathologic classification of lymphomas.

Dorfman, who co-chaired the Airlie House conference with Berard, further comments:

> To those who may question the propriety of the endeavors described previously, my response is to paraphrase Murphy, who, in his admirable text, *The Logic of Medicine* [96], emphasizes that the cardinal criterion of a classification is utility. It provides one means in an attempt to give order to what would otherwise be a hopeless jumble of disconnected facts. As such it is of the first importance in any field of scholarly endeavor.

Clinical Relevance of the Working Formulation

Most clinical studies of lymphomas that were published in major international journals during the 1980s and 1990s used the WF, as a free-standing classification or in addition to a local classification (50). The results of these studies are discussed in other chapters. Much of our current understanding of the clinical behavior and response to treatment of these disorders is based on studies that have used the WF.

Revised European-American Lymphoma and World Health Organization Classifications

In 1991, an international group of pathologists (International Lymphoma Study Group) was formed by Peter Isaacson and

Harald Stein to promote better understanding between European and American hematopathologists. At its third meeting, the group proposed a new classification of lymphoid neoplasms, which they called the "Revised European-American Classification of Lymphoid Neoplasms" (REAL) (97). This classification adopted most of the principles and many of the categories of the Kiel Classification but included extranodal lymphomas. It avoided the grouping of lymphoma entities according to their histopathologic grade of malignancy (Kiel Classification) or their prognosis (WF Classification). Only lymphomas that were considered to be well-defined entities were included. Diseases were defined by a combination of morphology, immunophenotype, and genetic and clinical features. The new classification offered the opportunity to be easily adapted to future progress in lymphoma research. A subsequent large clinical study showed the classification to be clinically and prognostically relevant, which was not surprising, because most of the entities had been recognized in the Kiel and other classifications and were known to be clinically distinctive (98,99). After a meeting between pathologists and oncologists in 1997 at Airlie House, where an agreement had so spectacularly failed in 1975, a consensus was reached on an improved and modified version of the REAL Classification, which was later published as the new official classification of the WHO (100). The introduction of the new WHO scheme marks the beginning of a new era in which all scientists and clinicians who are involved in lymphoma research and patient care can finally speak the same language. This long-awaited consensus is all the more remarkable in that many of the principal scientific elements of the REAL-WHO Classification had been recognized 25 years earlier in the Kiel Classification (see Chapter 4 for a more detailed discussion of the REAL and WHO classifications).

The formulation of the REAL Classification was accompanied by consequences in clinical research. The most striking experience was the rediscovery of mantle cell lymphoma, which had not been defined in the Rappaport scheme, the Lukes-Collins Classification, or the WF (109–111). These and subsequent studies not only confirmed the unique clinical and prognostic features of this lymphoma, but also showed that it is a biologic entity with characteristic cytogenetic and molecular properties. After a period of stagnation, new approaches to basic and clinical research in chronic lymphocytic leukemia have been made possible by the recent knowledge that this disorder is more heterogenous than was previously expected and that the presence or absence of somatic mutations in immunoglobulin variable region genes (101,102) and of chromosomal aberrations such as 11q and 17p deletions (103) are good predictors of the outcome of the disease.

Recent studies have begun to address the known heterogeneity of the lymphoma category that is defined as *diffuse large B-cell* lymphoma by the REAL-WHO Classification. Some studies had shown that the centroblastic (germinal center–derived) variant had a more favorable prognosis than the immunoblastic (presumed nongerminal center–derived) variant (104,105). Several groups (106–108) have recently begun to analyze the expression of large series of genes that are thought to be involved in lymphomagenesis by using the DNA microarray technique in which fragments of genes are hybridized with complementary DNA that is synthesized from lymphoma-derived messenger RNA. One group has identified three main gene expression subgroups of large B-cell lymphoma, among them germinal center and activated B-cell-like types. Retrospective clinical data suggest that patients with lymphomas of the germinal center B-cell-like subtype have a more favorable prognosis than patients with the other gene expression subgroups, a finding that correlates with previous observations that were based on morphology. It is likely that, in the near future, these new molecular techniques may contribute considerably to the understanding, the classification, and the treatment of non-Hodgkin's lymphomas.

REFERENCES

1. Kaplan HS. *Hodgkin's disease,* 2nd ed. Cambridge, MA: Harvard University Press, 1978.
2. Dorfman RF. Hematopathology: a crescendo of scholarly activity. *Mod Pathol* 1994:7:226–241.
3. Lennert K, Mohri N, Stein H, et al. Malignant lymphomas other than Hodgkin's disease. Histology-Cytology-Ultrastructure-Immunology. In: Uehlinger E, ed. *Handbuch der speziellen pathologischen Anatomie und Histologie,* vol 1. Berlin: Springer-Verlag, 1978.
4. Hodgkin T. On some morbid appearances of the absorbent glands and spleen. *Med-Chir Trans* 1832;17:68–114.
5. Aisenberg AC. *Malignant lymphoma: biology, natural history, and treatment.* Philadelphia: Lea & Febiger,1991.
6. Wilks S. Cases of lardaceous disease and some allied affections. With remarks. *Guy's Hosp Rep* 1856;2:103–132.
6a. Wilks S. Cases of enlargement of the lymphatic glands and spleen (or, Hodgkin's disease). With remarks. *Guy's Hosp Rep* 1865;11:56–67.
7. Fox H. Remarks on the presentation of microscopical preparations made from some of the original tissue described by Thomas Hodgkin, 1832. *Ann Med Hist* 1926;8:370–374.
7a. Virchow R. Die krankhaften Geschwülste. Dreißig Vorlesungen, gehalten während des Wintersemesters 1862–1863 an der Universität zu Berlin, vol. 2. Berlin: A. Hirschwald, 1864–1865.
7b. Virchow R. Weißes Blut. Neue Notizen aus dem Gebiete der Natur- und Heilkunde. 1845;36:151–156.
7c. Cohnheim J. Ein Fall von Pseudoleukämie. *Arch F Path Anat* 1865; 33:451–454.
7d. Billroth TH. Chirurgische Reminiscenzen aus dem Sommersemester 1871. V. Multiple Lymphome. Erfolgreiche Behandlung mit Arsenik. *Wien Med Wochnschr* 1871;21:1065–1068.
7e. Dreschfeld J. Clinical lecture on acute Hodgkin's disease. *BMJ* 1892;1:893–896.
8. Kundrat H. Ueber Lympho-Sarkomatosis. *Wien Klin Wochnschr* 1893;6:211–213;234–239.
9. Sternberg C. Über eine eigenartige unter dem Bilde der Pseudoleukämie verlaufende Tuberculose des lymphatischen Apparates. *Ztschr Heilk* 1898;19:21–90.
10. Reed DM. On the pathological changes in Hodgkin's disease, with especial reference to its relation to tuberculosis. *Johns Hopkins Hosp Rep* 1902;10:133–196.
11. Sternberg C. Ueber Leukosarkomatose. *Wien Klin Wschr* 1908;21:475–480.
12. Barcos MP, Lukes RJ. Malignant lymphoma of convoluted lymphocytes: a new entity of possible T-cell type. In: Sinks LF, Godden JO, eds. *Conflicts in childhood cancer. An evaluation of current management (progress in clinical and biological research),* vol. 4. New York: Alan R. Liss, 1975:147–177.
13. Jackson H Jr. The classification and prognosis of Hodgkin's disease and allied disorders. *Surg Gynec & Obst* 1937;64:465–467.
13a. Jackson H Jr, Parker F Jr. *Hodgkin's disease and allied disorders.* New York: Oxford University Press, 1947.

14. Ewing J. *Neoplastic diseases: a treatise on tumors,* 4th ed. Philadelphia: WB Saunders, 1928;335–433.

14a. Oberling C. Les réticulosarcomes et les réticulo-endothéliosarcomes de la moelle osseuse (sarcomes d'Ewing). *Bulletin de l'Association Française pour l'étude du Cancer* 1928;17:259–296.

15. Roulet F. Das primäre Retothelsarkom der Lymphknoten. *Virchows Arch F Pathol Anat* 1930;277:15–47.

16. Ghon A, Roman B. Über das Lymphosarkom. *Frankfurt Z Pathol* 1916;19:1–138.

17. Parker F Jr, Jackson H Jr. Primary reticulum cell sarcoma of bone. *Surg Gynecol Obstet* 1939;68:45–53.

18. Gall EA, Mallory TB. Malignant lymphoma. A clinico-pathologic survey of 618 cases. *Am J Pathol* 1942;18:381–429.

19. Brill NE, Baehr G, Rosenthal N. Generalized giant lymph follicle hyperplasia of the lymph nodes and spleen. A hitherto undescribed type. *JAMA* 1925;84:668–671.

20. Symmers D. Follicular lymphadenopathy with splenomegaly, a newly recognized disease of the lymphatic system. *Arch Pathol Lab Med* 1927;3:816–820.

21. Symmers D. Giant follicular lymphadenopathy with or without splenomegaly. Its transformation into polymorphous cell sarcoma of the lymph follicles and its association with Hodgkin's disease, lymphatic leukemia and an apparently unique disease of the lymph nodes and spleen—a disease entity believed heretofore undescribed. *Arch Pathol* 1938;26:603–647.

22. Gall EA, Morrison HR, Scott AT. The follicular type of malignant lymphoma: a survey of 63 cases. *Ann Intern Med* 1941;14:2073–2090.

23. Bence Jones, H. On a new substance occurring in the urine of a patient with mollities ossium. *Phil Trans R Soc Lond* 1848;138:55–62.

23a. Clamp JR. Some aspects of the first recorded case of multiple myeloma. *Lancet* 1967;2:1354–1356.

23b. Von Rustizky J. Multiples Myelom. *Deutsche Zeitschrift für Chirurgie* 1873;3:162–172.

24. Wright JH. A case of multiple myeloma. *Bull Johns Hopkins Hosp* 1900;9:359–366.

24a. Alibert JLM. Description des maladies de la peau observées à l'Hôpital St. Louis. Paris, Barrois L'aîné et Fils 1806.

24b. Sézary A, Bouvrain Y. Erythrodermie avec présence de cellules monstrueuses dans le derme et le sang circulant. *Bull Soc Franç Derm Syph* 1938;45:254–260.

24c. Waldenström J. Incipient myelomatosis or "essential" hyperglobulinemia with fibrinogenopenia—a new syndrome ? *Acta Med Scand* 1944;117:216–247.

25. Burkitt DP. A sarcoma involving the jaws in African children. *Br J Surg* 1958;46:218–223.

26. Burkitt DP, O'Conor GT. Malignant lymphoma in African children. I. A clinical syndrome. *Cancer* 1961;14:258–269.

27. O'Conor GT. Malignant lymphoma in African children. II. A pathological entity. *Cancer* 1961;14:270–283.

28. O'Conor GT, Rappaport H, Smith EB. Childhood lymphoma resembling "Burkitt tumor" in the United States. *Cancer* 1965;18:411–417.

29. Burkitt D. Burkitt's lymphoma. *JAMA* 1972;222:1164.

30. Burkitt D. The discovery of Burkitt's lymphoma. *Cancer* 1983;51:1777–1786.

31. Burkitt D. The beginnings of the Burkitt's lymphoma story. *IARC Sci Publ* 1985;60:11–15.

32. Epstein MA, Achong BG, Barr YM. Virus particles in cultured lymphoblasts from Burkitt's lymphoma. *Lancet* 1964;1:702–703.

33. Kafuko GW, Burkitt DP. Burkitt's lymphoma and malaria. *Int J Cancer* 1970;6:1–9.

34. de The G. The etiology of Burkitt's lymphoma and the history of the shaken dogmas. *Blood Cells* 1993;19:667–673; discussion, 674–675.

35. Burkitt DP, Kyalwazi SK. Spontaneous remission of African lymphoma. *Br J Cancer* 1967;21:14–16.

36. Burkitt D. African lymphoma. Observations on response to vincristine sulphate therapy. *Cancer* 1966;19:1131–1137.

37. Heilmeyer L, Begemann H. Das großfollikuläre Lymphoblastom (Brill-Symmerssche Krankheit). In: von Bergmann G, Frey W, Schwiegk H, eds. *Handbuch der inneren Medizin,* vol 2. Berlin: Springer-Verlag, 1951:704–705.

38. Bilger R. Über eine noch wenig bekannte Erkrankung des lymphatischen Systems: Das follikuläre Lymphoblastom (Brillsche Krankheit). *Klin Wschr* 1949;27:707–709.

39. Wright CJE. Macrofollicular lymphoma. *Am J Pathol* 1956;32:201–233.

40. Willis RA. The tumours of lymphoid tissue. In: *Pathology of tumours.* London: Butterworth, 1948;760–783.

41. Callender GR. Tumors and tumor-like conditions of the lymphocyte, the myelocyte, the erythrocyte and the reticulum cell. *Am J Pathol* 1934;10:443–465.

42. Robb-Smith AH. Reticulosis and reticulosarcoma: a histological classification. *J Pathol* 1938;47:457–480.

42a. Rössle R. Das Retothelsarkom der Lymphdrüsen. Seine Formen und Verwandtschaften. *Beitr Path Anatomie* 1939;103:385–415.

43. Gall EA, Rappaport H. Seminar on diseases of lymph nodes and spleen. In: McDonald JR (ed). *Proceedings of the twenty-third anatomic pathology seminar of the American Society of Clinical Pathologists.* Chicago: ASCP Press, 1958.

44. Rappaport H. Tumors of the hematopoietic system. In: *Atlas of tumor pathology,* 3rd section, fasc 8. Washington: Armed Forces Institute of Pathology, 1966.

45. Rappaport H, Winter WJ, Hicks EB. Follicular lymphoma. A re-evaluation of its position in the scheme of malignant lymphoma, based on a survey of 253 cases. *Cancer* 1956;9:792–821.

46. Nowell P. Phytohemagglutinin: an initiator of mitosis in cultures of normal human leukocytes. *Cancer Res* 1960;20:462–466.

47. Jones SE, Fuks Z, Bull M, et al. Non-Hodgkin's lymphomas IV. Clinicopathologic correlation in 405 cases. *Cancer* 1973;31:806–823.

48. Ezdinli EZ, Costello W, Wasser LP, et al. Eastern Cooperative Oncology Group experience with the Rappaport classification of non-Hodgkin's lymphomas. *Cancer* 1979;43:544–550.

49. DeVita VT Jr, Canellos GP, Chabner B, et al. Advanced diffuse histiocytic lymphoma, a potentially curable disease. *Lancet* 1975;1:248–250.

50. National Cancer Institute sponsored study of classifications of non-Hodgkin's lymphomas. Summary and description of a working formulation for clinical usage. The Non Hodgkin's Lymphoma Pathologic Classification Project. *Cancer* 1982;49:2112–2135.

51. Murphy SB. Management of childhood non-Hodgkin's lymphoma. *Cancer Treat Rep* 1977;61:1161–1173.

52. Cooper MD, Peterson RDA, Good RA. Delineation of the thymic and bursal lymphoid systems in the chicken. *Nature (Lond)* 1965;205:143–146.

53. Cooper MD, Peterson RDA, South MA, et al. The functions of the thymus system and the bursa system in the chicken. *J Exp Med* 1966;123:75–102.

54. Cooper MD, Peterson RDA, Gabrielsen AE, et al. Lymphoid malignancy and development, differentiation, and function of the lymphoreticular system. *Cancer Res* 1966;26:1165–1169.

55. Wilson JD, Nossal GJ. Identification of human T and B lymphocytes in normal peripheral blood and in chronic lymphocytic leukaemia. *Lancet* 1971;2:788–791.

56. Cooper MD, Schwartz ML, Good RA. Restoration of gamma globulin production in agammaglobulinemic chickens. *Science* 1966;151:471–473.

57. Dorfman R. Present concepts of the proliferative and malignant diseases of the lymphoreticular tissue. *The Leech* 1961;31:10–16.

58. DeVita VT, Rappaport H, Frei E. Announcement of the formation of The Lymphoma Task Force and Pathology Reference Center. *Cancer* 1968;22:1087–1088.

59. Jaffe E, Shevach E, Frank M, et al. Nodular lymphoma: evidence for origin from follicular B lymphocytes. *N Engl J Med* 1974;290:813–819.

60. Dorfman RF. The non-Hodgkin's lymphomas. In: Rebuck JW, Berard CW, Abell MR, eds. *The reticuloendothelial system. International Academy of Pathology Monographs in Pathology, no. 16.* Baltimore: Williams and Wilkins, 1975:262–281.

61. Dorfman RF. Classification of non-Hodgkin's lymphomas [Letter]. *Lancet* 1974;1:1295–1296.

61a. Dorfman RF. Classification of non-Hodgkin's lymphomas [Letter]. *Lancet* 1974;2:961–962.

62. Dorfman RF. Pathology of the non-Hodgkin's lymphomas: new classifications. *Cancer Treat Rep* 1977;61:945–951.

63. Bennett MH, Farrer-Brown G, Henry K, et al. Classification of non-Hodgkin's lymphomas [Letter]. *Lancet* 1974;2:405–406.

64. Gérard-Marchant R, Hamlin I, Lennert K, et al. Classification of non-Hodgkin's lymphomas [Letter]. *Lancet* 1974;2:406–408.

65. Lukes RJ, Collins RD. Immunologic characterization of human malignant lymphomas. *Cancer* 1974;34:1488–1503.

66. Kay HE. Classification of non-Hodgkin's lymphomas [Letter]. *Lancet* 1974;2:586.

67. Lennert K. Lymphknoten. Diagnostik in Schnitt und Ausstrich. Bandteil A: Cytologie und Lymphadenitis. In: Lubarsch O, Henke F, Rössle R, et al., eds. *Handbuch der speziellen pathologischen Anatomie und Histologie.* Berlin: Springer-Verlag, 1961.

68. Lennert K. Germinal centers and germinal center neoplasms. *Acta Haem Jap* 1969;32:495–500.

69. Lennert K. Classification of malignant lymphomas (European concept). In: Rüttimann A, ed. *Progress in lymphology.* Stuttgart, Germany: Thieme Medical Publishers,1967:103–109.

70. Lennert K, Mohri N, Stein H, et al. The histopathology of malignant lymphoma. *Br J Haematol* 1975;31[Suppl]:193–203.

71. Brittinger G, Bartels H, Common H, et al. Clinical and prognostic relevance of the Kiel classification of non-Hodgkin lymphomas: results of a prospective multicenter study by the Kiel Lymphoma Study Group. *Hematol Oncol* 1984;2:269–306.

72. Stansfeld AG, Diebold J, Kapanci Y, et al. Updated Kiel classification for lymphomas [Letter]. *Lancet* 1988;1:292–293;603.

73. Lennert K, Feller AC. *Histopathology of non-Hodgkin's lymphomas (according to the updated Kiel classification),* 2nd ed. New York: Springer-Verlag, 1992.

74. Meusers P, Engelhard M, Bartels H, et al. Multicentre randomized therapeutic trial for advanced centrocytic lymphoma: anthracycline does not improve the prognosis. *Hematol Oncol* 1989;7:365–380.

74a. Engelhard M, Brittinger G, Heinz R, et al. Chronic lymphocytic leukemia (B-CLL) and immunocytoma (LP-IC): clinical and prognostic relevance of this distinction. *Leuk Lymphoma* 1991;5[Suppl]:161–173.

75. Schlegelberger B, Zwingers T, Harder L, et al. Clinicopathogenetic significance of chromosomal abnormalities in patients with blastic peripheral B-cell lymphoma. *Blood* 1999;94:3114–3120.

76. Griesser H, Feller AC, Lennert K, et al. Rearrangement of the β chain of the T cell antigen receptor and immunoglobulin genes in lymphoproliferative disorders. *J Clin Invest* 1986;78:1179–1184.

77. A clinical evaluation of the International Lymphoma Study Group classification of non-Hodgkin's lymphoma. The Non-Hodgkin's Lymphoma Classification Project. *Blood* 1997;89:3909–3918.

78. Brittinger G, Bartels H, Bremer K, et al. Clinical aspects of malignant non-Hodgkin's lymphomas with reference to Kiel classification: centrocytic lymphoma, centroblastic-centrocytic lymphoma, lymphoblastic lymphoma, immunoblastic lymphoma. *Häematol Bluttransfus* 1976;18:211–223.

79. Brittinger G, Bartels H, Bremer K, et al. Retrospective analysis of the clinical relevance of the Kiel classification of malignant lymphomas [Author's transl]. *Strahlentherapie* 1977;153:222–228.

80. Parker JW, Wakasa H, Lukes RJ. The morphologic and cytochemical demonstration of lysosomes in lymphocytes incubated with phytohemagglutinin by electron microscopy. *Lab Invest* 1965;14:1736–1743.

81. Parker JW, Steiner J, Coffin A, et al. Blastomitogenic agents in *Leguminosae* and other families. *Experientia* 1969;25:187–188.

82. Rogers ER, Parker JW, Lukes RJ, et al. A simplified and modified methyl green pyronin stain. *Am J Clin Pathol* 1970;54:667–669.

83. Parker JW, Lukes RJ. A microculture method for lymphocyte transformation studies in the clinical laboratory. *Am J Clin Pathol* 1971;56:174–180.

84. Cramer AD, Rogers ER, Parker JW, et al. The Giemsa stain for tissue sections: an improved method. *Am J Clin Pathol* 1973;60:148–156.

85. Leech JH, Glick AD, Waldron JA, et al. Malignant lymphomas of follicular center cell origin in man. I. Immunologic studies. *J Natl Cancer Inst* 1975;54:11–21.

86. Glick AD, Leech JH, Waldron JA, et al. Maligant lymphomas of follicular center cell origin in man. II. Ultrastructural and cytochemical studies. *J Natl Cancer Inst* 1975;54:23–36.

87. Stein RS, Cousar J, Flexner JM, et al. Malignant lymphomas of follicular center cell origin in man. III. Prognostic features. *Cancer* 1979;44:2236–2243.

88. Oviatt DL, Cousar JB, Flexner JM, et al. Malignant lymphoma of follicular center cell origin in humans. IV. Small transformed (noncleaved) cell lymphoma of the non-Burkitt's type. *Cancer* 1983;52:1196–1201.

89. Stein RS, Magee MJ, Lenox RK, et al. Malignant lymphomas of follicular center cell origin in man. VI. Large cleaved cell lymphoma. *Cancer* 1987;60:2704–2711.

90. Stein RS, Greer JP, Cousar JB, et al. Malignant lymphomas of follicular center cell origin in man. VII. Prognostic features in small cleaved cell lymphoma. *Hematol Oncol* 1989;7:381–391.

91. Mathé, G, Rappaport H, O'Conor GT, et al. *Histological and cytological typing of neoplastic diseases of haematopoietic and lymphoid tissues (International Histological Classification of Tumours No. 14).* Geneva: World Health Organization, 1976.

92. Schein PS, Chabner B, Canellos G, et al. Potential for prolonged disease-free survival following combination chemotherapy of non-Hodgkin's lymphoma. *Blood* 1974;43:181–189.

93. Strauchen J, Young RC, De Vita VT Jr, et al. Clinical relevance of the histopathological subclassification of diffuse "histiocytic" lymphoma. *N Engl J Med* 1978;299:1382–1387.

94. Classification of non-Hodgkin's lymphomas. Reproducibility of major classification systems. NCI Non-Hodgkin's Lymphoma Classification Project Writing Committee. *Cancer* 1985;55:91–95.

95. Lennert K, Collins RD, Lukes RJ. Concordance of the Kiel and Lukes-Collins classifications of non-Hodgkin's lymphomas. *Histopathology* 1983;7:549–559.

96. Murphy EA. *The logic of medicine.* Baltimore: The Johns Hopkins University Press, 1976.

97. Harris NL, Jaffe ES, Stein H, et al. A revised European-American classification of lymphoid neoplasms: a proposal from the International Lymphoma Study Group. *Blood* 1994;84:1361–1392.

98. Hiddemann W, Longo DL, Coiffier B, et al. Lymphoma classification—the gap between biology and clinical management is closing. *Blood* 1996;88:4085–4089.

99. Armitage JO, Weisenburger DD, for the Non-Hodgkin's Lymphoma Classification Project. New approach to classifying non-Hodgkin's lymphomas: clinical features of the major histologic subtypes. *J Clin Oncol* 1998;16:2780–2795.

100. Jaffe ES, Harris NL, Stein H, et al. *World Health Organization Classification of tumours. Pathology and genetics of tumours of haematopoietic and lymphoid tissues.* Lyon, France: IARC Press, 2001.

101. Damle RN, Wasil T, Fais F, et al. Ig V gene mutation status and CD38 expression as novel prognostic indicators in chronic lymphocytic leukemia. *Blood* 1999;94:1840–1847.

102. Hamblin TJ, Orchard JA, Gardiner A, et al. Immunoglobulin V genes and CD38 expression in CLL. *Blood* 2000;95:2455–2457.

103. Döhner H, Stilgenbauer S, Benner A, et al. Genomic aberrations and survival in chronic lymphocytic leukemia. *N Engl J Med* 2000; 343:1910–1916.

104. Engelhard M, Brittinger G, Huhn D, et al. Subclassification of diffuse large B-cell lymphomas according to the Kiel classification: distinction of centroblastic and immunoblastic lymphomas is a significant prognostic risk factor. *Blood* 1997;89:2291–2297.

105. Schmits R, Glass B, Trümper L, et al. Therapeutic strategies for aggressive lymphomas: the trials of the DSHNHL. *Ann Hematol* 2001;80[Suppl 3]:B77–B83.

106. Alizadeh AA, Eisen MB, Davis RE, et al. Distinct types of diffuse large B-cell lymphoma identified by gene expression profiling. *Nature* 2000;403:503–511.

107. Shipp MA, Ross KN, Tamayo P, et al. Diffuse large B-cell lymphoma outcome prediction by gene-expression profiling and supervised machine learning. *Nat Med* 2002;8:68–74.

108. Rosenwald A, Wright G, Chan WC, et al. The use of molecular profiling to predict survival after chemotherapy for diffuse large-B-cell lymphoma. *N Engl J Med* 2002;346:1937–1947.

109. Zukerberg L, Medeiros L, Ferry J, et al. Diffuse low-grade B-cell lymphomas: four clinically distinct subtypes defined by a combination of morphologic and immunophenotypic features. *Am J Clin Pathol* 1993;100:373–385.

110. Banks P, Chan J, Cleary M, et al. Mantle cell lymphoma: a proposal for unification of morphologic, immunologic, and molecular data. *Am J Surg Pathol* 1992;16:637–640.

111. Rosenberg CL, Wong E, Petty EM, et al. PRAD1, a candidate BCL1 oncogene: mapping and expression in centrocytic lymphoma. *Proc Natl Acad Sci U S A* 1991;88:9638–9642.

CHAPTER 2

History of Chemotherapy of Lymphomas and Description of Early Trials

Joseph R. Bertino

In any historical review, events are colored by the bias of the writer. This writer has at least one advantage: he has had the privilege of personally witnessing the remarkable change in our ability to treat (or not to treat) patients with lymphoma. An extensive review of all of the early studies that led to this progress is beyond the scope of this review. Additional details of the early history of the therapy of lymphomas may be found in the book *Hodgkin's Disease*, by Kaplan (1); the reviews by Brookes (2) and Ultmann (3); the chapter on lymphomas by DeVita, Jaffe, and Hellman in *Cancer: Principles and Practice of Oncology* (4); and the chapter on Hodgkin's disease by Mauch and Armitage in *Cancer Medicine* (5). This review covers the period from the early 1900s to the mid 1970s.

ROOTS OF CHEMOTHERAPY

The first attempts to find drugs that are effective against neoplastic diseases are attributed to Paul Ehrlich, "the father of chemotherapy." His major efforts were directed at finding drugs to treat infectious diseases, and he was successful in finding drugs to treat trypanosome infections (salvarsan) and syphilis (arsphenamine) in 1910. Although effective anticancer drugs were not found, his use of rodent models to screen compounds to treat infectious diseases provided the basis for the pioneering work of Clowes in the early 1900s, who developed inbred rodent lines to bear transplanted tumors. These models were used by Clowes and, subsequently, others to screen for potential anticancer agents.

Although arsenicals, Fowler's solution in particular, were used to treat leukemias and lymphomas in the late nineteenth century and early 1900s, the usefulness of this treatment was uncertain. It is somewhat ironic that the first effective agent to treat lymphoma was derived from the development of poisonous gases, which were designed to kill and injure soldiers in World War I. *Mustard gas*, dichlorodiethyl sulfide, not only had local tissue-damaging effects, but also was found to have systemic effects on the marrow and gastrointestinal tract. The real-

ization that this compound had effects on cell division led investigators in the 1930s to study its effects on experimental tumors and in humans (6,7). This sulfur mustard was soon abandoned for clinical use because of its poor therapeutic index and the difficulties that were experienced in handling it.

World War II (1939–1945) again stimulated the search for compounds for chemical warfare, and attention was focused on a nitrogen mustard, tri-(2-chloroethyl)amine hydrochloride, HN3, which was synthesized by Ward in 1935 (8). During the war, this compound and other nitrogen mustards were actively investigated at Yale Medical School, the Army Chemical Center in Edgewood, Maryland and in Oxford, England, and at the Sloan-Kettering Institute (2).

The beginnings of modern chemotherapy may be attributed to the remarkable tumor response of the first patient who was treated with a nitrogen mustard (HN3), at Yale-New Haven Hospital, in 1942, although this treatment was not reported until 1946 (9) because of wartime security. This clinical trial was based on experiments in transplanted lymphosarcoma in mice by Dougherty and Gardner at Yale, which showed that the nitrogen mustards caused rapid disappearance of these tumors, albeit transiently. The following is a description of the first patient who was treated with nitrogen mustard (9a):

> At New Haven, when favorable results in animals with tumors of lymphoid tissue were reported, Dr. Alfred Gilman, in charge of the work there on the nitrogen mustards, decided to attempt control of similar tumors in man. A suitable case was made available by Dr. Gustaf Lindskog. This unfortunate patient had an extensive lymphosarcoma infiltrating widely the tissue of the neck and mediastinum as well as the other lymphoid organs of the body. The tumor was said to have become wholly resistant to the therapeutic effect of x-rays. Because of its rapid growth, the trachea was rapidly being compressed below a point where a tracheotomy could be done, to an extent which bade fair to strangle the patient. With the permission and complete understanding on the part of the subject, an amount of nitrogen mustard was administered by vein, which if given on a similar weight basis to an animal, would have resulted in dissolution of

a similar cellular structure. The mass in the neck melted away. Breathing became easier once more. Lymph nodes and spleen became smaller in size. But the effect on the bone marrow was extreme. Lymphopenia, leukopenia, granulocytopenia ensued, with severe and intractable purpura, and eventual aplastic anemia requiring repeated transfusions. The bone marrow depression was transient, however, and disappeared within a few weeks. No further treatment was given: the tumor grew again and eventually terminated the life of the patient.

A new fact had been established, however. A chemical compound was at hand which would affect adversely and cause dissolution of a lymphoid neoplasm reputedly resistant to x-rays.

Several other patients were treated, but the trials were put on hold when Gilman and his associates entered military service and continued their research on nitrogen mustards at the Edgewood Arsenal laboratories. In a prescient statement in his review in 1947 (9a), Rhoads commented: "It is wholly possible that chemotherapeutic substances specifically destructive to one of the other forms of cancer tissue might be developed. There is at least ample precedent for this possibility. Time only will tell whether the public wishes to have this sort of work done."

Following this lead, a Committee on Atypical Growth was established during wartime by the National Research Council, and work to establish these chemicals as therapeutic agents in civilian medicine was assigned to three institutions: the Memorial Hospital in New York, the Billings Hospital of the University of Chicago, and the Medical School of the University of Utah at Salt Lake. These investigators studied more than 150 patients and confirmed the antitumor activity of the nitrogen mustards in patients with Hodgkin's disease and in patients with other lymphomas (10,11).

These observations were soon confirmed by others (12) and, after the end of the war, stimulated extensive research on alkylating agents as anticancer agents (2). For example, Burchenal et al. (13,14) tested more than 50 different nitrogen mustards against mouse leukemias; Haddow (15), at the Chester Beaty Institute, synthesized and tested aromatic nitrogen mustards and sulphonic acid esters against the Walker 256 carcinosarcoma in the rat and discovered myleran, which was used to treat chronic myelocytic leukemia for many years and is still in clinical use as part of transplant regimens for leukemia. At approximately the same time as nitrogen mustards were being tested, Dougherty and White reported that adrenocorticotropic hormone caused lymphoid tissue to atrophy (16). This observation was followed by the report of Heilman and Kendall (17), in 1944, who showed that compound E (cortisone) treatment regressed lymphosarcoma in mice. When adrenocorticotropic hormone and cortisone became available for clinical use in 1949 to 1950, these drugs also proved to cause regressions in patients with lymphomas (18,19); however, similar to nitrogen mustard treatment, in most patients, these regressions were short lived. Other derivatives of cortisone were tested over the next two decades, thus leading to the discovery of other more potent corticosteroids,

including prednisone and dexamethasone, which are now widely used in the clinic.

By the end of the 1940s, the demonstration that regressions could be obtained with nitrogen mustard and cortisone, together with the development of folate antagonists for the treatment of childhood leukemia (20), accelerated the search for additional anticancer drugs. The National Cancer Institute's (NCI) Drug Development program was initiated and included large-scale screening for anticancer drugs by using transplanted mouse tumors.

HODGKIN'S DISEASE

Radiation Therapy: Evidence That a Cure Was Possible

After the description of Hodgkin's disease in 1832 by Thomas Hodgkin, various systemic remedies were tried in the ensuing decades, including arsenicals and iodides. When radiation therapy became available in the early 1900s, the treatment for all stages of Hodgkin's disease was radiation therapy, as the arsenicals were considered to have minimal effectiveness. Until the 1950s, it was believed that Hodgkin's disease was not curable, despite the sensitivity of this tumor to irradiation. The early studies of Gilbert elaborated the principles of radiation treatment of Hodgkin's disease, namely to treat all involved areas with the highest dose possible and to treat adjacent areas as well (21). Using these guidelines, Peters (22) reported that a small percentage of patients with limited disease could be cured, if the involved nodes with contiguous areas were treated. Reports from Eason and Russell (23) also indicated that early stage disease was curable, thus setting the stage for the definitive work of Kaplan at Stanford (1). Kaplan used supervoltage irradiation to show that it was possible to irradiate involved lymph nodes to tumoricidal levels as well as to treat contiguous lymph node areas with large fields, such as *mantle* and *inverted Y*, as well as *total nodal* irradiation. The result was the cure of early stage (stage I and II) Hodgkin's disease in the majority of patients (1).

Chemotherapy: Single-Agent Treatment

Stimulated by the demonstration that nitrogen mustard caused temporary regressions in the majority of patients with lymphomas, including Hodgkin's disease, the 1950s and the early 1960s saw the discovery of additional agents that had therapeutic effects in patients with cancer. In the early 1960s, two new drug classes, in addition to alkylating agents and corticosteroids, were found to have significant activity in the treatment of advanced Hodgkin's disease: the vinca alkaloids, vincristine and vinblastine (24,25), and the methylhydrazine derivative, procarbazine (26,27). The finding that vinca alkaloids, which are extracted from the periwinkle plant, an ornamental shrub (*Vinca rosea*), had anticancer activity was important for three reasons: namely, natural products could be a good source of new anticancer agents; they revealed a new target for drug development, tubulin; and responses were seen in patients who developed resistance to nitrogen mustard. The testing of periwinkle extracts (initially as folk medicine, as they were thought to be useful to treat diabetes) as anticancer agents was again based on the finding that they caused a decrease in granulocytes in experimental animals. The methylhydrazine derivative, procarbazine, which was initially called *ibenzamethyzin*, came from a program that was designed to find monoamine oxidase inhibitors.

In 1968, a randomized trial of two combined clinical cooperative groups (Acute Leukemia B and the Eastern Solid Tumor Group) reported that vinblastine was superior to cyclophosphamide for remission induction in patients with Hodgkin's disease, whereas cyclophosphamide was more effective than vincristine for remission induction for patients with non-Hodgkin's lymphoma (28). Another conclusion from this study was that patients who had a complete remission had longer response durations than patients with partial responses. Thus, the achievement of a complete remission became an important goal for future studies. In the 1950s and early 1960s, a large number of other drugs were tested for anticancer activity in the clinic and were found to cause regressions in patients with Hodgkin's disease, but the corticosteroids, nitrogen mustards, the vincas, and procarbazine emerged as the most promising of these drugs. Table 2.1 lists the drugs that were found effective as single agents in the 1950s and early 1960s for the treatment of Hodgkin's disease (29).

During the 1960s, an increase in the cure rate of early stage Hodgkin's disease was an outcome of the use of extended-field radiation therapy (*vide supra*), which was prompted by the studies from Rosenberg and Kaplan (30) showing that this disease spread in an orderly fashion to contiguous lymph nodes and that the risk of recurrence in the treatment field was related to the dose. The role of radiation therapy was further defined by the development of lymphangiography, which was described in 1952 (31) and made clinically useful with the use of oil-based iodine contrast materials (32). The use of exploratory laparotomy, which was pioneered at Stanford (33), also contributed to the clinical usefulness of lymphangiography; it showed that many patients with disease above the diaphragm also had previously unrecognized periaortic node and splenic involvement (34,35).

Basic Principles of Chemotherapy

The 1960s also saw the beginnings of combination chemotherapy for treatment of Hodgkin's disease. The use of drug combinations to treat cancer and treatment with maximally tolerated doses to attempt to achieve complete remissions and even cures was not obvious at this time. Goldin (36) and Skipper and Schmidt (37) used a sensitive, rapidly growing, transplanted murine leukemia L1210 to evaluate new drugs and combinations and to quantify tumor cell kill from chemotherapy. The Skipper studies showed that, in this sensitive tumor, there was a direct relationship between the dose of an

TABLE 2.1. *Single agents that were found to be effective in the treatment of Hodgkin's disease in the 1950s and early 1960s*

Alkylating agents
  Nitrogen mustard
  Trenimon
  Degranol
  Mannitol mustard
  N-Formyl sarcolysine
Antimetabolites
  6-Mercaptopurine
  Cytosine arabinoside
  5-Fluorouridine
  Methotrexate
Antibiotics
  Actinomycin C and D
  Streptonigrin
  Aurantin
Vinca alkaloids
  Vinblastine
  Vincristine
Miscellaneous agents
  Methylglyoxal-bisguanylhydrazone
  Desacetyl methylcolchine
  Procarbazine

Adapted from Hall TC. New chemotherapeutic agents in Hodgkin's disease. *Cancer Res* 1966;26:1297–1302.

effective drug and tumor cell kill, and the dose schedule and combinations of drugs were key to increasing tumor cell kill and preventing the development of drug resistance. By quantifying cell kill based on the relationship between survival and the number of tumor cells that were inoculated, this group showed that, in this model, every cell had to be killed to cure the animal and that a given dose of a chemotherapeutic agent kills a certain fraction of tumor cells. Thus, if an animal had 100,000 tumor cells, and the drug killed 5 logarithms (logs), some animals would be cured. If the tumor size was 1,000,000, a 5-log kill would still leave ten tumor cells, and the animal would not be cured. Furthermore, because a resistant mutant may arise every 10×5 or 10×6 doublings, a cure by a single agent, even with this low tumor burden, would not be likely—human tumors of 1 cm^3 are estimated to contain 109 cells. These considerations provided a strong rationale for the combination of drugs with different mechanisms of action. Another important series of experiments by Bruce et al. (38) showed that chemotherapeutic agents could be classified as *cycle active* or *non–cycle active*. The latter were the alkylating agents, nitrosoureas and radiation therapy, whereas cycle-active drugs were drugs such as methotrexate, which did not affect resting or G_0 cells. The non–cycle-active agents were less schedule dependent than the cycle-active drugs, thus total dose rather than schedule was important. The increased sensitivity of spleen lymphoma colonies to cycle-active drugs compared to normal hematopoietic splenic colonies was explained by the idea that all of the lymphoma cells were *in cycle*, whereas an appreciable number of normal colony-forming cells were temporarily out of cycle (G$_0$) and not affected by cell cycle-active agents. These experiments provided a rationale for the use of high doses of cycle-active drugs delivered in an intermittent fashion. One of the first combinations that was explored for the treatment of Hodgkin's disease was the combination of vinblastine and chlorambucil (39). Lacher and Durant (39) treated patients with weekly vinblastine and daily chlorambucil. In this small series, 10 of 16 patients had excellent responses, and three others had partial responses, lasting 1 to 2 years, but no long-term remissions were noted.

Combination Chemotherapy: Cure of Advanced Disease

The concepts that were derived from the experimental studies of Skipper were used by Freireich et al. (40) to develop combination chemotherapy programs to treat childhood leukemia, which led to increased remission rates and duration of remissions and initial evidence that a cure could be obtained in this disease. Stimulated by the Skipper concepts and the results of the combination studies of patients with childhood acute lymphocytic leukemia, investigators at the NCI began to explore combinations of four drugs for the treatment of Hodgkin's disease. A combination of cyclophosphamide, vincristine, prednisone, and methotrexate, together with irradiation, produced an 80% complete remission rate in 14 patients with Hodgkin's disease of stages I to III (41). Although this program only treated patients for 2.5 months, 12 of the 14 patients had rapid and complete regression of their disease, usually with the first course of chemotherapy, and ten of these patients enjoyed long-term disease-free remissions (more than 12 months). Longer-term follow-up has not been reported.

When it was shown that procarbazine was an active drug for the treatment of Hodgkin's disease, investigations substituted this drug for methotrexate in the four-drug combination, and the duration of treatment was extended to 6 months. This new combination [mechlorethamine, vincristine, procarbazine, and prednisone (MOPP)] was used to treat 43 patients with stage III and IV Hodgkin's disease from 1964 to 1967, and the results of this benchmark study were described in the *Annals of Internal Medicine* by DeVita et al. (42). This combination treatment of patients with Hodgkin's disease was not only tolerable, but also produced complete remissions in 80% of patients; 55% of these patients remained disease free at 5 years, thus raising, for the first time, the possibility of a cure of advanced Hodgkin's disease. Studies from other institutions duplicated these results and confirmed that many patients with advanced Hodgkin's disease could be cured with MOPP chemotherapy (43,44). During the next decade, many variations of MOPP were tried, including the substitution of cyclophosphamide for nitrogen mustard (cyclophosphamide, vincristine, procarbazine, and prednisone), the substitution of vinblastine for vincristine (mechlorethamine,

vinblastine, procarbazine, and prednisone), or the addition of bleomycin (bleomycin, mechlorethamine, vincristine, procarbazine, and prednisone). None of these combinations produced superior complete remission rates or improved survival (45). Intensive chemotherapy with nitrogen mustard as a single agent was compared to MOPP chemotherapy by Hugeley et al. (46); nitrogen mustard produced complete remissions in only 3 of 23 patients. The issue of whether sequential single-agent treatment with three drugs could achieve similar results to MOPP was tested by Monfardi et al. (47). This study used an alkylating agent first, followed by vinblastine and procarbazine. An overall median survival of only 24 months and less than 30% complete remissions were observed.

The role of maintenance chemotherapy in patients, after achieving a complete remission, was addressed by several groups. Additional cycles of MOPP or the use of other drugs after six cycles of MOPP (bischloroethylnitrosourea, chloroethylcyclohexylnitrosourea plus vinblastine or vinblastine plus procarbazine) did not improve cure rates in patients who had a documented complete remission (4). Interestingly, patients who relapsed after achieving a complete remission with MOPP chemotherapy were found to continue to be sensitive to this combination regimen. If patients relapsed within a year after achieving a complete remission, the remission rate was only 29%, whereas patients who relapsed after more than a year after a complete remission had a 93% complete remission rate; in many cases, this second remission was durable (49). Also of interest was that previous treatment with local radiation therapy did not compromise the chances of a patient achieving a complete remission with MOPP chemotherapy (48).

Combined Modality Therapy

The Yale program used three cycles of a combination of drugs that included nitrogen mustard, prednisone, and vincristine, followed by vinblastine and procarbazine, thus predating the concept of the use of sequential combinations. The rationale was to use an alkylating drug first to decrease the tumor mass, to convert the tumor-to-log phase growth, and to increase sensitivity to antimetabolites. In addition, low-dose radiation was added to all known sites of disease after completion of chemotherapy. Like MOPP, the complete remission rate with this program was approximately 80%; however, this study was important in that it showed that the addition of low-dose radiation therapy after 6 months of chemotherapy resulted in an improvement in the percent of patients who remained in a relapse-free remission (50). Other studies that compared MOPP alone to MOPP plus full-dose radiotherapy in stage IV patients did not show any survival advantage with the addition of x-rays (51).

Development of an Effective, Less Toxic Combination

In the early 1970s, several other drugs were shown to have significant activity in Hodgkin's disease, namely, bleomycin, dacarbazine, and doxorubicin. Bleomycin, which was isolated from the fungus *Streptomyces verticillus* by Umezawa et al. in Japan, is a mixture of small-molecular-weight peptides, which allow binding to DNA and subsequent strand breaks (52). This drug was of interest in that it caused regressions in patients with lymphoma with minimal marrow toxicity (53). The anthracyclines, doxorubicin (Adriamycin) and daunomycin, were antibiotics that were also produced by the *Streptomyces* species, and doxorubicin was shown to have a broad spectrum of activity against solid tumors, as well as lymphomas (54,55). Several combinations that used these drugs were studied in patients who relapsed from MOPP chemotherapy. Combinations that consisted of doxorubicin, bleomycin, vinblastine, and dacarbazine, which were reported by Santoro and Bonadonna (56) and by Lokich et al. (bleomycin, dacarbazine, vincristine, prednisone, and doxorubicin) (57), were shown to produce 60% complete remissions in patients who failed after MOPP, and many of these patients had durable remissions. The combination of doxorubicin, bleomycin, vinblastine, and dacarbazine proved to be less carcinogenic and to have less antifertility effects than MOPP (58). In the 1990s, it has also replaced MOPP as first-line treatment for advanced Hodgkin's disease.

NON-HODGKIN'S LYMPHOMA

The response to treatment of lymphomas other than Hodgkin's disease is related to the type of the lymphoma, and, as the recognition of the many types of non-Hodgkin's lymphoma has evolved, the role of chemotherapy to treat these lymphomas has been more delineated. Fortunately, like Hodgkin's disease, non-Hodgkin's lymphoma proved to be a chemosensitive tumor.

Single-Agent Chemotherapy

As in Hodgkin's disease, until the introduction of chemotherapy into the clinic in the late 1940s (see above), the only treatment available for patients with non-Hodgkin's lymphoma was palliative radiation therapy (1,59). When effective agents became available (alkylating agents, corticosteroids, vincristine), single-agent chemotherapy was used only after radiation failure, except for stage IV patients (60). Until the mid 1960s, the most widely used histologic classification of non-Hodgkin's lymphoma included three major groups: reticulum cell sarcoma, lymphosarcoma, and giant follicular lymphoma (60a). The classification of Rappaport et al. (61), which was described first in 1956 and later formalized in 1966 (61a), considered pattern (nodular or diffuse) and differentiation (poorly or well-differentiated lymphocyte, histiocytic, or a mixture of the two) in defining categories of lymphoma. This classification was used to ascertain the relationship between the histopathologic category of lymphoma and the results of single-agent chemotherapy by Jones et al. in 1972 (60). In this seminal study, it was found that patients with nodular lymphoma (now known as *follicular lymphoma*) had a higher response rate and longer survival after chemotherapy (alkylating agents or vin-

cristine) than patients with diffuse histiocytic lymphoma (now known as *diffuse large B-cell lymphoma*). Furthermore, patients with follicular lymphomas that were composed of large cells (nodular histiocytic in the Rappaport Classification, now known as *grade 3 follicular lymphoma*) had a shorter survival than patients with follicular lymphomas that were composed of small cells (poorly differentiated lymphocytic, now known as *grade 1 or 2 follicular lymphoma*).

With the availability of three effective agents to treat non-Hodgkin's lymphoma (cyclophosphamide, prednisone, and vincristine), trials of these combinations were initiated in the 1960s. These phase II trials demonstrated the effectiveness of these combinations for follicular lymphomas, but they were less effective for diffuse large-cell lymphoma (62,63). Surprisingly, when tested in a randomized trial against single-agent alkylating therapy in patients with follicular lymphomas, this combination did not prove to be better than single-agent treatment in regards to the response rate or to survival (64,65).What was also clear from these studies was that there was no plateau in the survival curve, and patients with follicular lymphomas that were composed of predominately small cells continued to relapse with time. Clinical and pathologic staging of these patients, including the use of staging laparotomies (66,67), showed that the follicular lymphomas were almost always disseminated at presentation, and chemotherapy was not curative. In the 5% to 10% of patients that had stage I disease, radiation therapy was curative (68). Another unique feature of follicular lymphomas was revealed by reports that indicated that many patients with this disease had indolent courses, and delay of therapy did not impact on survival; furthermore, 15% to 20% of these patients had evidence of spontaneous partial regressions, if they were followed over time (69–71). In contrast to the follicular lymphomas, 20% to 30% of patients with diffuse large-cell lymphoma were found to have stage I and II disease. Although cure rates were high in patients with stage I diffuse large-cell lymphomas that were treated with involved field irradiation, the cure rate in patients with stage II disease who received x-ray therapy alone was less than 40% (68).

Development of Curative Combination Regimens for Diffuse Histiocytic Lymphoma

Two important studies that used new combinations of drugs provided the first indication that diffuse large-cell lymphomas could be cured by combination chemotherapy. The Yale group used a five-drug program, sequencing cyclophosphamide, vincristine, methotrexate, leucovorin, and arabinosylcytosine (COMLA), to treat stage III and IV "reticulum cell sarcomas," with 9 of 15 complete responses (72). When the results were reexamined using the Rappaport Classification, it was found that six of the eight patients who were reclassified as diffuse histiocytic lymphoma had complete remissions and that five of these patients were still in remission 5 to 6 years after treatment, thus raising the possibility that diffuse large-cell lymphoma could be cured by combination chemotherapy (73). Other studies confirmed the activity of this combination for diffuse large-cell lymphoma (74). The NCI group used the regimens that were shown to be effective for the treatment of Hodgkin's disease (MOPP or cyclophosphamide, vincristine, procarbazine, and prednisone), and, although the complete response rate was lower than COMLA (45%), 70% of these patients with complete remissions had extended disease-free survival (75). Thus, these two early studies added diffuse large-cell lymphoma to the list of advanced cancers that could be cured with chemotherapy. The important finding that doxorubicin is an active drug for the treatment of diffuse large-cell lymphoma (76,77) led to its use in combination, and this drug was added to the combination of cyclophosphamide, prednisone, and vincristine, with and without bleomycin. After these studies, many other combinations of active drugs were evaluated in patients with advanced diffuse large-cell lymphoma, but, as of 2003, none have been shown to be more effective than the combination of cyclophosphamide, doxorubicin, vincristine, prednisone, which produces 5-year disease-free remissions in approximately 30% to 40% of cases (78).

Burkitt's Lymphoma

In 1959, Denis Burkitt described an unusual tumor that involved the jaw in African children (79). Histopathologic examination revealed it to be a malignant lymphoma that was composed of uniformly undifferentiated lymphoid cells and that was diffuse in its pattern, with other distinguishing features (80). What was remarkable about this tumor was that a single large dose of cyclophosphamide caused complete regressions in 80% of these children and long-term survival in one-fourth of these patients (81,82). Methotrexate was also found to be effective in the treatment of this disease, and combinations with both drugs increased the percentage of long-term survivors, depending on the clinical stage of the patient (83). Photos of large, disfiguring jaw tumors that regressed completely with even one dose of cyclophosphamide attested to the unique sensitivity of this tumor to certain chemotherapy drugs and stimulated the search for other tumors that could be effectively treated with chemotherapy. This entity was subsequently recognized in other countries, including the United States, and, although patients in this country were more likely to be Epstein-Barr virus negative and to present with large abdominal tumors rather than jaw tumors, the response to chemotherapy was also dramatic (84). Like African Burkitt's lymphoma, early stage disease was more curable than disseminated disease. Rapid tumor lysis after chemotherapy was found to cause uric acid nephropathy and electrolyte disturbances, thus requiring close monitoring and even temporary dialysis in some patients (85,86). Interestingly, this tumor, perhaps unlike any other, has a high growth fraction, which is similar to the L1210 leukemia, and, in part, this explains its sensitivity to chemotherapy agents.

High-Dose Chemotherapy and Bone Marrow Transplantation

Studies on the effects of whole-body irradiation, particularly in patients who were exposed to radiation from nuclear explosions or accidents, showed that marrow failure, as well as gastrointestinal toxicity, were the major causes of death (87). The pioneering work of Thomas et al. (88,89), which began in Cooperstown, using dogs as a model system, and then continued in Seattle, was first directed toward the reversal of bone marrow failure due to irradiation. The identification of various histocompatibility antigens in humans and the successful cryopreservation of bone marrow cells allowed clinical trials to be initiated in the late 1960s. When it became feasible to prevent marrow toxicity from not only x-rays, but also high doses of chemotherapy, this approach was used to treat patients who failed treatment with conventional doses of chemotherapy (90). Allogeneic transplants, initially in histocompatibility leukocyte antigen–identical twins, were followed by allogeneic transplants in histocompatibility leukocyte antigen–matched siblings. Marrow toxicity, as a limitation to the dose of many of the drugs that are used to treat lymphomas, and the information that response was a function of dose then led to autologous bone marrow transplants in patients with large-cell diffuse lymphoma that relapsed from conventional doses of chemotherapy in the late 1970s (91). Allogeneic and autologous transplantation after high doses of chemotherapy or irradiation, or both, has saved many lives, and many centers now carry out these procedures in patients with relapsed or even high-risk lymphoma (92).

CONCLUSION

Perhaps not apparent to the current generation is the sometimes agonizingly slow, step-by-step progress in our ability to treat lymphoma. It is hoped that this review illustrates how each advance builds on a previous observation. Those of my generation realize that these gains have been made without a large amount of input from basic science discoveries and, in a large measure, reflect the creativeness of the clinical scientist and the bedside as the laboratory. Clearly, chemists, pharmacologists, immunologists, pathologists, and toxicologists have played key roles in the understanding of this disease and drug development to date. There is great anticipation that progress in the future toward the even more successful and minimally toxic treatment of all lymphoma will be accelerated and aided by the increased molecular understanding of these diseases.

REFERENCES

1. Kaplan HS. *Hodgkin's disease,* 2nd ed. Cambridge: Harvard University Press, 1980.
2. Brookes P. The early history of the biological alkylating agents. *Mutat Res* 1990;233:3–14.
3. Ultmann JE. Current status: the management of lymphoma. *Semin Hematol* 1970;7:441–460.

4. DeVita VT, Jaffe ES, Hellman S. Hodgkin's disease and the non-Hodgkin's lymphomas. In: *Cancer: principles and practice of oncology,* 2nd ed. New York: Lippincott Williams & Wilkins, 1985:1623–1685.

5. Mauch P, Armitage JO. Hodgkin's disease. In: Bast R, ed. *Cancer medicine,* 5th ed. Hamilton, Ontario: BC Decker Inc, 2000:2010–2033.

6. Adair FE, Bogg HJ. Experimental and clinical studies on the treatment of cancer by dichloroethylsulphide (mustard gas). *Ann Surg* 1931;93:190–199.

7. Berenblum I. Experimental inhibition of tumor induction by mustard gas and other compounds. *J Pathol Bacteriol* 1935;40:549–558.

8. Ward K. The chlorinated ethylamines—a new type of vesicant. *J Am Chem Soc* 1935;57:914–916.

9. Goodman LS, Wintrobe MM, Dameshek W, et al. Nitrogen mustard therapy: use of methylbis(b-chloroethyl) amino hydrochloride for Hodgkin's disease, lymphosarcoma, leukemia and certain allied disorders. *JAMA* 1946;132:126–132.

9a. Rhoads CP. The sword and the plowshare. *J Mt Sinai Sch Med* 1947;13:299–309.

10. Jacobson LO, Spurr CL, Guzman Baron ES, et al. Nitrogen mustard therapy: studies on neoplastic disorders and allied diseases of the hematopoietic system. *JAMA* 1946;132:263–271.

11. Karnofsky DA, Carver LF, Rhoads CP, et al. An evaluation of methyl-bis-(b-chloroethyl) amine hydrochloride and tris-(b-chloroethyl)amine hydrochloride (nitrogen mustards) in the treatment of lymphomas, leukemia and allied diseases. In: Moulton FR, ed. *Approaches to tumor chemotherapy.* Washington, DC: American Association for the Advancement of Science, 1952:319–337.

12. Dameshek W, Weifuse L, Stein T. Nitrogen mustard therapy in Hodgkin's disease. Analysis of 50 consecutive cases. *Blood* 1949;4:338–379.

13. Burchenal JH, Lester RA, Riley JB, et al. Studies on the chemotherapy of leukemia. Effect of certain nitrogen mustards and carbamates on transmitted mouse leukemia. *Cancer* 1948;1:399–412.

14. Burchenal JH, Burchenal JR, Johnston SF. Chemotherapy of leukemia, III. Further studies on the effect of nitrogen mustards and related compounds on transmitted mouse leukemia. *Cancer* 1951;4:353–356.

15. Haddow A. On the biological alkylating agents. *Perspect Biol Med* 1973;16:503–524.

16. Dougherty TF, White A. Effect of pituitary adrenal adrenotrophic hormone on lymphoid tissue. *Proc Exp Biol Med* 1943;53:132–133.

17. Heilman FR, Kendall ED. The influence of 11-dehydro-17-hydroxy-corticosterone (compound E) on the growth of a malignant tumor in the mouse. *Endocrinology* 1944;34:416–420.

18. Pearson OH, Eliel LP. Use of pituitary adrenocorticotropic hormone (ACTH) and cortisone in lymphomas and leukemias. *JAMA* 1950;144:1349–1950.

19. Kyle RA, McParland CE, Dameshek W. Large doses of prednisone and prednisolone in the treatment of malignant lymphoproliferative disorders. *Ann Intern Med* 1962;57:717–731.

20. Farber S, Diamond LK, Mercer RD, et al. Temporary remissions in acute leukemia in children produced by the folic acid antagonist, 4-aminopteroylglutamic acid (aminopterin). *N Engl J Med* 1948;238:787–793.

21. Gilbert R. Radiotherapy in Hodgkin's disease (malignant granulomatosis): anatomic and clinical foundations: governing principles, results. *AJR Am J Roentgenol* 1939;41:198–241.

22. Peters MV, Middlemiss KC. A study of Hodgkin's disease treated by irradiation. *AJR Am J Roentgenol* 1958;79:114.

23. Easson EC, Russell MH. The cure of Hodgkin's disease. *Br Med J* 1963;1:1704–1707.

24. Johnson IS, Armstrong JG, Gorman M, et al. The vinca alkaloids, a new class of oncolytic agents. *Cancer Res* 1963;23:1390.

25. Costa G, Hreshchyshyn MD, Holland JF. Initial clinical studies with vincristine. *Cancer Chemother Rep* 1996;24:39–41.

26. Mathe G, Schweissguth O, Schneider M, et al. Methylhydrazine in the treatment of Hodgkin's disease. *Lancet* 1963;2:1077.

27. Bollag W. The tumor-inhibitory effects of the methyl hydrazine derivative Ro-4-6467/1 (NSC-77213). *Cancer Chemother Rep* 1963:331–334.

28. Carbone PP, Spurr C, Schneiderman M, et al. Management of patients with lymphoma, a comparative study with cyclophosphamide and vinca alkaloids. *Cancer Res* 1968;28:811–822.

29. Hall TC. New chemotherapeutic agents in Hodgkin's disease. *Cancer Res* 1966;26:1297–1302.

30. Rosenberg SA, Kaplan HS. Evidence for orderly progression in the spread of Hodgkin's disease. *Cancer Res* 1966;26:1225–1231.

31. Kinmonth JD. Lymphangiography in man. Method of outlining lymphatic trunks and operation. *Clin Sci* 1952;11:13–20.

32. Brunn S, Engeset A. Lymphadenography. A new method for the visualization of enlarged lymph nodes and lymphatic vessels. *Acta Radiol* 1956;45:389–395.

33. Glatstein E, Guerney JM, Rosenberg SA, et al. The value of laparotomy and splenectomy in the staging of Hodgkin's disease. *Cancer* 1969;24:709–718.

34. Lukes RJ, Butler JJ. Pathology and nomenclature of Hodgkin's disease. *Cancer Res* 1966;26:1063–1083.

35. Rosenberg SA. A report of the committee on staging of Hodgkin's disease. *Cancer Res* 1966;26:1310.

36. Goldin A. Factors pertaining to complete drug-induced remission of tumor in animals and man. *Cancer Res* 1969;29:2285–2291.

37. Skipper HE, Schmidt LH. A manual on quantitative drug evaluation in experimental tumor systems. *Cancer Chemother Rep* 1962;17:1–143.

38. Bruce WA, Meeker BE, Valeriote FA. Comparison of the sensitivity of normal hematopoietic and transplanted lymphoma colony-forming cells to chemotherapeutic agents administered in vivo. *J Natl Cancer Inst* 1966;32:233–245.

39. Lacher MJ, Durant JR. Combined vinblastine and chlorambucil therapy of Hodgkin's disease. *Ann Intern Med* 1965;62:468–476.

40. Freireich EJ, Karon M, Frei E III. Quadruple combination therapy (VAMP) for acute lymphocytic leukemia of childhood. *Proc Am Assoc Cancer Res* 1964;5:20.

41. Moxley JH III, DeVita VT, Brace K, et al. Intensive combination chemotherapy and x-irradiation for Hodgkin's disease. *Cancer Res* 1967;27:1258–1263.

42. DeVita VT, Serpick AA, Carbone PP. Combination chemotherapy in the treatment of advanced Hodgkin's disease. *Ann Intern Med* 1970;73:881–895.

43. Frei E III, Luce JK, Gamble GE, et al. Combination chemotherapy in advanced Hodgkin's disease: induction and maintenance of remission. *Ann Intern Med* 1973;79:376–382.

44. Moore MR, Jones SE, Bull JM, et al. MOPP chemotherapy for advanced Hodgkin's disease. Prognostic factors in 81 patients. *Cancer* 1973;32:52–60.

45. DeVita VT, Lewis BT, Rozencweig M, et al. The chemotherapy of Hodgkin's disease. Past experiences and future directions. *Cancer* 1978;42:979–990.

46. Hugeley CM Jr, Durant JR, Moores RR, et al. Comparison of nitrogen mustard, vincristine, procarbazine and prednisone (MOPP) to nitrogen mustard in advanced Hodgkin's disease. *Cancer* 1975;36:1227–1240.

47. Monfardi S, Tancini G, Gasparini M, et al. Response and survival in Hodgkin's disease after sequential chemotherapy employing a single agent. *Tumori* 1973;59:45–56.

48. DeVita VT, Simon RN, Hubbard SM, et al. Curability of advanced Hodgkin's disease with chemotherapy: long term follow up of patients treated at NCI. *Ann Intern Med* 1980;92:587–595.

49. Fisher RI, DeVita VT, Hubbard SP, et al. Prolonged disease-free survival in Hodgkin's disease with MOPP reinduction after first relapse. *Ann Intern Med* 1979;90:761–776.

50. Prosnitz LR, Farber LR, Fischer JJ, et al. Low dose radiation therapy and combination chemotherapy in the treatment of advanced Hodgkin's disease. *Radiology* 1973;107:187–193.

51. Rosenberg SA, Kaplan HS, Portlock CS, et al. Combined modality therapy of Hodgkin's disease, a report on the Stanford trials. *Cancer* 1978;42:991–1000.

52. Umezawa H. Bleomycin and other tumor antibiotics of high molecular weight. *Antimicrob Agents Chemother* 1965;17:1079–1085.

53. Kimura I, Onoshi T, Kunimasa I, et al. Treatment of malignant lymphomas with bleomycin. *Cancer* 1972;29:58–60.

54. Bonadonna G, Monfardini S, De Lena M, et al. Phase I and preliminary phase II evaluation of adriamycin (NSC 123127). *Cancer Res* 1970;30:2572–2582.

55. Gottlieb J, Gutterman J, McCredie K, et al. Chemotherapy of malignant lymphoma with adriamycin. *Cancer Res* 1973;33:3024–3028.

56. Santoro A, Bonadonna G. Prolonged disease free survival in MOPP resistant Hodgkin's disease after treatment with adriamycin, bleomy-

cin, vinblastine and dacarbazine (ABVD). *Cancer Chemother Pharmacol* 1979;2:101–105.

57. Lokich JJ, Frei E III, Jaffe N, et al. New multiple agent chemotherapy (B-DOPA) for advanced Hodgkin's disease. *Cancer* 1976;38:667–671.

58. Valagussa P, Santoro A, Fassati Bellani F, et al. Absence of treatment-induced second neoplasms after ABVD in Hodgkin's disease. *Blood* 1982;59:4388–4982.

59. Peckham MJ. Radiation therapy of the non-Hodgkin's lymphomas. *Semin Hematol* 1974;11:41–58.

60. Jones SE, Rosenberg SA, Kaplan HS, et al. Non-Hodgkin's lymphomas: single agent chemotherapy. *Cancer* 1972;30:31–38.

60a. Gall EA, Mallory TB. Malignant lymphoma: a clinicopathologic survey of 618 cases. *Am J Pathol* 1942;18:381–395.

61. Rappaport H, Winter WJ, Hicks EB. Follicular lymphoma: re-evaluation of its position in the scheme of malignant lymphomas, based on a survey of 253 cases. *Cancer* 1956;9:792–821.

61a. Rappaport H. Tumors of the hematopoietic system. In: *Atlas of tumor pathology,* 3rd ser., fasc 8. Section III. Washington, DC: Armed Forces Institute of Pathology, 1966.

62. Bagley CM, DeVita VT, Berard CW, et al. Advanced lymphosarcoma: intensive cyclic combination chemotherapy with cyclophosphamide, vincristine and prednisone. *Ann Intern Med* 1972;76:227–234.

63. Canellos GP, Lester A, Skarin AT. Chemotherapy of the non-Hodgkin's lymphomas. *Cancer* 1978;42:932–940.

64. Portlock CS, Rosenberg SA, Glatstein E, et al. Treatment of advanced non-Hodgkin's lymphomas with favorable histologies. Preliminary results of a prospective trial. *Blood* 1976;47:747–756.

65. Lister TA, Cullen MH, Beard ME, et al. Comparison of combined and single-agent chemotherapy in non-Hodgkin's lymphoma of favorable histologic type. *Br Med J* 1978;1:533–537.

66. Goffinet DR, Castellino RA, Kim H, et al. Staging laparotomies in unselected previously untreated patients with non-Hodgkin's lymphoma. *Cancer* 1973;32:672–681.

67. Lotz MJ, Chabner B, DeVita VT. Pathologic staging of 100 consecutive untreated patients with non-Hodgkin's lymphoma. *Cancer* 1976;37:266–270.

68. Fuks Z, Kaplan HS. Recurrence rates following radiation therapy of nodular and diffuse malignant lymphomas. *Radiology* 1973;108:675–684.

69. Gattiker HH, Wiltshaw E, Galton D. Spontaneous regression in non-Hodgkin's lymphoma. *Cancer* 1980;45:2627–2632.

70. Krikorian J, Portlock C, Cooney P, et al. Spontaneous regression in non-Hodgkin's lymphoma. *Cancer* 1980;45:2093–2099.

71. Horning S, Rosenberg S. The natural history of initially untreated low grade non-Hodgkin's lymphoma. *N Engl J Med* 1984;11:1471–1475.

72. Levitt M, Marsh JC, DeConti RC, et al. Combination sequential chemotherapy in advanced reticulum cell sarcoma. *Cancer* 1972;29:630–636.

73. Berd D, Cornog J, DeConti RC, et al. Long term remission in diffuse histiocytic lymphoma treated with combination sequential therapy. *Cancer* 1975;35:1050–1054.

74. Sweet DL, Golomb HM, Ultmann JE, et al. Cyclophosphamide, vincristine, methotrexate with leucovorin rescue, and cytarabine (COMLA) combination sequential chemotherapy for advanced diffuse histiocytic lymphoma. *Ann Intern Med* 1980;92:785–790.

75. Schein PS, Chabner BA, Canellos GP, et al. Potential for prolonged disease-free survival following combination chemotherapy of non-Hodgkin's lymphoma. *Blood* 1974;43:181–189.

76. Rodriguez V, Cabanillas R, Burgess MA, et al. Combination chemotherapy ("CHOP-Bleo") in advanced (non-Hodgkin) malignant lymphoma. *Blood* 1977;49:325–333.

77. Jones SE, Grozea PN, Metz EN, et al. Superiority of adriamycin-containing combination chemotherapy in the treatment of diffuse lymphoma. *Cancer* 1979;43:417–425.

78. Fisher RI, Gaynor ER, Dalberg S, et al. Comparison of a standard regimen (CHOP) with three intensive chemotherapy regimens for advanced non-Hodgkin's lymphoma. *N Engl J Med* 1993;328:1002–1006.

79. Burkitt DP. Sarcomas involving jaws in African children. *Br J Surg* 1969;46:218–223.

80. Berard C, O'Connor GT, Thomas LB, et al. Histopathological definition of Burkitt's lymphoma. *Bull* 1969;40:601–607.

81. Burkitt D. Long-term remissions following one and two dose chemotherapy for African lymphoma. *Cancer* 1967;20:756–759.

82. Burkitt D, Hutt MS, Wright DH. The African lymphoma: preliminary observations on response to therapy. *Cancer* 1965;18:399–410.

83. Ramirez I, Sullivan M, Wang Y-M, et al. Effective therapy for Burkitt's lymphoma: high dose cyclophosphamide + high dose methotrexate with coordinated intrathecal therapy. *Cancer Chemother Pharmacol* 1979;3:103–109.

84. Ziegler JL. Treatment results of 54 American patients with Burkitt's lymphoma are similar to the African experience. *N Engl J Med* 1977;3:75–80.

85. Arsenau JC, Bagley CM, Anderson T, et al. Hyperkalemia, a sequel to chemotherapy of Burkitt's lymphoma. *Lancet* 1973;1:10–14.

86. Cadman EC, Lunberg WB, Bertino JR. Hyperphosphatemia and hypocalcemia accompanying rapid lysis in a patient with Burkitt's lymphoma and Burkitt cell leukemia. *Am J Med* 1977;62:283–290.

87. Cronkite EP, Bond VP. *Radiation injury in man.* Springfield, IL: Charles C Thomas Publisher, 1960:138–139.

88. Thomas ED, Lochte HL Jr, Lu WC, et al. Intravenous infusion of bone marrow in patients receiving radiation and chemotherapy. *N Engl J Med* 1957;257:491–496.

89. Thomas ED, Lochte HL Jr, Cannon JH, et al. Supra-lethal whole body irradiation and isologous marrow transplantation in man. *J Clin Invest* 1959;38:1709–1716.

90. Thomas ED, Storb R, Clift RA, et al. Bone-marrow transplantation. *N Engl J Med* 1975;292:832–843,895–902.

91. Appelbaum FR, Herzig GP, Ziegler JL, et al. Successful engraftment of cryopreserved autologous bone marrow in patients with malignant lymphoma. *Blood* 1978;52:85–95.

92. Armitage JO, Vose JM. Bone marrow transplantation for malignant lymphoma. In: Canellos GP, Lister TA, Sklar JL, eds. *The lymphomas.* Philadelphia: WB Saunders, 1998:247–260.

CHAPTER 3

History of Radiation Therapy of Lymphomas and Description of Early Trials

Lena Specht

We undoubtedly have in the x-ray a therapeutic agent of immense value, one which in proper hands and in the hands of those who appreciate its limitation, is capable of doing an immense amount of good.

—Burnside Foster, M.D., 1906

FIRST 50 YEARS: THE KILOVOLT ERA

In December 1895, Wilhelm Conrad Röntgen first published his discovery of x-rays in a short communication to the Medical Physics Society of Würzburg, Germany, entitled "Über eine neue Art von Strahlen" ("On a new type of rays") (1–3). The news spread rapidly within the medical and scientific community on both sides of the Atlantic, the paper was translated into several languages, and, during the year 1896, more than 1,000 oral and written communications on x-rays were presented. It was soon discovered that the x-rays had biologic effects, and many started using them in dermatology and for superficial cancers. The first radiotherapy for cancer was probably given to a patient with pharyngeal cancer by Voight in Germany in January 1896 (4,5), possibly followed closely by Grubbé in Chicago (2,6–8). The first documented cure of cancer was a case of skin cancer on the nose that was treated by Stenbeck in Stockholm, Sweden, in 1899 (9). Shortly afterwards, cases of mycosis fungoides were treated with x-rays, which resulted in the healing of tumors as well as patches and plaques in the irradiated area (10,11). In 1903, Kienböck (12) further described the technique of irradiating mycosis fungoides (and other skin diseases), which, by then, already was apparently a fairly widely used treatment, at least in Vienna.

In Chicago, in 1902, Pusey published what appears to be the first documented cases of radiotherapy of extracutaneous lymphomas; he reported excellent local effect, at least in the short term (13). Figure 3.1 shows a 24-year-old man, who was treated by Pusey, with a "small round cell sarcoma" (undoubtedly a lymphoma, judging from the description of the clinical signs and response to radiation). The patient was treated in September 1901 with "21 x-ray exposures, with a hard tube and a weak light. The distance of the tube from the surface was maintained at 5 cm. And the length of the exposures varied from 10 to 15 minutes." The effect on the tumor was described as "almost magical." Two weeks after the end of treatment, "there was no trace of the disease left except a small, freely movable, painless gland not larger than an almond kernel." Equally impressive results were published by Senn (14), Williams (15), and others in the following couple of years (16,17). In 1904, Krause (18), from Breslau (now Wroclaw, Poland), gave an overview of the published cases of radiotherapy of lymphomas (and other hematologic diseases). In 1903 and 1905, in Leipzig, Germany, Heineke (19,20) published experimental and clinical data that showed the radiosensitivity of lymphoid cells, and he described some cases of lymphomas that were treated with x-rays, although with only transient responses. The optimism that was fostered by these early reports of what were regularly described as almost miraculous responses to x-ray therapy was soon to be tempered by reports of almost inevitable recurrences (21–24). In the words of Foster (25) (in 1906): "As has happened frequently before in the history of medicine, the world was doomed to a bitter disappointment."

The equipment for radiotherapy was, at first, rather primitive and difficult to control. The maximum energy that was available ranged from 50 to 100 kV, the x-ray tube was placed at a short distance from or in contact with the skin, and no filter was used (2,26). Gradually, better equipment was developed that could operate at 250 to 400 kV, filters were introduced, and the treatment distance increased, typically to 50 cm, thus allowing much larger volumes to be treated with better control of dosage (2,26). Still, for several decades, the treatment of lymphomas was considered palliative in all but a few exceptional cases, and radiation doses were limited to doses that did not cause too much discomfort for the patients (27–33). It was realized that most cases had advanced disease that could not be cured by radiotherapy,

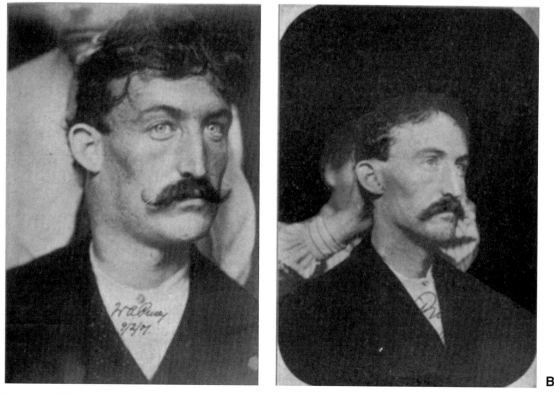

FIGURE 3.1. A case of lymphoma that was treated in September 1901 by W. A. Pusey, Professor of Dermatology in the Medical Department of the University of Illinois. **A:** The patient on September 2, before the start of radiotherapy. **B:** The patient on October 11, 2 weeks after the end of treatment. This seems to be the first documented case of radiotherapy for lymphoma. (From Pusey WA. Cases of sarcoma and of Hodgkin's disease treated by exposures to x-rays—a preliminary report. *JAMA* 1902;38:166–169, with permission.)

but these patients could often be effectively palliated with relatively small doses (32,34–39). In these circumstances, wide regional irradiation (the so-called x-ray bath) or total-body irradiation was regularly used with good palliative effect that lasted up to several years (33,36,40–43). It was noted that, with generalized body irradiation, a considerably smaller dose was required to cause tumor regression than was necessary for equal regression of tumors that were treated locally. A certain technique that was called the Heublein method, after its inventor, was developed at the Memorial Hospital in New York for continuously irradiating several patients at a time in a specially designed room with treatment times over 10 days (44). Patient safety was ostensibly ensured by monitoring the effect of the irradiation on a canary that was placed in the same room halfway between the x-ray tube and the patients. A series of 30 patients with widely disseminated lymphosarcoma who were treated with the Heublein method at the Memorial Hospital was published in 1942; it indicated some prolongation of survival in these patients (45). Total-body irradiation with radioactive isotopes, particularly radiophosphorus, was also tried but generally proved unsatisfactory (33).

The bewildering diversity within the lymphomas was recognized early, and attempts were made to determine the radiosensitivity of different lymphoma types (30,39,46,47). The striking radiosensitivity of the lymphoid tissue and lymphomatous lesions was acknowledged (20,32,39,47–50). Of the lymphomas, the follicular type and mycosis fungoides were found to be the most sensitive of all; complete regression was often seen after total doses of only 400 to 800 R (30,46,51–55). It was noticed that the tumor cells died soon after irradiation, often within the first 2 weeks (50), and Coutard (48), in Paris, observed that the daily repetition of irradiation in small doses and an increase in the number of days of treatment of these tumors "enable us mainly to achieve the preservation of the general tissues and to avoid early or late accidents." Radiotherapy in this era was the only effective treatment for patients with malignant lymphomas, however, treatment was regarded throughout as merely palliative in nearly all cases, and recommended radiation doses varied greatly: from 600 to 4,000 R (30,32,39,46,47,50). The techniques also varied, but it was recognized early on that even localized cases needed fairly large treatment volumes to encompass not only the overt lymphoma, but also occult disease in the adjacent areas. It thus became apparent that moderate- to high-voltage x-ray treatment was clearly superior to radium treatment, which has only rarely been used for lymphomas (29,32,47,49,50).

Despite the prevailing skepticism regarding the curative potential of radiotherapy, in 1932, Berven (56), in Stockholm, Sweden, had already reported 35 cases of lymphosarcoma of the tonsil that were treated with x-rays and local application of radium during the period 1916 to 1927, with a 5-year relapse-free survival of 37%. In the following years, other reports began to appear that documented the possibility of a cure for localized cases by repeated treatments and radical radiotherapy techniques with large fields. Some of these studies advised the inclusion of neighboring noninvolved regions (41,47,57,58), whereas others did not (50,59–61). Long-term survivors were seen in series that were treated with minimum doses of 2,000 to 3,500 R (skin dose) to all manifest lesions, in lymphosarcomas and reticulosarcomas, although more frequently in the former (48,50,54,61–69). Exceptional cases, even of reticulosarcoma, were reported to be cured with lower doses (70). The great prognostic impact of the size of the tumor on the outcome after radiotherapy was demonstrated (67). Combined treatment with operation followed by radiotherapy for localized cases was advocated by some (35,71), but this strategy did not ultimately seem to produce better results than radiotherapy alone in comparable cases (50,67). Still, most authorities questioned whether x-ray therapy alone appreciably prolonged life in patients with malignant lymphomas (27,29,35,72). A large series that was published by Rosenberg et al. (73) from the Memorial Center in New York, with more than 1,200 patients who were treated from the late 1920s to the early 1950s, showed a 5-year survival of 54% for giant follicle lymphosarcoma, 27% for lymphosarcoma, and 23% for reticulum cell sarcoma, with no indication of an improvement of results during the period that was covered. Rosenberg cautiously stated that "the comparative radiosensitivity of these tumors generally permits some degree of symptomatic improvement, but it is not known whether this treatment has significantly prolonged survival" (73). He rightly deplored the lack of randomized, well-controlled comparisons of different therapeutic regimens. Other studies were not quite so guarded. Easson and Russell (74) reported long-term follow-up (15 years) of 202 patients who were treated with large-field regional x-ray therapy in the Christie Hospital, Manchester, United Kingdom, during the period from 1933 to 1949. They concluded that, for patients with localized disease (over one-half of their patients), the definitive cure rate was 49% (74). Peters (75) reported that 414 patients from Toronto were treated during the period from 1934 to 1952 with fairly aggressive irradiation to tumor in doses of 2,000 to 6,500 rad, with prophylactic irradiation of uninvolved lymphatic regions in approximately one-half the patients. For patients with localized disease, Peters reported crude 5-, 10-, and 15-year survivals of 51%, 43%, and 36%, respectively, with no indication that prophylactic irradiation of uninvolved regions improved results (75). Fuller and Fletcher (76), from Houston, reported 278 patients who were treated from 1947 to 1959; the majority were treated with 250 kV, but some were treated with cobalt 60. Patients with localized disease had a 5-year survival of 47%. Van der Werf-Messing (77), from Rotterdam, the Netherlands, reported a series of 113 cases with localized disease; between 1953 and 1963, the patients were treated with orthovoltage x-rays to the clinically involved area with a fairly large margin. She reported a 5-year survival of greater than 50% in these patients (77). Hansen (78), from Copenhagen, Denmark, reported a series of patients who were treated during the period from 1940 to 1966; this series included 66 patients with localized disease who were treated with 180 or 250 kV, with a 5-year survival of 45%. Results from these and other series (79) of patients with localized disease who were treated with kilovolt irradiation are shown in Table 3.1. Results were best for giant follicular lymphomas and poorest for reticulum cell sarcoma, with results for lymphosarcoma in the middle of the result spectrum, but few of the studies split localized

TABLE 3.1. *Studies of primary radiotherapy for localized non-Hodgkin's lymphoma that was treated in the kilovolt era*

Reference	Number of patients	Histology	5-year survival (%)	10-year survival (%)	15-year survival (%)
Rosenberg et al. (73)	245	Lymphosarcoma	41	—	—
Easson and Russell (74)	107	Lymphoreticular sarcoma	52	49	49
Peters (75)	102	Lymphoma	51	43	36
Fuller and Fletcher (76)	131	Lymphoma	47	—	—
Van der Werf-Messing (77)	113	Reticulum cell sarcoma and lymphosarcoma	66 (1 region) 50 (2 contiguous regions)	—	—
Hansen (78)	66	Reticulum cell sarcoma	45	30	—
Cook et al. (79)	211	Lymphosarcoma and reticulum cell sarcoma	30	—	—

cases into the different histologic groups. Results for patients with widespread disease were, not unexpectedly, much poorer, with few long-term survivors.

NEXT 50 YEARS: THE MEGAVOLT ERA

Certain scientific and technologic developments before and during World War II created new opportunities for improvements in radiotherapy. Thus, the production of radionuclides in nuclear reactors made possible the construction of tele-gamma devices with cobalt 60 that produced x-rays of approximately 1.2 MV of high intensity, which represented a great technical improvement over conventional kilovolt x-ray tubes and teleradium cannons. Eventually, the construction of electron accelerators enabled the production of high-energy x-rays (4 to 50 MV) with high intensity from a small focus, thus allowing the treatment distance to be increased to 100 cm, with treatment times of a duration of typically less than 1 minute. The x-ray beam from these devices is characterized by high tissue penetration and dose homogeneity in the irradiated field and by sharp field boundaries. Electron accelerators have the added advantage of being able to deliver high-energy electron irradiation, as well. Because of the limited penetration of electron irradiation (depth depending on the energy of the electrons), it is particularly suitable for treating superficial lesions. Linear accelerators, which were based on microwave technology that was developed during World War II, became available in the early 1950s, and this device now dominates the market.

These huge advances in technology allowed for the treatment of all lymphoid tissues in the body with acceptable normal tissue toxicity. Many of the techniques that were used for nodal lymphomas are copied to a great extent from the techniques that were developed for the treatment of Hodgkin's disease. Treatment volumes may roughly be divided into involved-field radiotherapy, extended-field radiotherapy, or total lymphoid irradiation. Problems with the classification of non-Hodgkin's lymphomas, however, made analyses and trials more difficult than in Hodgkin's disease. In the following discussion, lymphomas have been roughly divided into the categories of favorable and unfavorable. In studies in which cases are subdivided according to follicular or diffuse histology, the former are considered favorable, the latter unfavorable.

The new technology was implemented in most large centers during the 1950s and 1960s. Some of the first linear accelerators were installed at Stanford University, and series of patients who were treated from the early 1960s were published by Kaplan, Rosenberg, Glatstein, Fuks, Jones, and Hoppe et al. (80–94). Patients with localized lymphomas were treated with involved-field radiotherapy, extended-field radiotherapy, or total lymphoid irradiation. In patients with favorable histology, total lymphoid irradiation resulted in superior relapse-free survival compared to extended-field radiotherapy and involved-field radiotherapy, but there was

no difference in overall survival (88,89,91). In patients with unfavorable histology and extranodal involvement, neither the extent of irradiation nor the addition of chemotherapy had a significant influence on outcome (92). Table 3.2 shows results of radiotherapy for localized lymphomas from Stanford and other centers. At Stanford, total lymphoid irradiation for favorable stage III patients, a group that was often considered incurable, was also tested, demonstrating that this treatment may be a potentially curative modality in these patients (89,90,93). Table 3.3 shows the results from Stanford and other centers of total lymphoid irradiation for stage III with favorable histology. Based on the data from Stanford, for patients in all stages, Fuks and Kaplan (80) made retrospective calculations on the dose-response relationship for the different types of lymphomas (Table 3.4), although they were aware of the pitfall that patients with relatively advanced disease (and, hence, an inherently poorer prognosis) tend to receive lower doses. These data were for a long time highly influential on the choice of dose levels.

Hellman et al. (95,96) and Mauch et al. (97), at Harvard, reported on patients who were treated at the Joint Center for Radiation Therapy in the late 1960s and 1970s. Their results for patients with localized disease who were treated with radiotherapy alone are shown in Table 3.2.

From the Princess Margaret Hospital in Toronto, Bush, Gospodarowicz, Sutcliffe and coworkers (98–101) published large series of patients with localized lymphomas who were treated with irradiation in the late 1960s and 1970s. The results are summarized in Table 3.2. They defined subgroups with high cure rates based on tumor bulk, age, and histology. Their large database allowed important analyses of the dose-response relationship; these are summarized in Table 3.4.

At the M.D. Anderson Hospital, Fuller et al. (103,104) and others (102,105–108), and later Cox, made several publications on their patients who were treated in the 1960s and 1970s. Summary results of two of their series of patients with localized disease who were treated with extended-field radiotherapy are shown in Table 3.2. Cox continued his interest in total lymphoid irradiation for favorable stage III patients (109–112), an interest he had previously entertained in Wisconsin when combining data from his own institution with data from other centers (Table 3.3) (113–116). This innovative treatment for an otherwise incurable group of patients is now receiving renewed interest (117). Cox et al. (118) and Kun et al. (119) also contributed data on the dose-response relationship in lymphomas (Table 3.4).

In Florida, Kamath et al. (120), Nathu et al. (121), De Los Santos et al. (122), and Mendenhall and Million (123) have reported series of patients who were treated from the mid 1960s with irradiation for localized disease (Table 3.2) (120,121) and with total lymphoid irradiation for stage III disease (Table 3.3) (122,123). They too contributed to our knowledge of the dose-response relationship (Table 3.4).

Other American centers also contributed series of patients who were treated with irradiation in the 1960s and 1970s.

TABLE 3.2. *Studies of primary radiotherapy for localized non-Hodgkin's lymphoma that was treated in the megavolt era*

Location of study (reference)	Number of patients	Histology	5-year RFS (%)	5-year OS (%)	10-year RFS (%)	10-year OS (%)	15-year RFS (%)	15-year OS (%)
Stanford (88)	177	F	55	82	44	64	40	44
Stanford (92)	111	U (extranodal)	49	46	49	36	—	—
Stanford (84)	35	U (Waldeyer)	50 (CS I)	50 (CS I)	—	—	—	—
			25 (CS II)	20 (CS II)	—	—	—	—
Harvard (97)	28	U	35	45	—	—	—	—
	26	F	47	91	—	—	—	—
Princess Margaret Hospital (101)	496	332 U, 143 F	54	62	49	49	—	—
M.D. Anderson (105)	113	U + F (Waldeyer)	37	47	26	32	—	—
M.D. Anderson (102)	45	F	48	—	45	—	35	53
Florida (120)	159	92 U	60	—	50	—	50	—
		67 F	80	—	80	—	—	—
Yale (124)	78	53 U	37	59	—	—	—	—
		25 F	83	100	—	—	—	—
Chicago (127)	31	U	78	80	54	58	—	—
Minnesota (131)	19	U	83	88	64	88	—	—
Freiburg (133)	39 CS I	U + F	75	75	65	65	65	60
	42 CS II		36	27	36	18	36	18
	35 CS IE, IIE		52	60	52	60	52	52
Institut Gustave Roussy (136)	134	123 U	—	40	—	—	—	—
		11F	—	60	—	—	—	—
European Organization for Research and Treatment of Cancer (139)	43 CS I	U + F	60	87	50	75	—	—
	21 CS II	F	62	75	—	—	—	—
	15 CS II	U	10	10	—	—	—	—
British National Lymphoma Investigation (141,144,146)	243 CS I	U	—	—	45	61	—	—
	208 CS I	F	—	—	47	64	—	—
	46 CS II	U	—	40	—	—	—	—
	43 CS II	F	—	75	—	60	—	—
The Royal Marsden Hospital (148,151)	12	U	—	83	—	—	—	—
	58	F	59	93	43	79	36	58
St. Bartholomew's Hospital (152)	57 CS I	U + F	68	78	58	64	—	—
	43 CS II	—	38	48	32	43	—	—
Sweden (154)	99 CS I	U + F	64	78	—	—	—	—
	48 CS II	U + F	8	30	—	—	—	—

CS, clinical stage; F, favorable; OS, overall survival; RFS, relapse-free survival; U, unfavorable.

Among them are Chen et al. (124), at Yale; Bitran et al. (125), Hallahan et al. (126), and Vokes et al. (127), in Chicago; and Levitt et al. (128–131) and Lee and Levitt (132), in Minnesota. Data from some of these studies are summarized in Table 3.2.

In Europe, Musshoff et al. (133), in Freiburg, Germany, published series of patients who were treated during the 1950s and 1960s, thus encompassing patients who were treated with kilovolt and megavolt equipment. He reported survival data on patients with localized disease, dividing them into patients with primary extranodal involvement and patients with primary nodal involvement. For stage I patients, survival was roughly the same for these two groups; for patients in stage II, survival was actually better for

TABLE 3.3. *Studies of primary radiotherapy for stage III patients with favorable histology*

Location of study (reference)	Number of patients	5-year RFS (%)	5-year OS (%)	10-year RFS (%)	10-year OS (%)	15-year RFS (%)	15-year OS (%)
Stanford (90)	66	57	76	42	48	37	38
Wisconsin (116)	34	58	70	40	50	40	28
Florida (122)	11	—	—	—	—	45	34

OS, overall survival; RFS, relapse-free survival.

patients with primary extranodal involvement. Altogether, prognosis for patients with localized extranodal involvement was much better than for patients with disseminated extranodal involvement, thus confirming the importance of the E stages that Musshoff had previously introduced in the staging classification for Hodgkin's disease. Data regarding localized disease are summarized in Table 3.2. Musshoff also contributed analyses of the dose-response relationship (Table 3.4) (134).

At the Institut Gustave Roussy in Paris, Brugere et al. (135) and Tubiana et al. (136) published large series of patients with localized disease treated in the late 1950s and the 1960s with involved-field radiotherapy to doses of 3,000 to 5,000 rad. Results are summarized in Tables 3.2 and 3.4. Tubiana was instrumental in creating the Lymphoma Group of the European Organization for Research and Treatment of Cancer, which has carried out important randomized trials in non-Hodgkin's lymphomas (137–139). Their results for patients with localized disease who were treated with irradiation alone are summarized in Table 3.2.

The British National Lymphoma Investigation, a large multiinstitutional collaboration that was based at the Middlesex Hospital in London and coordinated by Jelliffe and G. and B. Vaughan Hudson for many years, managed to gather together large numbers of patients in their many trials (140–146). Data from some of their series of patients with localized disease who were treated with irradiation are summarized in Table 3.2.

At the Royal Marsden Hospital, London, Horwich, Peckham, and coworkers (147–150) and Pendlebury et al. (151) have published series of patients with localized disease who were treated with irradiation alone in the 1970s and 1980s (Table 3.2). Their analyses of dose-response relationships are summarized in Table 3.4.

At St. Bartholomew's Hospital, London, Timothy et al. (152) and Richards et al. (153) also published data on patients with localized disease who were treated in the 1960s and 1970s with irradiation, which, in a few cases, was supplemented with adjuvant chemotherapy. Most of their cases had unfavorable histology. Results are summarized in Table 3.2.

TABLE 3.4. *Radiation doses recommended for local control in different studies*

Location of study (reference)	Histology	Minimum total dose (cGy)
Stanford (80)	U	— (No correlation found between 1,500 and 6,500)
	F	4,400
Princess Margaret Hospital (101)	U	3,000
	F	2,000
M.D. Anderson (105)	U + F	3,500
Wisconsin (119)	U	4,000
Walter Reed General Hospital (118)	U	4,200
	F	2,200
Florida (120)	U	4,000
	F	3,000
Freiburg (134)	F	2,500
Institut Gustave Roussy (136)	U + F	3,500 to 4,000
The Royal Marsden Hospital (150)	U	— (No correlation found between 3,500 and 5,500)
	F	3,000

F, favorable histology; U, unfavorable histology.

In Sweden, Hagberg et al. (154) published a series of patients who were treated in the 1970s, two-thirds of whom were in stage I (Table 3.2). A later series of 129 patients with stage I high-grade disease who were treated with radiotherapy showed a relapse rate of 29% (155).

The overall conclusion from these and other studies is that a significant number of patients with truly localized disease are cured with radiotherapy. This is true for indolent as well as aggressive subtypes of lymphoma, although it is true more frequently in the former.

Addition of Chemotherapy

With the advent of single-drug chemotherapy in the 1940s and 1950s and the development of combinations of drugs in the 1960s, the idea arose to combine radiotherapy and chemotherapy with the aim of further improving outcome. Early nonrandomized studies showed promising results for combined modality treatment in localized disease (97,156–158); however, the assessment of the true value of this novel approach had to await the results of randomized trials. A number of randomized trials of radiotherapy alone versus combined modality treatment in localized disease have since been carried out. Early trials that tested the addition of single-drug therapy, or combinations without anthracycline, to radiotherapy are summarized in Table 3.5 (143,145,159–165). Some of the trials that included patients with unfavorable histology showed a significant improvement in relapse-free survival, but only one trial showed an improvement in survival. Two randomized trials of adjuvant chemotherapy with the combination of cyclophosphamide, Adriamycin, vincristine, and prednisone in addition to radiotherapy for localized disease have been published (166,167); see Table 3.6. With effective modern chemotherapy, relapse-free and overall survival are improved with combined modality treatment for patients with aggressive localized lymphomas but not for patients with indolent localized lymphomas.

When chemotherapy was first introduced in the treatment of lymphomas, radiotherapy was the standard treatment. Consequently, chemotherapy was introduced as an adjuvant and was given after what was considered the standard treatment. In all except one of the previously mentioned randomized trials, radiotherapy was given initially, followed by chemotherapy after 4 to 8 weeks. However, in some series, relapses occurred in approximately 10% of patients in the interval between radiotherapy and chemotherapy (161,162). Consequently, Nissen et al. (163) introduced in their trial concurrent chemoradiotherapy, which improved the early

TABLE 3.5. *Early randomized studies of radiotherapy alone versus combined modality treatment in localized disease*

| Reference | Number of patients | Histology | Chemotherapy | RT alone | | RT + CT | | p value |
				5-year RFS (%)	5-year OS (%)	5-year RFS (%)	5-year OS (%)	RFS/OS
Landberg et al. (161)	55	U + F	CVP	41[a]	92[a]	86[a]	91[a]	0.02/NS
Monfardini et al. (162)	96	U + F	CVP	46	56	72	83	0.005/0.03
Kelsey et al. (143)	148	F	Chlorambucil	33[b]	52[b]	42[b]	42[b]	NS/NS
Phillips (145)	80	U	CVP	—	68	—	48	NS
Nissen et al. (163)	73	U + F	CVPS	49	58	90	71	0.001/NS
Kaminski et al. (160)	46	U	CVP	68	62	54	60	NS/NS
Gomez et al. (159)	21	F	BMCVP	—	—	—	—	NS/NS
Somers et al. (165)	124	U + F	CVP	55	86	75	84	0.002/NS
Panahon et al. (164)	63 (some stage III)	U + F —	BMCVP —	80[c] (CS I) 75[c] (CS II)	90[c] (CS I) 100[c] (CS II)	66[c] (CS I) 75[c] (CS II)	100[c] (CS I) 75[c] (CS II)	NS/NS —

B, bischloroethylnitrosourea; C, cyclophosphamide; CS, clinical stage; CT, chemotherapy; F, favorable; M, mechlorethamine; NS, not significant; OS, overall survival; P, prednisone; RFS, relapse-free survival; RT, radiotherapy; S, streptonigrin; U, unfavorable; V, vincristine.

[a]30-month figures only.
[b]10-year figures only.
[c]3-year figures only.

TABLE 3.6. *Randomized studies of radiotherapy alone versus combined modality treatment with cyclophosphamide, Adriamycin, vincristine, and prednisone (CHOP) in localized disease*

Reference	Number of patients	Histology	RT alone		RT + CT		p value
			5-year RFS (%)	5-year OS (%)	5-year RFS (%)	5-year OS (%)	RFS/OS
Yahalom et al. (167)	44	U + F	47[a]	66[a]	83[a]	88[a]	0.03/NS
Avilés et al. (166)	224	U	48	56	83	90	0.001/0.001

CT, chemotherapy; F, favorable; NS, not significant; OS, overall survival; RFS, relapse-free survival; RT, radiotherapy; U, unfavorable.
[a]7-year figures.

relapse rate, but at the expense of more toxicity. Furthermore, in some trials, radiotherapy was given to extended fields, which sometimes precluded full doses of chemotherapy afterwards (159). With the introduction in the 1980s of the more effective anthracycline-containing chemotherapy regimens, the sequence of combined modality in aggressive localized lymphomas has changed, with chemotherapy assuming a primary role for induction of response and with radiotherapy being used for consolidation (167). This approach has the added advantage of reducing disease bulk before radiotherapy, thus allowing the use of lower doses of irradiation.

Total-Body Irradiation

In the kilovolt era, irradiation of the whole body with low doses in patients with advanced disease had been used already with good palliative effect (see First 50 Years: the Kilovolt Era). In the 1960s, interest in low-dose total-body irradiation was renewed. The treatment was given with total doses of 100 to 300 cGy in 10 to 30 cGy fractions in various protocol schedules over several weeks. In America, Johnson et al. (168–170) at the National Cancer Institute, Carabell et al. (171) and Chaffey et al. (172–174) at the Joint Center for Radiation Therapy (171–174), Hoppe et al. (175) at Stanford, and Mendenhall et al. (176) and Thar and Million (177) in Florida published series of patients, some with aggressive and some with indolent lymphomas, who were treated in this way. In Europe, series were published by the British National Lymphoma Investigation (178), Pettingale (179) and Dobbs et al. (180) at the Royal Marsden Hospital, and De Neve et al. (181), Lybeert et al. (182), and Qasim (183) in Rotterdam. Results are summarized in Table 3.7. In aggressive lymphomas, the results of total-

TABLE 3.7. *Studies of total-body irradiation in advanced disease*

Location of study (reference)	Number of patients	Histology	5-year RFS (%)	5-year OS (%)	10-year RFS (%)	10-year OS (%)
National Cancer Institute (170)	13	U	8	27	—	—
	22	F	14	84	—	—
Harvard (171)	15	U	10	42	0[a]	42[a]
	43	F	23	65	15[a]	57[a]
Stanford (175)	17	F	34	95	—	—
Florida (176)	17	U	0	17	0	0
	27	F	28	56	12	32
British National Lymphoma Investigation (178)	48	U	0	0	—	—
The Royal Marsden Hospital[b] (180)	15	U	—	0	—	0
	22	F	—	30	—	30[a]
Rotterdam Radiotherapeutic Institute (182)	20	U	0	15	0	0
	25	F	32	48	27	35

CT, chemotherapy; F, favorable; OS, overall survival; RFS, relapse-free survival; RT, radiotherapy; U, unfavorable.
[a]7.5-year figures.
[b]13 patients previously treated.

TABLE 3.8. *Studies of total skin electron-beam therapy for mycosis fungoides*

Location of study (reference)	Number of patients	Subset	Complete remission (%)	5-year relapse-free survival (%)	5-year overall survival (%)
Stanford (196)	43	Limited plaques	98	50	80
	104	Generalized plaques	71	25	45
	47	Tumors	36	—	25
Lahey Clinic and Massachusetts Institute of Technology (200)	89	Generalized plaques	—	19	48
	54	Tumors	—	17	32
Ontario Cancer Foundation (198)	68	Limited plaques	88	38	93
	59	Generalized plaques	80	25	81
	13	Tumors	62	—	53
Montreal (197)	11	Generalized plaques	91	—	64
	21	Tumors	71	—	20
Henri Mondor University Hospital, France (199)	46	Plaques <50% of surface	100	62	93
	20	Plaques >50% of surface	44	19	79
		Tumors or Sézary syndrome	39	0	44
University Hospital Leiden, Netherlands (201)	30	Mixed	90	—	70

body irradiation were poor. In indolent lymphomas, approximately 30% of patients were recurrence free at 5 years. This result was similar to that which could be obtained with chemotherapy, which was substantiated by the results of the two randomized studies, from Stanford and National Cancer Institute, that compared total-body irradiation with the chemotherapy combination of cyclophosphamide, vincristine, and prednisone (170,175). The notion that a radiation dose as low as 2 Gy should be able to induce long-lasting remission remains something of a puzzle. This effect may possibly be mediated through mechanisms of immune modulation and induction of apoptosis. There is a revival of investigations of low-dose total-body irradiation in the treatment of lymphomas.

Total Skin Electron-Beam Therapy

Mycosis fungoides, or cutaneous T-cell lymphoma, was probably the first type of lymphoma ever to be treated with x-rays (11), and, as mentioned above, it was found to be an extremely radiosensitive disease. Local x-ray therapy remained the most effective palliative therapy for mycosis fungoides until the 1950s. The problem with conventional x-ray therapy is that, if it is administered over large areas, the dose to the underlying internal organs exceeds their tolerance. Electrons, by contrast, have a limited range of penetration and deposit their total energy within that range. The effect of electrons is therefore limited to superficial tissues, the depth depending on the energy of the electrons. The possibility of using artificially accelerated high-energy electrons (cathode rays) in radiotherapy was envisaged as far back as the 1920s and 1930s (184,185), but energies at the

time were not high enough. In the 1940s, Trump et al. (186), at the Massachusetts Institute of Technology, constructed a Van de Graaff generator that was able to produce a 1,500 keV electron beam; experiments were conducted, but this technique still only yielded a maximum range of electrons in tissue of approximately 7 mm. Trump et al. gradually improved their technology, and, by 1950, they were able to produce electron beams for therapy with energies of up to 2.5 MeV. They published the first two cases of mycosis fungoides that were treated with total skin electron-beam therapy by using a four-field technique, with the patient lying on a couch and moving under the machine (187). With the introduction of linear accelerators, it became possible to generate electrons for therapy with energies from 4 MeV to more than 20 MeV, and techniques were enhanced to yield a more uniform dose to the entire skin surface. At Stanford, Cox et al. (188) and Karzmark et al. (189) refined the physical aspects of the technique, and Fuks et al. (190–192) and Hoppe et al. (193–196) refined the clinical aspects of total skin electron-beam therapy, by using a six-field standing technique (190–196). The Stanford technique has gained wide acceptance, but other techniques have also been used with largely similar results. Published series from different centers are summarized in Table 3.8 (196–201). Complete remission is attained in 70% to 100% of patients with plaque disease and less often in patients with tumors. Most patients relapse within 5 years, but often with quite limited disease, which may be managed with limited irradiation or other topical therapies. When relapse is widespread in the skin, total skin electron beam therapy may be repeated (202). Although total skin electron-beam therapy is rarely curative, it offers significant palliation in most patients.

FUTURE

Radiotherapy is a highly effective treatment modality for lymphomas that, as demonstrated by the previous discussion, has been used to the benefit of vast numbers of lymphoma patients for more than a century. The benefit has depended on scientific and technologic ingenuity and the intelligent employment of specific innovations by oncologists with a profound knowledge of lymphomas. The coming years hold great promise for further significant advances in the use of radiotherapy for lymphomas. The new lymphoma classification defines far more disease entities with distinctive clinical features than before (203,204), thus enabling us to tailor treatment, including radiation fields and doses, more specifically to each recognized disease entity. The technical side of radiotherapy is also changing dramatically. Advances in computer hardware and software have led to the development of sophisticated three-dimensional treatment planning and computer-controlled radiation therapy delivery systems. This three-dimensional conformal radiation therapy and the even more sophisticated intensity-modulated radiation therapy allow us to shape the high-dose volume precisely to the tumor volume while minimizing the dose to the surrounding normal structures (205). The implementation of these techniques to the treatment of lymphomas is still in its early phase. However, these technical innovations already show significant potential for improving and expanding the use of radiotherapy, alone or in combination with chemotherapy or biologic therapies, with the aim of further optimizing the treatment that can be offered to lymphoma patients in the future.

ACKNOWLEDGMENTS

The author wishes to thank Copenhagen University Library, the Medical Library of Copenhagen University Hospital, and Professor Torsten Landberg for their generous assistance. The author received support from the Preben and Anna Simonsen Foundation.

REFERENCES

1. Röntgen WC. Über eine neue Art von Strahlen. *Sitzungsberichte Physikalisch-Medicinischen Gesellschaft zu Würzburg* 1895;30:132–141.
2. Lederman M. The early history of radiotherapy: 1895–1939. *Int J Radiat Oncol Biol Phys* 1981;7:639–648.
3. Dubois JB, Ash D. The discovery of x-rays and radioactivity. In: Bernier J, ed. *Radiation oncology: a century of progress and achievement.* Belgium: The European Society for Therapeutic Radiology and Oncology, 1995:77–98.
4. Case JT. History of radiation oncology. *Prog Radiat Ther* 1958;1:13–41.
5. McCarty PJ, Million R. History of radiation oncology. *J Florida Med Assoc* 1995;82:745–748.
6. Grubbé EH. Priority in the therapeutic use of x-rays. *Radiology* 1933;21:156–162.
7. Walstam R. A historical review on radiotherapeutic applications. In: Bernier J, ed. *Radiation oncology: a century of progress and achievement.* Belgium: The European Society for Therapeutic Radiology and Oncology, 1995:17–46.
8. Mould RF. Invited review: the early years of radiotherapy with emphasis on x-ray and radium apparatus. *Br J Radiol* 1995;68:567–582.
9. Berven E. The development and organization of therapeutic radiology in Sweden. *Radiology* 1962;79:829–841.
10. Riehl, Vereine, Kongresse. Gesellschaft der Ärzte in Wien. 1903. 15. Mai. *Fortschr Geb Röntgenstr* 1903;7:41.
11. Scholz W. Ueber den Einfluss der Röntgenstrahlen auf die Haut in gesundem und krankem Zustande. III. Klinischer Theil. *Archiv F Dermatol Syphilis* 1902;59:421–445.
12. Kienböck R. Der gegenwärtige Stand der Radiotherapie. *Fortschr Geb Röntgenstr* 1903;7:343–346.
13. Pusey WA. Cases of sarcoma and of Hodgkin's disease treated by exposures to x-rays—a preliminary report. *JAMA* 1902;38:166–169.
14. Senn N. The therapeutical value of the Röntgen ray in the treatment of pseudoleukemia. *N Y Med J* 1903;77:665–668.
15. Williams FH. The use of the x-rays in the treatment of diseases of the skin, of new-growths, of the glandular system, and of other diseases, and as a means of relieving pain. *Trans Assoc of Am Phys* 1903;18:89–96.
16. Chrysospathes JG. Erfolgreiche Behandlung eines inoperablen Sarkoms mittels Röntgenstrahlen. *Munch Med Wochenschr* 1903;50:2182–2185.
17. Cohn M. Die Bedeutung der Röntgenstrahlen für die Behandlung der lymphatischen Sarkome. *Berliner Klin Wochenschr* 1906;43:14–17.
18. Krause P. Zur Röntgenbehandlung von Bluterkrankungen (Leukaemie, Pseudoleukaemie, Lymphomatosis, perniciöse Anaemie, Anaemia splenica, Polycythaemia mi Milztumor). *Fortschr Geb Röntgenstr* 1904;8:209–235.
19. Heineke H. Experimentelle Untersuchungen über die Einwirkung der Röntgenstrahlen auf innere Organe. *Mitteilungen aus den Grenzgebieten der Medizin und Chirurgie* 1903;14.
20. Heineke H. Experimentelle Untersuchungen über die Einwirkung der Röntgenstrahlen auf das Knochenmark, nebst einigen Bemerkungen über die Röntgentherapie der Leukämie und Pseudoleukämie und des Sarcoms. *Dtsch Zeitschrift Chirurgie* 1905;78:196–230.
21. Ewald CA. Ein Fall von geheiltem Lymphosarkom, mit Röntgen und Arsen behandelt. *Berliner Klin Wochenschr* 1906;43:910–911.
22. Forssell G. Kort öfversikt öfver nyare rön inom Röntgenterapien. *Almänna Svenska Läkartidningen* 1904;1:481–509.
23. Coley WB. The present status of the x-ray treatment of malignant tumors. *Med Rec N Y* 1903;63:441–451.
24. Coley WB. Primary neoplasms of the lymphatic glands including Hodgkin's disease. In: Binnie JF, ed. *Transactions of the American Surgical Association.* Philadelphia: William J. Dornan, 1915:499–644.
25. Foster B. The present state of our knowledge concerning the therapeutic value of the x-ray. *J Minn State Med Assoc Northwest Lancet* 1906;26:23–26.
26. Ewing J. Early experiences in radiation therapy. Janeway memorial lecture. *AJR Am J Roentgenol* 1934;31:153–163.
27. Desjardins AU, Ford F. Hodgkin's disease and lymphosarcoma: clinical and statistical study. *JAMA* 1923;81:925–927.
28. Minot GR. Lymphoblastoma. *Radiology* 1926;7:119–120.
29. Desjardins AU. Radiotherapy for Hodgkin's disease and lymphosarcoma. *JAMA* 1932;99:1231–1236.
30. Craver LF. The treatment of the more important lymphadenopathies, with special reference to irradiation. *Med Clin North Am* 1934;18:703–726.
31. Desjardins AU, Habein HC, Watkins CH. Unusual complications of lymphoblastoma and their radiation treatment. *AJR Am J Roentgenol* 1936;36:169–179.
32. Arons I. Further studies on radiotherapy of lymphoblastoma. *Radiology* 1941;37:164–173.
33. Craver LF. Lymphomas and leukemias. *Bull N Y Acad Med* 1947;23:79–100.
34. Fabian E. Ueber die Behandlung des Lymphosarkoms. *Munch Med Wochenschr* 1913;43:1876–1878.
35. Minot GR, Isaacs R. Lymphoblastoma (malignant lymphoma). *JAMA* 1926;86:1185–1189.
36. Cutler M. Lymphosarcoma: a clinical, pathologic and radiotherapeutic study, with a report of thirty cases. *Arch Surg* 1935;30:405–441.
37. Scott RB. Some clinical aspects of the reticuloses. *Br J Radiol* 1951;24:475–478.
38. Elkins HB. Treatment of malignant lymphoma and blood dyscrasias by conventional roentgen therapy. *AJR Am J Roentgenol* 1956;76:960–964.
39. Gall EA, Mallory TB. Malignant lymphoma: a clinico-pathologic survey of 618 cases. *Am J Pathol* 1942;18:381–429.

40. Cottenot P, Sluys F. La Téléroentgenthérapie totale. *J Radiol Électrol* 1935;19:347–359.

41. Finzi NS. The Roentgen treatment of lymphadenoma. *AJR Am J Roentgenol* 1938;39:261–262.

42. Levitt WM. Regional x-ray baths in the treatment of lymphadenoma. *Br J Radiol* 1938;11:183–188.

43. Teschendorf W. Über Bestrahlung des ganzen menschlichen Körpers bei Blutkrankheiten. *Strahlentherapie* 1927;26:720–728.

44. Heublein AC. A preliminary report on continuous irradiation of the entire body. *Radiology* 1932;18:1051–1062.

45. Medinger FG, Craver LF. Total body irradiation with review of cases. *AJR Am J Roentgenol* 1942;48:651–671.

46. Gall EA, Morrison HR, Scott AT. The follicular type of malignant lymphoma: a survey of 63 cases. *Ann Intern Med* 1941;14:2073–2090.

47. Paterson R, Tod M. The reticuloendothelial system. In: Paterson R, ed. *The treatment of malignant disease by radium and x-rays.* London: Edward Arnold, 1948:414–437.

48. Coutard H. Principles of x-ray therapy of malignant diseases. *Lancet* 1934;2:1–8.

49. Ewing J. Radiosensitivity. *Radiology* 1929;13:313–318.

50. Sugarbaker ED, Craver LF. Lymphosarcoma. *JAMA* 1940;115:112–117.

51. Meyer OO. Follicular lymphoblastoma. *Blood* 1948;3:921–933.

52. Craver LF. Treatment of chronic forms of malignant lymphomas and leukemias. *Med Clin North Am* 1949;33:527–540.

53. Cocchi U. Die Therapie des grossfollikulären Lymphoblastoms (Brill-Symmersche Erkrankung). *Schweiz Med Wschr* 1950;17:440–442.

54. Gilbert RJ. Lymphogranulome, lymphosarcome, réticulosarcome; radiothérapie. *Radiol Clin (Basel)* 1951;20:313–336.

55. Bauer R. Die Strahlentherapie der Retikulosen unter besonderer Berücksichtigung der Lymphogranulomatose. *Strahlentherapie* 1953;91:65–80.

56. Berven E. Le traitement radiologique des tumeurs malignes de la cavité buccale. *Acta Radiologica* 1932;13:213–231.

57. Decker FH, Leddy ET, Desjardins AU. Leukopenia and leukocytosis in lymphoblastoma: their reaction to Roentgen therapy. *AJR Am J Roentgenol* 1938;39:747–766.

58. Hynes JF, Frelick RW. Roentgen therapy of malignant lymphoma with special reference to segmental radiation therapy. Results 1935–1945. *AJR Am J Roentgenol* 1953;70:247–257.

59. Catlin D. Lymphosarcoma of head and neck. *AJR Am J Roentgenol* 1948;59:354–358.

60. Oeser H. *Strahlenbehandlung der Geschwülste. Technik, Ergebnisse und Probleme.* München: Urban & Schwarzenberg, 1954.

61. Hilton G, Sutton PM. Malignant lymphomas: classification, prognosis, and treatment. *Lancet* 1962:283–287.

62. Baumann-Schenker R. Über das Rundzellensarkom. Lymphosarkom, Retothelsarkom, Rundzellensarkom im engeren Sinne. Zürcher Erfahrungen aus den Jahren 1919–1934. *Strahlentherapie* 1934;51:201–236.

63. Stout AP. Is lymphosarcoma curable? *JAMA* 1942;118:968–970.

64. Stout AP. The results of treatment of lymphosarcoma. *N Y J Med* 1947;47:158–164.

65. Gardini GF. La radioterapia dei reticulo-sarcomi. *Radiol Clin (Basel)* 1952;21:219–222.

66. Scheel A, Myhre E. Malignant lymphomata: a review of the pathology, clinic features and therapy. *Acta Radiologica* 1953;40:63–80.

67. Goes M. Zur Klinik der Lympho- und Retothelsarkome. *Strahlentherapie* 1953;89:554–566.

68. Hancock PE. Malignant tumours of the reticulo-endothelial system. In: Raven RW, ed. *Cancer,* vol 4, part VIII. London: Butterworth, 1958:411–441.

69. Levitt WM. Cancer of the reticulo-endothelial system. In: Raven RW, ed. *Cancer,* vol 5. London: Butterworth, 1959:363–374.

70. Lawrence KB, Lenson N. Reticulum cell sarcoma. Report of a thirteen-year survival following one thousand roentgens of x-ray therapy. *JAMA* 1952;149:361–362.

71. Verhagen A. Strahlenbehandlung bei Rerothelsarkomen. *Strahlentherapie* 1948;77:605–612.

72. Ross JF, Ebaugh FG. Current trends in the management of the leukemias and the malignant lymphomas. *Med Clin North Am* 1951;35:1381–1401.

73. Rosenberg SA, Diamond HD, Jaslowitz B, et al. Lymphosarcoma: a review of 1269 cases. *Medicine (Baltimore)* 1961;40:31–84.

74. Easson EC, Russell MH. *The curability of cancer in various sites.* London: Pitman Medical Publishing Company, 1968.

75. Peters MV. The contribution of radiation therapy in the control of early lymphomas. *AJR Am J Roentgenol* 1963;90:956–967.

76. Fuller LM, Fletcher GH. The radiotherapeutic management of the lymphomatous diseases. *Am J Roentgenol Radium Ther Nucl Med* 1962;88:909–923.

77. Van der Werf-Messing B. Reticulum cell sarcoma and lymphosarcoma. A retrospective study of potential survival in loco-regional disease. *Eur J Cancer* 1968;4:549–557.

78. Hansen HS. Reticulum cell sarcoma treated by radiotherapy. Significance of clinical features upon the prognosis. *Acta Radiol Ther Phys Biol* 1969;8:439–458.

79. Cook JC, Krabbenhoft KL, Leucutia T. Lymphosarcoma, reticulum cell sarcoma and giant follicular lymphoma; long term results following radiation therapy. *Am J Roentgenol Radium Ther Nucl Med* 1960;84:656–665.

80. Fuks Z, Kaplan HS. Recurrence rates following radiation therapy of nodular and diffuse malignant lymphomas. *Radiology* 1973;108:675–684.

81. Fuks Z, Glatstein E, Kaplan HS. Patterns of presentation and relapse in the non-Hodgkin's lymphomata. *Br J Cancer* 1975;31:286–297.

82. Glatstein E, Fuks Z, Goffinet DR, et al. Non-Hodgkin's lymphomas of stage III extent. Is total lymphoid irradiation appropriate treatment? *Cancer* 1976;37:2806–2812.

83. Goffinet DR, Glatstein E, Fuks Z, et al. Abdominal irradiation in non-Hodgkin's lymphomas. *Cancer* 1976;37:2797–2805.

84. Hoppe RT, Burke JS, Glatstein E, et al. Non-Hodgkin's lymphoma: involvement of Waldeyer's ring. *Cancer* 1978;42:1096–1104.

85. Jacobs C, Hoppe RT. Non-Hodgkin's lymphomas of head and neck extranodal sites. *Int J Radiat Oncol Biol Phys* 1985;11:357–364.

86. Jones SE, Kaplan HS, Rosenberg SA. Non-Hodgkin's lymphomas. III. Preliminary results of radiotherapy and a proposal for new clinical trials. *Radiology* 1972;103:657–662.

87. Jones SE, Fuks Z, Kaplan HS, et al. Non-Hodgkin's lymphomas. V. Results of radiotherapy. *Cancer* 1973;32:682–691.

88. Mac-Manus MP, Hoppe RT. Is radiotherapy curative for stage I and II low-grade follicular lymphoma? Results of a long-term follow-up study of patients treated at Stanford University. *J Clin Oncol* 1996;14:1282–1290.

89. Mac-Manus MP, Hoppe RT. Overview of treatment of localized low-grade lymphomas. *Hematol Oncol Clin North Am* 1997;11:901–918.

90. Murtha AD, Knox SJ, Hoppe RT, et al. Long-term follow-up of patients with stage III follicular lymphoma treated with primary radiotherapy at Stanford University. *Int J Radiat Oncol Biol Phys* 2001;49:3–15.

91. Paryani SB, Hoppe RT, Cox RS, et al. Analysis of non-Hodgkin's lymphomas with nodular and favorable histologies, stages I and II. *Cancer* 1983;52:2300–2307.

92. Paryani S, Hoppe RT, Burke JS, et al. Extralymphatic involvement in diffuse non-Hodgkin's lymphoma. *J Clin Oncol* 1983;1:682–688.

93. Paryani SB, Hoppe RT, Cox RS, et al. The role of radiation therapy in the management of stage III follicular lymphomas. *J Clin Oncol* 1984;2:841–848.

94. Rosenberg SA, Dorfman RF, Kaplan HS. A summary of the results of a review of 405 patients with non-Hodgkin's lymphoma at Stanford University. *Br J Cancer* 1975;31:168–173.

95. Hellman S, Rosenthal DS, Moloney WC, et al. The treatment of non-Hodgkin's lymphoma. *Cancer* 1975;36:804–808.

96. Hellman S, Chaffey JT, Rosenthal DS, et al. The place of radiation therapy in the treatment of non-Hodgkin's lymphomas. *Cancer* 1977;39:843–851.

97. Mauch P, Leonard R, Skarin A, et al. Improved survival following combined radiation therapy and chemotherapy for unfavorable prognosis stage I–II non-Hodgkin's lymphomas. *J Clin Oncol* 1985;3:1301–1308.

98. Bush RS, Gospodarowicz M, Sturgeon J, et al. Radiation therapy of localized non-Hodgkin's lymphoma. *Cancer Treat Rep* 1977;61:1129–1136.

99. Bush RS, Gospodarowicz M. The place of radiation therapy in the management of patients with localized non-Hodgkin's lymphoma. In: Rosenberg SA, Kaplan HS, eds. *Malignant lymphomas. Etiology, immunology, pathology, treatment.* Orlando, FL: Academic Press, 1982:485–502.

100. Gospodarowicz MK, Bush RS, Brown TC, et al. Prognostic factors in nodular lymphomas: a multivariate analysis based on the Princess Margaret Hospital experience. *Int J Radiat Oncol Biol Phys* 1984;10:489–497.

101. Sutcliffe SB, Gospodarowicz MK, Bush RS, et al. Role of radiation therapy in localized non-Hodgkin's lymphoma. *Radiother Oncol* 1985;4:211–223.

102. Besa PC, McLaughlin PW, Cox JD, et al. Long term assessment of patterns of treatment failure and survival in patients with stage I or II follicular lymphoma. *Cancer* 1995;75:2361–2367.

103. Fuller LM, Banker FL, Butler JJ, et al. The natural history of non-Hodgkin's lymphomata stages I and II. *Br J Cancer* 1975;31:270–285.

104. Fuller LM, Gamble JF, Butler JJ, et al. Team approach to management of non-Hodgkin's lymphomas: past and present. *Cancer Treat Rep* 1977;61:1137–1148.

105. Kong JS, Fuller LM, Butler JJ, et al. Stages I and II non–Hodgkin's lymphomas of Waldeyer's ring and the neck. *Am J Clin Oncol* 1984; 7:629–639.

106. McLaughlin P, Fuller LM, Velasquez WS, et al. Stage I-II follicular lymphoma. Treatment results for 76 patients. *Cancer* 1986;58:1596–1602.

107. Seymour JF, McLaughlin P, Fuller LM, et al. High rate of prolonged remissions following combined modality therapy for patients with localized low-grade lymphoma. *Ann Oncol* 1996;7:157–163.

108. Wong DS, Fuller LM, Butler JJ, et al. Extranodal non-Hodgkin's lymphomas of the head and neck. *Am J Roentgenol Radium Ther Nucl Med* 1975;123:471–481.

109. Ha CS, Cabanillas F, Lee MS, et al. Serial determination of the bcl-2 gene in the bone marrow and peripheral blood after central lymphatic irradiation for stages I-III follicular lymphoma: a preliminary report. *Clin Cancer Res* 1997;3:215–219.

110. Ha CS, Tucker SL, Blanco AI, et al. Salvage central lymphatic irradiation in follicular lymphomas following failure of chemotherapy: a feasibility study. *Int J Radiat Oncol Biol Phys* 1999;45:1207–1212.

111. Ha CS, Tucker SL, Lee MS, et al. The significance of molecular response of follicular lymphoma to central lymphatic irradiation as measured by polymerase chain reaction for t(14;18)(q32;q21). *Int J Radiat Oncol Biol Phys* 2001;49:727–732.

112. Ha CS, Tucker SL, Blanco AI, et al. Hematologic recovery after central lymphatic irradiation for patients with stage I-III follicular lymphoma. *Cancer* 2001;92:1074–1079.

113. Cox JD. Total central lymphatic irradiation for stage III nodular malignant lymphoreticular tumors. *Int J Radiat Oncol Biol Phys* 1976;1:491–496.

114. Cox JD. Central lymphatic irradiation to low dose for advanced nodular lymphoreticular tumors (non-Hodgkin's lymphoma). *Radiology* 1978;126:767–772.

115. Cox JD, Komaki R, Kun LE, et al. Stage III nodular lymphoreticular tumors (non-Hodgkin's lymphoma): results of central lymphatic irradiation. *Cancer* 1981;47:2247–2252.

116. Jacobs JP, Murray KJ, Schultz CJ, et al. Central lymphatic irradiation for stage III nodular malignant lymphoma: long-term results. *J Clin Oncol* 1993;11:233–238.

117. Yahalom J. Radiation therapy for stage III follicular lymphoma—often ignored, but still effective. *Int J Radiat Oncol Biol Phys* 2001;49:1–2.

118. Cox JD, Koehl RH, Turner WM, et al. Irradiation in the local control of malignant lymphoreticular tumors (non-Hodgkin's malignant lymphoma). *Radiology* 1974;112:179–185.

119. Kun LE, Cox JD, Komaki R. Patterns of failure in treatment of stage I and II diffuse malignant lymphoid tumors. *Radiology* 1981;141:791–794.

120. Kamath SS, Marcus RB, Lynch JW, et al. The impact of radiotherapy dose and other treatment-related and clinical factors on in-field control in stage I and II non-Hodgkin's lymphoma. *Int J Radiat Oncol Biol Phys* 1999;44:563–568.

121. Nathu RM, Mendenhall NP, Almasri NM, et al. Non-Hodgkin's lymphoma of the head and neck: a 30-year experience at the University of Florida. *Head Neck* 1999;21:247–254.

122. De Los Santos JF, Mendenhall NP, Lynch JW. Is comprehensive lymphatic irradiation for low-grade non-Hodgkin's lymphoma curative therapy? Long-term experience at a single institution. *Int J Radiat Oncol Biol Phys* 1997;38:3–8.

123. Mendenhall NP, Million RR. Comprehensive lymphatic irradiation for stage II-III non-Hodgkin's lymphoma. *Am J Clin Oncol* 1989;12:190–194.

124. Chen MG, Prosnitz LR, Gonzalez-Serva A, et al. Results of radiotherapy in control of stage I and II non-Hodgkin's lymphoma. *Cancer* 1979;43:1245–1254.

125. Bitran JD, Kinzie J, Sweet DL, et al. Survival of patients with localized histiocytic lymphoma. *Cancer* 1977;39:342–346.

126. Hallahan DE, Farah R, Vokes EE, et al. The patterns of failure in patients with pathological stage I and II diffuse histiocytic lymphoma treated with radiation therapy alone. *Int J Radiat Oncol Biol Phys* 1989;17:767–771.

127. Vokes EE, Ultmann JE, Golomb HM, et al. Long-term survival of patients with localized diffuse histiocytic lymphoma. *J Clin Oncol* 1985;3:1309–1317.

128. Levitt SH, Bloomfield CD, Lee CK, et al. Extended field radiotherapy in non-Hodgkin's lymphoma. *Radiology* 1976;118:457–459.

129. Levitt SH. The treatment of non-Hodgkin's lymphoma with radiation therapy. *Prog Clin Biol Res* 1978;25:27–31.

130. Levitt SH, Bloomfield CD, Frizzera G, et al. Curative radiotherapy for localized diffuse histiocytic lymphoma. *Cancer Treat Rep* 1980;64:175–177.

131. Levitt SH, Lee CK, Bloomfield CD, et al. The role of radiation therapy in the treatment of early stage large cell lymphoma. *Hematol Oncol* 1985;3:33–37.

132. Lee CK, Levitt SH. Long-term follow-up of pathologic stage I large cell non-Hodgkin's lymphoma patients after primary radiotherapy. *Am J Clin Oncol* 1996;19:93–98.

133. Musshoff K, Schmidt-Vollmer H. Prognostic significance of primary site after radiotherapy in non-Hodgkin's lymphomata. *Br J Cancer* 1975;31:425–434.

134. Musshoff K, Leopold H. On the question of the tumoricidal dose in non-Hodgkin's lymphomas. In: Mathé G, Seligmann M, Tubiana M, eds. *Lymphoid neoplasias II. Clinical and therapeutic aspects.* Berlin: Springer-Verlag, 1978:203–206.

135. Brugere, Schlienger M, Gerard-Marchant R, et al. Non-Hodgkin's malignant lymphomata of upper digestive and respiratory tract: natural history and results of radiotherapy. *Br J Cancer* 1975;31[Suppl 2]:435–440.

136. Tubiana M, Pouillart P, Hayat M, et al. Resultats de la radiotherapie dans les stades I et II des lymphosarcomes et reticulosarcomes [Results of radiotherapy in stage I and II lymphosarcomas and reticulosarcomas]. *Bull Cancer* 1974;61:93–110.

137. Carde P, Burgers JM, van Glabbeke M, et al. Combined radiotherapy-chemotherapy for early stages non-Hodgkin's lymphoma: the 1975–1980 EORTC controlled lymphoma trial. *Radiother Oncol* 1984;2:301–312.

138. Tubiana M, Carde P, Burgers JM, et al. Non-Hodgkin's lymphoma. *Cancer Surv* 1985;4:377–398.

139. Tubiana M, Carde P, Burgers JM, et al. Prognostic factors in non-Hodgkin's lymphoma. *Int J Radiat Oncol Biol Phys* 1986;12:503–514.

140. Denham JW, Denham E, Dear KB, et al. The follicular non-Hodgkin's lymphomas—I. The possibility of cure. *Eur J Cancer* 1996;32A:470–479.

141. Vaughn Hudson B, Vaughn Hudson G, Maclennan KA, et al. Clinical stage 1 non-Hodgkin's lymphoma: long-term follow-up of patients treated by the British National Lymphoma Investigation with radiotherapy alone as initial therapy. *Br J Cancer* 1994;69:1088–1093.

142. Vaughn Hudson B. The BNLI: past and present. British National Lymphoma Investigation. *Clin Oncol (R Coll Radiol)* 1998;10:212–218.4

143. Kelsey SM, Newland AC, Vaughn Hudson G, et al. A British National Lymphoma Investigation randomised trial of single agent chlorambucil plus radiotherapy versus radiotherapy alone in low grade, localised non-Hodgkins lymphoma. *Med Oncol* 1994;11:19–25.

144. Lamb DS, Vaughn Hudson G, Easterling MJ, et al. Localised grade 2 non-Hodgkin's lymphoma: results of treatment with radiotherapy (BNLI Report No. 24). *Clin Radiol* 1984;35:253–260.

145. Phillips DL. Radiotherapy in the treatment of localised non-Hodgkin's lymphoma (Report no 16). *Clin Radiol* 1981;32:543–546.

146. Spry NA, Lamb DS, Vaughn Hudson G, et al. Localized grade I non-Hodgkin's lymphoma: results of treatment with radiotherapy alone in 88 patients. *Clin Oncol (R Coll Radiol)* 1989;1:33–38.

147. Horwich A, Peckham M. "Bad risk" non-Hodgkin's lymphomas. *Semin Hematol* 1983;20:35–56.

148. Horwich A, Catton CN, Quigley M, et al. The management of early-stage aggressive non-Hodgkin's lymphoma. *Hematol Oncol* 1988;6:291–298.

149. Peckham MJ. Radiation therapy of the non-Hodgkin's lymphomas. *Semin Hematol* 1974;11:41–58.

150. Peckham MJ, Guay JP, Hamlin IM, et al. Survival in localized nodal and extranodal non-Hodgkin's lymphomata. *Br J Cancer* 1975;31:413–424.

151. Pendlebury S, el Awadi M, Ashley S, et al. Radiotherapy results in early stage low grade nodal non-Hodgkin's lymphoma. *Radiother Oncol* 1995;36:167–171.
152. Timothy AR, Lister TA, Katz D, et al. Localized non-Hodgkin's lymphoma. *Eur J Cancer* 1980;16:799–807.
153. Richards MA, Gregory WM, Hall PA, et al. Management of localized non-Hodgkin's lymphoma: the experience at St. Bartholomew's Hospital 1972–1985. *Hematol Oncol* 1989;7:1–18.
154. Hagberg H, Glimelius B, Sundstrom C. Radiation therapy of non-Hodgkin's lymphoma stages I and II. *Acta Radiol Oncol* 1982;21:145–150.
155. Osterman B, Cavallin-Stahl E, Hagberg H, et al. High-grade non-Hodgkin's lymphoma stage I. A retrospective study of treatment, outcome and prognostic factors in 213 patients. *Acta Oncol* 1996;35:171–177.
156. Ossenkoppele GJ, Mol JJ, Snow GB, et al. Radiotherapy versus radiotherapy plus chemotherapy in stages I and II non-Hodgkin's lymphoma of the upper digestive and respiratory tract. *Cancer* 1987;60:1505–1509.
157. Taylor RE, Allan SG, McIntyre MA, et al. Influence of therapy on local control and survival in stage I and II intermediate and high grade non-Hodgkin's lymphoma. *Eur J Cancer Clin Oncol* 1988;24:1771–1777.
158. Toonkel LM, Fuller LM, Gamble JF, et al. Laparotomy staged I and II non-Hodgkin's lymphomas: preliminary results of radiotherapy and adjunctive chemotherapy. *Cancer* 1980;45:249–260.
159. Gomez GA, Barcos M, Krishnamsetty RM, et al. Treatment of early—stages I and II—nodular, poorly differentiated lymphocytic lymphoma. *Am J Clin Oncol* 1986;9:40–44.
160. Kaminski MS, Coleman CN, Colby TV, et al. Factors predicting survival in adults with stage I and II large-cell lymphoma treated with primary radiation therapy. *Ann Intern Med* 1986;104:747–756.
161. Landberg TG, Hakansson LG, Moller TR, et al. CVP-remission-maintenance in stage I or II non-Hodgkin's lymphomas: preliminary results of a randomized study. *Cancer* 1979;44:831–838.
162. Monfardini S, Banfi A, Bonadonna G, et al. Improved five year survival after combined radiotherapy-chemotherapy for stage I–II non-Hodgkin's lymphoma. *Int J Radiat Oncol Biol Phys* 1980;6:125–134.
163. Nissen NI, Ersboll J, Hansen HS, et al. A randomized study of radiotherapy versus radiotherapy plus chemotherapy in stage I–II non-Hodgkin's lymphomas. *Cancer* 1983;52:1–7.
164. Panahon A, Kaufman JA, Grasso JA, et al. A randomized study of radiation therapy (RT) vs. RT and chemotherapy (CT) in stage IA–IIIB non-Hodgkin's lymphoma. *Proc Am Assoc Cancer Res Am Soc Clin Oncol* 1977;18:321.
165. Somers R, Burgers JM, Qasim M, et al. EORTC trial non-Hodgkin lymphomas. *Eur J Cancer Clin Oncol* 1987;23:283–293.
166. Avilés A, Delgado S, Ruiz H, et al. Treatment of non-Hodgkin's lymphoma of Waldeyer's ring: radiotherapy versus chemotherapy versus combined therapy. *Eur J Cancer B Oral Oncol* 1996;32B:19–23.
167. Yahalom J, Varsos G, Fuks Z, et al. Adjuvant cyclophosphamide, doxorubicin, vincristine, and prednisone chemotherapy after radiation therapy in stage I low-grade and intermediate-grade non-Hodgkin's lymphoma. Results of a prospective randomized study. *Cancer* 1993;71:2342–2350.
168. Johnson RE. Total body irradiation (TBI) as primary therapy for advanced lymphosarcoma. *Cancer* 1975;35:242–246.
169. Johnson RE. Management of generalized malignant lymphomata with "systemic" radiotherapy. *Br J Cancer* 1975;31:450–456.
170. Johnson RE, Canellos GP, Young RC, et al. Chemotherapy (cyclophosphamide, vincristine, and prednisone) versus radiotherapy (total body irradiation) for stage III–IV poorly differentiated lymphocytic lymphoma. *Cancer Treat Rep* 1978;62:321–325.
171. Carabell SC, Chaffey JT, Rosenthal DS, et al. Results of total body irradiation in the treatment of advanced non-Hodgkin's lymphomas. *Cancer* 1979;43:994–1000.
172. Chaffey JT, Rosenthal DS, Pinkus G, et al. Advanced lymphosarcoma treated by total body irradiation. *Br J Cancer* 1975;31[Suppl 2]:441–449.
173. Chaffey JT, Rosenthal DS, Moloney WC, et al. Total body irradiation as treatment for lymphosarcoma. *Int J Radiat Oncol Biol Phys* 1976;1:399–405.
174. Chaffey JT, Hellman S, Rosenthal DS, et al. Total-body irradiation in the treatment of lymphocytic lymphoma. *Cancer Treat Rep* 1977;61:1149–1152.
175. Hoppe RT, Kushlan P, Kaplan HS, et al. The treatment of advanced stage favorable histology non-Hodgkin's lymphoma: a preliminary report of a randomized trial comparing single agent chemotherapy, combination chemotherapy, and whole body irradiation. *Blood* 1981;58:592–598.
176. Mendenhall NP, Noyes WD, Million RR. Total body irradiation for stage II–IV non-Hodgkin's lymphoma: ten-year follow-up. *J Clin Oncol* 1989;7:67–74.
177. Thar TL, Million RR. Total body irradiation in non-Hodgkin's lymphoma. *Cancer* 1978;42:926–931.
178. British National Lymphoma Investigation Report. A prospective comparison of combination chemotherapy with total body irradiation in the treatment of advanced non-Hodgkin's lymphoma. *Clin Oncol* 1981;7:193–200.
179. Pettingale KW. The management of generalised Grade 2 non-Hodgkin's lymphomas (Report No 18). *Clin Radiol* 1981;32:553–556.
180. Dobbs HJ, Barrett A, Rostom AY, et al. Total-body irradiation in advanced non-Hodgkin's lymphoma. *Br J Radiol* 1981;54:878–881.
181. De Neve WJ, Lybeert ML, Meerwaldt JH. Low-dose total body irradiation in non-Hodgkin lymphoma: short- and long-term toxicity and prognostic factors. *Am J Clin Oncol* 1990;13:280–284.
182. Lybeert ML, Meerwaldt JH, Deneve W. Long-term results of low dose total body irradiation for advanced non-Hodgkin lymphoma. *Int J Radiat Oncol Biol Phys* 1987;13:1167–1172.
183. Qasim MM. Total body irradiation as a primary therapy in non-Hodgkin lymphoma. *Clin Radiol* 1979;30:287–289.
184. Brasch A, Lange F. Aussichten und Möglichkeiten einer Therapie mit schnellen Kathodenstrahlen. *Strahlentherapie* 1934;51:119–128.
185. Coolidge WD, Moore CN. Some experiments with high voltage cathode rays outside of the generating tube. *J Franklin Inst* 1926;202:722–735.
186. Trump JG, van de Graaff RJ, Cloud RW. Cathode rays for radiation therapy. *Am J Roentgenol Radium Ther Nucl Med* 1940;43:728–734.
187. Trump JG, Wright KA, Evans WW, et al. High energy electrons for the treatment of extensive superficial malignant lesions. *AJR Am J Roentgenol* 1953;69:623–629.
188. Cox RS, Heck RJ, Fessenden P, et al. Development of total-skin electron therapy at two energies. *Int J Radiat Oncol Biol Phys* 1990;18:659–669.
189. Karzmark CJ, Loevinger R, Steele RE, et al. A technique for large-field, superficial electron therapy. *Radiology* 1960;74:633–644.
190. Fuks Z, Bagshaw MA. Total-skin electron treatment of mycosis fungoides. *Radiology* 1971;100:145–150.
191. Fuks Z, Bagshaw MA, Farber EM. New concepts in the management of mycosis fungoides. *Br J Dermatol* 1974;90:355–356.
192. Fuks Z, Hoppe T, Bagshaw MA. The role of total skin irradiation with electrons in the management of mycosis fungoides. *Bull Cancer* 1977;64:291–304.
193. Hoppe RT, Fuks Z, Bagshaw MA. The rationale for curative radiotherapy in mycosis fungoides. *Int J Radiat Oncol Biol Phys* 1977;2:843–851.
194. Hoppe RT, Cox RS, Fuks Z, et al. Electron-beam therapy for mycosis fungoides: the Stanford University experience. *Cancer Treat Rep* 1979;63:691–700.
195. Hoppe RT, Fuks Z, Bagshaw MA. Radiation therapy in the management of cutaneous T-cell lymphomas. *Cancer Treat Rep* 1979;63:625–632.
196. Hoppe RT, Wood GS, Abel EA. Mycosis fungoides and the Sézary syndrome: pathology, staging, and treatment. *Curr Probl Cancer* 1990;14:295–361.
197. Freeman CR, Suissa S, Shenouda G, et al. Clinical experience with a single field rotational total skin electron irradiation technique for cutaneous T-cell lymphoma. *Radiother Oncol* 1992;24:155–162.
198. Jones GW, Tadros A, Hodson DI, et al. Prognosis with newly diagnosed mycosis fungoides after total skin electron radiation of 30 or 35 GY. *Int J Radiat Oncol Biol Phys* 1994;28:839–845.
199. Kirova YM, Piedbois Y, Haddad E, et al. Radiotherapy in the management of mycosis fungoides: indications, results, prognosis. Twenty years experience. *Radiother Oncol* 1999;51:147–151.
200. Lo TC, Salzman FA, Moschella SL, et al. Whole body surface electron irradiation in the treatment of mycosis fungoides. An evaluation of 200 patients. *Radiology* 1979;130:453–457.
201. van Vloten WA, de Vroome H, Noordijk EM. Total skin electron beam irradiation for cutaneous T-cell lymphoma (mycosis fungoides). *Br J Dermatol* 1985;112:697–702.
202. Becker M, Hoppe RT, Knox SJ. Multiple courses of high-dose total

skin electron beam therapy in the management of mycosis fungoides. *Int J Radiat Oncol Biol Phys* 1995;32:1445–1449.

203. Harris NL, Jaffe ES, Diebold J, et al. World Health Organization classification of neoplastic diseases of the hematopoietic and lymphoid tissues: report of the Clinical Advisory Committee meeting—Airlie House, Virginia, November 1997. *J Clin Oncol* 1999;17:3835–3849.

204. Jaffe ES, Harris NL, Stein H, et al. *World Health Organization classification of tumours. Pathology and genetics of tumours of haematopoietic and lymphoid tissues.* Lyon, France: IARC Press, 2001.

205. Intensity-modulated radiotherapy: current status and issues of interest. *Int J Radiat Oncol Biol Phys* 2001;51:880–914.

SECTION II

Diagnosis, Staging, and Initial Evaluation

CHAPTER 4

Revised European-American and World Health Organization Classifications of Non-Hodgkin's Lymphomas

Nancy Lee Harris

LYMPHOMA CLASSIFICATION: ISSUES AND CONTROVERSIES

Classification is the language of medicine. Diseases need to be defined and named before they can be diagnosed and treated. Classification has two aspects: disease definition (class discovery) and disease diagnosis (class prediction). Disease definition, or class discovery, is the process of determining what diseases exist and how to define them: when applied to a large group of diseases, this can be called the *development of a classification*. Disease diagnosis, or class prediction, is the act of deciding which category of disease a given patient has. A wide variety of parameters may be combined to define a given disease; a smaller number of parameters may be required to assign a given specimen or patient to a particular category.

Controversy in lymphoma classification dates back to the first attempts to organize the variety of described neoplasms into a comprehensive scheme (see Chapter 1) (1–15). This controversy stems from several factors: among them, the large variety of tumors that arise from cells of the lymphoid system, the relative insensitivity of the techniques of routine histopathology that are useful in other organ systems in the recognition of defining features of lymphoid cells and their tumors, and the assumption of many authorities that there had to be a single guiding principle—a gold standard—for lymphoma classification. Many classifications were based purely on morphology [Gall and Mallory, Jackson and Parker, Rappaport, World Health Organization (WHO)], others used primarily clinical features [American Registry of Pathology, Working Formulation (WF)], and still others were based primarily on cell lineage and differentiation, in the belief that each neoplasm corresponded to a recognizable normal cell or differentiation stage (Robb-Smith, Kiel, Lukes-Collins).

In the 1980s and early 1990s, the WF was the most commonly used classification worldwide. Despite the fact that it was based largely on clinical survival data, however, clinicians typically modified its categories in practice. Reflecting the fact that the prognostic groups that were defined by the WF did not accurately predict the behavior of the tumors, many clinical trials of so called *low-grade* lymphoma included diffuse, small cleaved cell lymphoma and follicular large-cell lymphoma, although these are considered intermediate grade in the WF (16). Trials of aggressive lymphoma usually included some but not all intermediate-grade lymphomas (diffuse mixed and large cell but not diffuse small cleaved and follicular large cell) and some but not all high-grade lymphomas (immunoblastic and sometimes small noncleaved cell but not usually lymphoblastic) (17,18). Some entities, which were already recognized to have distinctive features, such as Burkitt's lymphoma, lymphoblastic lymphoma, hairy-cell leukemia, and B-cell chronic lymphocytic leukemia, were typically treated according to disease-specific protocols.

Because of the demographics of non-Hodgkin's lymphoma in the United States, clinical trials of treatment of *WF low-grade lymphoma* were essentially trials of follicular lymphoma, which were contaminated by a small number of cases of mantle cell, small lymphocytic, and marginal zone lymphoma of mucosa-associated lymphoid tissue (MALT); trials of *WF intermediate- and high-grade lymphoma* were trials of diffuse large B-cell lymphoma, which were contaminated by small numbers of peripheral T-cell lymphomas and other rare diseases. Lumping diverse entities into these broad prognostic groups distorted the data on the common entities and obscured the distinctive features of rare entities.

An additional result of the adoption of the WF, with its letter designations of categories and its clinical grades, was a growing disregard among oncologists for the pathologic classification of lymphomas. Thus, instead of *follicular lymphoma*, the terms "WF B-D" were used, and rather than asking for a histologic diagnosis, many practicing oncologists simply wanted to know whether a tumor was low, intermediate, or high grade in the

WF. The crutch of the WF prognostic groups gave oncologists a sense of security, but it delayed the recognition and development of new therapies for diseases, such as extranodal low-grade MALT B-cell lymphoma, mantle cell lymphoma, and peripheral T-cell lymphomas.

Although the WF represented a consensus among the participating pathologists, Robert Lukes and Karl Lennert published critical commentaries along with its initial publication (14), and many American and European pathologists continued to use the Lukes-Collins or Kiel classifications, respectively. Thus, the lack of consensus on lymphoma classification and terminology persisted, with the WF being the standard in the United States and several other countries, and the Kiel Classification being the standard in many European countries. This situation caused continued problems for pathologists and clinicians and created difficulty in the interpretation of published studies. In addition, in the 1980s and 1990s, many new disease entities were described that were not included in either classification, leading to confusion among pathologists and oncologists about which were "real" diseases that they should recognize in daily practice. Finally, the introduction of the new techniques of immunophenotyping and molecular genetic analysis led to confusion about what, if anything, should be the modern gold standard for defining disease entities.

In the late 1980s and early 1990s, most experienced hematopathologists began to modify both the WF and the Kiel Classification to address these issues. This led to even more confusion, because not only were there differences between American and European classifications, but each institution also developed idiosyncratic internal classification schemes. In the United States, consideration was given to updating the WF, and, in Europe, the Kiel Classification had been updated in 1987; there were discussions about the adoption of one as the new international standard. However, both classifications had limitations that made this impractical. As stated in Chapter 1, the WF was not intended to be a free-standing classification, and its categories were intentionally broad and imprecise. In addition, the clinical data that were thought to give it validity were based on the original study patients; thus, a similar large-scale clinical study would theoretically be required to provide an updated version with similar clinical relevance. The Kiel Classification was intended for use on primary nodal lymphomas only; thus, the issue of MALT extranodal lymphomas and their relationship to other lymphomas was not clarified, and other primary extranodal lymphomas other than mycosis fungoides were not addressed. In addition, the scheme for classifying peripheral T-cell lymphomas was based on morphologic criteria that were difficult to reproduce, and the histologic grades did not appear to correlate well with clinical behavior (19,20).

REVISED EUROPEAN-AMERICAN LYMPHOMA CLASSIFICATION OF LYMPHOID NEOPLASMS

The International Lymphoma Study Group (ILSG) was formed in 1991 by Harald Stein of the Free University of Berlin and Peter Isaacson of University College Hospital, London to promote better communication between American and European hematopathologists. This informal group included 19 hematopathologists from the United States, Europe, and Asia and began meeting annually to review interesting cases, to present unpublished research data, and to discuss issues in classification and diagnosis of lymphomas. It soon became clear that there was general agreement among the members on diseases that they recognized in their daily practice with a combination of morphology, immunophenotyping, and genetic techniques and that appeared to be distinct clinical entities. It was also clear, however, that there was no uniform approach to the definition and diagnosis of these entities at different centers around the world and that a consensus was needed on the definitions and criteria for diagnosis, as well as nomenclature for these diseases.

In the first 2 years of its existence, the group published consensus papers on definitions, diagnostic criteria, and nomenclature for two diseases that were controversial or poorly understood: mantle cell lymphoma and nodular lymphocyte-predominant Hodgkin's lymphoma (21,22). By the time of their third meeting, the group was ready to approach the idea of a new lymphoma classification. Given the difficulty of defining an overarching principle for the classification of all lymphoid neoplasms, the group agreed that the best approach for the present was to try to reach a consensus on a list of distinct disease entities, including defining criteria, diagnostic criteria, and nomenclature. The diseases could then be grouped according to a variety of principles, depending on the needs of the user, but each disease could stand alone as an entity to be understood, diagnosed, and treated using currently available methods. As one of the group members, David Mason, said: the classification should reflect what pathologists do, not what they should do (22).

The ILSG approach to lymphoma classification was novel. In this approach, *all* available information—morphology, immunophenotype, genetic features, and clinical features—is used to define a disease entity. The relative importance of each of these features varies among diseases, and there is no one gold standard. Morphology is always important, and some diseases are primarily defined by morphology—follicular lymphoma, angioimmunoblastic T-cell lymphoma, nodular sclerosis Hodgkin's disease—with immunophenotype as backup in difficult cases. Some diseases have a virtually specific immunophenotype, such as mantle cell lymphoma, small lymphocytic lymphoma, and anaplastic large-cell lymphoma, such that one would hesitate to make the diagnosis in the absence of the immunophenotype. In a few lymphomas, a specific genetic abnormality is an important defining criterion, such as t(11;14) in mantle cell lymphoma, t(8;14) in Burkitt's lymphoma, and t(14;18) in follicular lymphoma, whereas others lack specific genetic abnormalities, such as MALT lymphoma and diffuse large B-cell lymphoma. Still others require a knowledge of clinical features as well, such as nodal versus extranodal presentation in marginal zone lymphoma and peripheral T-cell lymphomas, and mediastinal location in

TABLE 4.1. *The Revised European-American Lymphoma Classification (1994)*

B-cell neoplasms	T-cell and putative natural killer–cell neoplasms
Precursor B-cell neoplasm	Precursor T-cell neoplasm
Precursor B-lymphoblastic leukemia and lymphoma	Precursor T-lymphoblastic lymphoma and leukemia
Peripheral B-cell neoplasms	Peripheral T-cell and natural killer–cell neoplasms
B-cell chronic lymphocytic leukemia, prolymphocytic leukemia, and small lymphocytic lymphoma	T-cell chronic lymphocytic leukemia and prolymphocytic leukemia
Lymphoplasmacytoid lymphoma or immunocytoma	Large granular lymphocyte leukemia
Mantle cell lymphoma	T-cell type
Follicle center lymphoma, follicular	Natural killer–cell type
Provisional cytologic grades: 1 (small cell), 2 (mixed small and large cell), 3 (large cell)	Mycosis fungoides or Sézary syndrome
Provisional subtype: diffuse, predominantly small cell type	Peripheral T-cell lymphomas, unspecified[a]
Marginal zone B-cell lymphoma, extranodal mucosa-associated–lymphoid tissue (MALT) type (± monocytoid B cells)	Provisional cytologic categories: medium-sized cell, mixed medium and large cell, large cell, lymphoepithelioid cell
Provisional subtype: nodal marginal zone lymphoma (± monocytoid B cells)	Provisional subtype: hepatosplenic gamma-delta T-cell lymphoma
Provisional entity: splenic marginal zone lymphoma (± villous lymphocytes)	Provisional subtype: subcutaneous panniculitic T-cell lymphoma
Hairy-cell leukemia	Angioimmunoblastic T-cell lymphoma (angioimmunoblastic lymphadenopathy with dysproteinemia)
Plasmacytoma or plasma cell myeloma	Angiocentric lymphoma
Diffuse large B-cell lymphoma[a]	Intestinal T-cell lymphoma (± enteropathy-associated)
Subtype: primary mediastinal (thymic) B-cell lymphoma	Adult T-cell lymphoma or leukemia (ATLL)
Burkitt's lymphoma	Anaplastic large-cell lymphoma (ALCL), CD30⁺, T- and null-cell types
Provisional entity: high-grade B-cell lymphoma, Burkitt-like[a]	Provisional entity: anaplastic large-cell lymphoma, Hodgkin's-like

[a]These categories are thought likely to include more than one disease entity.
Reproduced with permission from Harris NL, Jaffe ES, Stein H, et al. A revised European-American classification of lymphoid neoplasms: a proposal from the International Lymphoma Study Group. *Blood* 1994;84:1361–1392.

mediastinal large B-cell lymphoma. The inclusion of clinical criteria was one of the most novel aspects of the ILSG approach. The emphasis on defining "real" disease entities, rather than focusing on subtleties of morphology or immunophenotype or primarily on patient survival, represented a new paradigm in lymphoma classification.

In 1993, the ILSG undertook to develop a consensus on a list of diseases that its members recognized in daily practice, by using a combination of available morphologic, immunologic, and genetic information, and that appeared to be distinct clinical entities. This consensus approach represented the second major departure from previous classifications, most of which represented the work of one or a few individuals. The ILSG recognized that the complexity of the field in the 1990s made it impossible for a single person or small group to be completely authoritative and that broad agreement was necessary, if the result were to be used by multiple pathologists, even if it required compromise. After a 3-day meeting in Berlin, a list of diseases on which a consensus had been reached was developed. The group held a joint meeting with an international group of hematologic oncologists at the National Cancer Institute in Bethesda, Maryland, in the spring of 1994, to get input from clinicians on the proposal, and a number of changes were made at their suggestions. The ILSG consensus list of well-defined "real" diseases was published in 1994 (Table 4.1) (23). Because it represented a revision of current or prior European and American lymphoma classifications (Table 4.2), it was called the *Revised European-American Lymphoma (REAL) Classification.* Although its initial publication incited considerable controversy, experience over the intervening years has shown that it can be used by most pathologists and that the entities it describes have distinctive clinical features, thus making it a useful and practical classification, despite its apparent complexity (24–27).

WORLD HEALTH ORGANIZATION CLASSIFICATION OF NEOPLASMS OF HEMATOPOIETIC AND LYMPHOID TISSUES

In 1993, the WHO decided to update the "blue book" on neoplasms of hematopoietic and lymphoid tissues, which had last been published in 1975 and which was virtually never used clin-

TABLE 4.2. *Comparison of the original Revised European-American Lymphoma Classification with the Kiel Classification and the Working Formulation*[a]

Kiel Classification	Revised European-American Lymphoma Classification	Working Formulation
B-lymphoblastic	Precursor B-lymphoblastic lymphoma or leukemia	Lymphoblastic
B-Lymphocytic, CLL	B-cell chronic lymphocytic leukemia, prolymphocytic leukemia, small lymphocytic lymphoma	**Small lymphocytic, consistent with CLL**
B-Lymphocytic, prolymphocytic leukemia		Small lymphocytic, plasmacytoid
Lymphoplasmacytoid immunocytoma		
Lymphoplasmacytic immunocytoma	Lymphoplasmacytoid lymphoma	**Small lymphocytic, plasmacytoid**
		Diffuse, mixed small and large cell
Centrocytic	Mantle cell lymphoma	Small lymphocytic
Centroblastic, centrocytoid subtype		**Diffuse, small cleaved cell**
		Follicular, small cleaved cell
		Diffuse, mixed small and large cell
		Diffuse, large cleaved cell
Centroblastic-centrocytic, follicular	Follicle center lymphoma, follicular	
	Grade 1	**Follicular, predominantly small cleaved cell**
	Grade 2	**Follicular, mixed small and large cell**
	Grade 3	**Follicular, predominantly large cell**
Centroblastic, follicular	Follicular center lymphoma, diffuse, small cell (provisional)	**Diffuse, small cleaved cell**
Centroblastic-centrocytic, diffuse		Diffuse, mixed small and large cell
—	Extranodal marginal zone B-cell lymphoma [low-grade B-cell lymphoma of mucosa-associated–lymphoid tissue (MALT) type]	**Small lymphocytic**
		Diffuse, small cleaved cell
		Diffuse, mixed small and large cell
Monocytoid, including marginal zone Immunocytoma	Nodal marginal zone B-cell lymphoma (provisional)	**Small lymphocytic**
		Diffuse, small cleaved cell
		Diffuse, mixed small and large cell
		Unclassifiable
—	Splenic marginal zone B-cell lymphoma (provisional)	**Small lymphocytic**
		Diffuse small cleaved cell
Hairy-cell leukemia	Hairy-cell leukemia	—
Plasmacytic	Plasmacytoma and myeloma	Extramedullary plasmacytoma
Centroblastic (monomorphic, polymorphic, and multilobated subtypes)	Diffuse large B-cell lymphoma	**Diffuse, large cell**
		Large cell immunoblastic
		Diffuse, mixed small and large cell
B-Immunoblastic		
B–Large cell anaplastic (Ki–1+)		
—	Primary mediastinal large B-cell lymphoma	**Diffuse, large cell**
		Large cell immunoblastic
Burkitt's lymphoma	Burkitt's lymphoma	**Small noncleaved cell, Burkitt's**
? Some cases of centroblastic and immunoblastic	High-grade B-cell lymphoma, Burkitt-like (provisional)	**Small noncleaved cell, non-Burkitt's**
		Diffuse, large cell
		Large cell immunoblastic
T-lymphoblastic	Precursor T-lymphoblastic lymphoma or leukemia	Lymphoblastic
T-lymphocytic, CLL type T-lymphocytic, prolymphocytic leukemia	T-cell chronic lymphocytic leukemia or prolymphocytic leukemia	**Small lymphocytic**
		Diffuse small cleaved cell
T-lymphocytic, CLL type	Large granular lymphocytic leukemia	**Small lymphocytic**
—	T-cell type	Diffuse, small cleaved cell
	Natural killer–cell type	

continued

TABLE 4.2. *Continued*

Kiel Classification	Revised European-American Lymphoma Classification	Working Formulation
Small cell cerebriform (mycosis fungoides, Sézary syndrome)	Mycosis fungoides or Sézary syndrome	Mycosis fungoides
T-zone	Peripheral T-cell lymphomas, unspecified (including provisional subtype: subcutaneous panniculitic T-cell lymphoma)	Diffuse, small cleaved cell
Lymphoepithelioid		**Diffuse, mixed small and large cell**
Pleomorphic, small T-cell		Diffuse, large cell
Pleomorphic, medium-sized and large T cell		**Large cell immunoblastic**
T-immunoblastic		
—	Hepatosplenic gamma-delta T-cell lymphoma (provisional)	—
Angioimmunoblastic (angioimmunoblastic lymphadenopathy with dysproteinemia, lymphogranulomatosis X)	Angioimmunoblastic T-cell lymphoma	**Diffuse, mixed small and large cell** Diffuse, large cell
		Large cell immunoblastic
—b	Angiocentric lymphoma	Diffuse, small cleaved cell
		Diffuse, mixed small and large cell
		Diffuse, large cell
		Large cell immunoblastic
—	Intestinal T-cell lymphoma	Diffuse, small cleaved cell
		Diffuse, mixed small and large cell
		Diffuse, large cell
		Large cell immunoblastic
Pleomorphic small T-cell	Adult T-cell lymphoma/leukemia, **human T-cell leukemia virus type I+**	Diffuse, small cleaved cell
		Diffuse, mixed small and large cell
Pleomorphic medium-sized and large T-cell		Diffuse, large cell
		Large cell immunoblastic
T-large cell anaplastic (Ki–1+)	Anaplastic large-cell lymphoma, T- and null-cell types	**Large cell immunoblastic**

CLL, chronic lymphocytic leukemia.

aEntries in bold comprise the majority of the cases. The REAL classification is shown in the center. Synonyms in the Kiel Classification and Working Formulation are shown on either side.

bNot listed in classification, but discussed as rare or ambiguous type.

ically (11). This was initially undertaken as a project of the Society for Hematopathology, which is based largely in the United States, and then reconfigured as a joint project with the European Association of Hematopathologists. The project, which began in earnest in 1995, was an opportunity to update and obtain a broader consensus on the REAL Classification for lymphomas and to apply the principles of the REAL Classification to the classification of myeloid and histiocytic neoplasms (28,29). The WHO project included more than 50 pathologists from around the world. In addition, building on the experience of the ILSG and the REAL Classification, the Steering Committee of the WHO project formed a Clinical Advisory Committee of more than 30 international expert hematologists and oncologists to advise the pathologists on clinical issues that were related to the classification (30). The final classification was published in 2001 (Table 4.3) (31). Proponents of all existing classifications—WF, Kiel, REAL, and French-American-British—agreed that the final WHO consensus would replace existing classifications. Thus, it represents the first true international consensus on the classification of hematologic malignancies.

Principles of the Revised European-American Lymphoma and World Health Organization Classification of Lymphoid Neoplasms

The REAL-WHO classification is a list of distinct disease entities, which are defined by a combination of morphology, immunophenotype, and genetic features and which have distinct clinical features. The classification includes all lymphoid neoplasms: Hodgkin's disease, non-Hodgkin's lymphomas, lym-

TABLE 4.3. *Updated Revised European-American–World Health Organization Classification of lymphoid neoplasms*

B-cell neoplasms	T- and NK-cell neoplasms
Precursor B-cell neoplasm	Precursor T-cell neoplasm
Precursor B-lymphoblastic leukemia and lymphoma (precursor B-cell acute lymphoblastic leukemia)	Precursor T-lymphoblastic lymphoma and leukemia (precursor T-cell acute lymphoblastic leukemia)
Mature (peripheral) B-cell neoplasms	Mature (peripheral) T-cell and NK-cell neoplasms
Chronic lymphocytic leukemia and B-cell small lymphocytic lymphoma	T-cell prolymphocytic leukemia
B-cell prolymphocytic leukemia	T-cell granular lymphocytic leukemia
Lymphoplasmacytic lymphoma	Aggressive NK-cell leukemia
Splenic marginal zone B-cell lymphoma (± villous lymphocytes)	Adult T-cell lymphoma or leukemia (human T-cell leukemia virus type I+)
Hairy-cell leukemia	Extranodal NK- and T-cell lymphoma, nasal type
Plasma cell myeloma and plasmacytoma	Enteropathy-type T-cell lymphoma
Extranodal marginal zone B-cell lymphoma of mucosa-associated–lymphoid tissue (MALT) type	Hepatosplenic T-cell lymphoma
Nodal marginal zone B-cell lymphoma (± monocytoid B cells)	Subcutaneous panniculitis-like T-cell lymphoma
Follicular lymphoma	Mycosis fungoides and Sézary syndrome
Mantle cell lymphoma	Primary cutaneous anaplastic large-cell lymphoma
Diffuse large B-cell lymphoma	Peripheral T-cell lymphoma, not otherwise specified
Mediastinal large B-cell lymphoma	Angioimmunoblastic T-cell lymphoma
Primary effusion lymphoma	Primary systemic anaplastic large-cell lymphoma
Intravascular large B-cell lymphoma	T-cell neoplasm of uncertain lineage and differentiation stage
Burkitt's lymphoma/ Burkitt's cell leukemia	Blastic NK-cell lymphoma
B-cell neoplasms of uncertain malignant potential	T-cell neoplasm of uncertain malignant potential
Lymphomatoid granulomatosis	CD30+ cutaneous lymphoproliferative disorder (lymphomatoid papulosis)
Posttransplant lymphoproliferative disease, polymorphous	

NK, natural killer.

phoid leukemias, and plasma cell neoplasms. Both lymphomas and lymphoid leukemias are included because solid and circulating phases are present in many lymphoid neoplasms, and distinction between them is artificial. Thus, B-cell chronic lymphocytic lymphoma and B-cell small lymphocytic lymphoma are simply different manifestations of the same neoplasm, as are lymphoblastic lymphomas and acute lymphoblastic leukemias. In addition, Hodgkin's disease and plasma cell myeloma are now recognized as lymphoid neoplasms of B lineage and therefore belong in a compilation of lymphoid neoplasms. Immunodeficiency-associated lymphomas are classified according to the basic lymphoma classification; a separate classification of the posttransplant lymphoid proliferations that do not fulfill criteria for lymphoma is also given (Table 4.4). The classification also includes a category of lymphoid proliferations of "uncertain malignant potential"—clonal proliferations of T cells or B cells that may be self limited, such as lymphomatoid papulosis and polymorphous posttransplant lymphoproliferative disorders. Many of the neoplasms that are recognized in the classification have morphologic variants or clinical subtypes, or both, which are shown in Tables 4.5 through 4.7.

In the REAL and WHO classifications, morphology, immunophenotype, and genetic and clinical features are understood to be surrogates or approximations for whatever the true, defining abnormality of a disease may be. Because we do not understand the basic pathophysiology of most malignancies, continued research and experience is needed to continue to improve the definition of these diseases. Furthermore, the important *defining* criteria may vary, depending on what preventive or therapeutic measures exist. In current clinical practice, morphology remains the first and most basic approach for classification of lymphoid neoplasms and is sufficient for diagnosis and classification in many typical cases of lymphoma. Immunophenotyping and, particularly, molecular genetic studies are not needed in all cases; however, they are an important part of the definition of a disease entity, are useful in the diagnosis of difficult cases, and improve interobserver reproducibility. It is the availability of these more objective methods that make a consensus on lymphoma classification possible now, whereas it was impossible in the 1970s, when classification was based purely on subjective morphologic features.

TABLE 4.4. *Categories of posttransplant lymphoproliferative disorders*

Early lesions
  Reactive plasmacytic hyperplasia
  Infectious mononucleosis–like
Posttransplant lymphoproliferative disorders: polymorphic
  Polyclonal (rare)
  Monoclonal
Posttransplant lymphoproliferative disorders: monomorphic
  (classified according to lymphoma classification)
  B-cell lymphomas
    Diffuse large B-cell lymphoma (immunoblastic, centro-blastic, anaplastic)
    Burkitt's or Burkitt-like lymphoma
    Plasma cell myeloma
  T-cell lymphomas
    Peripheral T-cell lymphoma, not otherwise categorized
    Other types (hepatosplenic T cell and natural killer cell)
Other types (rare)
  Hodgkin's disease–like lesions (associated with metho-trexate therapy)
  Plasmacytoma-like lesions

Normal Counterparts of Neoplastic Cells

The attempt to understand the normal counterpart of the neo-plastic cell is an important component of any tumor clas-sification. At present, the normal counterpart—lineage and differentiation stage—of many hematologic malignancies can be postulated with reasonable certainty; however, our under-standing of the immune system is insufficient to permit this to be done in all cases, and, therefore, rigid adherence to classifica-tion by normal counterpart is not feasible at this time. Diseases must be defined, diagnosed, and treated, even if the normal counterpart is not known or is controversial. Three major lin-eages of lymphoid malignancies can be defined, corresponding to normal lymphocyte subsets: B-cell neoplasms, T-cell neo-plasms, and natural killer (NK)–cell neoplasms. It is sometimes difficult to distinguish between T-cell and NK-cell neoplasms, however, and some well-defined clinical entities, such as nasal-type lymphoma, appear to be of T-cell lineage in some cases and NK-cell in others. For this reason, T- and NK-cell neoplasms are lumped into one category in the REAL and WHO classifica-tions. Hodgkin's disease, or, as we now prefer to call it, *Hodgkin's lymphoma*, is now known to be a B-cell neoplasm in virtually all the cases, but both types (nodular lymphocyte-pre-dominant and classical Hodgkin's lymphoma) differ morpho-logically and clinically from other B-cell lymphomas and have morphologic and clinical similarities with one another; for these reasons, Hodgkin's lymphoma is still considered a distinct category. Within the B- and T- and NK-cell neoplasms, two major categories are recognized—precursor neoplasms, which correspond to the earliest (lymphoblastic) stages of differentiation (lymphoblastic lymphomas and acute lympho-

blastic leukemias), and peripheral or mature neoplasms, which correspond to more differentiated B- and T-cell stages.

Classification according to the normal counterpart of the malignant cell has limitations. For example, a clinically iden-tical neoplasm may be composed, in some cases, of gamma-delta T cells and, in other cases, of alpha-beta T cells (hepatosplenic T-cell lymphoma and subcutaneous T-cell lymphoma are two examples). Conversely, neoplasms of the same apparent cell type or differentiation stage may be clini-cally different, depending on their site of origin. For example, marginal zone B-cell lymphomas of extranodal, nodal, and splenic types appear to be distinct, unrelated diseases, as are anaplastic large T-cell lymphomas of cutaneous and systemic types and diffuse large B-cell lymphomas of cutaneous and systemic origin. This fact should not be surprising when we consider that nonlymphoid neoplasms of similar cell types have distinctive clinical behavior in different sites: for exam-ple, squamous cell carcinomas of cutaneous versus pulmonary or uterine cervical origin or adenocarcinomas of various sites.

Grading and Prognostic Groups

The final classification includes more than 30 distinct entities. These diseases are in most cases unrelated to one another; that is, we can no longer talk about *lymphoma* or *non-Hodgkin's lymphoma* as a single disease with a range of histologic grades and clinical aggressiveness. Now that lymphomas can be defined more precisely with the aid of immunophenotype and genetic features, we find that many malignant lymphomas have—within the same disease entity—a spectrum of mor-phologic features and clinical aggressiveness. This has been known for years for follicular lymphoma, but it is also proba-bly true for B-cell chronic lymphocytic lymphoma, mantle cell lymphoma, and MALT lymphoma. Thus, histologic grade is just one of many prognostic factors that should be applied *within* a disease entity not across the whole range of lymphoid neoplasms. Another corollary of the definition of distinct lym-phoma entities is that it is neither possible nor helpful to sort them broadly according to histologic grade or clinical aggres-siveness. For example, although it is true that many lympho-mas that are composed of relatively small cells with a low proliferation fraction have a generally indolent course, at least one of them—mantle cell lymphoma—is rather aggressive. In addition, they each have a distinctive set of presenting features and, often, different treatments—for example, hairy-cell leu-kemia versus B-cell chronic lymphocytic lymphoma versus MALT lymphoma. Thus, the pathologist and the oncologist must get to know each disease entity, its spectrum of morphol-ogy and clinical behavior, and its peculiarities of occurrence and response to therapy.

Although a group of oncologists published a suggested clinical grouping of the entities in the REAL Classification in 1996 (32), they have since recognized its impracticality. The WHO Clinical Advisory Committee agreed that clinical groupings of lymphoid neoplasms are of no practical value and may be misleading (30). In practice, treatment of a spe-

TABLE 4.5. *B-cell neoplasms: variants*

Chronic lymphocytic leukemia and B-cell small lymphocytic lymphoma

    Variant: with monoclonal gammopathy or plasmacytoid differentiation

Hairy-cell leukemia

    Variant: hairy-cell leukemia variant

Follicular lymphoma

    Grades:

        Grade 1: 0 to 5 centroblasts per hpf

        Grade 2: 6 to 15 centroblasts per hpf

        Grade 3: >15 centroblasts per hpf

            Grade 3a: >15 centroblasts, but centrocytes are still present

            Grade 3b: centroblasts form solid sheets with no residual centrocytes

    Variant:

        Cutaneous follicle center lymphoma

Diffuse follicle center lymphoma

    Grade 1: 0 to 5 centroblasts per hpf

    Grade 2: 6 to 15 centroblasts per hpf

Mantle cell lymphoma

    Variant: blastoid

Diffuse large B-cell lymphoma, morphologic variants:

    Centroblastic

    Immunoblastic

    T-cell or histiocyte-rich

    Anaplastic large B-cell

        Plasmablastic

Diffuse large B-cell lymphoma, subtypes:

    Mediastinal (thymic) large B-cell lymphoma

    Primary effusion lymphoma

    Intravascular large B-cell lymphoma

    Lymphomatoid granulomatosis–type large B-cell lymphoma

Burkitt's lymphoma

    Morphologic variants:

        Atypical Burkitt's or Burkitt-like

        Plasmacytoid

    Clinical and genetic subtypes

        Endemic

        Sporadic

        Immunodeficiency-associated

Plasma cell disorders: subtypes and variants

    Monoclonal gammopathy of undetermined significance

    Plasma cell myeloma variants:

        Indolent myeloma

        Smoldering myeloma

        Osteosclerotic myeloma [polyneuropathy, organomegaly, endocrinopathy, M protein, and skin changes (POEMS) syndrome]

        Plasma cell leukemia

        Nonsecretory myeloma

    Plasmacytoma variants:

        Solitary plasmacytoma of bone

        Extramedullary plasmacytoma

hpf, high-power field.

TABLE 4.6. *T-cell neoplasms: variants*

T-cell prolymphocytic leukemia, morphologic variants:

    Small cell

    Cerebriform cell

Adult T-cell leukemia and lymphoma (human T-cell leukemia virus type I+), clinical variants:

    Acute

    Lymphomatous

    Chronic

    Smoldering

    Hodgkin's-like

Mycosis fungoides variants

    Pagetoid reticulosis

    Mycosis fungoides–associated follicular mucinosis

    Granulomatous slack skin disease

Primary cutaneous CD30+ T-cell lymphoproliferative disorders

    Lymphomatoid papulosis (type A and B)

    Primary cutaneous anaplastic large-cell lymphoma

    Borderline lesions

Peripheral T-cell lymphoma (not otherwise specified), variants

    Lymphoepithelioid (Lennert's lymphoma)

    T zone

Anaplastic large-cell lymphoma T- and null-cell type, variants

    Lymphohistiocytic

Small cell

TABLE 4.7. *Differences between the original Revised European-American and the World Health Organization classifications*

World Health Organization B-cell neoplasms: differences from Revised European-American Lymphoma Classification

Nomenclature

    Follicular lymphoma

    Lymphoplasmacytic lymphoma

Provisional entities now "real" entities

    Nodal marginal zone lymphoma

    Splenic marginal zone lymphoma

New, separated, or deleted entities

    Separation of B-prolymphocytic leukemia from B-cell chronic lymphocytic leukemia

    Immunodeficiency-associated lymphomas

    Burkitt-like type is a variant of Burkitt's lymphoma

World Health Organization T-cell neoplasms: differences from Revised European-American Lymphoma Classification

Nomenclature

    T-prolymphocytic leukemia (versus T-cell chronic lymphocytic leukemia)

    Extranodal natural killer– and T-cell lymphoma, nasal-type (versus angiocentric)

Provisional entities now "real" entities

    Hepatosplenic gamma-delta T-cell lymphoma

    Subcutaneous panniculitis-like T-cell lymphoma

New, separated, or deleted entities

    Natural killer–cell leukemia

    Primary cutaneous ALCL

    ALCL Hodgkin's-like is either Hodgkin's disease or ALCL

ALCL, anaplastic large-cell lymphoma.

TABLE 4.8. *Reproducibility of lymphoma diagnosis*

Reproducibility	Contribution of immunophenotype (%)
Reproducibility >85% (86% to 96%)	
B-cell chronic lymphocytic leukemia and small lymphocytic lymphoma	3
Mantle cell lymphoma	10
Follicular lymphoma	0
MALT lymphoma	2
Diffuse large B-cell lymphoma	15
T-lymphoblastic lymphoma	40
Anaplastic large-cell lymphoma	39
Peripheral T-cell lymphoma, unspecified	41
Mycosis fungoides	—
Reproducibility 80%	
Angioimmunoblastic T-cell lymphoma	—
Extranodal natural killer– and T-cell lymphoma	—
Reproducibility <50%	
Burkitt-like lymphoma	6
Lymphoplasmacytic lymphoma	—

MALT, mucosa-associated lymphoid tissue.

From A clinical evaluation of the International Lymphoma Study Group classification of non-Hodgkin's lymphoma. *Blood* 1997;89:3909–3918 and Armitage JO, Weisenburger DD. New approach to classifying non-Hodgkin's lymphomas: clinical features of the major histologic subtypes. *J Clin Oncol* 1998;16: 2780–2795.

relevance, because there appear to be important biologic differences between primary nodal and primary extranodal lymphomas, particularly in the T- and NK-cell diseases. However, any principle of sorting these neoplasms is artificial, and the lists can be regrouped in different ways for different purposes.

CLINICAL IMPLICATIONS OF THE REVISED EUROPEAN-AMERICAN LYMPHOMA AND WORLD HEALTH ORGANIZATION CLASSIFICATION

An initial criticism of the REAL Classification was that it had not been tested in a clinical study (34), although it only included diseases that had been previously published and for which the clinical features were known (35). To address this issue, an international group of oncologists and pathologists devised a clinical study of the classification, in which five expert pathologists reviewed more than 1,300 cases of non-Hodgkin's lymphoma at centers around the world (26,27). The aims of the study were (a) to see whether the classification could be used in practice, (b) to test its interobserver reproducibility, (c) to determine the need for immunophenotyping in diagnosis, (d) to determine whether the categories of disease that were identified in the classification were clinically distinctive at presentation or in outcome, and (e) to determine the relative frequency of these diseases in the populations studied.

cific patient should be determined not by the broad prognostic group into which the patient's neoplasm falls but by the specific *type* of neoplasm, with the addition of grade *within* the tumor type, if applicable, and *clinical prognostic factors*, such as stage, age, performance status, and the International Prognostic Index (IPI), or a combination of these (33).

Organization of the World Health Organization Classification

Because of the impracticality of arranging the list of B and T lymphoid neoplasms according to prognostic groups, the final WHO classification lists them, first, according to differentiation stage (precursor followed by mature or peripheral) and, second, according to predominant clinical presentation (predominantly disseminated or leukemic, primary extranodal, and predominantly nodal or systemic). This approach is intended for convenience and ease of learning by placing diseases that are likely to resemble one another clinically and histologically in proximity to each other in the list and in a text. It also has some biologic

TABLE 4.9. *Presenting features of common B- and T-cell neoplasms*

Neoplasm	Frequency (%)	Age (yr)	Male (%)	Stage				B symptoms (%)	Any extranodal site, including bone marrow (%)	Bone marrow (%)	Gastrointestinal tract (%)	International Prognostic Index		
				I (%)	II (%)	III (%)	IV (%)					0/1 (%)	2/3 (%)	4/5 (%)
Large B-cell	31	64	55	25	29	13	33	33	71	16	18	35	46	19
Mediastinal	2	37	34	10	56	3	31	38	56	3	0	52	37	11
Follicular	22	59	42	18	15	16	51	28	64	42	4	45	48	7
Small lymphocytic lymphoma or chronic lymphocytic leukemia	6	65	53	4	5	8	83	33	80	72	3	23	64	13
Mucosa-associated lymphoid tissue	8	60	48	39	28	2	31	19	98	14	50	44	48	8
Mantle cell	6	63	74	13	7	9	71	28	81	51	9	23	54	23
Peripheral T-cell	7	61	55	8	12	15	65	50	82	36	15	17	52	31
Anaplastic large-cell lymphoma	2	34	69	19	32	10	39	53	59	13	9	61	18	21

TABLE 4.10A. *Immunohistologic and genetic features of common B-cell neoplasms*

Neoplasm	Surface immunoglobulin; intracytoplasmic immunoglobulin	CD5	CD10	CD23	CD43	CD103	Cyclin D1	Genetic abnormality	Immunoglobulin genes[a]
B-cell chronic lymphocytic leukemia and small lymphocytic lymphoma	+; –/+	+	–	+	+	–	–/+	trisomy 12; 13q	R, U
Lymphoplasmacytic lymphoma	+; +	–	–	–	–/+	–	–	t(9;14); del 6(q23)	R, M
Hairy-cell leukemia	+;–	–	–	–	+	++	+/–	none known	R, M
Splenic marginal zone lymphoma	+; –/+	–	–	–	–	+	–	7q21-32	R, M
Follicle center lymphoma	+; –	–	+/–	–/+	–	–	–	t(14;18); bcl-2	R, M, O
Mantle cell lymphoma	+; –	+	–	–	+	–	+	t(11;14); bcl-1	R, U
Mucosa-associated–lymphoid tissue lymphoma	+; +/–	–	–	–/+	–/+	–	–	trisomy 3, t(11;18) t(1;10)	R, M, O
Diffuse large B-cell lymphoma	+/–	–	–/+	NA	–/+	NA	–	t(14;18), t(8;14), 3q; bcl-2, myc, bcl-6	R, M
Burkitt's lymphoma	+	–	+	–	–	NA	–	t(8;14), t(2;8), t(8;22); c-myc; EBV–/+	R, M

+, >90% positive; +/–, > 50% positive; –/+, < 50% positive; –, < 10% positive; NA, not applicable; M, mutated variable region; O, ongoing (indicating germinal center stage); R, rearranged; U, unmutated.
[a]Mutations in the immunoglobulin gene V region indicate exposure to antigen.

This study convincingly demonstrated that the classification could be used by expert hematopathologists: more than 95% of the cases with adequate material could be classified into one or another of the categories. The interobserver reproducibility was substantially better than that for other classifications and was better than 85% for most diseases (Table 4.8). Immunophenotyping was helpful in some diseases, such as mantle cell lymphoma and diffuse large B-cell lymphoma, in which it improved accuracy by 10% to 15%, and was essential for all types of T-cell lymphoma, as it improved reproducibility from approximately 50% to more than 90%. It was not required for many diseases, such as follicular lymphoma, B-cell small lymphocytic lymphoma, and MALT lymphoma (26).

The relative frequency of the different B- and T- and NK-cell lymphomas in the study population was similar to previous patterns that were reported in the literature (Table 4.9). The most common lymphoma was diffuse large B-cell lymphoma, followed by follicular lymphoma; together, these comprised 50% of the lymphomas in the study. New entities that were not specifically recognized in the WF accounted for 27% of the cases: MALT lymphoma, 8%; mantle cell, 7%; peripheral T cell, 6%; nodal marginal zone, 2%; mediastinal large B cell, 2%; and anaplastic large T and null cell, 2%. These results are reassuring,

confirming that the majority of the cases that are encountered by oncologists and pathologists are only a few subtypes with which they are already familiar. However, these results also underscore the need for recognition of the more recently described entities, which, although less common, have important clinical differences. The study also found differences in geographic distribution of the lymphoma types, with follicular lymphoma being more common in North America and western Europe, T-cell lymphomas more common in Hong Kong, and mediastinal large B-cell lymphoma and mantle cell lymphoma more common in Ticino (the Italian-speaking canton), Switzerland (36).

The different entities that were recognized by the classification had significantly different clinical presentations and survivals. For example, diffuse aggressive lymphomas, which would be lumped as intermediate and high grade in the WF, include diffuse large B-cell lymphoma, mediastinal large B-cell lymphoma, peripheral T-cell lymphoma, and anaplastic large T- or null-cell lymphoma. The clinical features at presentation were strikingly different, with a younger age group for mediastinal large T-cell lymphoma and anaplastic large T or null lymphoma, and striking differences in male to female ratios, thus suggesting that these are distinctive biologic entities (Table 4.10A). When overall survivals were analyzed, entities that would have been

TABLE 4.10B. *Immunohistologic and genetic features of common T-cell neoplasms*

Neoplasm	CD3, S;C	CD5	CD7	CD4	CD8	CD30	T-cell receptor genes	Natural killer (16, 56)	Cytotox granule[a]	Epstein-Barr virus	Genetic abnormality	T-cell receptor genes
T-cell prolymphocytic leukemia	+	–	+	+/–	–	–	αβ	–/+	–	–	inv 14, trisomy 8q	R
T-cell large granular lymphocytic leukemia	+	–	+	–	+	–	αβ	+, –	+	–	None known	R
Natural killer–cell large granular lymphocytic leukemia	–	–	+	–	+/–	–	–	–, +	+	+	None known	G
Extranodal natural killer– and T-cell lymphoma	–; +	–	–/+	–	–	–	–	+	+	++	None known	G
Hepatosplenic T-cell lymphoma	+	–	+	–	–	–	γδ	+, –/+	+	–	Iso 7q	R
Enteropathy-type T-cell lymphoma	+	+	+	–	+/–	+/–	αβ	–	+	–	None known	R
Subcutaneous panniculitis-like T-cell	+	+	+	+	–	–/+	αβ	–	+	–	None known	R
Peripheral T-cell lymphoma, NOS	+/–	+/–	+/–	+/–	–/+	–, +	αβ>γδ	–/+	–/+	–/+	inv 14; complex	R
Angioimmunoblastic	+	+	+	+/–	–	–	αβ	–	NA	+/–	None known	R
Anaplastic large-cell lymphoma, primary systemic	+/–	+/–	NA	–/+	–/+	+/+	αβ	–	+	–	t(2;5); NPM/ALK	R
Anaplastic large-cell lymphoma, cutaneous	+/–	+/–	+/–	–	–	+/+	αβ	–	–/+	–	None known	R

+, >90% positive; +/–, > 50% positive; –/+, < 50% positive; –, < 10% positive; C, cytoplasmic; G, germline; NA, not applicable; NPM/ALK, nucleophosmin/anaplastic lymphoma kinase; NOS, not otherwise specified; R, rearranged; S, surface.

[a]Cytotox granule is TIA-1, perforin, or granzyme, or a combination of these.

lumped together as *low grade* or *intermediate or high grade* in the WF showed marked differences in survival, again confirming that they need to be recognized and treated as distinct entities.

A critical finding in this study was that classification is not the only predictor of clinical outcome. Patients with any of these diseases could be stratified into better and worse prognostic groups according to the IPI (33). For example, although patients with follicular lymphoma typically have IPI scores of 1 to 3, those patients with scores of 4 or 5 had a predicted median overall survival of only 18 months. Thus, to plan treatment for an individual patient, the oncologist must know not only the diagnosis, but also the clinical prognostic factors that influence that patient's course.

USE OF SPECIAL STUDIES IN THE DIAGNOSIS OF LYMPHOID NEOPLASMS

Each of the lymphoid neoplasms has a characteristic morphology, which may be sufficient in a given case to permit diagnosis and classification on morphologic grounds alone, if well-prepared sections are available; thus, most cases of lymphoma can be diagnosed and classified with reasonable certainty on the basis of routine histologic sections alone. However, there are many pitfalls in the histologic diagnosis of malignant lymphoma, and immunophenotyping or, less often, genetic studies can be useful in resolving major differential diagnostic problems (Table 4.10B). Details of the performance, interpretation, and usefulness of these studies are found in chapters 5, 49, and 50. Problems that can be resolved by these techniques include (a) differentation of reactive versus neoplastic lymphoid infiltrates, (b) differentation of lymphoid versus nonlymphoid malignancies, and (c) subclassification of lymphoma. In a given case, if the morphology is typical of a given entity, but the immunophenotypic or genetic features are unusual, the histologic sections should be reexamined; however, the case may still be accepted as an example of the entity that is suggested by the morphologic features. If the morphology is atypical, but the immunophenotype and genetic features are classic for a given entity, these features may override morphology in classification. If the morphology and the immunophenotype or genetic features are atypical, then the case is best regarded as unclassifiable or borderline.

Increasingly, immunophenotyping and genetic analysis may be important in the prediction of prognosis and response to treatment, as is now the case in some myeloid neoplasms with specific translocations that lead to therapeutic targets, such as acute promyelocytic leukemia and chronic myelogenous leukemia with the BCR/ABL translocation. Although no such targets currently exist for lymphoid neoplasms, they should be the subject of future study.

FUTURE DIRECTIONS IN LYMPHOMA CLASSIFICATION

Any classification of diseases must be considered a work in progress. The diseases that are recognized in the REAL-WHO classification and their definitions represent our cur-

rent best approximation; the list will need to be updated periodically as long as there continues to be progress in our understanding of the biology of the immune system and cancer in general. Important new technologies, such as DNA microarrays for the assessment of gene expression in hematologic and other malignancies, should improve our understanding of these neoplasms and should provide additional markers for classification and diagnosis (37,38). On an ongoing basis, joint committees of the major hematopathology societies will periodically review and update the classification of lymphoid and other hematologic neoplasms, together with clinical colleagues.

REFERENCES

1. Callendar GR. Tumors and tumor-like conditions of the lymphocyte, the myelocyte, the erythrocyte, and the reticulum cell. *Am J Pathol* 1934;10:443–465.
2. Robb-Smith AH. Reticulosis and reticulosarcoma. A histological classification. *J Pathol Bacteriol* 1938;47:457–480.
3. Gall EA, Mallory TB. Malignant lymphoma. A clinicopathologic survey of 618 cases. *Am J Pathol* 1942;18:381–395.
4. Rappaport H, Winter W, Hicks E. Follicular lymphoma. A re-evaluation of its position in the scheme of malignant lymphoma, based on a survey of 253 cases. *Cancer* 1956;9:792–821.
5. Rappaport H. Tumors of the hematopoietic system. In: *Atlas of tumor pathology.* Washington, DC: Armed Forces Institute of Pathology, 1966.
6. Dorfman RF. Classification of non-Hodgkin's lymphomas [Letter]. *Lancet* 1974;2:961–962.
7. Bennett M. Classification of non-Hodgkin's lymphomas [Letter]. *Lancet* 1974;2:405–408.
8. Lukes R, Collins R. Immunologic characterization of human malignant lymphomas. *Cancer* 1974;34:1488–1503.
9. Gerard-Marchant R. Classification of non-Hodgkin's lymphomas. *Lancet* 1974;2:406–408.
10. Kay HE. Classification of non-Hodgkin's lymphomas [Letter]. *Lancet* 1974;2:586.
11. Mathe G. Histological and cytological typing of neoplastic diseases of hematopoietic and lymphoid tissues. In: *World Health Organization international histological classification of tumors,* vol 14. Lyon: IARC Press, 1976.
12. Lennert K. The histopathology of malignant lymphoma. *Br J Haematol* 1975;31[Suppl]:193–203.
13. Lennert K. Malignant lymphomas other than Hodgkin's disease. New York: Springer-Verlag, 1978.
14. Non-Hodgkin's lymphoma pathologic classification project. National Cancer Institute sponsored study of classifications of non-Hodgkin's lymphomas: summary and description of a Working Formulation for clinical usage. *Cancer* 1982;49:2112–2135.
15. Lennert K, Feller A. *Histopathology of non-Hodgkin's lymphomas,* 2nd ed. New York: Springer-Verlag, 1992.
16. Fisher RI, Dahlberg S, Nathwani BN, et al. A clinical analysis of two indolent lymphoma entities: mantle cell lymphoma and marginal zone lymphoma (including the mucosa-associated lymphoid tissue and monocytoid B-cell subcategories): a Southwest Oncology Group study. *Blood* 1995;85:1075–1082.
17. Fisher RI, Gaynor ER, Dahlberg S, et al. Comparison of a standard regimen (CHOP) with three intensive chemotherapy regimens for advanced non-Hodgkin's lymphoma. *N Engl J Med* 1993;328:1002–1006.
18. Longo DL. Lymphocytic lymphomas. In: DeVita VT, Hellman S, Rosenberg S, eds. *Principles and practice of oncology.* Philadelphia: Lippincott Williams & Wilkins, 1993:1859–1927.
19. Hastrup N, Hamilton-Dutoit S, Ralfkiaer E, et al. Peripheral T-cell lymphomas: an evaluation of reproducibility of the updated Kiel classification. *Histopathology* 1991;18:99–105.
20. Chott A, Augustin I, Wrba F, et al. Peripheral T-cell lymphomas—a clinicopathologic study of 75 cases. *Hum Pathol* 1990;21:1117–1125.

21. Banks P, Chan J, Cleary ML, et al. Mantle cell lymphoma: a proposal for unification of morphologic, immunologic, and molecular data. *Am J Surg Pathol* 1992;16:637–640.
22. Mason DY, Banks PM, Chan J, et al. Nodular lymphocyte predominance Hodgkin's disease: a distinct clinico-pathological entity. *Am J Surg Pathol* 1994;18:526–530.
23. Harris NL, Jaffe ES, Stein H, et al. A revised European-American classification of lymphoid neoplasms: a proposal from the International Lymphoma Study Group. *Blood* 1994;84:1361–1392.
24. Weisenburger D. The International Lymphoma Study Group (ILSG) Classification of non-Hodgkin's lymphoma (NHL): pathology findings from a large multi-center study. *Mod Pathol* 1997;10:136A.
25. Weisenburger D. The International Lymphoma Study Group (ILSG) Classification of non-Hodgkin's lymphoma (NHL): clinical findings from a large multi-center study. *Mod Pathol* 1997;10:136A.
26. A clinical evaluation of the International Lymphoma Study Group classification of non-Hodgkin's lymphoma. *Blood* 1997;89:3909–3918.
27. Armitage JO, Weisenburger DD. New approach to classifying non-Hodgkin's lymphomas: clinical features of the major histologic subtypes. *J Clin Oncol* 1998;16:2780–2795.
28. Jaffe ES. Proposed World Health Organization classification of neoplastic diseases of hematopoietic and lymphoid tissues. *Am J Surg Pathol* 1997;21:114–121.
29. Jaffe ES, Harris NL, Diebold J, et al. World Health Organization Classification of lymphomas: a work in progress. *Ann Oncol* 1998;9 [Suppl 5]:S25–S30.
30. Harris NL, Jaffe ES, Diebold J, et al. The World Health Organization Classification of hematological malignancies. Report of the Clinical Advisory Committee Meeting—Airlie House, Virginia, November 1997. *J Clin Oncol* 1999;17:3835–3849.
31. Jaffe ES, Harris NL, Stein H, Vardiman JW. Pathology and genetics of tumors of hematopoietic and lymphoid tissues. In: Kleihues P, Sobin L, eds. World Health Organization classification of tumors, vol 3. Lyon: IARC Press, 2001.
32. Hiddemann W, Longo DL, Coiffier B, et al. Lymphoma classification—the gap between biology and clinical management is closing. *Blood* 1996;88:4085–4089.
33. A predictive model for aggressive non-Hodgkin's lymphoma. The International non-Hodgkin's Lymphoma Project. *N Engl J Med* 1993;329:987–994.
34. Rosenberg SA. Classification of lymphoid neoplasms. *Blood* 1994;84:1359–1360.
35. Harris NL, Jaffe ES, Stein H, et al. Lymphoma classification proposal: clarification. *Blood* 1995;85:857–860.
36. Anderson JR, Armitage JO, Weisenburger DD. Epidemiology of the non-Hodgkin's lymphomas: distributions of the major subtypes differ by geographic locations. Non-Hodgkin's Lymphoma Classification Project. *Ann Oncol* 1998;9:717–720.
37. Alizadeh AA, Eisen MB, Davis RE, et al. Distinct types of diffuse large B-cell lymphoma identified by gene expression profiling. *Nature* 2000;403:503–511.
38. Shipp MA, Ross KN, Tamayo P, et al. Diffuse large B-cell lymphoma outcome prediction by gene-expression profiling and supervised machine learning. *Nat Med* 2002;8:68–74.

CHAPTER 5

Immunophenotyping in Lymphoma Diagnosis and Classification

Patricia Aoun and Timothy C. Greiner

Immunophenotyping of lymphoid neoplasms is a required element in the morphologic evaluation of the tissue for proper classification of the disease. The importance of immunophenotyping is emphasized by the following statement: "Some diseases have a virtually specific immunophenotype, such that one would hesitate to make the diagnosis in the absence of the immunophenotype" (1). The Revised European and American Lymphoma classification system and the subsequent World Health Organization Classification of Tumors of the Hematopoietic and Lymphoid Tissues are the first classification systems to use both immunophenotyping and molecular characteristics as cardinal elements in developing the systems (1,2). The two methods that are most frequently used to phenotype lymphomas are flow cytometry of cell suspensions and immunohistochemistry of paraffin-embedded tissue.

USE OF FLOW CYTOMETRY

Flow cytometry is an automated fluorescence detection method used for measuring the physical and fluorescent properties of large numbers of cells in a relatively short time (3). The availability of a broad array of monoclonal antibodies that permit the characterization of various cellular populations in patient samples has made possible the transformation of flow cytometry from a research tool to a tool that is indispensable in routine clinical practice. Immunophenotyping by flow cytometry is highly sensitive and reproducible. The methods and procedures used can be standardized, and the data generated can be quantified (3,4). Furthermore, large numbers of cells can be studied, and the ability to perform multiparameter analysis makes it possible to detect simultaneously the presence of more than one property on any given cell population (5,6). Instruments currently available for clinical use can detect as many as five parameters simultaneously on each cell. Features that are routinely analyzed include cellular viability; physical properties such as cell size and complexity; expression of surface, cytoplasmic, or nuclear antigens; and DNA content.

Together, these features can establish the lineage and state of differentiation of various populations in a patient sample.

Clinical Indications

Current indications for immunophenotyping by flow cytometry are varied, and, because immunophenotyping can be accomplished using a variety of techniques, the decision to use flow cytometry is dependent on the sample being studied and the disease being evaluated. The most common clinical applications include the detection and characterization of lymphoma cells, determination of the lineage in acute leukemia, detection of minimal residual disease, determination of lymphocyte subsets for monitoring immune status in immunodeficiency states or after bone marrow transplantation, enumeration of CD34$^+$ stem cells, and cell-cycle analysis in solid tumors (7). Immunophenotyping by flow cytometry is not useful in assessment of the bone marrow or lymph node for involvement by Hodgkin's disease, or as a screening test on peripheral blood from patients who do not have a sustained lymphocytosis, morphologically suspicious lymphocytes on a peripheral smear, or splenomegaly (7).

Principles of Flow Cytometry

The basic principle of flow cytometry is that cells in suspension are made to flow singly through the path of a monochromatic light source, resulting in light scatter and fluorescence emission (3). The light source in a clinical flow cytometer is usually a gas laser. The light that is emitted and scattered by each cell that passes through the laser light beam is separated by optical filters and focused onto individual detectors. The latter generate analog electrical signals, which are converted into digital signals that in turn are stored in and displayed by a computer.

Analysis of the patterns of light scattered by cells allows determination of physical properties such as cell size and cytoplasmic complexity. These properties alone are sufficient to separate reproducibly for further analysis the different cellular populations present in a sample. Much more specific information about the different populations is derived with the use of fluorescent-labeled monoclonal antibodies directed against specific cellular protein or carbohydrate structures present on the cell surface or in the cytoplasm or nucleus. Although most standard clinical assays depend on the detection of antigens expressed on the surface, the detection of intracellular antigens is useful in many clinical settings, including the detection of cytoplasmic immunoglobulin in myeloma cells and of Tdt in lymphoblastic lymphomas or acute leukemia.

Specimen Collection and Transportation

Immunophenotyping by flow cytometry can be routinely performed on peripheral blood, bone marrow aspirate, serosal fluids, cerebrospinal fluid, cell suspensions prepared from tissue biopsies, and fine-needle aspirates of tumors (Table 5.1) (4,8). The most common specimens analyzed are peripheral blood and bone marrow aspirates. These specimens should be collected in ethylenediamine tetra-acetate (EDTA), sodium heparin, or acid citrate dextrose and maintained at room temperature. At least 5 cc of peripheral blood and 2 cc of bone marrow are usually required to obtain sufficient numbers of cells for analysis. Anticoagulant is not necessary for other body fluids. Tissue specimens should be submitted fresh, in a sterile container, and covered with sterile saline or tissue culture media for transportation to the flow cytometry laboratory. Unlike blood or bone marrow, tissue specimens are better preserved during transportation if refrigerated (4°), but care should be taken to prevent freezing.

Although short-term storage (24–48 hours) of specimens is acceptable in many situations, immediate transportation to the laboratory is optimal to preserve the maximum number of viable cells in any specimen. A large proportion of dead cells in a specimen can alter phenotyping results. Specimens older than 48 hours are generally suboptimal or inadequate for analysis by flow cytometry due to decreased viability, degradation of antigens, and increased autofluorescence. Large-cell lymphomas are especially susceptible to rapid degeneration, resulting in frequent false-negative immunophenotyping results for specimens delayed in transport. However, because specimens other than peripheral blood

TABLE 5.1. *Specific recommendations for flow cytometry*

5 cc peripheral blood

2 cc bone marrow

Ethylenediamine tetra-acetate, heparin, or acid citrate dextrose anticoagulant

Submit fresh in saline or tissue culture media

<48 hr shipping

TABLE 5.2. *Limitations of flow cytometry*

Problem	Example
Cell loss (during shipping delays)	Large-cell lymphoma
Inadequate sample	Limited antibodies performed
Nonrepresentative sample	False negative
Poor sensitivity	Hodgkin's disease
No aberrant pattern	Some peripheral T-cell lymphomas

cannot easily be recollected, flow cytometry laboratories often attempt to derive whatever useful information can be obtained from any given specimen. Limited panels that are directed at answering specific questions posed by the patient's clinical history can sometimes be performed with specimens that yield few cells (Table 5.2). Specimens in which an insufficient number of cells are present for any immunophenotyping by flow cytometry often can be redirected for cytogenetic, molecular, or immunohistochemical studies.

Specimen Processing

The detection by flow cytometry of normal and abnormal populations in patient specimens often requires the removal and isolation of various populations in a sample to enhance the detection of the population of interest (4,8). At a minimum, removal of erythrocytes is performed and is generally accomplished by lysis. Density gradient separation is also frequently used and has the additional advantage of enriching mononuclear cells while removing dead cells and granulocytes along with red blood cells. Morphologic review of smears prepared directly from the original specimen and of cytospins prepared from the cell suspension is critical to ensuring that the cellular population of interest has not been lost as a result of specimen processing (8,9). Once cell suspensions have been prepared from the submitted specimen, staining with the various antibodies is performed. The concentration of commercially available antibodies determines the number of cells needed for each test. This number is generally in the range of 100,000 to 200,000 cells for each antibody combination tested.

Antigens that are frequently analyzed by flow cytometry when evaluating a sample for the presence of lymphoma are summarized in Table 5.3. Although attempts have been made to identify a universal strategy for selection of antibodies to be included in immunophenotyping panels (6,10), the selection of antibodies varies between laboratories. In some laboratories, the choice of specific antibodies depends at least in part on the clinical history communicated with the specimen and on a preliminary morphologic review. The applications of flow cytometric analysis in characterizing hematopoietic malignancies developed with the recognition

TABLE 5.3. *Cellular markers useful in the identification and classification of lymphoproliferative disorders*

Antigen	Target	Major normal hematopoietic cellular distribution
CD1a	Transmembrane antigen-presenting polypeptide	Cortical thymocytes (CD4+, CD8+), Langerhan's cells
CD2	E-rosette receptor, lymphocyte function–associated antigen-2	Thymocytes, T cells, NK cells
CD3	T-cell receptor complex component	Thymocytes, T cells
CD4	HLA class II transmembrane coreceptor	Thymocytes, T-helper/inducer cells, stem cells, monocytes, granulocytes
CD5	Transmembrane receptor	Thymocytes, T cells, mature B-cell subset
CD7	Costimulatory membrane protein	Thymocytes, T cells, NK cells, stem cells
CD8	HLA class I coreceptor	Thymocytes, T-cytotoxic/suppressor cells, NK cells
CD10	Zinc metallopeptidase	Lymphoid precursors, germinal center B-cells, mature neutrophils
CD11c	Transmembrane receptor and adhesion molecule	T-cell subset, B-cell subset, monocytes, macrophages, NK cells, granulocytes
CD16	IgG Fc receptor	NK cells, granulocytes, macrophages
CD19	Transmembrane signal transduction glycoprotein	B cells, follicular dendritic cells
CD20	Membrane phosphoprotein	B cells, some activated T cells
CD22	Adhesion and signaling membrane protein	B cells
CD23	IgE Fc receptor	B cells, monocytes, dendritic cells
CD25	Interleukin-2 receptor	Activated T cells, B cells, monocytes
CD34	Transmembrane sialomucin adhesion protein	Stem cells, endothelial cells
CD38	Transmembrane enzyme	Plasma cells and most hematopoietic cells during early differentiation and activation
CD45	Transmembrane receptor costimulatory molecules	All hematopoietic cells
CD56	Neural cell adhesion molecule	NK cells, T-cell subset
CD57	Glycoprotein	NK cells, T-cell subset
CD79a	B-cell receptor component	Mature B cells, plasma cells
CD103	Transmembrane protein (integrin chain family)	Intraepithelial lymphocytes, small subset of peripheral blood lymphocytes
Kappa	Ig light chain	B cells, plasma cells
Lambda	Ig light chain	B cells, plasma cells
Tdt	Nuclear protein	Lymphoid precursors

HLA, human lymphocyte antigen; Ig, immunoglobulin; NK, natural killer.
Adapted from Jaffe ES, Harris NL, Stein H, et al. The pathology and genetics of tumours of haematopoietic and lymphoid tissues. In: Kleihauer Psorion L, ed. *World Health Organization classifications of tumors*, 1st ed. Lyon: IARC Press, 2001; Carey JL. Immunophenotyping in diagnosis and prognosis of mature lymphoid leukemias and lymphomas. In: Keren DF, McCoy P, Carey JL, eds. *Flow cytometry in clinical diagnosis*, 3rd ed. Chicago: ASCP Press, 2002:227–338; and Pirruccello S, Aoun P. Hematopoietic cell differentiation: monoclonal antibodies and cluster designation (CD)-defined hematopoietic cell antigens. In: Keren DF, McCoy JP, Carey JL, eds. *Flow cytometry in clinical diagnosis*, 3rd ed. Chicago: ASCP Press, 2001:65–97.

that malignant cells express antigens in patterns similar to those present in normal, precursor, and mature cells. It is important to note that for flow cytometry, as for other immunophenotyping methods, the detection of abnormal populations relies on the ability to detect *abnormal patterns* of antigen expression (Tables 5.4 and 5.5). No single marker is sufficiently specific to definitively classify a lymphoproliferative disorder. The broader the panel, the better it will discriminate between normal and abnormal populations and subclassify lymphoproliferative disorders. Regardless of which antibodies are included in a panel, the selection should be sufficiently broad so as to separate populations reliably.

For non-Hodgkin's lymphomas, the *minimum* panel should include a general marker such as CD45 that allows separation of the different hematopoietic populations present in a specimen (5,11); pan T-cell markers, such as CD3, CD4, CD5, CD7, and CD8; pan B-cell markers, such as CD19 and CD20; CD10; and kappa and lambda light chains.

B-cell lymphoproliferative disorders are generally identified by the detection of clonal kappa and lambda light chain distributions. A minority of B-cell lymphoproliferative disorders do not express detectable surface light chains, and, in these cases, cytoplasmic staining for light chains may be helpful. In addition, abnormal coexpression of antigens such

TABLE 5.4. *Markers useful in the classification by flow cytometry of low-grade B-cell lymphoproliferative disorders*

Antigen	Chronic lymphocytic leukemia	Prolymphocytic leukemia	Mantle cell lymphoma	Hairy-cell leukemia	Splenic lymphoma/ villous lymphocytes	Follicular lymphoma	Marginal zone lymphoma
CD5	+	+/–	+	–	–	–	–
CD10	–	–	–/+	–	–	+/–	–
CD11c	+dim/–	+dim/–	–	+bright	–/+	–	+/–
CD19	+	+	+	+	+	+	+
CD20	+dim	+	+	+	+	+	+
CD23	+	+	–	–	–	–/+	–
CD25	+dim/–	+dim/–	–	+bright/–	–	–	–
CD103	–	–	–	+	–	–	–
sIg	+dim	+bright	+bright	+	+	+	+

sIg, surface immunoglobulin; +, positive; –, negative.

as CD5 can help distinguish malignant from benign populations in cases in which surface light chains are not detectable. Detection of neoplastic T-cell populations is more difficult, as no direct markers of T-cell clonality comparable to kappa and lambda staining are available. Instead, absent or abnormal expression of expected T-cell antigens is relied on. However, antigen loss is not sufficiently diagnostic, and gene rearrangement studies should be performed to confirm clonality.

Analysis of the immunophenotypic information generated includes review of the frequency distributions generated by the flow cytometer and correlation of the findings with morphologic assessment of cytospins and smears prepared from the sample. Flow cytometry reports should include not only a listing of the antibodies used for analysis, but also a descriptive summary of the phenotype of the abnormal cells, the fraction of abnormal cells present in the samples, and an interpretation of the phenotype

with a differential diagnosis (12). Application of the World Health Organization classification requires the integration of clinical, morphologic, cytogenetic, molecular, and immunophenotypic features for characterization of lymphoproliferative disorders; therefore, it is important that all available clinical and diagnostic information related to a specimen be made available to the pathologist interpreting the results of flow cytometry data (Table 5.6).

USE OF IMMUNOHISTOCHEMISTRY

Development of Antibodies Reactive in Paraffin

Early immunophenotyping by direct and indirect immunofluorescent studies on cell surface markers required the existence of frozen tissues or cell suspensions. Initially, in the 1980s, followed by an explosion in the 1990s, a wide variety of antibodies reactive in paraffin-embedded tissue

TABLE 5.5. *Markers useful in the classification by flow cytometry of mature T-cell and natural killer–cell lymphoproliferative disorders with leukemic presentation*

Antigen	T-cell prolymphocytic leukemia	T-cell large granular lymphocytic leukemia	Natural killer–cell large granular lymphocytic leukemia	Adult T-cell lymphoma/ leukemia	Mycosis fungoides/Sézary syndrome
CD2	+	+	+	+	+
CD3	+	+	–	+	+
CD4	+	–	–	+	+
CD5	+	+	–	+	+
CD7	+	+	+	–	–/+
CD8	–	+	+/–	–	–
CD16	–	+	+	–	–
CD25	–	–	–	+	–/+
CD56	–	–	+/–	–	–

TABLE 5.6. *Critical clinical information for flow cytometry*

Site of specimen

Date and time obtained

Complete blood count and differential, if blood or bone marrow submitted

Clinical diagnosis in new patients

History of specific lymphoma/leukemia subtype

became available for the cluster-designated (CD) markers and many other antigens. Thus, although this section will focus only on phenotyping paraffin-embedded tissue, be aware that some antibodies still require frozen tissue for best results. However, for those antibodies reactive in paraffin-embedded tissues, the requirements for good performance necessitate optimally fixed tissues. Different reactivities can occur in formalin-fixed tissue versus B5- or other heavy metal–fixed tissue. Excellent antigen retention is often seen in B5-fixed tissue for many cytoplasmic/membrane antigens, with less favorable results seen in nuclear-based antigens (13).

Tissue Recommendations

Good lines of communication are necessary between primary care physicians, oncologists, surgeons, and pathologists to obtain proper tissue allocation and fixation in the work-up of lymphoid neoplasms. To our referring laboratories, we recommend that a lymph node be submitted promptly to the surgical pathology laboratory and immediately processed on receipt in the laboratory. A lymphoid specimen will degenerate rapidly compared to solid tumor neoplasms. This can result in the nonviability of tumor cells, particularly large-cell lymphoma for flow cytometry, and artifactual staining results in immunohistochemistry as the cells undergo autolysis. Portions of the specimen should be set aside for cytogenetics, a minimum of 200 mm^3 frozen for molecular studies or immunohistochemistry, and thin 2-mm slices fixed in formalin and B5 fixatives. Fixation in formalin allows for possible gene rearrangement analysis by polymerase chain reaction methodology. Despite the excellent morphologic detail it provides, the use of B5 (mercuric chloride) fixative has declined because of the cost and safety of waste disposal.

Methodology

The most commonly used protocol for immunohistochemistry in paraffin-embedded tissue is a five-step procedure incorporating a variation of the avidin-biotin-conjugate (ABC) method. The major steps include: (a) deparaffinization of the tissue on the slides, (b) antigen retrieval, (c) incubation with primary antibody, (d) incubation with secondary antibody linked with biotin, (e) incu-

bation with streptavidin/biotin complex linked with peroxidase substrate for detection by various chromogen labels, of which diaminobenzidine is most common. Antigen retrieval is the technique of unmasking antigens bound by the formaldehyde fixation. The two major approaches include protein digestion and heating in a buffer solution. Various enzymes have been used to digest tissue, including pepsin, trypsin, and protease. The most common buffers used in heat-induced antigen retrieval include citrate buffer at pH 6 and ethylenediamine tetra-acetate buffer at pH 8–10. The choice of buffer is established empirically within laboratories for each antibody. Heating instrumentation may include water baths, microwave, steam cooker, or autoclave. These options provide many ways for variability to occur in antigen profiles identified between laboratories.

Identification of Benign Lymphoid Hyperplasias

Immunohistochemistry is of immense value in assessing the CD20$^+$ B-cell and CD3$^+$ T-cell architecture of lymphoid biopsies. In addition, kappa and lambda antibodies are used to demonstrate polyclonal plasma cells in benign tissues. CD5 or CD43 coexpression with CD20 is frequently used to identify the presence of low-grade B-cell lymphomas (14).

Differential Diagnosis of Subtypes of Lymphoma

The expected pattern of reactivities of key antibodies is incorporated into the interpretation of immunohistochemical results. Few antigens are pathognomonic for a particular subtype of lymphoma, and rarely is an antigen seen in 100% of cases in a subtype of lymphoma (15). For example, bcl-2 is positive in 90% of follicular lymphomas; however, it is negative in 25% of grade 3 follicular lymphomas (16) and is positive in most diffuse low- to intermediate-grade lymphomas. Positivity with the nuclear antigen bcl-6 is seen largely in diffuse large-cell and follicular lymphomas. Cyclin D-1/PRAD-1/bcl-1 (parathyroid adenoma-1/B-cell lymphoma-1) overexpression is not seen exclusively in mantle cell lymphoma. Cyclin D-1 may be seen in a small percentage of multiple myeloma/plasmacytoma, hairy-cell leukemia, and lymphoplasmacytic lymphomas (17). Anaplastic lymphoma kinase is one of the few specific antibodies used to diagnose the subtype of anaplastic large-cell lymphoma, but it is not expressed in many elderly or cutaneous cases (18). However, anaplastic lymphoma kinase is also expressed in some inflammatory myofibroblastic tumors (19). CD5 is useful for separating small lymphocytic and mantle cell lymphomas from the lack of expression in mucosa-associated lymphoid tissue, lymphoplasmacytic and follicular lymphomas (20,21), the last of which typically express CD10 (22). The expression of Tdt is restricted to lymphoblastic lymphoma; however, rare cases of biphenotypic or mixed-

TABLE 5.7. *Antibodies reactive in paraffin-embedded tissue in low-grade B-cell lymphomas[a]*

Antigen	Small lymphocytic lymphoma	Mantle cell lymphoma	Mucosa-associated lymphoid tissue lymphoma	Marginal zone lymphoma	Follicular lymphoma
CD5	+	+	−	−	−
CD10	−	−/+	−	−	+
CD20	+	+	+	+	+
CD21	+	+/−	−	+/−	+
CD22	+	+	+	+	+
CD23	+	−	−	−	−
CD30	−	−	−	−	−
CD43	+	+	−/+	−/+	−
CD79a	+	+	+	+	+
ALK-FL	−	−	−	−	−
PRAD-1	−	+	−	−	−
bcl-2	+	+	+	+	+/−
bcl-6	−	−	−	−	+
c-myc	−	−	−	−	−/+
Tdt	−	−	−	−	−

[a]The expression patterns are based largely on a compilation of results in the WHO classification (1).

lineage extramedullary myeloid tumors may be positive. The expected antigen expression profiles in paraffin-embedded tissue useful in the differential diagnosis of the low-grade B-cell, high-grade B-cell, and T-cell lymphomas are listed in Tables 5.7, 5.8, and 5.9, respectively. The key advantage of immunohistochemistry in paraffin-embedded tissue is the correlation with the morphology of the lymphoma cells. In addition, antibodies to anaplastic

TABLE 5.8. *Antibodies reactive in paraffin-embedded tissue in high-grade B-cell neoplasms[a]*

Antigen	Diffuse large-cell lymphoma	Anaplastic large-cell lymphoma	Burkitt's lymphoma	Lymphoblastic lymphoma	Plasma-cell myeloma
CD5	−/+	−	−	−	−
CD10	+/−	−	+	+/−	−
CD20	+	+/−	+	−/+	−
CD21	+/−	+/−	+/−	−	−
CD22	+	+	+	+/−	−
CD23	−	−	−	−	−
CD30	−/+	+/−	−	−	+/−
CD43	−/+	−/+	−/+	+	−
CD79a	+	+/−	+	−/+	+/−
ALK-FL	−	+	−	−	−
PRAD-1	−	−	−	−	−/+
bcl-2	+/−	−/+	−	+/−	+
bcl-6	+	+/−	+	−	−
c-myc	−/+	−	+	−	−
Tdt	−	−	−	+	−

[a]The expression patterns are based largely on a compilation of results in the WHO classification (1).

TABLE 5.9. *Antibodies reactive in paraffin-embedded tissue in T-cell and natural killer–cell lymphomas[a]*

Antigen	Peripheral T-cell lymphoma (not otherwise specified)	Peripheral T-cell lymphoma (angioimmunoblastic type)	Lymphoblastic lymphoma	Mycosis fungoides	Anaplastic large-cell lymphoma	Natural killer–cell lymphoma	Nasal T-cell lymphoma
CD2	+	+	+/–	+	+/–	–/+	+
CD3s	+	+	+/–	+	–/+	–	–
CD3c	+/–	+	+	–/+	+/–	+/–	+
CD4	+	+/–	+	+	+/–	+	–
CD5	–/+	+/–	–/+	+	–/+	–	–
CD7	–/+	–/+	+	–	–/+	–/+	–/+
CD8	–	–/+	+	–	–	–	–
CD10	–	+	+/–	–	–	–	–
CD30	–/+	–/+	–	–	+	–	–/+
CD43	+	+	+	+	+/–	–/+	–
CD34	–	–	–/+	–	–	–/+	–
TIA-I	–/+	–	–	–	+/–	–/+	+
Gran B	–/+	–	–	–	+/–	–/+	+
ALK	–	–	–	–	+/–	–	–
CD56	–/+	–	–	–	–	+	+
Tdt	–	–	+	–	–	–/+	–
TCRB	+/–	+/–	+	+/–	–	–	+/–
CD45	+	+/–	+	+	+/–	+/–	+/–

[a]The expression patterns are based largely on a compilation of results in the WHO classification (1).

lymphoma kinase, PRAD1, bcl-6, c-myc, TIA-I, granzyme B, and CD30 are not routinely used in flow cytometry.

Differential Diagnosis from Hodgkin's Disease

In many cases of classical Hodgkin's disease, a straightforward immunophenotype to support the diagnosis is obtained (Table 5.10). This includes positivity for CD30 and CD15 and negativity for CD3, CD20, and CD45 (23,24). However, there are some cases of Hodgkin's disease where the Reed-Sternberg cells are sheeting out, and a variant phenotype is obtained, which makes the diagnosis difficult to differentiate from anaplastic large-cell lymphoma, or diffuse large B-cell lymphoma. Also, it is known that CD15 is negative in 10% to 15% of cases of classical Hodgkin's disease (25). To compound matters, CD20 is positive in a significant number of cases of classical Hodgkin's disease, although the cellular expression is usually variable. The reactivity of CD45 and the presence of immunoglobulin gene

TABLE 5.10. *Differential diagnosis of classical Hodgkin's disease, lymphocyte-predominant Hodgkin's disease, and non-Hodgkin's lymphoma*

Antigen	Classical Hodgkin's disease	Lymphocyte-predominant Hodgkin's disease	B-cell non-Hodgkin's lymphoma
CD3	–	–	–
CD20	–/+	+	+
CD15	+/–	–	–
CD30	+	–	–/+
CD45	–	+	+
EMA	–	+	–
EBERS	+/–	–	–/+

EMA, epithelial membrane antigen; EBERS, Epstein-Barr virus, early RNA sequences.

TABLE 5.11. *Factors affecting immunohistochemistry–in situ hybridization results*

Problem	Result
Delay in processing	Autolysis; RNA loss
Inadequate fixation	Distortion, poor antigen preservation
Overfixation	Poor antigen retrieval
Different antibody clones	Variant results between labs
Different fixative	Variant performance of antibody

rearrangements assist in the diagnosis of non-Hodgkin's lymphoma. In lymphocyte-predominant Hodgkin's disease, the variant L and H cells are expected to be CD20+, along with CD45 positivity (26). Epithelial membrane antigen, which is seen in approximately 50% of cases, aids in the diagnosis of lymphocyte-predominant Hodgkin's disease.

Variation in Immunohistochemistry Results

Discrepancies in immunohistochemical results between laboratories can occur for at least four reasons: (a) choice of a formalin-fixed tissue block by one laboratory and a B5- (or heavy metal–) fixed tissue by a second laboratory, (b) use of an inadequately fixed tissue in one lab and overfixed tissue in the second lab, (c) use of antibodies that target different epitopes, and (d) suboptimal immunohistochemistry protocols (Table 5.11). These variations could lead to different interpretations of immunophenotypic results, thus resulting in a difference in the subclassification of the lymphoma. Fortunately, the common antibodies used for routine B- and T-cell phenotyping are robust reagents.

Selection of Immunophenotyping Techniques

Some of the advantages and disadvantages of each of the different approaches to immunophenotyping are summarized in Table 5.12. In any given case, the best approach depends on the size and type of specimen submitted for analysis, the suspected or known disease process, and the antigens being examined. In some cases, the different techniques will be complementary. Close communication between the oncologist, surgeon, and pathologist is critical to ensuring that the best use of the tissue available for diagnosis is made.

TABLE 5.12. *Advantages and disadvantages of immunophenotyping techniques*

	Flow cytometry	Frozen immunohistochemistry	Fixed, paraffin-embedded immunohistochemistry
Advantages	Greatest sensitivity Large numbers of cells analyzed Rapid Reproducible Quantitative Methods are standardized Can easily analyze multiple features simultaneously on the same cell Automated method	Architectural and cytologic features of stained cells are preserved Sensitive Most antigens are well preserved during freezing More antibodies are available than for fixed tissues Can be automated for improved reproducibility	Fixed tissue is routinely available Can be performed on archival tissue Architectural and cytologic features are well preserved Special retrieval techniques can be used to enhance the identification of some antigens Can be automated for improved reproducibility
Disadvantages	Requires fresh viable tissue for phenotyping Architectural features are not preserved Inadequate sampling of partially involved tissues can lead to false negatives Low cellular viability in large-cell lymphoma can result in false negatives Not useful for Hodgkin's disease	Frozen tissue is not always preserved at the time of biopsy Cytologic features are not as well preserved as in paraffin-embedded tissue Double-staining is relatively difficult to interpret Difficult to standardize Data are difficult to quantitate	Fewer antibodies reactive in paraffin-embedded tissues are available Reactivity of some antibodies is fixative-dependent Antigen preservation is less than in fresh or frozen tissue due to antigen loss during fixation and processing Double-staining is relatively difficult to perform and interpret Difficult to standardize Data are difficult to quantitate

REFERENCES

1. Jaffe ES, Harris NL, Stein H, et al. The pathology and genetics of tumours of haematopoietic and lymphoid tissues. In: Kleihauer Psorion L, ed. *World Health Organization classifications of tumors*, 1st ed. Lyon: IARC Press, 2001.
2. Harris NL, Jaffe ES, Stein H, et al. A revised European-American classification of lymphoid neoplasms: a proposal from the International Lymphoma Study Group. *Blood* 1994;84:1361–1392.
3. McCoy P. Basic principles in clinical flow cytometry. In: Kern DF, McCoy P Jr, Carey JL, eds. *Flow cytometry in clinical diagnosis*, 3rd ed. Chicago: ASCP Press, 2002:31–97.
4. Stelzer GT, Marti G, Hurley A, et al. U.S.–Canadian Consensus recommendations on the immunophenotypic analysis of hematologic neoplasia by flow cytometry: standardization and validation of laboratory procedures. *Cytometry* 1997;30:214–230.
5. Stelzer GT, Shults KE, Loken MR. CD45 gating for routine flow cytometric analysis of human bone marrow specimens. *Ann N Y Acad Sci* 1993;677:265–280.
6. Stewart CC, Behm FG, Carey JL, et al. U.S.–Canadian Consensus recommendations on the immunophenotypic analysis of hematologic neoplasia by flow cytometry: selection of antibody combinations. *Cytometry* 1997;30:231–235.
7. Davis BH, Foucar K, Szczarkowski W, et al. U.S.–Canadian Consensus recommendations on the immunophenotypic analysis of hematologic neoplasia by flow cytometry: medical indications. *Cytometry* 1997;30:249–263.
8. Carey JL. Immunophenotyping in diagnosis and prognosis of mature lymphoid leukemias and lymphomas. In: Keren DF, McCoy P, Carey JL, eds. *Flow cytometry in clinical diagnosis*, 3rd ed. Chicago: ASCP Press, 2002:227–338.
9. Borowitz MJ, Bray R, Gascoyne R, et al. U.S.–Canadian Consensus recommendations on the immunophenotypic analysis of hematologic neoplasia by flow cytometry: data analysis and interpretation. *Cytometry* 1997;30:236–244.
10. Rothe G, Schmitz G. Consensus protocol for the flow cytometric immunophenotyping of hematopoietic malignancies. Working Group on Flow Cytometry and Image Analysis. *Leukemia* 1996;10:877–895.
11. Rainer RO, Hodges L, Seltzer GT. CD45 gating correlates with bone marrow differential. *Cytometry* 1995;22:139–145.
12. Braylan RC, Atwater SK, Diamond L, et al. U.S.–Canadian Consensus recommendations on the immunophenotypic analysis of hematologic neoplasia by flow cytometry: data reporting. *Cytometry* 1997;30:245–248.
13. Taylor CR. The current role of immunohistochemistry in diagnostic pathology. In: *Advances in pathology and laboratory medicine*, vol. 7. St. Louis: Mosby–Year Book, 1994:59–105.
14. Dorfman DM, Pinkus GS. Utility of immunophenotypic studies in the diagnosis of low-grade lymphoma of mucosa-associated lymphoid tissue (MALT) and other low-grade non-Hodgkin's lymphomas of extranodal sites. *Appl Immunohistochem* 1995;3:160–167.
15. Gelb AB, Rouse RV, Dorfman RF, et al. Detection of immunophenotypic abnormalities in paraffin-embedded B-lineage non-Hodgkin's lymphomas. *Am J Clin Pathol* 1994;102:825–834.
16. Weisenburger DD, Gascoyne RD, Bierman PJ, et al. Clinical significance of the t(14;18) and BCL2 overexpression in follicular large cell lymphoma. *Leuk Lymphoma* 2000;36:513–523.
17. Zukerberg LR, Yang WI, Arnold A, et al. Cyclin D1 expression in non-Hodgkin's lymphomas. Detection by immunohistochemistry. *Am J Clin Pathol* 1995;103:756–760.
18. Gascoyne RD, Aoun P, Wu D, et al. Prognostic significance of anaplastic lymphoma kinase (ALK) protein expression in adults with anaplastic large cell lymphoma. *Blood* 1999;93:3913–3921.
19. Griffin CA, Hawkins AL, Dvorak C, et al. Recurrent involvement of 2p23 in inflammatory myofibroblastic tumors. *Cancer Res* 1999;59:2776–2780.
20. Jaffe ES, Raffeld M, Medeiros LJ. Histopathologic subtypes of indolent lymphomas: caricatures of the mature B-cell system. *Semin Oncol* 1993;20:3–30.
21. de Leon ED, Alkan S, Huang JC, et al. Usefulness of an immunohistochemical panel in paraffin-embedded tissues for the differentiation of B-cell non-Hodgkin's lymphomas of small lymphocytes. *Mod Pathol* 1998;11:1046–1051.
22. Jaffe ES, Raffeld M, Medeiros LJ, et al. An overview of the classification of non-Hodgkin's lymphomas: an integration of morphological and phenotypical concepts. *Cancer Res* 1992;52:5447s–5452s.
23. Hsu SM, Jaffe ES. Leu M1 and peanut agglutinin stain the neoplastic cells of Hodgkin's disease. *Am J Clin Pathol* 1984;82:29–32.
24. Stein H, Mason DY, Gerdes J, et al. The expression of the Hodgkin's disease associated antigen Ki-1 in reactive and neoplastic lymphoid tissue: evidence that Reed-Sternberg cells and histiocytic malignancies are derived from activated lymphoid cells. *Blood* 1985;66:848–858.
25. Vasef MA, Alsabeh R, Medeiros LJ, et al. Immunophenotype of Reed-Sternberg and Hodgkin's cells in sequential biopsy specimens of Hodgkin's disease: a paraffin-section immunohistochemical study using the heat-induced epitope retrieval method. *Am J Clin Pathol* 1997;108:54–59.
26. Pinkus GS, Said JW. Hodgkin's disease, lymphocyte predominance type, nodular—a distinct entity? Unique staining profile for L&H variants of Reed-Sternberg cells defined by monoclonal antibodies to leukocyte common antigen, granulocyte-specific antigen, and B-cell-specific antigen. *Am J Pathol* 1985;118:1–6.

CHAPTER 6

Gray Zone, Synchronous, and Metachronous Lymphomas: Diseases at the Interface of Hodgkin's and Non-Hodgkin's Lymphomas

Elaine S. Jaffe and Wyndham H. Wilson

Considerable progress has been made regarding the origin of the neoplastic cell in classical Hodgkin's disease, *the Reed-Sternberg cell*. Recent evidence shows it is a B cell in all or nearly all cases. If Hodgkin's disease is derived from an altered B lymphocyte, it is not surprising that areas of overlap with B-cell non-Hodgkin's lymphoma should occur both biologically and clinically (Fig. 6.1) (1). The Reed-Sternberg cell is a crippled B cell incapable of immunoglobulin secretion. The biologic and molecular events leading to this state are complex and not fully resolved (2,3). These events may occur in the context of a relatively normal immune system, as seen in most patients with Hodgkin's disease, or in the setting of immunodeficiency (4–8). In addition, cells resembling Reed-Sternberg cells and variants may be observed in disease states not meeting all diagnostic criteria for Hodgkin's disease and may represent early steps in the transformation to Hodgkin's disease (7,9). The study of lymphomas at the interface of Hodgkin's disease and non-Hodgkin's lymphoma may provide insight into the pathogenesis of *de novo* Hodgkin's disease and the molecular and cellular events distinguishing it from lymphoma.

Gray zone lymphoma is defined as a process at the histologic interface between Hodgkin's lymphoma and non-Hodgkin's lymphomas. Similarly, *synchronous lymphomas* of discordant histologies can involve a combination of Hodgkin's disease and non-Hodgkin's lymphoma. Some of the first *metachronous lymphomas* described involved the late presentation of lymphoma after Hodgkin's disease; however, the opposite sequence also occurs. Hodgkin's disease and non-Hodgkin's lymphoma have long been regarded as distinct disease entities based on differences in pathology, immunophenotype, clinical features, and response to therapy. Recent observations, however, suggest that these disorders may be more closely related than previously thought and provide insight into the biology of gray zone and synchronous/metachronous lymphomas.

We limit the use of the term *gray zone lymphoma* to those cases in which morphologic, biologic, and clinical features

suggest overlap between Hodgkin's disease and non-Hodgkin's lymphoma (10). Disorders in which a biologic interface is proposed are classical Hodgkin's disease with T-cell–rich large B-cell lymphomas and diffuse large B-cell lymphomas. A second category of gray zone lymphoma involves nodular lymphocyte–predominant Hodgkin's lymphoma and T-cell–rich large B-cell lymphoma. This topic is covered elsewhere (see Chapter 27). A similar but unrelated diagnostic issue involves those cases in which there may be diagnostic uncertainty but not true biologic overlap. The interface between anaplastic large cell lymphoma and classical Hodgkin's disease may be ambiguous histologically and immunophenotypically, but it does not represent a biologic gray zone (Fig. 6.2). This chapter discusses the pathobiology of these infrequent but important lymphoma disease states and provides clinical guidelines for treatment decisions.

Other benign and malignant conditions contain Reed-Sternberg-like cells that may mimic Hodgkin's disease. These conditions are best discussed in the context of differential diagnosis and, for the most part, are not covered here.

PATHOBIOLOGY AND DIAGNOSIS

Gray Zone Lymphomas—Interface between Classical Hodgkin's Disease and Large B-Cell Lymphoma

Hodgkin's and Mediastinal Large B-Cell Lymphoma

One of the more common gray zone lymphomas, which also may present as a composite lymphoma, involves mediastinal (thymic) large B-cell lymphoma and nodular sclerosis Hodgkin's disease (11–13). Nodular sclerosis Hodgkin's disease and mediastinal large B-cell lymphoma share a number of common clinical features: They both show a female predominance; present in young adults, albeit at a slightly older age in mediastinal large B-cell lymphoma; and involve the anterior mediastinum, thymus gland, and supraclavicular lymph nodes (14–16).

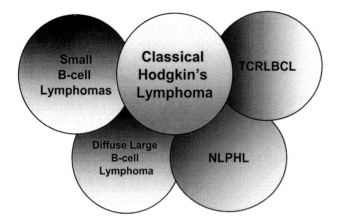

FIG. 6.1. Biologic gray zones in Hodgkin's (HL) and non-Hodgkin's lymphomas. HL is derived from an altered B lymphocyte. The precise molecular events that result in the Reed-Sternberg cell are not fully elucidated; however, it is likely that these events can occur *de novo*, in a normal B cell, or secondarily, in a neoplastic B cell. Therefore, biologic interfaces are identified between HL and diverse subtypes of B-cell lymphoma. NLPHL, nodular lymphocyte–predominant HL; TCRLBCL, T-cell–rich B-cell lymphoma.

In gray zone lymphoma cases, the histologic and immunophenotypic features are transitional between nodular sclerosis Hodgkin's disease and mediastinal large B-cell lymphoma. Clusters of cells akin to lacunar cells or even classical Reed-Sternberg cells may be seen in a background resembling mediastinal large B-cell lymphoma. In some cases, the histology is composite, with some areas resembling nodular sclerosis Hodgkin's disease and other areas showing sheets of large B cells characteristic of mediastinal large B-cell lymphoma. The

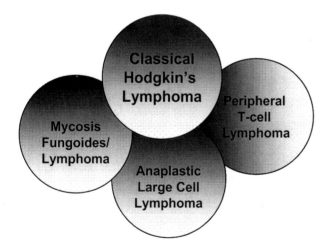

FIG. 6.2. Morphologic gray zones in Hodgkin's (HL) and non-Hodgkin's (NHL) lymphomas. In contrast to true biologic interfaces, morphologic interfaces occur between HL and other non-Hodgkin's lymphomas. These morphologic interfaces may cause problems in differential diagnosis, but they do not reflect an underlying biologic relationship.

inflammatory background and pattern of sclerosis usually corresponds to the appearance of the neoplastic cells, resembling nodular sclerosis Hodgkin's disease or mediastinal large B-cell lymphoma, respectively. Immunophenotypically, the features also are intermediate. Scattered Reed-Sternberg-like cells are CD30+, but CD15 positivity is more inconsistent. Interestingly, the CD30 antigen is often expressed in mediastinal large B-cell lymphoma (17). The majority of the infiltrating cells are usually CD20+, sometimes with variable staining intensity. Nodular sclerosis Hodgkin's disease and mediastinal large B-cell lymphoma are negative for immunoglobulin expression; thus, studies of immunoglobulin are noninformative (18,19).

Mediastinal large B-cell lymphoma has been reported following Hodgkin's disease, but in contrast to most lymphomas that typically present 10 years or longer after the diagnosis of Hodgkin's disease, mediastinal large B-cell lymphoma presents early, frequently within 1 year (12). This close association suggests a different pathogenesis for secondary mediastinal large B-cell lymphoma compared to the late-occurring lymphomas, and it raises the likely possibility that these cases are clonally related to the Hodgkin's disease (20). Nodular sclerosis Hodgkin's disease and mediastinal large B-cell lymphoma also share a number of molecular characteristics, such as REL amplification and gains on chromosome 9, suggesting molecular overlap as well (21,22). Studies have identified the MAL gene as aberrantly expressed in mediastinal large B-cell lymphoma, but expression of MAL has not been investigated in nodular sclerosis Hodgkin's disease (23).

At a workshop exploring the interrelationship of Hodgkin's disease and non-Hodgkin's lymphoma, several cases were presented that relate to a possible association of mediastinal large B-cell lymphoma and nodular sclerosis Hodgkin's disease (10). Five cases had a transitional histologic appearance, showing features of Hodgkin's disease and mediastinal large B-cell lymphoma. The histology in these cases most closely resembled a diffuse large cell lymphoma with sheeting out of malignant cells, a sparse inflammatory background, and infiltration of adjacent soft tissue. Fibrous bands were absent (three cases) or focal (two cases). Necrosis, which is usually a prominent feature in histologically aggressive nodular sclerosis Hodgkin's disease (grade II), was absent or focal. Most of the cases, however, did show some vague nodularity reminiscent of that seen in nodular sclerosis Hodgkin's disease.

The immunohistochemical phenotype of these cases was also "transitional." Although all cases were CD30+ and four of the five cases were CD15+, CD20 and CD79a were expressed on the neoplastic cells in the majority of cases. The neoplastic cells were frequently positive for leukocyte-common antigen as well. Thus, the immunologic phenotype was intermediate between that of a diffuse large cell lymphoma and Hodgkin's disease. All cases were negative for Epstein-Barr virus (EBV), arguing against a role for EBV in the process.

The clinical course in these patients was generally aggressive, and many had relapsed after conventional treatment for Hodgkin's disease. In addition, relapse often occurred at distant sites that are common for mediastinal large B-cell lymphoma, such as kidneys or central nervous system. An unexpected finding based on review of the literature and the cases presented at the workshop is that most of these cases presented in males (10 of 11). This fact is surprising because both nodular sclerosis Hodgkin's disease and mediastinal large B-cell lymphoma are more common in females than males. Whether mediastinal large B-cell lymphoma represents an unusual evolution of nodular sclerosis Hodgkin's disease in these patients is purely speculative.

Hodgkin's Lymphoma and T-Cell–Rich Large B-Cell Lymphoma

Since 1991, several groups have reported cases that histologically resemble Hodgkin's disease but have an immunophenotype of T-cell–rich large B-cell lymphoma (24–27). The neoplastic cells are strongly CD20+ but negative for CD30 and CD15. These cases may resemble classical Hodgkin's disease or, more often, lymphocyte-predominant Hodgkin's disease (28). Epithelial membrane antigen is typically expressed in those T-cell–rich large B-cell lymphoma cases resembling nodular lymphocyte–predominant Hodgkin's lymphoma but is negative in many other cases (27,29).

Modern biologic studies of Hodgkin's disease have suggested that classical Hodgkin's disease may in fact be a form of T-cell–rich large B-cell lymphoma (30). In both diseases, the malignant cell is a B lymphocyte, and both have an inflammatory background comprised mostly of T cells (31). They usually have qualitative differences, however. Classical Hodgkin's disease, for example, shows significant variation among the Reed-Sternberg cells in B-cell antigen expression, and in morphologically borderline cases in which all neoplastic cells are strongly CD20+, the diagnosis of T-cell–rich large B-cell lymphoma is favored (32,33). Clinically, T-cell–rich large B-cell lymphoma has a more aggressive course than Hodgkin's disease and frequently does not adequately respond to conventional therapy for Hodgkin's disease (26,28). Interestingly, the expression of B-cell antigens by >20% of malignant cells in Hodgkin's disease was found to be an adverse prognostic factor by the German Hodgkin Study Group (34). Other immunophenotypic markers may be of value in this differential diagnosis. Positivity for BCL-6, CD79a, and leukocyte-common antigen favors T-cell–rich large B-cell lymphoma, whereas staining for CD30, CD15, or latent membrane protein–1 favors Hodgkin's disease. A common clonal origin has been identified in rare cases of Hodgkin's disease and T-cell–rich large B-cell lymphoma occurring in the same patient, further suggesting that the distinction between classical Hodgkin's disease and T-cell–rich large B-cell lymphoma is a biologic gray zone (35,36).

Hodgkin's Lymphoma and Epstein-Barr Virus–Positive Lymphoproliferative Disorders

Patients with rheumatologic disorders on long-term methotrexate immunosuppression are at increased risk of developing EBV-positive lymphoproliferative disorders that may resemble Hodgkin's disease and non-Hodgkin's lymphoma (7,37,38).

Their etiology is most likely from chronic immunosuppression, rather than direct oncogenic effects, because the atypical lymphoproliferations may regress when immunosuppression is withdrawn (7,37). These cases may present as a spectrum of EBV-positive B-cell proliferations ranging from polymorphic B-cell lymphomas, as seen in solid-organ transplantation, to lymphomas resembling Hodgkin's disease and diffuse large cell lymphoma (39). The cases of lymphoproliferative disorders that resemble Hodgkin's disease often occur in soft tissue or other nonnodal sites, whereas cases with more typical Hodgkin's disease features tend to present in lymph nodes. Immunohistochemical studies may help to distinguish typical Hodgkin's disease from lymphoproliferative disorders; the atypical cells in lymphoproliferative disorders are usually negative for CD15, although as in Hodgkin's disease, CD30 may be positive, with antigenic expression induced by EBV (40–42). It is of interest that classical Hodgkin's disease is relatively uncommon following solid-organ transplantation; however, an increased risk of Hodgkin's disease following allogeneic bone marrow transplantation has been observed, and virtually all cases are EBV positive (43).

Interface between Classical Hodgkin's Disease and Anaplastic Large Cell Lymphoma

Classical Hodgkin's disease and anaplastic large cell lymphoma share some immunophenotypic features such as CD30 antigen expression, which led to early speculation that they were related (44,45). Subsequent studies, however, showed them to be distinct diseases without true biologic or clinical overlap. The neoplastic cells of anaplastic large cell lymphoma usually express one or more T-cell–associated antigens and have a cytotoxic phenotype, whereas the malignant cells of Hodgkin's disease usually lack cytotoxic antigens, such as TIA-1, granzyme B, and perforin (46,47). One early report suggested that the t(2;5)(p23;q35) characteristic of anaplastic large cell lymphoma, could be detected by a sensitive reverse transcription–polymerase chain reaction (PCR) method in some cases of classical Hodgkin's disease (48), but this finding could not be confirmed by subsequent genetic or immunophenotypic studies (49–53).

Hodgkin's-related anaplastic large cell lymphoma was initially described as a form of anaplastic large cell lymphoma closely resembling Hodgkin's disease (54,55). Patients were often young males with mediastinal masses who responded poorly to conventional therapy for Hodgkin's disease but appeared to respond to third-generation lymphoma chemotherapy regimens. It is now apparent that most of these cases are aggressive forms of Hodgkin's disease, probably within the spectrum of grade II nodular sclerosis Hodgkin's disease (39,50,56–58). The sheeting out of large numbers of CD30+ cells, often without CD15 positivity, led investigators to favor anaplastic large cell lymphoma. The poor prognosis associated with these cases may be related to the known poorer prognosis of massive mediastinal Hodgkin's disease and grade II nodular sclerosis Hodgkin's disease (59,60).

By contrast, some cases of anaplastic large cell lymphoma histologically resemble nodular sclerosis Hodgkin's disease, having a vaguely nodular growth pattern and areas of fibrosis. Anaplastic large cell lymphoma, however, usually lacks a prominent inflammatory background of eosinophils, neutrophils, and plasma cells, although histiocytes may be abundant. Moreover, careful immunophenotypic evaluation usually reveals an absence of CD15, expression of epithelial membrane antigen, and some T-cell associated antigens. Positivity for the ALK tyrosine kinase may further confirm the diagnosis of anaplastic large cell lymphoma (53,56). Finally, mediastinal involvement is rare in anaplastic large cell lymphoma, in contrast to its prevalence in nodular sclerosis Hodgkin's disease.

Synchronous Lymphomas

Synchronous lymphomas may be defined as the simultaneous occurrence of two lymphoma subtypes within a single patient. These may be further distinguished by presentations within the same anatomic site, termed *composite lymphoma*, and presentations in different sites, termed *discordant lymphoma*. Although the definition of composite lymphoma historically has been broadly applied to the presence of two variants of lymphoma, in most cases, phenotypic and genotypic studies have indicated that the two histologies are clonally related. For example, diffuse large cell lymphoma that occurs with follicular lymphomas is considered evidence of histologic progression within the same B-cell clone (61). As such, the term *composite lymphoma* has been more narrowly defined to situations in which the clonal relationship of the two neoplasms is more ambiguous. As with the B-cell lymphoma, an analysis of composite Hodgkin's disease and non-Hodgkin's lymphoma may shed light on the nature of molecular events associated with both malignancies.

Hodgkin's and B-Cell Non-Hodgkin's Lymphomas

Composite lymphoma may be more narrowly defined as the simultaneous occurrence of Hodgkin's disease and non-Hodgkin's lymphoma in the same anatomic site or biopsy specimen (62,63). Composite Hodgkin's disease and non-Hodgkin's lymphoma most often represents a B-cell lymphoma in association with classical Hodgkin's disease, usually of the nodular sclerosis or mixed cellularity subtype. The type of B-cell lymphoma involved reflects the incidence of B-cell lymphoma subtypes in the population, such that most composite lymphomas involve Hodgkin's disease with follicular lymphoma or diffuse large cell lymphoma (11,35,36,64,65). Uncommonly, other types of B-cell lymphoma may be seen in association with classical Hodgkin's disease, including marginal zone B-cell lymphoma and mantle cell lymphoma (66). The association of chronic lymphocytic leukemia with Hodgkin's disease has some distinctive features and is discussed separately.

Biopsy specimens usually show a segregation of the two histologic patterns within the lymph node. In some instances, however, the Hodgkin's disease and non-Hodgkin's lym-

phoma may be more intertwined, such as some cases involving follicular lymphoma in which the Hodgkin's disease may be found in the interfollicular paracortical regions. Immunohistochemical studies are usually required for the diagnosis of a composite lymphoma. The neoplastic cells of the Hodgkin's disease component should retain the classical phenotype of Hodgkin's disease: CD30$^+$, CD15$^+$, and negative for leukocyte-common antigen and B-cell–associated and T-cell–associated antigens. A minority of the Reed-Sternberg cells in a composite lymphoma also may be CD20$^+$, as seen in other cases of classical Hodgkin's disease (32). Studies to show a clonal relationship are difficult to perform, as it is difficult to isolate the Reed-Sternberg cells. In rare cases employing single-cell microdissection, however, a clonal relationship has been demonstrated (35,67).

EBV has been implicated in the pathogenesis of many cases of Hodgkin's disease and is most often associated with the mixed cellularity and lymphocyte-depleted subtypes. EBV also has been investigated in composite lymphomas, and in most cases studied, it was concordantly expressed or not in both components (Tables 6.1 and 6.2) (68). Overall, approximately 33% of composite lymphomas are positive for EBV sequences in the neoplastic cells. In all EBV-positive cases, the lymphoma component was an aggressive B-cell lymphoma, either diffuse large cell lymphoma or Burkitt-like lymphoma, whereas all composite follicular lymphoma and Hodgkin's disease cases were EBV negative. Only limited

TABLE 6.1. *Interrelationship between classical Hodgkin's lymphoma and non-Hodgkin's lymphomas*

	NHL subtypes (%)[a]	Associated with EBV
NHL following cHL	Large B cell (45)	14% of all B-cell subtypes
	Burkitt/Burkitt-like (45)	(Mainly in high-grade subtypes)
	Other B cell (10)	
Composite cHL/NHL	Follicular (45)	No
	Large B cell (45)	50% (in both HL and NHL)
	Other B cell (10)	No
cHL following NHL[b]	CLL	90% (in HL)
	Follicular lymphoma	No
	Large B-cell	No
	Mycosis fungoides	ND
	Other PTL (rare)	Yes

cHL, classical Hodgkin's lymphoma; CLL, chronic lymphocytic leukemia; EBV, Epstein-Barr virus; HL, Hodgkin's lymphoma; ND, not determined; NHL, non-Hodgkin's lymphoma; PTL, peripheral T-cell lymphomas.

[a](%) Approximate distribution of associated lymphomas and lymphocytic leukemias based on published data.

[b]Accurate relative incidence figures for cHL following NHL are not available; only most common associations are shown.

TABLE 6.2. *Summary of antigen expression in classical Hodgkin's lymphoma, T-cell–rich large B-cell lymphoma, and mediastinal large B-cell lymphoma*

	CD30	CD20	CD79a	CD15	EBV	BCL-6
Classical HL	+	–/+	–	+	+/–	–
TCRLBCL	–	+	+	–	–/+	+/–
M-LBCL	–/+	+	–/+	–	–	+/–

HL, Hodgkin's lymphoma; M-LBCL, mediastinal large B-cell lymphoma; TCRLBCL, T-cell–rich large B-cell lymphoma.

molecular studies have been applied to composite lymphomas. With the advent of techniques permitting the microdissection of individual tumor cells, it is likely that future studies will shed more light on the interrelationship of Hodgkin's disease and non-Hodgkin's lymphoma in composite lymphomas.

The coexistence of classical Hodgkin's disease with nodular lymphocyte–predominant Hodgkin's lymphoma also has been observed. Since the early 1990s, nodular lymphocyte–predominant Hodgkin's lymphoma has been considered a distinct entity, separable from classical Hodgkin's disease in virtually all cases on morphologic, immunophenotypic, and clinical grounds (69,70). Nodular lymphocyte–predominant Hodgkin's lymphoma has a mature B-cell phenotype and contains functional, rather than crippled, immunoglobulin genes (71,72). Just as classical Hodgkin's disease may occur in the setting of a lymphoma of B-cell phenotype, classical Hodgkin's disease has also been reported in association with rare cases of nodular lymphocyte–predominant Hodgkin's lymphoma (73–75).

Clinically, composite lymphomas present in an older age group, with a median age of 63 years in one study (11). This clinical presentation is more typical of the underlying lymphoma, and it coincides with the second "peak" seen in epidemiologic studies of Hodgkin's disease, which features a bimodal age distribution. The prognosis for patients with composite Hodgkin's disease and non-Hodgkin's lymphoma is most dependent on the histologic subtype of the lymphoma identified.

A situation closely related to composite lymphoma is discordant lymphomas in which Hodgkin's disease and non-Hodgkin's lymphoma simultaneously present in different anatomic sites (1). Only a small number of cases have been identified, perhaps because few patients undergo multiple simultaneous diagnostic biopsies at different sites. Although the true frequency of discordant Hodgkin's disease and non-Hodgkin's lymphoma is difficult to assess, it nevertheless appears to be a rare phenomenon. The distribution of the lymphoma subtypes encountered is similar to that of composite lymphoma, with follicular lymphomas and diffuse large cell lymphoma being the most frequent.

Metachronous Lymphomas

Patients with a history of lymphoma are at increased risk of developing a second, clonally unrelated lymphoma. Although the risk is low across all lymphoma subtypes, it is mostly confined to specific lymphoma subtypes, such as lymphoma after Hodgkin's disease and EBV-positive diffuse large cell lymphoma after angioimmunoblastic T-cell lymphoma, in which case the risk is not insignificant.

Non-Hodgkin's Lymphoma after Hodgkin's Lymphoma

Krikorian and colleagues were the first to report an increased incidence of lymphoma in patients successfully treated for Hodgkin's disease with an actuarial risk of 4.4% (76). Generally, these are late-occurring events, typically at least 5 years after Hodgkin's disease diagnosis, with a reported range of 1–26 years. Their etiology has been postulated to be related to the underlying defects in cell-mediated immunity that persist after treatment of Hodgkin's disease, and interestingly, their risk appears higher in patients with evidence of underlying immunodeficiency or immune suppression, such as low peripheral blood lymphocyte counts, advanced clinical stage, or systemic symptoms (12,77,78). Histologically, diffuse large cell lymphoma or high-grade B-cell lymphomas, such as Burkitt-like lymphoma, are most commonly seen, although low-grade lymphomas can also rarely occur, and the histology does not appear to be related to Hodgkin's disease subtype or treatment (12,78,79). Virtually all cases are of B-cell phenotype, and most patients present with intraabdominal disease with pathologic and clinical features similar to aggressive B-cell lymphomas seen in other immunodeficiency states, such as AIDS. Based on these findings, one might expect these secondary lymphomas to be EBV positive, but this is an uncommon finding; EBER1 mRNA was only found in two of 14 (14%) lymphoma cases by *in situ* hybridization, and two cases of simultaneous Hodgkin's disease and diffuse large cell lymphoma were also EBV negative (68). The absence of EBV, however, does not preclude the etiologic role of immune deficiency. Parallels may be drawn with AIDS-related lymphomas in which EBV-negative Burkitt's lymphomas with c-myc oncogene rearrangements are observed (80). Indeed, a similar pathogenesis may be operative in secondary lymphoma in which Burkitt-like lymphoma is also observed, along with evidence of polyclonal B-cell hyperplasia and plasmacytosis, similar to HIV-positive patients. Although these findings are of interest, they do not shed light on the clonal relationship between the Hodgkin's disease and secondary non-Hodgkin's lymphoma. One case study, however, has provided evidence for two distinct B-cell clones in the tumors using a single-cell microdissection assay and PCR amplification (81).

Hodgkin's Disease after Non-Hodgkin's Lymphoma

Compared to the risk of lymphoma after Hodgkin's disease, the risk of Hodgkin's disease after lymphoma is rare. Carrato and colleagues reported five cases occurring 5 to 23 years after a primary diagnosis of lymphoma (82). Travis et al. reviewed the experience of the national Surveillance, Epidemiology, and End Results Cancer Registry and found Hodgkin's disease to be the most common cancer after lymphoma, with an observed-to-expected risk ratio of 4.16:1, even more common than treatment-related leukemias (83). In a study expanding on

Hodgkin's disease after non-Hodgkin's lymphoma, all cases involved a B-cell lymphoma, mostly follicular lymphoma or diffuse large cell lymphoma, with presentation at a median patient age of 54 years (12). The median interval between non-Hodgkin's lymphoma and Hodgkin's disease was 5 years, and most patients had received chemotherapy alone or in combination with radiation therapy. Nodular sclerosis Hodgkin's disease was the most common histologic subtype in this study, with lymph node presentation in all cases, and most patients responded to treatment. Hodgkin's disease has also been reported in association with T-cell malignancies, most commonly mycosis fungoides and chronic lymphocytic lymphoma.

Expectedly, the immunologic phenotypes of the Hodgkin's disease and non-Hodgkin's lymphoma were discordant. In one study of bcl-2 rearrangements investigated by PCR in 32 unselected cases of Hodgkin's disease, only two showed bcl-2 rearrangements, and both occurred in patients with a prior follicular lymphoma (84). In one case, identical chromosomal breakpoints were identified in the Hodgkin's disease and the follicular lymphoma, suggesting a clonal relationship between the two tumors. Given the sensitivity of PCR, however, it is difficult to rule out the presence of small numbers of contaminating follicular lymphoma B-cells in the lymph node. In a separate study that investigated EBV in Hodgkin's disease after non-Hodgkin's lymphoma, no EBV was found in the Reed-Sternberg cells, a somewhat unexpected finding given the role of EBV in Hodgkin's disease after chronic lymphocytic lymphoma (68).

Hodgkin's Lymphoma and Chronic Lymphocytic Leukemia

The development of lymphomas resembling Hodgkin's disease in patients with chronic lymphocytic lymphoma is well recognized and had been considered a form of *Richter's transformation* (85,86). It was often assumed that these cases represented pleomorphic non-Hodgkin's lymphoma resembling Hodgkin's disease, rather than true Hodgkin's disease (87–89). More recently, however, several groups have histologically and immunophenotypically documented the association of Hodgkin's disease and chronic lymphocytic lymphoma (90,91). Two histologic patterns have been observed (92,93). In one, the Hodgkin's disease is histologically segregated from the chronic lymphocytic lymphoma, involving a different lymph node or anatomic site or occurring within a single lymph node (92,94). In these cases, Reed-Sternberg cells and variants are found in the usual cellular milieu of Hodgkin's disease with numerous T lymphocytes, plasma cells, eosinophils, and other inflammatory cells. The Reed-Sternberg cells display a typical phenotype for classical Hodgkin's disease and are usually EBV positive by *in situ* hybridization, and CD20 is often expressed by some Reed-Sternberg cells.

The second pattern, which is more frequently encountered, shows Reed-Sternberg cells and variants in a background of otherwise typical chronic lymphocytic lymphoma without the cellular background of Hodgkin's disease (64,90). Although the Reed-Sternberg cells are surrounded by small lymphocytes, closer inspection using immunohistochemical studies shows they are rosetted by T cells, as is typical of Hodgkin's disease, with the surrounding B cells showing a classical chronic lymphocytic lymphoma phenotype and monoclonality (90). This process is considered a form of composite lymphoma, because both diseases are present in the same anatomic site. Immunohistochemical studies show an unusual phenotype in the Reed-Sternberg cells with CD30 and CD15 expression, and variable expression of some B-cell antigens. EBV appears to play a major role in the development of Hodgkin's disease in this setting, with more than 90% of cases studied showing EBV by *in situ* hybridization or staining for latent membrane protein–1 (95). Although most of the background chronic lymphocytic lymphoma cells are negative for EBV, a small number of EBV-positive cells are often found. In one study, EBV was identified in a small population of lymphocytes in the underlying chronic lymphocytic lymphoma several years before the development of Hodgkin's disease, suggesting EBV infection of chronic lymphocytic lymphoma B lymphocytes may be an initial step in lymphomagenesis (93). Rare cases of EBV-negative Hodgkin's disease have been described, indicating other mechanisms of lymphomagenesis (96).

One study examined the clonal relationship between chronic lymphocytic lymphoma and Hodgkin's disease using microdissection techniques and PCR amplification of immunoglobulin heavy chain genes (IgH) in two cases and found identical IgH CDRIII sequences in the Reed-Sternberg and chronic lymphocytic lymphoma cells (97). This study provides further evidence that the Reed-Sternberg cells in chronic lymphocytic lymphoma and classical Hodgkin's disease are derived from transformed B lymphocytes.

Clinically, the development of Hodgkin's disease in a patient with chronic lymphocytic lymphoma usually portends an aggressive clinical course that is associated with advanced and poorly responsive disease (92,95). The median survival is <2 years after the diagnosis of Hodgkin's disease. It is interesting to speculate on the role of immune deficiency in the development of Hodgkin's disease after chronic lymphocytic lymphoma. Patients with chronic lymphocytic lymphoma typically display defects in cellular and humoral immunity and have an increased risk of viral infections. Perhaps an increased EBV viral load is associated with the secondary development of Hodgkin's disease. In this regard, it has been suggested that treatment with fludarabine, which leads to profound lymphopenia, may increase the risk of secondary Hodgkin's disease (98).

Hodgkin's and T-Cell Lymphomas

T-cell lymphomas are much less often reported in association with Hodgkin's disease than B-cell lymphomas (99). The relative risk of secondary Hodgkin's disease may be equivalent in both B- and T-cell lymphomas but T-cell lymphomas are much less common, or the biology of T-cell lymphomas may not predispose to secondary Hodgkin's disease. Alternatively, the difficulty in distinguishing Hodgkin's disease from peripheral T-cell lymphoma may lead to underreporting. Peripheral T-cell lymphoma is associated with a prominent inflammatory background and may contain pleomorphic cells resembling Reed-Sternberg cells that might incorrectly be considered a manifestation of the T-cell malignancy instead of Hodgkin's disease. However, if the association of Hodgkin's disease with non-Hodgkin's lymphoma is an indication of the clonal relationship of these disorders, as a B-cell origin is likely for most cases of Hodgkin's disease, it is not surprising that Hodgkin's disease is rarely found with T-cell lymphomas. In one well-documented case, cytogenetic studies were performed on the Hodgkin's disease and the associated peripheral T-cell lymphoma, and two distinct clones were found (100).

The most common association is that of Hodgkin's disease and mycosis fungoides, with more than 20 well-documented reports since 1979 (101–106). Moreover, some reports employing molecular techniques found distinct clonal origins for Hodgkin's disease and mycosis fungoides (105), showing in one instance a B-cell origin for the malignant cells of Hodgkin's disease and a T-cell origin for mycosis fungoides (106).

In cases of mycosis fungoides and Hodgkin's disease, the diagnosis of mycosis fungoides usually precedes Hodgkin's disease by months to years, further supporting the view that some of these cases represent pleomorphic T-cell lymphomas simulating Hodgkin's disease. In other cases, however, the diagnosis of Hodgkin's disease may precede mycosis fungoides or the two disorders may present simultaneously (101,107–109). A true association of mycosis fungoides and Hodgkin's disease is further supported by the diagnosis of Hodgkin's disease in the relatives of patients with mycosis fungoides (110). In a large epidemiological study of 526 patients with mycosis fungoides or Sézary syndrome, 21 had first-degree relatives with lymphoma or leukemia, one-third of which was Hodgkin's disease. Such observations suggest these disorders may share genetically influenced pathways of oncogenesis.

Cells resembling Reed-Sternberg cells both morphologically and immunophenotypically have been reported in a number of T-cell lymphoproliferative disorders, including mycosis fungoides, lymphomatoid papulosis, adult T-cell leukemia/lymphoma, and peripheral T-cell lymphoma unspecified (111–116). Studies of an association between mycosis fungoides, lymphomatoid papulosis, and Hodgkin's disease are complicated by the existence of common morphologic and immunophenotypic characteristics, such as CD15 and CD30, making it difficult to distinguish Hodgkin's disease from Hodgkin's-like lymphoproliferations (111,117–120). In one case studied with molecular techniques, a common clonal T-cell gene rearrangement was found in tissues involved by lymphomatoid papulosis, mycosis fungoides, and Hodgkin's disease, suggesting that these were all different manifestations of a single neoplastic clone (121).

A relationship between Hodgkin's disease and mycosis fungoides, lymphomatoid papulosis, and primary cutaneous anaplastic large cell lymphoma is further complicated by controversy as to whether a T-cell form of Hodgkin's disease

exists (117,122). Although it is generally agreed that the vast majority of cases of Hodgkin's disease are of B-cell origin, cases of Hodgkin's disease with a T-cell immunophenotype and, more rarely, genotype have been described (123–125). A T-cell form of Hodgkin's disease raises certain conceptual issues, because lineage is generally considered one of the defining features of a disease entity. Do classical Hodgkin's disease and "T-cell Hodgkin's disease" share common pathogenetic mechanisms, or are the shared similarities more superficial in nature?

Reed-Sternberg-like cells have also been observed in angioimmunoblastic T-cell lymphoma and adult T-cell leukemia/lymphoma (113,114). A Hodgkin's disease histologic pattern appears to precede the development of acute adult T-cell leukemia/lymphoma in the few published cases, with one report suggesting the Reed-Sternberg-like cells were EBV-positive transformed B cells and not part of the neoplastic T-cell process. In contrast to the neoplastic T cells, the Reed-Sternberg-like cells lacked HTLV-I–associated sequences. A similar basis appears to underlie the Reed-Sternberg-like cells in angioimmunoblastic T-cell lymphomas (114). In these cases, the Reed-Sternberg-like cells contained EBV sequences and expressed CD20 and did not express T-cell antigens. Notably, both adult T-cell leukemia/lymphoma and angioimmunoblastic T-cell lymphoma are malignancies associated with immune suppression and an increased risk of opportunistic infections, and the presence of EBV-transformed B-cell blasts may be secondary to the underlying immunodeficiency. EBV-positive B-cell immunoblastic lymphomas also are seen in this setting (126).

CLINICAL MANAGEMENT

Proper histologic classification is fundamental to the selection of appropriate clinical treatment for lymphomas (127). In some circumstances, however, the histology may bridge two lymphoma diagnoses that would otherwise indicate different treatment approaches. Gray zone lymphomas contain immunophenotypic and histologic features that are shared or intermediate between two different lymphoma subtypes (10). For clinical considerations, gray zone lymphomas should be differentiated from composite lymphomas, in which two distinct histologic subtypes of lymphoma are seen. Divergent histologies can also simultaneously present in different lymph nodes, known as *discordant lymphomas*, and may or may not be clonally related. The metachronous occurrence of different lymphoma subtypes raises different biologic and clinical issues from gray zone and synchronous lymphomas (76). These usually arise in patients with known risk factors for a second lymphoma, such as non-Hodgkin's lymphoma after Hodgkin's disease or Hodgkin's disease in patients with chronic lymphocytic lymphoma. They may be temporally separated by months to years, and treatment decisions are generally directed toward the most recent histology.

Virtually any combination of lymphomas can occur synchronously, and the subtypes have a variable impact on treatment decisions. Foremost is the need to identify the treatment options for each lymphoma subtype and its stage, and to determine its curative potential and effect on survival. Treatment decisions should generally be guided by maximizing curative potential and the optimal treatment of the more aggressive subtype.

Gray Zone Lymphomas

Morphologic gray zone lymphomas, that is, cases with an indeterminate diagnosis due to ambiguous histologic or immunophenotypic features, do not present a clinical dilemma if the diagnosis can ultimately be resolved. These diagnostic problems can result from an inadequate or small biopsy specimen, or lack of available diagnostic techniques. Such cases, although they present a diagnostic challenge, do not represent a true biologic gray zone. They can, however, present a serious clinical problem if incorrectly diagnosed, such as can occur when distinguishing classical Hodgkin's disease from anaplastic large cell lymphoma; the treatments of which are very different. The inclusion of immunophenotype and genetics into modern lymphoma classification systems such as the Revised European-American Lymphoma Classification (128) and its descendent, the World Health Organization system (39), has reduced classification errors (14). Nevertheless, some cases continue to present a diagnostic challenge, and a diagnosis may be changed after disease evolution and/or larger tissue biopsies.

The impact of misdiagnosis of morphologic gray zone lymphoma was recently addressed by a study from the Groupe d'Etude des Lymphomes de l'Adulte through a retrospective pathology review of 2,855 cases entered on the LNH85 lymphoma protocol between 1987 and 1993 (58). Employing contemporary pathologic definitions and immunohistochemistry, 77 (2.7%) of the cases were reclassified as classical Hodgkin's disease, with the most common previous diagnosis of anaplastic large cell lymphoma (primarily Hodgkin's disease-like) (38 cases) or peripheral T-cell lymphoma unspecified (25). The reclassification of the anaplastic large cell lymphoma Hodgkin's disease-like cases (30) to classical Hodgkin's disease reflects the current consensus that these cases represent grade 2 nodular sclerosis Hodgkin's disease (129). The interface between some cases of classical Hodgkin's disease and anaplastic large cell lymphoma or peripheral T-cell lymphoma, however, can still present a diagnostic dilemma and requires the appropriate use of immunophenotype and genetic analyses. Clinically, the 5-year event-free survival of these misdiagnosed Hodgkin's disease cases was inferior to that reported by the International Database of Hodgkin Disease and might suggest the inferior efficacy of lymphoma regimens over those developed for Hodgkin's disease. This conclusion is far from certain, given the retrospective nature of the study, and it could equally likely reflect the poorer prognosis of grade 2 nodular sclerosis Hodgkin's disease (59).

Biologic gray zone lymphomas present a different clinical problem because they do not fit into a known histologic subgroup, and their rarity has precluded clinical studies (10). Many of these cases contain biologic and histologic features intermediate between nodular sclerosis Hodgkin's disease and medias-

tinal large B-cell lymphoma. Treatment recommendations for gray zone lymphomas must be derived from an understanding of their biology and natural history, due to the lack of prospective clinical trials. Clinically, many of these cases present in mediastinal nodes, and as such, the clinical presentation is not particularly helpful in the differential diagnosis of nodular sclerosis Hodgkin's disease and mediastinal large B-cell lymphoma (13,130). A superior vena caval syndrome is more common in mediastinal large B-cell lymphoma.

Both the morphology and immunophenotype of these cases may be ambiguous, with extensive sclerosis, scattered lacunar-type and Reed-Sternberg-like cells, and focal CD30 positivity. The majority of the cells, however, are generally CD20$^+$. Clinically, these lymphomas often reach large size in the mediastinum before spreading outside the anatomic region, similar to both nodular sclerosis Hodgkin's disease and mediastinal large B-cell lymphoma. They have an aggressive clinical behavior.

Based on these findings, we favor doxorubicin-based regimens developed for aggressive diffuse large cell lymphoma, but with the inclusion of rituximab (131). We have had successful experience with the dose-adjusted infusional etoposide, vincristine, doxorubicin, bolus cyclophosphamide, and prednisone (EPOCH)-rituximab regimen without radiation in mediastinal gray zone lymphoma and mediastinal large B-cell lymphoma (132,133). Among five patients with gray zone lymphoma, four achieved durable complete remissions, and all nine patients with mediastinal large B-cell lymphoma achieved durable complete remissions. Methotrexate-leucovorin, Adriamycin, cyclophosphamide, Oncovin, prednisone, and bleomycin (MACOP-B) is an alternative chemotherapy regimen with activity in mediastinal large B-cell lymphoma (134). Zinzani and colleagues, however, reported that 70% of cases treated with MACOP-B in their study were persistently gallium-avid at the end of chemotherapy and before receiving radiation therapy, compared to only one of eleven (9%) patients treated with dose-adjusted EPOCH alone (132,134). These results suggest that radiation may not be necessary with the dose-adjusted EPOCH-rituximab regimen, although it is unknown whether radiation can be avoided with MACOP-B and rituximab. Nonetheless, we have encountered occasional cases of gray zone lymphoma that have weak or variable expression of CD20 and believe such cases would likely benefit from radiation consolidation. Clearly, radiation consolidation should be used in all cases with localized disease in which there is an inadequate response to chemotherapy, as judged by CT and PET scans.

The mediastinal gray zone lymphomas serve as a good clinical model from which to base treatment recommendations for other types of gray zone lymphomas. In the authors' experience, the anatomic distribution of other gray zone lymphomas, such as those in the mediastinum, reflects the distribution of the associated histologic subtypes (10). Hence, gray zone lymphomas intermediate between classical Hodgkin's disease and T-cell–rich large B-cell lymphoma tend to occur in peripheral lymph nodes. Similar to the mediastinal gray zone lymphomas, we recommend doxorubicin-based regimens designed for aggressive lymphomas, with the addition of rituximab.

The role of radiation consolidation is more uncertain in these lymphomas and we suggest its use be restricted to patients with early stage disease and an inadequate response.

The clinical management of gray zone lymphomas in the setting of chronic immunosuppression presents a different set of complex issues. Clearly, in cases that resemble EBV-positive lymphoproliferative disorders in the posttransplant setting, immunosuppression should be withdrawn and the patient observed for spontaneous regression. A similar approach might be followed in patients with lymph node involvement resembling more typical Hodgkin's disease or even non-Hodgkin's lymphoma, because some cases will spontaneously regress. If the lesions persist, however, conventional therapy is recommended and should be guided by the histologic diagnosis.

Synchronous Lymphomas

Composite or discordant lymphomas raise different biologic issues compared to gray zone lymphomas, but they are clinically more straightforward. Transformation of low-grade lymphoma to an aggressive large B-cell lymphoma, best illustrated by follicular lymphomas, comprises the majority of composite or discordant lymphomas and reflects the natural history of these diseases (135,136). In such circumstances, treatment is directed toward controlling the most aggressive lymphoma subtype and frequently calls for a doxorubicin-based regimen (137). Less common is the synchronous presentation of lymphoma subtypes that do not appear to share a common histologic root, although many of these cases are clonally related. The principle of treatment is similar to transformed lymphomas, but the atypical histologic presentations suggest these tumors are biologically unique. Of course, histologically and clonally unrelated lymphomas do synchronously occur, some of which reflect risk factors associated with the underlying disease process, whereas others are simply sporadic. An example of the former includes the occurrence of EBV large B-cell lymphoma in patients with angioimmunoblastic T-cell lymphoma, whereas the latter can include virtually any combination of lymphoma subtypes (126,138,139).

Metachronous Lymphomas

It is well recognized that lymphoma patients are at increased risk of developing a second lymphoma subtype, usually many years after the first presentation (76). Most common is the late development of non-Hodgkin's lymphomas after the curative treatment of Hodgkin's lymphoma, although the converse occurs as well (82,83,140). Clinically, treatment is directed toward the most recent lymphoma, and should entail standard treatment regimens. Anecdotally, however, the clinical outcome of these late lymphomas appears worse than similar histologies that present de novo and raises the question of whether more aggressive treatment should be used, such as stem cell transplant consolidation. In the absence of controlled trials, clinical decisions must be individualized and based on established clinical and biologic precepts.

CONCLUSION

From the above observations, we may draw the following conclusions: (a) Hodgkin's disease and non-Hodgkin's lymphoma occur together with greater frequency than would be expected by chance alone; (b) the association supports a lymphoid origin for the malignant cell of Hodgkin's disease, and given the predominance of B-cell lymphoma, it would be consistent with a B-cell origin in the majority of cases; (c) a clonal relationship may exist between certain forms of classical Hodgkin's disease and non-Hodgkin's lymphoma, most likely follicular lymphoma, diffuse large cell lymphoma, and chronic lymphocytic lymphoma; (d) data support the concept that typical Hodgkin's disease may be an altered lymphoid malignancy, with secondary transformation by a virus such as EBV and/or other candidates yet to be identified; and (e) late-occurring lymphomas in patients in remission for Hodgkin's disease are rarely EBV positive and may have a similar pathogenesis to the Burkitt-like lymphomas seen in association with HIV infection.

Clearly, the cases of Hodgkin's disease occurring in association with non-Hodgkin's lymphoma, either as composite lymphomas or as secondary Hodgkin's disease, differ clinically from typical Hodgkin's disease. The patients are elderly, and the clinical behavior of the Hodgkin's disease is usually aggressive, especially in the context of chronic lymphocytic lymphoma. The question may be posed: Are such cases truly Hodgkin's disease, or do they represent a Hodgkin's disease–like transformation induced by EBV or other unknown causes? Until the molecular events that cause classical Hodgkin's disease are fully elucidated, this question cannot be addressed; however, it is important for both the pathologist and clinician to be aware of these transformations, as they impact the clinical management of the patient. Study of such cases also may yield clues to the pathogenesis of usual Hodgkin's disease.

Clinically, metachronous lymphomas tend to have a worse outcome and more aggressive clinical course compared to de novo presentations. Their biology, however, appears to be distinct from their de novo counterparts in many cases and likely accounts for many of the differences in clinical outcome, above and beyond the effects of prior treatment exposure. Biologic gray zone lymphomas appear to have a particularly aggressive clinical course and represent a unique biologic entity among lymphomas.

REFERENCES

1. Jaffe ES, Zarate-Osorno A, Medeiros LJ. The interrelationship of Hodgkin's disease and non-Hodgkin's lymphomas—lessons learned from composite and sequential malignancies. *Semin Diagn Pathol* 1992;9(4):297–303.
2. Kanzler H, Kuppers R, Hansmann ML, et al. Hodgkin and Reed-Sternberg cells in Hodgkin's disease represent the outgrowth of a dominant tumor clone derived from (crippled) germinal center B cells. *J Exp Med* 1996;184(4):1495–1505.
3. Stein H, Marafioti T, Foss HD, et al. Down-regulation of BOB.1/OBF.1 and Oct2 in classical Hodgkin disease but not in lymphocyte predominant Hodgkin disease correlates with immunoglobulin transcription. *Blood* 2001;97(2):496–501.

4. Andrieu JM, Roithmann S, Tourani JM, et al. Hodgkin's disease during HIV1 infection: the French registry experience. French Registry of HIV-associated Tumors. *Ann Oncol* 1993;4(8):635–641.

5. Levine AM. Hodgkin's disease in the setting of human immunodeficiency virus infection. *J Natl Cancer Inst Monogr* 1998;(23):37–42.

6. Bellas C, Santon A, Manzanal A, et al. Pathological, immunological, and molecular features of Hodgkin's disease associated with HIV infection. Comparison with ordinary Hodgkin's disease. *Am J Surg Pathol* 1996;20(12):1520–1524.

7. Kamel OW, Weiss LM, van de Rijn M, et al. Hodgkin's disease and lymphoproliferations resembling Hodgkin's disease in patients receiving long-term low-dose methotrexate therapy. *Am J Surg Pathol* 1996;20(10):1279–1287.

8. Kumar S, Fend F, Quintanilla-Martinez L, et al. Epstein-Barr virus-positive primary gastrointestinal Hodgkin's disease: association with inflammatory bowel disease and immunosuppression. *Am J Surg Pathol* 2000;24(1):66–73.

9. Poppema S, van Imhoff G, Torensma R, et al. Lymphadenopathy morphologically consistent with Hodgkin's disease associated with Epstein-Barr virus infection. *Am J Clin Pathol* 1985;84(3):385–390.

10. Rudiger T, Jaffe ES, Delsol G, et al. Workshop report on Hodgkin's disease and related diseases ('grey zone' lymphoma). *Ann Oncol* 1998;9[Suppl 5]:S31–S38.

11. Gonzalez CL, Medeiros LJ, Jaffe ES. Composite lymphoma. A clinicopathologic analysis of nine patients with Hodgkin's disease and B-cell non-Hodgkin's lymphoma. *Am J Clin Pathol* 1991;96:81–89.

12. Zarate-Osorno A, Medeiros LJ, Longo DL, et al. Non-Hodgkin's lymphomas arising in patients successfully treated for Hodgkin's disease. A clinical, histologic, and immunophenotypic study of 14 cases. *Am J Surg Pathol* 1992;16(9):885–895.

13. Perrone T, Frizzera G, Rosai J. Mediastinal diffuse large-cell lymphoma with sclerosis. A clinicopathologic study of 60 cases. *Am J Surg Pathol* 1986;10(3):176–191.

14. The Non-Hodgkin's Lymphoma Classification Project. A clinical evaluation of the International Lymphoma Study Group classification of non-Hodgkin's lymphoma. *Blood* 1997;89(11):3909–3918.

15. Lamarre L, Jacobson J, Aisenberg A, et al. Primary large cell lymphoma of the mediastinum. *Am J Surg Pathol* 1989;13:730–739.

16. Moller P, Moldenhauer G, Momburg F, et al. Mediastinal lymphoma of clear cell type is a tumor corresponding to terminal steps of B cell differentiation. *Blood* 1987;69:1087–1095.

17. Higgins JP, Warnke RA. CD30 expression is common in mediastinal large B-cell lymphoma. *Am J Clin Pathol* 1999;112(2):241–247.

18. Kanavaros P, Gaulard P, Charlotte F, et al. Discordant expression of immunoglobulin and its associated molecule mb-1/CD79a is frequently found in mediastinal large B-cell lymphomas. *Am J Pathol* 1995;146(3):735–741.

19. Pileri SA, Gaidano G, Zinzani PL, et al. Primary mediastinal B-cell lymphoma: high frequency of BCL-6 mutations and consistent expression of the transcription factors OCT-2, BOB.1, and PU.1 in the absence of immunoglobulins. *Am J Pathol* 2003;162(1):243–253.

20. Addis B, Isaacson P. Large cell lymphoma of the mediastinum: a B-cell tumor of probable thymic origin. *Histopathology* 1986;10:379–390.

21. Barth TF, Leithauser F, Moller P. Mediastinal B-cell lymphoma, a lymphoma type with several characteristics unique among diffuse large B-cell lymphomas. *Ann Hematol* 2001;80[Suppl 3]:B49–B53.

22. Joos S, Menz CK, Wrobel G, et al. Classical Hodgkin lymphoma is characterized by recurrent copy number gains of the short arm of chromosome 2. *Blood* 2002;99(4):1381–1387.

23. Copie-Bergman C, Gaulard P, Maouche-Chretien L, et al. The MAL gene is expressed in primary mediastinal large B-cell lymphoma. *Blood* 1999;94(10):3567–3575.

24. Chittal S, Brousset P, Voigt J, et al. Large B-cell lymphoma rich in T-cells and simulating Hodgkin's disease. *Histopathology* 1991;19:211–220.

25. Delabie J, Vandenberghe E, Kennes C, et al. Histiocyte-rich B-cell lymphoma. A distinct clinicopathologic entity possibly related to lymphocyte predominant Hodgkin's disease, paragranuloma subtype. *Am J Surg Pathol* 1992;16:37–48.

26. McBride JA, Rodriguez J, Luthra R, et al. T-cell rich B large-cell lymphoma simulating lymphocyte rich Hodgkin's disease. *Am J Surg Pathol* 1996;20:193–201.

27. Lim MS, Beaty M, Sorbara L, et al. T-cell/histiocyte-rich large B-cell lymphoma: a heterogeneous entity with derivation from germinal center B cells. *Am J Surg Pathol* 2002;26(11):1458–1466.

28. Achten R, Verhoef G, Vanuytsel L, et al. T-cell/histiocyte–rich large

29. Achten R, Verhoef G, Vanuytsel L, et al. Histiocyte-rich, T-cell-rich B-cell lymphoma: a distinct diffuse large B-cell lymphoma subtype showing characteristic morphologic and immunophenotypic features. *Histopathology* 2002;40(1):31–45.

30. Schwartz RS. Hodgkin's disease—time for a change [editorial; comment]. *N Engl J Med* 1997;337(7):495–496.

31. Gruss HJ, Pinto A, Duyster J, et al. Hodgkin's disease: a tumor with disturbed immunological pathways. *Immunol Today* 1997;18(4):156–163.

32. Schmid C, Pan L, Diss T, et al. Expression of B-cell antigens by Hodgkin's and Reed-Sternberg cells. *Am J Pathol* 1991;139(4):701–707.

33. Zukerberg L, Collins A, Ferry J, et al. Coexpression of CD15 and CD20 by Reed-Sternberg cells in Hodgkin's disease. *Am J Pathol* 1991;139:475–483.

34. von Wasielewski R, Mengel M, Fischer R, et al. Classical Hodgkin's disease. Clinical impact of the immunophenotype. *Am J Pathol* 1997;151(4):1123–1130.

35. Brauninger A, Hansmann ML, Strickler JG, et al. Identification of common germinal-center B-cell precursors in two patients with both Hodgkin's disease and non-Hodgkin's lymphoma. *N Engl J Med* 1999;340(16):1239–1247.

36. Bellan C, Lazzi S, Zazzi M, et al. Immunoglobulin gene rearrangement analysis in composite Hodgkin disease and large B-cell lymphoma: evidence for receptor revision of immunoglobulin heavy chain variable region genes in Hodgkin-Reed-Sternberg cells? *Diagn Mol Pathol* 2002;11(1):2–8.

37. Georgescu L, Quinn GC, Schwartzman S, et al. Lymphoma in patients with rheumatoid arthritis: association with the disease state or methotrexate treatment. *Semin Arthritis Rheum* 1997;26(6):794–804.

38. Kamel OW, van de Rijn M, Weiss LM, et al. Brief report: reversible lymphomas associated with Epstein-Barr virus occurring during methotrexate therapy for rheumatoid arthritis and dermatomyositis. *N Engl J Med* 1993;328(18):1317–1321.

39. Jaffe ES, Harris NL, Stein H, et al. *Pathology and genetics of tumours of haematopoietic and lymphoid tissues.* Lyon, France: IARC Press, 2001.

40. Andreesen R, Osterholz J, Lohr GW, et al. A Hodgkin cell-specific antigen is expressed on a subset of auto- and alloactivated T (helper) lymphoblasts. *Blood* 1984;63(6):1299–1302.

41. Ansieau S, Scheffrahn I, Mosialos G, et al. Tumor necrosis factor receptor-associated factor (TRAF)-1, TRAF-2, and TRAF-3 interact in vivo with the CD30 cytoplasmic domain; TRAF-2 mediates CD30-induced nuclear factor kappa B activation. *Proc Natl Acad Sci U S A* 1996;93(24):14053–14058.

42. Kanavaros P, Jiwa NM, de Bruin PC, et al. High incidence of EBV genome in CD30-positive non-Hodgkin's lymphomas. *J Pathol* 1992;168(3):307–315.

43. Rowlings PA, Curtis RE, Passweg JR, et al. Increased incidence of Hodgkin's disease after allogeneic bone marrow transplantation. *J Clin Oncol* 1999;17(10):3122–3127.

44. Leoncini L, Del Vecchio M, Kraft R, et al. Hodgkin's disease and CD30-positive anaplastic large cell lymphomas: a continuous spectrum of malignant disorders. *Am J Pathol* 1990;137:1047–1057.

45. Stein H, Mason D, Gerdes J, et al. The expression of the Hodgkin's disease associated antigen Ki-1 in reactive and neoplastic lymphoid tissue: evidence that Reed-Sternberg cells and histiocytic malignancies are derived from activated lymphoid cells. *Blood* 1985;66:848–858.

46. Foss HD, Anagnostopoulos I, Araujo I, et al. Anaplastic large-cell lymphomas of T-cell and null-cell phenotype express cytotoxic molecules. *Blood* 1996;88(10):4005–4011.

47. Krenacs L, Wellmann A, Sorbara L, et al. Cytotoxic cell antigen expression in anaplastic large cell lymphomas of T- and null-cell type and Hodgkin's disease: evidence for distinct cellular origin. *Blood* 1997;89(3):980–989.

48. Orscheschek K, Merz H, Hell J, et al. Large-cell anaplastic lymphoma-specific translocation (t[2;5] [p23;q35]) in Hodgkin's disease: indication of a common pathogenesis? *Lancet* 1995;345(8942):87–90.

49. Wellman A, Otsuki T, Vogelbruch M, et al. Analysis of the t(2;5) (p23;q35) translocation by reverse transcription-polymerase chain reaction in CD 30+ anaplastic large-cell lymphomas, in other non-

Hodgkin's of T-cell phenotype, and in Hodgkin's disease. *Blood* 1995;86:2321–2328.

50. Nakamura S, Shiota M, Nakagawa A, et al. Anaplastic large cell lymphoma: a distinct molecular pathologic entity. A reappraisal with special reference to p80(NPM/ALK) expression. *Am J Surg Pathol* 1997;21(12):1420–1432.

51. Chittal SM, Delsol G. The interface of Hodgkin's disease and anaplastic large cell lymphoma. *Cancer Surv* 1997;30:87–105.

52. Weber-Matthiesen K, Deerberg-Wittram J, Rosenwald A, et al. Translocation t(2;5) is not a primary event in Hodgkin's disease. Simultaneous immunophenotyping and interphase cytogenetics. *Am J Pathol* 1996;149(2):463–468.

53. Pittaluga S, Wlodarska I, Pulford K, et al. The monoclonal antibody ALK1 identifies a distinct morphological subtype of anaplastic large cell lymphoma associated with 2p23/ALK rearrangements. *Am J Pathol* 1997;151(2):343–351.

54. Pileri S, Bocchia M, Baroni C, et al. Anaplastic large cell lymphoma (CD30+/Ki-1+): results of a prospective clinicopathologic study of 69 cases. *Br J Haematol* 1994;86:513–523.

55. Zinzani PL, Bendandi M, Martelli M, et al. Anaplastic large-cell lymphoma: clinical and prognostic evaluation of 90 adult patients. *J Clin Oncol* 1996;14(3):955–962.

56. Benharroch D, Meguerian-Bedoyan Z, Lamant L, et al. ALK-positive lymphoma: a single disease with a broad spectrum of morphology. *Blood* 1998;91(6):2076–2084.

57. MacLennan K, Bennett M, Tu A, et al. Relationship of histopathologic features to survival and relapse in nodular sclerosing Hodgkin's disease. *Cancer* 1989;64:1686–1693.

58. Cazals-Hatem D, Andre M, Mounier N, et al. Pathologic and clinical features of 77 Hodgkin's lymphoma patients treated in a lymphoma protocol (LNH87): a GELA study. *Am J Surg Pathol* 2001;25(3):297–306.

59. Bennett MH, MacLennan KA, Easterling MJ, et al. The prognostic significance of cellular subtypes in nodular sclerosing Hodgkin's disease: an analysis of 271 non-laparotomised cases (BNLI report no. 22). *Clin Radiol* 1983;34(5):497–501.

60. DeVita VT Jr, Simon RM, Hubbard SM, et al. Curability of advanced Hodgkin's disease with chemotherapy. Long-term follow-up of MOPP-treated patients at the National Cancer Institute. *Ann Intern Med* 1980;92(5):587–595.

61. Sander CA, Yano T, Clark HM, et al. p53 mutation is associated with progression in follicular lymphomas. *Blood* 1993;82(7):1994–2004.

62. Custer R, Bernard W. The interrelationship of Hodgkin's disease and other lymphatic tumors. *Am J Med Sci* 1948;216:625–642.

63. Kim H, Hendrickson R, Dorfman RF. Composite lymphoma. *Cancer* 1977;40(3):959–976.

64. Hansmann ML, Fellbaum C, Hui PK, et al. Morphological and immunohistochemical investigation of non-Hodgkin's lymphoma combined with Hodgkin's disease. *Histopathology* 1989;15(1):35–48.

65. Paulli M, Rosso R, Kindl S, et al. Nodular sclerosing Hodgkin's disease and large cell lymphoma. Immunophenotypic characterization of a composite case. *Virchows Arch A Pathol Anat Histopathol* 1992;421(3):271–275.

66. Aguilera NS, Howard LN, Brissette MD, et al. Hodgkin's disease and an extranodal marginal zone B-cell lymphoma in the small intestine: an unusual composite lymphoma. *Mod Pathol* 1996;9(10):1020–1026.

67. Kuppers R, Sousa AB, Baur AS, et al. Common germinal-center B-cell origin of the malignant cells in two composite lymphomas, involving classical Hodgkin's disease and either follicular lymphoma or B-CLL. *Mol Med* 2001;7(5):285–292.

68. Kingma DW, Medeiros LJ, Barletta J, et al. Epstein-Barr virus is infrequently identified in non-Hodgkin's lymphomas associated with Hodgkin's disease. *Am J Surg Pathol* 1994;18(1):48–61.

69. Pinkus G, Said J. Hodgkin's disease, lymphocyte predominance type, nodular: further evidence for a B cell derivation: L & H variants of Reed-Sternberg cells express L26, a pan B cell marker. *Am J Pathol* 1988;133:211–217.

70. Mason D, Banks P, Chan J, et al. Nodular lymphocyte predominance Hodgkin's disease: a distinct clinico-pathological entity. *Am J Surg Pathol* 1994;18:528–530.

71. Marafioti T, Hummel M, Anagnostopoulos I, et al. Origin of nodular lymphocyte-predominant Hodgkin's disease from a clonal expansion of highly mutated germinal-center B cells. *N Engl J Med* 1997;337(7):453–458.

72. Ohno T, Stribley JA, Wu G, et al. Clonality in nodular lymphocyte-predominant Hodgkin's disease. *N Engl J Med* 1997;337(7):459–465.

73. Gelb AB, Dorfman RF, Warnke RA. Coexistence of nodular lymphocyte predominance Hodgkin's disease and Hodgkin's disease of the usual type. *Am J Surg Pathol* 1993;17(4):364–374.

74. Hansmann M, Stein H, Fellbaum C, et al. Nodular paragranuloma can transform into high-grade malignant lymphoma of B type. *Hum Pathol* 1989;20:1169–1175.

75. Miettinen M, Franssila KO, Saxen E. Hodgkin's disease, lymphocytic predominance nodular. Increased risk for subsequent non-Hodgkin's lymphomas. *Cancer* 1983;51(12):2293–2300.

76. Krikorian JG, Burke JS, Rosenberg SA, et al. Occurrence of non-Hodgkin's lymphoma after therapy for Hodgkin's disease. *N Engl J Med* 1979;300(9):452–458.

77. Levy R, Kaplan HS. Impaired lymphocyte function in untreated Hodgkin's disease. *N Engl J Med* 1974;290(4):181–186.

78. Bennett M, MacLennan K, Hudson G, et al. Non-Hodgkin's lymphoma arising in patients treated for Hodgkin's disease in the BNLI: a 20-year experience. *Ann Oncol* 1991;2[Suppl 2]:83–92.

79. Shimizu K, Hara K, Kunii A. Non-Hodgkin's lymphoma following Hodgkin's disease. A case report and immunohistochemical corroboration. *Am J Clin Pathol* 1986;86(3):370–374.

80. Gaidano G, Carbone A, Dalla-Favera R. Pathogenesis of AIDS-related lymphomas: molecular and histogenetic heterogeneity. *Am J Pathol* 1998;152(3):623–630.

81. Ohno T, Trenn G, Wu G, et al. The clonal relationship between nodular sclerosis Hodgkin's disease with a clonal Reed-Sternberg cell population and a subsequent B-cell small non-cleaved cell lymphoma. *Mod Pathol* 1998;11:485–490.

82. Carrato A, Filippa D, Koziner B. Hodgkin's disease after treatment of non-Hodgkin's lymphoma. *Cancer* 1987;60(4):887–896.

83. Travis LB, Gonzalez CL, Hankey BF, et al. Hodgkin's disease following non-Hodgkin's lymphoma. *Cancer* 1992;69(9):2337–2342.

84. LeBrun DP, Ngan BY, Weiss LM, et al. The bcl-2 oncogene in Hodgkin's disease arising in the setting of follicular non-Hodgkin's lymphoma. *Blood* 1994;83(1):223–230.

85. Richter M. Generalized reticular cell sarcoma of lymph nodes associated with lymphocytic leukemia. *Am J Pathol* 1928;4:285–292.

86. Choi H, Keller RH. Coexistence of chronic lymphocytic leukemia and Hodgkin's disease. *Cancer* 1981;48(1):48–57.

87. Dick F, Maca R. The lymph node in chronic lymphocytic leukemia. *Cancer* 1978;41:283–292.

88. Foucar K, Rydell RE. Richter's syndrome in chronic lymphocytic leukemia. *Cancer* 1980;46(1):118–134.

89. Caveriviere P, Mallem O, Al Saati T, et al. Reed-Sternberg-like cells in Richter's syndrome express granulocytic- associated-antigen (Leu-M1) [letter]. *Am J Clin Pathol* 1986;85(6):755–757.

90. Williams J, Schned A, Cotelingam JD, et al. Chronic lymphocytic leukemia with coexistent Hodgkin's disease: Implications for the origin of the Reed-Sternberg cell. *Am J Surg Pathol* 1991;15:33–42.

91. Brecher M, Banks P. Hodgkin's disease variant of Richter's syndrome: report of eight cases. *Am J Clin Pathol* 1990;93:333–339.

92. Fayad L, Robertson LE, O'Brien S, et al. Hodgkin's disease variant of Richter's syndrome: experience at a single institution. *Leuk Lymphoma* 1996;23(3–4):333–337.

93. Rubin D, Hudnall SD, Aisenberg A, et al. Richter's transformation of chronic lymphocytic leukemia with Hodgkin's-like cells is associated with Epstein-Barr virus infection. *Mod Pathol* 1994;7(1):91–98.

94. Weisenberg E, Anastasi J, Adeyanju M, et al. Hodgkin's disease associated with chronic lymphocytic leukemia. Eight additional cases, including two of the nodular lymphocyte predominant type. *Am J Clin Pathol* 1995;103(4):479–484.

95. Momose H, Jaffe ES, Shin SS, et al. Chronic lymphocytic leukemia/small lymphocytic lymphoma with Reed-Sternberg-like cells and possible transformation to Hodgkin's disease. Mediation by Epstein-Barr virus. *Am J Surg Pathol* 1992;16(9):859–867.

96. Cha I, Herndier BG, Glassberg AB, et al. A case of composite Hodgkin's disease and chronic lymphocytic leukemia in bone marrow. Lack of Epstein-Barr virus. *Arch Pathol Lab Med* 1996;120(4):386–389.

97. Ohno T, Smir BN, Weisenburger DD, et al. Origin of the Hodgkin/Reed-Sternberg cells in chronic lymphocytic leukemia with "Hodgkin's transformation." *Blood* 1998;91(5):1757–1761.

98. Giles FJ, O'Brien SM, Keating MJ. Chronic lymphocytic leukemia in (Richter's) transformation. *Semin Oncol* 1998;25(1):117–125.

99. Jaffe ES, Zarate-Osorno A, Kingma DW, et al. The interrelationship between Hodgkin's disease and non-Hodgkin's lymphomas. *Ann Oncol* 1994;5[Suppl 1]:7–11.

100. Wlodarska I, Delabie J, De Wolf-Peeters C, et al. T-cell lymphoma

developing in Hodgkin's disease: evidence for two clones. *J Pathol* 1993;170(3):239–248.

101. Simrell CR, Boccia RV, Longo DL, Jaffe ES. Coexisting Hodgkin's disease and mycosis fungoides. Immunohistochemical proof of its existence. *Arch Pathol Lab Med* 1986;110(11):1029–1034.

102. Hawkins KA, Schinella R, Schwartz M, et al. Simultaneous occurrence of mycosis fungoides and Hodgkin disease: clinical and histologic correlations in three cases with ultrastructural studies in two. *Am J Hematol* 1983;14(4):355–362.

103. Clement M, Bhakri H, Monk B, et al. Mycosis fungoides and Hodgkin's disease. *J R Soc Med* 1984;77(12):1037–9103.

104. Kaufman D, Gordon LI, Variakojis D, et al. Successfully treated Hodgkin's disease followed by mycosis fungoides: case report and review of the literature. *Cutis* 1987;39(4):291–296.

105. Brousset P, Lamant L, Viraben R, et al. Hodgkin's disease following mycosis fungoides: phenotypic and molecular evidence for different tumour cell clones. *J Clin Pathol* 1996;49(6):504–507.

106. Kremer M, Sandherr M, Geist B, et al. Epstein-Barr virus-negative Hodgkin's lymphoma after mycosis fungoides: molecular evidence for distinct clonal origin. *Mod Pathol* 2001;14(2):91–97.

107. Caya JG, Choi H, Tieu TM, et al. Hodgkin's disease followed by mycosis fungoides in the same patient. Case report and literature review. *Cancer* 1984;53(3):463–467.

108. Park CS, Chung HC, Lim HY, et al. Coexisting mycosis fungoides and Hodgkin's disease as a composite lymphoma: a case report. *Yonsei Med J* 1991;32(4):362–369.

109. Lipa M, Kunynetz R, Pawlowski D, et al. The occurrence of mycosis fungoides in two patients with preexisting Hodgkin's disease. *Arch Dermatol* 1982;118(8):563–567.

110. Greene MH, Pinto HA, Kant JA, et al. Lymphomas and leukemias in the relatives of patients with mycosis fungoides. *Cancer* 1982;49(4):737–741.

111. van der Putte SC, Toonstra J, Go DM, et al. Mycosis fungoides. Demonstration of a variant simulating Hodgkin's disease. A report of a case with a cytomorphological analysis. *Virchows Arch B Cell Pathol Incl Mol Pathol* 1982;40(2):231–247.

112. Picard F, Dreyfus F, Le Guern M, et al. Acute T-cell leukemia/lymphoma mimicking Hodgkin's disease with secondary HTLV I seroconversion. *Cancer* 1990;66(7):1524–1528.

113. Ohshima K, Kikuchi M, Yoshida T, et al. Lymph nodes in incipient adult T-cell leukemia-lymphoma with Hodgkin's disease-like histologic features. *Cancer* 1991;67(6):1622–1628.

114. Quintanilla-Martinez L, Fend F, Moguel LR, et al. Peripheral T-cell lymphoma with Reed-Sternberg-like cells of B-cell phenotype and genotype associated with Epstein-Barr virus infection. *Am J Surg Pathol* 1999;23(10):1233–1240.

115. Paulli M, Berti E, Rosso R, et al. CD30/Ki-1-positive lymphoproliferative disorders of the skin--clinicopathologic correlation and statistical analysis of 86 cases: a multicentric study from the European Organization for Research and Treatment of Cancer Cutaneous Lymphoma Project Group. *J Clin Oncol* 1995;13(6):1343–1354.

116. Kaudewitz P, Stein H, Plewig G, et al. Hodgkin's disease followed by lymphomatoid papulosis. Immunophenotypic evidence for a close relationship between lymphomatoid papulosis and Hodgkin's disease. *J Am Acad Dermatol* 1990;22(6 Pt 1):999–1006.

117. Kadin ME, Drews R, Samel A, et al. Hodgkin's lymphoma of T-cell type: clonal association with a CD30+ cutaneous lymphoma. *Hum Pathol* 2001;32(11):1269–1272.

118. Ralfkiaer E, Bosq J, Gatter KC, et al. Expression of a Hodgkin and Reed-Sternberg cell associated antigen (Ki-1) in cutaneous lymphoid infiltrates. *Arch Dermatol Res* 1987;279(5):285–292.

119. Wieczorek R, Suhrland M, Ramsay D, et al. Leu-M1 antigen expression in advanced (tumor) stage mycosis fungoides. *Am J Clin Pathol* 1986;86(1):25–32.

120. Scheen SRd, Banks PM, Winkelmann RK. Morphologic heterogeneity of malignant lymphomas developing in mycosis fungoides. *Mayo Clin Proc* 1984;59(2):95–106.

121. Davis T, Morton C, Miller-Cassman R, et al. Hodgkin's disease, lymphomatoid papulosis, and cutaneous T-cell lymphoma derived from a common T-cell clone. *N Engl J Med* 1992;326:1115–1122.

122. Willenbrock K, Ichinohasama R, Kadin ME, et al. T-cell variant of classical Hodgkin's lymphoma with nodal and cutaneous manifestations demonstrated by single-cell polymerase chain reaction. *Lab Invest* 2002;82(9):1103–1109.

123. Kadin ME, Muramoto L, Said J. Expression of T-cell antigens on Reed-Sternberg cells in a subset of patients with nodular sclerosing and mixed cellularity Hodgkin's disease. *Am J Pathol* 1988;130(2):345–353.

124. Seitz V, Hummel M, Marafioti T, et al. Detection of clonal T-cell receptor gamma-chain gene rearrangements in Reed-Sternberg cells of classic Hodgkin disease. *Blood* 2000;95(10):3020–3024.

125. Muschen M, Rajewsky K, Brauninger A, et al. Rare occurrence of classical Hodgkin's disease as a T cell lymphoma. *J Exp Med* 2000; 191(2):387–394.

126. Abruzzo LV, Schmidt K, Weiss LM, et al. B-cell lymphoma after angioimmunoblastic lymphadenopathy: a case with oligoclonal gene rearrangements associated with Epstein-Barr virus. *Blood* 1993; 82(1):241–246.

127. Jaffe ES, Harris NL, Diebold J, et al. World Health Organization classification of neoplastic diseases of the hematopoietic and lymphoid tissues. A progress report. *Am J Clin Pathol* 1999;111[1 Suppl 1]:S8–S12.

128. Harris NL, Jaffe ES, Stein H, et al. A revised European-American classification of lymphoid neoplasms: a proposal from the International Lymphoma Study Group. *Blood* 1994;84(5):1361–1392.

129. Harris NL, Jaffe ES, Diebold J, et al. World Health Organization classification of neoplastic diseases of the hematopoietic and lymphoid tissues: report of the Clinical Advisory Committee meeting, Airlie house, Virginia, November 1997. *J Clin Oncol* 1999;17(12):3835–3849.

130. Yonetani N, Kurata M, Nishikori M, et al. Primary mediastinal large B-cell lymphoma: a comparative study with nodular sclerosis-type Hodgkin's disease. *Int J Hematol* 2001;74(2):178–185.

131. Coiffier B, Lepage E, Briere J, et al. CHOP chemotherapy plus rituximab compared with CHOP alone in elderly patients with diffuse large-B-cell lymphoma. *N Engl J Med* 2002;346(4):235–242.

132. Wilson WH, Grossbard ML, Pittaluga S, et al. Dose-adjusted EPOCH chemotherapy for untreated large B-cell lymphomas: a pharmacodynamic approach with high efficacy. *Blood* 2002;99(8):2685–2693.

133. Wilson WH, Gutierrez M, O'Connor P, et al. The role of rituximab and chemotherapy in aggressive B-cell lymphoma: a preliminary report of dose-adjusted EPOCH-R. *Semin Oncol* 2002;29[1 Suppl 2]:41–47.

134. Zinzani PL, Martelli M, Magagnoli M, et al. Treatment and clinical management of primary mediastinal large B-cell lymphoma with sclerosis: MACOP-B regimen and mediastinal radiotherapy monitored by (67)Gallium scan in 50 patients. *Blood* 1999;94(10):3289–3293.

135. Zelenetz AD, Chen TT, Levy R. Histologic transformation of follicular lymphoma to diffuse lymphoma represents tumor progression by a single malignant B cell. *J Exp Med* 1991;173(1):197–207.

136. Oviatt DL, Cousar JB, Collins RD, et al. Malignant lymphomas of follicular center cell origin in humans. V. Incidence, clinical features, and prognostic implications of transformation of small cleaved cell nodular lymphoma. *Cancer* 1984;53(5):1109–1114.

137. Gutierrez M, Chabner BA, Pearson D, et al. Role of a doxorubicin-containing regimen in relapsed and resistant lymphomas: an 8-year follow-up study of EPOCH. *J Clin Oncol* 2000;18(21):3633–3642.

138. Matsue K, Itoh M, Tsukuda K, et al. Development of Epstein-Barr virus-associated B cell lymphoma after intensive treatment of patients with angioimmunoblastic lymphadenopathy with dysproteinemia. *Int J Hematol* 1998;67(3):319–329.

139. Abruzzo LV, Rosales CM, Medeiros LJ, et al. Epstein-Barr virus-positive B-cell lymphoproliferative disorders arising in immunodeficient patients previously treated with fludarabine for low-grade B-cell neoplasms. *Am J Surg Pathol* 2002;26(5):630–636.

140. Zarate-Osorno A, Medeiros LJ, Kingma DW, et al. Hodgkin's disease following non-Hodgkin's lymphoma. A clinicopathologic and immunophenotypic study of nine cases. *Am J Surg Pathol* 1993;17(2):123–132.

CHAPTER 7

Procedures for the Primary Diagnosis and Follow-Up of Patients with Lymphoma

Andrew S. Jack and Alan K. Burnett

The approach to the diagnosis and follow-up of patients with lymphomachronic lymphocytic leukemia differs in a number of important respects from the investigation of epithelial malignancies, and it is important that these differences are fully recognized in the design of protocols for the investigation and management of these patients. Diagnosis of most types of epithelial malignancy involves the identification of malignant cells using cytomorphologic criteria at a particular anatomic site. In many instances, this can be accomplished with a high degree of accuracy using minimally invasive techniques, such as fine-needle aspiration cytology. In contrast, accurate diagnosis and classification of lymphoproliferative disorders requires the coordinated use of a wide range of diagnostic techniques, and this places greater constraints on the type of specimen that is suitable for diagnosis. Unlike epithelial malignancies at a given site, lymphoproliferative disorders are diverse, and accurate classification is essential for good patient care. It is important that all those concerned in the management of patients with lymphoma fully understand the strengths and weaknesses of the various types of diagnostic biopsy specimens that may be taken in the course of primary investigation and staging. If a diagnosis of an epithelial malignancy is made by cytology or on a needle biopsy, it is usually validated on a subsequent surgical resection specimen. Surgical resection of lymphomas is rare, and it is essential that the scope of investigations performed on a diagnostic biopsy specimen is sufficiently broad to provide high levels of confidence in the diagnosis before treatment begins.

Designing effective protocols for the investigation of lymphoma is made more complicated by the wide range of possible clinical presentations. Lymphomas can effectively present at any anatomic site, and at many of these sites, there may be special problems associated with surgical biopsy. The wide range of presentations also means that patients with lymphoma may be referred to almost any medical specialist, some of whom may rarely encounter this type of problem. There is, therefore, a potential difficulty in the dissemination of practice guidelines across an entire institution rather than within a single department.

Finally, as therapeutic strategies develop, there is increasing need for diagnostic procedures to monitor the effects of therapy or detect disease progression. This requires a coordinated approach involving the use of imaging, biopsy of suspicious lesions, and techniques designed to detect minimal levels of residual disease.

PRINCIPLES OF LABORATORY DIAGNOSIS

Accurate Diagnosis of Lymphoproliferative Disorders Requires Integration of a Range of Laboratory Techniques

Accurate diagnosis and precise classification of lymphoproliferative disorders is the essential starting point for effective patient care. Fortunately, the tools needed to achieve this, in terms of classification and laboratory methods, have improved greatly. The Revised European-American Lymphoma Classification, published in 1994, and more recently, the World Health Organization (WHO) classification are based on the definition of clinicopathologic entities. These are defined using a combination of morphologic, immunophenotypic, molecular cytogenetic, and clinical criteria (1,2). It is remarkable that the large number of variables within each of these categories cluster together, leading to the definition of relatively few common entities. If these variables had been randomly associated, this approach to classification would have been impossible. This has important consequences for the laboratory investigation of suspected lymphoproliferative disorders. The demonstration that results of morphologic examination, immunophenotypic studies, molecular cytogenetics, and clinical staging investigations are internally consistent for any given diagnosis is the mainstay of quality assurance (Fig. 7.1). Diagnostic protocols in each of these areas need to be designed so that they provide effective cross-checking of the results of other investigations. This also implies that investigation must be performed systematically rather than on an ad hoc basis; with systematic investigation, high levels of diagnostic accuracy can be achieved. This

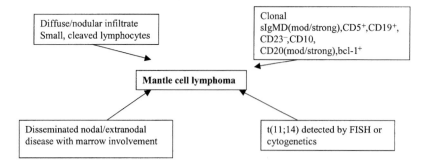

FIG. 7.1. Accurate diagnosis of lymphoma depends on a systematic approach to laboratory and clinical investigations. Immunophenotypic, molecular, cytogenetic, and clinical investigations should be performed using predetermined protocols, rather than on an ad hoc basis, to confirm a presumptive morphologic diagnosis. As illustrated by the example of mantle cell lymphoma, demonstrating that the results of these independent investigative techniques are mutually consistent is a key element in assuring the quality of the final diagnosis. FISH, fluorescent *in situ* hybridization.

represents an important advance, given that many studies have shown that in a significant number of cases, the diagnosis of lymphoma is inaccurate or sometimes completely incorrect, with serious consequences for patient care (3–7). It is also important to identify clearly cases in which it has not been possible to carry out a full set of investigations and the degree of confidence in the accuracy of the diagnosis is consequently reduced. In such cases, a decision on the need for further biopsy needs to be considered in the light of the patient's clinical state. A systematic approach to diagnosis is also essential in the collection of uniform data sets for each institution that are suitable for comparison of clinical outcomes and for epidemiologic purposes.

Accurate classification of lymphoproliferative disorders, according to the WHO criteria, is only one part of the diagnostic process. Although many of the WHO entities are precisely defined and can be diagnosed reproducibly using the approach described above, a single entity may still encompass a wide range of clinical outcomes. Diffuse large B-cell lymphoma is a single entity, but only approximately 40% of patients will be cured of their disease using standard combination chemotherapy. Similarly, B-cell chronic lymphocytic leukemia can be accurately diagnosed in a high proportion of cases, but the clinical spectrum ranges from occult subclinical disease to progressive disease that is refractory to treatment. Within many of the WHO entities, including B-cell chronic lymphocytic leukemia and diffuse large B-cell lymphoma, there are a growing number of biologic prognostic factors that can be used to risk-stratify patients. These include immunophenotypic characteristics, cytogenetic abnormalities, and molecular abnormalities, such as immunoglobulin heavy chain (IgH) mutational patterns (8–18). Although there is as yet no general international consensus on the use of biologic prognostic factors, it is clear that it is already feasible to use a variety of approaches to accurately predict clinical outcome from biologic data in many cases. The development of new approaches to diagnosis is also being driven by the development of new therapeutic agents, including enzyme inhibitors and monoclonal antibodies (19–23). Finally, as effec-

tive therapies are developed, it will become more important to have sensitive systems of response monitoring to allow dose titration and therapy duration to be tailored to individual patient needs. This is a rapidly changing area, and the need to provide prognostic data and information on the likely response to particular agents will further alter the approach to the primary investigation of patients with lymphoma.

Excision Biopsies of Lymph Nodes Are the Specimens of Choice for the Diagnosis of Lymphoma

To carry out the full range of investigations required for accurate diagnosis, it is clear that an adequate volume of tissue is required, and this usually means an excision biopsy. There are other reasons, however, for suggesting that excision biopsy is the technique of choice. A key component in the diagnosis of lymphoma is the assessment of tissue architecture. Replacement of the normal architecture of a lymph node is a key feature of all types of lymphoproliferative disorders and probably reflects a fundamental property of the malignant cell. The microarchitecture of lymph nodes has a number of major components, and each of these should be assessed systematically. These include the capsule and sinus structure; the demarcation of T- and B-cell zones; and the assessment of the structure of the B-cell follicle, including the germinal center, mantle, and marginal zones. This is achieved by examining routinely stained sections and demonstrating these key components using lineage-specific antibodies. The degree to which normal nodal architecture is lost may vary widely. Lymphoproliferative disorders may diffusely replace the normal architecture of the node, but often, only part of the node is infiltrated. A specific segment of the node may be involved, as in diffuse large B-cell lymphoma or Hodgkin's lymphoma, or the tumor may be largely confined to specific structures within the node, such as the B-cell marginal zone. The ability to demonstrate that a tumor has breached the capsule of the node or is replacing the sinus structure of the node is also an important diagnostic feature. Therefore, to allow adequate assessment of architecture and to provide sufficient tissue for the full range of diagnostic investigation, it is clear that an excision biopsy of lymph node is the diagnostic technique of choice. There are clinical situations in which this statement needs to be qualified by the risks of open surgical biopsy or inconvenience to the patient, as discussed in Suspected Lymphoma Presenting in the Thorax and Mediastinum. In some cases, the relatively limited range of types of lymphoma encountered at a particular site may compensate for less than optimal biopsy material.

It Is Essential That Lymph Node Biopsy Specimens Are Sent Unfixed to the Laboratory

It is essential that diagnostic lymph node biopsies taken from patients with suspected lymphoma are sent unfixed to the laboratory (Fig. 7.2). Placing an intact lymph node in fixative in the operating room can seriously affect all subsequent stages of the diagnostic process. Routine fixatives may penetrate pathologic lymph nodes relatively slowly, and morphologic preservation at the center of the lymph node may be very poor. In some cases, this may render accurate diagnosis almost impossible. Poor initial fixation also has a serious effect on the quality of immunocytochemistry performed on paraffin sections, to the extent that false-negative results may be obtained with a range of key antibodies, such as anti-CD5 or CD10. To avoid these problems, a lymph node should be sliced as soon as possible after removal from the patient, and 1- to 2-mm slices, preferably cut along the long axis, should be placed in 10% buffered formalin. Lymphoid tissue requires fixation for 24 hours, followed by routine paraffin processing and sectioning. Attempting to accelerate this process may be counterproductive in terms of loss of diagnostic quality. In cases in which unfixed tissue is available, there may be other options if an urgent diagnosis is required. In the past, many special fixatives have been recommended. These offer no advantage over formalin when modern immunocytochemical techniques are used, and those that contain mercuric salts may be a hazard to staff and the environment.

Flow cytometry is a powerful investigative technique in the diagnosis of lymphoproliferative disorders, and this is only possible if a piece of unfixed tissue is available. Lymphoid tissue can be easily disaggregated to a single-cell suspension by simple mechanical methods. Although custom-made equipment is available, this is not essential for good results. Flow cytometry used in conjunction with Giemsa-stained touch preparations can allow a rapid diagnosis to be made in cases of clinical urgency, with results available in a few hours. Again, this opportunity is lost if the tissue is fixed.

In centers using metaphase cytogenetics for the demonstration of chromosomal translocations and other abnormalities, it is clearly essential to have access to unfixed tissue for culture. Fluorescent *in situ* hybridization (FISH) and polymerase chain reaction (PCR) can be performed on fresh- and fixed-tissue samples, but fixation greatly reduces the effectiveness of both techniques. Touch preparations are an excellent substrate for interphase FISH studies. These are simple to prepare and, when air dried, can be stored until required. If only fixed material is available, there are two main options for carrying out FISH studies: normal histologic sections can be used, or nuclei can be extracted from the paraffin block. In sections, individual nuclei are cut in multiple planes, and evaluation of the number of FISH signals can be difficult The use of isolated nuclei is an effective technique but is labor intensive (46–48). Both techniques require well-fixed tissue, and the ability to carry out these techniques may be lost if whole lymph nodes are placed in formalin before dissection. There are many studies using PCR on DNA extracted from fixed tissue (49–51); however, a major limitation is the fragmentation of DNA by fixation. In material that has been well fixed, the fragment size is approximately 400 base pairs (bp) (52) and will be much less in poorly processed tissue. For example, in the case of IgH PCR, this means that in most cases in which DNA is extracted from fixed and pro-

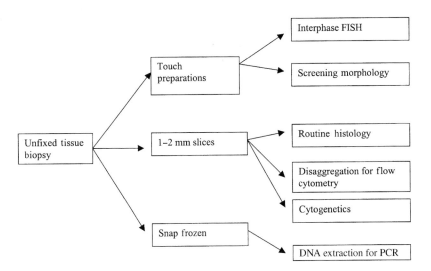

FIG. 7.2. Outline protocol for handling unfixed lymph node or other biopsy specimens taken for diagnosis of lymphoma. The use of unfixed tissue not only expands the range of possible investigations but also improves the quality of routine histology and immunocytochemistry by allowing greater control of the fixation process. FISH, fluorescent *in situ* hybridization; PCR, polymerase chain reaction.

cessed tissue, only FR3/JH primers will produce a PCR product, and it will only be possible to demonstrate monoclonality in approximately 50% of lymphoma specimens, compared to approximately 90% of cases in which fresh tissue is available. A similar effect is seen with T-cell receptor gamma and bcl-2/IgH PCR. A high false-negative rate means that these techniques are of limited value in primary diagnosis in the absence of fresh tissue. In the absence of fresh tissue, the only technique available for the demonstration of clonality in many cases is light-chain restriction by immunocytochemistry, and this is prone to artefact when fixation is in any way suboptimal.

The two main problems that arise from the use of fresh tissue are the need for efficient transport and safety considerations. When the specimen is being sent within the same institution or only a short delay of 1 to 2 hours is expected, it is acceptable to send it in a dry, sterile container. If the specimen is small or there may be a slightly longer delay, it can be placed in any one of a wide range of transport media. Also note that some patients with lymphadenopathy may have unsuspected infection, and fresh lymph nodes need to be handled with appropriate precautions to ensure the safety of laboratory staff.

An Effective Hematopathology Laboratory Needs Access to a Full Range of Diagnostic Technologies

Morphologic interpretation of cytology smears and histologic sections remains an important, although probably a declining, aspect of the diagnosis of leukemia and lymphoma. To provide accurate diagnostic and prognostic information, an effective hematopathology laboratory requires the ability to carry out detailed immunophenotyping for cell surface and cytoplasmic antigens, to demonstrate the presence of a range of cytogenetic abnormalities, and to identify clonal populations of lymphocytes. There are many ways in which an individual laboratory can achieve these aims, and the exact choice of technique used depends on factors such as local expertise and cost effectiveness. It is important that all those involved in the diagnosis and treatment of patients are fully aware of the methods used and their strengths and limitations.

Immunophenotyping by Flow Cytometry and Immunocytochemistry

Immunophenotypic analysis is performed using a combination of flow cytometry and immunocytochemistry, and all hematopathology laboratories need to have broad expertise in these techniques, even though the way they are applied in individual institutions may vary. Flow cytometry is used to determine the immunophenotype of cells in suspension. In the hematopathology laboratory, this includes peripheral blood, bone marrow aspirates, serous effusions, and solid-tissue specimens that have been disaggregated. Flow cytometry is a powerful and

versatile technique that allows very large numbers of cells to be analyzed in a short time. It is now standard practice to use three- or four-color flow cytometric techniques, which allow much higher resolution of cellular populations in complex samples; single-color methods are obsolete (24,25). Successful flow cytometry depends on identifying cells of interest using their physical properties and expression of one or more antigens that define a cell lineage. Additional antibodies are then used to characterize the cell further. The scope of the technique has been expanded by the development of fixation and permeabilization methods that allow a combination of cell-surface, nuclear, and cytoplasmic antigens to be studied simultaneously (26). Advanced gating strategies using four antibodies in combination can now be used to identify a very small population in complex samples, such as bone marrow (27,28). The usefulness of flow cytometry is likely to be further enhanced by developments in antibody and instrument technology. For these reasons, flow cytometry is now the method of choice for most diagnostic applications in hematopathology (Tables 7.1 and 7.2).

TABLE 7.1. *Core flow cytometry panel for the investigation of surface antigen expression in suspected mature B-cell malignancies in bone marrow, peripheral blood, or solid-tissue specimens[a]*

Surface immunoglobulin-heavy and -light chains CD79a	Strength of expression of CD79 and surface immunoglobulin is important in diagnosis of CLL. Kappa:lambda ratio is used to determine clonality. Expression of sIgG is found mainly in germinal center–type B-cell lymphoma.
CD10	Expressed on germinal center–type lymphoma/follicular lymphoma and subset of diffuse large B-cell lymphoma.
CD5	CD5 is expressed on CLL, mantle cell lymphoma, and a subset of follicular and diffuse large B-cell lymphoma.
CD23	Important for the distinction between chronic lymphocytic leukemia and mantle cell lymphoma.
	Also expressed on normal mantle zone B-cell and some germinal center lymphoma.
CD22	Additional pan–B-cell marker, very high expression in hairy-cell leukemia.
CD38	Expressed in follicular lymphoma and most diffuse large B-cell lymphoma. Prognostic marker in CLL.

CLL, chronic lymphocytic leukemia; sIgG, surface IgGs.
[a]For effective results, three-color technique is required with cells gated according to CD19 expression and physical characteristic.

TABLE 7.2. *Additional antibodies used for investigation of mature B-cell malignancies*[a]

CD138	Identification of plasma cells
CD56	Characterization of plasma cells
CD11c	Identification of hairy-cell leukemia and variants
CD103	
CD25	

[a]The identification of plasma-cells requires a four-color technique. Normal and neoplastic (myeloma) type plasma cells can be distinguished using patterns of CD19 and CD56 expression.

Immunocytochemistry has also witnessed major developments with the introduction of antigen retrieval and amplification methods that have allowed the use of a much greater range of antibodies in fixed-tissue specimens (29–32). Extensive immunophenotypic studies can now be performed when only fixed tissue is available. All immunocytochemical techniques are based on the correlation between cellular morphology and antigen expression; this is analogous to gating in flow cytometry. Dual-color techniques are only beginning to be used in diagnostic applications. Even when flow cytometry is performed, immunocytochemistry has an important role in delineating tissue architecture; identifying minor subpopulations, such as Reed-Sternberg cells; and allowing distinction between cytoplasmic and nuclear antigen expression. This will have increasing importance in the investigation of

TABLE 7.3. *Suggested minimum immunocytochemistry antibody panel for investigation of suspected mature B-cell malignancies in fixed tissue specimens*[a]

CD20 CD79a (Pax-5)	Pan B-cell marker to define B-cell population
CD10 Bcl-6	Identification of germinal center B cell; may be the neoplastic population or residual B-cell follicles
CD5	Identification of CLL, mantle cell lymphoma, and subset of germinal center B-cell lymphoma; must be interpreted in conjunction with CD3
CD23	Identification of normal mantle zone B cell and follicular dendritic cells; essential for the differential diagnosis of CLL and mantle cell lymphoma
Bcl-2	Essential for diagnosis of follicular lymphoma and important prognostic marker in diffuse large B-cell lymphoma
Bcl-1	Essential for the diagnosis of mantle cell lymphoma
Ki67	Important for distinction between diffuse large B-cell lymphoma and other types of lymphoma; useful for identification of residual normal germinal centers

CLL, chronic lymphocytic leukemia.
[a]When the differential diagnosis includes Hodgkin's lymphoma, additional antibodies (CD30, CD15, Bob-1, Oct-2) are required. The demonstration of surface immunoglobulin in fixed tissue sample is frequently unreliable.

TABLE 7.4. *Suggested minimum immunocytochemistry panel for the diagnosis of mature T-cell malignancies*[a]

CD2 CD3 CD4 CD5 CD7 CD8	Most mature T-cell lymphomas have an "abnormal" phenotype with loss of one or more pan–T-cell markers. Caution is required in interpretation, as some normal transformed T-cells may slow down regulation of CD3 or CD7 in particular.
CD30 Alk-1	Essential for the diagnosis and subclassification of anaplastic large-cell lymphoma of T-cell type.
CD56 CD57	Essential for the diagnosis of tumors with NK or T/NK phenotype.
CD23 CD138 CD68 CD20	Identification of normal B cells, plasma cells, macrophages, and follicular dendritic cells is an integral part of the diagnosis of T-cell lymphoma.

[a]Additional markers are required when the differential diagnosis includes T-cell–rich B-cell lymphoma or Hodgkin's lymphoma.

key proteins, such as NfkappaB, in which the intracellular localization of the protein is an indicator of its activation state (33) (Tables 7.3 and 7.4).

Demonstration of Chromosomal Abnormalities

The demonstration of chromosomal abnormalities can be performed using metaphase cytogenetics with conventional staining, *in situ* hybridization techniques (34), interphase FISH methods, PCR, or by antibody methods. Conventional metaphase-based cytogenetics techniques are often considered the gold standard, but these have a number of major disadvantages, including high cost and the need for dividing cells. Many indolent lymphoproliferative disorders do not grow well in culture, and there is the possibility that the cells that grow may not be representative of the tumor as a whole. In most situations, there is only a limited range of key abnormalities that are relevant to validating the diagnosis or assessing prognosis. For these reasons, many laboratories use interphase FISH or PCR as the first-choice methods for demonstration of chromosomal translocations or numerical abnormalities (35,36). In the investigation of lymphomas, PCR is mainly used for the identification of t(14;18). RT-PCR techniques are sometimes used for the t(11;18) (37). Routine PCR-based techniques are much less successful for the demonstration of other key abnormalities, such as t(11;14) or t(8;14), because of variability of breakpoints. Interphase FISH using multicolor probes is a highly versatile method for detecting chromosomal translocations and a wide range of other numerical and structural abnormalities (38–40). In presentation specimens, it is almost certainly the method of choice, although it is not sensitive enough to detect small residual disease populations in follow-up samples. A number of antibody-based methods can also be used for the detection of genetic abnormalities, including bcl-1 in t(11;14)–containing mantle cell lymphomas and Alk-1 in t(2;5)–containing anaplastic large-cell lymphomas. This area is also likely to expand with increasing knowledge of patterns of gene expression associated with particular abnormalities (41). The use of microarray technology will enhance the ability to describe the patterns of gene expression associated with particular genetic abnormalities, and this may in turn allow such abnormalities to be identified through discordant patterns of antigen expression demonstrated by flow cytometry or immunocytochemistry (Table 7.5).

Demonstration of Monoclonality

The demonstration of monoclonality is a key part of the diagnosis of lymphomas. In most B-cell malignancies, monoclonality can be demonstrated using light-chain restriction and flow cytometry. Equivalent immunocytochemical techniques are less reliable. T-cell monoclonality can be identified using anti-Vbeta family antibodies, but this is a complex technique that is difficult to use routinely (42). For all T-cell malignancies and for B-cell malignancies in which clonality cannot be demonstrated by light-chain restriction, PCR is the method of choice. Technical development in primer design and the use of extended panels or primers in multiplex techniques have increased the proportion of lymphomas in which monoclonality can be detected to approximately 90%. This means that the presence of monoclonality can now be used as a critical test of the validity of a diagnosis of lymphoma. The absence of monoclonality in these circumstances should prompt a reassessment of the diagnosis. It should, however, be stressed that monoclonality alone in the absence of other features required to make a diagnosis of malignancy should not be regarded as diagnostic of lymphoma (43–45).

TABLE 7.5. *Key cytogenetic features used in the diagnosis of mature B-cell malignancies[a]*

t(14;18)	Essential for diagnosis of follicular lymphoma and major prognostic factor in diffuse large B-cell lymphoma. Strongly correlates with bcl-2 expression in germinal center cells.
t(8;14) and variants	Essential for diagnosis of Burkitt's lymphoma.
t(11;14)	Essential for diagnosis of mantle cell lymphoma. Correlates with bcl-1 expression.
3q27 rearrangements (bcl–6)	Poor prognostic factor in diffuse B-cell lymphoma and progression of follicular lymphoma.
13q,17p, and 11q deletions	Prognostic factors in chronic lymphocytic leukemia. 17p deletions are frequently associated with mutation/inactivation of p53.

[a]All can be demonstrated using interphase fluorescent *in situ* hybridization or conventional cytogenetics.

APPROACH TO DIAGNOSIS DEPENDS ON THE SITE OF DISEASE

Peripheral Lymphadenopathy

Peripheral lymphadenopathy is very common and exceeds the incidence of lymphoma or metastatic epithelial malignancy by a very large margin. For family practitioners or general physicians, identification of the very small number of patients who may have malignant disease and require further investigation is a complex problem (Table 7.6). It is possible to produce only the most general guidance to assist in identification of such patients. This would include enlarged nodes that are persistent or progressive without apparent cause, infiltration and tethering to surrounding structures, and weight loss and classical *B symptoms*. When a decision has been made to refer a patient for further investigation, it is highly desirable that this is performed efficiently. To facilitate this, there is a strong case for the use of assessment clinics within hematologic oncology departments, rather than simply referring patients to a surgeon for a biopsy. A specialized clinic is able to coordinate all the necessary investigations and has established relationships with designated surgeons to ensure that biopsies are performed without delay and that tissue is handled appropriately. In this setting, the patient can be given appropriate advice on the likely diagnosis, its consequences, and arranging necessary urgent treatment.

For the reasons detailed above, in patients who present with peripheral lymphadenopathy a formal excision biopsy of lymph node should be performed, unless there is a strong reason to do otherwise. The discomfort and inconvenience of a short general anesthetic are trivial in comparison with chemotherapy or radiotherapy, and any risks are outweighed by the benefits of a secure and confident diagnosis. Before a lymph node biopsy is carried out, however, it is essential to review the results of a full blood count in all patients. Many patients with B-cell chronic lymphocytic leukemia and a few patients with acute leukemia have unnecessary lymph node biopsies each year when the diagnosis could have been

TABLE 7.6. *Guidelines for urgent referral of patients for further investigation of possible hematologic malignancy[a]*

Lymphadenopathy >1 cm persisting for >6 wk

Hepatosplenomegaly

Bone pain with anemia and raised erythrocyte sedimentation rate or plasma viscosity

Blood film or count suggestive of leukemia

Three or more of the following symptoms: fatigue, night sweats, weight loss, itching, breathlessness, bruising, recurrent infection, or bone pain

[a]This is modified from guidance to family practitioners issued by the U.K. Department of Health (www.doh.gov.uk/cancer) with the aim of reducing delays in diagnosis and access to care. The nonspecific clinical features of many types of lymphoma make it difficult to produce guidelines likely to operate with a high degree of sensitivity and specificity.

readily made on examination of the blood and bone marrow. One other possible pitfall is the presence of a large granular lymphocytosis in the peripheral blood. This may be due to active viral infections but is also associated with some B-cell lymphomas (53). This finding should not lead to the assumption that the patient has a reactive cause of lymphadenopathy.

Patients who present with cervical lymphadenopathy may have metastatic squamous carcinoma arising in the head and neck. This is an important differential diagnosis, because excision biopsy of a lymph node may compromise the possibility of carrying out a subsequent radical neck dissection, which constitutes an important aspect of the treatment of epithelial malignancy. However, this may be at variance with studies suggesting the importance of sentinel node biopsy in the management of carcinoma of the head and neck (54). In young patients, head and neck cancer is unlikely, although occasional cases of nasopharyngeal carcinoma are seen in children (55,56). Most lymphomas occur in age groups in which epithelial malignancy is most common. It is, therefore, good practice for a detailed examination of the upper aerodigestive tract to be performed by the surgeon before lymph node biopsy. It is not known how many patients who have no abnormality detected by a specialist examination of the mouth, pharynx, and larynx will still be found to have a metastatic carcinoma in a cervical lymph node. In nonsmokers, in particular, it is likely to be a very rare occurrence; however, in many centers, a fine-needle aspiration of cervical nodes is routinely performed as a screening test before formal node biopsy. This can exclude metastatic carcinoma with a high degree of confidence, assuming that adequate specimens are taken, but it should never be used to exclude the possibility of lymphoma (57,58).

In female patients who present with enlarged axillary lymph nodes, the main differential diagnosis is carcinoma of the breast. It is, therefore, usual to perform breast examination and mammography before lymph node biopsy. If these examinations are normal, the possibility of lymphadenopathy being due to carcinoma of the breast are low.

Suspected Lymphoma Presenting in the Thorax and Mediastinum

Almost all patients with lymphoma who present with a mediastinal mass will have Hodgkin's lymphoma or mediastinal B-cell lymphoma. A few younger patients will have T-cell–precursor lymphoblastic leukemia/lymphoma. Although other types of lymphoproliferative disorders, such as follicular lymphoma and mantle cell lymphoma, may involve the mediastinum, this generally is in the context of generalized disease, and the diagnosis should be made on peripheral node biopsy. The main differential diagnosis in patients with a mediastinal mass is metastatic carcinoma, reactive lymph node, tuberculosis or sarcoidosis, and in a few cases, thymoma. It is generally not considered an acceptable level of risk to perform a thoracotomy, and open biopsy in most

patients presenting with a mediastinal mass and mediastinoscopy is the technique of first choice (59). This involves taking biopsies under direct vision using an endoscope inserted through the suprasternal notch or sometimes through an intercostal space. Unfortunately, from the viewpoint of lymphoma diagnosis, this technique has significant limitations. It is only possible to biopsy the upper mediastinum, and the biopsy may consist mainly of displaced reactive lymphoid tissue or thymus or fibrous tissue, rather than lymphoma. The biopsy fragments may be small and have significant crushing artefact, and although it is usually possible to make suitable touch preparation, which can be used for FISH or as a source of DNA for PCR, the tissue is often insufficient for flow cytometry. Fortunately, the range of differential diagnosis in patients with a localized mediastinal mass is fairly limited, and in most cases, it is possible to make a confident diagnosis using a combination of morphology and immunocytochemistry. In young patients with T-cell precursor acute lymphoblastic leukemia who present with a mediastinal mass, bone marrow and blood may be uninvolved at presentation. This possibility should be considered before proceeding to mediastinal biopsy, however. A small number of patients exist in whom an open surgical biopsy is required to make a confident diagnosis of lymphoma.

A small number of patients with lymphoma present with pleural effusion as a sole abnormality, although the pleura is a common site of relapsed disease (60). The classical example of a lymphoma localized to the pleural space is primary effusion lymphoma (61); this is exceptionally rare, and in most cases, patients who present with a pleural effusion have extension from a mediastinal mass. Examination of pleural fluid specimens by flow cytometry is often sufficient to diagnose relapsed disease. In some cases in which only the visceral pleura is infiltrated with lymphoma, however, the pleural fluid may contain only reactive cells. The ability to detect small numbers of neoplastic cells in the pleural fluid depends on the sensitivity of the flow cytometry technique used. Modern pleural biopsy techniques carried out under video guidance produce good-quality specimens suitable for the full range of laboratory investigations (62–64).

Lymphoma localized to the lung parenchyma is rare. Most cases are indolent marginal zone lymphoma, but a few cases of diffuse large B-cell lymphoma and aggressive T-cell lymphomas present in this way (65–69). In many cases, the diagnosis may not be suspected preoperatively, and the patient will have a presumptive diagnosis of carcinoma. The diagnosis is usually made using an open surgical approach with a wedge biopsy or lobectomy, depending on surgical considerations. In cases in which the lesion involves the pleura, an adequate specimen may be obtained under direct video-guided pleural biopsy. It is possible to make a diagnosis of pulmonary marginal zone lymphoma on a percutaneous computed tomography (CT)-guided biopsy, especially when an aspirate sample is available for flow cytometry, although there are no studies of the sensitivity of this technique. As in the mediastinum, the limited range of diagnostic possibilities may compensate for a less than ideal specimen.

Lymphoma Presenting in the Abdomen and Retroperitoneum

Patients who present with an abdominal mass are more likely to have disseminated carcinoma than lymphoma. In some cases, it is possible to demonstrate a primary site of the tumor by imaging studies and endoscopy. In the remainder, a biopsy is essential to establish the diagnosis. Using CT guidance, it is possible to carry out a percutaneous biopsy safely on all but a small proportion of deep abdominal masses. The major contraindication to this procedure is patients in whom there is a risk of bleeding. When an adequate sample is obtained, a percutaneous core biopsy and a fine-needle aspiration sample are effective in making the diagnosis of metastatic epithelial malignancy in a high proportion of cases. The diagnosis of lymphoma can be more difficult. In cases in which the diagnosis of lymphoma is suspected, multiple core biopsies and a fine-needle aspirate specimen should be taken. The core biopsies should be processed for morphology and immunohistology, and the aspirate specimen can be used for flow cytometry and as a source of DNA (70,71). One problem with this approach is that often only sparse aspirate samples are obtained, and these can be heavily contaminated with blood; this may be a reflection of the dead space in the long needles required for this procedure. Depending on local facilities, it may be possible to assess the adequacy of the aspirate sample by performing automated cell counts with the needle still *in situ*. Another problem with this approach is nonhomogenous lesions, which can include the presence of necrosis, fibrosis, or normal lymphoid tissue, or transformed elements within an indolent lymphoma. A small needle core may be difficult to interpret or give a misleading assessment of the tumor. This can be partly overcome by taking multiple cores, but this is not always possible. Given these limitations, it is especially important to critically review the diagnosis made on this type of specimen against the radiologic and clinical features. The majority of lymphomas found in the abdomen or retroperitoneum are follicular lymphomas or diffuse large B-cell lymphomas; Hodgkin's lymphoma presenting in the abdomen is rare (72). In cases in which the diagnosis of follicular lymphoma cannot be made with certainty on a CT-guided biopsy, it is worthwhile to perform a bone marrow examination before attempting a second biopsy or a laparotomy. In approximately 60% of cases of follicular lymphoma, marrow involvement will be detected, and this can be used to validate the diagnosis made on the abdominal biopsy. This is much less likely to be helpful for other types of lymphoma.

At present, a lower standard of diagnostic accuracy and quality assurance in comparison to that achieved in the biopsy of peripheral nodes appears to be accepted as the price for using low-invasive and convenient biopsy techniques. This balance may be altered by the rapid development of powerful prognostic markers and by the need to identify patients who are suitable for novel biologic therapies. It is unlikely that current CT-guided methods will be able to provide sufficient tissue for these purposes. One possible alternative that appears to have been little used is laparoscopic lymph node biopsy (73,74). This has the advantage of providing large samples of lymph node and allowing a direct inspection of the extent of disease in the abdominal cavity, which may be a useful adjunct to cross-sectional imaging in establishing the stage of disease. The major disadvantage is the need for a skilled surgical team willing to provide this service.

Suspected Lymphoma in the Gastrointestinal Tract

Lymphomas occur in any part of the gastrointestinal tract, but the majority present in the stomach. In general, patients with gastric marginal zone lymphoma have the same range of symptoms as the much larger group of patients with gastritis, and there are no specific features that lead to a suspected diagnosis of lymphoma before endoscopy. Patients with diffuse large B-cell lymphomas may present with the symptoms of ulceration and bleeding, and again, there are no specific characteristics that distinguish this group from patients with peptic ulceration or gastric adenocarcinoma. The primary mode of diagnosis is upper gastrointestinal endoscopy and biopsy. This is an effective technique for the diagnosis of lymphoma, but there are a number of specific issues that need to be considered. Endoscopic biopsies are very small in comparison to the overall area of the gastric mucosa. It is important that the endoscopist takes multiple biopsies (6–8) of any suspicious lesion to reliably establish the diagnosis and confidently exclude malignancy. If only one or two biopsies are taken and these are normal, a repeat endoscopy may be required. Many patients with gastric marginal zone lymphoma are treated with anti-*Helicobacter* therapy and then followed-up (75–77). It is, therefore, essential to accurately document the extent of the lesion at presentation, so the regression can be monitored. This requires multiple biopsies, including sampling of apparently unaffected mucosa and assessment of the depth of tumor infiltration using endoscopic ultrasound. Depth of invasion is a predictor of lack of response to anti-*Helicobacter* therapy alone (78,79). More recently, the importance of molecular cytogenetics in predicting outcome of gastric marginal zone lymphoma has been described (80–83). The t(11;18), in particular, appears to be a powerful marker of tumors that are unlikely to regress following anti-*Helicobacter* treatment (84). It may be possible to infer the presence of this abnormality by nuclear expression of bcl-10 in paraffin sections, but this has not been fully validated (85). The alternative methods are RT-PCR or FISH; the former is easier to apply to small biopsy specimens. Although suitable RNA can sometimes be extracted from paraffin sections, RT-PCR generally requires fresh tissue (86). If current data on the value of the t(11;18) are confirmed, it may justify a repeat endoscopy in some patients to obtain tissue for RNA extraction.

Lymphomas of the small intestine are more diverse in pathologic type and clinical presentation. Marginal zone lymphomas of the more distal small intestine may grow to a considerable size, with extensive infiltration of the bowel wall leading to obstruction. In many cases, the diagnosis is made on a resection specimen. This is also the case for diffuse large B-cell lymphoma, which is typically found around the ileocecal junction (87). Mantle cell lymphoma can affect any part of the gastrointestinal tract but classically causes a polypoid pattern of infiltration of the small intestinal or colonic mucosa (88,89). Patients frequently have involvement of tonsils, peripheral nodes, marrow, and peripheral blood, and this allows the diagnosis to be made by means other than direct biopsy of the intestine. In patients with suspected intestinal lymphoma, this option should be considered as an alternative to direct intestinal biopsy.

Enteropathy-associated T-cell lymphoma is a specific entity found in the small intestine. The classical form of this condition presents with bleeding or perforation, and diagnosis is made on a surgical resection (90). Recently, this type of tumor was recognized as having a broad clinical spectrum that includes some patients with celiac disease that is refractory to treatment and patients with apparently nonspecific ulceration of the small intestine (91). The prognosis of all forms of this condition appears poor, and there is little consensus on treatment. As criteria for making this diagnosis on random biopsies of the duodenum remain provisional, it is essential that great caution is exercised. Key features are intestinal villous atrophy with morphologically atypical intraepithelial T cells. These cells should have an atypical phenotype, either $CD4^-$, $CD8^-$, or $CD56^+$, and should be monoclonal by PCR. This requires optimum biopsy specimens, including fresh tissue for PCR. If there is any doubt, the examination should be repeated to obtain further tissue.

Lymphoma Presenting at Other Extranodal Sites

Lymphomas can present with a lesion involving any anatomic site, and the type of biopsy that can be obtained varies. After the gastrointestinal tract, the skin is the next commonest site of extranodal lymphomas. T-cell lymphomas of mycosis fungoides type present as a rash, and other T- and B-cell lymphomas present as a lump. Biopsy of skin lesions presents little difficulty and can be readily repeated in case of diagnostic difficulty. In investigating patients with skin lymphomas, note that a significant number—possibly up to one third—have systemic disease.

The thyroid and salivary glands are also common sites of lymphoma presentation. Again, both sites are readily accessible to surgical biopsy, and this should be performed wherever possible. Almost all primary salivary or thyroid lymphomas are marginal zone lymphomas, and many thyroid tumors also have a large-cell component. However, patients may also present with salivary or thyroid enlargement caused by infiltration of the gland by lymphoma spreading from adjacent lymph nodes. This is usually follicular lymphoma, diffuse large B-cell lymphoma, or Hodgkin's lymphoma and is seldom the only site of disease. Before taking a surgical biopsy of the thyroid or salivary gland, it is important to assess whether there are more accessible lymph nodes that could be sampled.

A much more difficult diagnostic problem is the patient with primary cerebral lymphoma. Most primary brain lymphomas arise in the white matter of the cerebral cortex, and the differential diagnosis includes infective lesions, gliomas, and metastatic tumors. There is little alternative in these cases to direct surgical biopsy, although it should be obvious that this is performed only after imaging studies have been used to exclude generalized disease that could be more easily biopsied. Unless the tumor involves the meninges, it is very unlikely that a diagnosis will be made on a specimen of cerebrospinal fluid (CSF). Even when there is direct evidence of meningeal disease, CSF specimens are often uninformative. In cases in which a lymphocytosis is detected, it is essential that immunophenotyping is performed to reliably distinguish lymphoma from inflammatory or infective disorders. Precursor acute lymphoblastic leukemia, Burkitt's lymphoma, and diffuse large B-cell lymphoma of the testis (92,93) are regarded as being at high risk of secondary central nervous system involvement. In these patients, it is routine to examine the CSF by microscopy and, where appropriate, flow cytometry; however, the proportion of patients with involved CSF at presentation is low.

ATTEMPTED SURGICAL RESECTION OF LYMPHOMA IS RARELY INDICATED

It is generally recognized that nodal lymphomas are part of systemic disease and that surgical excision is not a curative therapy, even when tumors appear to be localized. In contrast, it has been suggested that some extranodal B-cell lymphomas may be localized to their organ of origin and may, therefore, be amenable to surgical resection. This approach has been most commonly applied to lymphomas arising in the skin, stomach, and lung.

B-cell lymphomas of the skin often arise as relatively small, localized lesions. If complete surgical excision is feasible as a simple procedure, then it is reasonable to do this. The diagnosis of cutaneous B-cell lymphoma may be difficult, and having access to the whole tumor, rather than a small punch biopsy, allows the full range of diagnostic techniques to be performed. An excision biopsy allows the whole lesion to be morphologically examined and a proper assessment made of the microarchitecture of the lymphoid tissue. Some B-cell lymphomas in the skin may be focal within a reactive background population, and examination of the entire lesion increases the probability that an accurate diagnosis is made. Finally, the diagnosis in most cases usually is uncertain before the biopsy is taken, and complete excision is also appropriate for the management of epithelial or melanocytic lesions. However, although the data are relatively sparse, there is evidence that surgical excision is not a curative procedure for any type of B-cell lymphoma of the skin, and prevention of recurrence requires treatment with chemotherapy (94). For this reason, there would appear to be little justification for undertaking complex surgery to fully excise a large lesion or attempting to fully excise a tumor that has been incompletely removed at the time of the initial biopsy.

Many patients with gastric marginal zone lymphoma or diffuse large B-cell lymphoma have been treated by surgical resection alone or in combination with chemotherapy or radiotherapy (76,95–97). Examination of surgical resection specimens has shown that marginal zone lymphoma is a multifocal disease in the stomach, and the only procedure likely to be curative is total gastrectomy (95). This is a major procedure and has a significant mortality and long-term morbidity (98,99). This needs to be set against the very low mortality of patients with marginal zone lymphoma treated with *Helicobacter* eradication or simple oral chemotherapy (100–102). In addition, studies have shown that many patients with marginal zone lymphoma have evidence of marrow involvement at presentation, and recurrences in the lung or other sites are well described (103). There would, therefore, appear to be little justification for carrying out major surgery on this group of patients. A similar argument can be used for gastric diffuse large B-cell lymphoma, in which the results of cyclophosphamide, hydroxydaunomycin, Oncovin (vincristine), and prednisone–type chemotherapy in patients with early stage localized disease are good (104).

Most lymphomas originating in the lung are marginal zone B-cell lymphomas. In some cases, a lobectomy has been carried out at diagnosis. This should not be regarded as a curative procedure in itself, and recurrence may occur in other parts of the lungs, even when the initial lesion appears to be completely excised. If the diagnosis is made on a wedge biopsy or other type of specimens, there would appear to be little justification for performing additional surgery to attempt to completely remove the tumor.

EXAMINATION OF BONE MARROW IN PRIMARY DIAGNOSIS AND STAGING OF LYMPHOMA

Examination of bone marrow in patients with known or suspected lymphoproliferative disorders always requires a marrow aspirate sample for morphology, flow cytometry, molecular studies, and a trephine biopsy. Conventional cytogenetic studies in these patients have a poor yield and are probably not cost effective. Translocations central to diagnosis and monitoring can best be identified by PCR or interphase FISH. The initial handling and processing of bone marrow specimens is as important as the processing of lymph node biopsies (as previously described) to assure accurate results. If the results of PCR studies or flow cytometry are to be valid, it is clearly important that the aspirate sample is not hemodilute. This can be assessed by morphologic examination of fresh aspirate smear prepared at the bedside. The trephine must be of adequate size (at least 10 mm) and should be intact. There are many ways to process trephine biopsies, but a particularly successful method is to fix the specimen in 10% formalin and then embed in methyl methacrylate resin. This provides excellent morphology and allows a wide range of cell markers to be performed, similar to those used on paraffin embedded samples of lymph node (105).

Primary Diagnosis of Lymphoproliferative Disorders in Bone Marrow

Bone marrow is usually the primary means of diagnosis in patients who present with lymphocytosis, a paraprotein, splenomegaly, pancytopenia, or less commonly, neutropenia. Most of these patients will have B-cell chronic lymphocytic leukemia, mantle cell lymphoma, splenic marginal zone lymphoma/Waldenström's macroglobulinemia, or myeloma/monoclonal gammopathy of uncertain significance. In each of these cases, a definitive diagnosis is possible on a bone marrow specimen without recourse to a lymph node biopsy. These are primarily immunophenotypic diagnoses supported by molecular cytogenetics. In the case of mantle cell lymphoma, the t(11;14) is the defining abnormality, and in B-cell chronic lymphocytic leukemia, a variety of abnormalities, most notably deletion of 11q, 13q and 17p, are of major prognostic significance. The presence of an IgM paraprotein does not imply any particular diagnosis, and PCR or FISH should be used to distinguish marginal zone from follicular lymphoma in all cases in which the immunophenotype is indeterminate (106). A small number of patients with diffuse large B-cell lymphoma or Burkitt's lymphoma present with marrow infiltration and consequent cytopenia. Again, this diagnosis can be readily made on a bone marrow examination without additional tissue biopsy.

A more difficult problem is the diagnosis of a monoclonal B-cell infiltrate found in the course of investigation of other clinical problems. Among the most common situations is the discovery of a small clonal B-cell population, usually with a marginal zone–type phenotype, in the investigation of immune-mediated hemolysis and, less commonly, in other immune cytopenias. Often, this is not detectable on examination of routinely stained bone marrow sections and smears. This is of uncertain significance for the pathogenesis or treatment of the condition.

Two lymphoproliferative disorders are specifically associated with selective neutropenia. A very small number of patients with neutropenia have hairy-cell leukemia. This has a highly distinctive morphology and immunophenotype and should be readily diagnosed. The second, probably larger, group has neutropenia in association with a large granular lymphocyte proliferation. In some patients with neutropenia in whom there are no dysplastic features in the bone marrow, immunocytochemistry sometimes shows a $CD8^+$ bone marrow lymphocytosis. The diagnosis can be confirmed on a peripheral blood sample by demonstrating an expanded population of $CD8^+$ large granular lymphocytes with expression of varying combinations of CD16, CD56, and CD57. Some of these are monoclonal, but this finding does not appear to have specific prognostic importance (53,107).

Lymphoid aggregates are a frequent incidental finding in bone marrow biopsy specimens. In most of these, the lymphocytes appear to be reactive T and B cell, but some may be monoclonal B-cell populations. A more difficult problem is the finding of a small peritrabecular aggregate with morphologic features suggestive of follicular lymphoma. Often, the infiltrate is too sparse to have been detected by flow cytometry. Even if a clonal B-cell population is detected by PCR, caution should be exercised in making a diagnosis of lymphoma. If the patient has lymphadenopathy, a node biopsy should be taken. In assessing the likely significance of lymphoid aggregates, it is important to compare the flow cytometric data with the trephine biopsy appearance to determine whether the flow cytometric results match the extent of the lymphoid infiltrate seen in the trephine biopsy. It appears likely that occult lymphoproliferative disorders are common in the general population, and most are of no significance. This is also the case for B-cell chronic lymphocytic leukemia, which may be found relatively frequently in marrow specimens taken for unrelated clinical problems and is common in healthy adults (108). Incidental finding of bone marrow lymphoid aggregates needs to be treated with great caution and requires corroborating evidence before a diagnosis of lymphoma is made.

Use of Bone Marrow Examination in Staging Patients with Lymphoproliferative Disorders

Almost all patients with lymphoma will have a bone marrow examination as part of routine staging. The incidence of bone marrow infiltration and its significance varies according to the type of lymphoma. Patients with radiologic stage I and II Hodgkin's lymphoma have a very low incidence of marrow involvement; this may be as low as 1 to 2% of cases (109–111). In patients with more advanced disease, the incidence increases but remains relatively low. Given that marrow infiltration is likely to be focal, the extent to which the detection of Hodgkin's lymphoma in routine bone marrow biopsies reflects the true incidence of marrow involvement is not clear (112). It is very rare for Hodgkin's lymphoma to be seen in an aspirate sample alone, and this diagnosis should never be made in the absence of other corroborating evidence. Given these circumstances, it is debatable whether routine bone marrow examination is justified in those with early stage disease. The contrary argument is that the detection of marrow involvement identifies a group of high-risk patients, and this is important given the trend toward less intensive treatment in early stage disease. In addition, it can be argued that marrow involvement detected in patients with apparently early stage disease should lead to a review of the diagnosis and imaging findings and consideration of alternative diagnoses, such as T-cell–rich B-cell lymphoma (113). In diffuse large B-cell lymphoma, marrow involvement is more common and less clearly related to radiologic stage. The incidence at a given center depends on the techniques used to assess bone marrow. Where routine three- or four-color flow cytometry and immunocytochemistry are used, more cases are detected than by morphology alone. There are few published data on the effect on outcome of the degree of marrow infiltration, which may range from a few cells to marrow replacement. A relatively frequent finding in patients with diffuse large B-cell lymphoma is the presence of marrow involvement by follicular lymphoma. If the presenting tumor has a germinal center phenotype, this can be taken as strong evidence that the patient has a transformed follicular lymphoma rather than *de novo* diffuse large B-cell lymphoma. Conversely, if the diagnosis of follicular lymphoma is made initially on a bone marrow specimen, the possibility of nodal diffuse large B-cell lymphoma should be considered if the patient has rapidly enlarging lymph nodes.

In contrast to Hodgkin lymphoma and diffuse large B-cell lymphoma, the incidence of marrow involvement in most types of indolent lymphoma is high. In the case of B-cell chronic lymphocytic leukemia and mantle cell lymphoma, it is effectively 100%, and in follicular lymphoma, it is approximately 60 to 70%. One important difference between these conditions is that it is rare to find chronic lymphocytic leukemia or mantle cell lymphoma in a trephine biopsy with negative flow cytometry on the corresponding aspirate sample; this is much more common with follicular lymphoma. A positive trephine biopsy may also be found with a negative PCR. These differences probably reflect differences in the propensity of different types of lymphoma cells to be aspirated, and emphasize the need for a multiple technique–based approach to marrow staging.

MONITORING LYMPHOMA PATIENTS DURING TREATMENT AND DIAGNOSIS OF RELAPSE

In B-cell chronic lymphocytic leukemia and follicular lymphoma, evidence suggests that achieving a negative bone marrow through treatment is a favorable prognostic factor, although it is not usually an indication that the patient has been cured of the disease. In patients in whom the aim of treatment is to achieve a clear marrow, it is important to use effective methods for the detection of very small amounts of residual disease. In the case of B-cell chronic lymphocytic leukemia, there are highly effective flow cytometric methods for the detection and monitoring of residual disease. These are quantitative to a level of approximately 0.05% of leucocytes and are unaffected by reactive B-cell populations (108). This technique can be used on peripheral blood samples until no disease is detected and then used to monitor sequential bone marrow samples. The detection of follicular lymphoma at presentation and follow-up is more complex. Most recent studies have used PCR for IgH or t(14;18) as the gold standard; however, a variety of PCR methods have been used and as the, there can be a wide variation in sensitivity. Some additional cases, including the 5% that lack a t(14;18), are detected by flow cytometry. As at primary diagnosis and staging, flow cytometry and PCR are limited by the quality of an aspirate sample, and there are patients with no evidence of lymphoma on PCR or flow cytometry who have evidence of disease on the trephine biopsy. For this reason, in circumstances in which the detection of low levels of follicular lymphoma is critical, it is important that all three approaches are used.

When a patient who has previously been in complete remission has symptoms or imaging findings suggestive of relapse, the question arises: Should the suspicious lesion be biopsied, or is the relapse evidence sufficiently conclusive to allow treatment to be commenced? The main argument in favor of rebiopsy is that indolent lymphomas may have transformed to large-cell lymphoma with important consequences for subsequent treatment or prognosis. Imaging studies are not infallible, and there are patients with recurrent lymphadenopathy who have reactive hyperplasia, infections, such as tuberculosis, or unrelated metastatic disease. In the case of diffuse large B-cell lymphoma, in particular, the consequences of relapsed disease for a patient previously in complete remission are so severe that the diagnosis should be made definitively. When additional treatment, particularly high-dose or relape-type chemotherapy is going to be given, the argument that relapse should be confirmed by biopsy would appear to be compelling, as long as this does not involve undue risk to the patient.

DEVELOPMENTS IN THE LABORATORY DIAGNOSIS OF LYMPHOMA

Knowledge of the cellular mechanisms responsible for the pathogenesis of lymphoma is expanding rapidly and is likely to lead to the development of lymphoma classifications based on pathogenesis rather than empirically derived morphologic or immunophenotypic features. This process will be driven by the development of therapeutic agents designed to target the abnormally expressed gene products that confer a survival or proliferative advantage on the tumor cells. These developments will require a new approach to the laboratory diagnosis of patients with lymphoma. Inevitably, the role of morphologic assessment will decline and be replaced by the need to interpret increasingly complex biologic information and translate this into an assessment of the likely efficacy of particular types of therapy.

Many of the techniques in current use, such as flow cytometry or FISH, are highly versatile and are likely to remain key elements of hematopathology laboratories in the future; however, a number of newer technologies are likely to play an increasing role in clinical practice. One major development has been the introduction of DNA microarrays that offer the ability to screen tissue specimens for the expression of very large numbers of genes. DNA arrays are powerful tools for identifying genes of potential diagnostic value but have a number of inherent limitations that are likely to restrict their direct application in the diagnostic laboratory, including the need for relatively pure samples of tumor cells and the uncertain relationship between mRNA and protein expression. Until recently, understanding of the pathogenesis of tumors was largely driven by identification of genes that are aberrantly expressed as a consequence of chromosomal rearrangements. The focus is now turning to the detection of mutated proteins, which in B-cell malignancies may be a consequence

of somatic hypermutation in the germinal center (114). This will mean that the ability to rapidly and accurately sequence DNA may become an essential technique in diagnosis. This is already the case in a number of specialist applications, such as the generation of allele-specific oligonucleotides used in residual disease monitoring (115). Finally, it is likely to be increasingly important to be able to identify not only the presence of a particular protein but also to determine its activation state or ability to interact with other molecules. A simple example already widely used is the detection of mutated p53 by the discordant expression of p53 and p21 (116). A new generation of monoclonal antibodies and other reagents able to discriminate between activated and nonactivated proteins is being produced, and techniques are being developed to allow heterodimers to be identified.

These conceptual and technologic developments are already having an impact on the diagnosis of lymphomas, and major changes can be confidently expected in coming years. This process of change will have important implications for the way that diagnostic services are organized and delivered. Realizing the full potential for improving clinical outcomes will require closer integration of the various diagnostic and clinical services involved in the care of patients with hematologic malignancies.

ROLE OF A MULTIDISCIPLINARY TEAM IN THE DIAGNOSTIC PROCESS

As has been described above, accurate diagnosis and follow-up of patients with lymphoma depends on a properly constituted laboratory and procedures to ensure that correct specimens are taken and handled appropriately. An equally important aspect of this process, however, is the way that information obtained from these investigations is communicated and interpreted. The approach to laboratory diagnosis has been described, particularly the use of protocols designed to cross-check the results of the various diagnostic techniques. An important extension of this process is the comparison of the pathologic diagnosis with imaging and other clinical information. Most of the entities of the WHO classification include a defined set of clinical features, and ensuring that these are consistent with the proposed pathologic diagnosis adds a further level of quality assurance. When inconsistencies occur, it is important that these are investigated and resolved before the patient is treated. In cases in which it has not been possible to perform a full range of investigations because of a poor-quality specimen, it is essential that the significance of this information and its effect on diagnostic confidence are fully discussed. At a more general level, the investigation, diagnosis, and treatment of lymphoma patients is a complex matter, and development of effective and rational protocols requires contributions from a range of specialists in both diagnostic and clinical areas. Protocols developed in this way need to be vigorously disseminated within the institution as a whole, and stringent audit systems need to be in place to monitor their effectiveness. These important objectives can be most easily achieved by creation of multidisciplinary teams that systematically review individual patients and provide a forum for the development of protocols within the institution. This may be problematic if important aspects of the diagnostic process are provided at remote locations; however, it should be recognized that the benefits of a sophisticated laboratory and imaging service can be negated if the results of these investigations are not effectively communicated. Equally, the accuracy of laboratory diagnosis may be compromised if it is performed without regard to the patient's clinical state.

REFERENCES

1. Harris NL, Jaffe ES, Stein H, et al. A revised European-American classification of lymphoid neoplasms: a proposal from the International Lymphoma Study Group. *Blood* 1994;84:1361–1392.
2. Jaffe ES. Hematopathology: integration of morphologic features and biologic markers for diagnosis. *Mod Pathol* 1999;12(2):109–115.
3. Wakely SL, Baxendine-Jones JA, Gallagher PJ, et al. Aberrant diagnoses by individual surgical pathologists. *Am J Surg Pathol* 1998;22(1):77–82.
4. Prescott RJ, Wells S, Bisset DL, et al. Audit of tumor histopathology reviewed by a regional oncology centre [see comments]. *J Clin Pathol* 1995;48(3):245–249.
5. Georgii A, Fischer R, Hubner K, et al. Classification of Hodgkin's disease biopsies by a panel of four histopathologists. Report of 1,140 patients from the German National Trial. *Leuk Lymphoma* 1993;9(4–5):365–370.
6. Santucci M, Biggeri A, Feller AC, Burg G. Accuracy, concordance, and reproducibility of histologic diagnosis in cutaneous T-cell lymphoma: an EORTC Cutaneous Lymphoma Project Group study. European Organization for Research and Treatment of Cancer. *Arch Dermatol* 2000;136(4):497–502.
7. Taylor PR, Angus B, Owen JP, et al. Hodgkin's disease: a population-adjusted clinical epidemiology study (PACE) of management at presentation. Northern Region Lymphoma Group. *QJM* 1998;91(2):131–139.
8. Kipps TJ. Genetics of chronic lymphocytic leukanemia. *Hematol Cell Ther* 2000;42(1):5–14.
9. Brito-Babapulle V, Garcia-Marco J, Maljaie SH, et al. The impact of molecular cytogenetics on chronic lymphoid leukanemia. *Acta Haematol* 1997;98(4):175–186.
10. Damle RN, Wasil T, Fais F, et al. Ig V gene mutation status and CD38 expression as novel prognostic indicators in chronic lymphocytic leukemia. *Blood* 1999;94(6):1840–1847.
11. Hamblin TJ, Davis Z, Gardiner A, et al. Unmutated Ig V(H) genes are associated with a more aggressive form of chronic lymphocytic leukemia. *Blood* 1999;94(6):1848–1854.
12. Alizadeh A, Eisen M, Davis RE, et al. The lymphochip: a specialized cDNA microarray for the genomic-scale analysis of gene expression in normal and malignant lymphocytes. *Cold Spring Harb Symp Quant Biol* 1999;64:71–78.
13. Alizadeh AA, Eisen MB, Davis RE, et al. Distinct types of diffuse large B-cell lymphoma identified by gene expression profiling. *Nature* 2000;403(6769):503–511.
14. Capello D, Vitolo U, Pasqualucci L, et al. Distribution and pattern of BCL-6 mutations throughout the spectrum of B-cell neoplasia. *Blood* 2000;95(2):651–659.
15. Chaganti SR, Chen W, Parsa N, et al. Involvement of BCL6 in chromosomal aberrations affecting band 3q27 in B-cell non-Hodgkin lymphoma. *Genes Chromosomes Cancer* 1998;23(4):323–327.
16. Barrans SL, Carter I, Owen RG, et al. Germinal center phenotype and bcl-2 expression combined with the International Prognostic Index improves patient risk stratification in diffuse large B-cell lymphoma. *Blood* 2002;99(4):1136–1143.
17. Leroy K, Haioun C, Lepage E, et al. p53 gene mutations are associated with poor survival in low and low–intermediate risk diffuse large B-cell lymphomas. *Ann Oncol* 2002;13(7):1108–1115.
18. Gronbaek K, de Nully BP, Moller MB, et al. Concurrent disruption of p16INK4a and the ARF-p53 pathway predicts poor prognosis in aggressive non-Hodgkin's lymphoma. *Leukemia* 2000;14(10):1727–1735.
19. Lundin J, Osterborg A, Brittinger G, et al. CAMPATH-1H monoclonal antibody in therapy for previously treated low-grade non-Hodgkin's lymphomas: a phase II multicenter study. European Study Group of CAMPATH-1H Treatment in Low-Grade Non-Hodgkin's Lymphoma. *J Clin Oncol* 1998;16(10):3257–3263.
20. Foran JM, Rohatiner AZ, Cunningham D, et al. European phase II study of rituximab (chimeric anti-CD20 monoclonal antibody) for patients with newly diagnosed mantle-cell lymphoma and previously treated mantle-cell lymphoma, immunocytoma, and small B-cell lymphocytic lymphoma [published erratum appears in *J Clin Oncol* 2000;18(9):2006]. *J Clin Oncol* 2000;18(2):317–324.
21. Mauro MJ, Druker BJ. Sti571: a gene product-targeted therapy for leukemia. *Curr Oncol Rep* 2001;3(3):223–227.
22. L'Allemain G. Update on the proteasome inhibitor PS341. *Bull Cancer* 2002;89(1):29–30.
23. Dumont FJ. CAMPATH (alemtuzumab) for the treatment of chronic lymphocytic leukemia and beyond. *Expert Rev Anticancer Ther* 2002;2(1):23–35.
24. Ormerod MG, Tribukait B, Giaretti W. Consensus report of the task force on standardisation of DNA flow cytometry in clinical pathology. DNA Flow Cytometry Task Force of the European Society for Analytical Cellular Pathology. *Anal Cell Pathol* 1998;17(2):103–110.
25. Lucio P, Gaipa G, van Lochem EG, et al. BIOMED-I concerted action report: flow cytometric immunophenotyping of precursor B-ALL with standardized triple-stainings. BIOMED-1 Concerted Action Investigation of Minimal Residual Disease in Acute Leukemia: International Standardization and Clinical Evaluation. *Leukemia* 2001;15(8):1185–1192.
26. Kappelmayer J, Gratama JW, Karaszi E, et al. Flow cytometric detection of intracellular myeloperoxidase, CD3 and CD79a. Interaction between monoclonal antibody clones, fluorochromes and sample preparation protocols. *J Immunol Methods* 2000;242(1–2):53–65.
27. Sanchez ML, Almeida J, Vidriales B, et al. Incidence of phenotypic aberrations in a series of 467 patients with B chronic lymphoproliferative disorders: basis for the design of specific four-color stainings to be used for minimal residual disease investigation. *Leukemia* 2002;16(8):1460–1469.
28. Rawstron AC, Fenton JA, Ashcroft J, et al. The interleukin-6 receptor alpha-chain (CD126) is expressed by neoplastic but not normal plasma cells. *Blood* 2000;96(12):3880–3886.
29. Brown RW, Chirala R. Utility of microwave-citrate antigen retrieval in diagnostic immunohistochemistry. *Mod Pathol* 1995;8(5):515–520.
30. Evers P, Uylings HB. Microwave-stimulated antigen retrieval is pH and temperature dependent. *J Histochem Cytochem* 1994;42(12):1555–1563.
31. Sale GE, Beauchamp M, Myerson D. Immunohistologic staining of cytotoxic T and NK cells in formalin-fixed paraffin-embedded tissue using microwave TIA-1 antigen retrieval. *Transplantation* 1994;57(2):287–289.
32. Erber WN, Gibbs TA, Ivey JG. Antigen retrieval by microwave oven heating for immunohistochemical analysis of bone marrow trephine biopsies. *Pathology* 1996;28(1):45–50.
33. Li X, Stark GR. NFkappaB-dependent signaling pathways. *Exp Hematol* 2002;30(4):285–296.
34. Aamot H, Micci F, Holte H, et al. M-FISH cytogenetic analysis of non-Hodgkin lymphomas with t(14;18)(q32;q21) and add(1)(p36) as a secondary abnormality shows that the extra material often comes from chromosome arm 17q. *Leuk Lymphoma* 2002;43(5):1051–1056.
35. Matutes E, Carrara P, Coignet L, et al. FISH analysis for BCL-1 rearrangements and trisomy 12 helps the diagnosis of atypical B cell leukemias. *Leukemia* 1999;13(11):1721–1726.
36. Kluin PH, Schuuring E. FISH and related techniques in the diagnosis of lymphoma. *Cancer Surv* 1997;30:3–20.
37. Luthra R, Sarris AH, Hai S, et al. Real-time 5'→3' exonuclease-based PCR assay for detection of the t(11;14)(q13;q32). *Am J Clin Pathol* 1999;112(4):524–530.
38. Vaandrager JW, Schuuring E, Raap T, et al. Interphase FISH detection of BCL2 rearrangement in follicular lymphoma using breakpoint-flanking probes. *Genes Chromosomes Cancer* 2000;27(1):85–94.

39. Kluin PH, Schuuring E. FISH and related techniques in the diagnosis of lymphoma. *Cancer Surv* 1997;30:3–20.
40. Bienz N, Cardy DL, Leyland MJ, et al. Trisomy 12 in B-cell chronic lymphocytic leukanemia: an evaluation of 33 patients by direct fluorescence in situ hybridization (FISH). *Br J Haematol* 1993;85(4):819–822.
41. Falini B, Mason DY. Proteins encoded by genes involved in chromosomal alterations in lymphoma and leukemia: clinical value of their detection by immunocytochemistry. *Blood* 2002;99(2):409–426.
42. Summerfield GP, Carey PJ, Galloway MJ, et al. An audit of delays in diagnosis and treatment of lymphoma in district hospitals in the northern region of the United Kingdom. *Clin Lab Haematol* 2000;22(3):157–160.
43. Calvert RJ, Evans PA, Randerson JA, et al. The significance of B-cell clonality in gastric lymphoid infiltrates. *J Pathol* 1996;180(1):26–32.
44. Wundisch T, Thiede C, Alpen B, et al. Are lymphocytic monoclonality and immunoglobulin heavy chain (IgH) rearrangement premalignant conditions in chronic gastritis? *Microsc Res Tech* 2001;53(6):414–418.
45. Klemke CD, Dippel E, Dembinski A, et al. Clonal T cell receptor gamma-chain gene rearrangement by PCR-based GeneScan analysis in the skin and blood of patients with parapsoriasis and early-stage mycosis fungoides. *J Pathol* 2002;197(3):348–354.
46. Barrans SL, O'Connor SJ, Evans PA, et al. Rearrangement of the BCL6 locus at 3q27 is an independent poor prognostic factor in nodal diffuse large B-cell lymphoma. *Br J Haematol* 2002;117(2):322–332.
47. Liehr T, Grehl H, Rautenstrauss B. FISH analysis of interphase nuclei extracted from paraffin-embedded tissue. *Trends Genet* 1995;11(10):377–378.
48. Johnson KL, Zhen DK, Bianchi DW. The use of fluorescence in situ hybridization (FISH) on paraffin-embedded tissue sections for the study of microchimerism. *Biotechniques* 2000;29(6):1220–1224.
49. Stanta G, Bonin S, Lugli M. Quantitative RT-PCR from fixed paraffin-embedded tissues by capillary electrophoresis. *Methods Mol Biol* 2001;163:253–258.
50. Akalu A, Reichardt JK. A reliable PCR amplification method for microdissected tumor cells obtained from paraffin-embedded tissue. *Genet Anal* 1999;15(6):229–233.
51. Hughes J, Weston S, Bennetts B, et al. The application of a PCR technique for the detection of immunoglobulin heavy chain gene rearrangements in fresh or paraffin-embedded skin tissue. *Pathology* 2001;33(2):222–225.
52. Chan PK, Chan DP, To KF, et al. Evaluation of extraction methods from paraffin wax–embedded tissues for PCR amplification of human and viral DNA. *J Clin Pathol* 2001;54(5):401–403.
53. Scott CS, Richards SJ. Classification of large granular lymphocyte (LGL) and NK-associated (NKa) disorders. *Blood* Rev 1992;6(4):220–233.
54. Ross GL, Shoaib T, Soutar DS, et al. The First International Conference on Sentinel Node Biopsy in Mucosal Head and Neck Cancer and adoption of a multicenter trial protocol. *Ann Surg Oncol* 2002;9(4):406–410.
55. Casanova M, Ferrari A, Gandola L, et al. Undifferentiated nasopharyngeal carcinoma in children and adolescents: comparison between staging systems. *Ann Oncol* 2001;12(8):1157–1162.
56. Sahraoui S, Acharki A, Benider A, et al. Nasopharyngeal carcinoma in children under 15 years of age: a retrospective review of 65 patients. *Ann Oncol* 1999;10(12):1499–1502.
57. Bhatia A, Singh N, Arora VK, Gupta K. Prospective peer review in fine needle aspiration cytology. Another step toward quality assurance. *Acta Cytol* 1998;42(4):865–868.
58. Das DK. Value and limitations of fine-needle aspiration cytology in diagnosis and classification of lymphomas: a review. *Diagn Cytopathol* 1999;21(4):240–249.
59. Glick RD, Pearse IA, Trippett T, et al. Diagnosis of mediastinal masses in pediatric patients using mediastinoscopy and the Chamberlain procedure. *J Pediatr Surg* 1999;34(4):559–564.
60. Elis A, Blickstein D, Mulchanov I, et al. Pleural effusion in patients with non-Hodgkin's lymphoma: a case-controlled study. *Cancer* 1998;83(8):1607–1611.
61. Boulanger E, Agbalika F, Maarek O, et al. A clinical, molecular and cytogenetic study of 12 cases of human herpesvirus 8–associated primary effusion lymphoma in HIV-infected patients. *Hematol J* 2001;2(3):172–179.
62. Hermansson U, Konstantinov IE, Aren C. Video-assisted thoracic surgery (VATS) lobectomy: the initial Swedish experience. *Semin Thorac Cardiovasc Surg* 1998;10(4):285–290.
63. Stoica SC, Ferguson T, Monaghan H, Walker WS. Video-assisted thoracoscopic management of primary pericardial Hodgkin's lymphoma. *Eur J Surg Oncol* 2001;27(3):325–326.
64. Alifano M, Guggino G, Gentile M, et al. Management of concurrent pleural effusion in patients with lymphoma: thoracoscopy a useful tool in diagnosis and treatment. *Monaldi Arch Chest Dis* 1997;52(4):330–334.
65. Kurtin PJ, Myers JL, Adlakha H, et al. Pathologic and clinical features of primary pulmonary extranodal marginal zone B-cell lymphoma of MALT type. *Am J Surg Pathol* 2001;25(8):997–1008.
66. Wilson WH, Kingma DW, Raffeld M, et al. Association of lymphomatoid granulomatosis with Epstein-Barr viral infection of B lymphocytes and response to interferon-alpha 2b. *Blood* 1996;87(11):4531–4537.
67. Koss M, Zeren EH. Low-grade B-cell lymphomas of lung and lymphomatoid granulomatosis. *Pathology (Phila)* 1996;4(1):125–139.
68. Ferraro P, Trastek VF, Adlakha H, et al. Primary non-Hodgkin's lymphoma of the lung. *Ann Thorac Surg* 2000;69(4):993–997.
69. Bolton-Maggs PH, Colman A, Dixon GR, et al. Mucosa associated lymphoma of the lung. *Thorax* 1993;48(6):670–672.
70. Aiello A, Delia D, Giardini R, et al. PCR analysis of IgH and BCL2 gene rearrangement in the diagnosis of follicular lymphoma in lymph node fine-needle aspiration. A critical appraisal. *Diagn Mol Pathol* 1997;6(3):154–160.
71. Jeffers MD, Milton J, Herriot R, McKean M. Fine needle aspiration cytology in the investigation on non-Hodgkin's lymphoma. *J Clin Pathol* 1998;51(3):189–196.
72. Cutuli B, Petit T, Hoffstetter S, et al. Treatment of subdiaphragmatic Hodgkin's disease: long-term results and side effects. *Oncol Rep* 1998;5(6):1513–1518.
73. Walsh RM, Heniford BT. Role of laparoscopy for Hodgkin's and non-Hodgkin's lymphoma. *Semin Surg Oncol* 1999;16(4):284–292.
74. Mann GB, Conlon KC, LaQuaglia et al. Emerging role of laparoscopy in the diagnosis of lymphoma. *J Clin Oncol* 1998;16(5):1909–1915.
75. Steinbach G, Ford R, Glober G, et al. Antibiotic treatment of gastric lymphoma of mucosa-associated lymphoid tissue. An uncontrolled trial. *Ann Intern Med* 1999;131(2):88–95.
76. Levy M, Copie-Bergman C, Traulle C, et al. Conservative treatment of primary gastric low-grade B-cell lymphoma of mucosa-associated lymphoid tissue: predictive factors of response and outcome. *Am J Gastroenterol* 2002;97(2):292–297.
77. Urakami Y, Sano T, Begum S, et al. Endoscopic characteristics of low-grade gastric mucosa-associated lymphoid tissue lymphoma after eradication of *Helicobacter pylori*. *J Gastroenterol Hepatol* 2000;15(10):1113–1119.
78. Pavlick AC, Gerdes H, Portlock CS. Endoscopic ultrasound in the evaluation of gastric small lymphocytic mucosa-associated lymphoid tumors. *J Clin Oncol* 1997;15(5):1761–1766.
79. Fusaroli P, Buscarini E, Peyre S, et al. Interobserver agreement in staging gastric malt lymphoma by EUS. *Gastrointest Endosc* 2002;55(6):662–668.
80. Sugiyama T, Asaka M, Nakamura T, et al. API2-MALT1 chimeric transcript is a predictive marker for the responsiveness of *H. pylori* eradication treatment in low-grade gastric MALT lymphoma. *Gastroenterology* 2001;120(7):1884–1885.
81. Liu H, Ruskon-Fourmestraux A, Lavergne-Slove A, et al. Resistance of t(11;18) positive gastric mucosa-associated lymphoid tissue lymphoma to *Helicobacter pylori* eradication therapy. *Lancet* 2001;357(9249):39–40.
82. Starostik P, Greiner A, Schultz A, et al. Genetic aberrations common in gastric high-grade large B-cell lymphoma. *Blood* 2000;95(4):1180–1187.
83. Du MQ, Isaccson PG. Gastric MALT lymphoma: from aetiology to treatment. *Lancet Oncol* 2002;3(2):97–104.
84. Baens M, Maes B, Steyls A, et al. The product of the t(11;18), an API2-MLT fusion, marks nearly half of gastric MALT type lymphomas without large cell proliferation. *Am J Pathol* 2000;156(4):1433–1439.
85. Liu H, Ye H, Dogan A, et al. T(11;18)(q21;q21) is associated with advanced mucosa-associated lymphoid tissue lymphoma that expresses nuclear BCL10. *Blood* 2001;98(4):1182–1187.

86. Inagaki H, Okabe M, Seto M, et al. API2-MALT1 fusion transcripts involved in mucosa-associated lymphoid tissue lymphoma: multiplex RT-PCR detection using formalin-fixed paraffin-embedded specimens. *Am J Pathol* 2001;158(2):699–706.

87. Foss HD, Stein H. Pathology of intestinal lymphomas. *Recent Results Cancer Res* 2000;156:33–41.

88. Hashimoto Y, Nakamura N, Kuze T, et al. Multiple lymphomatous polyposis of the gastrointestinal tract is a heterogenous group that includes mantle cell lymphoma and follicular lymphoma: analysis of somatic mutation of immunoglobulin heavy chain gene variable region. *Hum Pathol* 1999;30(5):581–587.

89. Oinonen R, Franssila K, Teerenhovi L, et al. Mantle cell lymphoma: clinical features, treatment and prognosis of 94 patients. *Eur J Cancer* 1998;34(3):329–336.

90. Gale J, Simmonds PD, Mead GM, et al. Enteropathy-type intestinal T-cell lymphoma: clinical features and treatment of 31 patients in a single center. *J Clin Oncol* 2000;18(4):795–803.

91. Bagdi E, Diss TC, Munson P, et al. Mucosal intra-epithelial lymphocytes in enteropathy-associated T-cell lymphoma, ulcerative jejunitis, and refractory celiac disease constitute a neoplastic population. *Blood* 1999;94(1):260–264.

92. Fenaux P, Bourhis JH, Ribrag V. Burkitt's acute lymphocytic leukemia (L3ALL) in adults. *Hematol Oncol Clin North Am* 2001;15(1):37–50.

93. Seymour JF, Solomon B, Wolf MM, et al. Primary large-cell non-Hodgkin's lymphoma of the testis: a retrospective analysis of patterns of failure and prognostic factors. *Clin Lymphoma* 2001;2(2):109–115.

94. Pandolfino TL, Siegel RS, Kuzel TM, et al. Primary cutaneous B-cell lymphoma: review and current concepts. *J Clin Oncol* 2000;18(10):2152–2168.

95. Bozer M, Eroglu A, Unal E, et al. Survival after curative resection for stage IE and IIE primary gastric lymphoma. *Hepatogastroenterology* 2001;48(40):1202–1205.

96. Mafune KI, Tanaka Y, Suda Y, et al. Outcome of patients with non-Hodgkin's lymphoma of the stomach after gastrectomy: clinicopathologic study and reclassification according to the revised European-American lymphoma classification. *Gastric Cancer* 2001;4(3):137–143.

97. Blair S, Shah S, Tamim W, et al. Surgical resection improves survival in the treatment of early gastric lymphomas. *J Gastrointest Surg* 2000;4(3):304–309.

98. Mariette C, Castel B, Toursel H, et al. Surgical management of and long-term survival after adenocarcinoma of the cardia. *Br J Surg* 2002;89(9):1156–1163.

99. Damhuis RA, Meurs CJ, Dijkhuis CM, et al. Hospital volume and post-operative mortality after resection for gastric cancer. *Eur J Surg Oncol* 2002;28(4):401–405.

100. Fischbach W, Dragosics B, Kolve-Goebeler ME, et al. Primary gastric B-cell lymphoma: results of a prospective multicenter study. The German-Austrian Gastrointestinal Lymphoma Study Group. *Gastroenterology* 2000;119(5):1191–1202.

101. Nathwani BN, Anderson JR, Armitage JO, et al. Marginal zone B-cell lymphoma: A clinical comparison of nodal and mucosa-associated lymphoid tissue types. Non-Hodgkin's Lymphoma Classification Project. *J Clin Oncol* 1999;17(8):2486–2492.

102. Pinotti G, Zucca E, Roggero E, et al. Clinical features, treatment and outcome in a series of 93 patients with low-grade gastric MALT lymphoma. *Leuk Lymphoma* 1997;26(5–6):527–537.

103. Thieblemont C, Berger F, Dumontet C, et al. Mucosa-associated lymphoid tissue lymphoma is a disseminated disease in one-third of 158 patients analyzed. *Blood* 2000;95(3):802–806.

104. Raderer M, Valencak J, Osterreicher C, et al. Chemotherapy for the treatment of patients with primary high grade gastric B-cell lymphoma of modified Ann Arbor Stages IE and IIE. *Cancer* 2000;88(9):1979–1985.

105. Blythe D, Hand NM, Jackson P, et al. Use of methyl methacrylate resin for embedding bone marrow trephine biopsy specimens. *J Clin Pathol* 1997;50(1):45–49.

106. Owen RG, Parapia LA, Higginson J, et al. Clinicopathological correlates of IgM paraproteinemias. *Clin Lymphoma* 2000;1(1):39–43.

107. Sivakumaran M, Richards SJ, Hunt KM, et al. Patterns of CD16 and CD56 expression in persistent expansions of CD3$^+$NKa$^+$ lymphocytes are predictive for clonal T-cell receptor gene rearrangements. The Yorkshire Leukaemia Group. *Br J Haematol* 1991;78(3):368–377.

108. Rawstron AC, Green MJ, Kuzmicki A, et al. Monoclonal B lymphocytes with the characteristics of "indolent" chronic lymphocytic leukemia are present in 3.5% of adults with normal blood counts. *Blood* 2002;100(2):635–639.

109. Taylor PR, Angus B, Owen JP, et al. Hodgkin's disease: a population-adjusted clinical epidemiology study (PACE) of management at presentation. Northern Region Lymphoma Group. *QJM* 1998;91(2):131–139.

110. Sutcliffe SB, Timothy AR, Lister TA. Staging in Hodgkin's disease. *Clin Haematol* 1979;8(3):593–609.

111. Mahoney DH Jr, Schreuders LC, Gresik MV, et al. Role of staging bone marrow examination in children with Hodgkin disease. *Med Pediatr Oncol* 1998;30(3):175–177.

112. Varan A, Cila A, Buyukpamukcu M. Prognostic importance of magnetic resonance imaging in bone marrow involvement of Hodgkin disease. *Med Pediatr Oncol* 1999;32(4):267–271.

113. Skinnider BF, Connors JM, Gascoyne RD. Bone marrow involvement in T-cell-rich B-cell lymphoma. *Am J Clin Pathol* 1997;108(5):570–578.

114. Pasqualucci L, Neumeister P, Goossens T, et al. Hypermutation of multiple proto-oncogenes in B-cell diffuse large-cell lymphomas. *Nature* 2001;412(6844):341–346.

115. Chim JC, Coyle LA, Yaxley JC, et al. The use of IgH fingerprinting and ASO-dependent PCR for the investigation of residual disease (MRD) in ALL. *Br J Haematol* 1996;92(1):104–115.

116. Jezersek-Novakovic B, Frkovic-Grazio S, Novakovic S. The immunohistochemical and serological determination of p53 protein in patients with malignant lymphomas. *Neoplasma* 2002;49(1):16–20.

CHAPTER 8

Initial Evaluation: Staging and Prognostic Factors

Kerry J. Savage and Margaret A. Shipp

STAGING IN NON-HODGKIN'S LYMPHOMA

The initial evaluation of the lymphoma patient serves to establish the correct diagnosis and extent of disease. Information is assembled through a history, physical examination, relevant radiographic studies, laboratory investigations, and necessary invasive procedures to identify the sites of disease, estimate prognosis, and develop a rational treatment approach. In contrast to the prognostic importance of stage in nonhematologic malignancies, advanced stage in non-Hodgkin's lymphoma does not always correlate with poor outcome. This is particularly true of indolent lymphomas, which often present with bone marrow involvement but have a long natural history. Nevertheless, a uniform staging system allows for the development of rational treatment strategies and for accurate study comparisons.

ANN ARBOR STAGING SYSTEM

The Ann Arbor staging classification (1), which was originally designed in 1971 for Hodgkin's lymphoma, is the recommended staging classification for all non-Hodgkin's lymphomas (Table 8.1). This classification emphasizes the number and location of involved nodal and extranodal regions with subcategories based on the presence of B symptoms. The spleen, thymus, Waldeyer's ring, appendix, and Peyer's patch are all considered lymphoid organs. Localized extralymphatic disease is designated as an E lesion; however, diffuse extranodal involvement is indicative of stage IV disease. The Ann Arbor staging originally included pathologic information obtained from invasive procedures such as bone marrow biopsy, staging laparotomy, and splenectomy. Today, only bone marrow biopsies are routinely performed.

Several limitations become apparent when the Ann Arbor classification is applied to non-Hodgkin's lymphoma. Unlike Hodgkin's lymphoma, which has a contiguous pattern of lymphatic involvement, non-Hodgkin's lymphomas have a tendency to spread hematogenously and involve noncontiguous lymph node sites (2). In addition, the Ann Arbor staging system does not reflect the unique natural history of specific lymphoma subtypes or the consequences of lymphomatous involvement of certain extranodal disease sites (e.g., sinus, central nervous system, testicular) (3–5). Finally, important factors reflecting tumor burden [e.g., lactate dehydrogenase (LDH), number of nodal or extranodal sites involved, tumor bulk, β_2-microglobulin, and B symptoms] and the physiologic reserve of the patient (e.g., age and performance status) are not included in this conventional staging system.

To more fully incorporate additional relevant prognostic features, more broadly relevant models have been developed in the most common lymphomas—diffuse large cell lymphoma (6–19) and follicular lymphoma (20–25). The most widely used model is the International Prognostic Index (IPI), which was originally developed for diffuse large-cell lymphoma (26) and is discussed in more detail later in the chapter. Alternate staging systems have also been adapted for other specific disease entities and sites. For example, in gastrointestinal lymphoma, a modified version of the Ann Arbor staging system (27), which distinguishes between local (gastric or mesenteric) and distant (abdominal) nodal disease, has been demonstrated to have prognostic significance (28–30). With the availability of endoscopic ultrasound, a tumor, node, metastasis (TNM) system has also been used to address the depth of gastric-wall invasion. An alternate staging system that was adapted from the pediatric population is often used in Burkitt's lymphoma (31). In this disease, the Ann Arbor classification is less precise because it does not include specific extranodal disease sites.

RECOMMENDED STUDIES FOR INITIAL EVALUATION

The diversity of lymphoma subtypes and the unique involvement of specific extranodal disease sites make it difficult to apply a uniform method of staging for all patients. Nevertheless, a general strategy can be followed for most lymphoma patients, with selected additional studies when there are suspicious clinical findings or disease-specific characteristics, or

TABLE 8.1. *Ann Arbor staging system*[a]

Stage	Definition[b]
I	Involvement of a single lymph node or of a single extranodal organ or site (IE)
II	Involvement of two or more lymph node regions on the same side of the diaphragm, or localized involvement of an extranodal site or organ (IIE) and one or more lymph node regions on the same side of the diaphragm
III	Involvement of lymph node regions on both sides of the diaphragm, which may also be accompanied by localized involvement of an extranodal organ or site (IIIE) or spleen (IIIS), or both (IIISE)
IV	Diffuse or disseminated involvement of one or more distant extranodal organs with or without associated lymph node involvement

[a]Fever > 38°C, night sweats, and/or weight loss >10% of body weight in the 6 months preceding admission are defined as systemic symptoms.
[b]The spleen is considered nodal.

both. The National Comprehensive Cancer Network recently proposed guidelines for staging the most common subtypes of lymphoma; these recommendations are incorporated here and outlined in Table 8.2 (32).

CLINICAL EVALUATION

A careful history and physical examination are critical in evaluating a new patient with lymphoma to delineate the extent of disease, guide further diagnostic imaging or procedures, and assist in treatment decisions.

History

Approximately two-thirds of patients with lymphoma present with painless lymph node enlargement. The most frequently involved disease sites include the cervical, supraclavicular, inguinal, and axillary regions. The duration and growth rate of suspected adenopathy should also be noted.

The presence of systemic symptoms, including fever (temperature higher than 38°C), night sweats, and unexplained weight loss (more than 10% of body weight over the past 6 months) (B symptoms) should also be determined. These B symptoms are adverse prognostic factors in patients with aggressive lymphoma, and their resolution is one measure of treatment response. In patients with indolent lymphoma, the onset of B symptoms may indicate transformation into a more aggressive histology.

Focal symptoms may arise from an obstructing nodal mass in the thorax or abdomen. Patients with mediastinal lymphadenopathy can develop cough, chest discomfort, and, occasionally, superior vena caval syndrome. Retroperitoneal adenopathy is usually asymptomatic; however, extensive disease may lead to abdominal discomfort, early satiety, and

TABLE 8.2. *Recommended studies for initial evaluation*

Biopsy of lesion with review by an experienced hematopathologist

History: Including B symptoms, performance status, duration and growth rate of lymph node enlargement, symptoms to suggest extranodal involvement, risk factors for lymphoma, comorbid illnesses

Physical examination: General examination with attention to node-bearing areas, including Waldeyer's ring and liver and spleen span, inspection of skin

Laboratory studies
  Mandatory:
    Complete blood cell count, differential, peripheral blood smear
    Lactate dehydrogenase, β_2-microglobulin
    Blood urea nitrogen, creatinine, albumin, serum glutamic-oxaloacetic transaminase, total bilirubin, alkaline phosphatase, calcium and uric acid (aggressive histologies)
    Serum protein electrophoresis
  In select patients:
    Hepatitis B, HIV, human T-cell leukemia virus type I
    Hepatitis C (lymphoplasmacytic lymphoma)

Bone marrow aspirate and biopsy

Radiologic studies and special procedures
  Mandatory:
    Chest radiograph (posteroanterior and lateral)
    CT chest scan in majority, particularly if abnormality in chest radiography
    CT abdomen and pelvis scans
    Gallium scan (where expertise in interpretation is available)
  In select patients:
    PET scan (optional/study purposes)
    MRI (to detect bone marrow involvement)
    Ear, nose, and throat examination (to detect preauricular, thyroid, gastrointestinal, or testicular involvement)
    Slit-lamp examination (to detect central nervous system and ocular lymphoma)
    Testicular ultrasound (contralateral testis in testicular lymphoma)
    Gastrointestinal evaluation [endoscopy or barium studies and endoscopic ultrasound (study purposes)] for Waldeyer's ring involvement or if suggestive symptoms
    Skeletal evaluation [e.g., plain bone radiographs, MRI, bone scan, or PET scan (optional)]
    Head CT scan or MRI if neurologic signs or symptoms
    Lumbar puncture and cerebrospinal fluid analysis if neurologic signs or symptoms, high-grade histologies, HIV-associated lymphomas, high-risk extranodal sites [e.g., bone marrow, central nervous system, ocular, sinus, epidural, testicular, ovary, or bilateral breast (aggressive histology)]
    Bilateral mammograms (to detect breast lymphoma)
    Multiple-gated cardiac blood pool scintigraphy or echocardiogram
    Pulmonary function tests

CT, computed tomography; HIV, human immunodeficiency virus; MRI, magnetic resonance imaging; PET, positron emission tomography.

obstructive uropathy. Mesenteric or pelvic adenopathy rarely results in visceral obstruction or perforation.

Although lymphoma is primarily a disorder of lymph nodes, extranodal disease often occurs and results in symptoms referable to the particular system (e.g., bone pain, gastrointestinal complaints, neurologic symptoms, cutaneous involvement, or pulmonary symptoms). In some cases, an extranodal site may be the only area of disease involvement. The skin and gastrointestinal tract were the most frequent sites of extranodal disease in patients included in the Non-Hodgkin's Lymphoma Classification Project (33).

Several primary extranodal lymphomas involve specific disease sites. For example, more than 50% of extranodal, marginal zone, B-cell lymphomas of mucosa-associated lymphoid tissue (MALT lymphoma) involve the gastrointestinal tract (34). Less frequent sites of MALT lymphoma include lung, head and neck, ocular adnexa, skin, thyroid, and breast (35). Gastric MALT lymphoma has been linked to a preceding infection by *Helicobacter pylori*, and patients often report chronic dyspeptic symptoms (36,37). In the World Health Organization (WHO) classification, specific subtypes of peripheral T-cell lymphoma also fall into the primary extranodal category: extranodal natural killer/T-cell lymphoma, nasal and nasal type, enteropathy-type T-cell lymphoma, hepatosplenic γδ T-cell lymphoma, and subcutaneous panniculitis-like T-cell lymphoma, as well as the cutaneous T-cell neoplasms (mycosis fungoides, Sézary syndrome, primary cutaneous anaplastic large-cell lymphoma, and lymphomatoid papulosis) (38). Patients exhibit a spectrum of symptoms specific to these entities.

Rarely, patients present with neurologic symptoms reflecting parenchymal central nervous system, leptomeningeal, or paraneoplastic disease. Space-occupying masses can result in headache, nausea, vomiting, and focal neurologic deficits. Leptomeningeal involvement may result in multiple cranial nerve palsies, headache, changes in mental status, back or radicular pain, incontinence, lower motor neuron weakness, and/or sensory abnormalities.

Other rare extranodal sites of involvement at presentation include the testes, sinus, eye, epidural space, kidney, prostate, bladder, ovary, heart, breast, and salivary, thyroid and adrenal glands.

Risk factors for lymphoma should be reviewed, including a history of human immunodeficiency virus (HIV) infection, immunosuppressive medications, and autoimmune disorders such as rheumatoid arthritis, Hashimoto's thyroiditis, and celiac sprue. Inherited disorders, such as severe combined immunodeficiency, hypogammaglobulinemia, common variable immunodeficiency, Wiskott-Aldrich syndrome, and ataxia-telangiectasia, are associated with an increased incidence of lymphoma. Epidemiologic studies suggest that environmental factors may also play an etiologic role in non-Hodgkin's lymphoma. Thus, an inquiry into potential environmental and occupational exposures should be made (39). Occupations that have been associated with an increased risk of non-Hodgkin's lymphoma include farmers; pesticide workers; cosmetologists; chemists; workers in the petro-

TABLE 8.3. *Eastern Cooperative Oncology Group (ECOG) Performance Status Scale*

ECOG Scale	Description
0	Asymptomatic: Normal activity
1	Symptomatic: Fully ambulatory, able to carry out activities of daily living
2	Symptomatic: In bed less than 50% of the day
3	Symptomatic: In bed more than 50% of the day
4	Bedridden: May need hospitalization

leum, rubber, plastics, and synthetics industries; and forestry workers (39).

Functional capacity based on the Eastern Cooperative Oncology Group Performance Status Scale (Table 8.3) has prognostic value (26). Performance status reflects the disease's impact on the patient and frequently predicts an individual's tolerance for therapy. Comorbid respiratory, cardiac, or renal disease that might influence treatment delivery should also be identified from the initial history.

Physical Examination

The physical examination should include all peripheral (i.e., cervical, supraclavicular, axillary, epitrochlear, inguinal, femoral, and popliteal) and intra-abdominal (i.e., mesenteric, retroperitoneal, and pelvic) lymph node–bearing areas. The site and size of all abnormal lymph nodes should be recorded. Waldeyer's ring (the tonsils and nasopharynx) is best assessed by indirect laryngoscopy or direct fiberoptic examination. This disease site is particularly important in individuals with high neck nodes or thyroid, testicular, or gastrointestinal involvement. Splenic and hepatic enlargement should be assessed, although this is not always indicative of lymphomatous involvement (40–44). With cutaneous disease, multiple remote areas may be affected simultaneously. Thus, the skin should be thoroughly inspected and any suspicious lesions biopsied. A complete neurologic and cardiorespiratory examination to assess for disease involvement and the presence of comorbid illnesses that may limit treatment delivery should be undertaken.

LABORATORY STUDIES

Laboratory studies should include a complete blood cell count with examination of the peripheral smear to assess for circulating lymphoma cells. Peripheral blood involvement is seen most commonly with the indolent lymphomas, which have a greater propensity for bone marrow involvement (45). Although abnormalities in the hematologic parameters may reflect bone marrow involvement (46,47), peripheral blood counts are not reliable indicators of bone marrow disease (48). Thrombocytopenia and neutropenia are more consistently associated with bone marrow involvement than anemia (46,49).

LDH and β_2-microglobulin are indirect measurements of tumor burden that have independent prognostic value (9,50). If elevated at presentation, these serologic parameters may also be useful in assessing treatment response. Serum creatinine and uric acid are important in identifying patients at risk of tumor lysis syndrome, particularly in aggressive lymphomas. Impaired renal function may signal ureteral obstruction or, rarely, indicate lymphomatous kidney involvement. Liver chemistries assess both hepatic function and organ involvement, although abnormalities in liver tests do not correlate well with hepatic infiltration (51–53). An isolated elevation in alkaline phosphatase should prompt an evaluation of the skeletal system. Hypercalcemia can occur in aggressive lymphomas, and, in particular, human T-cell lymphotrophic virus type I (HTLV-I)–associated adult T-cell leukemia/lymphoma. A serum protein electrophoresis may reveal monoclonal gammopathy, most notably in lymphoplasmacytic lymphoma or chronic lymphocytic leukemia/small lymphocytic lymphomas (54,55).

Viral serologies are performed in those patients who are at risk for exposure or who have a compatible clinical picture. Patients with HIV-related lymphomas are more likely to have aggressive B-cell tumors, B symptoms, and advanced-stage disease with multiple extranodal sites of involvement (56). Human herpes virus 8 is recovered from virtually all cases of body cavity–associated or primary effusion lymphoma (57,58). HTLV-I is a retrovirus that is endemic to regions of Southern Japan and the Caribbean basin and sporadic elsewhere. It is transmitted in intact lymphocytes by blood transfusion, sexual contact, and breast-feeding (59). Patients infected in infancy can rarely develop a T-cell leukemia/lymphoma associated with peripheral blood involvement, skin and central nervous system infiltration, and hypercalcemia (60). Epstein-Barr virus (EBV) is present in almost all cases of Burkitt's lymphoma from Africa and in many HIV- or transplant-associated lymphoproliferative disorders. Hepatitis C is seen in approximately 30% of patients with lymphoplasmacytic lymphoma and should be evaluated in this lymphoma subtype (61). Although hepatitis B virus (HBV) is not causally related to any of the lymphomas, reactivation is a well-recognized complication in patients with chronic HBV infection who receive cytotoxic chemotherapy (62). Thus, patients who are in high-risk groups or from endemic areas (e.g., Asia, the Middle East, or Mediterranean) should be screened for chronic infection and considered for prophylactic therapy with lamivudine (63).

RADIOGRAPHIC STAGING

Plain Films, Computed Axial Tomography, and Magnetic Resonance Imaging

A standard posterior-anterior and lateral chest radiograph will detect the majority of abnormalities affecting the mediastinal and hilar lymph nodes, lung parenchyma, and pleura. Pleural effusions are found in approximately 10% of patients, usually in association with mediastinal adenopathy (64). Pathologic verification is required because pleural effusions are often benign. The chest radiograph is less accurate in defining disease extent, detecting adenopathy in the subcarinal and cardiophrenic

spaces, and determining chest wall and pericardial involvement (65–67). A computed tomography (CT) scan of the chest more accurately delineates the extent of mediastinal disease and evaluates the aforementioned regions missed by radiography (68). The recent National Comprehensive Cancer Network practice guidelines recommend that in the initial staging of a lymphoma patient, a chest CT scan is indicated for all patients with aggressive histology as well as the majority of indolent lymphomas (32). Furthermore, a chest CT scan should be obtained if there are any abnormalities on chest radiograph or further assessment of a poorly visualized region is needed. In addition, if radiotherapy is to be used for mediastinal disease, CT is required for accurate determination of treatment portals. Finally, for patients with disease outside the thorax in whom radiotherapy is being considered as the only mode of therapy (e.g., follicular lymphoma with localized disease), a CT scan may be useful in detecting thoracic lymphadenopathy that is not otherwise appreciated on the standard chest radiograph.

Staging laparotomies were previously performed to provide information regarding intraabdominal involvement with non-Hodgkin's lymphoma. With improvements in imaging studies as well as the widespread use of systemic chemotherapy, there are currently no indications for staging laparotomies in non-Hodgkin's lymphoma. Lymphangiography and ultrasonography were used before CT for the evaluation of intraabdominal disease. CT has replaced lymphangiography as the preferred method for evaluating disease below the diaphragm because lymphangiography is difficult to perform and insensitive in certain nodal regions. Abdominal CT scans have also replaced ultrasonography because CT scans more effectively image continuous lymph node regions.

Lymphomatous involvement of the liver or spleen may be subtle. Although diffuse organ infiltration may not be apparent on CT scan, this pattern is typically associated with subdiaphragmatic lymphadenopathy, and management is unaltered. In a patient with otherwise localized disease, abnormalities in liver function tests or suspicious lesions on imaging are an indication for biopsy. Genitourinary involvement is established by CT, with the exception of testicular masses, which are best assessed by ultrasonography (69–71). Intrinsic gastrointestinal tract involvement or extension from adjacent nodal disease may occur, particularly with aggressive lymphoma subtypes. In the presence of extensive disease, abnormalities are often apparent on CT, and extraluminal tumor extension can be quantified. However, clinical symptoms suggestive of gastrointestinal lymphoma should also prompt an endoscopic or barium study because isolated luminal disease may not be detected by CT. The role of endoscopic ultrasound of the stomach may be useful to establish depth of lymphomatous penetration, but requires prospective validation (72–74).

Magnetic resonance imaging (MRI) has a limited role in the staging of non-Hodgkin's lymphoma. Compared with CT, MRI is more costly and has limited availability and a longer imaging time. Nevertheless, MRI is preferable in selected settings. For example, MRI is the modality of choice to characterize bone disease because the technique is more sensitive than bone scintigraphy or conventional radiographs (75,76). MRI can also detect lymphomatous bone marrow involvement (77) and more specifically evaluate disease of the chest wall or pericardium (78). In addition, MRI is superior to CT scan for the detection of central nervous system disease; when gadolinium is used, meningeal enhancement may indicate leptomeningeal involvement.

Functional Imaging

Gallium-67 Scintigraphy

Gallium-67 (^{67}Ga) scintigraphy was the first whole-body, noninvasive imaging modality used for the diagnosis and staging of lymphoma. This technique depends on the binding of ^{67}Ga to transferrin receptors in the tumor (79) and provides additional information regarding tumor viability (80). Thus, ^{67}Ga scintigraphy can be useful in determining treatment response and evaluating residual masses posttherapy.

Detection of lymphoma using ^{67}Ga scintigraphy depends on the imaging technique as well as tumor type, size, and location. Current methods use 8 to 11 mCi gallium, delayed 72-hour imaging, and single-photon emission computed tomography. These methods are highly sensitive in detecting sites of viable tumor (81–83) in aggressive non-Hodgkin's lymphomas (84,85). In contrast, only approximately 50% of indolent lymphomas are ^{67}Ga-avid (85–89). Earlier reports demonstrated a lower sensitivity of ^{67}Ga scintigraphy in detecting intraabdominal disease compared to mediastinal disease [60% and 96%, respectively (89)]. However, the routine use of additional delayed (96- and 120-hour) views and single-photon emission computed tomography has significantly increased the sensitivity of detection of infradiaphragmatic disease.

[67]Ga uptake is not specific for lymphoma; the radionuclide may also localize to sites of infection or inflammation (80). In addition to the liver, ^{67}Ga also localizes in the spleen; bone marrow; mammary, lacrimal, and salivary glands; as well as at sites of increased bone formation (80). Thymic ^{67}Ga uptake is not uncommon after treatment with either chemotherapy or radiotherapy. Knowledge of these physiologic and posttherapy uptake patterns is critical for correct interpretation of ^{67}Ga scintigraphy results. In addition, ^{67}Ga scans should be read in association with concurrent CT scans.

In aggressive lymphomas, ^{67}Ga scintigraphy can complement CT in identifying initial disease sites (90,91), assessing response to therapy (83,91,92), and detecting early recurrences (93). Documenting ^{67}Ga avidity before treatment provides a baseline for comparison in follow-up during and after the completion of therapy. Early (mid-treatment) re-staging ^{67}Ga scintigraphy provides important additional information regarding rapidity of response and the likelihood of attaining a durable remission (94,95).

Positron Emission Tomography

[^{18}F]-2-fluoro-2-deoxy-D-glucose (FDG-PET) is a glucose analog labeled with a short-lived positron emitter that can be used to image lymphoid neoplasms using positron emission tomography (PET). ^{18}F-FDG uptake is proportional to the glycolytic metabolic rate of viable tumor cells (96), providing information on the functional status of the tumor (97–102). Malignant lymphocytes have a high metabolic activity and thus display avidity for ^{18}F-FDG. Increased ^{18}F-FDG uptake is seen in the kidneys and bladder as well as tissues with relatively active glucose metabolism such as skeletal and cardiac muscle (80). Like ^{67}Ga, physiologic uptake of ^{18}F-FDG occurs in organs such as the thymus after therapy, and in benign disorders such as granulomatous disease (103,104).

Although indolent and aggressive lymphomas can be visualized by PET (100,105–108), aggressive lymphomas with high proliferative activity have the greatest ^{18}F-FDG uptake (99,100,106,109,110). FDG-PET does not appear to be as useful to visualize the MALT-type lymphomas (111).

Several studies have evaluated the role of FDG-PET in the staging of non-Hodgkin's lymphoma. There is little information comparing FDG-PET to ^{67}Ga scintigraphy (91,102,108,112,113). However, preliminary studies suggest that FDG-PET may be more sensitive than ^{67}Ga scintigraphy and, possibly, CT scan in the staging of lymphoma (97,98,105,107–109,112–123). Like ^{67}Ga scintigraphy, FDG-PET provides functional information, whereas CT scans rely entirely on anatomic features.

Limited data indicate that FDG-PET is able to accurately detect splenic, gastrointestinal, and hepatic disease (101,116,119,121,124–126). Although physiologic hepatic uptake remains problematic, FDG-PET is able to detect liver lesions with high glycolytic activity (127). FDG-PET may also be superior to CT or endoscopy at defining the extent of lymphomatous involvement of the stomach (101) or small bowel (126). Furthermore, FDG-PET appears to be superior to bone scan in detecting skeletal lymphomatous lesions (125); this technique is able to demonstrate, to some degree, bone marrow involvement with lymphoma, as described below (128,129). FDG-PET has also been useful in distinguishing central nervous system lymphoma from toxoplasmosis in patients with acquired immunodeficiency syndrome (130,131).

Overall, the available literature suggests at least equivalence of FDG-PET to CT and ^{67}Ga scintigraphy and possible superiority in the pre- and posttreatment evaluation of non-Hodgkin's lymphoma. Although these preliminary reports are encouraging, large prospective studies with long-term follow-up will be necessary to define the precise role of FDG-PET in lymphoma staging and to determine how this technique compares with other dynamic and anatomic imaging studies.

BONE MARROW ASPIRATION AND BIOPSY

Bone marrow disease assessment should include both an aspirate and a biopsy. An aspirate may be useful for morphologic analysis, as well as special studies such as cytogenetics and flow cytometry; however, it does not replace a biopsy for establishing disease involvement. For optimal accuracy, bone marrow biopsies should be 2.0 cm in aggregate (132). For the majority of patients, unilateral bone marrow aspirate and biopsy are sufficient (133–135).

Bone marrow infiltration varies with histologic subtype (2,135). Among indolent lymphomas, the small lymphocytic lymphoma/chronic lymphocytic leukemias and follicular lymphomas frequently exhibit bone marrow involvement (2). Mantle cell lymphoma commonly involves the bone marrow. In contrast, bone marrow disease is an infrequent occurrence in diffuse large B-cell lymphoma (diffuse large B-cell lymphoma) (2). However, the presence of large cells in the bone marrow correlates with an increased risk of central nervous system involvement in diffuse large B-cell lymphoma (49).

Bone Marrow Flow Cytometry

The role of routine flow cytometry in detecting bone marrow involvement is not clearly defined, with the majority of studies suggesting that flow cytometry is redundant in most circumstances (132,136–138). However, flow cytometry may be more sensitive than morphologic examination for the detection of minimal bone marrow disease (less than 5%) (139). Disease-specific, long-term follow-up studies are required to determine the prognostic significance of bone marrow involvement that is only detected by flow cytometry.

Magnetic Resonance Imaging for Bone Marrow Involvement

Recent studies suggest that MRI may be more sensitive than biopsy in detecting bone marrow infiltration, particularly occult disease (140–147). On T1-weighted images, fatty marrow is depicted by a homogeneous signal; therefore, lymphomatous involvement is readily detectable. As MRI is able to readily assess large portions of the bone marrow, it may direct bone marrow sampling. However, the diagnostic yield of MRI is lower in indolent lymphomas and in younger patients who tend to have a higher proportion of red marrow. Clinical information, such as constitutional symptoms, bone pain, and increased alkaline phosphatase, may be helpful in selecting patients with normal bone marrow biopsies who should undergo MRI (143). Although MRI may have a role in individual cases, whole-body MRI is an impractical and an expensive modality for establishing lymphomatous bone marrow involvement in the majority of patients.

Positron Emission Tomography for Bone Marrow Involvement

The utility of FDG-PET to detect bone marrow involvement in lymphoma is not yet known. Both physiologic uptake and diffuse posttherapy uptake in reactive marrow have been described. Abnormal FDG-PET marrow findings include uptake equal to greater than that in liver, uptake in the distal long bones, and heterogeneous or focal uptake (128,129). Thus far, the reported false-positive rate of FDG-PET bone

marrow is 10% to 15%, and the false-negative rate is approximately 5%, although specific lymphoma subtypes may also influence these findings (128,129).

ADDITIONAL PROCEDURES: SITES OF INVOLVEMENT AND PATTERNS OF PRESENTATION OF LYMPHOMA

Specific procedures, which are not routinely performed in asymptomatic individuals, may be indicated in the presence of specific clinical symptoms. For example, certain neurologic symptoms should prompt a lumbar puncture and cerebrospinal fluid examination. Similarly, complaints of bone pain may warrant additional imaging of the skeletal system. Furthermore, some extranodal disease sites and certain lymphoma subtypes require additional staging studies because site-specific lymphomatous involvement may alter prognosis and treatment (Table 8.2). The following disease sites deserve special attention due to their predictive pattern of involvement, even in the absence of clinical findings.

Waldeyer's Ring

The coexistence of large-cell lymphoma of Waldeyer's ring and the stomach was first described in the early 1970s (148) and repeatedly confirmed thereafter (149–151). Patients with Waldeyer's ring involvement are at increased risk of gastrointestinal tract involvement either at presentation or at relapse. Waldeyer's ring involvement has also been reported in patients with thyroid, testicular, and preauricular lymph node disease. Thus, patients with Waldeyer's ring disease should have an upper gastrointestinal evaluation with contrast or endoscopic studies, and, conversely, patients with the other aforementioned disease sites should have evaluation of the Waldeyer's ring.

Gastrointestinal Tract

The gastrointestinal tract represents the most frequent extranodal site of non-Hodgkin's lymphomas (2). The stomach is the most common site of lymphomatous involvement in the gastrointestinal tract (152). Gastric lymphomas are typically either extranodal marginal zone, MALT-type, or diffuse large B-cell lymphomas, most commonly on a background of MALT lymphoma (152). Endoscopic ultrasound may be helpful to establish depth of intramural penetration (72–74), although it is suboptimal in distinguishing benign versus malignant lymph nodes (72–74). The development of gastric MALT lymphoma in the presence of *Helicobacter pylori* gastritis is well established, and pathologic evaluation should include tests to document underlying infection (153), as eradication of the organism often leads to lymphoma regression (153–156).

In addition to the customary staging evaluation, as described above, patients with gastrointestinal lymphomas should also be carefully evaluated for Waldeyer's ring involvement (149).

Sinus Lymphoma

The frontal, maxillary, ethmoid, and sphenoid sinuses can all become involved with lymphoma, resulting in local symptoms of pain, nasal obstruction, facial swelling, or rhinorrhea. Sinus lymphomas are usually of aggressive histology (157–159); in North America, the majority are B-cell malignancies (157) whereas in Asia, T- or natural killer–cell tumors predominate (160). Due to the porous nature of the bony sinus walls, there is a high propensity for central nervous system spread (158,161–163). Thus, all patients with lymphomatous sinus involvement should have a lumbar puncture and cerebrospinal fluid analysis followed by central nervous system chemoprophylaxis.

Central Nervous System and Ocular Lymphoma

Primary central nervous system lymphoma represents 2% of all lymphomas and more than 90% are aggressive B-cell malignancies (164). Central nervous system lymphomas are frequently multifocal, with an increased risk of concomitant leptomeningeal and ocular involvement. Initial analysis should include a CT or MRI (preferred) of the head with gadolinium enhancement, lumbar puncture with analysis of the cerebrospinal fluid, and an ophthalmologic evaluation with a slit-lamp examination. Although cerebrospinal fluid cytology often appears benign, specific immunohistochemical studies may reveal a monoclonal population. Elevation of LDH and/or β_2-microglobulin in the cerebrospinal fluid may also provide indirect evidence of lymphomatous involvement (165).

Ocular, as opposed to periorbital, lymphomatous involvement occurs in less than 1% of patients and is often incorrectly diagnosed as chronic uveitis (166). Lymphomas involving the optic nerve, retina, and vitreous are most often associated with central nervous system involvement (164). In contrast, lymphomas involving the uveal tract (choroids, ciliary body, and iris) are more commonly associated with visceral involvement (167). A thorough ophthalmologic examination will often identify ocular involvement; however, a vitrectomy is usually required for confirmation. Bilateral ocular involvement is possible, and concurrent brain or leptomeningeal disease is not uncommon. Thus, the initial evaluation of a patient with primary ocular non-Hodgkin's lymphoma should include a slit-lamp examination of the contralateral eye, CT scan or MRI of the brain, and cytologic examination of the cerebrospinal fluid.

Testicular

Non-Hodgkin's lymphoma is the most common cause of a testicular mass in men older than 60 years. Testicular lymphomas are almost exclusively aggressive B-cell tumors (168). Approximately 30% to 40% of patients with testicular lymphoma present with advanced-stage disease. Contralateral testicular involvement is common, either at presentation or later in the disease course (169–171). There is also frequent involvement of the skin and Waldeyer's ring as well as central nervous system sites, including the meninges, epidural space, and cerebrum (172–175). Thus, patients with testicular lymphoma should have an ultrasound of the contralateral testis, assessment of Waldeyer's ring, and cerebrospinal fluid examination for malignant cells in addition to standard staging procedures. Furthermore, with any clinical suspicion of central nervous system parenchymal disease, a CT scan or MRI of the head is required.

Other

Patients with diffuse large-cell lymphomas with bone marrow involvement may have an increased risk of leptomeningeal disease and require a lumbar puncture as part of their initial staging, and patients should be given central nervous system prophylaxis (176–179). Highly aggressive lymphomas (lymphoblastic lymphoma and small noncleaved-cell lymphoma) and acquired immunodeficiency syndrome–related B-cell lymphomas also have a predilection for leptomeningeal disease. In these lymphoma subtypes, cerebrospinal fluid analysis at diagnosis is mandatory, regardless of the presence of symptoms or other risk factors (176–178,180).

Lymphoma of the bone is not uncommon in advanced-stage disease; however, it represents less than 5% of localized extranodal presentations (181,182). Bone pain or isolated elevation in alkaline phosphatase should prompt further studies. In addition, approximately 30% of patients with primary lymphoma of the bone have more than one site involved (183). There does not appear to be a propensity for central nervous system relapse. A bone scan is highly sensitive in demonstrating bone abnormalities; however, findings are nonspecific and should be confirmed with either a CT scan or standard radiograph and biopsy. As described, MRI (75,76) or FDG-PET (125) may be superior in detecting lymphoma of the bone and planning additional directed radiation therapy.

In women, lymphomas may infrequently involve the ovaries and breasts. Breast lymphoma can present bilaterally, particularly in younger women with aggressive lymphoma subtypes, necessitating evaluation of the contralateral breast (184–188). Similarly, lymphomas of the ovary are typically aggressive lymphoma subtypes with an increased incidence of bilateral involvement (167,189,190).

EVALUATION OF COMORBID DISEASE

In patients who are scheduled to receive anthracyclines as part of their treatment regimen, baseline cardiac function should be assessed with either a multiple-gated cardiac blood pool scintigraphy or an echocardiogram. In patients with a history of respiratory disease who are candidates for thoracic radiotherapy, pulmonary function tests may be needed to identify significant obstructive or restrictive lung pathology.

EVALUATION OF THE RESIDUAL MASS POSTTREATMENT

A major clinical challenge in the management of lymphoma patients is the evaluation of residual masses posttherapy. Persistent abnormalities are often detected by physical examination, CT scan, or plain radiographs (191). However, these studies cannot reliably distinguish fibrotic tissue from active lymphoma. Stability over time provides indirect evidence of fibrosis; nevertheless, it is often advantageous to identify persistent tumor early to optimize further curative treatment. There is poor correlation between the size of a residual mass on CT and risk of relapse (116,192). MRI has not proven to be more effective in this setting than CT (193).

[67]Ga scintigraphy has been used to detect persistent viable tumor in patients with a residual mass posttherapy (83,90,193–199). One study evaluating patients with residual mediastinal masses posttreatment found the specificity of [18]Ga scintigraphy to be superior (95%) to CT (57%) or chest radiograph (55%) (198). A new technique called *transmission emission tomography*, which simultaneously registers Ga uptake with CT findings, appears promising for differentiating residual tissue from active disease (91).

FDG-PET is also able to detect viable tumor within a residual mass (105,114,116,200,201) with greater accuracy than CT (105,116,200). In a recent analysis, the positive predictive values of FDG-PET and CT in detecting persistent lymphoma in a residual mass were 100% and 42%, respectively (116). Of interest, the majority of relapses in FDG-PET negative patients occurred outside the residual mass site (116). Although FDG-PET shares some of the limitations of ^{67}Ga scintigraphy, preliminary studies suggest that FDG-PET may be superior for the detection of residual disease and more accurate for the evaluation of intraabdominal masses (114). Larger prospective studies are required before FDG-PET can be routinely recommended; however, it is strongly recommended that every attempt should be made to correlate conventional imaging with functional imaging in the evaluation of the residual mass.

RECOMMENDED STUDIES FOR FOLLOW-UP AFTER TREATMENT

Patient surveillance after treatment of lymphoma should address both long-term complications of therapy and disease recurrence. Long-term effects of therapy depend on the type of treatment and whether radiotherapy was also administered. Radiotherapy to the head and neck region leads to decreased salivation with dental caries; consequently, patients who have received such therapy need careful dental follow-up. Additionally, if the thyroid was included in the radiation field, a large proportion of patients may eventually become hypothyroid. Long-term survivors are also at risk of second malignancies (202–205). In an earlier survey of 6,171 lymphoma patients who survived for 2 or more years, second cancers were seen in 541 subjects with significant

excesses for all solid tumors, acute myelogenous leukemia, melanoma, and Hodgkin's lymphoma as well as cancers of the lung, brain, kidney, and bladder (205). In addition, after high-dose therapy with autologous bone marrow transplant, myelodysplasia and acute leukemia have been reported at an increased frequency (206–209).

However, the greatest risk to patients treated for lymphoma is relapse of their disease. In patients with aggressive B- and T-cell lymphomas, a minority are cured of their disease, leaving most patients at risk for relapse. In aggressive lymphoma, the majority of recurrences are seen within 2 years of completing therapy; however, late relapses can occur in both limited (210,211) and advanced-stage disease (212–217). Patients with indolent lymphomas are continuously at risk of relapse, and late relapses are not uncommon.

There is limited information regarding the use of routine imaging in the follow-up of lymphoma patients after treatment (91,95,218–220). On completion of treatment, a set of baseline studies is warranted to provide a basis for future comparisons. The value of performing routine surveillance studies rather than responding to new clinical symptoms is not clearly established. In lymphoma subtypes that can potentially be cured with salvage high-dose therapy, there is a theoretical advantage to early detection of recurrence (218,221,222). One group assessed the sensitivity of various procedures for the detection of relapse in aggressive lymphoma patients who attained a complete response after cyclophosphamide, hydroxydaunomycin, Oncovin (vincristine), and prednisone (CHOP) chemotherapy (218). The majority of relapsed patients (89%) were diagnosed at an unscheduled evaluation prompted by new clinical symptoms. Similar results were obtained in another study in which the majority of relapses were suspected after an interim history or physical examination, or both (220). Other studies have also demonstrated that [18]Ga scintigraphy has a high sensitivity (95%) and specificity (89%) for the detection of relapse (91,95). In some cases, [18]Ga scintigraphy was abnormal before the emergence of clinical or radiographic abnormalities, but the impact on clinical outcome is unknown.

The role of abdominopelvic CT in stage I–III follicular lymphoma relative to standard clinical and hematologic studies was recently evaluated (223). Only 14% of relapses were detected solely on the basis of imaging, and only 4% of those patients who achieved a complete remission benefited from abdominopelvic CT (223). β_2-microglobulin has been assessed as an early indicator of relapse in aggressive lymphomas with approximately 50% of patients having elevated marker levels before the onset of clinical symptoms (224).

FDG-PET has not been evaluated in the follow-up setting; however, given its apparent superiority to [18]Ga scintigraphy in non-Hodgkin's lymphoma staging, FDG-PET may have a role in the detection of early disease relapse.

Current recommendations for the follow-up of lymphoma patients completing their induction therapy include visits every 3 to 4 months for the first 2 years, every 6 months until 5 years, and annually thereafter. The recommended follow-

TABLE 8.4. *Recommended follow-up procedure for patients with non-Hodgkin's lymphoma*

History and physical examination: Same as for initial evaluation, including assessment for secondary organ toxicity from treatment

Laboratory studies: Complete blood cell count and differential, lactate dehydrogenase, β_2-microglobulin (optional), thyroid-stimulating hormone (neck radiation)

Imaging: Chest x-ray if initially involved; gallium scan if initially positive and available; computed tomography scans of chest, abdomen, and pelvis (consider periodic evaluation); positron emission tomography scan (optional)

Frequency of surveillance: Every 3–4 mo for 2 yr, every 6 mo to 5 yr, annually thereafter

up evaluation is shown in Table 8.4. At each visit, the following should be performed: a thorough history and physical examination and a laboratory evaluation, including a complete blood cell count and LDH. CT scans of previously involved disease sites should be strongly considered in patients with aggressive lymphomas who may be candidates for curative salvage treatment. Furthermore, in patients with aggressive lymphomas, follow-up dynamic imaging (^{67}Ga scintigraphy or [18]FDG-PET) may be useful for identifying relapsed disease before clinical signs or symptoms. The use of any further imaging should be directed by clinical or laboratory findings.

RECOMMENDED STUDIES FOR RECURRENT DISEASE

Once a patient is confirmed to have recurrent disease, appropriate restaging, including repeat bone marrow aspirate and biopsy, should be undertaken. Additional investigations should be guided by the presence of any new signs or symptoms. In addition, re-evaluation of the cardiorespiratory status as well as hepatic and renal function should be carried out to assess a patient's suitability for more aggressive salvage therapy.

PROGNOSTIC FACTORS IN LYMPHOMA

The lymphomas are a heterogeneous group of diseases with highly variable clinical behavior and outcome. Over the years, a number of variables have been identified that impact prognosis, including clinical factors, treatment-related variables, and biologic features. Clinical prognostic models, such as the IPI, have been developed to identify patient groups that are unlikely to be cured with standard therapy. However, these risk models are based on clinical features that are likely surrogate markers of underlying molecular heterogeneity. Recent advances in cytogenetics and molecular analysis have identified specific genes and gene products that influence disease pathogenesis, prognosis, or both. More recently, genome-wide approaches based on gene expression profiling have characterized the molecular signatures of distinct lymphoid neoplasms and relevant prognostic subgroups. The following section reviews prognostic features in lymphoma with the greatest clinical relevance and outlines recent advances in further elucidating the molecular basis for disease heterogeneity.

Clinical Prognostic Factors

Initial Presenting Clinical Features

As previously described, the Ann Arbor staging system poses many limitations in non-Hodgkin's lymphoma. For this reason, investigators have attempted to identify clinical prognostic factors that more accurately reflect the behavior of lymphomas. A number of pretreatment clinical features have been associated with the achievement of a complete remission and long-term survival in patients with lymphomas. The factors reflect either tumor burden and invasive potential (e.g., LDH, β_2-microglobulin, localized versus advanced stage, number of nodal and extranodal disease sites, B symptoms, tumor size, and bone marrow involvement), the patient's response to the tumor (e.g., performance status and B symptoms), and the patient's ability to tolerate treatment (e.g., performance status, bone marrow involvement, and age) (6–18,225–229).

Age is a particularly important prognostic factor that has been linked to poor outcome in a number of studies (230–235). Patients older than 60 years have lower response rates and higher rates of relapse (230,231,236,237). The prognosis for patients older than 70 years of age appears to be worse than that for patients 60 to 69 years of age (236). Many factors may contribute to poor outcome in elderly patients, including differences in disease biology, altered drug pharmacokinetics, and underlying comorbid disease that may complicate treatment decisions. As a result, dose reductions are often carried out to avoid toxicity. Elderly patients who receive reduced doses of CHOP-type chemotherapy have lower rates of complete remission and more frequent relapses (238). However, with full-dose treatment, survival of elderly patients approaches that of younger patients (230). Recent studies also suggest that treatment-related toxicity is more influenced by poor performance status than chronological age (239).

The clinical pretreatment variables that retain independent significance in multivariate analyses of survival have been used to develop prognostic factor models that predict a patient's risk for death (12,14–16,26,227,240,241). All of the previously described prognostic factor models incorporate measures of tumor burden and extent of disease. Each model calculates risk based on the number of risk factors present at diagnosis.

International Prognostic Index

The most widely used system to stratify patients with aggressive lymphomas is the IPI (26). Sixteen institutions from the United States, Canada, and Europe all provided information on patients with aggressive lymphomas (by the Working Formulation and Kiel and Rappaport classifications) to determine which pretreatment variables predict relapse-free and overall survival after treatment with doxorubicin-containing combination chemotherapy (26). Clinical features independently associated with survival were age (≤60 vs. >60), LDH (abnormal vs. normal), performance status (<2 vs. ≥2), stage (I/II vs. III/IV), and number of extranodal sites (≤1 vs. >1). Each factor was determined to have an approximately equal impact on outcome and, thus, the risk for death was estimated by adding up the number of adverse prognostic factors present at diagnosis. Four risk groups were identified: low risk (none to one factor), low-intermediate risk (two factors), high-intermediate risk (three factors), and high risk (four to five factors). When the model was applied to 2,031 patients with aggressive lymphoma, the four risk groups had 5-year survivals of 73%, 51%, 43%, and 26%, respectively (Table 8.5 and Fig. 8.1A) (26).

In the same study, 1,274 patients 60 years of age or younger were evaluated in an age-adjusted model with the notion that these patients were more likely to be candidates for experimental therapy. In this simplified age-adjusted model, only stage, LDH, and performance status remained independently predictive of survival, and a model based on these three features again identified four risk groups with predicted survivals of 83% (no factors), 69% (one factor), 46% (two factors), and 32% (three factors) (26). When the age-adjusted IPI is applied to patients older than 60 years, clear survival differences are seen in the low and low-intermediate risk patients, further emphasizing the importance of age in clinical outcome in aggressive lymphoma (Table 8.5 and Fig. 8.1B).

A stage-modified IPI has been developed for limited-stage diffuse large-cell lymphomas using age, nonbulky stage II, LDH, and performance status to define subgroups that should be treated more aggressively (211). The 5-year survival in the corresponding risk categories are 82% (no to one risk factor), 71% (two risk factors), and 48% (three risk factors) (211).

Although the IPI was originally developed in aggressive lymphomas, numerous studies have validated its use in almost all subtypes of lymphoma (2,25,33,242–244). The subtypes of aggressive lymphomas in the updated Revised European-American Lymphoma (REAL) and WHO classifications prompted additional analysis of the IPI in specific disease categories. The Non-Hodgkin's International Classification Project and others have also found the IPI to be prognostic in mantle cell lymphoma and Burkitt-like lymphoma (2,33). In contrast, IPI risk categories were less useful in small series of patients with lymphoblastic lymphoma and Burkitt's lymphoma (2,33).

The IPI has not been rigorously applied to peripheral T-cell lymphomas due to disease rarity and heterogeneity and the relatively recent advent of routine immunophenotyping. In recent studies of patients with T-cell lymphoma as defined by either the Kiel or the REAL classifications, IPI-defined risk groups had significantly different outcomes (242,245–248). The Non-Hodgkin's Lymphoma Classification Project investigators were unable to distinguish different risk categories of peripheral T-cell lymphomas in their original report (2,33). However, in a more recent expanded analysis of peripheral T-cell lymphomas (n = 96), Non-Hodgkin's Lym-

TABLE 8.5. *Outcome according to risk group defined by the International Prognostic Index and the Age-Adjusted International Prognostic Index*

Risk group	Risk factors (#)	Distribution of cases (%)	Complete remission rate (%)	5-yr overall survival (%)
All ages				
Low	0, 1	35	87	73
Low-intermediate	2	27	67	51
High-intermediate	3	22	55	43
High	4, 5	16	44	26
Age-adjusted index (≤60 yr)				
Low	0	22	92	83
Low-intermediate	1	32	78	69
High-intermediate	2	32	57	46
High	3	14	46	32
Age-adjusted index (>60 yr)				
Low	0	18	91	56
Low-intermediate	1	31	71	44
High-intermediate	2	35	56	37
High	3	16	36	21

Adapted from Shipp M, Harrington D. A predictive model for aggressive non-Hodgkin's lymphoma: the International NHL Prognostic Factors Project. *N Engl J Med* 1993;329:987–994.

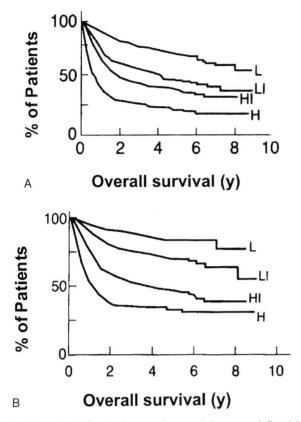

A

Overall survival (y)

B

Overall survival (y)

FIGURE 8.1. A: Survival according to risk group defined by the International Prognostic Index. Overall survival for four risk groups. **B:** Survival among patients ≤60 years according to risk group defined by the Age-Adjusted International Prognostic Index. H, high-risk group; HI, high-intermediate risk; L, low risk; LI, low-intermediate risk. (Adapted from Shipp M, Harrington D. A predictive model for aggressive non-Hodgkin's lymphoma: the International NHL Prognostic Factors Project. *N Engl J Med* 1993;329:987–994.)

phoma Classification Project investigators reported a difference in both failure-free survival and overall survival when patients with no to two factors are compared with those with three to five IPI risk factors (249). In a larger series of patients with peripheral T-cell lymphoma not otherwise classified (based on the REAL classification) (242), investigators identified a low-risk group (IPI zero to one) with a 5-year overall survival approaching that of comparable low-risk diffuse large B-cell lymphoma patients. More recently, the IPI was applied to peripheral T-cell lymphomas, unspecified, as defined by the WHO classification, and found to be useful in distinguishing prognostic subgroups (250).

There have been conflicting reports regarding the predictive value of the IPI in anaplastic large-cell lymphoma. The Non-Hodgkin's Lymphoma Classification Project did not find that the IPI separated anaplastic large-cell lymphoma patients into different risk groups because the majority of patients had an excellent outcome (2,33,251). However, in more recent larger studies, anaplastic large-cell lymphomas could be stratified into relevant prognostic groups using the

IPI (252,253). It also has become clear that in anaplastic large-cell lymphoma, it is critical to evaluate the expression of anaplastic lymphoma kinase (ALK) in addition to traditional clinical prognostic factors because patients with ALK-positive tumors have more favorable outcomes (252–254).

The IPI has also been shown to predict survival in some studies of patients with follicular lymphoma (2,33,244,255–257), transformed low-grade lymphoma (258), and subtypes of non-Hodgkin's lymphoma described as small lymphocytic, follicular small cleaved, and follicular mixed lymphoma (Working Formulation) (243). However, the IPI is less useful in indolent non-Hodgkin's lymphomas because few patients present with "high-risk" disease (2,33). For this reason, other prognostic models have been proposed in indolent lymphomas (20–25,225,259,260) although none have been widely accepted.

Treatment-Related Prognostic Factors

In subtypes of lymphoma that are potentially curable with current induction therapy, the rapidity of response to treatment may have prognostic significance (191,261,262). In one of the earliest studies to demonstrate the importance of rapidity of response, patients with aggressive lymphomas who failed to achieve a remission by the third cycle of chemotherapy had an inferior outcome (261). In an additional large series of patients with aggressive lymphoma, time to complete remission was the single most important predictor of overall survival (94,263).

One of the challenges in assessing for complete remission is the high frequency of residual abnormalities with conventional CT imaging, particularly in patients with bulky disease. A number of reports have shown a failure of CT to predict outcome after treatment in aggressive lymphoma (83,192,194,198,264,265), presumably because a residual mass may represent either scar or persistent disease.

[67]Ga scintigraphy has been used to distinguish residual viable tumor from scar tissue at the end of induction therapy (193,194,266,267). In addition, the technique has been used for an early (mid-course) assessment of response to treatment (94,195,268–271). In an initial series of aggressive lymphoma patients who received serial ^{67}Ga scintigraphy monitoring, only 24% of patients with persistent ^{67}Ga uptake midway through treatment obtained durable long-term remissions; in contrast, 70% of patients who became ^{67}Ga negative midway through therapy obtained durable complete remissions (94). In a subsequent report of 118 patients with aggressive non-Hodgkin's lymphoma, there was a significant difference between the failure-free survivals of patients with negative and positive ^{67}Ga scintigraphy midway through therapy (268). In contrast, CT findings were not predictive of relapse (268). In a similar study, the predictive value of early restaging ^{67}Ga scintigraphy and CT was evaluated in patients with newly diagnosed bulky or advanced-stage aggressive lymphoma treated with high-dose CHOP chemotherapy (269). Although residual mass size on CT was

not predictive of subsequent relapse, early restaging ^{67}Ga scintigraphy was highly predictive; 94% of patients with a negative early restaging ^{67}Ga scintigraphy remained free from progression, whereas only 18% of patients with a positive early restaging ^{67}Ga remained free from progression (269). In a recent analysis, persistent ^{67}Ga uptake midway through therapy identified patients who ultimately relapsed or progressed (271).

More recently, important prognostic information has been attained from FDG-PET analysis of tumor response. As described previously, FDG-PET differentiates between fibrosis and active lymphoma by measuring glucose uptake (97) and provides additional information regarding the nature of a residual mass (105,114,116,200,201,272). There are several technical advantages of FDG-PET over ^{67}Ga scintigraphy, including superior resolution, 1-day protocol, and more precise imaging of splenic abnormalities. Several small studies have confirmed the predictive value of FDG-PET in the posttreatment evaluation of lymphomas (116,272–275), and studies are ongoing to determine the predictive value of FDG-PET midway through planned induction therapy (276–278). In a small study, FDG-PET was used to monitor response to chemotherapy in patients with aggressive lymphoma at 1 week and 6 weeks after treatment initiation (276); the later time point was more predictive of long-term outcome (276).

In a large, more recent study of 70 newly diagnosed patients with aggressive lymphoma, no patients with persistent abnormalities on repeat scanning mid-treatment remained in complete remission (279). Furthermore, the majority of patients with negative mid-treatment FDG-PET scans (84%) had durable complete remissions (279). The same group of investigators evaluated the predictive value of FDG-PET after completion of induction treatment and found that all patients with a positive scan relapsed, and 79% of patients with a normal FDG-PET remained in complete remission (275). Taken together, these studies strongly suggest that persistent abnormal ^{18}F-FDG uptake either during or after chemotherapy is highly predictive of residual or recurrent disease.

Prognostic Factors in Refractory and Relapsed Disease

The management of patients with relapsed lymphoma remains a challenge. Approximately 5% to 10% of patients with aggressive lymphoma fail initial induction, and 20% to 40% who achieve an initial complete remission develop recurrent disease.

Chemosensitivity to Salvage Therapy

Although at least 50% of patients with relapsed aggressive lymphomas remain chemosensitive, less than 10% have durable remissions with second-line chemotherapy regimens (222,280–286). However, a subset of patients with chemosensitive recurrent disease are cured with high-dose chemother-

apy and autologous bone marrow transplant or stem cell transplant (285,287–290). Patients who achieve a complete remission to standard salvage therapy have more favorable outcomes after high-dose chemotherapy and stem cell transplant (291). In contrast, patients whose relapsed disease is resistant to conventional second-line chemotherapy have a poor outcome with high-dose chemotherapy and stem cell transplant, with an event-free survival similar to that observed with salvage regimens (222,285,286).

Failure to Achieve Complete Remission to Induction Therapy

Patients with primary progressive aggressive lymphoma have a dismal prognosis, faring much worse than those who relapse after attaining a complete remission (292–294). Clinical features that are associated with shortened overall survival in non-Hodgkin's lymphoma are also linked to a lower likelihood of attaining an initial complete remission (293). However, a small proportion of patients with primary progressive or refractory disease who demonstrate chemosensitivity to salvage regimens may benefit from high-dose chemotherapy and stem cell transplant (290,294,295).

Duration of First Remission

The duration of remission is the single most important predictor of outcome in patients with recurrent aggressive lymphoma (296). Patients with early relapses (<1 year) have a much poorer outcome than those with late relapses (>1 year) (296). The duration of first remission is also related to overall survival in patients with indolent non-Hodgkin's lymphoma (297). Patients younger than 60 years of age with a complete remission or partial remission of less than 1 year had a median survival of 2.4 years, whereas those with remissions lasting longer than 1 year had a median survival of 5.9 years (297).

Clinical Features

Factors reflecting tumor burden (e.g., bulky disease, advanced stage at relapse, the number of extranodal sites, and increased LDH) and patient tolerance for additional therapy (e.g., performance status and primary refractory disease) are also predictive of outcome in relapsed disease (298,299). The IPI has also been found to be predictive of outcome at relapse. The second-line IPI (sIPI) was first analyzed in relapsed aggressive lymphoma patients who were randomized to receive additional dexamethasone, high-dose Ara-C, cisplatin (DHAP) therapy or high-dose chemotherapy and autologous bone marrow transplant in the PARMA trial (300). In patients receiving conventional salvage DHAP therapy, the age-adjusted sIPI was highly correlated with 5-year overall survival; patients with one, two, or three risk factors had 5-year overall survival of 33%, 21%, and 0%, respectively. However, the sIPI did not correlate with 5-year survival in the autologous bone marrow transplant arm, suggesting that transplant overcame the poor outcome of patients with one or more risk factors (300). Of interest, patients with no risk factors who were treated with DHAP or high-dose chemotherapy and stem cell transplant had comparable outcomes (300). In a similar study, the predictive value of the sIPI was evaluated in relapsed or refractory lymphoma patients before receiving ifosfamide, carboplatin, etoposide chemotherapy followed by stem cell transplant. The sIPI defined two groups: no to two risk factors, 2.5-year failure-free survival of 45%; and three to five risk factors, 2.5-year failure-free survival of 9% (301). The same investigators applied the age-adjusted sIPI to a group of patients with primary refractory aggressive lymphoma and found that patients with two and three risk factors had poor response rates to salvage treatment (30%) and a dismal 3-year survival rate (7.4%) (295).

Disease-Related Prognostic Factors

The Working Formulation divides the non-Hodgkin's lymphomas into three groups (or grades) based on growth pattern, cell size, and untreated natural history: (a) low, (b) intermediate, and (c) high grade (302). The more recent REAL and the WHO classifications incorporate more subtle morphologic distinctions, immunophenotypic signatures, and hallmark genetic abnormalities and define several unique biologic entities (38,303) with characteristic natural histories. For example, mantle cell lymphoma was recognized as having unique phenotypic (CD5$^+$, CD23$^-$) and genotypic features [e.g., t(11;14)(q13;32)] and a natural history characterized by frequent relapses and lack of curative potential. In diffuse large B-cell lymphoma, several disease subtypes are recognized on the basis of (a) clinical characteristics and cell of origin (primary mediastinal large B-cell lymphoma), (b) histologic appearance (intravascular lymphoma), and (c) viral pathogenesis (primary effusion lymphoma and lymphomatoid granulomatosis). These distinctions are of prognostic relevance because certain newly identified entities have much less favorable natural histories.

The International Lymphoma Study Group further assessed the frequency of the various subtypes defined by the REAL classification and the clinical course of the most prevalent disease entities. This comprehensive study emphasized the differences in both clinical presentation and overall survival in discrete lymphoma subtypes and characterized the impact of IPI risk groups in each entity (2,33).

Biologic Prognostic Factors

The IPI remains the most useful prognostic tool for the identification of patients who are unlikely to be cured with standard therapies. However, it has become clear that the clinical features that define high-risk disease are likely to be surrogate variables for intrinsic cellular and molecular heterogeneity. Immunophenotypic, cellular, immune, and molecular markers are being increasingly used in diagnosis, disease characterization, and initial risk assessment. More recent genome-wide approaches to risk assessment are even more promising (304,305).

Immunophenotypic Characteristics

B- versus T-Cell Phenotype

Approximately 12% to 15% of all lymphomas have a T-cell phenotype (2). The T-cell lymphomas are a heterogeneous group of diseases with diverse clinical behavior, immunophenotypic features, and prognosis. The peripheral T-cell lymphomas are defined as being post-thymic in origin. Initial studies failed to reveal a prognostic difference between aggressive B- and T-cell lymphomas (306–308). However, treatment regimens were nonuniform, and these reports were before the recognition of specific disease entities with unique natural histories. Recent studies support the notion that peripheral T-cell lymphomas have a worse outcome than diffuse large B-cell lymphomas (2,33,245,246,309–313). The IPI may define a subgroup of the peripheral T-cell lymphomas with a more favorable prognosis (242,245–248,250). In contrast, the T-cell or null-cell anaplastic large-cell lymphomas have a more favorable natural history and additional biologic heterogeneity; those patients expressing the t(2;5) ALK fusion protein have a superior survival compared to those who are ALK negative (252–254). Many of the rare subtypes (e.g., nasal and nasal-type, enteropathy-type, HTLV-I associated, and hepatosplenic) of peripheral T-cell lymphoma have an extremely poor prognosis, emphasizing the heterogeneity of peripheral T-cell lymphoma and the need to consider these diseases separately.

CD Antigens

Immunophenotypic analysis of non-Hodgkin's lymphoma is useful in diagnosing discrete disease entities. Combined with morphologic features, specific immunophenotypic signatures distinguish previously unidentified entities. In addition, the expression of specific cell surface antigens has demonstrated prognostic significance.

CD38

CD38 is a transmembrane glycoprotein originally characterized as a T-cell differentiation antigen (314). Subsequent studies revealed that CD38 expression was more widely distributed in lymphoid cells, depending on maturation and activation stage (315). Recently, relative levels of CD38 expression have been used to divide chronic lymphocytic leukemia into two subgroups (316) and to link overexpression of CD38 with adverse clinical features and shorter survival (317–319). However, others have questioned the use of CD38 as a prognostic marker (320), suggesting that CD38 expression may vary at specific time points in the disease (319).

CD5

CD5 is a glycoprotein expressed by most T cells and a subset of B cells. CD5 is expressed by the majority of chronic lymphocytic leukemias and mantle cell lymphomas and a subset of diffuse large B-cell lymphomas. Recent studies suggest that CD5⁺ diffuse large B-cell lymphoma is a rare but well-recognized subtype that may have an inferior prognosis (321,322).

Cellular Prognostic Factors

A number of cellular features have emerged over the years as having prognostic value in non-Hodgkin's lymphoma, including the expression of specific serologic parameters (e.g., LDH and β_2-microglobulin), proliferative indices (e.g., Ki-67), adhesion molecules [e.g., major histocompatibility complex (MHC), CD44, and intercellular adhesion molecule], angiogenic peptides [e.g., vascular endothelial growth factor (VEGF)], matrix metalloproteinases, tissue inhibitors of metalloproteinase, cytokines [tumor necrosis factor (TNF) and interleukin-6 (IL-6)], and modulators of cellular migration (e.g., BAL) and apoptosis (e.g., bcl-2, survivin, and NF-κB). The majority of factors evaluated in these single-parameter studies were selected on the basis of their observed role in other malignancies or in normal lymphocyte development. As additional information regarding comprehensive molecular signatures emerges (304,305), it is likely that individual parameters will be viewed in the context of the larger gene signatures.

Major Histocompatibility Complex Molecules

It has been postulated that the absence of MHC-encoded recognition structures may limit the ability of the host to mount an immune response against specific tumor antigens. In earlier studies of patients with aggressive lymphomas, tumors lacking HLA-DR were associated with shorter survivals than tumors with intact HLA-DR expression (323). Further tumor expression of class I and class II MHC determinants was found to correlate with the number of CD8⁺ T-tumor infiltrating lymphocytes in patients with aggressive non-Hodgkin's lymphoma (324). Taken together, these reports suggest that an impaired host immune system may be implicated in both disease pathogenesis and poor response to treatment.

Adhesion Molecule Expression

The expression of cell adhesion molecules (e.g., CD44, intercellular adhesion molecule-1, and CD11a/18) on lymphoma cells has been linked to tumor spread and poor outcome (325,326). Unlike B- and T-cell markers, adhesion molecules are not routinely assessed in the diagnostic workup. The CD44 adhesion molecule facilitates lymphocyte binding to the vascular endothelium with subsequent migration to nodal areas (327). Normal B cells have high CD44 expression before germinal center entry, weak expression in the germinal center, and increased expression after germinal center exit (328,329). Compared to patients whose tumors have low levels of CD44, those with CD44-high diffuse large B-cell lymphomas are more likely to present with advanced-stage disease and have an inferior outcome (329–331). In localized diffuse large B-cell lymphoma, CD44 expression is a strong predictor of tumor-related death, independent of IPI risk factors (332).

An alternatively spliced variant of CD44 (CD44-6v) has been shown to be preferentially expressed in aggressive B-cell lymphomas (333–335). In diffuse large B-cell lymphoma, the expression of specific CD44 variant isoforms, exon 3v or 6v, has been linked with widespread metastasis and shortened survival (336,337). In analyses of both the standard and variant isoforms, CD44-6v expression retains independent prognostic significance, suggesting that this isoform may be a stronger predictor of poor outcome (336,338).

More recently, serum CD44 has also been correlated with disseminated disease and shortened survival (325,339–342) independent of clinical parameters (325,341). For example, patients with early stage chronic lymphocytic leukemia and elevated serum CD44 have an increased risk of rapid disease progression (342).

Serologic Factors

Lactate Dehydrogenase

LDH was one of the first serologic factors to emerge as a prognostic factor in lymphoma (8,9,343). It is a consistent and reproducible risk factor across studies of both indolent and aggressive non-Hodgkin's lymphomas.

β_2-Microglobulin

β_2-microglobulin is a small extracellular protein that associates with the β chain of the class I MHC; the protein is also detectable in the serum of patients with lymphoid malignancies (229). It is not clear whether β_2-microglobulin is shed due to alterations of the cell surface or due to the lack of synthesis of other co-associated MHC components. Elevated β_2-microglobulin levels have been correlated with high tumor burdens and reduced survival in patients with aggressive (50,344–346) and indolent lymphomas (347). In one small study, added serum β_2-microglobulin levels improved the sensitivity of the IPI in predicting failure to standard chemotherapy (348). An earlier serologic staging system based on β_2-microglobulin and LDH levels also had predictive value in aggressive lymphomas (50).

Tumor Necrosis Factor

Elevated levels of TNF and its soluble receptors p55 and p75 have been correlated with shorter freedom from progression and overall survival in aggressive lymphomas (349,350). Information regarding TNF ligand and receptor status has been reported to increase the predictive value of the IPI (350).

Interleukin-6

IL-6 is a potent growth and differentiation factor in both benign and malignant B cells. Circulating IL-6 levels at diagnosis have been correlated with poor outcome in diffuse large B-cell lymphoma and additional indolent lymphoid malignancies (351–353).

nm23-H1

More recently, nm23-H1 protein, a differentiation inhibitory factor involved in tumor metastasis, has been identified as an important prognostic factor in diffuse large B-cell lymphoma as well as in peripheral T-cell lymphoma (354). Protein levels correlate well with traditional IPI risk factors and maintain prognostic significance in multivariate analysis. The worst outcome was observed in patients with levels greater than 80 ng/mL regardless of their IPI score (354). Furthermore, combining nm23-H1 levels with other serologic prognostic factors (e.g., sIL-2R and sCD44) increased the accuracy of serologic outcome prediction (354).

Antiapoptosis Proteins

Abnormalities in the balance between cell death and cell viability are critical in the pathogenesis and prognosis of a number of malignancies, including non-Hodgkin's lymphoma. Many investigators have studied the prognostic significance of proteins that regulate cell cycle (e.g., Rb, p27, p21, and p53) and apoptosis (e.g., p53, bcl-2, survivin, and NF-κB) in lymphoid malignancies.

Bcl-2

Bcl-2 was the first described member of a family of apoptosis regulators that homo- or heterodimerize. The antiapoptotic protein is widely expressed in both hematopoietic and nonhematopoietic cells; however, it is absent from the germinal centers of B-cell follicles and from cortical thymocytes (355–358). Bcl-2 overexpression inhibits cell death (359,360) and confers both chemotherapy and radiation resistance (361). Overexpression of bcl-2 occurs in approximately 80% to 90% of follicular lymphomas, often in association with a t(14;18), which brings the bcl-2 gene under the control of the immunoglobulin heavy chain promoter. In diffuse large-cell lymphomas, overexpression of the bcl-2 protein is associated with decreased disease-free and overall survival (362–367). In aggressive B-cell lymphomas, bcl-2 protein is often elevated in the absence of the t(14;18), suggesting that there are other mechanisms of bcl-2 protein overexpression in these tumors (355,362–365,368).

In a recent large series of patients with nodal diffuse B-cell lymphomas, bcl-2 expression was combined with the IPI to increase the predictive value of the IPI (369). Both bcl-2 expres-

sion and the IPI were independent poor prognostic factors. Using the IPI alone, only 8% of nodal diffuse large B-cell lymphomas were identified as being high risk. However, intermediate-risk group patients whose tumors expressed high levels of bcl-2 had inferior overall survivals, comparable to that of the high-risk group (369).

p53

p53 is a tumor suppressor gene located on chromosome 17 that induces cell cycle arrest or apoptosis, or both, in response to a variety of stimuli. Loss of function of p53 can occur through deletions or point mutations, which can generate dominant-negative forms of the protein (370). p53 mutation can prevent apoptosis and confer resistance to chemotherapy and radiation treatment (371). Wild-type p53 has a short half-life and is not generally detectable by routine immunohistochemistry (311). In contrast, mutated p53 has a prolonged half-life, making it detectable by immunostaining techniques. However, p53 immunostaining is complicated by the high frequency of mutations inducing stop codons in the open reading frame and the occasional detection of background wild-type protein (311).

p53 mutations in lymphoma appear limited to the late stages of indolent lymphomas (372–375), aggressive lymphoid malignancies (376–382), and relapsed disease (371). In follicular lymphoma, p53 mutations and increased protein expression are associated with higher grades and transformed disease (372,373). Mantle cell lymphomas with p53 mutations and immunopositivity have poorer prognoses than those tumors with wild-type p53 (380,381). In aggressive B-cell lymphoma, the correlation between p53 mutations and immunopositivity and outcome is less consistent, although mutational analysis has not been consistently performed (364,382). Mutated p53 has been described more frequently in aggressive lymphomas (diffuse large-cell and mantle cell lymphoma), with or without abnormalities in 17p. Such p53 mutations have been associated with complex karyotypic abnormalities, p53 protein expression, and poor outcome (383).

Survivin

Survivin is a recently identified member of the inhibitor of apoptosis gene family expressed in several solid tumors and many aggressive lymphomas (384). In contrast, survivin is absent in normal, terminally differentiated adult tissue (384). Survivin appears to inhibit cell death in B-lymphoid precursors that have been deprived of growth factors. In a large series of patients with diffuse large B-cell lymphoma treated with CHOP-type chemotherapy, 60% of tumors expressed survivin, and overall survival was significantly worse in patients with survivin-positive tumors (385). Survivin expression maintained prognostic significance in multivariate analysis independent of IPI clinical risk factors (385). Residual survivin-positive tumor cells may have a growth advantage because the protein is known to inhibit apoptosis at the G2/M checkpoint (385).

NF-κB

NF-κB is a member of the Rel protein family that plays a prominent role in lymphocyte development, activation and the prevention of apoptosis (386). High levels of NF-κB are required for B-cell proliferation and survival in response to mitogens. NF-κB transcriptional activity is governed by homo- and heterodimerization of the NF-κB family members and by interactions with members of the IκB family of inhibitors, which retain NF-κB dimers in the cytoplasm (386). Phosphorylation of IκB by IκB kinase (IκK) targets IκB for ubiquitination and degradation, allowing NF-κB to translocate to the nucleus and activate transcription of a number of targets, including members of the bcl-2 family (e.g., bcl-2, bfl-1/A1, and bcl-xL) (386–392). Recent studies suggest that a subset of diffuse large B-cell lymphoma and diffuse large B-cell lymphoma cell lines may exhibit constitutive NF-κB activity (386).

Proliferative Indices

Ki-67 is a nuclear antigen expressed by dividing tumor cells. The percentage of cells expressing Ki-67 reflects the number of cells that are cycling. In patients with aggressive lymphomas, high Ki-67 expression (>80%) has been correlated with poor prognosis (18% survival at 1 year), whereas low Ki-67 expression has been linked with favorable outcome (82% at 1 year) (393,394).

Tumor Invasiveness

A number of factors in lymphoma have been linked to the invasive potential of the tumor, including overexpression of matrix metalloproteinases, angiogenic peptides, and proteins that influence cellular migration. For example, overexpression of a major matrix metalloproteinase, gelatinase B, has been linked with shortened survival in patients with a subtype of diffuse large B-cell lymphoma (immunoblastic lymphoma) (395).

Tumor angiogenesis is critical for local growth and distant spread of hematologic malignancies (396). In earlier analyses of microvessel densities, aggressive lymphomas had more prominent evidence of a tumor vasculature (397,398). VEGF is a potent angiogenic peptide with demonstrated prognostic significance in multiple tumor types (399–401). In a recent study, VEGF serum levels were elevated in a subset of patients with non-Hodgkin's lymphoma and correlated with clinical IPI risk factors (402). In an additional broad-based analysis of molecular prognostic factors in diffuse large B-cell lymphoma, increased VEGF transcripts were associated with fatal or refractory disease (304). Furthermore, high pretreatment levels of another angiogenic peptide, basic fibroblast growth factor, have also been correlated with inferior survival in diffuse large B-cell lymphoma (403).

In additional recent studies, a novel risk-related gene family, BAL1 and 2, was identified and found to be highly expressed in fatal or refractory diffuse large B-cell lymphomas (404,405). Overexpression of cloned BAL1 complementary DNAs (cDNAs) increased the migratory potential of diffuse large B-cell lymphoma cell lines (404) in classic transwell assays, suggesting that BAL family members may promote tumor dissemination (404).

Host Immune Response

The presence of tumor-infiltrating T lymphocytes has been consistently observed in patients with non-Hodgkin's lymphoma, suggesting that the host immune response may be a critical factor in determining patient outcome (310,324,406–410). This is in keeping with earlier observations correlating the absence of HLA-DR on tumors with an impaired immune response and worse outcome (323). Studies in murine models and some human tumors suggest that the presence of tumor-infiltrating lymphocytes is a manifestation of a specific antitumor immune response (411,412) and that relapse and survival from B-cell lymphoma may be directly related to the type, number, and activation state of specific infiltrating T-cell subsets (406,408,410,413,414).

Reports focusing on cytotoxic T cells (CD8+) have suggested that low levels are correlated with patient relapse or reduced survival, or both, in some lymphoproliferative disorders (414,415). However, helper T-cell (CD4+) levels may be even more critical in determining patient outcome. In a recent study, patients with diffuse large B-cell lymphoma who had low levels of tumor-infiltrating memory CD4+ cells had a poorer outcome than patients with higher levels of comparable T cells (406). The significance of the percentage of CD4+ infiltration was maintained, along with the IPI, in multivariate analysis (406). More recently, the gene expression profiles of T-cell–rich and T-cell–poor diffuse large B-cell lymphoma have been evaluated (416). Transcripts that were more abundant in the T-cell–rich group included certain class II MHC molecules and chemokines. In contrast, adhesion molecules and proliferative markers, such as c-myc, were underrepresented in the T-cell–rich group (416).

Other reports have suggested antigen-specific infiltrating T-cells may actually be supporting tumor growth in tumors such as MALT lymphomas (417). A specific subtype of diffuse large B-cell lymphoma, T-cell-rich B-cell lymphoma, may have a worse prognosis (418) than standard diffuse large B-cell lymphoma. This could reflect an important distinction between T cells involved in an inflammatory reaction and those clearly participating in the host immune response to the malignant cells.

Genetic and Molecular Abnormalities

Hematologic malignancies are characterized by translocations, deletions, and other nonrandom genetic alterations (419–421). Conventional cytogenetics is limited to the analysis of metaphase chromosomes. Fluorescence *in situ* hybridization has enabled the detection of chromosomal aberrations in interphase nuclei using probes that span the immunoglobulin locus (422). The recent introduction of spectral karyotyping has provided even more precise identification of rearrangements in lymphoid malignancies (423).

t(14;18) and bcl-2

The t(14;18)(q32;q21) translocation is the most common translocation in lymphoid tumors. As a result of the translocation, the bcl-2 gene on chromosome 18 is juxtaposed to the promoter region of the immunoglobulin heavy chain region on chromosome 14, resulting in constitutive expression of the bcl-2 proto-oncogene. The t(14;18) is found in up to 90% of follicular lymphomas (424) and approximately 20% to 33% of aggressive non-Hodgkin's lymphomas (362). It is unclear whether the presence of a t(14;18) in diffuse large B-cell lymphoma is a marker of histologic transformation of a previous follicular lymphoma or reflects an early transforming event in a subset of *de novo* diffuse large B-cell lymphoma (311). Although bcl-2 protein expression impacts outcome in diffuse large B-cell lymphoma, patients who harbor a t(14;18) do not appear to have a worse prognosis (362,365,425). The t(14;18) appears to be a more common occurrence in the centroblastic variant of diffuse large B-cell lymphoma (426) and diffuse large B-cell lymphomas with a germinal center B-cell gene expression profile (427).

Bcl-6

Chromosomal alterations involving the band 3q27 are the most common karyotypic abnormalities in diffuse large B-cell lymphoma (428). Chromosome rearrangements that substitute immunoglobulin regulatory elements or alternate promoters upstream of the bcl-6 coding region are found in approximately 40% of diffuse large B-cell lymphomas, except primary mediastinal large B-cell lymphomas (428). Subsequent cloning of the 3q27 breakpoints identified the involved gene to be bcl-6. The bcl-6 translocation can involve either an immunoglobulin or nonimmunoglobulin partner (429). The bcl-6 gene encodes a POZ/zinc finger sequence–specific transcriptional repressor, which is specifically expressed in normal germinal center B cells (430). Although 3q27 translocations are also found in a small fraction of follicular lymphomas (431), they are noticeably absent in other lymphoid neoplasms. Additional somatic point mutations that alter the bcl-6 5' regulatory region, independent of 3q27 translocations, are found in up to 70% of diffuse large B-cell lymphomas (432,433) and may accompany transformation of follicular lymphoma to diffuse large B-cell lymphoma (434).

To date, the prognostic significance of bcl-6 rearrangements and mutations is unclear. Although an earlier study suggested that tumors with bcl-6 gene rearrangements were associated with better clinical outcomes (435), the majority of studies has failed to demonstrate this benefit (436–438).

In a recent study, the expression of bcl-6 at both the messenger RNA and protein level was associated with improved overall survival in patients with diffuse large B-cell lymphoma (439). Patients with low or high clinical risk by the IPI were further stratified based on bcl-6 gene expression (439). Bcl-6 messenger RNA levels have been compared in diffuse large B-cell lymphomas, with bcl-6 translocations involving immunoglobulin or other partner genes. Of interest, bcl-6 transcripts were significantly more abundant in tumors with immunoglobulin/bcl-6 translocations, and these tumors were associated with a more favorable prognosis (440,441).

t(2;5) and Anaplastic Lymphoma Kinase in Anaplastic Large-Cell Lymphoma

Among the aggressive T-cell lymphomas, anaplastic large-cell lymphoma has a uniquely favorable outcome (2,33, 242,247,254). However, clear biologic heterogeneity exists within this disease entity. Many anaplastic large-cell lymphomas exhibit a characteristic cytogenetic abnormality t(2;5)(p23;q35) (254,442–444) and express a chimeric protein due to the fusion of the nucleophosmin gene on chromosome 5 to a portion of the ALK gene on chromosome 2 (445). Anaplastic large-cell lymphomas that lack expression of the ALK protein (ALK-negative) have a significantly worse 5-year overall survival when compared to anaplastic large-cell lymphomas that express the fusion protein (ALK-positive) (253,254,445–447). In one study, 5-year overall survival of ALK-positive cases was 93% compared with 37% in ALK-negative cases (252). Patients with ALK-negative anaplastic large-cell lymphoma are also more likely to be older with a poor performance status (252–254,448).

t(11;18) and t(1;14) in Gastric Mucosa-Associated Lymphoid Tissue–Type Lymphoma

The most common structural abnormality in MALT lymphoma is t(11;18)(q21;21), resulting in a fusion of API-2, a member of the inhibitor of apoptosis family on chromosome 11q21, with MALT-1 on chromosome 18q21. More recently, t(1;14) (p22;q14) was found to result in the overexpression of a newly characterized gene, bcl-10 (449,450). Both of these structural abnormalities lead to bcl-10 nuclear localization and constitutive NF-κB activation through independent mechanisms. In the former, the API/MALT fusion protein activates IκK, resulting in translocation of NF-κB into the nucleus and NF-κB–dependent transcription. In the latter, bcl-10 is overexpressed, binds to MALT-1 (normal partner), and together they increase the activity of IκK (450). As described previously, NF-κB has been implicated in other lymphoid neoplasms and likely plays a role in the pathogenesis of MALT lymphoma. Moreover, NF-κB activation may be a marker of more aggressive clinical disease and resistance to antibiotic therapy (450).

Immunoglobulin Heavy Chain Somatic Mutations

It is widely appreciated that germinal center B cells are subject to somatic hypermutation of the immunoglobulin heavy chain, which enhances immunoglobulin affinity for specific antigens (451). Somatically mutated variable region genes (along with bcl-6 mutations) are indicative of origin from the germinal center or post–germinal center (i.e., memory) B cells (451).

Many subtypes of non-Hodgkin's lymphoma, including diffuse large B-cell lymphoma, follicular lymphoma, and Burkitt's lymphoma, demonstrate somatic mutations of their immunoglobulin genes, suggesting that these tumors arise from germinal center or post–germinal center B cells.

More recently, subsets of chronic lymphocytic leukemia and marginal zone lymphoma have been identified with mutated immunoglobulin. In these indolent lymphomas, immunoglobulin mutations appear to have prognostic significance. In chronic lymphocytic leukemia, patients whose tumors have mutations in the immunoglobulin heavy chain have a more favorable prognosis (approximate median survival, 25 years), whereas those with tumors with unmutated immunoglobulin heavy chain tend to present with advanced stage, higher lymphocyte count, and diffuse bone marrow involvement and have reduced survivals (approximate median survival, 8 years) (318,452–454). Of note, initial reports linked the absence of CD38 expression with immunoglobulin somatic mutation and improved survival (318). However, other studies have found that CD38 expression and immunoglobulin mutations are independent prognostic variables that may identify different patient risk groups (319,455).

Recent studies in splenic marginal zone lymphoma suggest that, as with chronic lymphocytic leukemia, marginal zone lymphomas with an unmutated immunoglobulin gene have a worse outcome (5-year overall survival, 38%) compared to those with a mutated immunoglobulin (5-year overall survival, 86%) (456). The former were also more frequently associated with 7q deletions (456), suggesting that a gene associated with disease progression may be located at this locus.

Other

Recent studies in chronic lymphocytic leukemia have elucidated a number of genetic abnormalities with prognostic significance. The most frequent abnormalities include 13q14, 11p deletions, 12q trisomy, and 17p deletions (457). There is little information regarding the genes involved in these cytogenetic alterations. p53 is altered by 17p deletions, and 13q14 is postulated to contain a tumor suppressor gene. Alterations in 11p, 12q, and, particularly, 17p are associated with reduced survival; however, patients with isolated 13q14 abnormalities have a superior outcome (457).

Minimal Residual Disease

With the development of polymerase chain reaction (PCR)-based techniques, it has become possible to detect as few as 1 in 10^6 tumor cells with an amplifiable translocation or clonal immunoglobulin gene rearrangement (458–461). The detection of minimal residual disease after therapy may have prognostic implications. To date, the majority of studies have focused on the prognostic implications of PCR-detectable t(14;18) translocations in blood or marrow after induction, salvage, or high-dose consolidation therapy. Patients with indolent non-Hodgkin's lymphoma who demonstrated t(14;18) negativity in the bone marrow and peripheral blood have a significantly better disease-free survival than those who continue to demonstrate PCR-detectable disease after autologous bone marrow transplant (462). The inability to purge residual t(14;18) lymphoma cells in non-Hodgkin's lymphoma patients undergoing autologous bone marrow transplant has been cited as an important predictor of relapse posttransplant (462,463). Similar results have also been reported in aggressive non-Hodgkin's lymphoma after either autologous bone marrow or stem cell transplant (464). When minimal residual disease was assessed using PCR-based assays of bcl-2 rearrangements or clonal CDRIII (immunoglobulin H complementary determining region III) or T-cell receptors (464), PCR-positive patients had a reduced event-free survival (464).

There have been conflicting results regarding the prognostic implications of PCR-detectable t(14;18) after treatment with conventional therapy complicated by the fact that PCR-detectable t(14;18) have also been found in the peripheral blood of healthy individuals (465). Recent studies suggest that patients who achieve a PCR-determined molecular response after conventional treatment may have a reduced risk of relapse (466–468). However, the utility of molecular analysis of minimal residual disease may differ in specific lymphoma subtypes and may be treatment dependent. For example, in a recent study of minimal residual disease after induction therapy of newly diagnosed follicular lymphoma, patients who remained t(14;18) positive after CHOP treatment subsequently received rituximab, with the aim of increasing the proportion of patients who achieved a molecular response. The majority of such patients converted from t(14;18) positive to a t(14;18) negative state in blood or bone marrow. Furthermore, those patients who achieved a PCR-negative status had an excellent 3-year overall survival (95%), although follow-up was short (467).

More recently, the predictive value of PCR-determined molecular responses have been assessed in newly diagnosed patients with mantle cell lymphoma treated with CHOP and rituximab induction therapy (469). In this study, molecular responses were evaluated using PCR for both t(11;14) and clonal immunoglobulin gene rearrangements (469). Although a subset of patients obtained molecular complete remission in peripheral blood or bone marrow, or both, these molecular responses were not predictive for progression-free survival (469). The lack of correlation between molecular complete remissions in the peripheral blood or bone marrow and long-term progression-free survival in mantle cell lymphoma may reflect the preferential clearing of tumor cells from peripheral blood or bone marrow in rituximab-treated patients and the relative insensitivity of mantle cell lymphoma to current therapy (469).

Gene Expression Signatures

Molecular analyses of clinical heterogeneity in lymphoid malignancies have largely focused on individual candidate genes, with particular emphasis on genes with known functions in other malignancies or in normal lymphocyte development. Although some of these candidate genes correlate with outcome, a comprehensive molecular approach to outcome prediction has been lacking. The recent development of DNA microarrays provides an opportunity to take a genome-wide approach to predicting treatment outcome in specific lymphoid neoplasms. In addition to providing molecular correlates of clinical outcome, genomic approaches may also improve diagnostic accuracy, identify new disease entities, and elucidate novel therapeutic targets.

Two major types of microarray platforms are currently in use: cDNA and oligonucleotide microarrays. In brief, cDNA arrays are comprised of PCR-amplified cDNA clones that have been systematically deposited onto glass slides or nitrocellulose filters (470). In the most commonly used protocols, sample and reference RNAs are used to generate fluorescently labeled cDNAs, which are then simultaneously hybridized to the arrays (470). In contrast, oligonucleotide microarrays are generated by depositing previously synthesized oligonucleotide probes onto slides or directly synthesizing these probes on the surface of silicon wafers (470). This approach offers the advantage of uniform probe length, more precise information regarding specific splice variants, and the capacity for analyzing approximately 60,000 human genes and expressed sequence tags in a single experiment.

There are two main computational approaches to analyzing the data generated by gene expression profiling: unsupervised and supervised learning. Unsupervised learning algorithms [e.g., hierarchical clustering and self-organizing maps (96)] cluster samples according to similarities in their gene expression profiles without a priori assumptions regarding the basis for the designated clusters (470). However, due to the complexity of gene expression profiles, many different relationships may exist in a data set, and an unsupervised learning algorithm may not directly address a specific clinical question. In contrast, supervised learning methods can be used to develop gene expression profiles reflective of specific, predetermined differences (i.e., cured vs. fatal or refractory disease) (470).

Recently, unsupervised and supervised learning techniques have been used to explore molecular signatures of the most common lymphoid malignancy, diffuse large B-cell lymphoma (304,471). Using an unsupervised approach (hierarchical clustering), investigators identified similarities in the gene expression profiles of certain normal B cells (germinal center B cells and in vitro activated B cells) and diffuse large B-cell lymphoma subsets. They postulated that diffuse large B-cell lymphoma subsets might derive from different types of normal B cells and that the putative cell of origin may impact outcome (471). In a larger follow-up study, the authors refined and simplified the cell-of-origin signature and identified a third tumor group unrelated to cell of origin (305).

In another recent analysis, investigators used a supervised learning method to directly characterize signatures of outcome in cured vs. fatal or refractory diffuse large B-cell lymphoma (304). A large number of genes were identified as differentially expressed in the cured and fatal or refractory subgroups. Genes implicated in diffuse large B-cell lymphoma outcome included ones that regulate responses to B-cell receptor signaling, critical serine/threonine phosphorylation pathways, and apoptosis, suggesting new potential rational targets for therapy (304).

Chronic lymphocytic leukemia expression profiles have recently been evaluated by two different groups (472,473). As described previously, two clinically relevant subsets of chronic lymphocytic leukemia have been defined on the basis of the presence or absence of hypermutated immunoglobulin variable regions (318,452–454,474). However, in unsupervised analyses, the gene expression profiles of chronic lymphocytic leukemia with and without hypermutated immunoglobulin variable regions are similar (472,473). In contrast, supervised analyses can be used to identify a small group of genes that are differentially expressed in the mutated and unmutated immunoglobulin groups (Color Plate 1) (472,473).

In summary, early studies of gene expression profiles in lymphoid malignancies suggest that this approach holds great promise for improved diagnosis, prognostication, and identification of rational therapeutic targets. In the future, such studies will be coupled with concurrent analyses of the molecular changes in associated genes and protein products, providing comprehensive molecular signatures of specific tumors.

REFERENCES

1. Carbone P, Kaplan H, Musshoff K, et al. Report of the Committee on Hodgkin's disease staging. *Cancer Res* 1971;31:1860–1861.
2. Armitage J. For The Non-Hodgkin's Lymphoma Classification Project. A clinical evaluation of the International Lymphoma Study Group classification of non-Hodgkin's lymphoma. *Blood* 1997;89:3909–3918.
3. d'Amore F, Christensen BE, Brincker H, et al. Clinicopathological features and prognostic factors in extranodal non-Hodgkin lymphomas. Danish LYFO Study Group. *Eur J Cancer* 1991;27(10):1201–1208.
4. Zucca E, Roggero E, Bertoni F, et al. Primary extranodal non-Hodgkin's lymphomas. Part 2: Head and neck, central nervous system and other less common sites. *Ann Oncol* 1999;10(9):1023–1033.
5. Zucca E, Roggero E, Bertoni F, Cavalli F. Primary extranodal non-Hodgkin's lymphomas. Part 1: Gastrointestinal, cutaneous and genitourinary lymphomas. *Ann Oncol* 1997;8(8):727–737.
6. Fisher R DV, Johnson BL, Simon R, Young RC. Prognostic factors for advanced diffuse histiocytic lymphoma following treatment with combination chemotherapy. *Am J Med* 1977;63:177.
7. Cabanillas F, Burke JS, Smith TL, et al. Factors predicting for response and survival in adults with advanced non-Hodgkin's lymphoma. *Arch Intern Med* 1978;138:413.
8. Ferraris AM, Giuntini P, Gaetani GF. Serum lactic dehydrogenase as a prognostic tool for non-Hodgkin lymphomas. *Blood* 1979;54(4):928–932.
9. Schneider RJ, Siebert K, Passe S, et al. Prognostic significance of serum lactate dehydrogenase in malignant lymphoma. *Cancer* 1980;46:139.
10. Armitage JO, Dick FR, Corder MP, et al. Predicting therapeutic outcome in patients with diffuse histiocytic lymphoma with cyclophosphamide, adriamycin, vincristine and prednisone (CHOP). *Cancer* 1982;50:1695.
11. Fisher RI, Hubbard SM, DeVita VT, et al. Factors predicting long-term survival in diffuse mixed, histiocytic, or undifferentiated lymphoma. *Blood* 1981;58:45.
12. Jagannath S, Velasquez S, Tucker S, et al. Tumor burden assessment and its implication for a prognostic model in advanced diffuse large-cell lymphoma. *J Clin Oncol* 1986;4(6):859–865.
13. Jagannath S, Velasquez WS, Tucker SL, et al. Stage IV diffuse large-cell lymphoma: a long-term analysis. *J Clin Oncol* 1985;3(1):39–47.
14. Shipp M, Harrington D, Klatt M, et al. Identification of major prognostic subgroups of patients with large-cell lymphoma treated with m-BACOD or M-BACOD. *Ann Intern Med* 1986;104:757–765.
15. Danieu L, Wong G, Koziner B, Clarkson B. Predictive model for prognosis in advanced diffuse histiocytic lymphoma. *Cancer Res* 1986;46(10):5372–5379.

16. Velasquez WS, Jagannath S, Tucker SL, et al. Risk classification as the basis for clinical staging of diffuse large-cell lymphoma derived from 10-year survival data. *Blood* 1989;74(2):551–557.
17. Jones S, Miller T, Connors J. Long-term follow-up and analysis for prognostic factors for patients with limited-stage diffuse large-cell lymphoma treated with initial chemotherapy with or without adjuvant radiotherapy. *J Clin Oncol* 1989;7:1186–1191.
18. Hoskins P, Ng V, Spinelli J, Klimo P, Connors J. Prognostic variables in patients with diffuse large-cell lymphoma treated with MACOP-B. *J Clin Oncol* 1991;9(2):220–226.
19. Coiffier B, Gisselbrecht C, Vose J, et al. Prognostic factors in aggressive malignant lymphomas: description and validation of a prognostic index that could identify patients requiring a more intensive therapy. *J Clin Oncol* 1991;9(2):211–219.
20. Gospodarowicz M, Bush R, Brown T, Chua T. Prognostic factors in nodular lymphomas: a multivariate analysis based on the Princess Margaret Hospital experience. *Int J Radiat Oncol Biol Phys* 1984;10:489–497.
21. Romaguera J, McLaughlin P, North L, et al. Multivariate analysis of prognostic factors in stage IV follicular low-grade lymphoma: a risk model. *J Clin Oncol* 1991;9(5):762–769.
22. Soubeyran P, Eghbali H, Bonichon F, et al. Low-grade follicular lymphomas: analysis of prognosis in a series of 281 patients. *Eur J Cancer* 1991;27:1606–1613.
23. Bastion Y, Berger F, Bryon PA, et al. Follicular lymphomas: assessment of prognostic factors in 127 patients followed for 10 years. *Ann Oncol* 1991;2[Suppl 2]:123–129.
24. Federico M, Vitolo U, Zinzani PL, et al. Prognosis of follicular lymphoma: a predictive model based on a retrospective analysis of 987 cases. Intergruppo Italiano Linfomi. *Blood* 2000;95(3):783–789.
25. Decaudin D, Lepage E, Brousse N, et al. Low-grade stage III–IV follicular lymphoma: multivariate analysis of prognostic factors in 484 patients—a study of the Groupe d'Etude des Lymphomes de l'Adulte. *J Clin Oncol* 1999;17(8):2499–2505.
26. Shipp M, Harrington D. A predictive model for aggressive non-Hodgkin's lymphoma: The International NHL Prognostic Factors Project. *N Engl J Med* 1993;329:987–994.
27. Musshoff K. [Clinical staging classification of non-Hodgkin's lymphomas (author's transl)]. *Strahlentherapie* 1977;153(4):218–221.
28. Rohatiner A, d'Amore F, Coiffier B, et al. Report on a workshop convened to discuss the pathological and staging classifications of gastrointestinal tract lymphoma. *Ann Oncol* 1994;5(5):397–400.
29. d'Amore F, Brincker H, Gronbaek K, et al. Non-Hodgkin's lymphoma of the gastrointestinal tract: a population-based analysis of incidence, geographic distribution, clinicopathologic presentation features, and prognosis. Danish Lymphoma Study Group. *J Clin Oncol* 1994;12(8):1673–1684.
30. Gospodarowicz M, Bush R, Brown T, Chua T. Curability of gastrointestinal lymphoma with combined surgery and radiation. *Int J Radiat Oncol* 1983;9:3–9.
31. Murphy SB, Hustu HO. A randomized trial of combined modality therapy of childhood non-Hodgkin's lymphoma. *Cancer* 1980;45(4):630–637.
32. Shipp M, Ambinder R, Appelbaum F, et al. NCCN preliminary non-Hodgkin's lymphoma practice guidelines. *Oncology* 1997;11:281–346.
33. Armitage JO, Weisenburger DD. New approach to classifying non-Hodgkin's lymphomas: clinical features of the major histologic subtypes. Non-Hodgkin's Lymphoma Classification Project. *J Clin Oncol* 1998;16(8):2780–2795.
34. Radaskiewicz T, Brigitte D, Bauer P. Gastrointestinal malignant lymphomas of the mucosa-associated lymphoid tissue: factors relevant to prognosis. *Gastroenterology* 1992;101:1159–1170.
35. Thieblemont C, Bastion Y, Berger F, et al. Mucosa-associated lymphoid tissue gastrointestinal and nongastrointestinal lymphoma behavior: analysis of 108 patients. *J Clin Oncol* 1997;15(4):1624–1630.
36. Isaacson P. Gastric lymphoma and *Helicobacter pylori*. *N Engl J Med* 1994;330:1310–1311.
37. Nakamura S, Yao T, Aoyagi K, et al. *Helicobacter pylori* and primary gastric lymphoma. A histopathologic and immunohistochemical analysis of 237 patients. *Cancer* 1997;79(1):3–11.
38. Harris NL, Jaffe ES, Diebold J, et al. World Health Organization classification of neoplastic diseases of the hematopoietic and lymphoid tissues: report of the Clinical Advisory Committee meeting-Airlie House, Virginia, November 1997. *J Clin Oncol* 1999;17(12):3835–3849.
39. Weisenburger DD. Epidemiology of non-Hodgkin's lymphoma: recent findings regarding an emerging epidemic. *Ann Oncol* 1994;5[Suppl 1]:S19–24.
40. Goffinet D, Warnke R, Dunnick N, et al. Clinical and surgical (laparotomy) evaluation of patients with non-Hodgkin's lymphomas. *Cancer Treat Rep* 1977;61:981–992.
41. Chabner B, Johnson R, DeVita V, et al. Sequential staging in non-Hodgkin's lymphoma. *Cancer Treat Rep* 1977;61:993–997.
42. Bitran J, Golomb H, Ultmann J, et al. Non-Hodgkin's lymphoma, poorly differentiated lymphocytic and mixed cell types: results of sequential staging procedures, response to therapy, and survival of 100 patients. *Cancer* 1978;42:88–95.
43. Lotz MJ, Chabner B, DeVita VT Jr, et al. Pathological staging of 100 consecutive untreated patients with non-Hodgkin's lymphomas: extramedullary sites of disease. *Cancer* 1976;37(1):266–270.
44. Moran EM, Ultmann JE, Ferguson DJ, et al. Staging laparotomy in non-Hodgkin's lymphoma. *Br J Cancer* 1975;31[Suppl 2]:228–236.
45. McKenna RW, Bloomfield CD, Brunning RD. Nodular lymphoma: bone marrow and blood manifestations. *Cancer* 1975;36(2):428–440.
46. Bloomfield CD, McKenna RW, Brunning RD. Significance of haematological parameters in the non-Hodgkin's malignant lymphomas. *Br J Haematol* 1976;32(1):41–46.
47. Conlan MG, Armitage JO, Bast M, Weisenburger DD. Clinical significance of hematologic parameters in non-Hodgkin's lymphoma at diagnosis. *Cancer* 1991;67(5):1389–1395.
48. Stein RS, Ultmann JE, Byrne GE Jr, et al. Bone marrow involvement in non-Hodgkin's lymphoma: implications for staging and therapy. *Cancer* 1976;37(2):629–636.
49. Conlan M, Bast M, Armitage J, Weisenburger D. Bone marrow involvement by non-Hodgkin's lymphoma: the clinical significance of morphologic discordance between the lymph node and bone marrow. *J Clin Oncol* 1990;8(7):1163–1172.
50. Swan F Jr, Velasquez W, Tucker S, et al. A new serologic staging system for large-cell lymphomas based on initial β_2-microglobulin and lactate dehydrogenase levels. *J Clin Oncol* 1989;7:907.
51. Chabner BA, Johnson RE, Chretien PB, et al. Percutaneous liver biopsy, peritoneoscopy and laparotomy: an assessment of relative merits in the lymphomata. *Br J Cancer* 1975;31[Suppl 2]:242–7.
52. Belloc C, lu H, Soria C, et al. The effect of platelets on invasiveness and protease production of human mammary tumor cells. *Int J Cancer* 1995;60:413–417.
53. Veronesi U, Musumegi R, Pizzetti F, et al. The value of staging laparotomy in non-Hodgkin's lymphomas. *Cancer* 1974;33(2):446–459.
54. Gandara DR, Mackenzie MR. Differential diagnosis of monoclonal gammopathy. *Med Clin North Am* 1988;72(5):1155–1167.
55. Kyle RA, Therneau TM, Rajkumar SV, et al. A long-term study of prognosis in monoclonal gammopathy of undetermined significance. *N Engl J Med* 2002;346(8):564–569.
56. Ioachim HL, Dorsett B, Cronin W, et al. Acquired immunodeficiency syndrome–associated lymphomas: clinical, pathologic, immunologic, and viral characteristics of 111 cases. *Hum Pathol* 1991;22(7):659–673.
57. Nador RG, Milligan LL, Flore O, et al. Expression of Kaposi's sarcoma-associated herpesvirus G protein-coupled receptor monocistronic and bicistronic transcripts in primary effusion lymphomas. *Virology* 2001;287(1):62–70.
58. Arvanitakis L, Mesri EA, Nador RG, et al. Establishment and characterization of a primary effusion (body cavity-based) lymphoma cell line (BC-3) harboring Kaposi's sarcoma-associated herpesvirus (KSHV/HHV-8) in the absence of Epstein-Barr virus. *Blood* 1996;88(7):2648–2654.
59. Yamaguchi F, Saya H, Bruner JM, Morrisson RS. Differential expression of two fibroblast growth factor-receptor genes is associated with malignant progression in human astrocytomas. *Proc Natl Acad Sci U S A* 1994;91:484–488.
60. Hollsberg P, Hafler DA. Seminars in medicine of the Beth Israel Hospital, Boston. Pathogenesis of diseases induced by human lymphotropic virus type I infection. *N Engl J Med* 1993;328(16):1173–1182.
61. Silvestri F, Baccarani M. Hepatitis C virus-related lymphomas. *Br J Haematol* 1997;99(3):475–80.
62. Lok AS, Liang RH, Chiu EK, et al. Reactivation of hepatitis B virus replication in patients receiving cytotoxic therapy. Report of a prospective study. *Gastroenterology* 1991;100(1):182–188.

63. Rossi G, Pelizzari A, Motta M, Puoti M. Primary prophylaxis with lamivudine of hepatitis B virus reactivation in chronic HbsAg carriers with lymphoid malignancies treated with chemotherapy. *Br J Haematol* 2001;115(1):58–62.

64. Celikoglu F, Teirstein AS, Krellenstein DJ, Strauchen JA. Pleural effusion in non-Hodgkin's lymphoma. *Chest* 1992;101(5):1357–1360.

65. Castellino RA, Hilton S, O'Brien JP, Portlock CS. Non-Hodgkin lymphoma: contribution of chest CT in the initial staging evaluation. *Radiology* 1996;199(1):129–132.

66. Salonen O, Kivisaari L, Standertskjold-Nordenstam CG, et al. Chest radiography and computed tomography in the evaluation of mediastinal adenopathy in lymphoma. *Acta Radiol* 1987;28(6):747–750.

67. Romano M, Libshitz HI. Hodgkin disease and non-Hodgkin lymphoma: plain chest radiographs and chest computed tomography of thoracic involvement in previously untreated patients. *Radiol Med (Torino)* 1998;95(1–2):49–53.

68. Khoury MB, Godwin JD, Halvorsen R, et al. Role of chest CT in non-Hodgkin lymphoma. *Radiology* 1986;158(3):659–662.

69. Phillips G, Kumari-Subaiya S, Sawitsky A. Ultrasonic evaluation of the scrotum in lymphoproliferative disease. *J Ultrasound Med* 1987;6(4):169–175.

70. Mazzu D, Jeffrey RB Jr, Ralls PW. Lymphoma and leukemia involving the testicles: findings on gray-scale and color Doppler sonography. *AJR Am J Roentgenol* 1995;164(3):645–647.

71. Charnsangavej C. Lymphoma of the genitourinary tract. *Radiol Clin North Am* 1990;28(4):865–877.

72. Tio TL, den Hartog Jager FC, Tijtgat GN. Endoscopic ultrasonography of non-Hodgkin lymphoma of the stomach. *Gastroenterology* 1986;91(2):401–408.

73. Caletti GC, Ferrari A, Bocus P, et al. Endoscopic ultrasonography in gastric lymphoma. *Schweiz Med Wochenschr* 1996;126(19):819–825.

74. Fujishima H, Misawa T, Maruoka A, et al. Staging and follow-up of primary gastric lymphoma by endoscopic ultrasonography. *Am J Gastroenterol* 1991;86(6):719–724.

75. Hermann G, Klein MJ, Abdelwahab IF, Kenan S. MRI appearance of primary non-Hodgkin's lymphoma of bone. *Skeletal Radiol* 1997;26(11):629–632.

76. White LM, Schweitzer ME, Khalili K, et al. MR imaging of primary lymphoma of bone: variability of T2-weighted signal intensity. *AJR Am J Roentgenol* 1998;170(5):1243–1247.

77. Hoane BR, Shields AF, Porter BA, Shulman HM. Detection of lymphomatous bone marrow involvement with magnetic resonance imaging. *Blood* 1991;78(3):728–738.

78. Berliner N, Ault K, Martin P, Weinberg S. Detection of clonal excess in lymphoproliferative disease by kappa/gamma analysis: correlation with immunoglobulin gene DNA rearrangement. *Blood* 1986;67:80–85.

79. Nejmeddine F, Caillat-Vigneron N, Escaig F, et al. Mechanism involved in gallium-67 (Ga-67) uptake by human lymphoid cell lines. *Cell Mol Biol* 1998;44(8):1215–1220.

80. Rehm PK. Radionuclide evaluation of patients with lymphoma. *Radiol Clin North Am* 2001;39(5):957–978.

81. Bekerman C, Szidon JP, Pinsky S. The role of gallium-67 in the clinical evaluation of sarcoidosis. *Semin Roentgenol* 1985;20(4):400–409.

82. Anderson K, Leonard R, Canellos G, et al. High-dose gallium imaging in lymphoma. *Am J Med* 1983;75:327–331.

83. Front D, Israel O, Epelbaum R, et al. Ga-67 SPECT before and after treatment of lymphoma. *Radiology* 1990;175(2):515–519.

84. Sandrock D, Lastoria S, Magrath IT, Neumann RD. The role of gallium-67 tumour scintigraphy in patients with small, non-cleaved cell lymphoma. *Eur J Nucl Med* 1993;20(2):119–22.

85. Nejmeddine F, Raphael M, Martin A, et al. 67Ga scintigraphy in B-cell non-Hodgkin's lymphoma: correlation of 67Ga uptake with histology and transferrin receptor expression. *J Nucl Med* 1999;40(1):40–45.

86. Andrews GA, Hubner KF, Greenlaw RH. Ga-67 citrate imaging in malignant lymphoma: final report of cooperative group. *J Nucl Med* 1978;19(9):1013–1019.

87. Brown ML, O'Donnell JB, Thrall JH, et al. Gallium-67 scintigraphy in untreated and treated non-Hodgkin lymphomas. *J Nucl Med* 1978;19(8):875–879.

88. Hoffer P. Status of gallium-67 in tumor detection. *J Nucl Med* 1980;21(4):394–398.

89. Bekerman C, Hoffer PB, Bitran JD. The role of gallium-67 in the clinical evaluation of cancer. *Semin Nucl Med* 1984;14(4):296–323.

90. Delcambre C, Reman O, Henry-Amar M, et al. Clinical relevance of gallium-67 scintigraphy in lymphoma before and after therapy. *Eur J Nucl Med* 2000;27(2):176–184.

91. Bar-Shalom R, Mor M, Yefremov N, Goldsmith SJ. The value of Ga-67 scintigraphy and F-18 fluorodeoxyglucose positron emission tomography in staging and monitoring the response of lymphoma to treatment. *Semin Nucl Med* 2001;31(3):177–190.

92. Israel O, Front D, Lam M, et al. Gallium 67 imaging in monitoring lymphoma response to treatment. *Cancer* 1988;61:2439–2443.

93. Seto M, Jaeger U, Hockett R, et al. Alternative promoters and exons, somatic mutation and deregulation of the Bcl-2—Ig fusion gene in lymphoma. *EMBO J* 1988;7:123.

94. Kaplan W, Jochelson M, Herman T, et al. Gallium-67 imaging: a predictor of residual tumor viability and clinical outcome in patients with diffuse large-cell lymphoma. *J Clin Oncol* 1990;8:1966–1970.

95. Front D, Bar-Shalom R, Epelbaum R, et al. Early detection of lymphoma recurrence with gallium-67 scintigraphy. *J Nucl Med* 1993;34:2101–2104.

96. Som P, Atkins HL, Bandoypadhyay D, et al. A fluorinated glucose analog, 2-fluoro-2-deoxy-D-glucose (F-18): nontoxic tracer for rapid tumor detection. *J Nucl Med* 1980;21(7):670–675.

97. Paul R. Comparison of fluorine-18-2-fluorodeoxyglucose and gallium-67 citrate imaging for detection of lymphoma. *J Nucl Med* 1987;28(3):288–292.

98. Okada J, Yoshikawa K, Imazeki K, et al. The use of FDG-PET in the detection and management of malignant lymphoma: correlation of uptake with prognosis. *J Nucl Med* 1991;32(4):686–691.

99. Lapela M, Leskinen S, Minn HR, et al. Increased glucose metabolism in untreated non-Hodgkin's lymphoma: a study with positron emission tomography and fluorine-18-fluorodeoxyglucose. *Blood* 1995;86(9):3522–3527.

100. Leskinen-Kallio S, Ruotsalainen U, Nagren K, et al. Uptake of carbon-11-methionine and fluorodeoxyglucose in non-Hodgkin's lymphoma: a PET study. *J Nucl Med* 1991;32(6):1211–1218.

101. Rodriguez M, Ahlstrom H, Sundin A, et al. [18F] FDG PET in gastric non-Hodgkin's lymphoma. *Acta Oncol* 1997;36(6):577–584.

102. Jerusalem G, Warland V, Najjar F, et al. Whole-body 18F-FDG PET for the evaluation of patients with Hodgkin's disease and non-Hodgkin's lymphoma. *Nucl Med Commun* 1999;20(1):13–20.

103. Bakheet SM, Powe J, Ezzat A, Rostom A. F-18-FDG uptake in tuberculosis. *Clin Nucl Med* 1998;23(11):739–742.

104. Vesselle HJ, Miraldi FD. FDG PET of the retroperitoneum: normal anatomy, variants, pathologic conditions, and strategies to avoid diagnostic pitfalls. *Radiographics* 1998;18(4):805–823; discussion 823–824.

105. Stumpe KD, Urbinelli M, Steinert HC, et al. Whole-body positron emission tomography using fluorodeoxyglucose for staging of lymphoma: effectiveness and comparison with computed tomography. *Eur J Nucl Med* 1998;25(7):721–728.

106. Rodriguez M, Rehn S, Ahlstrom H, et al. Predicting malignancy grade with PET in non-Hodgkin's lymphoma. *J Nucl Med* 1995;36(10):1790–1796.

107. Kostakoglu L, Leonard JP, Kuji I, et al. Comparison of fluorine-18 fluorodeoxyglucose positron emission tomography and Ga-67 scintigraphy in evaluation of lymphoma. *Cancer* 2002;94(4):879–888.

108. Newman JS, Francis IR, Kaminski MS, Wahl RL. Imaging of lymphoma with PET with 2-[F-18]-fluoro-2-deoxy-D-glucose: correlation with CT. *Radiology* 1994;190(1):111–116.

109. Cremerius U, Fabry U, Kroll U, et al. [Clinical value of FDG PET for therapy monitoring of malignant lymphoma—results of a retrospective study in 72 patients]. *Nuklearmedizin* 1999;38(1):24–30.

110. Rodriguez M. Computed tomography, magnetic resonance imaging and positron emission tomography in non-Hodgkin's lymphoma. *Acta Radiol Suppl* 1998;417:1–36.

111. Hoffmann M, Kletter K, Diemling M, et al. Positron emission tomography with fluorine-18-2-fluoro-2-deoxy-D-glucose (F18-FDG) does not visualize extranodal B-cell lymphoma of the mucosa-associated lymphoid tissue (MALT)-type. *Ann Oncol* 1999;10(10):1185–1189.

112. Moog F, Bangerter M, Diederichs CG, et al. Lymphoma: role of whole-body 2-deoxy-2-[F-18]fluoro-D-glucose (FDG) PET in nodal staging. *Radiology* 1997;203(3):795–800.

113. Kotzerke J, Guhlmann A, Moog F, Frickhofen N, Reske SN. Role of attenuation correction for fluorine-18 fluorodeoxyglucose positron

emission tomography in the primary staging of malignant lymphoma. *Eur J Nucl Med* 1999;26(1):31–38.

114. Kostakoglu L, Goldsmith SJ. Fluorine-18 fluorodeoxyglucose positron emission tomography in the staging and follow-up of lymphoma: is it time to shift gears? *Eur J Nucl Med* 2000;27(10):1564–1578.

115. Lin P, Delaney G, Chu J, Kiat H, Pocock N. Fluorine-18 FDG dual-head gamma camera coincidence imaging of radiation pneumonitis. *Clin Nucl Med* 2000;25(11):866–869.

116. Jerusalem G, Beguin Y, Fassotte MF, et al. Whole-body positron emission tomography using 18F-fluorodeoxyglucose for posttreatment evaluation in Hodgkin's disease and non-Hodgkin's lymphoma has higher diagnostic and prognostic value than classical computed tomography scan imaging. *Blood* 1999;94(2):429–433.

117. Hoh CK, Glaspy J, Rosen P, et al. Whole-body FDG-PET imaging for staging of Hodgkin's disease and lymphoma. *J Nucl Med* 1997;38(3): 343–348.

118. Mainolfi C, Maurea S, Varrella P, et al. [Positron-emission tomography with fluorine-18-deoxyglucose in the staging and control of patients with lymphoma. Comparison with clinico-radiologic assessment]. *Radiol Med (Torino)* 1998;95(1–2):98–104.

119. Thill R, Neuerburg J, Fabry U, et al. [Comparison of findings with 18-FDG PET and CT in pretherapeutic staging of malignant lymphoma]. *Nuklearmedizin* 1997;36(7):234–239.

120. Bangerter M, Kotzerke J, Griesshammer M, et al. Positron emission tomography with 18-fluorodeoxyglucose in the staging and follow-up of lymphoma in the chest. *Acta Oncol* 1999;38(6):799–804.

121. Moog F, Bangerter M, Diederichs CG, et al. Extranodal malignant lymphoma: detection with FDG PET versus CT. *Radiology* 1998;206(2): 475–481.

122. Shah N, Hoskin P, McMillan A, et al. The impact of FDG positron emission tomography imaging on the management of lymphomas. *Br J Radiol* 2000;73(869):482–487.

123. Buchmann I, Moog F, Schirrmeister H, Reske SN. Positron emission tomography for detection and staging of malignant lymphoma. *Recent Results Cancer Res* 2000;156:78–89.

124. Talbot JN, Haioun C, Rain JD, et al. [18F]-FDG positron imaging in clinical management of lymphoma patients. *Crit Rev Oncol Hematol* 2001;38(3):193–221.

125. Moog F, Kotzerke J, Reske SN. FDG PET can replace bone scintigraphy in primary staging of malignant lymphoma. *J Nucl Med* 1999;40(9): 1407–1413.

126. Ullerich H, Franzius CH, Domagk D, et al. 18F-Fluorodeoxyglucose PET in a patient with primary small bowel lymphoma: the only sensitive method of imaging. *Am J Gastroenterol* 2001;96(8):2497–2499.

127. Bangerter M, Moog F, Griesshammer M, et al. Usefulness of FDG-PET in diagnosing primary lymphoma of the liver. *Int J Hematol* 1997;66(4):517–520.

128. Carr R, Barrington SF, Madan B, et al. Detection of lymphoma in bone marrow by whole-body positron emission tomography. *Blood* 1998;91(9):3340–3346.

129. Moog F, Bangerter M, Kotzerke J, et al. 18-F-fluorodeoxyglucose-positron emission tomography as a new approach to detect lymphomatous bone marrow. *J Clin Oncol* 1998;16(2):603–609.

130. Hoffman JM, Waskin HA, Schifter T, et al. FDG-PET in differentiating lymphoma from nonmalignant central nervous system lesions in patients with AIDS. *J Nucl Med* 1993;34(4):567–575.

131. Heald AE, Hoffman JM, Bartlett JA, Waskin HA. Differentiation of central nervous system lesions in AIDS patients using positron emission tomography (PET). *Int J STD AIDS* 1996;7(5):337–346.

132. Cheson B, Horning S, Coiffier B, et al. Report of an international workshop to standardize response criteria for non-Hodgkin's lymphomas. *J Clin Oncol* 1999;17:1244.

133. Luoni M, Declich P, De Paoli Ap, et al. Bone marrow biopsy for the staging of non-Hodgkin's lymphoma: bilateral or unilateral trephine biopsy? *Tumori* 1995;81(6):410–413.

134. Juneja SK, Wolf MM, Cooper IA. Value of bilateral bone marrow biopsy specimens in non-Hodgkin's lymphoma. *J Clin Pathol* 1990;43(8):630–632.

135. Coller HA, Grandori C, Tamayo P, et al. Expression analysis with oligonucleotide microarrays reveals MYC regulates genes involved in growth, cell cycle, signaling, and adhesion. *Proc Natl Acad Sci U S A* 2000;97(7):3260–3265.

136. Fineberg S, Marsh E, Alfonso F, et al. Immunophenotypic evaluation of the bone marrow in non-Hodgkin's lymphoma. *Hum Pathol* 1993;24(6):636–642.

137. Naughton MJ, Hess JL, Zutter MM, Bartlett NL. Bone marrow staging in patients with non-Hodgkin's lymphoma: is flow cytometry a useful test? *Cancer* 1998;82(6):1154–1159.

138. Dunphy CH. Combining morphology and flow cytometric immunophenotyping to evaluate bone marrow specimens for B-cell malignant neoplasms. *Am J Clin Pathol* 1998;109(5):625–630.

139. Duggan PR, Easton D, Luider J, Auer IA. Bone marrow staging of patients with non-Hodgkin lymphoma by flow cytometry: correlation with morphology. *Cancer* 2000;88(4):894–899.

140. Hoane B, Shields A, Porter B, Shulman H. Detection of lymphomatous bone marrow involvement with magnetic resonance imaging. *Blood* 1991;78(3):728–738.

141. Altehoefer C, Blum U, Bathmann J, et al. Comparative diagnostic accuracy of magnetic resonance imaging and immunoscintigraphy for detection of bone marrow involvement in patients with malignant lymphoma. *J Clin Oncol* 1997;15(5):1754–1760.

142. Tsunoda S, Takagi S, Tanaka O, Miura Y. Clinical and prognostic significance of femoral marrow magnetic resonance imaging in patients with malignant lymphoma. *Blood* 1997;89(1):286–290.

143. Tardivon AA, Munck JN, Shapeero LG, et al. Can clinical data help to screen patients with lymphoma for MR imaging of bone marrow? *Ann Oncol* 1995;6(8):795–800.

144. Tardivon AA, Vanel D, Munck JN, Bosq J. Magnetic resonance imaging of the bone marrow in lymphomas and leukemias. *Leuk Lymphoma* 1997;25(1–2):55–68.

145. Ozguroglu M, Esen Ersavasti G, Demir G, et al. Magnetic resonance imaging of bone marrow versus bone marrow biopsy in malignant lymphoma. *Pathol Oncol Res* 1999;5(2):123–128.

146. Takagi S, Tsunoda S, Tanaka O. Bone marrow involvement in lymphoma: the importance of marrow magnetic resonance imaging. *Leuk Lymphoma* 1998;29(5–6):515–522.

147. Linden A, Zankovich R, Theissen P, et al. Malignant lymphoma: bone marrow imaging versus biopsy. *Radiology* 1989;173(2):335–339.

148. Banfi A, Bonadonna G, Ricci SB, et al. Malignant lymphomas of Waldeyer's ring: natural history and survival after radiotherapy. *BMJ* 1972;3(819):140–143.

149. Gospodarowicz M, Sutcliffe S, Brown T, et al. Patterns of disease in localized extranodal lymphomas. *J Clin Oncol* 1987;5(6):875–880.

150. Jacobs C, Hoppe R. Non-Hodgkin's lymphomas of head and neck extranodal sites. *Int J Radiat Oncol Biol Phys* 1985;11:357–364.

151. Saul S, Kapadia S. Primary lymphoma of Waldeyer's ring: clinicopathologic study of 68 cases. *Cancer* 1985;56:157–166.

152. Crump M, Gospodarowicz M, Shepherd FA. Lymphoma of the gastrointestinal tract. *Semin Oncol* 1999;26(3):324–337.

153. Wotherspoon A, Doglioni C, Diss T, et al. Regression of primary low-grade B-cell gastric lymphoma of mucosa-associated lymphoid tissue type after eradication of *Helicobacter pylori*. *Lancet* 1993;342:575–577.

154. Bayerdorffer E, Neubauer A, Rudolph B, et al. Regression of primary gastric lymphoma of mucosa-associated lymphoid tissue type after cure of *Helicobacter pylori* infection. MALT Lymphoma Study Group. *Lancet* 1995;345(8965):1591–1594.

155. Roggero E, Zucca E, Pinotti G, et al. Eradication of *Helicobacter pylori* infection in primary low-grade gastric lymphoma of mucosa-associated lymphoid tissue. *Ann Intern Med* 1995;122(10):767–769.

156. Savio A, Franzin G, Wotherspoon A, et al. Diagnosis and posttreatment follow-up of *Helicobacter pylori*–positive gastric lymphoma of mucosa-associated lymphoid tissue: histology, polymerase chain reaction, or both? *Blood* 1996;87:1255–1260.

157. Abbondanzo SL, Wenig BM. Non-Hodgkin's lymphoma of the sinonasal tract. A clinicopathologic and immunophenotypic study of 120 cases. *Cancer* 1995;75(6):1281–1291.

158. Logsdon MD, Ha CS, Kavadi VS, et al. Lymphoma of the nasal cavity and paranasal sinuses: improved outcome and altered prognostic factors with combined modality therapy. *Cancer* 1997;80(3):477–488.

159. Liang R. Diagnosis and management of primary nasal lymphoma of T-cell or NK-cell origin. *Clin Lymphoma* 2000;1(1):33–37; discussion 38.

160. Jaffe E. Classification of natural killer (NK) cell and NK-like T-cell malignancies. *Blood* 1996;87:1207–1210.

161. Johnson CD, Kent DM, Varjabedian GC, Lepoudre C. Malignant lymphoma of the maxillary sinus. *J Am Osteopath Assoc* 1993;93(2):252, 255–258.
162. Frierson HF Jr, Mills SE, Innes DJ Jr. Non-Hodgkin's lymphomas of the sinonasal region: histologic subtypes and their clinicopathologic features. *Am J Clin Pathol* 1984;81(6):721–727.
163. Juman S, Robinson P, Balkissoon A, Kelly K. B-cell non-Hodgkin's lymphoma of the paranasal sinuses. *J Laryngol Otol* 1994;108(3):263–265.
164. Fine HA, Mayer RJ. Primary central nervous system lymphoma. *Ann Intern Med* 1993;119(11):1093–1104.
165. Lossos IS, Breuer R, Intrator O, Lossos A. Cerebrospinal fluid lactate dehydrogenase isoenzyme analysis for the diagnosis of central nervous system involvement in hematooncologic patients. *Cancer* 2000;88(7):1599–1604.
166. Whitcup SM, de Smet MD, Rubin B, et al. Intraocular lymphoma. Clinical and histopathologic diagnosis. *Ophthalmology* 1993;100(9):1399–1406.
167. Sutcliffe S, Gospodarowicz M. Primary extranodal lymphomas. In: Canellos GP, Lister TA, Sklar JL, eds. *The lymphomas*. Philadelphia: WB Saunders, 1998.
168. Ferry J, Harris, N, Young, R, et al. Malignant lymphoma of the testis, epididymis and spermatic cord: a clinicopathologic study of 69 cases with immunophenotypic analysis. *Cancer* 1994;18:376–390.
169. Seymour JF, Solomon B, Wolf MM, et al. Primary large-cell non-Hodgkin's lymphoma of the testis: a retrospective analysis of patterns of failure and prognostic factors. *Clin Lymphoma* 2001;2(2):109–115.
170. Shahab N, Doll DC. Testicular lymphoma. *Semin Oncol* 1999;26(3):259–269.
171. Fonseca R, Habermann TM, Colgan JP, et al. Testicular lymphoma is associated with a high incidence of extranodal recurrence. *Cancer* 2000;88(1):154–161.
172. Tondini C, Ferreri AJ, Siracusano L, et al. Diffuse large-cell lymphoma of the testis. *J Clin Oncol* 1999;17(9):2854–2858.
173. Touroutoglou N, Dimopoulos MA, Younes A, et al. Testicular lymphoma: late relapses and poor outcome despite doxorubicin-based therapy. *J Clin Oncol* 1995;13(6):1361–1367.
174. Crellin AM, Hudson BV, Bennett MH, et al. Non-Hodgkin's lymphoma of the testis. *Radiother Oncol* 1993;27(2):99–106.
175. Moller MB, d'Amore F, Christensen BE. Testicular lymphoma: a population-based study of incidence, clinicopathological correlations and prognosis. The Danish Lymphoma Study Group, LYFO. *Eur J Cancer* 1994;12(4):1760–1764.
176. Bunn PA Jr, Schein PS, Banks PM, DeVita VT Jr. Central nervous system complications in patients with diffuse histiocytic and undifferentiated lymphoma: leukemia revisited. *Blood* 1976;47(1):3–10.
177. Young RC, Howser DM, Anderson T, et al. Central nervous system complications of non-Hodgkin's lymphoma. The potential role for prophylactic therapy. *Am J Med* 1979;66(3):435–443.
178. Mackintosh F, Colby T, Podolsky W, et al. Central nervous system involvement in non-Hodgkin's lymphoma: an analysis of 105 cases. *Cancer* 1982;49:586–595.
179. Levitt L, Aisenberg A, Harris N, et al. Primary non-Hodgkin's lymphoma of the mediastinum. *Cancer* 1982;50:2486–2492.
180. Litam JP, Cabanillas F, Smith TL, et al. Central nervous system relapse in malignant lymphomas: risk factors and implications for prophylaxis. *Blood* 1979;54(6):1249–1257.
181. Rathmell AJ, Gospodarowicz MK, Sutcliffe SB, Clark RM. Localised lymphoma of bone: prognostic factors and treatment recommendations. The Princess Margaret Hospital Lymphoma Group. *Br J Cancer* 1992;66(3):603–606.
182. Baar J, Burkes RL, Gospodarowicz M. Primary non-Hodgkin's lymphoma of bone. *Semin Oncol* 1999;26(3):270–275.
183. Ostrowski ML, Unni KK, Banks PM, et al. Malignant lymphoma of bone. *Cancer* 1986;58(12):2646–2655.
184. Mambo NC, Burke JS, Butler JJ. Primary malignant lymphomas of the breast. *Cancer* 1977;39(5):2033–2040.
185. Cleary M, Mecker T, Levy S, et al. Clustering of extensive somatic mutations in the variable region of an immunoglobulin heavy chain gene from a human B cell lymphoma. *Cell* 1986;44:97–106.
186. Nazario AC, Tanaka CI, de Lima GR, et al. Primary lymphoma of the breast. *Rev Paul Med* 1992;110(4):177–179.
187. Wong WW, Schild SE, Halyard MY, Schomberg PJ. Primary non-Hodgkin lymphoma of the breast: The Mayo Clinic experience. (This work was presented at the Radiologic Society of North America 86th Annual Meeting, Chicago, IL, November 26–December 1, 2000.) *J Surg Oncol* 2002;80(1):19–25.
188. Domchek SM, Hecht JL, Fleming MD, et al. Lymphomas of the breast: primary and secondary involvement. *Cancer* 2002;94(1):6–13.
189. Monterroso V, Jaffe ES, Merino MJ, Medeiros LJ. Malignant lymphomas involving the ovary. A clinicopathologic analysis of 39 cases. *Am J Surg Pathol* 1993;17(2):154–170.
190. Dimopoulos MA, Daliani D, Pugh W, et al. Primary ovarian non-Hodgkin's lymphoma: outcome after treatment with combination chemotherapy. *Gynecol Oncol* 1997;64(3):446–450.
191. Coiffier B. How to interpret the radiological abnormalities that persist after treatment in non-Hodgkin's lymphoma patients? *Ann Oncol* 1999;10(10):1141–1143.
192. Canellos GP. Residual mass in lymphoma may not be residual disease. *J Clin Oncol* 1988;6(6):931–933.
193. Zinzani PL, Zompatori M, Bendandi M, et al. Monitoring bulky mediastinal disease with gallium-67, CT-scan and magnetic resonance imaging in Hodgkin's disease and high-grade non-Hodgkin's lymphoma. *Leuk Lymphoma* 1996;22(1-2):131–135.
194. Front D, Israel O. The role of Ga-67 scintigraphy in evaluating the results of therapy of lymphoma patients. *Semin Nucl Med* 1995;(1):60–71.
195. Gasparini M, Bombardieri E, Castellani M, et al. Gallium-67 scintigraphy evaluation of therapy in non-Hodgkin's lymphoma. *J Nucl Med* 1998;39(9):1586–1590.
196. DeRisi J, Penland L, Brown PO, et al. Use of a cDNA microarray to analyse gene expression patterns in human cancer [see comments]. *Nat Genet* 1996;14(4):457–460.
197. Ionescu I, Brice P, Simon D, et al. Restaging with gallium scan identifies chemosensitive patients and predicts survival of poor-prognosis mediastinal Hodgkin's disease patients. *Med Oncol* 2000;17(2):127–134.
198. Israel O, Front D, Epelbaum R, et al. Residual mass and negative gallium scintigraphy in treated lymphoma. *J Nucl Med* 1990;31(3):365–368.
199. Drossman SR, Schiff RG, Kronfeld GD, et al. Lymphoma of the mediastinum and neck: evaluation with Ga-67 imaging and CT correlation. *Radiology* 1990;174(1):171–175.
200. Cremerius U, Fabry U, Neuerburg J, et al. Positron emission tomography with 18F-FDG to detect residual disease after therapy for malignant lymphoma. *Nucl Med Commun* 1998;19(11):1055–1063.
201. Miki Y, Swensen J, Shattuck-Eidens D, et al. A strong candidate for the breast and ovarian cancer susceptibility gene BRCA1. *Science* 1995;266:66–71.
202. Zarrabi MH. Association of non-Hodgkin's lymphoma and second neoplasms. *Semin Oncol* 1990;17(1):120–132.
203. Travis LB, Gospodarowicz M, Curtis RE, et al. Lung cancer following chemotherapy and radiotherapy for Hodgkin's disease. *J Natl Cancer Inst* 2002;94(3):182–192.
204. Travis L, Curtis R, Boice J, et al. Second cancers following non-Hodgkin's lymphoma. *Cancer* 1991;67(7):2002–2009.
205. Travis LB, Curtis RE, Glimelius B, et al. Second cancers among long-term survivors of non-Hodgkin's lymphoma. *J Natl Cancer Inst* 1993;85(23):1932–1937.
206. Travis L, Weeks J, Curtis R, et al. Leukemia following low-dose total body irradiation and chemotherapy for non-Hodgkin's lymphoma. *J Clin Oncol* 1996;14:565–571.
207. Friedberg JW, Neuberg D, Stone RM, et al. Outcome in patients with myelodysplastic syndrome after autologous bone marrow transplantation for non-Hodgkin's lymphoma. *J Clin Oncol* 1999;17(10):3128–3135.
208. Stone RM. Myelodysplastic syndrome after autologous transplantation for lymphoma: the price of progress. *Blood* 1994;83(12):3437–3440.
209. Darrington DL, Vose JM, Anderson JR, et al. Incidence and characterization of secondary myelodysplastic syndrome and acute myelogenous leukemia following high-dose chemoradiotherapy and autologous stem-cell transplantation for lymphoid malignancies. *J Clin Oncol* 1994;12(12):2527–2534.
210. Shenkier TN, Voss N, Fairey R, et al. Brief chemotherapy and involved-region irradiation for limited-stage diffuse large-cell lymphoma: an 18-year experience from the British Columbia Cancer Agency. *J Clin Oncol* 2002;20(1):197–204.

211. Miller T, Dahlberg S, Cassady J, et al. Chemotherapy alone compared with chemotherapy plus radiotherapy for localized intermediate- and high-grade non-Hodgkin's lymphoma. *N Engl J Med* 1998;339:21–26.

212. Dumontet C, Bastion Y, Felman P, et al. Long-term outcome and sequelae in aggressive lymphoma patients treated with the LNH-80 regimen. *Ann Oncol* 1992;3(8):639–644.

213. Cabanillas F, Velasquez W, Hagemeiester F, et al. Clinical, biologic, and histologic features of late relapses in diffuse large cell lymphoma. *Blood* 1992;79(4):1024–1028.

214. Coltman CJ, Dahlberg S, Jones S, et al. CHOP is curative in 30% of patients with large cell lymphoma: a 12-year Southwest Oncology Group follow-up. In: Skarin A, ed. *Advances in cancer chemotherapy: update on treatment for diffuse large cell lymphoma.* New York: Park Row, 1986.

215. Sanz L, Lopez-Guillermo A, Martinez C, et al. Risk of relapse and clinico-pathological features in 103 patients with diffuse large-cell lymphoma in complete response after first-line treatment. *Eur J Haematol* 1998;61(1):59–64.

216. Shipp MA, Klatt MM, Yeap B, et al. Patterns of relapse in large-cell lymphoma patients with bulk disease: implications for the use of adjuvant radiation therapy. *J Clin Oncol* 1989;7(5):613–618.

217. Mead GM, Mackintosh FR, Burke JS, Rosenberg SA. Late relapse from complete remission in nodular and diffuse histiocytic lymphoma. *Cancer* 1983;52(8):1356–1359.

218. Weeks J, Yeop B, Canellos G, Shipp M. Value of follow-up procedures in patients with large-cell lymphoma who achieve a complete remission. *J Clin Oncol* 1991;9:1196–1203.

219. Shioyama Y, Nakamura K, Kunitake N, et al. Relapsed non-Hodgkin's lymphoma: detection and treatment. *Radiat Med* 2000;18(6):369–375.

220. Elis A, Blickstein D, Klein O, et al. Detection of relapse in non-Hodgkin's lymphoma: role of routine follow-up studies. *Am J Hematol* 2002;69(1):41–44.

221. Vose J. High-dose chemotherapy and hematopoietic stem cell transplantation for relapsed or refractory diffuse large-cell non-Hodgkin's lymphoma. *Ann Oncol* 1998;9[Suppl 1]:S1–S3.

222. Velasquez WS, Cabanillas F, Salvador P, et al. Effective salvage therapy for lymphoma with cisplatin in combination with high-dose ara-C and dexamethasone (DHAP). *Blood* 1988;71(1):117–122.

223. Oh YK, Ha CS, Samuels BI, et al. Stages I–III follicular lymphoma: role of CT of the abdomen and pelvis in follow-up studies. *Radiology* 1999;210(2):483–486.

224. Aviles A, Narvaez BR, Diaz-Maqueo JC, et al. Value of serum beta 2 microglobulin as an indicator of early relapse in diffuse large cell lymphoma. *Leuk Lymphoma* 1993;9(4–5):377–380.

225. Coiffier B, Bastion Y, Berger F, et al. Prognostic factors in follicular lymphomas. (46 Refs). *Semin Oncol* 1993;20[5 Suppl 5]:89–95.

226. Velasquez WS, Fuller LM, Jagannath S, et al. Stages I and II diffuse large cell lymphomas: prognostic factors in long-term results with CHOP-BLEO and radiotherapy. *Blood* 1991;77(5):942–947.

227. Hayward RL, Leonard RC, Prescott RJ. A critical analysis of prognostic factors for survival in intermediate and high grade non-Hodgkin's lymphoma. Scotland and Newcastle Lymphoma Group Therapy Working Party. *Br J Cancer* 1991;63(6):945–952.

228. Kirn D, Mauch P, Shaffer K, et al. Large-cell and immunoblastic lymphoma of the mediastinum: prognostic features and treatment outcome in 57 patients. *J Clin Oncol* 1993;11:1336–1343.

229. Shipp MA. Prognostic factors in aggressive non-Hodgkin's lymphoma: who has "high-risk" disease? *Blood* 1994;83(5):1165–1173.

230. Dixon D, Neilan B, Jones S, et al. Effect of age on therapeutic outcome in advanced diffuse histiocytic lymphoma: the Southwest Oncology Group experience. *J Clin Oncol* 1986;4(3):295–305.

231. Vose J, Armitage J, Weisenburger D, et al. The importance of age in survival of patients treated with chemotherapy for aggressive non-Hodgkin's lymphoma. *J Clin Oncol* 1988;6(12):1838–1844.

232. d'Amore F, Brincker H, Christensen BE, et al. Non-Hodgkin's lymphoma in the elderly. A study of 602 patients aged 70 or older from a Danish population-based registry. The Danish Lyeo-Study Group. *Ann Oncol* 1992;3(5):379–386.

233. Grogan L, Corbally N, Dervan PA, Byrne A, Carney DN. Comparable prognostic factors and survival in elderly patients with aggressive non-Hodgkin's lymphoma treated with standard-dose adriamycin-based regimens. *Ann Oncol* 1994;5[Suppl 2]:47–51.

234. O'Reilly SE, Connors JM, Macpherson N, et al. Malignant lymphomas in the elderly. *Clin Geriatr Med* 1997;13(2):251–263.

235. Greil R. Prognosis and management strategies of lymphatic neoplasias in the elderly. I. Aggressive non-Hodgkin's lymphomas. *Oncology* 1998;55(3):189–217.

236. Effect of age on the characteristics and clinical behavior of non-Hodgkin's lymphoma patients. The Non-Hodgkin's Lymphoma Classification Project. *Ann Oncol* 1997;8(10):973–978.

237. Maartense E, Kluin-Nelemans HC, le Cessie S, et al. Different age limits for elderly patients with indolent and aggressive non-Hodgkin lymphoma and the role of relative survival with increasing age. *Cancer* 2000;89(12):2667–2676.

238. Coiffier B. What treatment for elderly patients with aggressive lymphoma? *Ann Oncol* 1994;5(10):873–875.

239. Gomez H, Mas L, Casanova L, et al. Elderly patients with aggressive non-Hodgkin's lymphoma treated with CHOP chemotherapy plus granulocyte-macrophage colony-stimulating factor: identification of two age subgroups with differing hematologic toxicity. *J Clin Oncol* 1998;16(7):2352–2358.

240. Coiffier B, Lepage E. Prognosis of aggressive lymphomas: a study of five prognostic models with patients included in the Lnh-84 regimen. *Blood* 1989;74(2):558–564.

241. Rodriguez J, Cabanillas F, McLaughlin P, et al. A proposal for a simple staging system for intermediate grade lymphoma and immunoblastic lymphoma based on the 'tumor score'. *Ann Oncol* 1992;3(9):711–717.

242. Lopez-Guillermo A, Cid J, Salar A, et al. Peripheral T-cell lymphomas: initial features, natural history, and prognostic factors in a series of 174 patients diagnosed according to the R.E.A.L. Classification. *Ann Oncol* 1998;9:849.

243. Hermans J vGK, Kluin-Nelemans KJC, et al. International prognostic index for aggressive non-Hodgkin's lymphoma is valid for all malignancy grades. *Blood* 1995;86:1460–1463.

244. Bastion Y, Coiffier B. Is the International Prognostic Index for aggressive lymphoma patients useful for follicular lymphoma patients? *J Clin Oncol* 1994;12(7):1340–1342.

245. Melnyk A, Rodriguez A, Pugh W, Cabannillas F. Evaluation of the Revised European-American Lymphoma classification confirms the clinical relevance of immunophenotype in 560 cases of aggressive non-Hodgkin's lymphoma. *Blood* 1997;89:4514–4520.

246. Ansell S, Habermann T, Kurtin P, et al. Predictive capacity of the International Prognostic Factor Index in patients with peripheral T-cell lymphoma. *J Clin Oncol* 1997;15:2296–2301.

247. Gisselbrecht C, Gaulard P, Lepage E, et al. Prognostic significance of T-cell phenotype in aggressive non-Hodgkin's lymphomas. Groupe d'Etudes des Lymphomes de l'Adulte (GELA). *Blood* 1998;92(1):76–82.

248. Kim K, Kim WS, Jung CW, et al. Clinical features of peripheral T-cell lymphomas in 78 patients diagnosed according to the Revised European-American Lymphoma (REAL) classification. *Eur J Cancer* 2002;38(1):75–81.

249. Rudiger T, Weisenburger DD, Anderson JR, et al. Peripheral T-cell lymphoma (excluding anaplastic large-cell lymphoma): results from the Non-Hodgkin's Lymphoma Classification Project. *Ann Oncol* 2002;13(1):140–149.

250. Savage KJ, Gascoyne RD, Chhanabhai M, et al. T cell lymphoproliferative disorders (LPD) in a single institution: a 20 year experience. *Blood* 2000;96(11):469a.

251. Weisenburger DD, Anderson JR, Diebold J, et al. Systemic anaplastic large-cell lymphoma: results from the non-Hodgkin's lymphoma classification project. *Am J Hematol* 2001;67(3):172–178.

252. Gascoyne R, Aoun P, Wu D, et al. Prognostic significance of anaplastic lymphoma kinase (ALK) protein expression in adults with anaplastic large cell lymphoma. *Blood* 1999;93:3913.

253. Falini B, Pileri S, Zinzani PL, et al. ALK+ lymphoma: clinico-pathological findings and outcome. *Blood* 1999;93(8):2697–2706.

254. Stein H, Foss HD, Durkop H, et al. CD30(+) anaplastic large cell lymphoma: a review of its histopathologic, genetic, and clinical features. *Blood* 2000;96(12):3681–3695.

255. Kondo E, Ogura M, Kagami, et al. Assessment of prognostic factors in follicular lymphoma patients. *Int J Hematol* 2001;73(3):363–368.

256. Lopez-Guillermo A, Montserrat E, Bosch F, et al. Applicability of the International Index for Aggressive Lymphomas to patients with low-grade lymphoma. *J Clin Oncol* 1994;12:1343–1348.

257. Foussard C, Desablens B, Sensebe L, et al. Is the International Prognostic Index for aggressive lymphomas useful for low-grade lym-

phoma patients? Applicability to stage III–IV patients. The GOELAMS Group, France. *Ann Oncol* 1997;8[Suppl 1]:49–52.

258. Micallef IN, Remstein ED, Ansell SM, et al. International Prognostic Index (IPI) predicts outcome after histological transformation of low grade non-Hodgkin's lymphoma. *Blood* 2001;98 (11):336a.

259. Cameron DA, Leonard RC, Mao JH, Prescott RJ. Identification of prognostic groups in follicular lymphoma. The Scotland and Newcastle Lymphoma Group Therapy Working Party. *Leuk Lymphoma* 1993;10(1-2):89–99.

260. Denham JW, Denham E, Dear KB, Hudson GV. The follicular non-Hodgkin's lymphomas—II. Prognostic factors: what do they mean? *Eur J Cancer* 1996;32A(3):480–490.

261. Armitage J, Weisenburger D, Hutchins M, et al. Chemotherapy for diffuse large-cell lymphoma-rapidly responding patients have more durable remissions. *J Clin Oncol* 1986;4(2):160–164.

262. Haw R, Sawka CA, Franssen E, Berinstein NL. Significance of a partial or slow response to front-line chemotherapy in the management of intermediate-grade or high-grade non-Hodgkin's lymphoma: a literature review. *J Clin Oncol* 1994;12(5):1074–1084.

263. Engelhard M, Meusers P, Brittinger G, et al. Prospective multicenter trial for the response-adapted treatment of high-grade malignant non-Hodgkin's lymphomas: updated results of the COP-BLAM/IMVP-16 protocol with randomized adjuvant radiotherapy. *Ann Oncol* 1991;2 [Suppl 2]:177–180.

264. Vose J, Byar K, Anderson J, Bierman P, et al. SPECT gallium (GS) imaging: more predictive than computed tomography (CT) of clinical outcome following high-dose chemotherapy and transplant (ABMT) for diffuse large cell (DLC) non-Hodgkin's lymphoma (NHL). *Proc Annu Meet Am Soc Clin Oncol* 1994;13:1259a.

265. Surbone A, Longo D, DeVita V, et al. Residual abdominal masses in aggressive non-Hodgkin's lymphoma after combination chemotherapy: significance and management. *J Clin Oncol* 1988;6:1832–1837.

266. Gasparini M, Balzarini L, Castellani M, et al. Current role of gallium scan and magnetic resonance imaging in the management of mediastinal Hodgkin lymphoma. *Cancer* 1993;72:577–582.

267. Setoain FJ, Pons F, Herranz R, et al. 67Ga scintigraphy for the evaluation of recurrences and residual masses in patients with lymphoma. *Nucl Med Commun* 1997;18(5):405–411.

268. Front D, Bar-Shalom R, Mor M, et al. Aggressive non-Hodgkin lymphoma: early prediction of outcome with 67Ga scintigraphy. *Radiology* 2000;214(1):253–257.

269. Shipp M, Neuberg D, Janicek M, et al. High-dose CHOP as initial therapy for patients with poor-prognosis aggressive non-Hodgkin's lymphoma: a dose-finding pilot study. *J Clin Oncol* 1995;13:2916–2923.

270. Janicek M, Kaplan W, Neuberg D, et al. Early restaging gallium scans predict outcome in poor prognosis patients with aggressive non-Hodgkin's lymphoma who are treated with high dose CHOP chemotherapy. *J Clin Oncol* 1997;15:1631–1637.

271. Israel O, Mor M, Epelbaum R, et al. Clinical pretreatment risk factors and Ga-67 scintigraphy early during treatment for prediction of outcome of patients with aggressive non-Hodgkin lymphoma. *Cancer* 2002;94(4):873–878.

272. Spaepen K, Stroobants S, Dupont P, et al. Prognostic value of positron emission tomography (PET) with fluorine-18 fluorodeoxyglucose ([18F]FDG) after first-line chemotherapy in non-Hodgkin's lymphoma: is [18F]FDG-PET a valid alternative to conventional diagnostic methods? *J Clin Oncol* 2001;19(2):414–419.

273. de Wit M, Bumann D, Beyer W, et al. Whole-body positron emission tomography (PET) for diagnosis of residual mass in patients with lymphoma. *Ann Oncol* 1997;8[Suppl 1]:57–60.

274. Zinzani PL, Magagnoli M, Chierichetti F, et al. The role of positron emission tomography (PET) in the management of lymphoma patients. *Ann Oncol* 1999;10(10):1181–1184.

275. Spaepen K, Stroobants S, Dupont P, et al. Can positron emission tomography with [(18)F]-fluorodeoxyglucose after first-line treatment distinguish Hodgkin's disease patients who need additional therapy from others in whom additional therapy would mean avoidable toxicity? *Br J Haematol* 2001;115(2):272–278.

276. Romer W, Hanauske AR, Ziegler S, et al. Positron emission tomography in non-Hodgkin's lymphoma: assessment of chemotherapy with fluorodeoxyglucose. *Blood* 1998;91(12):4464–4471.

277. Hoekstra OS, Ossenkoppele GJ, Golding R, et al. Early treatment response in malignant lymphoma, as determined by planar fluorine-

18-fluorodeoxyglucose scintigraphy. *J Nucl Med* 1993;34(10):1706–1710.

278. Barth TF, Dohner H, Werner CA, et al. Characteristic pattern of chromosomal gains and losses in primary large B-cell lymphomas of the gastrointestinal tract. *Blood* 1998;91(11):4321–4330.

279. Spaepen K, Stroobants S, Dupont P, et al. Early restaging positron emission tomography with (18)F-fluorodeoxyglucose predicts outcome in patients with aggressive non-Hodgkin's lymphoma. *Ann Oncol* 2002;13(9):1356–1363.

280. Velasquez W, Hagemeister F, McLaughlin P, et al. E-SHAP: an effective treatment for refractory and relapsing lymphoma. a long follow-up (meeting abstract). *Proc Annu Meet Am Soc Clin Oncol* 1992;11:A1111.

281. Velasquez WS, McLaughlin P, Tucker S, et al. ESHAP—an effective chemotherapy regimen in refractory and relapsing lymphoma: a 4-year follow-up study. *J Clin Oncol* 1994;12(6):1169–1176.

282. Cabanillas F, Hagemeister FB, McLaughlin P, et al. Results of MIME salvage regimen for recurrent or refractory lymphoma. *J Clin Oncol* 1987;5(3):407–412.

283. Cabanillas F, Hagemeister FB, Bodey G, Freireich EJ. IMVP-16: an effective regimen for patients with lymphoma who have relapsed after initial combination chemotherapy. *Blood* 1982;60:693.

284. Chao NJ, Rosenberg SA, Horning SJ. CEPP(B): an effective and well-tolerated regimen in poor-risk, aggressive non-Hodgkin's lymphoma. *Blood* 1990;76(7):1293–1298.

285. Philip T, Guglielmi C, Hagenbeek A, et al. Autologous bone marrow transplantation as compared with salvage chemotherapy in relapses of chemotherapy-sensitive non-Hodgkin's lymphoma. *N Engl J Med* 1995;333:1540–1545.

286. Wilson WH, Bryant G, Bates S, et al. EPOCH chemotherapy: toxicity and efficacy in relapsed and refractory non-Hodgkin's lymphoma. *J Clin Oncol* 1993;11(8):1573–1582.

287. Freedman A, Takvorian T, Anderson K, et al. Autologous bone marrow transplantation in B-cell non-Hodgkin's lymphoma: very low treatment-related mortality in 100 patients in sensitive relapse. *J Clin Oncol* 1990;8:784–791.

288. Petersen FB, Appelbaum FR, Hill R, et al. Autologous marrow transplantation for malignant lymphoma: a report of 101 cases from Seattle. *J Clin Oncol* 1990;8(4):638–647.

289. Philips G, Fay J, Herzig R, Lazarus H, et al. The treatment of progressive non-Hodgkin's lymphoma with intensive chemotherapy and autologous marrow transplantation. *Blood* 1990;75:831–838.

290. Stiff PJ, Dahlberg S, Forman SJ, et al. Autologous bone marrow transplantation for patients with relapsed or refractory diffuse aggressive non-Hodgkin's lymphoma: value of augmented preparative regimens—a Southwest Oncology Group trial. *J Clin Oncol* 1998;16(1):48–55.

291. Prince HM, Imrie K, Crump M, et al. The role of intensive therapy and autologous blood and marrow transplantation for chemotherapy-sensitive relapsed and primary refractory non-Hodgkin's lymphoma: identification of major prognostic groups. *Br J Haematol* 1996;92(4):880–889.

292. Josting A, Reiser M, Rueffer U, et al. Treatment of primary progressive Hodgkin's and aggressive non-Hodgkin's lymphoma: is there a chance for cure? *J Clin Oncol* 2000;18(2):332–339.

293. Villela L, Lopez-Guillermo A, Montoto S, et al. Prognostic features and outcome in patients with diffuse large B-cell lymphoma who do not achieve a complete response to first-line regimens. *Cancer* 2001;91(8):1557–1562.

294. Vose JM, Zhang MJ, Rowlings PA, et al. Autologous transplantation for diffuse aggressive non-Hodgkin's lymphoma in patients never achieving remission: a report from the Autologous Blood and Marrow Transplant Registry. *J Clin Oncol* 2001;19(2):406–413.

295. Kewalramani T, Zelenetz AD, Hedrick EE, et al. High-dose chemoradiotherapy and autologous stem cell transplantation for patients with primary refractory aggressive non-Hodgkin lymphoma: an intention-to-treat analysis. *Blood* 2000;96(7):2399–2404.

296. Guglielmi C, Gomez F, Philip T, et al. Time to relapse has prognostic value in patients with aggressive lymphoma enrolled onto the PARMA trial. *J Clin Oncol* 1998;16(10):3264–3269.

297. Weisdorf D, Anderson J, Glick J, Oken M. Survival after relapse of low-grade non-Hodgkin's lymphoma: implications for marrow transplantation. *J Clin Oncol* 1992;10(6):942–947.

298. Moskowitz C, Bertino J, Glassman J, et al. Ifosfamide, carboplatin, and etoposide: a highly effective cytoreduction and peripheral-blood

progenitor-cell mobilization regimen for transplant-eligible patients with non-Hodgkin's lymphoma. *J Clin Oncol* 1999;17:3776.

299. de Kreuk M, Ossenkoppele GJ, Meijer CJ, Huijgens PC. Prognostic factors for survival of non-Hodgkin's lymphoma patients treated with high-dose chemotherapy and autologous bone marrow transplantation. *Bone Marrow Transplant* 1996;17(6):963–971.

300. Blay J, Gomez F, Sebban C, et al. The International Prognostic Index correlates to survival in patients with aggressive lymphoma in relapse: analysis of the PARMA trial. Parma Group. *Blood* 1998;92(10):3562–3568.

301. Moskowitz CH, Nimer SD, Glassman JR, et al. The International Prognostic Index predicts for outcome following autologous stem cell transplantation in patients with relapsed and primary refractory intermediate-grade lymphoma. *Bone Marrow Transplant* 1999;23(6):561–567.

302. Non-Hodgkin's Lymphoma Pathologic Classification Project. National Cancer Institute sponsored study of classifications of non-Hodgkin's lymphomas: summary and description of a Working Formulation for clinical usage. *Cancer* 1982;49:2112–2135.

303. Harris N, Jaffe E, Stein H, et al. A revised European-American classification of lymphoid neoplasms: a proposal from the International Lymphoma Study Group. *Blood* 1994;84(5):1361–1392.

304. Shipp MA, Ross KN, Tamayo P, et al. Diffuse large B-cell lymphoma outcome prediction by gene-expression profiling and supervised machine learning. *Nat Med* 2002;8(1):68–74.

305. Rosenwald A, Wright G, Chan WC, et al. The use of molecular profiling to predict survival after chemotherapy for diffuse large-B-cell lymphoma. *N Engl J Med* 2002;346(25):1937–1947.

306. Kwak LW, Wilson M, Weiss LM, et al. Similar outcome of treatment of B-cell and T-cell diffuse large-cell lymphomas: the Stanford experience. *J Clin Oncol* 1991;9(8):1426–1431.

307. Cheng AL, Chen YC, Wang CH, et al. Direct comparisons of peripheral T-cell lymphoma with diffuse B-cell lymphoma of comparable histological grades—should peripheral T-cell lymphoma be considered separately? *J Clin Oncol* 1989;7(6):725–731.

308. Karakas T, Bergmann L, Stutte HJ, et al. Peripheral T-cell lymphomas respond well to vincristine, adriamycin, cyclophosphamide, prednisone and etoposide (VACPE) and have a similar outcome as high-grade B-cell lymphomas. *Leuk Lymphoma* 1996;24(1–2):121–129.

309. Armitage J, Greer J, Levine A, et al. Peripheral T-cell lymphoma. *Cancer* 1989;63:158–163.

310. Lippman S, Miller T, Spier C, Slymen D, Grogan T. The prognostic significance of the immunotype in diffuse large-cell lymphoma: a comparative study of the T-cell and B-cell phenotype. *Blood* 1988;72:436–441.

311. Gascoyne RD. Pathologic prognostic factors in diffuse aggressive non-Hodgkin's lymphoma. *Hematol Oncol Clin North Am* 1997;11(5):847–862.

312. Coiffier B, Brousse N, Peuchmaur M, et al. Peripheral T-cell lymphomas have a worse prognosis than B-cell lymphomas: a prospective study of 361 immunophenotyped patients treated with the LNH-84 regimen. *Ann Oncol* 1990;1:45–50.

313. Campo E, Gaulard P, Zucca E, et al. Report of the European Task Force on Lymphomas: workshop on peripheral T-cell lymphomas. *Ann Oncol* 1998;9(8):835–843.

314. Mehta K, Shahid U, Malavasi F. Human CD38, a cell-surface protein with multiple functions. *FASEB J* 1996;10(12):1408–1417.

315. Funaro A, Spagnoli GC, Ausiello CM, et al. Involvement of the multilineage CD38 molecule in a unique pathway of cell activation and proliferation. *J Immunol* 1990;145(8):2390–2396.

316. Zupo S, Isnardi L, Megna M, et al. CD38 expression distinguishes two groups of B-cell chronic lymphocytic leukemias with different responses to anti-IgM antibodies and propensity to apoptosis. *Blood* 1996;88(4):1365–1374.

317. Ibrahim S, Keating M, Do KA, et al. CD38 expression as an important prognostic factor in B-cell chronic lymphocytic leukemia. *Blood* 2001;98(1):181–186.

318. Damle RN, Wasil T, Fais F, et al. Ig V gene mutation status and CD38 expression as novel prognostic indicators in chronic lymphocytic leukemia. *Blood* 1999;94(6):1840–1847.

319. Hamblin TJ, Orchard JA, Ibbotson RE, et al. CD38 expression and immunoglobulin variable region mutations are independent prognostic variables in chronic lymphocytic leukemia, but CD38 expression

may vary during the course of the disease. *Blood* 2002;99(3):1023–1029.

320. Thunberg U, Johnson A, Roos G, et al. CD38 expression is a poor predictor for VH gene mutational status and prognosis in chronic lymphocytic leukemia. *Blood* 2001;97(6):1892–1894.

321. Yamaguchi M, Seto M, Okamoto M, et al. De novo CD5+ diffuse large B-cell lymphoma: a clinicopathologic study of 109 patients. *Blood* 2002;99(3):815–821.

322. Harada S, Suzuki R, Uehira K, et al. Molecular and immunological dissection of diffuse large B cell lymphoma: CD5+, and CD5- with CD10+ groups may constitute clinically relevant subtypes. *Leukemia* 1999;13(9):1441–1447.

323. Miller TP, Lippman SM, Spier CM, et al. HLA-DR (Ia) immune phenotype predicts outcome for patients with diffuse large cell lymphoma. *J Clin Invest* 1988;82(1):370–372.

324. List A, Spier C, Miller T, Grogan T. Deficient tumor-infiltrating T-lymphocyte response in malignant lymphoma: relationship to HLA expression and host immunocompetence. *Leukemia* 1993;7:398.

325. Drillenburg P, Pals S. Cell adhesion receptors in lymphoma dissemination. *Blood* 2000;95:1900–1910.

326. Angelopoulou MK, Kontopidou FN, Pangalis GA. Adhesion molecules in B-chronic lymphoproliferative disorders. *Semin Hematol* 1999;36(2):178–197.

327. Ristamaki R, Joensuu H, Jalkanen S. Serum CD44 in non-Hodgkin's lymphoma. *Leuk Lymphoma* 1999;33(5–6):433–440.

328. Koppman G, Heider K-H, Horst E, et al. Activated human lymphocytes and aggressive non-Hodgkin's lymphomas express a homologue of the rat metastasis-associated variant of CD44. *J Exp Med* 1993;177:897–904.

329. Horst E, Meijer C, Radaszkiewicz T, et al. Adhesion molecules in the prognosis of diffuse large-cell lymphoma: expression of a lymphocyte homing receptor (CD44). LFA-1 (CD11a/18). and ICAM-1 (CD54). *Leukemia* 1990;4:595.

330. Jalkanen S, Joensuu H, Klemi P. Prognostic value of lymphocyte homing receptor and S phase fraction in non-Hodgkin's lymphoma. *Blood* 1990;75:1549–1556.

331. Jalkanen S, Joensuu H, Soderstrom KO, Klemi P. Lymphocyte homing and clinical behavior of non-Hodgkin's lymphoma. *J Clin Invest* 1991;87(5):1835–1840.

332. Drillenburg P, Wielenga VJ, Kramer MH, et al. CD44 expression predicts disease outcome in localized large B cell lymphoma. *Leukemia* 1999;13(9):1448–1455.

333. Pals ST, Koopman G, Heider KH, et al. CD44 splice variants: expression during lymphocyte activation and tumor progression. *Behring Inst Mitt* 1993(92):273–277.

334. Koopman G, Taher TE, Mazzucchelli I, et al. CD44 isoforms, including the CD44 V3 variant, are expressed on endothelium, suggesting a role for CD44 in the immobilization of growth factors and the regulation of the local immune response. *Biochem Biophys Res Commun* 1998;245(1):172–176.

335. Terpe HJ, Koopmann R, Imhof BA, Gunthert U. Expression of integrins and CD44 isoforms in non-Hodgkin's lymphomas: CD44 variant isoforms are preferentially expressed in high-grade malignant lymphomas. *J Pathol* 1994;174(2):89–100.

336. Stauder R, Eisterer W, Thaler J, Gunthert U. CD44 variant isoforms in non-Hodgkin's lymphoma: a new independent prognostic factor. *Blood* 1995;85:2885–2899.

337. Sasaki K, Niitsu N. Elevated serum levels of soluble CD44 variant 6 are correlated with shorter survival in aggressive non-Hodgkin's lymphoma. *Eur J Haematol* 2000;65(3):195–202.

338. Inagaki H, Banno S, Wakita A, et al. Prognostic significance of CD44v6 in diffuse large B-cell lymphoma. *Mod Pathol* 1999;12(5):546–552.

339. Ristamaki R, Joensuu H, Salmi M, Jalkanen S. Serum CD44 in malignant lymphoma: an association with treatment response. *Blood* 1994;84:238–243.

340. Ristamaki R, Joesuu H, Lappalainen K, et al. Elevated serum CD44 level is associated with unfavorable outcome in non-Hodgkin's lymphoma. *Blood* 1997;90:4039–4045.

341. Niitsu N, Iijima K. High serum soluble CD44 is correlated with a poor outcome of aggressive non-Hodgkin's lymphoma. *Leuk Res* 2002;26(3):241–248.

342. Molica S, Vitelli G, Levato D, et al. Elevated serum levels of soluble CD44 can identify a subgroup of patients with early B-cell chronic

lymphocytic leukemia who are at high risk of disease progression. *Cancer* 2001;92(4):713–719.

343. Ridgway D, Smiley S, Neerhout RC. The prognostic value of presenting serum LDH in non-Hodgkin lymphoma. *J Pediatr* 1981;99(4):611–613.

344. Pavlidis AN, Kalef-Ezra J, Bourantas LC, et al. Serum tumor markers in non-Hodgkin's lymphomas and chronic lymphocytic leukemia. *Int J Biol Markers* 1993;8(1):14–20.

345. Suki S, Swan F, Jr, Tucker S, et al. Risk classification for large cell lymphoma using lactate dehydrogenase, beta-2 microglobulin, and thymidine kinase. *Leuk Lymphoma* 1995;18(1–2):87–92.

346. Aviles A, Diaz-Maqueo JC, Rodriguez L, et al. Prognostic value of serum beta 2 microglobulin in primary gastric lymphoma. *Hematol Oncol* 1991;9(2):115–21.

347. Litam P, Swan F, Cabanillas F, et al. Prognostic value of serum β-2 microglobulin in low-grade lymphoma. *Ann Int Med* 1991;114:855–860.

348. Conconi A, Zucca E, Roggero E, et al. Prognostic models for diffuse large B-cell lymphoma. *Hematol Oncol* 2000;18(2):61–73.

349. Warzocha K, Salles G, Bienvenu J, et al. Prognostic significance of TNFα and its p55 soluble receptor in malignant lymphomas. *Blood* 1998;91:3574–3581.

350. Warzocha K, Salles G, Bienvenu J, et al. Tumor necrosis factor ligand-receptor system can predict treatment outcome in lymphoma patients. *J Clin Oncol* 1997;15:499–508.

351. Preti H, Cabanillas F, Talpaz M, et al. Prognostic value of serum interleukin-6 in diffuse large-cell lymphoma. *Ann Intern Med* 1997;127:186–194.

352. Seymour JF, Talpaz M, Cabanillas F, et al. Serum interleukin-6 levels correlate with prognosis in diffuse large-cell lymphoma. *J Clin Oncol* 1995;13(3):575–582.

353. Fayad L, Cabanillas F, Talpaz M, et al. High serum interleukin-6 levels correlate with a shorter failure-free survival in indolent lymphoma. *Leuk Lymphoma* 1998;30(5–6):563–571.

354. Niitsu N, Okabe-Kado J, Okamoto M, et al. Serum nm23-H1 protein as a prognostic factor in aggressive non-Hodgkin lymphoma. *Blood* 2001;97(5):1202–1210.

355. Pezzella F, Tse A, Cordell J, et al. Expression of the Bcl-2 oncogene protein is not specific for the 14-18 chromosomal translocation. *Am J Pathol* 1990;137:225–232.

356. Fujii Y, Okumura M, Takeuchi Y, et al. Bcl-2 expression in the thymus and periphery. *Cell Immunol* 1994;155(2):335–344.

357. Krajewski S, Bodrug S, Gascoyne R, et al. Immunohistochemical analysis of Mcl-1 and Bcl-2 proteins in normal and neoplastic lymph nodes. *Am J Pathol* 1994;145(3):515–525.

358. Wang T, Lasota J, Hanau CA, Miettinen M. Bcl-2 oncoprotein is widespread in lymphoid tissue and lymphomas but its differential expression in benign versus malignant follicles and monocytoid B-cell proliferations is of diagnostic value. *APMIS* 1995;103(9):655–662.

359. Hockenbery D, Nunez G, Milliman C, et al. BCL-2 is an inner mitochondrial membrane protein that blocks programmed cell death. *Nature* 1990(348):334–336.

360. Yang E, Korsmeyer SJ. Molecular thanatopsis: a discourse on the BCL2 family and cell death. *Blood* 1996;88(2):386–401.

361. Reed JC. Bcl-2 family proteins: regulators of apoptosis and chemoresistance in hematologic malignancies. *Semin Hematol* 1997;34[4 Suppl 5]:9–19.

362. Gascoyne R, Adomat S, Krajewski S, et al. Prognostic significance of bcl-2 protein expression and bcl-2 gene rearrangement in diffuse aggressive non-Hodgkin's lymphoma. *Blood* 1997;90:244–251.

363. Hermine O, Haioun C, Lepage E, et al. Bcl-2 protein expression in aggressive non-Hodgkin's lymphoma (NHL). A new adverse prognostic factor? Proceedings of the Fifth International Conference on Malignant Lymphoma, 1993:28.

364. Kramer M, Hermans J, Parker J, et al. Clinical significance of bcl2 and p53 protein expression in diffuse large B-cell lymphoma: a population-based study. *J Clin Oncol* 1996;14:2131–2138.

365. Hill ME, MacLennan KA, Cunningham DC, et al. Prognostic significance of BCL-2 expression and bcl-2 major breakpoint region rearrangement in diffuse large cell non-Hodgkin's lymphoma: a British National Lymphoma Investigation Study. *Blood* 1996;88(3):1046–51.

366. Sanchez E, Chacon I, Plaza MM, et al. Clinical outcome in diffuse large B-cell lymphoma is dependent on the relationship between different cell-cycle regulator proteins. *J Clin Oncol* 1998;16(5):1931–1939.

367. Sarris A, Ford R. Recent advances in the molecular pathogenesis of lymphomas. *Curr Opin Oncol* 1999;11(5):351–363.

368. Monni O, Franssila K, Joensuu H, Knuutila S. BCL2 overexpression in diffuse large B-cell lymphoma. *Leuk Lymphoma* 1999;34:45–52.

369. Barrans SL, Carter I, Owen RG, et al. Germinal center phenotype and bcl-2 expression combined with the International Prognostic Index improves patient risk stratification in diffuse large B-cell lymphoma. *Blood* 2002;99(4):1136–1143.

370. Hollstein M, Sidransky D, Vogelstein B, Harris CC. p53 mutations in human cancers. *Science* 1991;253(5015):49–53.

371. Wilson W, Teruya-Feldstein J, Fest T, et al. Relationship of p53, bcl-2, and tumor proliferation to clinical drug resistance in non-Hodgkin's lymphomas. *Blood* 1997;89:601–609.

372. Sander CA, Yano T, Clark HM, et al. p53 mutation is associated with progression in follicular lymphomas. *Blood* 1993;82:1994–2004.

373. Lo Coco F, Gaidano G, Louie DC, et al. p53 mutations are associated with histologic transformation of follicular lymphoma. *Blood* 1993;82(8):2289–2295.

374. Gaidano G, Pastore C, Capello D, et al. Molecular pathways in low grade B-cell lymphoma. *Leuk Lymphoma* 1997;26[Suppl 1]:107–113.

375. Du M, Peng H, Singh N, Isaacson PG, Pan L. The accumulation of p53 abnormalities is associated with progression of mucosa-associated lymphoid tissue lymphoma. *Blood* 1995;86(12):4587–4593.

376. Ichikawa A, Kinoshita T, Watanabe T, et al. Mutations of the p53 gene as a prognostic factor in aggressive B-cell lymphoma. *N Engl J Med* 1997;337:529–534.

377. Ballerini P, Gaidano G, Gong J, et al. Multiple genetic lesions in AIDS-related non-Hodgkin lymphoma. *Blood* 1993;81:166–176.

378. Piris MA, Villuendas R, Martinez JC, et al. p53 expression in non-Hodgkin's lymphomas: a marker of p53 inactivation? *Leuk Lymphoma* 1995;17(1–2):35–42.

379. Matsushima AY, Cesarman E, Chadburn A, Knowles DM. Post-thymic T cell lymphomas frequently overexpress p53 protein but infrequently exhibit p53 gene mutations. *Am J Pathol* 1994;144(3):573–584.

380. Hernandez L, Fest T, Cazorla M, et al. p53 gene mutations and protein overexpression are associated with aggressive variants of mantle cell lymphomas. *Blood* 1996;87(8):3351–3359.

381. Louie DC, Offit K, Jaslow R, et al. p53 overexpression as a marker of poor prognosis in mantle cell lymphomas with t(11;14)(q13;q32). *Blood* 1995;86(8):2892–2899.

382. Piris MA, Pezzella F, Martinez-Montero JC, et al. p53 and bcl-2 expression in high-grade B-cell lymphomas: correlation with survival time. *Br J Cancer* 1994;69(2):337–341.

383. Koduru PR, Raju K, Vadmal V, et al. Correlation between mutation in P53, p53 expression, cytogenetics, histologic type, and survival in patients with B-cell non-Hodgkin's lymphoma. *Blood* 1997;90(10):4078–4091.

384. Ambrosini G, Adida C, Altieri D. A novel anti-apoptosis gene, survivin, expressed in cancer and lymphoma. *Nat Med* 1997;3:917–921.

385. Adida C, Haioun C, Gaulard P, et al. Prognostic significance of survivin expression in diffuse large B-cell lymphomas. *Blood* 2000;96(5):1921–1925.

386. Davis RE, Brown KD, Siebenlist U, Staudt LM. Constitutive nuclear factor kappaB activity is required for survival of activated B cell-like diffuse large B cell lymphoma cells. *J Exp Med* 2001;194(12):1861–1874.

387. Wang CY, Guttridge DC, Mayo MW, Baldwin AS Jr. NF-kappaB induces expression of the Bcl-2 homologue A1/Bfl-1 to preferentially suppress chemotherapy-induced apoptosis. *Mol Cell Biol* 1999;19(9):5923–5929.

388. Chen C, Edelstein LC, Gelinas C. The Rel/NF-kappaB family directly activates expression of the apoptosis inhibitor Bcl-x(L). *Mol Cell Biol* 2000;20(8):2687–2695.

389. Cheng Q, Lee HH, Li Y, Parks TP, Cheng G. Upregulation of Bcl-x and Bfl-1 as a potential mechanism of chemoresistance, which can be overcome by NF-kappaB inhibition. *Oncogene* 2000;19(42):4936–4940.

390. D'Souza B, Rowe M, Walls D. The bfl-1 gene is transcriptionally upregulated by the Epstein-Barr virus LMP1, and its expression promotes the survival of a Burkitt's lymphoma cell line. *J Virol* 2000;74(14):6652–6658.

391. Lee H, Dadgostar H, Cheng Q, et al. NF-kappaB-mediated up-regulation of Bcl-x and Bfl-1/A1 is required for CD40 survival signaling in B lymphocytes. *Proc Natl Acad Sci U S A* 1999;96:9136–9141.
392. Zong W, Edelstein L, Chen C, Bash J, Gelinas C. The prosurvival Bcl-2 homolog Bfl-1/A1 is a direct transcriptional target of NF-kappaB that blocks TNFalpha-induced apoptosis. *Genes Devel* 1999;13:382–387.
393. Miller T, Grogan T, Dahlberg S, et al. Prognostic significance of the Ki-67-associated proliferative antigen in aggressive non-Hodgkin's lymphomas: a prospective Southwest Oncology Group trial. *Blood* 1994;83:1460–1466.
394. Grogan T, Kippman S, Spier C, et al. Independent prognostic significance of a nuclear proliferation antigen in diffuse large cell lymphomas as determined by the monoclonal antibody Ki-67. *Blood* 1988; 71:1157.
395. Kossakowska A, Urbanski S, Huchcroft S, Edwards D. Relationship between the clinical aggressiveness of large cell immunoblastic lymphomas and expression of 92 kDa gelatinase (type IV collagenase) and tissue inhibitor of metalloproteinases-1 (TIMP-1) RNAs. *Oncol Res* 1992;4:233–240.
396. Salven P. Angiogenesis in lymphoproliferative disorders. *Acta Haematol* 2001;106(4):184–189.
397. Ribatti D, Urbinati C, Nico B, et al. Endogenous basic fibroblast growth factor is implicated in the vascularization of the chick embryo chorioallantoic membrane. *Dev Biol* 1995;170:39–49.
398. Vacca A, Ribatti D, Iurlaro M, et al. Human lymphoblastoid cells produce extracellular matrix-degrading enzymes and induce endothelial cell proliferation, migration, morphogenesis, and angiogenesis. *Int J Clin Lab Res* 1998;28(1):55–68.
399. Salven P, Teerenhovi L, Joensuu H. A high pretreatment serum vascular endothelial growth factor concentration is associated with poor outcome in non-Hodgkin's lymphoma. *Blood* 1997;90:3167–3172.
400. Dvorak HF, Sioussat TM, Brown LF, et al. Distribution of vascular permeability factor (vascular endothelial growth factor) in tumors: concentration in tumor blood vessels. *J Exp Med* 1991;174(5):1275–1278.
401. Yamamoto Y, Toi M, Kondo S, et al. Concentrations of vascular endothelial growth factor in the sera of normal controls and cancer patients. *Clin Cancer Res* 1996;2(5):821–826.
402. Salven P, Teerenhovi L, Joensuu H. A high pretreatment serum vascular endothelial growth factor concentration is associated with poor outcome in non-Hodgkin's lymphoma. *Blood* 1997;90(8):3167–3172.
403. Salven P, Teerenhovi L, Joensuu H. A high pretreatment serum basic fibroblast growth factor concentration is an independent predictor of poor prognosis in non-Hodgkin's lymphoma. *Blood* 1999;94(10):3334–3339.
404. Aguiar R, Yakushijin Y, Kharbanda S, et al. BAL is a novel risk-related gene in diffuse large B-cell lymphomas which enhances cellular migration. *Blood* 2000;96:4328–4334.
405. Aguiar R, Kreinbrink K, Shipp M. Cloning and characterization of BAL2, a novel member of a risk-related gene family in diffuse large B-cell lymphomas. *Blood* 2000;96:505a.
406. Ansell SM, Stenson M, Habermann TM, et al. Cd4+ T-cell immune response to large B-cell non-Hodgkin's lymphoma predicts patient outcome. *J Clin Oncol* 2001;19(3):720–726.
407. Bashir R, Freedman A, Harris N, et al. Immunophenotypic profile of CNS lymphoma: a review of 18 cases. *J Neurooncol* 1989;7:249–254.
408. Grogan TM, Miller TP. Immunobiologic correlates of prognosis in lymphoma. *Semin Oncol* 1993;20[5 Suppl 5]:58–74.
409. Jacob MC, Piccinni MP, Bonnefoix T, et al. T lymphocytes from invaded lymph nodes in patients with B-cell-derived non-Hodgkin's lymphoma: reactivity toward the malignant clone. *Blood* 1990;75(5):1154–1162.
410. Medeiros L, Picker L, Gelb A, et al. Numbers of host "helper" T cells and proliferating cells predict survival in diffuse small-cell lymphomas. *J Clin Oncol* 1989;7:1009–1017.
411. Rosenberg SA, Spiess P, Lafreniere R. A new approach to the adoptive immunotherapy of cancer with tumor-infiltrating lymphocytes. *Science* 1986;233(4770):1318–1321.
412. Muul LM, Spiess PJ, Director EP, Rosenberg SA. Identification of specific cytolytic immune responses against autologous tumor in humans bearing malignant melanoma. *J Immunol* 1987;138(3):989–995.
413. Bashir R, Chamberlain M, Ruby E, Hochberg FH. T-cell infiltration of primary CNS lymphoma. *Neurology* 1996;46(2):440–444.
414. Lippman SM, Spier CM, Miller TP, et al. Tumor-infiltrating T-lymphocytes in B-cell diffuse large cell lymphoma related to disease course. *Mod Pathol* 1990;3(3):361–367.
415. Hoppe RT, Medeiros LJ, Warnke RA, Wood GS. CD8-positive tumor-infiltrating lymphocytes influence the long-term survival of patients with mycosis fungoides. *J Am Acad Dermatol* 1995;32(3):448–453.
416. Chan WC, Huang JZ. Gene expression analysis in aggressive NHL. *Ann Hematol* 2001;80[Suppl 3]:B38–41.
417. Koulis A, Diss T, Isaacson PG, Dogan A. Characterization of tumor-infiltrating T lymphocytes in B-cell lymphomas of mucosa-associated lymphoid tissue. *Am J Pathol* 1997;151(5):1353–1360.
418. Achten R, Verhoef G, Vanuytsel L, De Wolf-Peeters C. T-cell/histiocyte-rich large B-cell lymphoma: a distinct clinicopathologic entity. *J Clin Oncol* 2002;20(5):1269–1277.
419. Rabbitts TH, Boehm T, Mengle-Gaw L. Chromosomal abnormalities in lymphoid tumours: mechanism and role in tumour pathogenesis. *Trends Genet* 1988;4(11):300–304.
420. Look AT, Downing JR. Molecular biology of leukemia and lymphoma. *Rev Invest Clin* 1994;[Suppl]:124–134.
421. Willis TG, Dyer MJ. The role of immunoglobulin translocations in the pathogenesis of B-cell malignancies. *Blood* 2000;96(3):808–822.
422. Taniwaki M, Nishida K, Ueda Y, et al. Interphase and metaphase detection of the breakpoint of 14q32 translocations in B-cell malignancies by double-color fluorescence in situ hybridization. *Blood* 1995;85(11):3223–3228.
423. Nanjangud G, Rao PH, Hegde A, et al. Spectral karyotyping identifies new rearrangements, translocations, and clinical associations in diffuse large B-cell lymphoma. *Blood* 2002;99(7):2554–2561.
424. Horsman DE, Gascoyne RD, Coupland RW, et al. Comparison of cytogenetic analysis, southern analysis, and polymerase chain reaction for the detection of t(14; 18) in follicular lymphoma. *Am J Clin Pathol* 1995;103(4):472–478.
425. Armitage JO, Sanger WG, Weisenburger D, et al. Correlation of secondary cytogenetic abnormalities with histologic appearance in non-Hodgkin's lymphomas bearing t(14;18)(q32;q21). *J Natl Cancer Inst* 1988;80(8):576–580.
426. Schlegelberger B. Cytogenetic subtyping of diffuse large B-cell lymphomas. *Ann Hematol* 2001;80[Suppl 3]:B32–34.
427. Huang JZ, Sanger WG, Greiner TC, et al. The t(14;18) defines a unique subset of diffuse large B-cell lymphoma with a germinal center B-cell gene expression profile. *Blood* 2002;99(7):2285–2290.
428. Capello D, Vitolo U, Pasqualucci L, et al. Distribution and pattern of BCL-6 mutations throughout the spectrum of B-cell neoplasia. *Blood* 2000;95(2):651–659.
429. Ohno H, Fukuhara S. Significance of rearrangement of the BCL6 gene in B-cell lymphoid neoplasms. *Leuk Lymphoma* 1997;27(1-2):53–63.
430. Cattoretti G, Chang CC, Cechova K, et al. BCL-6 protein is expressed in germinal-center B cells. *Blood* 1995;86(1):45–53.
431. Lo Coco F, Ye BH, Lista F, et al. Rearrangements of the BCL6 gene in diffuse large cell non-Hodgkin's lymphoma. *Blood* 1994;83(7):1757–1759.
432. Pasqualucci L, Migliazza A, Fracchiolla N, et al. BCL-6 mutations in normal germinal center B cells: evidence of somatic hypermutation acting outside Ig loci. *Proc Natl Acad Sci U S A* 1998;95(20):11816–11821.
433. Migliazza A, Martinotti S, Chen W, et al. Frequent somatic hypermutation of the 5' noncoding region of the BCL6 gene in B-cell lymphoma. *Proc Natl Acad Sci U S A* 1995;92(26):12520–12524.
434. Lossos IS, Levy R. Higher-grade transformation of follicle center lymphoma is associated with somatic mutation of the 5' noncoding regulatory region of the BCL-6 gene. *Blood* 2000;96(2):635–639.
435. Offit K, Lo Coco F, Louie D, et al. Rearrangement of the BCL-6 gene as a prognostic marker in diffuse large-cell lymphoma. *N Engl J Med* 1994;331:74–80.
436. Kramer M, Hermans J, Wijburg E, et al. Clinical relevance of BCL2, BCL6, and MYC rearrangements in diffuse large B-cell lymphoma. *Blood* 1998;92:3152–3162.
437. Ye B, Lista F, Lo Coco F, et al. Alterations of BCL-6, a novel zinc-finger gene, in diffuse large cell lymphoma. *Science* 1993;262:747–750.
438. Bastard C, Deweindt C, Kerckaert JP, et al. LAZ3 rearrangements in non-Hodgkin's lymphoma: correlation with histology, immunophe-

notype, karyotype, and clinical outcome in 217 patients. *Blood* 1994;83:2423–2427.

439. Lossos IS, Jones CD, Warnke R, et al. Expression of a single gene, BCL-6, strongly predicts survival in patients with diffuse large B-cell lymphoma. *Blood* 2001;98(4):945–951.

440. Ueda C, Uchiyama T, Ohno H. Immunoglobulin (Ig)/BCL6 versus non-Ig/BCL6 gene fusion in diffuse large B-cell lymphoma corresponds to a high- versus low-level expression of BCL6 mRNA. *Blood* 2002;99(7):2624–2625.

441. Akasaka T, Ueda C, Kurata M, et al. Nonimmunoglobulin (non-Ig)/BCL6 gene fusion in diffuse large B-cell lymphoma results in worse prognosis than Ig/BCL6. *Blood* 2000;96:2907–2909.

442. Morris SW, Kirstein MN, Valentine MB, et al. Fusion of a kinase gene, ALK, to a nucleolar protein gene, NPM, in non-Hodgkin's lymphoma [letter]. *Science* 1995;267(5196):316–317.

443. Rimokh R, Magaud J-P, Berger F, et al. A translocation involving a specific breakpoint on chromosome 5 is characteristic of anaplastic large-cell lymphoma. *Br J Haematol* 1989;71:31–36.

444. Kaneko Y, Frizzera G, Edamura S, et al. A novel translocation, t(2;5)(p23;q35), in childhood phagocytic large T-cell lymphoma mimicking malignant histiocytosis. *Blood* 1989;73(3):806–813.

445. Shiota M, Nakamura S, Ichinohasama R, et al. Anaplastic large cell lymphomas expressing the novel chimeric protein p80NPM/ALK: a distinct clinicopathologic entity. *Blood* 1995;86(5):1954–1960.

446. Gascoyne R, Krajewska M, Krajewski S, et al. Prognostic significance of Bax protein expression in diffuse aggressive non-Hodgkin's lymphoma. *Blood* 1997;90:3173–3178.

447. Nakamura S, Shiota M, Nakagawa A, et al. Anaplastic large cell lymphoma: a distinct molecular pathologic entity. *Am J Surg Pathol* 1997;21:1420–1432.

448. Shiota M, Fujimoto J, Takenaga M, et al. Diagnosis of t(2;5)(p23;q35)-associated Ki-1 lymphoma with immunohistochemistry. *Blood* 1994;84(11):3648–3652.

449. Gascoyne RD. The Molecular Biology of MALT Lymphomas. *ASH Education Program Book* 2001:244–248.

450. Liu H, Ye H, Ruskone-Fourmestraux A, et al. T(11;18) is a marker for all stage gastric MALT lymphomas that will not respond to *H. pylori* eradication. *Gastroenterology* 2002;122(5):1286–1294.

451. Hummel M, Stein H. Clinical relevance of immunoglobulin mutation analysis. *Curr Opin Oncol* 2000;12(5):395–402.

452. Hamblin TJ, Davis Z, Gardiner A, et al. Unmutated Ig V(H) genes are associated with a more aggressive form of chronic lymphocytic leukemia. *Blood* 1999;94(6):1848–1854.

453. Maloum K, Davi F, Merle-Beral H, et al. Expression of unmutated VH genes is a detrimental prognostic factor in chronic lymphocytic leukemia. *Blood* 2000;96(1):377–379.

454. Naylor M, Capra JD. Mutational status of Ig V(H) genes provides clinically valuable information in B-cell chronic lymphocytic leukemia. *Blood* 1999;94(6):1837–1839.

455. Hamblin TJ, Orchard JA, Gardiner A, et al. Immunoglobulin V genes and CD38 expression in CLL. *Blood* 2000;95(7):2455–2457.

456. Algara P, Mateo MS, Sanchez-Beato M, et al. Analysis of the IgV(H) somatic mutations in splenic marginal zone lymphoma defines a group of unmutated cases with frequent 7q deletion and adverse clinical course. *Blood* 2002;99(4):1299–1304.

457. Dohner H, Stilgenbauer S, Benner A, et al. Genomic aberrations and survival in chronic lymphocytic leukemia. *N Engl J Med* 2000;343(26):1910–1916.

458. Gribben J, Freedman A, Sunhee D, et al. All advanced stage non-Hodgkin's lymphomas with a polymerase chain reaction amplifiable breakpoint of *bcl-2* have residual cells containing the *bcl-2* rearrangement at evaluation and after treatment. *Blood* 1991;78:3275–3280.

459. Lee M, Chang K, Cabanillas F, et al. Detection of minimal residual cells containing t(14;18) by DNA sequence amplification. *Science* 1987;237:175–178.

460. Corradini P, Astolfi M, Cherasco C, et al. Molecular monitoring of minimal residual disease in follicular and mantle cell non-Hodgkin's lymphomas treated with high-dose chemotherapy and peripheral blood progenitor cell autografting. *Blood* 1997;89(2):724–731.

461. van Belzen N, Hupkes PE, Doekharan D, et al. Detection of minimal disease using rearranged immunoglobulin heavy chain genes from intermediate- and high-grade malignant B cell non-Hodgkin's lymphoma. *Leukemia* 1997;11(10):1742–1752.

462. Gribben JG, Neuberg D, Freedman AS, et al. Detection by polymerase chain reaction of residual cells with the bcl-2 translocation is associated with increased risk of relapse after autologous bone marrow transplantation for B-cell lymphoma. *Blood* 1993;81(12):3449–3457.

463. Hardingham JE, Kotasek D, Sage RE, et al. Significance of molecular marker-positive cells after autologous peripheral-blood stem-cell transplantation for non-Hodgkin's lymphoma. *J Clin Oncol* 1995;13(5):1073–1079.

464. Vose JM, Sharp G, Chan WC, et al. Autologous transplantation for aggressive non-Hodgkin's lymphoma: results of a randomized trial evaluating graft source and minimal residual disease. *J Clin Oncol* 2002;20(9):2344–2352.

465. Limpens J, Stad R, Vos C, et al. Lymphoma-associated translocation t(14;18) in blood B cells of normal individuals. *Blood* 1995;85(9):2528–2536.

466. Lopez-Guillermo A, Cabanillas F, McLaughlin P, et al. Molecular response assessed by PCR is the most important factor predicting failure-free survival in indolent follicular lymphoma: update of the MDACC series. *Ann Oncol* 2000;11[Suppl 1]:137–140.

467. Rambaldi A, Lazzari M, Manzoni C, et al. Monitoring of minimal residual disease after CHOP and rituximab in previously untreated patients with follicular lymphoma. *Blood* 2002;99(3):856–862.

468. Colombat P, Salles G, Brousse N, et al. Rituximab (anti-CD20 monoclonal antibody) as single first-line therapy for patients with follicular lymphoma with a low tumor burden: clinical and molecular evaluation. *Blood* 2001;97(1):101–106.

469. Howard O, Gribben J, Neuberg D, et al. Rituximab and CHOP induction therapy for newly diagnosed mantle-cell lymphoma: molecular complete responses are not predictive of progression-free survival. *J Clin Oncol* 2002;20(5):1288–1294.

470. Ramaswamy S, Golub TR. DNA microarrays in clinical oncology. *J Clin Oncol* 2002;20(7):1932–1941.

471. Alizadeh A, Elsen M, Davis R, et al. Distinct types of diffuse large B-cell lymphoma identified by gene expression profiling. *Nature* 2000;4051:503–511.

472. Rosenwald A, Alizadeh AA, Widhopf G, et al. Relation of gene expression phenotype to immunoglobulin mutation genotype in B cell chronic lymphocytic leukemia. *J Exp Med* 2001;194(11):1639–1647.

473. Klein U, Tu Y, Stolovitzky GA, et al. Gene expression profiling of B cell chronic lymphocytic leukemia reveals a homogeneous phenotype related to memory B cells. *J Exp Med* 2001;194(11):1625–1638.

474. Fais F, Ghiotto F, Hashimoto S, et al. Chronic lymphocytic leukemia B cells express restricted sets of mutated and unmutated antigen receptors. *J Clin Invest* 1998;102(8):1515–1525.

CHAPTER 9

Diagnostic Radiology

Kitt Shaffer and Liangge Hsu

Non-Hodgkin's lymphoma presents particular challenges for imaging due to the heterogeneity of appearance and site of involvement in this complex group of diseases. Approximately 55,000 new cases of non-Hodgkin's lymphoma are diagnosed annually (compared to approximately 7,500 cases of Hodgkin's disease), with approximately 25,000 deaths expected per year (1,2). Overall, non-Hodgkin's lymphoma involves more different sites and can have more varied imaging appearance than Hodgkin's disease, which is typically a bulky anterior mediastinal mass with contiguous spread to adjacent nodal groups (3,4). Classification schemes for non-Hodgkin's lymphoma have not always correlated with imaging findings, because older systems were based on somewhat subjective histopathologic findings. Newer classifications, such as the REAL (Revised European-American Lymphoma) Classification, may correlate better with imaging because this system integrates histologic, genetic, and molecular biologic features of the disease to provide a more accurate reflection of pathophysiology (1,5).

For imaging of non-Hodgkin's lymphoma, a variety of radiologic modalities are used. Plain films are inexpensive and give a quick, painless overview of large areas of anatomy at relatively low radiation dose to the patient. Ultrasound can be useful in selected situations, particularly in imaging the breast or superficial sites such as cervical nodes, guiding interventional procedures, or renal imaging. Computed tomography (CT) is widely used in imaging all parts of the body involved in lymphoma but is more expensive than plain films, has a higher radiation dose, and often requires injection of intravenous contrast material with concomitant risk of allergic reaction or renal damage (6,7). However, for most parts of the body, CT offers a clearer look at tissues due to its cross-sectional format and superior resolution of different tissue densities compared to plain films or ultrasound. Magnetic resonance (MR) imaging offers advantages over CT in some parts of the body, particularly the central nervous system. In general, MR costs slightly more than CT, uses no ionizing radiation, and may require injection of very small amounts of contrast agents with much less risk of systemic effects or allergic reaction than for CT contrast agents (8). Nuclear medicine imaging is gaining in importance in imaging of lymphoma, and is discussed in Chapter 10 (9).

All of these imaging modalities may be used in initial evaluation or follow-up of non-Hodgkin's lymphoma. No single follow-up scheme can be recommended for non-Hodgkin's lymphoma, because there is such a wide variety of sites of involvement as well as a range of aggressiveness, from indolent to rapidly progressive disease. Follow-up intervals will vary depending on the nature of the particular type of lymphoma being evaluated. For assessment of residual masses after treatment, more functional imaging, such as gallium or positron emission tomography (PET) scanning, provides better differentiation between fibrosis and residual active tumor than the anatomic methods, such as CT and MR. Each imaging modality is considered separately, with examples of typical and atypical cases as well as a brief discussion of the expected appearance of treatment effects and common complications. For research protocols, accurate measurement of sites of disease is crucial, and the strengths and weaknesses of each modality in this regard are discussed in each section. Because techniques for neurologic imaging are extremely specialized, separate sections discuss the use of CT and MR in this area.

BODY IMAGING

It is important in considering the role of imaging in any oncologic situation to understand what the goals and purposes of the studies are in any given patient. Different imaging protocols are used in the initial workup of an unknown abnormality than for staging of a known malignancy, evaluation of response to treatment, and detection of recurrence. In the case of non-Hodgkin's lymphoma, a wide variety of imaging studies are potentially useful, and no single recommendation can be made that will be applicable to all of the diverse diseases grouped under this name. Some studies have suggested that modern nuclear medicine techniques, such as PET, may actually be the most cost-effective single study for use in follow-up of lymphoma (10).

The interval that is appropriate for follow-up also varies depending on the aggressiveness of disease. Follow-up at 3 or 6 months may be appropriate for a highly aggressive diffuse large B-cell lymphoma, whereas yearly follow-up may be sufficient for an indolent small follicular lymphoma. In some studies, any routine imaging follow-up has been questioned for certain types of non-Hodgkin's lymphoma, in which imaging only as clinically directed may actually be more cost-effective (11). In some cases, such as mediastinal large B-cell lymphoma, imaging limited to the likeliest area for recurrence (the chest) may be sufficient, rather than routine follow-up scanning of the neck, chest, abdomen, and pelvis (12). In one study of routine CT compared to clinical follow-up for follicular lymphoma, only 4% of patients benefited from routine CT scanning, and only 14% of all recurrences were detected with CT alone (13). For patients on investigational treatment protocols, more detailed imaging may be appropriate to include even asymptomatic areas of possible disease as well as to monitor for unexpected treatment effects.

An area where imaging can play a large role is in planning of radiation fields. CT in particular can be very helpful in determining whether key regions (such as the left anterior descending coronary artery) can be excluded from the field safely. For such regions as the deep axilla, where clinical examination may be misleading, CT can play a large role in detection of clinically unsuspected sites of disease. However, in certain areas, CT can be misleading, as in central lung masses with postobstructive pneumonia. In this case, the lack of tissue specificity of CT can hamper the ability to accurately demonstrate where disease ends and inflammation begins in terms of radiation planning. Follow-up studies after optimal treatment of presumed infection can sometimes give a more accurate estimation of extent of disease.

It is important at the time of initial imaging to realize that baseline information, even in areas of no current disease, may be helpful for future comparisons. In non-Hodgkin's lymphoma, comparison to prior studies is particularly important, especially for patients on investigational treatment protocols. Access to experienced oncoradiologists can be particularly helpful in these complex patients, as early detection of recurrence can be essential in successful salvage therapy. It is also important to choose the type of imaging that is the most sensitive and specific for the type of disease present. For example, detection of marrow involvement is best with MR (14), whereas assessment of cortical bone integrity is best with CT. Measurement of areas of disease is also not a trivial matter, and methods for this are far from standardized. In a study comparing one-, two-, and three-dimensional measures of nodal involvement in non-Hodgkin's lymphoma, there were no significant differences in staging, although the three-dimensional methods were most accurate and reproducible (15). Again, such time-consuming methods are probably best reserved for patients on investigational treatment protocols.

Plain Films

The plain chest film remains a mainstay of evaluation of non-Hodgkin's lymphoma because it is inexpensive and gives a broad overview of the entire chest in a very short examination time with relatively low radiation dose.

Approximately 40% to 50% of non-Hodgkin's lymphoma overall involves the mediastinum, with more pulmonary involvement at presentation than for Hodgkin's disease (3,16), so a chest radiograph is often helpful as an initial rough assessment of the extent of disease and is also a very simple way to observe known chest disease for response to treatment. In the past, the bulk of disease has been estimated on chest radiographs by comparing the transverse diameter of the largest tumor mass to the total chest diameter. Such crude measurements are better replaced by chest CT evaluation of nodes, because transverse diameter on chest radiograph may be confounded by inclusion of intervening normal tissues and may also miss substantial disease in other sites (17). However, as an overall estimate of extent, the chest radiograph still has a definite role in the imaging of non-Hodgkin's lymphoma (Fig. 9.1).

Plain films of bones also have some role in skeletal lymphoma; however, the lesions of lymphoma often involve primarily the marrow cavity and may be better seen with MR (Fig. 9.2). Most bony lymphoma has a large extraosseous soft tissue component (Fig. 9.3), which may not be well demonstrated on plain films (18). In general, lesions that are well seen on plain films will also be well seen on CT, which shows cortical bone best. Lesions that are subtle or invisible on plain films may be best seen on MR, which shows effects of marrow infiltration with relative preservation of cortical bone. CT and MR are better than plain films at showing associated soft tissue masses adjacent to bony lesions. For multiple myeloma, because bone scans do not typically show any activity in the purely lytic disease present, skeletal surveys (plain films of selected bones) are still the mainstay of detection of disease and follow-up of response to treatment.

Most academic radiology departments are switching from analog to digital acquisition for plain films (19). Digital images actually have slightly poorer spatial resolution than analog images, but this disadvantage is outweighed by the advantages of postprocessing and image transmission. Images that are slightly too dark or too light can be corrected, and special image processing can be done to enhance edges and make certain structures (such as support lines) easier to see. With Picture Archiving and Communication Systems (PACS), images can be transmitted over a computer network linked to other hospital clinical computing systems and the electronic medical record. PACS systems are very expensive to implement but in the long run should be more cost-effective than film systems because of savings on processing and storage costs (20,21).

Assessment of organomegaly is possible on plain films of the abdomen (KUB—kidney, ureter, and bladder film) in some cases (Fig. 9.4), but in general, assessment of solid abdominal structures is extremely limited with plain films. Obtaining only indirect evidence of bowel wall abnormalities is possible if there is alteration of the contour of luminal gas (Fig. 9.5). Severe complications, such as perforation or pneumatosis coli, can be detected with plain films but are much better seen with CT (Fig. 9.6). Even detection of

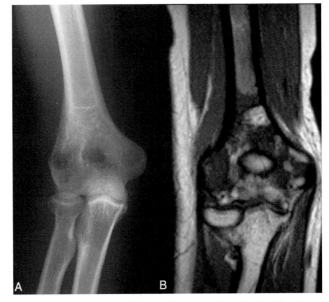

FIG. 9.2. Elbow film **(A)** in a 44-year-old patient with elbow pain. No bony abnormality is evident. T1-weighted magnetic resonance image in the coronal plane **(B)** demonstrates marked heterogeneity of signal in the marrow, indicating extensive infiltration with non-Hodgkin's lymphoma.

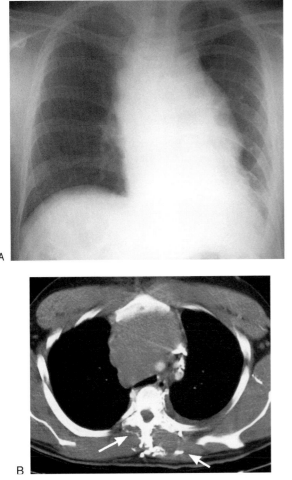

FIG. 9.1. Chest x-ray **(A)** in a 28-year-old patient with chest pain found to have mediastinal large B-cell non-Hodgkin's lymphoma. Mass is obvious on plain film, and extent of overall bulk is well demonstrated, along with small left pleural effusion. Computed tomographic image **(B)** just above the level of the aortic arch shows typical homogenous soft tissue mass in the anterior mediastinum with marked displacement of vascular structures and compression of the trachea. Collateral vessels in the posterior body wall (*arrows*) suggest hemodynamically significant obstruction of venous return.

obstruction with kidney, ureter, and bladder film is limited in the early stages, when dilated bowel loops may be filled with fluid rather than gas and are therefore relatively invisible on plain films. Most cases of gastrointestinal lymphoma will have some abnormal imaging, but findings are rarely specific, and pathologic confirmation is generally needed to reach a diagnosis (22).

Computed Tomography

CT is one of the mainstays of imaging in non-Hodgkin's lymphoma. To detect small hilar nodes in the chest or abdomen, intravenous contrast should be used. Most mediastinal nodes can be detected without intravenous contrast but may be more easily measured after intravenous contrast administration

(23,24). Slice thickness between 5 and 10 mm is usually adequate to delineate nodes in the chest. Lung windows are best viewed after reconstruction with an edge-enhancing or sharp algorithm, which brings out fine details of the lung interstitium. Detection of small lung nodules is actually easier on thicker slices, because they are more easily discriminated from vascular structures when their branching can be seen. For CT of the abdomen, adequate opacification of the gastrointestinal structures is essential, requiring several hours of preparation with oral contrast material. If transit time is slow, rectal contrast may be needed to fill distal colonic structures. Because non-Hodgkin's lymphoma lesions in general are not vascular enough to show more than minimal enhancement on CT, there is usually no need to do multiphase imaging, and a single scan during the portal phase after intravenous contrast administration is generally adequate to demonstrate renal, liver, and splenic lesions in most cases (25).

Spiral CT has become the standard for most large imaging centers (26,27). In this technique, the radiation generator can spin continuously in the CT gantry due to development of a specialized electrical coupling called a *slip-ring*, which obviates the need for an electrical cable. With a continuously rotating generator, a spiral ring of data can be obtained over a large volume of tissue. The entire chest, abdomen, and pelvis can be scanned with this technique in less than 2 minutes. The continuous motion of the scanner degrades the spatial resolution of the images slightly, but the advantages of elimination of respiratory motion and speed of scanning more than balance this minor disadvantage. Another advantage of spiral scanning's speed is that a large volume of the body can be scanned during peak contrast enhancement, improving

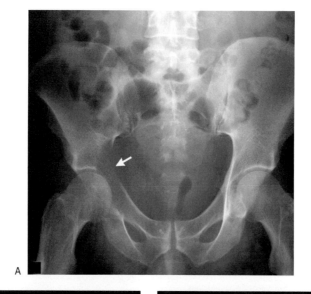

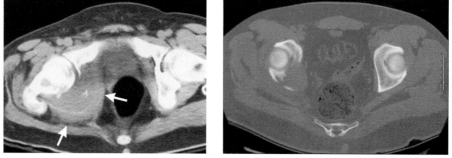

FIG. 9.3. Pelvis film **(A)** in a 37-year-old man with right hip pain. Lytic disease is present in the medial acetabulum (*arrow*) with extensive bone destruction. Computed tomographic scan displayed with soft-tissue windows **(B)** demonstrates a large associated soft-tissue mass (*arrows*). Bone destruction is better demonstrated on computed tomography displayed with bone windows **(C)**.

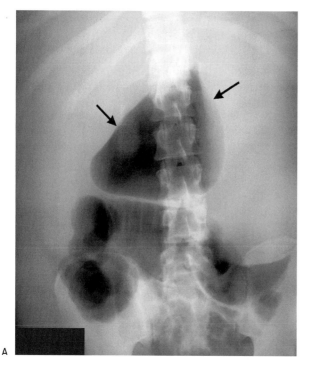

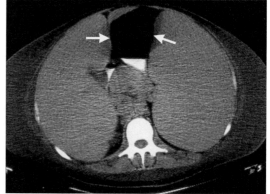

FIG. 9.4. Kidney, ureter, bladder film **(A)** of a patient with abdominal fullness and early satiety. The gastric air bubble (*arrows*) is displaced by markedly enlarged liver and spleen. On a computed tomographic image through the upper abdomen **(B)**, the organomegaly and compression of the stomach (*arrows*) are more evident.

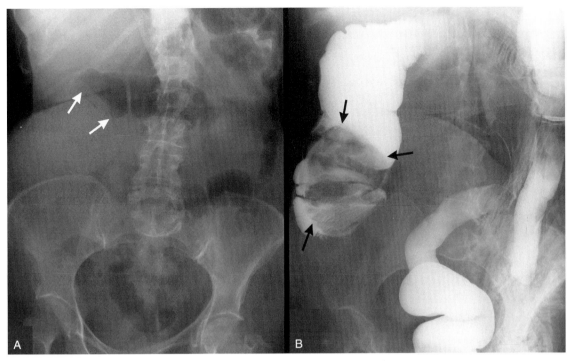

FIG. 9.5. Kidney, ureter, bladder film **(A)** in a middle-aged patient with abdominal pain. No air is visible in the right colon, and the transverse colon shows a suggestion of a large intraluminal filling defect (*arrows*). On single-contrast barium enema **(B)**, a large filling defect is visible in the cecum (*arrows*), which was due to an intussusception of a region of focal involvement of the terminal ileum by non-Hodgkin's lymphoma.

visualization of some abdominal lesions. The latest development in CT scan technology is *multidetector scanning* (28), which in effect combines several adjacent spiral scanners all running simultaneously to acquire even more data in a short

time. Another recent technological development is in units that combine PET and CT, allowing immediate superimposition of the functional PET images with the anatomic CT images to better localize disease (29,30).

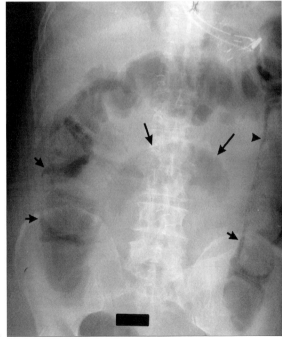

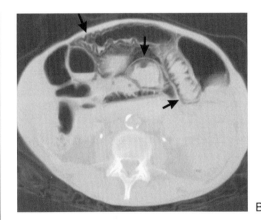

FIG. 9.6. Kidney, ureter, bladder film **(A)** in a patient with abdominal pain after resection of a left abdominal mass that demonstrated non-Hodgkin's lymphoma on pathologic analysis. A dilated loop of small bowel is present in the mid-abdomen (*arrows*), and there are streaks of gas in the wall of the colon (*arrowheads*) representing pneumatosis, in this case due to ischemia. Image **B** is a different patient with abdominal pain showing the appearance of pneumatosis (*arrows*) due to mesenteric vein thrombosis.

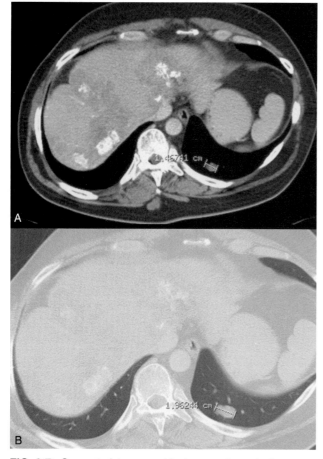

FIG. 9.7. Computed tomographic images through the upper abdomen in a patient with metastatic colon carcinoma displayed at soft tissue **(A)** and lung **(B)** windows. A lung lesion is measured on both images, revealing apparent diameter of 1.5 cm in image **A** but 2.0 cm in image **B** for the same lesion. Conspicuity of liver lesions is much higher in image **A** than in image **B**.

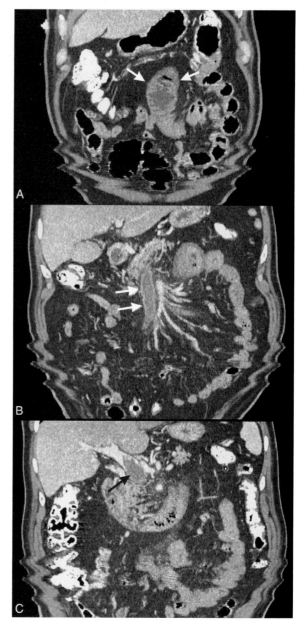

FIG. 9.8. Coronal reconstructions from a multidetector helical abdominal computed tomographic study with intravenous contrast of a middle-aged patient with abdominal pain. Reconstruction in the anterior portion of the abdomen **(A)** reveals a distended small bowel loop with thickened wall (*arrows*), which could represent ischemia or infiltration with tumor. Reconstruction in the plane of the superior mesenteric vessels **(B)** reveals a normal superior mesenteric artery, but clot (*arrows*) within the superior mesenteric vein. Reconstruction in the plane of the portal vein **(C)** reveals thrombus occluding this vessel (*arrow*).

Several technical factors are important when using CT to measure response to therapy, particularly in the setting of investigational treatment protocols. It is very important to be sure that the same lesion is being measured and that the same diameters are used each time. Differences in slice thickness or other technical factors such as use of intravenous contrast can alter the appearance of lesions and may make comparison of measurements difficult. It is also important to be sure lesions are measured on the same window/level settings each time, as changes in brightness and contrast of the image can alter apparent diameter, particularly for lung lesions (Fig. 9.7). Ideally, measurements should be saved in the PACS workstation so that the next radiologist can duplicate the measurements on follow-up scans as accurately as possible. For mesenteric masses, measurement can be particularly problematic, as they may move in position, making determination of the identical level for measurement between scans difficult.

Areas for which MR may be preferable to CT include evaluation of small adrenal masses, characterization of liver and renal lesions, and examination of pelvic organs. The lung apices and diaphragms may also be better examined with MR than with CT, as the axial plane is not the optimal view for visualizing these horizontally oriented structures. However, with spiral and particularly multidetector scanning, very clear sagittal and coronal reconstructions are now pos-

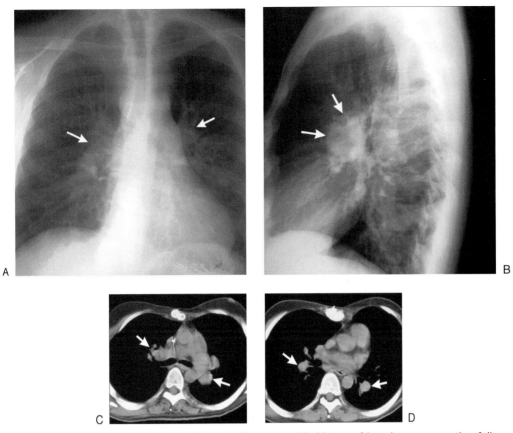

FIG. 9.9. Frontal chest x-ray **(A)** in a 39-year-old patient with history of lymphoma on routine follow-up. The hila bilaterally appear enlarged (*arrows*), also confirmed on the lateral view **(B)**, where marked central opacity is evident (*arrows*). Computed tomographic images at the level of the hilum **(C)** and descending pulmonary arteries **(D)** reveal that these central opacities represent enlarged pulmonary arteries (*arrows*). The patient also had a history of atrial septal defect, and this appearance represents shunt vascularity rather than adenopathy.

sible, which may eliminate these indications for MR in some cases (Fig. 9.8). In the case of interventional procedures, MR, CT, and ultrasound may all have roles. For guidance of lung fine-needle aspiration, CT is preferable. For ablation of tumors in lung or liver, either CT or MR can be used (31,32). For guidance of pleurodesis or paracentesis, ultrasound is usually the most cost-effective.

When using CT for staging and restaging of non-Hodgkin's lymphoma, it is important to keep in mind the possibility that patients may have more than one process at a given time. In a study of prostate cancer patients with retroperitoneal adenopathy, concomitant non-Hodgkin's lymphoma was actually more likely than metastatic disease from the primary prostate tumor (33). The pulmonary vasculature must be carefully evaluated for unsuspected embolism or abnormal flow patterns that may indicate unsuspected cardiac abnormalities (Fig. 9.9). Lung lesions may represent infection, atelectasis, or nonneoplastic inflammatory processes as well as non-Hodgkin's lymphoma (Fig. 9.10). Changes of radiation therapy are usually characteristic, with sharp nonanatomic borders, but occasionally can be more nodular or atypical in appearance (Fig. 9.11). Most increased

density in the lung due to radiation appears within 3 months of completion of treatment and stabilizes with characteristic fibrosis, retraction, and traction bronchiectasis within 18 months (34). Vascular anomalies, such as left superior vena cava, left inferior vena cava, or double inferior vena cava can also be confusing in evaluation of adenopathy unless intravenous contrast is used (Fig. 9.12).

CT is an excellent modality for detection of many common complications of treatment, such as radiation fibrosis, drug toxicity, opportunistic infections, or development of second malignancies. It is important to keep in mind when using CT for measurement of disease that CT is a purely anatomic modality. Because CT is often performed after intravenous contrast administration, it is important to consider the kinetics of contrast within the circulatory system. If contrast is administered rapidly in a bolus, and scanning is performed too soon, the liver and spleen may have a very atypical appearance (Fig. 9.13) due to inhomogeneous vascular distribution early in the injection (35). Therefore, it is important to look at other areas of the scan, which can give clues as to the timing of the injection. Presence of excreted contrast within the renal collecting systems is a good indica-

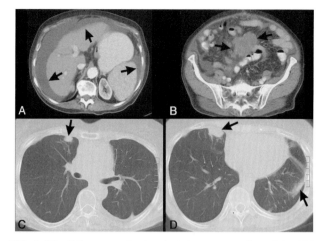

FIG. 9.10. CT scan at the level of the upper poles of the kidneys **(A)** in a 59-year-old patient with non-Hodgkin's lymphoma shows ascites (*arrows*) surrounding liver and spleen. Image at the level of the sacral promontory **(B)** shows a mesenteric mass (*arrows*) proven to represent recurrence on biopsy. Images through the mid- **(C)** and lower **(D)** chest show multiple rounded masses (*arrows*) initially felt to represent lung involvement with non-Hodgkin's lymphoma. However, on comparison to films from 5 years earlier, these had not changed. On closer inspection, these masses have features suggestive of rounded atelectasis, an infolding of lung in regions of pleural thickening most often due to fibrosis or asbestos exposure.

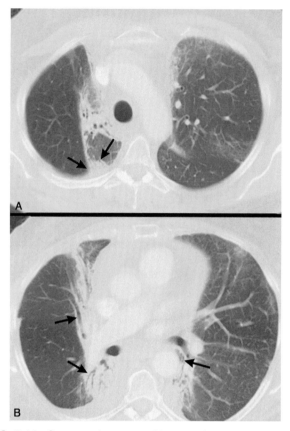

FIG. 9.11. Computed tomographic scan in the upper chest **(A)** in a patient after chemotherapy and radiation for mediastinal large B-cell non-Hodgkin's lymphoma. A rounded mass posteriorly on the right (*arrows*) might be considered possible recurrent disease, but examination of lower images **(B)** confirms that this opacity lies within the margins of radiation, as shown by straight lateral borders and extensive traction bronchiectasis (*arrows*). Findings remained stable on follow-up scans and are most consistent with focal radiation fibrosis.

tor of relatively long delay between injection and scanning. Dense contrast in the aorta with little contrast in the inferior vena cava indicates scanning early after injection.

CT is the primary modality for imaging of the lung parenchyma. Routine imaging is sufficient for most purposes, but when there is a question of interstitial involvement, high-resolution imaging may be needed. High-resolution CT consists of thin sections and reconstruction with an edge-enhancing algorithm and is generally used in assessment of interstitial processes. With multidetector spiral CT scanning, reconstruction of overlapping sections may increase detection of tiny nodules (36). Either CT or MR can be used to evaluate suspected vascular compromise by non-Hodgkin's lymphoma, such as superior vena cava syndrome (Fig. 9.14). MR in this setting has the advantage of having no requirement for intravenous contrast, but CT is best for patients who are clinically unstable.

CT is often used to guide biopsy in the setting of non-Hodgkin's lymphoma. There is some controversy about the best methods for use—coaxial needles or core biopsy guns (37,38)—but with enough of a sample, sensitivities and specificities of more than 90% are generally possible, and histologic subclassification using special studies can be performed on core samples. However, in the setting of residual masses after treatment, open procedures are probably preferable to percutaneous techniques due to the increased risk of false-negative results due to sampling error within fibrotic tissue (39). In the case of mural or serosal involvement of the gastrointestinal tract with non-Hodgkin's lymphoma, CT

can guide biopsies of lesions that are inaccessible to endoscopic biopsy (40).

Ultrasound

Ultrasound has much to offer in the workup and treatment of patients with non-Hodgkin's lymphoma. Although ultrasound is rarely a primary staging modality, it can be used to solve specific problems as well as guide interventional procedures. It has the advantage of being portable, using no ionizing radiation, and offering real-time visualization of structures. Using Doppler and color flow imaging, vascular structures can be assessed, as in suspected deep venous thrombosis (Fig. 9.15). As a modality for guidance of fine-needle aspiration, ultrasound has many advantages, including direct visualization of the needle entering the lesion (Fig. 9.16). Limitations of ultrasound are primarily related to physical limitations of the transmission of sound waves, which are blocked by air (lungs, bowel) and bone. The field

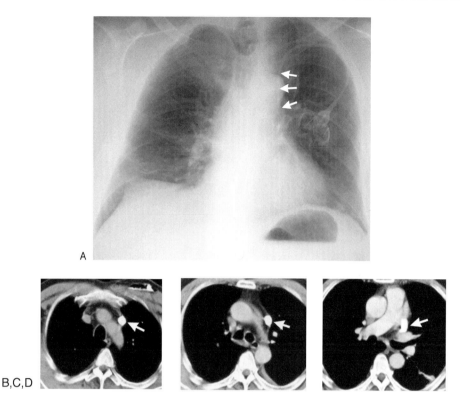

FIG. 9.12. Frontal chest x-ray **(A)** of a patient with non-Hodgkin's lymphoma after placement of Port-A-Cath for chemotherapy infusion. The course of the catheter is abnormal (*arrows*), passing downward to the left of the aortic arch. Chest computed tomographic images at the level of the aortic arch **(B)**, carina **(C)**, and left main pulmonary artery **(D)** show an aberrant vessel passing to the left of the aorta and extending downward to join the coronary sinus (*arrows*). This is the most common course of a persistent left superior vena cava, a relatively common venous anomaly.

of view of most ultrasound images is somewhat limited, making accurate measurement of the size of enlarged organs such as the liver and spleen problematic. Ultrasound is also the most operator-dependent of the imaging modalities, leading to wide variation in the quality of images depending on experience of the operator, which may be an ultrasonographic technologist or a radiologist. The limited sampling obtained with ultrasound is very important to keep in mind when considering this modality for follow-up of lesions.

Manipulation of the ultrasound transducer can be thought of as shining a flashlight into a dark storeroom. Images are obtained only of the areas where the beam is shined. This does not always guarantee a complete sampling of a large organ, such as the liver or spleen. For such uses, CT or MR is more appropriate for initial and follow-up studies. It is also important to keep in mind that the very different physical parameters used to image with ultrasound may lead to differences in apparent size of lesions when compared to other modalities such as CT. In observing lesions closely for treatment protocols, it is best to use the same modality each time to allow more accurate comparisons.

Ultrasound is particularly useful in superficial locations, such as breast or axilla, neck, or extremities, because the depth of penetration of sound waves is limited, and transducers designed for deep penetration have much lower spatial resolu-

tion. For guidance of superficial biopsies, detection of cystic collections or abscesses, or evaluation of peripheral vascular structures, therefore, ultrasound is very useful. Newer methods, such as ultrasound contrast agents (41), may increase the utility of ultrasound in the liver. For nodal imaging, use of color flow and Doppler may allow discrimination between lymphoma and other causes of enlarged nodes using analysis of hilar morphology and vascular patterns (42,43).

In the spleen, focal non-Hodgkin's lymphoma can sometimes appear cystic, but, again, use of color flow analysis to confirm avascularity can help in this setting (44), and modern power Doppler techniques may even allow detection of more diffuse infiltration in the spleen by analysis of regional flow (45). Imaging of the kidneys and biliary tree is also very useful, although the imaging of the right kidney is often better than the left, because the solid parenchyma of the liver offers a better acoustic window than the spleen in most patients. Because the images in ultrasound are not standardized, and the imaging plane depends entirely on how the operator is holding the transducer, comparison of lesions for measurement purposes with ultrasound can be problematic. Because ultrasound visualizes tissues based on their sound transmission characteristics rather than density (as in CT or radiography), lesions may sometimes be better seen with ultrasound, as can occur with breast cancer or

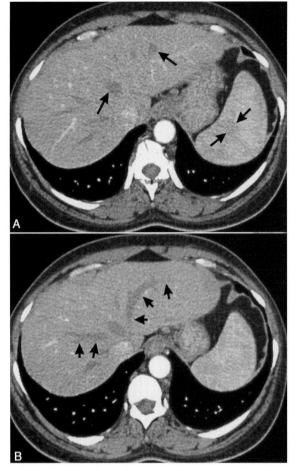

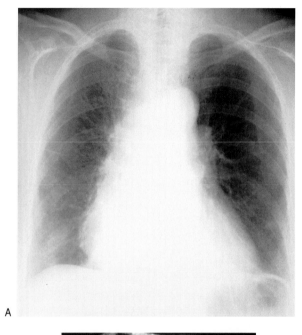

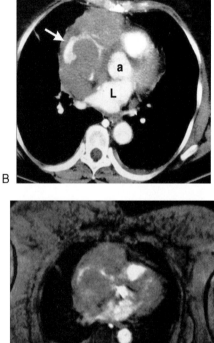

FIG. 9.13. Computed tomographic scan of a patient with abnormal liver function tests and history of non-Hodgkin's lymphoma, follicular cell type. On the upper image **(A)**, several areas of vague low attenuation are visible in the liver and spleen (*arrows*). On the lower image **(B)**, these low-attenuation areas are more clearly branching and tubular in shape (*arrows*), representing unopacified portal vessels. These scans were obtained very soon after contrast injection, and only the hepatic arterial branches in the liver are filled with contrast. Scans performed 20 to 40 seconds later reveal the expected uniform enhancement pattern of both liver and spleen.

breast lymphoma (Fig. 9.17). Even with use of ultrasound in the breast, however, a specific diagnosis of lymphoma can rarely be made on imaging alone, and biopsy is generally needed (46). Ultrasound can sometimes determine the fluid-filled nature of lesions that are indeterminate on CT due to high protein content or blood in the fluid. For any procedure in a superficial location near a vascular structure, the color flow capabilities of ultrasound make it an ideal imaging method to guide biopsies and aspirations, as long as no bone or lung intervenes to block the sound waves.

Magnetic Resonance Imaging

MR has both strengths and limitations for oncologic patients. For lesions requiring repeated study, the lack of ionizing

FIG. 9.14. Imaging in a 66-year-old patient with mediastinal large B-cell non-Hodgkin's lymphoma and chest pain. Chest x-ray **(A)** shows only a slightly wide mediastinum and enlarged cardiac silhouette. Computed tomographic scan **(B)** shows tumor infiltration along the right mediastinal border invading and filling the right atrium. Only a trace of intravenous contrast passes through the tumor mass (*arrow*). The aortic root (a) and left atrium (L) are displaced slightly by the mass. Magnetic resonance scan **(C)** with bright blood technique shows similar features, but without the need for intravenous contrast. Small bilateral pleural effusions are more evident on the magnetic resonance scan (*arrows*).

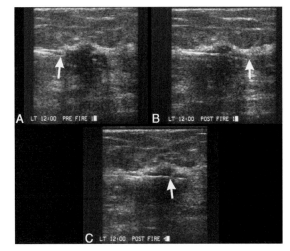

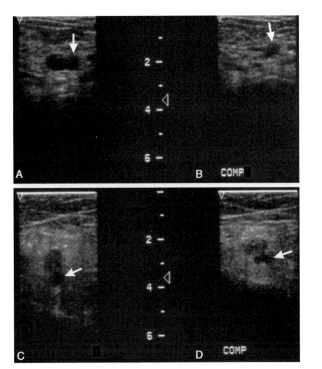

FIG. 9.15. Lower-extremity ultrasound in a 50-year-old patient with lung cancer and left leg swelling. Anechoic oval regions in the region of the superficial femoral vessels represent the normal right artery and vein with light pressure from the transducer **(A)**. The artery is indicated by the white arrow. When increasing pressure is applied, the vein disappears, as is normal when blood flow is unimpaired **(B)**. The artery is unchanged in appearance, as indicated by the white arrow. On the left, with light pressure from the transducer, the artery (*arrow*) and vein are again visible, although the vein contains some internal echoes, suggesting the presence of a clot. On deep compression with the transducer, the vein does not disappear, in spite of sufficient pressure to flatten the artery (*arrow*), confirming the presence of an occluding clot.

FIG. 9.16. Ultrasound-guided core biopsy of a focal breast mass noted on mammography and found to represent invasive breast cancer. When lesions are visible on ultrasound, this is the fastest and easiest approach to tissue sampling. Image **(A)** shows the position of the core needle with its tip (*arrow*) touching the proximal margin of the hypoechoic mass. Image **(B)** shows the image after the core needle has been fired through the mass, with the tip (*arrow*) passing through the entire mass. Image **(C)** shows the image after the fourth pass, confirming that the needle tip (*arrow*) is still passing through the mass. The ability to watch the actual biopsy in real time is a major advantage of ultrasound in sampling of small lesions.

radiation is advantageous. Compared to CT, MR has poorer spatial resolution but better tissue discrimination. The cost of MR is generally more than that of CT, but this difference is decreasing with technical advances. Patient motion is a larger problem in MR than in CT, because multiple slices may be obtained simultaneously in some sequences, so that motion during a limited period of time may degrade the entire study, rather than a single image, as in CT. Patient claustrophobia is more of a problem in standard MR units than with CT, but open magnet design is becoming more common (47). MR takes longer to perform than CT, so in patients with pain who are unable to lie still for longer than an hour, MR may be limited. However, newer and faster imaging sequences for MR are constantly being developed.

The physical basis of MR depends on the local magnetic properties of hydrogen atoms in the patient's body, mainly in the form of water but also present in lipids and other organic molecules. Liquid water, water tightly bound to hydrophilic molecules, interstitial fluid, and intracellular fluid all have slightly different magnetic properties and yield different characteristic MR signals. Because the physical basis for MR is not based on density or sound transmission, certain lesions may be better visualized on MR than on CT, plain films, or ultrasound. However, MR has limited value in detection of abnormalities of cortical bone or calcifications, because densely calcified tissue contains little hydrogen. A relatively high signal is obtained from fat on most MR sequences, which can be useful in delineating other structures, as in the abdomen or mediastinum. However, in the breast, the large amount of fat signal actually interferes with detection of small parenchymal lesions. In this setting, there are specialized sequences that can be used to dampen the signal from fat, leaving only signal from water (48). Such sequences are called *fat suppressed* sequences and are also useful in detection of fat-containing lesions elsewhere in the body.

Theoretically, MR can be performed with other atoms besides hydrogen, such as carbon or phosphorus, but such imaging requires a very high field strength and thus far has only experimental application (49,50). Contrast agents exist for MR and are based on perturbation of local magnetic environment rather than increased tissue density, as in iodinated contrast used for CT. The main contrast agents for MR contain gadolinium in a chelated form. Iron-containing agents are sometimes used to change the signal in liver parenchyma and increase conspicuity of abnormal areas, such as metastases (51,52). MR spectroscopy is a method for more specifically

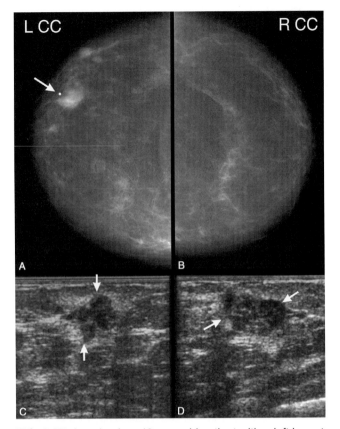

FIG. 9.17. Imaging in a 40-year-old patient with a left breast lump. Routine left **(A)** and right **(B)** craniocaudal (CC) mammograms show fatty breasts with a group of nodules in the outer left breast corresponding to the palpable finding, as indicated by a metallic marker placed on the patient's skin (*arrow*). Ultrasound is useful in this setting to rule out cystic lesions that require no further workup. Ultrasound of the more lateral lesion **(C)** shows that it is not cystic but hypoechoic, with a relatively "tall" appearance (*arrows*) indicating that it is crossing transverse tissue planes of the breast. This appearance is more often seen in malignancies than in benign solid breast lesions such as fibroadenomas. The larger lesion is more elongated on ultrasound (*arrows*) **(D)** but still does not demonstrate cystic features. Biopsy confirmed non-Hodgkin's lymphoma of the breast, but breast carcinoma would have a similar appearance.

characterizing the structure of hydrogen-containing compounds within a small defined area of a scan, and can sometimes be useful in discriminating among different disease entities, particularly in the central nervous system.

Another advantage of MR is the ability to perform imaging in any mathematically definable plane. Image planes may be sagittal, coronal, or oblique, and can even follow the curves of a structure such as the aorta. Because flowing blood leads to displacement of magnetic effects, vascular flow can be detected and even quantified without use of contrast agents. By altering the type of input to the system, flowing blood can be set to appear either black or white on MR images. The choice of "bright blood" or "dark blood"

technique depends on the signal of surrounding structures. If the vascular structures to be examined are surrounded by low signal (as in the lungs, where the air in the parenchyma gives virtually no signal), bright blood shows up best. In fatty areas, dark blood shows up best. For cardiac imaging, MR has many advantages over CT both in the ability to demonstrate blood flow without use of intravenous contrast as well as in the ability to demonstrate complex structures such as the heart and great vessels in several imaging planes (Fig. 9.18).

MR has limitations due to the strength of the magnetic field required to generate images. Many metallic devices, such as pacemakers or cochlear implants, cannot be brought into the scanner. Large, well-seated metallic objects such as spinal rods or hip replacements are not a problem. Smaller objects, however, such as vascular aneurysm clips or recent surgical clips, are unsafe in the magnetic field, which may cause them to move within the body. Certain types of tattoos may heat up in the magnet, leading to skin burns (53). Most MR suites have metal detectors on entry, and patients must fill out a detailed questionnaire before being allowed inside the scanner room.

In the oncologic setting, there are several areas in which MR may give complementary or additional information relative to CT. In the liver, characterization of cystic lesions, hemangiomas, and other types of nodular liver disease may be better with MR than with CT (54,55). However, for routine follow-up of liver metastases, CT offers lower cost and better spatial resolution. In the adrenal, MR's ability to characterize the presence or absence of fat can be particularly useful in evaluation of small adrenal masses, which are often due to benign adenomas (56,57). These adenomas often contain enough intracytoplasmic lipid to allow a specific diagnosis to be made with MR, unlike CT. In the breast, mammography, ultrasound, and MR are somewhat complementary, but in the setting of the postoperative breast or in patients with dense breasts, MR can sometimes show lesions that are invisible on mammography and ultrasound (58,59).

Imaging Specific Anatomic Areas

Thoracic Imaging

The chest is one of the commonest areas of the body involved in non-Hodgkin's lymphoma. The chest radiograph remains a simple, quick, and cost-effective way to follow thoracic involvement with lymphoma. Areas on the chest film in which abnormalities may be missed include the cardiophrenic region, the subcarinal area, and the posterior mediastinum (3,60,61). The cardiophrenic angle is a particularly important site to examine carefully on chest films as well as on CT, because this is often the region of the edge of a radiation field and may be an early site for recurrence after treatment with a mantle field (Fig. 9.19). Subtle diffuse lung abnormalities, particularly interstitial findings, may be missed on plain films

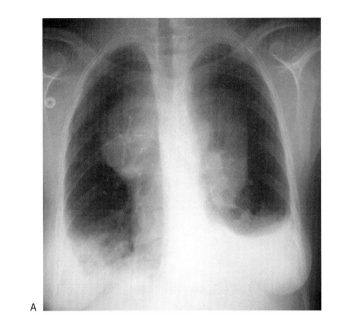

A

FIG. 9.18. 33-year-old woman with neck swelling and chest x-ray **(A)** showing large lobular anterior mediastinal mass and bilateral pleural effusions. Biopsy revealed mediastinal large B-cell non-Hodgkin's lymphoma. Coronal magnetic resonance image with bright blood technique **(B)** shows the lobular mass of intermediate signal intensity. Coronal image further posterior in the chest **(C)** shows dilated collateral vessels in the neck bilaterally (*arrows*) draining into an enlarged azygos vein (*arrowhead*). Sagittal magnetic resonance image **(D)** shows the entire course of the markedly dilated azygos providing collateral flow past the obstructed superior vena cava (*arrow*).

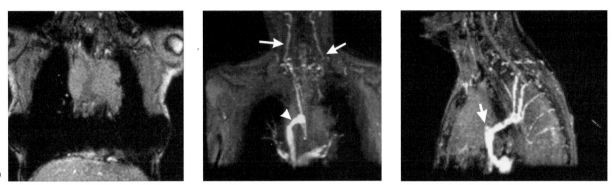

B,C,D

but are generally well demonstrated on CT (Fig. 9.20). Support lines that do not have obvious metallic markings may also be difficult to see on plain films. When assessing support lines, course, tip position, and contour must all be carefully assessed to exclude placement in aberrant locations (Fig. 9.21) or compromise of catheter lumen by bony structures (Fig.

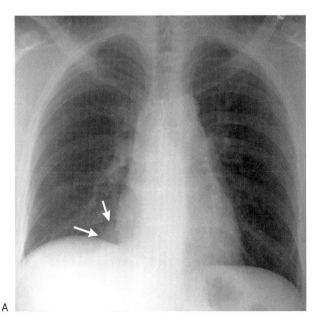

A

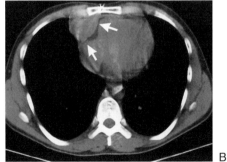

B

FIG. 9.19. Chest x-ray in a 25-year-old man 2 years after mediastinal irradiation for non-Hodgkin's lymphoma **(A)**. A rounded right cardiophrenic angle mass is evident (*arrows*), which represents a recurrence at the edge of the radiation field. The mass is more easily measured on computed tomography **(B)**, where it indents the right atrium (*arrows*).

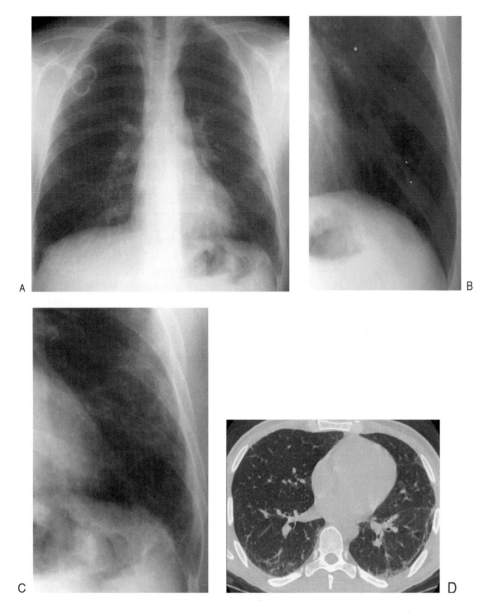

FIG. 9.20. Chest x-ray (A) in a patient after chemotherapy for stage 4B non-Hodgkin's lymphoma who had developed new shortness of breath. A Port-A-Cath is in place on the right. Subtle abnormal markings are present at the lung bases. Image B shows a close-up of the left lateral costophrenic region on a prior normal film for comparison to image C, which is a close-up of the left costophrenic region from the chest x-ray shown in A. Increased linear and reticular markings are evident that are suggestive of drug toxicity. Image D shows a high-resolution computed tomography scan at the lung bases, which confirms the subpleural linear and reticular findings in a bibasilar distribution that are characteristic of drug toxicity. Other differential possibilities include infiltration by lymphoma, bronchiolitis obliterans with organizing pneumonia, or viral infection.

9.22), which can ultimately result in breakage and embolization (62). Postprocessing of digital images to accentuate edges or to alter brightness and contrast may sometimes help visualize support lines in this setting.

Pulmonary lymphoma can have a variety of appearances, from nodules to interstitial thickening to dense airspace consolidation (63,64). Distribution of disease and specific patterns can sometimes help in the differential diagnosis of non-Hodgkin's lymphoma from infectious or inflammatory processes (65–67). Mosaic perfusion pattern in the lung parenchyma on high-resolution CT imaging can be seen in intravascular lymphoma (68) or bronchus-associated lymphoma (67), but can also be seen in pulmonary embolism or small airways disease related to drug toxicity. Pulmonary lymphoma can also present as ground-glass opacities or diffuse nodules, which are more common in lymphoma occurring in the setting of immune compromise (Fig. 9.23).

It is unusual for untreated non-Hodgkin's lymphoma nodes to contain calcification (Fig. 9.24), although calcification is not rare after treatment (69,70). Overall, calcification is seen more often in treated Hodgkin's disease than in non-Hodgkin's lymphoma. Whereas Hodgkin's disease most often is localized to the anterior mediastinum with contiguous spread to other nodal groups, non-Hodgkin's lymphoma often involves other sites in the chest in a discontinuous manner (Fig. 9.25). In particular, non-Hodgkin's lymphoma that develops in the setting of the acquired immunodeficiency syndrome (AIDS) or after transplant may involve unusual sites or be extranodal in location (71–73) or limited to serosal surfaces (74). Pulmonary involvement is common in the late stages of non-Hodgkin's lymphoma but is rare as an isolated presenting site (Fig. 9.26). Primary pulmonary non-Hodgkin's lymphoma may be identical in appearance to infection on both chest radiographs and CT, with air-bronchograms and ill-defined lobar or sublobar distribution.

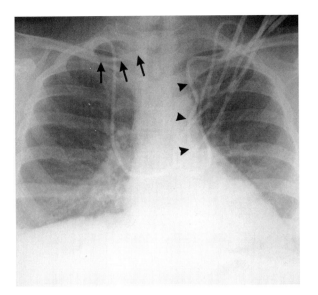

FIG. 9.21. Chest x-ray in a patient with non-Hodgkin's lymphoma after placement of bilateral Hickman catheters for chemotherapy. The catheter on the right has an unusual horizontal course toward the midline (*arrows*), most consistent with either extravascular placement or placement in a small tributary of the jugular system. The left catheter passes inferiorly to the left of midline (*arrowheads*), most likely lying in a left superior vena cava or a tributary of the left brachiocephalic vein. Contrast venography confirmed the right catheter to lie in the anterior jugular vein and the left to lie in the internal mammary vein, both requiring repositioning.

For imaging of chest wall involvement with lymphoma, MR or CT are similar in their ability to demonstrate extent of disease (75). For bony lesions, MR generally demonstrates marrow involvement better than CT at presentation (76), although signal abnormalities in the marrow cavity on MR after treatment may be more problematic. In patients with both bony and adjacent soft-tissue involvement with non-Hodgkin's lymphoma, soft-tissue masses may resolve with treatment, but MR abnormalities may remain in the marrow with no other evidence of persistent disease (18). For demonstration of both soft-tissue masses and marrow involvement, MR is preferred over CT (Fig. 9.27) and is also more useful in determining extent of disease in pure soft-tissue lymphoma for radiation treatment planning (Fig. 9.28).

Abdominal Imaging

Involvement of the abdomen with non-Hodgkin's lymphoma can be seen as enlarged nodes, most often retroperitoneal, or as involvement of parenchymal organs, serosal surfaces, or bony structures. Nodal involvement with non-Hodgkin's lymphoma is most often of uniform soft tissue density on CT but may be necrotic or of mixed attenuation in up to 25% of cases (Fig. 9.29) and probably indicates more aggressive disease and worse prognosis (77,78). Some studies have suggested that dynamic contrast-enhanced CT with spiral scanners may also allow classification of lym-

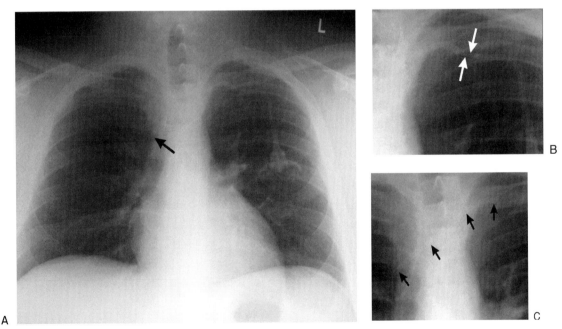

FIG. 9.22. Chest x-ray **(A)** in a patient with a left Port-A-Cath in place for chemotherapy of non-Hodgkin's lymphoma, with the tip in the expected position of the superior vena cava (*arrow*). Close-up view of the catheter **(B)** reveals that it is narrowed at the point of passage between the clavicle and the first anterior rib to enter the chest (*arrows*). After removal of the port, close-up of the same region on follow-up chest x-ray **(C)** shows that the catheter has separated at the narrowed region, with the more distal fragment remaining intravascularly (*arrows*), requiring interventional angiographic removal.

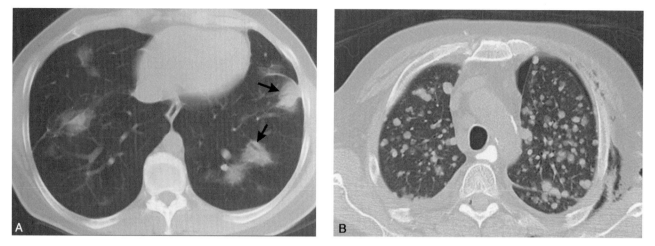

FIG. 9.23. High-resolution computed tomography scans of two different patients with pulmonary non-Hodgkin's lymphoma. In image **A**, ill-defined areas of ground-glass opacity are present, some with air-bronchograms (*arrows*). In image **B**, a patient after left lung transplantation, innumerable well-defined nodules are present, along with small left pneumothorax and subcutaneous emphysema from persistent air leak after the surgery.

phomatous nodes based on their vascularity and permeability (79). CT is preferable to ultrasound for assessment of liver and splenic disease, and calculation of splenic volume on serial scans may be used as a predictor of response and relapse in some cases (80). For involvement of the liver by non-Hodgkin's lymphoma, imaging is often done with a combination of CT, ultrasound, and MR, but none are generally specific, and pathologic confirmation is usually needed to establish the diagnosis (81). Spiral CT is the imaging modality of choice for pancreatic lymphoma (Fig. 9.30) as well as renal lymphoma (82), which can present as single or multiple masses, diffuse enlargement, or perinephric disease (Fig. 9.31). Mesenteric involvement is important to distinguish from retroperitoneal nodal involvement on CT, because this has significance for radiation planning and prognosis (Fig. 9.32).

Imaging of Head and Neck and Central Nervous System

Primary central nervous system lymphoma is a rare disease that has been on the rise in the last two decades partly but not entirely due to an increase in AIDS- and transplant-related

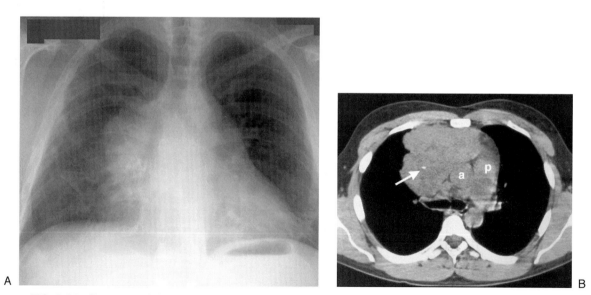

FIG. 9.24. Chest x-ray **(A)** in a 36-year-old patient with mediastinal large B-cell non-Hodgkin's lymphoma before treatment. Large lobular mass extends primarily to the right of midline. Computed tomography scan at the level of the carina **(B)** reveals slight heterogeneity in density of the mass with a tiny focal area of calcification (*arrow*). The mass displaces the ascending aorta (a) and pulmonary artery (p) posteriorly.

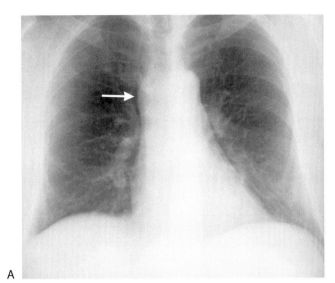

FIG. 9.25. Chest x-ray **(A)** in a middle-aged patient with follicular non-Hodgkin's lymphoma showing abnormal convexity (*arrow*) in the region of the ascending aorta. Computed tomography image in the upper chest **(B)** reveals large right axillary nodes (n) extending into the subpectoral region. Computed tomography image at the level of the aortic arch **(C)** reveals lower right axillary nodes (n) as well as right paratracheal adenopathy (*arrow*) corresponding to the chest radiographic finding and representing involvement of discontinuous nodal groups. Computed tomography image at the level of the diaphragms **(D)** reveals additional enlarged nodes in the anterior cardiophrenic regions bilaterally (*arrow*).

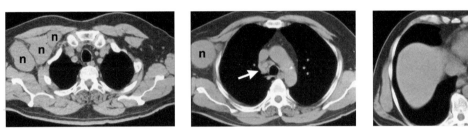

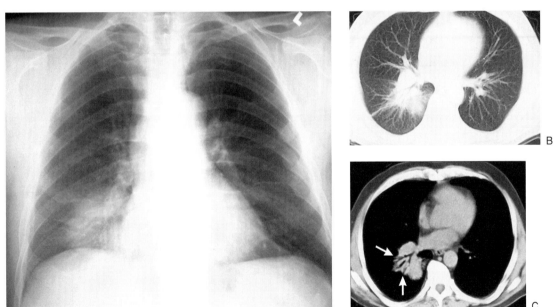

FIG. 9.26. Chest x-ray **(A)** in a 51-year-old patient with shortness of breath and night sweats. An ill-defined airspace opacity is present at the right base with an appearance suggestive of pneumonia; however, no change was noted in more than 1 month of antibiotic therapy. Chest computed tomography images viewed with lung **(B)** and mediastinal **(C)** windows show very ill-defined margins of the lesion and central air-bronchograms (*arrows*). The main differential diagnostic possibilities include infection (unlikely given the clinical scenario), bronchoalveolar carcinoma, alveolar sarcoid, or lymphoma. Transbronchial biopsy revealed non-Hodgkin's lymphoma.

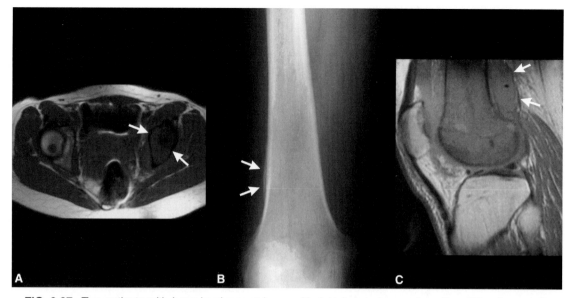

FIG. 9.27. Two patients with bony involvement by non-Hodgkin's lymphoma show the utility of magnetic resonance imaging. In image **A**, a 41-year-old patient with left hip pain who had a normal hip and pelvis on plain films underwent magnetic resonance imaging. This T1-weighted image shows normal high signal from marrow fat on the right, but low signal on the left (*arrows*) due to diffuse marrow infiltration that was not evident on plain films. In image **B**, a 56-year-old patient had severe right knee pain and a plain film showing only very subtle periosteal reaction (*arrow*) along the distal lateral border of the right femur. On knee magnetic resonance imaging **(C)**, the marrow signal throughout the femur is abnormal compared to the normal tibia and patella, with a large posterior soft-tissue mass (*arrows*), which was not evident on the plain films.

central nervous system lymphoma. It accounts for 6.6% to 15.4% of all primary brain tumors (83,84) and occurs in approximately 10% of the AIDS population. One-third of systemic lymphoma patients ultimately develop secondary brain and spine disease (85).

Central nervous system lymphoma is almost exclusively of the non-Hodgkin's type, the majority (>80%) of which are of B-cell phenotype. Histologically, these cases are identical to systemic extranodal non-Hodgkin's lymphoma and have similar classification. The origin of primary central nervous system lymphoma is unclear, as the central nervous system is devoid of lymphatic and lymphoid tissue. The microglia have been proposed as a source, although this also remains controversial. The immunocompromised population is at risk for the development of central nervous system lymphoma, including patients with prior organ transplantation and AIDS, and other immuno-deficient patients. It has been reported that Epstein-Barr virus appears to be primarily associated with central nervous system lymphoma patients in the AIDS population. One- and 3-year survival rates were 29% and 7.8%, respectively, and concurrent immunosuppression is the most important predictor of outcome (86). Immunocompromised patients are also younger (30s and 40s), often male, and tend to present with multiple lesions that are often of the diffuse large-cell subtype. In contrast immunocompetent patients are often older than 65, with an equal distribution of males and females, and with

lesions that are often periventricular in location (87), Primary central nervous system lymphoma almost always remains confined to nervous system with only occasional reports of systemic metastasis (88).

The most frequent locations of central nervous system lymphoma are supratentorial (85%), including cerebral hemispheres, followed by corpus callosum, basal ganglia, and, rarely, cerebellum. Other more unusual sites are ocu-

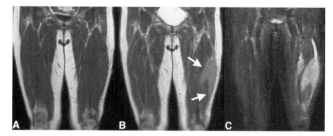

FIG. 9.28. Middle-aged patient with painless left thigh swelling, found on biopsy to represent high-grade B-cell non-Hodgkin's lymphoma. Plain films were normal. Image **A** shows the nonenhanced T1-weighted coronal image through the mid-thighs, with only subtle abnormality of signal in the left quadriceps region. Image **B** shows the appearance at the same level after intravenous administration of gadolinium. An enhancing mass (*arrows*) is now more evident. Image **C** shows the T2-weighted image, which demonstrates the extent of edema infiltrating through fascial planes from this mass.

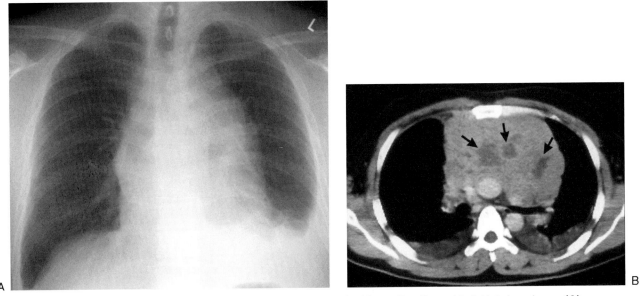

FIG. 9.29. Chest x-ray of 35-year-old man with mediastinal large B-cell non-Hodgkin's lymphoma **(A)**, showing large left pleural effusion and large mediastinal mass extending to the right and left of midline. On contrast-enhanced computed tomography image **(B)**, the mass contains areas of central necrosis (*arrows*) and displaces mediastinal vascular structures posteriorly.

lar and spinal cord (89). Subarachnoid space involvement is often seen in recurrent disease. Intracranial metastasis from systemic lymphoma may present as dural or leptomeningeal disease with or without parenchymal involvement. It is unusual for parenchymal lesions to occur in the absence of leptomeningeal disease (90). Tumor may also extend beyond the dura into the skull in rare instances. CT is adequate as the initial modality for detection of central nervous system lymphoma (Fig. 9.33). MR, however, is superior in delineating leptomeningeal involvement (both brain and spine), skull base disease, and small anatomic sites such as orbit, cavernous sinus, and cranial nerves (Fig. 9.34). On imaging, lymphoma often appears as high attenuation on CT and iso- or low signal on T2-weighted MR sequence (91), thought to be secondary to dense cellularity and cells having a high nuclear to cytoplasmic ratio. This is useful in distinguishing lymphoma from other brain tumors that are more likely to show T2 prolongation. Exceptions are other small round-cell tumors such as medulloblastoma, pinealoblastoma, and neuroblastoma.

With both CT and MR, most (92% to 100%) central nervous system lymphoma cases show contrast enhancement (91–93). Lack of enhancement has been reported in those patients who have received prior steroid therapy (93). There are reports of 74% homogeneous and approximately 12% ring-enhancing pattern in central nervous system lymphoma in the immunocompetent population. This is in contrast to approximately 50% rim enhancement with high T2 signal in immunocompromised patients due to a higher incidence of necrosis (87). This may be due in part to the

fact that central nervous system lymphoma often falls into the intermediate- to high-grade category, particularly the diffuse large-cell and immunoblastic subtypes in these patients (94).

Overall, approximately half of patients present with multiple lesions with a slightly higher rate of multifocal disease in AIDS patients (60%) (91,95,96). Contiguity to the ependymal and meningeal surfaces is also slightly more common in this population. Primary central nervous system lymphoma usually does not calcify or show hemorrhage and tends to have less edema when compared to primary glioma

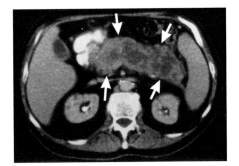

FIG. 9.30. Computed tomography at the level of the pancreas in a 69-year-old patient with abdominal pain and a history of treated follicular non-Hodgkin's lymphoma. The pancreas (*arrows*) is markedly enlarged and heterogeneous in density due to diffuse infiltration with non-Hodgkin's lymphoma, proven to be an aggressive large-cell type on biopsy. No retroperitoneal adenopathy or other sites of disease in the abdomen were present.

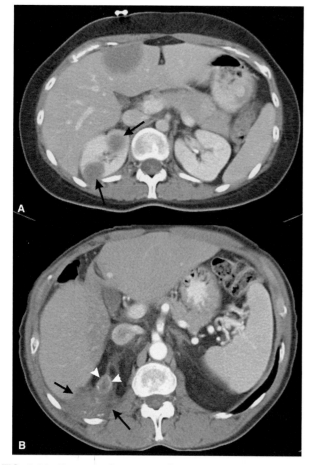

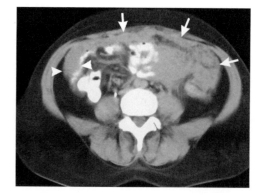

FIG. 9.32. Computed tomography scan without intravenous contrast in a middle-aged patient with non-Hodgkin's lymphoma and abdominal pain. Diffuse infiltration of the omentum is present (*arrows*), as well as more focal masses (*arrowheads*). A right ureteral stent is present due to hydronephrosis. No nodal disease is evident.

FIG. 9.31. Computed tomography scans of two patients with renal involvement by non-Hodgkin's lymphoma. In image **A**, multiple focal, relatively low-attenuation lesions are present in the right kidney (*arrows*) without hydronephrosis or retroperitoneal adenopathy. There is also a large area of focal infiltration of the liver by non-Hodgkin's lymphoma. In image **B**, non-Hodgkin's lymphoma is present in the perinephric tissues of the right kidney (*arrows*), infiltrating into the posterior abdominal wall and inferior tip of the right lobe of the liver. The top of the right kidney is indicated by the arrowheads.

or metastasis, perhaps due to their more infiltrative nature. It is also important to emphasize that areas of nonenhancement or "edema" do not necessarily exclude the presence of disease (97). In the immunocompromised population, a diffuse white matter disease involvement requires differentiation from similar imaging findings due to human immunodeficiency virus encephalopathy or progressive multifocal leukoencephalopathy. These two entities, however, tend not to exhibit enhancement. In cases of multiple enhancing lesions, toxoplasmosis should also be considered. Other diseases that need to be considered include sarcoidosis if there is meningeal enhancement of the basal cisterns, glioblastoma multiforme, and metastasis for corpus callosal involvement.

As mentioned above, a frequently encountered problem in AIDS patients is differentiating central nervous system lym-

phoma from toxoplasmosis. Due to the low sensitivity and specificity of the polymerase chain reaction test for toxoplasmosis (50% sensitivity in the central nervous system) and Epstein-Barr virus titers for lymphoma, patients are empirically treated with pyrimethamine and sulfadiazine for 2 to 4 weeks. Imaging characteristics can be similar in both, barring the classic description of toxoplasmosis as more often involving the basal ganglia and corticomedullary junction versus lymphoma with a more periventricular and callosal location. In recent years, both thallium 201 (a potassium analog taken up by active transport in growing cells) and MR perfusion imaging have been cited as potential methods to differentiate between these two diseases. Unlike toxoplasmosis, central nervous system lymphoma shows increased thallium 201 uptake as well as increased perfusion and blood volume due to hypercellularity (98,99). Another series showed that, even though the perfusion parameter in lymphoma is higher than in toxoplasmosis, it is still lower than that of glioblastoma multiforme (100). PET 18F-deoxyglucose imaging reflects metabolic activity and is shown to have increased uptake in lymphoma (101). Difficulty arises, however, when central nervous system lymphoma is necrotic or if the lesion is too small (6–8 mm) or in close proximity to large vessels, whereby these methods are rendered less effective (102). A more detailed description of the role of nuclear medicine in lymphoma can be found in Chapter 10.

With the recent advent of MR spectroscopy (Fig. 9.35) (a technique that generates a frequency spectrum making use of different resonant frequencies of protons subjected to different local magnetic fields), it has been shown that toxoplasmosis demonstrates elevated lactate and lipid (1.3 ppm) peaks due to an acellular and anaerobic environment as is seen in a necrotic abscess. Lymphoma, on the other hand, may reveal moderately elevated lactate and lipid peaks (areas of necrosis) but also demonstrate elevated choline level (high membrane turnover) due to hypercellularity (103).

Patients with untreated primary central nervous system lymphoma have an average survival of 1.5 months; average sur-

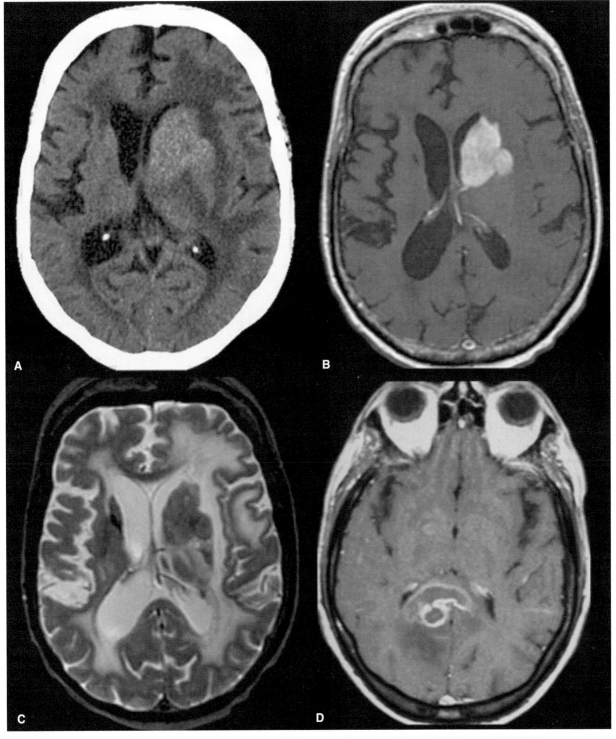

FIG. 9.33. Left basal ganglia lymphoma shows high attenuation on axial computed tomography **(A)**, homogeneous enhancement after gadolinium T1 **(B)**, and low signal on T2-weighted magnetic resonance images **(C)**. (Case courtesy of Dr. Alvand Hassankhani.) **D:** Typical irregular enhancement of lymphoma involving the splenium of corpus callosum on magnetic resonance imaging. FLAIR, fluid-attenuated inversion recovery; NEX, averages; TE, echo time; TR, repetition time.

Magnetic resonance imaging parameters for figures 9.33–9.38:

T1: TR 500 ms; TE 20 ms; 5 mm skip 0; 256 × 192; 2 NEX

T2: TR 2,900 ms; TE 96 ms; 5 mm skip 1 mm; 256 × 192; 2 NEX

FLAIR: TR 8,002 ms; TE 133 ms; 5 mm skip 1 mm; 256 × 160; 1 NEX

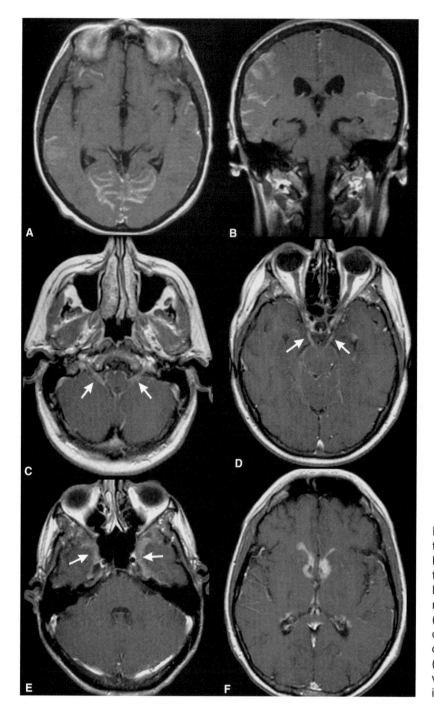

FIG. 9.34. A,B: Axial and coronal T1 postcontrast magnetic resonance images demonstrate linear sulcal enhancement consistent with leptomeningeal disease. Axial T1 postgadolinium lower **(C)** and higher **(D)** slices show enhancement of cranial nerves IX, X, XI (*arrows*), and III (*arrows*), respectively and bilaterally. **E:** Bilateral dural enhancement along the medial middle cranial fossa on post-contrast T1 MR image (*arrows*). **F:** Homogeneous ependymal and intraventricular enhancement from lymphomatous involvement.

vival for treated patients is approximately 45 months for those with solitary lesions, 9 months for those with multiple lesions, and 7.5 months for those with meningeal and subependymal disease. Steroid therapy has been shown to cause rapid regression of lesions within 8 hours after administration (93).

Both Hodgkin's and non-Hodgkin's lymphoma can occur in the head and neck region, including extranodal lymphatic sites. The most common site is Waldeyer's ring (adenoids, palatine, and lingual tonsils/tongue base), followed by sinus, nasal cavity, nodal sites, and, occasionally, salivary gland (parotid mostly) and orbit (Fig. 9.36). Cross-sectional imag-

ing can be particularly important in these areas for planning radiation fields, particularly in the orbit and parotid. The majority (approximately 75%) of head and neck lymphoma is of the non-Hodgkin's variety and, often, the histiocytic subtype for extranodal sites. It is second only to squamous cell carcinoma as the most common head and neck cancer. Almost 50% of extranodal lymphoma of head and neck patients has associated nodal disease, and 20% present with systemic symptoms (104). Painless nodal enlargement is a common presentation. Sex, age, and histology are not significant prognostic factors. Patients with disease in Waldeyer's

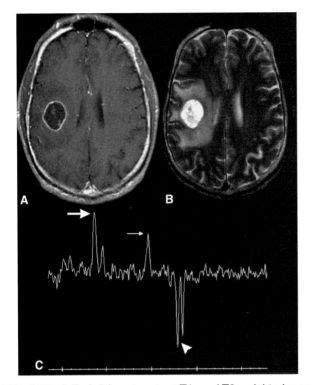

FIG. 9.35. A,B: Axial postcontrast T1- and T2-weighted magnetic resonance images show necrotic rim-enhancing high T2–signal lymphoma at the right posterior frontal lobe with surrounding edema. C: The corresponding single-voxel spectroscopy shows inversion of lactate/lipid peak at 1.3 ppm at TE (echo time) of 135 ms, reflecting necrosis (*arrowhead*). The choline peak at 3.25 ppm (*large arrow*) is also elevated relative to *N*-acetylaspartate peak at 2 ppm (*small arrow*).

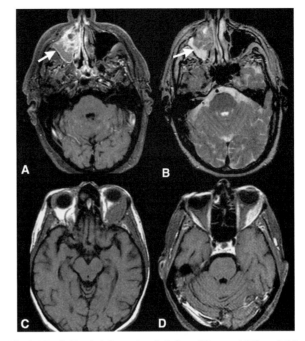

FIG. 9.36. A,B: Axial postgadolinium T1- and T2-weighted magnetic resonance images show lymphoma of right maxillary sinus (enhancing and low signal on T2) with postobstructive fluid (*arrow*) seen as nonenhancing area with high T2 signal. C,D: Pre- (without fat saturation) and post- (with fat saturation) gadolinium axial T1 images show left lateral intraorbital lymphoma. Intraorbital fat acts as intrinsic contrast to assist in disease localization on noncontrast image but can obscure enhancing lesion if fat saturation is not applied after gadolinium.

ring have less favorable staging and slightly worse overall survival (105). Tumor size may have prognostic significance (106), and CT and MR offer the most accurate measures of tumor diameter. Five-year survival for Hodgkin's disease in the head and neck is 73% versus 43% to 48% for non-Hodgkin's lymphoma. There may also be survival differences depending on nodal versus extranodal sites of involvement (107), and both CT and MR offer relatively accurate determination of nodal versus extranodal disease. Primary lymphoma of the maxilla and mandible has also been described (108) with the endemic form of Burkitt's lymphoma in central Africa associated with Epstein-Barr virus, whereas the nonendemic North American type has no such association. Radiation is often the primary treatment for localized low-grade disease, with combined chemotherapy and radiation reserved for advanced and high-grade lymphoma.

On imaging, nodal sizes are variable, although central necrosis may occur, but much less frequently than nodal metastasis from other primary cancers. Calcification is also rare in lymphomatous nodes and is usually a sequela to radiation. Otherwise, tuberculosis, thyroid cancer metastasis and mucin-producing nodal metastasis should be considered in

the differential diagnosis of cervical adenopathy. Nodal sites usually show mild to moderate homogeneous enhancement on CT and MR in non-Hodgkin's lymphoma. T1 post contrast with fat suppression MR sequence has proved useful in facilitating the identification of neck nodes. In general, neither CT nor MR can definitely differentiate lymphomatous nodal involvement from metastatic disease.

Lymphomatous involvement of the spine can be primary or secondary to systemic disease, comprising approximately 40% in an autopsy series (109). Bony changes are often of the lytic or moth-eaten variety with rare sclerotic lesions. MR is especially useful in detecting disease in the spine, particularly cord compression from bony disease and dural or epidural involvement (Fig. 9.37). As is often said, MR is sensitive but nonspecific for marrow involvement by lymphoma. Areas of involvement can appear as low signal on T1 with variable signal on T2 sequences. The heterogeneous spectrum of marrow signal can range from benign entities such as osteoporosis to hemangiomas to other metastases to marrow turnover secondary to posttreatment changes.

Finally, intravascular lymphomatosis, also known as *malignant angioendotheliomatosis*, is a rare but aggressive (average survival, 5 months) and high-grade non-Hodgkin's involve-

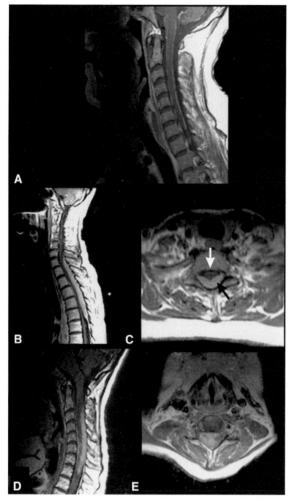

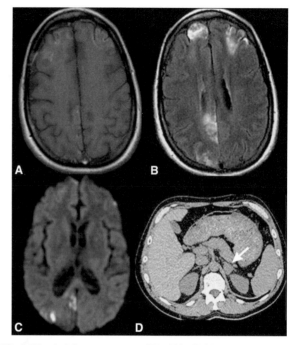

FIG. 9.38. Axial noncontrast T1 (A), fluid-attenuated inversion recovery (B), and diffusion (C) images show multiple areas of infarct at different stages (subacute in A, acute in C) in a patient with intravascular lymphoma. D: In the same patient, an axial computed tomography image of the abdomen shows disease involvement of the left adrenal gland (arrow).

FIG. 9.37. A: Linear enhancement (etching) along surface of spinal cord on sagittal postcontrast T1 image secondary to lymphomatous involvement of cerebrospinal fluid space. B,C: Sagittal and coronal postgadolinium T1 images show homogeneous epidural disease (black arrow) with anterior displacement and compression of the cord (white arrow). D,E: Sagittal and axial postcontrast T1 images demonstrate both intramedullary and intradural extramedullary lymphomatous involvement.

ment of the central nervous system (Fig. 9.38). Intravascular lymphomatosis was first described by Pfleger and Tappeiner in 1959 (110). It tends to occur in older patients (70s) and shows affinity for an endothelial membrane receptor. It is often (at least half of the time) diagnosed postmortem due to the very nonspecific clinical presentation (fever, malaise, weight loss, arthralgia, dementia, myelopathy, and neuropathy), imaging, and lab findings (anemia and elevated serum lactate dehydrogenase and erythrocyte sedimentation rate). Intravascular lymphomatosis is characterized by proliferation of large atypical lymphoid cells within the lumen of small vasculature (especially central nervous system and skin) causing narrowing and associated thrombosis and ischemic tissue changes. Intravascular lymphomatosis may involve other organs such as lung, kid-

ney, and adrenal glands with sparing of liver, spleen, lymph nodes, and bone marrow until the very late stages of disease. It is therefore not surprising that it is often difficult to differentiate intravascular lymphomatosis from central nervous system vasculitis, multiinfarct dementia, occult infection, and other entities in which vascular damage results in ischemic injury. To make diagnosis even more difficult, no circulating cells are present in the blood or cerebral spinal fluid. Both central nervous system vasculitis and intravascular lymphomatosis may involve small parenchymal and leptomeningeal vessels with multifocal ischemic lesions on imaging. In a large series of 79 patients by Domizio (111), 32% had central nervous system symptoms alone and 12% had both central nervous system and systemic findings with an average survival of 4 months.

On imaging of intravascular lymphomatosis, CT may show ischemic changes but is generally nonspecific. MR may show no abnormality, small-vessel ischemic pattern, or nonspecific white matter changes (112). Some authors have described a more diffuse deep white matter involvement in central nervous system vasculitis versus the subcortical and periventricular involvement of intravascular lymphomatosis (112–114). As is seen in acute infarct, areas of ischemic changes show bright signal on T2- and diffusion-weighted imaging, signifying cytotoxic edema and decreased apparent diffusion coefficient, respectively. Contrast MR does increase the sensitivity of brain and spine lesions, although enhancement can be patchy or linear and often subtle or small. Conventional arteriogram is also inadequate in the differentiation of central nervous system vasculitis from intravascular lymphomatosis, as both can be normal or show focal areas of stenosis or dilatation. Biopsy is often the only means for tissue diagnosis. Interestingly, in one series, approximately 60% of patients with intravascular lymphomatosis had involvement of the adrenal glands at autopsy (115). Due to the confounding clinical picture and rapid progression of intravascular lymphomatosis, many patients die before biopsy can even be performed. There can be a transient response to steroids, and there have been a few reports of favorable outcome after chemotherapy (113,116).

In summary, central nervous system lymphoma has a variable appearance on imaging both in distribution, signal characteristics, and enhancing pattern. In the brain, central nervous system lymphoma can be of different density and intensity on CT and T2-weighted MR sequences, although diagnosis is most specific if the tumor appears hyperdense on CT and hypointense on T2-weighted MR sequence. Enhancement is more homogeneous with fewer lesions and is more often periventricular in immunocompetent patients. In the AIDS population, central nervous system lymphoma is more often multiple and diffuse and with rim enhancement due to a higher tendency for necrosis. The rare intravascular lymphomatosis is even more difficult to diagnose with nonspecific imaging patterns resembling other entities such as central nervous system vasculitis, multiinfarct dementia, or other causes of ischemic injury. Finally, primary central nervous system lymphoma and secondary involvement from systemic disease are indistinguishable by imaging.

REFERENCES

1. Porcu P, Nichols CR. Evaluation and management of the "new" lymphoma entities: mantle cell lymphoma, lymphoma of mucosa-associated lymphoid tissue, anaplastic large-cell lymphoma and primary mediastinal B-cell lymphoma. Curr Probl Cancer 1998;22:283–368.
2. Baris D, Zahm SH. Epidemiology of lymphomas. Curr Opin Oncol 2000;12:383–394.
3. Romano M, Libshitz HI. Hodgkin disease and non-Hodgkin lymphoma: plain chest radiographs and chest computed tomography of thoracic involvement in previously untreated patients. Radiol Med 1998;95:49–53.
4. Diehl LF, Hopper KD, Giguere J, et al. The pattern of intrathoracic Hodgkin's disease assessed by computed tomography. J Clin Oncol 1991;9:438–443.
5. Young NA, Al-Saleem T. Diagnosis of lymphoma by fine-needle aspiration cytology using the revised European-American classification of lymphoid neoplasms. Cancer 1999;87:325–345.
6. Wang YX, Jia YF, Chen KM, et al. Radiographic contrast media induced nephropathy: experimental observations and the protective effect of calcium channel blockers. Br J Radiol 2001;74:1103–1108.
7. Morcos SK, Thomsen HS, Webb JA. Contrast Media Safety Committee of the European Society of Urogenital Radiology. Prevention of generalized reactions to contrast media: a consensus report and guidelines. Eur Radiol 2001;11:1720–1728.
8. Runge VM. Safety of magnetic resonance contrast media. Top Magn Reson Imaging 2001;12:309–314.
9. Bangerter M, Griesshammer M, Bergmann L. Progress in medical imaging of lymphoma and Hodgkin's disease. Curr Opin Oncol 1999;11:339–342.
10. Kostakoglu L, Goldsmith SJ. Positron emission tomography in lymphoma: comparison with computed tomography and Gallium-67 single photon emission computed tomography. Clin Lymphoma 2000; 1:67–74, discussion 75–66.
11. Elis A, Blickstein D, Klein O, et al. Detection of relapse in non-Hodgkin's lymphoma: role of routine followup studies. Am J Hematol 2002;69:41–44.
12. Boger-Megiddo I, Apter S, Spencer JA, et al. Is chest CT sufficient for follow-up of primary mediastinal B-cell lymphoma in remission? AJR Am J Roentgenol 2002;178:165–167.
13. Oh YK, Ha CS, Samuels BI, et al. Stages I-III follicular lymphoma: role of CT of the abdomen and pelvis in follow-up studies. Radiology 1999;210:483–486.
14. Takagi S, Tsunoda S, Tanaka O. Bone marrow involvement in lymphoma: the importance of marrow magnetic resonance imaging. Leuk Lymphoma 1998;29:515–522.
15. Sohaib SA, Turner B, Hanson JA, et al. CT assessment of tumour response to treatment: comparison of linear, cross-sectional and volumetric measures of tumour size. Br J Radiol 2000;73:1178–1184.
16. Bangerter M, Kotzerke J, Griesshammer M, et al. Positron emission tomography with 18-fluorodeoxyglucose in the staging and follow-up of lymphoma in the chest. Acta Oncol 1999;38:799–804.
17. Hopper KD, Diehl LF, Lynch JC, et al. Mediastinal bulk in Hodgkin disease. Method of measurement versus prognosis. Invest Radiol 1991;26:1101–1110.
18. Yuki M, Narabayashi I, Yamamoto K, et al. Multifocal primary lymphoma of bone: scintigraphy and MR findings before and after treatment. Radia Med 2000;18:305–310.
19. Bick U, Lenzen H. PACS: the silent revolution. Eur Radiol 1999;9:1152–1160.
20. Reiner B, Siegel E. Understanding financing options for PACS implementation. Picture archiving and communication systems. J Digit Imaging 2000;13:49–54.
21. Strickland NH. Review article: some cost-benefit considerations for PACS: a radiological perspective. Br J Radiol 1996;69:1089–1098.
22. Babu RD, Damodaran D. Primary malignant intestinal lymphoma. Trop Gastroenterol 2001;22:113–116.
23. Kuhns LR, Roubal S. Should intravenous contrast be used for chest CT in children with nonlymphomatous extrathoracic malignancies? Pediatr Radiol 1995;25:S184–S186.
24. Cascade PN, Gross BH, Kazerooni EA, et al. Variability in the detection of enlarged mediastinal lymph nodes in staging lung cancer: a comparison of contrast-enhanced and unenhanced CT. AJR Am J Roentgenol 1998;170:927–931.
25. Kuszyk BS, Bluemke DA, Urban BA, et al. Portal-phase contrast-enhanced helical CT for the detection of malignant hepatic tumors: sensitivity based on comparison with intraoperative and pathologic findings. AJR Am J Roentgenol 1996;166:91–95.
26. Kirchgeorg MA, Prokop M. Increasing spiral CT benefits with post-processing applications. Eur J Radiol 1998;28:39–54.
27. Brink JA. Technical aspects of helical (spiral) CT. Radiol Clin North Am 1995;33:825–841.
28. Fuchs T, Kachelriess M, Kalender WA. Technical advances in multi-slice spiral CT. Eur J Radiol 2000;36:69–73.
29. Charron M, Beyer T, Bohnen NN, et al. Image analysis in patients with cancer studied with a combined PET and CT scanner. Clin Nucl Med 2000;25:905–910.
30. Beyer T, Townsend DW, Brun T, et al. A combined PET/CT scanner for clinical oncology. J Nucl Med 2000;41:1369–1379.
31. Dupuy DE, Goldberg SN. Image-guided radiofrequency tumor ablation: challenges and opportunities—part II. J Vasc Interv Radiol 2001;12:1135–1148.
32. Cline HE, Hynynen K, Watkins RD, et al. Focused US system for MR imaging-guided tumor ablation. Radiology 1995;194:731–737.
33. Coakley FV, Lin RY, Schwartz LH, et al. Mesenteric adenopathy in patients with prostate cancer: frequency and etiology. AJR Am J Roentgenol 2002;178:125–127.
34. Theuws JC, Seppenwoolde Y, Kwa SL, et al. Changes in local pulmonary injury up to 48 months after irradiation for lymphoma and breast cancer. Int J Radiat Oncol Biol Phys 2000;47:1201–1208.
35. Berland LL. Slip-ring and conventional dynamic hepatic CT: contrast material and timing considerations. Radiology 1995;195:1–8.
36. Diederich S, Lentschig MG, Winter F, et al. Detection of pulmonary nodules with overlapping vs non-overlapping image reconstruction at spiral CT. Eur Radiol 1999;9:281-286.

37. Appelbaum AH, Kamba TT, Cohen AS, et al. Effectiveness and safety of image-directed biopsies. *South Med J* 2002;95:212–217.

38. Demharter J, Muller P, Wagner T, et al. Percutaneous core-needle biopsy of enlarged lymph nodes in the diagnosis and subclassification of malignant lymphomas. *Eur Radiol* 2001;11:276–283.

39. Gossot D, Girard P, de Kerviler E, et al. Thoracoscopy or CT-guided biopsy for residual intrathoracic masses after treatment of lymphoma. *Chest* 2001;120:289–294.

40. Fields S, Libson E. CT-guided aspiration core needle biopsy of gastrointestinal wall lesions. *J Comput Assist Tomogr* 2000;24:224–228.

41. Rickert D, Jecker P, Metzler V, et al. Color-coded duplex sonography of the cervical lymph nodes: improved differential diagnostic assessment after administration of the signal enhancer SH U 508A (Levovist). *Eur Arch Otorhinolaryngol* 2000;257:453–458.

42. Ahuja A, Ying M, King A, et al. Lymph node hilus: gray scale and power Doppler sonography of cervical nodes. *J Ultrasound Med* 2001;20:987–992.

43. Shirakawa T, Miyamoto Y, Yamagishi J, et al. Color/power Doppler sonographic differential diagnosis of superficial lymphadenopathy: metastasis, malignant lymphoma, and benign process. *J Ultrasound Med* 2001;20:525–532.

44. Ishida H, Konno K, Ishida J, et al. Splenic lymphoma: differentiation from splenic cyst with ultrasonography. *Abdom Imaging* 2001;26:529–532.

45. Restrepo-Schafer I, Wollenberg B, Riera-Knorrenschild J, et al. Partially reversed intrasplenic venous blood flow detected by color Doppler sonography in two patients with hematologic diseases and splenomegaly. *J Clin Ultrasound* 2001;29:294–297.

46. Lyons JA, Myles J, Pohlman B, et al. Treatment of prognosis of primary breast lymphoma: a review of 13 cases. *Am J Clin Oncol* 2000;23:334–336.

47. Kettenbach J, Silverman SG, Hata N, et al. Monitoring and visualization techniques for MR-guided laser ablations in an open MR system. *J Magn Reson Imaging* 1998;8:933–943.

48. Delfaut EM, Beltran J, Johnson G, et al. Fat suppression in MR imaging: techniques and pitfalls. *Radiographics* 1999;19:373–382.

49. Lee RF, Giaquinto R, Constantinides C, et al. A broadband phased-array system for direct phosphorus and sodium metabolic MRI on a clinical scanner. *Magn Reson Med* 2000;43:269–277.

50. Iriguchi N, Hasegawa J. Carbon-13 magnetic resonance imaging of a human arm. *Magn Reson Imaging* 1993;11:269–271.

51. Bellin MF, Beigelman C, Precetti-Morel S. Iron oxide-enhanced MR lymphography: initial experience. *Eur J Radiol* 2000;34:257–264.

52. Petersein J, Saini S, Weissleder R. Liver. II: Iron oxide-based reticuloendothelial contrast agents for MR imaging. Clinical review. *Magn Reson Imaging Clin N Am* 1996;4:53–60.

53. Kreidstein ML, Giguere D, Freiberg A. MRI interaction with tattoo pigments: case report, pathophysiology, and management. *Plast Reconstr Surg* 1997;99:1717–1720.

54. Martin DR, Semelka RC. Imaging of benign and malignant focal liver lesions. *Magn Reson Imaging Clin N Am* 2001;9:785–802, vi–vii.

55. Morrin MM, Rofsky NM. Techniques for liver MR imaging. *Magn Reson Imaging Clin N Am* 2001;9:675–696.

56. Siegelman ES. MR imaging of the adrenal neoplasms. *Magn Reson Imaging Clin N Am* 2000;8:769–786.

57. Weishaupt D, Debatin JF. Magnetic resonance: evaluation of adrenal lesions. *Curr Opin Urol* 1999;9:153–163.

58. Goscin CP, Berman CG, Clark RA. Magnetic resonance imaging of the breast. *Cancer Control* 2001;8:399–406.

59. Harms SE, Flamig DP. Breast MRI. *Clin Imaging* 2001;25:227–246.

60. Salonen O, Kivisaari L, Standertskjold-Nordenstam CG, et al. Chest radiography and computed tomography in the evaluation of mediastinal adenopathy in lymphoma. *Acta Radiol* 1987;28:747–750.

61. Sussman SK, Halvorsen RA Jr, Silverman PM, et al. Paracardiac adenopathy: CT evaluation. *AJR Am J Roentgenol* 1987;149:29–34.

62. Hinke DH, Zandt-Stastny DA, Goodman LR, et al. Pinch-off syndrome: a complication of implantable subclavian venous access devices. *Radiology* 1990;177:353–356.

63. Ooi GC, Chim CS, Lie AK, et al. Computed tomography features of primary pulmonary non-Hodgkin's lymphoma. *Clin Radiol* 1999;54:438–443.

64. King LJ, Padley SP, Wotherspoon AC, et al. Pulmonary MALT lymphoma: imaging findings in 24 cases. *Eur Radiol* 2000;10:1932–1938.

65. Honda O, Johkoh T, Ichikado K, et al. Differential diagnosis of lymphocytic interstitial pneumonia and malignant lymphoma on high-resolution CT. *AJR Am J Roentgenol* 1999;173:71–74.

66. Honda O, Johkoh T, Ichikado K, et al. Comparison of high resolution CT findings of sarcoidosis, lymphoma, and lymphangitic carcinoma: is there any difference of involved interstitium? *J Comput Assist Tomogr* 1999;23:374–379.

67. Lee IJ, Kim SH, Koo SH, et al. Bronchus-associated lymphoid tissue (BALT) lymphoma of the lung showing mosaic pattern of inhomogeneous attenuation on thin-section CT: a case report. *Korean J Radiol* 2000;1:159–161.

68. Walls JG, Hong YG, Cox JE, et al. Pulmonary intravascular lymphomatosis: presentation with dyspnea and air trapping. *Chest* 1999;115:1207–1210.

69. Cheng J, Castellino RA. Post-treatment calcification of mesenteric non-Hodgkin lymphoma: CT findings. *J Comput Assist Tomogr* 1989;13:64–66.

70. Lautin EM, Rosenblatt M, Friedman AC, et al. Calcification in non-Hodgkin lymphoma occurring before therapy: identification on plain films and CT. *AJR Am J Roentgenol* 1990;155:739–740.

71. Hamed KA, Hoffman MS. Primary esophageal lymphoma in AIDS. *AIDS Patient Care Stds* 1998;12:5–9.

72. Lin DW, Thorning DR, Krieger JN. Primary penile lymphoma: diagnostic difficulties and management options. *Urology* 1999;54:366.

73. Baschinsky DY, Weidner N, Baker PB, et al. Primary hepatic anaplastic large-cell lymphoma of T-cell phenotype in acquired immunodeficiency syndrome: a report of an autopsy case and review of the literature. *Am J Gastroenterol* 2001;96:227–232.

74. Ferrozzi F, Tognini G, Mulonzia NW, et al. Primary effusion lymphomas in AIDS: CT findings in two cases. *Eur Radiol* 2001;11:623–625.

75. Jeung MY, Gangi A, Gasser B, et al. Imaging of chest wall disorders. *Radiographics* 1999;19:617–637.

76. Altehoefer C, Blum U, Bathmann J, et al. Comparative diagnostic accuracy of magnetic resonance imaging and immunoscintigraphy for detection of bone marrow involvement in patients with malignant lymphoma. *J Clin Oncol* 1997;15:1754–1760.

77. Saito A, Takashima S, Takayama F, et al. Spontaneous extensive necrosis in non-Hodgkin lymphoma: prevalence and clinical significance. *J Comput Assist Tomogr* 2001;25:482–486.

78. Rodriguez M, Rehn SM, Nyman RS, et al. CT in malignancy grading and prognostic prediction of non-Hodgkin's lymphoma. *Acta Radiologica* 1999;40:191–197.

79. Dugdale PE, Miles KA, Bunce I, et al. CT measurement of perfusion and permeability within lymphoma masses and its ability to assess grade, activity, and chemotherapeutic response. *J Comput Assist Tomogr* 1999;23:540–547.

80. Daskalogiannaki M, Prassopoulos P, Katrinakis G, et al. Splenic involvement in lymphomas. Evaluation on serial CT examinations. *Acta Radiologica* 2001;42:326–332.

81. Maher MM, McDermott SR, Fenlon HM, et al. Imaging of primary non-Hodgkin's lymphoma of the liver. *Clin Radiol* 2001;56:295–301.

82. Urban BA, Fishman EK. Renal lymphoma: CT patterns with emphasis on helical CT. *Radiographics* 2000;20:197–212.

83. Eby NL, Grufferman S, Flannelly CM, et al. Increasing incidence of primary brain lymphoma in the US. *Cancer* 1988;62:2461–2465.

84. Schabet M. Epidemiology of primary CNS lymphoma. *J Neurooncol* 1999;43:199–201.

85. Barnard RO, Scott T. Patterns of proliferation in cerebral lymphoreticular tumours. *Acta Neuropathol* 1975;[Suppl]:125–130.

86. Nuckols JD, Liu K, Burchette JL, et al. Primary central nervous system lymphomas: a 30-year experience at a single institution. *Mod Pathol* 1999;12:1167–1173.

87. Johnson BA, Fram EK, Johnson PC, et al. The variable MR appearance of primary lymphoma of the central nervous system: comparison with histopathologic features. *AJR Am J Neuroradiol* 1997;18:563–572.

88. Brown MT, McClendon RE, Gockerman JP. Primary central nervous system lymphoma with systemic metastasis: case report and review. *J Neurooncol* 1995;23:207–221.

89. Buhring U, Herrlinger U, Krings, et al. MRI features of primary central nervous system lymphomas at presentation. *Neurology* 2001;57:393–396.

90. Russell DS, Rubinstein LJ. *Pathology of tumors of the nervous system*, 5th ed. Baltimore: Williams & Wilkins, 1989.

91. Roman-Goldstein SM, Goldman DL, Howieson J, et al. MR of primary CNS lymphoma in immunologically normal patients. *AJR Am J Neuroradiol* 1992;13:1207–1213.
92. Hochberg FH, Miller DC. Primary central nervous system lymphoma. *J Neurosurg* 1988;68:835–853.
93. Jack CR Jr, Reese DF, Scheithauer BW. Radiographic findings in 32 cases of primary CNS lymphoma. *AJR Am J Roentgenol* 1986;146: 271–276.
94. Cordoliani YS, Derosier C, Pharaboz C, et al. Primary brain lymphoma in AIDS. 17 cases studied by MRI before stereotaxic biopsies (French). *J Radiol* 1992;73:367–376.
95. Socie G, Piprot-Chauffat C, Schlienger M, et al. Primary lymphoma of the central nervous system. An unresolved therapeutic problem. *Cancer* 1990;65:322–326.
96. Goldstein JD, Zeifer B, Chao C, et al. CT appearance of primary CNS lymphoma in patients with acquired immunodeficiency syndrome. *J Comput Assist Tomogr* 1991;15:39–44.
97. Thomas M, MacPherson P. Computed tomography of intracranial lymphoma. *Clin Radiol* 1982;33:331–336.
98. Ernst TM, Chang L, Witt MD, et al. Cerebral toxoplasmosis and lymphoma in AIDS: perfusion MR imaging experience in 13 patients. *Radiology* 1998;208:663–669.
99. Ruiz A, Ganz WI, Post MJ, et al. Use of thallium-201 brain SPECT to differentiate cerebral lymphoma from toxoplasma encephalitis in AIDS patients. *AJR Am J Neuroradiol* 1994;15: 1885–1894.
100. Cha S, Knopp EA, Johnson G. Intracranial mass lesions: Dynamic contrast-enhanced susceptibility-weighted echo-planar perfusion MR imaging. *Radiology* 2002;223:1–29.
101. Hoffman JM, Waskin HA, Schifter T, et al. FDG-PET in differentiating lymphoma from nonmalignant central nervous system lesions in patients with AIDS. *J Nucl Med* 1993;34:567–575.
102. Kessler LS, Ruiz A, Donovan Post MJ, et al. Thallium-201 brain SPECT of lymphoma in AIDS patients: pitfalls and technique optimization. *AJR Am J Neuroradiol* 1998;19:1105–1109.
103. Chinn RJ, Wilkinson ID, Hall-Craggs MA, et al. Toxoplasmosis and primary central nervous system lymphoma in HIV infection: diagnosis with MR spectroscopy. *Radiology* 1995;197:649–654.
104. Hanna E, Wanamaker J, Adelstein D, et al. Extranodal lymphomas of the head and neck. A 20-year experience. *Arch Otolaryngol Head Neck Surg* 1997;123:1318–1323.
105. Economopoulos T, Asprou N, Stathakis N, et al. Primary extranodal non-Hodgkin's lymphoma of the head and neck. *Oncology* 1992;49:484–488.
106. Nathu RM, Mendenhall NP, Almasri NM, et al. Non-Hodgkin's lymphoma of the head and neck: a 30-year experience at the University of Florida. *Head Neck* 1999;21:247–254.
107. Rowley H, McRae RD, Cook JA, et al. Lymphoma presenting to a head and neck clinic. *Clin Otolaryngol* 1995;20:139–144.
108. Steg RF, Dahlin DC, Gores RJ. Malignant lymphoma of the mandible and maxillary region. *Oral Surg Oral Med Oral Pathol Oral Radiol Endod* 1959;2:128.
109. Fornasier VL, Horne JG. Metastases to the vertebral column. *Cancer* 1975;36:590–594.
110. Pfleger L, Tappeiner J. *Tappeiner J. Zur Kanntuis der Systemisierten Endotheliomatose der Cutanen Blutgefasse*. 1959:359–363.
111. Domizio P, Hall PA, Cotter F, et al. Angiotropic large cell lymphoma (ALCL): morphological, immunohistochemical and genotypic studies with analysis of previous reports. *Hematol Oncol* 1989;7:195–206.
112. Greenan TJ, Grossman RI, Goldberg HI. Cerebral vasculitis: MR imaging and angiographic correlation. *Radiology* 1992;182:65–72.
113. Calamia KT, Miller A, Shuster EA, et al. Intravascular lymphomatosis. A report of ten patients with central nervous system involvement and a review of the disease process. *Adv Exp Med Biol* 1999;455: 249–265.
114. Devlin T, Moll S, Hulette C, et al. Intravascular malignant lymphomatosis with neurologic presentation factors facilitating antemortem diagnosis. *South Med J* 1998;91:672–676.
115. Shimokawa M, Sato K, Michikawa M, et al. A case of angiotropic lymphoma diagnosed by adrenal biopsy (Japanese). *Rinsho Shinkeigaku* 1992;32:747–751.
116. Baumann TP, Hurwitz N, Karamitopolou-Diamantis E, et al. Diagnosis and treatment of intravascular lymphomatosis. *Arch Neurol* 2000;57:374–377.

CHAPTER 10

Nuclear Medicine

Annick D. Van den Abbeele, Stanislav Lechpammer, Richard J. Tetrault, and Ramsey D. Badawi

NUCLEAR MEDICINE APPLICATIONS IN ONCOLOGY

Nuclear medicine is an imaging modality that distinguishes itself from conventional radiologic imaging, such as x-ray, computed tomography (CT), and magnetic resonance imaging (MRI), by providing unique information on the metabolic function of the investigated organ, tissue, or system. Conventional imaging focuses on the anatomic structure and is dependent on structural changes in morphology or size. In nuclear medicine, subjects are injected or ingest radiopharmaceuticals designed to track a physiologic or pathophysiologic process. In this context, the radiopharmaceuticals may be described as radiotracers. The usefulness of nuclear medicine in investigating any particular organ or disease is based on the great diversity and biochemical properties of the available radiotracers. The majority of radiotracers consist of two distinct moieties: a carrying agent, which is responsible for the biodistribution of the tracer (e.g., [^{18}F]-2-fluoro-2-deoxy-D-glucose (FDG), a glucose analog), and a radioactive marker, which enables external detection (e.g., fluorine-18). Some radionuclide radiotracers, due to their biochemical properties, do not require a carrying agent (e.g., ^{67}Ga citrate, an iron analog, or ^{201}Tl thallous chloride, a potassium analog). Regardless of their structure, the common characteristic of all radiotracers is that they can be metabolized in certain physiologic or pathophysiologic processes that are correlated with physiologic or pathologic conditions of target organs or tissues (1–3).

To gain full insight into the role of nuclear medicine in the diagnosis and therapy of diseases, a basic knowledge of the specific methodology is required, as reviewed by Badawi (4). In brief, the simplest nuclear medicine imaging technique is planar imaging, which provides functional images in a two-dimensional format analogous to that obtained with plain film x-ray imaging. These are obtained on gamma camera systems equipped with scintillation detection material, typically sodium iodide scintillation crystals. Nuclear medicine imaging may also be performed using tomographic techniques, in which case the results are functional images in a three-dimensional format analogous to those obtained with CT or MRI (that is, cross-sectional slices throughout the body). This technique is known as *single-photon emission computed tomography* (SPECT). Finally, nuclear medicine imaging may also be performed using positron emission tomography (PET), which allows the use of positron-emitting radionuclides and a range of new radiotracers.

Nuclear oncology is a rapidly growing field within nuclear medicine. Its unique functional imaging capabilities are highly complementary to morphologic imaging, and it has become an integral part of the multidisciplinary clinical management of patients with cancer. Contemporary roles of nuclear oncology in the assessment of cancer patients are summarized in Table 10.1. The introduction of PET and its increasing use and application in various types of cancer has also shown that nuclear oncology is becoming a vehicle to extend functional imaging from the cellular to the molecular domain.

This chapter focuses on nuclear medicine imaging techniques and therapeutic procedures used in the management of patients with non-Hodgkin's lymphoma. Summarized are applications of nonspecific lymphoma radiotracers, such as ^{67}Ga citrate, ^{201}Tl thallous chloride, and ^{99m}Tc sestamibi. Part of the chapter is devoted to a review of the growing role of PET in the overall management of lymphomas. Details regarding the imaging protocols for each of these radiopharmaceuticals are listed in Table 10.2. The role of nuclear medicine in the context of radioimmunotherapy of lymphomas is also discussed.

^{67}GA CITRATE IMAGING

^{67}Ga citrate was initially developed as an agent for bone imaging and was also investigated and widely used to visualize infection and inflammation sites. However, ^{67}Ga citrate is known to accumulate in a variety of malignancies, including tumors of the lungs, soft tissues, and head and neck. ^{67}Ga citrate particularly reliable for the diagnosis of metastatic

TABLE 10.1. *Roles of nuclear oncology*

Characterization of lesions/masses
Staging and assessment of baseline tumor avidity
Restaging
Evaluation of therapeutic response
Radiation therapy planning
Follow-up
Prediction of clinical outcome

melanoma and hepatocellular carcinoma (1), but the predominant indications for ^{67}Ga citrate imaging today are the staging, restaging, and follow-up of patients with Hodgkin's and non-Hodgkin's lymphomas (5). The role of ^{67}Ga citrate citrate in lymphoma was reported as early as 1969 (6), and today it is recognized as a valuable functional tool for assessment of tumor viability. As such, ^{67}Ga citrate has been increasingly used for monitoring response to chemotherapy and radiotherapy, in addition to its uses in staging, restaging, and follow-up of patients with lymphomas (1,5,7).

Physical Properties and Pharmacokinetics

^{67}Ga citrate is a group IIIA metal that behaves as a ferric ion analog. The radionuclide is produced in a cyclotron by bombardment of zinc-68. It has a physical half-life of 78 hours and decays by electron capture, emitting a range of gamma rays from 93 to 300 keV (Table 10.3). *In vivo*, ^{67}Ga citrate binds to iron-binding proteins, such as transferrin, lactoferrin, haptoglobulin, ferritin, and bacterial siderophores. Although ^{67}Ga citrate competes with iron for binding to transferrin, it does not form heme because ^{67}Ga citrate cannot be reduced *in vivo* from its +3 oxidation state to interact with protoporphyrins (1,8). It is presumed that ^{67}Ga citrate penetrates into viable tumor cells by several diverse mechanisms, including tumor cell surface binding via the transfer-

rin receptor CD-71 and active transport into the cytoplasm. Once inside the tumor cells, ^{67}Ga citrate localizes in lysosomal-like granules. It is important to emphasize that due to its mechanisms of uptake, ^{67}Ga citrate accumulation reflects binding to live cells and not to necrotic or scar tissue.

Physiologic Distribution of ^{67}Ga Citrate

^{67}Ga citrate normal biodistribution includes liver, spleen, bone, and bone marrow. Splenic uptake is usually diffuse and mild, and it should be less intense than the uptake seen in the liver when imaging is performed on the third day postinjection. If imaging is performed later, diffuse physiologic increased uptake within the spleen will be seen. On days 7 to 14 postinjection, the splenic uptake is routinely higher than that seen in the liver. Focal uptake within the spleen at any time is an indication of splenic involvement.

Diffuse increased bone marrow uptake is commonly seen at presentation, in anemic patients, during chemotherapy, and with bone marrow expansion drugs. In the context of secondary hematopoiesis, the splenic uptake can be intense and higher than that seen in the liver, but it is not focal and is usually accompanied by diffuse bone marrow uptake. Focal increased bone marrow uptake is worrisome for pathologic bone marrow involvement. Radiotherapy may result in focal decreased bone marrow uptake within the radiation field.

Physiologic uptake of ^{67}Ga citrate is also seen in salivary and lacrimal glands, anterior nasopharynx, thymus and epiphyseal regions in children, soft tissues, external genitalia, and female breast tissue (particularly postpartum and during lactation due to ^{67}Ga citrate binding to lactoferrin). In the postpartum period, ^{67}Ga citrate scanning is contraindicated in women who wish to breast-feed, because ^{67}Ga citrate is excreted into the milk. Renal and urinary bladder activity is usually observed at 24 hours but decreases by 48 and 72 hours (9).

The large intestine is a critical organ with respect to radiation-absorbed dose from ^{67}Ga citrate (0.9 cGy/mCi), and the

TABLE 10.2. *Imaging parameters*

Study	Tracer	Imaging
Gallium scan	10 mCi (370 MBq) ^{67}Ga citrate-IV	Acquire planar and tomographic images 72 hr postinjection on a camera equipped with medium energy, parallel hole collimators, and three pulse-height analyzers centered at 93, 185, and 300 keV with 20% energy windows
Thallium scan	3 mCi (111 MBq) ^{201}Tl thallous chloride-IV (NPO 4 hr before injection)	Acquire planar and tomographic images 20 min postinjection on a camera equipped with low-energy, high-resolution, parallel hole collimators and two pulse-height analyzers centered at 75 and 167 keV with 20% energy windows
Sestamibi scan	25 mCi (925 MBq) ^{99m}Tc sestamibi IV (NPO 4 hr before injection)	Acquire planar and tomographic images 20 min postinjection on a camera equipped with low-energy, parallel hole collimators and one pulseheight analyzer centered at 140 keV with 15% energy window
FDG-PET scan	10–20 mCi (370–740 MBq) FDG IV (NPO 4 hr before injection)	Images acquired 45 min postinjection on a dedicated PET or PET/CT scanner from the base of the skull to the mid-thighs

CT, computed tomography; NPO, nothing by mouth; PET, positron-emission tomography.

TABLE 10.3. *Physical properties of some of the radiopharmaceuticals used in nuclear oncology*

Radiopharmaceutical	Physical half-life	Isotopic decay	Photopeaks		Patient dose (mCi)
			keV	Abundance (%)	
[67]Ga citrate	3.26 d	Electron capture	93.3	35.7	10
			184.6	19.7	
			300.2	16.0	
[201]Tl thallous chloride	3.04 d	Electron capture	68.9–80.3	94.4	3
			167.4	10.0	
			135.3	2.7	
[99m]Tc sestamibi	6 hr	Isomeric transition	140.5	89.07	25
[^{18}F]-2-fluoro-2-deoxy-D-glucose	109.8 min	Positron	511	193.46	10–20
Indium-111 anti-CD20 monoclonal antibody (Zevalin)	2.8 d	Electron capture	171.3	90.2	6
			245.4	94	

From Kocher DC. Radioactive decay tables. U.S. Dept. of Energy publication, 1981.

presence of activity within the bowel has been reported to interfere with the interpretation of ^{67}Ga citrate scans below the diaphragm on planar images (10). Large intestine preparation with laxatives and/or enemas has been used in some centers, whereas others have not found this practice helpful. When planar imaging was used alone, delayed images up to 14 days after the injection of ^{67}Ga citrate were often required to differentiate normal intestinal clearance from pathologic tumor accumulation. However, the introduction of SPECT and its routine use in clinical practice has substantially reduced the requirement for delayed views because the improved localization that SPECT provides allows differentiation of normal physiologic excretion within the bowel from pathologic uptake. The use of SPECT for evaluation of the abdomen and pelvis is particularly useful and increases both the sensitivity and the specificity of the scan, as it does in the chest. Negative SPECT has been reported to rule out disease in 81% to 96% of the cases (11–13). SPECT of the chest and abdomin/pelvis should be an integral component of routine ^{67}Ga citrate scanning (14).

[67]Ga Citrate Uptake in Lymphomas

In the majority of lymphomas, ^{67}Ga citrate scintigraphy is an effective method for staging and restaging of disease, evaluation of therapeutic response, radiotherapy planning, characterization of residual masses, and detection of relapse, and it has been reported to be predictive of outcome as discussed in Chapter 8. [67]Ga citrate has been found to be particularly sensitive in imaging intermediate- (>85%) and high-grade (>95%) non-Hodgkin's lymphomas (5,7,15). The indolent low-grade non-Hodgkin's lymphomas are, in general, far less ^{67}Ga citrate-avid than their intermediate- or high-grade counterparts. Although one study found ^{67}Ga citrate sensitivity in low-grade lymphoma to be 79% (16), the majority of studies report a sensitivity of approximately 50% (7,15,17–19). Sensitivity lower than 25% has also been reported in

mucosa-associated lymphoid tissue lymphoma and in lymphomas involving the skin, intestine, or testis (16).

[201]Tl thallous chloride or ^{99m}Tc sestamibi scintigraphy is more sensitive in staging low-grade lymphomas, with sensitivities reported in the range of 94% to 100% versus 56% to 60% for ^{67}Ga citrate scintigraphy (7,20). Paired ^{201}Tl thallous chloride and ^{67}Ga citrate scintigraphy has been used in the staging, restaging, and follow-up of patients with low-grade lymphomas, as discussed in the Clinical Applications section of this chapter under ^{201}Tl thallous chloride and ^{99m}Tc sestamibi.

Clinical Applications

Although CT remains the primary imaging modality used in the management of patients with lymphomas, functional imaging, such as ^{67}Ga citrate scintigraphy, plays an important complementary role and is an integral part of the clinical management of patients with lymphoma.

If ^{67}Ga citrate scintigraphy is being considered in the management of a patient with lymphoma, a baseline study before therapy is essential to demonstrate the initial tumor avidity for ^{67}Ga citrate, as well as the extent of the disease. Once ^{67}Ga citrate avidity has been demonstrated at baseline, ^{67}Ga citrate scintigraphy can be used as a functional imaging tool to determine the viability of that tissue in the course of therapy or in the follow-up. In addition, a baseline ^{67}Ga citrate study is also helpful in differentiating benign findings from malignant involvement. For example, it is common to see new bihilar uptake during therapy and in follow-up of patients who have received cyclophosphamide, hydroxydaunomycin (Adriamycin), Oncovin (vincristine), and prednisone (CHOP) therapy (21). Frohlich et al. have shown that as long as the intensity of ^{67}Ga citrate uptake in the hilum is symmetric and less intense than the original disease, the negative predictive value is very high; however, if it is asymmetric and equal to the baseline avidity within the tumor, the positive predictive value is high and thus, likely represents recurrence (21). Failure to inject ^{67}Ga citrate *before* initiation of therapy significantly increases the risk for subsequent false-negative scintigraphic findings (22,23). False-negative ^{67}Ga citrate scans at baseline may be seen if the patient has received steroid therapy, or if therapy was initiated before the injection of ^{67}Ga citrate. Therapy may be initiated a few hours, but preferably 24 to 48 hours, after the injection of ^{67}Ga citrate without resulting in a false-negative scan at 72 hours.

Several studies have pointed out the prognostic importance of ^{67}Ga citrate scans performed in lymphoma patients mid-treatment (23–26). In their report comparing the predictive capability of ^{67}Ga citrate scintigraphy and CT, Front and colleagues found a positive interim ^{67}Ga citrate scan to be an independent predictor of negative outcome in patients with aggressive lymphomas (23). In a similar series of patients with aggressive lymphoma histologies, 70% of patients who had negative interim ^{67}Ga citrate scans midway through standard induction therapy remained disease free, whereas only 25% of patients who were ^{67}Ga citrate positive at the same therapeutic point had a durable remission (26). When imaging patients with lymphoma mid-treatment, the recommendation is to perform the ^{67}Ga citrate scan just before the next cycle of chemotherapy.

Because ^{67}Ga citrate uptake within a mass reflects uptake within viable cancer cells, ^{67}Ga citrate scintigraphy has been shown to be a suitable indicator of complete response at the end of induction chemotherapy, particularly when a residual mass persists after treatment (Fig. 10.1). Several studies (18,23,25) have shown that early restaging ^{67}Ga citrate scans could differentiate patients with a high probability of prolonged disease-free survival from those who fail to respond to initial therapy and are likely to have a poor outcome. Persistent positive ^{67}Ga citrate scans in patients with intermediate- and, therefore, high-grade lymphomas can be used to identify patients who need more aggressive therapy.

Residual mediastinal or abdominal masses after radiation therapy or chemotherapy create a common dilemma when evaluating response to therapy in patients with lymphoma. The change in the size of a mass has not been proven to be a reliable indicator of responsiveness to treatment (7,23), and conventional imaging modalities, such as chest radiography and CT, are not necessarily reliable tools to distinguish between complete and partial remissions. [67]Ga citrate can help resolve this dilemma because it only binds to viable tumor cells and, therefore, will differentiate between residual disease and scar tissue. Several studies have demonstrated the high predictive value of both positive and negative ^{67}Ga citrate scintigraphy in the prediction of outcome in patients with intermediate- and high-grade lymphomas, whereas CT cannot be used to predict outcome after treatment in these cases (Fig. 10.2) (22,23).

MRI has been reported to discriminate signal characteristics originating from normal tissue, fibrosis, or malignant tissue. In fact, several studies have found similar sensitivity and specificity of MRI and ^{67}Ga citrate scintigraphy for assessing lymphoma tissue within residual masses (27–29). MRI is not routinely used in the management of patients with lympho-

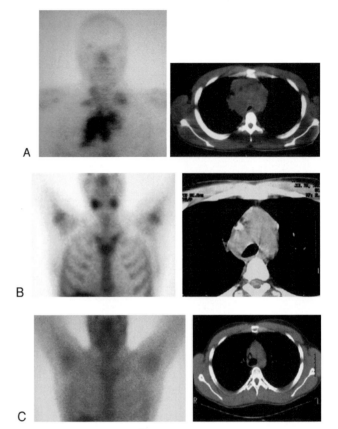

FIG. 10.1. A: Baseline ^{67}Ga citrate scan and CT scan in a patient with large-cell lymphoma showing high ^{67}Ga citrate avidity in the large mediastinal mass demonstrated on CT. **B:** Mid-treatment ^{67}Ga citrate scan and CT scan showing no correlation on ^{67}Ga citrate scan for the residual mediastinal mass seen on CT. **C:** Follow-up ^{67}Ga citrate scan and CT scan obtained 3.5 years later showing normal ^{67}Ga citrate distribution despite a small residual mass on CT (*black circle*) confirming the negative predictive value of the negative ^{67}Ga citrate scan at mid-treatment in this patient.

mas, however, with the exception of evaluation of bone marrow and skeletal involvement. PET with FDG has shown advantages over ^{67}Ga citrate scintigraphy in this case, particularly in the evaluation of therapeutic response, because ^{67}Ga citrate scintigraphy can be falsely positive in the context of skeletal repair and bone remodeling.

It should be noted that the methodology used in ^{67}Ga citrate scintigraphy has a significant impact on its effectiveness. In the adult population, ^{67}Ga citrate scans should be performed following the injection of 10 mCi (370 MBq) of ^{67}Ga citrate. Tomographic techniques (SPECT) of the chest and abdomen/pelvis should be mandatory, as should correlation with anatomic modalities, such as CT. SPECT may help to detect disease when planar images appear normal due to superimposition of organs on the two-dimensional images. Data suggest a 15% improvement in accuracy by SPECT over planar imaging, resulting in 92% sensitivity and 99% specificity of ^{67}Ga citrate scintigraphy in non-Hodgkin's lymphomas (7,12,13). SPECT

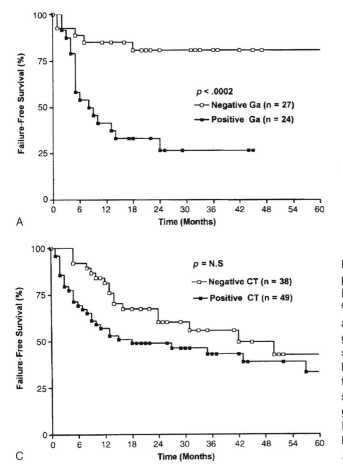

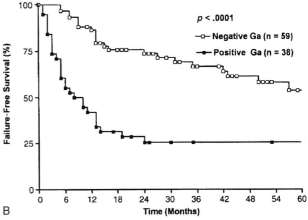

FIG. 10.2. Predictive diagnostic value of ^{67}Ga citrate scintigraphy and computed tomography (CT) in patients with non-Hodgkin's lymphomas. **A:** Patients who have positive or negative ^{67}Ga citrate scintigraphic findings after one cycle of chemotherapy. **B:** Patients who have positive or negative ^{67}Ga citrate scintigraphic findings at mid-treatment. In (**A**) and (**B**), there is a statistically significant (*p* < .001) difference in failure-free survival between the two groups. **C:** Patients who have positive or negative CT findings at mid-treatment. In (**C**), there is no statistically significant difference in failure-free survival between the two groups. Ga, ^{67}Ga citrate; NS, not significant. [Reprinted from Front D, Bar-Shalom R, Mor M, et al. Aggressive non-Hodgkin's lymphoma: early prediction of outcome with ^{67}Ga scintigraphy. *Radiology* 2000;214(1): 253–257, with permission.]

is also particularly valuable in differentiating normal physiologic ^{67}Ga citrate accumulation within soft tissues, bone, liver, or bowel from pathologic uptake.

[201]Tl THALLOUS CHLORIDE AND [99M]Tc SESTAMIBI-METOXYISOBUTYL ISONITRILE (SESTAMIBI) IMAGING

[201]Tl thallous chloride and ^{99m}Tc sestamibi have been developed and are predominantly used to evaluate myocardial perfusion; however, the potential use of both agents in nuclear oncology has been gradually recognized. [201]Tl thallous chloride was initially used for the differentiation between benign and malignant thyroid nodules, while today both agents are used in the diagnostic evaluation of several malignancies, including brain tumors, primary bone tumors, breast cancer, and lung cancers (5,30–32). Their role in imaging low grade lymphomas is reviewed here.

Physical Properties and Pharmacokinetics

[201]Tl thallous chloride is a metal in the IIIA group of the periodic table. It decays by electron capture and emits a cluster of x-rays between 69 and 80 keV (abundance of 94%) and gamma rays of 135 keV and 167 keV (abundance of 3% and 10%, respectively; see Table 10.3). Biologically, ^{201}Tl thallous chloride behaves similarly to potassium and after injection is distributed through-

out the body proportionally to the blood flow. Accordingly, tumor uptake of ^{201}Tl thallous chloride depends on several factors, such as tumor vascularization, capillary permeability, cell viability and activity of the ATPase sodium/potassium pump that maintains a high intracellular gradient of potassium and, consequently, ^{201}Tl thallous chloride. [201]Tl thallous chloride is accumulated by viable tumor cells and somewhat by connective tissue, but it does not penetrate into necrotic tissue (1,33).

[99m]Tc sestamibi builds up as a product of molybdenum-99 decay, and it is the most commonly used radionuclide in nuclear medicine. [99m]Tc sestamibi owes its vast utility to its convenient production method by means of a simple generator pack (4), together with its 6-hour half-life and the favorable energy of its principal gamma photon (140 keV; see Table 10.3). [99m]Tc sestamibi is a lipophilic cation, which diffuses into the cells in response to negative transmembrane potentials and mitochondrial content (31). Similarly to ^{201}Tl thallous chloride, uptake of ^{99m}Tc sestamibi is highly dependent on adequate blood supply (32,33).

Physiologic Distribution of [201]Tl Thallous Chloride and [99m]Tc Sestamibi

Normal uptake of ^{201}Tl thallous chloride is seen in salivary glands, thyroid, lungs, heart, liver, spleen, kidneys, skeletal muscles, and soft tissues, and is excreted primarily through the kidneys and partially through the hepatobiliary system. For the most part, ^{99m}Tc sestamibi follows the normal accumulation pattern of ^{201}Tl thallous chloride, with more intense hepatobiliary clearance. As opposed to ^{201}Tl thallous chloride, it is also taken up within the choroid plexus. It should be noted that high hepatobiliary and renal clearances may result in difficulties in interpreting tomographic acquisitions of ^{201}Tl thallous chloride or ^{99m}Tc sestamibi studies in the abdomen and pelvis because excretion is a dynamic process occurring throughout the tomographic acquisition (30–32,34).

Clinical Applications

^{67}Ga citrate is considered the standard nuclear medicine radiopharmaceutical for the evaluation of patients with lymphomas, and therefore, data on the use of ^{201}Tl thallous chloride are relatively modest. ^{201}Tl thallous chloride still has a limited role primarily in the management of low-grade lymphomas, in which it better defines disease sites above the diaphragm compared with ^{67}Ga citrate (7). Due to its intestinal clearance, ^{201}Tl thallous chloride should be used with caution in the evaluation of the disease sites within the abdomen and pelvis.

Paired ^{201}Tl thallous chloride and ^{67}Ga citrate scintigraphy may be helpful in the follow-up of patients with untreated low-grade lymphomas (Fig 10.3). In such cases, as long as the ^{67}Ga citrate scintigraphy is negative or shows lower avidity than that seen on ^{201}Tl thallous chloride scintigraphy, the disease is relatively indolent, and a watch-and-wait observation may be pursued. Patients may remain ^{201}Tl thallous chloride positive and ^{67}Ga citrate negative for several years. Sudden change in ^{67}Ga citrate uptake in one tumor site relative to the others reflects a change in the biology of the tumor at that site; however, pathologic examination remains the gold standard to establish the histology of the disease and/or document transformation. Serial follow-up with paired studies may help document the changes in the biology in various tumor sites as demonstrated in Figure 10.4.

^{99m}Tc sestamibi has been used as an alternative to ^{201}Tl thallous chloride in the detection of low-grade lymphomas. Because ^{201}Tl thallous chloride and ^{99m}Tc sestamibi demon-

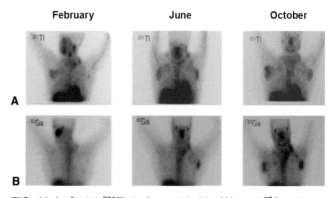

FIG. 10.4. Serial ^{201}Tl thallous chloride **(A)** and ^{67}Ga citrate scans **(B)** obtained 3 days apart in the same patient diagnosed with low-grade lymphoma over a 9-month period. In February, there is better delineation of disease sites in the neck and axillae on the ^{201}Tl thallous chloride scan compared with ^{67}Ga citrate scan. More intense focal avidity for ^{67}Ga citrate is seen in some sites in June, followed by matching ^{67}Ga citrate and ^{201}Tl thallous chloride avidity in all disease sites in October. A biopsy at that time was consistent with large-cell lymphoma.

ered equally suitable for monitoring of the therapy response in the disease sites above the diaphragm (5,7,30–32). Of note, the wider use of PET may significantly influence the way that these tracers will be used in the future.

[^{18}F]-2-FLUORO-2-DEOXY-D-GLUCOSE POSITRON EMISSION TOMOGRAPHY

FDG-PET is a rapidly evolving whole-body functional imaging technique. FDG-PET takes advantage of the fact, first observed by Warburg in 1931, that malignant tumors have an increased rate of aerobic glycolysis compared to normal tissues (35). Most tumors demonstrate an increase in glucose transporters, such as GLUT 1, as well as increased hexokinase and decreased glucose-6-phosphatase activity, resulting in the retention of the glucose analog FDG (4,36,37). Clinical studies with FDG have shown that PET imaging can detect most common types of cancers, often outperforming CT and MRI (35,38). FDG-PET has been proven to be useful in the characterization of tissues and residual masses, staging and restaging, evaluation of therapeutic response, and detection of recurrence in many human cancers (39). The Centers for Medicaid and Medicare Services have recognized the utility of FDG-PET in the management of patients with cancer and have approved reimbursement for the diagnosis, staging, and restaging of patients with lymphomas and other malignancies, such as non–small-cell lung, esophageal, colorectal, breast, head and neck cancers, as well as melanoma and solitary pulmonary nodule characterization (40). Cancer imaging with PET is one of the most dynamic and rapidly growing areas of contemporary nuclear medicine and clinical imaging.

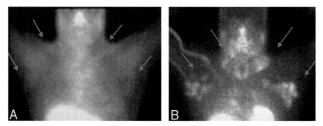

FIG. 10.3. ^{67}Ga citrate scan **(A)** and ^{201}Tl thallous chloride scan **(B)** in a patient with indolent low-grade lymphoma. The ^{201}Tl thallous chloride scan **(B)** was performed 3 days before the ^{67}Ga citrate scan **(A)** and demonstrated better delineation of disease sites in the neck and axillae (*arrows*) compared with the ^{67}Ga citrate scan.

TABLE 10.4. *Physical properties of the positron-emitting radionuclides used in positron emission tomography imaging*

Radionuclide	Physical half-life (min)	Maximum positron energy (MeV)
^{11}C	20.39	0.96
^{13}N	9.97	1.19
^{15}O	2.03	1.73
^{18}F	109.77	0.63
^{82}Rb	1.27	3.38

From Kocher DC. *Radioactive decay tables*. U.S. Department of Energy publication, 1981; Tilley DR, Weller HR, Cheves CM, Chasteler RM. Energy levels of light nuclei A=18-19. *Nucl Phys* 1995;A 595(1):1–170; Ajzenberg-Selove F. Energy levels of light nuclei A = 11-12. *Nucl Phys* 1990;A 506(1):1–158; Ajzenberg-Selove F. Energy levels of light nuclei A = 11-12. *Nucl Phys* 1991;A523(1)1–196; King MM and Chou WT. Nuclear data sheets update for A=82. *Nucl Data Sheets* 1995;76:285.

Physical Properties and Pharmacokinetics

The radionuclides used for radiolabeling in PET are positron emitters, whereas single-photon emitters are used in conventional nuclear medicine imaging. An emitted positron (a positively charged beta particle, signified by β+) will penetrate only a few millimeters in soft tissues before combining with an electron (β−). The particle pair then annihilates and their masses are entirely converted into energy. This energy takes the form of two 511 keV annihilation photons, emitted at approximately 180° to each other. Detection of both annihilation photons within a certain time frame (known as a *coincidence time window*) is termed *annihilation coincidence detection*, and this is the

principle by which PET tomographs operate. Dedicated full-ring high-end clinical PET scanners offer high spatial resolution (4 to 7 mm), as well as semiquantitative and quantitative information on radiotracer uptake. The semiquantitative information provided by measurements such as the standardized uptake value has shown independent value as a prognostic factor (1,35). It is important to realize that PET imaging performed on gamma-camera–based systems has lower effective resolution (approximately 15 mm vs. 5 to 7 mm on dedicated PET scanners) and may not be able to provide the quantitative information that can be obtained on high-end systems (35).

The positron-emitting radionuclides used for clinical imaging possess relatively short half-lives and are produced, for the most part, by a cyclotron (Table 10.4). The most widely used tracer in clinical PET applications is FDG. Fluorine-18 has a half-life of 109.8 minutes, allowing acquisition of images over 30 to 120 minutes at reasonable data rates (41).

The kinetics of FDG *in vivo* can be described by a three-compartment model as shown in Figure 10.5. Briefly, FDG is transported into viable cells by facilitative glucose transporter molecules (such as GLUT 1), where it is phosphorylated by hexokinase to FDG-6-phosphate, as glucose is phosphorylated to glucose-6-phosphate. Unlike glucose-6-phosphate, however, FDG-6-phosphate undergoes no further metabolism within the cell. Moreover, its dephosphorylation by glucose-6-phosphatase is a relatively slow process in comparison to that of glucose-6-phosphate. This, combined with the fact that FDG-6-phosphate cannot easily cross the cell membrane, results in an entrapment of FDG-6-phosphate within viable cells. The entrapment is further potentiated in malignant cells, which typically have a

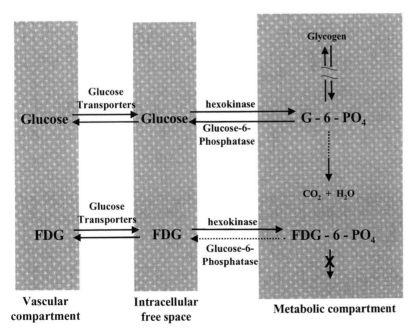

FIG. 10.5. Three-compartment model comparing the kinetics of [^{18}F]-2-fluoro-2-deoxy-D-glucose (FDG) and glucose *in vivo*. (Modified from Maisey MN, Wahl RL, Barrington SF. *Atlas of clinical positron emission tomography*. London: Arnold, 1999.)

greater number of glucose transport molecules at the cell surface, higher hexokinase activity, and low levels of glucose-6-phosphatase or lack it altogether (35–37).

Physiologic Distribution of [^{18}F]-2-Fluoro-2-Deoxy-D-Glucose

High uptake of FDG is typically found in the brain cortex, basal ganglia, and thalami. Even after the use of sedative or anesthetic drugs, the cortical activity (although depressed) remains higher than that seen in other normal tissues (41).

Normal myocardial uptake of FDG is variable, as myocardial metabolism physiologically depends on glucose and free fatty acids (42–44). In oncologic PET studies, intense myocardial FDG uptake may impair the detection of malignant lesions in the mediastinum and lungs. To mitigate this effect, a recommended fast for 4 to 6 hours before tracer administration results in enhanced myocardial fatty acid metabolism and reduced myocardial uptake of glucose and FDG. Normoglycemic status also helps minimize competition between circulating glucose and FDG at the cellular level. Diabetic patients and insulin-dependent patients need to be screened for excessive blood glucose concentration before the test. Performing the test in a hyperinsulinemic state results in intense striated muscle uptake and increase the risk of a false-negative scan.

Accumulation of FDG in skeletal muscle depends predominantly on its metabolic activity. Accordingly, skeletal muscle at rest usually shows low FDG uptake (43,44). Therefore, patients are asked to refrain from intense exercise 24 hours before and on the day of the scan. Simple methods aimed at optimizing patient comfort and controlling room temperature may also help reduce nonspecific striated muscle and fat uptake, which may impair the interpretation of the study, particularly if muscle and/or fat uptake is seen within the neck, pectoral, and axillary regions. Oral sedation with 5 mg of Valium may help reduce muscle and/or fat uptake if clinically indicated.

Unlike glucose, FDG is excreted by the kidneys, with resulting visualization of the renal collecting system, ureters, and urinary bladder. Low-grade uptake of FDG is usually seen in the abdomen, mostly in the liver and, to a lesser extent, in the spleen. This uptake is lower than the background uptake usually seen with ^{67}Ga citrate scintigraphy and is one reason for the increased sensitivity of PET scanning for detection of disease in these organs relative to ^{67}Ga citrate scintigraphy. Normal FDG accumulation in the stomach and intestine is variable. Bowel preparation can be used but requires procedures similar to those used before colonoscopy (35,44) and may be too invasive for the oncologic patient population.

Benign Pathologic Conditions Accumulating [^{18}F]-2-Fluoro-2-Deoxy-D-Glucose

Various benign diseases and conditions may mimic malignancy on FDG-PET scans, as reviewed by Cook and others (44) and are often related to infections or inflammatory changes. Conditions that may mimic lymphoma with widespread lymphadenopathy are granulomatous diseases, including tuberculosis, sarcoidosis, glandular fever, and Epstein-Barr virus infection. Nevertheless, in these cases PET can still be helpful in identifying disease foci that may be the most accessible for biopsy. Other false-positive FDG uptake can be seen in histoplasmosis, coccidioidomycosis, pyogenic infections, sites of inflammatory changes postradiation therapy, postoperative wound healing, and other inflammatory states (44).

FDG-PET was reported to correctly detect bone marrow involvement in the majority of lymphoma patients studied before the onset of therapy (45). However, diffuse benign homogenous bone marrow FDG uptake can be seen after treatment secondary to physiologic reactive changes and secondary to drugs resulting in bone marrow expansion (45). Familiarity with all the normal variants are important when interpreting these studies.

FDG-PET studies are usually able to distinguish between intracerebral lymphoma and toxoplasmosis in human immunodeficiency virus–positive patients due to generally greater uptake in lymphoma (35). However, lymphoma cannot be differentiated from generalized mycobacterial and human immunodeficiency virus–associated lymphadenopathy in autoimmune deficiency syndrome patients based on FDG-PET alone. The strength of FDG-PET resides in its overall high negative predictive values.

Clinical Applications

Most clinical series have shown that FDG-PET is superior to CT in the staging and restaging of patients with lymphoma and that FDG uptake declines promptly with effective therapy. A review of diagnostic performance of PET imaging alone and in comparison with other diagnostic modalities in patients with lymphoma is summarized in Table 10.5. In low-grade non-Hodgkin's lymphomas, FDG-PET scans may show low-level tracer uptake when the disease is indolent. However, the quality of FDG-PET images is generally better than with conventional gamma-camera based scintigraphy because of the higher effective spatial resolution that can be obtained with dedicated PET scanners compared with gamma cameras (35). PET can also be performed the same day, approximately 45 minutes after the injection of FDG, whereas there is a delay of 3 days after ^{67}Ga citrate injection before scanning is performed. FDG has a further advantage over ^{67}Ga citrate in terms of effective dose: FDG results in an effective patient dose of 27 μSv/MBq, or 5 to 20 mSv, depending on applied adult dose (5 to 20 mCi; 185 to 740 MBq). Due to its long half-life, ^{67}Ga citrate delivers a higher radiation dose of 120 μSv/MBq, or an average adult dose of 44 mSv per standard injection dose (10 mCi; 370 MBq) (58,59). FDG-PET can also be offered as an alternative to ^{67}Ga citrate scintigraphy to postpartum women who wish to continue breast-feeding. Although FDG is excreted into breast milk,

TABLE 10.5. *Diagnostic performance of positron emission tomography (PET) imaging in patients with lymphoma*

Study	Patients	Methods	Tx Alteration	Sens (%)	Spec (%)	PPV (%)	NPV (%)	DA (%)
Kostakoglu et al. 2002 (46)	Staging: NHL 17; HD 13	PET: after one cycle		82		90		
		PET: after Ch		45		83		
Bangerter et al. 1999 (47)	Initial staging: NHL 43 (LG 3, IG 4, HG 36); HD 45	PET: before Tx	6 pts (14%)	98	90	92	97	94
		PET: after Tx		86	96	75	98	95
Jerusalem et al. 1999 (48)	Restaging: IG/HG NHL 35; HD 19; Ch 41; Ch + RT 13	CT: res. malignancy		71	65	42	87	67
		PET: res. malignancy		43	100	100	83	85
Zinzani et al. 1999 (49)	Restaging: HG NHL 31; HD 13; Ch 15; Ch + RT 29	CT: res. malignancy		93	23	36	88	45
		PET: res. malignancy		93	100	100	97	98
Moog et al. 1999 (50)	Untreated: NHL 22 (LG 3, HG 19); HD 34	Bone scan		80	92	80	92	88
		PET: bone		100	100	100	100	100
Moog et al. 1998 (51)	Untreated: NHL 43 (LG 17, HG 26); HD 38	CT: extranodal	13 pts (16%)	63	93	90	70	45
		PET: extranodal		97	100	100	97	98
Stumpe et al. 1998 (52)	Restaging: NHL 15 (LG 6, HG 9)	CT		86	67	67	86	75
		PET		89	100	100	90	94
Cremerius et al. 1998 (53)	Restaging: NHL 17 (LG 5, HG 12); HD 8	CT		100	17			
		PET		100	92			
Carr et al. 1998 (45)	Staging: NHL 38; HD 12	PET: marrow		81	76	62	90	78
de Wit et al. 1997 (54)	Restaging: NHL 17 (LG 9, IG 1, HG 7); HD 17	PET: res. malignancy		100	71	59	100	79
Hoh et al. 1997 (55)	Staging/restaging: NHL 11 (LG 3, IG 5, HG 3); HD 7	CT/MRI	3 pts (17%)	89				
		PET		89				
Okada et al. 1994 (56)	Untreated: NHL 19 (LG 1, IG 17, HG 1); HD 2	PET		100				
Leskinen-Kallio et al. 1991 (57)	NHL 13 (LG 5, IG 5, HG 3)	PET: all grades		62				
		PET: LG		60				
		PET: IG		40				
		PET: HG		100				

Ch, chemotherapy; DA, diagnostic accuracy; HD, Hodgkin's disease; HG, high grade; IG, intermediate grade; LG, low grade; NHL, non-Hodgkin's lymphoma; NPV, negative predictive value; PPV, positive predictive value; pts, patients; res, residual; RT, radiation therapy; sens, sensitivity; spec, specificity; Tx, therapy.

the shorter half-life of fluorine-18 (109.8 minutes) allows women to resume breast-feeding within 24 to 48 hours.

The increase in the number of reimbursable indications by the Centers for Medicaid and Medicare Services (40) has resulted in the rapid expansion of this functional imaging technique, not only in academic centers but in community hospitals as well. FDG-PET scanning in lymphomas is being used for staging and restaging, prediction of outcome, and evaluation of residual masses seen on CT after treatment (Table 10.5). Figure 10.6 illustrates the use of FDG-PET in the staging and restaging of a patient

with lymphoma. Figure 10.7 and Color Plate 2 illustrate the use of the technology at staging, restaging, and in the follow-up of a patient with lymphoma. Recurrence in the spleen, as suggested by the FDG-PET scan performed at the 6-month follow-up, was confirmed at surgery.

In a prospective study, Buchmann et al. have demonstrated that FDG-PET is an efficient and noninvasive method for the primary staging of patients with untreated lymphomas (60). They evaluated 52 patients with untreated malignant lymphoma and 1,297 anatomic regions (lymph nodes, organs, and bone marrow). FDG-PET, CT, and

Staging   End of therapy

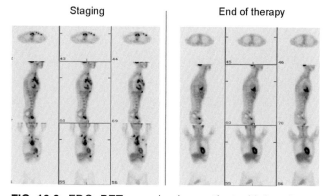

FIG. 10.6. FDG–PET scanning in a patient with lymphoma at baseline and at the end of chemotherapy. The staging scan shows multiple sites of intense FDG uptake in the neck, mediastinum, pectoral, axillary, and diaphragmatic regions. The scan at the end of chemotherapy shows resolution in all sites. Normal myocardial uptake is seen on both scans.

bone marrow biopsy were performed to investigate lymph node/extranodal manifestations and bone marrow infiltration. FDG-PET and CT scans were compared by receiver operating characteristic (ROC) curve analysis, which indicated that the accuracy of FDG-PET was significantly superior to CT in detecting lymph node and extranodal lymphoma involvement ($p < .05$). FDG-PET provided significantly more information than CT regarding the subdivision of supradiaphragmatic and infradiaphragmatic spread of lymphomas, according to the Ann Arbor Classification (61). In detecting bone marrow infiltration, FDG-PET also outperformed CT and was equivalent to bone

Baseline   End-Treatment   6-month Follow-up

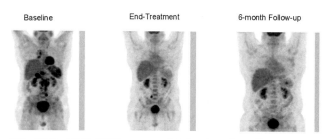

FIG. 10.7. FDG–PET scans obtained at baseline, at the end of therapy, and 6 months after the end of therapy in a patient with lymphoma. The baseline study shows extensive disease above and below the diaphragm, including splenic involvement. The scan performed at the end of chemotherapy shows resolution in all sites. The focus seen to the right of the lumbar spine at that time represents physiologic urinary excretion in the right ureter. The scan obtained at the 6-month follow-up shows uptake within the spleen that may indicate recurrent disease. Normal urinary activity is seen in the bladder on all scans and normal myocardial uptake is seen on the baseline scan. (See Color Plate 2.)

marrow biopsy. Finally, FDG-PET led to changes in the therapy regimen in 8% of patients (60).

As described earlier in this chapter, ^{67}Ga citrate scintigraphy is routinely used in many clinical centers to complement CT for staging, response assessment, and confirmation of relapse; however, few studies have compared FDG-PET to ^{67}Ga citrate scintigraphy in a prospective manner in the same group of patients. The authors recently conducted a prospective study comparing both modalities in 36 patients with Hodgkin's disease at staging, mid-therapy, and at the end of treatment. The results show that FDG-PET and ^{67}Ga citrate scintigraphy findings are largely concordant , however, only FDG-PET detected splenic disease, resulting in the upstaging of three out of five patients who demonstrated splenic involvement on PET alone. Positive FDG-PET findings at mid-treatment and at the end of therapy had a higher sensitivity for predicting subsequent relapse than ^{67}Ga citrate scintigraphy (62).

Wirth et al. reviewed the medical records of 50 patients who had FDG-PET, ^{67}Ga citrate scintigraphy, or conventional staging of indolent and aggressive non-Hodgkin's lymphomas (63). Both modalities led to upstaging in 11% of patients classified as stage I or II by conventional assessment. The treatment approach was altered by FDG-PET in 18% of patients and by ^{67}Ga citrate scans in 14% of cases. FDG-PET was shown to have 13% higher sensitivity than ^{67}Ga citrate scintigraphy in the detection of additional sites of disease (63).

Schoder et al. surveyed 54 referring physicians by standardized questionnaires to determine the impact of FDG-PET imaging results in influencing clinical staging and therapeutic decision-making in patients with lymphomas (64). Treatment modifications, when present, were classified as intermodality (e.g., medical to surgical, surgical to radiation, medical to no treatment) or intramodality (e.g., altered medical, surgical, or radiotherapy approach) changes. Physicians indicated that FDG-PET led to a change in the clinical stage in 44% of patients, of whom 21% were upstaged and 23% were downstaged. Findings of the FDG-PET examination resulted in intermodality treatment changes in 42% of patients, in intramodality modifications in 10%, and in a combination of the two in 10% of cases. Nonspecified treatment adjustments were reported in an additional 6% of patients, whereas FDG-PET did not affect clinical approach in only 32% of patients. This survey-based study highlights the major impact of FDG-PET scanning on the clinical management of lymphoma patients (64).

Use of posttreatment FDG-PET to identify patients who are at high risk of recurrent disease might be of equal clinical importance as the primary staging of lymphoma. Correlation of FDG-PET and CT scans with relapse data in 49 adult patients with aggressive lymphomas showed that FDG-PET is more accurate than CT in assessing remission and in predicting relapse-free survival (59). Results of posttreatment FDG-PET scans were highly predictive of disease outcome, with relapse rates of 100% for positive and 17% for negative FDG-PET, compared to 41% and 25% for patients with positive and negative CT, respectively (Fig. 10.8). Interim FDG-PET scans after two to three cycles of chemotherapy also provided valuable information regarding early assessment of response and long-term prognosis. No relapses were recorded in patients with no or minimal residual uptake, in contrast to an 87.5% relapse rate in patients with persistent FDG accumulation. With such a high negative predictive value (100%), FDG-PET may therefore assist in the early identification of patients who are likely to be cured with standard chemotherapy versus those with poorer prognosis who require alternative additional treatment (59).

Jerusalem et al. compared FDG-PET with CT in patients with aggressive lymphomas who underwent PET scanning 1 to 3 months after completion of chemotherapy. Relapse occurred in all six patients with positive FDG-PET scans, 26% of patients with residual CT masses but negative FDG-PET, and 10% with negative CT and FDG-PET. One-year disease-free survival was 86% for patients with negative FDG-PET versus 0% for those with positive scans (48).

In a similar series of patients with aggressive lymphoma histology who underwent FDG-PET scanning 1 to 3 months after the end of chemotherapy and before radio-

therapy, Spaepen et al. found that out of 67 patients with negative FDG-PET, 53 were also CT negative. With a median follow-up of 653 days, there were ten recurrences (20%) in this group and only one recurrence among the 14 with positive CT and negative FDG-PET. All 26 patients with positive posttreatment FDG-PET relapsed, including 14 with negative posttreatment CT scans. The 2-year progression-free survival rate for FDG-PET-negative patients was 85%, compared with 4% for those who were FDG-PET positive (65).

In their study, Naumann et al. semiquantitatively analyzed FDG uptake by using regions of interest and standardized uptake values (66). The patient population consisted of 43 Hodgkin's disease patients and 15 non-Hodgkin's lymphoma cases with posttherapeutic complete remission and residual masses detected by CT. Analysis of 62 residual locations by FDG-PET was performed separately for the two pathologic entities. Patients with an FDG-PET–positive residual mass had a recurrence rate of 62.5%, whereas those with FDG-PET–negative residual mass showed a much lower recurrence rate of 4% (p = .004). A positive FDG-PET study correlated with a significantly poorer progression-free survival (p < .00001). No recurrence occurred in any of the patients with a negative FDG-PET scan, resulting in a nega-

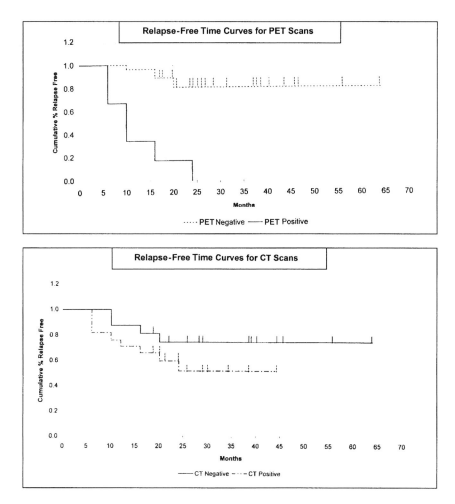

FIG. 10.8. Predictive diagnostic value, expressed as relapse-free survival, of [^{18}F]-2-fluoro-2-deoxy-D-glucose–positron-emission tomography (PET) and computed tomography (CT). [From Mikhaeel NG, Timothy AR, O'Doherty MJ, et al. 18-FDG-PET as a prognostic indicator in the treatment of aggressive non-Hodgkin's lymphoma: comparison with CT. *Leuk Lymphoma* 2000;39 (5–6):543–553, with permission.]

tive predictive value of 100%. All non-Hodgkin's lymphoma patients with a positive FDG-PET study relapsed (positive predictive value, 100%) (66).

These studies support the routine use of posttreatment FDG-PET in aggressive non-Hodgkin's lymphomas. The question of whether posttreatment FDG-PET should be reserved only for those cases with residual lesions detected by CT remains open; however, the study by Spaepen et al. suggests otherwise, because one-half of the patients with posttreatment positive FDG-PET and complete remission by CT subsequently relapsed (65). Although further evaluation of this approach awaits the results of new prospective studies, FDG-PET is well established as a valuable tool that can assist clinicians in the identification of patients with poor prognosis following the standard first-line treatment (67,68).

Fusion of Positron Emission Tomography and Computed Tomography

In clinical settings, fusion of images between separate modalities can be of considerable help in guiding patient management in numerous circumstances. This is especially true when anatomic images (e.g., CT or MRI) are fused with functional images (e.g., PET or SPECT). The hardware is available to acquire combined PET and CT scans in a single setting, and there are continuing efforts to develop combined PET and MRI systems (69–71).

It should be noted that although image fusion obtained on integrated scanners is less prone to error from body movement, some inaccuracies still exist due to, for example, differences in respiratory chest movement between fast CT and slower PET acquisitions (69). Nevertheless, early experiences show that PET/CT image fusion has the potential to improve patient diagnosis and follow-up, particularly in the field of oncology.

PET/CT combined scanners have been installed at multiple institutions. The first such system was developed at the University of Pittsburgh and consisted of a third-generation CT scanner and a rotating partial-ring PET scanner combined in a single gantry (72). Martinelli et al. reviewed the results from more than 100 patients studied on this scanner, covering a wide range of malignancies, including lung, colorectal, head and neck, and ovarian cancer, as well as lymphoma and melanoma (73). According to this study, the combined PET/CT modality resulted in improved distinction of pathology from normal physiologic uptake, more accurate localization of functional abnormalities, and improved efficacy in monitoring of response to therapy.

Aside from results obtained on fully integrated combined PET/CT scanners, reports on registration of independently performed PET and CT images are also available (70). These show that fused PET and CT images may improve the spatial localization of a wide range of foci with increased FDG uptake found within the thorax, abdomen, and pelvis, despite the added difficulties associated with registration of two images acquired noncontemporaneously (74,75). Such digi-

tally fused images were reported to be particularly helpful in the anatomic localization of pathologic FDG uptake in retroperitoneal masses and abdominal or pelvic wall lesions (75).

Residual masses are frequently seen in patients with lymphomas after treatment. The potential to characterize those masses in one setting on the same day of the tracer injection will have a major impact in the management of patients with lymphomas and is likely to become routine in the near future.

RADIOLABELED ANTIBODIES IN THE TREATMENT OF LYMPHOMAS

For many years, efforts have been made to develop clinically successful radioimmunotherapy agents through specific targeting of tumor antigens by antibodies serving as carriers for radioactivity (76). However, identification of the most beneficial combinations of monoclonal antibodies and radioactive isotopes, as well as definition of the diseases in which such novel combinations would have the highest efficacy, is a complicated multidisciplinary process. As accentuated by Nagle, nuclear medicine is at the forefront of the emerging field of radioimmunotherapy, and it is to be expected that nuclear medicine professionals will be members of the multidisciplinary team that is necessary to administer this form of therapy (77). Treatment of non-Hodgkin's lymphoma has been one of the first targets of the new technology, and during the last decade, progress in the radioimmunotherapy of low-grade lymphoma has been considerable (78). The radionuclides found to be the most appropriate for radiopharmaceutical development in radioimmunotherapy are yttrium-90 and iodine-131. The therapeutic effect of these radionuclides is mediated by high-energy beta particles, which have a short range in human tissues (76). Two radiolabeled antibody products utilizing each of these radionuclides attracted the attention of the medical community—one by receiving approval from the U.S. Food and Drug Administration (FDA) in the first quarter of 2002 and the other by receiving a recommendation for approval in December 2002 (79). Both agents are briefly described.

Radioimmunotherapy with Yttrium-90-Ibritumomab Tiuxetan (Zevalin)

In early 2002, yttrium-90-ibritumomab tiuxetan (Zevalin, IDEC Pharmaceuticals, San Diego, CA) became the first radioimmunotherapy agent to receive the FDA's product approval. Zevalin is approved for patients with refractory or relapsed low-grade, follicular, or transformed B-cell non-Hodgkin's lymphoma, including patients with rituximab-refractory follicular lymphoma (79,80). An integral part of Zevalin's therapeutic protocol is rituximab (Rituxan, Genentech, San Francisco, CA), an unlabeled anti-CD20 chimeric antibody that received FDA approval in 1998.

Zevalin consists of two moieties: a murine monoclonal antibody and a linker-chelator moiety. The antibody moiety of Zevalin is ibritumomab, a murine IgG₁ monoclonal antibody directed against the CD20 antigen, which is found on the surface of normal and malignant B lymphocytes. This antibody is covalently attached to a metal chelator, tiuxetan, which provides a high-affinity stable chelation site for radionuclide binding. Zevalin is designed for radiolabeling with two radioisotopes: indium-111 for imaging purposes and yttrium-90 for therapeutic purposes. As yttrium-90 is a pure beta emitter, a tracer dose of ibritumomab labeled with indium-111, which emits γ-radiation, is required before therapy to evaluate the biodistribution of the antibody before the subsequent administration of the therapeutic dose of Zevalin (80). Tumor sites are routinely visualized on images obtained at 48 hours. Predominant visualization of spleen, liver, and bone marrow may indicate impaired distribution, possibly secondary to immune complex formation and subsequent uptake by the reticuloendothelial system. This altered distribution may represent a contraindication for Zevalin therapy. All diagnostic and therapeutic administrations of the radiolabeled antibodies must be preceded by the infusion of rituximab, which requires close coordination between the nuclear medicine and oncologic clinics and the referring physician.

Physical Properties

Indium-111 decays by electron capture, with a physical half-life of 67 hours. The product of its decay is nonradioactive cadmium-111 (80). Radiation emission data for indium-111 are summarized in Table 10.3.

Yttrium-90 decays by emission of beta particles (β⁻) only, with a physical half-life of 64 hours (2.67 days). The product of radioactive decay is nonradioactive zirconium-90. The average energy of the principal beta particle of yttrium-90 is 934 keV, and 90% of this energy is absorbed within a radius of 5.3 mm. This pathlength corresponds to approximately 200 cell diameters, enabling irradiation of tumor cells that are not directly bound to the antibody and, thus, increasing the tumor-killing effect. This may be particularly beneficial for treatment of poorly vascularized and/or bulky tumors (80).

Clinical Applications

Zevalin was approved for clinical use on the basis of the overall response rates demonstrated in two multicenter trials that included a total of 197 subjects (81–84). The first study reported on 54 patients with relapsed follicular lymphoma who became refractory to the treatment rituximab. Of these patients, 15% achieved complete remission on Zevalin, and 74% showed clinical improvement (81). The second trial was a randomized, controlled, multicenter study that included 143 patients with relapsed or refractory low-grade or follicular lymphoma, or transformed B-cell lymphoma. The trial was designed to evaluate the efficacy and safety of Zevalin radioimmunotherapy compared to rituximab immunotherapy, with the secondary objective being to determine

if radiation dosimetry before Zevalin administration was required for safe treatment in this patient population (82,83). The patients treated with Zevalin showed an overall response rate of 80%, compared with 56% in patients treated with unlabeled antibodies. Complete remission was recorded in 30% of patients treated with Zevalin and in 16% of patients treated with rituximab, whereas unconfirmed complete remissions were reported in 4% of patients in both groups (84). Furthermore, for all patients with dosimetry data, radiation-absorbed doses from yttrium-90 were estimated to be below 300 cGy to red marrow and 2,000 cGy to normal organs (83). Based on these findings, researchers concluded that radioimmunotherapy with Zevalin was well tolerated and produced statistically and clinically significant higher overall and complete response rates compared with rituximab alone (84).

Radioimmunotherapy with Iodine-131-Tositumomab (Bexxar)

At the end of 2002, the FDA recommended approval of iodine-131-tositumomab (Bexxar, Corixa Corporation, Seattle, WA), another potential radioimmunotherapy agent utilizing antibodies directed against CD20-expressing lymphomas. Clinical trials including 229 patients have reported an overall response rate of 47% to 68% and complete response rate from 20% to 34% after at least 1 year (85,86). An earlier pivotal report on a phase III clinical trial by Kaminski et al. concluded that a single course of iodine-131-tositumomab applied in extensively pretreated patients with chemotherapy-refractory, low-grade, or transformed low-grade lymphomas was significantly more efficacious than the last qualifying chemotherapy (86). This agent seemed to also have an acceptable safety profile (87). The FDA emphasized that this drug will likely benefit patients with chemotherapy-refractory, low-grade and follicular non-Hodgkin's lymphoma with or without transformation. In addition, iodine-131-tositumomab may also benefit patients refractory to rituximab.

ACKNOWLEDGMENT

The authors gratefully acknowledge the valuable assistance of Leonid Syrkin, M.S., Senior Computer Engineer, Nuclear Medicine, Dana-Farber Cancer Institute, for his assistance in the preparation of the figures.

REFERENCES

1. Maisey M. Radionuclide imaging in cancer management. *J R Coll Physicians Lond* 1998;32(6):525–529.
2. Munley MT, Marks LB, Hardenbergh PH, et al. Functional imaging of normal tissues with nuclear medicine: applications in radiotherapy. *Semin Radiat Oncol* 2001;11(1):28–36.
3. Valdes Olmos RA, Hoefnagel CA. Nuclear medicine in tailoring treatment in oncology. *Nucl Med Commun* 2001;22(1):1–4.
4. Badawi RD. Nuclear medicine. *Physics Education* 2001;36(6):452–454.

5. Mansberg R, Wadhwa SS, Mansberg V. Tl-201 and Ga-67 scintigraphy in non-Hodgkin's lymphoma. *Clin Nucl Med* 1999;24(4):239–242.

6. Edwards CL, Hayes RL. Tumor scanning with ^{67}Ga citrate. *J Nucl Med* 1969;10(2):103–105.

7. Waxman AD, Eller D, Ashook G, et al. Comparison of gallium-67-citrate and thallium-201 scintigraphy in peripheral and intrathoracic lymphoma. *J Nucl Med* 1996;37(1):46–50.

8. Vallabhajosula S, Goldsmith SJ, Lipszyc H, et al. ^{67}Ga-transferrin and ^{67}Ga-lactoferrin binding to tumor cells: specific versus nonspecific glycoprotein-cell interaction. *Eur J Nucl Med* 1983;8(8):354–357.

9. Tsan MF, Scheffel U. Mechanism of gallium-67 accumulation in tumors. *J Nucl Med* 1988;29(12):2019–2020.

10. Chen DC, Scheffel U, Camargo EE, et al. The source of gallium-67 in gastrointestinal contents: concise communication. *J Nucl Med* 1980;21(12):1146–1150.

11. Even-Sapir E, Bar-Shalom R, Israel O, et al. Single-photon emission computed tomography quantitation of gallium citrate uptake for the differentiation of lymphoma from benign hilar uptake. *J Clin Oncol* 1995;13(4):942–946.

12. Holman BL, Tumeh SS. Single-photon emission computed tomography (SPECT). Applications and potential. *JAMA* 1990;263(4):561–564.

13. Tumeh SS, Rosenthal DS, Kaplan WD, et al. Lymphoma: evaluation with Ga-67 SPECT. *Radiology* 1987;164(1):111–114.

14. Van den Abbeele AD. Scintigraphy of neoplastic disease. Lymphoma. In: Donohoe KJ, Van den Abbeele AD, eds. *Teaching atlas of nuclear medicine*. New York: Thieme, 2000;199–217.

15. Sandrock D, Lastoria S, Magrath IT, et al. The role of gallium-67 tumour scintigraphy in patients with small, non-cleaved cell lymphoma. *Eur J Nucl Med* 1993;20(2):119–122.

16. Ben-Haim S, Bar-Shalom R, Israel O, et al. Utility of gallium-67 scintigraphy in low-grade non-Hodgkin's lymphoma. *J Clin Oncol* 1996;14(6):1936–1942.

17. Nejmeddine F, Raphael M, Martin A, et al. [67]Ga scintigraphy in B-cell non-Hodgkin's lymphoma: correlation of ^{67}Ga uptake with histology and transferrin receptor expression. *J Nucl Med* 1999;40(1):40–45.

18. Setoain FJ, Pons F, Herranz R, et al. [67]Ga scintigraphy for the evaluation of recurrences and residual masses in patients with lymphoma. *Nucl Med Commun* 1997;18(5):405–411.

19. Bekerman C, Hoffer PB, Bitran JD. The role of gallium-67 in the clinical evaluation of cancer. *Semin Nucl Med* 1984;14(4):296–323.

20. Arthur JE, Kehoe K, Van den Abbeele A. Thallium-201 scintigraphy in low grade non-Hodgkin's lymphoma. *J Nucl Med* 1996;37(5):258P.

21. Frohlich DE, Chen JL, Neuberg D, et al. When is hilar uptake of ^{67}Ga-citrate indicative of residual disease after CHOP chemotherapy? *J Nucl Med* 2000;41(2):269–274.

22. Israel O, Mor M, Epelbaum R, et al. Clinical pretreatment risk factors and Ga-67 scintigraphy early during treatment for prediction of outcome of patients with aggressive non-Hodgkin lymphoma. *Cancer* 2002;94(4):873–878.

23. Front D, Bar-Shalom R, Mor M, et al. Aggressive non-Hodgkin lymphoma: early prediction of outcome with ^{67}Ga scintigraphy. *Radiology* 2000;214(1):253–257.

24. Cheson BD, Horning SJ, Coiffier B, et al. Report of an international workshop to standardize response criteria for non-Hodgkin's lymphomas. NCI Sponsored International Working Group. *J Clin Oncol* 1999;17(4):1244.

25. Janicek M, Kaplan W, Neuberg D, et al. Early restaging gallium scans predict outcome in poor-prognosis patients with aggressive non-Hodgkin's lymphoma treated with high-dose CHOP chemotherapy. *J Clin Oncol* 1997;15(4):1631–1637.

26. Shipp MA, Mauch P, Harris NL. Non-Hodgkin's lymphomas. In: DeVita VTJ, Hellman S, Rosenberg SA, eds. *Cancer: Principles & Practice of Oncology*, 5th ed. Philadelphia: Lippincott–Raven, 1996;2165–2220.

27. Abrahamsen AF, Lien HH, Aas M, et al. Magnetic resonance imaging and [67]gallium scan in mediastinal malignant lymphoma: a prospective pilot study. *Ann Oncol* 1994;5(5):433–436.

28. Bendini M, Zuiani C, Bazzocchi M, et al. Magnetic resonance imaging and ^{67}Ga scan versus computed tomography in the staging and in the monitoring of mediastinal malignant lymphoma: a prospective pilot study. *Magma* 1996;4(3–4):213–224.

29. Zinzani PL, Zompatori M, Bendandi M, et al. Monitoring bulky mediastinal disease with gallium-67, CT-scan and magnetic resonance imaging in Hodgkin's disease and high-grade non-Hodgkin's lymphoma. *Leuk Lymphoma* 1996;22(1–2):131–135.

30. Fletcher BD, Xiong X, Kauffman WM, et al. Hodgkin disease: use of Tl-201 to monitor mediastinal involvement after treatment. *Radiology* 1998;209(2):471–475.

31. Aktolun C, Bayhan H, Kir M. Clinical experience with Tc-99m MIBI imaging in patients with malignant tumors. Preliminary results and comparison with Tl-201. *Clin Nucl Med* 1992;17(3):171–176.

32. Ohta M, Isobe K, Kuyama J, et al. Clinical role of Tc-99m-MIBI scintigraphy in non-Hodgkin's lymphoma. *Oncol Rep* 2001;8(4):841–845.

33. Biersack HJ, Briele B, Hotze AL, et al. The role of nuclear medicine in oncology. *Ann Nucl Med* 1992;6(3):131–136.

34. Maurea S, Acampa W, Varrella P, et al. Tc-99m sestamibi imaging in the diagnostic assessment of patients with lymphomas: comparison with clinical and radiological evaluation. *Clin Nucl Med* 1998;23(5):283–290.

35. Maisey MN, Wahl RL, Barrington SF. *Atlas of clinical positron emission tomography*. London: Arnold, 1999.

36. Brown RS, Wahl RL. Overexpression of Glut-1 glucose transporter in human breast cancer. An immunohistochemical study. *Semin Nucl Med* 1993;72(10):2979–2985.

37. Brown RS, Goodman TM, Zasadny KR, et al. Expression of hexokinase II and Glut-1 in untreated human breast cancer. *Nucl Med Biol* 2002;29(4):443–453.

38. Lacic M, Maisey MN, Kusic Z. Positron emission tomography in oncology: the most sophisticated imaging technology. *Acta Med Croatica* 1997;51(1):1–9.

39. Lechpammer S, Tetrault RJ, Badawi RD, et al. PET imaging and treatment evaluation in cancer patients. *Uptake* 2002;8(6):4–5.

40. Department of Health and Human Services. Coverage and related claims processing requirements for positron emission tomography (PET) scans. *Program Memorandum Intermediaries/Carriers* 2002;CMS-Pub. 60AB (AB-02-065):1–4.

41. Phelps ME, Mazziotta JC, Schelbert HR. *Positron emission tomography and autoradiography. Principles and applications for the brain and heart.* New York: Raven Press, 1986.

42. Choi Y, Brunken RC, Hawkins RA, et al. Factors affecting myocardial 2-[F-18]fluoro-2-deoxy-D-glucose uptake in positron emission tomography studies of normal humans. *Eur J Nucl Med* 1993;20(4):308–318.

43. Cook GJ, Fogelman I, Maisey MN. Normal physiological and benign pathological variants of 18-fluoro-2-deoxyglucose positron-emission tomography scanning: potential for error in interpretation. *Semin Nucl Med* 1996;26(4):308–314.

44. Cook GJ, Maisey MN, Fogelman I. Normal variants, artefacts and interpretative pitfalls in PET imaging with 18-fluoro-2-deoxyglucose and carbon-11 methionine. *Eur J Nucl Med* 1999;26(10):1363–1378.

45. Carr R, Barrington SF, Madan B, et al. Detection of lymphoma in bone marrow by whole-body positron emission tomography. *Blood* 1998;91(9):3340–3346.

46. Kostakoglu L, Coleman M, Leonard JP, et al. PET predicts prognosis after 1 cycle of chemotherapy in aggressive lymphoma and Hodgkin's disease. *J Nucl Med* 2002;43(8):1018–1027.

47. Bangerter M, Kotzerke J, Griesshammer M, et al. Positron emission tomography with 18-fluorodeoxyglucose in the staging and follow-up of lymphoma in the chest. *Acta Oncol* 1999;38(6):799–804.

48. Jerusalem G, Beguin Y, Fassotte MF, et al. Whole-body positron emission tomography using ^{18}F-fluorodeoxyglucose for posttreatment evaluation in Hodgkin's disease and non-Hodgkin's lymphoma has higher diagnostic and prognostic value than classical computed tomography scan imaging. *Blood* 1999;94(2):429–433.

49. Zinzani PL, Magagnoli M, Chierichetti F, et al. The role of positron emission tomography (PET) in the management of lymphoma patients. *Ann Oncol* 1999;10(10):1181–1184.

50. Moog F, Kotzerke J, Reske SN. FDG PET can replace bone scintigraphy in primary staging of malignant lymphoma. *J Nucl Med* 1999;40(9):1407–1413.

51. Moog F, Bangerter M, Diederichs CG, et al. Extranodal malignant lymphoma: detection with FDG PET versus CT. *Radiology* 1998;206(2):475–481.

52. Stumpe KD, Urbinelli M, Steinert HC, et al. Whole-body positron emission tomography using fluorodeoxyglucose for staging of lym-

phoma: effectiveness and comparison with computed tomography. *Eur J Nucl Med* 1998;25(7):721–728.

53. Cremerius U, Fabry U, Neuerburg J, et al. Positron emission tomography with 18F-FDG to detect residual disease after therapy for malignant lymphoma. *Nucl Med Commun* 1998;19(11):1055–1063.

54. de Wit M, Bumann D, Beyer W, et al. Whole-body positron emission tomography (PET) for diagnosis of residual mass in patients with lymphoma. *Ann Oncol* 1997;8(Suppl 1):57–60.

55. Hoh CK, Glaspy J, Rosen P, et al. Whole-body FDG-PET imaging for staging of Hodgkin's disease and lymphoma. *J Nucl Med* 1997;38 (3):343–348.

56. Okada J, Oonishi H, Yoshikawa K, et al. FDG-PET for predicting the prognosis of malignant lymphoma. *Ann Nucl Med* 1994;8(3):187–191.

57. Leskinen-Kallio S, Ruotsalainen U, Nagren K, et al. Uptake of carbon-11-methionine and fluorodeoxyglucose in non-Hodgkin's lymphoma: a PET study. *J Nucl Med* 1991;32(6):1211–1218.

58. Bartold SP, Donohoe KJ, Fletcher JW, et al. Procedure guideline for gallium scintigraphy in the evaluation of malignant disease. Society of Nuclear Medicine. *J Nucl Med* 1997;38(6):990–994.

59. Mikhaeel NG, Timothy AR, O'Doherty MJ, et al. 18-FDG-PET as a prognostic indicator in the treatment of aggressive non-Hodgkin's lymphoma: comparison with CT. *Leuk Lymphoma* 2000;39(5–6):543–553.

60. Buchmann I, Reinhardt M, Elsner K, et al. 2-(fluorine-18)fluoro-2-deoxy-D-glucose positron emission tomography in the detection and staging of malignant lymphoma. A bicenter trial. *Cancer* 2001;91(5): 889–899.

61. Finn WG, Kroft SH. New classifications for non-Hodgkin's lymphoma. *Cancer Treat Res* 1999;99:1–26.

62. Van den Abbeele A, Friedberg JW, Fischman A, et al. FDG-PET is superior to 67-Ga scintigraphy in the staging and follow-up of patients with Hodgkin disease: a prospective, blinded comparison. *J Nucl Med* 2002;43(5):30P.

63. Wirth A, Seymour JF, Hicks RJ, et al. Fluorine-18 fluorodeoxyglucose positron emission tomography, gallium-67 scintigraphy, and conventional staging for Hodgkin's disease and non-Hodgkin's lymphoma. *Am J Med* 2002;112(4):262–268.

64. Schoder H, Meta J, Yap C, et al. Effect of whole-body (18)F-FDG PET imaging on clinical staging and management of patients with malignant lymphoma. *J Nucl Med* 2001;42(8):1139–1143.

65. Spaepen K, Stroobants S, Dupont P, et al. Prognostic value of positron emission tomography (PET) with fluorine-18 fluorodeoxyglucose ([18F]FDG) after first-line chemotherapy in non-Hodgkin's lymphoma: is [18F]FDG-PET a valid alternative to conventional diagnostic methods? *J Clin Oncol* 2001;19(2):414–419.

66. Naumann R, Vaic A, Beuthien-Baumann B, et al. Prognostic value of positron emission tomography in the evaluation of post-treatment residual mass in patients with Hodgkin's disease and non-Hodgkin's lymphoma. *Br J Haematol* 2001;115(4):793–800.

67. Kaplan LD. Fluorine-18 fluorodeoxyglucose positron emission tomography for lymphoma: incorporating new technology into clinical care. *Am J Med* 2002;112(4):320–321.

68. Huic D, Dodig D. Fluorine-18-fluorodeoxyglucose positron emission tomography metabolic imaging in patients with lymphoma. *Croat Med J* 2002;43(5):541–545.

69. Cook GJ, Ott RJ. Dual-modality imaging. *Eur Radiol* 2001;11(10): 1857–1858.

70. Israel O, Keidar Z, Iosilevsky G, et al. The fusion of anatomic and physiologic imaging in the management of patients with cancer. *Semin Nucl Med* 2001;31(3):191–205.

71. Townsend DW, Cherry SR. Combining anatomy and function: the path to true image fusion. *Eur Radiol* 2001;11(10):1968–1974.

72. Beyer T, Townsend DW, Brun T, et al. A combined PET/CT scanner for clinical oncology. *J Nucl Med* 2000;41(8):1369–1379.

73. Martinelli M, Townsend D, Meltzer C, et al. 7. Survey of results of whole body imaging using the PET/CT at the University of Pittsburgh Medical Center PET Facility. *Clin Positron Imaging* 2000;3(4):161.

74. D'Amico TA, Wong TZ, Harpole DH, et al. Impact of computed tomography-positron emission tomography fusion in staging patients with thoracic malignancies. *Ann Thorac Surg* 2002;74(1):160–163; discussion, 163.

75. Schaffler GJ, Groell R, Schoellnast H, et al. Digital image fusion of CT and PET data sets—clinical value in abdominal/pelvic malignancies. *J Comput Assist Tomogr* 2000;24(4):644–647.

76. Colcher D. Centralized radiolabeling of antibodies for radioimmunotherapy. *J Nucl Med* 1998;39(8 Suppl):11S–13S.

77. Nagle C. From the Newsline editor. *J Nucl Med* 2002;43(4):11N.

78. Illidge TM, Bayne MC. Antibody therapy of lymphoma. *Expert Opin Pharmacother* 2001;2(6):953–961.

79. Knight N. Radioimmunotherapy and NHL: nuclear medicine on the oncology team. *J Nucl Med* 2002;43(4):11N–12N, 25N.

80. Wagner HN Jr, Wiseman GA, Marcus CS, et al. Administration guidelines for radioimmunotherapy of non-Hodgkin's lymphoma with (90)Y-labeled anti-CD20 monoclonal antibody. *J Nucl Med* 2002;43(2):267–272.

81. Wiseman GA, White CA, Stabin M, et al. Phase I/II 90Y-Zevalin (yttrium-90 ibritumomab tiuxetan, IDEC-Y2B8) radioimmunotherapy dosimetry results in relapsed or refractory non-Hodgkin's lymphoma. *Eur J Nucl Med* 2000;27(7):766–777.

82. Wiseman GA, White CA, Sparks RB, et al. Biodistribution and dosimetry results from a phase III prospectively randomized controlled trial of Zevalin radioimmunotherapy for low-grade, follicular, or transformed B-cell non-Hodgkin's lymphoma. *Crit Rev Oncol Hematol* 2001;39(1–2):181–194.

83. Wiseman GA, Leigh B, Erwin WD, et al. Radiation dosimetry results for Zevalin radioimmunotherapy of rituximab-refractory non-Hodgkin lymphoma. *Cancer* 2002;94(4 Suppl):1349–1357.

84. Gordon LI, Witzig TE, Wiseman GA, et al. Yttrium 90 ibritumomab tiuxetan radioimmunotherapy for relapsed or refractory low-grade non-Hodgkin's lymphoma. *Semin Oncol* 2002;29(1 Suppl 2):87–92.

85. Iodine-131 Tositumomab (Bexxar) in Relapsed/Refractory Non-Hodgkin's Lymphoma: Update from the 2001 American Society of Hematology Meeting. *Clin Lymphoma* 2002;2(4):209–211.

86. Kaminski MS, Zelenetz AD, Press OW, et al. Pivotal study of iodine I 131 tositumomab for chemotherapy-refractory low-grade or transformed low-grade B-cell non-Hodgkin's lymphomas. *J Clin Oncol* 2001;19(19):3918–3928.

87. Rutar FJ, Augustine SC, Kaminski MS, et al. Feasibility and safety of outpatient Bexxar therapy (tositumomab and iodine I 131 tositumomab) for non-Hodgkin's lymphoma based on radiation doses to family members. *Clin Lymphoma* 2001;2(3):164–172.

89. Tilley DR, Weller HR, Cheves CM, et al. Energy levels of light nuclei A = 18-19. *Nucl Phys* 1995;A595(1):1–170.

90. Ajzenberg-Selove F. Energy levels of light nuclei A = 11-12. *Nucl Phys* 1990;A506(1):1–158.

91. Ajzenberg-Selove F. Energy levels of light nuclei A = 13-15. *Nucl Phys* 1991;A523(1):1–196.

92. King MM, Chou WT. Nuclear data sheets update for A = 82. *Nucl Data Sheets* 1995;76:285.

Treatment Principles and Techniques

CHAPTER 11

Principles of Radiation Therapy

Peter M. Mauch, Andrea K. Ng, Elisa J. Wu, Richard T. Hoppe, Jorgen L. Hansen, Mary K. Gospodarowicz, and Joachim Yahalom

Patients newly diagnosed with lymphoma now have the potential for a longer survival with advances in diagnosis and treatment. Although many of the advances have been in immunotherapeutic and chemotherapeutic approaches, advances in technology have allowed the increasingly precise delivery of radiation therapy to involved sites while sparing normal tissues. Medical oncologists and radiation oncologists face a myriad of treatment choices in the management of lymphoma. Among indolent lymphomas, in which median survivals often exceed 10 years, these choices are increasingly influenced not only by the efficacy but also by the acute and late effects of treatment. Among aggressive lymphomas, of which many patients are cured, the intensity of treatment may be justified by improvements in survival, such as the addition of radiation therapy to chemotherapy in stage I to II patients.

Early trials in patients with indolent lymphomas demonstrated that for stage III to IV disease, more aggressive initial treatment resulted in an improved freedom from relapse but did not affect survival. In addition, more aggressive treatment was associated with increased toxicity and, in some cases, resulted in decreased survival (1). For these patients, tailored therapy has become an important concept; that is, to offer the best chance of a high quality of life with the least risk of toxicity. In many cases, this can be accomplished with the judicious use of modified chemotherapy or radiation therapy, or both. Radiation therapy in combined-modality regimens not only enhances disease control, but also may allow for reduction of the amount of chemotherapy. For effective treatment, radiation therapy and chemotherapy must be delivered with precision and according to standard guidelines. It is critical that the efficacy of radiotherapy be maximized through an understanding of the principles underlying appropriate field selection and design, dose prescription, and normal-tissue tolerance and protection.

HISTORY

Many of the early techniques and guidelines for treating non-Hodgkin's lymphoma with radiation therapy came from pioneering work in Hodgkin's disease. The discovery of x-rays by Roentgen, radioactivity by Becquerel, and radium by the Curies in the late nineteenth century led to the early treatment of Hodgkin's disease with crude x-rays in 1901. Within 1 to 2 years, there were reports of dramatic shrinkage of enlarged lymph nodes with x-ray treatments in patients with Hodgkin's disease and other lymphomas (2,3).

During the first two decades of the twentieth century, crude x-ray equipment was used to treat patients with lymphoma. Although there was initial shrinkage of nodes, the superficial characteristics of the radiation therapy deposited high doses in the skin and subcutaneous tissues, causing skin burns and ulceration, and underdosed deep nodes, resulting in less than optimal control.

Two technical advances in the 1920s, an improved cathode tube and deep-therapy transformers capable of delivering higher voltage x-rays, produced more deeply penetrating x-ray beams. Even with the more powerful x-rays, however, adequate treatment of tumors deep in the abdomen or chest frequently was associated with complications to the skin, muscles, heart, or bowel. Machines powerful enough to treat deep tumors without delivering excessive dose to more superficial normal tissues were not available until the late 1950s, when high-activity cobalt sources were produced.

The development of modern radiation therapy techniques for the treatment of Hodgkin's disease began with the work of Gilbert, a Swiss radiotherapist, in 1925 (4). Gilbert was one of the first physicians to point out specific clinical patterns in the spread of Hodgkin's disease. Initial treatment was concentrated on the regions involved by Hodgkin's disease; afterward, additional fields were used to encompass apparently healthy regions until low blood counts precluded further radiation. Gilbert and Babaiantz, in 1931, reported on 15 patients treated with fractionated and adjacent-site irradiation. Seven of the fifteen were still alive, with an average survival time of 4.3 years for all patients (5), a survival rate that was unprecedented for that time.

Vera Peters, in 1950, was the first physician to present definitive evidence that radiation therapy was a curative modality for early-stage Hodgkin's disease (6,7). She did this by identifying patients with limited-stage disease who were cured with high-dose, fractionated radiation therapy. Patients received 1,800 to 5,000 R to areas of involvement, with the highest dose given to patients with early-stage disease. She reported 5- and 10-year survival rates of 88% and 79%, respectively, for patients with stage I Hodgkin's disease—rates that were notably high for a disease in which virtually no one survived 10 years.

At Stanford, Henry S. Kaplan, building on the work of Rene Gilbert and Vera Peters, helped pioneer a new technology for cancer treatment: the linear accelerator. Kaplan became aware of the work in linear accelerator technology being conducted at the Stanford Microwave Laboratory by Edward Ginzton, William Hansen, and others. Kaplan and Ginzton realized that the features of the linear accelerator made it ideally suitable for cancer therapy (8). They secured funding from the U.S. Public Health Service, the Office of Naval Research, and the American Cancer Society to develop a linear accelerator suitable for clinical radiation therapy (9). The unit was completed in 1956.

Applying the treatments designed for Hodgkin's disease resulted in much less predictable outcomes for patients with lymphoma. Initial data from the 1930s suggested that follicular lymphoma appeared to be more sensitive to radiation than lymphosarcoma or reticulum-cell sarcoma. Sixty-five percent of patients with follicular lymphoma had complete regression of lymphadenopathy with 600 to 1,800 R delivered with a 200-kV machine, resulting in long intervals between treatments and a median survival of 3 to 4 years. Less than 10% of patients with more aggressive lymphomas had complete regression with these doses (10). The poor prognosis of patients with lymphoma as compared to Hodgkin's disease was apparent at the Paris conference of 1963, where clinical outcome was correlated with pathologic review. Patients with Hodgkin's disease often demonstrated long disease-free survivals; such results were unusual for patients with lymphoma.

EQUIPMENT

The linear accelerator is the machine of choice for radiotherapy of lymphomas. The desired energy is 6 megavolt (MV) for treatment of peripheral nodal sites, but higher energies, such as 15 MV, may be used for abdominal and thoracic tumors. A 6-MV beam is sufficiently penetrating to produce good dose homogeneity throughout the treatment field. The maximum dose point of 6 MV is close enough to the skin surface to avoid underdosing superficially located lymph nodes, such as cervical or inguinal nodes. The dose inhomogeneity measured in fields treated with a 6-MV beam may be as high as 10%, due primarily to differences in anterior-posterior distance (separation) within the field and to large separations in large patients. For patients with large nodes right at the skin, tissue-equivalent bolus may be needed to increase the subcutaneous dose.

Four-MV linear accelerators and cobalt-60 are less desirable than higher energy equipment. Greater inhomogeneity is seen with 4 MV energies within the field due to the less penetrating beam. Cobalt-60 units, although seldom utilized in the United States today, are still common in other areas of the world. With cobalt-60, the dose tends to fall off toward the edge of the field, so that there is a risk of underdosing the tumor (11). To compensate, a larger field size may be needed. With both 4-MV linear accelerators and cobalt-60, skin reactions are greater than with 6-MV energies. Also, field sizes and ability to treat at extended source-to-skin distance are more limited with cobalt-60.

RADIATION THERAPY TECHNIQUES

Dose, Dose Delivery, and Field Sizes: Historical Data

The relationship between radiation dose and probability of tumor control has been the subject of numerous reports extending back to the early 1970s. Because of the long-term survival of patients with early-stage disease and the association of tumor dose and field size to normal-tissue complications, it is important to define an optimal dose and field size for radiation therapy. A number of factors probably affect the relationship between dose and tumor control, including histopathology, tumor size, use of chemotherapy before radiation therapy, and responsiveness to chemotherapy. Unfortunately, there are no randomized trials evaluating the dose of radiation therapy in the management of lymphoma.

Two of the earliest retrospective papers on dose were published from Stanford University and the Princess Margaret Hospital in Toronto. Both series evaluated patients with early-stage diffuse large-cell lymphoma and follicular lymphoma. In the 1973 Stanford study, Fuks and Kaplan reported that doses of 25 Gy, 35 Gy, and 40 Gy achieved local control in 50%, 80%, and 90%, respectively, of patients with follicular lymphoma (estimated from curves) (12). For diffuse histiocytic lymphoma (similar to the current classification of diffuse large B-cell lymphoma), local control rates were 70% to 80%, regardless of the dose of radiotherapy delivered (from 20 to 50 Gy). The lack of a dose-response curve for diffuse large-cell lymphoma illustrates the potential problems of a retrospective analysis that is not able to control for stage, size, and site of disease. The Princess Margaret Hospital study evaluated histology, bulk of disease, and patterns of relapse (13,14). Patients with nodular lymphocytic poorly differentiated lymphoma (follicular lymphoma) had local or local-plus-distant recurrence rates of approximately 10% with 25 Gy or greater and 25% with less than 25 Gy. In contrast, patients with diffuse large-cell lymphoma had local or local-plus-distant recurrence rates of nearly 30%. Patients with medium- or large-bulk disease, defined as 2.5 to 5.0 cm in size and greater than 5 cm, respectively, had higher local or local-plus-distant recurrence rates than patients with smaller bulk disease. For example, in the small-bulk group with diffuse large-cell lymphoma treated with radiation therapy alone, the local or local-plus-distant recurrence rates were less

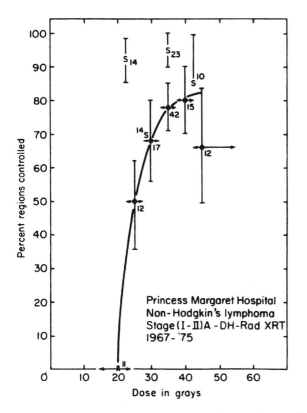

FIG. 11.1. Dose–regional control curve for patients with stage IA and IIA Hodgkin's lymphoma treated with radiation therapy alone. The main curve represents patients with medium (2.5 to 5.0 cm) or large disease (>5 cm). Data points for patients with small disease (S, <2.5 cm) are plotted separately. The total number of regions kept under control at each dose level is also shown. The dose range for each data point is illustrated by the horizontal arrows, and the 1 standard error is represented by the vertical bars. (From Bush R, Gospodarowicz M. The place of radiation therapy in the management of patients with localized non-Hodgkin's lymphoma. In: *Malignant lymphomas.* New York: Academic Press 1982:485–502, with permission.)

than 20% versus greater than 45% for patients with medium- and large-bulk tumors. The dose–regional control curve (Fig. 11.1) for diffuse large-cell lymphoma treated with radiation alone in patients with medium- or large-bulk disease showed 50% and 80% local control rates with 25 Gy and 40 Gy, respectively, with a plateau in the local-control curve after 40 Gy (13). Another retrospective study also shows the association of local control with tumor bulk (15). A total of 74 patients were treated with radiation therapy alone to a median dose of 50 Gy (all histologies). There were no in-field recurrences out of 51 patients with minimal disease and 10 in-field recurrences out of 23 patients (44%) with bulky disease.

Several other retrospective studies using radiation therapy alone and three randomized trials comparing radiation therapy with or without the addition of combination chemotherapy helped to establish early standards for the

technical use of radiation therapy, including guidelines for dose and field size. Two of the retrospective studies used a median dose of 50 Gy to the initial sites of involvement and treated extended fields to cover adjacent sites of disease (16–18). The randomized trials compared radiation therapy alone versus radiation therapy followed by chlorambucil, vincristine, and prednisone (CVP). Patients with indolent and aggressive histologies were included. For the diffuse lymphoma and large-cell lymphoma patients, there was an advantage in failure-free and overall survival favoring the use of adjuvant CVP (19–21). These trials somewhat reduced the dose of radiation therapy but continued to give prophylactic radiation therapy to uninvolved adjacent lymph node regions. In the Italian trial, 40 to 50 Gy were delivered to clinically involved areas, and proximal uninvolved lymph node–bearing areas received 35 to 45 Gy (20). Similar field sizes were used in the Danish trial, with the tumor receiving 37 to 43 Gy, with higher doses given for persistent disease (21). In this trial, there were six recurrences out of 36 patients (17%) in the radiation field with radiation therapy alone; none of the 46 patients recurred in the radiation field among patients receiving combined radiation therapy and chemotherapy. Data suggested that the addition of chemotherapy to radiation therapy not only reduced the incidence of distant relapse, but it also made the radiation therapy more effective for control of initial sites of involvement. In addition, approximately 10% of patients developed distant recurrences while on radiation therapy before chemotherapy was initiated. This suggested that the combination of the two modalities might be more effective with the chemotherapy given first.

Clinical Stage I to II Diffuse Large B-Cell Lymphoma Treated with Combined Adriamycin-Based Chemotherapy and Radiation Therapy

With the use of the more effective doxorubicin-based regimens, a number of retrospective trials reported good results using smaller radiation fields limited to the initial regions of involvement and given at somewhat reduced doses in patients with diffuse large-cell lymphoma. Table 11.1 shows selected retrospective studies using doxorubicin-based chemotherapy regimens and radiation therapy (22–30). The first six series used six to eight cycles of chemotherapy (22–27); the last three series gave three to four cycles (28–30). The median radiation doses ranged from 36 to 45 Gy in the first six studies and 35 to 40 Gy in the last three studies, except for some patients in the Rotterdam study who received 26 Gy. In one study, a greater number of cycles of chemotherapy was used for patients not achieving a complete remission (25). The M.D. Anderson Cancer Center study used 40 Gy for patients in complete remission after chemotherapy and 50 for a partial response/remission (27). Another study used a higher dose of radiation therapy (40 Gy) with three to four cycles of chemotherapy versus a

TABLE 11.1. *Multiagent chemotherapy and local radiation therapy for stage I to II intermediate- or high-grade lymphomas: selected retrospective trials*

Research site (reference)	No. of patients	Stage	Median RT dose (Gy)	Type and median no. cycles of CT	RT field size	MM/IF recur only	% FFR (yr)	% Survival (yr)
University of Florida (22)	121	I–II	NA	Nearly all ABR ≥4 cycles	NA	5/121 (4%)	63 (10)	44 (10)
Institute Gustave-Roussy (23)	96	I–II	45	CHVmP	NA	7/95 (7%)	NA	77 (5)
Stanford University (24)	23	I	40	ABR (85%)	IF (86%)	6/94 (6%)	78	81 (5)
	71	II		6 cycles			70	72 (5)
Milan (25)	183	I–II	40–44	CHOP × 4 cycles (CR) or 6 cycles (PR)	IF (41%); REG (59%)	9/183 (3%)	—	83 (5)
The Netherlands Multicenter Trial (26)	94	I–IE	36 (6–8 cycles CT); 40 (3–4 cycles CT)	92% ABR 3–8 cycles	IF (53%); EF (47%)	0/94, 3/94 local and distant	NA	70 (10)
MDACC (27)	57	I	40 (CR)	CHOP-Bleo	Gross disease + margin	5/147 (3%)	—	72 (10)
	90	II	50 (PR)				—	43 (10)
Rotterdam (28)	74	I–II	26 (CR)	CHOP × 4 cycles	IF	5/74 (7%)	69 DFS	76 (5)
	20		40 (CR)			1/20 (5%)	90	100 (5)
	34		40 (PR)			2/34 (6%)	75	75 (5)
British Columbia (29)	308	I–II	30/10 fx	ABR 3 cycles	IF	7/308 (2%)	—	80 (5)
			35/20 fx					63 (10)
National Cancer Institute (30)	47	I	40	ProMACE-MOPP 4 cycles	IF	2/47 (4%)	96	94 (5)
						0/45 (CR)		

ABR, adriamycin-based regimens; CHOP, cyclophosphamide, hydroxydaunomycin, Oncovin (vincristine), and prednisone; CHOP-Bleo, cyclophosphamide, hydroxydaunomycin, Oncovin, prednisone, and bleomycin; CHVmP, cyclophosphamide, hydroxorubicin, Vm-26, prednisone; CT, chemotherapy; CR, complete response; EF, extended field; FFR, freedom from recurrence: progression-free survival, disease-free survival (DFS), or recurrence/relapse-free survival noted when appropriate; MDACC, M.D. Anderson Cancer Center; MM/IF recur only, recurrences limited to within or on the edge of the radiation field; NA, information not available; PR, partial response; ProMACE-MOPP, prednisone, methotrexate, doxorubicin, cyclophosphamide, etoposide, mechlorethamine, vincristine, and prednisone; REG, regional radiation, usually the involved region and immediately adjacent uninvolved regions; RT, radiation therapy.

lower dose (36 Gy) with six to eight cycles of chemotherapy. Most of the studies used involved-field irradiation; in two series, approximately one half of the patients were treated to larger fields (25,26). The majority of patients in the studies had diffuse large-cell lymphoma, although diffuse undifferentiated, follicular large-cell, and diffuse poorly differentiated small cleaved–cell lymphomas were included in many of the series. Recurrences within or on the edge of the radiation field as the only site of relapse were rare (0% to 7%). Although the range of median doses was small, no differences in local control were seen in the different studies within this dose range. Similarly, no differences in local control were seen in studies that used six to eight cycles of chemotherapy versus four cycles.

Some additional dose/tumor control information not listed in Table 11.1 is presented below. In the University of Florida study, there were four local recurrences (7%) out of 59 patients receiving 30 to 40 Gy versus one local recurrence (2%) out of 51 patients when more than 40 Gy was used (22). In the Institute Gustave Roussy study, patients with nonbulky disease had a freedom-from-progression rate of 31% at 5 years versus 77% for patients with bulky presentations (23). Local recurrence rates were not analyzed by bulk in this study. In the Rotterdam study, a group of patients receiving 26 Gy (n = 74) was compared to a smaller group receiving 40 Gy (n = 20). Although significant differences were not seen in local control, the disease-free survival and overall survival rates were higher in the 40 Gy group (not significant).

Table 11.2 shows the two prospective randomized trials evaluating chemotherapy alone versus chemotherapy and radiation therapy. Both trials used involved-field irradiation.

TABLE 11.2. *Chemotherapy versus combined-modality therapy for stage I–II intermediate- or high-grade lymphomas: prospective randomized trials*

Author	No. of patients	Stage	CT	RT dose (Gy)	% CR or PR	% FFS	% Survival (yr)
ECOG (31)	173	CS I (EN–B) and all CS II	CHOP × 8 (CR)	—	61 (CR)	58	70 (6)
	172	CS I–II	CHOP × 8 (CR)	30 (IF)		73[a]	84 (6)[b]
			CHOP × 8 (PR)	40 (IF)	28 (PR)	60	64 (6)
SWOG (66)	201	CS I–IE (B–NB)	CHOP × 8	—	73	64	72 (5)
	200	and CS II (NB)	CHOP × 3	40–55	75	77[a]	82 (5)[a]

B, bulky disease; CHOP, cyclophosphamide, hydroxydaunomycin, Oncovin (vincristine), and prednisone; CR, complete response; CS, clinical stage; CT, chemotherapy; ECOG, Eastern Cooperative Oncology Group; EN, extranodal; FFS, failure-free survival; IF, involved field; NB, no bulky disease; PR, partial response; RT, radiation therapy; SWOG, Southwest Oncology Group.
[a]Significant difference between RT and no RT.
[b]Borderline significant difference between RT and no RT, p = .06.

The definition of involved fields in the Eastern Cooperative Oncology Group (ECOG) trial is detailed later (see Definition of Fields for Nodal Presentations). The Southwest Oncology Group trial used doses of 40 to 55 Gy based on physician preference and on the extent of residual disease after the three cycles of cyclophosphamide, doxorubicin, Oncovin, and prednisone (CHOP) chemotherapy. The ECOG trial used 30 Gy after eight cycles of CHOP for those patients who were in complete remission and 40 Gy for patients in partial remission. Although the results of the ECOG trial are only available in abstract form and details of location of relapse are not available, this is the first large trial to use the lower dose of 30 Gy with the full number of cycles of CHOP.

What can we conclude regarding the dose and field size of radiation therapy when combined with chemotherapy based on these retrospective and prospective trials? For diffuse large-cell lymphoma, radiation therapy alone is associated with a high distant-failure rate, as well as a 20% in-field recurrence rate, despite doses of 45 Gy or higher. The in-field recurrence rates appear to be higher for bulky disease than for patients with less bulky disease. In contrast, using doses of 35 to 45 Gy after a complete response to four to eight cycles of CHOP is associated with a low in-field/margin-of-field recurrence rate (0% to 7%; see Table 11.1). Furthermore, data do not appear to support the use of prophylactic adjacent nodal region irradiation. Similar local control data are seen in patients in complete response after chemotherapy before radiation therapy compared to a partial response before involved-field irradiation (28); however, studies suggest somewhat lower overall recurrence rates and survival rates in the patients with a partial response to chemotherapy (25,28,31). Exactly what doses to recommend for patients with initial bulk disease is still unclear, but following a complete remission after CHOP, data suggest that doses of 36 Gy should be sufficient (32).

Based on the above data, we recommend the following for diffuse large-cell lymphoma treated with combined modality therapy:

1. Use of involved fields
2. After a complete remission after six to eight cycles of CHOP: 36 Gy if initial bulky disease; 30 Gy for the remainder of patients
3. After three to four cycles of CHOP: 35 to 40 Gy
4. After a partial remission: 40 Gy

In the studies reported above, complete or partial remission are not always defined or defined consistently, especially because nuclear medicine imaging was not available for the majority of patients in these reports. Residual masses are common on computed tomography (CT) after chemotherapy, especially in patients with bulky mediastinal or abdominal disease. We do not have data on the success of radiation therapy (or the doses or field sizes needed) after a partial response based on a positive CT scan with a negative gallium or positron emission tomography (PET) scan versus both positive CT and positive nuclear medicine studies. The data that are available, using a variety of methods to define partial response, suggest that radiation therapy alone after a partial remission to chemotherapy allows for a very good freedom-from-treatment failure rate and long-term survival (31,33,34).

In the ECOG trial, patients with bulky or extranodal stage I and II intermediate-grade non-Hodgkin's lymphoma who achieved a complete response after eight cycles of CHOP were randomized to receive 30 Gy of radiation therapy versus no further treatment. All patients with a partial response to CHOP received radiation therapy to 40 Gy. Patients treated with radiation therapy after a partial remission had a 6-year disease-free survival rate of 54% and an overall survival rate of 64%. Another study from M.D. Anderson Cancer Center also demonstrated the effectiveness of radiation therapy in achieving a durable remission after a partial response to chemotherapy (33). Investigators reviewed 294 patients with large-cell lymphoma treated with CHOP-based chemotherapy. CT scans were obtained in every case to assess response to chemotherapy, using the International Working Group guidelines. An unconfirmed complete response or partial response was documented in 44 patients. At a median follow-up of 43 months, compared with patients who received salvage chemotherapy, those who received salvage radiation therapy had a significantly better 4-year local-control rate (86% vs. 53%, p = .009) and 4-year progression-free survival (67% vs. 8%, p < .0001). Using historical controls, the authors also noted that the 6-year progression-free survival and overall survival rates of 61% and 70%, respectively, were comparable to results achieved by high-dose therapy with autologous stem-cell rescue.

In a study by Zinzani and colleagues (34), 50 patients with primary mediastinal large B-cell lymphoma were prospectively treated with methotrexate, Adriamycin, cyclophosphamide, vincristine, prednisone, and bleomycin (MACOP-B), followed by radiation therapy. CT and ^{67}Ga citrate single-photon emission CT (GaSPECT) were obtained at diagnosis, at the end of chemotherapy, and 3 months after radiation therapy. Three patients with progressive disease during chemotherapy were excluded from the analysis. After chemotherapy, 31 out of 47 patients (66%) had a positive GaSPECT. Among these 31 patients, 22 became GaSPECT negative after radiation therapy. None of the patients with a negative GaSPECT posttreatment relapsed at a median follow-up of 39 months.

Clinical Stage III to IV Diffuse Large B-Cell Lymphoma

Although adjuvant radiation therapy is not generally used for stage III to IV diffuse large B-cell lymphoma, some studies have recommended its routine use or use in specific circumstances. In a retrospective study from the M.D. Anderson Cancer Center, use of radiation therapy after CHOP-based chemotherapy appeared to significantly improve freedom from progression and local control but not overall survival compared to chemotherapy alone (35). Another study from the same institution demonstrated that radiation therapy delivered to patients with clinical stage I to IV disease after a partial response or unconfirmed complete response significantly improved local control and progression-free survival compared to the use of alternative chemotherapy (33). These studies used 30 to 50 Gy to involved fields. Aviles and colleagues randomized patients with clinical stage IV diffuse large B-cell lymphoma after a complete remission to CHOP-bleomycin to radiation therapy to prior sites of bulk disease or no further treatment (36). Patients randomized to radiation therapy had a higher disease-free survival (72% vs. 35%) and overall survival (81% vs. 55%) compared to patients not receiving radiation therapy. An ECOG trial randomized 433 patients with stage III to IV disease to Adriamycin-based chemotherapy alone or combined with involved-field radiation therapy. There were no differences for stage IV patients, but there was an improved disease-free survival for stage III patients (36a).

Clinical Stage I to II Follicular Large-Cell Lymphoma

There are few data on follicular large-cell lymphoma, an unusual subtype of lymphoma. Current practice recom-

mends treatment similar to patients with diffuse large-cell lymphoma (see Diffuse Large B-Cell Lymphoma) (37). Some of the series on radiation therapy alone for early-stage follicular lymphoma included patients with follicular grade 3 disease (38–41), and one study from Japan reported good results in patients with stage I disease treated with radiation therapy alone using 40 Gy or greater (42).

Stage I to II Follicular Grade 1 to 2 Lymphoma

Radiation therapy alone is standard treatment for patients with clinical stage (CS) I to II follicular grade 1 to 2 lymphoma. Nine large series reporting results of treatment for follicular grade 1 to 2 are shown in Table 11.3 (22,33,38–41,43–45). The median radiation doses vary from 30 to 40 Gy in eight of the nine series, with the two largest series reporting a median dose of 35 Gy (38,39). In-field recurrences range from 0 to 11%, with higher percentages occurring in patients with bulky disease or those who received a radiation dose of less than 30 Gy (22,33,44). A variety of field sizes have been used, ranging from involved fields to total nodal irradiation. There are no differences in survival by field size utilized. Freedom from recurrence was better in the Stanford University study with total nodal irradiation (40) and in the Royal Marsden Hospital study with larger field sizes (45). In the other studies, older age, extensive stage II disease, and bulky disease are adverse features for recurrence risk. The most common fields used are involved or regional fields (including the immediate adjacent prophylactic nodal sites).

What can we conclude regarding the dose and field size of radiation therapy when used alone in the treatment of follicular lymphoma based on these retrospective trials? Although there are few data, doses under 30 Gy may be associated with a higher in-field (and overall) recurrence risk. The majority of studies report median doses of 35 to 40 Gy, with most patients treated to involved or regional fields (the involved nodal region plus one additional uninvolved region on each side of the involved nodes).

Based on all the above data, we recommend the following for early-stage follicular grade 1 and 2 lymphoma:

1. Use of involved or regional fields. Carefully planned radiation therapy to limited fields with modest doses can significantly reduce the risk of significant damage to the marrow reserve, the risk of developing a treatment-related malignancy, and the risk of long-term toxicity to other normal tissues, such as the salivary glands, lungs, heart, kidneys, and bowel.
2. The recommended dose is 30 to 36 Gy, with a boost to areas of initial involvement to 36 to 40 Gy. Bulky disease should be treated to the upper end of the range; 30 to 36 Gy should suffice for smaller disease. This approach provides a 40% to 50% probability of cure.

Use of smaller (involved or regional) fields preserves the ability to effectively treat patients who later recur with the

TABLE 11.3. *Radiation therapy alone for early-stage low-grade follicular non-Hodgkin's lymphoma (selected trials containing ≥50 patients)*

Report	No. of patients/ med FU/ % CT	Stage (%)	10-yr FFTF/OS (%)	Median RT dose to the tumor (Gy)	RT field size	MM/IF recur	Grade/stage distribution (%)	Adverse prognostic factors (FFTF)
Princess Margaret Hospital (38)	573/ 10.6 yr/ 27	I (64) II (36)	48/>60	35	IF	NA	FG1 (33) FG2 (32) FG3 (35)	Ext. CS II >2-cm disease
BNLI (39)	208/ NA/ 0	I (100)	47/64	35 (suggested)	NA	NA	FG1 (39) FG2 (35) FG3 (5) Other (21)	Age ≥50 yr
Stanford University (40)	177/ 7.7 yr/ 5	I (41) II (59)	44/64	35–50	IF/RF/EF (77%) TLI (23%)	NA/13.8	FG1 (57) FG2–3 (43)	Age >60 yr Extranodal site RT fields <TLI
Fondation Bergonie (43)	103/ 8.3 yr/ 70	I (44) II (56)	49/56	35–40	IF (54%) RF (46%)	NA	NA	Age >60 yr
M.D. Anderson Cancer Center (33)	80/ 19 yr/ 0	I (41) II (59)	41/43 at 15 yr	40	IF (9%) RF (54%) EF (37%)	<3 cm: 0/44 sites with 30 Gy <3 cm: 0/74 sites with 40 Gy >3 cm: 4/54 with 40 Gy	FG1 (63) FG2 (37)	CS IIA >3-cm disease
Edinburgh (44)	64/ 5 yr/ 2%	I (58) II (42)	49/78	30–40 (82%) >40 (18%)	NA	30–40 Gy: non-bulky-0/14 30–40 Gy: unk/ bulky-3/32 >40 Gy: unk/ bulky-1/9	FG1 (78) FG2 (3) Other (19)	NA
University of Florida (22)	72/ 8.5 yr/ 7	I (75) II (25)	46/59	NA	IF (53%) EF (43%) TNI/WA (4%)	With RT alone <30 Gy (4/41– 10%) ≥30 Gy (0/26)	NA	NA
National Cancer Institute (41)	54/ 9 yr/ 10	I (50) II (50)	48/69	36	IF (38%) EF (48%) TLI/TBI (14%)	1/48 (2%)		Age ≥45 yr
Royal Marsden Hospital (45)	58/ NA/ 0	I (69) II (31)	43/79	40	IF (52%) EF (48%)	3/54 (9%)	FG1 (64) FG2 (21) Other (15)	Field size not significant for recurrence

BNLI, British National Lymphoma Investigation; CT, chemotherapy; DFS, disease-free survival, or recurrence/relapse free survival; EF, extended field RT, mantle or whole abdominal fields (Wilder), mantle, whole abdominal, inverted Y (Pendlebury, McManus), mantle, inverted Y (Lawrence); Ext., extensive; FFTF, freedom from treatment failure, also, progression-free survival; FG, follicular grade; Med FU, median follow-up time; MM/IF, recurrences limited to within or on the edge of the radiation field; OS, overall survival (all causes); NA, not reported; RF, regional field RT, 1–3 adjacent nodal regions (Wilder); RT, radiation therapy; TBI, total-body irradiation; TLI, total lymphoid irradiation; TNI, total nodal irradiation; WA, whole abdominal.

same histology or who transform to a high-grade histology. More than one half of the patients with early-stage disease eventually develop recurrent disease, and increasingly, there will be new and more effective approaches for these patients.

Stage III to IV Follicular Grade 1 to 2 Lymphoma

Although less frequently used in current practice, data suggest that large-field irradiation may be effective in the treatment of patients with stage III disease. This treatment consists of total-lymph-node irradiation and, in some cases, whole-abdominal irradiation (to cover the mesenteric nodes). One of the largest series is from Stanford University (46). Sixty-six patients with stage III follicular lymphoma were treated with total-lymphoid (61 patients) or whole-body irradiation (5 patients) from 1963 to 1982. The failure-free survival was 35% at 15 years; cause-specific survival was 58%, and the overall survival was 35%. A small cohort of patients with a lower tumor burden, defined as fewer than five disease sites and no tumor mass greater than 10 cm, had a failure-free survival of 88% and a cause-specific survival of 100% at 15 years. There were few relapses beyond 10 years. Similar data have been reported from the University of Florida and the Medical College of Wisconsin (47,48).

Radiotherapy has also been advocated as consolidation therapy after chemotherapy for patients with advanced-stage follicular lymphoma. A phase III trial by Aviles and colleagues randomized 118 untreated patients with stage III or IV follicular lymphoma to receive CVP chemotherapy alone or the same chemotherapy followed by involved-field radiotherapy to initially involved nodal sites to doses of 35 to 45 Gy (49). The 7-year failure-free survival was 33% for patients treated with chemotherapy alone and 66% when receiving combined-modality therapy. The 7-year survival was also significantly higher in patients receiving adjuvant radiation therapy ($p = .06$).

Stage I to II Mucosa-Associated Lymphoid Tissue and Extranodal Marginal Zone Lymphoma

The indolent extranodal lymphomas associated with mucosa-associated lymphoid tissues (MALT) involve the gastrointestinal tract, salivary glands, breast, thyroid, orbit, conjunctiva, skin, lung, and, less commonly, other sites. As this subtype of lymphoma tends to remain localized for long periods of time, local treatment (surgery or local/regional irradiation) is very effective at long-term control of disease and provides the opportunity for cure. In particular, low doses of radiation therapy (30 Gy) to involved nodal regions or extranodal sites almost always control sites of disease. These doses are somewhat lower than those used for patients with localized follicular grade 1 to 2 disease. Three retrospective studies provide dose-control data for this type of lymphoma. Schechter and colleagues first reported in a small series of 17 patients with gastric MALT lymphomas that low doses of radiation (median 30 Gy, range 28.5–43.5 Gy) were associated with a 100% probability of local control (50). Tsang and colleagues reported local control data in 70 patients

with stage I (62) and stage II (8) MALT lymphomas presenting in the stomach and other sites treated to a median dose of 30 Gy (range, 17.5–35 Gy) (51). The most common doses used were 25 Gy (mostly orbit presentations) and 30 Gy. The overall local control rate was 97%. Of the two local recurrences, one occurred after 17.5 Gy, and the other occurred after 30 Gy. The 5-year disease-free and overall survival rates were 76% and 96%, respectively. In a report from Harvard Medical School by Hitchcock and colleagues, 66 patients with stage I to IV marginal zone lymphoma were evaluated (52). The median radiation dose was 33.5 Gy. All 35 stage I to II patients who received radiation therapy as initial treatment achieved local control. Among stage I to II patients, the 5-year progression-free and overall survival rates were 75% and 93%, respectively.

Based on all the above data, we recommend the following for early stage MALT or extranodal marginal zone lymphoma:

1. Use of radiation therapy alone to involved nodal regions or extranodal sites to 30 Gy (defined in more detail later in Defintion of Fields for Nodal Presentations). Doses of 30 Gy result in a near-100% local control rate. Although there are very few data with lower doses, such as 25 Gy (except for orbital MALT), there is a suggestion that local control rates are high with this dose as well. This should allow for modification of dose in settings in which normal involved field tissue risks are somewhat higher (orbit, salivary glands).
2. Although there are high complete-response rates with chemotherapy for marginal zone lymphoma, there is little evidence that it is curative (see Chapter 22) (53,54). Therefore, outside of clinical trials, chemotherapy should be reserved for patients with stage III to IV disease. Asymptomatic individuals with generalized disease may be considered for observation, similar to patients with generalized follicular lymphoma.

Mantle Cell Lymphoma

This newly designated disease has a poor prognosis, and patients with stage I to II disease are seldom encountered. The therapy of mantle cell lymphoma has been explored in a number of retrospective analyses, as well as prospective phase II and phase III trials utilizing a variety of chemotherapy programs (55,56). There is no evidence for the superiority of any one combination over any other or the ability of any regimen to cure patients with advanced-stage disease. There are very limited data suggesting that patients with stage I to II diffuse, poorly differentiated lymphocytic lymphoma (this category does not exist in the REAL classification; some of these patients would now be classified as mantle cell lymphoma) may be cured with local-regional radiation therapy often combined with chemotherapy (15). Extrapolating from other aggressive lymphomas, it appears reasonable to add radiation therapy to chemotherapy in patients with mantle cell lymphomas with stage I to II disease.

We have observed that advanced-stage patients with mantle cell lymphomas are very responsive to low doses of radiation therapy (20 to 25 Gy), allowing for large fields to be used for bulky disease not responsive to chemotherapy. Based on this limited information and extrapolating from the data for dose in diffuse large-cell lymphoma, we suggest doses of 30 to 36 Gy to involved fields.

Palliative Radiation Therapy for Advanced Disease

Radiation therapy is a very effective palliative approach in the management of advanced lymphomas. Some of the indications for palliative radiation therapy include

1. Alleviation of symptoms, including prevention or relief of symptoms from spinal cord or nerve root involvement; orbital or conjunctiva disease causing diplopia, partial loss of vision or irritation; and gastric or bowel irritation.
2. Cosmetic relief from large neck nodes.
3. Treatment of chemotherapy-resistant solitary masses, allowing longer remissions and an increased freedom from additional systemic treatment.
4. Avoidance of fracture of weight-bearing bones.

Recommended doses of radiation therapy are generally lower than those used for early-stage disease, given that the field sizes may be larger, patients have often received extensive prior treatment, and the risk of systemic relapse is generally higher than with stage I to II disease. Recommended doses are generally two-thirds to three-quarters of the curative dose. Adjustments in doses may also be needed due to prior radiation therapy (lower doses if re-irradiating a site), large field sizes (lower doses), or the presence of crucial normal tissues in the field. Two histologies, marginal zone and mantle cell lymphomas, appear especially sensitive to radiation therapy. Figure 11.2 shows the CT scans of a patient with marginal zone lymphoma with extensive thoracic involvement. A daily dose of 1.5 Gy given over 2 weeks to a total dose of 15 Gy resulted in complete disappearance of disease. This patient is in remission 4 years later. Figure 11.3 shows a patient with extensive mantle cell lymphoma. A dramatic and durable response was seen with a total dose of 22 Gy. Doses in the 15 to 20 Gy range allow use of large radiation fields that are usually within normal-tissue tolerance and can provide a significant improvement in the quality of life for these patients. Also, there are some data to suggest that even smaller doses of radiation can be effective. In a French study, Grinsky and colleagues treated patients with advanced-stage follicular lymphomas with doses of 4 Gy in two fractions, achieving an 81% objective response rate as well as a 2-year freedom-from-local-progression rate of 56% (56a).

Stage I to II Extranodal Presentations: Radiation Fields, Doses, and Dose Delivery

There is an extensive literature describing the pathology, staging, and treatment of patients with localized extranodal disease (see Chapter 43). As a general rule, however, it is the pathologic subtype and stage, rather than the extranodal disease location, that should determine the approach to therapy. The most common extranodal sites are discussed below. Primary lymphomas of the skin and central nervous system are discussed in separate chapters.

Gastric Lymphoma

Gastric lymphomas primarily are of two types, diffuse large B-cell and MALT lymphoma, occurring in approximately equal frequency. MALT lymphomas consist of both low- and high-grade subtypes, with the high-grade subtype consisting of large cells with low-grade elements as well. High-grade MALT lymphoma behaves like diffuse large-cell lymphoma and should be managed similarly to other aggressive lymphomas.

Patients with gastric lymphoma usually present with symptoms of abdominal pain (80%). Other common symptoms include loss of appetite (50%), weight loss (25%), bleeding (20%), and B symptoms (10%). The diagnosis of gastric lymphoma is usually established endoscopically, although in the past, laparotomy and partial or complete gastrectomy were utilized. Although surgical resection followed by adjuvant radiotherapy and/or chemotherapy has resulted in a high event-free and overall survival, the long-term morbidity of gastric resection is significant. The availability of other equally effective treatment strategies has reduced the role of surgery in this disease (57–60).

The treatment of localized diffuse large-cell lymphomas of the stomach without systemic therapy historically resulted in overall survivals of 25% to 50%, similar to results of radiation therapy alone in other sites. The use of systemic chemotherapy has resulted in considerable improvement. Multiple centers now report 5-year survivals ranging from 70% to 80% for patients with localized disease treated with chemotherapy with or without radiotherapy (61–65). Although some authors have suggested that chemotherapy alone is adequate treatment, most studies have employed a combination of chemotherapy and radiotherapy. In addition, the Southwest Oncology Group and ECOG CS I to II trials support this approach, demonstrating an advantage for combined chemotherapy and radiation therapy versus chemotherapy alone in freedom from progression and overall survival (31,66,67). There is no evidence to suggest that the number of cycles of chemotherapy and dose of radiation should differ from recommendations for stage I to II diffuse large-cell lymphomas in other sites. The response to chemotherapy should be assessed by repeating the imaging studies that were positive before the onset of chemotherapy. In addition, repeat endoscopy and biopsy may be useful for assessing the completeness of response.

Recommended radiation doses range from 30 to 40 Gy, as with other sites. Doses on the low side of the range should be used for minimal disease at presentation and a complete remission after full-course chemotherapy. Higher doses should be used for bulky disease at presentation, a partial response after chemotherapy, or after a limited number of cycles of chemotherapy (three to four cycles). For patients undergoing com-

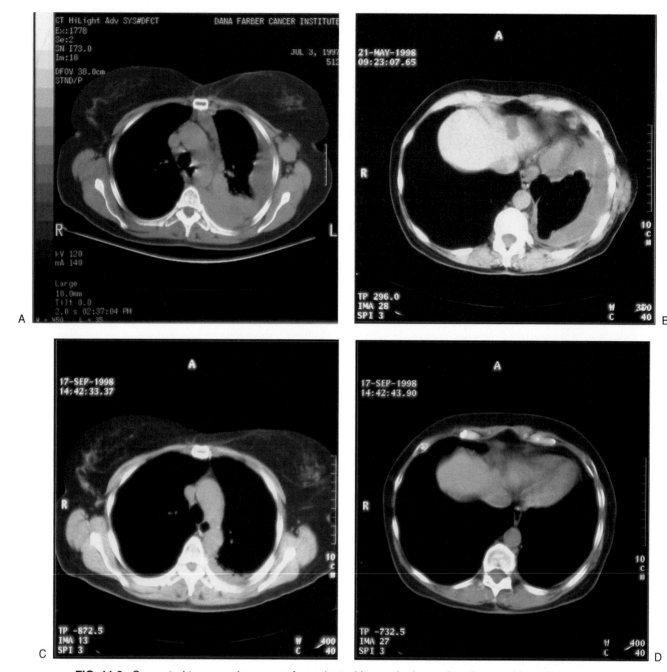

FIG. 11.2. Computed tomography scans of a patient with marginal zone lymphoma with extensive thoracic involvement. **A,B:** Axial cuts showing pretreatment disease involvement of the lung parenchyma, left axilla, diaphragm, and left lateral chest wall. **C,D:** Axial cuts of the same levels showing an excellent response after 15 Gy of radiation therapy to the left hemithorax. A, anterior; L, left; R, right.

plete resection with a partial or total gastrectomy before chemotherapy, radiation therapy may be omitted in some cases. The radiation field should encompass the entire stomach, immediately adjacent celiac axis nodes, and any other involved areas with a margin of several centimeters. A three- or four-field approach should be used, as it allows the left kidney to be protected by placing a posterior block on the lateral fields, thus keeping the kidney dose within tolerance levels (Fig. 11.4 and Color Plate 3).

A unique feature of gastric MALT lymphoma is the association with *H. pylori* infection (68–70). Treatment of *H. pylori* infection–associated gastric MALT lymphoma with antibiotics commonly results in tumor regression. The complete remission rate is approximately 75%, with most patients remaining in remission at the time of follow-up (71,72). Although a high response rate is achieved, the ultimate cure rate with antibiotic therapy alone is still not known. The largest series and the series with the longest

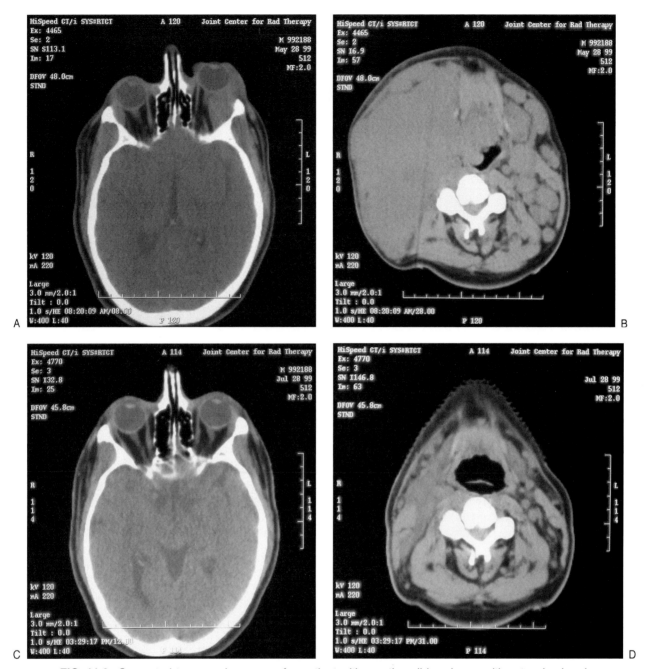

FIG. 11.3. Computed tomography scans of a patient with mantle cell lymphoma with extensive head and neck involvement. **A,B:** Axial cuts showing pretreatment disease involvement of the left neck and right retroorbital area causing proptosis. **C,D:** Axial cuts of the same levels showing an excellent response after 22 Gy of radiation therapy.

follow-up is from the German MALT Lymphoma Study Group (71). The authors describe 97 patients, 77 of whom achieved a complete endoscopic and histologic remission. Seven patients relapsed clinically; however, approximately 50% of patients with demonstrated monoclonality at diagnosis by polymerase chain reaction examination continued to display monoclonal bands on follow-up polymerase chain reaction analysis, despite the maintenance of a clinical remission. The significance of this observation is unclear.

Radiotherapy is the treatment of choice for patients who do not respond to antibiotics. Local control of MALT lymphoma is nearly 100% with doses of radiotherapy of 30 Gy (50–52). Patients who are *H. Pylori* negative may be less likely to respond to antibiotics than *H. Pylori*–positive patients; initial treatment of *H. Pylori*–negative patients with antibiotics remains under study (72). Data regarding the use of chemotherapy for gastric MALT lymphoma are sparse. The disease is chemotherapy responsive, and complete

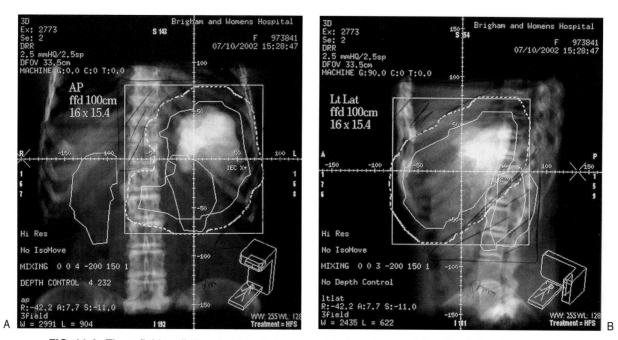

FIG. 11.4. Three-field radiation treatment for a gastric lymphoma. **A,B:** Simulation films showing anteroposterior (AP) and left lateral fields. Oral barium was given before the simulation for gastric opacification. The clinical target volume was outlined in solid line, and the planning target volume was outlined in broken line, with a 1.5-cm margin from the gross target volume. The kidneys were also outlined in solid line. Note that the majority of the left kidney was included in the AP field, but both kidneys were behind the stomach and were blocked in the lateral field. (See Color Plate 3.)

remission rates of 50% or better are described in a number of studies (53,73). However, data suggest that similar to other low-grade lymphomas, MALT lymphoma is responsive to chemotherapy, but recurrences are common and there is no evidence for cure. Thus, there is little role for chemotherapy in early-stage MALT lymphoma.

Extrapolating from the gastric data, intestinal MALT lymphomas are managed similarly to their counterparts in the stomach. The role of chemotherapy is limited. Crump and colleagues recommend whole-abdominal radiotherapy for intestinal MALT lymphomas after surgical resection, with a dose of 20 to 25 Gy in 1.0- to 1.25-Gy fractions. However, there are few data to support a large-field versus small-field approach for intestinal MALT lymphomas. If all apparent disease has been resected, chemotherapy alone or watchful waiting without radiation therapy is recommended.

Head and Neck Lymphomas

Head and neck lymphomas occur in a variety of sites, including Waldeyer's ring, the thyroid, salivary glands, nasal cavity, paranasal sinuses, and orbit with differing histologies and clinical characteristics, depending on the site of origin. Most appear to be of B-cell origin, and the three major subtypes are diffuse large-cell lymphoma, marginal zone lymphoma, and nasal natural killer/T-cell lymphoma.

Lymphomas presenting in Waldeyer's ring typically involve tonsil, base of tongue, or nasopharynx. The clinical

symptoms are those associated with epithelial tumors in those sites, such as dysphagia, sore throat, nasal congestion, and eustachian tube blockage. The lesions are frequently clinically apparent on thorough head and neck examination and are often associated with neck adenopathy.

For diffuse large-cell lymphoma, treatment guidelines are similar to those for nodal stage I to II disease. Historical series of radiotherapy alone for large-cell lymphoma of the head and neck region report 50% survival in stage I patients and lower survivals for stage II disease (74–76). Retrospective studies show significantly improved survivals with the use of combined-modality therapy (63,77–79).

Most lymphomas presenting in the paranasal sinuses are B-cell in origin. The outlook after treatment with radiotherapy alone is poor for both stage I and II patients (80,81). Some authors have described a predilection for central nervous system spread (81a). Overall, the outlook improves markedly when patients are treated with combined radiation therapy and chemotherapy (80–82). After chemotherapy, the involved sinus should be treated with a margin. CT planning with conformal radiation therapy or intensity-modulated radiation therapy should be employed whenever possible. Immobilization in this region is excellent (with an Aquaplast mask or removable head frame), and conformal treatment allows reduction of dose to normal crucial structures, such as the eye and salivary glands. Patients with low-grade lymphoma of the sinus can be treated with radiation therapy alone to doses of 35 to 40 Gy. For diffuse

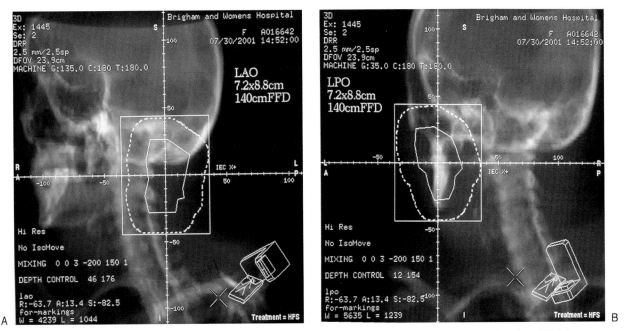

FIG. 11.5. Wedge pair radiation treatment for a parotid lymphoma. Simulation films showing **(A)** left anterior oblique (LAO) and **(B)** left posterior oblique (LPO) fields. The clinical target volume was outlined in solid line, and the planning target volume was outlined in broken line, with a 1.5-cm margin from the gross target volume. FFD, focus-film-distance. (See Color Plate 4.)

large-cell lymphoma after chemotherapy, a minimum dose of 40 Gy should be used. Although there are few specific data, it is often hard to evaluate complete versus partial responses in the sinuses after chemotherapy. In addition, concerns about tumor necrosis and poor oxygenation potentially making chemotherapy and radiation therapy less effective, as well as the difficulties with retreating this region, suggest that radiation-dose reduction should not be attempted for this site.

Nasal cavity lymphomas are usually natural killer/T-cell lymphomas and are seen more commonly in Asia. The disease appears to progress locally, with only a small risk of regional or systemic failure (83). Approximately two-thirds of patients achieve a complete remission with radiation therapy alone (83,84), but approximately one-half of these patients relapse. The contribution of chemotherapy in the management of natural killer/T-cell lymphoma is unclear, especially as complete response occurs in only a minority of patients after chemotherapy alone (84,85). Yet, the poor results with radiotherapy alone argue for use of the combined-modality approach. With the combination of chemotherapy, most studies suggest treating the nasal cavity to 40 to 44 Gy.

Salivary gland lymphomas are frequently of the marginal zone lymphoma type. Treatment usually consists of radiotherapy alone with an excellent prognosis. For ipsilateral parotid involvement, a wide-angled wedge pair treating the parotid and upper cervical nodes to 30 Gy should result in virtually 100% local control. This approach allows sparing of the opposite parotid and maintenance of salivary function (Fig. 11.5 and Color Plate 4).

The *preauricular field* includes the superficial lymph nodes just anterior to the tragus and, therefore, above or on the edge of a standard anterior-posterior neck field. This field may be used in a patient with disease limited to the preauricular/parotid nodes with or without upper neck involvement. Techniques include the use of photons to anterior-posterior or wide-angled wedge-paired fields. Sometimes, a three-field approach is used that includes a lightly weighted lateral field. Usually, the opposite salivary glands and some of the base of the tongue can be spared. Patients with ipsilateral tonsillar involvement who do not need full Waldeyer's ring irradiation are candidates for a modification of this field (upper and lower borders are slightly different). Simulation is done in an Aquaplast mask as described earlier in this section, and the bottom of the orbit is marked anteriorly to make sure that the posterior field does not diverge through the lower portion of the orbit. Some centers use a lateral *en face* electron field or combined electrons and photons as an alternative approach.

What about field and dose selection for other head and neck presentations? Involved fields after chemotherapy for diffuse large-cell lymphoma should include the ipsilateral cervical and supraclavicular nodes for ipsilateral neck presentations (see Specific Involved-Field Sites). Involvement of the ipsilateral tonsil with low-grade lymphoma requires treatment of the entire Waldeyer's ring region. The dose can be limited to 30 Gy, with a cone down to the initial site(s) of involvement if indicated. Ipsilateral tonsillar involvement with diffuse large-cell lymphoma should initially be treated with chemotherapy. If there is a complete

Set-Up Diagram

Harvard Joint Center for
Radiation Therapy

Graphic Plans

Therapy number: *983472*   Machine: *6BWH*

Orientation: SUPINE

Minimum target dose: 100%
Inhomogeneity:
Initials, TPC: ___
Date: *17-SEP-98*

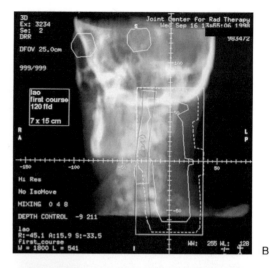

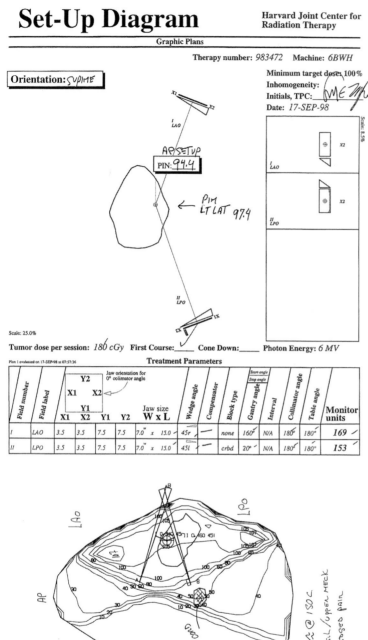

Tumor dose per session: *180 cGy*   First Course: ___   Cone Down: ___   Photon Energy: *6 MV*

Treatment Parameters

Field number	Field label	X1 X1	X2 X2	Y1 Y1	Y2 Y2	Jaw size W x L	Wedge angle	Compensator	Block type	Gantry angle	Interval	Collimator angle	Table angle	Monitor units
I	LAO	3.5	3.5	7.5	7.5	7.0" x 15.0	45r		none	160°	N/A	180°	180°	169
II	LPO	3.5	3.5	7.5	7.5	7.0" x 15.0	45l		crbd	20°	N/A	180°	180°	153

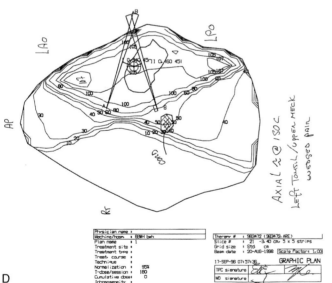

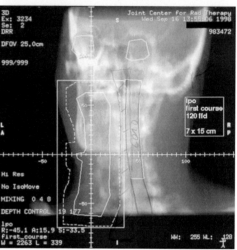

FIG. 11.6. Wedge pair radiation treatment for an ipsilateral tonsil lymphoma. **A:** Set-up diagram showing beam arrangements to the left tonsil and upper neck. **B,C:** Simulation films showing left anterior oblique (LAO) and left posterior oblique (LPO) fields. The left tonsillar and upper neck disease was outlined in solid line, and the planning target volume was outlined in broken line, with a 1.5-cm margin from the gross target volume. Note that the spinal cord was blocked in the LPO. **D:** Graphic plan for the wedge pair technique, showing isodose distribution to the clinical target volume and the spinal cord. AP, anteroposterior; LP, left posterior; LT LAT, left lateral; RA, right anterior; RT, right.

response, it may be feasible to treat the ipsilateral tonsil and neck to 30 to 40 Gy, depending on the initial size of the disease and number of cycles of chemotherapy (Fig. 11.6). Alternatively, one could treat Waldeyer's ring to 25 to 30 Gy, followed by a cone down to the tonsil. If there is a partial response to chemotherapy or if there is bilateral tonsillar involvement, the entire Waldeyer's ring must be treated

(Fig. 11.7). This approach can be associated with significant xerostomia.

Orbit and Globe

Lymphomas of the eye may involve the extraocular orbital tissues, such as the conjunctiva, retrobulbar region, or lacrimal

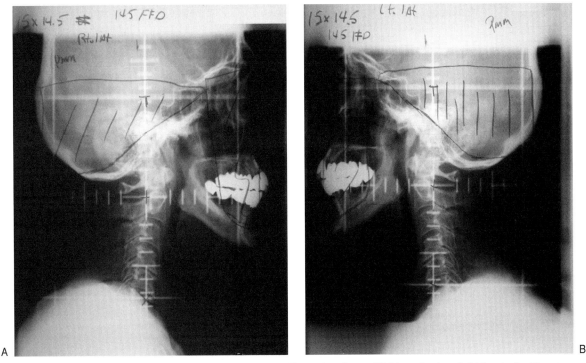

FIG. 11.7. Waldeyer's ring field. **A,B:** Simulation films showing a Waldeyer's ring field treated with an opposed-lateral technique. The nasopharynx is included in the treatment field superiorly. FFD, focus-film-distance.

gland, or may be primary within the tissues of the eye itself. The latter condition is referred to as *primary intraocular lymphoma* and is a subset of primary central nervous system lymphoma, in which lymphoma cells are initially present only in the eyes without evidence of disease in the brain or other central nervous system tissues. Patients with disease of the eye itself have a high risk of initial involvement of the central nervous system or subsequent relapse in that site. For this reason, these patients should be treated as if they have primary central nervous system lymphoma (see Chapter 41).

Orbital lymphomas comprise approximately 4% of all extranodal lymphomas. They typically arise in superficial tissues, such as conjunctiva and eyelids, or in the retrobulbar region. Mass lesions in the conjunctiva or lids are described typically in the literature as "salmon pink" in color. Tumors of the retrobulbar region may present with swelling and may disturb the function of the extraocular muscles, resulting in proptosis. Bilaterality occurs in approximately 10% of cases and should be assessed at the time of staging. In addition to the usual staging studies for systemic disease, a CT and/or magnetic resonance (MR) imaging of the orbit should be done to precisely delineate the anatomic extent of disease for radiotherapy planning purposes.

Histopathologically, approximately two-thirds of orbital lymphomas are of the marginal zone type (86). Most of the remaining cases are diffuse large-cell lymphoma. Marginal zone lymphoma of the orbit is treated with radiotherapy alone. No more than 30 Gy is required, with some reports using as little as 25 Gy with excellent results (51). Doses of 25 to 30 Gy

should be well tolerated by almost all eye tissues except the lens (51,86–89). Orbital lesions are best treated with a pair of narrow-angle wedged anterior fields. This allows for good dose coverage of the tumor without treating the opposite eye (Fig. 11.8 and Color Plate 5). In this circumstance, the lens cannot be protected without risking underdosing the lymphoma, and a high percentage of patients eventually develop a cataract, requiring surgical correction.

The treatment of choice of diffuse large-cell lymphoma is combined-modality therapy with CHOP chemotherapy followed by involved-field radiation. As in other sites, 30 to 36 Gy following a complete response to chemotherapy is probably sufficient (89).

Conjunctival lymphoma tends to be localized, but it may be associated with advanced disease. Due to its infiltrative nature, conjunctival lymphoma recurs with a high frequency after surgical excision alone. Surgery is used for diagnosis, but local radiation therapy to the entire conjunctiva is the definitive treatment of choice. Treatment of conjunctival lymphoma can be accomplished with electrons or photons. The advantage to electrons is that the lens can be protected with daily placement of a tungsten eye shield. Dunbar and colleagues used doses of 24 to 30 Gy for patients with conjunctival lymphoma. They saw no local recurrences in a series of 12 patients treated with electron beam radiation therapy (90). Sometimes, the involvement of the conjunctiva is extensive enough to risk blocking the tumor with the eye shield. In this circumstance, a single anterior photon field with a hanging eye block allows protection of the lens without compromising the efficacy of treatment. The central

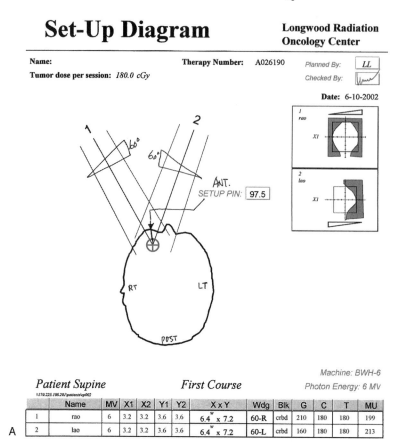

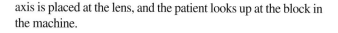

Set-Up Diagram

Longwood Radiation Oncology Center

Name: Therapy Number: A026190   *Planned By:* LL

Tumor dose per session: *180.0 cGy*   *Checked By:*

Date: 6-10-2002

ANT.
SETUP PIN: 97.5

RT   LT

POST

Patient Supine   *First Course*   *Machine:* BWH-6
Photon Energy: 6 MV

	Name	MV	X1	X2	Y1	Y2	X x Y	Wdg	Blk	G	C	T	MU
1	rao	6	3.2	3.2	3.6	3.6	6.4" x 7.2	60-R	crbd	210	180	180	199
2	lao	6	3.2	3.2	3.6	3.6	6.4" x 7.2	60-L	crbd	160	180	180	213

A

FIG. 11.8. Narrow-angle wedge pair radiation treatment for an orbital lymphoma. **A:** Set-up diagram showing beam arrangements to the right orbit. **B,C:** Simulation films showing right anterior oblique (RAO) and left anterior oblique (LAO) fields. The right orbit was outlined in solid line, and planning target volume was outlined in broken line, with a 1.5-cm margin from the gross target volume. The contralateral orbit outside of the treatment field was also outlined in solid line. ANT, anterior; LT, left; POST, posterior; RT, right. (See Color Plate 5.)

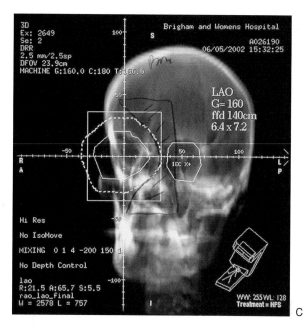

axis is placed at the lens, and the patient looks up at the block in the machine.

Extranodal Lymphomas of Other Sites

In addition to the areas described, non-Hodgkin's lymphoma may arise in almost any organ or tissue of the body, including, but not limited to, bone, testis, ovary, kidney, bladder, female genital tract, breasts, lymphoma, and lung. Lymphoma in any of these sites is quite uncommon. General principles of evaluation and management apply to these sites. Testicular, bone, and lung lymphomas are discussed below.

Testicular lymphoma is rare and presents typically in elderly males in their 60s and 70s. Most patients have localized disease on presentation. The histology is typically diffuse large B-cell type. The diagnosis is typically made by orchiectomy. Thus, the initial treatment is surgical, and often all disease is removed at diagnosis. In the past, surgery was frequently followed by radiotherapy to pelvic and paraaortic nodes in a fashion similar to that for testicular carcinoma or seminoma. This approach resulted in poor survivals. Although the introduction of CHOP chemotherapy combined with radiation and surgery improved survival somewhat, a high central nervous system and contralateral testis recurrence rate remained with this approach (91–93). More recent treatment programs have advocated the use of central nervous system prophylaxis with intrathecal methotrexate, as well as systemic high-dose methotrexate coupled with prophylactic radiation therapy to the contralateral testis, with much improved 5-year survivals (92). With the use of high-dose methotrexate, there is some debate whether contralateral testis irradiation is needed. If administered, a total dose of 30 Gy is delivered, often using electrons.

The long bones are primarily affected with extranodal *lymphoma of bone*. The presenting signs and symptoms are generally local bone pain, with or without soft-tissue swelling, occasionally a palpable mass lesion or a pathologic fracture. Histopathologically, 70% to 90% of patients have diffuse large B-cell lymphoma. Treatment has historically consisted of radiotherapy alone to doses of 40 to 50 Gy. Similar to other nodal and extranodal sites, approximately one-half of patients with stage IE bone disease are cured with this approach, with most relapses occurring distant to the initial region of involvement (94–96). Thus, the current approach is to use chemotherapy followed by radiation therapy as with other sites.

Objective assessment of response is often difficult for primary bone lymphomas. Radiographic response as manifested by bone healing is a slow process. Isotopic scanning studies, such as bone, gallium, or PET, may continue to be positive for significant periods of time and may represent healing of the bone in question, rather than persistent tumor. Thus, by radiologic criteria, patients will almost always have a partial remission after chemotherapy. Therefore, we recommend a dose of 40 Gy to patients with primary bone lymphoma after chemotherapy if the gallium or PET scan remains positive, or if there continue to be radiographic abnormalities on CT or MR imaging. Small reductions in dose (36 Gy) can be used if all the restaging studies are normal. In the literature, there is very little discussion of appropriate field size for this site of presentation. We recommend that the site of bone involvement, as defined by imaging studies obtained before chemotherapy, be covered with a margin of several centimeters. Irradiation of the entire bone is probably unnecessary given the use of systemic chemotherapy.

Most *pulmonary lymphomas* are marginal zone lymphomas, also known as *BALT lymphomas* from the involvement of bronchus-associated lymphoid tissue. The 5-year survival is excellent and similar to other presentations of marginal zone lymphoma (97,98). Patients usually present with an asymptomatic abnormality on chest x-ray. It may be hard to obtain sufficient tissue at bronchoscopy or by fine-needle

aspirate to establish the diagnosis, and an open procedure is usually required. Most of the studies have treated patients with surgical resection, sometimes followed by chemotherapy. There are few data on radiation therapy, alone or in combination with surgery and chemotherapy; however, excellent local tumor control would be predicted for radiotherapy with modest doses. Radiation therapy, therefore, is the treatment of choice in unresectable BALT lymphoma or cases in which the extent of pulmonary resection would significantly compromise lung function. In this situation, although the usual recommended doses are 25 to 30 Gy, lower doses within lung tolerance (less than 20 Gy) may be highly effective, as this disease is very sensitive to low doses of radiation therapy.

A small percentage of pulmonary lymphomas are of the diffuse large-cell type. These should be managed initially with chemotherapy. If the disease has been completely resected to establish the diagnosis, no additional radiotherapy is needed. If resection has not been accomplished, CHOP should be followed by radiotherapy, as long as the amount of lung irradiated is small enough to preserve a significant amount of the lung (50% or more).

Positioning and Immobilization

Increasingly, CT simulation is utilized in the treatment of patients with lymphoma, as it allows for optimizing the dose to the tumor and minimizing normal-tissue toxicity. One of the important lessons learned from three-dimensional treatment planning is that radiotherapy accuracy during a course of fractionated radiation is only as good as the immobilization of the patient. With Cerrobend blocks attached to a standard machine block-holding tray or automated multileaf collimator blocks, very small changes in patient position may result in considerable field variations. Accurate positioning requires reproducible neck and arm positioning, and reproducible alignment and rotation of the torso and pelvis. Reproducible knee and foot positioning may also be required under certain circumstances.

The following techniques can be used for immobilization of the head. Most patients are treated in the supine position. Although resting the head on a soft sponge (or alternatively in a head rest or cup) with tape used to fix the chin position allows good visualization of the light field and subtle adjustment of the head position, the authors increasingly recommend the use of an Aquaplast mask. This mask can be molded to the shape of the head and chin at treatment planning, and it is fixed to the table at simulation and treatment, allowing patient comfort but very little movement (see Color Plate 6). Furthermore, if the fields are limited to the head and neck region, marks can be placed on the mask, eliminating the need to permanently mark the patient. On occasion, with very large tumors, the patient may need to undergo a new simulation and mask mid-treatment to adjust for tumor shrinkage. One tremendous advantage of the mask is its ability to achieve the immobilization needed for the use of conformal fields or intensity-modulated radiation therapy designed to avoid irradiation of salivary glands and other crucial structures.

An alternative method of immobilization is a customized upper body Styrofoam mold or an alpha cradle in conjunction with a chin band. The patient is simulated and treated in the cradle. A disadvantage of this system is that some bolusing of the back results when the posterior field is treated through the cradle, resulting in an increase in the skin reaction posteriorly (99). Arm position varies according to the age of the patient and institutional preference. The akimbo arm position can be reproduced by simply having the patient place his or her thumbs in the waistband or belt or on the table at that level. The arms up position can be secured with an alpha cradle or customized upper body mold with hand grips for reproducible position (100), although in a cooperative patient, the arm position may be secured with a less rigorous setup. The arms up position should be used when treating the axilla, or when oblique or lateral thoracic field approaches are planned. An upper body mold is useful for the treatment of lower neck and thoracic fields.

Wall-mounted lasers in the simulation and treatment rooms can aid in reproducing torso and pelvic alignment and rotation. Leveling tattoos, one pair of lateral tattoos on each side of the central axis, aid in lining up with the side lasers.

Techniques to assure reproducibility of the knee and foot position are especially important for patients treated to fields below the diaphragm. One technique is to place a standard wedge under the knees that can be used each day. The ankles can be immobilized with tape or a bandage with a reproducible ankle separator that maintains ankle separation and thereby precludes knee or hip rotation. Many patients prefer a small amount of knee flexion for comfort.

If the patient is to be treated with sequential radiation fields, positioning for the two fields must be as consistent as possible to avoid inadvertent overlap with the previously treated field, created by shifts in patient position. The previous field position must be clearly documented. Inconspicuous tattoos placed at the field borders, use of the same patient position, radiographic documentation, and knowledge of previous field size and source-to-skin distance allow calculation of an appropriate skin gap, so that sequential fields may be treated safely. Although it is unusual to use matching fields in the initial treatment of patients with lymphoma, as the field size is often limited, often fields must be used that overlap a previously treated area in cases of recurrent lymphoma. In this case, the prior details of treatment and simulation films must be obtained, so that doses to crucial organs such as the spinal cord can be limited.

Custom Blocks

Custom shielding blocks are essential to the delivery of high-quality radiation therapy. Divergent blocks are generally cast from a low-melting-point alloy, such as Cerrobend, and mounted on the collimator of the linear accelerator. Most modern linear accelerators, as an alternative, have multileaf collimators, which allow blocking with the head of the machine itself. In either case, the blocks are of a thickness calculated

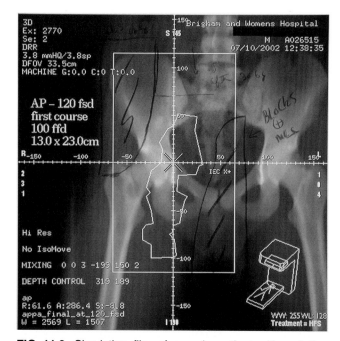

FIG. 11.9. Simulation film of a male patient with radiation treatment to the right external iliac, inguinal, and femoral region, combining Cerrobend blocks and multileaf collimator to limit radiation dose to the ipsilateral testes. AP, anteroposterior; ffd, focus-film distance; fsd, focus-skin distance.

to reduce the transmitted beam by five half-values, that is, to approximately 3% of the prescribed dose.

In addition to the 3% transmitted from the primary beam directly through the block, some dose is delivered to the shielded areas from radiation scattered internally from other tissues within the direct path of the radiation beam. The amount of scatter depends on the amount of surrounding tissue within the primary beam (width of the area contributing scatter), the width of the block, the radiation energy (less scatter with higher energy beams), and the distance from the edge of the protective block. Of the normal tissues, the testes are the most sensitive to low-dose fractionated radiation. A total of 300 to 350 cGy delivered over 20 treatments results in sterility in more than 50% of patients. Thus, the 3% received from the primary beam through the block may significantly add to the scattered dose and bring the total dose into this range. This is of importance in patients receiving external iliac, inguinal, and femoral irradiation in which the testes are within the radiation field borders but under the block. One way to reduce the primary beam dose to the testes is to utilize both the templated blocks and the multileaf collimators. This should provide ten half-layers of protection and reduce the primary dose component to 0.01% of the total dose (Fig. 11.9).

Definition of Fields for Nodal Presentations: Involved Fields

The lymphatic system is arbitrarily divided into lymph node regions for the purpose of field design. An *involved field*

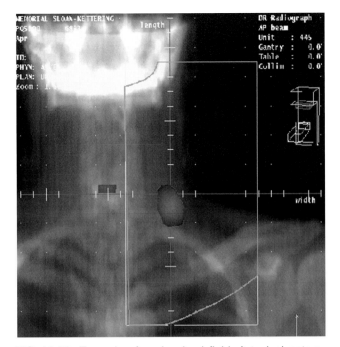

FIG. 11.10. Example of an involved field. A typical antero-posterior (AP) field used to radiate the involved field for unilateral neck disease with an anterior-posterior technique. For medially located lymph nodes, the medial border may be extended to the contralateral side of the vertebral bodies to allow adequate margin.

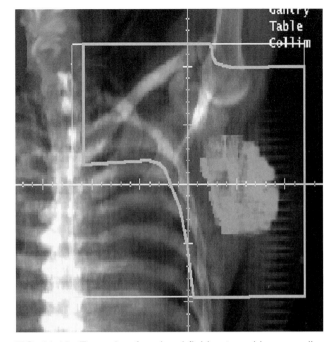

FIG. 11.11. Example of regional-field external-beam radiation therapy to treat a large axillary mass. The anteroposterior field, extended to include the ipsilateral supraclavicular fossa, is used in conjunction with a posterior field.

includes not only the individual clinically involved or enlarged nodes, but also the other lymph nodes within the same lymph node region [see discussion by Yahalom (101) and Fig. 11.10]. The involved field is the minimum radiation field size used for the treatment of early-stage nodal lymphomas. See Specific Involved-Field Sites later in this chapter for general guidelines for involved fields based on descriptions from clinical trials.

Regional Fields

Regional fields have been variously described in the literature to include the involved field and at least one adjacent noninvolved region in the initial treatment volume. Regional fields are designed to reduce the risk of a recurrence in the adjacent nodal region and were initially based on the patterns of failure observed in Hodgkin's disease when radiation therapy alone with limited fields was used as primary treatment (Fig. 11.11). In general, regional fields are currently used for the treatment of patients with stage I to II follicular lymphomas presenting in nodal sites. An example is the treatment of the ipsilateral external iliac, inguinal, and femoral nodes in a patient with stage I follicular grade 1 to 2 lymphoma of the inguinal region.

Extended Fields

The term *extended fields* has been used to describe treatment of all lymphoid groups on one side of the diaphragm and, in

some cases, the treatment of both mantle and paraaortic-splenic fields. Extended fields are rarely used today in the treatment of lymphoma.

Large-Field Irradiation

Total-lymphoid and total-nodal irradiation are synonymous and imply treatment of all the major lymph node regions above and below the diaphragm. Certain lymph node groups, including brachial, epitrochlear, and popliteal nodes, are rarely involved in lymphoma and are not included in these fields. Mesenteric and sacral nodes may be involved in patients with lymphoma, and the treatment of the abdomen and pelvis may need to be modified to include these groups. Total-nodal irradiation is rarely used in patients with lymphoma, although some physicians still advocate it for the treatment of patients with limited stage III follicular histology (102–104). It also has been used to prevent graft rejection in patients receiving mismatched T-depleted allogeneic grafts after high-dose therapy for recurrent lymphoma (105–107). Low-dose total-body irradiation has been used in the past for treatment of patients with advanced-stage follicular lymphoma and for chronic lymphocytic leukemia. Patients usually received 10 to 15 cGy two to three times per week to a total dose of 150 cGy (108–111). Given advances in treatment and the potential long-term consequences of wide-field irradiation (marrow toxicity, second cancers), this approach is rarely used today. High-dose total-body irradiation (12 to 14 Gy), given in multiple fractions, often at a low dose rate, is used in conjunction with high-dose chemotherapy in preparation for allogeneic and, in some cases, autologous transplantation. Several excellent reviews have been written on the subject (112–115).

Specific Involved-Field Sites

Involved fields can be used after combination chemotherapy to treat the initially involved lymph node region. By definition, these fields treat the region of initial nodal involvement. The technique of treating the enlarged node without treating the region should be avoided.

Waldeyer's Ring

Waldeyer's ring covers the lymphoid tissue of the nasopharynx, tonsil, and base of tongue. The typical Waldeyer field (see Fig. 11.7) includes extranodal lymphoid tissue in the nasopharynx, base of tongue, and tonsils, as well as retropharyngeal, preauricular, submandibular, and submental nodes. It is matched to the upper border of the neck fields if there are cervical nodes involved. The easiest method of matching fields is to set the central axis of each field at the field junction to eliminate divergence. Extra protection should be provided by placing a short (2-cm) block over the superior portion of the spinal cord on the anterior-posterior neck field. The most common energy chosen is 6 MV photons. Radiation therapy alone for early-stage follicular grade 1 to 2 lymphoma involving the tonsil, base of tongue, or nasopharynx results in treatment of all of Waldeyer's ring. Because this field is associated with significant xerostomia that may be permanent in older adults, the dose to this field should be limited to 25 to 30 Gy. A cone down field can then be used to a total dose of 30 to 36 Gy, which allows for blocking of some of the salivary tissue.

Cervical/Supraclavicular Fields

The *neck fields* include all nodal tissue from the base of the skull to the clavicles. The patient is positioned supine and treated with opposed anterior and posterior fields. The neck should be positioned so that the upper border of the field passes through mid-mandible, mid-tragus, and mastoid when the head is extended. The inferior border is 1 to 2 cm below the clavicles. The lateral border is set at the medial aspect of the acromion to encompass the supraclavicular and low neck nodes, and the beam tangentially irradiates the lateral neck skin and lower ear superiorly. The medial border for a single neck field is set at either the ipsilateral (cervical nodal involvement alone) or contralateral (with supraclavicular nodal involvement) vertebral pedicles (i.e., either including or excluding the entire width of the spinal cord). When the contralateral vertebral pedicles are used, the pharynx and larynx can be blocked to approximately C-5. Treatment should be given with 6 MV photons. If a higher energy is utilized, bolus should be applied, because

some of the nodes are located no more than 0.5 cm below the skin surface. Even with 6 MV photons, response of the supraclavicular or cervical nodes to radiation should be assessed midway into treatment. If the response is less than ideal, daily bolus over this region should be applied for the second half of the treatment.

Mediastinum

The *mediastinal field* includes anterior superior mediastinal, pretracheal, paratracheal, paraesophageal, hilar, internal mammary, and subcarinal nodes. The caudad/cephalad extent should cover from the top of T-1 to the bottom of T-7 or T-8 (varies with patient anatomy) to cover the hilar and subcarinal nodes (Fig. 11.12 and Color Plate 7). If the central cardiac and diaphragmatic nodes are involved, the field should extend to the level of the diaphragm. The superior border should encompass the T-1 vertebral body at the minimum. If there is extension into the deep supraclavicular fossa, the field should extend to the top of C-7. Laterally, the fields should encompass any clinically evident tumor with a 1- to 2-cm margin, as well as a 1- to 2-cm margin on the superior mediastinal shadow and the hila.

Epitrochlear Nodes

Epitrochlear involvement in lymphoma is rare. With the arms rotated outward, the nodes lie in the medial half of the arm. The easiest way to treat the epitrochlear nodes is to use a separate involved field. Usually, the lateral half of the arm can be blocked. In some cases, the ipsilateral axillary nodes are covered as well. With careful arm positioning and immobilization, the axilla and epitrochlear region can be treated in a single field.

Retroperitoneal Nodes

Retroperitoneal nodes are treated through equally weighted, opposed anterior and posterior portals with the patient supine. The superior border is usually at the top of T-10; however, the upper border may vary depending on the extent of nodal involvement. The inferior border is set at the bottom of L-4 (bifurcation of the aorta). The paraaortic nodes normally lie within the lattermost extent of the transverse processes of the vertebral bodies; however, CT planning should be used to determine the width of the lymphadenopathy, so that it can be covered with a 1.5-cm margin laterally. It is imperative that the location of each kidney be known and mapped, and that no more than one-third of the total renal volume is included in the paraaortic field. In most patients, a portion of the spleen abuts the diaphragm; inclusion of the diaphragm with a 0.5- to 1.0-cm border of lung ensures adequate splenic coverage that can be verified with routine port films. The spleen also typically abuts the lateral abdominal wall; inclusion of rib cage or the lateral abdominal wall ensures adequate lateral cov-

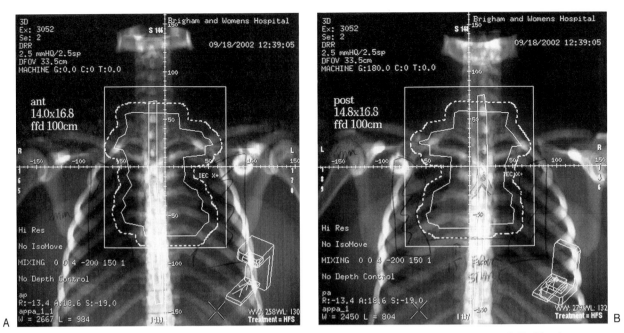

FIG. 11.12. A modified mantle field in a lymphoma patient with mediastinal involvement. **A,B:** Simulation films showing a modified mantle field treated with an anterior-posterior technique. Included in the treatment field were the bilateral supraclavicular fossa; mediastinum, including the subcarinal region; and the bilateral hila. The initially uninvolved axillae were excluded from the field. The bilateral mantle blocks were shaded, and the carina was outlined on the posterior field. ant, anterior; ffd, focus-film distance; post, posterior. (See Color Plate 7.)

erage. The medial and inferior borders of the spleen are determined by CT scanning. It is critical that the location of the kidneys be documented, as a portion of the spleen and the left kidney are frequently superimposed.

Mesenteric Nodal Irradiation

Mesenteric nodes are commonly involved in patients with lymphoma. Mesenteric nodes should be treated with lateral fields, so that the kidneys can be protected with blocking as they lie posteriorly to the mesentery. In some cases, a third anterior-posterior field is used to improve the dose distribution.

Inguinal/Pelvic Fields

The pelvic nodes are treated through opposed anterior and posterior fields with the patient supine. For ipsilateral external iliac nodal involvement, the ipsilateral common iliac nodes, external iliac nodes, and inguinal nodes are included in the field. In this case, the field extends superiorly to the top of L-5 and inferiorly to the bottom of the ischial tuberosities. If both the ipsilateral common and external iliac nodes are involved, then the opposite common iliac nodes are included in the field, and the top of the field extends to the top of L-4. For patients presenting with inguinal nodes, the ipsilateral femoral and external iliac nodes should be included in the field. The inferior border of the field extends inferiorly to include the palpa-

ble femoral triangle with a 1.5- to 2.0-cm margin, or approximately 5 cm below the inferior portion of the lesser trochanter (see Fig. 11.9). The superior border extends to the bifurcation of the internal and external iliac nodes or approximately middle of the sacroiliac joints. The lateral border may be set to the outer edge of the acetabulum with blocking of the iliac crests. A medial block extending superiorly to the bottom of the sacroiliac joints should be added to shield the symphysis pubis, central bladder, and rectum.

In the standard pelvic field, the testicles are not in the primary beam. Scattered irradiation from the pelvic and inguinal fields, however, may produce temporary oligospermia. The scattered dose received by the testicles depends on the total dose, the distance from the edge of the contributing fields to the testes, and the design and positioning of external testicular shielding devices. When the femoral nodes are treated, the testes are often in the primary beam and receive 3.1% through the central pelvic block, as well as increased scatter from the open fields that lie to the side of the testis; this results in a higher risk of sterility. The dose can be reduced with additional blocking of the primary beam as discussed in Custom Blocks earlier in this chapter.

To preserve fertility in the male patient treated with pelvic irradiation, the testicles must be shielded from as much internally scattered radiation as possible by using a special clamshell-like testicular shield (116–118). It is important that the testicles are positioned behind the front wall of the shield. These shields provide a three- to ten-fold reduction in scatter dose to the testes (117). Loss of fertility is significantly reduced by limiting the radiation field to one side of the pelvis. With bilateral pelvic nodal irradiation, the internal scatter component increases greatly.

Normally, the ovaries lie just medial to the external iliac nodes and within a standard pelvic radiation field. The tolerance of the ovaries to radiation is well below the doses employed for lymphoma. If preservation of ovarian function, including fertility, is desired, the ovaries must be transposed to a location outside the primary radiation beam, or to a location over which sufficient secondary shielding can be provided to prevent ovarian ablation. Surgical transposition or *oophoropexy* may be accomplished through a laparoscopic procedure. Careful coordination between surgeon and radiation oncologist is required, so that the surgeon understands exactly where the ovaries must be placed, marks them with radiopaque clips, and takes radiographs at the time of surgery on the operating room table to insure that placement is correct. With unilateral pelvic irradiation, one ovary should remain outside of the field and should have normal function. In many patients with lymphoma, the age at onset is beyond childbearing age. In the young patient receiving whole-pelvic irradiation, transposition of the ovaries is the only way to preserve hormonal function and fertility.

Three-Dimensional Treatment Planning

Image-driven treatment planning is the most precise means to maximize the dose to the tumor while minimizing dose to normal tissues. This should result in improved local control with less toxicity.

Three-dimensional treatment planning in Hodgkin's disease has been studied extensively at several institutions (119,120). Less information is available in the treatment of lymphoma. In a study by Cho and colleagues (121), 123 patients with Hodgkin's disease and 33 patients with non-Hodgkin's lymphoma underwent pretreatment chest CT. Seventeen patients were shown to have chest wall involvement that was not apparent on conventional x-ray and clinical examination. The results suggest the important role of CT scans in directing radiation therapy and support the usefulness of three-dimensional treatment planning in this patient population. In another study from Stanford University comparing the effect of MR imaging and CT scans on radiation therapy planning in 57 patients with thoracic lymphoma (122), MR studies were found to be more sensitive in detecting chest wall and pleural disease. The MR findings subsequently resulted in change in radiation portal and dose in 20% of patients. Investigators from Germany developed a planning technique for radiation therapy in patients with subdiaphragmatic malignant lymphoma (123). Coronal MR tomograms and MR angiograms of the abdominal vessels were obtained in 38 patients. The images were superimposed and projected onto the simulation film in correct scale. The technique was found to result in a 32% reduction in the treated kidney volume. The results demonstrate the impor-

tance of conformal radiation therapy in patients with lymphoma, because many patients present with disease in locations where optimal shielding of radiosensitive structures is crucial. The applicability of three-dimensional treatment planning for central lymphoid irradiation was investigated by Garcia and colleagues at M.D. Anderson (124). Compared with a standard two-dimensional treatment plan, the three-dimensional approach was found to have advantages of providing a single plan for each patient with multiple views of the data, including different planar cross-sections and dose-volume histograms of relevant structures.

Treatment Verification and Documentation

A number of studies have documented difficulty with accurate daily delivery of treatment (125–130). With the frequent use of imaging films, which document the volume of tissue actually exposed to radiation during a treatment, it is clear that both systematic errors and random errors may occur. Systematic errors result from a flawed simulation, perhaps because the patient was tense and later relaxed on the actual treatment table or because the initial simulation position was uncomfortable and not sustainable (125,127,129). Typically, systematic errors can be identified with an imaging film on the first day of treatment. Random errors are related to malposition of the patient or shielding blocks in daily treatment setups. The use of better positioning tools, such as immobilization devices and lasers, have aided in securing more accurate setups, and the use of frequent imaging films has focused attention on accuracy and identified systematic problems (125,127,128).

There is limited information specific to lymphoma cases on the accuracy of radiation treatment planning. In a study from the Netherlands, the accuracy of patient positioning was prospectively evaluated in 13 lymphoma patients receiving mantle radiation therapy (131). Patients were treated in the supine position for the anterior field and in the prone position for the posterior field. Larger discrepancies between simulation films and portal films were found in the posterior fields than the anterior fields. The authors concluded that attention should be directed to increasing the stability of patients in the prone position to minimize systemic and random error rates. Naida and colleagues from the University of Michigan evaluated the localization error rate of four experienced radiation oncologists on their lung blocks for mantle-field irradiation, with or without the diagnostic CT scans available (119). A three-dimensional treatment planning system displaying tumor volumes was used as reference. *Localization errors* were defined as touching or overlap of the shielding blocks onto tumors. The overall error rates in the absence and presence of the diagnostic CT were 18% and 13%, respectively ($p = .038$). The axillary region was found to be associated with the highest error rate, whereas the superior mediastinum had the lowest error rate. Localization errors were also more likely with increasing tumor volume. These results showed that even with the diagnostic CT available, the error rate can still be considerable, and that the use of three-dimensional planning in mantle-field definition may reduce the incidence of geographic misses.

QUALITY CONTROL AND ASSURANCE

Cooperative Group Trials: Accuracy of Delivery of Electron Beam Radiation Therapy and Outcome

Quality control and assurance is critical to the interpretation of clinical trial results and ensuring uniformly optimal patient care. The quality of radiation treatment depends on the successful completion of each of the following steps:

1. Identification of sites of involvement and sites at significant risk for microscopic disease. This requires an ability to perform an accurate and complete physical examination, to interpret the diagnostic images used in staging, and to understand the regions at risk and patterns of spread of lymphoma.
2. Selection and design of treatment fields that adequately cover all areas requiring treatment and adequately spare normal tissues.
3. Prescription of the optimal dose for disease control and normal-tissue preservation.
4. Meticulous delivery of the treatment plan.

Proper execution of each these steps is important in ensuring the quality and success of overall treatment. Quality control programs for radiation treatment have been established by European cooperative groups for Hodgkin's disease, although none are available specific to non-Hodgkin's lymphoma. In the European Organization for Research and Treatment of Cancer (EORTC) H8 protocol (132), a quality control program for verification of radiation technical files was implemented. Among 161 files reviewed, major deviations in radiation volumes and dose were observed in 13.6% and 39.7% of the cases, respectively. The number of major deviations were felt to justify such a radiation quality control program. In the German Hodgkin's Lymphoma Study Group (GHSG) HD4 trial (133), all planning and verification films, as well as dose charts, were prospectively reviewed. Cases with protocol violations were found to have a significantly lower 5-year freedom-from-treatment failure rate (70% vs. 82%, $p < .04$), illustrating the importance of quality assurance. Ongoing cooperative trials on non-Hodgkin's lymphoma treatment may provide an opportunity to collect similar data.

Patterns of Care

The Patterns of Care studies in the United States have reported extensively on Hodgkin's disease. The results demonstrated that patients with adequate portal margins had significantly fewer in-field or marginal recurrences, or relapses of any type (134). Furthermore, the experience of the treating radiation oncologists; use of a dedicated simulator; performance of routine port films to ensure set-up accuracy; and use of individually

shaped blocks, linear accelerators, and extended-field treatments were all associated with an improved treatment outcome (135,136). In the Patterns of Care study published in 1995, discrepancies between the consensus guidelines developed in 1993 and the surveyed U.S. practice were noted in a number of areas (137). The authors suggested that specific changes in treatment techniques and utilization of appropriate equipment and services may improve the quality of treatment planning and delivery. Although such studies are not available for non-Hodgkin's lymphoma, most of the findings are likely relevant to radiation treatment for non-Hodgkin's lymphoma as well, given the similarity in the typical radiation treatment sites and the dose used.

The National Comprehensive Cancer Network (NCCN) outcomes database measures the adherence of clinicians to NCCN guidelines and provides clinical and other outcomes data to evaluate the quality of cancer care (138). The first disease site studied was breast cancer; the final results have not yet been published. Non-Hodgkin's lymphoma is the next disease site to be measured by the NCCN outcomes database. The results, when available, will hopefully provide information on patterns of care and allow integration of quality control into improved care in patients with lymphoma.

NEW DEVELOPMENTS AND FUTURE DIRECTIONS

A radical decrease in radiation field size accompanied the evolution of radiation therapy from a single-modality therapy to its current role as consolidation therapy after chemotherapy in aggressive lymphomas. Even as the first-line treatment of limited stage indolent lymphomas, the current concept is of a limited radiation field, because systemic options are available for relapse. The conceptual change from large "extended-field" irradiation to more limited involved-field design requires better targeting and allows more consideration for the normal-tissue injury (101). Thus, in many cases, three-dimensional conformal treatment design is advisable and offers an advantage over the standard coplanar beam arrangement typically used in large classical lymphoma radiation fields, such as mantle or inverted Y.

The rapid increase in the availability of fluorine-18-fluoro-2-deoxy-D-glucose (FDG)–PET scanning has had a major impact on stage determination and disease response evaluation after systemic therapies (139–142). Although the prognostic implications of residual PET-avid lesions on consolidation or salvage local radiation considerations are rapidly evolving, PET scanning clearly provides important anatomic targeting information for involved-field design (143). Furthermore, the level of residual metabolic activity may be considered in determining the radiation dose (although no data are available yet to support this logically appealing approach). PET has several advantages over radioactive gallium in metabolic imaging of lymphomas (144,145): PET provides better resolution imaging and is particularly more accurate for infradiaphragmatic sites where gallium is often useless due to nonspecific uptake in the bowel and other abdominal organs. Furthermore, although gallium is rarely positive in low-grade lymphomas, PET uptake has been depicted in low-grade follicular lymphomas, as well as in mantle cell and some marginal zone lymphomas (140). Moreover, the new technology of PET-CT fusion increased the diagnostic accuracy of PET imaging, and three-dimensional dynamic display of the data is helpful in contemplating the radiation treatment options of complex cases.

The accuracy of radiation treatment volume selection could be improved by incorporating PET (or MR imaging in selected cases) information while determining the gross tumor volume. The fusion of PET (or MR imaging) data with CT-simulation information allows simultaneous outlining of the treatment volumes with higher anatomic accuracy (Color Plate 8). Future simulators are designed to include x-rays based CT and PET and will simplify multiple-source data acquisition.

Three-dimensional conformal treatment planning is often used for irradiation of lymphoma involving extranodal organs, such as orbits, parotid, or stomach, as well as mediastinal and abdominal nodal disease. Yet, in selected cases, more conformal design and improved dose homogeneity may be achieved using intensity-modulated radiation therapy (146). This new mode of radiation planning and delivery using powerful "inverse planning" and optimization programs together with dynamic multileaf-collimators automated radiation delivery systems allows "dose sculpting" and "dose painting." Intensity-modulated radiation therapy broadens the range of radiation treatment options, while minimizing the radiation dose to normal organs (Color Plates 8 and 9). Although the experience with this technology in lymphoma patients is still limited, intensity-modulated radiation therapy appears to be of benefit when bulky thoracic disease is present, particularly if the chest wall is also extensively involved. It also may be beneficial with difficult intraabdominal volumes (Fig. 11.12 and Color Plate 7), such as involvement of the lower esophagus, stomach, and duodenum with MALT lymphoma, and in situations in which re-irradiation is considered and cord tolerance is the dose-limiting organ.

Although the benefit from incorporating "biologic" imaging and intensity-modulated radiation therapy in lymphoma patients has not been subjected to prospective trial, and theoretical concerns regarding its long-term risk have been raised (147), it is unlikely that this subject be amenable in practice amenable to a randomized study type of evaluation, given the individual design aspect of many lymphoma cases. In selected cases, especially those previously irradiated, or when complex volumes are targeted, intensity-modulated radiation therapy provides the best chance for offering effective radiation therapy with reduced toxicity and, thus, should not be withheld for lack of comparative studies.

REFERENCES

1. Rosenberg S. The low-grade non-Hodgkin's lymphomas: challenges and opportunities. *J Clin Oncol* 1985;3:299–310.
2. Pusey W. Cases of sarcoma and of Hodgkin's disease treated by exposures to x-rays: a preliminary report. *JAMA* 1902;38:166–169.
3. Senn N. Therapeutical value of Röntgen ray in treatment of pseudo-leukemia. *New York Med J* 1903;7:665–668.
4. Gilbert R. La roentgentherapie de la granulomatose maligne. *J Radiol Electrol* 1925;9:509–514.
5. Gilbert R, Babaiantz L. Notre methode de roentgentherapie de la lymphogranulomatose (Hodgkin); resultats eloignes. *Acta Radiol* 1931;12:523–529.
6. Peters M. A study of survivals in Hodgkin's disease treated radiologically. *AJR Am J Roentgenol* 1950;63:299–311.
7. Peters M, Middlemiss K. A study of Hodgkin's disease treated by irradiation. *Am J Roentgenol* 1958;79:114–121.
8. Fuks Z, Feldman M. Henry S. Kaplan 1918–1984: a physician, a scientist, a friend. *Cancer Surveys* 1985;4:295–311.
9. Ginzton E, Mallory K, Kaplan H. The Stanford medical linear accelerator I: design and development. *Stanford Med Bull* 1957;15:123–140.
10. Gall E, Morrison H, Scott A. The follicular type of malignant lymphoma. A survey of 63 cases. *Ann Intern Med* 1941;14:2073–2090.
11. Gray L, Prosnitz L. Dosimetry of Hodgkin's disease therapy using a 4-MV linear accelerator. *Radiology* 1975;116:423–428.
12. Fuks Z, Kaplan H. Recurrence rates following radiation therapy of nodular and diffuse malignant lymphomas. *Radiol* 1973;108:675–684.
13. Bush R, Gospodarowicz M. The place of radiation therapy in the management of patients with localized non-Hodgkin's lymphoma. In: *Malignant lymphomas*. New York: Academic Press 1982:485–502.
14. Gospodarowicz M, Bush R, Brown T. Role of radiation in treatment of patients with localized intermediate and high grade non-Hodgkin's lymphoma. *Proc Amer Soc Clin Onc* 1984;3:C–922 (abstract).
15. Mauch P, Leonard R, Skarin A, et al. Improved survival following combined radiation therapy and chemotherapy for unfavorable prognosis stage I–II non-Hodgkin's lymphomas. *J Clin Oncol* 1985;3:1301–1308.
16. Hallahan D, Farah R, Vokes E, et al. The patterns of failure in patients with pathological stage I and II diffuse histiocytic lymphoma treated with radiation therapy alone. *Int J Radiation Onc Biol Phys* 1989;17:767–771.
17. Vokes E, Ultmann J, Golomb H, et al. Long-term survival of patients with localized diffuse histiocytic lymphoma. *J Clin Oncol* 1985;3:1309–1317.
18. Levitt S, Lee C, Bloomfield C, et al. The role of radiation therapy in the treatment of early stage large cell lymphoma. *Hematol Oncol* 1985;3:33–37.
19. Landberg T, Hakansson L, Moller T, et al. CVP remission maintenance in stage I or II non-Hodgkin's lymphomas: preliminary results of a randomized study. *Cancer* 1979;44:831–838.
20. Monfardini S, Banfi A, Bonadonna G, et al. Improved five-year survival after combined radiotherapy-chemotherapy for stage I–II non-Hodgkin's lymphoma. *Int J Rad Oncol Biol Phys* 1980;6:125–134.
21. Nissen N, Ersboll J, Hansen H, et al. A randomized study of radiotherapy versus radiotherapy plus chemotherapy in stage I–II non-Hodgkin's lymphomas. *Cancer* 1982;52:1–7.
22. Kamath S, Marcus RJ, Lynch J, et al. The impact of radiotherapy dose and other treatment-related and clinical factors on in-field control in stage I and II non-Hodgkin's lymphoma. *Int J Radiat Oncol Biol Phys* 1999;44:563–568.
23. Munck J, Dhermain F, Koscielny S, et al. Alternating chemotherapy and radiotherapy for limited-stage intermediate and high-grade non-Hodgkin's lymphomas: long-term results for 96 patients with tumors >5 cm. *Ann Oncol* 1996;7:925–931.
24. Prestige B, Horning S, Hoppe R. Combined modality therapy for stage I–II large cell lymphoma. *Int J Rad Oncol Biol Phys* 1988; 15:633–639.
25. Tondini C, Giardini R, Bozzetti F, et al. Combined modality treatment for primary gastrointestinal non-Hodgkin's lymphoma: The Milan Cancer Institute Experience. *Ann Oncol* 1993;4:831–837.
26. van der Maazen R, Noordijk E, Thomas J, et al. Combined modality treatment is the treatment of choice for stage I/IE intermediate and high grade non-Hodgkin's lymphomas. *Radiother Oncol* 1998;49:1–7.
27. Velasquez W, Fuller L, Jagannath S, et al. Stage I and II diffuse large cell lymphoma: prognostic factors and long-term results with CHOP-bleo and radiotherapy. *Blood* 1991;77:942–947.
28. Krol A, Berenschot H, Doekharan D, et al. Cyclophosphamide, doxorubicin, vincristine and prednisone chemotherapy and radiotherapy for stage I intermediate or high grade non-Hodgkin's lym-

phomas: results of a strategy that adapts radiotherapy dose to the response after chemotherapy. *Radiotherapy and Oncology* 2001; 58:251–255.

29. Shenkier T, Voss N, Fairey R, et al. Brief chemotherapy and involved-field irradiation for limited-stage diffuse large-cell lymphoma: an 18-year experience from the British Columbia Cancer Agency. *J Clin Oncol* 2001;20:197–204.

30. Longo D, Glatstein E, Duffey P, et al. Treatment of localized aggressive lymphomas with combination chemotherapy followed by involved-field radiation therapy. *J Clin Oncol* 1989;7:1295–1302.

31. Glick J, Kim K, Earle J, O'Connell M. An ECOG randomized phase III trial of CHOP vs. CHOP + radiotherapy for intermediate grade early stage non-Hodgkin's lymphoma. *Proc Amer Soc Clin Oncol* 1995;14:391.

32. Roy I, Yahalom J. Excellent local control with involved-field radiotherapy following CHOP chemotherapy: analysis of 145 patients with early-stage intermediate-grade non-Hodgkin's lymphoma. *Int J Radiat Oncol Biol Phys* 2001;51:362a–363a.

33. Wilder R, Rodriguez M, Tucker S, et al. Radiation therapy after a partial response to CHOP chemotherapy for aggressive lymphomas. *Int J Radiat Oncol Biol Phys* 2001;50:743–749.

34. Zinzani P, Martelli M, Magagnoli M, et al. Treatment and clinical management of primary mediastinal large B-cell lymphoma with sclerosis: MACOP-B regimen and mediastinal radiotherapy monitored by (67) Gallium scan in 50 patients. *Blood* 1999;94:3288–3293.

35. Schlembach P, Wilder R, Tucker S, et al. Impact of involved field radiotherapy after CHOP-based chemotherapy on stage III–IV, intermediate grade and large-cell immunoblastic lymphomas. *Int J Radiat Oncol Biol Phys* 2000;48:1107–1110.

36. Aviles A, Delgado S, Nambo M, et al. Adjuvant radiotherapy to sites of previous bulky disease in patients with stage IV diffuse large cell lymphoma. *Int J Radiat Oncol Biol Phys* 1994;30:799–803.

36a. O'Connell, et al. *Proceedings of the American Society for Clinical Oncology*, 1984.

37. Rodriguez J, McLaughlin P, Hagemeister F, et al. Follicular large cell lymphoma: an aggressive lymphoma that often presents with favorable prognostic features. *Blood* 1999;93:2202–2207.

38. Gospodarowicz M, Lippuner T, Pintilie M, et al. Stage I and II follicular lymphoma: long-term outcome and pattern of failure following treatment with involved field radiation therapy alone. *Int J Radiat Biol Oncol Phys* 1999;45:217a.

39. Vaughan Hudson B, Vaughan Hudson G, MacLennan KA, et al. Clinical stage 1 non-Hodgkin's lymphoma: long-term follow-up of patients treated by the British National Lymphoma Investigation with radiotherapy alone as initial therapy. *Br J Cancer* 1994;69:1088–1093.

40. MacManus M, Hoppe R. Is radiotherapy curable for stage I and II low-grade follicular lymphoma? Results of a long-term follow-up study of patients treated at Stanford University. *J Clin Oncol* 1996; 14:1282–1290.

41. Lawrence T, Urba W, Steinberg S, et al. Retrospective analysis of stage I and II indolent lymphomas at the National Cancer Institute. *Int J Radiat Oncol Biol Phys* 1988;14:417–424.

42. Hayabuchi N, Jingu K, Masaki N, et al. Nodular histiocytic lymphoma, emphasizing results of stage I disease treated by radiotherapy. *Amer J Clin Oncol* 1990;13:501–506.

43. Soubeyran P, Eghbali H, Bonichon F, et al. Localized follicular lymphomas: prognosis and survival of stages I and II in a retrospective series of 103 patients. *Radiother Oncol* 1988;13:91–98.

44. Taylor R, Allan S, McIntyre M, et al. Low-grade stage I and II non-Hodgkin's lymphoma: results of treatment and relapse pattern following therapy. *Clin Radiol* 1988;39:87–290.

45. Pendlebury S, el Awadi M, Ashley S, et al. Radiotherapy results in early stage low grade nodal non-Hodgkin's lymphoma. *Radiother Oncol* 1995;36:167–71.

46. Murtha A, Rupnow B, Hansson J, et al. Long-term follow-up of patients with stage III follicular lymphoma treated with primary radiotherapy at Stanford University. *Int J Radiat Oncol Biol Phys* 2001;49:3–15.

47. De Los Santos JF, Mendenhall NP, Lynch JW Jr. Is comprehensive lymphatic irradiation for low-grade non-Hodgkin's lymphoma curative therapy? Long-term experience at a single institution [Comment]. *Int J Radiat Oncol Biol Phys* 1997;38(1):3–8.

48. Jacobs J, Murray K, Schultz C, et al. Central lymphatic irradiation for stage III nodular malignant lymphoma: long-term result. *J Clin Oncol* 1993;11:233–238.

49. Aviles A, Diaz-Maqueo J, Sanchez E, et al. Long-term results in patients with low-grade nodular non-Hodgkin's lymphoma. A ran-

domized trial comparing chemotherapy plus radiotherapy with chemotherapy alone. *Acta Oncol* 1991;30:329–333.

50. Schechter N, Portlock C, Yahalom J. Treatment of mucosa-associated lymphoid tissue of the stomach with radiation alone. *J Clin Oncol* 1998;16:1916–1921.

51. Tsang RG, Pintilie MK, Bezjak A, et al. Stage I and II MALT lymphoma: results of treatment with radiotherapy. *Int J Radiat Oncol Biol Phys* 2001;50:1258–1264.

52. Hitchcock S, Ng A, Fisher D, et al. Treatment outcome of mucosa-associated lymphoid tissue/marginal zone non-Hodgkin's lymphoma. *Int J Radiat Oncol Biol Phys* 2002;52:1058–1066.

53. Hammel P, Haioun C, Chaumette M-T, et al. Efficacy of single-agent chemotherapy in low-grade B-cell mucosa-associated lymphoid tissue lymphoma with prominent gastric expression. *J Clin Oncol* 1995;13:2524–2529.

54. Fisher R, Dahlberg S, Nathwani B, et al. A clinical analysis of two indolent lymphoma entities: mantle cell lymphoma and marginal zone lymphoma (including the mucosa-associated lymphoid tissue and monocytoid B-cell subcategories): a Southwest Oncology Group study. *Blood* 1995;85:1075–1082.

55. Teodorovic I, Pittaluga SK-N, Meerwaldt JC, et al. Efficacy of four different regimens in 64 mantle-cell lymphoma cases: clinicopathologic comparison with 498 other non-Hodgkin's lymphoma subtypes. European Organization for the Research and Treatment of Cancer Lymphoma Cooperative Group. *J Clin Oncol* 1995;13:2819–2826.

56. Meusers P, Engelhard M, Bartels H, et al. Multicentre randomized therapeutic trial for advanced centrocytic lymphoma: anthracycline does not improve the prognosis. *Hematol Oncol* 1989;7:365–380.

56a. Girinsky T, Guillot-Vals D, Koscielny S. A high and sustained response rate in refractory or relapsing low-grade lymphoma masses after low-dose radiation: analysis of predictive parameters of response to treatment. *Int J Radiat Oncol Biol Phys* 2001;51(1):148–155.

57. Maor M, Maddux B, Osborne B, et al. Stages IE and IIE non-Hodgkin's lymphomas of the stomach: Comparison of treatment modalities. *Cancer* 1984;54:2330–2337.

58. Gobbi P, Dionigi P, Barbieri F, et al. The role of surgery in the multimodal treatment of primary gastric non-Hodgkin's lymphomas. A report of 76 cases and review of the literature. *Cancer* 1990;65:2528–2536.

59. Coiffier B, Salles G. Does surgery belong to medical history for gastric lymphomas? *Ann Oncol* 1997;8:419–421.

60. Willich N, Reinartz G, Horst E, et al. Operative and conservative management of primary gastric lymphoma: interim results of a German multicenter study. *Int J Radiat Oncol Biol Phys* 2000;46:895–901.

61. Salvagno L, Soraru M, Busetto M, et al. Gastric non-Hodgkin's lymphoma: analysis of 252 patients from a multicenter study. *Tumori* 1999;85:113–121.

62. Koch P, del Valle F, Berdel W, et al. Primary gastrointestinal non-Hodgkin's lymphoma: II. Combined surgical and conservative or conservative management only in localized gastric lymphoma—results of the prospective German Multicenter Study GIT NHL 01/92. *J Clin Oncol* 2001;19:3874–3883.

63. Ferreri A, Cordio S, Paro S. Therapeutic management of stage I–II high-grade primary gastric lymphomas. *Oncology* 1999;56:274–282.

64. Raderer M, Valencak J, Osterreicher C, et al. Chemotherapy for the treatment of patients with primary high grade gastric B-cell lymphoma of modified Ann Arbor Stages IE and IIE. *Cancer* 2000; 88:1979–1985.

65. Tondini C, Balzarotti M, Santoro A, et al. Initial chemotherapy for primary resectable large-cell lymphoma of the stomach. *Ann Oncol* 1997;8, 497–499.

66. Miller T, Dahlberg S, Cassady J, et al. Chemotherapy alone compared with chemotherapy plus radiotherapy for localized intermediate- and high-grade non-Hodgkin's lymphoma. *New Engl J Med* 1998;339:21–26.

67. Horning S, Glick J, Kim K, et al. Final report of E1484: CHOP v CHOP + radiotherapy for limited stage diffuse aggressive lymphoma. *Blood* 2001;98:724a.

68. Wotherspoon A, Doglioni C, Diss T, et al. Regression of primary low-grade B-cell gastric lymphoma of mucosa-associated lymphoid tissue type after eradication of *Helicobacter pylori*. *Lancet* 1993;342:575–577.

69. Wotherspoon A, Ortiz-Hidalgo C, Falzon M, et al. *Helicobacter pylori*-associated gastritis and primary B-cell lymphoma. *Lancet* 1991;338:1175.

70. Hussell T, Isaacson P, Crabtree J, et al. The response of cells from low-grade B-cell gastric lymphomas of mucosa-associated lymphoid tissue to *Helicobacter pylori*. *Lancet* 1993;342:571.

71. Thiede C, Wundisch T, Alpen B, et al. Long-term persistence of monoclonal B cells after cure of *Helicobacter pylori* infection and complete histologic remission in gastric mucosa-associated lymphoid tissue B-cell lymphoma. *J Clin Oncol* 2001;19:1600–1609.

72. Steinbach G, Ford R, Glober G, et al. Antibiotic treatment of gastric lymphoma of mucosa-associated lymphoid tissue. *Ann Intern Med* 1999;131:88–95.

73. Montalban C, Castrillo J, Abraira V, et al. Gastric B-cell mucosa-associated lymphoid tissue (MALT) lymphoma. Clinicopathological study and evaluation of the prognostic factors in 143 patients. *Ann Oncol* 1995;6:355–363.

74. Nathu R, Mendenhall N, Almasri N, Lynch J. Non-Hodgkin's lymphoma of the head and neck: a 30-year experience at the University of Florida. *Head Neck* 1999;21:247–254.

75. Jacobs C, Hoppe R. Non-Hodgkin's lymphomas of head and neck extranodal sites. *Int J Radiat Oncol Biol Phys* 1985;11:357–364.

76. Shimm D, Dosoretz D, Harris N, et al. Radiation therapy of Waldeyer's ring lymphoma. *Cancer* 1984;54:426–431.

77. Kondo M, Mikata A, Ogawa K, et al. Prognostic factors in stage I and II non-Hodgkin's lymphoma of Waldeyer's ring. *Acta Radiol Oncol* 1985;24:153–158.

78. Fujitani T, Takahara T, Hattori H, et al. Radiochemotherapy for non-Hodgkin's lymphoma in palatine tonsil. *Cancer* 1984;54:1288–1292.

79. Ezzat A, Ibrahim E, El Weshi A, et al. Localized non-Hodgkin's lymphoma of Waldeyer's ring: clinical features, management, and prognosis of 130 adult patients. *Head Neck* 2001;23:547–558.

80. Hausdorff J, Davis E, Long G, et al. Non-Hodgkin's lymphoma of the paranasal sinuses: clinical and pathological features, and response to combined-modality therapy. *Cancer J Sci Am* 1997;3:303–311.

81. Logsdon M, Ha C, Kavadi V, et al. Lymphoma of the nasal cavity and paranasal sinuses: improved outcome and altered prognostic factors with combined modality therapy. *Cancer* 1997;80:477–488.

81a. Burton GV, Atwater S, Borowitz MJ. Extranodal head and neck lymphoma. Prognosis and patters of recurrence. *Arch Otolaryngol Head Neck Surg* 1990;116:69–73.

82. Sasai K, Yamabe H, Kokubo M, et al. Head-and-neck stages I and II extranodal non-Hodgkin's lymphomas: Real classification and selection for treatment modality. *Int J Radiat Oncol Biol Phys* 2000;48:153–160.

83. Kim W, Song S, Ahn Y, et al. CHOP followed by involved field radiation: is it optimal for localized nasal natural killer/T-cell lymphoma? *Ann Oncol* 2001;12:349–353.

84. Liang R, Todd D, Chan T, et al. Treatment outcome and prognostic factors for primary nasal lymphoma. *J Clin Oncol* 1995;13:666–670.

85. Ribrag V, Ell Hajj M, Janot F, et al. Early locoregional high-dose radiotherapy is associated with long-term disease control in localized primary angiocentric lymphoma of the nose and nasopharynx. *Leukemia* 2001;15:1123–1126.

86. Auw-Haedrich CC, Kapp SE, Schmitt-Graff A, et al. Long-term outcome of ocular adnexal lymphoma subtyped according to the REAL classification. Revised European and American Lymphoma. *Br J Ophthalmol* 2001;85:63–69.

87. Bolek T, Moyses H, Marcus RJ, et al. Radiotherapy in the management of orbital lymphoma. *J Radiat Oncol Biol Phys* 1999;44:31–36.

88. Stafford S, Kozelsky T, Garrity J, et al. Orbital lymphoma: radiotherapy outcome and complications. *Radiother Oncol* 2001;35:139.

89. Pelloski C, Wilder R, Ha C, et al. Clinical stage IEA–IIEA orbital lymphomas: outcomes in the era of modern staging and treatment. *Radiother Oncol* 2001;59:145–151.

90. Dunbar S, Linggood R, Doppke K, et al. Conjunctival lymphoma: Results and treatment with a single anterior electron field. A lens sparing approach. *Int J Radiat Oncol Biol Phys* 1990;19:249–257.

91. Tondini C, Ferreri A, Siracusano L, et al. Diffuse large-cell lymphoma of the testis. *J Clin Oncol* 1999;17:2854–2858.

92. Visco C, Medeiros L, Mesina O, et al. Non-Hodgkin's lymphoma affecting the testis: is it curable with doxorubicin-based therapy? *Clin Lymphoma* 2001;2:40–46.

93. Seymour J, Solomon B, Wolf M, et al. Primary large-cell non-Hodgkin's lymphoma of the testis: a retrospective analysis of patterns of failure and prognostic factors. *Clin Lymphoma* 2001;2:109–115.

94. Baar J, Burkes R, Bell R, et al. Primary non-Hodgkin's lymphoma of bone. A clinicopathologic study. *Cancer* 1994;73:1194–1199.

95. Baar J, Burkes R, Gospodarowicz M. Primary non-Hodgkin's lymphoma of bone. *Semin Oncol* 1999;26:270–275.

96. Fairbanks R, Bonner J, Inwards C, et al. Treatment of stage IE primary lymphoma of bone. *Int J Radiat Oncol Biol Phys* 1994;28:363–372.

97. Ferraro P, Trastek V, Adlakha H, et al. Primary non-Hodgkin's lymphoma of the lung. *Ann Thorac Surg* 2000;69:993–997.

98. Cordier J, Chailleux E, Lauque D, et al. Primary pulmonary lymphomas. A clinical study of 70 cases in nonimmunocompromised patients. *Chest* 1993;103:201–208.

99. Bentel GC, Marks LB, Krishnamurthy R, Prosnitz LR. Comparison of two repositioning devices used during radiation therapy for Hodgkin's disease. *Int J Radiat Oncol Biol Phys* 1997;38:791–795.

100. Bentel G. Positioning and immobilization of patients undergoing radiation therapy for Hodgkin's disease. *Med Dosim* 1991;16:111–117.

101. Yahalom J. Changing role and decreasing size: current trends in radiotherapy for Hodgkin's disease. *Curr Oncol Rep* 2002;4:415–423.

102. Stuschke M, Hoederath A, Sack H, et al. Extended field and total central lymphatic radiotherapy in the treatment of early stage lymph node centroblastic-centrocytic lymphomas: result of a prospective multicenter study. Study Group NHL-frühe Stadien. *Cancer* 1997;80:2273–2284.

103. De Los Santos J, Mendenhall N, Lynch JJ. Is comprehensive lymphatic irradiation for low-grade non-Hodgkin's lymphoma curative therapy? Long-term experience at a single institution. *Int J Radiat Oncol Biol Rhys* 1997;38:3–8.

104. Ha C, Cabanillas F, Lee M, et al. Serial determination of the bcl-2 gene in the bone marrow and peripheral blood after central lymphatic irradiation for stages I–III follicular lymphomas: a preliminary report. *Clin Cancer Res* 1997;3:215–219.

105. Ganem G, Kuentz M, Beaujean F, et al. Additional total-lymphoid irradiation in preventing graft failure of T-cell-depleted bone marrow transplantation from HLA-identical siblings. Results of a prospective randomized study. *Transplantation* 1988;45:244–248.

106. Soiffer R, Mauch P, Tarbell N, et al. Total lymphoid irradiation to prevent graft rejection in recipients of HLA non-identical T-cell–depleted allogeneic marrow. *Bone Marrow Transplant* 1991;7:23–33.

107. Hale G, Waldmann H. Control of graft-versus-host disease and graft rejection by T cell depletion of donor and recipient with Campath-1 antibodies. Result of matched sibling transplants for malignant disease. *Bone Marrow Transplant* 1994;13:597–611.

108. Roncadin M, Arcicasa M, Bortolus R, et al. Feasibility of total body irradiation in chronic lymphocytic leukemia and low-grade non-Hodgkin's lymphomas. *Cancer Invest* 1991;9:403–407.

109. Meerwaldt J, Carde P, Burgers M, et al. Low-dose total body irradiation versus combination chemotherapy for lymphomas with follicular growth pattern. *Int J Radiat Oncol Biol Phys* 1991;21:1167–1172.

110. Richaud P, Soubeyran P, Eghabali H, et al. Place of low-dose total body irradiation in the treatment of localized follicular non-Hodgkin's lymphoma: result of a pilot study. *Int J Radiat Oncol Biol Phys* 1998;40:378–390.

111. Safwat A. The role of low-dose total body irradiation in treatment of non-Hodgkin's lymphoma: a new look at an old method. *Radiother Oncol* 2000;56:1–8.

112. Vitale V, Barra S, Franzone P. Total body irradiation in the conditioning regimen for hematological malignancies. *Bone Marrow Transplant* 1991;8 Suppl:28–29.

113. Appelbaum F. The influence of total dose, fractionation, dose rate, and distribution of total body irradiation on bone marrow transplantation. *Semin Oncol* 1993;20:3–10.

114. Santos G. Preparative regimens: chemotherapy versus chemoradiotherapy. A historical perspective. *Ann N Y Acad Sci* 1995;770:1–7.

115. Shank B. Total body irradiation for marrow or stem-cell transplantation. *Cancer Invest* 1998;16:397–404.

116. Fraass BA, van de Geijn J. Peripheral dose from megavolt beams. *Med Phys* 1983;10:809–818.

117. Fraass B, Kinsella T, Harrington F, Glatstein E. Peripheral dose to the testes: the design and clinical use of practical and effective gonadal shield. *Int J Radiat Biol Phys* 1985;11:609.

118. Kubo H, Shipley WU. Reduction of the scatter dose to the testicle outside the radiation treatment fields. *Int J Radiat Oncol Biol Phys* 1982;8:1741–1745.

119. Naida J, Eisbruch A, Schoeppel S, et al. Analysis of localization errors in the definition of the mantle field using a beam's eye view treatment-planning system. *Int J Radiat Oncol Biol Phys* 1996;35:377–382.

120. Brown A, Urie M, Barest G, et al. Three-dimensional photon treatment planning for Hodgkin's disease. *Int J Radiat Oncol Biol Phys* 1991;21:205–215.
121. Cho C, Blank N, Castellino R. Computerized tomography evaluation of chest wall involvement in lymphoma. *Cancer Invest* 1985;55:1892–1894.
122. Carlsen S, Bergin C, Hoppe R. MR imaging to detect chest wall and pleural involvement in patients with lymphoma: effect on radiation therapy planning. *AJR Am J Roentgenol* 1993;160:1191–1195.
123. Koster A, Kimmig B, Muller-Schimpfle M, et al. MR tomography and MR angiography—a new method for the planning of the irradiation of large abdominal fields. *Strahlenther Onkol* 1992;168:230–236.
124. Garcia J, Bryant C, Ha C, et al. Three-dimensional treatment for planning for central lymphoid irradiation. *Medical Dosimetry* 1999;24:395–400.
125. McCord DL, Million RR, Northrop MF, Kavanaugh HV. Daily reproducibility of lung blocks in the mantle technique. *Radiology* 1973;109:735–736.
126. Marks J, Haus A, Sutton H, Griem M. Localization error in the radiotherapy of Hodgkin's disease and malignant lymphoma with extended mantle fields. *Cancer* 1974;34:83–90.
127. Griffiths S, Pearcey R. The daily reproducibility of large complex-shaped radiotherapy fields to the thorax and neck. *Clin Radiol* 1986;37:39.
128. Taylor BW Jr, Mendenhall NP, Million RR. Reproducibility of mantle irradiation with daily imaging films. *Int J Radiat Oncol Biol Phys* 1990;19:149–151.
129. Hulshof M, Vanuytsel L, Van Den Bogaert W, Van Der Schueren E. Localization errors in mantle-field irradiation for Hodgkin's disease. *Int J Radiat Biol Phys* 1989;17:679–683.
130. Rabinowitz I, Broomberg J, Goitein M, et al. Accuracy of radiation field alignment in clinical practice. *Int J Radiat Oncol Biol Phys* 1985;11:1857–1867.
131. Creutzberg C, Visser A, De Porre P, et al. Accuracy of patient positioning in mantle field irradiation. *Radiother Oncol* 1992;23:257–264.
132. Hennequin C, Carrie C, Hofstetter S, Cosset J. A quality control program for radiotherapy in Hodgkin's disease. *Cancer Radiother* 1999;3:187–190.
133. Duhmke E, Diehl V, Loeffler M, et al. Randomized trial with early-stage Hodgkin's disease testing 30 Gy vs. 40 Gy extended field radiotherapy alone. *Int J Radiat Oncol Biol Phys* 1996;36:305–310.
134. Kinzie J, Hanks G, Maclean C, Kramer S. Patterns of Care study: Hodgkin's disease relapse rates and adequacy of portals. *Cancer* 1983;52:2223–2226.
135. Hanks G, Kinzie J, White R, et al. Patterns of Care outcome studies. Results of the national practice in Hodgkin's disease. *Cancer* 1983;51:569–573.
136. Hoppe R, Hanlon A, Hanks G, Owen J. Progress in the treatment of Hodgkin's disease in the United States, 1973 versus 1983: The Patterns of Care Study. *Cancer* 1994;74:3198–3203.
137. Hughes DB, Smith AR, Hoppe R, et al. Treatment planning for Hodgkin's disease: a Patterns of Care study. *Int J Radiat Oncol Biol Phys* 1995;33:519–524.
138. Weeks J. Outcomes assessment in the NCCN. *Oncology (Huntingt)* 1997;11:137–140.
139. de Wit M, Bohuslavizki K, Buchert R, et al. [18]FDG-PET following treatment as valid predictor for survival in Hodgkin's lymphoma. *Ann Oncol* 2001;12:29–37.
140. Jerusalem G, Beguin Y, Najjar F, et al. Positron emission tomography (PET) with ^{18}F-fluorodeoxyglucose (^{18}F-FDG) for the staging of low-grade non-Hodgkin's lymphoma (NHL). *Ann Oncol* 2001;12:825–830.
141. Spaepen K, Stroobants S, Dupont P, et al. Prognostic value of positron emission tomography (PET) with fluorine-18 fluorodeoxyglucose ([^{18}F]FDG) after first-line chemotherapy in non-Hodgkin's lymphoma: is [^{18}F]FDG-PET a valid alternative to conventional diagnostic methods? *J Clin Oncol* 2001;19:141–149.
142. Schoder H, Meta J, Yap C, et al. Effect of whole-body (18)F-FDG PET imaging on clinical staging and management of patients with malignant lymphoma. *J Nucl Med* 2001;42:1139–1143.
143. Erdi Y, Rosenzweig K, Erdi A, et al. Radiotherapy treatment planning for patients with non-small cell lung cancer using positron emission tomography (PET). *Radiother Oncol* 2002;62:51–60.
144. Wirth A, Seymour J, Hicks R, et al. Fluorine-18 fluorodeoxyglucose positron emission tomography, gallium-67 scintigraphy, and conventional staging for Hodgkin's disease and non-Hodgkin's lymphoma. *Am J Med* 2002;112:262–268.
145. Kostakoglu L, Leonard J, Kuji I, et al. Comparison of fluorine-18 fluorodeoxyglucose positron emission tomography and Ga-67 scintigraphy in evaluation of lymphoma. *Cancer* 2002;94:879–888.
146. Ling C, Humm J, Larson S, et al. Towards multidimensional radiotherapy (MD-CRT): biological imaging and biological conformality. *Int J Radiat Oncol Biol Phys* 2000;47:551–560.
147. Goffman T, Glatstein E. Intensity-modulated radiation therapy. *Radiat Res* 2002;158:115–117.1.

CHAPTER 12

Principles of Chemotherapy and Combined Modality Therapy

Joseph M. Connors

The evolution of our appreciation of the principles underlying effective treatment of human cancers has proceeded stepwise in parallel with our understanding of basic biology, especially at the molecular level. Crude concepts of direct cytotoxicity based on observations from antibacterial antibiotics gave way to more sophisticated linking of the chemical activity of specific drugs to metabolic pathways of varying importance to cellular integrity, only to be superseded by more interactive models based on cellular biology and molecular genetics, in which chemotherapeutic agents are seen as initiators of complex intracellular processes, such as apoptosis, that lead to cellular destruction or terminal differentiation. Only recently has the science of chemotherapy moved from being an essentially empiric process in which many thousands of candidates were laboriously screened for antineoplastic activity to the actual design of new agents targeted to specific cellular antigenic determinants or key metabolic pathways. This evolution will continue. Thus, any accounting of the principles and practice of chemotherapy is a description of work in progress. Not only will new agents continue to be discovered, but the process of discovery itself will also continue to evolve into an ever more rational pursuit of specifically targeted agents aimed at more and more carefully chosen pathways. In this chapter, we examine the major advances in our understanding of how chemotherapy works, the families of agents useful in treatment of lymphoproliferative neoplasms, the design of combination chemotherapy regimens, and the integration of chemotherapy and radiation therapy.

GENERAL PRINCIPLES OF CHEMOTHERAPY

Preclinical Models

The pioneering work by Skipper and others with the L1210 murine leukemia cell line provided the first major quantitative insights into how chemotherapy works (1,2). Mice injected with malignant cells reproducibly succumb to aggressive disease in a time frame determined by the number of leukemic cells injected and their doubling times (1,2). Small numbers of initially injected cells or long doubling times correlate with longer survival. With the chemotherapeutic agents available for testing at that time, primarily alkylating agents and antimetabolites, survivals of animals injected with L1210 cells could be extended or even restored to normal and the animals rendered free of evident tumor (3). This effect correlated with the dose of the chemotherapeutic agent and the fraction of neoplastic cells actively synthesizing DNA at the time of chemotherapy administration (1–3). This implied that, at least for these agents, cells actually replicating DNA were accessible to the chemotherapy, but those in resting phase were not. Additional insights included observations of dose-limiting toxicity in the form of myelotoxicity or gastrointestinal toxicity, primarily mucositis, that limited the amount of the chemotherapy drug that could be safely given before the treatment itself began to contribute to shortened animal survival (1,2). Another important observation was that although some chemotherapeutic agents can cure some tumors with a single dose, at other times, repeated doses of the chemotherapy are required (1,2). One reasonable explanation for this greater efficacy of repeated doses is that the cells become available to eradication by the chemotherapy as they move into the replicative phase of cell cycling. However, this is only a partial explanation, because some tumors can be eliminated completely, even though not every cell is in replicative phase of the times of drug administration. How this could occur awaited explanation until much later, when an understanding of programmed cell death was developed. The crucial observation that the fractional cell kill could be translated into cure of transplanted neoplasms provided a scientific underpinning for all later investigations of the mechanisms of chemotherapy action.

Dose Intensity

Building on the initial observations from models of mice injected with L1210 leukemia that prolongation of survival or cure was partially dependent on the dose of chemotherapy, later investigators established that the fractional cell kill and, therefore, likelihood of cure could be enhanced by increasing the chemotherapy drug dose. However, full understanding of the link between dose intensity and effectiveness of chemotherapy is still being acquired. Intuitively, it is obvious that tiny doses must be ineffective, and very large doses—doses that may be well above those that cause lethal toxicity—must always be able to eradicate the neoplasm. However, precise identification of the dose intensity that optimizes the balance between maximum effectiveness and acceptable levels of toxicity remains elusive. Figure 12.1 illustrates alternative models that fit the available data. Certain experiences with lymphoproliferative neoplasms fit the prediction of a continuously rising effect—for example, the ability to cure Hodgkin's lymphoma with a single course of very-high-dose chemotherapy supported by hematopoietic stem cell transplantation even when standard-dose chemotherapy has failed (4–7). On the other hand, the relative inability of the same approach to cure chemotherapy-refractory diffuse large B-cell lymphoma (8–10) argues that at least some human lymphoproliferative neoplasms behave according to a plateau effect whereby once a threshold has been exceeded, further increases in dose intensity contribute little, if anything, to increasing the cure rate. Although insights into the mechanisms that determine which model will apply for a given lymphoproliferative neoplasm are being derived from improved understanding of drug resistance, molecular genetics, and mechanisms of apoptosis, these insights are not fully reliable. We must still rely on empiric observation to identify those neoplasms that can be effectively treated with escalated doses and those that cannot.

Non–Cross-Resistance and Non-Overlapping Toxicity

Early in the development of chemotherapy, it became clear that different agents work via different mechanisms at the cel-

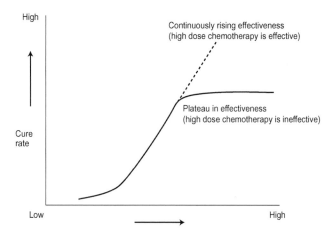

FIG. 12.1. Graph showing contrasting dose-response effects of high-dose chemotherapy for two types of neoplasms, one in which the likelihood of cure continues to increase as higher doses are employed and another in which the dose response plateaus and higher doses are not more effective.

lular level and impose differing toxicities on specific tissues. For example, alkylating agents, such as mechlorethamine and cyclophosphamide, cause interstrand DNA cross-linking and are associated with myelotoxicity (11,12). Vinca alkaloids, such as vincristine, on the other hand, cause inhibition of microtubular formation by inhibiting tubulin formation and are associated with neurologic toxicity (13,14). Alternatively, high-dose corticosteroids are potently lymphocytotoxic and exert toxicities consistent with hypercortisolism (15,16). It is reasonable to postulate that a combination of agents from each of these different classes might offer two highly desirable properties: non–cross-resistance and non-overlapping toxicity. The first, non–cross-resistance, occurs when neoplastic cells resistant to one agent can be killed by another from a different class. The second, non-overlapping toxicity, allows coincident administration of full doses of two or more agents, because their dose-limiting toxicities are different. In landmark studies now appreciated as classics of oncologic clinical investigation, the team of investigators at the United States National Cancer Institute in the 1960s, led by Dr. Vincent DeVita, demonstrated that two until-then incurable malignancies, advanced-stage Hodgkin's lymphoma and advanced-stage diffuse large-cell lymphoma, could be cured by combinations of alkylators, vinca alkaloids, and corticosteroids, using the MOPP [Mustargen (mechlorethamine), Oncovin (vincristine), procarbazine, and prednisone] (17–19) or C-MOPP [cyclophosphamide, Oncovin (vincristine), procarbazine and prednisone] (20) regimen, respectively. In both cases, this was accomplished by taking advantage of at least partial non–cross-resistance and non-overlapping toxicity.

Eventually, a more rigorous mathematic rationale was developed to account for the enhanced effectiveness of non–cross-resistant combinations in the form of the Goldie-Coldman hypothesis (21–23). These theoreticians provided an elegant mathematic model that quantitatively predicts that early introduction of genuinely non–cross-resistant drugs maximizes the likelihood of cure (23). The demonstration that curative combinations can be assembled from agents that are not curative on their own is predicted by this hypothesis. The usefulness of this model is not diminished by disappointment that elaborate seven- or eight-drug combinations are no more effective than three- or four-drug regimens (24–27) now that we realize that the more complex regimens did not include genuinely non–cross-resistant subgroups of drugs. The guiding principle that the best regimens incorporate as many definitely non–cross-resistant drugs as early as possible remains sound even as we venture into the era of increasingly potent biologic agents and targeted therapy.

Drug Resistance

Studies of resistance to antibacterial antibiotics provided the initial conceptual framework to study malignant cell resistance to antineoplastic chemotherapy. Microbial organisms become resistant to antibiotics by altering susceptibility of the target metabolic or synthetic pathways such that the drug can no longer exert its intended influence. The microbes accomplish this by altering cell influx of the drug, changing binding efficiency to target and enzymes, adopting alternative metabolic or synthetic pathways, or otherwise adapting so that growth and survival occur in the presence of a heretofore-lethal substance. The organism does not actually choose to express different proteins or bind drugs differently. Rather, within any population of organisms, there is differential, genetically controlled expression of proteins or other structural elements such that a few of the microbes may express a resistant phenotype. Exposure to an antimicrobial antibiotic alters the environment, causing death of all the microbes with the susceptible phenotype and conferring a strong survival advantage on the few microbes expressing the resistant phenotype. Conceptually, analogous processes appear to account for resistance to antineoplastic chemotherapy.

Neoplastic mammalian cells have acquired several broad behavioral characteristics distinguishing them from normal cells: loss of contact inhibition of growth and proliferation; metastatic capability allowing spread to and growth in abnormal body sites; enhanced ability to induce ingrowth of neovascular blood vessels; altered tolerance for genetic errors and damage, such that changes that would ordinarily induce apoptosis are ignored; and wide genetic and phenotypic variation across the malignant cell population leading to subpopulations with great variation in growth characteristics, metastatic potential, and drug resistance. This combination of acquired characteristics confers either a growth or survival advantage, or both, over normal cells and permits tumor progression leading to illness and death. Crucially, for consideration of the effects of chemotherapy, acquired changes within the malignant cells mimic conceptually those within resistant microbes. The genetic instability intrinsic to the malignant cells leads to variation in the structure of enzymes, membranes, and other structural elements. This, in turn, leads to differences in responsiveness to chemotherapeutic agents. Thus, just as a subpopulation of bacteria may be resistant to penicillin, a subpopulation of diffuse large B-cell lymphoma cells may be resistant to doxorubicin. In the first case, infection will worsen as penicillin proves ineffective and the resistant microbial population expands, replacing the now-absent sensitive population. In the second, relapse occurs as the doxorubicin-resistant clones grow and spread despite an initial clinical response to chemotherapy. The underlying problem in both cases is selection for the resistant clones of microbes or neoplastic cells, respectively.

There are many specific mechanisms by which neoplastic cells become resistant to chemotherapeutic drugs. Cells may express an effective efflux pump that actively removes drugs from the cell mediated by the mdr (multidrug resistance) gene family (28–32). Key enzymes, such as thymidylate synthase, may change in amino acid sequence and tertiary structure altering binding efficiency of the drug (33–35). Actual numbers of the rate-limiting enzyme molecules may be increased by gene amplification (36,37). Normal pathways to apoptosis, the final common effect of many chemotherapeutic drugs, may be blocked by loss of key initiators such as p53 (38) or elaboration of blocking factors such as bcl-2 protein (39,40). Inactivating

enzymes or pathways may be upregulated, as exemplified by glutathione S-transferase and other glutathione-associated enzymes that alter activity of alkylating agents (41). Alternative mechanisms of recruitment of essential microvascular blood vessels may be exploited after one or more specific angiogenesis factors is inhibited (42,43). Cell-surface antigens or receptors may be no longer expressed, may be shed into the extravascular fluids, or may become altered in configuration, in each case evading effective recognition and binding by monoclonal antibodies or receptor-specific small molecules (44,45). These and other mechanisms can confer a survival advantage on a clone of neoplastic cells. The net result is resistance to whole classes of agents that operate via common mechanisms and clinical progression with all of its consequences. In each case, whether one or more resistance mechanisms is exploited, the inherent genetic instability of the neoplastic cell has led to the presence of a stable clone of cells that can ignore the chemotherapeutic agent and continue to proliferate.

Induction of Apoptosis

Most older hematologists and oncologists can recall being taught in extensive detail how chemotherapeutic agents were thought to induce neoplastic cell death. These older models usually focused on mechanisms involving cumulative nucleic acid damage or interference with synthesis of crucial proteins, leading eventually to lethal cytotoxicity. Such models always encountered difficulty explaining differential effects on normal and neoplastic cells. Now, an increasingly comprehensive understanding of the process of apoptosis—programmed cell death—has transformed our thinking about how neoplastic cells are eliminated (46). Many neoplastic cells, especially those of lymphoid neoplasms, maintain a precarious survival based on blocking normal apoptotic pathways that, if unleashed, lead rapidly to cell death. Chemotherapy is now seen as shifting this balance. The neoplastic cells, with their precarious balance, succumb to the chemotherapy because the balance is perturbed, and normal apoptotic processes proceed. Most normal cells, with their much more robust and intact intracellular defenses against inappropriate apoptosis, survive therapeutic doses of antineoplastic agents. Thus, chemotherapy has come to be viewed as a way of facilitating normal, highly potent, natural cytotoxic mechanisms within already defective neoplastic cells rather than just a crude blunderbuss indiscriminately injuring all cells enough to kill the neoplastic ones while sparing the tougher normal cells. This more sophisticated model helps to explain why many antineoplastic drugs seem to have a biphasic dose-response curve in which increasing dose brings increasing effectiveness up to a threshold beyond which higher doses have little effect.

Targeted Therapies

A fundamental drawback of almost all chemotherapeutic agents developed until quite recently has been lack of specificity. Toxicity to nontarget tissue limits dose delivery, precludes the use of

TABLE 12.1. *Subclasses of targeted chemotherapeutic agents*

Subclass	Target	Example Agent	Target
Monoclonal antibodies	Cell antigens	Rituximab	CD20
Enzyme inhibitors	Metabolic or synthetic pathways	Imatinib mesylate	Bcr-abl tyrosine kinase
High-affinity receptor ligands	Over- or uniquely expressed high-affinity receptors	Denileukin diftitox	IL-2 receptor
Supportive tissue disrupters	Angiogenic or other factors essential to tumor survival	Angiostatin cell surface ATP synthase	Endothelial
Antisense oligonucleotides	Specific over-expressed gene products	Anti-BCL2	BCL-2 mRNA

some agents in the face of preexisting organ dysfunction, and forces patients to accept unpleasant or even life-threatening complications to maximize the potential for cure. For these reasons, specific agents that target only the neoplastic cells and spare all others have long been sought. The remarkable improvements in our understanding of the basic biology of neoplastic cells and the ability to craft potent man-made molecules achieved over the past two decades are finally yielding new therapeutics that come close to this goal of selective killing of neoplastic cells. This field promises to transform the practice of oncology.

The new targeted therapies can be divided into subclasses (Table 12.1). Monoclonal antibodies achieve their specificity by binding to cellular antigens displayed on the surface of the malignant cells and can act directly via signal transduction, indirectly by recruiting immune effector cells, or as vehicles to deliver radioactive isotopes or molecular toxins (47). Certain small molecules, often wholly synthesized to achieve a particular steric configuration, target specific enzyme-binding sites and, thus, block key metabolic or anabolic pathways crucial to survival of the neoplastic cells (48). Another approach has been to take advantage of high-affinity binding sites on the cell surface by constructing hybrid fusion molecules that contain two domains, one to bind to the high-affinity receptor and the other to act as a cellular poison after being internalized (49). Some new agents attempt to exert their influence by targeting not the neoplastic cells but rather the supportive tissues essential to tumor survival—for example, antiangiogenic agents (50,51). Finally, antisense oligonucleotides attempt to block the expression of the chosen genes by binding directly to specifically targeted mRNA, essentially performing individualized gene down-regulation (52,53). In each of these cases, the fundamental concept is that the therapeutic agent is chosen because it is aimed at a structural characteristic or metabolic pathway unique to the target neoplastic cell. When optimized, such agents achieve the long-sought goal of selectively killing neoplastic cells while sparing the normal cell population.

Late and Irreversible Toxicities

All chemotherapeutic agents have at least some undesirable side effects. However, many of these toxicities, for example, alopecia, are temporary, not life-threatening, and entirely reversible.

Even when the side effect is uncomfortable or modestly dangerous, such as vomiting, mucositis, or neutropenia, complete reversibility and supportive medications keep these toxicities within reasonably acceptable bounds for the treatment of a potentially lethal disease. On the other hand, some toxicities may linger for long periods or permanently after chemotherapy and prove troublesome or life-threatening well after the primary neoplasm was cured. The major classes of such late toxicities with the inducing agents are shown in Table 12.2. None of these late toxicities occurs in more than 5% to 10% of patients, and thus, they do not constitute absolute contraindications to the use of the potentially offending agent, especially if that use is associated with a high likelihood of cure. However, when equally effective choices are available—for example, ABVD [Adriamycin (doxorubicin), bleomycin, vinblastine, and dacarbazine] (54) or MOPPABV hybrid [mechlorethamine, Oncovin (vincristine), procarbazine, prednisone, Adriamycin (doxorubicin), bleomycin, vinblastine] (55)—for Hodgkin's lymphoma (26,27), reducing the risk of major late toxicity—in this example, infertility, premature menopause (56), or leukemia/myelodysplasia (57,58)—makes ABVD obviously more desirable.

TABLE 12.2. *Major late toxicities of chemotherapeutic agents*

Drug or drug class	Specific consequence
Anthracyclines	Cardiomyopathy
Bleomycin	Pulmonary fibrosis
Alkylating agents or nitrosoureas	Bone marrow failure
	Male oligospermic infertility
	Female anovulatory infertility, premature menopause and osteoporosis
Cisplatin	Renal dysfunction
Corticosteroids	Osteonecrosis, femoral or humeral
	Osteoporosis
Alkylating agents, nitrosoureas, epipodophyllotoxins, and anthracyclines	Acute leukemia, myelodysplasia
Vinca alkaloids	Distal peripheral neuropathy

CHEMOTHERAPEUTIC AGENTS

A list of chemotherapeutic drugs commonly used in the treatment of lymphoproliferative neoplasms is contained in Table 12.3, grouped by class of agent. In the discussion below, we focus on their known mechanisms of action and dose-limiting toxicities, characteristics that will prove important when we discuss multiagent chemotherapy protocols and combined modality treatment programs. This section is not meant to be exhaustive but rather to emphasize those aspects of the individual drugs important to understanding the potential for non–cross-resistance and non-overlapping toxicity.

Alkylating Agents and Nitrosoureas

Alkylating agents are widely useful in the treatment of lymphoproliferative neoplasms and are frequently incorporated in curative multiagent protocols (59). They induce covalent cross-linking of DNA strands and, thus, potentially disrupt all aspects of nucleic acid metabolism. Cyclophosphamide and ifosfamide require metabolic activation in the liver to the active metabolites acrolein and others, which, in turn, are responsible for a specific toxicity, cystitis and bladder fibrosis, that can be blocked by mercaptoethane-sulfate, mesna (60). Resistance to alkylating agents can be specific—for example, reduced cellular influx of mechlorethamine (61)—or more general, as in conjugation of active metabolites mediated by glutathione synthetase (41). Cyclophosphamide and chlorambucil can be given orally and are often used alone or with corticosteroids to control indolent lymphoproliferative diseases such as follicular lymphoma or chronic lymphocytic leukemia (62–66). Ifosfamide is always given with mesna, and this pair is usually used in combination regimens for relapsed aggressive histology lymphoma or in high-dose regimens to be followed by hematopoietic stem cell transplantation (67,68). Mechlorethamine, procarbazine, and lomustine are seldom used anymore but were commonly incorporated in combinations for Hodgkin's lymphoma in the 1970s through the early

TABLE 12.3. *Chemotherapeutic agents commonly used in the treatment of lymphoproliferative neoplasms*

Class	Agents	Usual dose-limiting toxicity	Standard dose range (mg/m^2)	Route	Treatment interval (wk)
Alkylating agents	Cyclophosphamide	Myelosuppression	600–1,500	IV	3–4
	Chlorambucil	Myelosuppression	16–20	PO	2
			40	PO	4
	Mechlorethamine	Myelosuppression	6	IV	2–4
	Ifosfamide	Myelosuppression	4,000–5,000	IV	3–4
	Procarbazine	Myelosuppression	100	PO daily × 7–14 d	2–4
	Dacarbazine	Myelosuppression	375	IV	2
	Lomustine	Myelosuppression	100–130	PO	6
Corticosteroids	Prednisone	None	40–80	PO daily × 5 d–12 wk	0–4
	Dexamethasone	None	4–20	PO daily × 4–5 d	2–4
Antimetabolites	Methotrexate	None[a]	400–8,000	IV	2–4
	Cytarabine	Cerebellar dysfunction	300-4,000	IV	2–4
Vinca alkaloids	Vincristine	Neuropathy	1.2–1.4	IV	2–4
	Vinblastine	Myelosuppression	6–8	IV	2–4
Anthracyclines	Doxorubicin	Myelosuppression	5–60	IV	3–4
Epipodophyllotoxins	Etoposide	Myelosuppression	50–100	PO daily × 10–21 d	2–6
			100–600	IV	3–4
Purine analogs and adenosine deaminase inhibitors	Fludarabine	Myelosuppression	20–25	IV daily × 5 d	4
	Cladribine	Myelosuppression	4–8	IV daily × 5–7 d	4–6
	Pentostatin	Myelosuppression	4	IV	2–4
Platinum derivatives	Cisplatin	Nephrotoxicity, neurotoxicity, ototoxicity	50–100	IV	3–4
	Carboplatin	Myelosuppression	200–300	IV	2–4
Monoclonal antibodies	Rituximab	None	375	IV	4
Other agents	Bleomycin	Pulmonary dysfunction	5–10 U	IV	1–4

[a]With leucovorin rescue.

1990s (17,18,69). Dacarbazine is currently only used in the ABVD program for Hodgkin's lymphoma (54).

The major and dose-limiting toxicity of the alkylating agents and nitrosoureas is myelosuppression. Relative lack of other toxicities and broad effectiveness across almost all lymphoproliferative neoplasms have led to the incorporation of cyclophosphamide into many high-dose protocols supported by hematopoietic stem cell transplantation. Additional acute side effects include moderate nausea and vomiting, mucositis, hair loss at higher doses, and bladder cystitis and hematuria. Alkylating agents cause dose-dependent risk of oligospermic infertility in men (70,71), anovulatory infertility and premature menopause in women (72–74), and leukemia with or without myelodysplasia in both genders (75–79). In general, longer courses of treatment and higher cumulative doses increase these risks. Thus, six to eight cycles of CHOP [cyclophosphamide, hydroxydaunomycin, Oncovin (vincristine), and prednisone)] with one alkylator at moderate dose seldom cause infertility (80), but six to eight or more courses of MOPP with two alkylators at full dose virtually always do so (56,81,82), and the induction of leukemia correlates with the cumulative lifetime dose (75,76).

Corticosteroids

Corticosteroids have two clinically useful effects in the management of lymphoproliferative neoplasms: first, they are directly lymphocytotoxic (83,84) and can often cause rapid cell lysis; second, they block the effects of lymphokines and cytokines, which mediate many of the distant effects of lymphoma such as fever, night sweats, anorexia, myalgias, and fatigue. Their cytotoxic effect appears to be induced by binding to specific corticosteroid receptors on the surface of the lymphoid cells, leading rapidly to apoptosis (83). Although this effect can, at times, be dramatic and cause such rapid cell lysis that the release of intracellular and membrane products induces tumor lysis syndrome with its electrolyte- and coagulation-based complications, the lymphocytotoxicity of corticosteroids is widely variable across lymphocyte populations and lymphoma subtypes. In addition, sole treatment with corticosteroids is virtually never curative, indicating that even the apparently sensitive lymphoma subtypes harbor some cell populations with corticosteroid resistance, often mediated by down-regulation of expression of corticosteroid receptors (85).

The toxicity profile of corticosteroids differs substantially from that of most antilymphoma antineoplastic agents. Corticosteroids do not cause alopecia, myelosuppression or direct gastrointestinal toxicity. Indeed they are highly effective anti-emetic medications. Acutely they are responsible for insomnia, flushing, tachycardia, palpitations, hyperglycemia, gastric hyperacidity and dyspepsia and proximal myopathy (86). An effective blocker of gastric acid secretion should always accompany prolonged or high-dose corticosteroids. Occasionally, corticosteroids can precipitate mania or psychosis and should be used very cautiously or avoided in patients with a history of manic-depressive or psychotic psychiatric disturbances. The most important short-term complication of corticosteroids is immunosuppression, an effect exploited in the treatment of autoimmune diseases, including hemolytic anemia or immune thrombocytopenia, that can accompany lymphoproliferative disease. However, prolonged courses of corticosteroids increase the risk of opportunistic infection with organisms such as varicella and *Pneumocystis carinii* (87,88). This can be doubly dangerous in the face of underlying immune dysfunction as is seen in patients with acquired immunodeficiency syndrome or when additional agents that induce prolonged lymphocytopenia such as the purine analog antagonists of adenosine deaminase are used (89,90).

The two major uses of corticosteroids in lymphoma treatment both capitalize on their broad lympholytic effects and their special spectrum of acute toxicities. These agents are often incorporated into multiagent programs because they work quickly; do not cause myelosuppression; ameliorate nausea, emesis, and anorexia; and rapidly reverse constitutional symptoms such as fever or night sweats. Corticosteroids are also very useful palliative agents when used judiciously as single agents in patients with late-stage incurable disease.

Antimetabolites

The classical antimetabolites currently have a very limited role in lymphoma management. Methotrexate is a folate antagonist that causes depletion of the intracellular pool of folate coenzymes and subsequent disruption of normal thymidylate and purine synthetic pathways (37). It is likely that this interference with necessary synthetic and repair processes increases the intracellular signals, encouraging apoptosis, and, thus, leads to cell death. The use of extremely high doses of methotrexate with resultant penetration of physiologic sanctuaries, such as the central nervous system (CNS) or chambers of the eye, can be accomplished with manageable risk and low toxicity by providing biochemical rescue with leucovorin that bypasses the folate depletion and restores normal folate coenzyme function (37). Cytarabine is converted intracellularly to ara-cytosine triphosphate, which, in turn, inhibits DNA repair and synthetic enzymes (91). Resistance to both methotrexate and cytarabine appears to primarily arise as cells ignore the competitive enzyme inhibition caused by these agents, either by altering the binding affinity of the enzyme for the antimetabolite or by producing larger quantities of the enzyme, thus eliminating its rate-limiting effect, an increased production often accomplished by gene amplification (37,91). The toxicity of high-dose methotrexate can be minimized with leucovorin rescue, but this requires meticulous attention to the rescue process. Leucovorin must be started within 24 to 42 hours of the methotrexate and continued until methotrexate blood levels have been verified to be below 0.05 μM (5×10^{-8}) (92). Methotrexate should not be given in the face of renal dysfunction or presence of third-space fluids such as pleural effusions, ascites, or extensive edema, because excretion is virtually entirely renal, and third-space fluids can act as a reservoir for the drug (37). Despite careful leucovorin rescue, some patients experience mucositis, transient elevation of serum creatinine, hepatic transaminitis, myelosuppression, or rash. Rarely, these toxicities can be severe or fatal. Cytarabine is very rapidly cleared from the circulation, and so its toxicity is dependent on both dose and duration of exposure. Bolus administration is much less toxic than infusional, but in both cases, myelosuppression is dose limiting (91). Higher-dose bolus administration can also be associated with neurologic, hepatic, or gastrointestinal toxicity, primarily mucositis (91). The neurologic toxicity usually takes the form of cerebellar dysfunction with ataxia, slurred speech, and confusion and is more likely in older patients or those with underlying renal dysfunction (91).

Previously, methotrexate with leucovorin rescue was incorporated into several commonly used multiagent programs for diffuse large-cell lymphoma; however, definitive randomized trials demonstrated that it does not add to the efficacy of standard regimens such as CHOP (24,25,93–96). Thus, methotrexate currently plays a role in lymphoma treatment only in two special circumstances. It is still often included in regimens for the treatment of Burkitt's lymphoma, in which it is combined with alkylators, vinca alkaloids, anthracyclines, and corticosteroids (97–99). Its other use takes advantage of its high penetrance into privileged areas. It is a useful agent for primary or secondary CNS lymphoma and for intraocular lymphoma. When the intention is to treat or prevent leptomeningeal disease, methotrexate may be given directly into the CNS via lumbar intrathecal injection or through an Ommaya reservoir into the intraventricular space. Intraparenchymal brain lymphoma and ocular lymphoma require intravenous administration. There is circumstantial evidence that very high doses, in the range of 8,000 mg per m^2, work better than do lower doses (100,101). Cytarabine is primarily used in secondary treatment regimens, often in combination with cisplatin because of possible synergistic antilymphoma activity (102,103). Whether such cytarabine-containing regimens are superior to other available secondary protocols is unknown and seems unlikely given the lack of any evidence that primary regimens incorporating cytarabine, such as ProMACE-CytaBOM [prednisone, methotrexate, Adriamycin (doxorubicin), cyclophosphamide, etoposide, cytarabine, bleomycin, Oncovin (vincristine), and methotrexate] (104) are any better than standard CHOP (24,94,105–107).

Vinca Alkaloids

Vincristine and vinblastine are the two vinca alkaloids widely used for lymphoma, the first primarily for non-Hodgkin's lymphoma and the latter for Hodgkin's lymphoma. These agents bind to tubulin, block polymerization, and disrupt microtubule formation (108). This interferes with mitotic spindle formation and possibly with other functions of microtubules within the cell, such as movement of organelles and macromolecules. The primary mode of resistance appears to be via one or more of the multidrug resistance efflux pumps (28,29,32).

The acute toxicity of vincristine is primarily neurologic. Almost all patients experience distal dysesthesias and numbness in the limbs, and loss of deep tendon reflexes is usual. Some patients develop transient jaw pain that resolves even though the drug is continued, and most develop at least mild constipation that can be partially prevented with stool softeners and cathartics. Motor dysfunction, severe constipation, hoarseness, or genuinely painful dysesthesias are uncommon but constitute grounds to reduce the dose substantially or discontinue the drug altogether. Vinblastine can cause all the same neuropathic toxicities as vincristine plus, at higher doses, severe myalgias, but these occur infrequently, because the dose is limited by myelosuppression. Newer vinca alkaloids, such as vindesine and vinorelbine (109,110) are active in lymphomas but have not been widely tested, nor do they appear to confer any advantage over the traditional two agents. Liposomal encapsulation of vincristine may reduce marrow toxicity and enhance efficacy; clinical trials are currently underway to explore its usefulness (111).

The major use of vinca alkaloids in lymphoma treatment has been the incorporation of vincristine into multidrug regimens, such as CHOP for diffuse large-cell and other aggressive histology lymphomas (112) and CVP (cyclophosphamide, vincristine, and prednisone) (113,114) for more indolent lymphomas. Its use as a single agent is limited both by only modest potency and by the cumulative nature of its neurotoxicity. Vinblastine is only used to treat Hodgkin's lymphoma among the lymphoid neoplasms. It is very useful for that disease both as a crucial element of the gold standard ABVD protocol (26,27,54) and in the single-agent palliation of late disease. The primary attractiveness of the vinca alkaloids, especially vincristine, for inclusion in multiagent programs is their minimal tendency to cause myelosuppression and lack of other overlapping toxicity with commonly included agents.

Anthracyclines

The anthracycline antibiotics are natural or semisynthetic antineoplastic agents that appear to act by two major mechanisms: complex formation with topoisomerase II and DNA, leading to DNA strand breaks and disruption of DNA transcription (115,116) and oxidative generation of free radicals that cause membrane deterioration (117). Both of these effects probably secondarily activate pathways leading to apoptosis. Resistance to anthracyclines is primarily mediated by the multidrug resistance efflux mechanism (28–32). Acutely, the anthracyclines cause alopecia, nausea, mucositis, and their dose–limiting toxicity, myelosuppression. Intravenous extravasation can lead to prolonged induration, pain, ulceration, and, in the extreme, tissue necrosis and must be avoided by using great care with intravenous administration and appropriate central venous devices. The major late toxicity of anthracyclines is cardiac. They induce a dose-dependent loss of cardiac myofibrils such that the risk of later cardiomyopathy rises from approximately 5% with cumulative doses of doxorubicin in the range of 400 to 450 mg per m^2 to more than 30% when the cumulative dose exceeds 700 to 750 mg per m^2 (118). Underlying cardiac disease, older age, and prior exposure of the heart to radiation increase this risk, and anthracyclines should be avoided in patients with preexisting cardiac failure (119,120).

Anthracyclines are the most broadly and potently effective antilymphoma agents currently in clinical use, rivaled only by the alkylating agents. Doxorubicin is a key component of the most widely used regimen for diffuse large-cell lymphoma—CHOP (24,112)—and for Hodgkin's lymphoma—ABVD (26,27,54). Anthracyclines are seldom used as single agents, because maximum allowable lifetime exposure has often been reached by the time such palliative use would be appropriate, but they can be very useful for selected patients. Doxorubicin is by far the most commonly used anthracycline for lymphoma. It is not clear that there is any therapeutic advantage gained in using one of the analogs of doxorubicin, such as daunorubicin, epirubicin, or idarubicin; the closely related anthracenedione, mitoxantrone; or the newer formulation, liposomal doxorubicin. In the few direct comparisons, these alternative agents have proven at best equal and sometimes inferior in efficacy to doxorubicin (121–124).

Epipodophyllotoxins

Etoposide is a semisynthetic derivative of the natural plant toxin podophyllotoxin and the major representative from the epipodophyllotoxins useful in lymphoma treatment. These drugs appear to act by directly inducing single-strand breaks in DNA and by inhibiting proper function of topoisomerase II, with resultant DNA damage and disruption of normal transcription (125–128). These cumulative injuries tip the intracellular balance in favor of apoptosis and lead to cell death. Resistance occurs either via the multidrug resistance efflux mechanism or via emergence of enhanced ability to repair DNA strand breaks (28–32,129). The toxicity of etoposide is primarily hematologic, with reversible myelosuppression occurring for 4 to 7 days starting approximately 1 week after intravenous dosing. Mild to moderate nausea, alopecia, and mucositis may occur but are seldom troublesome. This narrow toxicity profile has led to frequent use of etoposide in high-dose regimens followed by hematopoietic stem cell transplantation for lymphomas (130–134). Rarely, etoposide causes a treatment-related acute myeloid leukemia associated with a specific 11q23 chromosomal abnormality and a shorter latency than that seen with leukemia after alkylating agents (135–137).

Attempts to integrate etoposide into primary chemotherapy programs for lymphoma have been generally unsuccessful. Regimens such as VACOP-B [VP-16 (etoposide), Adriamycin (doxorubicin), cyclophosphamide, Oncovin (vincristine), prednisone, and bleomycin] (138), CHOPE (CHOP plus etoposide) (139), and ProMACE-CytaBOM (105–107,140,141)

are not superior to CHOP alone. Recently, preliminary results from a large German trial of CHOPE for diffuse large-cell lymphoma demonstrated a modest advantage over standard CHOP, but full details have not yet been published (142). Thus, the major roles for etoposide currently are in secondary regimens such as ICE (ifosfamide, carboplatin, and etoposide) (67), high-dose protocols supported by hematopoietic stem cell transplantation (4–7,143,144), and as a single agent for palliative purposes in late-stage disease, in which its well-tolerated oral formulation can be particularly convenient (145,146).

Purine Analogs and Inhibitors of Adenosine Deaminase

The first purine analogs that proved clinically useful were among the earliest of chemotherapeutic agents introduced into clinical practice and included 6-mercaptopurine and 6-thioguanine, both of which proved useful in the treatment of childhood acute lymphoblastic leukemia (147–149). Today these agents are of mostly historical interest as antineoplastic agents for lymphomas, although they continue to be used for immunomodulation and treatment of acute leukemias. Currently, the most clinically useful agents from the group of purine analogs are the halogenated derivatives of adenosine. This group of agents can be classed together, because their mechanisms of action, although different in detail, all focus on disruption of normal nucleic acid metabolism. Fludarabine, 2-fluro-ara-adenosine monophosphate, a fluorinated analog of adenosine, is metabolized to a fluorinated derivative of adenosine triphosphate that inhibits DNA polymerase and DNA prolongation and disrupts normal transcription (150,151). Cladribine, 2-chloro-2-deoxyadenosine, also leads to a halogenated form of adenosine triphosphate, with eventual blockage of DNA synthesis, strand breaks, and transcription errors (152). Pentostatin is a natural product derivative structurally related to deoxyadenosine. It binds irreversibly to the enzyme adenosine deaminase, an enzyme richly present in lymphoid cells. This leads to accumulation of unwanted nucleic acid metabolic products and inhibition of DNA and RNA synthesis (153). With all three drugs, the global effect is disruption of normal nucleic acid metabolism, interference with faithful DNA synthesis, the accumulation of DNA strand breaks, and blockage of normal transcription. These cumulative errors eventually reach the point at which the self-destruction pathways of apoptosis are initiated, and the cell dies. Resistance to these agents primarily takes the form of altered binding affinity in one or more of the crucial enzymes.

Fludarabine, cladribine, and pentostatin are very well tolerated in standard doses. Acute toxicity is unusual, although some patients report headache, lassitude, mild nausea, or fatigue. Higher-than-standard doses have been linked to severe, sometimes irreversible, neurologic toxicity and should not be used (154). The dose-limiting toxicity of all three is myelosuppression with reversible neutropenia and thrombocytopenia occurring 10 to 20 days after administration. However, the most important toxicity is immunosuppression (155). Severe lymphocytopenia occurs after several cycles of treatment and usually lasts for many months to several years. Opportunistic infections with *Pneumocystis carinii*, varicella, legionella, *Candida albicans*, and others may occur during or well after treatment (155). Coincident use of other lymphocytotoxic agents, such as corticosteroids, increases the risk of opportunistic infection (155).

The major impact of the purine analogs and adenosine deaminase inhibitors has been on indolent lymphoproliferative diseases. Fludarabine and cladribine are the most potent single agents available for lymphoplasmacytic lymphoma (156–159), follicular lymphoma (156,160–163), hairy-cell leukemia (164,165), and chronic lymphocytic leukemia (163,166–169). Pentostatin is also effective in the same conditions but is much less widely used, primarily because of greater myelotoxicity and expense. However, the cumulative myelotoxicity and long-term immunosuppression associated with these agents have led most clinicians to reserve them for secondary use after traditional alkylators no longer control disease. Ongoing investigations combining purine analogs or pentostatin with alkylators, anthracyclines, or newer targeted agents, such as rituximab, have produced impressive phase II results but await confirmation of superiority in randomized trials (162,170). Eventually, one of the most important contributions of this class of agents to lymphoma treatment may not come from their direct antilymphoma effects but rather from their potent ability to induce the immunosuppression required for nonmyeloablative hematopoietic stem cell transplantation, thus allowing that new immunotherapeutic approach to be used more widely (171) (also see Chapter 13).

Platinum Derivatives

The platinum derivatives have had a much larger impact on solid tumors, especially testicular, ovarian, and lung carcinoma, than they have on lymphoid neoplasms, for which they have mostly been incorporated in secondary treatment regimens for diffuse large-cell and other aggressive-histology lymphomas (67,102,172). They appear to work by forming inter- and intrastrand DNA-DNA and DNA-protein linkages (173). Once again, the theme emerges that DNA damage and transcriptional disruption lead to cumulative errors and eventual apoptotic cell death. Cisplatin causes significant nausea, vomiting, nephrotoxicity, sensory neuropathy, and ototoxicity but only mild myelosuppression (174). Carboplatin, on the other hand, causes dose-limiting myelosuppression but no or only mild versions of the other major cisplatin-associated toxicities (175).

Primarily based on its *in vitro* synergy with cytarabine, cisplatin continues to be used in several secondary regimens for lymphoma, such as DHAP [dexamethasone, high-dose arabinosyl cytosine (cytarabine), and cisplatin] (102,172), although its independent contribution has never been verified. Carboplatin is a major component of the ICE regimen that is used primarily as a secondary protocol for diffuse large-cell lymphoma before high-dose chemotherapy and hematopoietic stem cell transplantation (67). The multiorgan toxicity of cisplatin and marked cumulative myelosuppression of carboplatin, together with only minimal activity as single agents against lymphoma, are likely to keep the role of the platinum derivatives limited for the lymphoid malignancies.

Monoclonal Antibodies

The monoclonal antibodies with known or potential effectiveness for the treatment of lymphoid neoplasms are described in detail in Chapter 13. Originally, these agents were assumed to work by mobilizing the effector mechanisms of the immune system, as is described there. However, a growing body of information suggests that these agents may actually work by much more direct mechanisms, including signal transduction from cell surface–binding sites, which leads directly to apoptosis (176,177) or down-regulation of expression of apoptosis-blocking agents, such as bcl-2 protein (176). Thus, discussion with more classical chemotherapeutic agents is appropriate. The major currently available monoclonal antibodies for the treatment of lymphoid malignancy are rituximab (anti-CD20) and alemtuzumab (anti-CD52). Rituximab binds to the CD20 transmembrane protein antigen that is found on the surface of most B-cell lymphomas and normal mature B cells but minimally or not at all on precursor B cells and mature plasma cells. Once bound, the antibody may induce complement-mediated cell lysis, may recruit antibody-dependent cytotoxic T and NK cells, or may act via other immunologic mechanisms, even including induction of cytotoxic memory cells (178). However, rituximab also induces apoptosis directly without mediation of either complement or other cells (176,177) and has been shown to down-regulate expression of bcl-2 protein (176), thus potentially directly reversing that protein's inhibition of apoptosis. Alemtuzumab may work by any of the same mechanisms except that its target is the CD52 antigen that is found on B, T, and NK cells, macrophages, monocytes, and a minority of granulocytes. Resistance to monoclonal antibodies may occur by alteration in availability of the target antigen by shedding, modulation such that it is no longer displayed on the cell surface, mutation of the target protein, or by blockage of any signal-transduction pathway essential to the antibody's activity (178).

Monoclonal antibodies come much closer to the goal of selective targeting of neoplastic cells than do any previously developed chemotherapeutic agents. Thus, their toxicities are much more limited. All may induce a cytokine-release syndrome, in which neoplastic and normal cells systemically release active amounts of cytokines and lymphokines capable of causing chills, fever, hypotension, rash, bronchospasm, tachycardia, and, in the extreme, a fatal shock syndrome, which may also have some of the features of tumor lysis syndrome (179). This severe reaction is more likely in the presence of large numbers of neoplastic cells circulating in the peripheral blood (179). Other toxicities reflect the extent to which normal cells express the target antigen. Rituximab causes a profound drop in circulating B cells for approximately 6 months; however, immunoglobulin levels are maintained, and opportunistic infections are rare (180,181). No other late toxicity has been seen with this agent. Alemtuzumab causes myelosuppression and immunosuppression, with resultant increased risk of opportunistic infection (182). It is likely that future monoclonal antibodies will show this same narrowness of toxicity, reflecting distribution of the target antigen.

Rituximab was originally shown to be effective in follicular lymphoma and remains an important addition to the agents useful for this disease. More recently, it has been demonstrated to increase the effectiveness of CHOP chemotherapy for diffuse large B-cell lymphoma in older patients (183). It is likely that its usefulness in B-cell neoplasms will continue to expand as more investigations focus on its ability to potentiate standard chemotherapy. Alemtuzumab is now available for treatment of fludarabine-refractory chronic lymphocytic leukemia (182), but its spectrum of usefulness is also likely to be expanded as more diseases are tested and it is incorporated into combinations, a task that will be made more challenging by its overlapping myelotoxicity. The importance of the monoclonal antibodies, however, lies primarily in the demonstration that such targeted agents can be constructed, that their antineoplastic activity can be specified, and that they can be combined with standard agents in a manner that augments effectiveness without expanding toxicity.

Antisense Oligonucleotides

Although the antisense oligonucleotides have not yet reached clinical use, it is important to understand their potential. Neoplasms in general, and lymphoid malignancies in particular, exist because cells inappropriately express genes that should remain quiescent or fail to express genes required to suppress the malignant phenotype. Antisense oligonucleotides offer the potential to selectively block the first of these two broad mechanisms. In practice, therapeutic antisense oligonucleotides consist of oligomers of ten to 20 nucleotides, with a backbone stabilized by alterations that provide resistance to ubiquitous endonucleases. The nucleotide sequence is chosen to be complementary to that of a crucial stretch of nucleotides in the target gene's messenger RNA (mRNA). Hydrogen bond–mediated hybridization of the antisense oligonucleotide to the target mRNA leads to blockage of mRNA translation and may enhance the mRNA's destruction by endonucleases (52,53). In theory, any overexpressed gene can be blocked, allowing selective reversal of that gene's contribution to the malignant phenotype. In addition, if nonspecific effects from the stabilized backbone or certain key short nucleotide sequence motifs can be avoided, these agents should be exquisitely selective.

Antisense agents directed at bcl-2 protein expression are the most advanced in clinical testing (53,184,185); however, oligonucleotides to suppress bcl-1, c-myc, p53, and other oncogenes have also been synthesized and are entering clin-

ical development (186,187). Others are sure to follow as additional target genes are identified and specific oligomers synthesized. As with the other chemotherapeutic agents, it is likely that antisense oligonucleotides will achieve the most when combined with other drugs. Up-regulation of bcl-2 protein correlates with poor prognosis after CHOP chemotherapy for diffuse large B-cell lymphoma (188), suggesting that coincident administration of effective chemotherapy and down-regulation of target-gene over-expression mediated by antisense oligonucleotides should translate into improved disease control.

Other Agents, Including Camptothecins, Taxanes, and Bleomycin

The camptothecins are a class of agents that inhibit the action of topoisomerase I. Although they have shown useful activity in certain solid tumors, especially gastrointestinal cancer, they have been disappointingly inactive against lymphoproliferative diseases (189–192). Likewise, the taxanes, which work by causing microtubule polymerization, are useful in lung, breast, and ovarian carcinoma but minimally active for lymphomas. Much of the antilymphoma effectiveness noted in phase II trials of taxanes was probably due to the high-dose corticosteroids that were given to ameliorate the acute toxicity of these agents (193–196).

Bleomycin, a mixture of natural peptides with antineoplastic activity, forms a complex of itself, iron, and DNA that produces single- and double–strand breaks and disrupts DNA transcription and replication (197,198). Although modestly active as a single agent and widely included in older combinations, such as CHOP-bleo (199–201), MACOP-B [methotrexate-leucovorin, Adriamycin (doxorubicin), cyclophosphamide, Oncovin (vincristine), prednisone, and bleomycin] (202,203), ProMACE-CytaBOM (104,140,141), and M-BACOD [methotrexate, bleomycin, Adriamycin (doxorubicin), cyclophosphamide, Oncovin (vincristine), and dexamethasone] (24,25,204,205), bleomycin was shown not to add to the effectiveness of any of these regimens (24,25) and has mostly been dropped from protocols for non-Hodgkin's lymphoma. It remains in the standard ABVD program for Hodgkin's lymphoma, but its actual independent contribution to that regimen's efficacy has never been proven. Bleomycin retains appeal predominantly because its sole major toxicity, pulmonary fibrosis, occurs infrequently and does not overlap with any other antilymphoma agents.

MULTIAGENT CHEMOTHERAPY

Principles and Evolution

The observations that single-agent chemotherapy brought about both useful amelioration of symptomatic disease and objective tumor shrinkage combined with the experimental evidence that multiple agents could have at least an additive and at times synergistic effect on tumor burden led logically to the idea of combining chemotherapeutic agents for the treatment of human neoplasms. By the 1950s and early 1960s, new drugs had become available that could clearly modify the course of advanced, widely disseminated lymphoproliferative neoplasms: corticosteroids, vinca alkaloids, and antimetabolites for acute lymphoblastic leukemia in children (13,15,147,148); mechlorethamine, vinca alkaloids, and prednisone for Hodgkin's lymphoma (17,18); melphalan and prednisone for myeloma (206,207); and alkylating agents and corticosteroids for non-Hodgkin's lymphomas (13,16,208). Initially, these agents were used alone, often repeatedly or sequentially, eventually establishing that multiple responses could be seen as the same drugs were repeated or when new ones were introduced. However, few, if any, patients were cured with this approach. With the experimental observation that some lymphoproliferative neoplastic cell lines could be eradicated by using multiple drugs at the same time (1,3) and the empiric observation that drugs from different classes of agents could have non- or only partially overlapping toxicity, investigators were emboldened to attempt to combine multiple agents. Remarkably, three previously incurable lymphoid neoplasms yielded to the use of such combinations. Childhood acute lymphoblastic leukemia responded to combinations of aminopterin (an early antifolate antimetabolite), vincristine, prednisone, and 6-mercaptopurine (an early antineoplastic purine analog) (16,147,209). Hodgkin's lymphoma, incurable with irradiation or single chemotherapeutic drugs, was cured with mechlorethamine, vincristine, procarbazine, and prednisone (17,18). Finally, diffuse large-cell lymphoma (then called *diffuse histiocytic lymphoma*), a disease characterized before this development by a median survival of shorter than 6 months, proved curable in at least 30% to 40% of patients with mechlorethamine or cyclophosphamide, vincristine, procarbazine, and prednisone (20). These observations transformed the field of oncology and established unequivocally that disseminated human neoplasms could be cured when effective drugs were crafted into combinations capitalizing on non–cross-resistance and non-overlapping toxicity.

Fundamental Role of Clinical Trials

The original clinical trials demonstrating the effectiveness of multiagent chemotherapy were modest in size and conducted at single centers (17,20,112). Concurrent controls were unnecessary, because these protocols changed the posttreatment natural history of their target diseases from relentlessly relapsing to permanently cured. However, once this alteration in natural history had been achieved, further advances required comparison to controls to produce unambiguous results. In addition, a rapidly expanding list of potentially effective agents required an orderly screening process to identify those with the greatest effectiveness. Although clinical trials had already been widely used across many fields of medicine, few specialties have come to use them as widely or fundamentally as does medical

oncology. A series of orderly developmental steps has been developed to move effective new drugs from preclinical promise to established treatments. Phase I trials identify the safe dose to be used in further testing and provide initial information about pharmacokinetics and specific organ toxicity. Phase II trials determine response rates for individual cancers and give an indication of relative effectiveness. Phase III trials confirm effectiveness of new agents and combinations relative to current best standards and require comparison to a control population, most often but not always a randomized concurrently managed group. This orderly approach to drug development has been quite productive for the treatment of lymphoid malignancies and underpins the array of effective regimens currently available for these diseases.

An excellent example of how serial clinical trials came to define current treatment is that of diffuse large B-cell lymphoma, the most common single type of lymphoma seen in the Western world. By the early 1970s, investigators had established that advanced diffuse large B-cell lymphoma could be cured in a minority of patients with MOPP or C-MOPP (20). Soon, new drugs, such as bleomycin, doxorubicin, and high-dose methotrexate, were discovered and found effective in phase I and II trials. The moderate toxicity and marked efficacy of doxorubicin as a single agent in multiple cancers, especially hematolymphoid neoplasms, made it a particularly attractive agent to add to the previously developed combinations of corticosteroids, vinca alkaloids, and alkylating agents. Phase II trials indicated that new combinations, such as CHOP (112), BACOP [bleomycin, Adriamycin (doxorubicin), cyclophosphamide, Oncovin (vincristine), and prednisone] (210,211), and M-BACOD (204,205), were also curative for this disease. By the end of the 1970s, several groups had demonstrated that CHOP could cure patients of diffuse large-cell lymphoma (diffuse histiocytic lymphoma) regardless of stage, without maintenance therapy, without additional radiation, within acceptable bounds of toxicity, and even after prior treatment with radiation had failed (112,212–214). Based on its ease of administration, tolerance across a wide range of ages, and convenience of scheduling, CHOP became the most widely accepted regimen in standard practice.

After this era in which CHOP emerged as the standard, the next two eras of clinical investigation proved frustrating. Complex, dose-intense protocols with as many as nine or ten drugs such as MACOP-B (202,203) and ProMACE-CytaBOM (104,140,141) failed to prove superior to CHOP when tested in definitive randomized trials (24,25,93–96,106,107). Attention then shifted to highly intensified programs with hematopoietic stem cell transplantation, anticipating that their ability to eliminate relapsed disease (215) would translate into more frequent cures when incorporated into primary management. Once again, a clear-cut improvement in outcome over what can be achieved with standard-dose chemotherapy has not been demonstrated. The modestly better results obtained in some trials (216,217) were counterbalanced by the clearly negative results in others (216,218–

220). Finally, with the advent of effective immunotherapy, we seem to be emerging into a more productive era, with new regimens building on the platform of CHOP chemotherapy augmented by the additive, if not synergistic, impact of the monoclonal antibody rituximab (183). These important observations, both positive and negative, could only be made through the mechanism of large, prospective, concurrently randomized, comparative clinical trials.

INTEGRATION OF CHEMOTHERAPY AND RADIATION

Building on Strengths

A full discussion of the role of radiation of the treatment of lymphoid neoplasms is provided in Chapter 11. This section will concentrate on its potential contribution to combined modality treatment. Radiation may contribute in one or more important ways. Understanding each of these potential roles is essential to the best integration of radiation and chemotherapy.

The most obvious way in which radiation might add to the effectiveness of chemotherapy is by providing non–cross-resistant killing of chemotherapy-resistant cells. Thus, disease persistent despite the best chemotherapy may, in theory, be eradicated by adding radiation. Another important role is to permit reduction of the chemotherapy. Indeed, this strategy plays to the strengths of both modalities. Chemotherapy works best against small bulk areas of systemically disseminated disease; radiation, by its nature a local treatment, may contribute the most by controlling regional disease. In combination, the radiation may allow minimization of the duration or dose intensity of the chemotherapy by controlling local disease and keeping the need for chemotherapy to the minimum required to eliminate systemic, low-bulk, micrometastatic disease. Another role for radiation is to deal with lymphoma present within sites not penetrated well by chemotherapy, such as the testes or CNS. Finally, radiation can play a very important role in providing palliative relief of symptoms due to localized tumors, even when cure is no longer possible, permitting continued high-quality survival without the undesirable systemic effects of chemotherapy. Incorporation of radiation into combined modality programs should attempt to capitalize on one or more of these special characteristics.

Avoiding Overlapping Toxicity

The acute toxic effects of radiation are predominantly local. Indeed, the areas of the body that can safely be treated with radiation are in large part defined by its local toxicity. Thus, disease within parenchymal organs such as the liver, lungs, or kidneys with limited tolerance for radiation is usually considered untreatable by this modality, because doses effective for lymphoma would be unacceptably toxic. On the other hand, most lymph node sites, bone metastases, and disease within the CNS can be quite successfully treated, because locally curative doses of radiation can be delivered within

the tolerance of the tissue surrounding the target lesion. Thus, in many circumstances, radiation can be added to chemotherapy with a minimum of overlapping toxicity. However, in addition to the necessity to avoid irradiation of organs that cannot tolerate exposure to full doses, in two cases, care must be taken because toxicity that overlaps with that of chemotherapy may be encountered. The first is seen in proportion to the extent that the field of radiation includes marrow-bearing bone. The greater the extent of marrow exposure, the greater will be the degree of marrow suppression and compromised blood counts. This effect of radiation is cumulative, such that increasingly extensive exposure of the marrow correlates with greater suppression of blood counts, and additive with chemotherapy, such that radiation fields that may have been tolerated well in isolation lead to exaggerated myelosuppression when given in addition to myelotoxic chemotherapy. The other cross-toxicity seen between radiation and chemotherapy is mucositis. Chemotherapeutic agents, such as doxorubicin and methotrexate and, to a lesser extent, alkylating agents and etoposide, can sensitize the mucosa, especially in the oropharyngeal, esophageal, or rectal areas. This potential for more severe mucosal toxicity must be anticipated when mucotoxic chemotherapy regimens and radiation to mucosal tissue are combined.

Integrating the Modalities

The major strength of radiation is that it can provide curative treatment for disease within the treatment field at a modest level of toxicity, sparing the rest of the body. On the other hand, the major strength of chemotherapy is that it treats disease throughout the body. For cure of lymphoproliferative neoplasms, the weaknesses of these modalities are also reciprocal. Radiation fails if disease lies outside the treatment field; chemotherapy, in local sites of highest tumor burden. Each modality's strength should compensate for the other's weakness and permit minimization of overall toxicity by reducing the required field size of the radiation or dose intensity or duration of the chemotherapy. In practice, capitalizing on these reciprocal strengths and weaknesses can be best accomplished when the lymphoid malignancy presents with apparently localized disease. In the case of lymphomas, even such localized presentations often come with a high risk of systemic micrometastases. An instructive example is localized diffuse large B-cell lymphoma. Here, the optimal approach is to give a brief course of chemotherapy—for example, three cycles of CHOP—followed by involved-field radiation (221). Such an approach produces progression-free survivals of 70% to 80% and sufficiently minimizes the overall toxicity to permit safe delivery even for elderly or frail patients. Several phase II and one large mature phase III trial have confirmed the usefulness of this approach (Table 12.4) (221–226). The usefulness of combined modality treatment for advanced-stage lymphoma has proven difficult to establish. As opposed to the goal in limited-stage disease, to be useful for advanced disease, the radiation must exert its effect on top of that

TABLE 12.4. *Effectiveness of brief chemotherapy and involved-field radiation for limited-stage aggressive-histology lymphoma*

Program	n	Progression-free survival (%)	Overall survival (%)	Reference
CHOP × 3 + IFRT	78	84	85	222
CHOP × 4 + IFRT	183	—	83	224
ProMACE-MOPP × 4 + IFRT	47	—	92	223
CHOP × 3/ACOB/ACOP-6 + IFRT	308	81	80	226
ACOP-6 + RT	84	—	90	225
CHOP × 3 + IFRT	200	77	82	221
vs.				
(CHOP × 8)[a]	201	64	72	

ACOB, doxorubicin, cyclophosphamide, vincristine and bleomycin; ACOP-6, doxorubicin, cyclophosphamide, vincristine and prednisone; CHOP, cyclophosphamide, doxorubicin, vincristine, and prednisone; IFRT, involved-field radiation therapy; ProMACE-MOPP, prednisone, methotrexate, doxorubicin, cyclophosphamide, etoposide, mechlorethamine, vincristine, and prednisone; RT, radiation therapy.

[a]CHOP × 8 included for comparison. This is the only randomized trial addressing the relative effectiveness of brief chemotherapy plus radiation versus chemotherapy alone.

already achieved by a full course of chemotherapy. Attempts to accomplish this for indolent lymphoma (227), diffuse large B-cell lymphoma (228), and Hodgkin's lymphoma (229–232) have failed. Whether specifically selected sets of patients, such as those with an initially bulky site of presentation; those with residual masses present by computed tomography (233), gallium (233), or positron emission scanning (234–238); or those with special types of lymphoma, such as mediastinal diffuse large B-cell lymphoma, with its tendency to present and relapse predominantly in one region of the body, would profit from targeted radiation remains an open question. Finally, radiation can play a very important role in the management of patients of all stages if there is a tendency for relapse to occur in specific sites despite otherwise effective systemic chemotherapy. The best example of such a situation is that of testicular lymphoma, in which relapse rates of up to 25% have been reported in the opposite testicle unless it is irradiated (239–242), which seems to reduce the risk to 5% or lower (243). Thus, in two circumstances—limited aggressive-histology lymphoma and lymphoma with a tendency to relapse in an irradiatable sanctuary site—radiation makes a clear contribution to the combined modality approach. However, addition of radiation to full-course chemotherapy as is used for advanced-stage disease has not been shown to improve outcome.

CONCLUSION

As we have come to understand that the non-Hodgkin's lymphomas are usually disseminated diseases, the need for effective chemotherapy has grown increasingly clear. Even when localized disease is well controlled by irradiation, the risk of relapse outside the treatment field is high. Thus, genuine control of these diseases has taken place in parallel with improvements in systemic chemotherapy. Over a period of

four decades from the 1960s to the 1990s, clinical investigators have acquired a large list of potentially effective chemotherapeutic agents, developed insight into their mechanisms of action, identified their dose-limiting toxicities, and conducted a large number of increasingly sophisticated clinical investigations that have established their potential to cure several lymphoproliferative neoplasms. Even when curative treatment has still not been discovered, highly effective palliative control can often be achieved for years. Chemotherapy is now the cornerstone of lymphoma treatment.

Radiation, the treatment modality first shown to be capable of curing lymphomas, albeit only occasionally, when the disease presented is confined to an irradiatable location, continues to make important contributions to the control of these neoplasms. By guaranteeing local control, radiation allows the chemotherapy necessary to eliminate micrometastatic disease to be kept to a short, and thus easily tolerated, duration. This permits use of curative combined modality treatment even for quite elderly or frail patients and holds unpleasant and debilitating therapy to a minimum for all patients. In addition, radiation can play a crucial role in eradicating disease in sanctuaries where chemotherapy is ineffective, such as the testis, or at sites where recurrence would be devastating, such as the epidural space. The integration of radiation into the combined modality program takes careful planning and coordination between the medical oncologist or hematologist and radiation oncologist, but this cooperation pays important dividends for the patient in terms of optimized disease control and minimized toxicity.

Future developments in the area of chemotherapy and combined modality treatment of non-Hodgkin's lymphoma will focus increasingly on targeted treatments. The use of monoclonal antibodies, antisense oligonucleotides, signal transduction–specific small molecules, enzyme-specific antagonists, high-affinity ligands, and antiangiogenic agents are all examples of such targeted treatments that are already in clinical testing. More will undoubtedly become available as knowledge and insight into the molecular characteristics of neoplastic lymphoid cells increase. The lessons learned over the past four decades will serve investigators and clinicians well, especially the need to attend to non-overlapping toxicity to assemble non–cross-resistant agents and modalities into combined modality programs.

REFERENCES

1. Skipper HE. The effects of chemotherapy on the kinetics of leukemic cell behavior. *Cancer Res* 1965;25(9):1544–1550.
2. Skipper HE, Perry S. Kinetics of normal and leukemic leukocyte populations and relevance to chemotherapy. *Cancer Res* 1970;30(6):1883–1897.
3. Skipper HE. Criteria associated with destruction of leukemia and solid tumor cells in animals. *Cancer Res* 1967;27(12):2636–2645.
4. Jagannath S, Dicke KA, Armitage JO, et al. High-dose cyclophosphamide, carmustine, and etoposide and autologous bone marrow transplantation for relapsed Hodgkin's disease. *Ann Intern Med* 1986;104(2):163–168.
5. Carella AM, Congiu AM, Gaozza E, et al. High-dose chemotherapy with autologous bone marrow transplantation in 50 advanced resistant Hodgkin's disease patients: an Italian study group report. *J Clin Oncol* 1988;6(9):1411–1416.
6. Gribben JG, Linch DC, Singer CR, et al. Successful treatment of refractory Hodgkin's disease by high-dose combination chemotherapy and autologous bone marrow transplantation. *Blood* 1989;73(1):340–344.
7. Phillips GL, Wolff SN, Herzig RH, et al. Treatment of progressive Hodgkin's disease with intensive chemoradiotherapy and autologous bone marrow transplantation. *Blood* 1989;73(8):2086–2092.
8. Hahn T, Wolff SN, Czuczman M, et al. The role of cytotoxic therapy with hematopoietic stem cell transplantation in the therapy of diffuse large cell B-cell non-Hodgkin's lymphoma: an evidence-based review. *Biol Blood Marrow Transplant* 2001;7(6):308–331.
9. Prince HM, Crump M, Imrie K, et al. Intensive therapy and autotransplant for patients with an incomplete response to front-line therapy for lymphoma. *Ann Oncol* 1996;7(10):1043–1049.
10. Vose JM, Zhang MJ, Rowlings PA, et al. Autologous transplantation for diffuse aggressive non-Hodgkin's lymphoma in patients never achieving remission: a report from the Autologous Blood and Marrow Transplant Registry. *J Clin Oncol* 2001;19(2):406–413.
11. Benson AJ, Martin CN, Garner RC. N-(2-hydroxyethyl)-N-[2-(7-guaninyl)ethyl]amine, the putative major DNA adduct of cyclophosphamide in vitro and in vivo in the rat. *Biochem Pharmacol* 1988;37(15):2979–2985.
12. Nissen-Meyer R, Host H. A comparison between the hematological side effects of cyclophosphamide and nitrogen mustard. *Cancer Chemother Rep* 1960;9:51–60.
13. Johnson IS, Armstrong JG, Gorman M. The vinca alkyloids: a new class of oncolytic agents. *Cancer Res* 1963;23:1390–1427.
14. Weiss HD, Walker MD, Weirnik PH. Neurotoxicity of commonly used antineoplastic agents. *N Engl J Med* 1974;291:127–133.
15. Dougherty T, White A. Influence of hormones on lymphoid tissue structure and function. Role of pituitary adrenotrophic hormone in regulation of lymphocytes and other cellular elements of the blood. *Endocrinology* 1944;35:1–35.
16. Rosenthal M, Saunders R, Schwartz L, et al. The use of adrenocorticotrophic hormone and cortisone in the treatment of leukemia and lymphosarcoma. *Blood* 1951;6:804–812.
17. Devita VT Jr, Serpick AA, Carbone PP. Combination chemotherapy in the treatment of advanced Hodgkin's disease. *Ann Intern Med* 1970;73(6):881–895.
18. Longo DL, Young RC, Wesley M, et al. Twenty years of MOPP therapy for Hodgkin's disease. *J Clin Oncol* 1986;4(9):1295–1306.
19. Lowenbraun S, DeVita VT, Serpick AA. Combination chemotherapy with nitrogen mustard, vincristine, procarbazine, and prednisone in lymphosarcoma and reticulum cell sarcoma. *Cancer* 1970;25(5):1018–1025.
20. DeVita VT Jr, Canellos GP, Chabner B, et al. Advanced diffuse histiocytic lymphoma, a potentially curable disease. *Lancet* 1975;1(7901):248–250.
21. Goldie JH, Coldman AJ. A mathematic model for relating the drug sensitivity of tumors to their spontaneous mutation rate. *Cancer Treat Rep* 1979;63(11–12):1727–1733.
22. Goldie JH, Coldman AJ. Quantitative model for multiple levels of drug resistance in clinical tumors. *Cancer Treat Rep* 1983;67(10):923–931.
23. Goldie JH, Coldman AJ, Gudauskas GA. Rationale for the use of alternating non-cross-resistant chemotherapy. *Cancer Treat Rep* 1982;66(3):439–449.
24. Fisher RI, Gaynor ER, Dahlberg S, et al. Comparison of a standard regimen (CHOP) with three intensive chemotherapy regimens for advanced non-Hodgkin's lymphoma. *N Engl J Med* 1993;328(14):1002–1006.
25. Gordon LI, Harrington D, Andersen J, et al. Comparison of a second-generation combination chemotherapeutic regimen (m-BACOD) with a standard regimen (CHOP) for advanced diffuse non-Hodgkin's lymphoma. *N Engl J Med* 1992;327(19):1342–1349.
26. Duggan D, Petroni G, Johnson J, et al. MOPP/ABV versus ABVD for advanced Hodgkin's disease. *Proc Am Soc Clin Oncol* 1997;16:13a (abstract 43).
27. Canellos GP, Anderson JR, Propert KJ, et al. Chemotherapy of advanced Hodgkin's disease with MOPP, ABVD, or MOPP alternating with ABVD. *N Engl J Med* 1992;327(21):1478–1484.
28. Shustik C, Dalton W, Gros P. P-glycoprotein-mediated multidrug resistance in tumor cells: biochemistry, clinical relevance and modulation. *Mol Aspects Med* 1995;16(1):1–78.
29. Gerlach JH, Kartner N, Bell DR, et al. Multidrug resistance. *Cancer Surv* 1986;5(1):25–46.
30. Kartner N, Riordan JR, Ling V. Cell surface P-glycoprotein associated with multidrug resistance in mammalian cell lines. *Science* 1983;221(4617):1285–1288.
31. Kartner N, Ling V. Multidrug resistance in cancer. *Sci Am* 1989;260(3):44–51.
32. Ling V, Gerlach J, Kartner N. Multidrug resistance. *Breast Cancer Res Treat* 1984;4(2):89–94.
33. Alexander HR, Grem JL, Hamilton JM, et al. Thymidylate synthase protein expression. *Cancer J Sci Am* 1995;1(1):49.
34. Barbour KW, Berger SH, Berger FG. Single amino acid substitution defines a naturally occurring genetic variant of human thymidylate synthase. *Mol Pharmacol* 1990;37(4):515–518.
35. Hughey CT, Barbour KW, Berger FG, et al. Genetic variation in thymidylate synthase confers resistance to 5-fluorodeoxyuridine. *Adv Exp Med Biol* 1993;339:67–76.
36. Berger SH, Jehn C-H, Johnson LF, et al. Thymidylate synthase overproduction and gene amplification in fluorodeoxyuridine-resistant human cells. *Mol Pharmacol* 1985;28:461–472.
37. Allegra CJ. Antifolates. In: Chabner B, Longo DL, eds. *Cancer Chemotherapy and Biotherapy: Principles and Practice*. Philadelphia: Lippincott-Raven, 1996:109–123.
38. Lowe SW, Ruley HE, Jacks T, et al. p53-dependent apoptosis modulates the cytotoxicity of anticancer agents. *Cell* 1993;74(6):957–967.
39. Miyashita T, Reed JC. Bcl-2 oncoprotein blocks chemotherapy-induced apoptosis in a human leukemia cell line. *Blood* 1993;81(1):151–157.
40. Reed JC, Kitada S, Takayama S, et al. Regulation of chemoresistance by the bcl-2 oncoprotein in non-Hodgkin's lymphoma and lymphocytic leukemia cell lines. *Ann Oncol* 1994;5(Suppl 1):61–65.
41. Tew KD. Glutathione-associated enzymes in anticancer drug resistance. *Cancer Res* 1994;54(16):4313–4320.
42. Eisterer W, Jiang X, Bachelot T, et al. Unfulfilled promise of endostatin in a gene therapy-xenotransplant model of human acute lymphocytic leukemia. *Mol Ther* 2002;5(4):352–359.
43. Pawliuk R, Bachelot T, Zurkiya O, et al. Continuous intravascular secretion of endostatin in mice from transduced hematopoietic stem cells. *Mol Ther* 2002;5(4):345–351.
44. Sung C, Shockley TR, Morrison PF, et al. Predicted and observed effects of antibody affinity and antigen density on monoclonal antibody uptake in solid tumors. *Cancer Res* 1992;52(2):377–384.
45. Meeker T, Lowder J, Cleary ML, et al. Emergence of idiotype variants during treatment of B-cell lymphoma with anti-idiotype antibodies. *N Engl J Med* 1985;312(26):1658–1665.

46. Reed JC. Apoptosis-regulating proteins as targets for drug discovery. *Trends Mol Med* 2001;7(7):314–319.
47. Multani PS, Grossbard ML. Monoclonal antibody-based therapies for hematologic malignancies. *J Clin Oncol* 1998;16(11):3691–3710.
48. Druker BJ. STI571 (Gleevec) as a paradigm for cancer therapy. *Trends Mol Med* 2002;8(4):S14–S18.
49. Olsen E, Duvic M, Frankel A, et al. Pivotal phase III trial of two dose levels of denileukin diftitox for the treatment of cutaneous T-cell lymphoma. *J Clin Oncol* 2001;19(2):376–388.
50. Folkman J. The role of angiogenesis in tumor growth. *Semin Cancer Biol* 1992;3(2):65–71.
51. Folkman J. Angiogenesis and angiogenesis inhibition: an overview. *EXS* 1997;79:1–8.
52. Magrath IT. Prospects for the therapeutic use of antisense oligonucleotides in malignant lymphomas. *Ann Oncol* 1994;5(Suppl 1):67–70.
53. Cotter FE. Antisense therapy for B cell lymphomas. *Cancer Surv* 1997;30:311–325.
54. Bonadonna G, Zucali R, Monfardini S, et al. Combination chemotherapy of Hodgkin's disease with Adriamycin, bleomycin, vinblastine, and imidazole carboxamide versus MOPP. *Cancer* 1975;36(1):252–259.
55. Klimo P, Connors JM. MOPP/ABV hybrid program: combination chemotherapy based on early introduction of seven effective drugs for advanced Hodgkin's disease. *J Clin Oncol* 1985;3(9):1174–1182.
56. Viviani S, Santoro A, Ragni G, et al. Gonadal toxicity after combination chemotherapy for Hodgkin's disease. Comparative results of MOPP vs ABVD. *Eur J Cancer Clin Oncol* 1985;21(5):601–605.
57. Valagussa P, Santoro A, Fossati-Bellani F, et al. Second acute leukemia and other malignancies following treatment for Hodgkin's disease. *J Clin Oncol* 1986;4(6):830–837.
58. Valagussa P, Bonadonna G. Hodgkin's disease and the risk of acute leukemia in successfully treated patients. *Haematologica* 1998;83(9):769–770.
59. Colvin M, Chabner BA. Alkylating agents. In: Chabner BA, Collins JM, eds. *Cancer Chemotherapy: Principles and Practice*. Philadelphia: J. B. Lippincott, 1990:276–313.
60. Andriole GL, Sandlund JT, Miser JS, et al. The efficacy of mesna (2-mercaptoethane sodium sulfonate) as a uroprotectant in patients with hemorrhagic cystitis receiving further oxazaphosphorine chemotherapy. *J Clin Oncol* 1987;5(5):799–803.
61. Goldenberg GJ, Vanstone CL, Israels LG, et al. Evidence for a transport carrier of nitrogen mustard in nitrogen mustard-sensitive and -resistant L5178Y lymphoblasts. *Cancer Res* 1970;30:2285–2291.
62. Rosenberg SA. Karnofsky memorial lecture. The low-grade non-Hodgkin's lymphomas: challenges and opportunities. *J Clin Oncol* 1985;3(3):299–310.
63. Lister TA, Cullen MH, Beard ME, et al. Comparison of combined and single-agent chemotherapy in non-Hodgkin's lymphoma of favourable histological type. *BMJ* 1978;1(6112):533–537.
64. Kennedy BJ, Bloomfield CD, Kiang DT, et al. Combination versus successive single agent chemotherapy in lymphocytic lymphoma. *Cancer* 1978;41(1):23–28.
65. Portlock CS, Rosenberg SA, Glatstein E, et al. Treatment of advanced non-Hodgkin's lymphomas with favorable histologies: preliminary results of a prospective trial. *Blood* 1976;47(5):747–756.
66. Dighiero G. Randomized trials: what do they teach us about chronic lymphocytic leukemia treatment. In: Cheson BD, ed. *Chronic Lymphoid Leukemia*. New York: Marcel Dekker, Inc., 2001:161–174.
67. Moskowitz CH, Bertino JR, Glassman JR, et al. Ifosfamide, carboplatin, and etoposide: a highly effective cytoreduction and peripheral-blood progenitor-cell mobilization regimen for transplant-eligible patients with non-Hodgkin's lymphoma. *J Clin Oncol* 1999;17(12):3776–3785.
68. Cabanillas F, Hagemeister FB, McLaughlin P, et al. Results of MIME salvage regimen for recurrent or refractory lymphoma. *J Clin Oncol* 1987;5(3):407–412.
69. Bloomfield CD, Pajak TF, Glicksman AS, et al. Chemotherapy and combined modality therapy for Hodgkin's disease: a progress report on Cancer and Leukemia Group B studies. *Cancer Treat Rep* 1982;66(4):835–846.
70. Miller DG. Alkylating agents and human spermatogenesis. *JAMA* 1971;217(12):1662–1665.
71. Richter P, Calamera JC, Morgenfeld MC, et al. Effect of chlorambucil on spermatogenesis in the human with malignant lymphoma. *Cancer* 1970;25(5):1026–1030.
72. Kumar R, Biggart JD, McEvoy J, et al. Cyclophosphamide and reproductive function. *Lancet* 1972;1(7762):1212–1214.
73. Koyama H, Wada T, Nishizawa Y, et al. Cyclophosphamide-induced ovarian failure and its therapeutic significance in patients with breast cancer. *Cancer* 1977;39(4):1403–1409.
74. Rose DP, Davis TE. Ovarian function in patients receiving adjuvant chemotherapy for breast cancer. *Lancet* 1977;1(8023):1174–1176.
75. Henry-Amar M. Second cancer after the treatment for Hodgkin's disease: a report from the International Database on Hodgkin's Disease. *Ann Oncol* 1992;3(Suppl 4):117–128.
76. Swerdlow AJ, Douglas AJ, Hudson GV, et al. Risk of second primary cancers after Hodgkin's disease by type of treatment: analysis of 2846 patients in the British National Lymphoma Investigation. *BMJ* 1992;304(6835):1137–1143.
77. van Leeuwen FE, Swerdlow AJ, Valagussa P, et al. Second cancers after treatment of Hodgkin's disease. In: Mauch PM, Armitage JO, Diehl V, et al., eds. *Hodgkin's Disease*. Philadelphia: Lippincott Williams & Wilkins, 1999:607–632.
78. Ng AK, Bernardo ME, Weller E, et al. Long-term survival and competing causes of death in patients with early-stage Hodgkin's disease treated at age 50 or younger. *J Clin Oncol* 2002;20(8):2101–2108.
79. Biti G, Cellai E, Magrini SM, et al. Second solid tumors and leukemia after treatment for Hodgkin's disease: an analysis of 1121 patients from a single institution. *Int J Radiat Oncol Biol Phys* 1994;29(1):25–31.
80. Pryzant RM, Meistrich ML, Wilson G, et al. Long-term reduction in sperm count after chemotherapy with and without radiation therapy for non-Hodgkin's lymphomas. *J Clin Oncol* 1993;11(2):239–247.
81. Waxman JH, Terry YA, Wrigley PF, et al. Gonadal function in Hodgkin's disease: long-term follow-up of chemotherapy. *BMJ (Clin Res Ed)* 1982;285(6355):1612–1613.
82. Horning SJ, Hoppe RT, Kaplan HS, et al. Female reproductive potential after treatment for Hodgkin's disease. *N Engl J Med* 1981;304(23):1377–1382.
83. Lippman ME, Yarbro GK, Leventhal BG. Clinical implications of glucocorticoid receptors in human leukemia. *Cancer Res* 1978;38(11 Pt 2):4251–4256.
84. Claman HN. Corticosteroids and lymphoid cells. *N Engl J Med* 1972;287(8):388–397.
85. Lippman M. Clinical implications of glucocorticoid receptors in human leukemia. *Am J Physiol* 1982;243(2):E103–E108.
86. Swain SM, Lippman ME. Endocrine therapies of cancer. In: Chabner BA, Collins JM, eds. *Cancer Chemotherapy: Principles and Practice*. Philadelphia: J. B. Lippincott, 1990:59–109.
87. Dale DC, Petersdorf RG. Corticosteroids and infectious diseases. *Med Clin North Am* 1973;57(5):1277–1287.
88. Hersh EV, Gutterman JU, Mavligit GM. Effect of haematological malignancies and their treatment on host defense factors. *Clin Haematol* 1976;5(2):425–448.
89. O'Brien S, Kantarjian H, Beran M, et al. Results of fludarabine and prednisone therapy in 264 patients with chronic lymphocytic leukemia with multivariate analysis-derived prognostic model for response to treatment. *Blood* 1993;82(6):1695–1700.
90. Betticher DC, Fey MF, von Rohr A, et al. High incidence of infections after 2-chlorodeoxyadenosine (2-CDA) therapy in patients with malignant lymphomas and chronic and acute leukaemias. *Ann Oncol* 1994;5(1):57–64.
91. Chabner B. Cytidine analogues. In: Chabner B, Longo DL, eds. *Cancer Chemotherapy and Biotherapy: Principles and Practice*. Philadelphia: Lippincott-Raven, 1996:213–260.
92. Stoller RG, Hande KR, Jacobs SA, et al. Use of plasma pharmacokinetics to predict and prevent methotrexate toxicity. *N Engl J Med* 1977;297(12):630–634.
93. Jerkeman M, Anderson H, Cavallin-Stahl E, et al. CHOP versus MACOP-B in aggressive lymphoma—a Nordic Lymphoma Group randomised trial. *Ann Oncol* 1999;10(9):1079–1086.
94. Sertoli MR, Santini G, Chisesi T, et al. MACOP-B versus ProMACE-MOPP in the treatment of advanced diffuse non-Hodgkin's lymphoma: results of a prospective randomized trial by the non-Hodgkin's Lymphoma Cooperative Study Group. *J Clin Oncol* 1994;12(7):1366–1374.
95. Cooper IA, Wolf MM, Robertson TI, et al. Randomized comparison of MACOP-B with CHOP in patients with intermediate-grade non-Hodgkin's lymphoma. The Australian and New Zealand Lymphoma Group. *J Clin Oncol* 1994;12(4):769–778.

96. Wolf M, Matthews JP, Stone J, et al. Long-term survival advantage of MACOP-B over CHOP in intermediate-grade non-Hodgkin's lymphoma. The Australian and New Zealand Lymphoma Group. *Ann Oncol* 1997;8(Suppl 1):71–75.

97. Sullivan MP, Ramirez I. Curability of Burkitt's lymphoma with high-dose cyclophosphamide-high-dose methotrexate therapy and intrathecal chemoprophylaxis. *J Clin Oncol* 1985;3(5):627–636.

98. McMaster ML, Greer JP, Greco FA, et al. Effective treatment of small-noncleaved-cell lymphoma with high-intensity, brief-duration chemotherapy. *J Clin Oncol* 1991;9(6):941–946.

99. Magrath I, Adde M, Shad A, et al. Adults and children with small noncleaved-cell lymphoma have a similar excellent outcome when treated with the same chemotherapy regimen. *J Clin Oncol* 1996;14(3):925–934.

100. Glass J, Gruber ML, Cher L, et al. Preirradiation methotrexate chemotherapy of primary central nervous system lymphoma: long-term outcome. *J Neurosurg* 1994;81(2):188–195.

101. Glantz MJ, Cole BF, Recht L, et al. High-dose intravenous methotrexate for patients with nonleukemic leptomeningeal cancer: is intrathecal chemotherapy necessary? *J Clin Oncol* 1998;16(4):1561–1567.

102. Velasquez WS, Cabanillas F, Salvador P, et al. Effective salvage therapy for lymphoma with cisplatin in combination with high-dose Ara-C and dexamethasone (DHAP). *Blood* 1988;71(1):117–122.

103. Machover D, Delmas-Marsalet B, Misra SC, et al. Dexamethasone, high-dose cytarabine, and oxaliplatin (DHAOx) as salvage treatment for patients with initially refractory or relapsed non-Hodgkin's lymphoma. *Ann Oncol* 2001;12(10):1439–1443.

104. Longo DL, DeVita VT Jr, Duffey PL, et al. Superiority of ProMACE-CytaBOM over ProMACE-MOPP in the treatment of advanced diffuse aggressive lymphoma: results of a prospective randomized trial. *J Clin Oncol* 1991;9(1):25–38.

105. Fisher RI, Gaynor ER, Dahlberg S, et al. A phase III comparison of CHOP vs. m-BACOD vs. ProMACE-CytaBOM vs. MACOP-B in patients with intermediate- or high-grade non-Hodgkin's lymphoma: results of SWOG-8516 (Intergroup 0067), the National High-Priority Lymphoma Study. *Ann Oncol* 1994;5(Suppl 2):91–95.

106. Federico M, Moretti G, Gobbi PG, et al. ProMACE-CytaBOM versus MACOP-B in intermediate and high grade NHL. Preliminary results of a prospective randomized trial. *Leukemia* 1991;5(Suppl 1):95–101.

107. Montserrat E, Garcia-Conde J, Vinolas N, et al. CHOP vs. ProMACE-CytaBOM in the treatment of aggressive non-Hodgkin's lymphomas: long-term results of a multicenter randomized trial. (PETHEMA: Spanish Cooperative Group for the Study of Hematological Malignancies Treatment, Spanish Society of Hematology). *Eur J Haematol* 1996; 57(5): 377–383.

108. Himes RH. Interactions of the catharanthus (Vinca) alkaloids with tubulin and microtubules. *Pharmacol Ther* 1991;51(2):257–267.

109. Rule S, Tighe M, Davies S, et al. Vinorelbine in the treatment of lymphoma. *Hematol Oncol* 1998;16(3):101–105.

110. Balzarotti M, Santoro A, Tondini C, et al. Activity of single agent vinorelbine in pretreated non-Hodgkin's lymphoma. *Ann Oncol* 1996;7 (9):970–972.

111. Sarris AH, Hagemeister F, Romaguera J, et al. Liposomal vincristine in relapsed non-Hodgkin's lymphomas: early results of an ongoing phase II trial. *Ann Oncol* 2000;11(1):69–72.

112. McKelvey EM, Gottlieb JA, Wilson HE, et al. Hydroxyldaunomycin (Adriamycin) combination chemotherapy in malignant lymphoma. *Cancer* 1976;38(4):1484–1493.

113. Steward WP, Crowther D, McWilliam LJ, et al. Maintenance chlorambucil after CVP in the management of advanced stage, low-grade histologic type non-Hodgkin's lymphoma. A randomized prospective study with an assessment of prognostic factors. *Cancer* 1988;61(3):441–447.

114. Hoogstraten B, Owens AH, Lenhard RE, et al. Combination chemotherapy in lymphosarcoma and reticulum cell sarcoma. *Blood* 1969;33(2):370–378.

115. Zunino F, Di Marco A, Zaccara A, et al. The interaction of daunorubicin and doxorubicin with DNA and chromatin. *Biochim Biophys Acta* 1980;607(2):206–214.

116. Zunino F, Gambetta R, Di Marco A, et al. A comparison of the effects of daunomycin and adriamycin on various DNA polymerases. *Cancer Res* 1975;35(3):754–760.

117. Bachur NR, Gordon SL, Gee MV. A general mechanism for microsomal activation of quinone anticancer agents to free radicals. *Cancer Res* 1978;38(6):1745–1750.

118. Alexander J, Dainiak N, Berger HJ, et al. Serial assessment of doxorubicin cardiotoxicity with quantitative radionuclide angiocardiography. *N Engl J Med* 1979;300(6):278–283.

119. Billingham ME, Bristow MR, Glatstein E, et al. Adriamycin cardiotoxicity: endomyocardial biopsy evidence of enhancement by irradiation. *Am J Surg Pathol* 1977;1(1):17–23.

120. Bristow MR, Billingham ME, Mason JW, et al. Clinical spectrum of anthracycline antibiotic cardiotoxicity. *Cancer Treat Rep* 1978;62(6): 873–879.

121. Guglielmi C, Gherlinzoni F, Amadori S, et al. A phase III comparative trial of m-BACOD vs m-BNCOD in the treatment of stage II-IV diffuse non-Hodgkin's lymphomas. *Haematologica* 1989;74(6):563–569.

122. Hollingshead LM, Faulds D. Idarubicin. A review of its pharmacodynamic and pharmacokinetic properties, and therapeutic potential in the chemotherapy of cancer. *Drugs* 1991;42(4):690–719.

123. Pavlovsky S, Santarelli MT, Erazo A, et al. Results of a randomized study of previously-untreated intermediate and high grade lymphoma using CHOP versus CNOP. *Ann Oncol* 1992;3(3):205–209.

124. Sonneveld P, de Ridder M, van der Lelie H, et al. Comparison of doxorubicin and mitoxantrone in the treatment of elderly patients with advanced diffuse non-Hodgkin's lymphoma using CHOP versus CNOP chemotherapy. *J Clin Oncol* 1995;13(10):2530–2539.

125. Loike JD, Horwitz SB. Effect of VP-16-213 on the intracellular degradation of DNA in HeLa cells. *Biochemistry* 1976;15(25):5443–5448.

126. Chen GL, Yang L, Rowe TC, et al. Nonintercalative antitumor drugs interfere with the breakage-reunion reaction of mammalian DNA topoisomerase II. *J Biol Chem* 1984;259(21):13560–13566.

127. Minocha A, Long BH. Inhibition of the DNA catenation activity of type II topoisomerase by VP16-213 and VM26. *Biochem Biophys Res Commun* 1984;122(1):165–170.

128. Ross W, Rowe T, Glisson B, et al. Role of topoisomerase II in mediating epipodophyllotoxin-induced DNA cleavage. *Cancer Res* 1984;44 (12 Pt 1):5857–5860.

129. Arnold AM, Whitehouse JM. Interaction of VP16-213 with the DNA repair antagonist chloroquine. *Cancer Chemother Pharmacol* 1982;7 (2–3):123–126.

130. Blume KG, Forman SJ, O'Donnell MR, et al. Total body irradiation and high-dose etoposide: a new preparatory regimen for bone marrow transplantation in patients with advanced hematologic malignancies. *Blood* 1987;69(4):1015–1020.

131. O'Donnell MR, Forman SJ, Levine AM, et al. Cytarabine, cisplatin, and etoposide chemotherapy for refractory non-Hodgkin's lymphoma. *Cancer Treat Rep* 1987;71(2):187–189.

132. Wheeler C, Antin JH, Churchill WH, et al. Cyclophosphamide, carmustine, and etoposide with autologous bone marrow transplantation in refractory Hodgkin's disease and non-Hodgkin's lymphoma: a dose-finding study. *J Clin Oncol* 1990;8(4):648–656.

133. Kessinger A, Bierman PJ, Vose JM, et al. High-dose cyclophosphamide, carmustine, and etoposide followed by autologous peripheral stem cell transplantation for patients with relapsed Hodgkin's disease. *Blood* 1991;77(11):2322–2325.

134. Crilley P, Lazarus H, Topolsky D, et al. Comparison of preparative transplantation regimens using carmustine/etoposide/cisplatin or busulfan/etoposide/cyclophosphamide in lymphoid malignancies. *Semin Oncol* 1993;20[4 Suppl 4]:50–54; quiz 55.

135. Nichols CR, Breeden ES, Loehrer PJ, et al. Secondary leukemia associated with a conventional dose of etoposide: review of serial germ cell tumor protocols. *J Natl Cancer Inst* 1993;85(1):36–40.

136. Bokemeyer C, Schmoll HJ, Kuczyk MA, et al. Risk of secondary leukemia following high cumulative doses of etoposide during chemotherapy for testicular cancer. *J Natl Cancer Inst* 1995;87(1):58–60.

137. Katato K, Flaherty L, Varterasian M. Secondary acute myelogenous leukemia following treatment with oral etoposide. *Am J Hematol* 1996;53(1):54–55.

138. O'Reilly SE, Hoskins P, Klimo P, et al. MACOP-B and VACOP-B in diffuse large cell lymphomas and MOPP/ABV in Hodgkin's disease. *Ann Oncol* 1991;2[Suppl 1]:17–23.

139. Celsing F, Widell S, Merk K, et al. Addition of etoposide to CHOP chemotherapy in untreated patients with high-grade non-Hodgkin's lymphoma. *Ann Oncol* 1998;9(11):1213–1217.

140. Fisher RI, Longo DL, DeVita VT Jr, et al. Long-term follow-up of ProMACE-CytaBOM in non-Hodgkin's lymphomas. *Ann Oncol* 1991;2[Suppl 1]:33–35.

141. Miller TP, Dahlberg S, Weick JK, et al. Unfavorable histologies of non-Hodgkin's lymphoma treated with ProMACE-CytaBOM: a groupwide Southwest Oncology Group study. *J Clin Oncol* 1990;8(12):1951–1958.

142. Pfreundschuh MG, Trumper L, Kloess M, et al. CHOEP (CHOP + etoposide): The new standard regimen for younger patients with low risk (low LDH) aggressive non-Hodgkin's lymphoma. *Blood* 2001;98:725a (abstract 3026).

143. Chopra R, Linch DC, McMillan AK, et al. Mini-BEAM followed by BEAM and ABMT for very poor risk Hodgkin's disease. *Br J Haematol* 1992;81(2):197–202.

144. Chopra R, McMillan AK, Linch DC, et al. The place of high-dose BEAM therapy and autologous bone marrow transplantation in poorrisk Hodgkin's disease. A single-center eight-year study of 155 patients. *Blood* 1993;81(5):1137–1145.

145. Hainsworth JD, Johnson DH, Frazier SR, et al. Chronic daily administration of oral etoposide in refractory lymphoma. *Eur J Cancer* 1990;26(7):818–821.

146. Greco FA. Oral etoposide in lymphoma. *Drugs* 1999;58(Suppl 3):35–41.

147. Krivit W, Brubaker C, Hartmann J, et al. Induction of remission in acute leukemia of childhood by combination of prednisone and either 6-mercaptopurine or methotrexate. *J Pediatr* 1966;68(6):965–968.

148. Sitarz AL, Brubaker C, Hartman J, et al. Induction of remission in childhood leukemia with vincristine and 6-mercaptopurine and methotrexate. Administration in sequence after prednisone. *Cancer* 1968;21(5):920–925.

149. Nelson JA, Carpenter JW, Rose LM, et al. Mechanisms of action of 6-thioguanine, 6-mercaptopurine, and 8-azaguanine. *Cancer Res* 1975;35(10):2872–2878.

150. Brockman RW, Schabel FM Jr, Montgomery JA. Biologic activity of 9-beta-D-arabinofuranosyl-2-fluoroadenine, a metabolically stable analog of 9-beta-D-arabinofuranosyladenine. *Biochem Pharmacol* 1977;26(22):2193–2196.

151. Brockman RW, Cheng YC, Schabel FM Jr, et al. Metabolism and chemotherapeutic activity of 9-beta-D-arabinofuranosyl-2-fluoroadenine against murine leukemia L1210 and evidence for its phosphorylation by deoxycytidine kinase. *Cancer Res* 1980;40(10):3610–3615.

152. Seto S, Carrera CJ, Kubota M, et al. Mechanism of deoxyadenosine and 2-chlorodeoxyadenosine toxicity to nondividing human lymphocytes. *J Clin Invest* 1985;75(2):377–383.

153. O'Dwyer PJ, Wagner B, Leyland-Jones B, et al. 2'-Deoxycoformycin (pentostatin) for lymphoid malignancies. Rational development of an active new drug. *Ann Intern Med* 1988;108(5):733–743.

154. Cheson BD, Vena DA, Foss FM, et al. Neurotoxicity of purine analogs: a review. *J Clin Oncol* 1994;12(10):2216–2228.

155. Cheson BD. Infectious and immunosuppressive complications of purine analog therapy. *J Clin Oncol* 1995;13(9):2431–2448.

156. Hoffman MA. Cladribine for the treatment of indolent non-Hodgkin's lymphomas. *Semin Hematol* 1996;33(1 Suppl 1):40–44.

157. Foran JM, Rohatiner AZ, Coiffier B, et al. Multicenter phase II study of fludarabine phosphate for patients with newly diagnosed lymphoplasmacytoid lymphoma, Waldenstrom's macroglobulinemia, and mantle-cell lymphoma. *J Clin Oncol* 1999;17(2):546–553.

158. Leblond V, Ben-Othman T, Deconinck E, et al. Activity of fludarabine in previously treated Waldenstrom's macroglobulinemia: a report of 71 cases. Groupe Cooperatif Macroglobulinemie. *J Clin Oncol* 1998;16(6):2060–2064.

159. Kantarjian HM, Alexanian R, Koller CA, et al. Fludarabine therapy in macroglobulinemic lymphoma. *Blood* 1990;75(10):1928–1931.

160. Solal-Celigny P, Brice P, Brousse N, et al. Phase II trial of fludarabine monophosphate as first-line treatment in patients with advanced follicular lymphoma: a multicenter study by the Groupe d'Etude des Lymphomes de l'Adulte. *J Clin Oncol* 1996;14(2):514–519.

161. Hagenbeek A, et al. Fludarabine vs conventional CVP in newly diagnosed patients with stage III or IV low grade non-Hodgkin's lymphoma. Preliminary results from a prospective randomized clinical trial in 381 patients. *Blood* 1998;92:315a(abstract 1294).

162. McLaughlin P, Hagemeister FB, Romaguera JE, et al. Fludarabine, mitoxantrone, and dexamethasone: an effective new regimen for indolent lymphoma. *J Clin Oncol* 1996;14(4):1262–1268.

163. Brugiatelli M, Holowiecka B, Dmoszynska A, et al. 2-Chlorodeoxyadenosine treatment in non-Hodgkin's lymphoma and B-cell chronic lymphocytic leukemia resistant to conventional chemotherapy: results of a multicentric experience. International Society for Chemo-Immunotherapy. *Ann Hematol* 1996;73(2):79–84.

164. Saven A, Burian C, Koziol JA, et al. Long-term follow-up of patients with hairy cell leukemia after cladribine treatment. *Blood* 1998;92(6):1918–1926.

165. Piro LD, Carrera CJ, Carson DA, et al. Lasting remissions in hairy cell leukemia induced by a single infusion of 2-chlorodeoxyadenosine. *N Engl J Med* 1990;322(16):1117–1121.

166. Boogaerts MA, Van Hoof A, Catovsky D, et al. Activity of oral fludarabine phosphate in previously treated chronic lymphocytic leukemia. *J Clin Oncol* 2001;19(22):4252–4258.

167. Johnson S, Smith AG, Loffler H, et al. Multicentre prospective randomised trial of fludarabine versus cyclophosphamide, doxorubicin, and prednisone (CAP) for treatment of advanced-stage chronic lymphocytic leukemia. The French Cooperative Group on CLL. *Lancet* 1996;347(9013):1432–1438.

168. Rai KR, Peterson BL, Appelbaum FR, et al. Fludarabine compared with chlorambucil as primary therapy for chronic lymphocytic leukemia. *N Engl J Med* 2000;343(24):1750–1757.

169. O'Brien S, del Giglio A, Keating M. Advances in the biology and treatment of B-cell chronic lymphocytic leukemia. *Blood* 1995;85(2):307–318.

170. Seymour JF, Grigg AP, Szer J, et al. Fludarabine and mitoxantrone: effective and well-tolerated salvage therapy in relapsed indolent lymphoproliferative disorders. *Ann Oncol* 2001;12(10):1455–1460.

171. Khouri IF, Keating M, Korbling M, et al. Transplant-lite: induction of graft-versus-malignancy using fludarabine-based nonablative chemotherapy and allogeneic blood progenitor-cell transplantation as treatment for lymphoid malignancies. *J Clin Oncol* 1998;16(8):2817–2824.

172. Velasquez WS, McLaughlin P, Tucker S, et al. ESHAP—an effective chemotherapy regimen in refractory and relapsing lymphoma: a 4-year follow-up study. *J Clin Oncol* 1994;12(6):1169–1176.

173. Harder HC, Rosenberg B. Inhibitory effects of anti-tumor platinum compounds on DNA, RNA and protein syntheses in mammalian cells in vitro. *Int J Cancer* 1970;6(2):207–216.

174. Loehrer PJ, Einhorn LH. Drugs five years later. Cisplatin. *Ann Intern Med* 1984;100(5):704–713.

175. Evans BD, Raju KS, Calvert AH, et al. Phase II study of JM8, a new platinum analog, in advanced ovarian carcinoma. *Cancer Treat Rep* 1983;67(11):997–1000.

176. Reed JC, Kitada S, Kim Y, et al. Modulating apoptosis pathways in low-grade B-cell malignancies using biological response modifiers. *Semin Oncol* 2002;29(1 Suppl 2):10–24.

177. Byrd JC, Kitada S, Flinn IW, et al. The mechanism of tumor cell clearance by rituximab in vivo in patients with B-cell chronic lymphocytic leukemia: evidence of caspase activation and apoptosis induction. *Blood* 2002;99(3):1038–1043.

178. LoBuglio AF, Saleh MN. Monoclonal antibody therapy of cancer. *Crit Rev Oncol Hematol* 1992;13(3):271–282.

179. Byrd JC, Waselenko JK, Maneatis TJ, et al. Rituximab therapy in hematologic malignancy patients with circulating blood tumor cells: association with increased infusion-related side effects and rapid blood tumor clearance. *J Clin Oncol* 1999;17(3):791–795.

180. Maloney DG, Grillo-Lopez AJ, White CA, et al. IDEC-C2B8 (rituximab) anti-CD20 monoclonal antibody therapy in patients with relapsed low-grade non-Hodgkin's lymphoma. *Blood* 1997;90(6):2188–2195.

181. McLaughlin P, Grillo-Lopez AJ, Link BK, et al. Rituximab chimeric anti-CD20 monoclonal antibody therapy for relapsed indolent lymphoma: half of patients respond to a four-dose treatment program. *J Clin Oncol* 1998;16(8):2825–2833.

182. Keating MJ, Flinn I, Jain V, et al. Therapeutic role of alemtuzumab (Campath-1H) in patients who have failed fludarabine: results of a large international study. *Blood* 2002;99(10):3554–3561.

183. Coiffier B, Lepage E, Briere J, et al. CHOP chemotherapy plus rituximab compared with CHOP alone in elderly patients with diffuse large-B-cell lymphoma. *N Engl J Med* 2002;346(4):235–242.

184. Smith MR, Abubakr Y, Mohammad R, et al. Antisense oligodeoxyribonucleotide down-regulation of bcl-2 gene expression inhibits growth of the low-grade non-Hodgkin's lymphoma cell line WSU-FSCCL. *Cancer Gene Ther* 1995;2(3):207–212.

185. Webb A, Cunningham D, Cotter F, et al. BCL-2 antisense therapy in patients with non-Hodgkin lymphoma. *Lancet* 1997;349(9059):1137–1141.

186. Wickstrom E. Antisense c-myc inhibition of lymphoma growth. *Antisense Nucleic Acid Drug Dev* 1997;7(3):225–228.

187. Bishop MR, Iversen PL, Bayever E, et al. Phase I trial of an antisense oligonucleotide OL(1)p53 in hematologic malignancies. *J Clin Oncol* 1996;14(4):1320–1326.

188. Gascoyne RD, Adomat SA, Krajewski S, et al. Prognostic significance of Bcl-2 protein expression and Bcl-2 gene rearrangement in diffuse aggressive non-Hodgkin's lymphoma. *Blood* 1997;90(1):244–251.

189. Sugiyama K, Omachi K, Fujiwara K, et al. Irinotecan hydrochloride for the treatment of recurrent and refractory non-Hodgkin lymphoma: a single institution experience. *Cancer* 2002;94(3):594–600.

190. Kraut EH, Balcerzak SP, Young D, et al. A phase II study of topotecan in non-Hodgkin's lymphoma: an Ohio State University phase II research consortium study. *Cancer Invest* 2002;20(2):174–179.

191. Sarris AH, Romaguera J, Hagemeister FB, et al. Irinotecan in relapsed or refractory non-Hodgkin's lymphoma. *Oncology (Huntingt)* 2001;15(7 Suppl 8):53–56.

192. Cabanillas F. The role of topoisomerase-I inhibitors in the treatment of non-Hodgkin's lymphoma. *Semin Hematol* 1999;36(4 Suppl 8):11–15.

193. Younes A. Paclitaxel for the treatment of lymphoma. *J Clin Oncol* 1998;16(6):2289–2290.

194. Miller TP, Chase EM, Dorr R, et al. A phase I/II trial of paclitaxel for non-Hodgkin's lymphoma followed by paclitaxel plus quinine in drug-resistant disease. *Anticancer Drugs* 1998;9(2):135–140.

195. Younes A, Ayoub JP, Sarris A, et al. Paclitaxel activity for the treatment of non-Hodgkin's lymphoma: final report of a phase II trial. *Br J Haematol* 1997;96(2):328–332.

196. Hopfinger G, Heinz R, Pfeilstöcker M, et al. Paclitaxel in the salvage treatment of Hodgkin's disease and non-Hodgkin's lymphoma. *Ann Oncol* 1996;7(4):423–424.

197. Blum RH, Carter SK, Agre K. A clinical review of bleomycin—a new antineoplastic agent. *Cancer* 1973;31(4):903–914.

198. Umezawa H, Maeda K, Takeuchi T, et al. New antibiotics, bleomycin A and B. J *Antibiot (Tokyo)* 1966;19(5):200–209.

199. Lubin A. CHOP-Bleo in advanced non-Hodgkin malignant lymphoma. *Blood* 1977;50(5):962–963.

200. Case DC Jr. Combination chemotherapy of advanced, diffuse, non-Hodgkin's lymphoma: results with cyclo-phosphamide, adriamycin, vincristine, prednisone, and bleomycin (CHOP-Bleo). *J Maine Med Assoc* 1979;70(9):348–350, 352, 368.

201. Lee R, Cabanillas F, Bodey GP, et al. A 10-year update of CHOP-Bleo in the treatment of diffuse large-cell lymphoma. *J Clin Oncol* 1986;4(10):1455–1461.

202. Klimo P, Connors JM. MACOP-B chemotherapy for the treatment of diffuse large-cell lymphoma. *Ann Intern Med* 1985;102(5):596–602.

203. Connors JM, Klimo P. MACOP-B chemotherapy for malignant lymphomas and related conditions: 1987 update and additional observations. *Semin Hematol* 1988;25[2 Suppl 2]:41–46.

204. Dana BW, Dahlberg S, Miller TP, et al. m-BACOD treatment for intermediate- and high-grade malignant lymphomas: a Southwest Oncology Group phase II trial. *J Clin Oncol* 1990;8(7):1155–1162.

205. Shipp MA, Yeap BY, Harrington DP, et al. The m-BACOD combination chemotherapy regimen in large-cell lymphoma: analysis of the completed trial and comparison with the M-BACOD regimen. *J Clin Oncol* 1990;8(1):84–93.

206. Bergsagel DE, Sprague CC, Austin C, et al. Evaluation of new chemotherapeutic agents in the treatment of multiple myeloma. IV. L-phenylalanine mustard (NSC-8806). *Cancer Chemotherapy Rep* 1962;21:87–99.

207. Myeloma Trialists' Collaborative Group. Combination chemotherapy versus melphalan plus prednisone as treatment for multiple myeloma: an overview of 6,633 patients from 27 randomized trials. Myeloma Trialists' Collaborative Group. *J Clin Oncol* 1998;16(12):3832–3842.

208. Brunner KW, Young CW. A methylhydrazine derivative in Hodgkin's disease and other malignant neoplasms. *Ann Intern Med* 1965;62:69–86.

209. Farber S, Diamond LK, Mercer RD, et al. Temporary remissions in acute leukemia in children produced by folic antagonist 4-amethopteroylglutamic acid (aminopterin). *N Engl J Med* 1948;238:787–798.

210. Schein PS, DeVita VT Jr, Hubbard S, et al. Bleomycin, adriamycin, cyclophosphamide, vincristine, and prednisone (BACOP) combination chemotherapy in the treatment of advanced diffuse histiocytic lymphoma. *Ann Intern Med* 1976;85(4):417–422.

211. Skarin AT, Rosenthal DS, Moloney WC, et al. Combination chemotherapy of advanced non-Hodgkin lymphoma with bleomycin, adriamycin, cyclophosphamide, vincristine, and prednisone (BACOP). *Blood* 1977;49(5):759–770.

212. Elias L, Portlock CS, Rosenberg SA. Combination chemotherapy of diffuse histiocytic lymphoma with cyclophosphamide, adriamycin, vincristine and prednisone (CHOP). *Cancer* 1978;42(4):1705–1710.

213. Armitage JO, Corder MP, Leimert JT, et al. Advanced diffuse histiocytic lymphoma treated with cyclophosphamide, doxorubicin, vincristine, and prednisone (CHOP) without maintenance therapy. *Cancer Treat Rep* 1980;64(4–5):649–654.

214. Comella P, Abate G, Comella G, et al. Combination chemotherapy with cyclophosphamide, adriamycin, vincristine and prednisone (CHOP) for non-Hodgkin's lymphomas with unfavorable histology: preliminary results. *Tumori* 1980;66(6):749–756.

215. Philip T, Guglielmi C, Hagenbeek A, et al. Autologous bone marrow transplantation as compared with salvage chemotherapy in relapses of chemotherapy-sensitive non-Hodgkin's lymphoma. *N Engl J Med* 1995;333(23):1540–1545.

216. Gianni AM, Bregni M, Siena S, et al. High-dose chemotherapy and autologous bone marrow transplantation compared with MACOP-B in aggressive B-cell lymphoma. *N Engl J Med* 1997;336(18):1290–1297.

217. Haioun C, Lepage E, Gisselbrecht C, et al. Benefit of autologous bone marrow transplantation over sequential chemotherapy in poor-risk aggressive non-Hodgkin's lymphoma: updated results of the prospective study LNH87-2. Groupe d'Etude des Lymphomes de l'Adulte. *J Clin Oncol* 1997;15(3):1131–1137.

218. Haioun C, Lepage E, Gisselbrecht C, et al. Comparison of autologous bone marrow transplantation with sequential chemotherapy for intermediate-grade and high-grade non-Hodgkin's lymphoma in first complete remission: a study of 464 patients. Groupe d'Etude des Lymphomes de l'Adulte. *J Clin Oncol* 1994;12(12):2543–2551.

219. Santini G, Salvagno L, Leoni P, et al. VACOP-B versus VACOP-B plus autologous bone marrow transplantation for advanced diffuse non-Hodgkin's lymphoma: results of a prospective randomized trial by the non-Hodgkin's Lymphoma Cooperative Study Group. *J Clin Oncol* 1998;16(8):2796–2802.

220. Verdonck LF, van Putten WL, Hagenbeek A, et al. Comparison of CHOP chemotherapy with autologous bone marrow transplantation for slowly responding patients with aggressive non-Hodgkin's lymphoma. *N Engl J Med* 1995;332(16):1045–1051.

221. Miller TP, Dahlberg S, Cassady JR, et al. Chemotherapy alone compared with chemotherapy plus radiotherapy for localized intermediate- and high-grade non-Hodgkin's lymphoma. *N Engl J Med* 1998;339(1):21–26.

222. Connors JM, Klimo P, Fairey RN, et al. Brief chemotherapy and involved field radiation therapy for limited-stage, histologically aggressive lymphoma. *Ann Intern Med* 1987;107(1):25–30.

223. Longo DL, Glatstein E, Duffey PL, et al. Treatment of localized aggressive lymphomas with combination chemotherapy followed by involved-field radiation therapy. *J Clin Oncol* 1989;7(9):1295–1302.

224. Tondini C, Zanini M, Lombardi F, et al. Combined modality treatment with primary CHOP chemotherapy followed by locoregional irradiation in stage I or II histologically aggressive non-Hodgkin's lymphomas. *J Clin Oncol* 1993;11(4):720–725.

225. Freilone R, Botto B, Vitolo U, et al. Combined modality treatment with a weekly brief chemotherapy (ACOP-B) followed by locoregional radiotherapy in localized-stage intermediate- to high-grade non-Hodgkin's lymphoma. *Ann Oncol* 1996;7(9):919–924.

226. Shenkier TN, Voss N, Fairey R, et al. Brief chemotherapy and involved-region irradiation for limited-stage diffuse large-cell lymphoma: an 18-year experience from the British Columbia Cancer Agency. *J Clin Oncol* 2002;20(1):197–204.

227. Gill KK, Klasa RJ, Hoskins PJ, et al. BP-VACOP and extensive lymph node irradiation (RT) in the treatment of advanced stage low grade non-Hodgkin's lymphoma (NHL) at diagnosis. *Blood* 2000;96:134a(abstract 579).

228. Wilder RB, Rodriguez MA, Tucker SL, et al. Radiation therapy after a partial response to CHOP chemotherapy for aggressive lymphomas. *Int J Radiat Oncol Biol Phys* 2001;50(3):743–749.

229. Behar RA, Hoppe RT. Radiation therapy in the management of bulky mediastinal Hodgkin's disease. *Cancer* 1990;66(1):75–79.

230. Fabian CJ, Mansfield CM, Dahlberg S, et al. Low-dose involved field radiation after chemotherapy in advanced Hodgkin disease. A Southwest Oncology Group randomized study. *Ann Intern Med* 1994;120(11):903–912.

231. Mauch P. What is the role for adjuvant radiation therapy in advanced Hodgkin's disease? *J Clin Oncol* 1998;16(3):815–817.

232. Yahalom J, Ryu J, Straus DJ, et al. Impact of adjuvant radiation on the patterns and rate of relapse in advanced-stage Hodgkin's disease treated with alternating chemotherapy combinations. *J Clin Oncol* 1991;9(12):2193–2201.

233. Zinzani PL, Zompatori M, Bendandi M, et al. Monitoring bulky mediastinal disease with gallium-67, CT-scan and magnetic resonance imaging in Hodgkin's disease and high-grade non-Hodgkin's lymphoma. *Leuk Lymphoma* 1996;22(1–2):131–135.

234. Zinzani PL, Magagnoli M, Chierichetti F, et al. The role of positron emission tomography (PET) in the management of lymphoma patients. *Ann Oncol* 1999;10(10):1181–1184.

235. Mikhaeel NG, Timothy AR, Hain SF, et al. 18-FDG-PET for the assessment of residual masses on CT following treatment of lymphomas. *Ann Oncol* 2000;11(Suppl 1):147–150.

236. Jerusalem G, Beguin Y, Fassotte MF, et al. Whole-body positron emission tomography using 18F-fluorodeoxyglucose for posttreatment evaluation in Hodgkin's disease and non-Hodgkin's lymphoma has higher diagnostic and prognostic value than classical computed tomography scan imaging. *Blood* 1999;94(2):429–433.

237. Spaepen K, Stroobants S, Dupont P, et al. Prognostic value of positron emission tomography (PET) with fluorine-18 fluorodeoxyglucose ([18F]FDG) after first-line chemotherapy in non-Hodgkin's lymphoma: is [18F]FDG-PET a valid alternative to conventional diagnostic methods? *J Clin Oncol* 2001;19(2):414–419.

238. Mikhaeel NG, Timothy AR, O'Doherty MJ, et al. 18-Fdg-PET as a prognostic indicator in the treatment of aggressive non-Hodgkin's lymphoma-comparison with CT. *Leuk Lymphoma* 2000;39(5–6):543–553.

239. Touroutoglou N, Dimopoulos MA, Younes A, et al. Testicular lymphoma: late relapses and poor outcome despite doxorubicin-based therapy. *J Clin Oncol* 1995;13(6):1361–1367.

240. Doll DC, Weiss RB. Malignant lymphoma of the testis. *Am J Med* 1986;81(3):515–524.

241. Tondini C, Ferreri AJ, Siracusano L, et al. Diffuse large-cell lymphoma of the testis. *J Clin Oncol* 1999;17(9):2854–2858.

242. Kiely JM, Massey BD Jr, Harrison EG Jr, et al. Lymphoma of the testis. *Cancer* 1970;26(4):847–852.

243. Connors JM, Klimo P, Voss N, et al. Testicular lymphoma: improved outcome with early brief chemotherapy. *J Clin Oncol* 1988;6(5):776–781.

CHAPTER 13

Biologic Therapy of Lymphoma

Kenneth A. Foon and Malek M. Safa

Lymphomas are very responsive to chemotherapy and radiation therapy. Many patients who do not respond or relapse after standard therapy can be treated by intensive therapy and stem cell transplantation. However, tumor cell resistance remains a problem, and the toxicity of chemotherapy and radiation therapy limits their potential. Important advances in molecular biology over the last decade have led to new, promising immunotherapies for the treatment of non-Hodgkin's lymphomas.

UNLABELED MONOCLONAL ANTIBODIES

Enthusiasm for antibodies as targeted therapy for cancer was rejuvenated by the hybridoma technology (1). Unlabeled monoclonal antibodies have been studied for their therapeutic potential since the early 1980s (2–12). They must bind to a receptor that mediates apoptosis (cell death) or must activate effector mechanisms, such as complement-mediated cytotoxicity and antibody-dependent cellular cytotoxicity. These murine monoclonal antibodies generate human anti-mouse antibody responses in most patients and are not very effective in activating human effector systems. To overcome these limitations, murine antibodies may be chimerized, humanized, or fully human.

Murine antibodies targeted to CD5, CD19, CD20, CD25, CD52, anti-HLA-DR, and antiidiotypes were used to treat T- and B-cell lymphomas. Responses ranging from 10% to 15% were typically transient, except for some unusually durable responses to antiidiotype antibodies. Immunoglobulin (Ig) contains two variable regions that serve as recognition sites for foreign antigens. These variable regions are formed by the rearrangement of germ-line Ig genes, and the genetic rearrangement allows for the diversity of human Igs. When B cells undergo malignant transformation, they create "clonal" populations of cells that express the same unique receptor, or "idiotype." Antibodies that target the idiotype are referred to as *antiidiotype* antibodies and represent a putative tumor-specific therapy. Forty-five patients with low-grade B-cell lymphoma were treated with 52 courses of antiidiotype antibodies that were tailor-made for each patient. The antiidio-

type antibody was infused alone or in combination with interferon alfa, chlorambucil, or interleukin-2 (IL-2); the response rate was 66%, and the complete-response rate was 18% (13–17). Many of these remissions were durable; however, some patients experienced recurrences with idiotype-negative tumors (18). These same investigators discovered that some idiotypes were "shared" between patients (19,20), so that all patients would not require a custom-tailored antibody; however, despite this finding, antiidiotype monoclonal antibody therapy has not been pursued.

Most current therapeutic studies with unlabeled monoclonal antibodies in lymphoma patients include humanized murine and chimeric human-murine antibodies (Table 13.1). They have the advantage of a human crystalizable fragment for complement-mediated cytotoxicity and antibody-dependent cellular cytotoxicity and are less immunogenic than are murine antibodies.

RITUXIMAB

CD20 does not shed, modulate, or internalize and is, therefore, an excellent target antigen for unlabeled antibody therapy. It may function as a calcium channel regulating a step in B-cell activation that is required for cell cycling and differentiation. Rituximab is a chimeric anti-CD20 antibody that was the first monoclonal antibody approved by the U.S. Food and Drug Administration (FDA) for the treatment of low-grade B-cell lymphoma patients who have not responded or have relapsed after standard therapy (21–24).

Low-Grade Follicular Lymphoma

In a multicenter phase II trial, 166 patients with previously treated low-grade lymphoma (follicular and small lymphocytic lymphoma) were treated with the standard dosing regimen of 375 mg per m² per week for 4 weeks. A 50% response rate was reported in assessable patients (181 total), with a median follow-up of 12 months. The projected median time to progression was 13 months (25) (Table 13.2). Toxicity included fever, chills, headache, asthenia, angioedema, and nausea, most com-

221

TABLE 13.1. *Therapeutic unlabeled antibodies*

Generic name (manufacturer)	Trade name	Species	Isotype	Antigen target	U.S. Food and Drug Administration approval
Rituximab (IDEC/Genentech)	Rituxan	Human-mouse (chimeric)	IgG1	CD20	Yes
Alemtuzumab (Millennium/ILEX)	Campath-1H	Human-rat (humanized)	IgG1	CD52	Yes
Epratuzumab (Immunomedics/Amgen)	LymdroCide	Human-mouse (humanized)	IgG1	CD22	No
Apolizumab (Protein Design Labs)	Remitogen	Human-mouse (humanized)	IgG1	HLA-DR-β chain	No

monly during the first infusion. Depletion of circulating B cells lasted for 3 to 6 months. Measurable levels of rituximab remained in the serum for several months after completion of therapy in most patients. Responses were predominantly in patients with follicular lymphoma (60%); the response rate was lower in patients with small lymphocytic lymphoma (13%). This might be related to the low antigen expression of CD20 on small lymphocytic lymphoma cells. Small lymphocytic lymphoma is also discussed below with chronic lymphocytic leukemia. Patients who had previously undergone high-dose chemotherapy followed by stem cell transplant demonstrated higher response rates (78%). In another study, 31 patients with previously treated bulky (larger than 10-cm lesion) low-grade lymphoma were treated with 4 weeks of 375-mg-per-m² rituximab. They reported a 43% response rate in assessable patients (28 total), with a median time to progression of 8.1 months (26). In another study (27), 30 patients with previously

TABLE 13.2. *Rituximab monotherapy for patients with lymphoma and chronic lymphocytic leukemia*

Disease	No. of patients	Prior therapy	Dose level of rituximab	No. of doses of rituximab	Complete response (%)	Any response (%)	Duration of response (mo)	Reference
Low-grade lymphoma	151	Yes	375 mg/m²	4	9 (6)	76 (50)	13	25
Bulky low-grade lymphoma	28	Yes	375 mg/m²	4	1 (4)	12 (43)	8.1	26
Follicular lymphoma	30	Yes	375 mg/m²	4	5 (17)	14 (47)	6.7	27
Low-grade lymphoma	60	No	375 mg/m²	4[a]	22 (37)	44 (73)	34	28,29
Follicular lymphoma	50	No	375 mg/m²	4	13 (26)	37 (73)	N/A	30
Low-grade lymphoma	37	Yes	375 mg/m²	8	5 (14)	22 (60)	19.4+	31
Follicular lymphoma	17	Yes	375 mg/m²	6	8 (47)	13 (76)	N/A	32
Aggressive lymphoma	54	Yes[b]	375 mg/m² / 500 mg/m²	8	5 (9)	17 (31)	8.2+	39
Chronic lymphocytic leukemia/small lymphocytic lymphoma	33	Yes	250 mg/m²/ 375 mg/m²	12[c]	1 (3)	15 (45)	10	46
Chronic lymphocytic leukemia and B-cell leukemia	40	Yes	500 mg/m²– 2,250 mg/m²	4	0	14 (36)	8	47
Mantle cell lymphoma, prolymphocytic leukemia, marginal zone lymphoma	10	Yes	500 mg/m²– 2,250 mg/m²	4	0	6 (60)	8	47
Waldenström's macroglobulinemia	27	Mixed	375 mg/m²	4[d]	—	12 (44)	16	58

N/A, not available.
[a]This protocol included maintenance rituximab at 6-month intervals in responders.
[b]Selected patients were older than 60 years and had no prior therapy.
[c]Rituximab was infused three times weekly.
[d]Repeat 4-week courses were given to patients without progressive disease.

treated advanced follicular lymphoma were treated with 4 weeks of 375-mg-per-m^2 rituximab. Five patients achieved a complete response (17%) and nine patients a partial response (30%). Median response duration was 6.7 months. Bulky disease or bone marrow involvement, or both, was associated with poor response.

Should rituximab be considered a first line therapy, particularly in patients for whom "watch and wait" may appear to be a superior option to chemotherapy? Studies to begin to address this question have been initiated. Patients with previously untreated indolent lymphoma (follicular and small lymphocytic lymphoma) received four weekly intravenous infusions of 375 mg per m^2 of rituximab and were restaged at week 6 for response (28,29). Stable or responding patients received maintenance rituximab at 6-month intervals for a maximum of four courses or until progression. Sixty patients (97%) completed the first course of therapy and were evaluable for response. Thirty-six (58%) received four courses at the 6-month interval. Forty-seven percent of patients had objective responses at 6 weeks, and 45% had stable disease. The final response rate after maintenance therapy was 73%, with 37% complete responses. Responses were similar in patients with follicular versus small lymphocytic lymphoma. Median progression-free survival was 34 months. In another study, 50 previously untreated patients with follicular lymphoma and low tumor burden were treated with four weekly doses of rituximab at 375 mg per m^2 (30). The response rate 1 month after therapy was 73% (13 complete remissions, 23 partial remissions, ten stable, and three progressed). Progressive disease at 1 year was seen in one of 13 complete responders, nine of 23 partial responders, and five of ten with stable disease. Using a polymerase chain reaction (PCR) for the bcl-2-J rearrangement, they reported a high correlation between progression-free survival and molecular responses ($p < .0001$).

Another issue is the duration of rituximab therapy. The standard dose of 4 weekly infusions at 375 mg per m^2 has been compared to more prolonged therapy in patients with previously treated low-grade lymphoma (follicular and small lymphocytic). In one study, 37 patients were treated with eight consecutive weekly doses of 375 mg per m^2 (31). Sixty percent responded to treatment (14% complete and 46% partial), with a median time to progression of 19.4+ months. They concluded that the safety profile and efficacy achieved in this pilot study compared favorably with the four weekly doses. In another study, 17 patients with refractory follicular lymphoma were treated with six weekly doses of 375 mg per m^2 of rituximab, with a total response rate of 76%, with eight (47%) complete responses (32). In conclusion, the issue of more extensive therapy beyond the standard four weekly infusions will have to be addressed in prospective randomized trials.

Should rituximab be combined with other biologic agents (Table 13.3)? In one study, rituximab was combined with interleukin-12, a cytokine that facilitates cytolytic T-cell responses, enhances the lytic activity of natural killer cells, and induces both T cells and natural killer cells to secrete interferon-γ (33). Therefore, this combination therapy theo-

retically could enhance rituximab cell–mediated toxicity. Forty-three patients with B-cell lymphoma (low, intermediate, and high grade) were treated with four weekly infusions of 375 mg per m^2 of rituximab and twice-weekly subcutaneous injections of interleukin-12 (30 mg per kg escalated through 500 mg per kg). A greater than 20-fold increase in serum levels of interferon-γ and 2.5- to fivefold increase in inducible protein 10 was seen at interleukin-12 doses of 100 mg per kg or greater. Objective responses were reported in 29 of 43 (69%) patients, with eight of 11 complete responses seen at interleukin-12 doses of 300 mg per kg or greater. These interesting results suggest that this is an active combination, and further studies are warranted.

Combination therapy of rituximab and interferon-α has been studied in patients with previously treated low-grade lymphoma. In one study, 64 patients were treated with standard-dose rituximab and interferon-α. The overall response rate was 70%, with 33% complete responses and a median duration of responses of 19 months (34). Standard side effects of interferon-α, including neutropenia, fever, and hypotension, were noted. In another study, 38 patients with previously treated follicular or small lymphocytic lymphoma were treated with subcutaneous interferon-α (2.5 or 5 million units) given three times weekly for 12 weeks (35). On the fifth week of treatment, rituximab was infused at 375 mg per m^2 weekly for four doses. Side effects of asthenia, chills, fever, headache, nausea, and myalgia were noted. The overall response rate was 45% (11% complete responses and 34% partial responses). Median time to progression was 25.2 months. Prospective trials will be required to prove whether interleukin-12 or interferon-α enhances the activity of rituximab.

Another important question is the combination of rituximab with chemotherapeutic agents in patients with indolent lymphoma. The combination of cyclophosphamide, hydroxydaunomycin, Oncovin (vincristine), and prednisone (CHOP) combined with rituximab (an infusion of 375 mg per m^2 before each course of CHOP, up to six courses) demonstrated a 95% response rate (55% complete response and 40% partial remission) among 40 patients with indolent lymphomas. Seven of seven patients with follicular histology who achieved complete remission also had molecular clearing of bcl-2 from blood and bone marrow (36,37). The median duration of response and time to progression had not been reached after a median observation of 29+ months, with 28 of 38 assessable patients (74%) in remission during this follow-up period. In another study, 128 previously untreated follicular lymphoma patients were treated with CHOP. Patients who achieved a complete remission but were positive for bcl-2/IgH–positive cells in the blood or bone marrow, or both, were eligible to receive 375 mg per m^2 of weekly rituximab for 4 weeks (38). Seventy-seven patients received rituximab, and at 12 weeks follow-up, 59% converted to bcl-2/IgH negativity in peripheral blood and marrow, with 74% converting to bcl-2/IgH negativity at 28 weeks and 63% at 44 weeks. Patients who achieved bcl-2/IgH negativity after CHOP and were, therefore, not eligible to receive rituximab, had a freedom from

TABLE 13.3. *Rituximab combination therapy for patients with lymphoma and chronic lymphocytic leukemia*

Disease	No. of patients	Prior therapy	Combination therapy	Complete response (%)	Any response (%)	Duration of response (mo)	Reference
Low intermediate and high-grade lymphoma	43	Yes	Interleukin-12 + rituximab	11 (26)	29 (69)	8+	33
Low-grade lymphoma	64	Yes	Interleukin-α + rituximab	21 (33)	45 (70)	19	34
Low-grade lymphoma	38	Yes	Interleukin-α + rituximab	4 (11)	17 (45)	25.2	35
Low-grade lymphoma	40	Mixed	CHOP + rituximab	22 (55)	38 (95)	29+	36, 37
Diffuse large B-cell lymphoma	197	No	CHOP	124 (63)[a]	—	13	40
	202	No	CHOP + rituximab	153 (76)[a]	—	26+	—
Aggressive lymphoma	33	No	CHOP + rituximab	20 (61)	31 (94)	26+	41
Aggressive lymphoma	20	No	Etoposide, vincristine, cyclophosphamide, prednisone and rituximab	17 (85)	17 (85)	12+	42
Aggressive lymphoma	14	Yes	Etoposide, vincristine, cyclophosphamide, prednisone and rituximab	9 (64)	12 (88)	N/A	42
Mantle cell lymphoma	40	No	CHOP + rituximab	19 (48)	38 (95)	16.6	43
Chronic lymphocytic leukemia	31	Mixed	Fludarabine + rituximab	—	27 (87)	19	55
Chronic lymphocytic leukemia	51	No	Fludarabine + rituximab	24 (47)	46 (90)	—	56
	53	No	Fludarabine followed by rituximab	15 (28)	41 (77)	—	—
Chronic lymphocytic leukemia	35	No	Cyclophosphamide, fludarabine + rituximab	20 (57)	33 (94)	N/A	57

N/A, not available; +, plus.
[a]$p = .005$ between the two arms.

recurrence of 52%. Patients treated with rituximab with a durable bcl-2/IgH–negative status had a freedom from recurrence of 57%, compared with 20% for those who never achieved or lost the molecular negativity ($p < .001$)

Aggressive Lymphoma

Rituximab has been evaluated as a single agent in more aggressive lymphoma histologies. Patients with diffuse large B-cell lymphoma, mantle cell lymphoma, or other intermediate- or high-grade B-cell lymphomas were included in a prospective phase II study. All patients were either in first or second relapse, were refractory to initial therapy, progressed after a partial response to initial therapy, or were older than 60 years and not previously treated (39). They received eight weekly infusions of rituximab at 375 mg per m^2 in arm A or one infusion of 375

mg per m^2 followed by seven weekly infusions of 500 mg per m^2 in arm B. Fifty-four patients were randomized, with a total of five complete responses and 12 partial responses, with no differences between the two doses. Responses were lower in patients with refractory disease and patients with tumors larger than 5 cm in diameter. Diffuse large-cell lymphoma and mantle cell lymphoma patients had response rates of 37% and 33%, respectively. The median time to progression among 17 responding patients was 246+ days.

Rituximab has also been studied in combination with chemotherapy in aggressive lymphoma. In a phase III trial, previously untreated elderly patients (60 to 80 years old) with diffuse large B-cell lymphoma were randomly assigned to receive either eight cycles of CHOP (197 patients) or eight cycles of CHOP plus rituximab (R-CHOP, 202 patients) given on day 1 of each cycle (40).

The rate of complete responses was significantly higher in the group that received R-CHOP than in the group that received CHOP (76% vs. 63%, p = .005). At a 2-year median follow-up, the event-free and overall survival times were significantly superior for the R-CHOP cohort over the CHOP cohort (p < .001 and p = .007, respectively). The authors concluded that there was minimal added toxicity with R-CHOP, with improved responses and survival.

In another study, 33 patients with previously untreated aggressive B-cell lymphoma received six infusions of 375 mg per m² of rituximab on the first day of each cycle of CHOP (41). They reported 20 complete responses (61%) and 11 partial responses (33%), with only two patients with progressive disease. Median duration of response and time to progression was 26+ months. Twenty-nine of 31 responders remained in remission during the follow-up period, including 15 of 16 patients with International Prognostic Index scores greater than or equal to 2. The bcl-2 rearrangement in blood or bone marrow converted to negative in all 11 patients who were studied, and only one reconverted to bcl-2 positivity. This promising combination is currently under investigation in randomized studies.

Rituximab was combined with etoposide, vincristine, doxorubicin, cyclophosphamide, and prednisone in 38 untreated or relapsed patients with poor-prognosis aggressive B-cell lymphoma (42). Complete remissions were achieved in 85% and 64% of untreated and previously treated patients, respectively. At a median of 12 months' follow-up, progression-free and overall survival rates in the untreated group were 85% and 79%, respectively, and none of the complete responders had relapsed. The authors concluded that these data suggest that rituximab may increase the sensitivity of these lymphomas to combination chemotherapy.

Forty previously untreated patients with mantle cell lymphoma were treated with six cycles of R-CHOP. There were 19 complete responses (48%) and 19 partial responses (48%) (43). Twenty-eight of 40 patients relapsed, with a median progression-free survival of 16.6 months. Nine of 25 patients who had bcl-1/IgH or clonal IgH detected by PCR before therapy had no detectable molecular disease after therapy. However, patients who achieved molecular remissions did not have an improved progression-free survival. These authors concluded that favorable clinical and molecular responses associated with R-CHOP did not translate into prolonged progression-free survival in patients with mantle cell lymphoma. Furthermore, they observed five patients in this study who had clinical evidence of persistent lymphoma at a time when their peripheral blood and bone marrow did not show evidence of molecular disease. They suggested that if R-CHOP transiently clears peripheral blood and bone marrow of mantle cell lymphoma cells, in spite of measurable disease, R-CHOP may provide *in vivo* purging for a better source of autologous stem cells for subsequent high-dose therapy.

Rituximab has also been used with high-dose chemotherapy before stem cell transplant. In one study, rituximab was combined with ifosfamide, mitoxantrone, and etoposide to produce a tumor-free graft (44). Twenty-two patients with aggressive B-cell lymphoma were treated with this high-dose regimen, with 11 complete responses and nine partial responses (40%). They reported only a single relapse post–stem cell transplant. In another study, 32 patients with advanced high-risk B-cell lymphoma either at disease onset (14 patients) or with relapsed or progressive disease (18 patients) received rituximab either concurrently with high-dose chemotherapy or immediately after (before harvesting stem cells) to target minimal residual disease (45). Thirteen of 14 previously untreated patients achieved a complete remission, and ten of 18 previously treated patients achieved a complete remission. Nine of nine patients with follicular lymphoma had bcl-2–negative cell harvests. In another study, 32 lymphoma patients (12 diffuse large-cell, six follicular, four mantle cell, and one small lymphocytic) were treated with high-dose chemotherapy and rituximab. Thirteen of 14 patients treated up front and ten of 18 previously treated patients achieved complete remission (46).

Chronic Lymphocytic Leukemia and Small Lymphocytic Lymphoma

Chronic lymphocytic leukemia and small lymphocytic lymphoma cells have a lower density of CD20 than do most other B-cell malignancies. Chronic lymphocytic leukemia also has the disadvantage of a large pool of circulating tumor cells. In one study, an alternate treatment schedule of rituximab was designed to optimize pharmacokinetics and decrease initial toxicity for patients with chronic lymphocytic leukemia and small lymphocytic lymphoma (46). Thirty-three patients were treated with the first dose of rituximab reduced to 100 mg over 4 hours. In cohort 1 (n = 3; 250 mg per m²) and cohort 2 (n = 7; 375 mg per m²), rituximab was infused on day 3 and thereafter three times weekly for 4 weeks using a standard administration schedule. Cohort 3 (n = 23; 375 mg per m²) was treated similarly to cohort 2 for the first two treatments and then over 1 hour thereafter. Only one patient discontinued therapy due to infusion-related toxicity. The overall response rate was 45% (3% complete responses and 42% partial responses), with a median response duration of 10 months. Infusion-related events appeared to be cytokine mediated and resolved by the third infusion, allowing for a more rapid administration of rituximab.

In another study, 40 patients with chronic lymphocytic leukemia and ten with other mature B-cell leukemia were treated with four weekly infusions of rituximab (47). The first dose was 375 mg per m² for all patients, and dose escalation began with dose 2 but was held constant for each patient. Doses escalated from 500 mg per m² to 2,250 mg per m². Toxicity was predominately seen with the first dose, including fever, chills, dyspnea, hypoxia, hypotension, and hypertension. Partial responses were seen in 36% of patients with chronic lymphocytic leukemia and 60% with other B-cell leukemias. There was a dose response, with responses in 22% of patients treated at 500 to 825 mg per m^2, 43% of those treated at 1,000 to 1,500 mg per m^2, and 75% of those treated at 2,250 mg per m^2. Median time to progression was 8 months. These data suggest that rituximab has significant activity in patients with chronic lymphocytic leukemia treated at the high dose levels. These investigators noted that severe first-dose reactions were uncommon in patients with chronic lymphocytic leukemia even with high circulating white counts but were more frequent in patients with other B-cell leukemias in which CD20 expression was greater.

The mechanisms of toxicity of rituximab in chronic lymphocytic leukemia have been addressed. Eleven patients with relapsed fludarabine-resistant chronic lymphocytic leukemia or leukemia variants of lymphoma were treated with rituximab (48). During the first infusion of rituximab, patients with circulating white blood cell counts exceeding 50×10^9 per L experienced a severe cytokine-release syndrome. Ninety minutes after the onset of infusion, serum levels of tumor necrosis factor-α and interleukin-6 peaked in all patients, and this was associated with fever, chills, nausea, vomiting, hypotension, and dyspnea. There was a 50% to 75% drop of platelets and lymphocytes within 12 hours from the start of infusion and a five- to tenfold increase of liver enzymes, D-dimers, and lactate dehydrogenase, as well as a prolongation of the prothrombin time. The frequency and severity of first-dose toxicity correlated with circulating white blood cell counts greater than 50×10^9 per L. These investigations proposed different infusion schedules (dividing the first dose over 3 days) or combination regimens, or both, with chemotherapy agents to reduce tumor burden before rituximab treatment. These data contrasted with the toxicity data reported in the above study, in which severe first-dose reactions were not prominent in chronic lymphocytic leukemia patients with high white blood cell counts (47).

The mechanism of tumor cell clearance in chronic lymphocytic leukemia has also been addressed. Rituximab likely has immunologic activity, including antibody-dependent cytotoxicity and complement-mediated cytotoxicity. A proportion of patients treated with rituximab were reported to have in vivo activation of caspase-9, caspase-3, and poly-(adenosine diphosphate–ribose) polymerase cleavage in circulating leukemia cells immediately after rituximab infusion (49). This suggests that apoptosis is involved in the elimination of leukemia cells after rituximab therapy. They reported that patients having caspase-3 activation and poly- (adenosine diphosphate–ribose) polymerase cleavage in vivo had a significantly lower circulating leukemia count after treatment with rituximab. They also noted downregulation of the antiapoptotic proteins XIAP and Mcl-1. They hypothesize that this may be in part the mechanism of how rituximab sen-

sitizes leukemia cells to chemotherapeutic agents. In other studies, rituximab downregulated bcl-2 through inhibition of interleukin-10 (50,51).

Combining rituximab with chemotherapeutic agents to treat patients with chronic lymphocytic leukemia has been studied. Fludarabine is perhaps the most active single agent in chronic lymphocytic leukemia, with responses ranging from 50% to 60% in previously treated patients to 80% in previously untreated patients, with 35% complete responses (52,53). However, all patients ultimately relapse. In vitro studies suggest synergy between fludarabine and rituximab (54). In a clinical study, 31 patients with chronic lymphocytic leukemia (20 previously untreated and 11 relapsed) were treated with standard-dose fludarabine (25 mg per m^2) on days 1 to 5, 29 to 33, 57 to 61, and 85 to 89 and rituximab (375 mg per m^2) given on days 57, 85, 113, and 151 (55). Neutropenia and thrombocytopenia were the predominant hematologic toxicity (grade 1 or 2 in 26% and grade 3 or 4 in 45%). The overall response rate was 87% (27 of 31 evaluable patients). In the 20 previously untreated patients, 17 (85%) responded with ten complete remissions. The median duration of response was 19 months.

A randomized phase 2 study was carried out to determine the efficacy, safety, and optimal administration schedule of rituximab with fludarabine in previously untreated patients with chronic lymphocytic leukemia (56). Patients were randomized to receive either six monthly courses of fludarabine combined with rituximab, followed 2 months later with four weekly doses of rituximab, or they received sequential fludarabine alone, followed 2 months later by four weekly doses of rituximab. One hundred four patients were randomized to concurrent (n = 51) or sequential (n = 53) regimens. Toxicities were similar in the two arms except for more grade 3 or 4 neutropenia (74% vs. 41%) and grade 3 or 4 infusion-related toxicity (20% vs. 0%) during the induction portion of treatment in the combined-therapy arm. The overall response rate on the combined-therapy arm was 90% (47% complete responses, 43% partial responses; 95% confidence interval, 0.82–0.98) compared to 77% overall response (28% complete responses, 49% partial responses; 95% confidence interval, 0.66–0.99) in the sequential arm. The combined-regimen arm had a significantly higher complete-response rate (p = .48). Median progression-free survival and overall survival have not been reached in either arm. After a median of 23 months of follow-up, 18 patients (35%) have experienced a relapse on the combined-treatment arm and 15 (28%) on the sequential regimen. The 2-year progression-free survival is 70% for each regimen. These data suggest that combining fludarabine and rituximab leads to a higher complete-response rate than does sequential therapy, although the long-term benefit of this therapy will require continued follow-up.

In another study, patients were treated with a combination of fludarabine, 25 mg per m^2 daily for 3 days; cyclophosphamide, 250 mg per m^2 daily for 3 days; and rituximab at 375 mg per m^2 1 day before the first course of therapy and at 500 mg per m^2 with chemotherapy in all subsequent courses (57). Therapy was given every 4 weeks for six courses. Thirty-five previously untreated patients were evaluable after six courses, with 57% complete responses, 20% nodular complete remissions and 27% partial remissions, for an overall response rate of 94%. The same regimen has been given to previously treated patients with chronic lymphocytic leukemia. Forty-three patients were evaluable after three courses. Complete response was 14%, and partial response was 56%. Infections were more common in the previously treated group of patients.

Other Lymphomas

Twenty-seven patients with Waldenström's macroglobulinemia were treated with 375 mg per m^2 of rituximab weekly for 4 weeks, followed by repeat 4-week courses in patients without progressive disease (58). Responses occurred in six (40%) of 15 previously untreated patients and in six (50%) of 12 pretreated patients. The median time to progression was 16 months, and nine of 12 responding patients continued free of progression at 15.7 months' follow-up. Rituximab appears active in Waldenström's macroglobulinemia in previously treated and untreated patients. The added benefit of repeat 4-week courses of rituximab requires confirmation in randomized studies.

Ten patients with primary cutaneous B-cell lymphoma (three follicular, and seven large B-cell) were treated with rituximab (59). Two complete responses, five partial responses, and one mixed response were reported. Histologic examination of biopsy specimens from two regressing tumors showed necrotic tumor cells with CD8$^+$ T-cell infiltration. Rituximab appears to be an effective treatment for primary cutaneous lymphoma.

ALEMTUZUMAB

Alemtuzumab is a humanized IgG1 monoclonal antibody (60) that targets the CD52 antigen, which is expressed on all B- and T-cell malignancies and normal leukocytes but not on hematopoietic progenitor cells (61) and has been approved by the FDA for the treatment of relapsed or refractory chronic lymphocytic leukemia. The mechanism of action of this antibody is unclear, but it has been shown *in vitro* to mediate complement lysis, antibody-dependent cellular cytotoxicity, and cell apoptosis. It has been evaluated in different settings, including autoimmune diseases such as rheumatoid arthritis and multiple sclerosis, solid-organ transplantation, graft-versus-host disease, and B- and T-cell malignancies. As with other monoclonal antibodies, its use has been associated with infusion-related reactions, including fever, rigors, rash, nausea, hypotension, and angioedema due to the release of cytokines and tumor necrosis factor (62). Prophylactic therapy with acetaminophen and diphenhydramine can reduce the severity of these reactions. The regimen includes a loading dose of 3 mg intravenously on day 1 and 10 mg on day 2,

followed by a maintenance dose of 30 mg per day three times per week for up to 12 weeks. Alemtuzumab has been associated with prolonged immunosuppression due to rapid depletion of T and B cells, which may last for many months and can result in opportunistic infections. Prophylaxis against pneumocystis carinii and herpes simplex virus infections is recommended for all patients treated with alemtuzumab.

In a multicenter trial, patients with chronic lymphocytic leukemia refractory to fludarabine were treated with alemtuzumab (63). The overall response rate was 33% (predominantly partial responses), with time to progression longer than 9 months. Infections occurred in 56% of patients, with 25% opportunistic and 20% fatal. Additional studies in relapsed or refractory chronic lymphocytic leukemia have demonstrated similar responses (64,65). Alemtuzumab has activity as first-line treatment of chronic lymphocytic leukemia (66). Activity has also been reported in patients with low-grade lymphoma and T and B prolymphocytic leukemia (67–69). Trials combining alemtuzumab with chemotherapy and rituximab are ongoing.

EPRATUZUMAB

Epratuzumab is a humanized IgG1 monoclonal antibody that targets the CD22 antigen, which is broadly expressed on both normal and malignant B cells (70,71). In a phase I/II single-center trial using this agent in relapsed or refractory low- and high-grade lymphoma, 114 patients were treated with 120 to 1,000 mg per m^2 once weekly for four doses. There was no dose-limiting toxicity and favorable infusion-related toxicity (72). Mean serum half-life was 23 days. Twenty of 51 evaluable indolent lymphoma patients (39%) had stable disease and nine (17.6%) had objective responses (three complete and six partial responses). Twelve of 52 (23%) patients with aggressive disease had stable disease, and there were five (10%) objective responses (three complete and two partial responses). In a phase II trial, 21 rituximab-naïve patients with B-cell lymphoma were treated with four weekly infusions of rituximab (375 mg per m^2) and epratuzumab (360 mg per m^2) (73). The treatment was well tolerated, and 19 patients were evaluable for response. Two of three patients with diffuse large B-cell lymphoma responded with one complete response. Eight of 16 patients with indolent lymphoma responded with 44% complete responses (one unconfirmed) and 6% partial responses. Responses were ongoing in nine of ten responders at 13+ months' follow-up.

APOLIZUMAB

Hu1D10 (Apolizumab) is a humanized IgG1 monoclonal antibody that binds to the HLA-DR β chain (74). This antigen is expressed on the surface of circulating B lymphocytes in 70% of normal individuals. This antibody induces antibody-dependent cellular cytotoxicity and complement-mediated lysis in lymphoma-cell lines. In a phase I trial

TABLE 13.4. *Therapeutic radiolabeled antibodies*

	Iodine-131 tositumomab (Corixa)	Yttrium-90 ibritumomab tiuxetan (IDEC)	Yttrium-90 (Immunomedics)	Lym-1 (Peregrine)
Trade name	Bexxar	Zevalin	Not applicable	Oncolym
Antigen target	CD20	CD20	CD22	HLA-DR10 (β-subunit)
Species	Murine	Murine	Human/murine (humanized)	Murine
Imaging isotope	Iodine-131	Indium-111	Indium-111	131-Iodine or 67-Copper
Therapeutic isotope	Iodine-131	Yttrium-90	Yttrium-90	131-Iodine or 67-Copper
U.S. Food and Drug Administration approved	No	Yes	No	No

using HuD10 in lymphoma, toxicity was limited to fever, chills, rigors, nausea, vomiting, and hypotension (75,76). The half-life of this antibody was shorter than other antibody reagents measured at a median of 11 days. Objective responses were seen in four of eight patients with follicular lymphoma with delayed time to response ranging from 105 to 296 days. HuD10 is currently under investigation in randomized trials in indolent lymphoma and chronic lymphocytic leukemia.

RADIOLABELED MONOCLONAL ANTIBODIES

To enhance the tumoricidal activity of monoclonal antibodies, they may be conjugated to radionuclides. The two most widely used radionuclides are Iodine-131 (I-131) and Yttrium-90 (Y-90) (Table 13.4). I-131 and Y-90 emit beta particles by the decaying radioisotope that penetrate through

several cell layers, allowing radioactive "cross-fire" from antigen-positive cells to antigen-negative cells or to cells that were not directly bound to antibody. This differs from unlabeled antibodies or immunotoxins, in which cell death is likely dependent on cell binding. An additional benefit is that lymphomas are among the most radiosensitive tumors. The primary disadvantage is toxicity to normal tissues. Excellent responses have been reported after radiolabeled-antibody treatment of lymphoma (Table 13.5). Radiolabeled-antibody therapy of lymphoma has recently been reviewed (77,78).

Iodine-131 Tositumomab

I-131 tositumomab is a murine I-131-labeled monoclonal antibody. Due to individual variability in clearance of I-131 tositumomab, a dosimetric dose of 10 mg of antibody labeled with 5mCi of I-131 was first infused. Total-body

TABLE 13.5. *Radiolabeled-antibody therapy of lymphoma*

Therapeutic agent	Disease	No. of patients	Prior therapy	Complete response (%)	Any response (%)	Duration of response (mo)	Reference
I-131 tositumomab	Low- and intermediate-grade	59	Yes	20 (34)	42 (75)	12	83
I-131 tositumomab	Low- and intermediate-grade	47	Yes	15 (32)	47 (57)	19.9	84
I-131 tositumomab	Follicular	76	No	56 (74)	76 (95)	Not available	85
I-131 tositumomab	Low-grade and transformed	60	Yes	12 (20)	39 (65)	6.5	86
Y-90 ibritumomab tiuxetan	Follicular	44	Yes	7 (15)	33 (74)	6.8	92
Y-90 ibritumomab tiuxetan	Follicular and transformed	30	Yes	11 (37)	25 (83)	9.4	93
Y-90 ibritumomab tiuxetan	Low-grade and transformed	73	Yes	22 (30)	58 (80)	14.2	94

I, iodine; Y, yttrium.

clearance was measured to calculate the mCi required for a therapeutic dose. The maximum tolerated total-body radiation was 75 c Gy, based on bone marrow toxicity (79–84). It was determined that a 457-mg dose of unlabeled tositumomab before the dosimetric dose increased the terminal half-life of the radiolabeled antibody (83). The therapeutic dose was delivered at least 1 week after the dosimetric dose. Each therapeutic dose consisted of a patient-specific mCi amount of I-131 tositumomab adjusted to deliver a total-body–radiation dose up to 75 cGy. Similar to the dosimetric dose of I-131 tositumomab, a dose of 475 mg of unlabeled tositumomab was given before the therapeutic dose. Forty-two (75%) of 59 previously treated patients responded, with 20 (34%) complete responses. Thirty-five (83%) of 42 patients with low-grade or transformed lymphoma responded, versus seven (41%) of 17 with de novo intermediate-grade lymphoma. The median progression-free survival was 12 months for all responding patients and 20.3 months for complete responders. Seven patients remained in complete remission at 5.7 years. Sixteen patients were retreated after progression, and nine responded, with five complete responses. Reversibly hematologic toxicity was dose limiting. Ten patients developed human antimouse antibodies. Five patients developed elevated thyroid-stimulating hormone levels, five developed myelodysplasia, and three developed solid tumors.

In a multicenter phase II trial for patients with previously treated low- and intermediate-grade lymphoma, 27 of 47 (57%) patients responded, including 15 (32%) patients with complete responses (84). The median duration of complete response was 19.9 months. Only one patient developed human antimouse antibodies. Seventy-six previously untreated patients with follicular lymphoma were treated with I-131 tositumomab (85). Seventy-two of 76 (95%) patients responded, with 56 (74%) complete responses. Forty-five of these 57 (79%) patients remain in complete remission from 30 to 66 months. The median duration of response and progression-free survival were not reached.

A multicenter pivotal trial enrolled 60 patients with refractory low-grade or transformed low-grade B-cell lymphoma (86). Patients were treated with I-131 tositumomab, and efficacy was compared to the patients' last qualifying chemotherapy regimen. All 60 patients were treated with at least two protocol-specified qualifying chemotherapy regimens and had not responded or progressed within 6 months after their last qualifying chemotherapy regimen before receiving a single course of I-131 tositumomab. Responses were observed in 39 patients (65%) after I-131 tositumomab, compared with 17 patients (28%) after their last qualifying chemotherapy regimen (p < .001). The median duration of response was 6.5 months after I-131 tositumomab, compared with 3.4 months after the last qualifying chemotherapy regimen (p < .001). Two patients (3%) had a complete response after their last qualifying chemotherapy regimen, compared with 12 (20%) after I-131 tositumomab (p < .001). The median duration of response for complete responders was 6.1 months after the last qualifying chemotherapy regimen and was not reached with follow-up of longer than 47 months after I-131 tositumomab. Only one patient was hospitalized for neutropenia, and five (8%) developed human antimouse antibodies. They concluded that a single course of I-131 tositumomab was significantly more efficacious than the last qualifying chemotherapy regimen.

I-131 tositumomab has also been combined with fludarabine (87). Three sequential cycles of fludarabine were followed 6 to 8 weeks later by I-131 tositumomab in 38 patients with previously untreated follicular and transformed lymphoma. Fourteen patients were assessable for response at the publication of this interim analysis. Four of 11 partial responders after fludarabine became complete responders after I-131 tositumomab, and one patient with stable disease became a partial responder.

Myeloablative doses of I-131 tositumomab have been used in combination with stem cell transplantation in patients with relapsed and refractory lymphoma (Table 13.6). Long-term follow-up was reported in 1998 (88) on the

TABLE 13.6. *Myeloablative therapy with iodine-131 tositumomab in combination with stem cell transplantation*

Disease	No. of patients	Prior therapy	Chemotherapy	Complete response (%)	Any response (%)	Progression-free survival (%)	Reference
Low- and intermediate-grade lymphoma	29	Yes	No	23 (79)	25 (86)	42[a]	89
Low- and intermediate-grade lymphoma	52	Yes	Etoposide, cyclophosphamide	24 (77)[b]	27 (87)	88[c]	90
Mantle cell lymphoma	16	Yes	Etoposide, cyclophosphamide	14 (90)	16 (100)	61[d]	91

[a]Progression-free survival at 42 months.
[b]Thirty-one of the 52 patients were evaluable for response by conventional measurements.
[c]Progression-free survival at 24 months.
[d]Progression-free survival at 36 months.

patients first reported in 1995 (89). Patients were first treated with trace-labeled doses of I-131 tositumomab for biodistribution studies. Based on these biodistribution studies, 29 patients were eligible to receive therapeutic infusions of single-agent I-131 tositumomab labeled with 280 to 785 mCi of I-131 calculated to deliver specific absorbed radiation doses to normal organs, followed by stem cell rescue. There were 25 (86%) major responses, with 23 (79%) complete responses. Nonhematopoietic dose-limiting toxicity was reversible cardiopulmonary insufficiency in two patients who received greater than or equal to 27 Gy to the lungs. At 42 months' median follow-up, the estimated overall and progression-free survival were 68% and 42%, respectively. Fourteen of 29 patients remained in unmaintained complete remissions for 27+ to 87+ months after treatment. Late toxicities included elevated thyroid-stimulating hormone levels in 60% of patients, and two patients developed second malignancies; neither developed myelodysplasia. These data suggest that myeloablative therapy with I-131 tositumomab with stem cell rescue is well tolerated, with prolonged remissions and few late toxicities.

In another study, myeloablative doses of I-131 tositumomab were combined with etoposide and cyclophosphamide, followed by autologous stem cell transplantation in 52 patients with relapsed B-cell lymphoma (90). Patients received trace-labeled infusions of 1.7 mg per kg I-131 tositumomab for biodistribution studies and, 10 days later, received a therapeutic dose of I-131 tositumomab labeled with a calculated dose to deliver 20 to 27 Gy to normal organs. Patients were maintained in radiation isolation until their total-body radioactivity was less than 0.07 mSv per hour at 1 m. They then received chemotherapy followed by stem cell rescue. Thirty-one patients were evaluable for response by conventional measurements with 24 (77%) complete responses and two (6%) partial responses. The estimated overall and progression-free survival rates for all 52 patients at 2 years were 83% and 88%, respectively. These results compared favorably with those in nonrandomized control patients who received external-beam total-body radiation and the same chemotherapy over the same period. Sixteen patients with refractory or relapsed mantle cell lymphoma were treated with I-131 tositumomab and etoposide and cyclophosphamide, as described above (91). There were no therapy-related deaths. Eleven patients had conventionally measurable disease at the time of treatment, and overall and complete responses were 100% and 90%, respectively. Fifteen patients were alive and 12 were progression free at 6 to 57 months from transplantation and 16 to 97 months from diagnosis. Estimated overall survival at 3 years from transplantation was 93%, and progression-free survival was 61%. This combined radioimmunotherapy and chemotherapy appeared to be highly effective in patients with relapsed and refractory mantle cell lymphoma.

Ibritumomab Tiuxetan

Y-90 ibritumomab tiuxetan was approved as a radioimmunotherapeutic by the FDA for the treatment of patients with relapsed or refractory low-grade, follicular, or transformed B-cell lymphoma. Ibritumomab tiuxetan consists of a murine anti-CD20 monoclonal antibody (ibritumomab) linked with a chelating agent (tiuxetan) to the radioisotope Y-90. Patients were pretreated with 250 mg per m^2 of rituximab on days 1 and 8 to deplete circulating B cells, then Y-90 ibritumomab tiuxetan (0.4 mCi per kg; maximum, 32 mCi) was given intravenously on day 8 (92). An imaging/dosimetry dose of In-111 ibritumomab tiuxetan (5 mCi) was injected after rituximab in 28 patients. Fifty-four patients with heavily pretreated refractory follicular lymphoma were treated. The overall response rate was 74% (15% complete responses, 59% partial responses), with time to progression of 6.8 months for all patients and 8.7 months for responders. Adverse events were primarily hematologic, with the incidence of grade 4 neutropenia, thrombocytopenia, and anemia 35%, 9%, and 4%, respectively. Only one patient developed a human antihuman mouse antibody response, and none of the patients developed a human antichimeric antibody response. The estimated radiation-absorbed doses were within acceptable levels in all 28 patients who underwent imaging and dosimetry with In-111 ibritumomab tiuxetan.

Thirty patients with relapsed or refractory low-grade follicular or transformed B-cell lymphoma with mild thrombocytopenia (100 to 149×10^9 platelets per L) were treated with a reduced dose of Y-90 ibritumomab tiuxetan (0.3 mCi per kg; maximum, 32 mCi) (93). All patients received rituximab (250 mg per m^2) and In-111 ibritumomab tiuxetan (5 mCi) on day 1, followed 1 week later with rituximab (250 mg per m^2) and Y-90 ibritumomab tiuxetan (0.3 mCi per kg). Estimated radiation-absorbed doses were well below the maximum allowed for all 30 patients. The overall response rate was 83% (37% complete responses, 6.7% unconfirmed complete responses, and 40% partial responses). Estimated time to progression was 9.4 months and 22.6 months in responders. The incidence of grade 4 neutropenia, thrombocytopenia, and anemia was 33%, 13%, and 3%, respectively.

A randomized trial of Y-90 ibritumomab tiuxetan versus rituximab was performed in relapsed or refractory low-grade, follicular, or transformed B-cell lymphoma patients (94). The radioimmunotherapy group was treated with rituximab (250 mg per m^2) on days 1 and 8, followed by Y-90 ibritumomab tiuxetan (0.4 mCi per kg; maximum, 32 mCi). A total of 143 patients were enrolled, 73 randomized to Y-90 ibritumomab tiuxetan and 70 to rituximab. The overall response rate for the Y-90 ibritumomab tiuxetan cohort was 80% and for the rituximab cohort 56% ($p = .0002$). Complete responses were seen in 30% and 16% of the Y-90 ibritumomab tiuxetan and rituximab cohorts, respectively ($p = .04$). Median duration of response was 14.2 months in the Y-90 ibritumomab tiuxetan group versus 12.1 months in the rituximab group ($p = .6$), and time to progression was 11.2 versus 10.1 months ($p = .173$). These investigators concluded that Y-90 ibritumomab tiuxetan produces significantly better overall and complete responses compared with rituximab alone.

Radiolabeled hLL2

Epratuzumab is the humanized unlabeled hLL2 that targets CD22. The antibody is rapidly internalized (95), allowing a higher residence time dose delivered for the attachment of radiometals (96). In early trials using murine LL2 labeled with I-131, responses were seen at very low doses of I-131 (97–100). Subsequent studies with Y-90–labeled hLL2 demonstrated clinical responses at very low doses of Y-90, and a comparison of dosimetry and pharmacokinetics of Y-90– and I-131–labeled hLL2 demonstrated superiority of Y-90–labeled hLL2 (101). A phase I/II study with myeloablative doses of Y-90–labeled hLL2 in patients with predominately aggressive lymphoma demonstrated that a single injection with a protein dose of 100 mg had excellent biodistribution, without the need of predosing with unlabeled epratuzumab (102). Similar to 90-Y ibritumomab tiuxetan, it did not appear that 90-Y–labeled hLL2 would require individualized patient dosimetry (101). Another phase I trial of hLL2 labeled with Re-186 allowed simultaneous imaging and therapy, with antitumor activity noted at the initial doses (103).

Lym-1

Lym-1 is a murine antibody that targets the HLA-DR10-β subunit expressed on most malignant B cells (104). Clinical responses have been reported with I-131– or Copper-67 (Cu-67)–labeled Lym-1 (104–106). Thirty patients with B-cell lymphoma were treated with fractionated low-dose Lym-1 in a phase I trial, with 17 of 30 (57%) patients with durable responses, including three complete responses (105). Thrombocytopenia was the dose-limiting toxicity. Cu-67–labeled Lym-1 demonstrated seven of 12 (58%) responses in B-cell lymphoma patients (107). Lym-1, similar to tositumomab and ibritumomab tiuxetan, is a murine antibody, and 28% of patients treated with multiple doses of antibody developed human antimouse antibody responses, without anaphylactoid or related toxicity (108). Prolonged survival was noted in the patients who developed human antimouse antibodies, suggesting that the immune response to Lym-1 may have had a survival advantage (109).

IMMUNOTOXINS

Monoclonal antibodies may also be conjugated to a highly potent toxin. The toxins are typically derived from a plant or bacteria that disrupts protein synthesis at picomolar concentrations. The immunotoxin must bind to the cell, translocate into the cytosol, and then irreversibly inhibit protein synthesis. Ricin and diphtheria toxin consist of two polypeptide chains (A chain and B chain). The B chain binds to the cell membrane and facilitates internalization of the A chain. The ricin A chain cleaves a specific adenine residue of the 60S ribosomal subunit, and the A chain of diphtheria toxin inactivates elongation factor 2. *Pseudomonas* exotoxin is a single-chain polypeptide containing three domains that serve the respective functions of toxicity, binding, and translocation. The B chains typically bind nonspecifically to cell membranes. To produce clinically useful reagents, either the A chain must be isolated by biochemical methods or recombinant DNA or the galactose-binding site of the B chain must be blocked with affinity ligands. Although the "blocked" ricin B chain weakly binds, it is capable of facilitating the A chain translocation into the cytosol. Deglycosylation of the ricin A chain minimizes nonspecific hepatic uptake and decreases toxicity.

Phase I trials with anti-CD19 and anti-CD22 immunotoxins for B-cell lymphoma patients have been reported (110–114). In these trials, deglycosylated ricin A (dgA) was linked to RFB4 (IgG-RFB4-dgA) or to Fab' fragments of the antibody (Fab'-RFB4-dgA). In one study (113), patients were treated with a bolus or continuous infusion regimen of the HD37 murine anti-CD19 monoclonal antibody linked to deglycosylated ricin A chain (IgG-HD37-SMPT-dgA). They reported one complete response (4%) lasting more than 40 months, one partial response (1%) among 23 evaluable patients treated on the bolus schedule, and one partial response (11%) among nine evauable patients treated on the continuous-infusion regimen. Twenty-five percent of the patients on the bolus regimen and 30% on the continuous-infusion regimen made antibody against mouse Ig or ricin A chain, or both. The major toxicity observed was vascular leak syndrome manifested by hypoalbuminemia, hyponatremia, and weight gain. Three patients developed delayed acrocyanosis that resembled a resolving vasoconstriction phase of Raynaud's phenomenon. Similar results were reported with an alternative immunotoxin approach using the "blocked" ricin linked to anti-B4 (anti-CD19; anti-B4-bR) (115–117), but hepatotoxicity was dose-limiting. In a phase II trial of 16 patients with relapsed B-cell lymphoma treated with five daily single-bolus doses of anti-CD19-bR at the maximum tolerated dose, no clinical responses were reported (118).

Smaller molecules with higher affinity and greater specificity should have better tumor penetration and less toxicity. Cytokine molecules, rather than antibodies, have been one approach. The native cell surface-binding sequences of the diphtheria toxin were substituted by human IL-2, restricting binding of the fusion toxin to cells that express the p55 or p75 subunits of IL-2. Conjugation (fusion) of a plant or bacterial toxin gene to a specific receptor ligand can guide the toxin gene to the target cell, where it can be internalized via receptor-mediated endocytosis and translocated into a toxic moiety in the cytosol (119). The early version of the ligand fusion-protein, DAB_{486} IL-2, was well tolerated and had antitumor activity in patients with advanced hematologic malignancies (120–125). In one study (125), there was one partial response and two additional patients with major cutaneous improvement of disease among 14 patients with cutaneous T-cell lymphoma (Table 13.7). Denileukin diftitox (DAB_{389} IL-2) differs from DAB_{486} IL-2 in the deletion of 97 amino acids from a portion of the native receptor-binding

TABLE 13.7. *Immunotoxin therapeutics*

Disease	Immunotoxin	Number of patients	Prior therapy	Complete response (%)	Any response (%)	Reference
Cutaneous T-cell lymphoma	DAB_{486} IL-2	14	Yes	0	1 (7)[a]	125
Cutaneous T-cell lymphoma	DAB_{389} IL-2	35	Yes	5 (14)	13 (37)	127
Hodgkin's disease	DAB_{389} IL-2	21	Yes		0	127
Lymphoma	DAB_{389} IL-2	17	Yes	1 (6)	3 (18)	127
CD25+ hematologic malignancies	LMB-2	35	Yes			132
Hairy-cell leukemia	BL22	16	Yes	11 (69)	13 (81)	133

[a]Two additional patients had major cutaneous responses without a change in circulating tumor cells.

domain. The resulting protein has a lower molecular weight and has a fivefold improved affinity and tenfold increased potency compared to DAB_{486} IL-2 (126). Seventy-three patients with previously treated IL-2R–positive hematologic malignancies were treated (35 cutaneous T-cell lymphoma, 21 Hodgkin's disease, 17 lymphoma). The dose-limiting toxicity was asthenia, establishing the maximum tolerated dose of 2.7 µg per kg per day. Half of the patients had antibodies against diphtheria toxin or to denileukin diftitox at the time of enrollment and 92% at the end of treatment. There were five complete responses and eight partial responses in patients with cutaneous T-cell lymphoma and one complete response and two partial responses in lymphoma patients. The duration of response was 2 to 39+ months. None of the patients with Hodgkin's disease responded. In another study, 35 patients with previously treated cutaneous T-cell lymphoma were treated with denileukin diftitox, with 13 (37%) responses, including five complete responses (14%) (127). Denileukin diftitox, which is the DAB_{389} IL-2 fusion toxin, has been approved for the treatment of cutaneous T-cell lymphoma by the FDA.

The first recombinant immunotoxin contained a single Fv fragment of anti-Tac monoclonal antibody to the IL-2–receptor alpha subunit (also referred to as *Tac*, *p55*, or *CD25*) fused to a truncated form of the bacterial toxin *Pseudomonas exotoxin* (128). This recombinant toxin was cytotoxic to malignant cells from patients with adult T-cell leukemia/lymphoma (129–131). A smaller derivative of this immunotoxin, anti-Tac (Fv)-PE38 (LMB-2), was developed for clinical testing. LMB-2 was administered to 35 patients with CD25+ hematologic malignancies for whom prior therapies had not worked (132). Dose-limiting toxicity at 63 µg per kg every other day was reversible transaminases in one patient and diarrhea and cardiomyopathy in another. Six patients developed neutralizing antibodies after the first three doses. The median half-life was 4 hours. One patient with hairy-cell leukemia achieved a complete remission, which was ongoing at 20 months. Several partial responses were observed in patients with cutaneous T-cell lymphoma, three with hairy-cell leukemia, one with chronic lymphocytic leukemia, and one patient with Hodgkin's disease. In

another study, 16 patients with cladribine-resistant hairy-cell leukemia were treated with BL-22 (133). Eleven patients had complete responses, and two patients had partial responses. Three of these patients relapsed at 10 to 23 months and had second remissions. Two patients had a reversible hemolytic-uremic syndrome.

Alternative approaches to immunotoxin therapy include toxins that are less immunogenic, including toxins that act at the cell surface, nonprotein toxins, and conjugates with agents such as myatansinoids (134) and calicheamicins (135), which are more potent than conventional chemotherapy agents. Immunotoxins may be combined with conventional chemotherapy agents to exploit *in vitro* and preclinical data that suggest synergy (136,137). Prodrugs are pharmacodynamically inert chemicals that may be conjugated to monoclonal antibodies and targeted directly to tumors and are converted by enzymes into active drug at the tumor site (138). Extremely toxic agents that cannot be used for conventional therapy may be exploited by this technology. Once converted at the tumor site, the active drug can diffuse into cells that are not bound to antibody. In summary, there appear to be many theoretic advantages to immunotoxins. Current limitations in the clinical setting include their immunogenicity, their unique toxicity of vascular leak syndrome, and their lack of ability to kill bystander cells.

BISPECIFIC ANTIBODIES

Bispecific antibodies bind to two different antigens. Typically, one arm binds to a tumor-associated antigen and the other arm to a cytotoxic cell. Anti-CD16/CD30 is a bispecific antibody that binds to CD16 found on natural killer cells and monocytes and CD30 found on Reed-Sternberg and anaplastic large-cell lymphoma cells (139). Fifteen patients with refractory Hodgkin's disease were treated in a phase I trial with HRS-3/A9, and the maximum tolerated dose was 64 mg per m^2. Human antimouse antibody was identified in nine patients, and four had allergic reactions. The CD3xCD19 bispecific antibody targets the CD3 T-cell receptor and the CD19 B-cell antigen. Preliminary data in three patients with B-cell lymphoma suggested efficacy with minimal toxicity

(140). Numerous additional bispecific antibodies that target lymphomas are in preclinical development.

VACCINE THERAPY

Specific active immunotherapy differs from nonspecific immune-based therapies in that the goal is specific activation of the immune system to eliminate tumor cells. Theoretically, these vaccines activate a unique lymphocyte (B- or T-cell, or both) response, which has an immediate antitumor effect as well as a memory response against future tumor challenge. B-cell malignancies present a unique opportunity for vaccine therapy. Malignant B lymphocytes clonally express Ig molecules, and because of their molecular structure, immunoglobulins represent tumor-specific antigens. The surface Ig displays antigenic determinants within the variable regions of the Ig heavy and light chains, termed *idiotypes*, which are uniquely expressed on the malignant cells. The harvest of sufficient quantities of lymphoma Ig for the production of an idiotype protein vaccine is accomplished by creating somatic cell hybrids between the lymphoma B cell and a non–Ig-producing myeloma cell. In the first clinical trial of idiotype vaccination for follicular non-Hodgkin's B-cell lymphoma (141), nine patients with minimal residual disease or a complete remission after chemotherapy received a series of subcutaneous injections of the Ig derived from tumor cells, which had been conjugated to keyhole limpet hemocyanin and emulsified in an immunologic adjuvant. Seven of the nine patients developed idiotype-specific immunologic responses: two humoral, four cell-mediated, and one both. Two patients with measurable disease had partial responses. Toxicity of the idiotype vaccine was minimal and limited to local reactions at the site of injections. In a subsequent update of the study (142), 41 patients were treated with the same idiotype vaccine. Twenty patients (49%) generated specific immune responses against the idiotypes of their tumor Ig. Two patients with residual disease, who developed immune responses, had complete responses. At a median follow-up from diagnosis of 7.3 years, the overall and disease-free survival of all 20 patients who mounted antiidiotype immune responses were significantly prolonged compared to patients who did not develop an immune response. In another trial, 20 patients with follicular lymphoma in first complete remission after chemotherapy were vaccinated with the idiotype protein coupled to keyhole limpet hemocyanin plus locally administered granulocyte-monocyte colony-stimulating factor (143). Eleven patients had positive PCR for the translocation (14,18) in their peripheral blood. After vaccination, eight of the 11 patients converted to negative PCR for t(14;18) in the peripheral blood. Tumor-specific cytotoxic CD8$^+$ and CD4$^+$ T cells were found in 19 of 20 patients. Antibodies were demonstrated in some patients but were not necessary for molecular responses. Prospective randomized trials are in progress to confirm the clinical benefit of idiotype vaccines.

One approach to stimulate the effective processing and presentation of antigens to the immune system is the use of antigen-presenting cells; the most immunologically powerful are dendritic cells. Dendritic cells, derived from the bone marrow, are present in most tissues, including skin, liver, lung, spleen, and lymphoid organs. They express high levels of major histocompatibility complex class I and II antigens and are capable of presenting antigens for days, stimulating naive T cells to respond to antigens, inducing protective immunity against tumor challenge, and producing IL-12, a potent cytokine that induces the development of interferon-γ producing cells. Methods have been developed to isolate dendritic cells from the peripheral blood. These cells can be cocultured or pulsed with antigens and reinfused intravenously as a vaccine. In a clinical trial (144), 35 patients with follicular non-Hodgkin's lymphoma were vaccinated with four intravenous infusions of dendritic cells pulsed with idiotype protein, followed 2 weeks later by subcutaneous injection of the soluble idiotype protein. In the first ten treated patients with relapsed measurable lymphoma, antiidiotype cellular proliferative responses were measured in eight, whereas antiidiotype humoral responses were not detected. Clinical responses included two complete remissions, one partial remission, and one molecular response. Twenty-five additional patients were vaccinated after chemotherapy. Fifteen of 23 (65%) who completed the vaccination schedule generated cellular or humoral antiidiotype responses. Among 18 patients with residual tumor at the time of vaccination, four (22%) had tumor regression, and 16 of 23 patients (70%) remain without tumor progression at a median of 43 months after chemotherapy. These results are encouraging and suggest clinical activity of idiotype-pulsed dendritic cell vaccination in follicular non-Hodgkin's lymphoma; larger trials are necessary to confirm this benefit.

In T-cell malignancies, tumor-specific T-cell receptor can serve as a target for active immunotherapy. In a murine model, vaccination with T-cell receptor protected mice from a subsequent lethal dose of tumor cells (145). Only vaccines containing adjuvants that induced Th1-type immune responses favored tumor protection. Based on these results, future T-cell receptor vaccines are designed to maintain T-cell receptor conformation and induce a strong Th1-type immune response.

In conclusion, vaccine therapy for lymphoma is a very promising adjunct to conventional therapies. The tumor-specific idiotype serves as an ideal target for B-cell lymphoma vaccine development because of its specificity and therapeutic potentials. In addition, T-cell malignancies could be targeted with tumor-specific T-cell receptor determinants. Future studies would likely focus on integration of these vaccine approaches with current standard therapies.

INTERFERON

Interferon-α is a biologic agent that influences the proliferation of lymphocytes and has been shown to be active in low-grade follicular lymphoma, with objective responses in 30% to 50%

TABLE 13.8. *Randomized studies of interferon-α treatment in follicular lymphomas*

Chemotherapy	No. of patients	Percent response	Time to progression	Overall survival	Reference
COPA[a]	147	86	20 mo (median)	5.7 yr (median)	152,153
vs.					
COPA with IFN-α 6 MU/m² d 22–26 of each cycle	141	86 (NS)	30 mo (median) ($p = .001$)	7.8 yr (median) ($p = .04$)	
CHVP[b]	119	69	1.5 yr (median)	5.6 yr (median)	154, 155
vs.					
CHVP with IFN-α 5 MU 3×/wk × 18 mo	123	86 ($p = .006$)	2.9 yr (median) ($p = .0002$)	Not reached ($p = .008$)	
C[c]	531 (total in both arms)	89	40% at 3 yr	80% at 3 yr	156
vs.					
C as above with IFN-α 2 MU/m² 3d/wk		84 (NS)	37% at 3 yr (NS)	78% at 3 yr (NS)	
CVP[d]	120	79	22 mo (median)	80% at 5 yr	157
vs.					
CVP with IFN-α 3 MU 3×/wk × 12 mo	122	80 (NS)	33 mo (median) ($p = .12$)	80% at 5 yr (NS)	

IFN, interferon-α; MU, million units; NS, not significant.
[a]COPA: cyclophosphamide, 600 mg/m² on day 1; vincristine, 1.2 mg/m² on day 1; prednisone, 100 mg/m² on days 1-5; doxorubicin, 50 mg/m² on day 1, × 8 to 10 cycles. CHVP: cyclophosphamide, 600 mg/m² on day 1; teniposide (VM-26), 60 mg/m² on day 1; prednisone, 40 mg/m² on days 1 to 5; adriamycin, 25 mg/m² on day 1, × 8 to 10 cycles.;
[b]CHVP: cyclophosphamide, 600 mg/m² on day 1; doxorubicin, 25 mg/m² on day 1; teniposide (VM26), 60 mg/m² on day 1; prednisone, 40 mg/m² days 1 to 5.
[c]C: cyclophosphamide, 100 mg/m²/day.
[d]CVP: cyclophosphamide, 300 mg/m² days 1 to 5; vincristine, 1.2 mg/m² day 1; prednisone, 40 mg/m² days 1 to 5.

of patients with relapsed follicular lymphoma (146–151). It has been used alone or in combination with chemotherapy during either induction or maintenance treatment. The use of interferon concurrently with chemotherapy in remission induction and maintenance has been evaluated in randomized studies (Table 13.8) (152–157). The two studies that used anthracycline-based chemotherapy showed an improvement in disease-free and overall survival (152–155). Two studies evaluated the use of interferon as maintenance treatment for patients who had achieved a remission with chemotherapy. One study showed an improvement in disease-free survival but not in overall survival (157). The other study showed improved disease-free survival, although overall survival duration was not reached in either arm (158). In another study, 127 patients with low-grade stage IV lymphoma were treated with CHOP and bleomycin for 9 to 18 months followed by interferon alfa-n-1 maintenance therapy for 24 months for those patients who had achieved a complete remission (159). Compared to 96 historical patients treated with only CHOP and bleomycin with similar pretreatment features, the relapse-free survival for the complete responses was significantly improved in the interferon cohort.

A metaanalysis was performed based on published data from nine separate studies adding interferon-α to chemotherapy regimens (160). Patients receiving interferon in either induction or maintenance therapy had significantly increased overall and progression-free survival rates at 3 and 5 years compared with concurrent controls. The advantages of interferon therapy were most marked in studies using anthracycline-containing induction chemotherapy; patients who received interferon had approximately 20% increased progression-free survival rates compared with controls. In intermediate and high-grade lymphoma, a prospective randomized study of CHOP versus CHOP plus interferon showed no response or survival advantage by adding interferon to chemotherapy (161).

In summary, the majority of data indicates a role for interferon in the treatment of follicular lymphoma. It appears most active in patients who have received anthracycline-based chemotherapy. However, interferon is not routinely used in the treatment of follicular lymphoma, likely because of its toxicity and only modest improvement in clinical benefit.

Antisense Oligonucleotides

Antisense oligonucleotides have been proposed as therapeutic agents in oncology for over two decades (162). Preclinical data suggest that translation of mRNA into proteins can be blocked by sequences of antisense RNA (163). Based on the specification of base pairing of Watson and Crick, it provides a rationale for oligonucleotides as anticancer drugs. Proteins whose overexpression contributes to the malignant phenotype are putative targets for downregulation through binding and destruction of mRNA. Antisense sequences of RNA from high-affinity covalent bands with mRNA should inhibit splicing and, therefore, impede translation, allowing the complex to be degraded by RNaseH (164,165). Substituting a sulfur atom for a nonbridging oxygen in the phosphate backbone of oligonucleotides confers nuclease resistance with favorable pharmacokinetic properties (166). The effect of downregulating mRNA encoding bcl-2 is an obvious target for follicular lymphoma. *In vitro* and *in vivo* studies have demonstrated the antitumor activity of antisense oligonucleotides to bcl-2 (167–170).

Twenty-one patients with bcl-2 positive lymphoma were treated with 14 daily subcutaneous doses of an antisense oligonucleotide against the bcl-2 oncogene designated oblimersen sodium (G3139, Genasense) (171). Dose-limiting toxicity was thrombocytopenia, hypotension, fever, and asthenia. One of three patients at an intermediate dose had a complete response. There were two minor responses and nine stable diseases, and seven of 16 patients had a reduction in the bcl-2 protein levels assessed in lymph nodes, peripheral blood, and bone marrow.

Twenty patients with chronic lymphocytic leukemia who relapsed after fludarabine or were refractory to fludarabine were treated in a phase II monotherapy trial with oblimersen sodium at 3 mg per kg per day for 5 to 7 days every 3 to 4 weeks (172). Thirteen patients were evaluable at this interim report, plus six additional patients from a phase I trial treated at the same dose. Of the 19 patients evaluable for response who received at least two cycles of therapy, two achieved a partial response, nine had stable disease, and eight progressed. The therapy was well tolerated, with low-grade fever as the most common adverse event. These results suggest that bcl-2 antisense therapy for lymphoma and chronic lymphocytic leukemia is feasible, has potential antitumor activity, and specifically downregulates bcl-2 protein.

REFERENCES

1. Kohler G, Milstein C. Continuous cultures of fused cells secreting antibody of predefined specificity. *Nature* 1975;256:495–497.
2. Nadler LM, Stashenko P, Hardy R, et al. Serotherapy of a patient with a monoclonal antibody directed against a human lymphoma-associated antigen. *Cancer Res* 1980;40:3147–3154.
3. Dyer MJ, Hale G, Hayhoe FG, et al. Effects of CAMPATH-1 antibodies in vivo in patients with lymphoid malignancies: influence of antibody isotype. *Blood* 1989;73:1431–1439.
4. Scheinberg DA, Straus DJ, Yeh SD, et al. A phase I toxicity, pharmacology, and dosimetry trial of monoclonal antibody OKB7 in patients with non-Hodgkin's lymphoma: effects of tumor burden and antigen expression. *J Clin Oncol* 1990;8:792–803.
5. Foon KA, Schroff RW, Bunn PA, et al. Effects of monoclonal antibody therapy in patients with chronic lymphocytic leukemia. *Blood* 1984;64:1085–1093.
6. Dillman RO, Beauregard J, Shawler DL, et al. Continuous infusion of T101 monoclonal antibody in chronic lymphocytic leukemia and cutaneous T-cell lymphoma. *J Biol Response Mod* 1986;5:394–410.
7. Hu E, Epstein AL, Naeve GS, et al. A phase 1a clinical trial of LYM-1 monoclonal antibody serotherapy in patients with refractory B cell malignancies. *Hematol Oncol* 1989;7:155–166.
8. Press OW, Appelbaum F, Ledbetter JA, et al. Monoclonal antibody 1F5 (anti-CD20) serotherapy of human B cell lymphomas. *Blood* 1987;69:584–591.
9. Waldmann TA, Goldman CK, Bongiovanni KF, et al. Therapy of patients with human T-cell lymphotrophic virus I-induced adult T-cell leukemia with anti-Tac, a monoclonal antibody to the receptor for interleukin-2. *Blood* 1988;72:1805–1816.
10. Miller RA, Oseroff AR, Stratte PT, et al. Monoclonal antibody therapeutic trials in seven patients with T-cell lymphoma. *Blood* 1983;62:988–995.
11. Multani PS, Grossbard ML. Monoclonal antibody-based therapies for hematologic malignancies. *J Clin Oncol* 1998;16:3691–3710.
12. Press OW. Prospects for the management of non-Hodgkin's lymphomas with monoclonal antibodies and immunoconjugates. *Cancer J Sci Am* 1998;4[Suppl 2]:S19–S26.
13. Davis TA, Maloney DG, Czerwinski DK, et al. Anti-idiotype antibodies can induce long-term complete remissions in non-Hodgkin's lymphoma without eradicating the malignant clone. *Blood* 1998;92:1184–1190.
14. Miller RA, Maloney DG, Warnke R, et al. Treatment of B-cell lymphoma with monoclonal anti-idiotype antibody. *N Engl J Med* 1982;306:517–522.
15. Meeker TC, Lowder J, Maloney DG, et al. A clinical trial of anti-idiotype therapy for B cell malignancy. *Blood* 1985;65:1349–1363.
16. Maloney DG, Brown S, Czerwinski DK, et al. Monoclonal anti-idiotype antibody therapy of B-cell lymphoma: the addition of a short course of chemotherapy does not interfere with the antitumor effect nor prevent the emergence of idiotype-negative variant cells. *Blood* 1992;80:1502–1510.
17. Brown SL, Miller RA, Horning SJ, et al. Treatment of B-cell lymphomas with anti-idiotype antibodies alone and in combination with alpha interferon. *Blood* 1989;73:651–661.
18. Meeker T, Lowder J, Cleary ML, et al. Emergence of idiotype variants during treatment of B-cell lymphoma with anti-idiotype antibodies. *N Engl J Med* 1985;312:1658–1665.
19. Chatterjee M, Barcos M, Han T, et al. Shared idiotype expression by chronic lymphocytic leukemia and B-cell lymphoma. *Blood* 1990;76:1825–1829.
20. Swisher EM, Shawler DL, Collins HA, et al. Expression of shared idiotypes in chronic lymphocytic leukemia and small lymphocytic lymphoma. *Blood* 1991;77:1977–1982.
21. Maloney DG, Grillo-Lopez AJ, White CA, et al. IDEC-C2B8 (Rituximab) anti-CD20 monoclonal antibody therapy in patients with relapsed low-grade non-Hodgkin's lymphoma. *Blood* 1997;90:2188–2195.
22. Maloney DG, Grillo-Lopez AJ, Bodkin DJ, et al. IDEC-C2B8: results of a phase I multiple-dose trial in patients with relapsed non-Hodgkin's lymphoma. *J Clin Oncol* 1997;15:3266–3274.
23. Berinstein NL, Grillo-Lopez AJ, White CA, et al. Association of serum Rituximab (IDEC-C2B8) concentration and anti-tumor response in the treatment of recurrent low-grade or follicular non-Hodgkin's lymphoma. *Ann Oncol* 1998;9:995–1001.
24. Walewski J, Kraszewska E, Mioduszewska O, et al. Rituximab (Mabthera, Rituxan) in patients with recurrent indolent lymphoma: evaluation of safety and efficacy in a multicenter study. *Med Oncol* 2001;18:141–148.
25. McLaughlin P, Grillo-Lopez AJ, Link BK, et al. Rituximab chimeric anti-CD20 monoclonal antibody therapy for relapsed indolent lymphoma: half of patients respond to a four-dose treatment program. *J Clin Oncol* 1998;16:2825–2833.
26. Davis TA, White CA, Grillo-Lopez AJ, et al. Single-agent monoclonal antibody efficacy in bulky non-Hodgkin's lymphoma: results of a phase II trial of rituximab. *J Clin Oncol* 1999;17:1851–1857.
27. Feuring-Buske M, Kneba M, Unterhalt M, et al. IDEC-C2B8 (Rituximab) anti-CD20 antibody treatment in relapsed advanced-stage follicular lymphomas: results of a phase-II study of the German Low-Grade Lymphoma Study Group. *Ann Hematol* 2000;79:493–500.
28. Hainsworth JD, Burris HA III, Morrissey LH, et al. Rituximab monoclonal antibody as initial systemic therapy for patients with low-grade non-Hodgkin lymphoma. *Blood* 2000;95:3052–3056.
29. Hainsworth JD, Litchy S, Burris HA III, et al. Rituximab as first-line and maintenance therapy for patients with indolent non-Hodgkin's lymphoma. *J Clin Oncol* 2002;20:4261–4267.
30. Colombat P, Salles G, Brousse N, et al. Rituximab (anti-CD20 monoclonal antibody) as single first-line therapy for patients with follicular lymphoma with a low tumor burden: clinical and molecular evaluation. *Blood* 2001;97:101–106.

31. Piro LD, White CA, Grillo-Lopez AJ, et al. Extended rituximab (anti-CD20 monoclonal antibody) therapy for relapsed or refractory low-grade or follicular non-Hodgkin's lymphoma. *Ann Oncol* 1999;10:655–661.

32. Aviles A, Leon MI, Diaz-Maqueo JC, et al. Rituximab in the treatment of refractory follicular lymphoma—six doses are better than four. *J Hematother Stem Cell Res* 2001;10:313–316.

33. Ansell SM, Witzig TE, Kurtin PJ, et al. Phase 1 study of interleukin-12 in combination with rituximab in patients with B-cell non-Hodgkin lymphoma. *Blood* 2002;99:67–74.

34. Sacchi S, Federico M, Vitolo U, et al. Clinical activity and safety of combination immunotherapy with IFN-alpha 2a and rituximab in patients with relapsed low grade non-Hodgkin's lymphoma. *Haematologica* 2001;86:951–958.

35. Davis TA, Maloney DG, Grillo-Lopez AJ, et al. Combination immunotherapy of relapsed or refractory low-grade or follicular non-Hodgkin's lymphoma with rituximab and interferon-alpha-2a. *Clin Cancer Res* 2000;6:2644–2652.

36. Czuczman MS, Grillo-Lopez AJ, White CA, et al. Treatment of patients with low-grade B-cell lymphoma with the combination of chimeric anti-CD20 monoclonal antibody and CHOP chemotherapy. *J Clin Oncol* 1999;17:268–276.

37. Czuczman MS. CHOP plus rituximab chemoimmunotherapy of indolent B-cell lymphoma. *Semin Oncol* 1999;26:88–96.

38. Rambaldi A, Lazzari M, Manzoni C, et al. Monitoring of minimal residual disease after CHOP and rituximab in previously untreated patients with follicular lymphoma. *Blood* 2002;99:856–862.

39. Coiffier B, Haioun C, Ketterer N, et al. Rituximab (anti-CD20 monoclonal antibody) for the treatment of patients with relapsing or refractory aggressive lymphoma: a multicenter phase II study. *Blood* 1998; 92:1927–1932.

40. Coiffier B, Lepage E, Briere J, et al. CHOP chemotherapy plus rituximab compared with CHOP alone in elderly patients with diffuse large-B-cell lymphoma. *N Engl J Med* 2002;346:235–242.

41. Vose JM, Link BK, Grossbard ML, et al. Phase II study of rituximab in combination with CHOP chemotherapy in patients with previously untreated, aggressive non-Hodgkin's lymphoma. *J Clin Oncol* 2001; 19:389–397.

42. Wilson WH, Gutierrez M, O'Connor P, et al. The role of rituximab and chemotherapy in aggressive B-cell lymphoma: a preliminary report of dose-adjusted EPOCH-R. *Semin Oncol* 2002;29[1 Suppl 2]: 41–47.

43. Howard OM, Gribben JG, Neuberg DS, et al. Rituximab and CHOP induction therapy for newly diagnosed mantle-cell lymphoma: molecular complete responses are not predictive of progression-free survival. *J Clin Oncol* 2002;20:1288–1294.

44. Joyce RM, Kraser CN, Tetrealt JC, et al. Rituximab and ifosfamide, mitoxantrone, etoposide (RIME) with Neupogen support for B-cell non-Hodgkin's lymphoma prior to high-dose chemotherapy with autologous haematopoietic transplant. *Eur J Haematol Suppl* 2001; 56–62.

45. Ladetto M, Zallio F, Vallet S, et al. Concurrent administration of high-dose chemotherapy and rituximab is a feasible and effective chemo/immunotherapy for patients with high-risk non-Hodgkin's lymphoma. *Leukemia* 2001;15:1941–1949.

46. Byrd JC, Murphy T, Howard RS, et al. Rituximab using a thrice weekly dosing schedule in B-cell chronic lymphocytic leukemia and small lymphocytic lymphoma demonstrates clinical activity and acceptable toxicity. *J Clin Oncol* 2001;19:2153–2164.

47. O'Brien SM, Kantarjian H, Thomas DA, et al. Rituximab dose-escalation trial in chronic lymphocytic leukemia. *J Clin Oncol* 2001; 19:2165–2170.

48. Winkler U, Jensen M, Manzke O, et al. Cytokine-release syndrome in patients with B-cell chronic lymphocytic leukemia and high lymphocyte counts after treatment with an anti-CD20 monoclonal antibody (rituximab, IDEC-C2B8). *Blood* 1999;94:2217–2224.

49. Byrd JC, Kitada S, Flinn IW, et al. The mechanism of tumor cell clearance by rituximab in vivo in patients with B-cell chronic lymphocytic leukemia: evidence of caspase activation and apoptosis induction. *Blood* 2002;99:1038–1043.

50. Alas S, Bonavida B. Rituximab inactivates signal transducer and activation of transcription 3 (STAT3) activity in B-non-Hodgkin's lymphoma through inhibition of the interleukin 10 autocrine/paracrine loop and results in down-regulation of Bcl-2 and sensitization to cytotoxic drugs. *Cancer Res* 2001;61:5137–5144.

51. Di Gaetano N, Xiao Y, Erba E, et al. Synergism between fludarabine and rituximab revealed in a follicular lymphoma cell line resistant to the cytotoxic activity of either drug alone. *Br J Haematol* 2001; 114:800–809.

52. O'Brien S, Kantarjian H, Beran M, et al. Results of fludarabine and prednisone therapy in 264 patients with chronic lymphocytic leukemia with multivariate analysis-derived prognostic model for response to treatment. *Blood* 1993;82:1695–1700.

53. Keating MJ, O'Brien S, Kantarjian H, et al. Long-term follow-up of patients with chronic lymphocytic leukemia treated with fludarabine as a single agent. *Blood* 1993;81:2878–2884.

54. Alas S, Emmanouilides C, Bonavida B. Inhibition of interleukin 10 by rituximab results in down-regulation of bcl-2 and sensitization of B-cell non-Hodgkin's lymphoma to apoptosis. *Clin Cancer Res* 2001;7:709–723.

55. Schulz H, Klein SK, Rehwald U, et al. Phase 2 study of a combined immunochemotherapy using rituximab and fludarabine in patients with chronic lymphocytic leukemia. *Blood* 2002;100:3115–3120.

56. Byrd JC, Peterson BL, Morrison VA, et al. Randomized phase 2 study of fludarabine with concurrent versus sequential treatment with rituximab in symptomatic, untreated patients with B-cell chronic lymphocytic leukemia: results from Cancer and Leukemia Group B 9712 (CALGB 9712). *Blood* 2003;101:6–14.

57. Keating MJ, O'Brien S, Albitar M. Emerging information on the use of rituximab in chronic lymphocytic leukemia. *Semin Oncol* 2002;29:70–74.

58. Dimopoulos MA, Zervas C, Zomas A, et al. Treatment of Waldenström's macroglobulinemia with rituximab. *J Clin Oncol* 2002;20: 2327–2333.

59. Heinzerling LM, Urbanek M, Funk JO, et al. Reduction of tumor burden and stabilization of disease by systemic therapy with anti-CD20 antibody (rituximab) in patients with primary cutaneous B-cell lymphoma. *Cancer* 2000;89:1835–1844.

60. Riechmann L, Clark M, Waldmann H, et al. Reshaping human antibodies for therapy. *Nature* 1988;332:323–327.

61. Gilleece MH, Dexter TM. Effect of Campath-1H antibody on human hematopoietic progenitors in vitro. *Blood* 1993;82:807–812.

62. Dyer MJS, Hale G, Marcus R, et al. Remission induction in patients with lymphoid malignancies using unconjugated CAMPATH-1 monoclonal antibodies. *Leuk Lymphoma* 1990;2:179–193.

63. Osterborg A, Dyer MJ, Bunjes D, et al. Phase II multicenter study of human CD52 antibody in previously treated chronic lymphocytic leukemia. European Study Group of CAMPATH-1H Treatment in Chronic Lymphocytic Leukemia. *J Clin Oncol* 1997;15: 1567–1574.

64. Keating MJ, Flinn I, Jain V, et al. Therapeutic role of alemtuzumab (Campath-1H) in patients who have failed fludarabine: results of a large international study. *Blood* 2002;99:3554–3561.

65. Rai KR, Freter CE, Mercier RJ, et al. Alemtuzumab in previously treated chronic lymphocytic leukemia patients who also had received fludarabine. *J Clin Oncol* 2002;20:3891–3897.

66. Osterborg A, Fassas AS, Anagnostopoulos A, et al. Humanized CD52 monoclonal antibody Campath-1H as first-line treatment in chronic lymphocytic leukaemia. *Br J Haematol* 1996;93:151–153.

67. Pawson R, Dyer MJ, Barge R, et al. Treatment of T-cell prolymphocytic leukemia with human CD52 antibody. *J Clin Oncol* 1997;15:2667–2672.

68. Lundin J, Osterborg A, Brittinger G, et al. CAMPATH-1H monoclonal antibody in therapy for previously treated low-grade non-Hodgkin's lymphomas: a phase II multicenter study. European Study Group of CAMPATH-1H Treatment in Low-Grade Non-Hodgkin's Lymphoma. *J Clin Oncol* 1998;16:3257–3263.

69. Khorana A, Bunn P, McLaughlin P, et al. A phase II multicenter study of CAMPATH-1H antibody in previously treated patients with non-bulky non-Hodgkin's lymphoma. *Leuk Lymphoma* 2001;41:77–87.

70. Clark EA. CD22, a B cell-specific receptor, mediates adhesion and signal transduction. *J Immunol* 1993;150:4715–4718.

71. Pawlak-Byczkowska EJ, Hansen HJ, Dion AS, et al. Two new monoclonal antibodies, EPB-1 and EPB-2, reactive with human lymphoma. *Cancer Res* 1989;49:4568–4577.

72. Leonard JP, Coleman M, Matthews JC. Phase I/II trial of epratuzumab (humanized anti-CD22 antibody) in non-Hodgkin's lymphoma (NHL). *Blood* 2002;100:358a(abstract).

73. Leonard JP, Coleman M, Matthews JC. Epratuzumab (anti-CD22) and rituximab (anti-CD20) combination immunotherapy for non-

Hodgkin's lymphoma: preliminary response data. *Proc Am Soc Clin Oncol* 2002;21:266a(abstract).

74. Kostelny SA, Link BK, Tso JY, et al. Humanization and characterization of the anti-HLA-DR antibody 1D10. *Int J Cancer* 2001;93:556–565.

75. Link BK, Wang H, Byrd JC. Phase I study of Hu1D10 monoclonal antibody in patients with B-cell lymphoma. *Proc Am Soc Clin Oncol* 2001;20:244a(abstract).

76. Link BK, Wang H, Byrd JC. A phase II study of RemitogenT (Hu1D10), a humanized monoclonal antibody in patients with relapsed or refractory follicular, small lymphocytic, or marginal zone/MALT B-cell lymphoma. *Blood* 2001;98:2540a(abstract).

77. Goldenberg DM. Targeted therapy of cancer with radiolabeled antibodies. *J Nucl Med* 2002;43:693–713.

78. Dillman RO. Radiolabeled anti-CD20 monoclonal antibodies for the treatment of B-cell lymphoma. *J Clin Oncol* 2002;20:3545–3557.

79. Kaminski MS, Zasadny KR, Francis IR, et al. Radioimmunotherapy of B-cell lymphoma with [131I]anti-B1 (anti-CD20) antibody. *N Engl J Med* 1993;329:459–465.

80. Kaminski MS, Zasadny KR, Francis IR, et al. Iodine-131-anti-B1 radioimmunotherapy for B-cell lymphoma. *J Clin Oncol* 1996;14:1974–1981.

81. Gates VL, Carey JE, Siegel JA, et al. Nonmyeloablative iodine-131 anti-B1 radioimmunotherapy as outpatient therapy. *J Nucl Med* 1998;39:1230–1236.

82. Wahl RL, Zasadny KR, MacFarlane D, et al. Iodine-131 anti-B1 antibody for B-cell lymphoma: an update on the Michigan Phase I experience. *J Nucl Med* 1998;39:21S–27S.

83. Kaminski MS, Estes J, Zasadny KR, et al. Radioimmunotherapy with iodine (131)I tositumomab for relapsed or refractory B-cell non-Hodgkin lymphoma: updated results and long-term follow-up of the University of Michigan experience. *Blood* 2000;96:1259–1266.

84. Vose JM, Wahl RL, Saleh M, et al. Multicenter phase II study of iodine-131 tositumomab for chemotherapy-relapsed/refractory low-grade and transformed low-grade B-cell non-Hodgkin's lymphomas. *J Clin Oncol* 2000;18:1316–1323.

85. Kaminski MS, Zelenetz AD, Press OW. High response rates and durable remissions in patients with previously untreated, advanced-stage, follicular lymphoma treated with tositumomab and iodine I-131 tositumomab (Bexxarr). *Blood* 2002;100:356a(abstract).

86. Kaminski MS, Zelenetz AD, Press OW. Pivotal study of iodine I 131 tositumomab for chemotherapy-refractory low-grade or transformed low-grade B-cell non-Hodgkin's lymphomas. *J Clin Oncol* 2001;19:3918–3928.

87. Leonard JP, Coleman M, Kostakoglu L. Fludarabine monophosphate followed by iodine I 131 tositumomab for untreated low-grade and follicular non-Hodgkin's lymphomas (NHL). *Blood* 1999;94:90a(abstract).

88. Liu SY, Eary JF, Petersdorf SH, et al. Follow-up of relapsed B-cell lymphoma patients treated with iodine-131-labeled anti-CD20 antibody and autologous stem-cell rescue. *J Clin Oncol* 1998;16:3270–3278.

89. Press OW, Eary JF, Appelbaum FR, et al. Phase II trial of 131I-B1 (anti-CD20) antibody therapy with autologous stem cell transplantation for relapsed B cell lymphomas. *Lancet* 1995;346:336–340.

90. Press OW, Eary JF, Gooley T, et al. A phase I/II trial of iodine-131-tositumomab (anti-CD20), etoposide, cyclophosphamide, and autologous stem cell transplantation for relapsed B-cell lymphomas. *Blood* 2000;96:2934–2942.

91. Gopal AK, Rajendran JG, Petersdorf SH, et al. High-dose chemoradioimmunotherapy with autologous stem cell support for relapsed mantle cell lymphoma. *Blood* 2002;99:3158–3162.

92. Witzig TE, Flinn IW, Gordon LI, et al. Treatment with ibritumomab tiuxetan radioimmunotherapy in patients with rituximab-refractory follicular non-Hodgkin's lymphoma. *J Clin Oncol* 2002;20:3262–3269.

93. Wiseman GA, Gordon LI, Multani PS, et al. Ibritumomab tiuxetan radioimmunotherapy for patients with relapsed or refractory non-Hodgkin lymphoma and mild thrombocytopenia: a phase II multicenter trial. *Blood* 2002;99:4336–4342.

94. Witzig TE, Gordon LI, Cabanillas F, et al. Randomized controlled trial of yttrium-90-labeled ibritumomab tiuxetan radioimmunotherapy versus rituximab immunotherapy for patients with relapsed or refractory low-grade, follicular, or transformed B-cell non-Hodgkin's lymphoma. *J Clin Oncol* 2002;20:2453–2463.

95. Shih LB, Lu HH, Xuan H, et al. Internalization and intracellular processing of an anti-B-cell lymphoma monoclonal antibody, LL2. *Int J Cancer* 1994;56:538–545.

96. Sharkey RM, Behr TM, Mattes MJ, et al. Advantage of residualizing radiolabels for an internalizing antibody against the B-cell lymphoma antigen, CD22. *Cancer Immunol Immunother* 1997;44:179–188.

97. Goldenberg DM, Horowitz JA, Sharkey RM, et al. Targeting, dosimetry, and radioimmunotherapy of B-cell lymphomas with iodine-131-labeled LL2 monoclonal antibody. *J Clin Oncol* 1991;9:548–564.

98. Juweid M, Sharkey RM, Markowitz A, et al. Treatment of non-Hodgkin's lymphoma with radiolabeled murine, chimeric, or humanized LL2, an anti-CD22 monoclonal antibody. *Cancer Res* 1995;55:5899s–5907s.

99. Vose JM, Colcher D, Gobar L, et al. Phase I/II trial of multiple dose 131Iodine-MAb LL2 (CD22) in patients with recurrent non-Hodgkin's lymphoma. *Leuk Lymphoma* 2000;38:91–101.

100. Linden O, Tennvall J, Cavallin-Stahl E, et al. Radioimmunotherapy using 131I-labeled anti-CD22 monoclonal antibody (LL2) in patients with previously treated B-cell lymphomas. *Clin Cancer Res* 1999;5:3287s–3291s.

101. Juweid ME, Stadtmauer E, Hajjar G, et al. Pharmacokinetics, dosimetry, and initial therapeutic results with 131I- and (111)In-/90Y-labeled humanized LL2 anti-CD22 monoclonal antibody in patients with relapsed, refractory non-Hodgkin's lymphoma. *Clin Cancer Res* 1999;5:3292s–3303s.

102. Juweid M, Schuster SL, Czuczman M. Updated results of radioimmunotherapy of relapsed refractory non-Hodgkin's lymphoma with conventional and stem cell supported doses of 90Y-labeled humanized LL2 anti-CD22 monoclonal antibody. *Cancer Biother Radiopharm* 2000;15:408(abstract).

103. Postema EJ, Mandigers CM, Oyen WJ. Radioimmunotherapy of patients with non-Hodgkin's lymphoma with 186Re-hLL2. *Cancer Biother Radiopharm* 2000;15:407(abstract).

104. Lewis JP, DeNardo GL, Denardo SJ. Radioimmunotherapy of lymphoma: a UC Davis experience. *Hybridoma* 1995;14:115–120.

105. DeNardo GL, DeNardo SJ, Goldstein DS, et al. Maximum-tolerated dose, toxicity, and efficacy of (131)I-Lym-1 antibody for fractionated radioimmunotherapy of non-Hodgkin's lymphoma. *J Clin Oncol* 1998;16:3246–3256.

106. DeNardo GL, DeNardo SJ, Lamborn KR, et al. Low-dose, fractionated radioimmunotherapy for B-cell malignancies using 131I-Lym-1 antibody. *Cancer Biother Radiopharm* 1998;13:239–254.

107. O'Donnell RT, DeNardo GL, Kukis DL, et al. 67Copper-2-iminothiolane-6-[p-(bromoacetamido)benzyl-TETA-Lym-1 for radioimmunotherapy of non-Hodgkin's lymphoma. *Clin Cancer Res* 1999;5:3330s–3336s.

108. DeNardo GL, Kroger LA, Mirick GR, et al. Analysis of antiglobulin (HAMA) response in a group of patients with B-lymphocytic malignancies treated with 131I-Lym-1. *Int J Biol Markers* 1995;10:67–74.

109. DeNardo SJ, Kroger LA, MacKenzie MR, et al. Prolonged survival associated with immune response in a patient treated with Lym-1 mouse monoclonal antibody. *Cancer Biother Radiopharm* 1998;13:1–12.

110. Vitetta ES, Stone M, Amlot P, et al. Phase I immunotoxin trial in patients with B-cell lymphoma. *Cancer Res* 1991;51:4052–4058.

111. Amlot PL, Stone MJ, Cunningham D, et al. A phase I study of an anti-CD22-deglycosylated ricin A chain immunotoxin in the treatment of B-cell lymphomas resistant to conventional therapy. *Blood* 1993;82:2624–2633.

112. Sausville EA, Headlee D, Stetler-Stevenson M, et al. Continuous infusion of the anti-CD22 immunotoxin IgG-RFB4-SMPT-dgA in patients with B-cell lymphoma: a phase I study. *Blood* 1995;85:3457–3465.

113. Stone MJ, Sausville EA, Fay JW, et al. A phase I study of bolus versus continuous infusion of the anti-CD19 immunotoxin, IgG-HD37-dgA, in patients with B-cell lymphoma. *Blood* 1996;88:1188–1197.

114. Farah RA, Clinchy B, Herrera L, et al. The development of monoclonal antibodies for the therapy of cancer. *Crit Rev Eukaryot Gene Expr* 1998;8:321–356.

115. Grossbard ML, Freedman AS, Ritz J, et al. Serotherapy of B-cell neoplasms with anti-B4-blocked ricin: a phase I trial of daily bolus infusion. *Blood* 1992;79:576–585.

116. Grossbard ML, Lambert JM, Goldmacher VS, et al. Anti-B4-blocked ricin: a phase I trial of 7-day continuous infusion in patients with B-cell neoplasms. *J Clin Oncol* 1993;11:726–737.

117. Grossbard ML, Multani PS, Freedman AS, et al. A phase II study of adjuvant therapy with anti-B4-blocked ricin after autologous bone

marrow transplantation for patients with relapsed B-cell non-Hodgkin's lymphoma. *Clin Cancer Res* 1999;5:2392–2398.

118. Multani PS, O'Day S, Nadler LM, et al. Phase II clinical trial of bolus infusion anti-B4 blocked ricin immunoconjugate in patients with relapsed B-cell non-Hodgkin's lymphoma. *Clin Cancer Res* 1998;4:2599–2604.

119. Williams DP, Parker K, Bacha P, et al. Diphtheria toxin receptor binding domain substitution with interleukin-2: genetic construction and properties of a diphtheria toxin-related interleukin-2 fusion protein. *Protein Eng* 1987;1:493–498.

120. LeMaistre CF, Meneghetti C, Rosenblum M, et al. Phase I trial of an interleukin-2 (IL-2) fusion toxin (DAB486IL-2) in hematologic malignancies expressing the IL-2 receptor. *Blood* 1992;79:2547–2554.

121. Hesketh P, Caguioa P, Koh H, et al. Clinical activity of a cytotoxic fusion protein in the treatment of cutaneous T-cell lymphoma. *J Clin Oncol* 1993;11:1682–1690.

122. Kuzel TM, Rosen ST, Gordon LI, et al. Phase I trial of the diphtheria toxin/interleukin-2 fusion protein DAB486IL-2: efficacy in mycosis fungoides and other non-Hodgkin's lymphomas. *Leuk Lymphoma* 1993;11:369–377.

123. LeMaistre CF, Craig FE, Meneghetti C, et al. Phase I trial of a 90-minute infusion of the fusion toxin DAB486IL-2 in hematological cancers. *Cancer Res* 1993;53:3930–3934.

124. Tepler I, Schwartz G, Parker K, et al. Phase I trial of an interleukin-2 fusion toxin (DAB486IL-2) in hematologic malignancies: complete response in a patient with Hodgkin's disease refractory to chemotherapy. *Cancer* 1994;73:1276–1285.

125. Foss FM, Borkowski TA, Gilliom M, et al. Chimeric fusion protein toxin DAB486IL-2 in advanced mycosis fungoides and the Sezary syndrome: correlation of activity and interleukin-2 receptor expression in a phase II study. *Blood* 1994;84:1765–1774.

126. LeMaistre CF, Saleh MN, Kuzel TM, et al. Phase I trial of a ligand fusion-protein (DAB389IL-2) in lymphomas expressing the receptor for interleukin-2. *Blood* 1998;91:399–405.

127. Saleh MN, LeMaistre CF, Kuzel TM, et al. Antitumor activity of DAB389IL-2 fusion toxin in mycosis fungoides. *J Am Acad Dermatol* 1998;39:63–73.

128. Chaudhary VK, Queen C, Junghans RP, et al. A recombinant immunotoxin consisting of two antibody variable domains fused to Pseudomonas exotoxin. *Nature* 1989;339:394–397.

129. Kreitman RJ, Chaudhary VK, Waldmann T, et al. The recombinant immunotoxin anti-Tac(Fv)-Pseudomonas exotoxin 40 is cytotoxic toward peripheral blood malignant cells from patients with adult T-cell leukemia. *Proc Natl Acad Sci U S A* 1990;87:8291–8295.

130. Kreitman RJ, Chaudhary VK, Waldmann TA, et al. Cytotoxic activities of recombinant immunotoxins composed of Pseudomonas toxin or diphtheria toxin toward lymphocytes from patients with adult T-cell leukemia. *Leukemia* 1993;7:553–562.

131. Saito T, Kreitman RJ, Hanada S, et al. Cytotoxicity of recombinant Fab and Fv immunotoxins on adult T-cell leukemia lymph node and blood cells in the presence of soluble interleukin-2 receptor. *Cancer Res* 1994;54:1059–1064.

132. Kreitman RJ, Wilson WH, White JD, et al. Phase I trial of recombinant immunotoxin anti-Tac(Fv)-PE38 (LMB-2) in patients with hematologic malignancies. *J Clin Oncol* 2000;18:1622–1636.

133. Kreitman RJ, Wilson WH, Bergeron K, et al. Efficacy of the anti-CD22 recombinant immunotoxin BL22 in chemotherapy-resistant hairy-cell leukemia. *N Engl J Med* 2001;345:241–247.

134. Liu C, Tadayoni BM, Bourret LA, et al. Eradication of large colon tumor xenografts by targeted delivery of maytansinoids. *Proc Natl Acad Sci U S A* 1996;93:8618–8623.

135. Hinman LM, Hamann PR, Wallace R, et al. Preparation and characterization of monoclonal antibody conjugates of the calicheamicins: a novel and potent family of antitumor antibiotics. *Cancer Res* 1993;53:3336–3342.

136. Yokota S, Hara H, Luo Y, et al. Synergistic potentiation of in vivo antitumor activity of anti-human T-leukemia immunotoxins by recombinant alpha-interferon and daunorubicin. *Cancer Res* 1990;50:32–37.

137. O'Connor R, Liu C, Ferris CA, et al. Anti-B4-blocked ricin synergizes with doxorubicin and etoposide on multidrug-resistant and drug-sensitive tumors. *Blood* 1995;86:4286–4294.

138. Bagshawe KD. Antibody directed enzymes revive anti-cancer pro-drugs concept. *Br J Cancer* 1987;56:531–532.

139. Hartmann F, Renner C, Jung W, et al. Treatment of refractory Hodgkin's disease with an anti-CD16/CD30 bispecific antibody. *Blood* 1997;89:2042–2047.

140. Weiner GJ, De Gast GC. Bispecific monoclonal antibody therapy of B-cell malignancy. *Leuk Lymphoma* 1995;16:199–207.

141. Kwak LW, Campbell MJ, Czerwinski DK, et al. Induction of immune responses in patients with B-cell lymphoma against the surface-immunoglobulin idiotype expressed by their tumors. *N Engl J Med* 1992;327:1209–1215.

142. Hsu FJ, Caspar CB, Czerwinski D, et al. Tumor-specific idiotype vaccines in the treatment of patients with B-cell lymphoma—long-term results of a clinical trial. *Blood* 1997;89:3129–3135.

143. Bendandi M, Gocke CD, Kobrin CB, et al. Complete molecular remissions induced by patient-specific vaccination plus granulocyte-monocyte colony-stimulating factor against lymphoma. *Nat Med* 1999;5:1171–1177.

144. Timmerman JM, Czerwinski DK, Davis TA, et al. Idiotype-pulsed dendritic cell vaccination for B-cell lymphoma: clinical and immune responses in 35 patients. *Blood* 2002;99:1517–1526.

145. Wong CP, Okada CY, Levy R. TCR vaccines against T cell lymphoma: QS-21 and IL-12 adjuvants induce a protective CD8+ T cell response. *J Immunol* 1999;162:2251–2258.

146. Horning SJ, Merigan TC, Krown SE, et al. Human interferon alpha in malignant lymphoma and Hodgkin's disease. Results of the American Cancer Society trial. *Cancer* 1985;56:1305–1310.

147. Louie AC, Gallagher JG, Sikora K, et al. Follow-up observations on the effect of human leukocyte interferon in non-Hodgkin's lymphoma. *Blood* 1981;58:712–718.

148. Quesada JR, Hawkins M, Horning S, et al. Collaborative phase I-II study of recombinant DNA-produced leukocyte interferon (clone A) in metastatic breast cancer, malignant lymphoma, and multiple myeloma. *Am J Med* 1984;77:427–432.

149. Foon KA, Roth MS, Bunn PA Jr. Interferon therapy of non-Hodgkin's lymphoma. *Cancer* 1987;59:601–604.

150. O'Connell MJ, Colgan JP, Oken MM, et al. Clinical trial of recombinant leukocyte A interferon as initial therapy for favorable histology non-Hodgkin's lymphomas and chronic lymphocytic leukemia. An Eastern Cooperative Oncology Group pilot study. *J Clin Oncol* 1986;4:128–136.

151. Foon KA, Sherwin SA, Abrams PG, et al. Treatment of advanced non-Hodgkin's lymphoma with recombinant leukocyte A interferon. *N Engl J Med* 1984;311:1148–1152.

152. Smalley RV, Andersen JW, Hawkins MJ, et al. Interferon alfa combined with cytotoxic chemotherapy for patients with non-Hodgkin's lymphoma. *N Engl J Med* 1992;327:1336–1341.

153. Andersen JW, Smalley RV. Interferon alfa plus chemotherapy for non-Hodgkin's lymphoma: five-year follow-up. *N Engl J Med* 1993;329:1821–1822.

154. Solal-Celigny P, Lepage E, Brousse N, et al. Recombinant interferon alfa-2b combined with a regimen containing doxorubicin in patients with advanced follicular lymphoma. Groupe d'Etude des Lymphomes de l'Adulte. *N Engl J Med* 1993;329:1608–1614.

155. Solal-Celigny P, Lepage E, Brousse N, et al. A doxorubicin containing regimen with or without interferon-α 2b (IFNα 2b) in advanced follicular lymphomas. Final analysis of survival, toxicity and quality of life of the GELF86 trial. *Blood* 88:453a(abstract).

156. Peterson BA, Petrioni G, Oken MM. Cyclophosphamide versus cyclophosphamide plus interferon alfa-2b in follicular low-grade lymphomas: a preliminary report from an Intergroup trial (CALGB 8691 and EST 7486). *Proc Am Soc Clin Oncol* 1993;12:366(abstract).

157. Hagenbeek A, Carde P, Meerwaldt JH, et al. Maintenance of remission with human recombinant interferon alfa-2a in patients with stages III and IV low-grade malignant non-Hodgkin's lymphoma. European Organization for Research and Treatment of Cancer Lymphoma Cooperative Group. *J Clin Oncol* 1998;16:41–47.

158. Aviles A, Duque G, Talavera A, et al. Interferon-α 2b as maintenance therapy in low grade malignant lymphoma improves duration of remission and survival. *Leuk Lymphoma* 1996;20:495–499

159. McLaughlin P, Cabanillas F, Hagemeister FB, et al. CHOP-Bleo plus interferon for stage IV low-grade lymphoma. *Ann Oncol* 1993;4:205–211.

160. Allen IE, Ross SD, Borden SP, et al. Meta-analysis to assess the efficacy of interferon-alpha in patients with follicular non-Hodgkin's lymphoma. *J Immunother* 2001;24:58–65.
161. Giles FJ, Shan J, Advani SH, et al. A prospective randomized study of CHOP versus CHOP plus Alpha-2B interferon in patients with intermediate and high grade non-Hodgkin's lymphoma: The International Oncology Study Group NHL1 study. *Leuk Lymphoma* 2001;40:95–103.
162. Flaherty KT, Stevenson JP, O'Dwyer PJ. Antisense therapeutics: lessons from early clinical trials. *Curr Opin Oncol* 2001;13:499–505.
163. Miyashita T, Reed JC. bcl-2 gene transfer increases relative resistance of S49.1 and WEHI7.2 lymphoid cells to cell death and DNA fragmentation induced by glucocorticoids and multiple chemotherapeutic drugs. *Cancer Res* 1992;52:5407–5411.
164. McDonnell TJ, Nunez G, Platt FM, et al. Deregulated Bcl-2-immunoglobulin transgene expands a resting but responsive immunoglobulin M and D-expressing B-cell population. *Mol Cell Biol* 1990;10:1901–1907.
165. McDonnell TJ, Korsmeyer SJ. Progression from lymphoid hyperplasia to high-grade malignant lymphoma in mice transgenic for the t(14;18). *Nature* 1991;349:254–256.
166. Hermine O, Haioun C, Lepage E, et al. Prognostic significance of bcl-2 protein expression in aggressive non-Hodgkin's lymphoma. Groupe d'Etude des Lymphomes de l'Adulte (GELA). *Blood* 1996;87:265–272.
167. Kitada S, Miyashita T, Tanaka S, et al. Investigations of antisense oligonucleotides targeted against bcl-2 RNAs. *Antisense Res Dev* 1993;3:157–169.
168. Kitada S, Takayama S, De Riel K, et al. Reversal of chemoresistance of lymphoma cells by antisense-mediated reduction of bcl-2 gene expression. *Antisense Res Dev* 1994;4:71–79.
169. Cotter FE, Johnson P, Hall P, et al. Antisense oligonucleotides suppress B-cell lymphoma growth in a SCID-hu mouse model. *Oncogene* 1994;9:3049–3055.
170. Mohammad R, Abubakr Y, Dan M, et al. Bcl-2 antisense oligonucleotides are effective against systemic but not central nervous system disease in severe combined immunodeficient mice bearing human t(14;18) follicular lymphoma. *Clin Cancer Res* 2002;8:1277–1283.
171. Waters JS, Webb A, Cunningham D, et al. Phase I clinical and pharmacokinetic study of bcl-2 antisense oligonucleotide therapy in patients with non-Hodgkin's lymphoma. *J Clin Oncol* 2000;18:1812–1823.
172. Rai KR, O'Brien S, Cunningham C. Genasense (Bcl-2 antisense) monotherapy in patients with relapsed or refractory chronic lymphocytic leukemia: phase 1 and 2 results. *Blood* 2002;100:384a(abstract).

Pathology, Biology, Clinical Evaluation, and Treatment Selection

Small B-Cell Lymphocytic Lymphoma/ Chronic Lymphocytic Leukemia and Prolymphocytic Leukemia

John G. Gribben, Nancy Lee Harris, and Riccardo Dalla-Favera

DEFINITIONS OF CHRONIC LYMPHOCYTIC LEUKEMIA AND SMALL LYMPHOCYTIC LYMPHOMA

Although historically chronic lymphocytic leukemia (CLL) was considered a different disease from small B-cell lymphocytic lymphoma (SLL), they are now believed to be simply different clinical manifestations of the same disease. In the World Health Organization Classification, B-cell SLL is considered as the tissue infiltrate of CLL (1). B-cell CLL/ SLL is a neoplasm of small, round B lymphocytes accompanied by larger cells known as *prolymphocytes*, expressing B-cell antigens and CD5 and CD23. When the disease involves the peripheral blood and bone marrow, it is called *CLL*, and when lymph nodes or other tissues are infiltrated by cells having identical morphologic and immunophenotypic features to CLL, but in which there are no leukemic manifestations of the disease, it is called *SLL*.

Etiology and Epidemiology

More than 7,000 cases of B-cell CLL/SLL are newly diagnosed in the United States every year, and recent data suggest that the incidence may be higher than that reported within the tumor registries (2). Only 5% of CLL/SLL patients present with clinical features of SLL without the leukemic component. The male to female ratio is 1.7:1.0. Although a higher incidence has been reported for whites compared to African-Americans (3), data from the National Cancer Institute's Surveillance, Epidemiology and End Results program (http://seer.cancer.gov/statistics) now suggest a more similar incidence pattern in these groups. CLL/SLL is considered to be mainly a disease of the elderly, with a median age at diagnosis of 70 years. It is extremely rare at younger than 30 years of age, but the incidence increases with increasing age. The Sur-

veillance, Epidemiology and End Results incidence crude rates in the nine registries program data for 1973 through 1999 show an incidence of 21 per 100,000 population in the age group 65 to 69 years and 33 in the age group 75 to 79 years (http://seer.cancer.gov/statistics). Younger patients do not have a worse prognosis than do older patients (4). Although younger and older patients have a similar survival, analysis of the relative survival rates showed that the disease had a greater adverse effect on the expected survival probability of the younger population, because the older patients often die of causes unrelated to their CLL.

The variation in international incidence patterns among the leukemias and lymphomas is most marked for B-cell CLL/SLL, and there is a 26-fold increase in incidence for men in Canada compared to those in Japan and a 38-fold increase for women between the United States and Japan (5). Genetic rather than environmental factors most likely explain these differences, because the disease is rare among Japanese-Americans (6).

Although occupational exposures can be linked to an excess occurrence of many cancers, there are no clearly discernible occupational or environmental risk factors that predispose to B-cell CLL/SLL. In particular, there is no evidence linking the disease to exposure to ionizing radiation (7). Although there have been reports of increased incidence among farm workers, this has not been substantiated (8,9). A report from the Institute of Medicine by a panel set up at the request of the Department of Veterans Affairs reexamined six separate studies on the possible link between Agent Orange and B-cell CLL/SLL and published findings in *Committee to Review the Health Effects in Vietnam Veterans of Exposure to Herbicides (Fourth Biennial Update)*. This report supported the idea that people exposed to Agent Orange, a pesticide used for defoliation in Vietnam, have a higher risk of B-cell CLL/SLL. Exposure to petrochemicals does not appear to increase the incidence of CLL/SLL (10). Similarly, whereas exposure to hair dyes has been suggested to be associated with an increased incidence of some types of non-Hodgkin's lymphoma, this was not the case for CLL/SLL (11).

Among the strongest risk factors for the development of B-cell CLL/SLL is a family history of this or other lymphoid malignancies. A number of familial clusters of B-cell CLL/SLL have been reported (12). More than 50 years ago, Videbaek reported that in familial cases of leukemia, the incidence of lymphoid leukemias was almost double that of myelogenous leukemias (13). In a report from the National Cancer Institute Familial Registry, the mean age at diagnosis among familial cases was 58 years, more than 12 years younger than the mean age of presentation observed in sporadic cases (14). A higher percentage of second primary tumors (16.0% vs. 8.8%) was also observed among familial than among sporadic CLL/SLL cases. Genetic anticipation, the process whereby the median age at onset in a child of a multigeneration family with malignancy is younger than that of the parent generations, has been observed in CLL/SLL (15–17). The risk of transformation to more aggressive non-Hodgkin's lymphomas does not appear to be different in familial cases from that reported for sporadic cases. Although there are some differences between familial and sporadic cases, it is not clear whether any of these characteristics affect survival time or severity of disease. However, it is highly likely that the study of families with multiple B-cell CLL/SLL cases will aid in delineating the genes and environmental factors that may play a role in the development of both forms of B-cell CLL/SLL.

Diagnosis

Morphology

The diagnosis of B-cell CLL/SLL is made by the detection of a clonal population of small B lymphocytes in the peripheral blood or bone marrow or by lymph node biopsy showing cells expressing the characteristic morphology and immunophenotype. The diagnostic criteria are shown in Table 14.1. In peripheral blood and bone marrow smears, the cells are monomorphic, small, round B lymphocytes, with only rare large cells with prominent nucleoli (prolymphocytes) seen. The bone marrow infiltrate may be nodular, interstitial, or diffuse or may show a combination of these patterns. The lymph node infiltrate of CLL/SLL is composed of predominantly small lymphocytes with condensed chromatin, round nuclei, and occasionally a small nucleolus (18). Larger lymphoid cells known as *prolymphocytes* and *paraimmunoblasts* with more prominent nucleoli and more dispersed chromatin are always present and are clustered in aggregates known as *proliferation centers* or *pseudofollicles* (Color Plate 10).

Immunophenotype

The cells in B-cell CLL/SLL express CD19, dim CD20, dim CD5, CD23, CD43, CD79a, and weakly express surface

TABLE 14.1. *Diagnosis of chronic lymphocytic leukemia*

Lymphocytosis (small, mature lymphocytes ≥5,000/µL)
Bone marrow involvement of ≥30% lymphocytes
≤55% atypical/immature lymphoid cells in peripheral blood
Clonal expansion of abnormal B lymphocytes
Low density of surface Ig (IgM or IgD) with κ or λ light chains
B-cell surface antigens [CD19, CD20 (dim), CD23]
CD5 surface antigen

Ig, immunoglobulin.

immunoglobulin (Ig) M and IgD. Immunophenotypic analysis of a case of CLL is shown in Color Plate 11. Cytoplasmic Ig is detectable in approximately 5% of cases. Occasional cases of CLL/SLL lack expression of CD23, and this can lead to a differential diagnosis of mantle cell lymphoma. Dim expression of CD20 and surface Ig is highly characteristic of CLL/SLL, and this can be useful in distinguishing CLL/SLL from mantle cell lymphoma. Expression of CD38 is variable and has been reported to have prognostic significance in this disease (19,20). For this reason, CD38 should continue to be included in the immunophenotypic panel of antigens assessed in this disease.

Immunophenotypic features are required to make the diagnosis of B-cell CLL/SLL. In difficult cases, particularly those in which there is an atypical immunophenotype, the detection of specific cytogenetic and molecular features can be helpful in making the definitive diagnosis. The immunophenotypic and genetic features of B-cell CLL/SLL and other small B-cell neoplasms are shown in Table 14.2.

Pathogenesis

Understanding the pathogenesis of CLL/SLL remains a major challenge. Unlike many of the other low-grade B-cell malignancies, nonrandom reciprocal chromosomal translocations occur rarely in CLL/SLL. However, a number of cytogenetic abnormalities have been identified. Using fluorescent *in situ* hybridization (FISH) techniques, one or more of these cytogenetic abnormalities can be found in more than 80% of patients with B-cell CLL/SLL, and as described below in the Cytogenetic and Molecular Analysis section of this chapter, these have important prognostic significance (21).

The most common abnormality is deletion of the long arm of chromosome 13. Deletions at 13q14 occur in more than 50% of cases of CLL/SLL and in a proportion of cases of mantle cell lymphoma and myeloma, suggesting that a tumor suppressor gene at this locus could be involved in the pathogenesis of these diseases. Considerable work has been performed attempting to identify the location and nature of this putative tumor suppressor gene (22–26), but its precise nature remains to be elucidated.

The next most common cytogenetic abnormality is deletion of the long arm of chromosome 11. Deletions at 11q22-23 occur in up to 20% of cases of B-cell CLL/SLL and are

TABLE 14.2. *Small B-cell neoplasms: immunophenotypic and genetic features*

Neoplasm	SIg; cIg	CD5	CD10	CD23	CD43	Cyclin D1	Bcl-6 protein[a]	Genetic abnormality	IgV region genes
B-cell chronic lympho-cytic leukemia/small lymphocytic lym-phoma	+; –/+	+	–	+	+	–	–	13q deletions (50%), trisomy 12 (20%)	50% unmutated
Lymphoplasmacytic lym-phoma	+; +	–	–	–	–/+	–	–	t(9;14)–PAX5R	Mutated
Mantle cell lymphoma	+; –	+	–	–	+	+	–	t(11;14)–BCL1R	Unmutated
Follicle center lym-phoma	+; –	–	+	–/+	–	–	+	t(14;18)–BCL2R	Mutated, ongoing
Extranodal and nodal marginal zone lym-phoma	+; –/+	–	–	–/+	–/+	–	–	Trisomy 3, t(11;18)–API2/MLT, t(1;14)–BCL10R	Mutated, ?ongoing
Splenic marginal zone lymphoma	+; –/+	–	–	–	–	–	–	Del 7q21-32 (40%)	50% mutated

+, ≥90% positive; +/–, ≥50% positive; –/+, <50% positive; –, ≤10% positive.
[a]Residual germinal center may be + in marginal zone lymphoma and mantle cell lymphoma.

associated with patients with a distinct clinical presentation, including younger age, male sex, extensive adenopathy, and poor prognosis (27). The ATM gene is located within the minimal region of loss at 11q23, suggesting that alterations in this gene may be involved in the pathogenesis of the disease. This is further supported by the finding that loss of functional atm is associated with poor outcome (28). The mechanism whereby loss of atm function is involved in leukemogenesis is not clear. However, atm binds to p53 and induces serine phosphorylation (29,30), thereby inhibiting the interaction of p53 with mdm2 as well as increasing transcription of p53 target genes. This results in arrest of the cell cycle. The pattern of atm inactivation of B-cell CLL/SLL with loss of one allele and functional inactivation of the other is suggestive of a tumor-suppressor inactivation mechanism. Again, the mechanism whereby this occurs has yet to be elucidated.

Deletions in the short arm of chromosome 17 occur in less than 10% of cases of CLL/SLL but are associated with rapid progression of disease, poor response to therapy, and short survival (21,31). The deletions involve the p53 locus at 17p13, and it is clear that mutations in the p53 gene can contribute to disease progression and alter the sensitivity of CLL/SLL cells to chemotherapy agents.

Trisomy 12 (Color Plate 12) occurs in up to 20% of cases of CLL/SLL, but the molecular mechanism by which this genetic abnormality contributes to leukemogenesis is unknown.

Therefore, although a number of genes, including bcl-2, ATM, and p53 are known to play a role in disease progression, the genes involved in the pathogenesis of the disease remain to be identified.

In addition to the heterogeneity of genetic abnormalities, CLL/SLL is also heterogeneous in its level of differentiation,

as evidenced by the status of the Ig genes. Although initial studies had suggested that CLL/SLL was derived from naïve B1 cells, more recent studies have clearly demonstrated that CLL/SLL can be divided into two subgroups based on the presence or absence of somatic hypermutation of the Ig heavy-chain variable (IgV) region (32). As discussed in more detail below, this finding has prognostic significance (19,33). This has led to the hypothesis that there are two subsets of B-cell CLL/SLL based on different cells of origin. In this hypothesis, cases with unmutated IgV regions are derived from naïve cells that are pregerminal center in origin, whereas those that have mutated IgV regions arise from a cell that has encountered antigen and is postgerminal center in origin. However, gene-expression profiling studies from two independent analyses have demonstrated that both subtypes of CLL/SLL display a common and distinct gene-expression profile, suggesting that both groups share a common mechanism of transformation (34,35). These findings are not in keeping with two distinct disease entities arising from different cells of origin. However, the gene-profiling studies did identify a restricted number of genes that are capable of distinguishing IgV-mutated versus -unmutated cases (34,35). Most attention has focused on expression of zap70, which is found in most unmutated but not mutated cases (36).

Clinical Presentation

In approximately 25% of cases, B-cell CLL/SLL is diagnosed in asymptomatic patients at the time of a routine blood count, when a lymphocytosis leads to the subsequent diagnosis. The National Cancer Institute–sponsored study group recommended that the threshold for diagnosis of CLL/SLL should require a lymphocytosis of greater than 5,000 per μL (37).

TABLE 14.3. *Rai Classification of chronic lymphocytic lymphoma*

Stage	Simplified three-stage system	Clinical features	Median survival (yr)
0	Low risk	Lymphocytosis in blood and marrow only	>10
I	Intermediate risk	Lymphadenopathy	7
II		Splenomegaly ± hepatomegaly	
III	High risk	Anemia	0.75–4.00
IV		Thrombocytopenia	

However, this criterion is likely outdated, and if diagnostic immunophenotypic features are clearly those of typical CLL/SLL, the diagnosis can be made in the presence of a blood lymphocyte count of less than 5,000 per µL. In the remaining cases, there is a wide range of initial presenting features.

The most consistent physical finding is painless lymphadenopathy, most frequently in the cervical, supraclavicular, or axillary regions, followed by splenomegaly or hepatomegaly, or both. Only 5% of patients present with lymphadenopathy without evidence of leukemic infiltration. Although CLL/SLL can involve virtually every tissue, involvement of other organs is rare, particularly at the time of initial diagnosis. Skin is the most commonly involved nonlymphoid organ, but this is present in less than 5% of cases (38). In contrast to other B-cell malignancies, gastrointestinal involvement is extremely rare in CLL/SLL. Meningeal involvement, although reported, is also extremely rare (39,40).

Up to 20% of cases present with *B symptoms*, which have been defined by the National Cancer Institute–sponsored working group as unintentional weight loss of greater than or equal to 10% of body weight over the previous 6 months, fevers greater than 38°C for longer than 2 weeks without evidence of infection, night sweats, or extreme fatigue [Eastern Cooperative Group (ECOG) performance status 2 or greater] (37). Anemia and thrombocytopenia may be present at the time of initial presentation. In 20% of cases, anemia less than 11 g per dL and thrombocytopenia less than 100,000 per µL are present and are associated with a poor prognosis (see Staging, below).

Unique Aspects of Staging

The natural history of CLL/SLL is extremely variable, and until the mid 1970s, there were no reliable methods to assess outcome. The two widely used staging systems that are now in place are based on their prognostic implications for survival (41,42). The Rai staging system (Table 14.3) is based on the premise that there is a progressive accumulation of neoplastic cells manifested by increasing lymphocytosis, progressive lymphadenopathy, splenomegaly, and hepatomegaly, followed by bone marrow replacement with development of anemia and thrombocytopenia (41). At the time of initial diagnosis, 25% of patients are stage 0, 50% stage I to II, and 25% stage III to IV.

The Binet system (Table 14.4) takes into consideration five potential sites of involvement: cervical, axillary, and inguinal lymph nodes (either unilateral or bilateral counts as one site), the spleen, and the liver (42). Patients are staged according to the number of involved sites plus the presence of anemia with hemoglobin less than 10 g per dL or thrombocytopenia with platelets less than 100,000 per µL. The International Workshop on CLL recommends that in practice, an integrated system using both methods (Table 14.5) should be used for uniformity in reporting clinical trials (43). Although this should be used in reports of clinical trials, it has not been widely accepted by clinicians in their everyday practice who prefer to use the more simple Rai or Binet systems, and it is often difficult to extract International Workshop on CLL staging in multicenter studies. A number of other staging systems have been proposed but have not received widespread acceptance (44–47).

Prognostic and Predictive Factors

Clinical Stage

A number of prognostic factors have been identified in CLL/SLL. The Rai and Binet staging systems were based on their prognostic significance, and the stage of disease remains perhaps the most important prognostic factor in CLL/SLL, although there are increasing attempts to correlate prognosis with biologic markers. The median survival from the time of diagnosis based on the Rai Classification was 150 months for stage 0, 71 to 101 months for stages I and II, and 9 months for stages III and IV (41). Although the original Rai staging system comprised five stages (stage 0 through IV), there were only three distinct survival patterns: stage 0, stages I and II combined, and stages III

TABLE 14.4. *Binet staging system of chronic lymphocytic leukemia*

Group	Clinical features	Median survival (yr)
A	<3 areas of lymphadenopathy; no anemia or thrombocytopenia	12
B	≥3 involved node areas; no anemia or thrombocytopenia	7
C	Hemoglobin <10 g/dL and/or platelets <100,000/µL	2–4

TABLE 14.5. *International Workshop on Chronic Lymphocytic Leukemia staging system and prognosis in chronic lymphocytic leukemia*

Stage	Description	Median survival (yr)
A	Lymphocytosis with clinical involvement of fewer than 3 lymph node groups; no anemia or thrombocytopenia	8–12+
	A(0) no nodes enlarged	
	A(I) nodes enlarged	
	A(II) hepatomegaly or splenomegaly	
B	Three or more lymph node groups involved, no anemia or thrombocytopenia	5+
	B(I) nodes enlarged	
	B(II) hepatomegaly or splenomegaly	
C	Anemia or thrombocytopenia regardless of number of lymph node groups involved	2.5
	C(III) anemia	
	C(IV) thrombocytopenia	

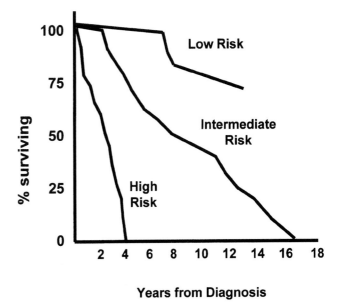

FIG. 14.1. Survival in chronic lymphocytic leukemia by modified Rai stage.

and IV combined. As a result, a modified Rai staging system recognizes three groups: low risk (Rai stage 0), intermediate risk (Rai stages I and II combined), and high risk (Rai stages III and IV combined) (48). The survival of patients using this modified Rai staging system is shown in Figure 14-1. Survival of the three groups within the Binet system is similar to that observed in the three groups of the modified Rai staging system.

Although the majority of patients with high-risk disease (Rai stages III and IV and Binet stage C) have a rapidly progressive clinical course and short survival, the course of disease is less uniform in the other groups, with some patients, particularly those with Rai stage 0, or Binet stage A, with a benign or "smoldering" course. (Smoldering CLL/SLL cases refer to those cases that show little or no evidence of progression over time and do not appear to affect survival.) Therefore, a number of other factors have been evaluated for their prognostic significance and have shown limited usefulness in their ability to predict the course of disease (Table 14.6).

Prognostic Markers

Although bone marrow biopsies are not needed to make the diagnosis of CLL/SLL, the pattern of bone marrow involvement (diffuse versus nodular or interstitial) has been shown to have prognostic significance (49). An atypical morphology with increased number of prolym-

phocytes is also an independent factor associated with an adverse prognosis (50). Not surprisingly, a lymphocyte doubling time shorter than 12 months in an untreated patient predicts a progressive course (51,52). Several other factors have been used to correlate tumor cell proliferation with clinical outcome, including Ki67 (53), p27 (54), and thymidine kinase (sTK) (55). Most useful clinically has been measurement of serum levels of sTK, an enzyme that reflects cellular division. Elevated sTK levels have been shown to add independent prognostic information to differentiate progressive from "smoldering" CLL/SLL (55).

TABLE 14.6. *Prognostic factors in chronic lymphocytic leukemia*

Advanced stage at diagnosis

Diffuse pattern of bone marrow infiltration

Short lymphocyte doubling time

Expression of Ki67, p27

High serum levels of thymidine kinase, β_2-microglobulin, soluble CD23, and tumor necrosis factor-α

Poor risk cytogenetics—17p, 11q deletions and complex abnormalities

Immunoglobulin V mutational status

CD38 expression

Advanced age

Male sex

Response to therapy

TABLE 14.7. *Cytogenetic abnormalities in 325 patients with chronic lymphoctyic leukemia*

Abnormality	No. of patients	%
13q deletion	178	55
11q deletion	58	18
Trisomy 12	53	16
17p deletion	23	7

Adapted from Dohner H, Stilgenbauer S, Benner A, et al. Genomic aberrations and survival in chronic lymphocytic leukemia. *N Engl J Med* 2000;343:1910, with permission.

Beta-2 Microglobulin

A number of studies have evaluated the prognostic value of measurement of serum beta-2 microglobulin (β2M) in CLL/SLL. In a prospective study of 113 patients with early stage disease, β2M in addition to sTK, performance status and platelet count were independent prognostic factors (56). Reports from the M.D. Anderson Cancer Center have also stressed the important prognostic significance of elevated levels of serum β2M. In 150 patients with CLL/SLL, elevated serum levels of interleukin-6 and interleukin-10 were adverse prognostic factors and were correlated with serum β2M levels. In a multivariate analysis, serum β2M was the most important independent prognostic factor (57).

Tumor Necrosis Factor

Tumor necrosis factor-alpha (TNFα) is produced by CLL/SLL cells and acts as an autocrine and paracrine growth factor in this disease. In 150 patients with CLL/SLL, TNFα levels were measured and correlated with disease characteristics, prognostic factors, and survival (58). Patients having an elevated TNFα level had more advanced Rai and Binet stage disease, higher serum β2M, a greater percentage of cells expressing CD38, and lower hemoglobin and platelet levels. The TNFα level remained predictive of survival in multivariate analysis, independent ($p = .005$) of Rai staging and β2M, hemoglobin, prior therapy, white cell count, and platelet level (58). Among 41 patients in Binet stage A, progression-free survival was significantly shorter in those patients whose vascular endothelial growth factor serum concentrations were elevated (59).

Cytogenetic and Molecular Analysis

Although conventional cytogenetic analyses only detected chromosome aberrations in 40% to 50% of cases, new molecular cytogenetic methods, such as fluorescent *in situ* hybridization, have greatly enhanced our ability to detect chromosomal abnormalities in B-cell CLL/SLL. In the most comprehensive study published to date, chromosomal abnormalities were detected in 268 of 325 B-cell CLL/SLL patients studied (82%) (21). In this study, Dohner and colleagues have convincingly demonstrated that genomic aberrations in B-cell CLL/SLL are important independent predictors of disease progression and survival (Table 14.7). The most frequent changes observed

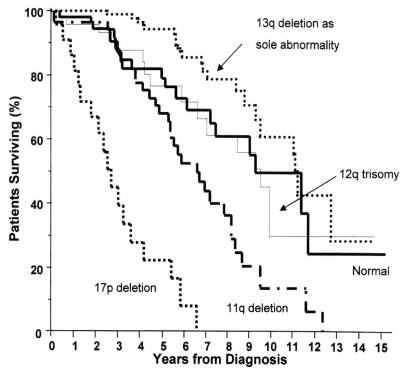

FIG. 14.2. Survival from time of diagnosis in chronic lymphocytic leukemia by cytogenetic abnormalities detected by fluorescent *in situ* hybridization. (Adapted from Dohner H, Stilgenbauer S, Benner A, et al. Genomic aberrations and survival in chronic lymphocytic leukemia. *N Engl J Med* 2000;343:1910, with permission.)

were deletion in 13q, deletion in 11q, trisomy 12q, and deletion in 17p. The median survival time for patients with 17p deletion was 32 months; for 11q deletion, 79 months; for 12q trisomy, 114 months; for normal karyotype, 111 months; and for 13q deletion as the sole abnormality, 133 months (Fig. 14.2). Patients in the 17p- and 11q-deletion groups had more advanced disease than those in the other three groups. Patients with 17p deletions had the shortest median treatment-free interval (9 months), and those with 13q deletions had the longest (92 months). Ongoing studies are assessing the impact of specific cytogenic abnormalities on response to particular therapeutic approaches. However, the presence of 17p deletion predicts for treatment failure with alkylating agents and fludarabine and short survival times. In multivariate analysis, 11q and 17p deletions provided independent adverse prognostic information. These findings have implications for the design of risk-adapted treatment strategies (60).

Immunoglobulin Gene Mutation Status and CD38 Expression

Recently, it has been demonstrated that those patients with CLL/SLL who have unmutated IgV-region genes have poor prognosis compared to those whose Ig genes are mutated (Fig. 14.3) (19,33). This finding led to the hypothesis that B-cell CLL/SLL might represent not a single disease entity but two different diseases with similar morphologic features arising from two separate cells of origin. As discussed in the Pathogenesis section of this chapter above, this was not supported by gene microarray analysis studies (34,35). It has been suggested

that higher levels of expression of CD38 are associated with unmutated IgV genes (19). In multivariate analysis, high levels of expression of CD38 on B-cell CLL/SLL cells were associated with more rapid progression of disease and poor response to therapy (61,62). However, there can be discordance between IgV status and CD38 expression, which may be partly explained by the finding that the level of expression of CD38 may vary over time (63). A multivariate analysis examined the prognostic significance of genetic abnormalities (detected at or shortly after presentation), clinical stage, lymphocyte morphology, CD38 expression, and IgV gene status in 205 patients with CLL/SLL (64). Deletion of chromosome 11q23, absence of a deletion of chromosome 13q14, atypical lymphocyte morphology, and more than 30% CD38 expression were significantly associated with the presence of unmutated IgV genes. Advanced stage, male sex, atypical morphology, more than 30% CD38 expression, trisomy 12, deletion of chromosome 11q23, loss or mutation of the p53 gene, and unmutated IgV genes were all poor prognostic factors in the univariate analysis in this study. However, IgV gene mutational status, loss or mutation of the p53 gene, and clinical stage retained prognostic significance in a multivariate analysis (64).

Treatment

In all other leukemias, early treatment is optimal. This is not the case in CLL/SLL for two main reasons. First, a proportion of cases of CLL/SLL have a smoldering clinical course, with no difference in survival compared to age-matched controls, and these patients do not require therapy.

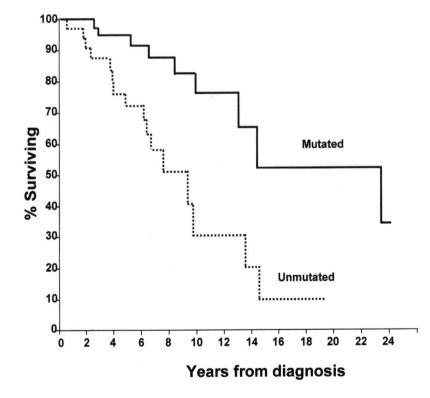

FIG. 14.3. Survival from time of diagnosis of chronic lymphocytic leukemia by presence of mutated versus unmutated immunoglobulin gene rearrangements. [Adapted from Hamblin TJ, Davis Z, Gardiner A, et al. Unmutated Ig V(H) genes are associated with a more aggressive form of chronic lymphocytic leukemia. *Blood* 1999;94:1848–1854, with permission.]

TABLE 14.8. *National Cancer Institute Working Group recommendations for indications to treat chronic lymphoctyic leukemia*

Progressive marrow failure—high-risk patients (Rai stages III and IV, Binet stage C)

Constitutional symptoms referable to chronic lymphocytic leukemia, including weakness, night sweats, and fatigue

Massive or progressive splenomegaly

Massive or progressive lymphadenopathy

Rapid lymphocyte doubling time (shorter than 6 mo)

Autoimmune anemia and/or thrombocytopenia poorly responsive to corticosteroids

TABLE 14.9. *National Cancer Insitute Working Group recommendations for response to therapy in chronic lymphocytic leukemia*

Parameter	Complete remission	Partial remission
Lymphocytes	≤4,000/μL	≥50% decrease
Lymph nodes	No palpable disease	≥50% decrease (liver/ spleen)
Neutrophils	≥1,500/μL	≥1,500/μL or ≥50% improvement
Platelets	>100,000/μL	>100,000/μL or >50% improvement
Hemoglobin	>11 g/dL	>11 g/dL or ≥50% improvement
Bone marrow	<30% lymphocytes	± Nodules (nodular partial response)
Symptomatology	None	Variable

Second, the disease remains incurable using standard treatment approaches, and previous trials have demonstrated no survival advantage of early treatment versus an initial "watch and wait" approach. More than 2,000 patients with early disease have been enrolled in trials of immediate versus deferred chemotherapy, all performed using alkylating agents. In a metaanalysis of these studies, there was no statistically significant difference in survival between early and deferred therapy (65). There was a trend toward a worse outcome for early treatment (10-year survival with immediate chemotherapy was 44% versus 47% for those whose therapy was deferred). Therefore, the most important treatment decision to be made in CLL/SLL is whether the patient requires therapy at a given time. Guidelines have been established recommending treatment for patients with active disease (Table 14.8) (37,66,67). The traditional goal of therapy for CLL/SLL has been palliation, and patients were usually treated until symptoms resolved. The availability of newer therapies has resulted in increased awareness of the importance of achieving a complete remission in CLL/SLL. Formal criteria for achievement of complete and partial remissions have been established for CLL/SLL by the National Cancer Institute Working Group (Table 14.9) (37,66,67).

Chemotherapy

Alkylating Agents

The main agent used in the treatment of B-cell CLL/SLL has been the alkylating agents chlorambucil and cyclophosphamide with or without corticosteroids. Chlorambucil is rapidly absorbed from the gastrointestinal tract, and peak plasma concentrations occur within 1 hour of ingestion. Metabolism is primarily hepatic and excretion of metabolites via renal clearance. There has been great variability in dosage and schedule of administration, but the two commonly used approaches are low-dose continuous therapy using a continuous dose of 0.08 mg per kg (usual dose, 4 to 8 mg orally) or a pulsed intermittent dosage of 0.8 mg per kg (usual dose, 40 to 80 mg) given in a single oral dose every 3 to 4 weeks. Chlorambucil is often given in combination with corticosteroids. Results of randomized trials of alkylators alone or with steroids, with the alkylator schedule, are shown in Table 14.10. There was no difference in survival

when chlorambucil therapy alone was compared to chlorambucil plus prednisone, but those patients treated with chlorambucil and prednisone had higher complete (20% vs. 9%) and overall response rates (87% vs. 45%) (68). In addition, the hematologic toxicity was less in the combination therapy group. A Cancer and Leukemia Group B study compared prednisone alone to prednisone and chlorambucil and evaluated two doses of chlorambucil (69). Ninety-six patients with stage III and stage IV CLL were randomized into one of three treatment schedules. Prednisone was given to all patients daily. One group received prednisone plus chlorambucil given as a once-a-month dose of 0.4 to 0.8 mg per kg; a second group also received both drugs, but the chlorambucil was given as a daily dose of 0.08 mg per kg, and the third group received prednisone alone. The overall response rate was 47% for schedule I, 38% for schedule II, and 11% for schedule III. Patients who responded (complete plus partial responses) in each of the treatment schedules survived longer than the nonresponders. There were complete responders in both chlorambucil treatment schedules, but not with the prednisone-alone regimen. There was no significant difference in survival time among the three treatment schedules, and toxicity was minimal. Augmentation of the intermittent monthly chlorambucil, even to 1.5 and 2.0 mg per kg, was tolerated without undue marrow toxicity.

A number of randomized trials have compared the efficacy of chlorambucil alone or in combination with prednisone to that of combinations of cyclophosphamide, vincristine (Oncovin), and prednisone (CVP or COP) or to combinations including hydroxydaunorubicin (CHOP) (Table 14.11). There was no difference in the 5-year survival (48% in both cases) of chlorambucil with or without steroids compared to combination chemotherapy alone. Six trials involved an anthracycline-containing regimen, but again, there was no difference in overall survival with chlorambucil compared to anthracycline-based regimens. The CLL-80 trial from the French Cooperative Group compared daily continuous chlorambucil

TABLE 14.10. *Selected randomized trials of alkylator therapy alone or with steroids*

Treatment arm	No. of patients	Complete remission (%)	Overall response (%)	Survival difference	Reference
Chlorambucil	11	9	45	No difference	Han et al. 1973 (68)
Chlorambucil plus prednisone	15	20	87		
I Chlorambucil (qm) plus prednisone	38	8	47	No difference	Sawitsky et al. (69)
II Chlorambucil (qd) plus prednisone	39	8	38		
III Prednisone	19	0	11		

with 12 monthly cycles of COP in 291 patients with Binet stage B disease and demonstrated no difference in overall response or survival (70). Similar studies were performed by the ECOG (71) and the Medical Research Council (72). A number of trials, not all of which have been published in peer-reviewed journals, have also compared chlorambucil with CHOP and failed to find any survival advantage, although response rates were generally higher with CHOP. One exception is the CLL-80 trial of the French Cooperative Group, which randomized patients with Binet stage C disease to receive COP versus CHOP (using a low dose of hydroxy-daunorubicin) (73). Median survival in the CHOP group was superior at 62 months to COP (*p* = .0005). However, the outcome of the COP arm in this study was inferior to that seen using COP in an ECOG trial that evaluated COP versus chlorambucil (71). In particular, the outcome of the COP arm in the ECOG study was similar to that seen with CHOP in the CLL-80 study. In a metaanalysis, there was no survival advantage for CHOP in all patients or even when analysis was restricted to Binet stage C patients, the setting in which the French study had shown an advantage for CHOP (65).

Taken together, the trials of alkylator therapy support a conservative treatment strategy for CLL, with no chemotherapy given for the most patients with early-stage disease, and single-agent chlorambucil as the first line of treatment for most patients with advanced disease as symptoms appear, with no evidence of benefit from early inclusion of an anthracycline. This strategy will need to be reconsidered as mature results become available from trials of other agents, notably the purine analogs in combination, as discussed below.

Purine Analogs

Recently, the purine analogs—fludarabine, cladribine, and pentostatin—have demonstrated major activity against CLL/SLL (Table 14.12). Each of these agents has been used in previously treated patients (74–83) and, more recently, in previously untreated patients (76,80,84–88). A number of studies have demonstrated the efficacy of fludarabine in patients with previously treated CLL/SLL (76,81,89).

A number of phase II studies have evaluated the combination of fludarabine with cyclophosphamide in previously untreated CLL/SLL with overall response rates of 79% to 100%, and with complete response rates ranging from 16% in a German multicenter study (90) to 90% to 100% in single-center studies (90–92). A number of studies that have evaluated cladribine in treatment of alkylator-resistant CLL/SLL have demonstrated response rates of 31% to 67% (79,93,94). In untreated CLL/SLL, cladribine demonstrated responses in 60%, with 25% achieving a complete response (87). Pentostatin has also demonstrated responses in 16% to 35% of patients with previously treated CLL/SLL, but complete responses have rarely been observed (81).

Three large randomized trials have been performed comparing fludarabine with alkylator-based therapies. In a European study, patients were randomized to receive fludarabine (106 patients) or CAP [cyclophosphamide, Adriamycin (doxorubi-

TABLE 14.11. *Randomized trials of chlorambucil alone compared to combination chemotherapy*

	No. of patients	Survival	Reference
Eastern Cooperative Oncology Group			71
Chlorambucil plus prednisone	60	48% 5 yr	
Cyclophosphamide, vincristine, and prednisone	62	48% 5 yr, no difference	
CLL-80—French Cooperative Group Binet Group B			70
Chlorambucil	151	44% 5 yr	
Cyclophosphamide, Oncovin (vincristine), and prednisone	150	43% 5 yr, no difference	
CLL-80—French Cooperative Group Binet Group C			73
Cyclophosphamide, Oncovin (vincristine), and prednisone	35	28% 3 yr	
Cyclophosphamide, hydroxydaunorubicin, Oncovin (vincristine), and prednisone	35	71% 5 yr, *p* = .0001	

TABLE 14.12. *Purine analogs as treatment for chronic lymphocytic leukemia*

	No. of patients	Complete remission (%)	Overall response (%)	Reference
Previously treated				
Fludarabine				
	32	3	13	Grever et al. 1988 (74)
	68	13	57	Keating et al. 1989 (75)
	169[a]	12	52	O'Brien et al. 1993 (76)
	56	5	73	Fenchel et al. 1995 (77)
	68	4	28	Montserrat et al. 1996 (78)
Cladribine (2-CdA)				
	26	0	31	Tallman et al. 1995 (79)
	184[b]	13	48	Robak et al. 2000 (80)
Pentostatin				
	26	4	15	Dillman et al. 1989 (81)
	26	0	27	Ho et al. 1990 (82)
	24	8	29	Johnson et al. 1998 (83)
Previously untreated				
Fludarabine				
	33	33	79	Keating et al. 1991 (84)
	95[a]	30	79	O'Brien et al. 1993 (76)
	170	20	63	Rai et al. 2000 (85)
	341	40	71	Leporrier et al. 2001 (86)
Cladribine (2-CdA)				
	20	25	85	Saven et al. 1995 (87)
	63	38	75	Juliusson et al. 1996 (88)
	194[c]	45	83	Robak et al. 2000 (80)
Pentostatin				
	13	0	46	Dillman et al. 1989 (81)

[a]Fludarabine plus prednisone.
[b]One hundred four patients also received prednisone.
[c]One hundred fifty-one patients also received prednisone.

TABLE 14.13. *Randomized phase II trial of fludarabine versus cyclophosphamide, Adriamycin (doxorubicin), and prednisone (CAP)*

	Fludarabine[a]	CAP[b]	p value
All			
No. of patients	100	96	
Overall response	60%	44%	p = .023
Previously treated			
No. of patients	48	48	
Overall response	48%	27%	p = .036
Previously untreated			
No. of patients	52	48	
Overall response	71%	60%	p = .26

[a]Fludarabine, 25 mg/m^2/day on days 1–5.
[b]Cyclophosphamide, 750 mg/m^2 on day 1; doxorubicin, 50 mg/m^2 on day 1; prednisone, 40 mg/m^2/day on days 1–5.
Adapted from Johnson S, Smith AG, Loffler H, et al. Multicentre prospective randomised trial of fludarabine versus cyclophosphamide, doxorubicin, and prednisone (CAP) for treatment of advanced-stage chronic lymphocytic leukemia. The French Cooperative Group on CLL. *Lancet* 1996;347:1432–1438, with permission.

cin), and prednisone, 102 patients] (95). This study included both previously treated and untreated patients (Table 14.13). Remission rates were significantly higher after fludarabine than after CAP, with overall response rates of 60% versus 44%, respectively ($p = .023$), with a significantly higher response rate observed with fludarabine in previously treated patients (48% vs. 27%, $p = .036$). The response rate with fludarabine was not significantly higher in previously untreated patients (71% vs. 60%, $p = .26$). However, in the previously untreated patients, the duration of response and overall survival were significantly longer with fludarabine than with CAP. The French Cooperative Group evaluated fludarabine versus low-dose CHOP versus CAP in 938 previously untreated patients (Table 14.14), with randomization stratified for Binet stage B and C patients (86). Both CHOP and fludarabine had better response rates than CAP, but no difference in overall survival was observed. There were, however, an increased complete response rate and duration of response noted in patients treated with fludarabine.

In an Intergroup study sponsored by the National Cancer Institute (Table 14.15), 544 previously untreated patients with CLL were randomized to receive fludarabine, chlorambucil, or the combination of fludarabine and chlorambucil (85). The combination arm was closed to accrual early because of higher toxicity. In 509 evaluable patients, the complete response rate (20% vs. 4%, $p < .001$), overall response rate (63% vs. 37%, $p < .001$), and duration of response (25 months vs. 14 months, $p < .001$) were higher with fludarabine than with chlorambucil. The response rate to fludarabine in patients for whom chlorambucil was ineffective was high, most likely explaining the fact that there is no difference in overall survival among the three arms ($p = .21$).

TABLE 14.14. *French Cooperative Group on Chronic Lymphocytic Leukemia: randomized trial of fludarabine[a] versus cyclophosphamide, hydroxydaunorubicin, Oncovin (vincristine), and prednisone (CHOP)[b] versus cyclophosphamide, Adriamycin (doxorubicin), and prednisone (CAP)[c]*

	No. of patients	Complete remission (%)	Median time to progression (mo)	Median survival (mo)
Fludarabine	336	40[d]	32	69
CAP	237	15	28	70
CHOP	351	30	30	67

[a]Fludarabine, 25 mg/m^2/day IV days 1–5.
[b]Cyclophosphamide, 750 mg/m^2 IV day 1; doxorubicin, 50 mg/m^2 IV day 1; prednisone, 40 mg/m^2/day PO days 1–5.
[c]Cyclophosphamide, 300 mg/m^2 PO days 1–5; doxorubicin, 25 mg/m^2 IV day 1; vincristine, 1 mg/m^2 IV day 1; prednisone, 40 mg/m^2 PO days 1–5.
[d]$p < .01$ for Fludarabine versus CAP or CHOP.
Adapted from Leporrier M, Chevret S, Cazin B, et al. Randomized comparison of fludarabine, CAP, and CHOP in 938 previously untreated stage B and C chronic lymphocytic leukemia patients. *Blood* 2001;98:2319–2325, with permission.

Radiation Therapy

Because CLL/SLL is disseminated early in the disease course, radiation therapy is palliative. However, CLL/SLL cells are radiosensitive (96,97), and radiation therapy can provide symptomatic relief for large, bulky lymphadenopathy. Splenic radiation has been used to treat patients with bulky, painful splenomegaly and patients with pancytopenia due to hypersplenism (98–100). A number of studies have demonstrated benefit for splenectomy in CLL/SLL (101,102). The role of splenic radiation versus splenectomy has not been evaluated, particularly in advanced-stage patients. Low-dose total-body irradiation has demonstrated efficacy in the treatment of CLL/SLL (103) and was found to be comparable to chlorambucil in advanced-stage CLL/SLL patients in one study (104). However, in an ECOG study, the response rate to chemotherapy was higher than that observed with total-body irradiation (105), and this approach has subsequently been used less frequently. Total-body irradiation has been used in CLL/SLL but was not found to be superior to chemotherapy in randomized clinical trials (104,105). The toxicity associated with high-dose total-body irradiation was high, with 75% of patients experiencing severe thrombocytopenia or neutropenia. Therefore, radiation therapy has a palliative role to play in the management of patients with relapsed and refractory CLL who have bulky adenopathy or splenomegaly.

Immune Therapy

Immunotherapy is emerging as an exciting modality with significant potential to advance the treatment of CLL. Immunotherapy includes passive immunotherapy with monoclonal antibodies against antigens on CLL/SLL B cells, including CD20 and CD52. Active immunotherapy by vaccination with tumor antigens or with genetically modified autologous leukemia cells is being evaluated in clinical trials. Humanized monoclonal antibodies have been developed that target antigens on the surface of CLL/SLL cells, and two agents have been approved for use in CLL/SLL. Rituximab, an anti-CD20 monoclonal antibody, is approved for use in relapsed B-cell non-Hodgkin's lymphoma. A number of

TABLE 14.15. *Intergroup study of fludarabine[a] versus chlorambucil[b] versus fludarabine plus chlorambucil[c] for previously untreated chronic lymphocytic leukemia*

	No. of patients	Evaluable	Complete remission (%)	Overall response (%)		Median duration of response (mo)	
Fludarabine	179	170	20	63	$p < .001$	25	$p < .001$
Chlorambucil	193	181	4	37		14	
Fludarabine plus chlorambucil[d]	137	123	24	75		—	

[a]Fludarabine, 25 mg/m^2 × 5 days.
[b]Chlorambucil, 40 mg/m^2 on day 1.
[c]Fludarabine, 20 mg/m^2/day × 5 days plus chlorambucil 20 mg/m^2 on day 1.
[d]Closed early to accrual due to increased toxicity.
Adapted from Rai KR, Peterson BL, Appelbaum FR, et al. Fludarabine compared with chlorambucil as primary therapy for chronic lymphocytic leukemia. *N Engl J Med* 2000;343:1750–1757, with permission.

studies have demonstrated low response rates in patients with CLL/SLL compared to other B-cell lymphomas (106,107). In a study of 28 patients with relapsed or refractory CLL/SLL, the overall response rate to rituximab therapy was 25%, with no complete responses noted, and the duration of response was short (108). However, two approaches have demonstrated improvement in response rate by the use of rituximab in CLL/SLL, by either increasing the dose (109) or the frequency (110) of administration of the antibody. Care has to be taken when administering rituximab to patients with CLL/SLL, because tumor lysis syndrome and deaths have been reported, likely because of high levels of cytokines released in these patients with a high circulating tumor load (108).

Alemtuzumab (Campath-1H), an anti-CD52 monoclonal antibody, is approved for CLL/SLL patients who are fludarabine refractory and may have activity in cases that are unresponsive to chemotherapy due to the presence of p53 mutations (111). Alemtuzumab demonstrated an overall response rate of 38% in a pilot study in previously treated patients (112). In a subsequent pivotal study of 93 patients with fludarabine-refractory CLL/SLL, Alemtuzumab demonstrated an overall response rate of 33% and improved survival in those patients who responded (113). Alemtuzumab has less activity against bulky lymphadenopathy but demonstrates impressive efficacy in clearing the peripheral blood and bone marrow compartments of disease. In previously untreated patients, Alemtuzumab has demonstrated increased response rates and has been administered subcutaneously in this clinical setting (114,115). Ongoing studies are evaluating new monoclonal antibody therapies used with chemotherapy either in combination or sequentially.

Active immunotherapy approaches involve vaccination strategies to induce an immune response in the tumor-bearing patient. CLL/SLL cells are very poor antigen-presenting cells, but one way to increase their antigen-presenting capacity is to stimulate the cells through their surface receptor CD40 (116). CLL/SLL cells can be made to express recombinant CD40-ligand (CD154) by transduction with a replication-defective adenovirus vector (Ad-CD154). Ad-CD154–transduced and bystander leukemia cells become highly effective antigen-presenting cells that can induce CLL/SLL-specific autologous cytotoxic T lymphocytes *in vitro*. After a one-time bolus infusion of autologous Ad-CD154–transduced leukemia cells, there was increased or *de novo* expression of immune accessory molecules on bystander noninfected CLL/SLL cells *in vivo* (117). Treated patients also developed high plasma levels of interleukin-12 and interferon-γ. This approach may provide a novel and effective form of gene therapy for patients with this disease and is currently in phase II trials.

Stem Cell Transplantation

For patients with intermediate-grade non-Hodgkin's lymphoma, autologous stem cell transplantation has been shown to result in improved outcome compared to conventional salvage therapy for patients with chemosensitive disease (118).

In CLL/SLL, no studies have been reported that directly compare the outcome after standard therapy compared to stem cell transplantation. However, a number of studies examining the outcome after autologous stem cell transplantation for CLL/SLL have been reported to date. In a pilot study from Dana-Farber Cancer Institute, 12 patients underwent autologous stem cell transplantation (119). These patients had been heavily pretreated and received an intensive conditioning regime. Eligibility criteria for entry into this study included documented chemosensitivity, and patients had to achieve protocol-eligible minimal-disease status before stem cell transplantation. After a median follow-up of 12 months, a complete response was achieved in six out of nine patients. More than 150 patients have currently undergone this treatment at Dana-Farber Cancer Institute. Initial results of autologous stem cell transplantation from the M.D. Anderson Cancer Center were less encouraging (120). These patients were also heavily pretreated and underwent autologous stem cell transplantation, not at a time of minimal tumor burden, but after subsequent relapse. Seven patients received stem cells purged by immunomagnetic depletion; however, in five patients, residual clonal B cells were detectable. The outcome for these patients was poor. Three underwent a Richter's transformation, two died in complete remission, and two relapsed. Only two achieved a complete remission and one a partial response. In a Finnish study, eight heavily pretreated patients received autologous stem cell transplantation with partially purged CD34$^+$ peripheral blood stem cells, and although four patients remained in complete remission, the median follow-up is very short at only 9 months (121). The potential role of autologous stem cell transplantation was evaluated in 20 heavily pretreated patients with advanced CLL/SLL (122). The majority of patients were not eligible for stem cell transplantation because of the lack of sufficient mobilization of CD34$^+$ cells, disease progression, or pretransplant therapy–related deaths. Of the remaining eight patients, six achieved a complete response with a median duration of 33 months. A high relapse rate after autologous stem cell transplantation in CLL/SLL has also been observed by Pavletic and colleagues (123). After a median follow-up of 41 months, eight of 16 patients had relapsed, and six had died (three from progressive malignancy). Other groups observed better results. Dreger et al. investigated 18 patients with CLL/SLL, including early-stage disease (124). Transplantation was performed in 13 patients. Only one patient had relapsed at the time of publication. In a study by Esteve and colleagues, five patients underwent autologous stem cell transplantation (125). Four of these patients achieved a complete molecular remission. The median follow-up in this study was 13 months. In another study, ten patients undergoing autologous stem cell transplantation were investigated, and at follow-up of 22 months, five patients remained in complete molecular remission (126). However, there does appear to be a higher incidence of opportunistic infections in patients undergoing autologous stem cell transplantation for CLL/SLL compared to other patient populations. Whether this is due to a greater degree of immune incompetence in patients with CLL/SLL or is secondary to the immune-suppressive effects of fludarabine and other therapy remains to be determined (127–129). The use of prophylactic antimicrobial therapy appears to be indicated in CLL/SLL patients after stem cell transplantation (130).

Allogeneic Stem Cell Transplantation

Allogeneic stem cell transplantation is associated with significant morbidity and mortality, both from regimen-related toxicity and from graft-versus-host disease and infection. In a report of registry data, treatment-related mortality after allogeneic stem cell transplantation was 46% in patients with CLL/SLL, with the mortality from graft-versus-host disease being 20% (131). In this report, patients with Rai stages 0, I, and II disease were included. Clearly, this level of mortality is worrisome, especially in patients who may have survived for many years without therapy. In a study from the M.D. Anderson Cancer Center, outcome after allogeneic bone marrow transplant in 14 patients with CLL/SLL that was refractory to, or had relapsed after, chemotherapy with fludarabine was reported. Thirteen (87%) achieved a complete response posttransplant. At the time of reporting, nine patients (53%) remained alive and in complete response, with a median follow-up of 36 months (132). These data compared favorably to published reports of patients with other forms of leukemia, as well as to the results in patients with CLL/SLL who had received comparable prior therapy but without fludarabine exposure. These data indicate that allogeneic hematopoietic transplantation can induce durable remission even in patients with CLL/SLL refractory to fludarabine. The authors suggested that prior exposure to fludarabine may decrease the incidence of severe acute graft-versus-host disease, possibly through its immunosuppressive effects (132). The outcomes of 25 patients with CLL/SLL who underwent allogeneic stem cell transplantation at the Fred Hutchinson Cancer Center were reported (133). Twenty-one donors were human lymphocyte antibody–matched siblings, one was a partially mismatched sibling, and three were syngeneic. Fourteen patients developed grades 2 to 4 acute graft-versus-host disease, and ten developed clinical, extensive, chronic graft-versus-host disease. Late clearance of CLL/SLL cells was associated with the development of chronic graft-versus-host disease in one patient. Two patients had recurrent CLL/SLL. Nonrelapse mortality at day 100 was unacceptably high at 57% for the seven patients conditioned with busulfan and cyclophosphamide and 17% for the 18 patients conditioned with total-body irradiation–containing regimens. Actuarial survival at 5 years for the 25 patients was 32%. All patients who received busulfan and cyclophosphamide died within 3 years of transplant. For the 14 patients transplanted since 1992 who received total-body irradiation, actuarial 5-year survival is 56%, suggesting that long-term disease-free survival might be achieved in this disease.

The major advantage of the use of allogeneic stem cell transplantation appears to be the potential for a graft-versus-leukemia effect. This effect can potentially be exploited by infusion of donor lymphocytes after allografting. A number of case reports in patients with CLL/SLL have suggested that a graft-versus-leukemia effect is operative in this malignancy, either after infusion of donor lymphocytes (134) or after cessation of immunosuppressive therapy (135). In a patient with persistent lymphocytosis and lymphadenopathy after allogeneic transplantation, infusion of donor lymphocytes on day 87 posttransplant resulted in attainment of complete response after development of chronic graft-versus-host disease (134). A number of studies are under way addressing the issue of the number of lymphocytes required and the optimal timing of donor lymphocyte infusions after allogeneic stem cell transplantation in this and other hematologic malignancies. In addition, preclinical studies are attempting to develop strategies to exploit maximal graft-versus-leukemia effect without concomitant graft-versus-host disease.

Nonmyeloablative Stem Cell Transplantation for Chronic Lymphocytic Leukemia/B-Cell Small Lymphocytic Lymphoma

A major advance in reducing the short-term morbidity and mortality has come from the introduction of nonmyeloablative conditioning regimens to allow engraftment of allogeneic stem cells. Although these procedures are commonly known as *mini–stem cell transplantation*, this misnomer significantly underestimates the risks of such procedures that are due to graft-versus-host disease. Frequently, these regimens include fludarabine in the conditioning regimen and exploit the immunosuppressive as well as antileukemic properties of this agent. In this setting, the majority of the antilymphoma effect results from the graft-versus-lymphoma effect and not from the chemotherapy (136,137). The patients were often heavily pretreated and therapy refractory. Despite this, the majority of patients demonstrated donor engraftment, and the complete response rate was high. Survival appeared to be improved in patients transplanted while they still had sensitive disease. These studies provide perhaps the strongest direct evidence to date for a graft-versus-lymphoma effect and demonstrate the presence of a potentially powerful graft-versus-leukemia effect that can be exploited in the management of CLL/SLL. A major focus of ongoing research is the amount of pretransplant and posttransplant immunosuppression required to establish stable mixed chimerism and eventual full donor chimerism after nonmyeloablative stem cell transplantation. It should be stressed that these procedures are currently investigational in nature, and although the acute morbidity and mortality appear significantly lower compared to high-dose conditioning regimens with allogeneic transplantation, the longer-term results with regard to the morbidity of chronic graft-versus-host disease and disease control are currently lacking.

Unique Complications of Chronic Lymphocytic Leukemia/Small Lymphocytic Lymphoma

CLL/SLL is frequently associated with autoimmune phenomena, the most common being autoimmune hemolytic anemia and immune thrombocytopenia. The direct anti-globulin test may be positive in up to one-third of cases during the course of disease, and overt autoimmune hemolytic anemia occurs in 11% of cases (138). In a comprehensive report of 1,203 consecutive patients with CLL/SLL reported from a single institution, 52 (4.3%) cases of autoimmune hemolytic anemia were observed (139). Nineteen cases were observed at the time of diagnosis and 33 during subsequent follow-up. Ninety percent of the patients with autoimmune hemolytic anemia had active CLL, and 25% occurred when the patient had been treated previously. The autoantibody was IgM in 13% and an IgG in 87% of cases. A lymphocyte count more than 60×10^9 per L ($p < .00001$), age older than 65 years, and male gender emerged as independent factors that correlated significantly with an increased rate of autoimmune hemolytic anemia at CLL diagnosis. Patients previously treated with chlorambucil plus prednisone or with fludarabine showed a similar rate of autoimmune hemolytic anemia (1.8% and 2.5%, respectively). In this study, the presence of autoimmune hemolytic anemia was not associated with poor prognosis. Autoimmune thrombocytopenia based on the presence of an adequate number of megakaryocytes with a low platelet count in peripheral blood occurs more rarely and is present in 2% to 3% of patients (138). This complication has been reported more frequently after therapy with fludarabine (140). Pure red-cell aplasia is rare but may occur early in the disease course. Although the etiology of this disorder is unclear, it has been reported that it responds to therapy with immune-modulating agents, including rituximab, fludarabine, and cyclosporin A (141–143). Neutropenia is common, but although agranulocytosis may be encountered, this is rare.

Infections are the major cause of morbidity and mortality in patients with CLL/SLL. Predisposition to infection in CLL/SLL is mediated through various abnormalities, including both the immune defects inherent in the primary disease (impairment in humoral and cellular immunity) and in the further immunosuppression related to the management of CLL/SLL. Hypogammaglobulinemia is probably the most important immune defect in terms of risk of severe bacterial infections, its frequency and severity progressing with the duration of the disease. In a randomized crossover study among patients with severe hypogammaglobulinemia, the incidence and severity of infections were less in the months when patients received Ig-replacement therapy (144). The frequency of infections may also be increased and altered after therapy (145). Although bacterial infections are most common, the purine analogs, especially when used in previously treated patients or in combination, may be associated with a wide spectrum of opportunistic infections, including *Listeria monocytogenes*, *Pneumocystis carinii*, cytomegalovirus, herpes simplex virus, and mycobacteria, because of the resulting T-cell dysfunction (76,146). Long-term follow-up of fludarabine-treated patients suggests that although the purine analogs have an impact on opportunistic infections,

complications of infection are more common in those patients with incomplete response to therapy or with progressive disease, suggesting that the disease itself has more impact than the therapy (147). Although opportunistic infections are also seen after therapy with Alemtuzumab (113), patients treated with this agent were fludarabine refractory, and serious infectious complications are high in this patient population. Serious infectious complications in patients with fludarabine-refractory disease occurred in 89% of patients, with infections being bacterial in 78.5%, viral in 12.5%, fungal in 4.5%, and opportunistic in 4.5% (148).

Future Directions

For many years, the treatment of CLL/SLL has been palliative rather than curative and has not resulted in improved survival in patients with CLL/SLL. Although stem cell transplantation may offer the possibility of cure in a small subset of patients, this approach is not applicable to the vast majority of more elderly patients. The median survival of patients with CLL/SLL from diagnosis ranges from months to several decades, and the decision whether to treat and, in particular, when to treat cannot be made without an assessment of the patient's underlying prognosis. It, therefore, seems most likely that we will continue to use "risk-adjusted" approaches to manage patients with CLL/SLL and that what is changing is what is used to assess prognosis. Disease stage remains important, but biologic markers (and in particular cytogenetics), Ig gene mutation status, CD38 expression, and, potentially, gene array may be capable of identifying patients who would benefit from more aggressive therapy. Although early results of combination chemotherapy and monoclonal antibody therapy appear encouraging, longer follow-up will be required to determine whether these combinations are curative in any patients. Although still premature, it will soon be timely to examine in the clinical trial setting the use of aggressive combination chemo-immunotherapy at the time of diagnosis and reexamine whether the era of "watch and wait" is over for patients with "high-risk" disease.

PROLYMPHOCYTIC LEUKEMIA

Prolymphocytic leukemia (PLL) was originally described as a variant of CLL, characterized by its distinct clinical and laboratory features. There is clonal proliferation of medium-sized prolymphocytes involving peripheral blood, bone marrow, and spleen. In this disease, prolymphocytes comprise greater than 55% of the cells in blood and bone marrow and typically more than 90% of the neoplastic cells. It is now apparent that this disease represents a separate entity from CLL. PLL can be B cell or T cell in type. Although both of these entities occur with almost equal frequency, the disease is rare and accounts for only 2% of cases with malignant lymphocytosis. Although B-cell and T-cell PLL are discussed together, they are also distinct diseases, based on their molecular pathogenesis.

B-Cell Prolymphocytic Leukemia

Morphology

In B-cell PLL (B-PLL), prolymphocytes comprise greater than 55% of the cells in blood and bone marrow and typically more than 90% of the neoplastic cells. The bone marrow is usually infiltrated with prolymphocytes, most often in an interstitial manner. The spleen shows extensive white- and red-pulp infiltration by prolymphocytes. Lymph node involvement may demonstrate nodularity, but proliferation centers or pseudofollicles are absent. Peripheral blood prolymphocytes are medium sized and approximately twice the size of small lymphocytes, with moderately condensed chromatin and a single prominent vesicular nucleolus. The nucleus is typically round, and the cytoplasm is usually scant to moderate and weakly basophilic.

Immunophenotype

The cells express bright surface IgM and IgD and bright CD20, as well as other B-cell markers, including CD19, CD21, CD22, CD24, and FMC7. In contrast to CLL/SLL, they do not express CD23, and more than two-thirds of cases do not express CD5. The differential diagnosis includes CLL, the leukemic form of mantle cell lymphoma, and other lymphomas. B-PLL may also be confused with hairy-cell–leukemia variants. The diagnosis requires histologic assessment and extended immunophenotype, with genetic and molecular analysis. Input from expert hematopathologists with experience in these diseases is often required to make a definitive diagnosis.

Genetics

Chromosome abnormalities in B-PLL are often complex, involving a number of different chromosomes. Deletions of 13q14 and 11q23 are frequent chromosome aberrations in B-PLL and, in contrast to CLL, there is a preferential loss of RB1, suggesting that allelic loss of the RB1 gene may play a role in the pathogenesis of B-PLL (149). More recent data have suggested that many of the cases with 11q23 abnormalities may represent variant cases of mantle cell lymphoma. Staining with cyclin D1 may be important to differentiate mantle cell variants from B-PLL. There is also a very high frequency of p53 mutation (53%) in B-PLL, and this may be responsible for the frequent resistance to therapy of this disease. In addition, the pattern of p53 mutation was different from that observed in CLL and other hematologic malignancies and may indicate a distinct pathogenesis in this disease (150). B-PLL cells express a skewed repertoire characterized by predominant use of the V3 family members and preferential use of the V3-23 gene. The IgV genes are mutated, suggesting expansion of postgerminal center cells that have undergone antigen-driven selection (151).

Clinical Presentation

Features distinguishing PLL from CLL/SLL include hyperlymphocytosis and massive splenomegaly, although the presenting features can be indistinguishable, and diagnosis depends on the distinct morphologic and immunophenotypic characteristics of this disease. Patients typically present with a high white count, with one-third of patients having a white blood cell count greater than 200×10^9 per L. Anemia and thrombocytopenia are common. In contrast to CLL, autoimmune phenomena are rare in B-PLL. Although in some cases the disease can remain stable for months or even years, progression is inevitable. The median survival in a series of 35 patients with B-PLL was 65 months (152). Response to alkylating agents is poor, and addition of anthracyclines appears to offer benefit. Treatment with purine analogs has resulted in response rates higher than those seen in historical controls (152,153).

T-Cell Prolymphocytic Leukemia

Morphology

In T-cell PLL (T-PLL), the majority of the circulating cells are prolymphocytes, which are typically smaller than B-PLL cells and have less abundant cytoplasm. In 20% of cases, the cells are small but have the typical immunophenotypic and genetic features described below. The pattern of bone marrow infiltration is interstitial or diffuse, or both, and often extensive. Histology of the spleen reveals infiltration of both the white and red pulp. Lymph node histology reveals infiltration of the paracortical area with residual follicular centers.

Immunophenotype

Immunologic markers show a postthymic T-cell phenotype with failure to express terminal deoxynucleotidyl transferase or CD1a. Most cases express CD2 and CD5 but do not express CD3. There is particularly strong expression of CD7. A CD4$^+$, CD8$^-$ phenotype is seen in two-thirds of cases. CD4 and CD8 are coexpressed in 25%, and a CD4$^-$, CD8$^+$ phenotype is rare. All cases exhibit rearrangement of the T-cell receptor alpha and beta genes.

Genetics

T-PLL is characterized by complex karyotypes with recurrent chromosomal abnormalities. The most common abnormality, seen in 75% of cases, includes translocations involving TCL1 at 14q32.1. Other abnormalities involve the MTCP1 at Xq28; inactivation of the ATM gene by deletion, mutation, or both; and isochromosome 8 (154). Deletion of the 11q is frequent and further analysis has revealed absence, premature truncation, or alteration of the ATM gene product on the other allele, suggesting that ATM functions as a tumor-suppressor gene and has a role in the pathogenesis of T-PLL (155). Deletions at 13q14.3, with additional loss of tumor-suppressor function, could further contribute to the development of overt disease (156).

Diagnosis and Treatment

Differential diagnosis between T-PLL and other T-cell malignancies is based on a constellation of their clinical and laboratory features. Generally, T-PLL patients are refractory to the therapy used in lymphoid disorders (157). Median survival is short (7.5 months). Although T-PLL is generally chemotherapy resistant, encouraging results have been observed with Alemtuzumab. In a series of 39 patients with T-PLL, all but two were heavily pretreated, and none had achieved a previous complete response. Alemtuzumab was administered three times weekly until maximal response (158). The overall response rate was 76%, with a 60% complete-response rate and a 16% partial-response rate. The median disease-free survival was 7 months and ranged from 4 to 45 months. Survival was prolonged significantly in patients achieving complete response. In another series of 76 T-PLL patients similarly treated, the overall response rate was 51%, with 39% achieving complete repsonse. The median duration of response was 8.7 months. The median overall survival was 7.5 months and 14.8 months for patients in complete remission (159). Alemtuzumab is now being explored as first-line therapy in this disease.

Stem Cell Transplantation for Prolymphocytic Leukemia

A small number of cases of PLL has been treated by allogeneic, hematopoietic, stem cell transplantation (158,160). Seven patients who had been treated with Alemtuzumab subsequently received high-dose therapy with autologous stem cell support, three of whom remain alive in complete remission 5, 7, and 15 months after autograft (158). Stem cell harvests in these patients were uncontaminated with T-PLL cells, as demonstrated by dual-color flow cytometry and polymerase chain reaction analysis. Four patients underwent allogeneic stem cell transplants, three from siblings and one from a matched unrelated donor. Two had nonmyeloablative conditioning. Three are alive in complete remission up to 24 months after allogeneic stem cell transplant (158).

Future Directions

The treatment of PLL has also been palliative. Better responses are seen with purine analogs, and Alemtuzumab is being used increasingly as first-line therapy. Combination therapies, including monoclonal antibodies, are being explored. With more durable responses, stem cell transplant approaches are being used in selected younger patients and may be associated with improved outcome for these previously incurable diseases.

REFERENCES

1. Harris NL, Jaffe ES, Diebold J, et al. World Health Organization classification of neoplastic diseases of the hematopoietic and lymphoid tissues: report of the Clinical Advisory Committee meeting-Airlie House, Virginia, November 1997. *J Clin Oncol* 1999;17:3835–3849.
2. Zent CS, Kyasa MJ, Evans R, et al. Chronic lymphocytic leukemia incidence is substantially higher than estimated from tumor registry data. *Cancer* 2001;92:1325–1330.
3. Hernandez JA, Land KJ, McKenna RW. Leukemias, myeloma, and other lymphoreticular neoplasms. *Cancer* 1995;75:381–394.
4. Mauro FR, Foa R, Giannarelli D, et al. Clinical characteristics and outcome of young chronic lymphocytic leukemia patients: a single institution study of 204 cases. *Blood* 1999;94:448–454.
5. Parkin DM, Muir CS. Cancer incidence in five continents. Comparability and quality of data. *IARC Sci Publ* 1992;(120):45–173.
6. Haenszel W, Kurihara M. Studies of Japanese migrants. I. Mortality from cancer and other diseases among Japanese in the United States. *J Natl Cancer Inst* 1968;40:43–68.
7. Ron E. Ionizing radiation and cancer risk: evidence from epidemiology. *Radiat Res* 1998;150:S30–S41.
8. Brandt L. Environmental factors and leukaemia. *Med Oncol Tumor Pharmacother* 1985;2:7–10.
9. Nanni O, Amadori D, Lugaresi C, et al. Chronic lymphocytic leukaemias and non-Hodgkin's lymphomas by histological type in farming-animal breeding workers: a population case-control study based on a priori exposure matrices. *Occup Environ Med* 1996;53:652–657.
10. Huebner WW, Chen VW, Friedlander BR, et al. Incidence of lympho-haematopoietic malignancies in a petrochemical industry cohort: 1983–94 follow up. *Occup Environ Med* 2000;57:605–614.
11. Zahm SH, Weisenburger DD, Babbitt PA, et al. Use of hair coloring products and the risk of lymphoma, multiple myeloma, and chronic lymphocytic leukemia. *Am J Public Health* 1992;82:990–997.
12. Yuille MR, Matutes E, Marossy A, et al. Familial chronic lymphocytic leukaemia: a survey and review of published studies. *Br J Haematol* 2000;109:794–799.
13. Videbaek A. Familial leukemia. *Acta Medica Scand* 1947;127:26–52.
14. Ishibe N, Sgambati MT, Fontaine L, et al. Clinical characteristics of familial B-CLL in the National Cancer Institute Familial Registry. *Leuk Lymphoma* 2001;42:99–108.
15. Horwitz M, Goode EL, Jarvik GP. Anticipation in familial leukemia. *Am J Hum Genet* 1996;59:990–998.
16. Yuille MR, Houlston RS, Catovsky D. Anticipation in familial chronic lymphocytic leukemia. *Leukemia* 1998;12:1696–1698.
17. Goldin LR, Sgambati M, Marti GE, et al. Anticipation in familial chronic lymphocytic leukemia. *Am J Hum Genet* 1999;65:265–269.
18. Ben-Ezra J, Burke JS, Swartz WG, et al. Small lymphocytic lymphoma: a clinicopathologic analysis of 268 cases. *Blood* 1989;73:579–587.
19. Damle RN, Wasil T, Fais F, et al. Ig V gene mutation status and CD38 expression as novel prognostic indicators in chronic lymphocytic leukemia. *Blood* 1999;94:1840–1847.
20. Hamblin TJ, Orchard JA, Ibbotson RE, et al. CD38 expression and immunoglobulin variable region mutations are independent prognostic variables in chronic lymphocytic leukemia, but CD38 expression may vary during the course of the disease. *Blood* 2002;99:1023–1029.
21. Dohner H, Stilgenbauer S, Benner A, et al. Genomic aberrations and survival in chronic lymphocytic leukemia. *N Engl J Med* 2000;343:1910–1916.
22. Stilgenbauer S, Leupolt E, Ohl S, et al. Heterogeneity of deletions involving RB-1 and the D13S25 locus in B-cell chronic lymphocytic leukemia revealed by fluorescence in situ hybridization. *Cancer Res* 1995;55:3475–3477.
23. Bullrich F, Veronese ML, Kitada S, et al. Minimal region of loss at 13q14 in B-cell chronic lymphocytic leukemia. *Blood* 1996;88:3109–3115.
24. Kalachikov S, Migliazza A, Cayanis E, et al. Cloning and gene mapping of the chromosome 13q14 region deleted in chronic lymphocytic leukemia. *Genomics* 1997;42:369–377.
25. Bullrich F, Fujii H, Calin G, et al. Characterization of the 13q14 tumor suppressor locus in CLL: identification of ALT1, an alternative splice variant of the LEU2 gene. *Cancer Res* 2001;61:6640–6648.
26. Mabuchi H, Fujii H, Calin G, et al. Cloning and characterization of CLLD6, CLLD7, and CLLD8, novel candidate genes for leukemogenesis at chromosome 13q14, a region commonly deleted in B-cell chronic lymphocytic leukemia. *Cancer Res* 2001;61:2870–2877.
27. Dohner H, Stilgenbauer S, James MR, et al. 11q deletions identify a new subset of B-cell chronic lymphocytic leukemia characterized by extensive nodal involvement and inferior prognosis. *Blood* 1997;89:2516–2522.
28. Bullrich F, Rasio D, Kitada S, et al. ATM mutations in B-cell chronic lymphocytic leukemia. *Cancer Res* 1999;59:24–27.

29. Banin S, Moyal L, Shieh S, et al. Enhanced phosphorylation of p53 by ATM in response to DNA damage. *Science* 1998;281:1674–1677.

30. Canman CE, Lim DS, Cimprich KA, et al. Activation of the ATM kinase by ionizing radiation and phosphorylation of p53. *Science* 1998;281:1677–1679.

31. Dohner H, Fischer K, Bentz M, et al. p53 gene deletion predicts for poor survival and non-response to therapy with purine analogs in chronic B-cell leukemias. *Blood* 1995;85:1580–1589.

32. Fais F, Ghiotto F, Hashimoto S, et al. Chronic lymphocytic leukemia B cells express restricted sets of mutated and unmutated antigen receptors. *J Clin Invest* 1998;102:1515–1525.

33. Hamblin TJ, Davis Z, Gardiner A, et al. Unmutated Ig V(H) genes are associated with a more aggressive form of chronic lymphocytic leukemia. *Blood* 1999;94:1848–1854.

34. Klein U, Tu Y, Stolovitzky GA, et al. Gene expression profiling of B cell chronic lymphocytic leukemia reveals a homogeneous phenotype related to memory B cells. *J Exp Med* 2001;194:1625–1638.

35. Rosenwald A, Alizadeh AA, Widhopf G, et al. Relation of gene expression phenotype to immunoglobulin mutation genotype in B cell chronic lymphocytic leukemia. *J Exp Med* 2001;194:1639–1647.

36. Chen L, Widhopf G, Huynh L, et al. Expression of ZAP-70 is associated with increased B-cell receptor signaling in chronic lymphocytic leukemia. *Blood* 2002;100:4609–4614.

37. Cheson BD, Bennett JM, Rai KR, et al. Guidelines for clinical protocols for chronic lymphocytic leukemia: recommendations of the National Cancer Institute-sponsored Working Group. *Am J Hematol* 1988;29:152–163.

38. Cerroni L, Zenahlik P, Hofler G, et al. Specific cutaneous infiltrates of B-cell chronic lymphocytic leukemia: a clinicopathologic and prognostic study of 42 patients. *Am J Surg Pathol* 1996;20:1000–1010.

39. Garicochea B, Cliquet MG, Melo N, et al. Leptomeningeal involvement in chronic lymphocytic leukemia. *Modern Pathology* 1997;10:500–503.

40. Miller K, Budke H, Orazi A. Leukemic meningitis complicating early stage chronic lymphocytic leukemia. *Arch Pathol Lab Med* 1997;121:524–527.

41. Rai KR, Sawitsky A, Cronkite EP, et al. Clinical staging of chronic lymphocytic leukemia. *Blood* 1975;46:219–234.

42. Binet JL, Auquier A, Dighiero G, et al. A new prognostic classification of chronic lymphocytic leukemia derived from a multivariate survival analysis. *Cancer* 1981;48:198–206.

43. Chronic lymphocytic leukaemia: proposals for a revised prognostic staging system. Report from the International Workshop on CLL. *Br J Haematol* 1981;48:365–367.

44. Rundles RW, Moore JO. Chronic lymphocytic leukemia. *Cancer* 1978;42:941–945.

45. Jaksic B, Vitale B. Total tumour mass score (TTM): a new parameter in chronic lymphocyte leukaemia. *Br J Haematol* 1981;49:405–413.

46. Mandelli F, De Rossi G, Mancini P, et al. Prognosis in chronic lymphocytic leukemia: a retrospective multicentric study from the GIMEMA group. *J Clin Oncol* 1987;5:398–406.

47. Lee JS, Dixon DO, Kantarjian HM, et al. Prognosis of chronic lymphocytic leukemia: a multivariate regression analysis of 325 untreated patients. *Blood* 1987;69:929–936.

48. Rai KR. A critical analysis of staging in CLL. In: *Chronic lymphocytic leukemia: recent progress and future directions. UCLA Symposia on Molecular and Cellular Biology*, vol. 59. New York: Alan R Liss, 1987:253–264.

49. Rozman C, Montserrat E, Rodriguez-Fernandez JM, et al. Bone marrow histologic pattern—the best single prognostic parameter in chronic lymphocytic leukemia: a multivariate survival analysis of 329 cases. *Blood* 1984;64:642–648.

50. Oscier DG, Matutes E, Copplestone A, et al. Atypical lymphocyte morphology: an adverse prognostic factor for disease progression in stage A CLL independent of trisomy 12. *Br J Haematol* 1997;98:934–939.

51. Montserrat E, Sanchez-Bisono J, Vinolas N, et al. Lymphocyte doubling time in chronic lymphocytic leukaemia: analysis of its prognostic significance. *Br J Haematol* 1986;62:567–575.

52. Molica S, Alberti A. Prognostic value of the lymphocyte doubling time in chronic lymphocytic leukemia. *Cancer* 1987;60:2712–2717.

53. Cordone I, Matutes E, Catovsky D. Monoclonal antibody Ki-67 identifies B and T cells in cycle in chronic lymphocytic leukemia: correlation with disease activity. *Leukemia* 1992;6:902–906.

54. Vrhovac R, Delmer A, Tang R, et al. Prognostic significance of the cell cycle inhibitor p27Kip1 in chronic B-cell lymphocytic leukemia. *Blood* 1998;91:4694–4700.

55. Hallek M, Langenmayer I, Nerl C, et al. Elevated serum thymidine kinase levels identify a subgroup at high risk of disease progression in early, nonsmoldering chronic lymphocytic leukemia. *Blood* 1999;93:1732–1737.

56. Hallek M, Wanders L, Ostwald M, et al. Serum beta(2)-microglobulin and serum thymidine kinase are independent predictors of progression-free survival in chronic lymphocytic leukemia and immunocytoma. *Leuk Lymphoma* 1996;22:439–447.

57. Fayad L, Keating MJ, Reuben JM, et al. Interleukin-6 and interleukin-10 levels in chronic lymphocytic leukemia: correlation with phenotypic characteristics and outcome. *Blood* 2001;97:256–263.

58. Ferrajoli A, Keating MJ, Manshouri T, et al. The clinical significance of tumor necrosis factor-alpha plasma level in patients having chronic lymphocytic leukemia. *Blood* 2002;100:1215–1219.

59. Molica S, Vitelli G, Levato D, et al. Increased serum levels of vascular endothelial growth factor predict risk of progression in early B-cell chronic lymphocytic leukaemia. *Br J Haematol* 1999;107:605–610.

60. Stilgenbauer S, Bullinger L, Lichter P, et al. Genetics of chronic lymphocytic leukemia: genomic aberrations and V(H) gene mutation status in pathogenesis and clinical course. *Leukemia* 2002;16:993–1007.

61. Del Poeta G, Maurillo L, Venditti A, et al. Clinical significance of CD38 expression in chronic lymphocytic leukemia. *Blood* 2001;98:2633–2639.

62. Ibrahim S, Keating M, Do KA, et al. CD38 expression as an important prognostic factor in B-cell chronic lymphocytic leukemia. *Blood.* 2001;98:181–186.

63. Hamblin TJ, Orchard JA, Gardiner A, et al. Immunoglobulin V genes and CD38 expression in CLL. *Blood* 2000;95:2455–2457.

64. Oscier DG, Gardiner AC, Mould SJ, et al. Multivariate analysis of prognostic factors in CLL: clinical stage, IGVH gene mutational status, and loss or mutation of the p53 gene are independent prognostic factors. *Blood* 2002;100:1177–1184.

65. Chemotherapeutic options in chronic lymphocytic leukemia: a meta-analysis of the randomized trials. CLL Trialists' Collaborative Group. *J Natl Cancer Inst* 1999;91:861–868.

66. Chronic lymphocytic leukemia: recommendations for diagnosis, staging, and response criteria. International Workshop on Chronic Lymphocytic Leukemia. *Ann Intern Med* 1989;110:236–238.

67. Cheson BD, Bennett JM, Grever M, et al. National Cancer Institute-sponsored Working Group guidelines for chronic lymphocytic leukemia: revised guidelines for diagnosis and treatment. *Blood* 1996;87:4990–4997.

68. Han T, Ezdinli EZ, Shimaoka K, et al. Chlorambucil vs. combined chlorambucil-corticosteroid therapy in chronic lymphocytic leukemia. *Cancer* 1973;31:502–508.

69. Sawitsky A, Rai KR, Glidewell O, et al. Comparison of daily versus intermittent chlorambucil and prednisone therapy in the treatment of patients with chronic lymphocytic leukemia. *Blood* 1977;50:1049–1059.

70. A randomized clinical trial of chlorambucil versus COP in stage B chronic lymphocytic leukemia. The French Cooperative Group on Chronic Lymphocytic Leukemia. *Blood* 1990;75:1422–1425.

71. Raphael B, Andersen JW, Silber R, et al. Comparison of chlorambucil and prednisone versus cyclophosphamide, vincristine, and prednisone as initial treatment for chronic lymphocytic leukemia: long-term follow-up of an Eastern Cooperative Oncology Group randomized clinical trial. *J Clin Oncol* 1991;9:770–776.

72. Catovsky D, Fooks J, Richards S. MRC working party on leukemia in adults. Prognostic factors in chronic lymphocytic leukemia: the importance of age, sex and response to treatment in survival. *Br J Haematol* 1989;72:141–149.

73. Long-term results of the CHOP regimen in stage C chronic lymphocytic leukaemia. French Cooperative Group on Chronic Lymphocytic Leukaemia. *Br J Haematol* 1989;73:334–340.

74. Grever MR, Kopecky KJ, Coltman CA, et al. Fludarabine monophosphate: a potentially useful agent in chronic lymphocytic leukemia. *Nouv Rev Fr Hematol* 1988;30:457–459.

75. Keating MJ, Kantarjian H, Talpaz M, et al. Fludarabine: a new agent with major activity against chronic lymphocytic leukemia. *Blood* 1989;74:19–25.

76. O'Brien S, Kantarjian H, Beran M, et al. Results of fludarabine and prednisone therapy in 264 patients with chronic lymphocytic leukemia with multivariate analysis-derived prognostic model for response to treatment. *Blood* 1993;82:1695–1700.

77. Fenchel K, Bergmann L, Wijermans P, et al. Clinical experience with fludarabine and its immunosuppressive effects in pretreated chronic lymphocytic leukemias and low-grade lymphomas. *Leuk Lymphoma* 1995;18:485–492.

78. Montserrat E, Hallek M. Current strategies for the treatment of CLL. *Leuk Lymphoma* 1996;2:65–68. [review]

79. Tallman MS, Hakimian D, Zanzig C, et al. Cladribine in the treatment of relapsed or refractory chronic lymphocytic leukemia. *J Clin Oncol* 1995;13:983–988.

80. Robak T, Blonski JZ, Kasznicki M, et al. Cladribine with or without prednisone in the treatment of previously treated and untreated B-cell chronic lymphocytic leukaemia—updated results of the multicentre study of 378 patients. *Br J Haematol* 2000;108:357–368.

81. Dillman RO, Mick R, McIntyre OR. Pentostatin in chronic lymphocytic leukemia: a phase II trial of Cancer and Leukemia Group B. *J Clin Oncol* 1989;7:433–438.

82. Ho AD, Thaler J, Stryckmans P, et al. Pentostatin in refractory chronic lymphocytic leukemia: a phase II trial of the European Organization for Research and Treatment of Cancer. *J Natl Cancer Inst* 1990;82:1416–1420.

83. Johnson SA, Catovsky D, Child JA, et al. Phase I/II evaluation of pentostatin (2'-deoxycoformycin) in a five day schedule for the treatment of relapsed/refractory B-cell chronic lymphocytic leukaemia. *Invest New Drugs* 1998;16:155–160.

84. Keating MJ, Kantarjian H, O'Brien S, et al. Fludarabine: a new agent with marked cytoreductive activity in untreated chronic lymphocytic leukemia. *J Clin Oncol* 1991;9:44–49.

85. Rai KR, Peterson BL, Appelbaum FR, et al. Fludarabine compared with chlorambucil as primary therapy for chronic lymphocytic leukemia. *N Engl J Med* 2000;343:1750–1757.

86. Leporrier M, Chevret S, Cazin B, et al. Randomized comparison of fludarabine, CAP, and CHOP in 938 previously untreated stage B and C chronic lymphocytic leukemia patients. *Blood* 2001;98:2319–2325.

87. Saven A, Lemon RH, Kosty M, et al. 2-Chlorodeoxyadenosine activity in patients with untreated chronic lymphocytic leukemia. *J Clin Oncol* 1995;13:570–574.

88. Juliusson G, Liliemark J. Long-term survival following cladribine (2-chlorodeoxyadenosine) therapy. *Ann Oncol* 1996;7:373–379.

89. Keating MJ, O'Brien S, Kantarjian H, et al. Long-term follow-up of patients with chronic lymphocytic leukemia treated with fludarabine as a single agent. *Blood* 1993;81:2878–2884.

90. Hallek M, Schmitt B, Wilhelm M, et al. Fludarabine plus cyclophosphamide is an efficient treatment for advanced chronic lymphocytic leukaemia (CLL): results of a phase II study of the German CLL Study Group. *Br J Haematol* 2001;114:342–348.

91. Flinn IW, Byrd JC, Morrison C, et al. Fludarabine and cyclophosphamide with filgrastim support in patients with previously untreated indolent lymphoid malignancies. *Blood* 2000;96:71–75.

92. O'Brien SM, Kantarjian HM, Cortes J, et al. Results of the fludarabine and cyclophosphamide combination regimen in chronic lymphocytic leukemia. *J Clin Oncol* 2001;19:1414–1420.

93. Saven A. The Scripps Clinic experience with cladribine (2-CdA) in the treatment of chronic lymphocytic leukemia. *Semin Hematol* 1996;33:28–33.

94. Juliusson G, Liliemark J. High complete remission rate from 2-chloro-2'-deoxyadenosine in previously treated patients with B-cell chronic lymphocytic leukemia: response predicted by rapid decrease of blood lymphocyte count. *J Clin Oncol* 1993;11:679–689.

95. Johnson S, Smith AG, Loffler H, et al. Multicentre prospective randomised trial of fludarabine versus cyclophosphamide, doxorubicin, and prednisone (CAP) for treatment of advanced-stage chronic lymphocytic leukaemia. The French Cooperative Group on CLL. *Lancet* 1996;347:1432–1438.

96. Thomson AE, Vaughan-Smith S, Peel WE, et al. The intrinsic radiosensitivity of lymphocytes in chronic lymphocytic leukaemia, quantitatively determined independently of cell death rate factors. *Int J Radiat Biol Relat Stud Phys Chem Med* 1985;48:943–961.

97. Thomson AE, Wetherley-Mein G, O'Connor TW, et al. Simplified quantitative estimation in vitro of lymphocyte radiosensitivity applied to patients with chronic lymphocytic leukaemia. *Leuk Res* 1991;15:577–589.

98. Weinmann M, Becker G, Einsele H, et al. Clinical indications and biological mechanisms of splenic irradiation in chronic leukaemias and myeloproliferative disorders. *Radiother Oncol* 2001;58:235–246.

99. Terstappen LW, de Grooth BG, van Berkel W, et al. The effects of splenic irradiation on lymphocyte subpopulations in chronic B-lymphocytic leukemia. *Eur J Haematol* 1988;41:496–505.

100. Chisesi T, Capnist G, Dal Fior S. Splenic irradiation in chronic lymphocytic leukemia. *Eur J Haematol* 1991;46:202–204.

101. Seymour JF, Cusack JD, Lerner SA, et al. Case/control study of the role of splenectomy in chronic lymphocytic leukemia. *J Clin Oncol* 1997;15:52–60.

102. Cusack JC Jr, Seymour JF, Lerner S, et al. Role of splenectomy in chronic lymphocytic leukemia. *J Am Coll Surg* 1997;185:237–243.

103. Johnson RE. Treatment of chronic lymphocytic leukemia by total body irradiation alone and combined with chemotherapy. *Int J Radiat Oncol Biol Phys* 1979;5:159–164.

104. Jacobs P, King HS. A randomized prospective comparison of chemotherapy to total body irradiation as initial treatment for the indolent lymphoproliferative diseases. *Blood* 1987;69:1642–1646.

105. Rubin P, Bennett JM, Begg C, et al. The comparison of total body irradiation vs chlorambucil and prednisone for remission induction of active chronic lymphocytic leukemia: an ECOG study. Part I: total body irradiation-response and toxicity. *Int J Radiat Oncol Biol Phys* 1981;7:1623–1632.

106. McLaughlin P, Grillo-Lopez AJ, Link BK, et al. Rituximab chimeric anti-CD20 monoclonal antibody therapy for relapsed indolent lymphoma: half of patients respond to a four-dose treatment program. *J Clin Oncol* 1998;16:2825–2833.

107. Foran JM, Rohatiner AZ, Cunningham D, et al. European phase II study of rituximab (chimeric anti-CD20 monoclonal antibody) for patients with newly diagnosed mantle-cell lymphoma and previously treated mantle-cell lymphoma, immunocytoma, and small B-cell lymphocytic lymphoma. *J Clin Oncol* 2000;18:317–324.

108. Huhn D, von Schilling C, Wilhelm M, et al. Rituximab therapy of patients with B-cell chronic lymphocytic leukemia. *Blood* 2001;98:1326–1331.

109. O'Brien SM, Kantarjian H, Thomas DA, et al. Rituximab dose-escalation trial in chronic lymphocytic leukemia. *J Clin Oncol* 2001;19:2165–2170.

110. Byrd JC, Murphy T, Howard RS, et al. Rituximab using a thrice weekly dosing schedule in B-cell chronic lymphocytic leukemia and small lymphocytic lymphoma demonstrates clinical activity and acceptable toxicity. *J Clin Oncol* 2001;19:2153–2164.

111. Stilgenbauer S, Dohner H. Campath-1H-induced complete remission of chronic lymphocytic leukemia despite p53 gene mutation and resistance to chemotherapy. *N Engl J Med* 2002;347:452–453.

112. Osterborg A, Dyer MJ, Bunjes D, et al. Phase II multicenter study of human CD52 antibody in previously treated chronic lymphocytic leukemia. European Study Group of CAMPATH-1H treatment in CLL. *J Clin Oncol* 1997;15: 1567–1574.

113. Keating MJ, Flinn I, Jain V, et al. Therapeutic role of alemtuzumab (Campath-1H) in patients who have failed fludarabine: results of a large international study. *Blood* 2002;99:3554–3561.

114. Osterborg A, Fassas AS, Anagnostopoulos A, et al. Humanized CD52 monoclonal antibody Campath-1H as first-line treatment in chronic lymphocytic leukaemia. *Br J Haematol* 1996;93:151–153.

115. Lundin J, Kimby E, Bjorkholm M, et al. Phase II trial of subcutaneous anti-CD52 monoclonal antibody alemtuzumab (Campath-1H) as first-line treatment for patients with B-cell chronic lymphocytic leukemia (B-CLL). *Blood* 2002;100:768–773.

116. Ranheim EA, Kipps TJ. Activated T cells induce expression of B7/BB1 on normal or leukemic B cells through a CD40-dependent signal. *J Exp Med* 1993;177:925–935.

117. Wierda WG, Cantwell MJ, Woods SJ, et al. CD40-ligand (CD154) gene therapy for chronic lymphocytic leukemia. *Blood* 2000;96:2917–2924.

118. Philip T, Armitage JO, Spitzer G, et al. High-dose therapy and autologous bone marrow transplantation after failure of conventional chemotherapy in adults with intermediate-grade or high-grade non-Hodgkin's lymphoma. *N Engl J Med* 1987;316:1493–1498.

119. Rabinowe SN, Soiffer RJ, Gribben JG, et al. Autologous and allogeneic bone marrow transplantation for poor prognosis patients with B-cell chronic lymphocytic leukemia. *Blood* 1993;82:1366–1376.

120. Khouri IF, Keating MJ, Vriesendorp HM, et al. Autologous and allogeneic bone marrow transplantation for chronic lymphocytic leukemia: preliminary results. *J Clin Oncol* 1994;12:748–758.

121. Itala M, Pelliniemi TT, Rajamaki A, et al. Autologous blood cell transplantation in B-CLL: response to chemotherapy prior to mobilization predicts the stem cell yield. *Bone Marrow Transplant* 1997; 19:647–651.

122. Sutton L, Maloum K, Gonzalez H, et al. Autologous hematopoietic stem cell transplantation as salvage treatment for advanced B cell chronic lymphocytic leukemia. *Leukemia* 1998;12:1699–1707.

123. Pavletic ZS, Bierman PJ, Vose JM, et al. High incidence of relapse after autologous stem-cell transplantation for B-cell chronic lymphocytic leukemia or small lymphocytic lymphoma. *Ann Oncol* 1998; 9:1023–1026.

124. Dreger P, von Neuhoff N, Kuse R, et al. Early stem cell transplantation for chronic lymphocytic leukaemia: a chance for cure? *Br J Cancer* 1998;77:2291–2297.

125. Esteve J, Villamor N, Colomer D, et al. Hematopoietic stem cell transplantation in chronic lymphocytic leukemia: a report of 12 patients from a single institution [see comments]. *Ann Oncol* 1998;9:167–172.

126. Schey S, Ahsan G, Jones R. Dose intensification and molecular responses in patients with chronic lymphocytic leukaemia: a phase II single centre study. *Bone Marrow Transplant* 1999;24:989–993.

127. Griffiths H, Lea J, Bunch C, et al. Predictors of infection in chronic lymphocytic leukaemia (CLL). *Clin Exp Immunol* 1992;89:374–377.

128. Robertson LE, Huh YO, Butler JJ, et al. Response assessment in chronic lymphocytic leukemia after fludarabine plus prednisone: clinical, pathologic, immunophenotypic, and molecular analysis. *Blood* 1993;80:29–36.

129. Zomas A, Mehta J, Powles R, et al. Unusual infections following allogeneic bone marrow transplantation for chronic lymphocytic leukemia. *Bone Marrow Transplantation* 1994;14:799–803.

130. Mehta J, Powles R, Singhal S, et al. Antimicrobial prophylaxis to prevent opportunistic infections in patients with chronic lymphocytic leukemia after allogeneic blood or marrow transplantation. *Leuk Lymphoma* 1997;26:83–88.

131. Michallet M, Archimbaud E, Bandini G, et al. HLA-identical sibling bone marrow transplantation in younger patients with chronic lymphocytic leukemia. European Group for Blood and Marrow Transplantation and the International Bone Marrow Transplant Registry. *Ann Internal Med* 1996;124:311–315.

132. Khouri IF, Przepiorka D, van Besien K, et al. Allogeneic blood or marrow transplantation for chronic lymphocytic leukemia: timing of transplantation and potential effect of fludarabine on acute graft-versus-host disease. *Br J Haematol* 1997;97:466–473.

133. Doney KC, Chauncey T, Appelbaum FR. Allogeneic related donor hematopoietic stem cell transplantation for treatment of chronic lymphocytic leukemia. *Bone Marrow Transplant* 2002;29:817–823.

134. Rondon G, Giralt S, Huh Y, et al. Graft-versus-leukemia effect after allogeneic bone marrow transplantation. *Bone Marrow Transplant* 1996;18:669–672.

135. deMagalhaes-Silverman M, Donnenberg A, Hammert L, et al. Induction of graft-versus-leukemia effect in a patient with chronic lymphocytic leukemia. *Bone Marrow Transplant* 1997;20:175–177.

136. Khouri IF, Keating M, Korbling M, et al. Transplant-lite: induction of graft-versus-malignancy using fludarabine-based nonablative chemotherapy and allogeneic blood progenitor cell transplantation as treatment for lymphoid malignancies. *J Clin Oncol* 1998;16:2817–2824.

137. Khouri IF, Saliba RM, Giralt SA, et al. Nonablative allogeneic hematopoietic transplantation as adoptive immunotherapy for indolent lymphoma: low incidence of toxicity, acute graft-versus-host disease, and treatment-related mortality. *Blood* 2001;98:3595–3599.

138. Diehl LF, Ketchum LH. Autoimmune disease and chronic lymphocytic leukemia: autoimmune hemolytic anemia, pure red cell aplasia, and autoimmune thrombocytopenia. *Semin Oncol* 1998;25:80–97.

139. Mauro FR, Foa R, Cerretti R, et al. Autoimmune hemolytic anemia in chronic lymphocytic leukemia: clinical, therapeutic, and prognostic features. *Blood* 2000;95:2786–2792.

140. Leach M, Parsons RM, Reilly JT, et al. Autoimmune thrombocytopenia: a complication of fludarabine therapy in lymphoproliferative disorders. *Clin Lab Haematol* 2000;22:175–178.

141. Ghazal H. Successful treatment of pure red cell aplasia with rituximab in patients with chronic lymphocytic leukemia. *Blood* 2002; 99:1092–1094.

142. Ribeiro I, Tsatalas C, Catovsky D. Treatment of red cell aplasia in CLL with fludarabine. *Leukemia* 1999;13:1897.

143. Shimoni A, Shvidel L, Klepfish A, et al. Refractory pure red cell aplasia associated with B-CLL: successful treatment with a combination of fludarabine, cyclosporin A and erythropoietin. *Leukemia* 1999; 13:142–143.

144. Griffiths H, Brennan V, Lea J, et al. Crossover study of immunoglobulin replacement therapy in patients with low-grade B-cell tumors. *Blood* 1989;73:366–368.

145. Morrison VA. Update on prophylaxis and therapy of infection in patients with chronic lymphocytic leukemia. *Expert Rev Anticancer Ther* 2001;1:84–90.

146. Morrison VA, Rai KR, Peterson BL, et al. Impact of therapy with chlorambucil, fludarabine, or fludarabine plus chlorambucil on infections in patients with chronic lymphocytic leukemia: Intergroup Study Cancer and Leukemia Group B 9011. *J Clin Oncol* 2001; 19:3611–3621.

147. Keating MJ, O'Brien S, Lerner S, et al. Long-term follow-up of patients with chronic lymphocytic leukemia (CLL) receiving fludarabine regimens as initial therapy. *Blood* 1998;92:1165–1171.

148. Perkins JG, Flynn JM, Howard RS, et al. Frequency and type of serious infections in fludarabine-refractory B-cell chronic lymphocytic leukemia and small lymphocytic lymphoma: implications for clinical trials in this patient population. *Cancer* 2002;94:2033–2039.

149. Lens D, Matutes E, Catovsky D, et al. Frequent deletions at 11q23 and 13q14 in B cell prolymphocytic leukemia (B-PLL). *Leukemia* 2000;14:427–430.

150. Lens D, De Schouwer PJ, Hamoudi RA, et al. p53 abnormalities in B-cell prolymphocytic leukemia. *Blood* 1997;89:2015–2023.

151. Davi F, Maloum K, Michel A, et al. High frequency of somatic mutations in the VH genes expressed in prolymphocytic leukemia. *Blood* 1996;88:3953–3961.

152. Shvidel L, Shtalrid M, Bassous L, et al. B-cell prolymphocytic leukemia: a survey of 35 patients emphasizing heterogeneity, prognostic factors and evidence for a group with an indolent course. *Leuk Lymphoma* 1999;33:169–179.

153. Saven A, Lee T, Schlutz M, et al. Major activity of cladribine in patients with de novo B-cell prolymphocytic leukemia. *J Clin Oncol* 1997;15:37–43.

154. Soulier J, Pierron G, Vecchione D, et al. A complex pattern of recurrent chromosomal losses and gains in T-cell prolymphocytic leukemia. *Genes Chromosomes Cancer* 2001;31:248–254.

155. Stilgenbauer S, Schaffner C, Litterst A, et al. Biallelic mutations in the ATM gene in T-prolymphocytic leukemia. *Nat Med* 1997;3:1155–1159.

156. Brito-Babapulle V, Baou M, Matutes E, et al. Deletions of D13S25, D13S319 and RB-1 mapping to 13q14.3 in T-cell prolymphocytic leukaemia. *Br J Haematol* 2001;114:327–332.

157. Matutes E, Brito-Babapulle V, Swansbury J, et al. Clinical and laboratory features of 78 cases of T-prolymphocytic leukemia. *Blood* 1991;78:3269–3274.

158. Dearden CE, Matutes E, Cazin B, et al. High remission rate in T-cell prolymphocytic leukemia with CAMPATH-1H. *Blood* 2001;98:1721–1726.

159. Keating MJ, Cazin B, Coutre S, et al. Campath-1H treatment of T-cell prolymphocytic leukemia in patients for whom at least one prior chemotherapy regimen has failed. *J Clin Oncol* 2002;20:205–213.

160. Collins RH, Pineiro LA, Agura ED, et al. Treatment of T prolymphocytic leukemia with allogeneic bone marrow transplantation. *Bone Marrow Transplant* 1998;21:627–628.

CHAPTER 15

Lymphoplasmacytic Lymphoma and Waldenström's Macroglobulinemia

Ama Z. S. Rohatiner, Nancy Lee Harris, Riccardo Dalla-Favera, and T. Andrew Lister

BACKGROUND

In 1944, Waldenström described two patients who presented with bleeding, lymphadenopathy, anemia, thrombocytopenia, low levels of serum albumin and fibrinogen, and increased numbers of lymphoid cells in the bone marrow (1). He drew attention to the differences between this illness and myeloma, specifically commenting on the fact that in contrast to myeloma, bone x-rays were normal, and bone pain was absent. The abnormal cells in the bone marrow were characterized as being lymphoid and not plasma cells. Both patients also had a high serum viscosity due to large amounts of a homogeneous globulin with a very high molecular weight. It was postulated that the protein consisted of a single giant molecule rather than an aggregation of smaller globulin molecules.

In subsequent studies, the tissue infiltrate accompanying Waldenström's macroglobulinemia came to be known by a variety of terms: In the Rappaport Classification (2), it was described as *well differentiated lymphocytic, plasmacytoid*; in the updated Kiel Classification (3), it was termed *lymphoplasmacytic immunocytoma*; and in the Working Formulation (4), it was included with small lymphocytic lymphomas and termed *plasmacytoid*. In addition, more sophisticated immunologic techniques have revealed serum paraproteins of varying levels in patients with other lymphomas, most typically in chronic lymphocytic leukemia and, more recently, in splenic marginal zone lymphoma (5) and rarely, in patients with extranodal marginal zone lymphoma of mucosa-associated lymphoid tissue type (6).

The current thinking in the World Health Organization (WHO) Classification (7) is that lymphoplasmacytic lymphoma is a specific disease entity made up of small B lymphocytes, plasmacytoid lymphocytes, and plasma cells, representing variable degrees of maturation toward the immunoglobulin-secreting plasma cell. The majority of patients with this lymphoma have a serum paraprotein, and many have the clinical syndrome of hyperviscosity described by Waldenström. Thus, Walden-ström's macroglobulinemia is considered to be a clinical syndrome associated with lymphoplasmacytic lymphoma, characterized by the presence of a monoclonal immunoglobulin (Ig) M serum paraprotein (greater than 3 g per dL), resulting in symptoms of hyperviscosity.

EPIDEMIOLOGY AND ETIOLOGY

Lymphoplasmacytic lymphoma is a rare disease, representing only 1.5% of all non-Hodgkin's lymphomas diagnosed by lymph node biopsy in the international study (8) conducted to validate the International Lymphoma Study Group's Revised European-American Lymphoma Classification (9), which preceded the WHO Classification (7). There was a slight male predominance (53%); the median age was 63 years.

In a study of the incidence of Waldenström's macroglobulinemia in 11 population-based cancer registries in the United States, a total of 624 cases were diagnosed over a 6-year period (1988 to 1994) (10). The male to female ratio was 1.4:1.0. The age-adjusted incidence for Waldenström's macroglobulinemia was 3.4 and 1.7 (per million person-years at risk) among men and women, respectively. There was a striking increase in incidence with age. The incidence was 17-fold less than that of multiple myeloma and 12-fold less than that of chronic lymphocytic leukemia (10). The disease was more common among whites than among blacks, in contrast to multiple myeloma.

Although the etiology is unknown, it has been suggested that occupational exposure to paints, leather, and rubber dyes may be implicated (11), although large-scale studies have not confirmed this (10), and the disease has been reported to occur in families, suggesting a degree of genetic susceptibility (10,12). An association with hepatitis C infection has also been reported (13–16), particularly in cases with mixed cryoglobulinemia; treatment with interferon to reduce viral load has been associated with regression of the lymphoma

(17). Thus, some cases of lymphoplasmacytic lymphoma may be antigen-driven, similar to mucosa-associated lymphoid tissue–type lymphomas.

DIAGNOSIS

Morphology

Lymphoplasmacytic lymphoma is defined in the WHO Classification as a neoplasm of small B lymphocytes, plasmacytoid lymphocytes, and plasma cells, involving bone marrow, lymph nodes, and spleen, lacking CD5, usually with a serum monoclonal protein, with hyperviscosity or cryoglobulinemia. Plasmacytoid variants of other neoplasms are excluded. The name, *lymphoplasmacytoid* lymphoma in the Revised European-American Lymphoma Classification was changed to *lymphoplasmacytic* in the WHO Classification, to avoid confusion with the Kiel Classification.

The tumor consists of a diffuse proliferation of small lymphocytes, plasmacytoid lymphocytes, and plasma cells, with variable numbers of immunoblasts. In lymph nodes, sinuses are often open and may contain histiocytes reacting to secreted PAS+ immunoglobulin (Color Plate 13). By definition, morphologic features of other lymphomas—particularly marginal zone lymphomas and small lymphocytic lymphoma—that may have plasmacytoid differentiation or a serum monoclonal paraprotein are absent. That is, the tumor does not have marginal zone B cells or a marginal zone pattern and, for the most part, does not involve extranodal sites. In the spleen, both red and white pulp may be infiltrated, but red pulp involvement is more prominent in contrast to splenic marginal zone lymphoma. The bone marrow infiltrate may be either diffuse or nodular and is often interstitial and rather subtle. Peripheral blood involvement is usually less prominent than in chronic lymphocytic leukemia, and the cells often have a plasmacytoid appearance.

Immunophenotype

The cells have surface and cytoplasmic (some cells) Ig, usually of IgM type, usually lack IgD, and strongly express B cell–associated antigens (CD19, CD20, CD22, CD79a). The cells are CD5−, CD10−, CD23−, and CD43+/−; CD25 or CD11c may be faintly positive in some cases (18–21). Lack of CD5 and CD23, strong surface Ig, and CD20 and the presence of cytoplasmic Ig are useful in distinguishing from B-cell chronic lymphocytic leukemia.

Genetic Features

Immunoglobulin heavy- and light-chain genes are rearranged, and Ig heavy-chain variable (IgV)-region genes show somatic mutations, suggesting that these cells arise from a population of B cells that have undergone antigen-driven selection in the germinal center (22–25). Translocation t(9;14)(p13;q32) and rearrangement of the PAX-5 gene

are reported in a proportion of the cases in the section on Pathogenesis below.

Postulated Normal Counterpart

It is postulated that the normal counterpart is a peripheral B lymphocyte stimulated to differentiate to a plasma cell, possibly corresponding to the primary immune response to antigen or to a postgerminal center cell that has undergone somatic mutation but not heavy-chain class switch.

PATHOGENESIS

The pathogenesis of lymphoplasmacytic lymphoma is largely unknown and, consistent with the phenotypic heterogeneity of these tumors, may involve distinct mechanisms in different cases. Approximately 50% of lymphoplasmacytic lymphomas display a specific chromosomal translocation, t(9;14)(p13;q32) (25a). This translocation is more frequent in cases associated with Waldenström's macroglobulinemia. The chromosomal breakpoints juxtapose the Ig heavy-chain locus on chromosome 14q32 to the PAX5 gene on chromosome 9p13 (25b,25c) (see Chapters 49 and 50 for additional details). The PAX5 gene encodes a transcription factor (also called *BSAP*) that is required for B-cell lineage commitment and is expressed in all B cells but is downregulated early during plasmacytoid differentiation (25d,26). As a consequence of the translocation, the PAX5 gene becomes constitutively expressed under the control of Ig transcriptional control elements, and its physiologic downregulation, associated with plasmacytoid differentiation, is prevented. This event is thought to contribute to lymphomagenesis by enforcing proliferation at the expense of differentiation, although a formal proof for this model is still lacking (25b,25c). No other genetic lesion has been detected recurrently in lymphoplasmacytic lymphoma cases lacking (9;14)(p13;q32) translocations.

CLINICAL FEATURES

Lymphoplasmacytic Lymphoma in General

Lymphoplasmacytic lymphoma is usually disseminated at presentation and characteristically involves the lymph nodes, bone marrow, and spleen (8,27–30). The majority of patients present with lymphadenopathy with or without splenomegaly. Extranodal infiltration may occur during the course of the disease, most commonly involving the lung (31) and gastrointestinal tract (32). However, localized extranodal presentations are uncommon, and this clinical feature should raise the question of an extranodal marginal zone lymphoma of mucosa-associated lymphoid tissue, which may have plasmacytoid differentiation. Most cases reported in the literature as *localized extranodal lymphoplasmacytic lymphoma* are in fact examples of mucosa-associated lymphoid tissue lymphoma. The bone marrow is usually involved, and most patients have a serum IgM paraprotein. Over a period of years, the illness is characterized by repeated but incomplete responsiveness to chemotherapy and is almost invariably fatal.

Waldenström's Macroglobulinemia

Approximately 30% of patients with lymphoplasmacytic lymphoma present with signs and symptoms due to hyperviscosity (33–46). Fifteen percent of patients with Waldenström's macroglobulinemia also have symptoms due to cryoglobulinemia and cold agglutinin anemia (33,35,40,42,43,47,48). A preceding monoclonal gammopathy of undetermined significance is seen in 5% to 10% of cases (34,40,49,50).

Hyperviscosity may be the *only* presenting symptom, manifest as dizziness, tiredness, and a propensity for bleeding from the oral or nasal mucous membranes (33–46). Symptoms do not usually supervene until the plasma viscosity is at least four times that of normal serum. Cryoglobulinemia may result in Raynaud's syndrome, purpura, joint pains, and peripheral neuropathy (33,37,39,47,48). Hemolysis can occur as a result of the abnormal and excess IgM reacting with specific red-cell antigens at temperatures lower than 37°C. The high levels of IgM may also result in symptoms due to tissue deposition; 5% to 10% of patients may have a demyelinating peripheral neuropathy, which can present with sensory or motor symptoms, or both (33,51–55). If there is renal involvement, this usually presents as nephrotic syndrome, which may be due to amyloidosis or can be the result of precipitation of IgM on the endothelial side of the glomerular basement membrane (56,57). In general, however, such complications are less severe and occur less frequently than in myeloma, perhaps in part due to the lower frequency and severity of hypercalcemia in Waldenström's macroglobulinemia.

In a retrospective analysis of patterns of clinical presentation, treatment, and outcome of 72 consecutive, newly diagnosed patients with Waldenström's macroglobulinemia referred to St. Bartholomew's Hospital, London, and the Karolinska Hospital, Stockholm (41), 45 of the patients were male, with a median age of 67 years. Approximately one-third had enlargement of the liver or spleen (or both) at the time of presentation, and approximately one-third presented with lymph node enlargement. In one-half of the patients, the paraprotein level was greater than 20 g per L at the time of referral (41).

A retrospective analysis from St. Bartholomew's Hospital (27) summarized the clinical characteristics and outcome of 126 patients with immunocytoma (Kiel Classification) treated over a 14-year period from 1972 to 1996. On review of the pathology (in light of the publication at that time of the International Lymphoma Study Group proposals), only 24 of the 126 patients had the lymphoplasmacytic subtype—that is, pathology consistent with what is currently described as *lymphoplasmacytic lymphoma* in the WHO Classification (7). Thirteen of the 24 patients had Waldenström's macroglobulinemia. The median age of the 24 patients was 62

TABLE 15.1. *Staging investigations*

Full blood count
Tests of renal and liver function
Serum uric acid
Protein electrophoresis and quantification of paraprotein, if present ("M" band)
Serum viscosity
Cold agglutinins/cryoglobulins
β_2-microglobulin
Bone marrow aspirate and trephine biopsy
Computed tomography scans

years (range, 46 to 80 years); 19 were men. At the time of presentation, 21 patients had bone marrow infiltration, the majority had B symptoms, and one-third presented with hepatosplenomegaly. All had a paraprotein; in 16, this was characterized as IgM; five and four patients were found to have IgG and IgA bands, respectively (27).

MANAGEMENT

A clinical history should be taken and physical examination should include examination of the optic fundi (to exclude retinal vein engorgement, hemorrhages, exudates, and papilledema).

Staging Investigations

Conventional baseline investigations comprising full blood count, tests of renal and liver function, serum uric acid, CT scans and a bone marrow aspirate and trephine biopsy need to be done, together with protein electrophoresis and characterization and quantification of a paraprotein, when present (Table 15.1). The serum viscosity should also be determined as a baseline value. The presence of cold agglutinins or cryoglobulins can affect the IgM level; testing for these should, therefore, be part of the initial evaluation. If either is present, serum should be retested under warm conditions. β_2-microglobulin level appears to be an important prognostic factor and should, therefore, also be measured.

General Considerations

The majority of patients are older, and in general, therefore, the aim of treatment will be to keep the person as well as possible for as long as possible. Specific treatment will depend on the person's age and on whether he or she is being treated in the context of a clinical trial. Other concurrent medical conditions need to be taken into account, as always. Lymphoplasmacytic lymphoma typically responds to treatment, but such responses are rarely complete and hardly ever more than temporary. Not all patients require treatment from the outset, and unless there is a specific indication for treatment, for example, pancytopenia or hyperviscosity, the person should be managed expectantly in the first instance. In the retrospective analysis from two centers mentioned above (41), 56% of patients referred to the British center received chemotherapy immediately after diagnosis, as compared to only 14% of those presenting in Sweden. This difference almost certainly relates to differences in referral patterns, patients in Sweden presenting (or being referred) earlier in the course of the illness.

Criteria for Starting Therapy

The absolute IgM level may not necessarily correlate with clinical symptoms. However, patients in whom the IgM level is rising should be considered for treatment. Treatment should also be started in patients who are anemic or whose platelet count is less than 100×10^9 per L, those who have uncomfortable lymph node enlargement or hepatosplenomegaly, and those who develop systemic B symptoms (i.e., fevers, night sweats, or weight loss). In patients with Waldenström's macroglobulinemia, treatment should also be started for symptoms relating to hyperviscosity and for those who develop neuropathy, renal impairment, or symptomatic cryoglobulinemia.

Response Criteria

At a recent Workshop Meeting in Athens, the following recommendations were made for definition of response:

Complete response
Complete disappearance of serum and urine IgM monoclonal protein as determined by immunofixation studies, with resolution of lymphadenopathy or splenomegaly, or both, and resolution of all other symptoms attributable to disease. In addition, histologic examination of the bone marrow should reveal no evidence of disease. Reconfirmation of complete remission status was suggested at 6 weeks.

Partial response
A greater than (or equal to) 50% reduction in serum IgM monoclonal protein levels, as determined by serum electrophoresis, with improvement in *at least one* of the signs, symptoms, or laboratory abnormalities attributable to disease for which treatment was initiated (e.g., anemia, thrombocytopenia, or both; bulky adenopathy or organomegaly; fevers; night sweats; weight loss; fatigue; or other symptomatic manifestations associated with Waldenström's macroglobulinemia, including symptoms of hyperviscosity, neuropathies, nephropathy, amyloidosis, or symptomatic cryoglobulinemia).

Minor response
A greater than (or equal to) 25% reduction in serum IgM monoclonal protein levels as determined by serum electrophoresis.

SPECIFIC TREATMENT

The two components of the illness need to be considered separately:

1. Treatment of hyperviscosity
   Plasmapheresis has historically been the quickest and most effective way of reducing the level of IgM; however, except in the small number of patients for whom chemotherapy is ineffective (or is deemed inappropriate, usually on account of age), who can be maintained on regular plasmapheresis—for example, once a month—it is not an end in itself and needs to be given together with effective treatment for the underlying lymphoma.
   As an emergency measure, daily plasmapheresis for 3 days is usually extremely effective in providing symptomatic relief. A single plasma exchange can reduce the IgM concentration by approximately 30% and the plasma viscosity by 50% to 60%. "Success" can be measured by a dramatic reduction in the level of IgM and a reduction in viscosity. While waiting for concurrent treatment of the underlying illness to be effective, it may be necessary to repeat the plasmapheresis until such time as a sustained reduction in IgM is achieved.
2. Treatment for lymphoma
   Lymphoplasmacytic lymphoma is generally considered an incurable lymphoproliferative disorder characterized by a chronic remitting and relapsing course. Significant responses can be achieved with most of the treatments that are generally used for chronic lymphocytic leukemia or for follicular lymphoma.

Alkylating Agents

Before the introduction of the purine analogs, standard treatment consisted of chlorambucil, with or without steroids, with treatment being continued to the point of maximum response (27,33,34,40) (Table 15.2). The response rate is of the order of 50%, daily administration having been shown to be as effective as intermittent use of the drug (58), with a median survival of approximately 5.5 years (8,27,33,37,39,40,42,43,50,58,59). There is seemingly no advantage to adding prednisolone (33) except in situations in which it clearly is useful—for example, in patients with immune hemolytic anemia, cold agglutinin disease, or cryoglobulinemia. The anthracycline-containing regimen of cyclophosphamide, hydroxydaunorubicin, Oncovin (vincristine), and prednisone (CHOP) has also been used but did not result in any improvement in survival (60), the median again being reported as approximately 5 years.

Thus, in many European centers, chlorambucil remains the treatment of choice, certainly in older patients, purine analogs generally being used in younger patients.

TABLE 15.2. *Response to alkylating agents in patients with Waldenström's macroglobulinemia*

Treatment	No. of patients	Response rate	Median survival (yr)	Reference
Chlorambucil	40	70%	—	59
Chlorambucil	46	(continuous 79%) (intermittent 68%)	5.4	58
Chlorambucil plus prednisolone	77	57%	5.0	33

Purine Analogs

Alkylating agents formed the mainstay of treatment until the introduction of fludarabine and 2-chlorodeoxyadenosine (2-CDA) (Tables 15.3 and 15.4). There are relatively few data for patients with lymphoplasmacytic lymphoma per se (in the new terminology) other than for those with Waldenström's macroglobulinemia.

Fludarabine

In newly diagnosed patients with Waldenström's macroglobulinemia, the response rate to fludarabine in a European study was 79% (61); however, the complete remission rate was only 5%. At a median follow-up of 1.5 years, the median time to progression was 3.5 years. Toxicity related mainly to myelosuppression and consequent infection. The response rate seen in this trial was considerably higher than that reported in a Southwest Oncology Group study (62) that was updated at a recent Workshop (63). A total of 231 patients had been entered into the study; 184 (64 previously treated, 120 newly diagnosed) received treatment with fludarabine (30 mg per m² for 5 days, repeated for four to eight cycles). The overall response rate was 33%, with a predicted 10-year survival of 43%. On multivariate regression analysis, factors associated with survival were β₂-microglobulin and IgM levels, hemoglobin at presentation, and prior therapy.

The reasons for the discrepancy in response rate are unclear but may relate to differences in response criteria or differences in patient selection, or both. In both studies, the treatment-related mortality was relatively high (5%), fludarabine being both myelosuppressive and immunosuppressive. However, it is clearly an active drug (Table 15.3) (64–66) and an appropriate treatment option for younger, newly diagnosed patients. Fludarabine has also been shown to be useful in patients considered resistant to alkylating-agent therapy (66–68). In a study from France (68), the response rate in 71 patients (with primary resistant disease or resistant recurrence despite one or more chemotherapy regimens) was 30% (ail partial responses).

The recommended dose of fludarabine used to be 25 mg per m² intravenously daily for 5 days, this regimen being administered every 4 weeks. More recently, with the availability of the oral formulation, the recommended dosage is 40 mg per m² orally daily for 5 days repeated every 4 weeks, as above.

There is one randomized trial comparing the efficacy of fludarabine with that of cyclophosphamide, doxorubicin,

and prednisolone (CAP) in patients treated at first recurrence or with Waldenström's macroglobulinemia deemed refractory to alkylating agents. The response rate to fludarabine was significantly higher than that observed with CAP, and the median time to progression and time to treatment failure were both significantly longer in patients treated with fludarabine. However, the median survival of patients in the two groups was similar, possibly because patients in whom CAP failed then went on to receive treatment with fludarabine (69).

2-Chlorodeoxyadenosine

The other nucleoside analog, 2-CDA (Cladribine), has also shown activity in Waldenström's macroglobulinemia. In newly diagnosed patients, administered intravenously by continuous infusion, or as a 2-hour intravenous infusion daily for 5 to 7 days every 4 weeks, 2-CDA has resulted in response rates ranging from 44% to 90% (70–77) (Table 15.4). The drug is also active in patients who have previously received other chemotherapy regimens, with response rates ranging from 38% to 54%. There does, however, appear to be cross resistance between the two purine analogs (78), as observed in chronic lymphocytic leukemia.

Although the purine analogs have not been directly, prospectively compared with chlorambucil, it may well be that they are more effective than the latter when a rapid response is required. However, this potential advantage needs to be balanced against their known myelosuppressive and immunosuppressive effects. Neutropenia is usually evident at approximately day 10 and may last for more than a week. There is also a profound and sus-

TABLE 15.3. *Response to fludarabine in patients with Waldenström's macroglobulinemia*

	Response rate	Reference
Newly diagnosed patients	(38%) 45/118	62
	(79%) 15/19	61
Previously treated patients	(40%) 4/10	65
	(31%) 8/26	66
	(61%) 8/13	67
	(30%) 21/71	68
	(33%) 21/64	62

TABLE 15.4. *Response to 2-chlorodeoxyadenosine in patients with Waldenström's macroglobulinemia*

	Response rate	Reference
Newly diagnosed patients	22/66 (85%)	79
	9/10 (90%)	75
	4/7 (57%)	76
	8/11 (73%)	84
	4/9 (44%)	72
Previously treated patients	20/46 (45%)	71
	7/13 (54%)	76
	8/16 (50%)	84
	9/24 (38%)	78
	5/13 (38%)	72

TABLE 15.5. *High-dose treatment in patients with Waldenström's macroglobulinemia*

No. of patients	Outcome	Reference
4	3 PRs, 1 treatment-related death	91
1	CR	89
7	2 PRs	88
6	1 CR, 5 PRs	86

CR, complete response; PR, partial response.

tained reduction of monocytes and of CD4+ and CD8+ lymphocytes (79), resulting in a significant risk of opportunistic infection, especially by *Pneumocystis carinii* (80–82). Prophylactic cotrimoxazole should always be given. Myelodysplasia has also been reported after treatment with both fludarabine (83) and 2-CDA (84), and fludarabine can make it difficult to collect sufficient numbers of autologous peripheral blood progenitor cells to support high-dose treatment (85).

In terms of efficacy overall, fludarabine and 2-CDA are not very different from chlorambucil. They do provide a useful alternative, however, particularly now that an oral formulation of the former is available. They should certainly be considered in patients who have been previously treated with an alkylating agent.

High-Dose Treatment with Hematopoietic Stem Cell Support

Because the majority of patients with lymphoplasmacytic lymphoma are older, and because complete remission is achieved in only a small proportion, the number of patients in whom high-dose therapy has been used is very small.

With regard to Waldenström's macroglobulinemia, treatment with high-dose melphalan (as for myeloma) has resulted in meaningful responses (86,87). Cyclophosphamide and total-body irradiation have also been used as the myeloablative regimen in several patients, resulting in long-term remissions (88). Follow-up for the latter and other similar reports (86,89,91) is still, however, relatively short (Table 15.5).

Allografting

There are occasional case reports of younger patients who have had an allograft, again with initially encouraging results (92,93) (Table 15.6). In view of the older age of most people

with Waldenström's macroglobulinemia, nonmyeloablative stem cell transplantation is now being considered (94).

Anti-CD20

Rituximab, the chimeric anti-CD20 monoclonal antibody, was administered to a small number of patients with *immunocytoma* (95) (as described in the Kiel Classification), but the data for anything other than Waldenström's macroglobulinemia predate the change in nomenclature.

With regard to Waldenström's macroglobulinemia, there is certainly evidence of clinical activity, partial responses being noted in six of 26 previously treated patients in a European trial (95), with similar results being reported in other series (96,97). In a study from several centers in the United States, rituximab was administered to 30 previously treated patients, of whom 14 had received a nucleoside analog. The majority of patients received four weekly infusions of anti-CD20 given at the standard dose of 375 mg per m^2. The median IgM level decreased in all patients, with 27% and 60% of patients, respectively, showing a greater than 50% and greater than 25% decrease in IgM. A concomitant decrease in the degree of bone marrow infiltration was observed, and this was associated with improvements in the hemoglobin and platelet counts. The overall partial response rate was 27%, but no complete responses were seen. The median time to treatment failure for responding patients was 8 months (98).

Thus, rituximab appears to have some activity in Waldenström's macroglobulinemia (Table 15.7), with useful responses being seen in patients who were previously transfusion or erythropoietin dependent. On this basis, a study of anti-CD20 given in conjunction with fludarabine is currently in progress.

TABLE 15.6. *Allogeneic bone marrow transplantation in patients with Waldenström's macroglobulinemia*

No. of patients	Outcome	Reference
2	1 CR, 1 PR	92
1	PR	93
4	1 CR, 1 PR	94

CR, complete response; PR, partial response.

TABLE 15.7. *Response to anti-CD20 (rituximab) in patients with Waldenström's macroglobulinemia*

No. of patients	Outcome	Reference
30	8 PR	98
7	2 PR	96
26	6 PR	95

PR, partial response.

Other Drugs

Thalidomide has recently been reported to show activity in Waldenström's macroglobulinemia, as in myeloma. A report from Greece showed a 25% partial response rate in 20 elderly patients (median age, 74 years). However, only low doses could be tolerated by this patient population (99). Gemcitabine has also been investigated in small numbers of patients with resistant or recurrent lymphoplasmacytic lymphoma, but no responses were seen (100). Small numbers of patients have also been treated with interferon-α, with some evidence of antitumor response being demonstrated in 20% to 50% of patients (101).

TREATMENT RECOMMENDATIONS

Initial Therapy

As with any illness, treatment depends on the individual patient's situation (Fig. 15.1). Treatment options include chlorambucil, a nucleoside analog such as fludarabine or 2-CDA, and the monoclonal antibody anti-CD20 (rituximab). The data do not currently exist to recommend one treatment over another; however, the following need to be considered when making the decision:

1. The patient's age, vis à vis the myelosuppression and T-cell dysfunction associated with fludarabine.
2. Potential difficulty in collecting sufficient numbers of autologous hematopoietic peripheral blood progenitor cells after treatment with fludarabine (see section on 2-Chlorodeoxyadenosine).

There are currently no data to recommend the routine use of *combinations* of these drugs outside the clinical trial setting.

Treatment at Recurrence

For patients who have demonstrated a durable response after chlorambucil, it is entirely reasonable to use it again. In younger patients, a nucleoside analog should also be considered. If high-dose treatment supported by autologous hematopoietic progenitor cells is being considered, as mentioned above, fludarabine may result in insufficient cells being obtained. Anti-CD20 might, in that situation, be a justifiable alternative.

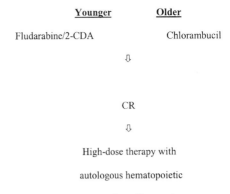

NEWLY DIAGNOSED PATIENTS

Younger	Older
Fludarabine/2-CDA	Chlorambucil

⇩

CR

⇩

High-dose therapy with
autologous hematopoietic
progenitor cell support

TREATMENT AT RECURRENCE

If initial treatment response lasting >1 yr, consider same treatment again

or

Chlorambucil (if fludarabine/2-CDA originally)

or

Fludarabine/2-CDA (if chlorambucil originally)

or

Anti-CD20

FIG. 15.1. Algorithm of treatment. 2-CDA, 2-chlorodeoxyadenosine; CR, complete response.

The data for high-dose treatment with autologous stem cell support and allogeneic bone marrow transplantation are limited and preliminary but encouraging. Younger patients (younger than the age of 60 years) should, therefore, be considered for high-dose treatment if (unusually) a complete remission has been achieved.

SURVIVAL

Lymphoplasmacytic Lymphoma

Again, there are very few data for patients with lymphoplasmacytic lymphoma as described in the WHO Classification, other than for those with Waldenström's macroglobulinemia. In the series from St. Bartholomew's Hospital (27), survival was evaluated for patients in the three Kiel subgroups separately; it is, therefore, possible to focus on the outcome of patients with the lymphoplasmacytic subtype (as described in Kiel), who would now fall into the lymphoplasmacytic lymphoma category (using WHO terminology). Essentially, their survival was not statistically different from that of a concurrent series of 159 patients with chronic lymphocytic leukemia/small lymphocytic lymphoma treated at the same hospital during the same period, although the *medians* are, in fact, different. The median survival for the group of patients with lymphoplasmacytic lymphoma was 5 years. This is similar to that reported in the international study conducted to validate the International Lymphoma Study Group proposals (8).

Waldenström's Macroglobulinemia

As mentioned above, there are considerably more data for patients with Waldenström's macroglobulinemia, the median survival generally being reported as averaging 5 years, but a number of people—at least 20%—may survive for longer than 10 years (35,41) (Color Plate 13B). Because this is predominantly a disease of older people, up to one-fifth may die of unrelated causes (35).

Most patients with Waldenström's macroglobulinemia die of progressive disease that has become resistant to treatment. Death usually occurs from infection as a consequence of pancytopenia due to bone marrow infiltration. A few patients die after transformation of the illness to large B-cell lymphoma. This is usually characterized by refractoriness to therapy and is often associated with the development of systemic B symptoms, rapidly enlarging lymph nodes, and often organ involvement. The outcome is almost always death (27,102,103). Although the incidence of transformation is low, its implications highlight the importance of rebiopsy at the time of each recurrence or progression during treatment (27).

Prognostic Factors

Because the illness is relatively rare, there have been few attempts to define prognostic factors. Moreover, some of the series included patients with asymptomatic Waldenström's macroglobulinemia as well as monoclonal gammopathy of undetermined significance with IgM paraproteinemia, and thus, it is difficult to be sure about the prognostic significance of certain variables. In the most recent series, however, there is consensus about advanced age being associated with an inferior prognosis (40,104,105), and in some, anemia has also consistently been found to be an adverse prognostic factor (104,105). Response to treatment, not surprisingly, has also been found to correlate with outcome, survival of 4 years being seen for patients who responded to chemotherapy as compared to only 2 years for those who did not (42). This has been confirmed in other series (40,105), but not in all (59).

Recently, Morel et al. (106) have proposed a prognostic scoring system based on the outcome of 232 patients with Waldenström's macroglobulinemia. This was then validated on data from 253 other patients. The following were deemed to be the most significant prognostic factors: age, albumin level at presentation, and degree of cytopenia. When taken in combination, these three parameters separated patients into those considered to be at low, intermediate, and high risk, with 5-year survival rates of 92%,

TABLE 15.8. *Prognostic scoring system according to Morel and colleagues*

Prognostic factor		Score
Age		
≥65 yr		1
<65 yr		0
Albumin		
<40		1
≥40		0
Number of cytopenias		
2 or 3		2
1		1
0		0
Prognostic group	Score	5-yr survival (%)
Low risk	0 or 1	87
Intermediate risk	2	62
High risk	3 or 4	25

Adapted from Morel P, Monconduit M, Jacomy D, et al. Prognostic factors in Waldenström's macroglobulinemia: a report on 232 patients with the description of a new scoring system and its validation on 253 other patients. *Blood* 2000;96:852.

63%, and 27% respectively (*p* < .0001) (106) (Tables 15.6 through 15.8) (Fig. 15.2).

The new scoring system thus defines subgroups of patients with Waldenström's macroglobulinemia who have significantly different probabilities of survival and confirms the strong prognostic value of older age. Taken together with albumin (40 g per L being the discriminating point) and the degree of cytopenia (i.e., none, anemia, neutropenia, thrombocytopenia, or any combination of these), it is possible to discriminate between different groups of patients very clearly. The scoring system was applied in the

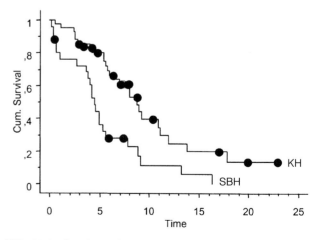

FIG. 15.2. Survival of patients with Waldenström's macroglobulinemia treated at St. Bartholomew's Hospital (SBH), London, and the Karolinska Hospital (KH), Stockholm.

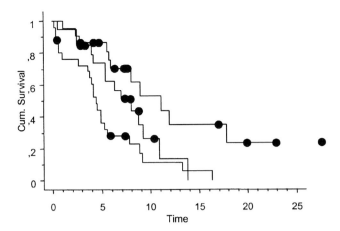

FIG. 15.3. Survival of patients with Waldenström's macroglobulinemia according to the prognostic scoring system of Morel and colleagues. (From Björkholm M, Johansson E, Papamichael D, et al. Patterns of clinical presentation, treatment and outcome in patients with Waldenström's macroglobulinemia. A two-institutional study. *Semin Oncol* 2003;30:226, with permission.)

recent analysis from St. Bartholomew's Hospital and the Karolinska Hospital (41) and was able to define three discrete groups of patients with quite different survival patterns (Fig. 15.3). The scoring system thus provides a basis for selecting patients for conventional or experimental therapy and could also be used to evaluate the results of new therapies, because it would make it possible to compare results for different prognostic groupings with greater validity. As a consequence of the Workshop Meeting on Waldenström's macroglobulinemia, a major international collaborative study has been initiated to construct a prognostic index (93).

FUTURE DIRECTIONS

Current and future studies are focusing on combinations of drugs given with the monoclonal antibody anti-CD20. It remains to be seen whether the use of these two treatment modalities will actually be superior to either one alone.

The combination of anti-CD20 and fludarabine is the subject of a current multicenter study, as is the combination of anti-CD20 and interferon.

A phase II trial of Campath-1H (anti-CD52) is currently in progress in patients with refractory Waldenström's macroglobulinemia. Anti-CD20 is also being combined with tumor necrosis factor-α (Etanercept) in patients with previously treated Waldenström's macroglobulinemia. Yttrium 90–labeled anti-CD20 (Zevalin) is also the subject of a phase I study in patients with Waldenström's macroglobulinemia.

In view of the similarities between Waldenström's macroglobulinemia and myeloma, there is also interest in investigating alternative treatment options such as thalidomide and the proteasome inhibitor PS-341, which have both shown promise in myeloma.

Wider use of the recently published prognostic scoring system should make it easier to compare new treatment modalities with those that have come before, particularly in view of the heterogeneity of presentation and prognosis in patients with Waldenström's macroglobulinemia.

ACKNOWLEDGMENTS

We are most grateful to Deirdre Byrne and Brenda Walsh for preparing the manuscript.

REFERENCES

1. Waldenström J. Incipient myelomatosis or essential hyperglobulinemia with fibrinogenopenia—a new syndrome? *Acta Med Scand* 1944;117:216.
2. Rappaport H. Tumors of the hematopoietic system. *Atlas of Tumor Pathology Section III* (Series I). Washington, DC: Armed Forces Institute of Pathology, 1966.
3. Stansfeld AG, Diebold J, Kapanci Y, et al. Updated Kiel classification for lymphomas. *Lancet* 1988;1:292.
4. Non-Hodgkin's lymphoma pathologic classification project. National Cancer Institute sponsored study of classifications of non-Hodgkin's lymphomas: summary and description of a Working Formulation for clinical usage. *Cancer* 1982;49:2112.
5. Berger F, Felman P, Thieblemont C, et al. Non-MALT marginal zone B-cell lymphomas: a description of clinical presentation and outcome in 124 patients *Blood* 2000;95:1950.
6. Nathwani BN, Anderson JR, Armitage JO, et al. Marginal zone B-cell lymphoma: a clinical comparison of nodal and mucosa-associated lymphoid tissue types. Non-Hodgkin's Lymphoma Classification Project. *J Clin Oncol* 1999;17:2486.
7. Jaffe ES, Harris NL, Stein H, eds. WHO Classification of Tumours. Tumours of haematopoietic and lymphoid tissues. Pathology & Genetics. JWIRAC Press, 2001.
8. A clinical evaluation of the International Lymphoma Study Group classification of non-Hodgkin's lymphoma. The Non-Hodgkin's Lymphoma Classification Project. *Blood* 1997;89:3909.
9. Harris NL, Jaffe ES, Stein H, et al. A revised European-American classification of lymphoid neoplasms: a proposal from the International Lymphoma Study Group. *Blood* 1994;84:1361.
10. Groves FD, Travis LB, Devesa SS, et al. Waldenström's macroglobulinemia: incidence patterns in the United States, 1988–1994. *Cancer* 1998;82:1078.
11. Tepper A, Moss C. Waldenström's macroglobulinemia: search for occupational exposure. *J Occup Med* 1994;36:133.
12. Fine JM, Mullier JY, Rochu D. Waldenström's macroglobulinemia in monozygotic twins. *Acta Med Scand* 1986;220:369.
13. Silvestri F, Barillari G, Fanin R, et al. Impact of hepatitis C virus infection on clinical features, quality of life and survival of patients with lymphoplasmacytoid lymphoma/immunocytoma. *Ann Oncol* 1998;9:499.
14. Zuckerman E, Zuckerman T, Levine AM, et al. Hepatitis C virus infection in patients with B-cell non-Hodgkin lymphoma. *Ann Intern Med* 1997;127:423.
15. Agnello V, Chung RT, Kaplan LM. A role for hepatitis C virus infection in type II cryoglobulinemia [see comments]. *N Engl J Med* 1992;327:1490.
16. Pozzato G, Mazzaro C, Crovatto M, et al. Low-grade malignant lymphoma, hepatitis C virus infection, and mixed cryoglobulinemia. *Blood* 1994;84:3047.
17. Mazzaro C, Franzin F, Tulissi P, et al. Regression of monoclonal B-cell expansion in patients affected by mixed cryoglobulinemia responsive to alpha-interferon therapy. *Cancer* 1996;77:2604.
18. Stein H, Lennert K, Feller A, et al. Immunohistological analysis of human lymphoma: correlation of histological and immunological categories. *Adv Cancer Res* 1984;42:67.
19. Harris NL, Bhan AK. B-cell neoplasms of the lymphocytic, lymphoplasmacytoid and plasma cell types: immunohistologic analysis and clinical correlation. *Hum Pathol* 1985;16:829.

20. Lennert K, Tamm I, Wacker H-H. Histopathology and immunocytochemistry of lymph node biopsies in chronic lymphocytic leukemia and immunocytoma. *Leuk Lymphoma* 1991;[Suppl]:157.

21. Zukerberg L, Medeiros L, Ferry J, et al. Diffuse low-grade B-cell lymphomas: four clinically distinct subtypes defined by a combination of morphologic and immunophenotypic features. *Am J Clin Pathol* 1993;100:373.

22. Aoki H, Takishita M, Kosaka M, et al. Frequent somatic mutations in D and/or JH segments of Ig gene in Waldenström's macroglobulinemia and chronic lymphocytic leukemia (CLL) with Richter's syndrome but not in common CLL. *Blood* 1995;85:1913.

23. Crouzier R, Martin T, Pasquali JL. Monoclonal IgM rheumatoid factor secreted by CD5-negative B cells during mixed cryoglobulinemia. Evidence for somatic mutations and intraclonal diversity of the expressed VH region gene. *J Immunol* 1995;154:413.

24. Sahota SS, Garand R, Bataille R, et al. VH gene analysis of clonally related IgM and IgG from human lymphoplasmacytoid B-cell tumors with chronic lymphocytic leukemia features and high serum monoclonal IgG. *Blood* 1998;91:238.

25. Wagner SD, Martinelli V, Luzzatto L. Similar patterns of Vk gene usage but different degrees of somatic mutation in hairy cell leukemia, prolymphocytic leukemia, Waldenström's macroglobulinemia, and myeloma. *Blood* 1994;83:3647.

25a. Offit K, Parsa NZ, Filippa D, et al. t(9;14)(p13;q32) denotes a subset of low-grade non-Hodgkin lymphoma with plasmacytoid differentiation. *Blood* 1992;80:2594.

25b. Iida S, Rao PH, Nallasivam P, et al. The t(9;14)(p13;q32) chromosomal translocation associated with lymphoplasmacytoid lymphoma involves the PAX-5 gene. *Blood* 1996;88:4110.

25c. Busslinger M, Klix N, Pfeffer P, et al. Deregulation of PAX-5 by translocation of the Emu enhancer of the IgH locus adjacent to two alternative PAX-5 promoters in a diffuse large-cell lymphoma. *Proc Natl Acad Sci U S A* 1996;93:6129.

25d. Schebesta M, Heavey B, Busslinger M. Transcriptional control of B-cell development. *Curr Opin Immunol* 2002;14:216.

26. Krenacs L, Himmelmann AW, Quintanilla-Martinez L, et al. Transcription factor B-cell-specific activator protein (BSAP) is differentially expressed in B cells and in subsets of B-cell lymphomas. *Blood* 1998;92:1308.

27. Papamichael D, Norton AJ, Foran JM, et al. Immunocytoma: a retrospective analysis from St. Bartholomew's Hospital, 1972 to 1996. *J Clin Oncol* 1999;17:2847.

28. Brittinger G, Bartels H, Common H, et al. Clinical and prognostic relevance of the Kiel classification on non-Hodgkin's lymphomas: results of a prospective multi-centre study by the Keil Lymphoma Study Group. *Hematol Oncol* 1984;2:269.

29. Peuchmaur M, Scoazec JY, Gaulard P, et al. Analytical study of the different subtypes of non-Hodgkin's lymphoma: clinical, histological and immunohistochemical aspects. In: Non-Hodgkin's Lymphomas.

30. Richards MA, Hall PA, Gregory WM, et al. Lymphoplasmacytoid and small cell centrocytic non-Hodgkin's lymphoma—a retrospective analysis from St. Bartholomew's Hospital, 1972–1986. *Hematol Oncol* 1989;7:19.

31. Kyrtsonis M-C, Angelopoulou MK, Kontopidou FN, et al. Primary lung involvement in Waldenström's macroglobulinemia. *Acta Haematol* 2001;105:92.

32. Recine MA, Perez MT, Cabello-Inchausti B, et al. Extranodal lymphoplasmacytoid lymphoma (immunocytoma) presenting as small intestinal obstruction. *Arch Pathol Lab Med* 2001;125:677.

33. Dimopoulos MA, Alexanian R. Waldenström's macroglobulinemia. *Blood* 1994;83:1452.

34. Kranjny M, Pruzanski W. Waldenström's macroglobulinemia: review of 45 cases. *Can Med Assoc J* 1976;114:899.

35. Kyle RA, Garton JP. The spectrum of IgM monoclonal gammopathy in 430 cases. *Mayo Clin Proc* 1987;62:719.

36. Crawford J, Cox EB, Cohen HP. Evaluation of hyperviscosity in monoclonal gammopathies. *Am J Med* 1985;79:13.

37. Andriko JA, Aguilera NSI, Chu WS, et al. Waldenström's macroglobulinemia: a clinicopathologic study of 22 cases. *Am Can Soc* 1997;80:1926.

38. Dimopoulos MA, Galani E, Matsouka C. Waldenström's macroglobulinemia. *Hematol Oncol Clin North Am* 1999;13:1351.

39. Owen RG, Johnson SA, Morgan GJ. Waldenström's macroglobulinemia: laboratory diagnosis and treatment. *Hematol Oncol* 2000;18:41.

40. Dimopoulos MA, Panayiotidis P, Moulopoulos LA, et al. Waldenström's macroglobulinemia: clinical features, complications and management. *J Clin Oncol* 2000;18:214.

41. Björkholm M, Johansson E, Papamichael D, et al. Patterns of clinical presentation, treatment and outcome in patients with Waldenström's macroglobulinemia. A two-institutional study. *Semin Oncol* 2003;30:226.

42. MacKenzie MR, Fudenberg HH. Macroglobulinemia: an analysis of forty patients. *Blood* 1972;39:874.

43. McCallister BD, Bayrd ED, Harrison EG, et al. Primary macroglobulinemia. *Am J Med* 1967;43:394.

44. Garcia-Sanz R, Monoto S, Torrequebrada A, et al. Waldenström's macroglobulinemia: presenting features and outcome in a series with 217 cases. *Br J Haematol* 2001;115:575.

45. Kyrtsonis MC, Vassilakopoulos TP, Angelopoulou MK, et al. Waldenström's macroglobulinemia: clinical course and prognostic factors in 60 patients. *Ann Hematol* 2001;80:722.

46. Brouet JC, Clauvel JP, Seligmann M. Evolution et prognostic de la maladie de Waldenstrom: etude de 150 observations. *Act Haematol (Paris)* 1975;9:38.

47. Rosse WF, Adams J, Logue G. Hemolysis by complement and cold reaction antibody. *Am J Hematol* 1977;2:259.

48. Bianco P, Viallard J-F, Rivel J, et al. Unusual manifestations in type II cryoglobulinaemia associated with Waldenström's macroglobulinemia. *J Clin Pathol* 2000;53:882.

49. Owen RG, Lubenko A, Savage J, et al. Auto-immune thrombocytopenia in Waldenström's macroglobulinemia. *Am J Hematol* 2001;66:116.

50. Andriko JA, Swerdlow SH, Aguilera NSI, et al. Is lymphoplasmacytic lymphoma/immunocytoma a distinct entity? A clinicopathologic study of 20 cases. *Am J Surg Pathol* 2001;25:742.

51. Nobile-Orazio E, Marmireli P, Baldini L, et al. Peripheral neuropathy in macroglobulinemia. *Neurology* 1987;37:1506.

52. Kelly JJ, Adelman LS, Berkman E, et al. Polyneuropathies associated with IgM monoclonal gammopathies. *Arch Neurol* 1988;45:1355.

53. Monaco S, Bonetti B, Ferrari S, et al. Complement mediated demyelination in patients with IgM monoclonal gammopathy and polyneuropathy. *N Engl J Med* 1990;322:649.

54. Ropper AH, Gorson KC. Neuropathies associated with paraproteinemia. *N Engl J Med* 1998;338:1601.

55. Dellagi K, Dupouey P, Brouet JC, et al. Waldenström's macroglobulinemia and peripheral neuropathy: a clinical and immunologic study of 25 patients. *Blood* 1983;62:280.

56. Nifosi G. Renal involvement in Waldenström's macroglobulinemia: case report and review of the literature. *Minerva Med* 2001;92:133.

57. Wong PN, Mak S-K, Lo K-Y, et al. Acute tubular necrosis in a patient with Waldenström's macroglobulinemia and hyperviscosity syndrome. *Nephrol Dial Transplant* 2000;15:1684.

58. Kyle RA, Greiff PR, Morie AG, et al. Waldenström's macroglobulinemia: a prospective study comparing daily with intermittent oral chlorambucil. *Br J Haematol* 2000;108:737.

59. Ngan S, Rohatiner AZ, Matthews J, et al. Waldenström's macroglobulinemia: A retrospective analysis of 40 patients from 1972 to 2001. *Semin Oncol* 2003;30:236.

60. Dimopoulos M, Weber D, Delasalle K, et al. Primary therapy of Waldenström's macroglobulinemia. *Blood* 1993;82[Suppl 1]:562a [abstract 2234].

61. Foran JM, Rohatiner AZ, Coiffier B, et al. Multicentre phase II study of fludarabine phosphate for patients with newly diagnosed lymphoplasmacytoid lymphoma, Waldenström's macroglobulinemia and mantle cell lymphoma. *J Clin Oncol* 1999;17:546.

62. Dhodapkar MV, Jacobson JL, Gertz MA, et al. Prognostic factors and response to fludarabine therapy in patients in Waldenström's macroglobulinemia: results of United States intergroup trial (Southwest Oncology Group S9003). *Blood* 2001;98:41.

63. Kyle RA, Treon SP, Alexanian R, et al. Prognostic markers and criteria to initiate therapy in Waldenström's macroglobulinemia: consensus panel recommendations from the Second International Workshop on Waldenström's Macroglobulinemia. *Semin Oncol* 2003;30:116.

64. Thalhammer-Scherrer R, Geissler K, Schwarzinger I, et al. Fludarabine therapy in Waldenström's macroglobulinemia. *Ann Hematol* 2000;79:556.

65. Kantarjian HM, Alexanian R, Koller CA, et al. Fludarabine therapy in macroglobulinemic lymphoma. *Blood* 1990;75:1928.
66. Dimopoulos MA, O'Brien S, Kantarjian H, et al. Fludarabine therapy in Waldenström's macroglobulinemia. *Am J Med* 1993;95:49.
67. Zinzani PL, Gherlinzoni F, Bendandi M, et al. Fludarabine treatment in resistant Waldenström's macroglobulinemia. *Eur J Haematol* 1995; 54:120.
68. Leblond V, Ben-Othman T, Deconinck E, et al. Activity of fludarabine in previously treated Waldenström's macroglobulinemia: a report of 71 cases. *J Clin Oncol* 1998;16:2060.
69. Leblond V, Cazin B, Fermand JP, et al. Results of a multicentric randomized study comparing the efficacy of cyclophosphamide, doxorubicin and prednisone to that of fludarabine patients with Waldenström's macroglobulinemia in first relapse or primary refractory disease. *Ann Oncol*, 1999;10[Suppl 3]:66 [abstract 223].
70. Dimopoulos MA, Kantarjian HM, Estey EH, et al. Treatment of Waldenström macroglobulinemia with 2-chlorodeoxyadenosine. *Ann Intern Med* 1993;118:195.
71. Dimopoulos MA, Weber D, Delasalle KB, et al. Treatment of Waldenström's macroglobulinemia resistant to standard therapy with 2-chlorodeoxyadenosine: identification of prognostic factors. *Ann Oncol* 1995;6:49.
72. Hellmann A, Lewandowski K, Zaucha JM, et al. Effect of a 2-hour infusion of 2-chlorodeoxyadenosine in the treatment of refractory or previously untreated Waldenström's macroglobulinemia. *Eur J Haematol* 1999;63:35.
73. Lillimark J, Martinsson U, Cavallin E, et al. Cladribine for untreated or early low-grade non-Hodgkin's lymphoma. *Leuk Lymphoma* 1998;30:573.
74. Weber DM, Dimopoulos MA, Delasalle K, et al. 2-Clorodeoxyadenosine alone and in combination for previously untreated Waldenström's macroglobulinaemia *Semin Oncol* 2003;30:243.
75. Fridrik MA, Jager G, Baldinger C, et al. First-line treatment of Waldenström's disease with cladribine. *Ann Hematol* 1997;74:7.
76. Liu F, Burian C, Miller W, et al. Bolus administration of cladribine in the treatment of Waldenström's macroglobulinemia. *Br J Haematol* 1998;103:690.
77. Hellmann A, Lewandowski K, Zaucha JM, et al. Treatment of Waldenström's macroglobulinemia with 2-chlorodeoxyadenosine. *Eur J Haematol* 1999;103:690.
78. Betticher DC, Hsu Schmitz SF, Ratschiller D, et al. Cladribine (2-CDA) given as a subcutaneous bolus injection in active pretreated Waldenström's macroglobulinemia: Swiss Group for Clinical Cancer Research (SAKK). *Br J Haematol* 1997;99:358.
79. Dimopoulos MA, Kantarjian H, Weber D, et al. Primary therapy of Waldenström's macroglobulinemia with 2-chlorodeoxyadenosine. *J Clin Oncol* 1994;12:2694.
80. Cheson BD. Infections and immunosuppressive complications of purine analog therapy. *J Clin Oncol* 1995;13:2431.
81. Van Den Neste E, Delannoy A, Vanderscan B, et al. Infectious complications after 2-chlorodeoxyadenosine therapy. *Eur J Haematol* 1996;56:235.
82. Costa P, Luzzati R, Nicolato A, et al. Cryptococcal meningitis and intracranial tuberculoma in a patient with Waldenström's macroglobulinemia treated with fludarabine. *Leuk Lymphoma* 1998;28: 617.
83. Micallef INM, Lillington DM, Apostolidis J, et al. Therapy-related myelodysplasia (tMDS) and secondary acute myelogenous leukemia (sAML) following high-dose therapy (HDT) with autologous hematopoietic progenitor cell support for lymphoid malignancies. *J Clin Oncol* 2000;18:947.
84. Delannoy A, Van de Neste E, Michaux JL, et al. Cladribine for Waldenström's macroglobulinemia. *Br J Haematol* 1999;104:933.
85. Micallef IN, Apostolidis J, Rohatiner AZ, et al. Factors which predict unsuccessful mobilisation of peripheral blood progenitor cells in patients with non-Hodgkin's lymphoma. *Hematol J* 2000;1:367.
86. Desikan R, Dhodapkar M, Siegel D, et al. High dose therapy with autologous peripheral blood stem cell support for Waldenström's macroglobulinemia: a pilot study. *Br J Haematol* 1999;105:993.
87. Mustafa M, Powles R, Treleaven J, et al. Total therapy with VAMP/ CVAMP and high dose melphalan and autograft for IgM lymphoplasmacytoid disease. *Blood* 1998;92[Suppl 1]:28lb [abstract 4212].
88. Dreger P, Glass B, Kuse R, et al. Myeloablative radiochemotherapy followed by reinfusion of purged autologous stem cells for Waldenström's macroglobulinemia. *Br J Haematol* 1999;106:115.
89. Yang L, Wen BP, Li HM, et al. Autologous peripheral blood stem cell transplantation for Waldenström's macroglobulinemia. *Bone Marrow Transplant* 1999;24:929.
90. Reference deleted.
91. Anagnostopoulos A, Dimopoulos MA, Aleman A, et al. High-dose chemotherapy followed by stem cell transplantation in patients with resistant Waldenström's macroglobulinemia. *Bone Marrow Transplant* 2001;27:1027.
92. Martino R, Shah A, Romero P, et al. Allogeneic bone marrow transplantation for advanced Waldenström's macroglobulinemia. *Bone Marrow Transplant* 1999;23:747.
93. Anagnostopoulos A, Aleman A, Giralt S. Autologous and allogeneic stem cell transplantation in Waldenström's macroglobulinemia: review of the literature and future directions. *Semin Oncol* 2003;30:286
94. Tourmithac O, Lebland V, Tabrizi R, et al. Transplantation in Waldenström's macroglobulinemia—the French experience. *Semin Oncol* 2003;30:291.
95. Foran J, Rohatiner AZ, Cunningham D, et al. A European phase II study of rituximab (chimeric anti-CD20 monoclonal antibody) for patients with newly-diagnosed mantle cell lymphoma, and previously-treated mantle cell lymphoma, immunocytoma and small lymphocytic lymphoma. *J Clin Oncol* 2000;18:317.
96. Byrd JC, White CA, Link B, et al. Rituximab therapy in Waldenström's macroglobulinemia: preliminary evidence of clinical activity. *Ann Oncol* 1999;10:1525.
97. Weide R, Heymanns J, Köppler H. The polyneuropathy associated with Waldenström's macroglobulinemia can be treated effectively with chemotherapy and the anti-CD20 monoclonal antibody rituximab. *Br J Haematol* 2000;109:838.
98. Treon SP, Agus DB, Link B, et al. CD20-directed antibody-mediated immunotherapy induces responses and facilitates hematologic recovery in patients with Waldenström's macroglobulinemia. *J Immunother* 2001;24:272.
99. Dimopoulos MA, Zomas A, Viniou NA, et al. Treatment of Waldenström's macroglobulinemia with thalidomide. *J Clin Oncol* 2001;19: 3596.
100. Dumontet C, Morschhauser F, Solal-Celigny P, et al. Gemcitabine as a single agent in the treatment of relapsed or refractory low-grade non-Hodgkin's lymphoma. *Br J Haematol* 2001;113:772.
101. Legouffe E, Rossi J-F, Laporte J-P, et al. Treatment of Waldenström's macroglobulinemia with very low doses of alpha interferon. *Leuk Lymphoma* 1995;19:337.
102. Leonhard SA, Muhleman AF, Hurtubise PF, et al. Emergence of immunoblastic sarcoma in Waldenström's macroglobulinemia. *Cancer* 1980;45:3102.
103. Garcia R, Hernandez JM, Caballero, et al. Immunoblastic lymphoma and associated non-lymphoid malignancies following two cases of Waldenström's macroglobulinemia. *Eur J Haematol* 1993;50:299.
104. Gobbi PG, Bettini R, Montecucco C, et al. Study of prognosis in Waldenström's macroglobulinemia: a proposal for a simple binary classification with clinical and investigational utility. *Blood* 1994;83:2939.
105. Facon T, Brouillard M, Duhamel A, et al. Prognostic factors in Waldenström's macroglobulinemia. *J Clin Oncol* 1993;11:1553.
106. Morel P, Monconduit M, Jacomy D, et al. Prognostic factors in Waldenström's macroglobulinemia: a report on 232 patients with the description of a new scoring system and its validation on 253 other patients. *Blood* 2000;96:852.

CHAPTER 16

Splenic Marginal Zone Lymphoma

Miguel A. Piris, Manuela Mollejo, Ignacio Chacón, Juan F. García, Francisca I. Camacho, and Miguel A. Cruz

DEFINITION

The term *splenic marginal zone lymphoma* was coined by Schmid in 1992 (1) to describe a micronodular B-cell lymphoma involving the spleen and bone marrow, in which tumoral cells undergo phenotypic and morphologic adaptations to different microenvironments. The splenic histology of these tumors therefore shows preexisting lymphoid follicles replaced by tumoral aggregates in a micronodular pattern. The tumor is composed of a peripheral rim of marginal zone component, an inner small-cell component situated in the mantle zone, and a centrofollicular compartment where tumoral cells replace germinal center cells (1,2).

Most of the cases show a relatively characteristic clinical presentation characterized by prominent splenomegaly and bone marrow and peripheral blood infiltration. Cells in peripheral blood can frequently be recognized by villous cytology, which has led to some confusion about the relationship with the entity designated as *splenic lymphoma with villous lymphocytes* (3–5).

The limits and definition of this entity have been somewhat blurred by the term *marginal zone lymphoma*, which has been understood as presupposing a close relation with other marginal zone–derived tumors, such as marginal zone lymphoma in mucosa-associated lymphoid tissue (MALT) and nodal marginal zone lymphoma. Indeed, the clinical and molecular features of splenic marginal zone lymphoma are strongly different from those of other tumors that are called marginal zone lymphomas, which clearly argues against grouping them in the same family.

EPIDEMIOLOGY

The incidence of splenic marginal zone lymphoma seems to be underestimated due to the limitations in obtaining splenectomy specimens, which makes it difficult to precisely compare its real incidence with that of other B-cell lymphomas. Nevertheless, several different series indicate that the real frequency of splenic marginal zone lymphoma could be approximately 1% of all lymphoma types (2,5,6).

The median age in the published series is approximately 65 years, with a range from 30 to 90 years. A slight predominance in males (male/female, 63/37) was observed in the series by Chacón (7) et al., although this was not confirmed in the series by Berger, in which a proportion of 44% of males was observed (8).

ETIOLOGY

Molecular studies of splenic marginal zone lymphoma cases show a selection for precise VH1 regions, suggesting a hypothetical role for unknown antigens in the promotion of the growth of the tumoral cells (9). The hypothetical role of hepatitis C virus in the genesis of splenic marginal zone lymphoma is suggested by some preliminary observations indicating that a small fraction of type II cryoglobulinemia associated with hepatitis C virus may have overlapping features with those of splenic marginal zone lymphoma (10). The recent description of splenic lymphoma with villous lymphocytes remission of hepatitis C virus–positive patients after antiviral treatment also suggests this hypothetical role (11).

CLINICAL FEATURES

The symptoms at diagnosis most frequently recorded are B symptoms, which are present in a proportion that varies from 25% to 58% of cases, and abdominal discomfort or pain. Splenomegaly is the most frequent sign, observed in three-fourths of patients, whereas anemia, thrombocytopenia, or leukocytosis is reported in one-fourth of patients. Autoimmune hemolytic anemia is found in 10% to 15% of patients, and infections are found in 10% (6,8). The disease is usually symptomatic and is very infrequently diagnosed as a causal finding.

When the disease is restricted to cases diagnosed in the spleen, a large majority of patients have bone marrow involve-

TABLE 16.1. *Major diagnostic features*

Clinical features

Splenomegaly

Bone marrow involvement

Lymphocytosis with or without villous cells

Morphologic features

Spleen

    Micronodular pattern, biphasic cytology, follicular replacement, marginal differentiation

Peripheral blood

    Villous cells, small lymphocytes

Bone marrow

    Intrasinusoidal involvement, intertrabecular nodules

Lymph nodes

    Micronodular pattern, small lymphocytes, scattered blast, rare marginal differentiation

Immunophenotypic features

CD20$^+$, IgD$^+$, bcl-2$^+$, CD3$^-$, CD23$^-$, CD43$^-$, CD5$^-$, CD10$^-$, cyclin D1$^-$, bcl-6$^-$

MIB1 low (target pattern)

Genetic features

7q deletion: 40% (associated with tumoral progression)

p53 gene alterations: 0–20% (18,42) (associated with poor prognosis)

p16 gene alterations: rare

bcl-6 gene somatic mutations: 13% (29)

IgVH gene somatic mutations: 51% (9) (unmutated cases associated with poor prognosis)

Ig, immunoglobulin.

ment, and approximately one-third have liver involvement (Table 16.1). Tumor involvement of peripheral blood (defined as the presence of absolute lymphocytosis or more than 5% of tumor lymphocytes in peripheral blood) was detected in 68% of cases in the series by Chacón et al. (7) and in 57% in the series by Berger (8). Abdominal lymphadenopathies were observed in 25%, and peripheral lymphadenopathies were observed more rarely (17%). Because of the high frequency of bone marrow or liver involvement, most patients in the series were classified as Ann Arbor stage IV.

Serum paraproteinemia [more frequently immunoglobulin (Ig) M] is observed in a small but significant proportion of patients—approximately 10% in the series by Chacón (7), but 24% in the series by Berger (8), and 28% in the series by Troussard (6). Autoimmune hemolytic anemia has been described in 10% to 28% of patients (6,8), and other autoimmune phenomena, such as immune thrombocytopenia or the presence of lupus anticoagulant and cardiolipin antibodies, are occasionally observed (12).

Until recently, the diagnosis was mainly restricted to splenectomized patients, because the diagnostic criteria were based on the splenic morphology. Nevertheless, the conjunction of clinical features and morphology in the bone marrow biopsy usually allows a diagnosis with a reasonable level of confidence.

MORPHOLOGY

Splenic morphology is characterized by a micronodular lymphoid infiltrate of the white pulp, with partial red pulp infiltration, biphasic cytology, and follicular replacement by neoplastic cells. All cases have a conspicuous component of small lymphocytes centered in preexisting follicles, whereas the extent of the marginal zone component is more variable and is dependent on the microenvironment (1,2).

In some cases, a conspicuous component of larger lymphocytes can be observed in the marginal zone ring, as well as large cells scattered in the central nodules and red pulp. These large cells show round nuclei with prominent nucleoli and medium to large cytoplasm (13).

Lymph node involvement by splenic marginal zone lymphoma is common in splenic hilar nodes and infrequent in other locations. Nevertheless, in these lymph nodes, it is common to identify only the micronodular pattern and small-cell component, unless nodal infiltration is associated with disease progression (14).

Bone marrow infiltration is highly frequent in splenic marginal zone lymphoma, although occasionally morphologic examination fails to show this. CD20 staining helps to reveal the presence of intertrabecular polymorphic nodules and aggregates on intrasinusoidal small tumoral cells. These intertrabecular nodules mimic the architecture and cell composition of tumoral nodules in the spleen, with occasional presence of a reactive germinal center surrounded by tumoral cells. Very characteristically, CD20 staining reveals the quite constant presence of slender aggregates of intrasinusoidal B cells (15,16)

Peripheral blood involvement is less frequent than bone marrow infiltration, but, nevertheless, it is relatively common to find a low proportion of B cells in the peripheral blood, some of them displaying morphology typically described as villous. The main morphologic features are summarized in Table 16.1.

VARIANTS

Diffuse

The existence of a subset of cases of splenic B-cell lymphoma has been described recently with predominantly red pulp involvement, absence of follicular replacement, and a monomorphous population of tumoral cells resembling marginal zone B cells, with scattered nucleolated blast cells. Some cases have the particular feature of the presence of reactive hyperplastic follicles in the white pulp isolated in the middle of the diffusely spread tumoral cells. The immunophenotype (bcl-2$^+$, CD5$^-$, CD10$^-$, CD43$^-$, CD23$^-$, cyclin D1$^-$, IgD-3/4), bone marrow infiltration and peripheral blood involvement showed similar findings to those described for splenic marginal zone lymphoma in these locations, therefore suggesting that these tumors could constitute a diffuse variant of splenic marginal zone lymphoma (17).

Aggressive

A short series of cases characterized by massive splenomegaly and a morphologic picture of classical cases of splenic marginal zone lymphoma with increased large lymphocytes has been described (13). Unlike classical cases, a conspicuous component of larger lymphocytes was distributed in the marginal zone ring, occasionally overrunning it, with isolated presence of the same cells within the central small-cell component and also in the red pulp. The bone marrow and peripheral lymph nodes showed histologic findings similar to those described in these locations. The genetic and molecular study of these cases showed no alterations specific to other lymphoma types, such as t(14;18) and t(11;14). Instead of this, it showed 7q loss in three of five cases, p53 inactivation in two of six cases, cyclin D1 overexpression in two of six cases, and the presence of translocations involving the 1q32 region in two of four cases. The recognition of this aggressive variant, besides offering a prognostic indication, indicated that it would be prudent to identify a more suitable form of clinical management of these patients.

IMMUNOPHENOTYPE

Immunophenotypic features are summarized in Table 16.1. The most common profile is CD20+, CD3-, CD23-, CD43-, CD38-, CD5-, CD10-, bcl-6-, Bcl2+, cyclin D1-, IgD+, p27+. DBA44 expression has been described in a small fraction of cases (18). MIB1 staining shows a distinctive annular pattern, outlining the presence of an increased growth fraction in both the germinal center and marginal zone.

Low expression of p53 is the most common finding, although a small proportion of cases may show increased p53 expression that is commonly associated with p53 mutations.

GENETICS

Until recently, no characteristic genetic alterations had been described for this entity, thus rendering an exact diagnosis of splenic marginal zone lymphoma difficult in some cases (Table 16.1). The analysis of chromosome region 7q22-36 with loss of heterozygosity and karyotyping displayed a frequency of allelic loss in splenic marginal zone lymphoma of 40%, which is higher than is observed in other B-cell lymphoproliferative syndromes (8%) (19–21). The most frequently deleted microsatellite was D7S487. Surrounding this microsatellite, a small commonly deleted region of 5cM has been identified, defined between D7S685 and D7S514. These results provide a useful cytogenetic marker for this neoplasm, which may be used in conjunction with other morphologic, phenotypic, and clinical features. Cases with 7q

loss tend to show more aggressive behavior, with more frequent tumoral progression. Although these data suggest that the region could contain a tumor suppressor gene—the region is being intensively examined in other human cancers (22–25)—so far no identification of a specific gene alteration has been achieved.

Other clonal chromosome abnormalities detected are again of 3q (10% to 20%) and involvement of chromosomes 1, 8, and 14. No patient showed translocation t(11;14) (q13;q32) or t(14;18) (q21;q32). Occasional cytogenetic abnormalities involving 14q32, such as t(6;14) (p12;q32) (26), t(10;14) (q24;q32) (26), and t(7;14) (q21;q32) (with deregulation of CDK6) have been reported (27). Deletion of 17p13, p53 has been observed in proportions that vary from 3% to 17% of cases (18,26,28).

The frequency of IgVH somatic mutations has also been analyzed in splenic marginal zone lymphoma. The real frequency has only been clarified recently, after a thorough analysis of 35 cases displayed an unexpected molecular heterogeneity in this entity, with 49% unmutated cases (less than 2% somatic mutations), and with a higher frequency of 7q31 deletions and shorter overall survival. Additionally, a high percentage of cases (18 of 40 sequences) showed selective use of the VH1-2 segment, thereby emphasizing the singularity of this neoplasm and suggesting that this tumor derives from a highly selected B-cell population (9). Not surprisingly, cases with IgVH mutations also display somatic mutations in the 5' noncoding region of the bcl-6 gene, although at a lower frequency (29).

CELL ORIGIN

The debate on the cellular origin of splenic marginal zone lymphoma has been fueled by the paradoxic situation created by a definition of the disease and a morphology implying marginal zone origin and conflicting morphologic and molecular findings. Thus, it seems that a large proportion of tumoral cells are IgD-positive small lymphocytes in which marginal zone differentiation is only produced in the microenvironment provided by the splenic marginal zone. The absence of somatic mutation in IgVH genes in half of the cases of splenic marginal zone lymphoma does not help to establish a close relationship with marginal zone B cells, which have been demonstrated to carry on somatic mutations (30). An alternative explanation for this situation could be provided by the presence in the primary lymphoid follicles of the spleen of a hitherto unknown small B-cell subpopulation. These cells would be able to differentiate into marginal zone B cells in a suitable environment and to acquire somatic mutations after exposure to antigens present in the germinal center.

CLINICAL COURSE

Splenic marginal zone lymphoma is a low-grade tumor with a survival probability at 5 years that varies from 65% (for

TABLE 16.2. *Prognostic factors*

	Parameters	Reference level	Overall survival	Author(s) (references)	Failure-free survival	Author (references)
Biologic	Somatic mutations IgVH	IgH mutated	$p<.05$	Algara (9)		
	7q31	Preservation		(7)	$p=.057$	Mateo (19)
	p53 gene alterations	Mutation	$p<.05$	Chacón, Baldini (43), Gruzcka (18)		
Clinical	ECOG 2–3	0–1	$p<.05$	Chacón (7)		
	Involvement of nonhematopoietic sites		$p<.05$	Chacón (7)		
	Response to therapy	Complete response	$p<.05$	Chacón (7)	$p<.05$	Thieblemont (44)
	Lymphocyte count	$>9\times10^3/\mu L$	$p<.05$	Thieblemont (44)		
		$<4\times10^3/\mu L$		Troussard (6)		
	Leukocyte count	$>20\times10^3/\mu L$	$p<.05$	Thieblemont (44)		
		$<30\times10^3/\mu L$		Troussard (6)		
	M component		$p<.05$	Thieblemont (44)	$p<.05$	Thieblemont (44)
	Use chemotherapy as the initial treatment		$p<.05$	Troussard (6)		
	β_2-microglobulin level	Elevated	$p<.05$	Thieblemont		
	Immunologic event	Presence			$p<.05$	Thieblemont (44)

ECOG, Eastern Cooperative Oncology Group; Ig, immunoglobulin.

patients diagnosed after splenectomy) to 78% (for patients diagnosed with splenic lymphoma with villous lymphocytes in peripheral blood). Differences in survival probability are likely dependent on imperfect overlapping between splenic marginal zone lymphoma and splenic lymphoma with villous lymphocytes, and on the poorer status of patients requiring splenectomy.

The few studies performed on relatively large series show that high tumored mass and poor general status are adverse clinical prognostic factors. The biologic parameters found to be associated with adverse outcome are p53 mutation or over-expression, 7q deletion and the absence of somatic mutation in IgVH genes (Table 16.2). Splenic marginal zone lymphoma cases therefore seem to behave in a similar pattern to those of chronic lymphocytic leukemia, which have also shown an unfavorable clinical course associated with p53 inactivation and naive IgVH.

Although very little information from clinical trials in splenic marginal zone lymphoma is available, some clear points are emerging. These include the lack of efficacy of 2-chlorodeoxyadenoside (31), the relatively favorable course of patients treated with splenectomy (6), and the potential interest of fludarabine as an efficient therapy for patients relapsing after splenectomy or for those who are resistant to chlorambucil (32).

Interestingly, the follow-up of splenic marginal zone lymphoma cases reveals a tendency (13% of splenic marginal zone lymphoma with adequate follow-up) toward histologic and clinical progression to large B-cell lymphomas. The incidence of large-cell transformation in splenic marginal zone lymphoma is thus lower than in follicular lymphoma (25% to 60%) and mantle cell lymphoma (11% to 39%), although it is roughly similar to the frequency of transformation in B-chronic lymphocytic lymphoma/small lymphocytic lymphoma (1% to 10%). In the few cases studied to date, it seems that progression in splenic marginal zone lymphoma is mainly independent of p53 or p16INK4a inactivation, and that it is preceded by a higher growth fraction and more frequent 7q deletion (28).

DIFFERENTIAL DIAGNOSIS

Differential diagnosis vis-à-vis other small B-cell lymphomas usually requires the integration of full clinical, morphologic, and molecular data (Tables 16.3 and 16.4). A micronodular pattern of splenic involvement with villous cells in the peripheral blood is not the hallmark of this entity and can be observed in other conditions, more specifically in follicular lymphoma and mantle cell lymphoma. The lack of cyclin D1, CD10, and bcl6 expression as well as the absence of t(11;14) and t(14;18) make it possible to rule out the most frequent entities included in differential diagnosis (33–36). Particularly helpful features are the intrasinusoidal pattern of involvement in the bone marrow (15,16), and IgD expression by tumoral cells (1,2).

Differential diagnosis in relation to lymphoplasmacytic lymphoma has been a controversial issue, because splenic

TABLE 16.3. *Differential diagnosis*

		SMZL	B-CLL	MCL	FL	LPL	MZL, MALT
Morphology	Cytology composition	Small cells Blasts cells Marginal cells	Small cells Prolympho-cytes Paraimmuno-blasts	Monomor-phous (centrocyte-like)	Centrocytes Centroblasts	Small cells Plasmacytoid cells Plasma cells	Small cells Blast cells Marginal cells
	Marginal zone pattern	+	−	−/+	+	−	+
Phenotype	IgD	+	+	+	−	−/+	−
	CD43	−	+	+	−	+/−	−/+
	CD5	−	+	+	−	−	−
	CD23	−	+	−	−	−	−
	CD10	−	−	−	+	−	−
	Cyclin D1	−	−	+	−	−	−
	bcl-6	−	−	−	+	−	−
	MIB1	Target pattern	Low	Low–medium	Low	Low	Low
Molecular findings	Trisomy 3 (%)	17	3	Rare	Rare	Rare	50–85
	Trisomy 12 (%)	10–50	20	5–15	—	—	5–15
	7q deletion (%)	40	Rare	Rare	Rare	Rare	Rare
	t(11;14)	−	−	+	−	−	−
	t14;18	−	−	−	+	−	−
	t11;18	−	−	−	−	−	−/+
	Somatic mutations IgVH (%)	51	54	10	90	100	100
Clinical findings	Splenomegaly	+	+	+	+	+	−
	Bone marrow involvement	+	+	25%	+	+	20%
	Peripheral blood involvement	+	+	20–58%	9%	+	−
	M-component	10–30%	−	−	−	+	Rare
	Peripheral lymph node	Rare	Rare	+	+	+	Rare
	Nonhematopoietic extranodal sites	Rare	−	Gastrointestinal Waldeyer's ring	Gastrointestinal	Rare	+

CLL, chronic lymphocytic leukemia; FL, follicular lymphoma; Ig, immunoglobulin; LPL, lymphoplasmacytic lymphoma; MCL, mantle cell lymphoma; MZL, MALT, marginal zone lymphoma, mucosa-associated lymphoid tissue; SMZL, splenic marginal zone lymphoma; +, positive; −, negative.

marginal zone lymphoma may show a gradient of plasmacytic differentiation with serum monoclonal paraproteinemia in up to 28% of cases in some series (6–8). It is reasonable to group these cases as bona fide splenic marginal zone lymphoma, indicating the existence of plasmacytic differentiation (37). This approach is consistent with that adopted in other B-cell lymphomas showing plasmacytic differentiation, such as marginal zone lymphoma, MALT type (38). Indeed, the splenic involvement by lymphoplas-

macytic lymphoma usually is distinguishable because of the presence of a mixed pattern of white and red pulp involvement by periarteriolar aggregates of plasmacytoid cells, small lymphocytes, and immunoblasts, with absence of marginal zone differentiation.

Differential diagnosis vis-à-vis MALT-type marginal zone lymphoma is occasionally necessary due to the existence of cases of marginal zone lymphoma, MALT type, that may infiltrate the spleen with a micronodular pattern. Two

TABLE 16.4. *Perils and pitfalls*

Specific findings	Comments
Follicular replacement (MIB1 and bcl-2 staining)	MIB1 shows a target pattern, and bcl-2$^+$ tumoral cells mixed with residual bcl-2$^-$ germinal center cells highlights follicular replacement. This contrasts with neoplastic follicles with homogenous bcl-2 staining and proliferating cells evenly distributed throughout the follicles in follicular lymphoma.
IgD staining	IgD is expressed in most cases of splenic marginal zone lymphoma. Residual mantle cells are absent from this lymphoma. In follicular lymphoma and marginal zone lymphoma, mucosa-associated lymphoid tissue type, preserved IgD$^+$ mantle cells could be observed.
Bone marrow infiltration	Bone marrow biopsy shows intertrabecular nodules of small lymphocytes and scattered blasts overrunning residual germinal centers. Intrasinusoidal involvement (demonstrated by CD20 staining) is quite characteristic of this entity.
Splenic hilar lymph node morphology	Lymph node involvement by splenic marginal zone lymphoma displays characteristic histologic and immunohistochemical features, with frequent loss of marginal zone differentiation.
7q deletion	7q31-32 loss is a relatively specific genetic marker of splenic marginal zone lymphoma and is present in 40% of cases.
IgVH somatic mutations	Analysis of somatic mutations in the IgVH gene reveals 49% of unmutated cases. This group is associated with shorter overall survival and 7q loss.
Marginal zone pattern	Marginal zone pattern can be observed in other small B-cell lymphomas when involving the spleen. Marginal zone differentiation in bone marrow and lymph node involvement by splenic marginal zone lymphoma are usually absent.
Villous cells in peripheral blood	Although splenic marginal zone lymphoma and splenic lymphoma with villous lymphocytes mostly overlap, not all splenic marginal zone lymphomas show villous cells in peripheral blood, and villous lymphocytes may appear in mantle cell lymphoma, follicular lymphoma, large B-cell lymphoma, and lymphoplasmacytic lymphoma.
Cyclin D1$^+$ cells	Scattered cyclin D1$^+$ cells independent of 11;14 translocation could be found in a few cases of splenic marginal zone lymphoma.

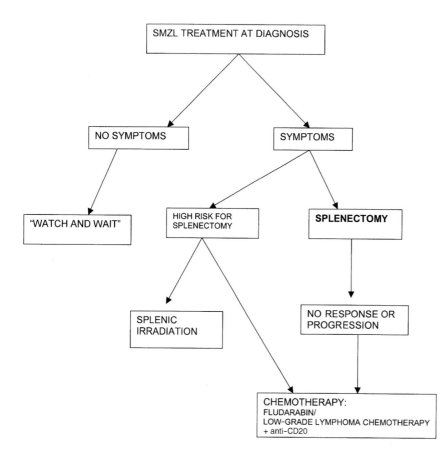

FIG. 16.1. Treatment algorithm for splenic marginal zone lymphoma (SMZL).

useful features are the absence of t11;18 in splenic marginal zone lymphoma cases (39) and the characteristic IgD expression in splenic marginal zone lymphoma, which is only rarely observed in marginal zone lymphoma, MALT type (Color Plate 14).

TREATMENT

Splenic marginal zone lymphoma is an indolent lymphoma, which explains the observation that in the larger series, a significant group of patients received no treatment for relatively long periods (6,8,40), and they did not seem to do worse than those initially treated. For this reason, a "watch and wait" conservative therapeutic approach has been recommended. In patients requiring therapy (e.g., due to cytopenias and/or huge symptomatic splenomegaly), splenectomy seems to be the treatment of choice. Patients treated by splenectomy show a reduction in or disappearance of atypical circulating cells or monoclonal bands and recover normal hematologic parameters.

The role of chemotherapy is still a matter of debate. No differences were found in overall survival in patients who received and did not receive chemotherapy. Because of this, chemotherapy probably should be reserved for selective use after clinical progression, for lack of response to splenectomy, or when splenectomy is contraindicated. Current treatment options for splenic marginal zone lymphoma include single-agent or combination chemotherapy, such as chlorambucil or cyclophosphamide/vincristine/prednisone or cyclophosphamide/doxorubicin/vincristine/prednisone. A potential role for fludarabine as an effective treatment for splenic marginal zone lymphoma has also been proposed (32). Radiotherapy could be considered an optional treatment for splenic marginal zone lymphoma when splenectomy is contraindicated. Recently, data have emerged to support the use of rituximab in combination with conventional chemotherapeutic regimens for the treatment of indolent lymphomas (Fig. 16.1) (41).

One of the most exciting pieces of information to emerge related to the treatment of splenic marginal zone lymphoma is the report of Hermine and colleagues (11) of clinical remission of the disease in a subset of hepatitis C virus–positive patients treated with antiviral therapy. If confirmed, this should constitute a clear indication of the potential interest of testing all the splenic marginal zone lymphoma patients for hepatitis C virus infection, treating the positive cases with antiviral therapy before taking another, more aggressive therapeutic decision.

REFERENCES

1. Schmid C, Kirkham N, Diss T, et al. Splenic marginal zone cell lymphoma. *Am J Surg Pathol* 1992;16:455–466.
2. Mollejo M, Menarguez J, Lloret E, et al. Splenic marginal zone lymphoma: a distinctive type of low-grade B-cell lymphoma. A clinicopathological study of 13 cases. *Am J Surg Pathol* 1995;19:1146–1157.
3. Matutes E, Morilla R, Owusu-Ankomah K, et al. The immunophenotype of splenic lymphoma with villous lymphocytes and its relevance to the differential diagnosis with other B-cell disorders. *Blood* 1994;83:1558–1562.
4. Catovsky D, Matutes E. Splenic lymphoma with circulating villous lymphocytes/splenic marginal-zone lymphoma. *Semin Hematol* 1999;36:148–154.
5. Melo JV, Robinson DS, Gregory C, et al. Splenic B cell lymphoma with "villous" lymphocytes in the peripheral blood: a disorder distinct from hairy cell leukemia. *Leukemia* 1987;1:294–298.
6. Troussard X, Valensi F, Duchayne E, et al. Splenic lymphoma with villous lymphocytes: clinical presentation, biology and prognostic factors in a series of 100 patients. Groupe Francais d'Hematologie Cellulaire (GFHC). *Br J Haematol* 1996;93:731–736.
7. Chacón JI, Mollejo M, Muñoz E, et al. Splenic marginal zone lymphoma: clinical characteristics and prognostic factors in a series of 60 splenectomized patients. *Blood* 2002;100:1648–1654.
8. Berger F, Felman P, Thieblemont C, et al. Non-MALT marginal zone B-cell lymphomas: a description of clinical presentation and outcome in 124 patients. *Blood* 2000;95:1950–1956.
9. Algara P, Mateo MS, Sanchez-Beato M, et al. Analysis of the IgV(H) somatic mutations in splenic marginal zone lymphoma defines a group of unmutated cases with frequent 7q deletion and adverse clinical course. *Blood* 2002;99:1299–1304.
10. De Vita S, De Re V, Gasparotto D, et al. Oligoclonal non-neoplastic B cell expansion is the key feature of type II mixed cryoglobulinemia: clinical and molecular findings do not support a bone marrow pathologic diagnosis of indolent B cell lymphoma. *Arthritis Rheum* 2000;43:94–102.
11. Hermine O, Lefrere F, Bronowicki JP, et al. Regression of splenic lymphoma with villous lymphocytes after treatment of hepatitis C virus infection. *N Engl J Med* 2002;347:89–94.
12. Murakami H, Irisawa H, Saitoh T, et al. Immunological abnormalities in splenic marginal zone cell lymphoma. *Am J Hematol* 1997;56:173–178.
13. Lloret E, Mollejo M, Mateo MS, et al. Splenic marginal zone lymphoma with increased number of blasts: an aggressive variant? *Hum Pathol* 1999;30:1153–1160.
14. Mollejo M, Lloret E, Menarguez J, et al. Lymph node involvement by splenic marginal zone lymphoma: morphological and immunohistochemical features. *Am J Surg Pathol* 1997;21:772–780.
15. Labouyrie E, Marit G, Vial JP, et al. Intrasinusoidal bone marrow involvement by splenic lymphoma with villous lymphocytes: a helpful immunohistologic feature. *Mod Pathol* 1997;10:1015–1020.
16. Franco V, Florena AM, Campesi G. Intrasinusoidal bone marrow infiltration: a possible hallmark of splenic lymphoma. *Histopathology* 1996;29:571–575.
17. Mollejo M, Algara P, Mateo MS, et al. Splenic small B-cell lymphoma with predominant red pulp involvement: a diffuse variant of splenic marginal zone lymphoma? *Histopathology* 2002;40:22–30.
18. Gruszka-Westwood AM, Hamoudi RA, Matutes E, et al. p53 abnormalities in splenic lymphoma with villous lymphocytes. *Blood* 2001;97:3552–3558.
19. Mateo M, Mollejo M, Villuendas R, et al. 7q31-32 allelic loss is a frequent finding in splenic marginal zone lymphoma. *Am J Pathol* 1999;154:1583–1589.
20. Sole F, Woessner S, Florensa L, et al. Frequent involvement of chromosomes 1, 3, 7 and 8 in splenic marginal zone B-cell lymphoma. *Br J Haematol* 1997;98:446–449.
21. Oscier DG, Gardiner A, Mould S. Structural abnormalities of chromosome 7q in chronic lymphoproliferative disorders. *Cancer Genet Cytogenet* 1996;92:24–27.
22. Inoue K, Kohno T, Takakura S, et al. Alterations of the PPP1R3 gene in hematological malignancies. *Int J Oncol* 2000;17:717–721.
23. Galbiati F, Volonte D, Liu J, et al. Caveolin-1 expression negatively regulates cell cycle progression by inducing G(0)/G(1) arrest via a p53/p21(WAF1/Cip1)-dependent mechanism. *Mol Biol Cell* 2001;12:2229–2244.
24. Tobias ES, Hurlstone AF, MacKenzie E, et al. The TES gene at 7q31.1 is methylated in tumours and encodes a novel growth-suppressing LIM domain protein. *Oncogene* 2001;20:2844–2853.
25. Zenklusen JC, Conti CJ, Green ED. Mutational and functional analyses reveal that ST7 is a highly conserved tumor-suppressor gene on human chromosome 7q31. *Nat Genet* 2001;27:392–398.

26. Sole F, Salido M, Espinet B, et al. Splenic marginal zone B-cell lymphomas: two cytogenetic subtypes, one with gain of 3q and the other with loss of 7q. *Haematologica* 2001;86:71–77.

27. Corcoran MM, Mould SJ, Orchard JA, et al. Dysregulation of cyclin dependent kinase 6 expression in splenic marginal zone lymphoma through chromosome 7q translocations. *Oncogene* 1999;18:6271–6277.

28. Camacho FI, Mollejo M, Mateo MS, et al. Progression to large B-cell lymphoma in splenic marginal zone lymphoma: a description of a series of 12 cases. *Am J Surg Pathol* 2001;25:1268–1276.

29. Mateo MS, Mollejo M, Villuendas R, et al. Molecular heterogeneity of splenic marginal zone lymphomas: analysis of mutations in the 5' non-coding region of the bcl-6 gene. *Leukemia* 2001;15:628–634.

30. Tierens A, Delabie J, Michiels L, et al. Marginal-zone B cells in the human lymph node and spleen show somatic hypermutations and display clonal expansion. *Blood* 1999;93:226–234.

31. Lefrere F, Hermine O, Francois S, et al. Lack of efficacy of 2-chlorodeoxyadenoside in the treatment of splenic lymphoma with villous lymphocytes. *Leuk Lymphoma* 2000;40:113–117.

32. Lefrere F, Hermine O, Belanger C, et al. An effective treatment in patients with splenic lymphoma with villous lymphocytes. *Leukemia* 2000;14:573–575.

33. Mollejo M, Lloret E, Solares J, et al. Splenic involvement by blastic mantle cell lymphoma (large cell/anaplastic variant) mimicking splenic marginal zone lymphoma. *Am J Hematol* 1999;62:242–246.

34. Savilo E, Campo E, Mollejo M, et al. Absence of cyclin D1 protein expression in splenic marginal zone lymphoma. *Mod Pathol* 1998; 11:601–606.

35. Piris MA, Mollejo M, Campo E, et al. A marginal zone pattern may be found in different varieties of non-Hodgkin's lymphoma: the morphology and immunohistology of splenic involvement by B-cell lymphomas simulating splenic marginal zone lymphoma. *Histopathology* 1998;33:230–239.

36. Schmid U, Cogliatti SB, Diss TC, et al. Monocytoid/marginal zone B-cell differentiation in follicle centre cell lymphoma. *Histopathology* 1996;29:201–208.

37. Van Huyen JP, Molina T, Delmer A, et al. Splenic marginal zone lymphoma with or without plasmacytic differentiation. *Am J Surg Pathol* 2000;24:1581–1592.

38. Jaffe ES, Harris NL, Stein H, et al. *Pathology and genetics of tumours of hematopoietic and lymphoid tissues. World Health Organization classification of tumours*. Lyon: IARC Press, 2001.

39. Remstein ED, James CD, Kurtin PJ. Incidence and subtype specificity of API2-MALT1 fusion translocations in extranodal, nodal, and splenic marginal zone lymphomas. *Am J Pathol* 2000;156:1183–1188.

40. Mulligan SP, Matutes E, Dearden C, et al. Splenic lymphoma with villous lymphocytes: natural history and response to therapy in 50 cases. *Br J Haematol* 1991;78:206–209.

41. Czuczman MS. Immunochemotherapy in indolent non-Hodgkin's lymphoma. *Semin Oncol* 2002;29:11–17.

42. Mateo MS, Mollejo M, Villuendas R, et al. Analysis of the frequency of microsatellite instability and p53 gene mutation in splenic marginal zone and MALT lymphomas. *Mol Pathol* 1998; 51:262–267.

43. Baldini L, Guffanti A, Cro L, et al. Poor prognosis in non-villous splenic marginal zone cell lymphoma is associated with p53 mutations. *Br J Haematol* 1997;99:375–378.

44. Thieblemont C, Felman P, Berger F, et al. Treatment of splenic marginal zone B-cell lymphoma: an analysis of 81 patients. *Clin Lymphoma* 2002;3:41–47.

CHAPTER 17

T-Cell Large Granular Lymphocytic Leukemia, T-Cell Prolymphocytic Leukemia, and Aggressive Natural Killer–Cell Leukemia/Lymphoma

Kathryn Foucar, Estella Matutes, and Daniel Catovsky

T-CELL LARGE GRANULAR LYMPHOCYTIC LEUKEMIA

Definition

T-cell large granular lymphocytic leukemia is a disorder characterized by the clonal expansion of mature T lymphocytes with a characteristic morphology and immunophenotype. In the 1970s and 1980s, the disease had been described under several designations, such as T γ lymphoproliferative disorder (1), chronic T-cell lymphocytosis (2), and T-cell chronic lymphocytic leukemia (3), until the term *large granular lymphocytic leukemia*, proposed by Loughran et al. (4), was widely adopted. Although the cells in cases presenting with large granular lymphocytes may have a T-cell or, rarely, a natural killer phenotype, the World Health Organization (WHO) Classification considers separately the cases derived from T-cells—for example, T-cell large granular lymphocytic leukemia (5)—from those derived from natural killer–cells, which are classified within the spectrum of aggressive natural killer–cell leukemias.

Etiology and Epidemiology

The etiology of T-cell large granular lymphocytic leukemia is unknown. There is no solid evidence that DNA or RNA viruses such as Epstein-Barr virus (EBV) or human T-cell leukemia viruses play a role in the pathogenesis of this disease (6,7). In contrast, large granular lymphocytic leukemia appears to be more common in patients with autoimmune disorders, particularly rheumatoid arthritis, suggesting that the immune system plays a role in the development of the disease. A history of rheumatoid arthritis is common and documented in 25% of patients (8,9); in some cases, T-cell large granular lymphocytic leukemia may precede the manifestations of rheumatoid arthritis, whereas in others, both

diseases manifest simultaneously. It has been shown that patients with large granular lymphocytic leukemia plus rheumatoid arthritis like Felty's syndrome have the DR4 haplotype with a significantly higher frequency than the normal population. This suggests a similar immunogenetic basis for these two conditions. (10).

T-cell large granular lymphocytic leukemia preferentially affects adult patients without sex predominance and is more common in Eastern than in Western countries. The disease has rarely been documented in childhood.

Diagnosis

Although T-cell large granular lymphocytic leukemia is often suspected in patients with a sustained increase in cells with large granular lymphocyte morphology, its diagnosis generally requires the integration of morphology, immunophenotyping, and, frequently, T-cell receptor gene rearrangement studies (11). Although most patients have sustained, $\geq 2 \times 10^9$ per L absolute large granular lymphocyte counts, some patients with confirmed clonal disease have substantially fewer circulating cells (5,12,13). Normally, large granular lymphocytes account for 10% to 15% of circulating lymphocytes, with absolute large granular lymphocyte counts in the range of 0.2 to 0.4×10^9 per L. Transient increases in circulating large granular lymphocytes are encountered in nonneoplastic conditions, especially viral infections, in which these cells are admixed with activated lymphocytes exhibiting heterogeneous morphology (11,14–16). Thus, a sustained large granular lymphocytosis is generally required for diagnosis.

By morphologic review of blood films, T-cell large granular lymphocytes have round nuclei with condensed chromatin, inconspicuous nucleoli, and abundant pale blue cytoplasm that contains sparse, coarse eosinophilic granules (Color Plate

15). Most patients with T-cell large granular lymphocytic leukemia also have neutropenia; anemia and thrombocytopenia are also fairly common (11,14,16).

Bone marrow involvement by T-cell large granular lymphocytic leukemia may be inconspicuous, consisting of poorly delineated interstitial or patchy infiltrates; these infiltrates may be particularly subtle in hypocellular specimens (Color Plate 16) (5,17). Immunohistochemical staining for CD3, CD8, and T-cell–restricted intracellular antigen (TIA-1) is very useful in highlighting these subtle infiltrates and for estimating the extent of infiltration by lymphocytes, which is generally more pronounced than suspected on hematoxylin-eosin–stained sections (Color Plates 17 and 18) (13,18). In addition, because some cases exhibit reticulin fibrosis, large granular lymphocytes may not be well represented on bone marrow aspirate films (17). Consequently, the successful diagnosis of T-cell large granular lymphocytic leukemia hinges on the recognition of increased numbers of large granular lymphocytes on blood films and a high index of suspicion prompting immunohistochemical assessment of core biopsy specimens. Other bone marrow/blood findings that should prompt immunohistochemical assessment for occult T-cell large granular lymphocytic leukemia include acquired pure red cell aplasia, neutropenia, and the very rare cases of adult-onset cyclic neutropenia (11).

Membrane marker studies by flow cytometry show in most cases a CD2, CD3, CD8, CD16, and CD57 immunophenotype. CD5 and CD7 are weakly expressed in 50% of cases; CD4 and CD56 are, as a rule, negative (Fig. 17.1) (5,15). Most cases represent expansions of T cells bearing

the T-cell receptor $\alpha\beta$ and a minority are derived from T-cell receptor $\gamma\delta$ positive cells.

The distinctive cytoplasmic granules of T-cell large granular lymphocytic leukemias are positive for TIA-1 and perforin. Criteria to diagnose this disease in bone marrow by immunohistochemical techniques vary, but, in general, substantially increased numbers of CD3[+], CD8[+], CD57[+], and TIA-1[+] T cells are evident diffusely or in at least eight cell clusters; intravascular/intrasinusoidal infiltrates may also be highlighted by immunohistochemical studies (Color Plates 17 and 18) (13,18). Spleen histology shows predominant red pulp involvement with atrophy or a reactive white pulp.

The diagnosis of T-cell large granular lymphocytic leukemia can be confirmed by documenting clonal T-cell receptor gene rearrangement of β or γ chains or both by either Southern blot or polymerase chain reaction (PCR) techniques. These gene rearrangement techniques are particularly useful in cases in which the absolute large granular lymphocyte count is not significantly increased (11,12).

Pathogenesis

Cytogenetic studies on T-cell large granular lymphocytic leukemias are limited, and clonal cytogenetics aberrations are infrequent, with no distinct genetic "markers" yet identified (4,5). However, in a recent study, clonal cytogenetics abnormalities were noted in two cases; both aberrations involved T-cell receptor gene loci at 7p14-p15 and 14q11, respectively (19).

Due to the frequent association of T-cell large granular lymphocytic leukemia with rheumatoid arthritis, a patho-

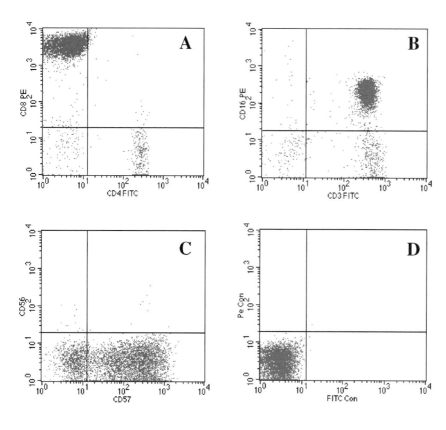

FIG. 17.1. Flow cytometry analysis of a peripheral blood sample from a patient with T-cell large granular lymphocytic leukemia: CD8[+], CD4[-], CD57[+], CD56[-], and coexpression of CD16[+] and CD3[+]. **A:** CD4 (–)Fitc / CD8 (+)Pe; **B:** CD3 (+)Fitc / CD16 (+)Pe; **C:** CD57 (+)Fitc / CD56 (–)Pe; **D:** Isotypic controls (–).

genic link has been suggested (8,9,11). Although the origin of this leukemia is unknown, recent authors suggest a multistep pathogenesis of this disorder beginning with chronic antigenic stimulation of large granular lymphocytes followed first by polyclonal, then eventual monoclonal, T-cell expansion (11). Even though these clonal large granular lymphocytes constitutively express both Fas (CD95) and Fas ligand, they are resistant to Fas-induced apoptosis due to a defective Fas apoptotic pathway (11,20).

The underlying mechanisms of the anemia may be multiple, including decrease or lack of erythroid precursors, Coomb's-positive hemolytic anemia, or inhibition of the burst-forming and erythroid colony–forming units by the leukemia (21,22). The mechanism responsible for the neutropenia is not well established, but it seems to be unrelated to hypersplenism or bone marrow infiltration; in a few cases, an inhibitory effect of these lymphocytes in the granular monocytes colony-forming has been documented. Although the presence of antineutrophil antibodies has been demonstrated in some cases, their pathogenic significance is uncertain, as these patients often have circulating immunocomplexes (11).

The postulated cell of origin of T-cell large granular lymphocytic leukemia is a postthymic immunocompetent (antigen-activated) cytotoxic T cell, including both memory and effector subsets (11,16,23).

Clinical and Laboratory Features

Approximately one-third of patients are asymptomatic at diagnosis, and the disease is discovered on a routine blood count that shows lymphocytosis or persistent neutropenia or both (14,24). The most frequent symptoms are fever due to recurrent bacterial infections or mouth ulcers; both are often related to neutropenia. Other symptoms are arthralgias and tiredness or fatigue, the latter unrelated to the degree of anemia. Other presenting features that occur in a minority of patients are thrombocytopenia, abdominal distension, a skin maculopapular rash, and severe anemia due to red cell hypoplasia.

Physical examination shows a moderate splenomegaly in 20% to 50% of patients, skin lesions in 20%, and hepatomegaly in a minority. Peripheral or intraabdominal lymphadenopathy is rare (<10% patients). In some cases, the spleen is noted to be enlarged only by ultrasound or computed tomography.

Laboratory investigations show a normal or mildly raised white blood cell count ranging from 5 to 20×10^9 per L. Even if the absolute lymphocyte count is normal, the majority of circulating cells are large granular lymphocytes; a few patients are lymphopenic but many develop lymphocytosis after splenectomy. Neutropenia (neutrophils $<0.5 \times 10^9$/L) is a frequent feature, and, as a rule, this cytopenia is unrelated to the degree of bone marrow infiltration or hypersplenism. Anemia and thrombocytopenia are less frequent and are detected in 30% and 20% of patients, respectively.

Liver biochemistry may show raised transaminases and alkaline phosphatase. Autoimmune screen may show a variety of immune abnormalities, such as the presence of rheumatoid factor, antinuclear antibodies, circulating immunocomplexes, and polyclonal hypergammaglobulinemia; rare patients may have severe hypogammaglobulinemia that relates to the suppressor activity of the large granular lymphocytes on the normal B lymphocytes (11).

Prognosis and Survival

The clinical course of T-cell large granular lymphocytic leukemia is chronic in the majority of patients. In a large series of 151 patients with a median follow-up of 26 months, only 17% of them died (25), and in another series of 68 patients, the median survival was greater than 10 years (26). Deaths are mainly due to infections with only a few with disease progression. There is a subgroup of patients in whom the disease pursues an aggressive clinical course, and it has been suggested that aggressive disease is associated with large granular lymphocytic leukemia coexpressing T-cell antigens and CD56 (27).

Although the vast majority of cases of T-cell large granular lymphocytic leukemia exhibit stable morphologic and immunophenotypic features, transformation to large-cell lymphoma has been rarely reported (28,29). T-cell large granular lymphocytic leukemia has a very chronic course, and quoted median survivals are 8 to 10 years (13,14,16).

Therapy

At least one-third of patients with T-cell large granular lymphocytic leukemia may never require therapy and have tolerable or minimal cytopenias. The main aim of treatment is to correct the neutropenia, which can be achieved without significant cytoreduction but by immunomodulation with agents like low-dose methotrexate once a week or cyclosporin A, daily in two divided doses. Indications for treatment are (a) recurrent infections caused by neutropenia or other cytopenias—for example, red cell aplasia; this is the most common indication; (b) progression with organomegaly and abnormal liver function tests; this is uncommon but may be seen in late stages; and (c) transformation to large-cell lymphoma; this is very rare (29).

Loughran et al. (30) reported good responses (correction of neutropenia, normalization of blood counts, and disappearance of circulating large granular lymphocytes) in five of ten patients treated with 10 mg/m² of weekly oral methotrexate; one further patient had a partial response. In three of the five responders, the peripheral blood clone was no longer detectable. There is no information on bone marrow changes, but it is likely to be persistence of infiltration, as the neutropenia, which improves in 1 to 4 months, tends to recur on discontinuation of therapy. In five of the ten patients, prednisolone was used initially with methotrexate and gradually tapered over several weeks. At the Royal Marsden Hospital we have used methotrexate in two patients (patient 3 and patient 8, Table 17.1) with good responses.

TABLE 17.1. *Response to treatment in T-cell large granular lymphocytic leukemia (Royal Marsden Hospital Series)*

Patient	Prednisolone	Cyclophosphamide	Pentostatin	Cyclosporin A	Methotrexate	EPO	G-CSF
1	—	CR (6+ yr)	MR	NR	—	—	Useful
2	NR	GPR (CHOP)	GPR (8 yr)	NR	—	NR	—
3[a]	MR	NR (high dose)	—	PR	PR	—	Useful
4[b]	—	—	CR (×3)	—	—	—	—
5	—	NR (COP)	—	GPR (8 yr)	—	—	—
6[c]	NR	—	MR	MR	—	Useful	Useful
7	—	—	—	NR	—	—	—
8	—	—	—	—	PR	—	—

CHOP, COP + doxorubicin; COP, cyclophosphamide, Oncovin (vincristine), and prednisolone; CR, complete response; EPO, erythropoietin; GPR, almost CR but not proven by bone marrow biopsy; G-CSF, granulocyte-colony stimulating factor; MR, minimal response; NR, no response; PR, partial response.

[a]No response to daunorubicin, cystosine arabinoside, and etoposide; CHOP, cyclophoshamide total-body irradiation; minimal response to DHAP; nodular partial response with Campath.
[b]CD4+, CD3+, CD16+, CD11b+.
[c]Natural killer phenotype: CD3−, CD2+, CD11b+, CD7+, CD16+.

Cyclosporin A was effective in two out of six patients (Table 17.1). One of them (patient 5) corrected the severe neutropenia (after not responding to cyclophosphamide, Oncovin [vincristine], and prednisolone and chlorambucil) and remained in clinical remission for 8 years on cyclosporin A, 4 mg/kg given in two divided doses. Neutrophils improved from 0.2 to 0.4×10^9 per L to 2.3 to 3.8×10^9 per L. The spleen reduced in size but remained palpable. This patient died of hepatocellular carcinoma, which may have been caused indirectly by the long-term immunosuppression. The overall survival since diagnosis was 18 years. As shown in Table 17.1, three patients (patients 1, 2, and 7) did not respond to cyclosporin A; patient 2 had red cell aplasia and responded instead to pentostatin (see below). Cyclosporin A needs continuous long-term maintenance treatment because there is always persistence of T-cell large granular lymphocytes despite clinical improvement (31–33).

Cytotoxic agents like cyclophosphamide and pentostatin (14,34,35) may induce good remissions, including reduction of bone marrow infiltration in some patients, and this may allow discontinuation of therapy. One of our patients (patient 2, Table 17.1) with red cell aplasia did not respond to splenectomy, prednisolone, erythropoietin, and cyclosporin A and achieved a good partial response with pentostatin (given at 4mg/m² every week for a total of ten injections) that lasted 8 years. A recent relapse was treated successfully with CHOP (cyclophosphamide, Oncovin, and prednisolone plus doxorubicin). Bone marrow tests were not done, thus we could not qualify the responses as complete responses (CRs). Patient 4, with atypical immunophenotype experienced three complete remissions over a 2-year period with pentostatin as single agent (Table 17.1).

A bone marrow complete remission was achieved in patient 1 (Table 17.1) with oral cyclophosphamide, 150 mg 3 times a week given for 10 months. Initially, granulocyte colony-stimulating factor was required to prevent accentuated neutropenia. This patient did respond minimally to pentostatin. The response continues unmaintained for 6 years.

Table 17.1 illustrates that the various treatment modalities useful in T-cell large granular lymphocytic leukemia are not always successful in every patient, and it is often necessary to try successive modalities until a response is obtained. Patient 3 (Table 17.1) best illustrates this problem. Having failed intensive chemotherapy given elsewhere on the basis of heavy bone marrow infiltration with T-cells, described initially as consistent with T-cell lymphoma, he responded twice to Campath-1H (Alemtuzumab) (to achieve nodular partial response), and this allowed harvest of sufficient peripheral blood stem cells for an autologous transplant. This was carried out using high-dose cyclophosphamide and total-body irradiation. Two months after the procedure, he remained profoundly neutropenic and with persistent interstitial bone marrow infiltration with CD8+ lymphocytes. He subsequently improved with prednisolone and cyclosporin A, which corrected the neutropenia. After 14 months, cyclosporin A was discontinued due to hypertension and rising creatinine. He continues to do well on oral methotrexate, 10 mg/m²/week, with normal neutrophils but still a moderate CD8+ lymphocytosis and the same moderate degree of bone marrow infiltration 2.5 years since the high-dose treatment and the autograft. The lack of response to intensive chemotherapy is a well-known feature of T-cell large granular lymphocytic leukemia, which may have its basis in findings by Lamy and Loughran (11) of high levels of P glycoprotein, the product of the multidrug-resistant gene.

The role of corticosteroids is uncertain, and they seem unlikely to improve given as single agent, but they may be useful as part of the initial treatment with methotrexate and cyclophosphamide. Growth factors are often useful as well (Table 17.1), but to facilitate more definitive therapy; granulocyte colony-stimulating factor alone did not correct the neutropenia in several patients. Similarly, erythropoietin may be a good adjuvant to therapy, but patients with red cell aplasia (such as patient 2) are unlikely to benefit.

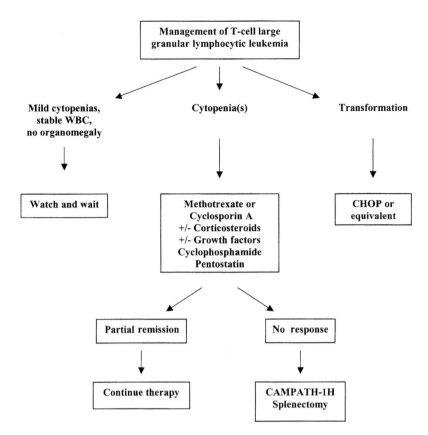

FIG. 17.2. Flow chart summarizing the management of large granular lymphocyte leukemia. CHOP, cyclophosphamide, Oncovin and prednisolone plus doxorubicin; WBC, white blood cell count.

In summary, on current evidence, the simple approach to treatment in T-cell large granular lymphocytic leukemia is to start with methotrexate with or without prednisolone; failing that, cyclosporin A may be the next option. Unfortunately, both therapies are required long term. Conversely, attempts to induce remissions with pentostatin (which is only mildly myelotoxic) and with cyclophosphamide with or without prednisolone may be justified in some patients and may induce durable unmaintained remissions. There is little information on the effect of Campath-1H and of other nucleoside analogs such as cladribine (36) in the treatment of T-cell large granular lymphocytic leukemia. A flow chart summarizing the management of large granular lymphocyte leukemia is shown in Figure 17.2.

Future Directions

T-cell large granular lymphocyte leukemia is a disease with an indolent clinical course. There is so far no effective therapy that achieves complete remission and can eradicate the disease. Future strategies should focus on blocking the release or production of cytokines by the clonal lymphocytes responsible for the cytopenias.

T-CELL PROLYMPHOCYTIC LEUKEMIA

Definition

T-cell prolymphocytic leukemia is an aggressive disorder characterized by the proliferation of small to medium-sized lymphocytes with a mature T-cell phenotype. The disease was first described in 1973 in a patient with prolymphocytic leukemia in whom the circulating cells were shown to be T lymphocytes by the formation of rosettes with sheep erythrocytes (37). The morphologic features, the recognition of a small cell variant and the cytogenetics were subsequently reported in the 1980s (38), and in the early 1990s, the clinical and laboratory features were documented enabling researchers to establish T-cell prolymphocytic leukemia as a distinct entity (39). T-cell prolymphocytic leukemia is now recognized as a disease entity in the WHO classification of lymphoid and hemopoietic tumors (40). Other designations used in the past to describe this condition are *"knobby-type" T-cell leukemia* and *T-cell chronic lymphocytic leukemia.*

Epidemiology, Frequency, and Etiology

Epidemiologic information on the disease is scanty. T-cell prolymphocytic leukemia has been described in Western and Eastern countries, including Japan and China (Hong Kong), the Caribbean, and South America (41). Although this form of leukemia is more common than B-cell prolymphocytic leukemia, both diseases are rare and account for 2% of leukemias of mature lymphocytes. There is no evidence that environmental factors play a role in its development, and a familial clustering has not been described. However, there is a higher prevalence of T-cell prolymphocytic leukemia in patients with ataxia telangiectasia in whom the disease has been described at a lower age of onset (42). Abnormalities of the ataxia telangiectasia mutated

(ATM) gene localized at 11q23 have been documented by molecular analysis in the sporadic form of T-cell prolymphocytic leukemia (43,44). This suggests that the ATM gene plays a role in disease initiation; however, an increased risk for developing T-cell prolymphocytic leukemia in those heterozygous for the ATM gene has not been demonstrated (43).

Diagnosis

The diagnosis of T-cell prolymphocytic leukemia is best achieved by the integration of morphology, immunophenotype, and genetic features with the greatest specificity provided by genotypic findings. However, the initial consideration of a diagnosis of T-cell prolymphocytic leukemia generally begins with the morphologic review of a blood film. Prototypic features of this leukemia include moderate to striking leukocytosis with variable anemia and thrombocytopenia (39,40). Although a spectrum of morphologic features has been described, most cases are characterized by small to intermediate-sized lymphocytes exhibiting regular or irregular nuclear outline, clumped chromatin, and generally distinct nucleoli (Color Plates 19 and 20). Cytoplasm is scant to moderate, agranular, and basophilic; blebbing/cytoplasmic protrusions are common (39,40,45). A minority of cases demonstrate morphologic features that overlap with B-cell prolymphocytic leukemia, chronic lymphocytic leukemia, Sézary syndrome, or even adult T-cell leukemia/lymphoma (46,47). The pattern of bone marrow infiltrates is diffuse (Color Plate 21) and often shows increased reticulin fibers, whereas lymph node sections show paracortical expansion by T-prolymphocytes with positivity for CD3 (Color Plate 22).

Flow cytometry immunophenotyping provides critical diagnostic information by confirming the mature T-cell nature of this disorder. The leukemic cells express pan T-cell antigens such as CD2, CD5, CD7, and CD3; membrane expression of CD3 may be weak or rarely negative (15,39,40). Immature markers such as CD34, TdT, and CD1a are negative, and most patients are also CD25 and HLA-DR negative (39,45,46). Experience with 150 patients tested by our group shows that T-cell prolymphocytic leukemia typically exhibits a CD4+/CD8− helper T-cell phenotype in 63% of patients; 23% demonstrate CD4, CD8 coexpression, which is a distinctive feature of the disease; 13% of patients are CD4−, CD8+, and 1% are negative for CD4 and CD8 (15,39,40).

Two morphologic variants of T-cell prolymphocytic leukemia have been recognized (40): the small-cell variant (approximately 20% of patients), in which the nucleoli may not be readily visible by light microscopy (38), and the cerebriform variant (5% of patients), in which the cells exhibit a morphology resembling Sézary cells (47).

Pathogenesis

T-cell prolymphocytic leukemia has distinct chromosome abnormalities. Studies in a large series show that 90% of patients have inv(14)(q11q32), and other translocations such as t(14;14)(q11;q32) are occasionally noted (39,40,48–50). Abnormalities of chromosome 8 are also very common (80% of cases) and include idic(8)p11, tri(8)q, and t(8;8)(p11-12;q12) (50). In addition, del(12)p13 is also commonly found by fluorescent in situ hybridization studies (51). Likewise, recent studies also describe del(13)q14.3 in some cases of T-cell prolymphocytic leukemia (52). As predicted by the phenotype, a clonal T-cell receptor gene rearrangement is documented by standard molecular techniques.

Either translocation or inversion involving the TCL1 (T-cell leukemia 1) locus at chromosome 14q32.1 results in activation of TCL1 due to rearrangements with the regulatory elements of T-cell receptor genes at 14q11, and this is the likely causal event in the pathogenesis of T-cell prolymphocytic leukemia (53,54). Four genes are present at the TCL1 locus, including TCL1, TCL1b, TNG1, and TNG2. Other less frequent translocations in T-cell prolymphocytic leukemia involve Xq28, the MTCP1 (mature T-cell proliferation) locus (50). Activation of either TCL1 or MTCP1 results in overexpression of either $p14^{TCL1}$ or $p13^{MTCP1}$, respectively, which share structural homology (53). Transgenic mice experiments with TCL1 and MTCP1 result in a T-cell leukemia after 15 months incubation but with a CD8+ CD4− phenotype (55,56).

In addition, other molecular genetic events likely to play a role in the pathogenesis and progression of T-cell prolymphocytic leukemia include the inactivation of the tumor suppressor gene ATM at 11q22-23. Indeed, ataxia telangiectasia patients often develop a variably indolent T-cell prolymphocytic leukemia-like picture (42,49), and knockout mice with an ataxia telangiectasia phenotype develop T-cell malignancies (57). T-cell prolymphocytic leukemia is the first sporadic cancer in which missense mutations in the ATM gene have been demonstrated (43,44). Other candidate tumor suppressor genes at 13q14.3 may also play a role in the pathogenesis of this disorder (53).

The postulated cell of origin in T-cell prolymphocytic leukemia is a mature (postthymic) T lymphocyte. The distinctive CD4, CD8 coexpression in conjunction with weak CD3 membrane expression suggests an intermediate stage of differentiation between the cortical thymocyte stage and a circulating mature T lymphocyte.

Clinical and Laboratory Features

T-cell prolymphocytic leukemia affects adults in the middle 60s and is slightly more frequent in males. In the series investigated at the Royal Marsden Hospital, the median age was 63 years and the male to female ratio was 1:3. The majority of patients are symptomatic at diagnosis and present with widespread disease. Main symptoms are abdominal distension often resulting from splenomegaly, bulky nodes, skin rash, and, less often, anemia or bleeding; initial manifestations such as a blurred vision due to infiltration of the retina by prolymphocytes are unusual, but we have seen this in two patients. A small number of patients, approximately 10%, are asymptomatic, and the diagnosis is made on a routine check-up that shows a low level of lymphocytosis. This group might be considered as a form of smoldering T-cell prolymphocytic leukemia (45), but, almost invariably, the disease progresses in terms of months or, more rarely, years.

Physical examination shows splenomegaly in more than two-thirds of the patients, hepatomegaly and lymphadenopathy in approximately half, and skin lesions in close to one-third of them. The latter are manifested as a localized or generalized maculopapular rash, nodules, and, more rarely, erythroderma similar to that seen in Sézary syndrome (58). Other less common signs at diagnosis are pleural or pericardial effusions and ascites, but these features are not rare in the relapse phase or during disease progression. Central nervous system involvement manifested by meningeal disease with the presence of prolymphocytes in the central spinal fluid or brain deposits is rare.

Peripheral blood counts show an elevated white blood cell count with values ranging between 10 and $1,000 \times 10^9$ per L, and more than 50% of patients have presenting counts greater than 100×10^9 per L. A normochromic normocytic anemia or thrombocytopenia is present in 25% and 45% of patients, respectively. Cytopenias usually result from a combination of bone marrow infiltration and a degree of hypersplenism. Renal and liver biochemistry may be normal or show a mild impairment, and the serum urate and lactate dehydrogenase levels are often raised. Serum immunoglobulins are, as a rule, normal. Serology for the human T-cell leukemia/lymphoma viruses types I and II is consistently negative, including patients of Japanese or Afro-Caribbean descent (39). The lack of involvement of these retroviruses in T-cell prolymphocytic leukemia has been confirmed by DNA analysis using a PCR with primers specific for the whole set of the human T-cell leukemia viruses types I and II (7).

Prognostic Factors

Information is scanty regarding the variables that may have an influence on survival or the response to therapy. Hepatomegaly seemed to be a strong predictor for survival in our original series (39) and a predictor for response to therapy with Campath-1H (59), whereas immunophenotype or molecular genetics do not appear to influence survival or response to therapy (34,59). In addition, response to therapy with either pentostatin or Campath-1H is a predictor for disease-free and overall survival (34,59). Thus, the median survival of the complete remitters with Campath-1H is close to 2 years, whereas in the partial responders it is 9 months (60).

Treatment

In the series of 78 cases reported in 1991 (39), the majority of patients were treated with alkylating agents, CHOP, and/or with the adenosine deaminase inhibitor pentostatin, but results were disappointing. Most patients did not respond to alkylating agents, and one-third experienced short-lived responses to CHOP. Pentostatin resulted in a higher response rate (45%), with few patients achieving a complete remission (39). The efficacy of pentostatin was further confirmed in a subsequent study that included 55 patients (34). These responses, however, were short lived. There is little information on the effect of other nucleoside analogs, such as cladribine and fludarabine, in T-cell prolymphocytic leukemia, but we have seen occasional response with the former.

Currently the best treatment for T-cell prolymphocytic leukemia is the monoclonal antibody Campath-1H. A recent update of our early results (59) shows that the complete remission rate is 63% in 44 patients, the highest with any single agent in this disease (60). The majority of patients treated with Campath-1H were previously treated and were resistant or had relapsed after first-line treatment with pentostatin (2-deoxycoformycin) or other agents. A strong case has been made for the use of Campath as first-line treatment (59–61): five patients in our series treated with this antibody as first-line treatment all achieved a complete response with 6 to 8 weeks of therapy (60).

Campath-1H is a humanized monoclonal antibody against the CD52 antigen, widely expressed in normal and neoplastic lymphocytes. The excellent results in T-cell prolymphocytic leukemia, better than in chronic lymphocytic leukemia and any other condition in which this reagent has been used, may relate to the high density of CD52 expression in the T prolymphocytes (62). The standard regimen is to start with 5 mg IV and increase daily to reach 30 mg, and this dose is given 3 times a week for 6 to 8 weeks, or longer if required, to clear the blood, bone marrow, and other tissues. Another series of T-cell prolymphocytic leukemia treated in a compassionate program (which included 18 of our patients) reported a 51% overall response rate with a 39% complete remission. Median duration of responses was 8.7 months with a median time to progression of 4.5 months (61). The main side effect of Campath-1H is immune suppression leading to opportunistic infections; the cytokine release syndrome can be well controlled with symptomatic treatment. Weekly monitoring of cytomegalovirus is recommended during this therapy because viral reactivation is not uncommon.

The disease course of T-cell prolymphocytic leukemia may be complicated with opportunistic infections and central nervous system involvement or effusions at the time of relapse.

Prognosis and Median Survival and Transformation

T-prolymphocytic leukemia has a poor prognosis. The median survival for patients treated with conventional therapy was 7 months (39). In 10% of T-cell prolymphocytic leukemia patients, the disease course may be initially stable or slowly progressive, but all patients finally show frank progression. The higher response rate with Campath-1H has not yet resulted in a survival benefit as shown in the updated survival of 45 patients treated with this antibody. Therefore, it is unlikely that Campath-1H will result in a cure for T-cell prolymphocytic leukemia. The median disease-free interval in our series was 10 months (60), and median survival from the start of therapy is 16 months for responders and 4 months for nonresponders.

Transformation into a large-cell lymphoma has not been reported in T-cell prolymphocytic leukemia. However, we have observed a patient who, after a 4-year remission with Campath-1H, relapsed with circulating blastoid cells and a rapid downward course suggestive of transformation. This was associated with immunophenotypic changes and down-regulation of CD52 (the Campath antigen). The blast cells were shown by cytogenetic analysis to correspond to the same clone as the original prolymphocytes (63). Another patient whose cells became CD52-negative after Campath-1H therapy did not respond any longer to the antibody (63). The downregulation of CD52 appears to be increasingly recognized as a mechanism of resistance to Campath-1H (64).

Future Directions

Despite the high complete remission rate to Campath-1H, ultimately all patients relapse, and thus new strategies are needed to consolidate responses. Preliminary data suggest a benefit from high-dose chemotherapy followed by an autologous transplantation or allogeneic transplant (or both) in patients younger than 65 years. The fact that it is possible to clear the bone marrow and produce remissions undetected by flow cytometry or PCR for the T-cell receptor suggests that the next step is to use this good complete remission as a first step for attempts at high-dose therapy with stem cell rescue. Because stem cells do not express CD52, it is possible to collect adequate numbers of CD34 cells after remission. We have observed nine patients with autografts and four others with allogeneic transplants; as of this writing, six of them remain alive up to 40 months after stem cell transplants, with a median survival post transplant of 18 months (61). Relapses still occur, but this strategy seems to prolong survival and disease-free interval in this aggressive form of T-cell leukemia.

Another attractive strategy in patients with an HLA-identical sibling and residual disease after Campath-1H is allogeneic transplant with nonmyeloablative conditioning with or without donor lymphocyte infusion according to the remaining recipient hematopoiesis or residual disease.

AGGRESSIVE NATURAL KILLER–CELL LEUKEMIA/LYMPHOMA

Definition

The natural killer–cell leukemias and lymphomas encompass a variety of neoplasms that arise from cells committed to the natural killer–cell lineage. They are considered in the WHO classification under the designations of *blastic natural killer lymphomas* and *aggressive natural killer leukemias* (65,66). There is overlap between natural killer–cell leukemias and lymphomas based on not only immunophenotype and the origin of the neoplastic cell, but also clinical features and disease course. The rare group of large granular lymphocytic leukemias with a natural killer phenotype is included within the aggressive natural killer–cell leukemias despite the fact that some patients have a benign and chronic clinical course (65). Furthermore, other neoplasms arising from natural killer–cells are considered in the WHO classification within distinct subgroups of lymphomas, such as nasal/angiocentric lymphoma (67). Indeed, it has been suggested that aggressive natural killer–cell leukemia may be the leukemic counterpart of the nasal-type natural killer/T-cell lymphoma. In this chapter we only discuss the aggressive natural killer–cell leukemias as per the WHO proposal (65).

Frequency, Epidemiology, and Etiology

The overall frequency of natural killer–cell leukemias is rare, but they are significantly more common in Eastern countries, where most of the cases have been reported. This geographic distribution suggests that a genetic background plays a role in disease development. In addition, the EBV has been shown to be the primary etiologic agent in a few patients (68–71); in some of these cases EBV has been shown to be integrated in a clonal (episomal) fashion. This disease affects adults almost exclusively and is extremely rare in childhood (65,71,72). There is no sex predominance, but it may be or it is slightly more common in males.

Diagnosis

Disorders of true natural killer–cells are uniquely problematic in hematopathologic diagnosis for a variety of reasons. First, natural killer–cells were originally defined and identified by functional properties; the transition to morphology/immunophenotype-based diagnostic definitions has been particularly challenging because neither morphology nor phenotype is specific for natural killer–cell disorders (72). For example, expression of CD56 (N-CAM) is the prototypic immunophenotypic "marker" for the natural killer–cell lineage (67). However, CD56 is also expressed on a variety of potential "look-alike" hematolymphoid disorders, including acute myeloid leukemias (especially monocytic/monoblastic), lymphoblastic lymphomas, various cytotoxic T-cell neoplasms, and the recently described CD4+, CD56+ dendritic cell malignancies (73–79). As both immunophenotype and morphology lack specificity, it is reasonable to presume that some cases originally classified as natural killer–cell neoplasms actually may be derived from other lineages (80). Further progress in subclassification is likely as techniques to define specific lineages improve.

Despite these caveats, sufficient evidence has been mounted to define rare subtypes of true natural killer–cell disorders. Aggressive natural killer–cell leukemias/lymphomas are natural killer–cell–derived neoplasms comprised of cells that retain many morphologic and immunophenotypic similarities to normal circulating large granular lymphocytes (65,81,82). The cells are medium to large and have abundant cytoplasm that contains distinct granules; nuclei are generally round to somewhat irregular with condensed chromatin. In some cases, greater cytologic atypia, immaturity, and larger cell size are evident (68,81) (Color Plate 23). Bone marrow infiltrates are variable and range from subtle to diffuse (Color Plate 24), with individual cell necrosis and apoptosis; hemophagocytosis by benign histiocytes may also be noted (65,79). Widespread disease is common, and interstitial leukemic infiltrates may be identified in many organs (Color Plate 25). The immunophenotypic profile of these systemic infiltrates is virtually identical to the extranodal nasal-type natural killer–cell lymphoma with expression of CD56, CD2, CD3ε (by immunoperoxidase with a polyclonal antibody) (Color Plate 26), TIA-1 (Color Plate 27), and granzyme. By *in situ* hybridization, EBV RNA can be detected (65,68,69) in the majority of patients (Color Plate 28). Based on both morphologic and immunophenotypic features, it is likely that this disorder may represent the leukemic phase of nasal type natural killer–cell lymphoma (67,68,83,84). T-cell receptor genes are unrearranged (germline).

Pathogenesis

Distinct chromosomal abnormalities have not been demonstrated and, thus, a specific gene involved in the pathogenesis (infiltration or progression) of this disease has not been identified. In contrast, the pathogenic role of EBV is strongly suggested in light of the consistent EBV-encoded small RNA positivity in the leukemia cells (65,68,69). A more aggressive disease course may also be linked to underlying immunosuppression.

Clinical Features

Systemic symptoms, such as fever and weight loss, multiorgan failure, and marked organomegaly, are common features at presentation. Skin lesions may be present in one-third to one-half of the patients, and in some patients, these lesions may precede the systemic manifestations. A few cases manifest with or develop extranodal involvement, such as pleural effusion, and in others the disease evolves with a hemophagocytic syndrome with profound pancytopenia (65,70,82). The latter may present diagnostic problems with a viral infection. Fever is a common symptom at presentation. Central nervous system involvement has been documented in a few patients during the disease course. Physical examination shows marked hepatosplenomegaly in the majority of cases, and in approximately half, lymphadenopathy. Anemia and thrombocytopenia and the presence of abnormal blood circulating cells are frequent findings. Biochemistry shows abnormal liver function tests and raised urate and lactate dehydrogenase in the majority of patients. A few patients may have a coagulopathy, particularly those with a rapid downhill course.

Therapy

There is little information about useful treatment modalities in this condition. Loughran (14) reported 11 cases with natural killer–cell leukemia, and nine died within 2 months from diagnosis. Loughran commented that combination chemotherapy was ineffective probably as a consequence of drug resistance caused by the multidrug resistance phenotype.

We have treated a man who presented with fever, pancytopenia, splenomegaly, and lactate dehydrogenase values above 3,000 U/L. His cells were morphologically large granular lymphocytes, and the markers were fairly typical of natural killer–cells. He had clinical improvement after splenectomy and minimal response to cyclosporin A. He continued to be managed with cyclosporin A and erythropoietin, and he remains clinically stable 2.5 years from diagnosis. His response to various therapies is summarized in Table 17.1 (patient 6) for comparison with cases of T-cell large granular lymphocytic leukemia. A flow chart summarizing the management of natural killer–cell leukemia is shown in Figure 17.3.

Survival

Natural killer–cell leukemia has a poor prognosis in most patients. The clinical course is aggressive and, as a rule, the disease is refractory to systemic chemotherapy; some patients die before starting chemotherapy from multiorgan failure. Survival ranges from weeks to a few months with only a few patients surviving more than 1 or 2 years (11,65,70,71,82,85).

Future Directions

Because this condition is rare, it will take some time to collect useful information on therapeutic options. The fact that the disease is recognized in the WHO classification (65) will facilitate case reporting and the description of treatment modalities that may change the extremely poor prognosis.

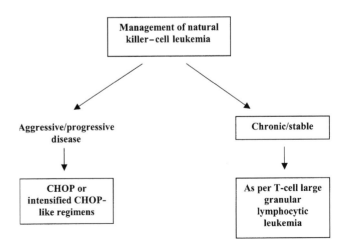

FIG. 17.3. Flow chart summarizing the management of natural killer–cell leukemia. CHOP, cyclophosphamine, hydroxydaunomycin, Oncovin (vincristine) and prednisone.

The role of monoclonal antibody therapy, such as anti-CD56, has not yet been considered.

REFERENCES

1. McKenna RW, Parkin J, Kersey JH, et al. Chronic lymphoproliferative disorder with unusual clinical, morphologic, ultrastructural and membrane surface marker characteristics. *Am J Med* 1977;62:588–596.
2. Newland AC, Catovsky D, Linch D, et al. Chronic T cell lymphocytosis: a review of 21 cases. *Br J Haematol* 1984;58:433–446.
3. Brouet JC, Sasportes M, Flandrin G, et al. Chronic lymphocytic leukaemia of T-cell origin. Immunological and clinical evaluation in eleven patients. *Lancet* 1975;2:890–893.
4. Loughran TP Jr, Kadin ME, Starkebaum G, et al. Leukemia of large granular lymphocytes: association with clonal chromosomal abnormalities and autoimmune neutropenia, thrombocytopenia, and hemolytic anemia. *Ann Intern Med* 1985;102:169–175.
5. Chan WC, Catovsky D, Foucar K, et al. T-cell large granular lymphocyte leukaemia. In: Jaffe ES, Harris NL, Stein H, et al., eds. *WHO classification of tumours: Tumours of haematopoietic and lymphoid tissues.* Lyon, France: IARC Press, 2001:197–198.
6. Loughran TP Jr, Sherman MP, Ruscetti FW, et al. Prototypical HTLV-I/II infection is rare in LGL leukemia. *Leuk Res* 1994;18:423–429.
7. Pawson R, Schulz TF, Matutes E, et al. The human T-cell lymphotropic viruses types I/II are not involved in T prolymphocytic leukemia and large granular lymphocytic leukemia. *Leukemia* 1997;11:1305–1311.
8. Wallis WJ, Loughran TP, Kadin ME, et al. Polyarthritis and neutropenia associated with circulating large granular lymphocytes. *Ann Intern Med* 1985;103:357–362.
9. Loughran TP Jr, Starkebaum G, Kidd P, et al. Clonal proliferation of large granular lymphocytes in rheumatoid arthritis. *Arthritis Rheum* 1988;31:31–36.
10. Starkebaum G, Loughran TP Jr, Gaur LK, et al. Immunogenetic similarities between patients with Felty's syndrome and those with clonal expansions of large granular lymphocytes in rheumatoid arthritis. *Arthritis Rheum* 1997;40:624–626.
11. Lamy T, Loughran TP Jr. Current concepts: large granular lymphocyte leukemia. *Blood Rev* 1999;13:230–240.
12. Semenzato G, Zambello R, Starkebaum G, et al. The lymphoproliferative disease of granular lymphocytes: updated criteria for diagnosis. *Blood* 1997;89:256–260.
13. Evans HL, Burks E, Viswanatha D, et al. Utility of immunohistochemistry in bone marrow evaluation of T-lineage large granular lymphocyte leukemia. *Hum Pathol* 2000;31:1266–1273.
14. Loughran TP Jr. Clonal diseases of large granular lymphocytes. *Blood* 1993;82:1–14.
15. Bartlett NL, Longo DL. T-small lymphocyte disorders. *Semin Hematol* 1999;36:164–170.
16. Kingreen D, Siegert W. Chronic lymphatic leukemias of T and NK cell type. *Leukemia* 1997;11(Suppl 2):S46–S49.
17. Foucar K. *Chronic lymphoproliferative disorders. Bone marrow pathology.* Chicago: ASCP Press, 2001:366–405.
18. Morice WG, Kurtin PJ, Tefferi A, et al. Distinct bone marrow findings in T-cell granular lymphocytic leukemia revealed by paraffin section immunoperoxidase stains for CD8, TIA-1, and granzyme B. *Blood* 2002;99:268–274.
19. Wong KF, Chan JCW, Liu HSY, et al. Chromosomal abnormalities in T-cell large granular lymphocyte leukaemia: report of two cases and review of the literature. *Br J Haematol* 2002;116:598–600.
20. Perzova R, Loughran TP Jr. Constitutive expression of Fas ligand in large granular lymphocyte leukaemia. *Br J Haematol* 1997;97:123–126.
21. Handgretinger R, Geiselhart A, Moris A, et al. Pure red-cell aplasia associated with clonal expansion of granular lymphocytes expressing killer-cell inhibitory receptors. *N Engl J Med* 1999;340:278–284.
22. Hoffman R, Kopel S, Hsu SD, et al. T cell chronic lymphocytic leukemia: presence in bone marrow and peripheral blood of cells that suppress erythropoiesis in vitro. *Blood* 1978;52:255–260.
23. Melenhorst JJ, Sorbara L, Kirby M, et al. Large granular lymphocyte leukaemia is characterized by a clonal T-cell receptor rearrangement

24. in both memory and effector CD8+ lymphocyte populations. *Br J Haematol* 2001;112:189–194.
24. Oshimi K, Yamada O, Kaneko T, et al. Laboratory findings and clinical courses of 33 patients with granular lymphocyte-proliferative disorders. *Leukemia* 1993;7:782–788.
25. Pandolfi F, Loughran TP Jr, Starkebaum G, et al. Clinical course and prognosis of the lymphoproliferative disease of granular lymphocytes. A multicenter study. *Cancer* 1990;65:341–348.
26. Dhodapkar MV, Li CY, Lust JA. Clinical spectrum of clonal proliferations of T-large granular lymphocytes: a T-cell clonopathy of undetermined significance? *Blood* 1994;84:620–627.
27. Gentile TC, Uner AH, Hutchison RE, et al. CD3+, CD56+ aggressive variant of large granular lymphocyte leukemia. *Blood* 1994;84:2315–2321.
28. Nowell P, Finan J, Glover D, et al. Cytogenetic evidence for the clonal nature of Richter's syndrome. *Blood* 1981;58:183–186.
29. Matutes E, Wotherspoon AC, Parker NE, et al. Transformation of T-cell large granular lymphocyte leukaemia into a high-grade large T-cell lymphoma. *Br J Haematol* 2001;115:801–806.
30. Loughran TP Jr, Kidd PG, Starkebaum G. Treatment of large granular lymphocyte leukemia with oral low-dose methotrexate. *Blood* 1994;84:2164–2170.
31. Sood R, Stewart CC, Aplan PD, et al. Neutropenia associated with T-cell large granular lymphocyte leukemia: long-term response to cyclosporine therapy despite persistence of abnormal cells. *Blood* 1998;91:3372–3378.
32. Brinkman K, van Dongen JJ, van Lom K, et al. Induction of clinical remission in T-large granular lymphocyte leukemia with cyclosporin A, monitored by use of immunophenotyping with Vbeta antibodies. *Leukemia* 1998;12:150–154.
33. Tura S, Finelli C, Bandini G, et al. Cyclosporin A in the treatment of CLL associated PRCA and bone marrow hypoplasia. *Nouv Rev Fr Hematol* 1988;30:479–481.
34. Mercieca J, Matutes E, Dearden C, et al. The role of pentostatin in the treatment of T-cell malignancies: analysis of response rate in 145 patients according to disease subtype. *J Clin Oncol* 1994;12:2588–2593.
35. Granjo E, Lima M, Correia T. CD8+/Vβ5.1+ large granular lymphocyte leukemia associated with autoimmune cytopenias, rheumatoid arthritis and vascular mammary skin lesions: successful response to 2-deoxycoformycin. *Hematol Oncol* 2002;20:87–93.
36. Edelman MJ, O'Donnell RT, Meadows I. Treatment of refractory large granular lymphocytic leukemia with 2-chlorodeoxyadenosine. *Am J Hematol* 1997;54:329–331.
37. Catovsky D, Galetto J, Okos A, et al. Prolymphocytic leukaemia of B and T cell type. *Lancet* 1973;2:232–234.
38. Matutes E, Garcia-Talavera J, O'Brien M, et al. The morphological spectrum of T-prolymphocytic leukaemia. *Br J Haematol* 1986;64:111–124.
39. Matutes E, Brito-Babapulle V, Swansbury J, et al. Clinical and laboratory features of 78 cases of T-prolymphocytic leukemia. *Blood* 1991;78:3269–3274.
40. Catovsky D, Ralfkiaer E, Müller-Hermelink HK. T-cell prolymphocytic leukaemia. In: Jaffe ES, Harris NL, Stein H, et al., eds. *WHO classification of tumours: Tumours of haematopoietic and lymphoid tissues.* Lyon, France: IARC Press, 2001:195–196.
41. Matutes E, Brito-Babapulle V, Yullie MR, et al. Prolymphocytic leukemia of B and T cell types. Biology and therapy. In: Cheson BD, ed. *Chronic lymphoid leukemias*, 2nd ed. New York: Marcel Dekker, 2001:525–541.
42. Taylor AMR, Metcalfe JA, Thick J, et al. Leukemia and lymphoma in ataxia telangiectasia. *Blood* 1996;87:423–438.
43. Vorechovsky I, Luo L, Dyer MJS, et al. Clustering of missense mutations in the ataxia-telangiectasia gene in a sporadic T-cell leukemia. *Nat Genet* 1997;17:96–99.
44. Stilgenbauer S, Schaffner C, Litterst A, et al. Biallelic mutations in the ATM gene in T-prolymphocytic leukemia. *Nat Med* 1997;3:1155–1159.
45. Garand R, Goasguen J, Brizard A, et al. Indolent course as a relatively frequent presentation in T-prolymphocytic leukemia. *Br J Haematol* 1998;103:488–494.
46. Hoyer JD, Ross CW, Li CY, et al. True T-cell chronic lymphocytic leukemia: a morphologic and immunophenotypic study of 25 cases. *Blood* 1995;86:1163–1169.

47. Brito-Babapulle V, Maljaie SH, Matutes E, et al. Relationship of T leukaemias with cerebriform nuclei to T-prolymphocytic leukaemia: a cytogenetic analysis with in situ hybridization. *Br J Haematol* 1997;96:724–732.

48. Brito-Babapulle V, Pomfret M, Matutes E, et al. Cytogenetic studies on prolymphocytic leukemia. II. T-cell prolymphocytic leukemia. *Blood* 1987;70:926–931.

49. Brito-Babapulle V, Catovsky D. Inversions and tandem translocations involving chromosome 14q11 and 14q32 in T-prolymphocytic leukemia and T-cell leukemias in patients with ataxia telangiectasia. *Cancer Genet Cytogenet* 1991;55:1–9.

50. Maljaie SH, Brito-Babapulle V, Hiorns LR, et al. Abnormalities of chromosomes 8, 11, 14 and X in T-prolymphocytic leukemia studied by fluorescence in situ hybridization. *Cancer Genet Cytogenet* 1998;103:110–116.

51. Salomon-Nguyen F, Brizard F, Le Coniat M, et al. Abnormalities of the short arm of chromosome 12 in T cell prolymphocytic leukemia. *Leukemia* 1998;12:972–975.

52. Brito-Babapulle V, Baou M, Matutes E, et al. Deletions of D13S25, D13S319 and RB-1 mapping to 13q14.3 in T-cell prolymphocytic leukaemia. *Br J Haematol* 2001;114:327–332.

53. Pekarsky U, Hallas C, Croce CM. Molecular basis of mature T-cell leukemia. *JAMA* 2001;286:2308–2314.

54. Pekarsky Y, Hallas C, Isobe M, et al. Abnormalities at 14q32.1 in T cell malignancies involve two oncogenes. *Proc Natl Acad Sci U S A* 1999;96:2949–2951.

55. Virgilio L, Lazzeri C, Bichi R, et al. Deregulated expression of TCL1 causes T cell leukemia in mice. *Proc Natl Acad Sci U S A* 1998;95:3885–3889.

56. Gritti C, Dastot H, Soulier J, et al. Transgenic mice for MTCP1 develop T-cell prolymphocytic leukemia. *Blood* 1998;92:368–373.

57. Stoppa-Lyonnet D, Soulier J, Lauge A, et al. Inactivation of the ATM gene in T-cell prolymphocytic leukemia. *Blood* 1998;91:3920–3926.

58. Mallett RB, Matutes E, Catovsky D, et al. Cutaneous infiltration in T-cell prolymphocytic leukaemia. *Br J Dermatol* 1995;132:263–266.

59. Dearden CE, Matutes E, Cazin B, et al. High remission rate in T-cell prolymphocytic leukemia with CAMPATH-1H. *Blood* 2001;98:1721–1726.

60. Dearden CE, Matutes E, Cazin B, et al. Longer follow up of T-prolymphocytic leukaemia patients treated with Alemtuzumab (CAMPATH-1H) shows improved survival and higher response rates in previously untreated patients. *Blood* 2002;100:364a.

61. Keating MJ, Cazin B, Coutre S, et al. Campath-1H treatment of T-cell prolymphocytic leukemia in patients for whom at least one prior chemotherapy regimen has failed. *J Clin Oncol* 2002;20:205–213.

62. Ginaldi L, De Martinis M, Matutes E, et al. Levels of expression of CD52 in normal and leukemic B and T cells: correlation with in vivo therapeutic responses to CAMPATH-1H. *Leuk Res* 1998;22:185–191.

63. Tuset E, Matutes E, Brito-Babapulle V, et al. Immunophenotype changes and loss of CD52 expression in two patients with relapsed T-cell prolymphocytic leukaemia. *Leuk Lymphoma* 2001;42:1379–1383.

64. Birhiray R, Shaw G, Guldan S, et al. Phenotypic transformation of CD52(+) to CD52(-) leukemic T-cells as a mechanism for resistance to CAMPATH-1H. *Leukemia* 2002;16:861–864.

65. Chan JKC, Wong KF, Jaffe ES, et al. Aggressive NK-cell leukemia. In: Jaffe ES, Harris NL, Stein H, et al., eds. *WHO classification of tumours: tumours of haematopoietic and lymphoid tissues*. Lyon, France: IARC Press, 2001:198–200.

66. Chan JKC, Jaffe ES, Ralfkiaer E. Blastic NK-cell lymphoma. In: Jaffe ES, Harris NL, Stein H, et al., eds. *WHO classification of tumours: tumours of haematopoietic and lymphoid tissues*. Lyon, France: IARC Press, 2001:214–215.

67. Chan JKC, Jaffe ES, Ralfkiaer E. Extranodal NK/T-cell lymphoma, nasal type. In: Jaffe ES, Harris NL, Stein H, et al., eds. *WHO classification of tumours: tumours of haematopoietic and lymphoid tissues*. Lyon, France: IARC Press, 2001:204–207.

68. Mori N, Yamashita Y, Tsuzuki T, et al. Lymphomatous features of aggressive NK cell leukaemia/lymphoma with massive necrosis, haemophagocytosis and EB virus infection. *Histopathology* 2000;37:363–371.

69. Hart DN, Baker BW, Inglis MJ, et al. Epstein-Barr viral DNA in acute large granular lymphocyte (natural killer) leukemic cells. *Blood* 1992;79:2116–2123.

70. Chan JKC, Sin VC, Wong KF, et al. Nonnasal lymphoma expressing the natural killer cell marker CD56: a clinicopathologic study of 49 cases of an uncommon aggressive neoplasm. *Blood* 1997;89:4501–4513.

71. Ohno T, Kanoh T, Arita Y, et al. Fulminant clonal expansion of large granular lymphocytes. Characterization of their morphology, phenotype, genotype, and function. *Cancer* 1988;62:1918–1927.

72. Nakamura MC. Natural killer cells and their role in disease. *Lab Med* 2002;33:278–282.

73. Koita H, Suzumiya J, Ohshima K, et al. Lymphoblastic lymphoma expressing natural killer cell phenotype with involvement of the mediastinum and nasal cavity. *Am J Surg Pathol* 1997;21:242–248.

74. Nakamura S, Koshikawa T, Yatabe Y, et al. Lymphoblastic lymphoma expressing CD56 and TdT. *Am J Surg Pathol* 1998;22:135–167.

75. Delgado J, Morado M, Jimenez MC, et al. CD56 expression in myeloperoxidase-negative FAB M5 acute myeloid leukemia. *Am J Hematol* 2002;69:28–30.

76. Feuillard J, Jacob M-C, Valensi F, et al. Clinical and biologic features of CD4+CD56+ malignancies. *Blood* 2002;99:1556–1563.

77. Petrella T, Dalac S, Maynadie M, et al. CD4+ CD56+ cutaneous neoplasms: a distinct hematological entity? Groupe Français d'Etude des Lymphomes Cutanes (GFELC). *Am J Surg Pathol* 1999;23:137–146.

78. Leroux D, Mugneret F, Callanan M, et al. CD4+, CD56+ DC2 acute leukemia is characterized by recurrent clonal chromosomal changes affecting 6 major targets: a study of 21 cases by the Groupe Français de Cytogénétique Hématologique. *Blood* 2002;99:4154–4159.

79. Natkunam Y, Warnke RA, Zehnder JL, et al. Aggressive natural killer-like T-cell malignancy with leukemic presentation following solid organ transplantation. *Am J Clin Pathol* 1999;111:663–671.

80. Di Giuseppe JA, Louie DC, Williams JE, et al. Blastic natural killer cell leukemia/lymphoma: a clinicopathologic study. *Am J Surg Pathol* 1997;21:1223–1230.

81. Sun T, Brody J, Susin M, et al. Aggressive natural killer cell lymphoma/leukemia. A recently recognized clinicopathologic entity. *Am J Surg Pathol* 1993;17:1289–1299.

82. Imamura N, Kusunoki Y, Kawa-Ha K, et al. Aggressive natural killer cell leukaemia/lymphoma: report of four cases and review of the literature. Possible existence of a new clinical entity originating from the third lineage of lymphoid cells. *Br J Haematol* 1990;75:49–59.

83. Mori KL, Egashira M, Oshimi K. Differentiation stage of natural killer cell-lineage lymphoproliferative disorders based on phenotypic analysis. *Br J Haematol* 2001;115:225–228.

84. Soler J, Bordes R, Ortuno F, et al. Aggressive natural killer cell leukaemia/lymphoma in two patients with lethal midline granuloma. *Br J Haematol* 1994;86:659–662.

85. Ohno Y, Amakawa R, Fukuhara S, et al. Acute transformation of chronic large granular lymphocyte leukemia associated with additional chromosome abnormality. *Cancer* 1989;64:63–67.

CHAPTER 18

Human T-Cell Leukemia Virus Type I–Associated Adult T-Cell Leukemia-Lymphoma

Kensei Tobinai, Toshiki Watanabe, and Elaine S. Jaffe

DEFINITION OF THE DISEASE

Adult T-cell leukemia-lymphoma was first recognized in Japan by Takatsuki et al. in 1977 (1). It is defined as a histologically or cytologically confirmed peripheral T-cell malignancy associated with a novel retrovirus, human T-cell leukemia virus type I (HTLV-I).

Retroviruses are unique among animal viruses in having a RNA genome that replicates through a DNA intermediate. The virally encoded reverse transcriptase converts the single-stranded RNA genome into a double-stranded DNA copy, which is irreversibly integrated into a host chromosome where it resides as a provirus. Retroviruses have been classified on the basis of pathogenetic roles into *Oncovirinae* (tumor viruses), *Lentivirinae* (genetically complex agents, including human immunodeficiency virus), and *Spumavirinae* (foamy viruses, not known to be associated with human diseases). *Oncovirinae* include the mammalian type C tumor viruses, the avian leukemia/sarcoma viruses, and HTLV-I and HTLV-II. HTLV-I is the first retrovirus that was found to be closely associated with human malignant neoplasm (Table 18.1).

FREQUENCY AND EPIDEMIOLOGY

Southwestern Japan is the district with the highest prevalence of HTLV-I infection and the highest incidence of patients with adult T-cell leukemia-lymphoma in the world. A high prevalence of HTLV-I infection is also found in the Caribbean islands, tropical Africa, South America, and northern Oceania. Many patients who have been diagnosed as having adult T-cell leukemia-lymphoma in Western countries are immigrants from the West Indies and tropical Africa.

A nationwide survey of HTLV-I seroprevalence in adult populations in Japan showed the characteristic geographic variations from 0.2% in low-endemic to 13% in high-endemic areas. It is estimated that approximately 1.2 million HTLV-I–infected individuals reside in Japan, and the annual

incidence of adult T-cell leukemia-lymphoma is estimated to be approximately 700 in Japan. The annual rate of adult T-cell leukemia-lymphoma development among HTLV-I carriers older than 40 years is estimated at 1.5 per 1,000 in males and 0.5 per 1,000 in females. The cumulative risk of the development of adult T-cell leukemia-lymphoma among the HTLV-I carriers is estimated to be 2.5% during a 70-year lifespan (2).

In a national survey in Japan, the mean age of patients with adult T-cell leukemia-lymphoma was 57.6 years, and this age appears to have increased with time. It was reported that the age of patients in areas outside Japan is somewhat lower, with an overall mean age in the mid-40s. There is a marked increase in HTLV-I prevalence with age until age 70 years and an increased prevalence in females compared with males. In addition to transmission by sexual and blood-borne routes, a major reason for the increase in seroprevalence with age appears to be the decreasing prevalence of HTLV-I in the population with time. This decrease in HTLV-I carriers among younger blood donors may be explained by the improvement in sanitation and changes in lifestyle in recent years in Japan, as well as by hepatitis B virus infection rates.

POTENTIAL STRATEGIES TO ELIMINATE ADULT T-CELL LEUKEMIA-LYMPHOMA

It has been shown that HTLV-I is transmitted via at least three routes: (a) mother-to-child transmission, mainly by HTLV-I–positive lymphocytes in breast milk; (b) sexual transmission, more commonly from males to females; and (c) blood-borne transmission, including blood transfusions and sharing needles by intravenous drug abusers. The overall infection rate of HTLV-I in children by seropositive mothers has been estimated to be 10% to 30%. However, HTLV-I infection has also been reported in children who had not been breast-fed, suggesting the possibility of intrauterine or transvaginal infection.

TABLE 18.1. *Diseases associated with human T-cell leukemia virus type I (HTLV-I) infection*[a]

Diseases	Association
Childhood diseases	
Infective dermatitis	++++
Persistent lymphadenopathy	++
Infant death	+
Adult T-cell leukemia-lymphoma	+++
HTLV-I–associated myelopathy	++++
Adult diseases	
Adult T-cell leukemia-lymphoma	++++
Tropical spastic paraparesis/HTLV-I–associated myelopathy	++++
Infective dermatitis	+++
Polymyositis	++
HTLV-I uveitis	+++
HTLV-I–associated arthritis	++
Pulmonary infiltrative pneumonitis	++

++++, proven association; +++, probable association; ++, likely association; +, possible association.

[a]The strength of association is based on epidemiologic studies as well as molecular data, animal models, and intervention trials.

Partially modified from Blattner WA, Gallo RC. Epidemiology of HTLV-I and HTLV-II infection. In: Takatsuki K, ed. *Adult T-cell leukaemia.* Oxford: Oxford University Press, 1994:45, with permission.

Several kinds of intervention trials have been conducted in some HTLV-I–endemic areas in Japan. Hino and colleagues investigated the influence of breast-feeding on HTLV-I transmission in an intervention study in Nagasaki, Japan during a 12-year period (3). More than 100,000 pregnant women in the third trimester were screened for anti-HTLV-I antibody since 1987. The seropositive mothers were advised to refrain from breast-feeding. Without any intervention, the prevalence of seropositive women decreased significantly, from 8% for those born in 1945 to below 2% for those born in 1975. Among the children born to carrier mothers, 18% of those breast-fed long-term were infected with HTLV-I, in contrast to 3% of those bottle-fed ($p < .001$). Considering the trend toward a decrease in maternal prevalence, the prevalence in the pregnant women born in 1987 is estimated to be 1%. The results confirm that breast-feeding plays the major role in the mother-to-child transmission of HTLV-I. It was also suggested that the intervention program has prevented approximately 800 new infections during the 12-year study period and is expected to prevent the development of 40 cases of adult T-cell leukemia-lymphoma in the future.

To prevent HTLV-I transmission through blood transfusions, serologic screening for HTLV-I in all blood donors has been conducted in Japan since 1986. Since then, no episodes of seroconversion in transfusion recipients have been recognized.

DIAGNOSIS

Pathology

The cytologic spectrum of adult T-cell leukemia-lymphoma is extremely diverse. Nevertheless, certain cytologic features are highly characteristic and may suggest the diagnosis, even if studies for HTLV-I are not provided (4). These features are best appreciated in the peripheral blood. Most patients are leukemic at some point in the clinical course, although peripheral blood involvement may not be evident at presentation.

The neoplastic cells in the peripheral blood are markedly polylobated and have been termed *flower cells* based on the petal-like appearance of the nuclear lobes, as shown in Color Plate 29 (5,6). The chromatin is condensed and usually hyperchromatic, although the flower cells usually do not manifest prominent nucleoli. The cytoplasm is basophilic, and cytoplasmic vacuoles may be seen. The basophilia of the cytoplasm and hyperchromasia are useful features in the differential diagnosis with Sézary syndrome (7). In addition, the nuclear irregularities in Sézary cells are much subtler, imparting the typical cerebriform appearance without separation into nuclear lobes.

These cytologic features are most evident in the acute type of adult T-cell leukemia-lymphoma. In the chronic and smoldering forms of the disease, atypical cells are relatively sparse in the peripheral blood, and cytologic atypia are less evident (8,9). In addition, there are epidemiologic differences in the frequency of peripheral blood involvement. For example, a leukemic phase is less common in the Caribbean basin than in Japan (10).

Lymph node involvement is present in most patients. Lymph nodes typically show diffuse architectural effacement. In keeping with a leukemic pattern of involvement, in some instances the sinuses may be preserved or may contain neoplastic cells similar to those of the blood.

The cytologic composition of the neoplastic infiltrate is very diverse (7). Small pleomorphic lymphoid cells equivalent to the flower cells of the peripheral blood may predominate or may be admixed with larger cells. The larger cells have vesicular nuclei and usually multiple eosinophilic or basophilic nucleoli. In some instances, the large transformed cells comprise the major population, and the process may mimic a diffuse large B-cell lymphoma. Alternatively, the transformed cells may have more pleomorphic nuclear features. Giant cells with convoluted or cerebriform nuclear contours may be present. Although it is important for the pathologist to be aware of the diverse cytology that can be encountered in adult T-cell leukemia-lymphoma, the cytologic composition does not impact the clinical course (7).

Some patients with the early or smoldering type may exhibit a Hodgkin's-lymphoma–like histology in the lymph nodes (11,12). This pattern is recognized in the WHO Classification as a morphologic variant (13). Involved lymph nodes show expanded paracortical areas with diffuse infiltrates of small to medium-sized lymphocytes with mild nuclear irregularities, indistinct nucleoli, and scant cytoplasm. There are interspersed Reed-Sternberg–like cells and giant cells with lobulated or convoluted nuclei. These cells are Epstein Barr virus–positive B lymphocytes that express CD30 and CD15. This variant of incipient disease usually progresses to overt disease within months. The expansion of Epstein Barr virus–positive B cells is felt to be secondary to the underlying immunodeficiency seen in patients with adult T-cell leukemia-lymphoma. Similar Reed-Sternberg–like cells have been described in other forms of peripheral T-cell lymphoma, most commonly angioimmunoblastic T-cell lymphoma (14).

Skin involvement is seen in more than 50% of patients with the disease. The dermis usually contains a superficial atypical lymphoid infiltrate, often with epidermotropism (15). Pautrier-like abscesses are common (7). However, in contrast to Sézary syndrome/mycosis fungoides, the neoplastic infiltrate is usually monomorphic, without numerous histiocytes or eosinophils. The smaller neoplastic cells predominate in the skin, and blastic forms are uncommon. In the smoldering and chronic types, cytologic atypia may be minimal. Hyperparakeratosis is variably present in the overlying epidermis.

Bone marrow involvement is typically not prominent. The marrow may contain patchy atypical lymphoid infiltrates. However, the degree of bone marrow infiltration is less than that expected, given the very marked lymphocytosis that may be present. Correlating with the clinical finding of hypercalcemia, one often sees evidence of bone resorption and osteoclastic activity (16). Bone trabeculae may show evidence of remodeling, and in some patients, lytic bone lesions can be present, even in the absence of tumoral bone infiltration (7,17).

Other frequent sites of involvement include lung and cerebrospinal fluid. Correlating with a leukemic phase, the pulmonary infiltrates are generally patchy and interstitial, without formation of tumor nodules. Similarly, involvement of the central nervous system is manifested as meningeal infiltration without nodular parenchymal lesions.

Immunophenotype

The neoplastic cells, regardless of cytologic subtype, are CD4+ T cells that strongly express the interleukin-2 receptor (IL-2R), CD25 (4). High levels of soluble IL-2R can also be found in the serum and correlate with disease activity (18). CD7 is nearly always absent, but CD3 and other mature T-cell antigens (CD2, CD5) are usually expressed. CD30 can be expressed in the larger blastic cells. As many peripheral T-cell lymphomas have a CD3+, CD4+, CD7– immunophenotype, the most specific feature is the presence of strong CD25 positivity.

Mechanisms of Pathogenesis

The onset of adult T-cell leukemia-lymphoma is preceded by a long period of latency, frequently lasting longer than four decades. In addition, less than 5% of all infected individuals with HTLV-I develop adult T-cell leukemia-lymphoma. As the leukemogenic mechanism, the promoter insertion model was rejected, because integration sites of the provirus were random depending on the patient (19). Consequently, a transacting viral factor, Tax (20,21), was proposed to be responsible for leukemogenesis. Roles of Tax in the multistep leukemogenesis of adult T-cell leukemia-lymphoma are shown in Figure 18.1. Tax is a 40-kDa phosphoprotein mainly located in the nucleus. Tax mediates potent activation of viral transcription through interaction with three 21-bp repeats in the long terminal repeat, each containing a cyclic adenosine monophosphate (AMP) response element core flanked by 5' G-rich and 3' C-rich sequences. The cyclic AMP response elements are bound by the cellular basic domain-leucine zipper transcription factors—cyclic AMP response element binding protein (CREB) and activating transcription factor –1—which, in turn, recruit Tax into stable ternary complexes (22).

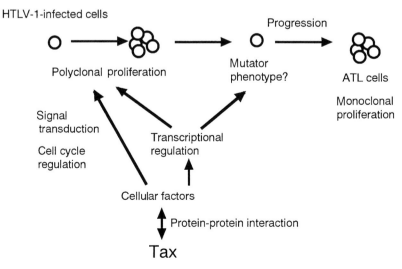

FIG. 18.1. Roles of human T-cell leukemia virus type I (HTLV-I) transactivating viral factor (Tax) in the multistep leukemogenesis of adult T-cell leukemia-lymphoma. Tax mainly exerts its biologic effects through protein–protein interaction, resulting in deregulation of transcription, cell cycle control, and signal transduction. It also impairs the cell's ability to repair DNA damage, which may lead to the mutator phenotype of the infected cells. ATL, adult T-cell leukemia.

Tax further recruits the coactivators CREB binding protein (CBP), p300, and a CBP-associated factor for potent transcriptional activation. Tax also transcriptionally regulates cellular genes by interaction with enhancer-binding proteins such as CREB (23), nuclear factor (NF)-κB (24), and serum response factor (25) and by tethering coactivators to the DNA-bound transcription factors (26,27). However, if Tax shows a low affinity with a specific transcription factor, it represses the gene expression driven by that factor through interaction competition with coactivators (28).

Among the cellular genes that are the targets of Tax, those with growth-promoting capacities are found among those transactivated, such as IL-6 (29) and lymphokine receptors such as IL-2 receptor-α (30), and oncogenes such as c-fos (31). However, those with growth-retarding functions are included among those transrepressed, such as p18INK4c (32) and Lck (33). Thus, transcriptional deregulation by Tax leads to efficient proliferation of infected cells (34).

Tax interacts with and activates specific components of growth factor signal–transduction pathways, such as IkappaB kinase (IKK)-IκB-NF-κB, Ras/mitogen-activated protein kinase (35), and protein kinases A and C (36). Interaction with IKKγ, a component of IKK complex, results in constitutive activation of this kinase complex (37). Constitutive activation of the JAK-STAT pathway in HTLV-I–transformed cells was also reported (38). Thus, HTLV-I infection results in aberrant activation of growth-promoting signaling pathways. Tax also induces cell cycle progression by inhibiting negative cell cycle regulators, such as p53, p16 and INK4A, and stimulates positive cell cycle regulators, such as cdk4/6, D-type cyclins, and E2F (39). The effects of Tax on apoptosis depend on the particular experimental system; Tax has been shown to both induce and inhibit apoptosis. Tax-induced resistance to apoptosis supports its role as a transforming factor. The oncogenic capacity of Tax was reported in various systems. However, cellular transformation by HTLV-I *in vivo* is a multistage process, and viral gene expression is absent in adult T-cell leukemia-lymphoma cells *in vivo* (40,41). Moreover, proviruses integrated in adult T-cell leukemia-lymphoma cells are frequently defective (42) or have mutations in the coding region of Tax, or both, or are methylated in the 5' region and 5' long terminal repeat (43,44). Thus, in addition to direct growth promotion, Tax should endow the infected T cells with capacities that help to progress to transformed phenotypes in the absence of Tax. In this context, induction of a mutator phenotype (45) by Tax in the infected cells appears to be important. Tax impairs the cell's ability to repair DNA damage. Tax appears to suppress base excision repair through repression of human DNA polymerase-β (46,47) and inhibit cellular nucleotide excision repair by suppression of DNA polymerase-δ activity (48). Induction of BclxL by Tax may also contribute to suppression of homologous recombination through inhibition of the RAD51 recombination pathway (49,50). Functional inactivation of p53 by Tax (51,52) allows HTLV-I–infected cells to survive and proliferate in the presence of unrepaired genomic damage. Thus, Tax not only stimulates proliferation of cells but also induces DNA damage in HTLV-I–infected cells, which may constitute a basis for multistep leukemogenesis.

Presentation, Unique Aspects of Staging, and Unusual Syndromes

Based on the nationwide survey of 854 patients with adult T-cell leukemia-lymphoma who were newly diagnosed between 1983 and 1987 in Japan, the Lymphoma Study Group proposed the diagnostic criteria of the four clinical subtypes of adult T-cell leukemia-lymphoma (5). The leukemic subtypes include the *acute type*, with a rapidly progressive clinical course and most of the characteristic features of adult T-cell leukemia-lymphoma: generalized lymphadenopathy, hepatomegaly, splenomegaly, skin involvement, hypercalcemia, and organ infiltration. The symptoms and signs include abdominal pain, diarrhea, ascites, pleural effusion, cough, sputum, and chest x-ray abnormalities. The *smoldering type* shows an indolent clinical course and only a small percentage of leukemic cells but may also include skin involvement. The *chronic type*, with a high percentage of leukemic cells, is occasionally associated with skin involvement, lymphadenopathy, and hepatosplenomegaly and also shows an indolent clinical course. The *lymphoma type* is comprised of patients who present with the manifestations of lymphoma without circulating malignant cells in the peripheral blood. When patients with adult T-cell leukemia-lymphoma are staged according to the Ann Arbor staging classification, most patients are categorized as stage intravenous, because leukemic cells are recognized even in clinically indolent forms. Therefore, in adult T-cell leukemia-lymphoma, the clinical subtype is more important than the Ann Arbor stage for predicting prognosis and deciding treatment in each patient.

Adult T-cell leukemia-lymphoma, particularly the aggressive forms (acute and lymphoma types), has been found to infiltrate the stomach in 29% and the intestine in 25% of patients at autopsy (53). Patients with adult T-cell leukemia-lymphoma experience a variety of abdominal symptoms, such as nausea, vomiting, abdominal fullness, and diarrhea, which may be attributable to the infiltration by neoplastic cells, but because of the associated immunodeficiency, various opportunistic infections, such as *Strongyloidiasis*, may complicate the course.

Hepatic involvement of neoplastic cells may be found in up to one-fourth of patients with the acute or the lymphoma type and is not infrequently manifested by jaundice and hepatic enzyme elevations. One hundred one patients with the acute type or the lymphoma type were analyzed for hepatic involvement and compared with 106 patients with non-Hodgkin's lymphoma other than adult T-cell leukemia-lymphoma (54). There was more frequent palpable hepatomegaly, and higher total bilirubin, hepatic transaminase, lactate dehydrogenase, and alkaline phosphatase values than among other non-Hodgkin's lymphoma patients ($p < .0001$). Autopsy liver samples disclosed that the portal area was most frequently infiltrated with adult T-cell leukemia-lymphoma cells.

Pulmonary complications are due to leukemic infiltration in one half of the patients and to infections with a variety of bacterial and opportunistic organisms in the other one half (55). Twenty-six percent of 854 Japanese patients with adult T-cell leukemia-lymphoma had active infections at diagnosis (5). The incidence was highest in the chronic and smoldering types (36%) and lower in the acute (27%) and lymphoma subtypes (11%). The encountered infections were bacterial (pneumonias, sepsis, and tuberculosis) in 43%, fungal in 31%, protozoal in 18%, and viral in 8% of patients with adult T-cell leukemia-lymphoma. The immunodeficiency at presentation in adult T-cell leukemia-lymphoma can be exacerbated by neutropenia produced by cytotoxic chemotherapy, leading to an extremely high risk of infection throughout therapy. Infections are responsible for the patient's death in approximately half of the cases.

Central nervous system involvement, mostly leptomeningeal involvement, occurs in approximately 10% of patients with adult T-cell leukemia-lymphoma (56). The initial symptoms include muscle weakness, altered mental status, paresthesia, headache, and urinary incontinence. Signs include nuchal rigidity and cranial nerve palsies. Hyponatremia secondary to the syndrome of inappropriate secretion of antidiuretic hormone is observed in some patients.

Laboratory Findings

Laboratory findings also depend on the clinical subtype (5). Leukocytosis is found in patients with the acute or the chronic type at presentation, exhibiting characteristic atypical lymphoid cells with marked polymorphic nuclei, so-called flower cells. Most patients with the acute or the lymphoma type have elevated serum lactate dehydrogenase levels.

The most striking laboratory finding in patients with adult T-cell leukemia-lymphoma is hypercalcemia, which was found in 32% (5). Lytic bone lesions have been described in some patients; however, examinations of bone obtained at autopsy or from bone marrow biopsies usually reveal activated osteoclasts with increased bone resorption; infiltrating

neoplastic T cells are rarely found. Patients with adult T-cell leukemia-lymphoma have low phosphates, hypercalciuria, high levels of nephrogenous cyclic AMP, and low levels of 1,25-dihydroxyvitamin D. The following factors have been suggested to have roles in the hypercalcemia: parathyroid hormone-related peptide, osteoclast-activating factor, tumor necrosis factors-α and -β, IL-1α, IL-1β, and overexpression of the receptor activator of the NF-κB ligand gene.

Prognostic Factors

In all cases of adult T-cell leukemia-lymphoma, age (40 years or older), poor performance status (greater than or equal to 2), high lactate dehydrogenase, hypercalcemia and four or more involved lesions are unfavorable prognostic factors (57,58). For patients with the chronic type, the major prognostic factors are the serum values of lactate dehydrogenase, albumin, and blood urea nitrogen. Patients with the chronic type and normal values for the three factors have a prognosis as good as those with the smoldering type and account for 30% of the patients with the chronic type. In contrast, patients with the unfavorable chronic type, having an abnormal value in at least one of the three factors, would be targets for cytotoxic chemotherapy.

TREATMENT

Patients with the favorable chronic or smoldering type should be carefully monitored for the development of infectious complications and for signs of disease progression to the acute or lymphoma type.

Most previously untreated patients with aggressive forms (acute or lymphoma type) die within weeks or months of the diagnosis without treatment. Figure 18.2 shows the survival curves of 818 patients with adult T-cell leukemia-lymphoma in Japan according to the four clinical subtypes (5). Most of the patients with the smoldering type lived well without chemotherapy for a long time. Approximately two-thirds of the chronic-type patients died within approximately 2.5 years from

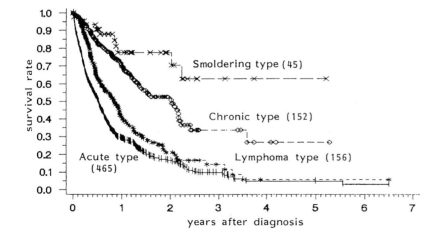

FIG. 18.2. Survival curves of 818 patients with adult T-cell leukemia-lymphoma, according to four clinical subtypes defined by the diagnostic criteria. Numbers in parentheses indicate the number of patients. [From Shimoyama M. Diagnostic criteria and classification of clinical subtypes of adult T-cell leukaemia-lymphoma. A report from the Lymphoma Study Group (1984–87). *Br J Haematol* 1991;79:428–437, with permission.]

TABLE 18.2. *Results of important clinical trials of untreated patients with adult T-cell leukemia-lymphoma*

Protocol	Drugs/regimen	No. of eligible patients	Complete-response rate (%)	Median survival time (mo)	Survival rate (%)	Reference
LSG1-VEPA	VCR, CPA, PSL, DOX	18	17 (3/18)	NA	NA	59
JCOG8101		54	28 (15/54)	7.5	8.3 (4-yr)	60, 61
LSG1-VEPA	VCR, CPA, PSL, DOX	24	17 (4/24)	NA	NA	
LSG2-VEPAM	VCR, CPA, PSL, DOX, MTX	30	37 (11/30)	NA	NA	
JCOG8701	VCR, CPA, PSL, DOX, BLM, MTX, VDS, ETP, PCZ	43	42 (18/43)	8.0	11.6 (4-yr)	62
JCOG9109	VCR, DOX, ETP, PSL, DCF	60	28 (17/60)	7.4	15.5 (2-yr)	63
JCOG9303	VCR, CPA, PSL, DOX, MCNU,VDS,ETP, CBDCA	93	35 (33/93)	13	31 (2-yr)	64
Gill et al.	IFN-α, AZT	12	25 (3/12)	4.8	NA	70

AZT, zidovudine; BLM, bleomycin; CBDCA, carboplatin; CPA, cyclophosphamide; DCF, 2'-deoxycoformycin; DOX, doxorubicin; ETP, etoposide; IFN, interferon; MCNU, nimustine; MTX, methotrexate; NA, not applicable; PCZ, procarbazine; PSL, prednisolone; VCR, vincristine; VDS, vindesine.

diagnosis. Patients with the lymphoma type had poor prognoses, with a median survival time of 10.2 months. The most aggressive type of adult T-cell leukemia-lymphoma was acute-type, with a median survival time of 6.2 months. The projected 4-year survival rates of patients with the lymphoma and acute types were only 5%. The clinical subtype clearly determines the prognosis of each patient with adult T-cell leukemia-lymphoma.

Clinical Trials by the Japan Clinical Oncology Group

Six chemotherapy trials have been consecutively conducted by the Lymphoma Study Group (LSG) of the Japan Clinical Oncology Group (JCOG) since 1978 (59–64) (Table 18.2). The first trial, LSG1 protocol (1978 to 1980), used VEPA therapy, which consisted of vincristine, cyclophosphamide, prednisolone, and Adriamycin (doxorubicin). In this study, patients with non-Hodgkin's lymphoma at an advanced stage, including adult T-cell leukemia-lymphoma, were enrolled. The complete response rate was lowest (18%) in adult T-cell leukemia-lymphoma, intermediate (36%) in peripheral T-cell lymphoma, and highest (64%) in B-cell lymphoma (59). Between 1981 and 1983, JCOG conducted a randomized phase III trial, LSG1-VEPA versus LSG2-VEPA-M (VEPA + methotrexate), for patients with advanced non-Hodgkin's lymphoma, including adult T-cell leukemia-lymphoma (60,61). The complete response rate of LSG2-VEPA-M for adult T-cell leukemia-lymphoma (37%) was higher than that of LSG1-VEPA (17%) ($p = .09$). In the LSG1/LSG2 trial, however, the complete response rate was significantly lower for adult T-cell leukemia-lymphoma than for B-cell lymphoma and peripheral T-cell lymphoma ($p < .001$). The median survival time of the 54 patients with adult T-cell leukemia-lymphoma treated with LSG1/LSG2 was 6 months, and the estimated 4-year survival rate was only 8%.

In 1987, against advanced aggressive non-Hodgkin's lymphoma, including adult T-cell leukemia-lymphoma, the JCOG initiated a phase II study (JCOG8701) of a multiagent combination chemotherapy called *LSG4*, consisting of three different regimens: (a) VEPA-B (i.e., VEPA and bleomycin), (b) M-FEPA (i.e., methotrexate, vindesine, cyclophosphamide, prednisolone, and doxorubicin), and (c) VEPP-B, (i.e., vincristine, etoposide, procarbazine, prednisolone, and bleomycin) (61). The overall complete response rate (72%) of the LSG4 protocol in aggressive non-Hodgkin's lymphoma was significantly higher than that of the LSG1/LSG2 trial (57%) ($p < .05$). The complete response rate for adult T-cell leukemia-lymphoma was improved from 28% (LSG1/LSG2) to 43% (LSG4). However, the complete response rate was significantly lower in adult T-cell leukemia-lymphoma than in B-cell lymphoma and peripheral T-cell lymphoma ($p < .01$). The patients with adult T-cell leukemia-lymphoma still showed a poor prognosis, with a median survival time of 8 months and a 4-year survival rate of 12%. However, the continued complete response rate was increased to 12% (5 of 43) compared with 4% (2 of 54) in the LSG1/LSG2 trial ($p = .13$). A multivariate analysis of the 267 eligible patients with advanced aggressive non-Hodgkin's lymphoma demonstrated that the clinical diagnosis of adult T-cell leukemia-lymphoma was the most significant unfavorable prognostic factor (relative risk, 3.185; $p = .0001$).

The disappointing results in adult T-cell leukemia-lymphoma patients treated with standard chemotherapies have led to the search for new active agents. Deoxycoformycin, which is an inhibitor of adenosine deaminase, has been shown to be effective in a number of lymphoid malignancies. Based on the promising results of some single-institution studies, multicenter phase I and II studies of deoxycoformycin were conducted against adult T-cell leukemia-lymphoma in Japan (58,65). The phase II study revealed a response rate of 32% (10 of 31) in relapsed or refractory adult T-cell leukemia-lymphoma using the weekly intravenous administration of 5 mg per m². Two patients achieved a complete response, and eight achieved a partial response. These encouraging results prompted us to conduct a deoxycoformycin-containing combination phase II trial (JCOG9109; LSG11 protocol) as the initial chemotherapy for adult T-cell leukemia-lymphoma (63). In this trial, patients with the acute, lymphoma and unfavorable chronic types were eligible. Between 1991 and 1993, 62 previously untreated patients with adult T-cell leukemia-lymphoma (34 acute, 21 lymphoma, and seven chronic types) were enrolled, but two of them were ineligible, because they were judged to be of the favorable chronic type. Vincristine, 1 mg per m² intravenous on days 1 and 8; doxorubicin, 40 mg per m² intravenous on day 1; etoposide, 100 mg per m² intravenous on days 1 to 3; prednisolone, 40 mg per m² orally on days 1 and 2; and deoxycoformycin 5 mg per m² intravenous on days 8, 15, and 22 were administered every 28 days for ten cycles unless disease progression occurred. Among the 61 patients evaluable for toxicity, four patients (7%) died of fatal infections. In the 60 eligible patients, there were 17 complete responses (28%) and 14 partial responses (overall response rate, 52%). After a median observation time of 27 months, the median survival time was 7.4 months, and the estimated 2-year survival was 17%, findings that were identical to those of the 43 patients with adult T-cell leukemia-lymphoma who were treated with the previous LSG4 protocol (JCOG8701). The prognosis of the patients with adult T-cell leukemia-lymphoma remained poor, even though they were treated with a deoxycoformycin-containing combination chemotherapy.

In 1994, JCOG initiated a new multiagent combination phase II trial (JCOG9303; LSG15 protocol), an eight-drug regimen consisting of vincristine, cyclophosphamide, doxorubicin, prednisolone, nimustine, vindesine, etoposide, and carboplatin for untreated patients with adult T-cell leukemia-lymphoma (64). In this trial, the elevation of relative dose intensity was attempted with the prophylactic use of granulocyte colony–stimulating factor. In addition, non–cross-resistant agents, such as nimustine and carboplatin, were incorporated. Ninety-six previously untreated patients with aggressive adult T-cell leukemia-lymphoma were enrolled: 58 acute type, 28 lymphoma type, and ten unfavorable chronic type. Eighty-one percent of the 93 eligible patients responded (75 of 93), with 33 patients obtaining a complete response (35%) and 42 obtaining a partial response (45%). Patients with the lymphoma type showed a better complete-response rate (67%, 18 of 27) than the the acute-type patients (20%, 11 of 56) and the unfavorable chronic-type patients (40%, 4 of 10). The overall survival of 93 eligible patients at 2 years was estimated to be 31% (Fig. 18.3). The median survival time was 13 months, and the median follow-up duration of the 20 surviving patients was 4.2 years. A trend toward better survival for lymphoma-type patients (median survival time, 20 months) compared with acute-type patients (median survival time, 11 months) was recognized (hazard ratio, 1.65). Grade 4 hematologic toxicities of neutropenia and thrombocytopenia were observed in 65% and 53% of the patients, respectively, but grade 4 nonhematologic toxicity was observed in only one patient. It was concluded that the LSG15 protocol is feasible with mild nonhematologic toxicity and improved the clinical outcome of patients with adult T-cell leukemia-lymphoma. To confirm whether the LSG15 is a new standard for the treatment of patients with aggressive adult T-cell leukemia-lymphoma, JCOG is presently conducting a randomized phase III study comparing the LSG15 with biweekly CHOP [cyclophosphamide, doxorubicin, Oncovin (vincristine), and prednisolone].

New-Agent Development for Adult T-Cell Leukemia-Lymphoma

Irinotecan hydrochloride (CPT-11) is a semisynthetic analog of camptothecin with inhibitory activity against topoisomerase I. CPT-11 has definitive activity against various kinds of solid

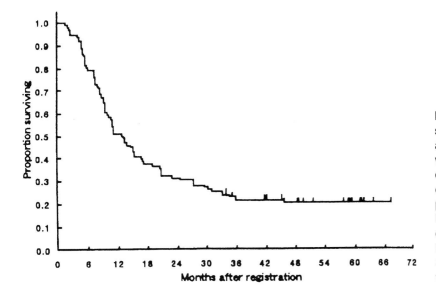

FIG. 18.3. Kaplan-Meier estimate of the overall survival for 93 eligible patients with aggressive adult T-cell leukemia-lymphoma. Overall survival was defined as the time from registration until death from any cause or until the last follow-up evaluation for patients who were still alive (20 patients). (From Yamada Y, Tomonaga M, Fukuda H, et al. A new G-CSF-supported combination chemotherapy, LSG15, for adult T-cell leukaemia-lymphoma: Japan Clinical Oncology Group Study 9303. *Br J Haematol* 2001;114:375–382, with permission.)

tumors, including colorectal cancer and lung cancer. Multicenter, early and late phase II studies of CPT-11 were conducted against relapsed or refractory non-Hodgkin's lymphoma in Japan (66,67). The study revealed nine complete responses and 17 partial responses [response rate 38% (26 of 69)], using weekly intravenous administration of 40 mg per m² per day for 3 consecutive days. Among them, five (38%) of 13 patients with adult T-cell leukemia-lymphoma showed a response to CPT-11 (one complete response and four partial responses). The major toxicities of CPT-11 were leukopenia, diarrhea, and nausea and vomiting. To develop a new effective chemotherapy regimen against non-Hodgkin's lymphoma and adult T-cell leukemia-lymphoma, we conducted two kinds of phase I/II study of CPT-11 in combination with carboplatin or etoposide for relapsed or refractory non-Hodgkin's lymphoma (68,69). However, in both studies, dose escalation was halted because of hematologic toxicity when combined with carboplatin and hepatotoxicity when combined with etoposide.

Based on the preliminary documentation of the efficacy of interferon-α against adult T-cell leukemia-lymphoma, two kinds of phase II trials of high-dose interferon-α (intravenous administration and subcutaneous administration) were conducted; however, the results were not promising. In 1995, Gill et al. in the United States reported that 11 of 19 patients with acute or lymphomatous adult T-cell leukemia-lymphoma achieved major responses (five complete responses and six partial responses) by the combination therapy of interferon-α and zidovudine (70). The therapeutic efficacy of this combination was also observed in a French study; major objective responses were obtained in all five patients with adult T-cell leukemia-lymphoma who were treated with this combination (71). However, the median survival of previously untreated patients with adult T-cell leukemia-lymphoma in the U.S. study was rather short (4.8 months) (70,72) compared with those in the JCOG studies (7 to 13 months). Furthermore, the complete response rate in previously untreated patients (25%, 3 of 12) was not superior to the complete response rates in those treated with the JCOG8701, JCOG9109 regimens, and JCOG9303 (28% to 42%). To evaluate the optimal role of this combination in the treatment of adult T-cell leukemia-lymphoma, further large-scale studies are needed.

Cladribine (2-chlorodeoxyadenosine, 2-CdA) is a chlorinated purine analog that is resistant to degradation by adenosine deaminase. Cladribine has been found to be effective against hairy-cell leukemia, B chronic lymphocytic leukemia, indolent B-cell non-Hodgkin's lymphoma, and cutaneous T-cell lymphoma. In a Japanese phase I study of cladribine, one relapsed patient with adult T-cell leukemia-lymphoma achieved a partial response (73). A multicenter phase II study of cladribine against adult T-cell leukemia-lymphoma was conducted in Japan (74). Cladribine was administered as 0.09 mg per kg per day by 7-day continuous intravenous infusion every 28 days up to three courses. However, because the interim analysis revealed that only one of the 15 eligible patients showed a partial response (overall response rate, 7%; 90% confidence interval, 0% to 28%), the phase II study was discontinued.

Because most adult T-cell leukemia-lymphoma cells express the α-chain of IL-2R (CD25), Waldmann et al. have treated patients with adult T-cell leukemia-lymphoma using monoclonal antibodies to CD25 (75). Six (32%) of 19 patients who were treated with anti-Tac showed a partial response (four) or complete response (two) lasting from 9 weeks to longer than 3 years. One of the impediments to this approach is that a quantity of soluble IL-2R is shed by the tumor cells into the circulation. The soluble IL-2R can bind to anti-Tac and inhibit binding to the tumor cell.

Another strategy using the IL-2R as a target for the treatment of adult T-cell leukemia-lymphoma is conjugation with an immunotoxin (*Pseudomonas* exotoxin) or radioisotope (90-yttrium). Anti-Tac coupled with *Pseudomonas* exotoxin, which inhibits protein synthesis, has been administered to patients with adult T-cell leukemia-lymphoma, and tumor regressions were observed in some patients. The action of immunotoxins depends on the expression of the target antigen on all malignant cells and on the cell's ability to internalize the antigen-antibody complex containing the toxin. To circumvent findings that not all malignant cells express the target antigen and not all cells internalize bound substances, radiolabeled monoclonal antibodies were developed. Waldmann et al. developed a stable conjugate of anti-Tac with 90-yttrium (76). Among the 16 patients with adult T-cell leukemia-lymphoma who received 5- to 15-mCi doses, nine (56%) showed major objective responses (two complete responses and seven partial responses). The response duration was longer than the previous results with unconjugated anti-Tac antibody. Grade 3 or greater toxicities were largely limited to hematologic toxicities. They concluded that radioimmunotherapy with 90-yttrium–labeled anti-Tac may provide a useful approach for the treatment of adult T-cell leukemia-lymphoma.

Hematopoietic Stem Cell Transplantation

The results of allogeneic hematopoietic stem cell transplantation in ten patients with adult T-cell leukemia-lymphoma were reported by Utsunomiya et al. (77). The patients tolerated well the conditioning regimens containing total-body irradiation, and engraftment occurred in all cases. Median disease-free survival after allogeneic hematopoietic stem cell transplantation was 17.5+ months (range, 3.7 to 34.4+). Six of ten patients developed acute graft-versus-host disease (one case each with grade I, III, or intravenous and three cases with grade II), and three patients developed extensive chronic graft-versus-host disease. Four patients died during the study period from either acute graft-versus-host disease (grade intravenous), pneumonitis, gastrointestinal bleeding, or renal insufficiency. Two of ten cases with no symptoms of graft-versus-host disease relapsed. These results suggest that allogeneic hematopoietic stem cell transplantation may improve the survival in adult T-cell leukemia-lymphoma if graft-versus-host disease can be controlled. In addition to the conventional allogeneic hematopoietic stem cell transplantation, a prospective, multicenter study of nonmyeloablative, allogeneic, hematopoietic stem cell transplantation against adult T-cell leukemia-lymphoma is presently being conducted in Japan.

FUTURE DIRECTIONS

Despite the consecutive clinical trials by the JCOG to develop more effective chemotherapy regimens, most patients with adult T-cell leukemia-lymphoma remain incurable with current chemotherapies. Further efforts to incorporate new innovative treatment modalities are needed, such as new anticancer agents, monoclonal antibody therapy, and allogeneic hematopoietic stem cell transplantation, including nonmyeloablative, allogeneic, hematopoietic stem cell transplantation.

Management Approach for Patients with Adult T-Cell Leukemia-Lymphoma

An algorithm summarizing management approaches for patients with adult T-cell leukemia-lymphoma is shown in Figure 18.4. When oncologists diagnose patients suspected of lymphoid malignancy, it is important to consider the possibility of adult T-cell leukemia-lymphoma at any time. Routine check for serum HTLV-I antibody is recommended at initial diagnosis. The following three points are essential for the diagnosis of adult T-cell leukemia-lymphoma: (a) cytologically or histologically proven lymphoid malignancy, (b) mature T-cell phenotype, mostly CD4+, determined by flow cytometry or immunohistochemistry, and (c) testing positive for anti–HTLV-I antibody. When a patient is diagnosed as having adult T-cell leukemia-lymphoma, it is important to make an accurate diagnosis of clinical subtype for the treatment decisions. For patients with the smoldering or chronic type, close observation is recommended. Careful monitoring for opportunistic infections, including bacterial infection, fungal infection, or *Pneumocystis carinii* infection, is also needed. For patients with the acute or lymphoma type, the serum calcium level should be checked immediately. For those complicated with hypercalcemia, prompt management, including fluid therapy, bisphosphonate, and chemotherapy, is needed. For patients with the acute or lymphoma type requiring therapy, enrollment in a clinical trial, if available, is recommended. When there is no active trial or the patient is ineligible for the trial, chemotherapy used for aggressive lymphoma should be considered. For such patients, we usually give biweekly CHOP therapy, consisting of CHOP every 2 weeks with the prophylactic use of granulocyte colony–stimulating factor and prophylactic intrathecal methotrexate. Because most patients with adult T-cell leukemia-lymphoma are not curable with current chemotherapy regimens, it is reasonable to consider the applicability of allogeneic stem cell transplantation in patients who show responses to chemotherapy. For relapsed or refractory patients, the possibility of enrollment in a new-agent trial should be considered in addition to allogeneic stem cell transplantation.

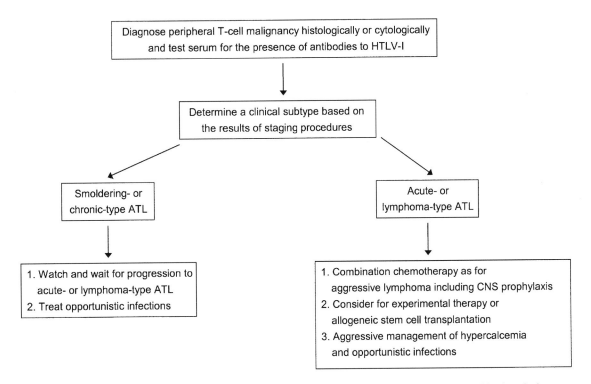

FIG. 18.4. Approach to the patient with adult T-cell leukemia-lymphoma. ATL, adult T-cell leukemia-lymphoma; CNS, central nervous system; HTLV-I, human T-cell leukemia virus type I.

REFERENCES

1. Uchiyama T, Yodoi J, Sagawa K, et al. Adult T-cell leukemia: clinical and hematologic features of 16 cases. *Blood* 1977;50:481–492.
2. Tajima K. The 4th nation-wide study of adult T-cell leukemia/lymphoma (ATL) in Japan: estimates of risk of ATL and its geographical and clinical features. The T- and B-cell Malignancy Study Group. *Int J Cancer* 1990;45:237–243.
3. Hino S. Updated results of an intervention study against the mother-to-child transmission of human T-cell leukemia virus type-I. Proceedings of the 15th International Symposium of Foundation for Promotion of Cancer Research 2002;15:43–44.
4. Levine PH, Cleghorn F, Manns A, et al. Adult T-cell leukemia/lymphoma: a working point-score classification for epidemiological studies. *Int J Cancer* 1994;59:491–493.
5. Shimoyama M. Diagnostic criteria and classification of clinical subtypes of adult T-cell leukaemia-lymphoma: a report from the Lymphoma Study Group (1984–87). *Br J Haematol* 1991;79:428–437.
6. Hanaoka M, Sasaki M, Matsumoto H, et al. Adult T cell leukemia. Histological classification and characteristics. *Acta Pathol Jpn* 1979;29:723–738.
7. Jaffe ES, Blattner WA, Blayney DW, et al. The pathologic spectrum of adult T-cell leukemia/lymphoma in the United States. *Am J Surg Pathol* 1984;8:263–275.
8. Kawano F, Yamaguchi K, Nishimura H, et al. Variation in the clinical courses of adult T-cell leukemia. *Cancer* 1985;55:851–856.
9. Yamaguchi K, Nishimura H, Kohrogi H, et al. A proposal for smoldering adult T-cell leukemia: a clinicopathologic study of five cases. *Blood* 1983;62:758–766.
10. Levine PH, Manns A, Jaffe ES, et al. The effect of ethnic differences on the pattern of HTLV-I-associated T-cell leukemia/lymphoma (HATL) in the United States. *Int J Cancer* 1994;56:177–181.
11. Ohshima K, Suzumiya J, Kato A, et al. Clonal HTLV-I-infected CD4+ T-lymphocytes and non-clonal non-HTLV-I-infected giant cells in incipient ATLL with Hodgkin-like histologic features. *Int J Cancer* 1997;72:592–598.
12. Duggan D, Ehrlich G, Davey F, et al. HTLV-I induced lymphoma mimicking Hodgkin's disease. Diagnosis by polymerase chain reaction amplification of specific HTLV-I sequences in tumor DNA. *Blood* 1988;71:1027–1032.
13. Jaffe ES, Harris NL, Stein H, et al. *Pathology and genetics of tumours of haematopoietic and lymphoid tissues. World Health Organization Classification of Tumours.* Lyon, France: IARC Press, 2001.
14. Quintanilla-Martinez L, Fend F, Moguel LR, et al. Peripheral T-cell lymphoma with Reed-Sternberg-like cells of B-cell phenotype and genotype associated with Epstein-Barr virus infection. *Am J Surg Pathol* 1999;23:1233–1240.
15. Mukai K, Sato Y, Watanabe S, et al. Non-Hodgkin lymphoma of the skin excluding mycosis fungoides and cutaneous involvement of adult T-cell leukemia/lymphoma. *J Cutan Pathol* 1988;15:193–200.
16. Yamaguchi K. Human T-lymphotropic virus type I in Japan. *Lancet* 1994;343:213–216.
17. Bunn PA Jr, Schechter GP, Jaffe E, et al. Clinical course of retrovirus-associated adult T-cell lymphoma in the United States. *N Engl J Med* 1983;309:257–264.
18. Marcon L, Rubin LA, Kurman CC, et al. Elevated serum levels of soluble Tac peptide in adult T-cell leukemia: correlation with clinical status during chemotherapy. *Ann Intern Med* 1988;109:274–279.
19. Seiki M, Eddy R, Shows TB, et al. Nonspecific integration of the HTLV provirus genome into adult T-cell leukaemia cells. *Nature* 1984;309:640–642.
20. Cann AJ, Rosenblatt JD, Wachsman W, et al. Identification of the gene responsible for human T-cell leukaemia virus transcriptional regulation. *Nature* 1985;318:571–574.
21. Sodroski JG, Rosen CA, Haseltine WA. Trans-acting transcriptional activation of the long terminal repeat of human T lymphotropic viruses in infected cells. *Science* 1984;225:381–385.
22. Wagner S, Green MR. HTLV-I Tax protein stimulation of DNA binding of bZIP proteins by enhancing dimerization. *Science* 1993;262:395–399.
23. Zhao LJ, Giam CZ. Human T-cell lymphotropic virus type I (HTLV-I) transcriptional activator, Tax, enhances CREB binding to HTLV-I 21-base-pair repeats by protein-protein interaction. *Proc Natl Acad Sci U S A* 1992;89:7070–7074.
24. Suzuki T, Hirai H, Yoshida M. Tax protein of HTLV-1 interacts with the Rel homology domain of NF-kappa B p65 and c-Rel proteins bound to the NF-kappa B binding site and activates transcription. *Oncogene* 1994;9:3099–3105.
25. Fujii M, Tsuchiya H, Chuhjo T, et al. Interaction of HTLV-1 Tax1 with p67SRF causes the aberrant induction of cellular immediate early genes through CArG boxes. *Genes Dev* 1992;6:2066–2076.
26. Giebler HA, Loring JE, van Orden K, et al. Anchoring of CREB binding protein to the human T-cell leukemia virus type 1 promoter: a molecular mechanism of Tax transactivation. *Mol Cell Biol* 1997;17:5156–5164.
27. Kwok RP, Laurance ME, Lundblad JR, et al. Control of cAMP-regulated enhancers by the viral transactivator Tax through CREB and the co-activator CBP. *Nature* 1996;380:642–646.
28. Van Orden K, Yan JP, Ulloa A, et al. Binding of the human T-cell leukemia virus Tax protein to the coactivator CBP interferes with CBP-mediated transcriptional control. *Oncogene* 1999;18:3766–3772.
29. Mori N, Shirakawa F, Shimizu H, et al. Transcriptional regulation of the human interleukin-6 gene promoter in human T-cell leukemia virus type I-infected T-cell lines: evidence for the involvement of NF-kappa B. *Blood* 1994;84:2904–2911.
30. Inoue J, Seiki M, Taniguchi T, et al. Induction of interleukin 2 receptor gene expression by p40x encoded by human T-cell leukemia virus type 1. *Embo J* 1986;5:2883–2888.
31. Fujii M, Sassone-Corsi P, Verma IM. c-fos promoter trans-activation by the tax1 protein of human T-cell leukemia virus type I. *Proc Natl Acad Sci U S A* 1988;85:8526–8530.
32. Suzuki T, Narita T, Uchida-Toita M, et al. Down-regulation of the INK4 family of cyclin-dependent kinase inhibitors by tax protein of HTLV-1 through two distinct mechanisms. *Virology* 1999;259:384–391.
33. Lemasson I, Robert-Hebmann V, Hamaia S, et al. Transrepression of lck gene expression by human T-cell leukemia virus type-1-encoded p40tax. *J Virol* 1997;71:1975–1983.
34. Yoshida M. Multiple viral strategies of HTLV-1 for dysregulation of cell growth control. *Annu Rev Immunol* 2001;19:475–496.
35. Pozzatti R, Vogel J, Jay G. The human T-lymphotropic virus type I tax gene can cooperate with the ras oncogene to induce neoplastic transformation of cells. *Mol Cell Biol* 1990;10:413–417.
36. Kadison P, Poteat HT, Klein KM, et al. Role of protein kinase A in tax transactivation of the human T-cell leukemia virus type I long terminal repeat. *J Virol* 1990;64:2141–2148.
37. Harhaj EW, Sun SC. IKKgamma serves as a docking subunit of the IkappaB kinase (IKK) and mediates interaction of IKK with the human T-cell leukemia virus Tax protein. *J Biol Chem* 1999;274:22911–22914.
38. Migone TS, Lin JX, Cereseto A, et al. Constitutively activated Jak-STAT pathway in T cells transformed with HTLV-I. *Science* 1995;269:79–81.
39. Mesnard JM, Devaux C. Multiple control levels of cell proliferation by human T-cell leukemia virus type 1 Tax protein. *Virology* 1999;257:277–284.
40. Franchini G, Wong-Staal F, Gallo RC. Human T-cell leukemia virus (HTLV-I) transcripts in fresh and cultured cells of patients with adult T-cell leukemia. *Proc Natl Acad Sci U S A* 1984;81:6207–6211.
41. Kozuru M, Uike N, Takeichi N, et al. The possible mode of escape of adult T-cell leukaemia cells from antibody-dependent cellular cytotoxicity. *Br J Haematol* 1989;72:502–506.
42. Tamiya S, Matsuoka M, Etoh K, et al. Two types of defective human T-lymphotropic virus type I provirus in adult T-cell leukemia. *Blood* 1996;88:3065–3073.
43. Kitamura T, Takano M, Hoshino H, et al. Methylation pattern of human T-cell leukemia virus in vivo and in vitro: pX and LTR regions are hypomethylated in vivo. *Int J Cancer* 1985;35:629–635.
44. Koiwa T, Usami-Hamano A, Ishida T, et al. 5'-LTR-selective CpG methylation of latent HTLV-1 provirus in vitro and in vivo. *J Virol* 2002;76:9389–9397.
45. Loeb LA. A mutator phenotype in cancer. *Cancer Res* 2001;61:3230–3239.
46. Jeang KT, Widen SG, Semmes OJT, et al. HTLV-I trans-activator protein, tax, is a trans-repressor of the human beta-polymerase gene. *Science* 1990;247:1082–1084.
47. Philpott SM, Buehring GC. Defective DNA repair in cells with human T-cell leukemia/bovine leukemia viruses: role of tax gene. *J Natl Cancer Inst* 1999;91:933–942.
48. Kao SY, Marriott SJ. Disruption of nucleotide excision repair by the human T-cell leukemia virus type 1 Tax protein. *J Virol* 1999;73:4299–4304.

49. Nicot C, Mahieux R, Takemoto S, et al. Bcl-X(L) is up-regulated by HTLV-I and HTLV-II *in vitro* and in *ex vivo* ATLL samples. *Blood* 2000;96:275–281.

50. Saintigny Y, Dumay A, Lambert S, et al. A novel role for the Bcl-2 protein family: specific suppression of the RAD51 recombination pathway. *Embo J* 2001;20:2596–2607.

51. Cereseto A, Diella F, Mulloy JC, et al. p53 functional impairment and high p21waf1/cip1 expression in human T-cell lymphotropic/leukemia virus type I-transformed T cells. *Blood* 1996;88:1551–1560.

52. Reid RL, Lindholm PF, Mireskandari A, et al. Stabilization of wild-type p53 in human T-lymphocytes transformed by HTLV-I. *Oncogene* 1993;8:3029–3036.

53. Utsunomiya A, Hanada S, Terada A, et al. Adult T-cell leukemia with leukemia cell infiltration into the gastrointestinal tract. *Cancer* 1988; 61:824–828.

54. Yamada Y, Kamihira S, Murata K, et al. Frequent hepatic involvement in adult T-cell leukemia: comparison with non-Hodgkin's lymphoma. *Leuk Lymphoma* 1997;26:327–335.

55. Yoshioka R, Yamaguchi K, Yoshinaga T, et al. Pulmonary complications in patients with adult T-cell leukemia. *Cancer* 1985;55:2491–2494.

56. Teshima T, Akashi K, Shibuya T, et al. Central nervous system involvement in adult T-cell leukemia/lymphoma. *Cancer* 1990;65:327–332.

57. Lymphoma Study Group. Major prognostic factors of patients with adult T-cell leukemia-lymphoma: a cooperative study. *Leuk Res* 1991;15:81–90.

58. Shimoyama M. Chemotherapy of ATL. In: Takatsuki K, ed. *Adult T-cell leukaemia*. Oxford: Oxford University Press, 1994:221–237.

59. Lymphoma Study Group. Final results of cooperative study of VEPA [vincristine, cyclophosphamide (Endoxan), prednisolone and adriamycin] therapy in advanced adult non-Hodgkin's lymphoma: relation between T- or B-cell phenotype and response. *Jpn J Clin Oncol* 1982;12:227–238.

60. Shimoyama M, Ota K, Kikuchi M, et al. Chemotherapeutic results and prognostic factors of patients with advanced non-Hodgkin's lymphoma treated with VEPA or VEPA-M. *J Clin Oncol* 1988;6:128–141.

61. Shimoyama M, Ota K, Kikuchi M, et al. Major prognostic factors of adult patients with advanced T-cell lymphoma/leukemia. *J Clin Oncol* 1988;6:1088–1097.

62. Tobinai K, Shimoyama M, Minato K, et al. Japan Clinical Oncology Group phase II trial of second-generation "LSG4 protocol" in aggressive T- and B-lymphoma: a new predictive model for T- and B-lymphoma. *Proc Am Soc Clin Oncol* 1994;13:378 [abstract].

63. Tsukasaki K, Tobinai K, Shimoyama M, et al. Deoxycoformycin-containing combination chemotherapy for adult T-cell leukemia-lymphoma: Japan Clinical Oncology Group study (JCOG9109). *Int J Hematol* 2003;77:164–170.

64. Yamada Y, Tomonaga M, Fukuda H, et al. A new G-CSF-supported combination chemotherapy, LSG15, for adult T-cell leukemia-lymphoma (ATL): Japan Clinical Oncology Group (JCOG) Study 9303. *Br J Haematol* 2001;113:375–382.

65. Tobinai K, Shimoyama M, Inoue S, et al. Phase I study of YK-176 (2'-deoxycoformycin) in patients with adult T-cell leukemia-lymphoma. *Jpn J Clin Oncol* 1992;22:164–171.

66. Ohno R, Okada K, Masaoka T, et al. An early phase II study of CPT-11: a new derivative of camptothecin, for the treatment of leukemia and lymphoma. *J Clin Oncol* 1990;8:1907–1912.

67. Tsuda H, Takatsuki K, Ohno R, et al. Treatment of adult T-cell leukemia-lymphoma with irinotecan hydrochloride. *Br J Cancer* 1994;70: 771–774.

68. Tobinai K, Hotta T, Saito H, et al. Combination phase I/II study of irinotecan hydrochloride and carboplatin in relapsed or refractory non-Hodgkin's lymphoma. *Jpn J Clin Oncol* 1996;26:455–460.

69. Ohtsu T, Sasaki Y, Igarashi T, et al. Unexpected hepatotoxicities in patients with non-Hodgkin's lymphoma treated with irinotecan (CPT-11) and etoposide. *Jpn J Clin Oncol* 1998;28:502–506.

70. Gill PS, Harrington W, Kaplan MH, et al. Treatment of adult T-cell leukemia-lymphoma with a combination of interferon alfa and zidovudine. *N Engl J Med* 1995;332:1744–1748.

71. Hermine O, Blouscary D, Gessain A, et al. Treatment of adult T-cell leukemia-lymphoma with zidovudine and interferon alfa. *N Engl J Med* 1995;332:1749–1751.

72. Tobinai K, Kobayashi Y, Shimoyama M, et al. Interferon alfa and zidovudine in adult T-cell leukemia-lymphoma. *N Engl J Med* 1995; 333:1285–1286 [correspondence].

73. Tobinai K, Ogura M, Hotta T, et al. Phase I study of cladribine (2-chlorodeoxyadenosine) in lymphoid malignancies. *Jpn J Clin Oncol* 1997;27:146–153.

74. Tobinai K, Uike N, Saburi Y, et al. Phase II study of cladribine in adult T-cell leukemia-lymphoma. *Proc Am Soc Clin Oncol* 2000;19 [abstract 149].

75. Waldmann TA. Multichain interleukin-2 receptor: a target for immunotherapy in lymphoma. *J Natl Cancer Inst* 1989;81:914–923.

76. Waldmann TA, White JD, Carrasquillo JA, et al. Radioimmunotherapy of interleukin-2Rα-expressing adult T-cell leukemia with yttrium-90-labeled anti-Tac. *Blood* 1995;86:4063–4075.

77. Utsunomiya A, Miyazaki Y, Takatsuka Y, et al. Improved outcome of adult T cell leukemia/lymphoma with allogeneic hematopoietic stem cell transplantation. *Bone Marrow Transplant* 2001;27:15–20.

CHAPTER 19

Mycosis Fungoides

Richard T. Hoppe, Jeff D. Harvell, and Youn H. Kim

Mycosis fungoides is a cutaneous lymphoma of mature, predominately CD4+ T cells. It is the most common type of cutaneous T-cell lymphoma and is distinguished from other cutaneous T-cell lymphomas by its unique clinical and histologic features. It is important to note that not all cutaneous T-cell lymphomas are mycosis fungoides. This term was introduced at a time when the immunoperoxidase characteristics of the entire spectrum of cutaneous lymphomas had not been defined, and only mycosis fungoides/Sézary syndrome was identified as being of T-cell origin. We now appreciate that other cutaneous T-cell lymphomas exist, including many cases of anaplastic large-cell lymphoma, peripheral T-cell lymphoma, and lymphoblastic lymphoma. Therefore, the terms *mycosis fungoides* and *cutaneous T-cell lymphoma* are not synonymous.

EPIDEMIOLOGY

The estimated annual incidence rate of mycosis fungoides and Sézary syndrome in the United States is 0.29 per 100,000 (1). It accounts for only 2% of new cases of non-Hodgkin's lymphoma. It commonly affects older adults (median age, 55 to 60 years), and there is a 2:1 male predominance without an established racial predilection.

The etiologies of mycosis fungoides and Sézary syndrome are unknown. Some retrospective studies have suggested a role for chemical exposure as a source of either chronic antigenic stimulation or toxic exposure. However, recent case-controlled studies refute this hypothesis (2,3). A viral etiology for mycosis fungoides was once proposed based on the isolation of human T-cell leukemia virus type 1 from the peripheral blood lymphocytes of a patient with a cutaneous lymphoma that resembled mycosis fungoides (4). However, it was later demonstrated that this patient actually had human T-cell leukemia virus type 1–associated T-cell lymphoma, a specific type of lymphoma that has now been described more precisely and is quite different from mycosis fungoides.

PATHOLOGY

Morphology

In patch lesions of mycosis fungoides, there is typically mild epidermal hyperplasia associated with a perivascular or band-like infiltrate of small- to medium-sized atypical lymphocytes with hyperchromatic and convoluted (cerebriform) nuclei. The atypical cells exhibit epidermotropism, with individual lymphocytes arranged along the dermal-epidermal junction in a single-file pattern or scattered throughout all layers of the epidermis in the absence of spongiosis (Color Plate 30). Small intraepidermal collections of neoplastic lymphocytes are known as *Pautrier's microabscesses* (Color Plate 31). Although such collections are virtually pathognomonic of mycosis fungoides, in early patch-stage lesions, Pautrier's microabscesses may not be present. As lesions evolve from patches to plaques, the density of neoplastic cells within the dermis increases, and the degree of epidermotropism becomes more exaggerated. In tumorous lesions, the dermal infiltrate is very dense, involving the full breadth of the dermis, often extending into the subcutaneous fat, and epidermotropism tends to diminish.

Biopsies of patients with erythroderma show very similar histology to that of patch mycosis fungoides, but the infiltrate is typically more sparse, and the diagnosis is more difficult to establish. By definition, in the Sézary syndrome, Sézary cells with cerebriform nuclei are seen within the peripheral blood (Color Plate 32). For a definitive diagnosis, they should number at least 1,000 per mm^3 (5). Additional ancillary tests, which help to refine the diagnosis, include an increased peripheral blood ratio of CD4 to CD8 T lymphocytes (greater than 10:1) and molecular evidence of a T-cell receptor gene rearrangement within either the peripheral blood or skin (5).

Involved lymph nodes in mycosis fungoides or Sézary syndrome show a range of histologic features (Table 19.1). The disease may cause regional nodes to develop the changes of dermatopathic lymphadenitis, with or without scattered individual atypical cerebriform lymphocytes (category I). Category II lymph nodes demonstrate dermatopathic lymphadenitis

TABLE 19.1. *Lymph node grading system for mycosis fungoides*

Category I (LN0-LN2)	Dermatopathic lymphadenopathy without atypical lymphocytes (LN0). Scattered atypical cerebriform lymphocytes (not in clusters), with or without dermatopathic lymphadenopathy (LN1). Atypical lymphocytes forming small clusters, not more than six cells per cluster, with or without dermatopathic lymphadenopathy (LN2).
Category II (LN3)	Clusters of ten or more cytologically atypical lymphocytes confined to the paracortex, with or without dermatopathic lymphadenopathy (LN3).
Category III (LN4)	Partial or complete effacement of lymph node architecture by cytologically atypical lymphocytes (LN4).

From Clendenning WE, Rappaport H. Report of the Committee on Pathology of Cutaneous T Cell Lymphomas. *Cancer Treat Rep* 1979;63:719–721, with permission.

with clusters of more than ten cytologically atypical lymphocytes confined to the paracortex. Category III is reserved for lymph nodes that demonstrate partial or total effacement of lymph node architecture by atypical lymphocytes (6–8). Because reactive lymph nodes can sometimes exhibit nonneoplastic lymphocytes with cerebriform nuclei, and because the diagnosis of early lymph node involvement by mycosis fungoides (i.e., category I) can be very difficult on histologic grounds alone, molecular methods for demonstrating T-cell clonality are gaining wide acceptance. Recent studies even suggest that patients with lymph nodes exhibiting rearranged T-cell receptor genes by molecular methods have a worse prognosis, regardless of the histologic grade (9).

Immunophenotype

Most cases of conventional mycosis fungoides exhibit the following immunophenotype: CD2+, CD3+, CD4+, CD8−, CD5+, CD7−, CD25−/+, CD30−, and T-cell receptor α/β+. Some cases exhibit a CD8+/CD4− immunophenotype, and rare ones exhibit surface T-cell receptor γ/δ rather than T-cell receptor α/β. Mycosis fungoides–associated follicular mucinosis and granulomatous slack skin generally exhibit the same immunophenotype as conventional mycosis fungoides (10,11). The immunophenotype in pagetoid reticulosis is variable: CD4+/CD8−, CD4−/CD8+, or CD4−/CD8−. As in conventional mycosis fungoides, CD7 is absent. The Ki-67 proliferation fraction in pagetoid reticulosis is higher than in conventional mycosis fungoides, usually greater than 30%, and unlike conventional mycosis fungoides, CD30 expression is common (12).

Genetics

T-cell receptor genes are clonally rearranged, but the ability to detect T-cell clonality in clinical material is variable.

Genetic aberrations that contribute to the development and progression of mycosis fungoides are becoming better elucidated. Cytogenetic studies have yet to disclose a consistent chromosomal change, but alterations to 10q, including loss of heterozygosity and microsatellite instability, are reported (13). These may result in the loss of function of a tumor suppressor gene (or genes) found in this region, such as PTEN. Other studies have found evidence that p16(INK4a), a tumor suppressor gene located on 9p, may be selectively inactivated with progression of mycosis fungoides from patch to tumor stage (14).

PATHOGENESIS

Cytokines have been implicated in the pathophysiology of mycosis fungoides and Sézary syndrome (15–17). However, whether cytokine abnormalities are primarily involved or are secondary processes in the pathogenesis is unclear. Studies have reported that soluble interleukin-2 (IL-2) receptor values in Sézary syndrome were significantly higher than for other malignant or inflammatory T-cell diseases and that the serum levels correlated with clinical course and Sézary cell count. The highest soluble IL-2 receptor levels were found in patients with advanced disease (17). Other investigators have shown that peripheral blood mononuclear cells from patients with the Sézary syndrome expressed higher levels of IL-4 and lower levels of IL-2 and interferon (IFN)-γ after phytohemagglutinin stimulation compared to normal controls (15).

A number of studies have suggested that the malignant T cells in Sézary syndrome account for aberrant cytokine production, with increased production of T-helper type 2 cytokines (e.g., IL-4, IL-5, IL-10) and decreased production of T-helper type 1 cytokines (e.g., IL-2 and IFN-γ) (18,19). Moreover, this aberrant cytokine production may be the cause for the immune abnormalities seen occasionally in Sézary syndrome. These immune abnormalities may include decreased T-cell responses to antigens and mitogens; impaired cell-mediated cytotoxicity, including natural killer–cell and lymphokine-activated killer-cell activities; increased levels of serum immunoglobulin E and immunoglobulin A; and peripheral eosinophilia.

Molecular Biology

Both Southern blot and polymerase chain reaction analyses are capable of detecting clonally rearranged T-cell receptor gene sequences in clinical material from patients with mycosis fungoides. In normal and neoplastic T-cell ontogeny, the γ region of the T-cell receptor gene is rearranged early on, such that most T-cell malignancies have detectable T-cell–receptor γ chain rearrangements, despite the fact that the α/β heterodimer is more often expressed at the cell surface. For various practical reasons, polymerase chain reaction analysis of the γ-chain region of the T-cell receptor (T-cell receptor γ) has proved more useful than Southern blot analysis in the evaluation of T-cell lymphoproliferative disorders. Polymerase chain reaction of T-cell receptor γ represents a very useful adjunct to the histopathologic diagnosis of various cutaneous T-cell malignancies, especially early patch-stage mycosis fungoides, and, at present, the sensitivity of the assay is approximately 70%. It is well established that non-neoplastic inflammatory dermatoses can exhibit detectable T-cell receptor gene rearrangements. The false-positive rate reported in the literature is quite variable, but the overall specificity is probably approximately 80% to 90% (20).

Postulated Cell of Origin

In most cases of mycosis fungoides and Sézary syndrome, the cell of origin is a clonal CD4+ T lymphocyte with skin homing (epidermotropic) properties.

Biology of Transformation

Histologically, transformation to large-cell lymphoma is defined on the basis of either an infiltrate of large atypical lymphocytes that comprise greater than 25% of the dermal infiltrate, or nodular expansile aggregates of atypical large lymphocytes (Color Plate 33) (21,22). In the majority of cases, increased mitotic activity is readily observed, and the Ki-67 proliferation rate by immunohistochemistry is greater than 25% (21). Immunophenotypically, the transformed large lymphocytes can exhibit variable loss of one or more T-cell–associated antigens such as CD3, CD5, CD4, CD8, CD45RO, or CD43 (21,22). Also, the large cells may express lymphocyte activation markers such as CD30 and CD25 (21). In some cases there are intermixed aggregates of small, medium, or large-sized B lymphocytes, which are presumably reactive and should not be erroneously interpreted as a secondary B-cell lymphoproliferative disorder (21). When CD30 expression is prominent among the transformed large lymphocytes, CD30+ lymphoproliferative disorders (especially CD30+ anaplastic large-cell lymphoma) must be considered in the differential diagnosis. Histologic findings that favor a diagnosis of transformed mycosis fungoides include an accompanying infiltrate of smaller-sized lymphocytes that exhibit epidermotropism (as seen in earlier-stage mycosis fungoides lesions), epidermotropism by CD30+ lymphocytes (which is usually not a feature of anaplastic large-cell lymphoma), and a relatively low percentage of CD30+ lymphocytes (as compared to cases of anaplastic large-cell lymphoma in which CD30+ large lymphocytes are greater than 75%). In some cases, correlation with the clinical findings is essential for a definitive diagnosis.

CLINICAL PRESENTATION

Mycosis fungoides often has a long natural history, and the median duration from the onset of skin symptoms to a diagnosis of mycosis fungoides may be 5 years or longer (5). In many patients, the disease presents initially in a premycotic phase with nonspecific, slightly scaling skin lesions that wax and wane over a period of years. Biopsies are generally nondiag-nostic during this phase of disease, and patients may respond to treatment with topical corticosteroids. Some of these patients will experience an evolution of their disease and develop more typical patches or infiltrated plaques, from which a definitive diagnostic biopsy may be obtained. Repeated biopsies must be obtained from patients suspected of having mycosis fungoides, even when an initial biopsy is negative.

The most common initial cutaneous presentation is patch and plaque disease; however, some patients may present with tumors or generalized erythroderma. There may be prominent poikiloderma (skin atrophy with telangiectasia) or associated alopecia or follicular mucinosis. Approximately 30% of patients present with limited patch and plaque disease (less than 10% of the skin surface involved, T1), 35% to 40% with generalized patch and plaque (greater than or equal to 10% of the skin surface involved, T2), 15% to 20% with tumorous (T3), and 15% with erythroderma (T4).

The typical patches of mycosis fungoides are slightly scaling and mildly erythematous (Color Plate 34). More infiltrated lesions evolve into palpable plaques (Color Plate 35). These plaques are erythematous and slightly scaling, with well-defined borders. The shape and distribution of lesions are variable. Many patients present with involvement in the "bathing trunk" distribution, although lesions may be present on any part of the body. Pruritus is the most common symptom even in the early phases of the disease and is often the problem that prompts a visit to the dermatologist.

Infiltrated plaques may evolve into ulcerating or fungating tumors (Color Plate 36). Tumors often become infected, and sepsis secondary to infection is often the cause of death in individuals so affected. Rare patients present *de novo* with tumors, so-called tumor *d'emblee*. Generalized dermal thickening from infiltrative disease may cause the classic but very unusual leonine facies of mycosis fungoides.

Another manifestation of skin involvement in mycosis fungoides is generalized erythroderma (Color Plate 37). The erythema may be accompanied by either atrophic or licheni-fied skin, and plaques or tumors may also be present. These patients are almost always intensely symptomatic from pruritus and scaling and often have lymphadenopathy due to diffuse and severe skin involvement. Cells may be present in the peripheral blood that have the same microscopic appearance and immunophenotypic and genotypic characteristics as the cells that infiltrate the epidermis. Patients with this complex of findings, generalized erythroderma, lymphadenopathy, and atypical T cells (Sézary cells) in the peripheral blood have Sézary syndrome (23). Patients with Sézary syndrome have a worse prognosis than erythrodermic patients with mycosis fungoides who do not have the other findings of the Sézary syndrome.

Mycosis fungoides may be associated with follicular mucinosis. In these cases, involvement of the hair follicles is clinically prominent, and biopsy shows a heavy infiltration of the hair follicle epithelium by atypical cerebriform lymphocytes. Often, the interfollicular epidermis is spared. In typical cases, there is expansion of the hair follicle epithelium by connective-tissue mucin, sometimes resulting in small pools of follicular mucin. However, mucin deposition can be variable, and because of this variability there has been a recent recommendation that cases of mycosis fungoides–associated follicular mucinosis be designated *follicular mycosis fungoides* (10,11).

Pagetoid reticulosis is a verrucous variant of mycosis fungoides that typically affects acral sites, such as the hands and feet, and features extensive epidermotropism by atypical lymphocytes. The degree of epidermotropism is greatly exaggerated as compared to conventional mycosis fungoides, to the point that atypical lymphocytes are almost exclusively confined to a markedly acanthotic epidermis.

Granulomatous slack skin is a variant of mycosis fungoides that results in pendulous folds of slack or lax skin. The laxity is due to macrophage-mediated destruction of the normal elastic fiber network of the dermis. Histologically, there is a diffuse granulomatous and lymphocytic infiltrate with well-formed granulomas containing multinucleated giant cells. Another distinctive feature is the finding of elastic fibers within the cytoplasm of multinucleated giant cells, a pathologic process known as *elastophagocytosis*. It is the histologic correlate of ongoing elastic fiber destruction, which in late stages of the disease results in near complete obliteration of dermal elastic tissue. Superimposed on the granulomatous infiltrate is an infiltrate of small cerebriform lymphocytes that display the typical epidermotropic changes encountered in conventional mycosis fungoides (24).

Many patients with mycosis fungoides have evidence of cutaneous disease only throughout the course of their disease. Only 15% to 20% of patients with mycosis fungoides develop clinical problems related to extracutaneous disease. The most commonly identified site of extracutaneous disease is the regional lymphatics, usually in areas that drain significant sites of skin involvement. Visceral disease may be identified subsequently. The most common visceral sites of involvement identified are the lungs, oral cavity/pharynx, and the central nervous system, but virtually any organ may be involved at autopsy in patients who have died of the disease.

STAGING

Conventional staging for patients with mycosis fungoides includes a comprehensive physical examination with careful examination of the skin (including the scalp, palms, soles, and perineum) and lymph nodes, a complete blood count with Sézary cell studies, screening chemistries (including lactate dehydrogenase), and chest x-ray. Additional imaging studies for patients with T1 or T2 skin involvement are not recommended unless the patient has lymphadenopathy. However, patients with T3 or T4 disease are at increased risk for extracutaneous involvement, and further imaging, such as a chest/abdomen/pelvis computed tomography scan, is appropriate. The usefulness of nuclear medicine scans, such as positron emission tomography, has not been established. Lymph node biopsies should be obtained if lymphadenopathy is present. Suspected sites of visceral involvement should be confirmed by appropriate biopsy. Bone marrow involvement may often be detected in patients who meet the clinical criteria for Sézary syndrome (25) but is extremely uncommon in classic mycosis fungoides. Therefore, a bone marrow biopsy is not routinely used as part of the initial staging.

A Tumor-Node-Metastasis-Blood (TNMB) staging system that has proved useful for mycosis fungoides was proposed at the Workshop on Mycosis Fungoides held at the National Cancer Institute in 1978 (26). Table 19.2 summarizes the TNMB categories and staging classification.

The T classification reflects the extent and type of skin involvement. The N category indicates the presence or

TABLE 19.2. *Tumor-node-metastasis-blood classification and clinical staging system for mycosis fungoides*

T (Skin)	
T1	Limited patch/plaque (<10% of total skin surface)
T2	Generalized patch/plaque (≥10% of total skin surface)
T3	Tumors
T4	Generalized erythroderma
N (Nodes)	
N0	Lymph nodes clinically uninvolved
N1	Lymph nodes enlarged, histologically uninvolved (includes "reactive" and "dermatopathic" nodes)
N2	Lymph nodes clinically uninvolved, histologically involved
N3	Lymph nodes enlarged and histologically involved
M (Viscera)	
M0	No visceral involvement
M1	Visceral involvement
B (Blood)	
B0	No circulating atypical (Sézary) cells (<5% of total lymphocytes)
B1	Circulating atypical (Sézary) cells (≥5% of total lymphocytes)

Clinical stages	Tumor node metastases classification[a]		
IA	T1	N0	M0
IB	T2	N0	M0
IIA	T1-2	N1	M0
IIB	T3	N0-1	M0
IIIA	T4	N0	M0
IIIB	T4	N1	M0
IVA	T1-4	N2-3	M0
IVB	T1-4	N0-3	M1

[a]The B classification does not alter clinical stage.

absence of lymph node involvement. The M category indicates visceral disease. In the B (blood) category, the absence or presence of a significant proportion of abnormal, cerebriform (Sézary) cells should be noted. Low levels of Sézary-like cells can be detected in the peripheral blood of patients with benign skin conditions. The current practice by many mycosis fungoides referral centers is to use a criterion of at least 20% of lymphocytes, an absolute Sézary count of at least 1,000 per mm^3, or a CD4:CD8 ratio greater than 10:1 to define peripheral blood involvement.

PROGNOSTIC AND PREDICTIVE FACTORS

The T classification and presence of extracutaneous disease are the most important predictors of survival in patients with mycosis fungoides (27,28). Among patients with T4 disease (erythroderma), age older than 60 years, peripheral blood involvement, and extracutaneous disease are independent adverse predictive factors for survival (29).

TREATMENT

The nonspecific, symptomatic treatment of mycosis fungoides and Sézary syndrome is an integral component of the overall therapeutic regimen. Pruritus and xerosis, either as a result of the disease or therapy, may be severe. Thus, supportive measures, such as aggressive emolliation, topical steroids, and oral antipruritics, should be used as necessary.

There are multiple therapeutic options for mycosis fungoides and the Sézary syndrome. Selection of treatment is based primarily on the clinical stage of the disease. However, other factors, such as access to special treatment approaches, the patient's age, and other social and medical problems, as well as the cost to benefit ratio, should be taken into consideration. For patients with patch or plaque skin involvement (T1 and T2) without extracutaneous disease, the treatment plan may be limited to topical therapeutic measures, whereas patients with any extracutaneous disease should receive systemic (cytotoxic or biologic) therapy as part of their management. It has been demonstrated in a prospective randomized clinical trial that there is no advantage to early aggressive combined modality therapy compared to conservative sequential therapies in the management of limited or advanced disease (30).

Topical Chemotherapy

Topical nitrogen mustard (mechlorethamine) is an effective topical therapy for mycosis fungoides (28,31,32). The mechanism of action when nitrogen mustard is applied topically is not well defined and may not be related simply to its alkylating agent properties. Its activity may be mediated by immune mechanisms or by interaction with the epidermal cell–Langerhan's cell–T cell axis.

Topical nitrogen mustard may be prepared as an aqueous solution or mixed in an ointment. Both preparations are generally applied at a concentration of 10 to 20 mg per 100 cc. The aqueous and ointment preparations have similar efficacy. The choice is often dependent on convenience, patient preference, or cost. The ointment preparation uses less nitrogen mustard for similar response. Also, the aqueous preparation is associated with a much higher incidence (greater than 30%) of hypersensitivity reaction compared with the low rate (less than 5%) reported with the ointment preparation.

Nitrogen mustard may be applied locally or to the entire skin. It is applied at least once daily during the clearing phase. Other areas of disease activity may become evident secondary to the inflammatory reaction provoked by the nitrogen mustard. After a period of several weeks, treatment may be limited to the affected region. Alternatively, if the disease is initially limited in distribution, the nitrogen mustard may be applied only to the affected anatomic region or regions, with careful follow-up to detect any new areas of involvement. Treatment is continued on a daily basis until skin clearance is complete. This may require 6 months or longer and is then followed by a variable duration of maintenance therapy (3 to 6 months). If response is particularly slow, the concentration of the topical nitrogen mustard may be increased, or the frequency of application may be increased. The complete response rate for topical nitrogen mustard for limited patch or plaque (T1) disease is 70% to 80%. The median time to skin clearance is 6 to 8 months. When treatment is discontinued, more than one-half of patients will relapse in the skin, but most will respond to a resumption of therapy. The proportion of patients treated with topical nitrogen mustard who have a durable complete response (longer than 10 years) is 20% to 25%. In patients with a discrete number of refractory lesions, treatment may be supplemented with local irradiation.

The primary acute complication of topical nitrogen mustard is a cutaneous hypersensitivity reaction. Desensitization may be achieved by a variety of topical or systemic desensitization programs. There is no systemic absorption of topical nitrogen mustard, thus systemic complications such as bone marrow suppression or sterility are not an issue. Occasional patients treated with topical nitrogen mustard develop secondary squamoproliferative lesions of the skin. This risk is the greatest among patients who have had long-term sequential therapy with multiple topical modalities.

Another topical chemotherapeutic agent that has been used for patients with limited disease is carmustine (BCNU) (33). The efficacy of topical BCNU is similar to topical nitrogen mustard; however, because of the systemic absorption of BCNU, the potential hematologic complications are greater, and the maximum duration of treatment is limited. In addition, patients treated with BCNU tend to develop significant telangiectasias in areas where the drug is applied.

Phototherapy

Phototherapy involves using ultraviolet (UV) radiation in the form of UVA or UVB wavelengths, which can be used alone, together, or with psoralen, a photosensitizing agent, as psoralen plus UVA, or PUVA. The long-wave UVA has the advantage over UVB in its greater depth of penetration into the dermal infiltrates of mycosis fungoides. For early limited disease, UVB alone (34) or home UV phototherapy (UVA plus UVB) (35) has been shown to be effective.

PUVA is the most commonly used form of phototherapy for mycosis fungoides and the Sézary syndrome. It was first used in the treatment of psoriasis but also has been shown to be effective for patients with mycosis fungoides (36–38). In the presence of UVA, the psoralen drug intercalates with DNA, forming both monofunctional and bifunctional adducts, which inhibit DNA synthesis.

During the clearing phase, which may require up to 6 months, patients are treated two to three times weekly. After this phase is completed, patients continue on a maintenance program with decreased frequency of treatment. If the disease begins to recur during the maintenance phase, then the frequency of treatment is increased in an effort to achieve better control.

With PUVA treatment, the complete clearance rate is 50% to 90% among patients with patch or plaque disease, and the likelihood of clearance is dependent on the initial extent of skin involvement. The response is less impressive among patients with erythrodermic or tumor disease.

The primary acute complications of PUVA therapy include nausea and phototoxic reactions such as erythroderma and blistering as well as skin dryness. Patients should shield their skin and eyes from the sun for at least 24 hours after psoralen ingestion. The potential long-term complications of PUVA therapy include cataract formation (requiring the use of UVA-opaque goggles during therapy) and secondary cutaneous malignancies. Among patients treated for mycosis fungoides, this risk is greatest for patients who have undergone long-term treatment with multiple topical therapies (39).

Topical Retinoids

Bexarotene (Targretin) 1% gel is the most commonly used topical retinoid for treating mycosis fungoides. The reported overall response rate is 63%, with a complete response rate of 21% (40). Due to the irritant effect of the retinoids, it is only feasible to use this agent when there are a discrete number of patches or plaques. It is not intended for generalized application. Bexarotene gel is applied with a thin application to the patches or plaques and is most effective when used twice daily. The most common toxicity is irritation at sites of gel application, which occurs in the majority of patients with variable intensity. Because of the erythema from the irritant reaction, it may be necessary to withhold therapy for a few weeks to assess for residual active disease.

Radiation Therapy

Mycosis fungoides is an exquisitely radiosensitive neoplasm, and irradiation may be exploited in several ways for its man-

agement (41). Individual plaques or tumors of mycosis fungoides may be treated to total doses of 15 to 25 Gy in 1 to 3 weeks, with a high likelihood of achieving long-term local control. For the unusual patient with unilesional or localized mycosis fungoides, local electron beam therapy achieves the most efficient and complete clearance of the disease.

Local disease may be treated with low-energy x-rays or electrons. Electrons have an intrinsic advantage over x-rays, because the depth of penetration of electrons can be controlled by the appropriate selection of electron energy. The relative dose contribution to the subcutaneous and deeper tissues is greater with even low-energy photons, compared to electrons. For treating individual lesions, an electron energy should be selected that provides an adequate depth of penetration through the entire depth of involvement by the patch, plaque, or tumor, with at least 0.5 cm of penetration beyond. For the typical patch or thin plaque, treatment with 6- to 9-MeV electrons usually suffices. However, with low-energy electrons, there is a "skin sparing" effect (i.e., the maximum dose is actually deep to the skin surface). Because the lesions of mycosis fungoides are so superficial, it is desirable to have the maximum dose at the skin surface. This can be achieved by the use of tissue-equivalent bolus material of 0.5- to 1.0-cm thickness. Exophytic tumors may require 9- to 12-MeV electrons. Peripheral margins of up to 2 cm are recommended but may be dependent on location and proximity to sensitive tissues.

Several centers have developed expertise in the use of total-skin electron beam therapy (42,43). Overall response rates are nearly 100%, with complete response rates ranging from 40% to 98% depending on the extent of skin involvement. As many as 50% of patients with limited plaque disease and 25% of patients with generalized plaque disease may remain free of disease for longer than 5 years after completion of a single course of electron beam therapy. Although the curative potential of this treatment remains disputed, there is no doubt that it provides an important palliative benefit, especially for patients with extensive disease. Often, when disease recurs, it is in a more limited distribution and may be controlled more readily with localized topical therapies.

The widespread use of total-skin electron beam therapy was facilitated by the development of the modern medical linear accelerator; the first adaptation of that device for total-skin treatment with electrons was at Stanford University (44). The basic concept used in the "Stanford technique" was to replace the target at the end of the linear accelerator with an electron-scattering foil to generate a diffuse electron beam. The patient stood approximately 10 ft from the end of the accelerator, and his or her entire surface could be treated with the broad electron beam. By using multiple field techniques, it was possible to irradiate the entire cutaneous surface.

In a typical contemporary set up, patients are treated in the standing position at a distance of 3.5 m from the isocenter (electron source). A 3/8-in. Lucite plate is placed as close as possible to the patient surface to degrade and further scatter the electrons. During treatment, the machine is angled upward or downward at an angle of 18 degrees. The combination of these two fields for treating each body surface results in a very homogeneous dose distribution at the patient's surface and minimizes photon contamination, which is greatest in the central axis of the beam.

Patients are treated with a six-field technique that includes anterior, posterior, and four opposed oblique fields (45). A full "cycle" of treatment is administered over a 2-day period. On the first day, the anterior and two posterior oblique fields are treated at each of the two accelerator angles. On the second day, the posterior and two anterior oblique fields are treated at each of the two accelerator angles. The dose administered with each cycle is 1.5 to 2.0 Gy. Most patients will tolerate 2.0 Gy per cycle, but lower doses are used for patients with erythroderma, atrophic skin, or a previous course of electron beam therapy. The prescribed total dose is 30 to 36 Gy administered over a 9- to 10-week period. A 1-week split may be used after a dose of 18 to 20 Gy has been delivered to provide some relief from the generalized skin erythema that usually accompanies treatment.

With this technique, certain portions of the body surface are "shadowed" and receive relatively lower total doses of irradiation (46). These areas include the top of the scalp, the perineum, and the soles of the feet. Other areas may be problematic in individual patients because of body habitus, such as underneath the breasts of some women and under the panniculus of obese individuals. To compensate for this effect, we routinely treat the perineum and soles of the feet using 6-MeV electrons (with 1-cm tissue-equivalent bolus) with daily fractions of 1 Gy to a total of 20 Gy. Supplemental treatment is provided to the vertex of the scalp only if there is scalp involvement, because permanent alopecia may result. Additional treatment also is administered underneath the breasts and panniculus of individual patients, as indicated. Also, some patients with a discrete number of tumorous lesions will receive boost treatment to these tumors at the outset of electron beam therapy to reduce their thickness and permit better penetration by the electrons. Usually, doses of 15.0 Gy in 1.5 to 3.0 Gy fractions using 6- to 9-MeV electrons is adequate for this purpose.

In the standard course of treatment, only the eyes are shielded. Internal lead eye shields with an inner coating of paraffin or dental acrylic are used whenever disease is present on the face or scalp (47). The shields are placed under the lids after the eyes have been anesthetized topically. If disease is absent from these areas, external lead eye shields, which are taped over the closed eyes, are used. In addition, in the absence of involvement of the scalp or face, scalp shielding is used after a dose of 25 Gy to facilitate adequate regrowth of scalp hair. Complete scalp shielding is contraindicated and may result in extension of disease to this area (48).

Individualized shielding is used as clinical circumstances demand. For example, some patients develop a more intense skin reaction on the fingers than on other surfaces. This may be minimized by the use of modified lead-lined fluoroscopic gloves. When increased skin reactions are observed in the feet or toes, footboards several inches in height may be placed behind the Lucite degrader to shield the feet from the electrons. The use of individualized shielding requires careful clinical judgment taking into account the extent and location of the patient's disease, inherent inhomogeneity of dose on different body surfaces, and the intensity of the local reactions.

The composite depth-dose distribution curve for total-skin electron beam therapy is affected by the extended treatment distance, the Lucite degrader near the patient surface, and the oblique angle of incidence. Using a 9-MeV beam and the six–dual-field technique, the 80% dose is located at a depth of 0.7 cm. The 50% depth dose is at 1.25 cm. These depth-dose characteristics are ideal for mycosis fungoides, in which the malignant infiltrates are generally limited to the epidermis and upper portions of the dermis. These depth-dose characteristics are markedly different from those of small *en face* electron fields.

The essentials of the Stanford technique have been adopted widely for the management of patients with mycosis fungoides. In addition, individual modifications have been introduced to suit local needs, such as treatment with a nonangulated electron beam (49), the use of a rotational patient platform (50), electron-arc therapy using a reclined patient position (51), and electron beams of varying energies (52).

Total-skin electron beam therapy should be considered as initial therapy for patients with very thickened plaques, because the effective depth of treatment of electron beam therapy is more substantial than either topical nitrogen mustard or phototherapy. It is also appropriate for patients with a recent history of rapid progression of disease and for those patients for whom topical nitrogen mustard, bexarotene gel, or phototherapy was not effective. Generally, after completion of total-skin electron beam therapy, adjuvant treatment with topical nitrogen mustard is indicated and may be continued for up to 6 months.

In patients who have lymph node involvement or in some situations of localized visceral disease, megavoltage (4 to 15 MeV) photon irradiation may be helpful in providing important additional palliation. Doses of 30 to 36 Gy in 3 to 4 weeks are often sufficient to achieve local control of lymph nodes or other extracutaneous sites of disease. This is often combined with systemic chemotherapy or biologic therapy (IFN-α or bexarotene), depending on the extent of the extracutaneous involvement.

The most common acute complications of total-skin electron-beam therapy are erythema and dry desquamation (45,48,53). Intermediate-term complications include alopecia, which is incomplete and only temporary if the scalp dose is limited to 25 Gy (53). Most patients also experience temporary loss of fingernails and toenails 2 to 4 months after completion of therapy. Most patients report the inability to sweat properly for 6 to 12 months after therapy (54) and chronically dry skin thereafter, which requires the regular use of emolliation. In long-term follow-up, evidence for chronic radiation dermatitis is uncommon (55). Although secondary malignancies, such as squamous cell and basal cell cancers of the skin, are increased after the use of total-skin electron beam therapy, the only patients in whom these have become problematic are those who have received repeated treatment with multiple therapies, including irradiation, topical nitrogen mustard, and PUVA (39).

Systemic Chemotherapy

Systemic chemotherapy is generally indicated only for patients with extracutaneous disease. With combination chemotherapy regimens, overall complete-response or partial-response rates can reach 80% to 100%; however, in most cases, the median duration of response is shorter than 1 year, and in many patients, shorter than several months (56,57). Virtually all drugs that have proved useful in the management of patients with non-Hodgkin's lymphomas have been tested in patients with mycosis fungoides. The most effective and commonly used combinations include cyclophosphamide, Oncovin (vincristine), and prednisone, with (CHOP) or without (CVP) hydroxydaunomycin (58). Other regimens used include cyclophosphamide, Adriamycin, vincristine, and etoposide (CAVE) and CVP with methotrexate (COMP) (30,59,60). Chemotherapy may be used alone or in combination with topical therapy (e.g., radiation) or biologic response modifiers (e.g., IFN-α). However, a randomized trial that compared electron beam radiation plus chemotherapy to sequential topical therapies in the initial treatment of mycosis fungoides did not demonstrate an improved survival with the more aggressive management approach (30).

Methotrexate, etoposide, bleomycin, vinblastine, or purine analogs (fludarabine, 2'-deoxycoformycin) are the most commonly used single-agent chemotherapy regimens in mycosis fungoides and Sézary syndrome (56,57). The overall clinical response and response duration tend to be less than those observed with combination chemotherapy regimens. The newer purine analogs show promise in early clinical trials, but complications related to immunosuppression are significant. Fludarabine, which causes profound decreases in peripheral T-cell counts, has demonstrated clinical activity against mycosis fungoides, chronic lymphocytic leukemia, and the low-grade lymphomas (61). Another drug that may be useful is 2'-deoxycoformycin, which inhibits adenosine deaminase, an enzyme with a high level of activity in T cells, and leads to inhibition of DNA synthesis. The response rate may be as high as 50% (62,63). Recently, single-agent gemcitabine has been reported to achieve complete and partial response rates of 12% and 59%, respectively, with median durations of 15 and 10 months (64). Another active single agent is liposomal doxorubicin.

In contrast to other non-Hodgkin's lymphomas, autologous bone marrow transplantation has not been actively investigated in mycosis fungoides and Sézary syndrome, and anecdotal experience in its use is limited (65,66). The ablative regimens used in these cases were combinations of total-skin electron beam therapy, total-body irradiation, and various combinations of cyclophosphamide, etoposide, BCNU, and cisplatin. Further studies are necessary to determine the role of autologous bone marrow transplantation in the treatment of this disease.

Extracorporeal Photopheresis

Photopheresis [extracorporeal photopheresis (ECPP) or systemic photochemotherapy] is a method of delivering PUVA systemically by using an extracorporeal technique (67). The patient's white blood cells are collected (leukapheresis), exposed to a photoactivating drug, and then irradiated with UVA. The irradiated cells then are returned to the patient. The mechanism of action of ECPP remains unclear. It is hypothesized that there may be a dual effect: a direct cytotoxic or antiproliferative effect on the neoplastic cells and an immune-enhancing effect on the competent lymphocytes against the neoplastic cells. Photopheresis is usually administered every 4 weeks, but in patients with severe disease, the frequency can be as often as every 2 to 3 weeks. Once complete clearance is achieved, the frequency can be gradually reduced and then discontinued.

Compared with other systemic therapies, ECPP has minimal adverse effects (67). Some patients may experience nausea, mostly due to the ingested psoralen, and some have a transient low-grade fever or slight malaise after treatment. There are no reports of organ injury or bone marrow or immune suppression.

Interferon-α

IFN-α is indicated primarily for the palliative management of refractory or advanced disease. It may be used alone or, more often, combined with topical or other systemic therapies. The dosage of IFN-α for mycosis fungoides is usually initiated at 3 to 5 million units daily or three times per week and is gradually increased, depending on the clinical response and the severity of adverse effects. Reported overall response rates when used as monotherapy are 53% to 74%, with complete response rates of 21% to 35% (68,69).

Retinoids

Systemic therapy with retinoids, most commonly bexarotene, has been shown to be beneficial in the management of mycosis fungoides and Sézary syndrome (70). The reported response rate is approximately 45%, with a 20% complete response rate (71). Systemic retinoids are indicated for palliative therapy for refractory or advanced disease, often in combination with other topical or systemic therapies, including PUVA (Re-PUVA), IFN-α, or total-skin electron beam therapy (72–75).

Bexarotene is administered orally. The initial dose is 300 mg per m^2 per day, which can be adjusted according to clinical response and the severity of adverse effects. The most common adverse effects include photosensitivity, xerosis, myalgia, arthralgia, headaches, and impaired night vision. The well-known teratogenic effects of retinoids must be carefully addressed in female patients. Because of its potential hepatotoxic and hyperlipidemic effects, liver function and serum lipid levels should be monitored in each patient during treatment. In addition, central hypothyroidism is often induced, so patients are routinely started on levothyroxine (Synthroid) immediately before or simultaneously with bexarotene.

Recombinant Fusion Proteins

Recombinant fusion protein therapy, such as the IL-2–diphtheria toxin fusion protein (Ontak, denileukin diftitox), involves the use of growth factor–diphtheria toxin fusion proteins designed specifically to kill defined neoplastic cell populations. Ontak has undergone a multicenter phase III trial in patients with IL-2 receptor (CD25+)-expressing mycosis fungoides (76). Patients with intermediate or advanced stages of disease were included in the phase III trial. The overall response rate was 30%, with complete-response and partial-response rates of 10% and 20%, respectively. The main complication is related to a "capillary leak" syndrome that may be ameliorated by pretreatment with corticosteroids.

Combined Modality Therapy

Patients who do not respond to a single-agent topical regimen can be treated with combined modality therapy. This may include multiple topical therapies, such as combinations of total-skin electron beam therapy, topical nitrogen mustard, PUVA, or bexarotene gel, or by combined topical and systemic biologic therapies, such as PUVA or total-skin electron beam therapy with IFN-α or systemic bexarotene (72,74,77).

The majority of patients with tumor-stage (stage IIB) mycosis fungoides has generalized involvement with tumor and plaque disease, and the greatest likelihood of a response is with total-skin electron beam therapy. However, in view of the high risk for relapse after irradiation, adjuvant therapy (e.g., topical nitrogen mustard) is generally used after completion of electron beam therapy. Topical nitrogen mustard in aquaphor provides the dual benefit of treatment for any residual disease and emolliation of the skin, often chronically dry after completion of electron beam therapy. Patients with a discrete number of tumors may be treated with topical nitrogen mustard or PUVA, combined with localized electron-beam therapy to individual tumors. Although topical (nitrogen mustard or PUVA) or systemic (IFN-α or photopheresis) adjuvant therapy after skin clearance with total-skin electron beam therapy may improve the disease-free interval, it does not improve survival (78–80).

Patients with recalcitrant disease may require a combination of systemic therapies, either with biologic therapies or a combination of biologic and chemotherapies, with or without topical therapy. IFN-α has been used in combination with systemic retinoids with variable results (73,81). Various chemotherapy regimens have been used in combination with total-skin electron-beam therapy (30,82). However, there is no evidence that an aggressive combination regimen using systemic chemotherapy at the outset results in superior survival (30).

PUVA can be given in combination with IFN-α. In one of the largest studies of this combination, a complete response rate of 33% and partial response rate of 50% were observed in patients with stage IIB disease (77). Studies using PUVA alone for erythrodermic (stage III) patients have reported complete response rates of 33% to 70% (36,38,83,84). Despite these good response rates, the majority of the patients relapses during maintenance therapy. In another study, the complete-response and partial-response rates for a combination regimen of PUVA plus IFN-α in stage III disease were 62% and 25%, respectively (77). It is thought that the combined regimen may improve clinical response or response duration beyond that observed with PUVA or IFN-α alone. However, there is no clear evidence that prolongation of response duration leads to improvement in the overall survival.

OUTCOME

Stage IA (Limited Patch or Plaque, T1) Disease

The primary therapy for patients with stage IA (T1) disease is topical. This may include topical chemotherapy (usually nitrogen mustard), phototherapy (UVB or PUVA), bexarotene gel, or localized radiation therapy. The complete-response rate to nitrogen mustard is 60% to 70% (85) and to total-skin electron beam therapy is 85% to 95% (86). However, there is no evidence that any one approach is superior to the others with respect to long-term disease control or survival. Treatment selection is often based on convenience and cost.

Patients with limited patch or plaque (T1, overall stage IA) disease who are treated with conventional therapies have an excellent prognosis, with an overall long-term life expectancy that is similar to an age-, gender-, and race-matched control population. In a retrospective study of 122 patients with stage IA disease at Stanford, the median survival was not reached at 33 years (87). Nearly all patients with stage IA disease who die will die from causes other than mycosis fungoides. Furthermore, only 9% of treated patients at this stage ever progress to a more advanced stage of disease. Early aggressive therapy with combination chemotherapy does not result in a more favorable survival outcome compared to patients managed more conservatively with sequential topical regimens (30).

Stage IB/IIA (Generalized Patch or Plaque, T2) Disease

Topical nitrogen mustard, PUVA, and total-skin electron beam therapy are commonly used for patients with T2 disease. Complete-response rates using topical nitrogen mustard are 50% to 70% (32,88,89), whereas the complete-response rate for total-skin electron beam therapy is 80%

to 90% (86,88). However, patients treated with total-skin electron beam therapy do not have an improved long-term survival compared to those who received topical nitrogen mustard as initial therapy, despite the superior complete-response rate (88). In patients treated with PUVA, the complete-response rate ranges from 50% to 80% (36,38,90).

Patients who do not respond to one topical therapy or who progress after an initial response may be treated with an alternative topical therapy. There is no evidence that development of resistance to one modality affects subsequent response to an alternative topical therapy (87,88). Combination topical or topical-plus-biologic therapies may also be used as initial therapy for patients with T2 disease. This may provide for better long-term control of disease, but the ultimate outcome is not usually affected (78,80,83). Patients who have generalized patch or plaque disease without evidence of extracutaneous involvement and who are treated with these modalities have a median survival longer than 11 years, but 25% of deaths in this group are attributable to mycosis fungoides (88).

Stage IIB (Tumorous) Disease

Patients who have a limited number of cutaneous tumors in the setting of generalized patch or plaque disease may be treated with local radiation to the tumors plus one of the topical therapies noted above. However, those who have generalized tumorous disease will be treated most effectively with total-skin electron beam therapy followed by maintenance therapy with nitrogen mustard (80) or combinations of PUVA with IFN-α (83) or PUVA plus oral bexarotene.

Secondary therapies for these patients include alternative topical or combination therapies, fusion proteins, or investigational treatment. Patients with cutaneous tumors have a median survival of 3.2 years, and the majority of these patients die of mycosis fungoides.

Stage III (Erythrodermic, T4) Disease

Patients with erythrodermic (T4) mycosis fungoides usually have very inflamed and itchy skin that may be irritated by topical therapies. Common treatments for these patients include extracorporeal photopheresis, PUVA, oral bexarotene, IFN-α, and single-agent methotrexate. With standard total-skin electron beam therapy techniques, these patients may experience severe desquamation with relatively low total doses. Therefore, total-skin electron beam therapy is generally not considered appropriate as the initial treatment. Treatment intent in these patients is almost always palliative, and most progress through several therapies or combinations of therapy during the course of their disease.

The long-term outcome for these patients is quite variable and is dependent on patient age at presentation (younger than 65 years vs. older than 65 years), overall stage (III vs. IV), and peripheral blood involvement (B0 vs. B1) (29). The median survival varies widely, depending on the number of independent adverse prognostic factors present: three distinct prognostic subgroups may be identified (favorable, intermediate, and unfavorable), with median survivals of 10.2, 3.7, and 1.5 years for patients with zero, one, or more than one unfavorable prognostic factor, respectively.

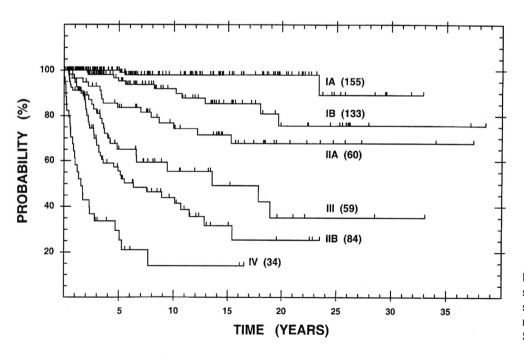

FIG. 19.1. Disease-specific survival by initial disease stage for 525 patients with mycosis fungoides treated at Stanford University.

Stage IV (Extracutaneous) Disease

Patients with extracutaneous disease have a poor prognosis. Appropriate management for these patients includes topical therapy suitable to the extent of skin involvement and, in addition, systemic therapy that may include biologicals as well as chemotherapy. Given the poor prognosis and lack of any truly effective treatment, these patients are also candidates for investigational therapies, such as monoclonal antibodies, vaccine trials, and stem cell transplants. Patients who have localized nodal disease as the only evidence of stage IV may benefit from treatment with involved-field irradiation (30 to 36 Gy) in addition to systemic management.

In a Stanford series, 77 patients either presented with or later developed extracutaneous (stage IV) disease (56 stage IVA, 21 stage IVB). The median survival of the 77 patients was only 13 months and was similar regardless of the extent of skin involvement (T2 vs. T3 vs. T4; $p = .69-.88$) or the site of extracutaneous disease (IVA vs. IVB) (28).

The outcome of 525 patients treated for mycosis fungoides at Stanford over a period of nearly 40 years is displayed in Figure 19.1.

REFERENCES

1. Weinstock MA, Horn JW. Mycosis fungoides in the United States. Increasing incidence and descriptive epidemiology. *JAMA* 1988;260:42–46.
2. Whittemore A, Holly E, Lee I, et al. Mycosis fungoides in relation to environmental exposures and immune response: a case-control study. *J Natl Cancer Inst* 1989;81:1560–1567.
3. Tuyp E, Burgoyne A, Aitchison T, et al. A case-control study of possible causative factors in mycosis fungoides. *Arch Dermatol* 1987;123:196–200.
4. Poiesz B. Detection and isolation of type C retrovirus particles from fresh and cultured lymphocytes of a patient with cutaneous T-cell lymphoma. *Proc Am Soc Clin Oncol* 1980;77:7415–7419.
5. Kim YH, Hoppe RT. Mycosis fungoides and the Sézary syndrome. *Semin Oncol* 1999;26:276–289.
6. Colby TV, Burke JS, Hoppe RT. Lymph node biopsy in mycosis fungoides. *Cancer* 1981;47:351–359.
7. Scheffer E, Meijer CJ, Van Vloten WA. Dermatopathic lymphadenopathy and lymph node involvement in mycosis fungoides. *Cancer* 1980;45:137–148.
8. Ralfkiaer E. Mycosis fungoides and Sézary syndrome. In: Jaffe ES, Harris NL, Stein H, et al., eds. *Pathology and genetics of tumours of haematopoietic and lymphoid tissues.* IARC Press: Lyon, 2001: 216–220.
9. Kern DE, Kidd PG, Moe R, et al. Analysis of T-cell receptor gene rearrangement in lymph nodes of patients with mycosis fungoides. Prognostic implications. *Arch Dermatol* 1998;134:158–164.
10. Van Doorn R, Scheffer E, Willemze R. Follicular MF, a distinct disease entity with or without associated follicular mucinosis. *Arch Dermatol* 2002;138:191–198.
11. Flaig MJ, Cerroni L, Schuhmann K, et al. Follicular mycosis fungoides. A histopathologic analysis of nine cases. *J Cutan Pathol* 2001;28:525–530.
12. Haghighi B, Smoller BR, LeBoit PE, et al. Pagetoid reticulosis (Woringer-Kolopp disease): an immunophenotypic, molecular, and clinicopathologic study. *Mod Pathol* 2000;13:502–510.
13. Scarisbrick JJ, Woolford AJ, Russell-Jones R, et al. Loss of heterozygosity on 10q and microsatellite instability in advanced stages of primary cutaneous T-cell lymphoma and possible association with homozygous deletion of PTEN. *Blood* 2000;95:2937–2942.
14. Inmaculada CN, Algara P, Mateo M, et al. p16(1NK4a) is selectively silenced in the tumoral progression of MF. *Lab Invest* 2002;82:123–132.
15. Vowels BR, Cassin M, Vonderheid EC, et al. Aberrant cytokine production by Sézary syndrome patients: cytokine secretion pattern resembles murine Th2 cells. *J Invest Dermatol* 1992;99:90–94.
16. Bernengo MG, Fierro MT, Novelli M, et al. Soluble interleukin-2 receptor in Sézary syndrome: its origin and clinical application. *Br J Dermatol* 1993;128:124.
17. Wasik MA, Vonderheid EC, Bigler RD, et al. Increased serum concentration of the soluble interleukin-2 receptor in cutaneous T-cell lymphoma. Clinical and prognostic implications. *Arch Dermatol* 1996;132:42–47.
18. Rook AH, Heald P. The immunopathogenesis of cutaneous T-cell lymphoma. *Hematol Oncol Clin North Am* 1995;9:997–1010.
19. Yoo EK, Cassin M, Lessin SR, et al. Complete molecular remission during biologic response modifier therapy for Sézary syndrome is associated with enhanced helper T type 1 cytokine production and natural killer cell activity. *J Am Acad Dermatol* 2001;45:208–216.
20. Kohler S, Jones CD, Warnke RA, et al. PCR-heteroduplex analysis of T-cell receptor gamma gene rearrangement in paraffin-embedded skin biopsies. *Am J Dermatopathol* 2000;22:321–327.
21. Cerroni L, Rieger E, Hodl S, et al. Clinicopathologic and immunologic features associated with transformation of mycosis fungoides to large-cell lymphoma. *Am J Surg Pathol* 1992;16:543–552.
22. Salhany KE, Cousar JB, Greer JP, et al. Transformation of cutaneous T cell lymphoma to large cell lymphoma: a clinicopathologic and immunologic study. *Am J Pathol* 1988;132:265–277.
23. Wieselthier JS, Koh HK. Sézary syndrome: diagnosis, prognosis, and critical review of treatment options. *J Am Acad Dermatol* 1990;22:381–401.
24. LeBoit PE. Granulomatous slack skin. *Dermatol Clin* 1994;12:375–389.
25. Salhany KE, Greer JP, Cousar JB, et al. Marrow involvement in cutaneous T-cell lymphoma. A clinicopathologic study of 60 cases. *Am J Clin Pathol* 1989;92:747–754.
26. Bunn PA, Lambert SI. Report of the Committee on Staging and Classification of Cutaneous T-Cell Lymphomas. *Cancer Treat Rep* 1979;63:725.
27. Sausville EA, Eddy JL, Makuch RW, et al. Histopathologic staging at initial diagnosis of mycosis fungoides and the Sézary syndrome. Definition of three distinctive prognostic groups. *Ann Intern Med* 1988; 109:372–382.
28. Kim YH, Liu HL, Mraz-Gernhard S, et al. Longterm outcome of 525 patients with mycosis fungoides and Sézary syndrome at Stanford: clinical prognostic factors and risks of disease progression and second cancer. *Arch Dermatol,* in press.
29. Kim YH, Bishop K, Varghese A, et al. Prognostic factors in erythrodermic mycosis fungoides and the Sézary syndrome [see comments]. *Arch Dermatol* 1995;131:1003–1008.
30. Kaye FJ, Bunn PA Jr, Steinberg SM, et al. A randomized trial comparing combination electron-beam radiation and chemotherapy with topical therapy in the initial treatment of mycosis fungoides. *N Engl J Med* 1989;321:1784–1790.
31. Ramsey D, Halperin P, Zeleniuch-Jacquotte A. Topical mechlorethamine therapy for early stage mycosis fungoides. *J Am Acad Dermatol* 1988;19:684–691.
32. Vonderheid EC, Tan ET, Kantor AF, et al. Long-term efficacy, curative potential, and carcinogenicity of topical mechlorethamine chemotherapy in cutaneous T cell lymphoma. *J Am Acad Dermatol* 1989;20:416–428.
33. Zackheim HS, Epstein EH Jr, Crain WR. Topical carmustine (BCNU) for cutaneous T cell lymphoma: a 15-year experience in 143 patients. *J Am Acad Dermatol* 1990;22:802–810.
34. Ramsay DL, Lish KM, Yalowitz CB, et al. Ultraviolet-B phototherapy for early-stage cutaneous T-cell lymphoma. *Arch Dermatol* 1992;128:931–933.
35. Resnik KS, Vonderheid EC. Home UV phototherapy of early mycosis fungoides: long-term follow-up observations in thirty-one patients. *J Am Acad Dermatol* 1993;29:73–77.
36. Honigsmann H, Brenner W, Rauschmeier W, et al. Photochemotherapy for cutaneous T cell lymphoma. A follow-up study. *J Am Acad Dermatol* 1984;10:238–245.
37. Abel EA, Sendagorta E, Hoppe RT, et al. PUVA treatment of erythrodermic and plaque-type mycosis fungoides. Ten-year follow-up study. *Arch Dermatol* 1987;123:897–901.
38. Herrmann JJ, Roenigk HH Jr, Hurria A, et al. Treatment of mycosis fungoides with photochemotherapy (PUVA): long-term follow-up. *J Am Acad Dermatol* 33:234–242, 1995.
39. Abel E. A, Sendagorta E, and Hoppe RT. Cutaneous malignancies and metastatic squamous cell carcinoma following topical therapies for mycosis fungoides. *J Am Acad Dermatol* 1986;14:1029–1038.
40. Breneman D, Duvic M, Kuzel T, et al. Phase 1 and 2 trial of bexaro-

tene gel for skin-directed treatment of patients with cutaneous T-cell lymphoma. *Arch Dermatol* 2002;138:325–332.

41. Hoppe RT, Wood GS, Abel EA. Mycosis fungoides and the Sézary syndrome: pathology, staging, and treatment. *Curr Probl Cancer* 1990;14:293–371.

42. Hoppe R. Total skin electron beam therapy in the management of mycosis fungoides. In: Vaeth J, Meyer J, eds. *Front Radiat Ther Oncol. The Role of High Energy Electrons in the Treatment of Cancer*, vol 25. Basel, Switzerland: S. Karger, 1991:80–89.

43. Jones GW, Tadros A, Hodson DI, et al. Prognosis with newly diagnosed mycosis fungoides after total skin electron radiation of 30 or 35 Gy. *Int J Radiat Oncol Biol Phys* 1994;28:839–845.

44. Karzmark CJ, Loevinger R, Steele RE, et al. A technique for large-field, superficial electron therapy. *Radiology* 1960;74:633–644.

45. Hoppe RT, Fuks Z, Bagshaw MA. Radiation therapy in the management of cutaneous T-cell lymphomas. *Cancer Treat Rep* 1979;63:625–632.

46. Antolak JA, Cundiff JH, Ha CS. Utilization of thermoluminescent dosimetry in total skin electron beam radiotherapy of mycosis fungoides. *Int J Radiat Oncol Biol Phys* 1998;40:101–108.

47. Asbell SO, Siu J, Lightfoot DA, et al. Individualized eye shields for use in electron beam therapy as well as low-energy photon irradiation. *Int J Radiat Oncol Biol Phys* 1980;6:519–521.

48. Tadros AA, Tepperman BS, Hryniuk WM, et al. Total skin electron irradiation for mycosis fungoides: failure analysis and prognostic factors. *Int J Radiat Oncol Biol Phys* 1983;9:1279–1287.

49. Tetenes PJ, Goodwin PN. Comparative study of superficial whole-body radiotherapeutic techniques using a 4-MeV nonangulated electron beam. *Radiology* 1977;122:219–226.

50. Podgorsak EB, Pla C, Pla M, et al. Physical aspects of a rotational total skin electron irradiation. *Med Phys* 1983;10:159–168.

51. Gerbi BJ, Khan FM, Deibel FC, et al. Total skin electron arc irradiation using a reclined patient position. *Int J Radiat Oncol Biol Phys* 1989;17:397–404.

52. Cox RS, Heck RJ, Fessenden P, et al. Development of total skin electron therapy at two energies. *Int J Radiat Oncol Biol Phys* 1990;18:659–669.

53. Desai KR, Pezner RD, Lipsett JA, et al. Total skin electron irradiation for mycosis fungoides: relationship between acute toxicities and measured dose at different anatomic sites. *Int J Radiat Oncol Biol Phys* 1988;15:641–645.

54. Price NM. Electron beam therapy. Effect on eccrine gland function in mycosis fungoides patients. *Arch Dermatol* 1979;115:1068–1070.

55. Price NM. Radiation dermatitis following electron beam therapy. An evaluation of patients ten years after total skin irradiation for mycosis fungoides. *Arch Dermatol* 1978;114:63–66.

56. Bunn PA Jr, Hoffman SJ, Norris D, et al. Systemic therapy of cutaneous T-cell lymphomas (mycosis fungoides and the Sézary syndrome). *Ann Intern Med* 1994;121:592–602.

57. Rosen ST, Foss FM. Chemotherapy for mycosis fungoides and the Sézary syndrome. *Hematol Oncol Clin North Am* 1995;9:1109–1116.

58. Grozoa P, Jones S, McKelvey E, et al. Combination chemotherapy for mycosis fungoides: a Southwest Oncology Group Study. *Cancer Treat Rep* 1979;63:647–653.

59. Braverman IM, Yager NB, Chen M, et al. Combined total body electron beam irradiation and chemotherapy for mycosis fungoides. *J Am Acad Dermatol* 1987;16:45–60.

60. Case DC Jr. Combination chemotherapy for mycosis fungoides with cyclophosphamide, vincristine, methotrexate, and prednisone. *Am J Clin Oncol* 1984;7:453–455.

61. Von Hoff D, Dahlberg S, Hartsock R, et al. Activity of fludarabine monophosphate in patients with advanced mycosis fungoides: a Southwest Oncology Group study. *J Natl Cancer Inst* 1990;82:1353–1355.

62. Mercieca J, Matutes E, Dearden C, et al. The role of pentostatin in the treatment of T-cell malignancies: analysis of response rate in 145 patients according to disease subtype. *J Clin Oncol* 1994;12:2588–2593.

63. Greiner D, Olsen EA, Petroni G. Pentostatin (2'-deoxycoformycin) in the treatment of cutaneous T-cell lymphoma. *J Am Acad Dermatol* 1997;36:950–955.

64. Zinzani PL, Baliva G, Magagnoli M, et al. Gemcitabine treatment in pretreated cutaneous T-cell lymphoma: experience in 44 patients. *J Clin Oncol* 2000;18:2603–2606.

65. Bigler RD, Crilley P, Micaily B, et al. Autologous bone marrow transplantation for advanced stage mycosis fungoides. *Bone Marrow Transplant* 1991;7:133–137.

66. Olavarria E, Child F, Woolford A, et al. T-cell depletion and autolo-

67. Edelson RL, Heald P, Perez M, et al. Photopheresis update. *Prog Dermatol* 1991;25:1–6.

68. Olsen EA, Rosen ST, Vollmer RT, et al. Interferon alfa-2a in the treatment of cutaneous T cell lymphoma. *J Am Acad Dermatol* 1989;20:395–407.

69. Vagna M, Papa G, Defazio D, et al. Interferon alpha-2a in cutaneous T-cell lymphoma. *Eur J Haematol* 1990;52:32–35.

70. Miller V, Benedetti F, Rigas J, et al. Initial clinical trial of a selective retinoid X receptor (RXR) ligand, 3-methyl TTNEB (LGD1069). *Proc Am Soc Clin Oncol* 1995;14:172.

71. Kessler JF, Jones SE, Levine N, et al. Isotretinoin and cutaneous helper T-cell lymphoma (mycosis fungoides). *Arch Dermatol* 1987;123:201–204.

72. Duvic M, Lemak NA, Redman JR, et al. Combined modality therapy for cutaneous T-cell lymphoma. *J Am Acad Dermatol* 1996;34:1022–1029.

73. Knobler RM, Trautinger F, Radaszkiewicz T, et al. Treatment of cutaneous T cell lymphoma with a combination of low-dose interferon alfa-2b and retinoids. *J Am Acad Dermatol* 1991;24:247–252.

74. Thomsen K, Hammar H, Molin L, et al. Retinoids plus PUVA (RePUVA) in mycosis fungoides, plaque stage. A report from the Scandinavian Mycosis Fungoides Group. *Acta Dermatol Venereol (Stockh)* 1989;69:217–222.

75. Jones G, McLean J, Rosenthal D, et al. Combined treatment with oral etretinate and electron beam therapy in patients with cutaneous T-cell lymphoma (mycosis fungoides and Sézary syndrome). *J Am Acad Dermatol* 1992;26:960–967.

76. Olsen EA, Duvic M, Martin A, et al. Pivotal phase III trial of two dose levels of DAB389IL-2 (Ontak) for the treatment of cutaneous T-cell lymphoma (CTCL). *J Invest Dermatol* 1998;110:678.

77. Kuzel TM, Roenigk HH Jr, Samuelson E, et al. Effectiveness of interferon alfa-2a combined with phototherapy for mycosis fungoides and the Sézary syndrome. *J Clin Oncol* 1995;13:257–263.

78. Quiros PA, Jones GW, Kacinski BM, et al. Total skin electron beam therapy followed by adjuvant psoralen/ultraviolet-A light in the management of patients with T1 and T2 cutaneous T-cell lymphoma (mycosis fungoides). *Int J Radiat Oncol Biol Phys* 1997;38:1027–1035.

79. Wilson LD, Licata A, Braverman IM, et al. Systemic chemotherapy and extracorporeal photochemotherapy to T3 and T4 cutaneous T-cell lymphoma patients who have achieved a complete response to total skin electron beam therapy. *Int J Radiat Oncol Biol Phys* 1995;32:987–995.

80. Chinn DM, Chow S, Kim YH, et al. Total skin electron beam therapy with or without adjuvant topical nitrogen mustard or nitrogen mustard alone as initial treatment of T2 and T3 mycosis fungoides. *Int J Radiat Oncol Biol Phys* 1999;15:951–958.

81. Dreno B. Roferon-A (interferon alpha 2a) combined with Tigason (etretinate) for treatment of cutaneous T cell lymphomas. *Stem Cells* 1993;11:269–275.

82. Winkler CF, Sausville EA, Ihde DC, et al. Combined modality treatment of cutaneous T cell lymphoma: results of a 6-year follow-up. *J Clin Oncol* 1986;4:1094–1100.

83. Roenigk HJ, Kuzel TM, Skoutelis A, et al. Photochemotherapy alone or combined with interferon alpha-2a in the treatment of cutaneous T-cell lymphoma. *J Invest Dermatol* 1990;95:198S–205S.

84. Herrmann JJ, Roenigk HH Jr, Honigsmann H. Ultraviolet radiation for treatment of cutaneous T-cell lymphoma. *Hematol Oncol Clin North Am* 1995;9:1077–1088.

85. Kim YH, Martinez G, Varghese A, et al. Management with topical nitrogen mustard in mycosis fungoides: update of the Stanford experience. *Arch Dermatol* submitted for publication, 2002.

86. Jones GW, Hoppe RT, Glatstein E. Electron beam treatment for cutaneous T-cell lymphoma. *Hematol Oncol Clin North Am* 1995;9:1057–1076.

87. Kim YH, Jensen RA, Watanabe GL, et al. Clinical stage IA (limited patch and plaque) mycosis fungoides. A long-term outcome analysis. *Arch Dermatol* 1996;132:1309–1313.

88. Kim YH, Chow S, Varghese A, et al. Clinical characteristics and long-term outcome of patients with generalized patch and/or plaque (T2) mycosis fungoides. *Arch Dermatol* 1999;135:26–32.

89. Ramsay DL, Zackheim HS. Topical treatment of early cutaneous T-cell lymphoma. *Hematol Oncol Clin North Am* 1995;9:1031–1056.

90. Abel EA, Deneau DG, Farber EM, et al. PUVA treatment of erythrodermic and plaque type mycosis fungoides. *J Am Acad Dermatol* 1981;4:423–429.

gous stem cell transplantation in the management of tumour stage mycosis fungoides with peripheral blood involvement. *Br J Haematol* 2001;114:624–631.

CHAPTER 20

Cutaneous B-Cell Lymphomas

Steven M. Horwitz, Lyn M. Duncan, Youn H. Kim, and Richard T. Hoppe

BACKGROUND AND DEFINITION

Primary cutaneous B-cell lymphomas are not distinct histologically from their nodal counterparts and may be defined simply as lymphomas with a B-cell phenotype that present in the skin and in which systemic or extracutaneous disease cannot be demonstrated, despite careful staging.

Some investigators have required that extracutaneous disease not be detected for a period of 3 to 6 months after diagnosis (1–5). Although a waiting period serves to minimize the inclusion of patients with undetected systemic lymphoma that has disseminated to the skin, it alters our understanding of the disease and is inconsistent with the approach to other extranodal lymphomas. The 3- to 6-month requirement includes no expectation for repeat staging studies to determine whether the patient remains free of extracutaneous disease. The impact of therapy is also ignored, because systemic treatment may decrease the likelihood that occult extracutaneous disease will become clinically apparent during the defined period. Finally, this requirement may bias series toward exclusion of an aggressive subset of cutaneous lymphoma that has a higher propensity for rapid growth and dissemination. This may create a false sense of the full spectrum of cutaneous lymphoma. Therefore, it is most logical to not incorporate an arbitrary time requirement into the definition and simply to require that there be no extracutaneous disease demonstrated by careful staging at presentation (6–8).

INCIDENCE AND EPIDEMIOLOGY

The incidence of skin lymphomas of all types is believed to be between 0.3 and 1.0 per 100,000 (9). Some reviews list skin as the second most common site of extranodal involvement after the gastrointestinal tract. However, if mycosis fungoides is excluded, the relative frequency of skin lymphomas is less and accounts for 2% of extranodal lymphomas in the Netherlands, 8% in the United States, and 11% in Denmark (9,10). In a series of stage I and II extranodal non-Hodgkin's lymphomas from the Princess Margaret Hospital, skin was involved in only 3.8% of cases, less frequently than the gastrointestinal tract, Waldeyer's ring, central nervous system, head and neck, thyroid, testis, and orbit (11). Primary cutaneous lymphomas are rare among children and not seemingly increased in the human immunodeficiency virus population (12).

The incidence of primary cutaneous B-cell lymphoma is even more challenging to define due to the small size of most series and significant geographic differences. A report from the Registry of the Dutch Cutaneous Lymphoma Working Group includes information on 626 evaluable patients with cutaneous lymphoma registered between 1986 and 1994. In this series, 19% had a B-cell phenotype (2). Similar frequencies of cutaneous B-cell lymphoma among all cutaneous lymphomas have been reported in series from India and Japan (13,14). The proportion of patients with a B-cell phenotype reported in series from the United States varies widely, likely due to referral patterns (15,16).

DIAGNOSIS

Appropriate biopsy of suspected sites of skin involvement is critical for the diagnosis and classification of cutaneous B-cell lymphoma. Whenever possible, one should perform a large incisional (elliptical) biopsy rather than small punch or shave biopsy. It is critical to obtain a sufficiently large specimen, including the subcutaneous fat, to facilitate optimal evaluation of the architecture, depth of involvement, and cell morphology. Fresh tissue may be needed for immunohistochemical or molecular studies to improve diagnostic accuracy. If the initial biopsy is of sufficient size, it may be bisected, or else one may take additional biopsies and preserve the frozen tissue for possible additional analyses. For optimal preservation (especially for molecular studies), freezing should be performed within 2 to 3 hours of tissue acquisition.

PATHOLOGY

Until recently, most cutaneous B-cell lymphomas were thought to represent dissemination of a primary nodal lymphoma. It is now known that there is a wide range of B-cell lymphomas that occur as primary tumors of the skin, and that not all of these tumors behave in an indolent fashion. The recognition of primary cutaneous B-cell lymphoma resulted in large part from the development of classification schemes that highlighted the similarities between extranodal lymphomas and their nodal counterparts.

In 1994, the Revised European-American Lymphoma classification scheme incorporated the ability of hematopathologists to recognize specific entities based on morphologic, immunologic, and genetic features (17). Subsequently, the European Organization for Research and Treatment of Cancer (EORTC) Cutaneous Lymphoma Program Project Group devised a classification scheme specifically for primary cutaneous lymphoma (2). The EORTC scheme used the foundation of the Revised European-American Lymphoma classification scheme while incorporating the clinical presentation and biologic behavior of these cutaneous tumors. One of the aims of the EORTC report was to define *primary cutaneous tumors* and draw attention to those lymphomas that have a clinical behavior that would not be predicted using classification schemes designed for nodal lymphomas. The World Health Organization (WHO) International Agency for Research and Cancer published the Pathology and Genetics of Tumours of Haematopoietic and Lymphoid Tissues that is the current template for the diagnosis of lymphoma (18).

In contrast to cutaneous T-cell lymphomas, most cutaneous B-cell lymphomas appear clinically similar to one another (19). There is some site predilection for various subtypes of tumors: follicular lymphomas more commonly arise on the scalp, marginal zone lymphomas usually occur on the trunk or upper extremities, and the aggressive large B-cell lymphoma often arises on the leg. Nevertheless, all types of cutaneous B-cell lymphoma can occur at any cutaneous site, such that the site of presentation is not particularly useful when approaching the diagnosis in an individual patient.

Cutaneous B-cell lymphomas are usually characterized by a dense superficial and deep dermal lymphoid infiltrate. Except for rare cases (20), the tumor cells spare the epidermis and are usually separated from it by a grenz zone of uninvolved papillary dermis (7,21–23). In the past, a top-heavy dermal infiltrate and lymphoid follicles were thought to support the diagnosis of benign reactive lymphoid infiltrate. It is now known that the two most common forms of cutaneous B-cell lymphoma, follicular lymphoma and low-grade B-cell lymphoma of mucosa-associated lymphoid tissue (MALT) type, are characterized by the presence of lymphoid follicles (23).

Immunohistochemical stains for κ and λ light chains may demonstrate light-chain restriction in these tumors. Because the responder cell in cutaneous inflammatory processes is usually a T cell, dense reactive T-cell infiltrates are frequently present in cutaneous B-cell lymphoma. Indeed, the neoplastic B cells may represent only a minor component in the lymphocytic infiltrate. On the other hand, an infiltrate composed of greater than 75% B lymphocytes strongly supports a diagnosis of cutaneous B-cell lymphoma.

The Southern blot method of detecting immunoglobulin gene rearrangements, although very specific, lacks sensitivity, and is of limited use in cases with a scant neoplastic infiltrate (24). If the tumor cells represent a small portion of the sample, molecular genetic techniques are likely to yield negative results. Polymerase chain reaction–based techniques are more sensitive and are reported to be positive in more than 50% of cases of cutaneous B-cell lymphoma (25,26). As with any diagnostic tool, the interpretation of the genetic results should be in the context of the clinical, histologic, and immunophenotypic findings of the case (27).

Follicular Lymphoma

Follicular lymphoma is likely the most common B-cell lymphoma to occur as a primary tumor of the skin and presents as multiple or solitary cutaneous nodules or plaques, often on the scalp or trunk (6,28–30). Follicular lymphoma is characterized by a dermal and subcuticular proliferation of centrocytes and centroblasts in a follicular pattern. Cutaneous follicular lymphomas are often low grade, with the centrocytes more plentiful than the centroblasts. This neoplastic proliferation of these follicle center cells often appears as expanded, irregularly shaped lymphoid follicles in the dermis (Color Plate 38). Occasionally, the neoplastic cells appear to spill out of the follicles and surround aggregates of benign small lymphocytes.

The neoplastic follicle center cells have a $CD10^{+/-}$, $CD5^-$, $CD43^-$, $bcl-6^+$ immunophenotype (31). In contrast to nodal follicular lymphomas, which are almost all $bcl-2^+$, cutaneous follicular lymphomas express the bcl-2 protein in less than 30% of cases (32,33). Bcl-2 protein is normally present on most T cells and B cells except for B cells in reactive follicle centers. Thus, bcl-2 may not be detected in cutaneous follicular lymphoma or in the follicle center cells in reactive follicles; a negative staining pattern of follicles does not exclude the diagnosis of follicular lymphoma. Likewise, primary cutaneous follicular lymphoma typically does not have the association of t(14;18) observed in nodal follicular lymphoma. Clonal rearrangement of immunoglobulin genes may be detected by polymerase chain reaction in most cases.

Marginal Zone Lymphoma

Marginal zone lymphomas are low-grade B-cell lymphomas in the skin that are classified by the recently published classification schemes as follows:

WHO: extranodal marginal zone lymphoma B-cell lymphoma of MALT
EORTC: marginal zone lymphoma (immunocytoma)

Primary cutaneous marginal zone lymphoma is a low-grade B-cell lymphoma that shares features with extranodal lymphomas of MALT type (7,34–39). There has been some controversy as to the terminology of these tumors; many observers consider that the cutaneous tumors termed *immunocytoma* may represent marginal zone lymphoma (2,19, 40–43). Marginal zone lymphoma likely represents the second most common form of primary cutaneous B-cell lymphoma after follicular lymphoma (21,30,44). Both follicular lymphoma and marginal zone lymphoma present a diagnostic challenge, because they share many histologic and clinical features with cutaneous lymphoid hyperplasia, a benign reactive proliferation of lymphocytes. Primary cutaneous marginal zone lymphoma is characterized by a dermal, and occasionally subcutaneous, proliferation of marginal zone (centrocyte-like) cells or monocytoid B cells, or both, often with zones of plasma cells. The neoplastic B cells surround reactive germinal centers, occasionally filling the interfollicular dermis (Color Plate 39) (7,23,35,37). Marginal zone B cells have small cleaved nuclei and variably abundant amphophilic cytoplasm. Zones of plasma cells, some with intranuclear inclusions of immunoglobulin termed *Dutcher bodies*, may be present. Marginal zone lymphomas arising at other extranodal sites characteristically display infiltration of glandular epithelium, termed *lymphoepithelial lesions*. This finding is less commonly observed in cutaneous marginal zone lymphoma and when present is observed in the epithelium of the hair follicles.

The presence of a diffuse proliferation of marginal zone cells, reactive germinal centers, zones of plasma cells, the absence of epidermal change, and a diffuse pattern of infiltration are more often seen in cutaneous marginal zone lymphoma than in cutaneous lymphoid hyperplasia (23). A dense infiltrate, bottom-heavy or top-heavy distribution, presence of eosinophils, and a grenz zone were seen equally often in both reactive and neoplastic disorders.

In cases with neoplastic plasma cells, light-chain restriction is identified with polyclonal antibodies against κ and λ light chains in formalin-fixed paraffin-embedded tissue. In this way, neoplastic plasma cells may be detected in 70% of cutaneous marginal zone lymphomas (7,23). Characteristically, in marginal zone lymphoma, one finds monotypic plasma cells and marginal zone cells in interfollicular regions, with polytypic follicle centers. The neoplastic marginal zone cells usually have a CD20+, CD22+, CD5−, CD10−, CD23−, Bcl-6 negative immunophenotype (31). Clonal rearrangement of immunoglobulin heavy-chain genes has been detected using polymerase chain reaction–based techniques in 70% of cutaneous marginal zone lymphomas (4).

Diffuse Large B-Cell Lymphoma

Large B-cell lymphoma may represent either diffuse large B-cell lymphoma or a grade III follicular lymphoma (e.g., a follicular lymphoma with a predominance of large B cells). The dermis is diffusely infiltrated by a proliferation of large B cells, predominantly centroblasts and immunoblasts, with scattered centrocytes (Color Plate 40). Epider-

motropism is absent, although the epidermis overlying the tumor may be ulcerated.

Monotypic surface immunoglobulin is identified along with a CD19+, CD20+, CD22+, CD79a+, CD5−/+, CD10−/+, bcl-2+ immunophenotype (45,46). Immunoglobulin genes have detectable clonal rearrangements; t(14:18) is usually absent (32,45,47).

Plasmacytoma

Extramedullary plasmacytoma of skin is an unusual neoplastic proliferation of plasma cells that occurs without underlying myeloma. These tumors have been reported to progress to myeloma (48–51). Plasmacytomas appear as a diffuse dermal nodule of mature plasma cells, multinucleate plasma cells, and occasional plasma cells with prominent eosinophilic macronucleoli and anaplastic nuclei. Monotypic expression of immunoglobulin light chains is observed; the plasma cells usually have a CD79a+, CD38+, CD43+, CD19−, CD20−, CD22− immunophenotype.

ISSUES IN CLASSIFICATION

The classification of primary cutaneous B-cell lymphoma is controversial. Two schemes that adopt fundamentally different approaches are in use. The WHO system classifies all of the hematopoietic and lymphoid tumors in a unified manner according to histologic and immunophenotypic characteristics, not differentiating between nodal or extranodal origin for identical histologic subtypes. The primary cutaneous B-cell lymphomas are defined according to their node-based counterparts. The most common entities include diffuse large B-cell lymphoma, follicular lymphoma, and extranodal marginal zone lymphoma of MALT type. The EORTC system is used exclusively for primary cutaneous lymphoma and includes immunophenotypic characteristics, clinical behavior, histologic appearance, and clinical presentation as components of its classification (2). The most common B-cell lymphomas in this system include two "indolent" diseases: follicle center cell lymphoma (which includes the WHO-follicular and most cases of WHO-diffuse large B-cell lymphomas) and immunocytoma/marginal zone lymphoma; and one "intermediate" prognosis disease: large B-cell lymphoma of the leg. Although this serves to emphasize the more indolent behavior of the majority of large B-cell lymphomas of the skin compared to other nodal or extranodal sites, knowledge of the natural history and clinical behavior of lymphomas at all sites is essential for proper clinical management. A separate classification system for each extranodal site cannot substitute for this knowledge.

PRESENTATION

Observations regarding the clinical presentation and behavior of cutaneous B-cell lymphomas are remarkably consistent over time. Long et al. reported 25 cases of malignant lymphoma of the skin in 1976, and Burke et al. published a series of 50 cases of cutaneous malignant lymphoma in 1981 (52,53). In these papers, they describe mostly solitary red or purplish nodules with rare ulceration. The disease had a strong predilection for the head and neck.

In the decade that followed, some reports described more specifically the cutaneous B-cell lymphomas. Patients often were in their 50s or 60s, with asymptomatic solitary or localized red to violaceous papules or nodules, with infrequent ulceration or epidermal changes, usually confined to the head and neck or trunk (6,28,54,55). The clinical appearance of these lesions was somewhat different from that of the cutaneous T-cell lymphomas, which were more clinically heterogeneous and more likely to present as plaques with epidermal changes, including ulceration.

The pace of development of the lesions of cutaneous B-cell lymphoma is variable and may range from months to years before a diagnosis is established (3,8). In general, lesions with an indolent histology (follicular or marginal zone) or with a low percentage of Ki-67[+] neoplastic cells tend to evolve over a longer period than those with a large-cell histology or a high proportion of Ki-67[+] cells.

Follicular Lymphoma

The follicular lymphomas of the WHO classification are included in the broader group of follicle center cell lymphomas in the EORTC system. In a series of patients from Stanford, follicular lymphomas accounted for 31% of cutaneous B-cell lymphoma (56), but they represented only 15% of cases of primary cutaneous B-cell lymphoma in the Scottish and Newcastle Lymphoma Group database (57).

Patients with follicular lymphoma typically present in the sixth or seventh decade of life, with a median age at diagnosis of 49 to 63 years (5,28,54,57–60). No children have been reported in any of these series. There is a male preponderance, with the ratio as high as 3:1 (6,19,28,54), although in one series, there was no gender predisposition (60).

Cutaneous follicular lymphoma most commonly presents on the head and neck and rarely the trunk, with the legs notably spared (Color Plate 41) (5,28,54,57–59,61). Lesions appear as erythematous nodules or tumors that develop slowly over months to years and rarely ulcerate (5,28,57–59,61). Papules and nodules may coalesce to form erythematous plaques occasionally, and these flatter plaques may predate the nodules by as long as 3 years (6,54). Although some patients may present with disseminated cutaneous disease, a solitary tumor or small group of papules or nodules is more common (5,28,54,57–59).

Marginal Zone Lymphoma

In the WHO classification, the cutaneous marginal zone lymphomas are included as extranodal marginal zone lymphomas. In the EORTC classification, marginal zone lymphomas are classified together with immunocytomas as an *indolent disease*. The median age of presentation for marginal zone lymphomas is generally in the late 40s or early 50s, with a wide range of 25 to 93 years (7,22,41,62). No consistent gender predilection has been reported (7,41). Marginal zone lymphomas represented 10% of cases of primary cutaneous B-cell lymphoma in a Dutch series (2), 19% of primary cutaneous B-cell lymphoma at Stanford University (56), and more than 50% of cutaneous B-cell lymphoma in a Danish series (63).

Patients with cutaneous marginal zone lymphoma present with erythematous papules, nodules, or tumors. Ulceration is rare; however, subcutaneous lesions are more often present than in follicular lymphoma (2,7,22,62,64). Marginal zone lymphomas can occur at any site but have a predilection for the extremities—particularly the upper extremities—and the trunk is also a common site of involvement (Color Plate 42) (2,7,22,62,64). Solitary, localized, and generalized presentations are all common (7,22,62,64). Lesions may present acutely or may be present for years before diagnosis (7).

Diffuse Large B-Cell Lymphoma

Primary cutaneous diffuse large B-cell lymphoma is one of the most common primary cutaneous B-cell lymphomas. In the EORTC system, these lymphomas are classified as either follicle center cell lymphoma or diffuse large-cell lymphoma of the leg, depending simply on the site of presentation. The follicle center cell lymphomas accounted for 71% of 118 cutaneous B-cell lymphomas in the Dutch Cutaneous Lymphoma Working Group registry (2). In the Stanford series, 42% of primary cutaneous B-cell lymphomas were diffuse large B-cell lymphomas (56), and in the Danish series, 33% of primary cutaneous B-cell lymphomas were diffuse large B-cell lymphomas (63).

The reported age range for this disease is similar to that for nodal diffuse large B-cell lymphoma, with a median in the mid to late 60s and a range of 18 to 92 years (1,3,6,65–67). Gender ratios vary in different series, but in general, there appears to be no gender preference (68).

The majority of patients with diffuse large B-cell lymphoma present with solitary or localized disease, including 83% of the 145 patients reported by Grange et al. (1,3,6,8,65,66). Like the other cutaneous lymphomas, diffuse large B-cell lymphoma may present as a red or violaceous nodule or tumor and less commonly as deep plaques and rarely with ulceration (Color Plate 43) (1,3,6,8,65,66). There may be adjacent papules or surrounding plaques, but an isolated plaque presentation is rare (1,8). Sites of presentation include the lower extremities followed by the trunk, head and neck region, and upper extremities (Color Plate 44) (1,3,6,65,66).

Cutaneous Plasmacytoma

Cutaneous plasmacytoma may occur in the setting of multiple myeloma or, more rarely, as a primary cutaneous tumor. In the context of myeloma, cutaneous plasmacytoma would not be considered a primary cutaneous lymphoma. However, extramedullary plasmacytoma may arise rarely as an isolated primary cutaneous lesion and accounts for 4% of extramedullary plasmacytomas. These lesions present as single or multiple erythematous nodules or plaques on any skin site (51,69). Ulceration and necrosis can be seen with large masses. There is a 4:1 male predominance (51,69). The prognosis is quite variable, with a long indolent course for some and rapid local or systemic progression to multiple myeloma in others (2,51,69). Patients with solitary lesions appear to have a favorable prognosis (2,69). However, patients with multiple lesions often develop multiple myeloma or other extramedullary plasmacytomas despite careful initial evaluation to exclude extracutaneous disease (51,69,70). Treatments with excision, radiation, and various chemotherapy regimens have been used, with long remissions generally confined to patients with solitary lesions (51,69).

T-Cell Rich B-Cell Lymphoma

T-cell rich B-cell lymphoma is an aggressive non-Hodgkin's lymphoma defined as a variant of diffuse large-cell lymphoma in the WHO classification (71). Nodal T-cell rich B-cell lymphoma has a propensity to involve the spleen and bone marrow and has a prognosis similar to other diffuse large-cell lymphomas. There are rare cutaneous presentations in which it seems to behave as other primary cutaneous diffuse large B-cell lymphomas. It may present as single or multiple cutaneous nodules or plaques on the head, trunk, or upper extremities (72,73) and also may present as erythema nodosum (74). The prognosis appears similar to other primary cutaneous diffuse large B-cell lymphomas, with a more aggressive course than observed with cutaneous follicular lymphoma or marginal zone lymphoma. In one series, five of six patients with disease confined to the skin were treated effectively with surgery, psoralen plus ultraviolet light of A wave length, or chlorambucil, although one patient with extracutaneous disease died despite chemotherapy (75).

Posttransplant Lymphoproliferative Disorders

Posttransplant lymphoproliferative disorders are often aggressive Epstein-Barr virus–induced lymphomas that arise secondary to the chronic immune suppression used to prevent graft rejection after organ transplantation. Posttransplant proliferative disorders usually have a B-cell phenotype but can rarely be T-cell diseases. These lymphomas have a predilection for extranodal sites, and some may arise as primary cutaneous lymphomas. Presentations include single or multiple nodules and plaques, often with ulceration (76). Posttransplant lymphoproliferative disorder often responds to a decrease in immunosuppression. In the skin, they may be treated effectively by excision, radiation, or both, although more aggressive treatments have also been described (76).

STAGING EVALUATION

Once a diagnosis of cutaneous B-cell lymphoma has been established, complete clinical staging is indicated. This should include a careful history and physical examination, with particular attention to the entire skin and lymphatic system. In patients with cutaneous marginal zone lymphoma, in which there are rare reports of concurrent involvement at other MALT sites, physical examination of the conjunctivae, parotids, thyroid, and breasts, as well as questions to elicit symptoms of occult gastrointestinal involvement, should be included (34,77). Laboratory evaluation should include complete blood counts and serum chemistries to evaluate kidney and liver function as well as measurement of serum lactate dehydrogenase. Routine imaging studies should include computed tomography of the chest, abdomen, and pelvis. The neck should be imaged as well for disease that presents in the head or neck region. Nuclear imaging, such as positron emission tomography and gallium scanning, is not considered routine but may prove to be valuable and require further clinical assessment (78,79). Additional evaluations should be guided by signs or symptoms that raise suspicion for involvement in other sites. A bone marrow biopsy also should be performed; however, given the infrequent involvement by large diffuse B-cell lymphoma in the absence of other extracutaneous disease, a unilateral biopsy is likely sufficient (30,80).

The staging system traditionally used for non-Hodgkin's lymphoma of all sites is the Ann Arbor system (81). This system was originally designed for Hodgkin's disease and has inadequacies with regard to extranodal lymphomas, particularly cutaneous lymphomas. The Ann Arbor system defines *stage IE* as localized involvement of a single extralymphatic organ or site. *Stages IIE and IIIE* imply lymph node as well as extralymphatic involvement and, therefore, do not fit into the definition of *primary cutaneous lymphoma*. *Stage IV* is defined as diffuse or disseminated involvement of one or more extralymphatic organ or tissue, with or without associated lymph node involvement. Certainly, by the Ann Arbor criteria, a solitary skin nodule represents stage IE disease or, more precisely, stage IE_D. The difficulty in cutaneous lymphomas relates to the concept of "diffuse or disseminated involvement" of the skin as a designation for stage IV. The arbiters of the Ann Arbor system likely never envisioned this problem, but varied interpretation makes comparison among series difficult.

Does disseminated involvement of the skin simply imply more than a single isolated lesion, or scattered lesions in multiple anatomic regions, or disease beyond certain dimensions? Various authors have addressed this issue differently. Some simply define *localized cutaneous disease* as stage IE and *generalized cutaneous involvement* as stage IV, without further defining *localized* (1,15,19,67,68). Others have defined localized or *circumscribed* disease to include an overall diameter of involvement smaller than 15 cm (1), restriction to "one anatomic site" (8), involvement of less than 10% of the total skin surface (67), or an overall disease surface area less than 100 cm². Other interpretations have been to define all patients with skin disease only (localized or disseminated) as stage IE (82) or to differentiate localized versus disseminated disease based on the number of body regions involved (8,83). Another alternative is to use a system based on tumor-node-metastases criteria, similar to that of mycosis fungoides (84). There may be prognostic importance to such distinction, because two of these studies showed a worse outcome for patients with "disseminated disease" (1,68). However, in another study, cutaneous dissemination did not adversely affect prognosis (67). Currently, there is no consistent interpretation of these definitions.

At the moment, it is appropriate to be consistent with other non-Hodgkin's lymphomas and use the Ann Arbor system for primary cutaneous lymphomas but to be clear regarding definitions for stage IE versus stage IV. A reasonable approach is to combine the concepts of size and anatomic distribution of disease. For example, a solitary lesion of any size would be stage IE. Multiple lesions encompassing an area smaller than or equal to 100 cm^2 and limited to one anatomic region (head or neck, an arm, anterior aspect of the trunk, posterior aspect of the trunk including the buttocks, a leg) also would be stage IE. Multiple lesions encompassing an area larger than 100 cm^2 or involving multiple anatomic regions would be stage IV. Further clarification may be added by including all details incorporated into the Ann Arbor system. For example, stage IV$_D$+$_M$– designates a patient with generalized cutaneous disease and a negative bone marrow biopsy.

PROGNOSTIC AND PREDICTIVE FACTORS

Beginning in the early 1980s, reports of a generally favorable prognosis for patients with lymphomas limited to the skin began to appear in the literature (19,52,80). General observations included a more favorable prognosis for patients who had involvement of the skin only versus skin plus extracutaneous disease; a propensity for relapse to occur primarily in the skin; and a good survival rate, even after relapse, with few patients ultimately dying from lymphoma.

More recent series have been larger and have examined variables of histology, stage, and so on in a more rigorous fashion. Grange et al. analyzed 158 patients with non–mycosis fungoides cutaneous lymphoma from the registry of the French Study Group on Cutaneous Lymphomas (68). Univariate analysis revealed a less successful outcome for those with a larger number, greater diameter, or generalized distribution of lesions; large B-cell lymphoma of the leg; CD30 negativity large T-cell lymphoma; elevated lactate dehydrogenase; or the presence of B symptoms. Age was predictive of overall survival but not disease-specific survival. Multivariate analysis found the EORTC classification and generalized versus localized disease to correlate with disease-specific survival. Others have also identified an elevated lactate dehydrogenase (1,83), disseminated cutaneous disease (1,65,67), and extracutaneous progression (1,52,80) as adverse prognostic factors.

Willemze et al. were the first to report a uniquely poor prognosis associated with large-cell lymphoma presenting

on the leg (6). Three of four patients with lesions on the lower extremities died; however, all of these patients were elderly, and one of the deaths was not due to lymphoma. Based on this observation as well as a subsequent study of 18 patients with lymphoma of the leg (46), the EORTC classification system proposed that *large B-cell lymphoma of the leg* be defined as a unique entity (2). This observation has not been confirmed in all studies (3,65,66).

The largest series examining prognostic factors for cutaneous large B-cell lymphoma was reported by Grange and colleagues, who analyzed 145 patients from the French Study Group on Cutaneous Lymphoma and the Dutch Cutaneous Lymphoma Working Group (8). A univariate analysis for disease-specific survival identified age older than 75 years, recent development of skin lesion (shorter than 10 months), presentation on the leg, disseminated skin lesions, elevated lactate dehydrogenase, and round cell morphology as negative predictors. Multivariate analysis identified only site of presentation and round cell morphology to be significant. The 5-year disease-specific survival for patients with disease presenting on the leg was 52%, compared to 94% for the remainder of cases. Further analysis of the patients with lymphoma involving the leg showed that all the deaths were among patients with multiple lesions. The 5-year survival was 100% among the 11 patients with solitary lesions.

TREATMENT

The selection of therapy for the primary cutaneous B-cell lymphomas is dependent on the histologic subtype of lymphoma and the stage. Assuming that staging has been thorough, as described earlier, patients may have either localized (stage IE$_D$) or disseminated skin involvement in the absence of extracutaneous disease (stage IV$_D$+$_M$–). Patients who have stage IIE or IIIE disease would not be considered to have primary cutaneous lymphoma and should be treated in a fashion analogous to the nodal-based variants of these diseases.

Radiation Therapy

Reports on the use of radiation therapy for patients with primary cutaneous B-cell lymphoma rarely provide sufficient detail to evaluate the variables of histology and radiotherapy dose, fractionation, and field size (85–87). Based on the data in the literature for both primary cutaneous and nodal-based B-cell lymphomas, as well as the authors' personal experiences, the following general recommendations can be made:

1. Cutaneous lesions should be treated with adequate margins, including at least 1 cm beyond the estimated depth of penetration of the disease. In most instances, electrons in the range of 6 to 9 MeV provide an ideal depth-dose distribution. However, due to the skin-sparing effects of low-energy electrons, up to 1 cm of tissue-equivalent bolus may be required. Particularly thick tumorous lesions may require higher-energy electrons,

and lesions on some curved surfaces may be treated most effectively with opposed tangential photon beams in the 4- to 6-MV range, again with the use of bolus.

2. The field size should be adequate to include the primary lesion and a 2-cm margin of apparently uninvolved skin. Clinical judgment may mandate narrower margins in certain situations—for example, in sites adjacent to sensitive structures, such as the eyelids.

3. The prescribed radiation dose depends on the histology and size of the lesion and may be modified depending on the rapidity of response. For diffuse large B-cell lymphoma, a dose of 36 Gy is likely sufficient if there has been a gross total excision, or a dose in the range of 40 to 44 Gy if there has simply been an incisional biopsy. For follicular lymphomas and marginal zone lymphomas, a dose of 30 Gy after total excision or doses in the range of 30 to 36 Gy generally suffice. Rare patients with cutaneous plasmacytoma should be treated to a dose of 40 Gy after complete excision, or 40 to 50 Gy if there is residual disease. Fractionation is usually at a rate of 1.8 to 2.0 Gy per day, 5 days per week. However, on skin surfaces that are more tolerant, such as the trunk or extremities, larger fractions may be used if cosmesis is not an issue.

Chemotherapy

There is little information regarding the optimal selection of chemotherapy for patients with cutaneous B-cell lymphoma. For indolent histologies, such as follicular lymphoma and marginal zone lymphoma, it is important to know that these patients have a good prognosis despite a propensity to relapse. For these indolent diseases, chemotherapy has been most often reserved for patients with disseminated cutaneous involvement. Various regimens have been used, including single-agent chlorambucil; CVP (cyclophosphamide, vincristine, and prednisone); CHOP [cyclophosphamide, hydroxydaunomycin, Oncovin (vincristine), prednisone]; cyclophosphamide, vincristine, procarbazine, and prednisone; and methotrexate, bleomycin, doxorubicin, cyclophosphamide, vincristine, and dexamethasone, all with reasonable activity. In a series of patients with cutaneous B-cell lymphoma by Rijlarsdam et al., CHOP provided superior freedom from relapse compared to cyclophosphamide, Oncovin (vincristine), and prednisone (COP)—100% versus 18%—but survival was not significantly different (86).

Brice et al. for the Groupe d'Etude des Lymphomes de L'Adulte analyzed 49 patients with primary cutaneous large-cell lymphoma (both B and T phenotypes), a subset of patients enrolled on a prospective trial evaluating polychemotherapy for high-grade lymphoma (67). Seventeen patients younger than 70 years received an anthracycline-containing regimen, either doxorubicin, cyclophosphamide, bleomycin, and prednisone or methotrexate, bleomycin, doxorubicin, cyclophosphamide, vincristine, and dexamethasone. The seven patients older than 70 years received either CVP or cyclophosphamide, teniposide, vincristine, and prednisone, with or without pirarubicin. Both relapse-free and overall survival were better in the group treated with anthracyclines. However, the median age was only 46 years (range, 18 to 65 years) in the anthracycline group and 73 years (range, 71 to 83 years) in the group treated with a non–anthracycline-containing regimen.

Fierro et al. evaluated their experience with chemotherapy in 46 patients with primary cutaneous B-cell lymphoma (88). Thirty-six were treated with COP and ten with CHOP. Eighty-nine percent of patients achieved a complete response. Fifteen relapses occurred, all in COP-treated patients. However, overall survival was not different based on treatment regimen. The authors recommended CHOP due to the lower relapse rates.

Based on these data alone, it is difficult to make a definitive recommendation. However, if one considers the large experience with combination chemotherapy for node-based lymphomas, it is reasonable to consider an anthracycline regimen as standard when systemic treatment is indicated for diffuse large B-cell lymphoma. However, other regimens, such as CVP or even single-agent chlorambucil, may suffice when systemic management is required for follicular and marginal zone lymphomas.

Surgery

Although there are no large series of excision only as a local therapy for primary cutaneous B-cell lymphoma, occasional patients in many series have been treated by surgery alone (5,7,57,58,61). This strategy has been used more frequently for patients with indolent histologies, and the results have been quite variable (5,58). However, despite frequent relapse in some series, the overall survival for indolent histologies is not compromised (5,30,57,58,60). Surgery alone has been used less often for large-cell lymphoma (1,3,66). Joly et al. reported frequent relapses in these patients and recommended against surgery as sole therapy for patients with large B-cell histology (1).

Rituximab

Primary cutaneous B-cell lymphomas almost universally express the CD20 antigen (2,64,69). Marginal zone lymphomas may have variable CD20 expression depending on the degree of plasmacytoid differentiation, and plasmacytomas, which have a mature plasma cell phenotype, do not generally express CD20 (2,4,30,64,69). The anti-CD20 monoclonal antibody rituximab is efficacious with minimal toxicity, both as a single agent for indolent systemic B-cell lymphomas and in combination with chemotherapy for more aggressive systemic B-cell lymphomas (89,90). There are anecdotal reports of its activity administered intralesionally or intravenously in primary cutaneous B-cell lymphoma (91,92). The indolent nature of many primary cutaneous B-cell lymphomas and the very favorable safety profile of single-agent rituximab compared to other systemic therapies make this an appealing agent for future study.

Interferon

Interferon-α, more commonly used in cutaneous T-cell lymphomas, has been used anecdotally with success in primary cutaneous B-cell lymphoma. A patient with low-grade cutaneous B-cell lymphoma, follicle center cell type, associated with *Borrelia burgdorferi*, was treated successfully with intralesional interferon α-2b, and another patient with marginal zone lymphoma was rendered disease free by intralesional interferon α-2a (93,94). In the large series by Santucci, two patients with multiple skin lesions received interferon as primary therapy (19). Both responded, one achieving a complete response.

Steroids

Rare patients with low-grade histology have been treated with mixed results with corticosteroids (19,30,59). The number of these patients is too small to support its use in anything but a palliative setting.

Antibiotics

Anecdotal reports exist of successful treatment of cutaneous marginal zone lymphomas with antibiotics (22,93). One patient treated with ceftriaxone and two patients treated with excision followed by unspecified antibiotics maintained complete responses in these reports (22,93).

PROGNOSIS

All reports of outcome in the literature are retrospective and many include patients with both B- and T-cell phenotypes. Treatments are usually variable, with very few reports limited to patients treated in a consistent fashion. There are no phase III randomized clinical trials testing different approaches to therapy. Historically, the majority of patients with localized primary cutaneous lymphoma have been treated by biopsy or excision, followed by local irradiation, with some patients also receiving chemotherapy (8,15,19,52,54,56,80,82,85–87,95). The general conclusion of these reports has been that patients with localized primary cutaneous B-cell lymphoma are often treated effectively by local radiation, and that relapses occur preferentially in the skin, rather than in extracutaneous sites. Patients with follicular lymphoma or marginal zone lymphoma, in particular, have an excellent prognosis.

Esche and Fitzpatrick (82) reported 43 patients with all histologies who had disease limited to the skin. Treatments were variable. Patients with stage IE_D or IV_D+_M- disease had a 10-year actuarial survival of 57%. The relapse-free survival was 65% for patients with small-bulk (smaller than 2.5 cm) and 20% for patients with larger-bulk disease. Among 11 patients treated by excision alone, it was unsuccessful for four in the initial skin site, one in a distant skin site, and two in extracutaneous sites. Among 22 patients treated by excision or biopsy plus radiation (25 to 35 Gy in 2 to 3 weeks),

it failed for none in the initial skin site, six in distant skin sites, and three in nodes or viscera. Among five patients treated with chemotherapy, it was unsuccessful for three in the original skin site, one in a distant skin site, and two in extracutaneous sites. Overall, 15 of 18 patients who relapsed had a component of relapse in the skin.

Santucci and associates reported on 72 patients with stage IE_D+ and 11 with stage IV_D+_M- primary cutaneous B-cell lymphoma (19). Among 65 patients with follow-up data, the majority (68%) was treated with radiation therapy alone and the remainder with a variety of therapies. Twenty-two patients relapsed, but only two of the relapses were in extracutaneous sites. Because many patients were treated with radiotherapy for relapse and continued to have an indolent course of disease, the authors concluded that local radiotherapy was the appropriate management for primary cutaneous B-cell lymphoma. Piccinno and associates (85) came to a similar conclusion based on their experience with 31 cases of cutaneous B-cell lymphoma.

Rijlaarsdam and colleagues reported outcome for 55 patients with primary cutaneous B-cell lymphoma (86). Forty patients were treated with radiotherapy and 15 with chemotherapy, usually CHOP. Among the 40 patients treated with radiation therapy, all achieved a complete response. Thirty-four of these patients had disease involving the head and neck or trunk, and four (12%) relapsed, in three cases in the skin. However, four of six patients with initial involvement of the leg relapsed, three with a systemic component of disease. Only three of 40 patients initially treated with radiotherapy died secondary to progressive lymphoma, and all of these had initial disease on the lower extremities.

Among the 15 patients treated with chemotherapy, 14 achieved a complete response. Thirteen of these patients had disease involving the head and neck or trunk, and five (38%) relapsed. In four of the five, relapse was in the skin. The relapse rate was much greater after COP chemotherapy (100%) than after CHOP (18%). Two of these patients had initial involvement of the leg, one did not achieve a complete response, and the other was disease free. There was one death from lymphoma among the 15 patients treated with chemotherapy. These authors concluded that localized primary cutaneous B-cell lymphoma of the head and neck or trunk was most reasonably treated with local radiation but recommended that patients with disease involving the legs or multiple anatomic regions of the skin be treated with CHOP.

Grange and associates from the French Study Group on Cutaneous Lymphomas and the Dutch Cutaneous Lymphoma Working Group reported the prognostic factors and outcome of treatment among 145 patients with primary cutaneous diffuse large B-cell lymphoma (8). Among 97 patients with disease limited to sites other than the legs, 11% developed extracutaneous disease, and 6% died of lymphoma. Among 48 patients with disease involving the legs, 50% developed extracutaneous disease, and 42% died of lymphoma. However, patients with lymphoma of the leg that was limited to a single lesion (11 of 48 patients) had a 5-year survival rate of 100%.

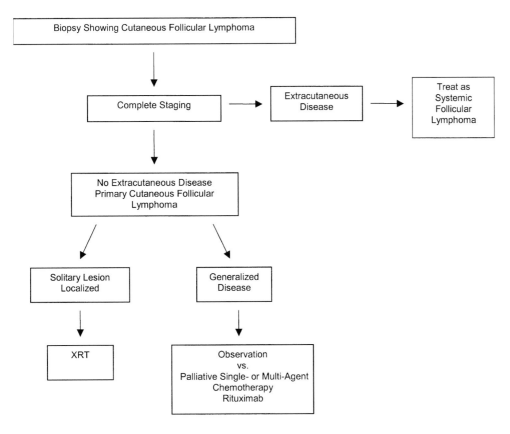

FIG. 20.1. Treatment of follicular cutaneous lymphoma. XRT, radiation therapy.

The 5-year disease-specific survival rates were 94% for patients with non–leg disease and 52% for those with leg disease. Based on their observations, they recommended radiotherapy as primary management for patients with localized disease of non-leg sites or solitary lesions of the leg, radiotherapy or combination chemotherapy for patients with generalized lesions in non-leg sites, and combination chemotherapy for patients with multiple lesions of the legs.

Follicular Lymphoma

There are occasional reports that provide outcome data for individual histologic subtypes of cutaneous B-cell lymphoma. Series of follicular lymphoma demonstrate an almost uniformly good prognosis. In two early series, the survival was 100% (28,54). All patients were treated with radiation alone or in combination with other therapies. A large proportion of patients in those series relapsed (63% to 67%), but the high relapse rate did not predict for poor survival. In more recent series of follicular lymphoma using the WHO criteria, 97% of 92 patients were alive, and two of the three deaths were unrelated to lymphoma (5,57–60). Nearly all patients had radiation or excision, or both, as their primary therapy, and relapse was not affected by type of therapy (Fig. 20.1).

Diffuse Large B-Cell Lymphoma

Joly and associates reported on 27 patients with stage IE cutaneous lymphoma, 23 of whom had a B-cell phenotype. Nine of 14 patents with intermediate- or high-grade lymphoma treated with radiation alone experienced a relapse, and in seven of these nine cases, it was in the skin outside of the initially involved site. In contrast, five of seven patients with intermediate- or high-grade lymphoma treated with ACVB combination chemotherapy (doxorubicin, cyclophosphamide, vindesine, bleomycin, and prednisolone) remained disease free (20 to 53 months). The conclusion of these investigators was that radiation therapy alone was inadequate for patients with intermediate- or high-grade primary cutaneous B-cell lymphoma and that chemotherapy was probably indicated.

Sarris and associates reported the outcome of treatment for 29 patients with primary cutaneous B-cell lymphoma (15). Among 19 with diffuse large B-cell lymphoma, all four patients treated with radiotherapy alone relapsed, versus only four of 14 patients treated with doxorubicin-based chemotherapy, with or without radiotherapy. Despite the small number of patients in their series treated with radiotherapy alone, they concluded that such treatment was inappropriate. Nine patients with follicular lymphoma were treated, usually with combined-modality therapy. Their 10-year progression-free survival was 89%, and overall survival was 70% (Fig. 20.2).

Marginal Zone Lymphoma

The prognosis for marginal zone lymphoma appears to be equally good. In four published series that included 60 patients, there was only a single death from lymphoma, also in a patient who had an extracutaneous relapse (7,22,41,62).

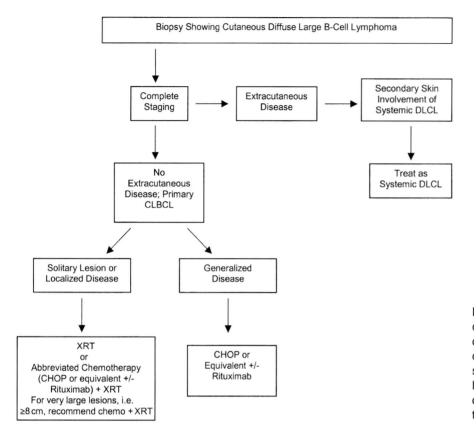

FIG. 20.2. Treatment of cutaneous diffuse large B-cell lymphoma. CHOP, cyclophosphamide, hydroxydaunomycin, Oncovin (vincristine), and prednisone; CLBCL, cutaneous large B-cell lymphoma; DLCL, diffuse large-cell cutaneous lymphoma; XRT, radiation therapy.

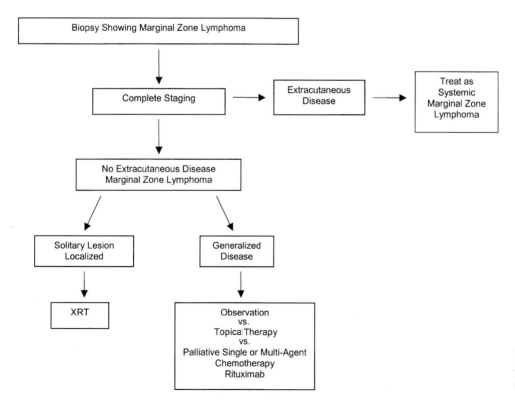

FIG. 20.3. Treatment of marginal zone cutaneous lymphoma. XRT, radiation therapy.

Patients were treated primarily by excision or radiation and occasionally with both. Relapse rates ranged from 19% to 71%, almost exclusively in the skin, although systemic relapse or relapse at other MALT sites has been reported (7,22,41,62,77). With the exception of the study from Denmark by Grobaek et al., no case of histologic transformation was reported for any patients with indolent cutaneous B-cell lymphoma, either follicular or marginal zone. In that series, three of 12 patients with marginal zone lymphoma underwent histologic transformation to a diffuse large-cell type (63). All three of these patients died of lymphoma. Two of these three patients had generalized skin disease at the time of initial diagnosis, and the authors postulate that this may be an adverse risk factor (Fig. 20.3).

REFERENCES

1. Joly P, Vasseur E, Esteve E, et al. Primary cutaneous medium and large cell lymphomas other than mycosis fungoides. An immunohistological and follow-up study on 54 cases. French Study Group for Cutaneous Lymphomas. Br J Dermatol 1995;132:506–512.
2. Willemze R, Kerl H, Sterry W, et al. EORTC classification for primary cutaneous lymphomas: a proposal from the Cutaneous Lymphoma Study Group of the European Organization for the Research and Treatment of Cancer. Blood 1997;90:354–371.
3. Fernandez-Vazquez A, Rodriguez-Peralto JL, Martinez MA, et al. Primary cutaneous large B-cell lymphoma: the relation between morphology, clinical presentation, immunohistochemical markers, and survival. Am J Surg Pathol 2001;25:307–315.
4. Cerroni L, Signoretti S, Hofler G, et al. Primary cutaneous marginal zone B-cell lymphoma: a recently described entity of low-grade malignant cutaneous B-cell lymphoma [see comments.]. Am J Surg Pathol 1997;21:1307–1315.
5. Mirza I, Macpherson N, Paproski S, et al. Primary cutaneous follicular lymphoma: an assessment of clinical, histopathologic, immunophenotypic, and molecular features. J Clin Oncol 2002;20:647–655.
6. Willemze R, Meijer CJLM, Sentis HJ, et al. Primary cutaneous large cell lymphomas of follicular center cell origin. J Am Acad Dermatol 1987;16:518.
7. Bailey EM, Ferry JA, Harris NL, et al. Marginal zone lymphoma (low-grade B-cell lymphoma of mucosa-associated lymphoid tissue type) of skin and subcutaneous tissue. Am J Surg Pathol 1996;8:1011–1023.
8. Grange F, Bekkenk MW, Wechsler J, et al. Prognostic factors in primary cutaneous large B-cell lymphomas: a European multicenter study. J Clin Oncol 2001;19:3602–3610.
9. Burg G, Kempf W, Haeffner A. Cutaneous lymphomas. Curr Probl Dermatol 1997;9:144–171.
10. Cavalli F. The non-Hodgkin's lymphomas. In: Mcgrath IT, ed. Extranodal lymphomas. London: Arnold, 1997:1007–1027.
11. Sutcliffe SB, Gospodarowicz M. Localized extranodal lymphomas. In: Keating A, Armitage J, Burnett A, et al., eds. Haematological Oncology. Cambridge, 1992:189–222.
12. de la Luz Orozco-Covarrubias M, Tamayo-Sanchez L, Duran-McKinster C, et al. Malignant cutaneous tumors in children. Twenty years of experience at a large pediatric hospital. J Am Acad Dermatol 1994; 30:243–249.
13. George R, Bhuvana S, Nair S, et al. Clinicopathological profile of cutaneous lymphomas—a 10 year retrospective study from south India. Indian J Cancer 1999;36:109–19.
14. Ishiji T, Takagi Y, Niimura M. Cutaneous lymphomas in Tokyo: analysis of 62 cases in a dermatology clinic. Int J Dermatol 2001;40:37–40.
15. Sarris AH, Braunschweig I, Medeiros LJ, et al. Primary cutaneous non-Hodgkin's lymphoma of Ann Arbor stage I: preferential cutaneous relapses but high cure rate with doxorubicin-based therapy. J Clin Oncol 2001;19:398–405.
16. Zackheim HS, Vonderheid EC, Ramsay DL, et al. Relative frequency of various forms of primary cutaneous lymphomas. J Am Acad Dermatol 2000;43:793–796.
17. Harris NL, Jaffe ES, Stein H, et al. A revised European-American classification of lymphoid neoplasms: a proposal from the International Lymphoma Study Group. Blood 1994;84:1361–1392.
18. Jaffe ES, Sander CA, Flaig MJ. Cutaneous lymphomas: a proposal for a unified approach to classification using the R.E.A.L./WHO Classification. Ann Oncol 2000;11(Suppl 1):17–21.
19. Santucci M, Pimpinelli N, Arganini L. Primary cutaneous B-cell lymphoma: a unique type of low-grade lymphoma. Clinicopathologic and immunologic study of 83 cases. Cancer 1991;67:2311–2326.
20. Chui CT, Hoppe RT, Kohler S, et al. Epidermotropic cutaneous B-cell lymphoma mimicking mycosis fungoides. J Am Acad Dermatol 1999; 41:271–274.
21. de la Fouchardiere A, Balme B, Chouvet B, et al. Primary cutaneous marginal zone B-cell lymphoma: a report of 9 cases. J Am Acad Dermatol 1999;41:181–188.
22. Cerroni L, Signoretti S, Hofler G, et al. Primary cutaneous marginal zone B-cell lymphoma: a recently described entity of low-grade malignant cutaneous B-cell lymphoma. Am J Surg Pathol 1997;21:1307–1315.
23. Baldassano MF, Bailey EM, Ferry JA, et al. Cutaneous lymphoid hyperplasia and cutaneous marginal zone lymphoma: comparison of morphologic and immunophenotypic features. Am J Surg Pathol 1999;23:88–96.
24. Bottaro M, Berti E, Biondi A, et al. Heteroduplex analysis of T-cell receptor gamma gene rearrangements for diagnosis and monitoring of cutaneous T-cell lymphomas. Blood 1994;83:3271–3278.
25. Veelken H, Wood GS, Sklar J. Molecular staging of cutaneous T-cell lymphoma: evidence for systemic involvement in early disease. J Invest Dermatol 1995;104:889–894.
26. Wood GS. Using molecular biologic analysis of T-cell receptor gene rearrangements to stage cutaneous T-cell lymphoma. Arch Dermatol 1998;134:221–223.
27. Wood GS, Haeffner A, Dummer R, et al. Molecular biology techniques for the diagnosis of cutaneous T-cell lymphoma. Dermatol Clin 1994;12:231–241.
28. Garcia CF, Weiss LM, Warnke RA, et al. Cutaneous follicular lymphoma. Am J Surg Pathol 1986;10:454.
29. Nagatani T, Miyazawa M, Matsuzaki T, et al. Cutaneous B-cell lymphoma-a clinical, pathological and immunohistochemical study. Clin Exp Dermatol 1993;18:530–536.
30. Bailey EM, Harris NL, Ferry JA, et al. Cutaneous B-cell lymphoma at the Massachusetts General Hospital, 1972–1994. Lab Invest 1996;74:39A.
31. de Leval L, Harris NL, Longtine J, et al. Cutaneous B-cell lymphomas of follicular and marginal zone types: use of Bcl-6, CD10, Bcl-2, and CD21 in differential diagnosis and classification. Am J Surg Pathol 2001;25:732–741.
32. Cerroni L, Volkenandt M, Rieger E, et al. Bcl-2 protein expression and correlation with the interchromosomal 14;18 translocation in cutaneous lymphomas and pseudolymphomas. J Invest Dermatol 1994;102:231–235.
33. Triscott JA, Ritter JH, Swanson PE, et al. Immunoreactivity for bcl-2 protein in cutaneous lymphomas and pseudolymphomas. J Cutan Pathol 1995;22:2.
34. Bailey EM, Ferry JA, Harris NL, et al. Primary low-grade B-cell lymphoma of skin and soft tissue resembling lymphoma of mucosa-associated lymphoid tissue type. J Cutan Pathol 1993;20:532.
35. Harris NL. Extranodal lymphoid infiltrates and mucosa-associated lymphoid tissue (MALT). A unifying concept [editorial]. Am J Surg Pathol 1991;15:879–884.
36. Harris NL. Low-grade B-cell lymphoma of mucosa-associated lymphoid tissue and monocytoid B-cell lymphoma. Related entities that are distinct from other low-grade B-cell lymphomas [editorial; comment]. Arch Pathol Lab Med 1993;117:771–775.
37. Isaacson P, Wright DH. Malignant lymphoma of mucosa-associated lymphoid tissue. A distinctive type of B-cell lymphoma. Cancer 1983;52:1410–1416.
38. Mattia AR, Ferry JA, Harris NL. Breast lymphoma. A B-cell spectrum including the low grade B-cell lymphoma of mucosa associated lymphoid tissue. Am J Surg Pathol 1993;17:574–587.
39. Pelstring RJ, Essel JH, Kurtin PJ, et al. Diversity of organ site involvement among malignant lymphomas of mucosa-associated tissues. Am J Clin Pathol 1991;96:738–745.
40. Duncan L, LeBoit P. Are primary cutaneous immunocytoma and marginal zone lymphoma the same disease? [editorial]. Am J Surg Pathol 1997;21:1368–372.

41. LeBoit PE, McNutt NS, Reed JA, et al. Primary cutaneous immuno-cytoma: a B-cell lymphoma that can easily be mistaken for cutaneous lymphoid hyperplasia. *Am J Surg Pathol* 1994;18:969–978.

42. Pimpinelli N, Santucci M. The skin-associated lymphoid tissue-related B-cell lymphomas. *Semin Cutan Med Surg* 2000;19:124–129.

43. Kerl H, Cerroni L. Primary B-cell lymphomas of the skin. *Ann Oncol* 1997;8(Suppl 2):29–32.

44. Pimpinelli N, Santucci M, Mori M, et al. Primary cutaneous B-cell lymphoma: a clinically homogeneous entity? *J Am Acad Dermatol* 1997;37:1012–1016.

45. Geelen FA, Vermeer MH, Meijer CJ, et al. Bcl-2 protein expression in primary cutaneous large B-cell lymphoma is site-related. *J Clin Oncol* 1998;16:2080–2085.

46. Vermeer MH, Geelen FA, van Haselen C, et al. Primary cutaneous large B-cell lymphomas of the legs. A distinct type of cutaneous B-cell lymphoma with an intermediate prognosis. Dutch Cutaneous Lymphoma Working Group. *Arch Dermatol* 1996;132:1304–1308.

47. Delia D, Borrello MG, Berti E, et al. Clonal immunoglobulin rearrangements and normal T-cell receptor, bcl-2 and c-myc in primary cutaneous B-cell lymphomas. *Cancer Res* 1989;49:4901–4905.

48. Chang YT, Wong CK. Primary cutaneous plasmacytomas. *Clin Exp Dermatol* 1994;19:177–180.

49. Llamas-Martin R, Postigo-Llorente C, Vanaclocha-Sebastian F, et al. Primary cutaneous extramedullary plasmacytoma secreting lambda IgG. *Clin Exp Dermatol* 1993;18:351–355.

50. Tuting T, Bork K. Primary plasmacytoma of the skin. *J Am Acad Dermatol* 1996;34:386–390.

51. Wong KF, Chan JK, Li LP, et al. Primary cutaneous plasmacytoma—report of two cases and review of the literature. *Am J Dermatopathol* 1994;16:392–397.

52. Burke JS, Hoppe RT, Cibull ML, et al. Cutaneous malignant lymphoma: a pathologic study of 50 cases with clinical analysis of 37. *Cancer* 1981;47:300–310.

53. Long JC, Mihm MC, Qazi R. Malignant lymphoma of the skin: a clinicopathologic study of lymphoma other than mycosis fungoides. *Cancer* 1976;38:1282–1296.

54. Pimpinelli N, Santucci M, Bosi A, et al. Primary cutaneous follicular centre-cell lymphoma—a lymphoproliferative disease with favourable prognosis. *Clin Exp Dermatol* 1989;14:12–19.

55. Santucci M, Pimpinelli N, Arganini L. Primary cutaneous B-cell lymphoma: a unique type of low-grade lymphoma. Clinicopathologic and immunologic study of 83 cases. *Cancer* 1991;67:2311–2326.

56. Mraz-Gernhard S, Horwitz S, Kim YH, et al. The clinical spectrum of cutaneous B-cell lymphomas (CBCL): excellent prognosis for patients with disease limited to the skin. American Society of Hematology, 42nd annual meeting. San Francisco, December 2000.

57. Goodlad JR, Krajewski AS, Batstone PJ, et al. Primary cutaneous follicular lymphoma: a clinicopathologic and molecular study of 16 cases in support of a distinct entity. *Am J Surg Pathol* 2002;26:733–741.

58. Cerroni L, Arzberger E, Putz B, et al. Primary cutaneous follicle center cell lymphoma with follicular growth pattern. *Blood* 2000;95:3922–3928.

59. Bergman R, Kurtin PJ, Gibson LE, et al. Clinicopathologic, immunophenotypic, and molecular characterization of primary cutaneous follicular B-cell lymphoma. [see comments]. *Arch Dermatol* 2001;137:432–439.

60. Franco R, Fernandez-Vazquez A, Mollejo M, et al. Cutaneous presentation of follicular lymphomas. *Mod Pathol* 2001;14:913–919.

61. Franco R, Fernandez-Vazquez A, Rodriguez-Peralto JL, et al. Cutaneous follicular B-cell lymphoma: description of a series of 18 cases. *Am J Surg Pathol* 2001;25:875–883.

62. Rijlaarsdam JU, van der Putte S, Berti E, et al. Cutaneous immunocytomas: a clinicopathologic study of 26 cases. *Histopathology* 1993;23:117–125.

63. Gronbaek K, Moller PH, Nedergaard T, et al. Primary cutaneous B-cell lymphoma: a clinical, histological, phenotypic and genotypic study of 21 cases. *Br J Dermatol* 2000;142:913–923.

64. LeBoit PE, McNutt NS, Reed JA, et al. Primary cutaneous immuno-cytoma. A B-cell lymphoma that can easily be mistaken for cutaneous lymphoid hyperplasia. *Am J Surg Pathol* 1994;18:969–978.

65. Kurtin PJ, DiCaudo DJ, Habermann TM, et al. Primary cutaneous large cell lymphomas. Morphologic, immunophenotypic, and clinical features of 20 cases. *Am J Surg Pathol* 1994;18:1183–1191.

66. Hembury TA, Lee B, Gascoyne RD, et al. Primary cutaneous diffuse large B-cell lymphoma: a clinicopathologic study of 15 cases. *Am J Clin Pathol* 2002;117:574–580.

67. Brice P, Cazals D, Mounier N, et al. Primary cutaneous large-cell lymphoma: analysis of 49 patients included in the LNH87 prospective trial of polychemotherapy for high grade lymphomas. Groupe d'Etude des Lymphomes de l'Adulte. *Leukemia* 1998;12:213–219.

68. Grange F, Hedelin G, Joly P, et al. Prognostic factors in primary cutaneous lymphomas other than mycosis fungoides and the Sezary syndrome. The French Study Group on Cutaneous Lymphomas. *Blood* 1999;93:3637–3642.

69. Kazakov DV, Belousova IE, Muller B, et al. Primary cutaneous plasmacytoma: a clinicopathological study of two cases with a long-term follow-up and review of the literature. *J Cutan Pathol* 2002;29:244–248.

70. Chan JK, Li LP, Yau TK, et al. Multiple primary cutaneous plasmacytomas. *Am J Dermatopathol* 1994;16:392–397.

71. Gatter K, Warnke R. Diffuse large B-cell lymphoma. In: Jaffe E, Harris N, Stein H, et al., eds. *World Health Organization: Pathology and Genetics of Tumors of Hematopoetic and Lymphoid Tissues.* Lyon: IARC Press, 2001:171–174.

72. Arai E, Sakurai M, Nakayama H, et al. Primary cutaneous T-cell-rich B-cell lymphoma. *Br J Dermatol* 1993;129:196–200.

73. Sander CA, Kaudewitz P, Kutzner H, et al. T-cell-rich B-cell lymphoma presenting in skin. A clinicopathologic analysis of six cases. *J Cutan Pathol* 1996;23:101–108.

74. Ribera JM, Vaquero M, Tuset E, et al. Erythema nodosum as a presenting feature of T-cell-rich B-cell lymphoma. *Ann Hematol* 1995;70:107–108.

75. Sander CA, Kaudewitz P, Schirren CG, et al. Immunocytoma and marginal zone B-cell lymphoma (MALT lymphoma) presenting in skin—different entities or a spectrum of disease? *J Cutan Pathol* 1996;23:59.

76. McGregor JM, Yu CC, Lu QL, et al. Posttransplant cutaneous lymphoma. Somatic mutations in c-myc intron I cluster in discrete domains that define protein binding sequences. *J Am Acad Dermatol* 1993;29:549–554.

77. Sangueza OP, Sanchez Yus E, Furio V. Primary cutaneous immunocytoma: report of an unusual case with secondary spreading to the gastrointestinal tract. *J Cutan Pathol* 1997;24:176–182.

78. Tsuyuguchi N, Hakuba A, Okamura T, et al. PET for diagnosis of malignant lymphoma of the scalp: comparison of [11C]methyl-L-methionine and [18F]fluoro-2-deoxyglucose. *J Comput Assist Tomogr* 1997;21:590–593.

79. Assassa GS, Siegel ME, Chen DC, et al. Ga-67 uptake in cutaneous B-cell lymphoma. *Clin Nucl Med* 1994;19:614–616.

80. Joly P, Charlotte F, Leibowitch M, et al. Cutaneous lymphomas other than mycosis fungoides: follow-up study of 52 patients. *J Clin Oncol* 1991;9:1994–2001.

81. Carbone PP, Kaplan HS, Musshoff K, et al. Report of the Committee on Hodgkin's Disease Staging Classification. *Cancer Res* 1971;31:1860–1861.

82. Esche B, Fitzpatrick P. Cutaneous malignant lymphoma. *Int J Radiat Oncol Biol Phys* 1986;12:2111–2115.

83. Visco C, Medeiros LJ, Jones D, et al. Primary cutaneous non-Hodgkin's lymphoma with aggressive histology: inferior outcome is associated with peripheral T-cell type and elevated lactate dehydrogenase, but not extent of cutaneous involvement. *Ann Oncol* 2002;13:1290–1299.

84. Burg G, Kerl H, Schmoeckel C. Differentiation between malignant B-cell lymphomas and pseudolymphomas of the skin. *J Dermatol Surg Oncol* 1984;10:271–275.

85. Piccinno R, Caccialanza M, Berti E, et al. Radiotherapy of cutaneous B-cell lymphomas: our experience in 31 cases. *Int J Radiat Oncol Biol Phys* 1993;27:385–389.

86. Rijlaarsdam JU, Toonstra J, Meijer OW, et al. Treatment of primary cutaneous B-cell lymphomas of follicle center cell origin: a clinical follow-up study of 55 patients treated with radiotherapy or polychemotherapy. *J Clin Oncol* 1996;14:549–555.

87. Kirova YM, Piedbois Y, Le Bourgeois JP. Radiotherapy in the management of cutaneous B-cell lymphoma. Our experience in 25 cases. *Radiother Oncol* 1999;52:15–18.

88. Fierro MT, Quaglino P, Savoia P, et al. Systemic polychemotherapy in the treatment of primary cutaneous lymphomas: a clinical follow-up study of 81 patients treated with COP or CHOP. *Leuk Lymphoma* 1998;31:583–588.

89. Coiffier B, Lepage E, Briere J. CHOP chemotherapy plus rituximab compared with CHOP alone in elderly patients with diffuse large B-cell lymphoma. *N Engl J Med* 2002;346:235–242.

90. McLaughlin P, Grillo-Lopez AJ, Link BK, et al. Rituximab chimeric anti-CD20 monoclonal antibody therapy for relapsed indolent lymphoma: half of patients respond to a four-dose treatment program. *J Clin Oncol* 1998;16:2825–2833.
91. Soda R, Costanzo A, Cantonetti M, et al. Systemic therapy of primary cutaneous B-cell lymphoma, marginal zone type, with rituximab, a chimeric anti-CD20 monoclonal antibody. *Acta Derm Venereol* 2001;81:207–208.
92. Paul T, Radny P, Krober SM, et al. Intralesional rituximab for cutaneous B-cell lymphoma. *Br J Dermatol* 2001;144:1239–1243.
93. Kutting B, Bonsmann G, Metze D, et al. Borrelia burgdorferi-associated primary cutaneous B cell lymphoma: complete clearing of skin lesions after antibiotic pulse therapy or intralesional injection of interferon alfa-2a. *J Am Acad Dermatol* 1997;36:311–314.
94. Zenone T, Catimel G, Barbet N, et al. Complete remission of a primary cutaneous B cell lymphoma treated with intralesional recombinant interferon alpha-2a. *Eur J Cancer* 1994;30A:246–247.
95. Eich H, Eich D, Stutzer H, et al. Radiotherapy of primary cutaneous B-cell lymphoma—a clinical followup study of 35 patients [abstract]. *Ann Oncol* 2002;13:134.

CHAPTER 21

CD30⁺ Cutaneous Lymphoproliferative Disease (Anaplastic Large-Cell Lymphoma) and Lymphomatoid Papulosis

Marshall E. Kadin, Howard L. Liu, Youn H. Kim, and Richard T. Hoppe

DEFINITION

CD30⁺ cutaneous lymphoproliferative diseases comprise a spectrum of disorders that arise in the skin from activated lymphocytes that express the CD30 antigen. *Primary cutaneous lymphomas* are defined as lymphomas without concurrent extracutaneous disease at the time of diagnosis, having a distinctive biology, clinical behavior, and prognosis that differ from those of corresponding nodal lymphomas. The skin lesions of CD30⁺ cutaneous lymphoproliferative disease range from papules and nodules up to 2 cm in lymphomatoid papulosis to tumors in anaplastic large-cell lymphoma (Color Plate 45). Borderline lesions are those that cannot be readily classified as *lymphomatoid papulosis* or *anaplastic large-cell lymphoma* (Color Plate 45). Spontaneous regression of skin lesions is the rule in lymphomatoid papulosis and may occur in up to 25% of cases in anaplastic large-cell lymphoma. Despite the spontaneous regression of lymphomatoid papulosis, the lesions appear malignant histologically. Hence, the original description of lymphomatoid papulosis by Macaulay as histologically malignant-clinically benign (1968). Because of this description of lymphomatoid papulosis as a recurrent proliferation of CD30⁺ lymphocytes in the skin, it was recognized that lymphomatoid papulosis is closely related to CD30⁺ cutaneous lymphomas and that a clear line of demarcation between the two entities cannot be easily drawn, leading to the concept of a continuous spectrum of CD30⁺ cutaneous lymphoproliferative disease (1,110).

Systemic anaplastic large-cell lymphoma originates in lymph nodes in most cases and often is positive for anaplastic lymphoma kinase, which confers a growth advantage on the lymphoma cells (2). Extranodal disease occurs in 40% of systemic anaplastic large-cell lymphoma, and the skin is the most common site (3,4). The skin lesions of systemic anaplastic large-cell lymphoma can be difficult if not impossible to distinguish from primary cutaneous anaplastic large-cell lymphoma. A thorough clinical evaluation, including imaging studies and staining for anaplastic lymphoma kinase, which is positive in most systemic anaplastic large-cell lymphoma and negative in most primary cutaneous anaplastic large-cell lymphomas, allows the distinction to be made in most cases.

FREQUENCY

Willemze estimated the frequency of CD30⁺ cutaneous lymphoproliferative disease in Europe to be approximately one-fifth of cutaneous T-cell lymphomas (5). Fink-Puches et al. determined CD30⁺ cutaneous lymphoproliferative disease to be approximately one-fifth as common as mycosis fungoides in a series of primary cutaneous lymphoma collected in Graz, Austria from 1960 to 1999 (6). Based on the 1980 census, the period prevalence rate of lymphomatoid papulosis was estimated to be 1.9 per 1,000,000 population (2.1 for male and 1.6 for female patients) for Massachusetts and 1.2 per 1,000,000 population (1.2 for both male and female patients) for Pennsylvania in a series of patients from the United States (7). Our estimate of 1.2 to 1.9 cases per 1,000,000 population should be considered a minimum estimate of the prevalence rate in the United States because of the difficulty of diagnosis and general lack of familiarity with these disorders among most dermatologists, oncologists, and pathologists. We predict that the incidence and prevalence of CD30⁺ cutaneous lymphoproliferative disease will appear to increase in the future as these disorders become more readily recognized.

Epidemiology

CD30⁺ cutaneous lymphoproliferative disease has been reported in all races and geographic regions. Lymphomatoid papulosis has a peak incidence in the fifth decade but also occurs in children, young adults, and the elderly. Only two

(3.5%) of the 57 patients with lymphomatoid papulosis in our initial epidemiologic study were black. This percentage was lower than the national average of blacks (12.3%) or the percentage of blacks (7.2%) in the two major contributing states (Massachusetts and Pennsylvania) (7). No overrepresentation of patients either born in or having lived in or traveled to endemic areas of human T-cell leukemia virus type 1 infection (e.g., Japan, the Caribbean basin, the southeastern United States, Central and South America, and equatorial Africa) was found in this selected sample of patients with lymphomatoid papulosis. Once diagnosed, lymphomatoid papulosis may persist as a life-long affliction whether or not treatment is administered.

Our first epidemiologic study revealed that lymphomatoid papulosis patients have an exaggerated response to mosquito bites compared with control subjects (7). Our recent study of children with lymphomatoid papulosis found a high frequency of atopy in this population group (101). Both studies suggest that lymphomatoid papulosis patients have exaggerated immune responses to environmental antigens.

Some series indicate that males are affected more often than females (6,8), whereas the Lymphomatoid Papulosis Registry at Beth Israel Deaconess Medical Center in Boston, Massachusetts, which contains data for more than 400 patients, indicates a slight female predominance for lymphomatoid papulosis. Patients with primary cutaneous anaplastic large-cell lymphoma tend to be slightly older, with a peak incidence in the sixth decade. There is a male predominance, with a male to female ratio of 1.5:1 to 3:1. Pediatric cases of primary cutaneous anaplastic large-cell lymphoma are less common than adult cases and should be distinguished from secondary skin involvement in systemic anaplastic large-cell lymphoma, which carries a poor prognosis (8–10).

Etiology

The etiology of CD30+ cutaneous lymphoproliferative disease is unknown. Early reports of a virus associated with the etiology of CD30+ cutaneous anaplastic large-cell lymphoma or lymphomatoid papulosis (11) have not been confirmed (12). The most interesting feature of lymphomatoid papulosis is its strong association with mycosis fungoides (13–15) and Hodgkin's disease (15–21). These diseases usually appear after recurrent lesions of lymphomatoid papulosis, but approximately 10% of patients with lymphomatoid papulosis have a prior diagnosis of mycosis fungoides or Hodgkin's disease (8). Interestingly, more than 20 patients with coexistent mycosis fungoides and Hodgkin's disease have been reported, indicating that mycosis fungoides, Hodgkin's disease, and lymphomatoid papulosis are all somehow related (22–24). A case in which all three diseases occurred in the same patient has been reported, leading to the hypothesis that a genetic event in an early precursor lymphocyte can link the three disorders (15). CD30 is a candidate gene for alteration in the lymphocyte precursor. Recent studies have revealed a polymorphic microsatellite repressor element in the CD30 promoter that can regulate CD30 expression (25,26). The transcription factor Sp1 and members of the Ets family induce CD30 expression. Sp1 is known to be upregulated by viral infection, so it is possible that viral infection of lymphocytes causes overexpression of CD30, which plays a role in the pathogenesis of Hodgkin's lymphoma (27). High expression of CD30 results in activation and nuclear translocation of nuclear factor (NF)-κB and survival of Hodgkin's cells (27,28), and NF-κB is constitutively overexpressed in tumor cells of mycosis fungoides (29). Thus, it is possible that the risk of developing Hodgkin's disease, lymphomatoid papulosis, and mycosis fungoides can be genetically determined, which is a subject for further research.

Diagnosis

Morphology

The histology of CD30+ cutaneous lymphoproliferative disease varies according to the size and age of the lesion (30). In general, lymphomatoid papulosis lesions contain relatively few CD30+ cells surrounded by many inflammatory cells, whereas anaplastic large-cell lymphoma contains more numerous CD30+ cells, with inflammatory cells concentrated at the periphery of the lesion. The infiltrate in lymphomatoid papulosis tends to remain in the superficial papillary and reticular dermis (Color Plate 46). In contrast, the infiltrate in anaplastic large-cell lymphoma extends throughout the dermis into the underlying subcutis.

Lymphomatoid Papulosis

Early lesions of lymphomatoid papulosis contain a predominantly perivascular and superficial dermal infiltrate of atypical lymphoid cells and smaller lymphocytes (30,31) (Color Plate 46). The vascular endothelium in the superficial capillaries and venules contain plump activated endothelial cells. Neutrophils accumulate and extravasate into the dermis, a feature that is highly characteristic of lymphomatoid papulosis and useful in making the diagnosis (32) (Color Plate 47). Eventually, neutrophils infiltrate the overlying epidermis, which then breaks down and ulcerates centrally. The epidermis does not show vacuolar change or necrosis of individual keratinocytes as in pityriasis lichenoides, which is a useful differential diagnostic feature (33,34). Blood vessels may become engorged with erythrocytes, but extravasation of erythrocytes is not prominent and contrasts lymphomatoid papulosis with pityriasis lichenoides, in which purpura is a constant feature (33). A vasculitis per se with fibrinoid change in the blood vessels is uncommon in lymphomatoid papulosis (33,34). Fully developed lesions of lymphomatoid papulosis contain abundant inflammatory cells, especially neutrophils, eosinophils, and small lymphocytes (tumor-infiltrating lymphocytes) (Color Plate 47). These cells are admixed with and infiltrate between the larger atypical lymphoid cells. The atypical lymphoid cells can resemble immunoblasts, with basophilic cytoplasm and conspicuous nucleoli (22,30). Some atypical cells appear bi- or multinucleated and can closely resemble Reed-Sternberg cells of Hodgkin's disease (Color Plate 47). Some of the atypical cells have irregular or convoluted nuclei, resembling Sézary cells or cerebriform mononuclear cells in mycosis fungoides (Color Plate 47). Individual lesions can have both cerebriform mononuclear cells and Reed-Sternberg cells, with forms in between, suggesting a transition between the two types of cells.

Mitoses are frequent in lymphomatoid papulosis and often appear atypical, with increased numbers of chromosomes. Apoptotic figures can be seen but usually are not numerous and, therefore, do not readily explain the spontaneous regression of lesions in lymphomatoid papulosis.

There are three principal histologic types of lymphomatoid papulosis (35) (Color Plate 47). Type A, the most common type, resembles Hodgkin's disease because of the predominance of large cells with prominent nucleoli, sometimes with Reed-Sternberg–like cells, surrounded by numerous inflammatory cells. Mitoses are frequent. Type B resembles mycosis fungoides because of a predominance of cerebriform mononuclear cells, few inflammatory cells, and some degree of epidermotropism. Mitoses are infrequent. Type B lesions are distinguished from mycosis fungoides by clinical features of spontaneous regression of papules rather than persistent patches or plaques, as seen in mycosis fungoides. Some patients have both lymphomatoid papulosis and mycosis fungoides, and in these individuals, distinction of lymphomatoid papulosis type B from mycosis fungoides may be difficult, if not controversial (13,14). Type C resembles large-cell lymphoma (anaplastic large-cell lymphoma) because of large clusters or sheets of anaplastic cells and few inflammatory cells. However, the distinction from anaplastic large-cell lymphoma depends on the superficial nature of the infiltrate, sparing of the subcutis, and the spontaneous regression of the lesion or lesions.

Anaplastic Large-Cell Lymphoma

In anaplastic large-cell lymphoma, large anaplastic cells predominate (Color Plate 48). Epidermotropism is not prominent, but some large cells can be found in the epidermis in a minority of cases. There may be a gradation of cell types in which cells with convoluted nuclei are predominant in the epidermis and papillary dermis, and larger immunoblasts and Reed-Sternberg–like cells are found in the reticular dermis and subcutis. Mitotic figures are frequent. Apoptosis may be more prominent in anaplastic large-cell lymphoma than in lymphomatoid papulosis. The cytology of tumor cells can vary from anaplastic with prominent nucleoli, frequent multinuclearity, and Reed-Sternberg–like cells to pleomorphic irregular nuclei without prominent nucleoli (9,36) (Color Plate 48). Less often, the predominant cell has a regular oval to round nucleus. Rarely, cells with convoluted nuclei predominate. Tumor cells can be found surrounding and sometimes within blood vessels. A distinguishing feature of anaplastic large-cell lymphoma is the extension of tumor cells into the subcutis.

Inflammatory cells are less numerous than in lymphomatoid papulosis and are concentrated around the periphery. However, some cases have a marked neutrophil infiltrate (37). The epidermis may become ulcerated. In some cases, the epidermis shows marked "pseudoepitheliomatous" hyperplasia (38).

Borderline Lesions

The distinction between lymphomatoid papulosis and anaplastic large-cell lymphoma becomes difficult in borderline lesions, which we define as *intermediate* in clinical appearance or histology between lymphomatoid papulosis and anaplastic large-cell lymphoma (1). It should be noted that the World Health Organization defines borderline lesions as those in which there is a *discrepancy* between the clinical features and histologic appearance and, as a consequence, are difficult to classify as lymphomatoid papulosis or anaplastic large-cell lymphoma (35). In the World Health Organization Classification, cases that mimic lymphoma histologically (confluent sheets of CD30⁺ atypical or anaplastic cells) but resemble lymphomatoid papulosis clinically are referred to as *lymphomatoid papulosis type C*, whereas solitary skin tumors that have the clinical features of lymphoma but are histologically similar to lymphomatoid papulosis are termed *anaplastic lymphoma, lymphomatoid papulosis–like*.

SKIN LESIONS OF SYSTEMIC ANAPLASTIC LARGE-CELL LYMPHOMA

"Metastatic" skin lesions in systemic anaplastic large-cell lymphoma can be difficult to distinguish from primary cutaneous anaplastic large-cell lymphoma. In secondary systemic anaplastic large-cell lymphoma, there is less likely to be epidermal involvement, and a gradation of cerebriform cells in the superficial portion to larger anaplastic cells in the deeper portion is less likely than in primary cutaneous anaplastic large-cell lymphoma. Secondary lesions of anaplastic large-cell lymphoma in the skin are usually deep nodular lesions with extensive involvement of the dermis and subcutis and may show contiguity with underlying lymph nodes. Staining of the neoplastic cells for anaplastic lymphoma kinase and clusterin is more common in secondary skin lesions of systemic anaplastic large-cell lymphoma but cannot be relied on for the distinction of skin lesions from primary cutaneous anaplastic large-cell lymphoma, which can express anaplastic lymphoma kinase and clusterin in a minority of cases (see the Immunophenotype section immediately below) (39,40).

Immunophenotype

The atypical cells in lymphomatoid papulosis have a phenotype of activated helper T cells expressing CD4 and some other T-cell antigens in 80% of cases (31,41,42). In 10% to 20% of cases, no specific T-cell antigens can be detected (31), but in at least some of these cases, clonal T-cell receptor–gene rearrangements are detected, indicating that the tumor cells are T cells that have deleted expression of some or all T-cell antigens, especially CD3 and CD7 (43). Most lymphomatoid papulosis cases analyzed show expression of cytotoxic molecules, Granzyme B, Perforin, and TIA-1 by the atypical cells (44). Similarly, most anaplastic large-cell lymphomas have the phenotype of activated T cells expressing cytotoxic molecules (45).

Expression of CD30 activation antigen is the hallmark of lymphomatoid papulosis and CD30 cutaneous lymphoproliferative disease (Color Plate 47) (31,41,42). However, CD30 is expressed by only few atypical cells in type B lymphomatoid papulosis. Some studies have used a criterion of greater than 75% of atypical lymphocytes staining positive for the CD30 antigen to define cases as type C lymphomatoid papulosis or anaplastic large-cell lymphoma (36). The atypical cells also express interleukin (IL)-2 receptor (CD25), transferrin receptor (CD71), and HLA-DR (31). In contrast to Hodgkin's disease, the atypical cells of lymphomatoid papulosis express leukocyte common antigen (CD45) and are usually negative for CD15 (31,46). Fascin, an actin-bundling protein expressed by Reed-Sternberg cells in Hodgkin's lymphoma (47), is also expressed by tumor cells in approximately 25% of lymphomatoid papulosis cases and 65% of primary cutaneous anaplastic large-cell lymphoma (48). Clusterin, a highly conserved glycoprotein implicated in intercellular and cell matrix interactions, was reported to be preferentially expressed in systemic anaplastic large-cell lymphoma but not in primary cutaneous anaplastic large-cell lymphoma (49), but this initial experience has not been confirmed (39).

Genetics

DNA cytophotometry and flow cytometry studies have revealed that lymphomatoid papulosis cells often are hyperdiploid, tetraploid, or aneuploid (30,50,51). Willemze et al. showed that the infiltrate in type A lesions was more likely to show marked aneuploidy than type B lesions, which were most often diploid (30). This was confirmed in a few studies in which cytogenetics with karyotyping could be performed (51–53). In some cases, only diploid karyotypes were seen, whereas in others both structural and numeric chromosome abnormalities could be found (53,54). Abnormalities found in lymphomatoid papulosis included trisomy 7 and structural abnormalities at 9p23 and 10q24 (52,53). Structural abnormalities found in primary cutaneous anaplastic large-cell lymphoma include add 1p36, add 10q26, del 6q, isochromosome 17q, allelic deletion at 9p21-22, and translocations involving 9q34 (55,56). The translocation (2;5)(p23;q35) or resulting nucleophosmin-anaplastic lymphoma kinase fusion protein characteristic of nodal or systemic anaplastic large-cell lymphoma has been found in only a few cases of primary cutaneous anaplastic large-cell lymphoma and not in lymphomatoid papulosis (40,55,57–59). Thus, detection of the t(2;5) or the anaplastic lymphoma kinase tyrosine kinase protein (anaplastic lymphoma kinase-1) resulting from the chimeric protein nucleophosmin-anaplastic lymphoma kinase in cutaneous lesions should lead to a search for extracu-

taneous disease, although some well-documented cases of primary cutaneous lymphoproliferative disease with the t(2;5) or anaplastic lymphoma kinase protein, or both, have been reported. It is particularly important to exclude the small-cell variant of systemic anaplastic large-cell lymphoma. The small-cell variant frequently occurs in children, involves the skin, and contains the t(2;5) and anaplastic lymphoma kinase protein in most cases (60). Unlike primary cutaneous anaplastic large-cell lymphoma, the prognosis for the small-cell variant of anaplastic large-cell lymphoma is poor.

Clonality

The clonality of lymphomatoid papulosis has been controversial. The report of Weiss et al. indicated that individual lesions contain T-cell clones, but the only case in which separate lesions were analyzed suggested that lymphomatoid papulosis is multiclonal (61). A report by Whittaker et al. suggested that some lymphomatoid papulosis lesions are clonal, but not pure type A lesions (62). The study of Chott et al. indicated that most lymphomatoid papulosis lesions are clonal and that separate lesions from the same patient are clonally related, regardless of histologic type (14). A recent study by Stein et al. in which T-cell clonality was analyzed by single-cell polymerase chain reaction confirmed that lymphomatoid papulosis is monoclonal and that separate lesions of the same patient are clonally related (63).

Our studies have shown that the regressing lymphomatoid papulosis lesions are clonally related to the T-cell lymphomas that some patients develop (14). We confirmed the clonal relationship between lymphomatoid papulosis and a subsequent cutaneous anaplastic large-cell lymphoma by cytogenetics. Others have shown a clonal relationship between lymphomatoid papulosis and anaplastic large-cell lymphoma by analysis of T-cell receptor genes (64–66). Similarly, a clonal relationship between individual lesions of lymphomatoid papulosis and mycosis fungoides has been demonstrated in several patients (13,66). We found a clonal relationship between lymphomatoid papulosis and a rare T-cell variant of Hodgkin's lymphoma (15). The relationship between lymphomatoid papulosis and the more common B-cell type of Hodgkin's lymphoma has yet to be proven.

Skin lesions of primary cutaneous anaplastic large-cell lymphoma and of secondary skin lesions in systemic anaplastic large-cell lymphoma are invariably monoclonal when assessed by T-cell receptor–gene rearrangement methods. The same gene rearrangements are found in secondary skin lesions and involved lymph nodes of systemic anaplastic large-cell lymphoma.

Postulated Cell of Origin

Possible Origin of Lymphomatoid Papulosis and Associated Lymphomas from an Early Lymphoid Stem Cell

The significant risk for Hodgkin's disease, mycosis fungoides, anaplastic large-cell lymphoma, and other lymphomas to develop before, after, or simultaneously with lymphomatoid papulosis led to the hypothesis that lymphomatoid papulosis and associated lymphomas are derived from a common early precursor lymphoid stem cell (15). An early genetic lesion in the lymphoid precursor may be the triggering event, and subsequent genetic lesions in subclones may determine the phenotype of the associated lymphoma.

Lymphomatoid Papulosis Cells Have a Th2 Cell Phenotype

The cytokines produced by several clones of lymphomatoid papulosis–associated lymphomas have been characterized. In these cases, the cytokine profile most closely resembles Th2 cells (67). These findings are in agreement with those of Yagi et al., who found expression of Th2 mRNAs in primary cutaneous CD30+ cutaneous lymphoproliferative disease and used this as a rationale for treatment with recombinant interferon-γ (68). These results are also consistent with the observation of Del Prete et al. that Th2 cells are the principal type of T cells that express CD30 antigen at the highest levels (69).

Regressing Lesions of CD30+ Cutaneous Lymphoproliferative Disease Contain High Levels of CD30 Ligand

Molecular analysis reveals that CD30 ligand is expressed at higher levels in regressing skin lesions than in growing ones, even of the same patient (70). By immunohistochemistry, CD30 ligand was detected in regressing lesions only. CD30 receptor cross-linking with recombinant CD30 ligand was found to inhibit proliferation of CD30+ cutaneous lymphoma cells (67). Hence, CD30 ligand may have a role in the regression of CD30+ cutaneous lymphoproliferative disease.

Transforming Growth Factor-β–Mediated Growth Inhibition is Lost in Advanced Disease

Transforming growth factor-β inhibits the growth of nonmalignant T lymphocytes (71). We found that CD30+ lymphoma cells clonally derived from lymphomatoid papulosis produce transforming growth factor-β, which acts as an inhibitory growth factor in early-stage disease (72,73). CD30+ cutaneous lymphoproliferative disease becomes resistant to transforming growth factor-β–mediated growth inhibition in late-stage disease, and this is due to receptor mutations that prevent binding of transforming growth factor-β (74,75). Because transforming growth factor-β upregulates cutaneous lymphocyte antigen (76), loss of response to transforming growth factor-β could lead to low expression of cutaneous lymphocyte antigen, facilitating extracutaneous spread of CD30+ lymphomas. Extracutaneous spread of CD30+ cutaneous lymphoproliferative disease is a significant adverse factor in survival (8,9).

Clinical Presentation

CD30+ cutaneous lymphoproliferative disease presents in the skin, without extracutaneous manifestations. Systemic symptoms of fever, weight loss, or night sweats are rare or absent in uncomplicated lymphomatoid papulosis and localized cutaneous anaplastic large-cell lymphoma but may be present in multifocal cutaneous anaplastic large-cell lymphoma. Lymphomatoid papulosis usually presents as multiple papules that last 4 to 6 weeks and then regress spontaneously, often with scarring and hyperpigmentation (or depigmentation). Lesions reappear without warning in most patients after varying intervals. For most patients, lymphomatoid papulosis is a disease of long duration that may be complicated by the development of lymphoma in 10% to 20% of cases. The most common types of secondary lymphoma are mycosis fungoides, anaplastic large-cell lymphoma, and Hodgkin's disease. The most serious complication is visceral spread of anaplastic large-cell lymphoma.

Female patients with lymphomatoid papulosis often report that their skin lesions are modified for better or worse by pregnancy and menstrual periods. This suggests that female hormones affecting the immune system have a modulating effect on the disease.

Primary cutaneous anaplastic large-cell lymphoma usually presents as a single or few clustered large lesions that form a tumor and frequently become ulcerated. Regression may occur in up to 25% of anaplastic large-cell lymphomas. Localized lesions can be treated with local excision and radiation. However, multifocal lesions or large recurrent lesions may require systemic management.

The most common extracutaneous site of spread by primary cutaneous anaplastic large-cell lymphoma is the regional lymph nodes; however, other organs may be involved as well, including the liver, spleen, and bones. Complications in the late stages may include infection secondary to immune suppression and cachexia.

Staging

An initial staging evaluation for patients with lymphomatoid papulosis should include a careful physical examination, screening laboratory studies, and a chest radiograph, due to the frequent association of lymphomatoid papulosis with other lymphomas. Patients with anaplastic large-cell lymphoma should also undergo a chest/abdomen/pelvis computed tomographic scan to further rule out extracutaneous disease. The value of a routine bone marrow biopsy is not known (8). There is no staging system recommended for CD30+ cutaneous lymphoproliferative disease. Because lymphomatoid papulosis lesions are usually multifocal and the prognosis is excellent, a staging system is not really required. The Ann Arbor staging system may be applied to primary cutaneous anaplastic large-cell lymphoma, or else the disease may simply be characterized as *localized* or *multifocal*.

Prognostic and Predictive Factors

The overall prognosis for patients with CD30$^+$ cutaneous lymphoproliferative disease is excellent. No patients die from lymphomatoid papulosis. However, as noted previously, 10% to 20% of patients with lymphomatoid papulosis may develop a lymphoma, such as mycosis fungoides, anaplastic large-cell lymphoma, or Hodgkin's disease. No factors have been identified that predict which patients with lymphomatoid papulosis are at greatest risk to develop lymphoma. Factors that have been investigated include age, ethnicity, gender, the extent of skin disease, histologic type of lymphomatoid papulosis (including type C), DNA flow cytometry, and T-cell receptor–gene rearrangement (77–81). However, a malignant clinical presentation, defined as evidence of tumorous lymphomatoid papulosis lesions and abnormal DNA-histograms, may be associated with a higher risk of developing lymphoma (82). The influence of lymphomatoid papulosis on the course of coexisting mycosis fungoides is unclear; however, one study of patients with lymphomatoid papulosis and patch or plaque mycosis fungoides suggests a less aggressive course for these patients (83). Development of primary cutaneous anaplastic large-cell lymphoma in patients with preexisting lymphomatoid papulosis does not signify a more aggressive course of disease than does *de novo* anaplastic large-cell lymphoma (84,85).

There are limited studies that have looked specifically at CD30$^+$ cutaneous lymphoproliferative disease borderline cases by histology, but it appears that they have a similar prognosis to lymphomatoid papulosis patients (9).

Primary cutaneous anaplastic large-cell lymphoma is defined by the presence of greater than 75% of the atypical lymphocytes positive for the CD30 antigen and no evidence of extracutaneous disease within 6 months of diagnosis. Primary cutaneous anaplastic large-cell lymphoma has been shown in several studies to have an overall excellent prognosis, with a 5-year disease-specific survival ranging from 85% to 100% (79,80,84–91), compared to a significantly worse 5-year survival seen in CD30$^-$ cutaneous T-cell lymphomas or systemic anaplastic large-cell lymphoma (86,92). Age younger than 60 years and the presence of spontaneous regression have been suggested by some to be associated with a more favorable prognosis (9); however, other studies have shown no significant differences in survival based on these same factors (84,86). Other factors, including ethnicity, gender, extent of skin disease, type of primary skin lesion, site of skin involvement, initial treatment or response to initial treatment, histologic morphology of the atypical lymphocytes, number of mitotic figures, and histologic epidermal changes have not been predictive of survival (86,90).

Lymphomatoid papulosis in the pediatric population is rare. The risk for children to develop a secondary lymphoma is similar to that of adults. Of 35 patients who developed lymphomatoid papulosis in childhood, three developed non-Hodgkin's lymphoma (101). Compared to the general population, patients with lymphomatoid papulosis have a significantly increased risk of developing lymphoma (relative risk = 226.2; 95%, CI = 73.4–697.0). Pediatric cases of primary cutaneous anaplastic large-cell lymphoma are rare, but the prognosis appears to remain favorable (87).

Treatment

The appropriate management of CD30$^+$ cutaneous lymphoproliferative disease depends on multiple factors, including the type and extent of disease and the goals of treatment (Fig. 21.1). For patients with primary cutaneous anaplastic large-cell lymphoma, the goal is likely to be cure, whereas for lymphomatoid papulosis, the goal may be palliative or cosmetic.

Most patients with lymphomatoid papulosis do not require therapy, unless their lesions are numerous or located on the face, hands, legs, genitalia, or other areas that cause discomfort or scarring. When therapy is needed, common treatment options include psoralen plus ultraviolet light of A wave length; low-dose methotrexate (93); and topical therapies, such as nitrogen mustard, carmustine, or corticosteroids (94,95). Other therapies may include retinoids, interferon (96–98), antibiotics, extracorporeal photopheresis (99), and FK 506 (100). Data are not available to define the clinical response or disease-free interval after these different therapies, and no single modality appears superior to the others. Frequent relapses are the norm, regardless of the treatment. There is no role for combination chemotherapy in the management of lymphomatoid papulosis, because recurrence of disease is likely despite aggressive intervention.

Topical corticosteroids may achieve some response of lymphomatoid papulosis lesions, but long-term use may be associated with skin atrophy, telangiectasias, and striae. There also may be systemic absorption, depending on the potency of the corticosteroid as well as the quantity and frequency of application. Topical chemotherapy agents, such as carmustine and mechlorethamine, are often used for patients who have concurrent lymphomatoid papulosis and mycosis fungoides, and regressions of the lymphomatoid papulosis lesions are commonly observed in this setting.

Psoralen plus ultraviolet light of A wavelength is another common therapy for lymphomatoid papulosis. Typically, psoralen plus ultraviolet light of A wavelength is administered two to three times per week at the outset. Although it may be quite effective in clearing generalized skin involvement, relapse is common, and sustained remissions are rare. The most serious potential complications of psoralen plus ultraviolet light of A wavelength include an increased risk for squamoproliferative lesions and cataracts.

Methotrexate has been used at low doses (10 to 25 mg weekly or biweekly) to treat lymphomatoid papulosis (93). The dose is titrated to the minimum that suppresses disease activity. Most patients will tolerate this treatment schedule well, but methotrexate is contraindicated in patients with impaired liver function or poor hematopoietic reserve. In addition, it is recommended that a liver biopsy be performed after a cumulative dose

Distinguish primary cutaneous lymphoproliferative disorders (LPD) from secondary manifestations of systemic ALCL and MF. Clinical evaluation, including imaging, as indicated, histopathology, including stains for ALK, clusterin, and fascin.

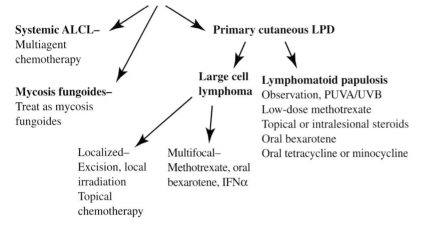

Systemic ALCL–
Multiagent
chemotherapy

Primary cutaneous LPD

Mycosis fungoides–
Treat as mycosis
fungoides

**Large cell
lymphoma**

Lymphomatoid papulosis
Observation, PUVA/UVB
Low-dose methotrexate
Topical or intralesional steroids
Oral bexarotene
Oral tetracycline or minocycline

Localized–
Excision, local
irradiation
Topical
chemotherapy

Multifocal–
Methotrexate, oral
bexarotene, IFNα

FIG. 21.1. Algorithm for diagnosis and treatment of CD30⁺ cutaneous lymphoproliferative disorders. ALCL, anaplastic large-cell lymphoma; ALK, anaplastic lymphoma kinase; IFNα, interferon-α; MF, mycosis fungoides; PUVA, psoralen plus ultraviolet light of A wave length; UVB, ultraviolet B.

of 1 g of methotrexate has been administered to rule out hepatic damage.

In pediatric cases of lymphomatoid papulosis, the most commonly used agents have been oral antibiotics or topical corticosteroids. Other agents have been avoided because of the systemic risks (111).

The treatment of primary cutaneous anaplastic large-cell lymphoma may be tailored to the extent of disease. For example, aggressive intervention may not be warranted when there is limited skin involvement only. Studies of outcome are not common, and none has shown a survival advantage for any specific therapy. Local therapy is the primary consideration for limited disease. Surgical excision and local radiation are the two most common forms of therapy. Complete excision with a 0.5-cm margin may be performed when technically appropriate. Local radiation is usually delivered as electron-beam therapy to a dose of 36 to 44 Gy, with a margin less than or equal to 2 cm. Complete response rates for local radiation are nearly 100%, but relapse in other skin sites is common and may occur in 30% to 40% of patients. Limited studies have compared excision with local radiation therapy; however, it appears that the relapse rates for both approaches are similar (84). Secondary therapies for localized skin involvement include topical chemotherapy, topical corticosteroids, and topical retinoids, but data on the efficacy of these agents are limited.

For generalized skin involvement by anaplastic large-cell lymphoma, systemic therapies are used, often in conjunction with local therapy. The important systemic therapies include single- or multiagent chemotherapy and biologic response modifiers. Because limited studies fail to show a significant benefit in disease-specific survival or relapse rates when comparing treatment interventions, systemic biologic response modifiers often are considered as first-line therapy. Interferon-2α and oral bexarotene are the two most commonly used biologic agents. Others include interferon-γ and IL-12. Combination therapy with biologic agents, such as

interferon combined with oral bexarotene, has been reported as well (112).

Single-agent drugs used for generalized cutaneous anaplastic large-cell lymphoma include methotrexate, doxorubicin, etoposide, pentostatin, and gemcitabine. The largest experience is with methotrexate. The most common multiagent chemotherapy regimen used is cyclophosphamide, doxorubicin, vincristine, and prednisone. Other doxorubicin-based regimens that have been used include Adriamycin, cyclophosphamide, vincristine, bleomycin, and prednisone and Adriamycin, cyclophosphamide, vincristine, bleomycin, prednisone, and methotrexate (88). No single regimen appears superior. Despite intensive chemotherapy, the relapse rates are reported to be 60% to 80% (84,86).

Primary cutaneous anaplastic large-cell lymphoma is relatively rare in the pediatric population; however, it appears that the clinical course is similar to that for adults. There is an overall good prognosis but a high rate of relapse in the skin even after aggressive interventions (87,113).

Extension of anaplastic large-cell lymphoma to extracutaneous sites warrants more aggressive therapy, and doxorubicin-based multiagent chemotherapy is used in almost all cases. Generally, treatment algorithms similar to those used for noncutaneous anaplastic large-cell lymphoma may be followed in these cases, often with the inclusion of biologic agents.

FUTURE DIRECTIONS

Clarification of Etiology

The etiology of lymphomatoid papulosis remains an enigma. Thus far, there is no evidence to support an infectious etiology for lymphomatoid papulosis. Epidemiologic studies are under way to identify clues to the etiology. The association of lymphomatoid papulosis with other lymphomas suggests a possible genetic alteration in an early lymphocyte precursor as an early event in the etiology of lymphomatoid papulosis.

Determination of Risk Factors for Development of Lymphoma

The study of Bekkenk and coworkers (8) failed to identify any risk factors for the development of lymphoma in lymphomatoid papulosis patients. We have found that progression of lymphomatoid papulosis to clonally related anaplastic large-cell lymphoma is associated with loss of tumor-cell growth inhibition by transforming growth factor-β (102). The loss of growth inhibition was due to inactivating mutations of the transforming growth factor-β–receptor complex (74,75).

Because anaplastic lymphoma kinase gene expression has not been observed in lymphomatoid papulosis but may occur in some primary cutaneous anaplastic large-cell lymphomas (40), anaplastic lymphoma kinase activation may be another risk factor for progression of lymphomatoid papulosis to anaplastic large-cell lymphoma.

The risks that lymphomatoid papulosis patients may develop Hodgkin's disease and mycosis fungoides are more puzzling, especially because approximately 10% of patients develop these lymphomas before clinical manifestations of lymphomatoid papulosis. A possible risk factor for development of Hodgkin's disease is abnormal regulation of CD30 expression, because high constitutive expression of CD30 is linked to the survival and proliferation of Hodgkin/Reed-Sternberg cells in Hodgkin's lymphoma (27,28). The survival of Hodgkin/Reed-Sternberg cells is mediated by activation and nuclear translocation of NF-κB, which also has been observed in tumor cells of mycosis fungoides (29). Therefore, a plausible hypothesis for the increased risk of lymphomatoid papulosis patients to develop Hodgkin's lymphoma and mycosis fungoides is via abnormal regulation of NF-κB by highly expressed CD30 or other pathways that activate NF-κB.

Biologic Treatments

Three major modes of biologic treatment are suggested from experimental data and previous experience. The first is the use of cytokines, which may have an antiproliferative effect on CD30+ lymphoma cells. The second is the use of CD30 agonistic antibodies, either alone or linked to a toxin. A third mode of treatment is the use of retinoids, such as bexarotene.

Yagi et al. demonstrated expression of Th2 cytokine mRNA in primary cutaneous CD30+ lymphoproliferative disorders (68). Based on this data, they studied the response of skin lesions to injections of interferon-γ, a type I cytokine. The numbers of skin-infiltrating CD30+ cells were decreased, and transcription of mRNA downregulated for Th2 cytokines IL-4 and IL-10 in one CD30+ anaplastic large-cell lymphoma and two lymphomatoid papulosis cases. In patients whose skin lesions responded to local injection of recombinant interferon-γ, the lesions objectively improved with reduction of CD30+ cells when interferon-γ was administered intravenously, whereas no improvement was observed in the patient who did not respond to a skin test.

Mori et al. discovered high concentrations of CD30 ligand in regressing lesions of CD30+ cutaneous lymphoproliferative disease (70). Based on this observation, we tested the effects of recombinant CD30 ligand on the proliferation of CD30+ anaplastic large-cell lymphoma lines clonally derived from lymphomatoid papulosis. The results showed an antiproliferative effect of immobilized CD30 ligand, suggesting that cross-linking of CD30 may provide a strategy for a biologic treatment for CD30+ anaplastic large-cell lymphoma (67). Moreover, Huhn and coworkers found that human angiogenin fused to human CD30 ligand exhibits specific cytotoxicity against CD30+ lymphoma (103). A related approach could target CD30 with a toxin covalently linked to an anti-CD30 antibody, such as has been used experimentally in systemic CD30+ anaplastic large-cell lymphoma (104). Thus, a variety of therapies targeting CD30 may ultimately be useful in the treatment of CD30+ cutaneous lymphoproliferative disease.

Bexarotene has been used for treatment of refractory advanced-stage cutaneous T-cell lymphomas (105). Chou and coworkers have shown that retinoids may induce regression of CD30+ anaplastic lymphomas (106). One patient with generalized skin lesions and two patients with CD30+ cutaneous anaplastic large-cell lymphoma that relapsed after intensive chemotherapy and radiotherapy experienced a complete durable remission after administration of oral 13-cis-retinoic acid, 1 mg per kg per day, followed by maintenance therapy with 0.5 mg per kg per day. Biopsy of the retinoic acid-indiced remission tumors showed "unequivocal evidence of cellular differentiation of the remitting tumors" (107). The mechanism of action of retinoic acids appears to be induction of apoptosis through interaction of RAR and RXR receptors (108,109). Further studies are indicated to determine the usefulness of retinoids in the treatment of lymphomatoid papulosis and other CD30+ cutaneous lymphoproliferative diseases.

REFERENCES

1. Kadin ME. The spectrum of Ki-1+ cutaneous lymphomas. In: van Vloten WA, Willemze R, Lange-Vejlsgaard G, eds. *Current Problems in Dermatology.* Farmington, Connecticut: Karger, 1990:132–143.
2. Morris SW, Kirstein M, Valentine M, et al. Fusion of a kinase gene, ALK, to a nucleolar protein gene, NPM, in non-Hodgkins lymphoma. *Science* 1994;263:1281–1284.
3. Kadin M. Primary Ki-1-positive anaplastic large-cell lymphoma: a distinct clinicopathologic entity. *Ann Oncol* 1994;5:S25–S30.
4. Kadin M, Sako E, Berliner N, et al. Childhood Ki-1 lymphoma presenting with skin lesions and peripheral lymphadenopathy. *Blood* 1986;68:1042–1049.
5. Willemze R, Meijer CJLM. Classification of cutaneous lymphomas: crosstalk between pathologist and clinician. *Curr Diagn Pathol* 1998;5:23–33.
6. Fink-Puches R, Zenahlik P, Back B, et al. Primary cutaneous lymphomas: applicability of current classification schemes (European Organization for Research and Treatment of Cancer, World Health Organization) based on clinicopathologic features observed in a large group of patients. *Blood* 2002;99:800–805.
7. Wang HH, Lach L, Kadin ME. Epidemiology of lymphomatoid papulosis. *Cancer* 1992;70:2951–2957.
8. Bekkenk MW, Geelen FA, van Voorst Vader PC, et al. Primary and secondary cutaneous CD30+ lymphoproliferative disorders: a report

from the Dutch Cutaneous Lymphoma Group on the long-term follow-up data of 219 patients and guidelines for diagnosis and treatment. *Blood* 2000;95:3653–3661.

9. Paulli M, Berti E, Rosso R, et al. CD30/Ki-1-positive lymphoproliferative disorders of the skin-clinicopathologic correlation and statistical analysis of 86 cases: a multicentric study from the European Organization for Research and Treatment of Cancer Cutaneous Lymphoma Project Group. *J Clin Oncol* 1996;13:1343–1354.

10. Reiter A, Schrappe M, Tiemann M et al. Successful treatment strategy for Ki-1 anaplastic large-cell lymphoma of childhood: a prospective analysis of 62 patients enrolled in three consecutive Berlin-Frankfurt-Munster Group Studies. *J Clin Oncol* 1994;12:899–908.

11. Anagnostopoulos I, Hummel M, Kaudewitz P, et al. Detection of HTLV-I proviral sequences in CD30+ large cell cutaneous T-cell lymphomas. *Am J Pathol* 1990;137:1317–1322.

12. Wood G, Schaffer JM, Boni R, et al. No evidence of HTLV-I proviral integration in lymphoproliferative disorders associated with cutaneous T-cell lymphoma. *Am J Pathol* 1997;150:667–673.

13. Basarab T, Fraser-Edwards EA, Orchard G, et al. Lymphomatoid papulosis in association with mycosis fungoides: a study of 15 cases. *J Am Acad Dermatol* 1998;139:630–638.

14. Chott A, Vonderheid EC, Olbricht S, et al. The same dominant T cell clone is present in multiple regressing lesions and associated T cell lymphomas of patients with lymphomatoid papulosis. *J Invest Dermatol* 1996;106:696–700.

15. Davis TH, Moron CC, Miller-Cassman R, et al. Hodgkin's disease, lymphomatoid papulosis, and cutaneous T cell lymphoma derived from a common T-cell clone. *N Engl J Med* 1992;326:1115–1122.

16. Sanchez NP, Pittelkow MR, Muller SA, et al. The clinicopathologic spectrum of lymphomatoid papulosis: study of 31 cases. *J Am Acad Dermatol* 1983;8:81–94.

17. Lederman NS, Sober AJ, Harrist TJ, et al. Lymphomatoid papulosis following Hodgkin's disease. *J Am Acad Dermatol* 1987;16:331–335.

18. Chen KT, Flam MS. Hodgkin's disease complicating lymphomatoid papulosis. *Am J Dermatopathol* 1985;7:555–561.

19. Kaudewitz P, Stein H, Plewig G, et al. Hodgkin's disease followed by lymphomatoid papulosis: immunophenotypic evidence for a close relationship between Hodgkin's disease and lymphomatoid papulosis. *J Am Acad Dermatol* 1990;22:999–1006.

20. Willemze R, van Vloten WA, Meijer CHLM. Lymphomatoid papulosis and Hodgkin's disease: how are they related? *Arch Dermatol Res* 1983;275:159–167.

21. Zackheim HS, LeBoit PE, Gordon BL, et al. Lymphomatoid papulosis followed by Hodgkin's lymphoma: differential response to therapy. *Arch Dermatol* 1993;129:86–91.

22. Kadin ME. Common activated T-cell origin of lymphomatoid papulosis, mycosis fungoides, and some types of Hodgkin's disease. *Lancet* 1985;2:864–865.

23. Chan WC, Griem ML, Grozea PN, et al. Mycosis fungoides and Hodgkin's disease occurring in the same patient: report of three cases. *Cancer* 1979;44:1408–1413.

24. Hawkins KA, Schinella R, Schwartz M, et al. Simultaneous occurrence of mycosis fungoides and Hodgkin's disease: clinical and histologic correlations in three cases with ultrastructural studies in two. *Am J Hematol* 1983;14:355–362.

25. Croager E, Gout AM, Abraham L. Involvement of Sp1 and microsatellite repressor sequences in the transcriptional control of the human CD30 gene. *Am J Pathol* 2000;156:1723–1731.

26. Durkop H, Oberbarnscheidt M, Latza U, et al. The restricted expression pattern of the Hodgkin's lymphoma-associated cytokine receptor CD30 is regulated by a minimal promoter. *J Pathol* 2000;192:182–193.

27. Horie R, Watanabe T, Morishita Y et al. Ligand-independent signaling by overexpressed CD30 drives NF-κB activation in Hodgkin-Reed Sternberg cells. *Oncogene* 2002;21:2493–2503.

28. Bargou RC, Emmerich F, Krappman D, et al. Constitutive nuclear factor-kappa B-RelA activation is required for proliferation and survival of Hodgkin's tumor cells. *J Clin Invest* 1997;100:2961–2969.

29. Izban KF, Ergin M, Qin J-Z, et al. Constitutive expression of NF-κB is a characteristic feature of mycosis fungoides: implications for apoptosis resistance and pathogenesis. *Hum Pathol* 2000;31:1482–1490.

30. Willemze R, Meyer CJ, van Vloten WA, et al. The clinical and histological spectrum of lymphomatoid papulosis. *Br J Dermatol* 1982;107:131–144.

31. Kadin ME, Nasu K, Sako D, et al. Lymphomatoid papulosis. A cutaneous proliferation of activated helper T cells expressing Hodgkin's disease associated antigens. *Am J Pathol* 1985;119:315–325.

32. Ackerman AB. *Histologic Diagnosis of Inflammatory Skin Diseases.* Philadelphia: Lea & Febiger, 1978.

33. McKee PH. Pityriasis lichenoides. In: *Vascular Diseases.* In: McKee PH, ed. *Pathology of the Skin with Clinical Correlations*, 2nd ed. London: Mosby-Wolfe, 1996:5.8–5.11.

34. Varga FJ, Vonderheid EC, Olbricht SM, et al. Immunohistochemical distinction of lymphomatoid papulosis and pityriasis et varioliformis acuta. *Am J Pathol* 1990;136:979–987.

35. Willemze R, Kerl H, Sterry W, et al. EORTC classification for primary cutaneous lymphomas: a proposal from the Cutaneous Lymphoma Study Group of the European Organization for Research and Treatment of Cancer. *Blood* 1997;90:354–371.

36. Beljaards RC, Meijer CHLM, Scheffer E, et al. Prognostic significance of CD30 (Ki-1/Ber-H2) expression in primary cutaneous large-cell lymphomas of T-cell origin. A clinicopathologic and immunohistochemical study in 20 patients. *Am J Pathol* 1989;135:1169–1178.

37. Mann KP, Hall B, Kamino H, et al. Neutrophil-rich, Ki-1-positive anaplastic large-cell malignant lymphoma. *Am J Surg Pathol* 1995;19:407–416.

38. Krishnan J, Tomaszewski MM, Kao GF. Primary cutaneous CD30-positive anaplastic large cell lymphoma. Report of 27 cases. *J Cutan Pathol* 1993;20:193–202.

39. Saffer H, Wahed A, Rassidakis G, et al. Clusterin expression in malignant lymphomas: a survey of 266 cases. *Mod Pathol* 2002;15:1221–1226.

40. Gould JW, Eppes RB, Gilliam AC, et al. Solitary primary cutaneous CD30+ large cell lymphoma of natural killer phenotype bearing the t(2;5)(p23;q35) translocation and presenting in a child. *Am J Dermatopathol* 2000;22:422–428.

41. Kaudewitz P, Stein H, Burg G, et al. Atypical cells in lymphomatoid papulosis express the Hodgkin cell-associated antigen Ki-1. *J Invest Dermatol* 1986;86:350–354.

42. Ralfkiaer E, Stein H, Lange-Wantzin G, et al. Lymphomatoid papulosis: characterization of skin infiltrates with monoclonal antibodies. *Am J Clin Pathol* 1985;84:587–593.

43. Kadin ME, Vonderheid EC, Sako D, et al. Clonal composition of T cells in lymphomatoid papulosis. *Am J Pathol* 1987;126:13–17.

44. Kummer JA, Vermeer MH, Dukers D, et al. Most primary cutaneous CD30-positive lymphoproliferative disorders have a CD4-positive cytotoxic T-cell phenotype. *J Invest Dermatol* 1997;109:636–640.

45. Krenacs L, Wellmann A, Sorbara L, et al. Cytotoxic cell antigen expression in anaplastic large cell lymphomas of T- and null cell type and Hodgkin's disease: evidence for a distinct cellular origin. *Blood* 1997;89:980–989.

46. Sioutos N, Kerl H, Murphy SB, et al. Primary cutaneous Hodgkin's disease. Unique clinical, morphologic, and immunophenotypic findings. *Am J Dermatopathol* 1994;16:2–8.

47. Pinkus GP, Pinkus JL, Langhoff E, et al. Fascin, a sensitive new marker for Reed-Sternberg cells of Hodgkin's disease. *Am J Pathol* 1997;150:543.

48. Kempf W, Levi E, Kamarashev J, et al. Fascin expression in CD30-positive cutaneous lymphoproliferative disorders. *J Cutan Pathol* 2002;29:295–300.

49. Wellmann A, Thieblemont C, Pittaluga S, et al. Detection of differentially expressed genes in lymphomas using cDNA arrays: identification of clusterin as a new diagnostic marker for anaplastic large-cell lymphomas. *Blood* 2000;96:398–404.

50. Wantzin GL, Thomsen K, Larsen JK, et al. DNA analysis by flow cytometry of lymphomatoid papulosis. *Clin Exp Dermatol* 1983;8:505–512.

51. Espinoza CG, Erkman-Balis B, Fenske NA. Lymphomatoid papulosis: a premalignant disorder. *J Am Acad Dermatol* 1985;13:736–743.

52. Harrington DS, Braddock SW, Blocher KS, et al. Lymphomatoid papulosis and progression to T cell lymphoma: an immunophenotypic and genotypic study. *J Am Acad Dermatol* 1989;21:951–957.

53. Peters K, Knoll JH, Kadin ME. Cytogenetic findings in regressing skin lesions of lymphomatoid papulosis. *Cancer Genet Cytogenet* 1995;80:13–16.

54. Parks JD, Synovec MS, Masih AS, et al. Immunophenotypic and genotypic characterization of lymphomatoid papulosis. *J Am Acad Dermatol* 1992;26:968–975.

55. Ott G, Katzenberger T, Siebert R, et al. Chromosomal abnormalities in nodal and extranodal CD30⁺ anaplastic large cell lymphomas: infrequent detection of the t(2;5) in extranodal lymphomas. *Genes Chromosomes Cancer* 1998;22:114–121.
56. Boni R, Xin H, Kamarashev J, et al. Allelic deletion at 9p21-22 in primary cutaneous CD30⁺ large cell lymphoma. *J Invest Dermatol* 2000;115:1104–1107.
57. DeCoteau J, Butmarc JR, Kinney MC, et al. The t(2;5) chromosomal translocation is not a common feature of primary cutaneous CD30⁺ lymphoproliferative disorders: comparison with anaplastic large-cell lymphoma of nodal origin. *Blood* 1996;87:3437.
58. Wood GS, Hardman DL, Boni R, et al. Lack of the t(2;5) or other mutations resulting in expression of anaplastic lymphoma kinase catalytic domain in CD30⁺ primary cutaneous lymphoproliferative disorders and Hodgkin's disease. *Blood* 1996;88:1765–1770.
59. Sarris AH, Luthra R, Papadimitracopoulou V, et al. Amplification of genomic DNA demonstrates the presence of the t(2;5)(p23;q35) in anaplastic large cell lymphoma, but not in other non-Hodgkin's lymphomas, Hodgkin's disease, or lymphomatoid papulosis. *Blood* 1996;88:1771–1779.
60. Kinney MC, Collins RD, Greer J, et al. A small cell predominant variant of Ki-1 (CD30⁺) T-cell lymphoma. *Am J Surg Pathol* 1993; 17:859–868.
61. Weiss LM, Wood GS, Trela M, et al. Clonal T-cell populations in lymphomatoid papulosis: evidence of a lymphoproliferative origin for a clinically benign disease. *N Engl J Med* 1986;315:475–479.
62. Whittaker S, Smith N, Hones RR, et al. Analysis of β, γ, and δ T-cell receptor genes in lymphomatoid papulosis: cellular basis of two distinct histologic subsets. *J Invest Dermatol* 1991;96:786–791.
63. Steinhoff M, Hummel M, Anagnostopoulos I, et al. Single cell analysis of CD30⁺ cells in lymphomatoid papulosis demonstrates a common T-cell origin. *Blood* 2002;100:578–584.
64. Amagai M, Kawakubo Y, Tsuyuk IA, et al. Lymphomatoid papulosis followed by Ki-1 positive anaplastic large cell lymphoma: proliferation of a common T-cell clone. *J Dermatol* 1995;22:743–746.
65. Kaudewitz P, Herbst H, Anagnostopoulos I, et al. Lymphomatoid papulosis followed by large-cell lymphoma: immunophenotypical and genotypical analysis. *Br J Dermatol* 1991;124:465–469.
66. Wood GS, Crooks CF, Uluer AZ. Lymphomatoid papulosis and associated cutaneous lymphoproliferative disorders exhibit a common clonal origin. *J Invest Dermatol* 1995;105:51–55.
67. Willers J, Dummer R, Kempf W, et al. Proliferation of CD30⁺ T helper 2 lymphoma cells can be inhibited by CD30 receptor cross-linking with recombinant CD30 ligand. *Clin Cancer Res in press.*
68. Yagi H, Tokura Y, Furukawa F, et al. Th2 cytokine mRNA expression in primary cutaneous CD30-positive lymphoproliferative disorders: successful treatment with recombinant interferon-γ. *J Invest Dermatol* 1996;107:827–832.
69. Del Prete G, De Carli M, Almeriogogna F, et al. Preferential expression of CD30 by human CD4⁺ T cells producing Th2-type cytokines. *FASEB J* 1995;9:81–86.
70. Mori M, Manuelli C, Pimpinelli N, et al. CD30-CD30 ligand interaction in primary cutaneous CD30⁺ T-cell lymphomas: a clue to the pathophysiology of clinical regression. *Blood* 1999;94:3077–3083.
71. Kehrl JH, Wakefield LM, Roberts AB, et al. Production of transforming growth factor beta by human T lymphocytes and its potential role in the regulation of T cell growth. *J Exp Med* 1986;163:3855–3860.
72. Newcom SR, Kadin ME, Ansari AA. Production of transforming growth factor-beta activity by Ki-1 positive lymphoma cells and analysis of its role in the regulation of Ki-1 positive lymphoma growth. *Am J Pathol* 1988;131:569–577.
73. Newcom SR, Tagra KK, Kadin ME. Neutralizing antibodies against transforming growth factor (TGF)-beta potentiate the proliferation of Ki-1 positive lymphoma cells: further evidence for negative autocrine growth regulation by TGF-beta. *Am J Pathol* 1992;140:709–718.
74. Knaus PI, Lindemann D, DeCoteau JF, et al. A dominant inhibitory mutant of the type II transforming growth factor β receptor in the malignant progression of a cutaneous T-cell lymphoma. *Mol Cell Biol* 1996;16:3480–3489.
75. Schiemann WP, Pfeifer WM, Levi E, et al. A deletion in the gene for transforming growth factor beta type I receptor abolishes growth regulation by transforming growth factor beta in a cutaneous T-cell lymphoma. *Blood* 1999;94:2854–2861.
76. Picker LJ, Treer JR, Ferguson-Darnell B, et al. Control of lymphocyte recirculation in man. II. Differential regulation of cutaneous lymphocyte-associated antigen, a tissue selective homing receptor for skin-homing T cells. *J Immunol* 1993;150:1122–1136.
77. Cabanillas F, Armitage J, Pugh WC, et al. Lymphomatoid papulosis: a T-cell dyscrasia with a propensity to transform into malignant lymphoma. *Ann Intern Med* 1995;122:210–217.
78. Beljaards RC, Willemze R. The prognosis of patients with lymphomatoid papulosis associated with malignant lymphomas. *Br J Dermatol* 1992;126:596–602.
79. Tomaszewski MM, Lupton GP, Krishnan J, et al. A comparison of clinical, morphological and immunohistochemical features of lymphomatoid papulosis and primary cutaneous CD30(Ki-1)-positive anaplastic large cell lymphoma. *J Cutan Pathol* 1995;22:310–318.
80. Krishnan J, Tomaszewski MM, Kao GF. Primary cutaneous CD30-positive anaplastic large cell lymphoma. Report of 27 cases. *J Cutan Pathol* 1993;20:193–202.
81. Christensen HK, Thomsen K, Vejlsgaard GL. Lymphomatoid papulosis: a follow-up study of 41 patients. *Semin Dermatol* 1994;13:197–201.
82. Thomsen K, Wantzin GL. Lymphomatoid papulosis. A follow-up study of 30 patients. *J Am Acad Dermatol* 1987;17:632–636.
83. Basarab T, Fraser-Andrews EA, Orchard G, et al. Lymphomatoid papulosis in association with mycosis fungoides: a study of 15 cases. *Br J Dermatol* 1998;139:630–638.
84. Lui H, Kim Y, Hoppe R. Largest single institution series of CD30⁺ cutaneous lymphoproliferative disorders in North America. *Am Acad Dermatol in press.*
85. Vergier B, Beylot-Barry M, Pulford K, et al. Statistical evaluation of diagnostic and prognostic features of CD30⁺ cutaneous lymphoproliferative disorders: a clinicopathologic study of 65 cases. *Am J Surg Pathol* 1998;22:1192–1202.
86. Reference deleted by author.
87. Tomaszewski MM, Moad JC, Lupton GP. Primary cutaneous Ki-1(CD30) positive anaplastic large cell lymphoma in childhood. *J Am Acad Dermatol* 1999;40:857–861.
88. Brice P, Cazals D, Mounier N, et al. Primary cutaneous large-cell lymphoma: analysis of 49 patients included in the LNH87 prospective trial of polychemotherapy for high-grade lymphomas. Groupe d'Etude des Lymphomes de l'Adulte. *Leukemia* 1998;12:213–219.
89. Paulli M, Berti E, Rosso R, et al. CD30/Ki-1-positive lymphoproliferative disorders of the skin—clinicopathologic correlation and statistical analysis of 86 cases: a multicentric study from the European Organization for Research and Treatment of Cancer Cutaneous Lymphoma Project Group. *J Clin Oncol* 1995;13:1343–1354.
90. Beljaards RC, Kaudewitz P, Berti E, et al. Primary cutaneous CD30-positive large cell lymphoma: definition of a new type of cutaneous lymphoma with a favorable prognosis. A European Multicenter Study of 47 patients. *Cancer* 1993;71:2097–2104.
91. Banerjee SS, Heald J, Harris M. Twelve cases of Ki-1 positive anaplastic large cell lymphoma of skin. *J Clin Pathol* 1991;44:119–125.
92. A clinical evaluation of the International Lymphoma Study Group classification of non-Hodgkin's lymphoma. The Non-Hodgkin's Lymphoma Classification Project. *Blood* 1997;89:3909–3918.
93. Vonderheid EC, Sajjadian A, Kadin ME. Methotrexate is effective therapy for lymphomatoid papulosis and other primary cutaneous CD30-positive lymphoproliferative diseases. *J Am Acad Dermatol* 1996;34:470–481.
94. Vonderheid EC, Tan E, Kantor A, et al. Long-term efficacy, curative potential and carcinogenicity of topical mechlorethamine chemotherapy in cutaneous T cell lymphoma. *J Am Acad Dermatol* 1989; 20:416–428.
95. Zackheim H, Epstein E Jr, Crain W. Topical carmustine therapy for lymphomatoid papulosis. *Arch Dermatol* 1985;121:1410–1414.
96. Proctor S, Jackson G, Lennerd A, et al. Lymphomatoid papulosis: response to treatment with recombinant interferon-alpha-2b. *J Clin Oncol* 1992;10:170.
97. Wyss M, Dummer R, Dommann S, et al. Lymphomatoid papulosis-treatment with recombinant interferon alfa-2a and etretinate. *Dermatology* 1995;190:288–291.
98. Schmuth M, Topar G, Illersperger B, et al. Therapeutic use of interferon-alpha for lymphomatoid papulosis. *Cancer* 2000;89:1603–1610.

99. Wollina U. Lymphomatoid papulosis treated with extracorporeal photochemotherapy. *Oncol Rep* 1998;5:57–59.

100. Siddiqui M, Sullivan S, al-Mofadhi A. Lymphomatoid papulosis and FK506. *Int J Dermatol* 1997;36:202–205.

101. Nijsten T, Curiel C, Kadin ME. Lymphomatoid papulosis in children: a retrospective study of 35 cases. *Arch Dermatol in press.*

102. Kadin ME, Cavaille-Coll MW, Gertz R, et al. Loss of receptors for transforming growth factor-β in human T cell malignancies. *Proc Natl Acad Sci U S A* 1994;91:6002–6006.

103. Huhn M, Sasse S, Tur MK, et al. Human angiogenin fused to human CD30 ligand (Ang-CD30L) exhibits specific cytotoxicity against CD30 positive lymphoma. *Cancer Res* 2001;61:8737–8742.

104. Pasqualucci L, Wasik MA, Teicher B, et al. Antitumor activity of anti-CD30 immunotoxin (Ber-H2/Saporin) in vitro and in severe combined immunodeficiency disease mice xenografted with human CD30+ anaplastic large cell lymphoma. *Blood* 1995;85:2139–2146.

105. Duvic M, Martin AG, Kim Y. Bexarotene is effective and safe treatment of refractory advanced-stage cutaneous T-cell lymphoma: multinational phase II-III trial results. *J Clin Oncol* 2001;19:2456–2471.

106. Chou W-C, Su I-J, Tien H-F, et al. Clinicopathologic, cytogenetic, and molecular studies of 13 Chinese patients with Ki-1 anaplastic large cell lymphoma. Special emphasis on the tumor response to 13-cis retinoic acid. *Cancer* 1996;78:1805–1812.

107. Cheng A-L, Su I-J, Chen C, et al. Use of retinoic acids in the treatment of peripheral T-cell lymphoma: a pilot study. *J Clin Oncol* 1994;12:1185–1192.

108. Szondy Z, Reichert U, Fesus L. Retinoic acids regulate apoptosis of T lymphocytes through an interplay between RAR and RXR receptors. *Cell Death Diff* 1998;5:4–10.

109. Wang K-C, Cheng A-L, Chuang S-E, et al. Retinoic acid-induced apoptotic pathway in T-cell lymphoma: Identification of four groups of genes with differential biological functions. *Exp Hematol* 2000;28:1441–1450.

110. Willemze R, Beljaards RC. Spectrum of primary cutaneous CD30 (Ki-1)-positive lymphoproliferative disorders. A proposal for classification and guidelines for management and treatment. *J Am Acad Dermatol* 1993;28:973–980.

111. Paul M, Krowchuck D, Hitchcock M, et al. Lymphomatoid papulosis: successful weekly pulse superpotent topical corticosteroid therapy in three pediatric patients. *Pediatr Dermatol* 1996;13:501–506.

112. French L, Shapiro M, Junkins-Hopkins J, et al. Regression of multifocal, skin-restricted, CD30-positive large T-cell lymphoma with interferon-alpha and bexarotene therapy. *J Am Acad Dermatol* 2001;45:914–918.

113. Vermeer MH, Bekkenk MW, Willemze R. Should primary cutaneous Ki-1 (CD30)-positive anaplastic large cell lymphoma in childhood be treated with multiple-agent chemotherapy? *J Am Acad Dermatol* 2001;45:638–640.

CHAPTER 22

Extranodal Marginal Zone B-Cell Lymphoma of Mucosa-Associated Lymphoid Tissue

Joachim Yahalom, Peter G. Isaacson, and Emanuele Zucca

DEFINITION

The extranodal marginal zone lymphoma of mucosa-associated lymphoid tissue (MALT lymphoma) is a distinct B-cell lymphoma that develops in extranodal sites and often has an indolent clinical course. MALT lymphoma was not identified as a separate pathologic entity in the Working Formulation or in lymphoma classifications preceding it. Cases that we currently classify as *mucosa-associated lymphoid tissue lymphoma* were included in the Working Formulation under the categories of *small lymphocytic*, *lymphoplasmacytoid*, and *diffuse small cleaved-cell lymphomas* (1). MALT lymphoma was first recognized as a separate clinical pathologic entity by Isaacson and Wright in 1983 (2,3) and is presently featured in the Revised European-American Lymphoma and World Health Organization classifications as a distinct lymphoma in the *mature B-cell neoplasms* category (1). Nodal marginal zone lymphoma and marginal zone lymphoma of the spleen have different clinical and pathologic features from MALT lymphoma and are discussed in Chapters 23 and 16, respectively (4–7).

INCIDENCE AND EPIDEMIOLOGY

MALT lymphoma is the third most common non-Hodgkin's lymphoma and accounts for approximately 8% of non-Hodgkin's lymphoma cases evaluated by the International Lymphoma Study Group (8,9). The most common and, thus, the best-studied organ involved by MALT lymphoma is the stomach; almost one-half of the lymphomas found in the stomach are MALT lymphoma (10). Yet, MALT lymphoma may have primary involvement of many other organs (Table 22.1). The most common extragastric MALT lymphoma sites are the salivary glands, skin, orbits and conjunctiva, lung, thyroid, upper airways, breast, other gastrointestinal sites, and liver (11). Most cases occur in adults, with a median age in the sixth decade and a slight female preponderance (male to female ratio of 1.0:1.2 to 1.0:1.6) (8,11). The highest incidence of gastric MALT lymphoma has been reported in northeastern Italy (13.2 per 100,000 per year, 13 times higher than in corresponding communities in the United Kingdom), suggesting the existence of important geographic variations (12). The incidence of primary gastric lymphomas is likely to be related to the rate of *Helicobacter pylori* infection observed in the population. Indeed, a very high prevalence (up to more than 90% of cases) of *H. pylori* infection has been reported in gastric MALT lymphomas (13). There is compelling evidence for a pathogenetic role of this infection in gastric lymphoma that is further discussed below. In the United States, the incidence of gastric MALT lymphoma has been estimated as between one in 30,000 and one in 80,000 in the *H. pylori*–infected population (14).

PATHOLOGY AND PATHOGENESIS OF B-CELL EXTRANODAL MARGINAL ZONE AND MUCOSA-ASSOCIATED LYMPHOID TISSUE LYMPHOMA

The nomenclature and classification of non-Hodgkin's lymphomas has, to a considerable extent, been based on the architectural, cytologic, and functional relationships between the various lymphomas and normal lymphoid tissue, as exemplified by the peripheral lymph node. The clinicopathologic features of many extranodal B-cell lymphomas, are, however, more closely related to the structure and function of mucosa-associated lymphoid tissue than of peripheral lymph nodes (2,3).

The anatomic distribution and structure of lymph nodes are adapted to deal with antigens carried to the node in the afferent lymphatics that drain sites at various distances from the node. Permeable mucosal sites, such as the gastrointestinal tract, are, however, particularly vulnerable, because they are in direct contact with the external environment, and spe-

TABLE 22.1. *Localization of mucosa-associated lymphoid tissue lymphoma*

Gastrointestinal tract
  Stomach
  Intestine (including immunoproliferative small intestinal disease)
Salivary glands
Respiratory tract
  Lung, pharynx, trachea
Ocular adnexa
  Conjunctiva, lacrimal gland, orbit[a]
Thyroid
Liver
Breast
Genitourinary tract
  Bladder, prostate, kidney
Rare sites

[a]Not mucosal.

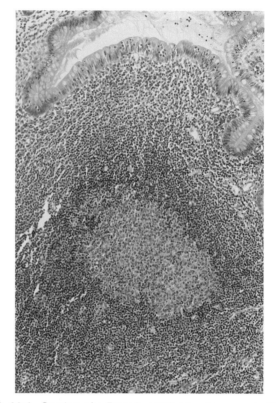

FIG. 22.1. Section of a Peyer's patch showing a central follicle surrounded by a marginal zone. Clusters of marginal zone cells are present in the dome epithelium.

cialized lymphoid tissue has evolved to protect them. This is known as *mucosa-associated lymphoid tissue.* Mucosa-associated lymphoid tissue comprises both B- and T-cell components; it is the former that we are concerned with here. The B-cell component of mucosa-associated lymphoid tissue comprises the B-cell compartment of Peyer's patches, the lamina propria plasma cells, and the B-cell compartment of mesenteric lymph nodes.

Peyer's Patches

There are concentrations of organized lymphoid nodules that are distributed throughout the small intestine, the appendix, and the colorectum. They are concentrated in the terminal ileum, where they collectively form the *Peyer's patches,* the generic term applied to this compartment of mucosa-associated lymphoid tissue (15–17). Peyer's patches are unencapsulated aggregates of lymphoid and accessory cells that in some respects resemble lymph nodes (Fig. 22.1). Each Peyer's patch consists of B- and T-cell areas and associated accessory cells. The B-cell area comprises a germinal center identical to that of reactive lymph nodes. The germinal center is surrounded by a mantle zone of small B lymphocytes that is broadest at the mucosal aspect of the follicle. Surrounding the mantle zone is a broad marginal zone in which most of the cells are small to intermediate-sized B lymphocytes with moderately abundant, pale, staining cytoplasm and nuclei with a slightly irregular outline, leading to a resemblance to centrocytes. The marginal zone extends toward the mucosal surface, and some marginal zone B cells are present within the overlying "dome" epithelium, where they may aggregate in small clusters. These intraepithelial B cells form the lymphoepithelium, which is one of the defining features of mucosa-associated lymphoid tissue. The

dome epithelium is a specialized structure containing microfold cells (18), which are thought to sample antigens in the intestinal contents that then interact with the underlying lymphoid tissue. It is possible, however, that some soluble antigens cross the dome epithelium directly.

The immunophenotype of Peyer's patches (15,16,18) is broadly similar to that of lymph nodes. The germinal center B cells express immunoglobulin (Ig) M and are surrounded by an IgD+, IgM+ mantle zone, which, in turn is surrounded by the IgM+, IgD− marginal zone. The marginal zone extends toward the dome epithelium wherein CD20+, IgM+ intraepithelial B cells can be seen. Lateral to the serosal aspect of the B-cell follicle, there is a T-cell zone containing prominent high endothelial venules equivalent to the paracortical T zone of the lymph node.

Lamina Propria

Few plasma cells are present in the Peyer's patch, in contrast to the lamina propria, where they comprise the principal B-cell component. The plasma cells secrete mainly IgA and IgM and are derived from memory B cells that migrate out of the Peyer's patch germinal centers (19–21). These cells leave the intestine via the efferent lymphatics of the Peyer's patches, pass through the sinuses of mesenteric lymph nodes, and enter the circulation via the thoracic duct, finally migrating out into the lamina propria from specialized venules. Here the majority complete their differentiation into plasma cells while a minority persist as small memory B lymphocytes.

Mesenteric Lymph Nodes

The basic structure of mesenteric lymph nodes is the same as that of peripheral lymph nodes, and in the presence of a breach in the intestinal mucosa, these nodes cannot be distinguished from reactive peripheral nodes. In normal circumstances, however, mesenteric nodes are distinguished by small, rather inactive B-cell follicles, which, in contrast to peripheral lymph nodes, are usually surrounded by a prominent marginal zone. Mesenteric lymph nodes have a poorly developed paracortex and prominent dilated sinuses containing transformed B blasts, most of which are synthesizing IgA.

THE MUCOSA-ASSOCIATED LYMPHOID TISSUE LYMPHOMA CONCEPT

In the early 1980s, Isaacson and Wright noted that just as low-grade nodal lymphomas exhibited the features of normal lymph nodes, certain low-grade B-cell lymphomas of the gastrointestinal tract recapitulated features of mucosa-associated lymphoid tissue Peyer's patches (2,3). MALT lymphomas tend to remain localized to their site of origin for long periods, less commonly disseminate to the bone marrow, and frequently respond favorably to local therapeutic measures. Lymphomas exhibiting these features arise at a wide variety of extranodal sites, not only the gastrointestinal tract. The stomach is by far the most common site of MALT lymphoma, and many of the data discussed in this section are derived from studies of gastric lymphoma.

Curiously, MALT lymphomas only rarely arise at sites of concentration of native mucosa-associated lymphoid tissue, such as the terminal ileum or the tonsils. On the contrary, they most commonly arise from acquired mucosa-associated lymphoid tissue at sites normally devoid of such tissue, such as the stomach, salivary glands, lung, and thyroid.

ACQUIRED MUCOSA-ASSOCIATED LYMPHOID TISSUE

MALT lymphomas of the salivary gland and thyroid, organs normally containing no lymphoid tissue, are always preceded, respectively, by lymphoepithelial (myoepithelial) sialadenitis, usually associated with Sjögren's syndrome, and Hashimoto's thyroiditis (22–24). Histologic and immunohistochemical studies of the heavy lymphoid infiltrate that characterizes these two conditions have shown a remarkable resemblance to mucosa-associated lymphoid tissue. This is most graphically illustrated with reference to lymphoepithelial (myoepithelial) sialadenitis.

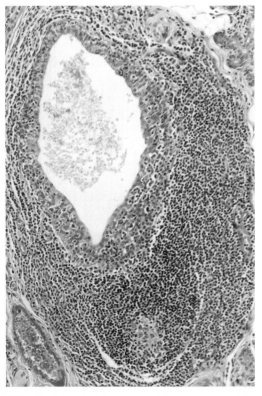

FIG. 22.2. Section of salivary gland from a case of lympho-epithelial sialadenitis. A lymphoid follicle is adjacent to a dilated salivary duct, which is infiltrated by B cells, resulting in a Peyer's patch–like structure.

In this condition, lymphoid tissue accumulates around dilated salivary gland ducts and forms, in effect, small Peyer's patches, complete with germinal center, mantle, a small marginal zone, and, significantly, collections of intraepithelial B cells (Fig. 22.2). This lymphoid tissue, which has become known as *acquired mucosa-associated lymphoid tissue*, is also a feature of Hashimoto's thyroiditis and has been identified in fetal and neonatal lung from infants with pulmonary infections of undetermined nature. It is also seen in a condition termed *follicular bronchiolitis*, which is associated with various autoimmune disorders, including Sjögren's syndrome. Here it is worth emphasizing that, despite claims to the contrary (25), mucosa-associated lymphoid tissue in the form of bronchus-associated lymphoid tissue cannot be found in normal lung (26). The absence of lymphoid tissue from normal stomach, the most common site of MALT lymphoma, is well documented, but here, too, mucosa-associated lymphoid tissue is commonly acquired as a result of the reaction to infection with *H. pylori* that precedes development of most cases of gastric MALT lymphoma (13).

There are certain common factors relating to the acquisition of mucosa-associated lymphoid tissue that may be relevant to development of lymphoma at these sites. In all instances, autoimmunity seems to play an important role in the underlying disease. Mucosa-associated lymphoid tissue accumulates in relation to columnar epithelium and appears to receive antigenic stimuli either from the epithelium itself or, like physiologic mucosa-associated lymphoid tissue, from antigens that enter the lymphoid tissue across the epithelium rather than from antigens carried in afferent lymphatics.

PATHOLOGY OF MUCOSA-ASSOCIATED LYMPHOID TISSUE LYMPHOMA

Macroscopic Appearances

Macroscopically, MALT lymphomas, although sometimes forming obviously tumorous masses, frequently are indistinguishable from the inflammatory lesion that underlies the acquisition of mucosa-associated lymphoid tissue from which the lymphoma arises. Thus, gastric MALT lymphoma, for example, at endoscopy is often indistinguishable from chronic gastritis. Although they may form a single dominant mass, MALT lymphomas are typically multifocal, with small, even microscopic foci of lymphoma scattered throughout the organ involved. All of these foci are clonally identical (27).

Histopathology

MALT lymphomas recapitulate the histologic features of Peyer's patches (28). Thus, the neoplastic B lymphocytes infiltrate around reactive B-cell follicles, external to a preserved follicular mantle, in a marginal zone distribution and spread out to form larger confluent areas that eventually overrun some or most of the follicles (Fig. 22.3). Like marginal zone B cells, the neoplastic cells have relatively abundant, pale cytoplasm with small to medium-sized, slightly irregularly shaped nuclei containing moderately dispersed chromatin and inconspicuous nucleoli. The accumulation of more abundant pale-staining cytoplasm may lead to a monocytoid appearance of the lymphoma cells, whereas in some cases, the cells more closely resemble small lymphocytes (Fig. 22.4). Large cells resembling centroblasts or immunoblasts are usually present but are in the minority. Plasma cell differentiation is present in up to one-third of cases and tends to be maximal beneath the surface gastric epithelium.

Glandular epithelium is often invaded and destroyed by discrete aggregates of lymphoma cells, resulting in the so-called *lymphoepithelial lesions* (Fig. 22.5). These are defined as aggregates of three or more neoplastic marginal zone lymphocytes within glandular epithelium, preferably associated with distortion or necrosis of the epithelium. In gastric MALT lymphoma, these lesions are often accompanied by eosinophilic degeneration of the epithelium. Lymphoepithelial lesions, although highly characteristic of MALT lymphoma, especially gastric lymphoma, are not pathognomonic.

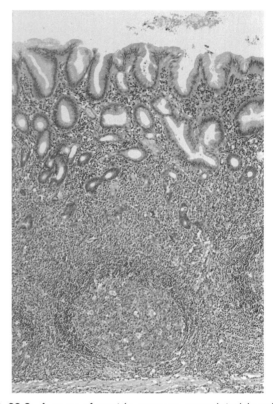

FIG. 22.3. A case of gastric mucosa–associated lymphoid tissue lymphoma. A reactive B-cell follicle is surrounded by an infiltrate of neoplastic marginal zone cells that form lymphoepithelial lesions with gastric glands.

The lymphoma cells sometimes specifically colonize germinal centers of the reactive follicles (Fig. 22.6) (29). Usually, this results in a vaguely nodular or follicular pattern to the lymphoma. In some cases, the plasma cell differentiation

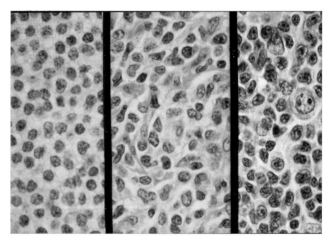

FIG. 22.4. Neoplastic marginal zone B cells from three cases of gastric mucosa–associated lymphoid tissue lymphoma. In the left-hand panel, the cells resemble small lymphocytes; in the center, they are "centrocyte-like"; and in the right-hand panel, they are monocytoid in appearance.

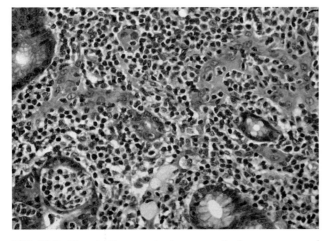

FIG. 22.5. Neoplastic marginal zone cells from a case of gastric mucosa–associated lymphoid tissue lymphoma forming lymphoepithelial lesions with gastric glands.

occurs within these reactive germinal centers and in others the intrafollicular marginal zone cells undergo blast transformation, which can lead to a close resemblance to follicular lymphoma.

Like other low-grade B-cell lymphomas, MALT lymphoma may undergo high-grade transformation (Fig. 22.7). Transformed centroblast or immunoblast-like cells may be present in larger numbers in MALT lymphoma, but only when solid or sheet-like proliferations of transformed cells are present should the lymphoma be considered to have transformed. The result is a tumor that currently cannot reliably be distinguished from other diffuse large B-cell lymphomas, particularly if the preceding MALT lymphoma has been overgrown. Thus, the current recommendation is that such cases be designated as *diffuse large B-cell lymphoma* and the presence of concurrent MALT lymphoma be documented (30).

MALT lymphomas preferentially disseminate to other sites where such lymphomas occur. Gastric MALT lym-

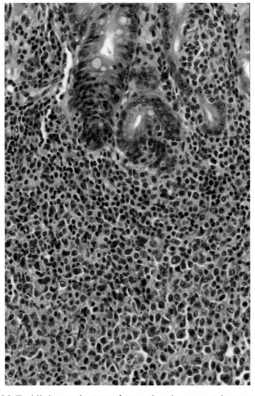

FIG. 22.7. High-grade transformation in a gastric mucosa–associated lymphoid tissue (MALT) lymphoma. A typical MALT lymphoma is present in the glandular epithelium, with transformation to a diffuse large-cell lymphoma below.

phomas, for example, tend to disseminate to the small intestine, salivary gland, and lung. When MALT lymphomas disseminate to lymphoid tissue, including lymph nodes and spleen, they specifically invade the marginal zone (Fig. 22.8). This can lead to a deceptively benign or reactive appearance, especially in mesenteric lymph nodes, in which a marginal zone is normally present. Subsequently, there is interfollicular expansion to form sheets of more obvious lymphoma. Cytologic heterogeneity is still a feature of disseminated disease.

Immunohistochemistry

The tumor cells typically express IgM, less often express IgA or IgG, and are IgD⁻. Their immunophenotype recapitulates that of marginal zone cells. They are CD20, CD79a, CD21, and CD35 positive and CD5, CD23, and CD10 negative. CD43 is expressed in approximately 50% of cases, and expression of CD11c is variable.

Differential Diagnosis

Because of differences in clinical behavior and management, it is important to differentiate MALT lymphoma from the other small B-cell lymphomas that may present in

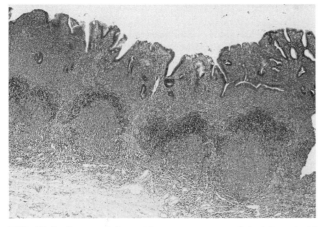

FIG. 22.6. A case of gastric mucosa–associated lymphoid tissue lymphoma with prominent follicular colonization.

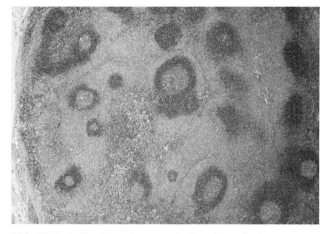

FIG. 22.8. Infiltration of a gastric lymph node by mucosa-associated lymphoid tissue lymphoma. The pale-staining infiltrate surrounds follicles and expands the interfollicular zones.

or involve extranodal sites. These include mantle cell lymphoma, lymphocytic lymphoma (chronic lymphocytic leukemia), and follicular lymphoma. The cytologic features of mantle cell lymphoma can closely simulate those of MALT lymphoma, even to the extent that occasional lymphoepithelial lesions may be present. However, absence of transformed blasts together with expression of CD5, IgD, and, importantly, intranuclear expression of cyclin D1, a consequence of t(11;14), serve to distinguish mantle cell lymphoma. Lymphocytic lymphoma is characterized by small, round lymphocytes, usually together with peripheral blood lymphocytosis. Expression of CD5, CD23, and IgD without nuclear cyclin D1 provide further distinction from MALT lymphoma. Finally, follicular lymphoma, which may arise extranodally, can be difficult to distinguish from MALT lymphoma with follicular colonization. The transformed MALT lymphoma cells within follicles may closely resemble centroblasts but typically are CD10[-] and bcl6[-] (nuclear), in contrast to the cells of follicular lymphoma, which usually express both antigens both within and between follicles.

Molecular Genetics

MALT lymphoma Ig heavy- and light-chain genes are rearranged and show somatic mutation of their variable regions, consistent with a postgerminal center memory B-cell derivation (31). Ongoing mutations are thought to occur in most cases (32). Because of the difficulty in distinguishing between acquired mucosa-associated lymphoid tissue and MALT lymphoma, there has been a tendency to rely on molecular evidence of monoclonality detected by polymerase chain reaction analysis for the diagnosis of lymphoma. This technique may fail to detect monoclonality in up to 15% of cases of overt lymphoma and, thus, produce false-negative results (33). There are also reports of apparently spurious monoclonality in biopsies of acquired mucosa-associated lymphoid tissue—for example, gastric biopsies showing only chronic gastritis (34–36) in which there is no histologic evidence of malignancy. The frequency of this spurious monoclonality varies between laboratories (37), which suggests that the technique may be a factor. These findings serve to emphasize that MALT lymphoma should not be diagnosed in the absence of clear histologic evidence.

Trisomy 3 has been reported in 60% of MALT lymphomas (38). T(11;18) has been observed in 25% to 40% of gastric MALT lymphoma cases and a similar proportion of pulmonary cases (39,40). However, the frequency of this translocation in other MALT lymphomas is much lower. Only 18% of conjunctival MALT lymphomas and 10% of orbital lymphomas carry the translocation, whereas it is not present in either salivary gland- or thyroid- MALT lymphomas. T(1:14) has been observed in a minority of MALT lymphomas arising in the stomach and the lung (41,42). There is an intriguing link between these two translocations, both of which appear to have the effect of activating NF-κB and, thus, promoting cell proliferation (43). They both result in intranuclear expression of a novel gene protein, bcl10 (44). Neither t(11;14) nor t(14;18) is present, although the latter has been reported in isolated cases. The clinical relevance of these translocations is in the section Treatment of Gastric Mucosa-Associated Lymphoid Tissue Lymphoma.

Normal Cell Counterpart

The tumor architecture and cytologic features, together with the immunophenotype, strongly suggest that the MALT lymphomas are related to the postgerminal-center marginal zone B cell.

CLASSIFICATION OF MUCOSA-ASSOCIATED LYMPHOID TISSUE LYMPHOMAS

MALT lymphoma could not be classified in either the Working Formulation or the Kiel Classification. With the advent of the Revised European-American Lymphoma and World Health Organization Classifications (45), MALT lymphoma is now formally classified as *extranodal marginal zone B-cell lymphoma of mucosa-associated lymphoid tissue (MALT lymphoma)* and defined as follows:

An extranodal lymphoma comprising morphologically heterogeneous small B cells including marginal zone (centrocyte-like) cells, monocytoid cells, small lymphocytes, and scattered immunoblast- and centroblast-like cells with plasma cell differentiation in a proportion of the cases. The infiltrate is in the marginal zone of reactive B-cell follicles and extends into the interfollicular region. In epithelial tissues the neoplastic cells typically infiltrate the epithelium forming lymphoepithelial lesions (46).

PATHOGENESIS OF MUCOSA-ASSOCIATED LYMPHOID TISSUE LYMPHOMA: THE *HELICOBACTER PYLORI* AND GASTRIC MUCOSA–ASSOCIATED LYMPHOID TISSUE LYMPHOMA MODEL

There are several lines of evidence that suggest that gastric MALT lymphoma arises from mucosa-associated lymphoid tissue acquired as a consequence of *H. pylori* infection (Fig. 22.9). *H. pylori* can be demonstrated in the gastric mucosa of the majority of cases of gastric MALT lymphoma (13). In the first study in which this association was examined, the organism was present in more than 90% of cases. Subsequent studies have shown a lower incidence (44) but also that the density and detectability of *H. pylori* decrease as lymphoma evolves from chronic gastritis (47). A case-control study showed an association between previous *H. pylori* infection and the development of primary gastric lymphoma (48). More direct evidence confirming the importance of *H. pylori* in the pathogenesis of gastric lymphoma has been obtained from studies that detected the lymphoma B-cell clone in the chronic gastritis that preceded the lymphoma (47,49) and from a series of *in vitro* studies showing that lymphoma growth could be stimulated in culture by *H. pylori* strain–specific T cells when crude lymphoma cultures were exposed to the organism (50). Finally, after the initial study by Wotherspoon et al. (51), several groups have confirmed that eradication of *H. pylori* with antibiotics results in regression of gastric MALT lymphoma in 75% of cases (52). The lymphoma may take up to 1 year or more to regress (53), and in up to 50% of cases, small monoclonal aggregates of lymphocytes may persist for some time without progression (54). Subsequent studies have shown well-documented regression of some cases of MALT lymphoma complicated by diffuse large-cell lymphoma (52).

Prediction of Regression of Gastric Mucosa–Associated Lymphoid Tissue Lymphoma after Eradication of *Helicobacter pylori*

The follow-up of MALT lymphoma patients after eradication of *H. pylori* is rather complex, requiring repeated gastroscopy, and it would be extremely useful to be able to identify the approximately 25% of cases of gastric MALT lymphoma that do not respond to eradication of *H. pylori*. Studies using endoscopic ultrasound have suggested that if the tumor has invaded beyond the submucosa, it will not respond (55,56). More recently, the two MALT lymphoma-associated translocations described above have been cloned (42,57) and have been shown to have a bearing on the response to *H. pylori* eradication. The first of these—t(1;14)(p22;q14)—which is present in rare cases, has been shown to involve a novel gene—bcl10—that is strongly expressed in the nucleus of the neoplastic lymphocytes (58). The second—t(11;18)(q21;q21)—is present in up to 40% of cases and is strongly associated with lack of response to eradication of *H. pylori* (59). Interestingly, t(11;18) is also associated with nuclear expression of bcl10, albeit more weakly than is t(1;14). Moreover, the frequency of both t(11;18)(q21;q21) and nuclear bcl10 expression is significantly higher in tumors that have disseminated beyond the stomach (78% and 93%, respectively) than in those confined to the stomach (10% and 38%) (60). These findings in part explain the results based on the use of endoscopic ultrasound and suggest that both t(11;18)(q21;q21) and bcl10 nuclear expression are associated with failure to respond to *H. pylori* eradication and with more advanced MALT lymphoma. This is in keeping with the observations of Lucas et al., who suggested that their oncogenic activities may be related (43).

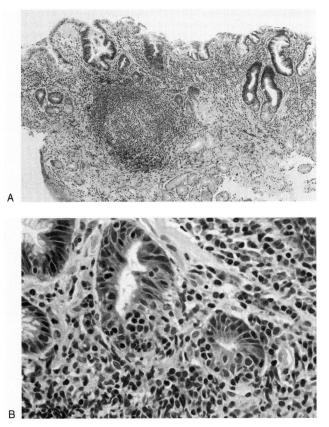

FIG. 22.9. A: Gastric mucosa from a case of *Helicobacter pylori*–positive chronic gastritis. A B-cell follicle is present, but the diffuse mucosal infiltrate is comprised by plasma cells and T lymphocytes. **B:** Two glands adjacent to the B-cell follicle are infiltrated by B cells, resulting in resemblance to a lymphoepithelial lesion.

CLINICAL ASPECTS OF GASTRIC MUCOSA–ASSOCIATED LYMPHOID TISSUE LYMPHOMA

The stomach is the most common organ involved with MALT lymphoma, and clinical aspects of diagnosis, staging,

TABLE 22.2. *Staging of gastric mucosa–associated lymphoid tissue lymphoma: comparison of different systems*

TMN stage	Lugano Staging System for gastrointestinal lymphomas (64)	TNM Staging System adapted for gastric lymphoma	Ann Arbor stage	Tumor extension
I	Confined to gastrointestinal tract (single primary or multiple, non-contiguous)	T1 N0 M0	IE	Mucosa, submucosa
		T2 N0 M0	IE	Muscularis propria
		T3 N0 M0	IE	Serosa
II	Extending into abdomen			
	II1 = local nodal involvement	T1–3 N1 M0	IIE	Perigastric lymph nodes
	II2 = distant nodal involvement	T1–3 N2 M0	IIE	More distant regional lymph nodes
IIE	Penetration of serosa to involve adjacent organs or tissues	T4 N0 M0	IE	Invasion of adjacent structures
IV	Disseminated extranodal involvement or concomitant supradiaphragmatic nodal involvement	T1–4 N3 M0	IIIE	Lymph nodes on both sides of the diaphragm/distant metastases (e.g., bone marrow or additional extranodal sites)
		T1–4 N0–3 M1	IVE	

TNM, tumor-node-metastasis.

and treatment of gastric MALT lymphoma is discussed separately from all other sites.

The most common presenting symptoms of gastric MALT lymphoma are nonspecific dyspepsia, epigastric pain, nausea, and chronic manifestations of gastrointestinal bleeding, such as anemia. B symptoms are rare. The upper gastrointestinal complaints often lead to an endoscopy, which usually reveals nonspecific gastritis or peptic ulcer, with mass lesions being unusual (61,62). Elevation of lactate acid dehydrogenase is also uncommon (62).

The question of the best staging system is still controversial (63). Most investigators of gastric MALT lymphoma use a modification of the Bleckledge staging system recommended at an international workshop (Lugano, 1993) (64). When ultrasound endoscopy is available, the tumor-node-metastases system can also be used, based on the echoendoscopic extent of the gastric wall involvement (65) (Table 22.2).

Diagnosis and Work-Up of Gastric Mucosa–Associated Lymphoid Tissue Lymphoma

The initial staging should include a gastroduodenal endoscopy with multiple biopsies from each region of the stomach, duodenum, and gastroesophageal junction and from any abnormal-appearing site. Fresh biopsy and washings material should be available for cytogenetic studies, in addition to routine histology and immunohistochemistry. The recommended immunophenotypings include paraffin panel for CD20 (L26/Pan B), CD3, CD5, CD10, cyclin D1, and kappa/lambda. Alternatively, flow cytometry for similar cell surface–marker analysis may provide adequate diagnostic information. A molecular-genetic analysis for detection of t(11;18) is strongly recommended for identifying disease that is unlikely to respond to antibiotic therapy

(59). The presence of active *H. pylori* infection must be determined by histology (Giemsa stain or Warthin-Starry stain of antral biopsy specimen); serology studies are recommended when the results of histology are negative (66). A repeat endoscopic biopsy is recommended if histology demonstrates atypical lymphoid infiltrates in the presence of *H. pylori*. Endoscopic ultrasound is highly recommended for evaluation of depth of infiltration and presence of perigastric lymph nodes (55,67). A deep infiltration of the gastric wall is associated with a higher risk of lymph node involvement (68) and a lower rate of lymphoma regression with antibiotic therapy alone (55,69). Other studies should include complete blood count; basic biochemical studies (including lactate acid dehydrogenase); computed tomography of the chest, abdomen, and pelvis; and bone marrow biopsy (Table 22.3).

Although systemic dissemination of gastric MALT lymphoma is uncommon, and the disease may remain localized in the stomach for a long period, systemic dissemination and bone marrow involvement should be excluded at presentation, because prognosis is worse with advanced-stage disease or with an unfavorable International Prognostic Index score (8,70,71). Patients with gastric MALT lymphoma were reported to have a better disease-free survival than patients with mucosa-associated lymphoid tissue in other sites (72,73).

Treatment of Gastric Mucosa–Associated Lymphoid Tissue Lymphoma

The role of *H. pylori* infection in the pathogenesis of gastric MALT lymphoma has been well established. Antibiotic eradication of *H. pylori* is the standard primary treatment for patients with gastric MALT lymphoma and concomitant evi-

TABLE 22.3. *Recommended staging procedures for gastric mucosa–associated lymphoid tissue lymphoma*

History (duration and presence of local or systemic symptoms)

Physical examination (careful evaluation of all lymph node regions, inspection of the upper airways and tonsils, clinical evaluation of the size of the liver and spleen, detection of any palpable mass)

Laboratory tests, including complete blood counts and peripheral blood smear, lactate acid dehydrogenase, evaluation of renal and liver function

Bone marrow biopsy

Standard posteroanterior and lateral chest radiographs

Abdominal and pelvic computed tomography scan

Gastroduodenal endoscopy with multiple gastric biopsies from all the visible lesions and the noninvolved areas, with a complete mapping of the organ

Gastric endoscopic ultrasound

Upper gastrointestinal series (in selected cases)

---

dence for the presence of the bacteria in the stomach. Multiple series documented histologic regression of the gastric MALT lymphoma after successful eradication of *H. pylori*, with a response ranging from 35% to 100%. Four relatively large series from Europe and North America documented responses of 50% to 80% (Table 22.4). A treatment algorithm for patients presenting with or without *H. pylori* is outlined in Figure 22.10.

Several effective anti–*H. pylori* programs are available (74). It is expected that after 10 to 14 days of antibiotic treatment, *H. pylori* will be eradicated in 85% to 90% of the patients. The regimen of choice is triple therapy with a proton pump inhibitor (e.g., lansoprazole, 30 mg twice daily; omeprazole, 20 mg twice daily; pantoprazole, 40 mg twice daily; rabeprazole, 20 mg twice daily; or esomeprazole, 40 mg once daily), amoxicillin (1 g twice daily), and clarithromycin (500 mg twice daily). Metronidazole (500 mg twice daily) can be substituted for amoxicillin, but only in penicillin-allergic individuals, because metronidazole resistance is common and can reduce the efficacy of treatment. Other regimens that include bismuth or histamine-2–receptor antagonists (rather than proton pump inhibitors) with antibiotics are also effective (74).

Several factors predict the likelihood of gastric MALT lymphoma regression after antibiotic therapy (Table 22.5). An obvious prerequisite for expecting a response to antibiotics is evidence of concomitant *H. pylori* infection. Indeed, in two series that included *H. pylori*–positive and –negative patients, none of the *H. pylori*–negative lymphomas (16 patients) responded to antibiotic therapy (65,69). Thus, it is highly questionable whether patients with no evidence of active *H. pylori* infection will benefit from a therapeutic trial with antibiotics (Fig. 22.10).

Other factors have been associated with a low response of gastric MALT lymphoma to antibiotic treatment alone. A study from the French Groupe d'Etude Lymphome Digestif (69) and M.D. Anderson Cancer Center (65) showed that in patients with *H. pylori*–positive gastric MALT lymphoma, the detection of nodal involvement by endoscopy with ultrasound or computed tomography was associated with a significantly lower rate of lymphoma remission (55). Likewise, penetration of lymphoma beyond the mucosa was also associated with a markedly decreased response (55). These two features are related, as deep involvement is linked to increased risk of nodal involvement (68). Furthermore, the

---

TABLE 22.4. *Response of gastric mucosa–associated lymphoid tissue lymphoma to* Helicobacter pylori *antibiotic therapy*

Group (reference)	Number of *H. pylori*–positive patients	CR (%)	Number of *H. pylori*–negative patients/number of CRs	Median follow-up (range) (mo)	Relapse (%)	CR patients remaining monoclonal (%)
Groupe d'Etude Lymphome Digestif (69)	34	56	10/0	6 (2–18)	11	42
M.D. Anderson Cancer Center (65)	28	50	6/0	41 (18–70)	0	N/A
LYO3 (International Extranodal Lymphoma Study Group, Groupe d'Etudes des Lymphomes de l'Adulte, United Kingdom Lymphoma Group) (81)	189	55	N/A	24 (6–72)	14	44
German Mucosa-Associated Lymphoid Tissue Study Group (54)	97	79	N/A	33 (0–65)	10	45

CR, complete remission; N/A, not applicable.

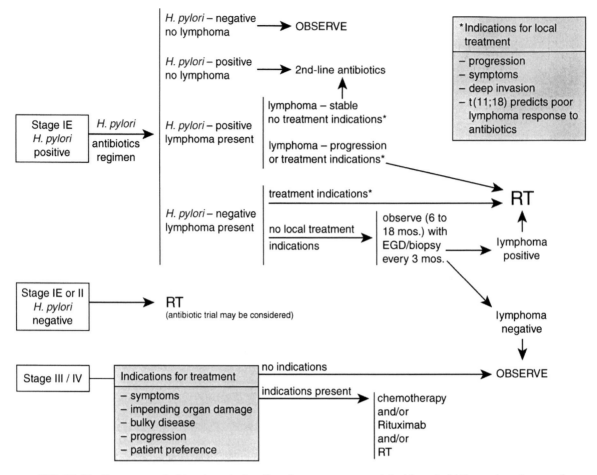

FIG. 22.10. Recommended treatment algorithm for mucosa-associated lymphoid tissue lymphoma of the stomach. RT, radiation therapy.

likelihood of *H. pylori* presence is smaller when lymphoma involvement is found beyond the submucosa (44). An additional (and not well-explained) finding of the M.D. Anderson group is that the regression rate of tumors located in the distal part of the stomach was better than that of proximally located disease (65). In a report from a German group, for four of six patients whose lymphoma had not regressed after eradication of *H. pylori,* surgical resection showed the presence of high-grade lymphoma in deeper sections that was not appreciated during endoscopy (75). This experience underlines the importance of multiple deep biopsies, particularly if endoscopy with ultrasound indicates deep penetration or lymph node enlargement. It also suggests that gastric MALT lymphoma with a high-grade component should be treated as intermediate-grade lymphoma with chemotherapy and involved-field radiotherapy.

Although endoscopy with ultrasound could identify locally advanced disease that is unlikely to respond to antibiotic treatment, there is still a significant number of patients (approximately 25%) with superficial lymphoma whose lymphoma will remain refractory even after *H. pylori* eradication. These antibiotic-resistant lymphomas are likely to demonstrate the chromosomal abnormality

t(11;18)(q21;q21), a translocation involving approximately 40% of MALT lymphomas (39,57,76,77). In analysis of biopsy material from 111 patients with *H. pylori*–positive gastric MALT lymphoma, only two of 48 (4%) patients whose lymphoma completely regressed after *H. pylori* eradication had t(11;18), whereas 42 of 63 (67%) of the nonresponding patients demonstrated the translocation (59). Thus, t(11;18) is a powerful indicator of response to *H. pylori* eradication, and its presence at diagnosis should

TABLE 22.5. *Predictors of poor response to antibiotic therapy (reference)*

Absence of *Helicobacter pylori* infection (65,69)
Perigastric node enlargement (by endoscopy with ultrasound or computed tomography) (65,69)
Infiltration beyond the mucosa layers (55,65,69)
Proximal location (65)
Presence of high-grade lymphoma component (75)
Translocation t(11;18) (q21;q21) (59)
Translocations involving bcl10 locus, nuclear localization of bcl10 protein (79)

suggest that an alternative treatment (e.g., radiotherapy) be administered early, rather than waiting for regression with repeated endoscopies (78). It has been suggested, however, that t(11;18)-negative tumors have a higher risk of transformation into diffuse large B-cell lymphoma. Therefore, t(11;18)-negative tumors that have not completely regressed after antibiotics should be closely monitored for early alternative therapeutic intervention.

It is estimated that in approximately one-third of cases, resistance of gastric MALT lymphoma to *H. pylori* eradication is not due to t(11;18). MALT lymphomas with translocations involving the bcl10 locus, such as t(1;14)(p22;q32) and t(1;2)(p22;p12), are typically at advanced stages and are unlikely to respond to antibiotics (79,80). Nuclear bcl10 expression is more commonly found in advanced MALT lymphomas and is associated with the above translocations as well as with t(11;18).

Several studies showed that polymerase chain reaction–detectable monoclonality may persist in almost one-half of patients who had histologic disappearance of gastric MALT lymphoma after antibiotic therapy (Table 22.4) (54,69,81), signifying that *H. pylori* eradication suppresses but does not completely obliterate the lymphoma clone. The implication of polymerase chain reaction–detected clonality in terms of relapse risk remains to be determined, and careful long-term follow-up of patients after successful antibiotic therapy is warranted (75,82). Minimal residual microscopic disease detected after macroscopic regression after antibiotic therapy may remain clinically dormant, and a watch-and-wait strategy could be considered for selected patients agreeable to frequent endoscopies (83). Yet, it should be acknowledged that lymphoma relapses in the absence of *H. pylori* reinfection have been described (75), and the projected risk of transformation of gastric MALT lymphoma into aggressive lymphoma has not been determined as yet.

Treatment of *Helicobacter pylori*–Independent Gastric Mucosa–Associated Lymphoid Tissue Lymphoma

Approximately 30% to 50% of patients with *H. pylori*–positive gastric MALT lymphoma show persistent or progressing lymphoma even after eradication of *H. pylori* with antibiotic therapy (Table 22.4). Of the complete responders, almost 15% will relapse within 3 years, suggesting that approximately one-half of patients with gastric MALT lymphoma will eventually be considered for additional therapies. Most of those will still have disease limited to the stomach. Patients who present with no evidence *H. pylori* infection are unlikely to respond to antibiotics and should be considered for alternative treatments (Fig. 22.10).

As a local therapy, surgery has been widely used in the past. Cogliatti et al. (84) reviewed 69 cases of low-grade gastric MALT lymphoma treated with surgery alone (45) or with surgery followed by either chemotherapy or radiother-

apy, or both (24). The 5-year overall survival was 91%, and no significant difference in survival was observed in patients selected for adjuvant therapy after surgery.

In recent years, the role of surgery in gastric MALT lymphoma has been questioned (10,85–87). Gastric MALT lymphoma is a multifocal disease (88), and adequate gastrectomy needs to be quite extensive, severely impairing quality of life, and yet residual disease at the margins may still require additional radiation, chemotherapy, or both.

Several institutions reported excellent results using involved-field radiotherapy of the stomach in *H. pylori*–independent gastric MALT lymphoma patients for whom antibiotic therapy was unsuccessful or who had no evidence of *H. pylori* infection (73,89–92). The recent update of the Memorial Sloan-Kettering Cancer Center experience included 51 patients with gastric MALT lymphoma (stage I: 39; stage II: 10; stage IV: 2) who were either *H. pylori*–negative (30 patients) or remained with persistent lymphoma after antibiotic therapies and adequate observation (21 patients) (93). All patients were treated with radiation to the stomach and perigastric nodes; the median total dose was 30 Gy in 4 weeks. All patients had regular follow-up endoscopic evaluations and biopsies. Forty-nine of 51 (96%) patients obtained a biopsy-proven complete response. Of three patients who relapsed, two were salvaged. Three patients died of other malignancies, all second tumors developed outside the radiation field. At a median follow-up of 4 years, freedom from treatment failure, overall survival, and cause-specific survival were 89%, 83%, and 100%, respectively. Treatment was well tolerated, with no significant acute or chronic side effects. The experiences from Toronto and Boston using the same radiation approach were equally successful (73,90,91), supporting the approach that modest-dose involved-field radiotherapy is the treatment of choice for patients with persistent gastric MALT lymphoma who have exhausted the antibiotic therapy approach or are unlikely to respond to it (*H. pylori*–negative patients) (94,95).

Patients with systemic disease should be considered for chemotherapy, immunotherapy (anti-CD20), or both. However, chemotherapy has never been adequately evaluated in gastric MALT lymphomas, because it was usually not administered or was given after surgery or radiotherapy. Only few compounds have been tested specifically in MALT lymphomas (96). A nonrandomized study of 24 patients (17 in stage I and seven in stage IV, most of them with primary gastric localization) reported that oral alkylating agents (either cyclophosphamide, 100 mg per day, or chlorambucil, 6 mg per day, with a median treatment duration of 1 year) can result in a high rate of disease control, with projected 5-year event-free and overall survival rates of 50% and 75%, respectively (96). A more recent phase II study of 19 patients with gastric and seven patients with nongastric MALT lymphoma demonstrated some antitumor activity of the purine analog, cladribine (2-CDA, given as a 2-hour intravenous infusion at a dose of 0.12 mg per kg of body weight on 5 consecutive days every 4 weeks), with a complete response rate of 84%. However, in this study, additional anti-*Helicobacter* treatment might have contributed to the very high remission rate in patients with gastric lymphoma, because only 43% of patients with extragastric presentation achieved a complete response (97).

In the presence of disseminated or advanced disease, chemotherapy may be an obvious choice. The activity of the anti-CD20 monoclonal antibody rituximab has also been shown in a phase II study (with a response rate of approximately 70%) and may represent an additional option for the treatment of systemic disease, but the efficacy of its combination with chemotherapy still needs to be explored in this histologic type (98). Depending on the response to systemic therapy, presence of bulky disease, and symptoms, selected patients with systemic disease may also benefit from irradiation of the stomach.

Nongastric Marginal Zone Lymphomas of the Mucosa-Associated Lymphoid Tissue Type

MALT lymphomas have also been described in various nongastric sites, such as salivary glands, skin, orbit, conjunctiva, lung, thyroid, larynx, breast, kidney, liver, bladder, prostate, urethra, small intestine, rectum, pancreas, and even in the intracranial dura (11,72,73,82,99–101). Nongastric MALT lymphomas have been difficult to characterize, because these tumors, numerous when considered together, are distributed so widely throughout the body that it is difficult to assemble adequate series of any given site. Yet, a few series have recently addressed the characteristics of nongastric MALT lymphomas (72,73,99). The International Extranodal Lymphoma Study Group (IELSG) published a retrospective survey of a large series of patients who were diagnosed as having nongastric MALT lymphoma, with the aim of better characterizing this disease entity (11). The IELSG study confirmed the indolent course of nongastric MALT lymphomas, despite the fact that one-quarter of cases presented with stage IV disease; regardless of treatment type, the 5-year survival was approximately 90% (Figs. 22.11 and 22.12) (11). The finding that dissemination to multiple mucosal sites does not change the outcome has also been demonstrated in other series (72,99). Nongastrointestinal MALT lymphoma patients seem to progress more often than do those with gastric MALT lymphoma (72,73), but whether different sites have a different natural history remains an open question. Location can be an important factor because of organ-specific problems, which result in particular management strategies. In the IELSG series, the patients with the disease initially presenting in the upper airways appeared to have a slightly poorer outcome, but their small number prevented any definitive conclusion (11).

The optimal management of nongastric MALT lymphomas has not yet been clearly established. Retrospective series included patients treated with surgery, radiotherapy, and chemotherapy alone or in combination (11,73, 82,90,95,99). In most patients, good disease control and excellent cause-specific and overall survival have been demonstrated independent of the treatment modality selected. In a multivariate analysis of the IELSG data, the minority of patients (17%) with International Prognostic Index intermediate-high or high risk scores had an inferior progression-free survival, and patients in stage IV due to disease at mucosa-associated lymphoid tissue sites plus bone marrow or lymph node involvement—but not those with multiple mucosal localizations only—had a lower overall survival rate. The presence of nodal involvement adversely affected cause-specific survival

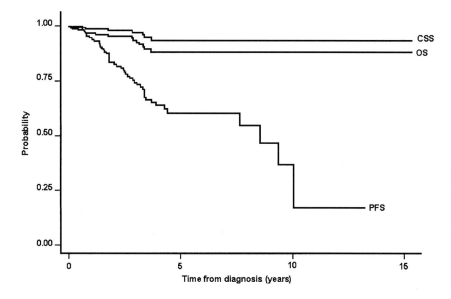

FIG. 22.11. Overall survival (OS), cause-specific survival (CSS), and progression-free survival (PFS) in primary nongastric mucosa–associated lymphoid tissue lymphomas. [From Zucca E, Conconi A, Pedrinis E, et al. Non-gastric marginal zone B-cell lymphoma of mucosa-associated lymphoid tissue. *Blood* 2003;101(7):2489–2495.]

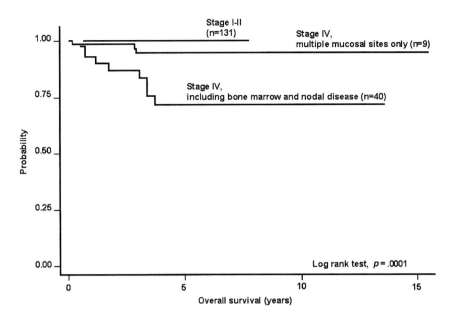

FIG. 22.12. Overall survival according to the Ann Arbor stage of disease in primary nongastric mucosa–associated lymphoid tissue lymphoma. [From Zucca E, Conconi A, Pedrinis E, et al. Non-gastric marginal zone B-cell lymphoma of mucosa-associated lymphoid tissue. *Blood* 2003;101 (7):2489–2495.]

(11). Thus, the treatment choice should be "patient-tailored," taking into account the site, stage, and clinical characteristics of the individual patient. In patients with localized disease, extensive surgery is unnecessary in most sites, because marginal zone lymphomas are exquisitely sensitive to relatively low doses of radiation. Specifically, MALT lymphoma in sites such as salivary glands, ocular adnexae, conjunctiva, thyroid, breast, and bladder have been successfully eradicated with involved-field radiation therapy encompassing the involved organ alone with a dose of 24 Gy to 36 Gy (73,90,95,102–109). Even unusual sites (e.g., the larynx, base of the skull, urethra, and prostate) not easily amenable to surgery have been well controlled by involved-field radiation therapy (100,101,110,111). Patients with extensive lung disease or involvement of multiple sites or the bone marrow are likely to respond to a variety of systemic chemotherapy regimens, although no specific chemotherapy regimen has been advocated (11,82,99). Because responses to rituximab have also been reported (98), the IELSG is planning a randomized trial to evaluate the benefit of the addition of rituximab to chlorambucil in either nongastric or gastric antibiotic-resistant mucosa-associated lymphoid tissue lymphoma.

Future Directions

For a disease that was defined as a separate entity only in the 1980s, extraordinary progress has been made in understanding the etiology and cellular and molecular pathologic events and identifying at least one easily treatable causative agent (*H. pylori*). Clinicians have also gathered encouraging experience in eradicating disease in sites that are unlikely to respond to antibiotics (extragastric MALT lymphoma) or in gastric MALT lymphomas that developed in the absence of *H. pylori*

or have become independent of it. Modest doses of limited-field radiation therapy have been shown to be effective in eradicating MALT lymphoma, allowing organ preservation without a need for surgery. The design of effective chemotherapy regimens and introduction of anti-CD20 therapy for appropriate clinical circumstances are in progress and will expand our treatment options. The recent identification of genetic and molecular events that predict response to treatment and risk of aggressive transformations will affect our therapeutic choices and the optimal timing for intervention. It may also help in developing future molecular targeted therapies. Finally, the establishment of national and international groups to retrospectively analyze patients with a relatively uncommon disease with involvement of a variety of sites has facilitated our clinical understanding of the disease. Groups like IELSG are moving now toward prospective studies with participation of groups from multiple countries. These studies and the close collaboration between pathologists and clinicians that have characterized the rapid progress in this disease in the last two decades are likely to further advance the understanding of this fascinating lymphoma, better define our treatment strategy, and expand our therapeutic options.

REFERENCES

1. Isaacson P, Berger F, Muller-Hermelink HK, et al. Extranodal marginal zone B-cell lymphoma of mucosa-associated lymphoid tissue (MALT lymphoma). In: Jaffe ES, Harris NL, Stein H, et al., eds. *Tumours of Haematopoietic and Lymphoid Tissues*. Lyon: IARC, 2001:157–160.
2. Isaacson P, Wright DH. Malignant lymphoma of mucosa-associated lymphoid tissue. A distinctive type of B-cell lymphoma. *Cancer* 1983;52:1410–1416.
3. Isaacson P, Wright DH. Extranodal malignant lymphoma arising from mucosa-associated lymphoid tissue. *Cancer* 1984;53:2515–2524.
4. Ott MM, Rosenwald A, Katzenberger T, et al. Marginal zone B-cell lymphomas (MZBL) arising at different sites represent different biological entities. *Genes Chromosomes Cancer* 2000;28:380–386.

5. Chacon JI, Mollejo M, Munoz E, et al. Splenic marginal zone lymphoma: clinical characteristics and prognostic factors in a series of 60 patients. *Blood* 2002;100:1648–1654.

6. Conconi A, Bertoni F, Pedrinis E, et al. Nodal marginal zone B-cell lymphomas may arise from different subsets of marginal zone B lymphocytes. *Blood* 2001;98:781–786.

7. Nathwani BN, Anderson JR, Armitage JO, et al. Marginal zone B-cell lymphoma: a clinical comparison of nodal and mucosa-associated lymphoid tissue types. Non-Hodgkin's Lymphoma Classification Project. *J Clin Oncol* 1999;17:2486–2492.

8. A clinical evaluation of the International Lymphoma Study Group classification of non-Hodgkin's lymphoma. The Non-Hodgkin's Lymphoma Classification Project. *Blood* 1997;89:3909–3918.

9. Fisher RI, Miller TP, Grogan TM. New REAL clinical entities. *Cancer J Sci Am* 1998;4(Suppl 2):S5–S12.

10. Zucca E, Bertoni F, Roggero E, et al. The gastric marginal zone B-cell lymphoma of MALT type. *Blood* 2000;96:410–419.

11. Zucca E, Conconi A, Pedrinis E, et al. Non-gastric marginal zone B-cell lymphoma of mucosa-associated lymphoid tissue. *Blood* 2003; 101(7):2489–2495.

12. Doglioni C, Wotherspoon AC, Moschini A, et al. High incidence of primary gastric lymphoma in northeastern Italy. *Lancet* 1992;339:834–835.

13. Wotherspoon AC, Ortiz-Hidalgo C, Falzon MR, et al. *Helicobacter pylori*-associated gastritis and primary B-cell gastric lymphoma. *Lancet* 1991;338:1175–1176.

14. Zaki M, Schubert ML. *Helicobacter pylori* and gastric lymphoma. *Gastroenterology* 1995;108:610–612.

15. Spencer J, Finn T, Isaacson PG. Human Peyer's patches: an immunohistochemical study. *Gut* 1986;27:405–410.

16. Spencer J, Finn T, Pulford KA, et al. The human gut contains a novel population of B lymphocytes which resemble marginal zone cells. *Clin Exp Immunol* 1985;62:607–612.

17. Spencer J, Finn T, Isaacson PG. Gut associated lymphoid tissue: a morphological and immunocytochemical study of the human appendix. *Gut* 1985;26:672–679.

18. Owen RL, Jones AL. Epithelial cell specialization within human Peyer's patches: an ultrastructural study of intestinal lymphoid follicles. *Gastroenterology* 1974;66:189–203.

19. Brandtzaeg P. Transport models for secretory IgA and secretory IgM. *Clin Exp Immunol* 1981;44:221–232.

20. Brandtzaeg P, Halstensen TS, Kett K, et al. Immunobiology and immunopathology of human gut mucosa: humoral immunity and intraepithelial lymphocytes. *Gastroenterology* 1989;97:1562–1584.

21. Brandtzaeg P, Valnes K, Scott H, et al. The human gastrointestinal secretory immune system in health and disease. *Scand J Gastroenterol Suppl* 1985;114:17–38.

22. Hyjek E, Isaacson PG. Primary B cell lymphoma of the thyroid and its relationship to Hashimoto's thyroiditis. *Hum Pathol* 1988;19:1315–1326.

23. Hyjek E, Smith WJ, Isaacson PG. Primary B-cell lymphoma of salivary glands and its relationship to myoepithelial sialadenitis. *Hum Pathol* 1988;19:766–776.

24. Harris NL, Isaacson PG. What are the criteria for distinguishing MALT from non-MALT lymphoma at extranodal sites? *Am J Clin Pathol* 1999;111:S126–S132.

25. Bienenstock J, Befus AD. Mucosal immunology. *Immunology* 1980; 41:249–270.

26. Pabst R. Compartmentalization and kinetics of lymphoid cells in the lung. *Reg Immunol* 1990;3:62–71.

27. Du MQ, Diss TC, Dogan A, et al. Clone-specific PCR reveals wide dissemination of gastric MALT lymphoma to the gastric mucosa. *J Pathol* 2000;192:488–493.

28. Isaacson PG, Spencer J. Malignant lymphoma of mucosa-associated lymphoid tissue. *Histopathology* 1987;11:445–462.

29. Isaacson PG, Wotherspoon AC, Diss T, et al. Follicular colonization in B-cell lymphoma of mucosa-associated lymphoid tissue. *Am J Surg Pathol* 1991;15:819–828.

30. Harris NL, Jaffe ES, Diebold J, et al. The World Health Organization classification of hematological malignancies: report of the Clinical Advisory Committee Meeting, Airlie House, Virginia, November 1997. *Mod Pathol* 2000;13:193–207.

31. Qin Y, Greiner A, Trunk MJ, et al. Somatic hypermutation in low-grade mucosa-associated lymphoid tissue-type B-cell lymphoma. *Blood* 1995;86:3528–3534.

32. Du M, Diss TC, Xu C, et al. Ongoing mutation in MALT lymphoma

33. Diss TC, Pan L. Polymerase chain reaction in the assessment of lymphomas. *Cancer Surv* 1997;30:21–44.

34. Hsi ED, Greenson JK, Singleton TP, et al. Detection of immunoglobulin heavy chain gene rearrangement by polymerase chain reaction in chronic active gastritis associated with *Helicobacter pylori*. *Hum Pathol* 1996;27:290–296.

35. Sorrentino D, Ferraccioli GF, DeVita S, et al. B-cell clonality and infection with *Helicobacter pylori*: implications for development of gastric lymphoma. *Gut* 1996;38:837–840.

36. Savio A, Franzin G, Wotherspoon AC, et al. Diagnosis and posttreatment follow-up of *Helicobacter pylori*-positive gastric lymphoma of mucosa-associated lymphoid tissue: histology, polymerase chain reaction, or both? *Blood* 1996;87:1255–1260.

37. de Mascarel A, Dubus P, Belleannee G, et al. Low prevalence of monoclonal B cells in *Helicobacter pylori* gastritis patients with duodenal ulcer. *Hum Pathol* 1998;29:784–790.

38. Wotherspoon AC, Finn TM, Isaacson PG. Trisomy 3 in low-grade B-cell lymphomas of mucosa-associated lymphoid tissue. *Blood* 1995;85: 2000–2004.

39. Ott G, Katzenberger T, Greiner A, et al. The t(11;18)(q21;q21) chromosome translocation is a frequent and specific aberration in low-grade but not high-grade malignant non-Hodgkin's lymphomas of the mucosa-associated lymphoid tissue (MALT-) type. *Cancer Res* 1997;57:3944–3948.

40. Remstein ED, Kurtin PJ, James CD, et al. Mucosa-associated lymphoid tissue lymphomas with t(11;18)(q21;q21) and mucosa-associated lymphoid tissue lymphomas with aneuploidy develop along different pathogenetic pathways. *Am J Pathol* 2002;161:63–71.

41. Wotherspoon AC, Pan LX, Diss TC, et al. Cytogenetic study of B-cell lymphoma of mucosa-associated lymphoid tissue. *Cancer Genet Cytogenet* 1992;58:35–38.

42. Willis TG, Jadayel DM, Du MQ, et al. Bcl10 is involved in t(1;14)(p22;q32) of MALT B cell lymphoma and mutated in multiple tumor types. *Cell* 1999;96:35–45.

43. Lucas PC, Yonezumi M, Inohara N, et al. Bcl10 and MALT1, independent targets of chromosomal translocation in MALT lymphoma, cooperate in a novel NF-kappa B signaling pathway. *J Biol Chem* 2001;276:19012–19019.

44. Nakamura S, Yao T, Aoyagi K, et al. *Helicobacter pylori* and primary gastric lymphoma. A histopathologic and immunohistochemical analysis of 237 patients. *Cancer* 1997;79:3–11.

45. Harris NL, Jaffe ES, Stein H, et al. A revised European-American classification of lymphoid neoplasms: a proposal from the International Lymphoma Study Group. *Blood* 1994;84:1361–1392.

46. Harris NL, Jaffe ES, Diebold J, et al. World Health Organization classification of neoplastic diseases of the hematopoietic and lymphoid tissues: report of the Clinical Advisory Committee meeting-Airlie House, Virginia, November 1997. *J Clin Oncol* 1999;17:3835–3849.

47. Nakamura S, Aoyagi K, Furuse M, et al. B-cell monoclonality precedes the development of gastric MALT lymphoma in *Helicobacter pylori*-associated chronic gastritis. *Am J Pathol* 1998;152:1271–1279.

48. Parsonnet J, Hansen S, Rodriguez L, et al. *Helicobacter pylori* infection and gastric lymphoma. *N Engl J Med* 1994;330:1267–1271.

49. Zucca E, Bertoni F, Roggero E, et al. Molecular analysis of the progression from *Helicobacter pylori*-associated chronic gastritis to mucosa-associated lymphoid-tissue lymphoma of the stomach. *N Engl J Med* 1998;338:804–810.

50. Hussell T, Isaacson PG, Crabtree JE, et al. The response of cells from low-grade B-cell gastric lymphomas of mucosa- associated lymphoid tissue to *Helicobacter pylori*. *Lancet* 1993;342:571–574.

51. Wotherspoon AC, Doglioni C, Diss TC, et al. Regression of primary low-grade B-cell gastric lymphoma of mucosa-associated lymphoid tissue type after eradication of *Helicobacter pylori*. *Lancet* 1993;342:575–577.

52. Stolte M, Bayerdorffer E, Morgner A, et al. *Helicobacter* and gastric MALT lymphoma. *Gut* 2002;50(Suppl 30):III19–III24.

53. Roggero E, Zucca E, Pinotti G, et al. Eradication of *Helicobacter pylori* infection in primary low-grade gastric lymphoma of mucosa-associated lymphoid tissue. *Ann Intern Med* 1995;122:767–769.

54. Thiede C, Wundisch T, Alpen B, et al. Long-term persistence of monoclonal B cells after cure of *Helicobacter pylori* infection and complete histologic remission in gastric mucosa-associated lymphoid tissue B-cell lymphoma. *J Clin Oncol* 2001;19:1600–1609.

55. Sackmann M, Morgner A, Rudolph B, et al. Regression of gastric MALT lymphoma after eradication of *Helicobacter pylori* is predicted by endosonographic staging. MALT Lymphoma Study Group. *Gastroenterology* 1997;113:1087–1090.
56. Nakamura S, Matsumoto T, Suekane H, et al. Predictive value of endoscopic ultrasonography for regression of gastric low grade and high grade MALT lymphomas after eradication of *Helicobacter pylori*. *Gut* 2001;48:454–460.
57. Dierlamm J, Baens M, Wlodarska I, et al. The apoptosis inhibitor gene API2 and a novel 18q gene, MLT, are recurrently rearranged in the t(11;18)(q21;q21)p6ssociated with mucosa-associated lymphoid tissue lymphomas. *Blood* 1999;93:3601–3609.
58. Ye H, Dogan A, Karran L, et al. BCL10 expression in normal and neoplastic lymphoid tissue. Nuclear localization in MALT lymphoma. *Am J Pathol* 2000;157:1147–1154.
59. Liu H, Ye H, Ruskone-Fourmestraux A, et al. T(11;18) is a marker for all stage gastric MALT lymphomas that will not respond to *H. pylori* eradication. *Gastroenterology* 2002;122:1286–1294.
60. Liu H, Ye H, Dogan A, et al. T(11;18)(q21;q21) is associated with advanced mucosa-associated lymphoid tissue lymphoma that expresses nuclear BCL10. *Blood* 2001;98:1182–1187.
61. Taal BG, Boot H, van Heerde P, et al. Primary non-Hodgkin lymphoma of the stomach: endoscopic pattern and prognosis in low versus high grade malignancy in relation to the MALT concept. *Gut* 1996;39:556–561.
62. Pinotti G, Zucca E, Roggero E, et al. Clinical features, treatment and outcome in a series of 93 patients with low-grade gastric MALT lymphoma. *Leuk Lymphoma* 1997;26:527–537.
63. de Jong D, Aleman BM, Taal BG, et al. Controversies and consensus in the diagnosis, work-up and treatment of gastric lymphoma: an international survey. *Ann Oncol* 1999;10:275–280.
64. Rohatiner A, d'Amore F, Coiffier B, et al. Report on a workshop convened to discuss the pathological and staging classifications of gastrointestinal tract lymphoma. *Ann Oncol* 1994;5:397–400.
65. Steinbach G, Ford R, Glober G, et al. Antibiotic treatment of gastric lymphoma of mucosa-associated lymphoid tissue. An uncontrolled trial. *Ann Intern Med* 1999;131:88–95.
66. Cutler AF, Havstad S, Ma CK, et al. Accuracy of invasive and noninvasive tests to diagnose *Helicobacter pylori* infection. *Gastroenterology* 1995;109:136–141.
67. Pavlick AC, Gerdes H, Portlock CS. Endoscopic ultrasound in the evaluation of gastric small lymphocytic mucosa-associated lymphoid tumors. *J Clin Oncol* 1997;15:1761–1766.
68. Eidt S, Stolte M, Fischer R. Factors influencing lymph node infiltration in primary gastric malignant lymphoma of the mucosa-associated lymphoid tissue. *Pathol Res Pract* 1994;190:1077–1081.
69. Ruskone-Fourmestraux A, Lavergne A, Aegerter PH, et al. Predictive factors for regression of gastric MALT lymphoma after anti-*Helicobacter pylori* treatment. *Gut* 2001;48:297–303.
70. Montalban C, Castrillo JM, Abraira V, et al. Gastric B-cell mucosa-associated lymphoid tissue (MALT) lymphoma. Clinicopathological study and evaluation of the prognostic factors in 143 patients. *Ann Oncol* 1995;6:355–362.
71. Fisher RI, Dahlberg S, Nathwani BN, et al. A clinical analysis of two indolent lymphoma entities: mantle cell lymphoma and marginal zone lymphoma (including the mucosa-associated lymphoid tissue and monocytoid B-cell subcategories): a Southwest Oncology Group study. *Blood* 1995;85:1075–1082.
72. Thieblemont C, Bastion Y, Berger F, et al. Mucosa-associated lymphoid tissue gastrointestinal and nongastrointestinal lymphoma behavior: analysis of 108 patients. *J Clin Oncol* 1997;15:1624–1630.
73. Tsang RW, Gospodarowicz MK, Pintilie M, et al. Stage I and II MALT lymphoma: results of treatment with radiotherapy. *Int J Radiat Oncol Biol Phys* 2001;50:1258–1264.
74. Walsh JH, Peterson WL. The treatment of *Helicobacter pylori* infection in the management of peptic ulcer disease. *N Engl J Med* 1995;333:984–991.
75. Neubauer A, Thiede C, Morgner A, et al. Cure of *Helicobacter pylori* infection and duration of remission of low-grade gastric mucosa-associated lymphoid tissue lymphoma. *J Natl Cancer Inst* 1997;89:1350–1355.
76. Auer IA, Gascoyne RD, Connors JM, et al. t(11;18)(q21;q21) is the most common translocation in MALT lymphomas. *Ann Oncol* 1997;8:979–985.
77. Akagi T, Motegi M, Tamura A, et al. A novel gene, MALT1 at 18q21,

is involved in t(11;18) (q21;q21) found in low-grade B-cell lymphoma of mucosa-associated lymphoid tissue. *Oncogene* 1999;18:5785–5794.
78. Starostik P, Patzner J, Greiner A, et al. Gastric marginal zone B-cell lymphomas of MALT type develop along 2 distinct pathogenetic pathways. *Blood* 2002;99:3–9.
79. Du MQ, Peng H, Liu H, et al. BCL10 gene mutation in lymphoma. *Blood* 2000;95:3885–3890.
80. Du MQ, Isaacson PG. Gastric MALT lymphoma: from aetiology to treatment. *Lancet Oncol* 2002;3:97–104.
81. Bertoni F, Conconi A, Capella C, et al. Molecular follow-up in gastric mucosa-associated lymphoid tissue lymphomas: early analysis of the LY03 cooperative trial. *Blood* 2002;99:2541–2544.
82. Cavalli F, Isaacson PG, Gascoyne RD, et al. MALT lymphomas. *Hematology (Am Soc Hematol Educ Program)* 2001:241–258. [review].
83. Fischbach W, Goebeler-Kolve M, Starostik P, et al. Minimal residual low-grade gastric MALT-type lymphoma after eradication of *Helicobacter pylori*. *Lancet* 2002;360:547–548.
84. Cogliatti SB, Schmid U, Schumacher U, et al. Primary B-cell gastric lymphoma: a clinicopathological study of 145 patients. *Gastroenterology* 1991;101:1159–1170.
85. Zucca E, Cavalli F. Gut lymphomas. *Baillieres Clin Haematol* 1996;9:727–741.
86. Schechter NR, Yahalom J. Low-grade MALT lymphoma of the stomach: a review of treatment options. *Int J Radiat Oncol Biol Phys* 2000;46:1093–1103.
87. Coiffier B, Salles G. Does surgery belong to medical history for gastric lymphomas? *Ann Oncol* 1997;8:419–421.
88. Wotherspoon AC, Doglioni C, Isaacson PG. Low-grade gastric B-cell lymphoma of mucosa-associated lymphoid tissue (MALT): a multifocal disease. *Histopathology* 1992;20:29–34.
89. Schechter NR, Portlock CS, Yahalom J. Treatment of mucosa-associated lymphoid tissue lymphoma of the stomach with radiation alone. *J Clin Oncol* 1998;16:1916–1921.
90. Hitchcock S, Ng AK, Fisher DC, et al. Treatment outcome of mucosa-associated lymphoid tissue/marginal zone non-Hodgkin's lymphoma. *Int J Radiat Oncol Biol Phys* 2002;52:1058–1066.
91. Fung CY, Grossbard ML, Linggood RM, et al. Mucosa-associated lymphoid tissue lymphoma of the stomach: long term outcome after local treatment. *Cancer* 1999;85:9–17.
92. Park HC, Park W, Hahn JS, et al. Low grade MALT lymphoma of the stomach: treatment outcome with radiotherapy alone. *Yonsei Med J* 2002;43:601–606.
93. Yahalom J, Gonzales M, et al. *H. Pylori*-independent MALT lymphoma of the stomach: excellent outcome with radiation alone. *Blood* 2002;100:160a [abstract].
94. Gospodarowicz MK, Pintilie M, Tsang R, et al. Primary gastric lymphoma: brief overview of the recent Princess Margaret Hospital experience. *Recent Results Cancer Res* 2000;156:108–115.
95. Yahalom J. MALT lymphomas: a radiation oncology viewpoint. *Ann Hematol* 2001;80:B100–B105.
96. Hammel P, Haioun C, Chaumette MT, et al. Efficacy of single-agent chemotherapy in low-grade B-cell mucosa-associated lymphoid tissue lymphoma with prominent gastric expression. *J Clin Oncol* 1995;13:2524–2529.
97. Jager G, Neumeister P, Brezinschek R, et al. Treatment of extranodal marginal zone B-cell lymphoma of mucosa-associated lymphoid tissue type with cladribine: a phase II study. *J Clin Oncol* 2002;20:3872–3877.
98. Conconi A, Thieblemont C, et al. IESLG Phase II Study of Rituximab in MALT Lymphomas. *Ann Oncol* 2002;13:81.
99. Zinzani PL, Magagnoli M, Galieni P, et al. Nongastrointestinal low-grade mucosa-associated lymphoid tissue lymphoma: analysis of 75 patients. *J Clin Oncol* 1999;17:1254.
100. Estevez M, Chu C, Pless M. Small B-cell lymphoma presenting as diffuse dural thickening with cranial neuropathies. *J Neurooncol* 2002;59:243–247.
101. Masuda A, Tsujii T, Kojima M, et al. Primary mucosa-associated lymphoid tissue (MALT) lymphoma arising from the male urethra. A case report and review of the literature. *Pathol Res Pract* 2002;198:571–575.
102. Suchy BH, Wolf SR. Bilateral mucosa-associated lymphoid tissue lymphoma of the parotid gland. *Arch Otolaryngol Head Neck Surg* 2000;126:224–226.

103. Jhavar S, Agarwal JP, Naresh KN, et al. Primary extranodal mucosa associated lymphoid tissue (MALT) lymphoma of the prostate. *Leuk Lymphoma* 2001;41:445–449.

104. Agulnik M, Tsang R, Baker MA, et al. Malignant lymphoma of mucosa-associated lymphoid tissue of the lacrimal gland: case report and review of literature. *Am J Clin Oncol* 2001;24:67–70.

105. Brogi E, Harris NL. Lymphomas of the breast: pathology and clinical behavior. *Semin Oncol* 1999;26:357–364.

106. Ansell SM, Grant CS, Habermann TM. Primary thyroid lymphoma. *Semin Oncol* 1999;26:316–323.

107. Galieni P, Polito E, Leccisotti A, et al. Localized orbital lymphoma. *Haematologica* 1997;82:436–439.

108. Balm AJ, Delaere P, Hilgers FJ, et al. Primary lymphoma of mucosa associated lymphoid tissue (MALT) in the parotid gland. *Clin Otolaryngol* 1993;18:528–532.

109. Le QT, Eulau SM, George TI, et al. Primary radiotherapy for localized orbital MALT lymphoma. *Int J Radiat Oncol Biol Phys* 2002; 52:657–663.

110. Sanjeevi A, Krishnan J, Bailey PR, et al. Extranodal marginal zone B-cell lymphoma of malt type involving the cavernous sinus. *Leuk Lymphoma* 2001;42:1133–1137.

111. de Bree R, Mahieu HF, Ossenkoppele GJ, et al. Malignant lymphoma of mucosa-associated lymphoid tissue in the larynx. *Eur Arch Otorhinolaryngol* 1998;255:368–3701.

CHAPTER 23

Nodal Marginal Zone B-Cell Lymphoma

Françoise Berger, Alexandra Traverse-Glehen, and Gilles A. Salles

DEFINITION

Nodal marginal zone B-cell lymphoma is a primary nodal B-cell lymphoma that shares morphologic, immunophenotypic, and genetic characteristics with extranodal and splenic marginal zone lymphoma, but without extranodal or splenic localization at presentation.

It was first described as *nodal monocytoid B-cell lymphoma* in 1986 by Sheibani (1,2), then as *parafollicular B-cell lymphoma* by Cousar in 1987 (3). The relationship with marginal zone B cells was established by Piris in 1988 (4). *Nodal monocytoid B-cell lymphoma* was introduced in the revised Kiel classification by Lennert in 1990 (5). *Nodal marginal zone lymphoma* (with or without monocytoid B cells) was considered as a provisional subtype in the Revised European-American Lymphoma Classification (6) and finally admitted as a distinct entity in the WHO Classification in 2001 (7). However, few series have been published, and discrepancies remain concerning the morphologic, biologic, and clinical characteristics of this disease (8–15).

FREQUENCY AND EPIDEMIOLOGY

Among other lymphomas, nodal marginal zone lymphoma is rare, representing respectively 1.5% and 1.8% of the cases analyzed within an international study and a single-center series (16,17). Two-thirds of the cases of the Southwest Oncology Group study (18) were described as "*composite lymphomas*" with concomitant follicular lymphoma and may include follicular lymphomas with marginal differentiation. Other series probably include cases corresponding to nodal spread of extranodal marginal zone lymphoma (19) or cases disseminated at diagnosis, with peripheral lymph nodes associated with extranodal or splenic involvement.

Association with hepatitis C virus infection has been reported (20), but the frequency of this association remains uncertain; some cases also appear to develop in patients presenting with Sjögren's syndrome (21) but may represent disseminated mucosa-associated lymphoid tissue (MALT) cases.

DIAGNOSIS

Morphology

Morphologic features of nodal marginal zone lymphoma are very heterogeneous, in terms of both architecture and cytology (15,17). The pattern of infiltration of lymph nodes may be perifollicular or "inverse follicular," interfollicular, perisinusoidal (Color Plate 49A), follicular by colonization of reactive follicles (less frequent than in MALT lymphomas) (Color Plate 49B), or diffuse. Particular patterns are often associated within the same lymph node. Residual atrophic, rarely, hyperplastic follicles are usually seen. Several cell types can be encountered in varying proportions: small cells with irregular nuclei, clumped chromatin, and clear cytoplasm; cells resembling small lymphocytes; small cells with a plasmacytoid differentiation; plasma cells; and a variable content of medium to large cells (centroblast- or immunoblast-like). Follicular dendritic cells, usually arranged in a nodular meshwork, are always present. "Monocytoid" B cells with more abundant and clear cytoplasm are not usually predominant, and pure monocytoid B-cell lymphomas are less frequent than are cases with a plasmacytoid or plasmacytic differentiation. Of note, the latter were considered in the past (and are probably still classified) as *immunocytoma*, and there is an important overlap between these two entities.

The proportion of large cells is often relatively high (more than 20%), as is the mitotic count index. Unlike extranodal and splenic marginal zone lymphoma, most nodal marginal zone lymphoma cannot, therefore, be considered a true low-grade B-cell lymphoma at presentation.

Differential diagnosis can be difficult with other small B-cell lymphomas, which sometimes have a marginal zone pattern or contain monocytoid B cells (marginal differentiation). These problems occur sometimes with small lymphocytic lymphoma and rarely with mantle cell lymphoma. Some aspects of nodal marginal zone lymphoma are also difficult to distinguish from folliclar lymphoma, especially when marginal cells colonize reactive follicles (Color Plate 49B). Immunophenotypic features (see below) are helpful to clarify these cases. In cases with plasmacytic differentiation, the differential diagnosis with lymphoplasmacytic lymphoma (immunocytoma) is probably semantic. In fact, as the contingent of large cells is often high, many cases were classified in the past as *diffuse mixed (F)* in the Working Formulation (22) or *polymorphic immunocytoma* in the Kiel Classification (23) and are perhaps sometimes considered among diffuse large B-cell lymphomas.

Immunophenotype

The phenotype, usually identical to extranodal (MALT) marginal zone lymphoma, is an important diagnostic feature that can help distinguish those cases from other small B-cell lymphomas (15,17): typically the lymphoma cells are sIgM/(G)$^+$; cIg$^{+/-}$; CD19$^+$; CD20$^+$; CD5$^-$; CD10$^-$; CD23$^-$; CD43$^{-/+}$; bcl2$^+$; and cyclinD1$^-$. The expression of immunoglobulin (Ig) D has been reported by Campo (24), who described a "splenic type" of nodal marginal zone lymphoma. An atypical phenotype (CD5$^+$, sometimes CD23$^+$, sometimes cyclinD1$^+$) has been reported (17,25), but "borderline" cases are rare with mantle cell lymphoma or small lymphocytic lymphoma. The use of a new differentiation antigen, such as IRTA1 (*Immune Receptor Translocation Associated*-1), which seems specific to marginal zone B cells, may prove to be useful in the future (26).

PATHOGENESIS

Cytogenetic and Molecular Features of Nodal Marginal Zone Lymphoma

The cytogenetic studies of marginal zone lymphomas have been presented in several series, usually including mostly splenic marginal zone lymphoma cases. However, Ott and coworkers reported that the different subsets of marginal zone lymphoma may differ according to their sites of origin. In their study, which included ten cases of nodal marginal zone lymphoma, clonal aberrations were found in six cases, with complex karyotypes in three of them. No specific recurrent abnormalities were found in this group, as opposed to splenic marginal zone lymphoma, in which trisomy 3, trisomy X, and del(10)(q22q24) appeared to be recurrent (27). Likewise, the t(11;18)(q21;q21) characteristic of MALT lymphomas has not been reported in nodal marginal zone lymphoma. In other series (28–30), +7 and 6q21-25 deletions, already associated with impaired outcome in other lymphoma entities, appeared to be more frequent (more than one-third of the cases) in nodal marginal zone lymphoma, whereas other changes, including trisomy 3, trisomy 18, trisomy 12, and structural aberrations involving 1p12-36 and 3q11-27, were found in all marginal zone lymphoma subgroups. Rare cases (less than 10%) of TP53 gene heterozygous deletions detected by fluorescence *in situ* hybridization analysis were reported (29,30), as well as 17p losses (16%) detected by comparative genomic hybridization analysis (31).

Postulated Cell of Origin

The Ig gene mutational status was investigated in small series. The majority of cases presented somatic mutations of Ig-heavy chain genes with evidence of antigen selection in some cases (32–34).

The normal counterpart of those lymphoma cells is not well characterized. Normal nodal marginal zones are only seen in mesenteric lymph nodes, and the relationship with monocytoid B cells observed in reactive lymph nodes (toxoplasmic lymphadenitis, human immunodeficiency virus infection) remains unclear (35,36).

PRESENTATION

Because the identification of this lymphoma is recent, only few reports present detailed clinical and evolutive data on nodal marginal zone lymphoma patients. The initial description of monocytoid B-cell lymphoma included elderly women, often with Sjögren's syndrome and extranodal lymphoma, probably corresponding at least in part to nodal spread of MALT lymphoma (9,10). Further reports identified patients within three large, different data sets (14,17,18), but only two of them, including, respectively, 20 and 37 patients (14,17), were restricted to nodal marginal zone lymphoma. The clinical characteristics were quite similar in both series (Table 23.1). The median age was 50 to 60 years, with a slight female predominance. The vast majority of patients presented with a peripheral lymph node, the neck being the predominant localization, and central lymph nodes were also frequently detected, predominantly in the paraaortic region (50% to 60%). Adverse prognostic features were relatively common, such as stage III or IV disease (68% to 71%), bone marrow involvement (28% to 49%), elevated lactate dehydrogenase (36% to 40%), and tumor mass greater than 5 (31%) or 10 (17%) cm , but B symptoms were uncommon (14%). Elevated β_2-microglobulin was found in one-third of

TABLE 23.1 *Clinical features of nodal marginal zone lymphoma*

	Nathwani (14)	Berger (17)
Number of patients	20	37
Median age	59	54
Performance status >1 (%)	0	13
Ann Arbor stage III/IV (%)	71	68
Bone marrow involvement (%)	28	43
Elevated serum lactate dehydrogenase (%)	36	40
Elevated β_2-microglobulin (%)	NA	33
Anemia (%)	NA	31

NA, not available.

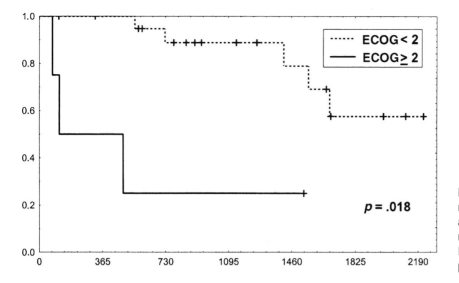

FIG. 23.1. Progression-free survival of nodal marginal zone lymphoma patients according to performance status at diagnosis (log-rank *p* value = .018). ECOG, Eastern Cooperative Oncology Group performance index score.

patients, and an M component was infrequently (8%) detected in patients' serum. Approximately half of the patients had a high-intermediate (36%) or high (7%) International Prognostic Index score. The analysis of 43 patients with stage III or IV diseases (approximately half of them being disseminated MALT lymphomas) that were included in Southwest Oncology Group trials showed an equilibrated sex ratio, a median age of approximately 50 years, a good performance status in 95% of cases, and bone marrow infiltration in one case out of two (18).

PROGNOSTIC AND PREDICTIVE FACTORS

Complete response to the first treatment is observed in 50% to 60% of the cases. In the International Lymphoma Study Group study, 5-year failure-free survival and overall survival were 28% and 56%, respectively, and this trend toward a poor prognosis was also found for patients with a low or intermediate International Prognostic Index

score. Of note, histologic progression toward large-cell lymphoma appeared at diagnosis in one out of five patients. In the Lyon series, time to progression was 1.3 years, and median overall survival was close to 5 years, indicating that this disease may remain indolent for several years. Given the small numbers of cases reported in these series, no specific prognostic factors were reported for this entity. A poor performance status at diagnosis was the only parameter significantly influencing the outcome (Fig. 23.1). Patients achieving a complete response to first-line treatment may also have a better prognosis (Fig. 23.2). At the time of relapse, nodal sites are usually predominantly encountered, although splenic or extranodal sites may occur, reminiscent of the other marginal zone lymphoma subtypes. However, histologic progression toward diffuse large-cell lymphomas appeared to occur quite frequently, and there was no evidence of plateau on survival curves to suggest that this disease is currently curable.

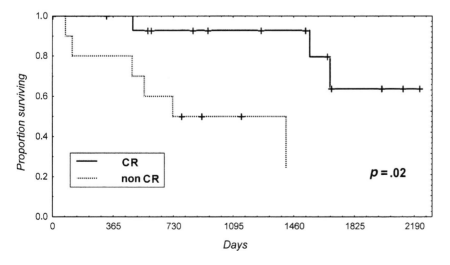

FIG. 23.2. Progression-free survival of nodal marginal zone lymphoma patients according to their responses to the first treatment (log-rank *p* value = .02). CR, complete response.

TREATMENT

Treatment options may include single-agent chemotherapy (chlorambucil or fludarabine) or a classical combination regimen such as cyclophosphamide, doxorubicin, vincristine, and prednisone. A more dose-intensive strategy, eventually including autologous bone marrow transplantation, was sometime applied to younger patients with a high number of large mitotic cells and adverse clinical prognostic factors. However, none of these approaches has been prospectively tested. Therefore, no specific therapeutic approach could be recommended at this time, and the clinician may decide based on the histologic and clinical characteristics of each patient. Monoclonal antibodies directed against the CD20 antigen appeared in some reports to have some efficacy in this setting (37).

FUTURE DIRECTIONS

This newly recognized entity is still incompletely understood, and its relationship with normal B cells as well as with other marginal zone lymphomas (splenic and MALT) remains to be further characterized. Overall, patients have a disseminated disease with some adverse clinical and biologic features and a short time to disease progression, although some patients may survive several years. A better recognition of nodal marginal zone lymphoma through new molecular and phenotypic markers may lead to a better identification of those patients to allow meaningful clinical studies.

REFERENCES

1. Sheibani K, Sohn C, Burke JS, et al. Monocytoid B-cell lymphoma: A novel B-cell neoplasm. *Am J Pathol* 1986;124:318.
2. Sheibani K, Burke JS, Swartz WG, et al. Monocytoid B cell lymphoma. Clinicopathological study of 21 cases of a unique type of low grade lymphoma. *Cancer* 1988;62:1531–1538.
3. Cousar JB, McGinn DL, Glick AD, et al. Report of an unusual lymphoma arising from parafollicular B-lymphocytes or so-called "monocytoid" lymphocytes. *Am J Clin Pathol* 1987;87:121–128.
4. Piris MA, Rivas C, Morente M, et al. Monocytoid B-cell lymphoma, a tumor related to the marginal zone. *Histopathology* 1988;12:383–392.
5. Lennert K, Feller AC. *Histopathologie der non Hodgkin's lymphome (nach der aktualisierten Kiel-klassifikation)*. Berlin: Springer Verlag, 1990.
6. Harris NL, Jaffe ES, Stein H, et al. A revised European-American classification of lymphoid neoplasms: a proposal from the International Lymphoma Study Group. *Blood* 1994;84:1361–1392.
7. Jaffe ES, Harris NL, Stein H, et al., eds. *WHO classification of tumours: pathology & genetics, tumours of haematopoietic and lymphoid tissues*. Lyon: IARC Press, 2001.
8. Ng CS, Chan JKC. Monocytoid B-cell lymphoma. *Hum Pathol* 1987; 18:1069–1071.
9. Cogliatti SB, Lennert K, Zwingers TL. Monocytoid B-cell lymphoma: clinical and prognostic features of 21 patients. *J Clin Pathol* 1990;43:619–625.
10. Ngan BY, Warnke RA, Wilson M, et al. Monocytoid B-cell lymphoma. A study of 36 cases. *Hum Pathol* 1991;22:409–421.
11. Nizze H, Cogliatti SB, von Schilling C, et al. Monocytoid B-cell lymphoma: morphological variants and relationship to low-grade B-cell lymphoma of mucosa-associated lymphoid tissue. *Histopathology* 1991;18:403–414.
12. Ortiz-Hidalgo C, Wright DH. The morphological spectrum of monocytoid B-cell lymphoma and its relationship to lymphoma of mucosa-associated lymphoid tissue. *Histopathology* 1992;21:555–561.
13. Fend F, Kraus-Huonder B, Muller-Hermelink HL, et al. Monocytoid B-cell lymphoma: its relationship to and possible cellular origin from marginal zone cells. *Hum Pathol* 1993;24:336–339.
14. Nathwani BN, Anderson JR, Armitage JO, et al. Marginal zone B-cell lymphoma: a clinical comparison of nodal and mucosa-associated lymphoid tissue types. Non-Hodgkin's Lymphoma Classification Project. *J Clin Oncol* 1999;17:2486–2492.
15. Nathwani BN, Drachenberg MR, Hernandez AM, et al. Nodal monocytoid B-cell lymphoma (nodal marginal-zone B-cell lymphoma). *Semin Oncol* 1999;36:128-138.
16. A clinical evaluation of the International Lymphoma Study Group classification of non-Hodgkin's lymphoma. The Non-Hodgkin's Lymphoma Classification Project. *Blood* 1997;89:3908–3918.
17. Berger F, Felman P, Thieblemont C, et al. Non-MALT marginal zone B-cell lymphomas: a description of clinical presentation and outcome in 124 patients. *Blood* 2000;95:1950–1956.
18. Fisher RI, Dahlberg S, Nathwani BN, et al. A clinical analysis of two indolent lymphoma entities: mantle cell lymphoma and marginal zone lymphoma (including the mucosa-associated lymphoid tissue and monocytoid B-cell subcategories): a Southwest Oncology Group study. *Blood* 1995;85:1075.
19. Piris MA, Rivas C, Morente M, et al. Monocytoid B-cell lymphoma, a tumour related to the marginal zone. *Histopathology* 1988;4:383–392.
20. Zuckerman E, Zuckerman T, Levine AM, et al. Hepatitis C virus infection in patients with B-cell non-Hodgkin lymphoma. *Ann Intern Med* 1997;127:423–428.
21. Royer B, Cazals-Hatem D, Sibilia J, et al. Lymphomas in patients with Sjogren's syndrome are marginal zone B-cell neoplasms, arise in diverse extranodal and nodal sites, and are not associated with viruses. *Blood* 1997;90:766–775.
22. Non-Hodgkin's Lymphoma Pathologic Classification Project. National Cancer Institute sponsored study of classifications of non-Hodgkin's lymphomas: Summary and description of a working formulation for clinical usage. *Cancer* 1982;49:2112–2135.
23. Lennert K. *Malignant lymphomas other than Hodgkin's disease*. New York: Springer Verlag, 1981.
24. Campo E, Miquel R, Krenacs L, et al. Primary nodal marginal zone lymphomas of splenic and MALT type. *Am J Surg Pathol* 1999;23: 59–68.
25. Swerdlow SH, Zukerberg LR, Yang WI, et al. The morphologic spectrum of non-Hodgkin's lymphomas with BCL1/cyclin D1 gene rearrangements. *Am J Surg Pathol* 1996;20:627–640.
26. Miller I, Hatzivassiliou G, Cattoretti G, et al. IRTAs: a new family of immunoglobulinlike receptors differentially expressed in B cells. *Blood* 2002;99:2662–2669.
27. Ott MM, Rosenwald A, Katzenberger T, et al. Marginal zone B-cell lymphomas (MZBL) arising at different sites represent different biological entities. *Genes Chromosomes Cancer* 2000;28:380–386.
28. Dierlamm J, Wlodarska I, Michaux L, et al. Genetic abnormalities in marginal zone B-cell lymphoma. *Hematol Oncol* 2000;18:1–13.
29. Dierlamm J, Pittaluga S, Wlodarska I, et al. Marginal zone B-cell lymphomas of different sites share similar cytogenetic and morphologic features. *Blood* 1996;87:299–307.
30. Callet-Bauchu E, Gazzo S, Poncet C, et al. Chromosomal analysis of marginal zone B-cell lymphomas may delineate cytogenetic profiles correlated with clinical characteristics and outcome: a study of 141 cases. Paper presented at: 44th Annual Meeting of the American Society of Hematology; December 6–10, 2002; Philadelphia.
31. Dierlamm J, Rosenberg C, Stul M, et al. Characteristic pattern of chromosomal gains and losses in marginal zone B cell lymphoma detected by comparative genomic hybridization. *Leukemia* 1997; 11:747–758.
32. Tierens A, Delabie J, Michiels L, et al. Marginal zone B cells in the human lymph node and spleen show somatic hypermutations and display clonal expansion. *Blood* 1999;93:226–234.
33. Conconi A, Bertoni F, Pedrinis E, et al. Nodal marginal zone B-cell lymphoma may arise from different subsets of marginal zone B lymphocytes. *Blood,* 2001;98:781–786.
34. Traverse-Glehen A, Berger F, Davi F, et al. Analysis of VH genes in 48 marginal zone lymphoma cases reveals marked heterogeneity

between splenic and nodal cases and suggest clonal selection. Paper presented at: 44th Annual Meeting of the American Society of Hematology. Philadelphia: December 6–10, 2002.

35. Stein K, Hummel M, Korbjuhn P, et al. Monocytoid B cells are distinct from splenic marginal zone cells and commonly derive from unmutated naive B cells and less frequently from postgerminal center B cells by polyclonal transformation. *Blood* 1999;94:2800–2808.

36. Camacho FI, Garcia JF, Sanchez-Verde L, et al. Unique phenotypic profile of monocytoid B cells: differences in comparison with the phenotypic profile observed in marginal zone B cells and so-called monocytoid B cell lymphoma. *Am J Pathol* 2001;158:1363–1369.

37. Koh LP, Lim LC, Thng CH. Retreatment with chimeric CD20 monoclonal antibody in a patient with nodal marginal zone B-cell lymphoma. *Med Oncol* 2000;17:225–228.

CHAPTER 24

Follicular Lymphoma

Arnold S. Freedman, Jonathan W. Friedberg, Peter M. Mauch, Riccardo Dalla-Favera, and Nancy Lee Harris

DEFINITION

Follicular lymphoma is defined as a lymphoma of follicle center B cells (centrocytes and centroblasts) that has at least a partially follicular pattern. This disorder was previously called *nodular lymphoma* and *follicle center lymphoma* (1). Follicular lymphoma is graded by the number of centroblasts (grades 1, 2, and 3).

FREQUENCY

Follicular lymphoma is the second most common lymphoma in the United States and Western Europe, comprising approximately 20% of all non-Hodgkin's lymphomas and up to 70% of "low-grade" lymphomas reported in American and European clinical trials (2,3). In contrast, follicular lymphoma is much less common in Asians and blacks than in whites in Western countries, including the United States, and is uncommon in Asia and developing countries (4). The risk was lower for first-generation migrants from China and Japan than for subsequent-generation migrants (5). Most cases are grade 1 or grade 2 (6). Follicular lymphoma most frequently presents in middle-aged individuals and the elderly, with a median age at diagnosis of 60 years and a slight female predominance (6,7). There are trends showing higher rates of follicular lymphoma in smokers (8). A lower incidence of bcl-2 translocations is seen within follicular lymphomas that occur in Asians as compared to follicular lymphoma in individuals from Western countries (9). This is in spite of similar rates of bcl-2 rearrangements detected in normal individuals from either Asian or Western countries. This suggests differences in the pathogenesis of follicular lymphoma in distinct geographic areas.

DIAGNOSIS

Morphology

Follicular lymphomas are composed of follicle center B cells, usually a mixture of centrocytes (cleaved follicle center cells,

"small cells") and centroblasts (large, noncleaved follicle center cells, "large cells"). Centrocytes typically predominate; centroblasts are usually in the minority but always present. Rarely, follicular lymphomas consist almost entirely of centroblasts. Occasional cases may show plasmacytoid differentiation or foci of marginal zone or monocytoid B cells (10).

The proportion of centroblasts is variable. Numerous criteria have been proposed for grading follicular lymphoma based on the number of large cells present in the neoplastic per high-power field (hpf). The current World Health Organization Classification includes grade 1 (zero to five centroblasts/hpf), grade 2 (six to 15 centroblasts/hpf), and grade 3 (more than 15 centroblasts/hpf) (1,2). The reproducibility of pathologic grading of follicular lymphoma has generally been poor. However, the clinical behavior and outcome of treatment of grades 1 and 2 follicular lymphomas are similar, and they are generally approached in the same manner: as indolent lymphomas (12). In contrast, grade 3 follicular lymphoma is generally approached as an aggressive disease. Thus, pathologic grading focuses on distinguishing low-grade (1 and 2) follicular lymphoma from the more aggressive grade 3.

Follicular lymphoma reproduces the architecture of normal germinal centers of secondary lymphoid follicles. Neoplastic follicles distort and replace the normal nodal architecture. The pattern may be entirely follicular, or diffuse components may be present. In contrast to normal follicles, neoplastic follicles contain a monomorphous population of centrocytes and often lack mantle zones, and tingible body (debris-laden) macrophages are typically absent (13). Neoplastic cells are often present in the interfollicular region. In the bone marrow, which is involved in 50% to 70% of patients affected, one sees characteristic paratrabecular lymphoid aggregates. Involvement of the peripheral blood is seen in approximately 30% of patients. These circulating malignant cells have nuclear clefts, in contrast to the cells of chronic lymphocytic leukemia.

Rare lymphomas composed of centrocytes, with a small proportion of centroblasts, have an entirely diffuse architecture and the same immunophenotype as nodal follicular lymphoma. These cases may represent diffuse areas of follicular lymphoma in which the follicular component is not represented in the biopsy. The term *diffuse follicle center–cell lymphoma* is used for these cases. Cases should be graded as for follicular lymphoma grades 1 and 2. If centroblasts predominate (grade 3), or if the small cells are T cells, the tumor is classified as diffuse large B-cell lymphoma. The clinical behavior of diffuse follicle center lymphoma has not been well clarified, because many of these cases would now be reclassified, often as mantle cell lymphoma.

Immunophenotype

The tumor cells in almost all cases of follicular lymphoma express monoclonal surface immunoglobulin (sIg+), with 50% to 60% immunoglobulin (Ig) M+, 40% IgG+, and rare cases IgA+ (14). Immunophenotyping studies have provided strong support that follicular lymphoma cells are derived from normal germinal center B cells. Virtually all cases express human leukocyte antigen-DR and pan–B-cell antigens (CD19, CD20, CD79a), complement receptors (CD21 and CD35), and CD10 (60%) as well as nuclear bcl-6 (15–18). However, in strong contrast to normal germinal center B cells, the cytoplasmic staining for bcl-2 protein in follicular lymphoma cells is strongly positive (19). The Ki-67+ fraction is lower than that of reactive follicles. Unlike small lymphocytic and mantle cell lymphomas, follicular lymphoma cells lack CD5 and CD43 (most cases); CD23 expression is variable. CD11a/CD18 is more frequently noted on tumor cells at initial diagnosis (60% to 90% of cases) than at relapse. Adhesion molecules, including CD44, ICAM-1 (CD54), L-selectin (CD62L), and CD58, are present in approximately one-half of the cases examined (20,21). CD4+ T cells and follicular dendritic cells are present in the malignant follicles in association with malignant B cells. When other tissues, such as liver or skin tissues, are involved, follicular dendritic cells and CD4+ T cells are generally present along with the follicular lymphoma cells.

Genetics

In follicular lymphoma, the Ig heavy- and light-chain genes are rearranged, and analysis of the Ig variable-region genes shows that most cases have extensive somatic mutations and a high frequency of intraclonal diversity, indicating ongoing mutations, similar to normal germinal center cells (22,23).

The genetic hallmark of follicular lymphoma is represented by chromosomal breaks at 18q21 and rearrangements of BCL-2, which are detected in 80% to 90% of cases (24,25). In this translocation, the BCL-2 gene on chromosome 18 is juxtaposed to the transcriptionally active Ig heavy-chain region on chromosome 14, forming the bcl-2/IgH rearrangement and upregulating the BCL-2 gene (26,27). Other chromosomal aberrations include gains of 7p, 7q, Xp, 12q, 18q, each occurring in 10% to 20% of patients (28). Deletions of chromosome 6q occur in 16% to 20% of cases (28,29). Although follicular non-Hodgkin's lymphomas with 3q27 (BCL-6 gene) abnormalities

are rare, the malignant cells express the BCL-6 gene and protein, which is a transcription factor involved in normal germinal center development (30).

Over time, a significant fraction of follicular lymphoma evolves into an aggressive lymphoma with a diffuse large-cell architecture (31). Cytogenetic analysis suggests that patients with follicular lymphoma whose tumor cells have deletions of chromosomes 6p, 17p, and 9p have significantly increased risk of histologic transformation. Specific genes have been identified as being altered in transformation, including deletions of the cyclin-dependent kinase inhibitors p15 and p16 and mutations of p53 and bcl-2, as well as of the noncoding regulatory region of the BCL-6 gene (32–36). Rearrangements of 1q21–23 have also been identified in a subset of follicular lymphoma during disease progression. In cases in which t(1;22)(q22;q11) was identified, the target gene is FCGR2B, which encodes for the IgG Fc receptor, FcgammaRIIB (37).

PATHOGENESIS

Chromosomal Translocations Involving BCL-2

The t(14;18)(q32;q21) is the most common translocation in human lymphoid malignancies (Color Plate 50). Virtually all follicular lymphomas and approximately 30% of diffuse large B-cell lymphomas carry breaks at 18q21. In t(14;18), the rearrangement joins the BCL-2 gene at its 3' untranslated region to an IgH J segment, resulting in deregulation of BCL-2 expression. The chromosomal breakpoints on BCL-2 cluster are at two main regions 3' to the bcl-2 coding region. The major breakpoint region is located within the 3' untranslated region, and the minor cluster region is located some 20 kb downstream. Both regions have been cloned and sequenced. The consequence of the translocation is the presence within the cells of constitutively high levels of bcl-2 protein, resulting from both enhanced transcription and, possibly, more efficient RNA processing (38,39).

The BCL-2 gene encodes a 26-kDa integral membrane protein that has been localized to mitochondria, endoplasmic reticulum, and perinuclear membrane (40). In contrast to most protooncogenes of lymphoid neoplasia, bcl-2 has little or no ability to promote cell-cycle progression or cell proliferation but rather controls the cellular apoptotic threshold by preventing programmed cell death. In normal cells, the topographic restriction of bcl-2 expression to germinal center zones of surviving B cells suggests that bcl-2 drives the emergence of long-surviving memory B cells. In fact, BCL-2 transgenic animals show markedly protracted secondary immune responses and an extended lifetime for memory B cells in the absence of antigen (41).

BCL-2 is only one member of a family of apoptotic regulators, which includes BAX and BCL-X (42,43). Bcl-2 exists as part of a high-molecular-weight complex generated through heterodimerization with bax (44). The inherent ratio of bcl-2 to bax determines the functional activity of Bcl-2 (44).

When bax is in excess, bax homodimers dominate, and cell death is accelerated. Conversely, when BCL-2 is in excess, as in lymphomas carrying BCL-2 rearrangements, bcl-2/bax heterodimers are the prevalent species, and cell death is repressed.

The pathogenetic contribution of BCL-2 lesions to follicular lymphoma development is complex. The observation that BCL-2–transgenic mice develop a pattern of polyclonal hyperplasia of mature, long-lived B cells resting in G0 suggests that BCL-2 activation is not sufficient for follicular lymphoma development and that other genetic lesions or host factors are required. Other evidence for this is the observation that complex karyotypic abnormalities are present in 34% of follicular lymphoma grade 1 and 62% of grade 2 cases (28). Chronic antigen stimulation and selection could also synergize with bcl-2 in driving follicular lymphoma expansion (45). With time—and analogous to the human disease—a fraction of BCL-2–transgenic mice develops aggressive, clonal, large-cell lymphomas that have additional genetic lesions, specifically c-myc translocations (46,47). However, these BCL-2–transgenic mice do not develop a disease analogous to indolent follicular lymphoma.

Further evidence that the bcl-2/IgH translocation alone is not causative for follicular lymphoma is provided by reports that B cells with t(14;18) are present in a substantial number of normal individuals (48–50). In peripheral blood, t(14;18)+ cells have been reported in 8% to 88% of normal subjects using polymerase chain reaction (PCR). The variability of these data is likely due to differing sensitivities of the assays used. Similarly, using fluorescent in situ hybridization techniques, B cells with t(14;18) have been detected in hyperplastic lymphoid tissues (tonsil, lymph nodes) in 12% to 54% of normal individuals (51). Similar to the risk of follicular lymphoma increasing with age, the detection of t(14;18) in the peripheral blood of normal humans appears to increase with age. In addition, t(14;18)+ cells have been detected by PCR in the peripheral blood of patients with localized follicular lymphoma who are in long-term remission (longer than 10 years) after radiation therapy (52). One interpretation of this finding is that these cells lack the other genetic changes necessary to develop into recurrent lymphoma. More recently, the expression of genes in follicular lymphoma has been compared to normal B cells (53,54). These gene expression profiling studies have provided support for the theory that follicular lymphomas are derived from normal germinal center B cells; however, a number of genes are clearly differentially expressed. These studies may provide insight into the other genetic events that contribute to the pathogenesis and pathophysiology of follicular lymphoma.

CLINICAL PRESENTATION AND STAGING

Follicular lymphoma (grades 1 and 2) usually presents in patients with painless peripheral adenopathy in cervical, axillary, inguinal, and femoral regions. Lymph node enlargement has often been present for long periods and is generally slowly progressive. Lymph nodes may wax and wane in size, including complete regressions followed by reappearance. Hilar and mediastinal nodes are often involved, but large mediastinal masses are rare. Some patients present with asymptomatic large abdominal masses with or without evidence of gastrointestinal or urinary tract obstruction. Central nervous system involvement is exceedingly rare, but peripheral nerve compression and epidural tumor masses causing cord compression may develop.

Although patients may present clinically with one or more sites of nodal disease, staging studies usually demonstrate widely disseminated disease with involvement of the spleen, liver, and bone marrow in 40%, 50%, and 60% to 70% of cases, respectively. Hepatosplenomegaly is diffuse rather than with discrete masses. Very few patients present with extranodal disease besides marrow involvement, and effusions (pleural, pericardial, ascites) are uncommon. Only 10% to 20% of patients present with B symptoms or increased serum concentrations of lactate dehydrogenase. There are no characteristic laboratory abnormalities specifically associated with follicular lymphoma, although elevation of β_2-microglobulin, which is seen in up to 25% of patients, can be a surrogate marker of the extent of disease (55,56). In addition to conventional imaging studies with computed tomography scans, gallium and positron emission tomography (PET) have been used to evaluate patients with follicular lymphoma. In contrast to aggressive non-Hodgkin's lymphomas, there is less evidence that gallium or PET scanning are useful tools. A false-negative rate of 60% for gallium scanning has been reported in follicular lymphoma. PET scans have been reported to detect 40% of nodal sites in follicular lymphoma patients, predominantly detecting peripheral and thoracic sites (57). There are very limited data on the value of PET scanning after completion of therapy. One study reported two relapses in two follicular lymphoma patients who were persistently PET positive and two relapses in six patients who had a negative PET scan (58).

Follicular lymphoma grade 3 is synonymous with what is often referred to as *follicular large-cell lymphoma* (12). In contrast to other follicular lymphomas, this histologic variant has less infiltration of the bone marrow and presents with larger lymphoid masses. Unlike follicular grade 1 or 2, follicular lymphoma grade 3 uncommonly circulates in the peripheral blood. Although the follicular morphology is preserved, the clinical presentation, behavior, and outcome with treatment more closely approximate those of diffuse large B-cell lymphoma, which is classified as an *aggressive lymphoma variant* (59,60).

An increasing number of cases of primary cutaneous B-cell lymphomas are reported to either have a follicular pattern or to be composed of cells that resemble centrocytes and centroblasts. These tumors often lack t(14;18), and their relationship to nodal follicular lymphoma is not known (61).

They tend to occur on the head and trunk and generally remain localized to the skin (62). In one study of 122 patients with this disorder, extracutaneous progression was noted in only seven cases (6%), three of which were in the central nervous system (63).

PROGNOSTIC AND PREDICTIVE FACTORS

A large number of pretreatment prognostic factors have been associated with an adverse prognosis in follicular lymphoma. These include age, sex, stage, presence of B symptoms, performance status, serum lactate dehydrogenase, serum β_2-microglobulin, hemoglobin, bulk disease, and extranodal involvement. Analogous to the International Prognostic Index (IPI) for aggressive lymphomas (64), a number of groups have attempted to apply the IPI to and create prognostic models for patients with follicular lymphoma (Table 24.1). The M.D. Anderson Cancer Center developed a tumor-burden model based on the number of extranodal sites, degree of marrow involvement, and lymph node size (65). Patients with a low tumor burden had a 10-year survival rate of 73% compared to 24% for those with a high tumor burden.

The IPI has been retrospectively applied to patients with follicular lymphoma and in general the model is predictive for progression-free and overall survival (66). In one report, the 10-year overall survivals were 74%, 45%, 54%, and 0% for the four IPI risk groups (low, low-intermediate, high-intermediate, and high risk). The limitations of the IPI in these patients are that some of the factors are not of prognostic significance and that a low number of patients (between 10% and 20%) are in the higher-risk groups (prognostic scores of 3 to 5).

Other predictive models for follicular lymphoma have been more recently reported. The Italian Lymphoma Intergroup model is based on the analysis of more than 900 patients (67). In this model, six adverse prognostic factors were identified: age older than 60, male sex, involvement of two or more extranodal sites, elevated serum lactate dehydrogenase, presence of B symptoms, and erythrocyte sedimentation rate greater than or equal to 30 mm per hour. Three risk groups were identified: low (no or one risk factor), intermediate (two risk factors), and high (three or more). Five and 10-year survivals were 90% and 65%, 75% and 54%, and 38% and 11% for the three risk groups, respectively. Patients at low risk had long survivals, those at intermediate risk had a continuous pattern of relapse with no suggestion of cure, and those at high risk had a poor outcome. The model was also predictive of survival in a subgroup of patients with follicular lymphoma treated uniformly with doxorubicin-containing regimens.

In a study of 484 patients with stage III or IV follicular lymphoma, three independent adverse risk factors were found: age older than 60 years, B symptoms, and the presence of at least three extranodal sites larger than 3 cm in diameter (68). Overall 5-year survival rates of patients with no, one to two, or three adverse factors were 74%, 66%, and 45%, respectively.

TABLE 24.1. *Selected prognostic and predictive factors for follicular non-Hodgkin's lymphoma*

Series	Factors	Overall survival (time)
International Prognostic Index (66)	Age >60 yr, stage III or IV, performance status >2, extranodal sites >2, LDH > normal	Low 73.6% (10 yr)
		Low intermediate 32% (10 yr)
		High intermediate 53.5% (10 yr)
		High 0% (10 yr)
M.D. Anderson Cancer Center (65)	Extranodal sites, degree of marrow involvement, lymph node size	Low 73% (10 yr)
		Intermediate 40% (10 yr)
		High 24% (10 yr)
Italian Lymphoma Intergroup (67)	Age >60 yr, male gender, extranodal sites ≥2, B symptoms, LDH > normal, Erythrocyte sedimentation rate >30	Low 65% (10 yr)
		Intermediate 54% (10 yr)
		High 11% (10 yr)
Groupe d'Etude des Lymphomas (68)	Age >60 yr, B symptoms, 3 nodal sites >3 cm	0 factors 74% (5 yr)
		1 factor 66% (5 yr)
		2–3 factors 45% (5 yr)

LDH, lactate dehydrogenase.
Data from Decaudin D, Lepage E, Brousse N, et al. Low-grade stage III-IV follicular lymphoma: multivariate analysis of prognostic factors in 484 patients—a study of the Groupe d'Etude des Lymphomes de l'Adulte. *J Clin Oncol* 1999;17:2499–2505; Federico M, Vitolo U, Zinzani PL, et al. Prognosis of follicular lymphoma: a predictive model based on a retrospective analysis of 987 cases. Intergruppo Italiano Linfomi. *Blood* 2000;95:783–789; Lopez-Guillermo A, Montserrat E, Bosch F, et al. Applicability of the International Index for aggressive lymphomas to patients with low-grade lymphoma. *J Clin Oncol* 1994;12:1343–1348; and Romaguera JE, McLaughlin P, North L, et al. Multivariate analysis of prognostic factors in stage IV follicular low-grade lymphoma: a risk model. *J Clin Oncol* 1991;9:762–769.

Histopathology has been controversial as a prognostic factor for patients with follicular lymphoma. The percentage of large cells has been observed to be an important prognostic factor of clinical behavior and response to therapy (59,60,69). It is generally agreed among pathologists and clinicians that grade 3 follicular lymphoma is a distinct histologic and clinical entity, whereas the distinction between grade 1 and 2 disease remains debated. Similarly, the architecture, specifically the degree of nodularity, has received attention as a prognostic factor in the literature (70–76). The presence of diffuse areas in follicular grades 1 and 2 has been reported in some series as a negative prognostic factor for survival, but in others it has not been found to be a significant factor. In one series from the Eastern Cooperative Oncology Group, patients with a purely follicular pattern, defined as greater than 75% of the cross sectional area of the tissue examined, had a median survival of 68 months (75). In contrast, patients with a significant diffuse component had a median survival of only 39 months. The impact of a mixed follicular and diffuse architecture was seen in both the grade 1 and grade 2 cases. A similar observation has been reported by Stanford University (74). An analysis of subdividing follicular lymphoma grade 3 (FL3a, FL3b, FLC), as suggested by the World Health Organization, and the impact of diffuse architecture has been reported from the University of Nebraska (76). No significant differences were seen in the clinical characteristics or outcome of patients with the different grades of follicular large-cell lymphoma. However, patients with a predominant diffuse component (greater than 50%) had a lower overall survival as compared to patients with a predominant follicular architecture.

TREATMENT

Clinical Course

The course of follicular lymphoma is quite variable. Some patients have waxing and waning disease for 5 years or longer without the need for therapy (77). Others present with more disseminated disease and rapid growth, and require treatment, because massive nodal or organ enlargement leads to pain, lymphatic obstruction, or organ obstruction.

Histologic transformation of follicular lymphoma from an indolent to a diffuse aggressive lymphoma occurs in 10% to 70% of patients and is associated with rapid progression of lymphadenopathy, infiltration of extranodal sites, development of systemic symptoms, elevated serum lactate dehydrogenase, and often a poor prognosis (78–84). The progression from follicular lymphoma to diffuse large B-cell lymphoma occurs regardless of whether follicular lymphoma is treated aggressively or conservatively at a rate of approximately 5% to 10% per year, depending on the magnitude of the large-cell component (31). At autopsy, 95% of patients with follicular lymphoma demonstrate some evidence of diffuse large B-cell lymphoma.

TABLE 24.2. *Treatment algorithm for newly diagnosed follicular lymphoma*[a]

Stage I, II
Locoregional or extended field XRT, or observation in selected cases
Bulky abdominal stage II, stage III and stage IV
No indication for therapy[b]
Observation
Options if there is indication for therapy
Local palliative XRT
Single-agent or combination chemotherapy
Antibody-based therapy with or without chemotherapy

XRT, radiation therapy.
[a]Clinical trial participation is always recommended.
[b]Indications for therapy: symptoms, threatened end-organ function, cytopenias, massive bulk, rapid progression.

Indications for Treatment

The indolent lymphomas are generally associated with survival measured in years, even if untreated (77,85). However, follicular lymphoma is usually not curable with conventional treatment. Therefore, in contrast to patients with curable aggressive lymphomas, in approaching patients with indolent lymphomas, one must consider the indications for treatment. Although the ultimate goal is to cure these diseases, currently the major reason for treatment is to alleviate symptoms. These include local symptoms due to progressive or bulky nodal disease; compromise of normal organ function due to progressive or bulky disease; B symptoms; symptomatic extranodal disease, such as effusions; and cytopenias due to extensive bone marrow infiltration or hypersplenism. Algorithms for management of previously untreated and relapsed patients are presented in Tables 24.2 and 24.3.

Therapy for Early-Stage Disease

Only 15% to 30% of patients have clinical stage I or II disease, and less than 10% has pathologic stage I or II disease (86). For this reason, limited studies are available concerning the treatment of early-stage indolent lymphoma.

Radiation therapy is the mainstay of treatment for limited-stage follicular grade 1 or 2 lymphoma. Some of the ongoing questions in the treatment of these patients are (a) What is the evidence that follicular grade 1 or 2 lymphoma is curative with radiation therapy alone? (b) What is the frequency of late recurrences (longer than 10 years after diagnosis and complete remission)? (c) What are the prognostic factors for recurrence? (d) What are the extent and dose of radiation therapy needed? (e) What is the role of chemotherapy in early-stage low-grade lymphoma? (f) What is the prognosis in patients who develop recurrent disease? and (g) What are potential areas for new investigation?

TABLE 24.3. *Treatment algorithm for relapsed follicular non-Hodgkin's lymphoma*[a]

No indication for treatment
  Observation
Options if there is indication for treatment at first relapse
  Single-agent or combination chemotherapy
  Monoclonal antibody-based therapy
  Chemotherapy with monoclonal antibody-based therapy
Options if there is indication for treatment at second or greater relapse
  Single-agent or combination chemotherapy
  Monoclonal antibody-based therapy
  Chemotherapy with monoclonal antibody-based therapy
  Radioimmunotherapy
  High-dose therapy and autologous or allogeneic stem cell transplantation
Histologic transformation
  Few prior therapies; localized
    Anthracycline-based combination chemotherapy, followed by observation, radiation, or consideration of high-dose therapy and autologous stem cell transplantation
  Options if there is widespread disease and multiple prior therapies
    Anthracycline-based combination chemotherapy
    Radioimmunotherapy
    Autologous stem cell transplantation for responding disease

[a]Clinical trial participation is always recommended.

Many published studies have demonstrated the efficacy of radiation therapy in the treatment of clinically staged patients with localized follicular grade 1 to 3 lymphoma. Table 24.4 summarizes data from nine published reports each containing 50 or more patients (87–94). All but one study contains both stage I and stage II patients (in approximately equal frequencies). The 10-year freedom from treatment failure in all nine studies ranged from 41% to 49%. The 10-year overall survival (all causes) ranged from 43% to 79%, with a median survival of 11.9 to 15.3 years. Nearly all patients were treated with radiation therapy alone, except in the Fondation Bergonie study, in which 70% of patients received some form of systemic treatment (90). The freedom from treatment failure and overall survival in this combined modality study were no better than in the primary radiation–alone studies. The majority of patients had follicular lymphoma grade 1 and grade 2; however, follicular lymphoma grade 3 and low-grade diffuse small-cell histologies were included in some of the series. The percentages are noted in Table 24.4 for each study.

Evidence that follicular grade 1 or 2 lymphoma is curable with radiation therapy alone is supported by the nearly 50% freedom from treatment failure (or progression-free, disease-free, or relapse-free survival) results at 10 years in all studies and by the low rates of recurrence after 10 years in patients who have remained continuously disease free since initial diagnosis and treatment (88,89,93,94). In the Stanford series, for example, only five of 47 patients in continuous remission for 10 years or longer have relapsed at longer intervals (89).

Adverse prognostic factors for freedom from treatment failure (or progression-free, disease-free, or relapse-free survival depending on the report) are analyzed by multivariate analysis in many of the studies. Age was the adverse factor most often reported and was seen in five of the nine studies (see Table 24.4). Follicular grade 3 histology, extensive clinical stage IIA disease, bulky disease (larger than 2 cm or larger than 3 cm), and extranodal presentations also were reported, but these adverse factors were seen in only one or two of the nine studies. There appears to be very little difference in outcome between follicular grade 1 and follicular grade 2 disease. Also, age was the most common significant adverse factor for overall survival. As the median age of patients was approximately 60 years of age in these studies, it is not surprising that age is a significant factor for survival in most of the analyses. Except for follicular lymphoma grade 3, which is treated similarly to diffuse large B-cell lymphoma, and extensive clinical stage II presentations that may be treated similarly to advanced-stage disease, none of the other factors is sufficiently adverse to alter the standard recommendation for curative local radiation therapy as the initial treatment approach.

The dose and field size of radiation therapy varied greatly within and between studies, and there are no randomized trials to evaluate optimal dose and field size. Clinical evidence for field-size and radiation-dose guidelines is discussed in detail in Chapter 11. The majority of studies do not report significant differences in the freedom from treatment failure (or progression-free, disease-free, or relapse-free survival) between local/regional and extensive/total-nodal fields. In the Stanford series (89), the data reporting the association of larger irradiated field sizes with an increased freedom from recurrence are confounded by the common use of staging laparotomy in this large-field group of patients. Thus, their improved results may be due to the exclusion of stage III and IV patients discovered on surgical staging but not appreciated with clinical staging. In addition, none of the studies that have reported improved freedom from treatment failure results with more aggressive treatment has demonstrated an improvement in survival. Of interest, in the Stanford study, late second tumors were noted in 6.8% of patients who received involved- or extended-field radiation and in 17% of those treated with extensive radiotherapy. In terms of dose, none of the studies show convincing evidence for improved local control above the 30 to 36 Gy.

We recommend the use of regional radiation therapy fields for patients with clinical stage I or II follicular lymphoma grade 1 or 2. This consists of irradiating the involved nodal region plus one additional uninvolved region on each side of the involved nodes. The recommended dose is 30 to 36 Gy with a boost to areas of initial involvement to 36 to 40 Gy.

TABLE 24.4. *Radiation therapy for early-stage low-grade follicular non-Hodgkin's lymphoma (selected trials containing 50 or more patients)*

Report (reference)	Number of patients/median follow-up time/CT	Stage (%)	10-yr FFTF/ OS (%)	Median RT dose to the tumor	RT field size (%)	Grade distribution (%)	Adverse prognostic factors (FFTF)
Princess Margaret Hospital (87)	573/10.6 yr/ 27%	I (64)	48/>60	35 Gy	IF	FG1 (33)	Ext CS II
		II (36)				FG2 (32)	>2 cm disease
						FG3 (35)	
British National Lymphoma Investigation (88)	208/NA/0%	I (100)	47/64	35 Gy (suggested)	NA	FG1 (39)	Age ≥50 yr
						FG2 (35)	
						FG3 (5)	
						Other (21)	
Stanford University (89)	177/7.7 yr/5%	I (41)	44/64	35–50 Gy	IF/RF/EF (77)	FG1 (57)	Age >60 yr
		II (59)			TLI (23)	FG2/3 (43)	Extranodal site RT fields < TLI
Foundation Bergonie (90)	103/8.3 yr/70%	I (44)	49/56	35–40 Gy	IF (54)	NA	Age >60 yr
		II (56)			RF (46)		
M.D. Anderson Cancer Center (91)	80/19 yr/0%	I (41)	41/43 at 15 yr	40 Gy	IF (9)	FG1 (63)	CS IIA
		II (59)			RF (54)	FG2 (37)	>3 cm disease
					EF (37)		
Edinburgh (92)	64/5 yr/2%	I (58)	49/78	30–40 Gy (82%)	NA	FG1 (78)	NA
		II (42)		>40 Gy (18%)		FG2 (3)	
						Other (19)	
University of Florida[a]	72/8.5 yr/7%	I (75)	46/59	NA	IF (53)	NA	NA
		II (25)			EF (43)		
					TNI/WA (4)		
NCI (93)	54/9 yr/10%	I (50)	48/69	36 Gy	IF (38)	NA	Age ≥45 yr
		II (50)			EF (48)		
					TLI/TBI (14)		
Royal Marsden Hospital (94)	58/NA/0%	I (69)	43/79	40 Gy	IF (52)	FG1 (64)	Field size not significant for recurrence
		II (31)			EF (48)	FG2 (21)	
						Other (15)	

CT, chemotherapy; DFS, disease free survival; EF, extended field radiation [mantle or whole abdominal (Wilder); mantle, whole abdominal, inverted Y (Pendlebury, McManus); mantle, inverted Y (Lawrence)]; FFTF, freedom from treatment failure; FG, follicular grade; NA, not reported; OS, overall survival (all causes); PFS, progression free survival; Prog, prognostic; RF, regional field radiation [1–3 adjacent nodal regions (Wilder)]; RFS, recurrence/relapse free survival; RT, radiation therapy; TBI, total-body irradiation; TLI, total-lymphoid irradiation; TNI, total-nodal irradiation.

[a]Data from Kamath SS, Marcus RB Jr, Lynch JW, et al. The impact of radiotherapy dose and other treatment-related and clinical factors on in-field control in stage I and II non-Hodgkin's lymphoma. *Int J Radiat Oncol Biol Phys* 1999;44:563–568.

This approach provides a 40% to 50% probability of cure. Carefully planned local radiation–therapy fields with modest doses can significantly reduce the risk of significant damage to the marrow reserve, the risk of developing a treatment-related malignancy, and the risk of long-term toxicity to the salivary glands, lungs, heart, kidneys, and bowel when in close proximity to the lymphoma. This less toxic approach (compared to larger-field irradiation) preserves the ability to effectively treat patients in whom the same histology later recurs or who transform to a higher-grade histology. For more than half of all patients, disease will recur at some point in their life, and increasingly, there will be new and more effective approaches for these patients. To maximize cure but reserve the option for effective treatment for relapse, the radiation and medical oncologists must work together to devise an optimum treatment approach.

The role of combination chemotherapy in the management of early-stage follicular lymphoma is unclear. At least three randomized studies conducted in the 1970s failed to demonstrate that a non–Adriamycin-containing combination chemotherapy regimen plus radiation therapy was superior to radiation therapy alone (94a,95,96). A more recent British National Lymphoma Investigation study randomized 148 patients to receive either radiation therapy alone or radiation therapy plus chlorambucil chemotherapy (97). There were no differences in freedom from recurrence or survival between the groups. A single-arm study of 91 stage I or II patients treated at the M.D. Anderson Cancer Center with COP [cyclophosphamide, Oncovin (vincristine), and prednisone] or CHOP-Bleo [cyclophosphamide, doxorubicin, Oncovin (vincristine), prednisone and bleomycin] chemotherapy in addition to radiation therapy demonstrated an improved freedom from recurrence compared to historical controls but no overall survival differences (98,99). In part, the choice of therapy may lie in the careful assessment of prognostic factors. Most patients with Ann Arbor clinical stage I or II follicular small cleaved-cell and follicular mixed lymphomas should have a good prognosis after local-regional radiation therapy alone. For patients whose prognosis is less certain, such as patients with stage II disease with multiple sites of involvement or bulky nodes or patients with follicular lymphoma grade 3 histology, chemotherapy followed by involved-field irradiation may provide more durable remissions. With a combined modality approach in follicular lymphoma grade 3, the failure-free survival and overall survival rates at 3 years are 61% and 76%, respectively (59).

There are few data on the outcome of patients who develop recurrent disease after radiation therapy for initial stage I or II presentations. In the Stanford study, most relapses were detected by physical examination (66%), with 76% of patients having stage I or II disease at relapse. Actuarial survival rates 5, 10, 15, and 20 years after relapse were 56%, 35%, 17%, and 17%, respectively (100). The progression-free survival rate for the entire group at 5 years was 44% and remained at 22% 10, 15, and 20 years after relapse. Therefore, approximately one-fifth of patients with early-stage follicular lymphoma have prolonged survival even after relapse from primary radiation therapy.

In summary, patients with early-stage follicular grade 1 or 2 lymphoma have a median survival of nearly 15 years. Local-regional radiation results in cure of approximately 40% of patients. There is a decreasing freedom from recurrence with age and extranodal involvement. There are no treatment outcome differences between grade 1 and grade 2 patients. There are a number of areas for ongoing investigation. Trials of field size and dose would allow better definition for the delivery of radiation therapy. Finally, the role of adjuvant chemotherapy and immunotherapy needs to be better defined.

Therapy of Advanced-Stage Disease

The long natural history of indolent lymphomas and the general lack of symptoms at diagnosis have fostered close observation as the initial approach for some patients. Because up to 23% of patients have spontaneous remissions lasting longer than 1 year, it is recommended that a period of observation is warranted for asymptomatic patients with low-volume disease (31,77,101,102). The most recent support for this approach is the randomized study from the National Cancer Institute (NCI) in advanced-stage patients. In that study, which compared no initial therapy to immediate combined modality treatment with ProMACE-MOPP [prednisone, methotrexate with leucovorin rescue, Adriamycin, Cytoxan (cyclophosphamide), and etoposide–Mustargen (mechlorethamine), Oncovin (vincristine), procarbazine, and prednisone] followed by total-lymphoid irradiation, there was no survival advantage to upfront therapy (31).

Withholding therapy in this situation requires an informed and cooperative patient and close follow-up. In a study from Stanford, patients were randomized to either receive therapy immediately or to defer treatment until the time of progressive symptomatic disease (103). In the latter group, the median time until therapy was administered was 3 years. However, for the three histologic subtypes, the median time to the need for therapy varied significantly, being 16 and 48 months for follicular lymphoma grade 2 (follicular mixed) and follicular lymphoma grade 1 (follicular small cleaved), respectively. Despite this, there was no difference in the 4-year actuarial survival between the two treatment groups.

Palliative Radiation Therapy

Localized radiation therapy can be very effective palliative treatment for patients with advanced-stage lymphomas. Indications for palliation include (a) treatment of a resistant localized mass in the setting of other chemotherapy-responsive disease to limit the need for additional cytotoxic treatment, (b) prevention or relief of neurologic signs from spinal cord involvement or nerve root compression, (c) relief of a superior vena cava syndrome or obstructive pneumonia, (d) reduction of the risk of fracture in involved weight-bearing bones, (e) alleviation of symptoms of localized involvement in areas such as the orbit or stomach, and (f) cosmetic reasons. The use of radiation therapy in these settings often focuses just on a single area, allowing the use of small fields with a low risk of acute and late effects from treatment. In addition, lower doses can be used than otherwise required for curative treatment. Several studies have advocated using very low doses for palliation, with good results (104,105).

Systemic chemotherapy is the mainstay of treatment for advanced-stage indolent lymphoma. However, radiation therapy has been used in some patients with stage III disease, with a complete response rate of 70% to 85% (103,106). In selected patients, mainly those with minimal stage III disease, total-lymphoid irradiation or total-body irradiation has led to prolonged relapse-free survival (107–109).

Chemotherapy

Indolent lymphomas are very sensitive to both alkylating agents (e.g., chlorambucil, cyclophosphamide) and combination chemotherapy, with complete-remission rates ranging from 30% to 60% for previously untreated patients (80,84). This variability in complete-remission rate is likely a function of the stringency of restaging. For example, the complete-remission rates were notably higher in studies before the advent of computed tomography scanning, when physical examination, ultrasound, and conventional radiography were used for restaging patients after treatment. As the sensitivity of modalities for restaging has increased, the complete-remission rates have decreased. However, the median duration of complete remission with either a single alkylating agent (e.g., cyclophosphamide) or combination chemotherapy [e.g., CVP (cyclophosphamide, vincristine, prednisone)] is only approximately 2.5 years.

A study from Stanford compared daily single-alkylating-agent treatment, combination chemotherapy (CVP), and total-body irradiation in patients with follicular lymphoma grade 1 or 2 and small lymphocytic lymphoma (103) (Table 24.5). Although the median time to achieve complete remission was 12, 5, and 3 months for single-agent therapy, CVP, and total-body irradiation, respectively, there were no significant differences in relapse-free or overall survival among the three regimens. In general, with either single-agent therapy or CVP, only 20% to 25% of patients remain disease-free at 4 years (80). After relapse, these diseases continue to be sensitive to single agents and CVP; however, the median relapse-free survival progressively decreases with each subsequent relapse, falling to a median of 13 months after the second remission (84).

In an attempt to improve the relapse-free and overall survival in patients with indolent non-Hodgkin's lymphoma, more aggressive combination chemotherapy regimens have been used (110–113). Regimens such as MOPP, BACOP [bleomycin, Adriamycin (doxorubicin), cyclophosphamide, Oncovin (vincristine), and prednisone], M-BACOD [methotrexate, bleomycin, Adriamycin (doxorubicin), cyclophosphamide, Oncovin (vincristine), and dexamethasone], CHOP, and BVCP (BCNU, vincristine, cyclophosphamide, prednisone) have been observed to give complete remission rates of 35% to 70%, but the median relapse-free survival remains similar to that seen with CVP, in the range of 1.5 to 3.9 years.

Studies from the 1970s suggested that patients with follicular lymphoma grade 2 treated with combination chemotherapy (e.g., C-MOPP [cyclophosphamide, mechlorethamine, Oncovin (vincristine), procarbazine, and prednisone],

CHOP-Bleo), had a high complete-remission rate with greater than 50% still in complete remission 5 to 7 years after treatment. This suggested that follicular lymphoma grade 2 might be curable with aggressive combination chemotherapy (114–116). However, a prospective randomized trial comparing cyclophosphamide/prednisone, C-MOPP, and BCVP failed to demonstrate significant long-term disease-free survival for patients with follicular lymphoma grade 2 (110). The World Health Organization classification conference consensus is that at the present time, the treatment approach to grade 1 and grade 2 follicular lymphoma should not differ (12).

Several randomized trials have looked at the impact of combination chemotherapy and specifically at the addition of doxorubicin in combination chemotherapy for patients with advanced-stage follicular lymphoma (Table 24.5) (117). In a comparison of cyclophosphamide and prednisone, BCVP, or CVPP (cyclophosphamide, vincristine, prednisone, and procarbazine), the 5-year progression-free survival was higher with CVPP, but no differences in overall survival were noted (118). When the role of Adriamycin was examined by comparing COP-Bleo to CHOP-Bleo (and CHOP-Bacillus Calmette-Guerin), no differences were seen (119). In a Cancer and Leukemia Group B study in which CHOP-Bleo was compared to cyclophosphamide alone in patients with follicular lymphoma grades 1 and 2, the complete remission rate and time to failure were not statistically different between the two arms for the entire patient population. However, in the 46 patients with follicular lymphoma grade 2, the failure-free and overall survival were better for combination chemotherapy (120). However, due to problems of reproducibility of histologic interpretation of follicular lymphoma grades 1 and 2 and the limited number of patients in this study, the use of Adriamycin-containing regimens for patients with follicular lymphoma remains controversial and not recommended as standard of care.

Advanced-stage follicular lymphoma grade 3 is generally treated like diffuse large B-cell lymphoma (59,60,69,76). With combination chemotherapy regimens, the complete-remission rates range from 50% to 75%. The 5- and 10-year failure-free survival rates were 34% and 67% and the overall survival rates were 61% and 72%, respectively. The IPI was useful in stratifying these patients, although 71% had either low or low-intermediate prognostic scores (60). The degree of follicularity has been examined by several groups and remains controversial. In a report from the University of Nebraska, the presence of a mixed follicular and diffuse architecture was significantly associated with survival; 3-year survival rates were 47% for patients with purely follicular architecture and 0% for patients with follicular and diffuse architecture (59).

Combined Modality Therapy

Studies from the National Cancer Institute and Stanford have failed to demonstrate an improved relapse-free or overall survival for patients treated with CVP with or without total-

TABLE 24.5. *Selected randomized therapeutic studies for follicular non-Hodgkin's lymphoma*

Series and number of patients	Arms	Conclusions
Previously untreated patients		
Hoppe et al., 1981 (n = 51)	Daily alkylating agent	No difference in RFS
	CVP	No difference in OS
	Total-body irradiation	
Ezdinli et al., 1980 (n = 252)	Cyclophosphamide/prednisone	PFS best with CVPP
	BCVP	No difference in OS
	CVPP	
Jones et al., 1979 (n = 443)	COP-Bleo	No differences in PFS
	CHOP-Bleo	No difference in OS
	CHOP-BCG	
Morrison, 1993	Cyclophosphamide	Survival advantage for grade 2 follicular lymphoma with CHOP-Bleo
	CHOP-Bleo	
Young et al., 1988 (n = 104)	Observation	No difference in OS
	ProMACE-MOPP/TLI	
Hagenbeek et al., 2001 (n = 381)	Fludarabine	Higher response rate/longer time to progression with fludarabine
	CVP	
		No difference in OS
Smalley et al., 1992	CHOP	OS at 2 yr not different
	CHOP-IFN	
Aviles et al., 1996 (n = 98)	Combination chemo	Improved OS with IFN
	Combination chemo–IFN maintenance	
Solal-Celigny et al., 1998	Combination chemo	Longer PFS with IFN
	Combination chemo-IFN	OS longer in certain subgroups
Fisher et al., 2000 (n = 571)	ProMACE-MOPP	No difference in PFS or OS
	ProMACE-MOPP-IFN	
	Additional randomization to maintenance	
Italian Cooperative Study Group on Lymphoma	Fludarabine/mitoxantrone/rituximab	Improved molecular complete-remission rate with FMR
	CHOP/rituximab	
German Low Grade Study Group	FCM	Improved response rate with rituximab
	FCM/rituximab	
Previously treated patients		
Klasa	Fludarabine	Similar response and OS
	CVP	PFS improved with fludarabine
Witzig et al. 2002 (n = 143)	Rituximab	Increased response rate with Zevalin
	Zevalin	No difference in time to progression

BCG, Bacillus Calmette-Guerin; BCVP, BCNU, vincristine, cyclophosphamide, prednisone; Bleo, bleomycin; CHOP, cyclophosphamide, doxorubicin, vincristine, prednisone; COP, cyclophosphamide, Oncovin (vincristine), prednisone; CVP, cyclophosphamide, vincristine, prednisone; CVPP, Cytoxan (cyclophosphamide), vinblastine, procarbazine, prednisone; FCM, fludarabine, cyclophosphamide, mitoxantrone; FMR, fludarabine, mitoxantrone, rituximab; IFN, interferon-α; OS, overall survival; PFS, progression-free survival; ProMACE-MOPP, prednisone, methotrexate, doxorubicin, cyclophosphamide, etoposide, leucovorin, mechlorethamine, vincristine, procarbazine, prednisone; RFS, relapse-free survival; TLI, total-lymphoid irradiation.

Data from Aviles A, Duque G, Talavera A, et al. Interferon alpha 2b as maintenance therapy in low grade malignant lymphoma improves duration of remission and survival. *Leuk Lymphoma* 1996;20:495–499; Ezdinli EZ, Costello WG, Silverstein MN, et al. Moderate versus intensive chemotherapy of prognostically favorable non-Hodgkin's lymphoma: a progress report. *Cancer* 1980;46:29–33; Fisher RI, Dana BW, LeBlanc M, et al. Interferon alpha consolidation after intensive chemotherapy does not prolong the progression-free survival of patients with low-grade non-Hodgkin's lymphoma: results of the Southwest Oncology Group randomized phase III study 8809. *J Clin Oncol* 2000;18:2010–2016; Hoppe RT, Kushlan P, Kaplan HS, et al. The treatment of advanced stage favorable histology non-Hodgkin's lymphoma: a preliminary report of a randomized trial comparing single agent chemotherapy, combination chemotherapy, and whole body irradiation. *Blood* 1981;58:592–598; Jones SE, Grozea PN, Metz EN, et al. Superiority of adriamycin-containing combination chemotherapy in the treatment of diffuse lymphoma: a Southwest Oncology Group study. *Cancer* 1979;43:417–425; Morrison VA, Peterson BA. Combination chemotherapy in the treatment of follicular low-grade lymphoma. *Leuk Lymphoma* 1993;10 Suppl:29–33; Smalley RV, Andersen JW, Hawkins MJ, et al. Interferon alfa combined with cytotoxic chemotherapy for patients with non-Hodgkin's lymphoma. *N Engl J Med* 1992;327:1336–1341; Solal-Celigny P, Lepage E, Brousse N, et al. Doxorubicin-containing regimen with or without interferon alfa-2b for advanced follicular lymphomas: final analysis of survival and toxicity in the Groupe d'Etude des Lymphomes Folliculaires 86 Trial. *J Clin Oncol* 1998;16:2332–2338; Witzig TE, Gordon LI, Cabanillas F, et al. Randomized controlled trial of yttrium-90-labeled ibritumomab tiuxetan radioimmunotherapy versus rituximab immunotherapy for patients with relapsed or refractory low-grade, follicular, or transformed B-cell non-Hodgkin's lymphoma. *J Clin Oncol* 2002;20:2453–2463; Young RC, Longo DL, Glatstein E, et al. The treatment of indolent lymphomas: watchful waiting v aggressive combined modality treatment. *Semin Hematol* 1988;25:11–16.

body irradiation or total-lymphoid irradiation. On the other hand, investigators at the M.D. Anderson Cancer Center reported an 81% complete-remission rate, 75% 5-year survival, and 52% relapse-free survival for patients with stage III follicular lymphoma treated with CHOP-Bleo and involved-field radiotherapy (121).

Although myelodysplasia and acute leukemia are uncommonly seen in patients with indolent lymphomas treated with chemotherapy alone, a 15-year cumulative incidence of myelodysplasia and secondary acute leukemia of 17% has been reported for the combination of low-dose total-body irradiation and cytotoxic chemotherapy (122). This suggests that combined modality therapy increases the incidence of hematopoietic stem cell disorders.

A randomized study from the National Cancer Institute attempted to address two issues: first, the role of aggressive combined modality therapy, and second, whether early institution of aggressive therapy affects the natural history of the disease. Patients with stage III or IV follicular lymphoma or small lymphocytic lymphoma were randomized to receive either no initial therapy or ProMACE-MOPP followed by total-lymphoid irradiation (Table 24.5) (123). Of 104 patients, 14% were not randomized but required initial treatment. For this group, there was a 71% complete-remission rate; only 33% were in unmaintained remission at a median follow-up of 23+ months. The patients who were randomized to initial aggressive treatment had a complete-remission rate of 78%; 86% of patients achieving complete remission were still in first complete remission at follow-up times ranging from 1 to 82+ months. Of the patients initially randomized to observation, 44% have crossed over to the treatment arm, with a lower complete-remission rate of 43%; 71% of those achieving complete remission remain in first complete remission at follow-up times ranging from 4 to 40+ months. To date, there is no difference in overall survival between patients treated initially and those treated after a period of observation, with over 75% of patients alive at 5 years. Therefore, although patients who have initial disease or progressive disease necessitating treatment have a lower complete-remission rate than those treated initially, there appears to be no difference in overall survival.

Purine Analogs

The purine analogs cladribine (2-chlorodeoxyadenosine, 2-CdA) and fludarabine are active against follicular lymphoma (124–130). Fludarabine and cladribine have been effective when given as single agents in previously untreated, as well as previously treated, patients. In previously untreated patients with follicular lymphoma, the overall-response rate to fludarabine was 65%, with 37% complete remission; the median progression-free survival was 13.6 months (131). Similar results were obtained with cladribine (132). Fludarabine was compared with CVP in a randomized study of 381 newly diagnosed patients with advanced-stage follicular lymphoma (Table 24.5). The overall response rates in the fludarabine and CVP arms were 68% (38% complete remission) versus 50% (15% complete remission), ($p = .001$). Significant cytopenias were more frequent in the fludarabine group. The median time to progression in the fludarabine group was 21 months versus 15 months in the CVP group. However, no differences in overall survival were detected (133).

In two studies, the overall-response rates of previously treated patients with follicular lymphoma to fludarabine ranged from 48% to 100%, with complete remission of less than 20% (125). In previously treated patients, 2-CdA induced responses in approximately 40% of patients, one-half of which were complete remissions, with a median duration of response of 5 months (126). A randomized trial has compared fludarabine to CVP in previously treated patients with follicular lymphoma. Although the response rates (62% vs. 52%) and 2-year overall survival (70% vs. 75%) appeared similar, 2-year progression-free survival was significantly improved with fludarabine (32% vs. 14%, $p = .03$) (Table 24.5) (134).

Fludarabine has been combined with other chemotherapeutic agents in previously untreated and previously treated patients with indolent lymphoma. In a phase I Eastern Cooperative Oncology Group trial of cyclophosphamide and fludarabine involving 27 patients with previously untreated indolent lymphoma, the overall-response and complete-remission rates were 100% and 89%, respectively. Estimated 5-year overall survival and disease-free survival rates were 66% and 53%, respectively. In this trial, grade 4 neutropenia was observed in 17% of all cycles and 31% of first cycles; grade 3 or 4 thrombocytopenia was seen in only 1% of all cycles (135). In a phase II multicenter trial, the combination of cyclophosphamide [600 mg/m^2 intravenously (IV) on day 1], fludarabine (20 mg/m^2 IV on days 1 through 5) and filgrastim (5 μg per kg per day subcutaneously starting on day 8) resulted in overall-response rates of 92% in patients with previously untreated follicular lymphoma (136). However, when this combination was brought to the intergroup setting, significant mortality from infection occurred, and the trial was closed early.

The combination of fludarabine and mitoxantrone was tested in 81 previously untreated patients with indolent lymphoma (follicular lymphoma and small lymphocytic lymphoma) (137). Overall- and complete-response rates were 91% and 43%, respectively, with 2-year progression-free and overall survival of 63% and 93%, respectively. Complete-remission rates (60% vs. 21%) and 2-year progression-free survival (82% vs. 47%) were better in patients with serum β$_2$-microglobulin levels less than 2.5 mg per dL as compared with patients with levels greater than 2.5 mg per dL. The addition of dexamethasone to fludarabine/mitoxantrone has been shown to be a highly effective regimen for patients with relapsed indolent lymphomas, with overall-response and complete-remission rates of 94% and 47%, respectively (138). The median failure-free survival was 14 months for all patients and 21 months for those attaining complete remission. Major toxicities were myelosuppression and infection, with nearly one-half being opportunistic infections, including pneumocystis pneumonia and dermatomal herpes zoster. Prophylactic use of trimethoprim-sulfamethoxazole is recommended with this regimen, and corticosteroids should be deleted in patients who develop opportunistic infections.

Interferon

Interferon-α has limited activity as a single agent in relapsed indolent non-Hodgkin's lymphoma, especially in follicular lymphoma (54% response rate, 17% complete-remission rate) (139). Several prospective randomized trials have examined the role of interferon when added to single-agent (140) or combination chemotherapy in advanced-stage disease patients (Table 24.5) (141–145). The latter studies have generally reported a significant effect on progression-free survival, particularly in patients with adverse prognostic factors and those treated with combination chemotherapy including an anthracycline. However, only two trials have observed a significant prolongation in overall survival, making the use of interferon controversial. In a multivariate analysis of an Eastern Cooperative Oncology Group study of cyclophosphamide, vincristine, doxorubicin, and prednisone with or without interferon-α, overall survival at 2 years was not significantly different between the two treatment arms (141). A study of patients with follicular lymphoma and small lymphocytic lymphoma treated with combination chemotherapy with or without 1 year of interferon-α 2b maintenance found improved survival for the interferon-α 2b–treated group (80% survival at 9 years, median survival not reached with interferon-α 2b, vs. a median survival of 6.2 years without interferon-α 2b) (146).

The Groupe d'Étude des Lymphomes Folliculaires 86 trial compared cyclophosphamide, teniposide, doxorubicin, and prednisone concurrently with or without interferon-α 2b in patients with follicular lymphoma (145). In addition to longer progression-free survival (median of 2.9 vs. 1.5 years), patients receiving interferon-α 2b had longer overall survival (at 6.0 years of follow-up, median overall survival not reached for interferon-α 2b vs. 5.6 years without interferon-α 2b). Patients with an IPI of low or low-intermediate risk had significantly longer progression-free survival and overall survival, whereas high- and high-intermediate–risk patients had prolonged survival only when receiving interferon-α 2b (Table 24.5). Toxicity due to concurrent chemotherapy and interferon-α 2b was significantly greater than in patients receiving chemotherapy alone. Moreover, the dose of interferon-α 2b was reduced, temporarily discontinued, or stopped completely in 38% of the patients.

A phase III Southwest Oncology Group trial randomized 571 patients with previously untreated stage III or IV low-grade lymphoma (small lymphocytic and follicular lymphomas) to receive six to eight cycles of intensive treatment with anthracycline-containing chemotherapy (ProMACE-MOPP) or chemotherapy plus involved-field radiation therapy (Table 24.5) (147). Responding patients were then randomized to observation alone or to consolidation therapy with interferon-α 2b (2 million units per m^2 subcutaneously three times/week for 2

years). Median progression-free survival was 4.1 and 3.2 years ($p = .25$), and 5-year overall survival was 78% and 77% ($p = .65$) for the interferon and observation groups, respectively.

Monoclonal Antibody–Based Therapies

A pivotal trial of the anti-CD20 monoclonal antibody rituximab, 375 mg per m^2 per week for 4 weeks, in 166 patients with relapsed or refractory follicular or low-grade lymphoma showed an overall response rate of 48%. There were complete responses in 6% of patients, and the subset of patients with follicular lymphoma had a response rate of 59%. Adverse events were brief and included fevers, rigors, and hypotension, usually related to the initial infusion. Only one patient developed an antichimeric antibody response. The median time to progression in this study was 13 months for responders. These promising results and favorable toxicity profile led to U.S. Food and Drug Administration approval for its use in patients with refractory or relapsed low-grade or follicular lymphoma. Post approval, a small number of severe mucocutaneous reactions, some with fatal outcomes, have been seen in patients treated with rituximab, although a direct link between these reactions and rituximab has not yet been made (148,149).

More recent studies have reported the safety of 375 mg per m^2 weekly for eight doses. There was no incidence of human antichimeric antibody response, and adverse events beyond the initial infusion were relatively mild (150). A phase II trial studied the safety and efficacy of retreatment with rituximab in 57 patients with relapsed, advanced, indolent lymphoma (small lymphocytic lymphoma and follicular lymphoma), all of whom had previously responded to treatment with this agent in one or more trials (151). The overall response rate was 40%, with 11% complete remissions; the estimated median time to progression after treatment was 18 months. Side effects were mild to moderate (grades 1 or 2) and self-limited and resembled those seen on initial treatment. No patient developed a human antichimeric antibody response.

Rituximab is currently approved for use in the treatment of relapsed or refractory low-grade or follicular CD20+ B-cell lymphoma, as well as for retreatment of such patients after an objective clinical response to an initial course of rituximab.

Two phase II trials have used rituximab (375 mg per m^2 IV per week for 4 consecutive weeks) as initial therapy in patients with indolent lymphoma (152,153). In one study of 41 patients, most patients had stage III or IV disease (71%), and none had received prior chemotherapy. Overall-response rates at 6 weeks and 6 months were 54% and 64%, with 5% and 15% complete remissions, respectively. Response rates at 6 weeks were similar in follicular lymphoma (52%) and small lymphocytic lymphoma/chronic lymphocytic leukemia (57%). Toxicity was mostly infusion related and of brief duration.

The second trial evaluated 50 patients with stage II to IV follicular lymphoma and a low tumor burden (no nodal or extranodal mass larger than 7 cm, B symptoms, splenomegaly, pleural effusion, ascites, organ compression, elevated serum lactate dehydrogenase, or β_2-microglobulin). The overall-response rate at 50 days was 73%, with 57% and 31% of informative patients negative by PCR for bcl-2 rearrangement in peripheral blood and bone marrow, respectively. Toxicity was minimal; the number and severity of adverse events decreased with subsequent infusions. It remains unclear what the role of rituximab will be in the early treatment of follicular lymphoma.

The role of maintenance therapy with rituximab remains unclear. Presently, there are randomized trials that are addressing that issue, which are ongoing or to date have limited follow-up. A recent study of 62 patients, 38 of whom had follicular lymphoma, evaluated a course of standard rituximab followed by four courses every 6 months (154). The final response rate was 73%, with 37% complete remission, and the median progression-free survival was 34 months. This suggests that additional doses of rituximab increase the response rate and duration of response, but the overall impact of this approach is unknown.

Rituximab Plus Chemotherapy

Rituximab has also been tested in combination with other forms of chemotherapy. As an example, rituximab has been combined with CHOP chemotherapy, with encouraging preliminary results in patients with indolent lymphoma with overall-response and complete-remission rates of 100% and 63%, respectively (155,156). At a follow-up of 36 to 54 months, 69% remain in remission. In a subset of eight patients with the bcl-2 translocation and t(14;18), seven attained complete remission and converted to PCR negativity at the end of treatment. After serial studies, six of these seven remain in complete remission, and five remain PCR negative (157).

The Southwest Oncology Group has conducted a study of rituximab after CHOP chemotherapy for the treatment of newly diagnosed follicular lymphoma (158). Of 104 patients enrolled in 49 institutions, 74 patients were treated with rituximab after CHOP. The overall-response rate was 72%, and rituximab converted 14 partial remissions to complete remissions. The 2-year progression-free survival in this study is 76%. Combinations of rituximab with chemotherapy are being explored further in randomized cooperative group trials.

Rituximab has also been combined with purine analog–based regimens. Preliminary analysis of an ongoing phase II study of 40 patients combining rituximab with fludarabine demonstrates an overall-response rate of 90% (159). Reactivation of varicella zoster occurred in six of these patients. The German Low Grade Study Group performed a randomized trial of fludarabine, cyclophosphamide, and mitoxantrone (FCM) with or without rituximab (Table 24.5) (160). In the group receiving FCM alone, a 53% response rate was observed, compared with a response rate of 89% for the combination. The Italian Cooperative Study Group on Lymphoma conducted a randomized trial of fludarabine and mitoxantrone plus rituximab versus CHOP plus rituximab for patients with follicular lymphoma (Table 24.5) (161). Rituximab was able to clear molecular disease in 71% of the fludarabine/mitoxantrone-treated patients compared with 44% of the CHOP-treated patients.

Radioimmunoconjugates

There are several anti-CD20 radioimmunoconjugates that are being investigated as treatment for the indolent lymphomas (Table 24.6). These agents deliver targeted radiotherapy to tumor-bearing areas (162). There is great enthusiasm for these radiolabeled monoclonal antibodies, which are efficacious in treating non-Hodgkin's lymphomas because lymphocytes and lymphoma cells are inherently sensitive to radiotherapy; the local emission of ionizing radiation by radiolabeled antibodies may kill cells in close proximity to the bound antibody. Patients with compromised effector cell function who have not responded to naked monoclonal antibodies may still respond to radioimmunoconjugates. These agents have more toxicities than does rituximab, with increased myelosuppression and possible human antimouse antibody formation, because they are murine antibodies.

Ibritumomab tiuxetan (Zevalin, IDEC Pharmaceuticals) is composed of the murine anti-CD20 monoclonal antibody ibritumomab, covalently bonded to the linker chelator tiuxetan. Zevalin can be radiolabeled with ^{90}Yttrium for therapy and ^{111}Indium for imaging or dosimetry, or both; however, dosimetry is not required for standard therapy, which is based on patient size and platelet count (163). In a phase III study, 143 patients with relapsed or refractory low-grade, follicular, or transformed CD20$^+$ lymphoma were randomized to receive either rituximab or Zevalin (164). Overall-

TABLE 24.6. *Comparison of radioimmunoconjugates used in the treatment of follicular non-Hodgkin's lymphoma*

	Ibritumomab tiuxetan (Yttrium-90)	Tositumomab (Iodine-131)
Half-life	64 h	192 h
Energy emitter	Beta (2.30 MeV)	Gamma (0.36 MeV), beta (0.60 MeV)
Path length	χ_{90} 5 mm	χ_{90} 0.8 mm
Nontumor distribution	Bone	Thyroid
Dosing	Based on weight and platelet count	Tracer dose and dosimetry used to customize dose
Administration	Outpatient	Inpatient or restrictions to protect family/environment

response rates to rituximab and Zevalin were 56% and 80%, respectively ($p = .002$). Interim results indicated that the response rates to the Zevalin combination were similar in the chemorefractory (77%) and chemosensitive (81%) patients. In a study of rituximab-refractory patients, the overall-response rate was 74%. The estimated median duration of response after Zevalin therapy (7.7+ months) was longer than that of the patients' prior rituximab therapy (4.0 months) and the patients' prior chemotherapy (6.5 months).

Adverse events associated with Zevalin are primarily hematologic, with grade 4 neutropenia occurring in 30% of patients. The incidence of human antimouse antibody/human antichimeric antibody is low, and a human antimouse antibody or human antichimeric antibody response did not result in unusual toxicity. Myelodysplasia has been reported for 1.4% of patients. Based on this data, the U.S. Food and Drug Administration has approved Zevalin for the treatment of patients with relapsed or refractory low-grade, follicular or transformed B-cell non-Hodgkin's lymphoma, including patients with rituximab-refractory follicular non-Hodgkin's lymphoma.

Bexxar (tositumomab) is another murine anti-CD20 mAb conjugated with radioactive Iodine-131. It has been used in 76 previously untreated patients with follicular lymphoma with overall-response and complete-remission rates of 97% and 63%, respectively, and a 3-year progression-free survival of 68% (165). Of the 34 patients in the study whose bone marrows were PCR positive for t(14;18) at baseline, 79% became PCR negative after B-cell recovery, with continuation of PCR negativity for as long as 36 months. In a phase II study of CHOP followed by Bexxar conducted by the Southwest Oncology Group in newly diagnosed patients with follicular lymphoma, the overall-response rate was 80%, including 50% complete remissions (166). A randomized trial is currently accruing to further define the role of this combination.

Radioimmunoconjugates have been used in high doses as part of the ablative regimen in stem cell–transplantation studies. In a phase I and II trial, tositumomab was combined with etoposide, cyclophosphamide, and autologous stem cell transplantation for patients with relapsed B-cell lymphoma, 73% of whom had follicular lymphoma. In this study, the estimated 2-year overall survival was 83% (167).

Bexxar appears to have a favorable effect in patients with relapsed disease, with a multicenter trial showing a 57% percent response rate, 27% complete remission, and median disease-free survival of 20 months (168). In a phase III study comparing unlabeled tositumomab with Bexxar, 17% of patients responded to the unlabeled murine antibody, compared to 55% of patients receiving Bexxar (169). Seventeen of 19 nonresponders in the unlabeled arm crossed over to Bexxar and subsequently responded. Unique toxicities associated with Bexxar, including thyroid dysfunction, may occur after Bexxar therapy, and thyroid blockade with Lugols solution, saturated solution of potassium iodide, or potassium iodide is indicated before radioimmunotherapy

with this agent. In a review of 773 patients who have been treated with Bexxar, 20 patients thus far have developed myelodysplasia or acute myelogenous leukemia (170). Further follow-up is needed to define the overall risk of this disorder; however, patients with abnormal bone marrow cytogenetics or clonal hematopoiesis should probably avoid radioimmunotherapy.

Autologous Stem Cell Transplantation

In contrast to relapsed aggressive lymphoma, relatively few patients with indolent lymphoma have undergone high-dose therapy followed by autologous bone marrow transplantation (ABMT) or stem cell transplantation. The high frequency of overt bone marrow and peripheral blood infiltration has been an obstacle due to contamination of the harvested marrow or peripheral blood stem cells with viable tumor cells and the theoretical concern of reinfusion of tumor cells. As an additional complication, many of these patients had disease resistant to conventional therapy before transplantation, a situation that is known to reduce effectiveness in other malignancies.

Autologous Bone Marrow or Stem Cell Transplantation for Relapsed Follicular Lymphoma

Studies of high-dose therapy and autologous stem cell transplants can be divided into those in which the stem cell product was unmanipulated and those in which efforts were made to potentially reduce the number of potential contaminating lymphoma cells (Table 24.7). The University of Nebraska reported 13 patients with indolent follicular lymphoma undergoing ABMT or autologous stem cell transplantation with unmanipulated marrow (171). The 4-year failure-free and overall survival rates in these patients were 62% and 76%, respectively. The use of peripheral blood stem cells has largely replaced the use of bone marrow. The University of Nebraska has reported on the results of 100 patients treated with peripheral blood progenitor cells. Four-year failure-free and overall survivals were 44% and 65%, respectively (172). There was no statistically significant difference in the outcome between patients receiving unpurged marrow and those receiving peripheral blood stem cells. Similar results using peripheral blood stem cells have been reported by others, with failure-free survival and overall survival ranging from 40% to 70% and 60% to 85%, respectively, at 4 to 8 years (173).

Although tumor cell contamination of peripheral blood stem cells is generally less than that of unpurged bone marrow, tumor cells can still be seen in peripheral blood stem cell preparations. It has been reported that 35% of peripheral blood stem cell harvests were contaminated with lymphoma cells (174). In other studies, patients whose peripheral blood stem cells had PCR-detectable tumor cells tended to remain PCR positive in the bone marrow and peripheral blood after transplant and have a higher risk of relapse (175,176).

TABLE 24.7. *Stem cell transplantation (SCT) in relapsed follicular non-Hodgkin's lymphoma*

Study (ref)	No. of patients	Stem cell source	Patients in complete remission at SCT (%)	Patients with BM at SCT (%)	Disease-free survival (%)	Overall survival (%)
Freedman et al., 1999 (177)	153	auto BM	30	47	42 (8 yr)	66 (8 yr)
Apostolidis et al., 2000 (178)	99	auto BM	38	13	63 (5.5 yr)	69 (5.5 yr)
Bierman et al., 1997 (172)	100	auto BM/ PBSC	9	—	48 (2 yr)	65 (4 yr)
Bastion et al., 1995 (173)	60	auto BM/ PBSC	17	65	53 (2 yr)	86 (2 yr)
van Besien et al., 1998 (199)	113	allo BM	40	—	49 (3 yr)	49 (3 yr)
Juckett et al., 1998 (200)	16	allo T-depleted BM	—	—	62 (5 yr)	—
Khouri et al., 2001 (203)	20	allo PBSC	60	5	84 (2 yr)	84 (2 yr)

allo, allogeneic; auto, autologous; BM, bone marrow; PBSC, peripheral blood stem cell.

Studies Using Tumor Cell Purging In Vitro

Several studies have focused on purged autologous bone marrow (Table 24.7). The Dana-Farber Cancer Institute treated 153 patients with follicular lymphoma in sensitive relapse or incomplete first remission with cyclophosphamide/total-body irradiation conditioning and anti–B-cell mAb-purged ABMT between 1985 and 1995 (177). Disease-free survival and overall survival at 8 years after ABMT were 42% and 66%, respectively. Overall survival from diagnosis for the entire group of patients was 69% at 12 years. Those patients whose bone marrow was purged of tumor cells and found to be PCR negative for t(14;18) had a significantly longer freedom from recurrence than did patients who were reinfused with bone marrow that remained PCR positive after purging. Moreover, continued PCR negativity in the bone marrow during long-term follow-up was strongly correlated with continued clinical remission.

Investigators at St. Bartholomew's Hospital have treated 99 patients with relapsed follicular lymphoma with anti-B1 mAb-purged ABMT (178,179). These patients were treated with a cyclophosphamide/total-body irradiation conditioning regimen similar to that used in the Dana-Farber Cancer Institute study. After high-dose therapy, 49 patients remained in continuous complete remission at a median follow-up of 5.5 years. The 5-year freedom from relapse and overall survival were 63% and 69%, respectively. Although no relationship between purging and outcome was found, continued PCR negativity was associated with a lower risk of recurrence.

Many of the studies of autologous stem cell transplantation in follicular lymphoma suggest a continuous pattern of relapse. It is unclear from these trials whether any patients are cured or whether survival is prolonged. In the St. Bartholomew's study, a retrospective analysis of 67 patients undergoing ABMT in second remission compared these patients to 34 patients in second remission who were treated with conventional therapy.

Patients undergoing ABMT had a significantly longer disease-free survival as compared to those undergoing standard therapy. However, there was no difference in overall survival between the two groups. In a nonrandomized study from the Groupe d'Étude des Lymphomes Folliculaires, patients who underwent autologous stem cell transplantation after first relapse had significantly longer freedom from progression (42% vs. 16%) and overall survival (58% vs. 38%) at 5 years than did patients treated with conventional therapy (180). In conclusion, in retrospective analysis and in the prospective randomized trials that have been preliminarily reported, patients who undergo autologous stem cell transplantation have a longer remission duration when compared to those who undergo conventional therapy; however, it remains uncertain if this will ultimately lead to longer survival or cure of the disease (181).

Several prognostic factors have been identified for patients undergoing high-dose therapy. Chemotherapy sensitivity before autologous stem cell transplantation is the most important prognostic variable for patients with follicular lymphoma (171,182–185). Extensive prior therapy is a negative prognostic factor (172,173,179). Patients with follicular small cleaved-cell lymphoma and those with follicular mixed histology appear to have similar outcomes (172,183). It is controversial whether patients with grade 3 follicular lymphoma have less favorable outcomes. Other negative prognostic factors that have been reported include male gender, involvement of more than eight sites, extranodal disease (exclusive of the marrow), and prior radiotherapy (186).

Rituximab Plus Chemotherapy for In Vivo Purging before Autologous Stem Cell Transplantation

Rituximab in combination with chemotherapy may be of value in preparing patients for autologous transplantation by clearing the bone marrow and blood (and the resulting leukapheresis product) of malignant cells (i.e., *in vivo* purging). Several studies have administered rituximab before peripheral blood stem cell collection (187–189). These pilot studies demonstrate that in patients with follicular lymphoma and t(14;18), the leukapheresis product became PCR negative for bcl-2/IgH after one or two courses of rituximab plus chemotherapy. This contrasts with PCR positivity in 74% of 47 patients treated with the same chemotherapy regimen without rituximab. In a similar approach in which rituximab was given after mobilization chemotherapy, the peripheral blood stem cells harvested from rituximab recipients were PCR negative for bcl2/IgH in 93% of cases compared to 40% of patients who did not receive rituximab (187). Furthermore, clinical and molecular remission was obtained in all 14 evaluable rituximab recipients, compared to 70% of controls, after high-dose therapy. Long-term follow-up will be required to see if this strategy has improved outcome in these patients.

Autologous Stem Cell Transplantation in First Remission

The absence of a definite plateau in disease-free survival after autologous stem cell transplantation for low-grade lymphoma has led to attempts at transplantation in first remission (190,191). At the Dana-Farber Cancer Institute, the actuarial 3-year disease-free survival and overall survival rates were 63% and 89%, respectively, after ABMT in first complete remission or with minimal disease after CHOP chemotherapy (190). Horning and coworkers at Stanford have reported results for patients transplanted in first complete or partial remission. With a median follow-up of 6.5 years, the estimated overall survival rates at 5 and 10 years were 92% and 86%, respectively. The estimated 10-year disease-specific survival was 97%, with overall survival of 86% (181). Other reports of autologous stem cell transplantation in first remission for low-grade lymphoma have shown a continuous pattern of treatment failure without evidence of cure (175,192). Analogous to studies in patients transplanted after conventional therapy relapse, remission duration is longer after autologous stem cell transplantation than after conventional therapy. Whether first remission transplant is superior to transplant for relapsed disease remains unclear. The overall survival from diagnosis for patients transplanted in first remission is similar to that seen in patients transplanted in second or greater remission (193).

Transplantation after Histologic Transformation

Histologic transformation from an indolent to an aggressive histology has been associated with a poor prognosis. There are several reports of autologous stem cell transplantation after histologic transformation of follicular lymphoma in patients with chemosensitive disease. At St. Bartholomew's Hospital, 19 patients received an anti–B-cell purged ABMT within 1 year of histologic transformation (194). The median

survival was 4.4 years, with three patients (16%) in remission with more than 4 years of follow-up. In the series from Dana-Farber Cancer Institute, 21 patients underwent anti–B-cell purged ABMT for follicular lymphoma transformed into diffuse large B-cell lymphoma (195). With follow-up from 12 to 120+ months, estimated 5-year disease-free survival was 46%. Patients who underwent histologic transformation within 18 months of diagnosis of follicular lymphoma had a significantly better overall survival when compared with patients who transformed later.

Similar results were reported by the European Bone Marrow Transplant Registry. In this analysis of 50 patients, the 5-year progression-free survival rate was 30% (196). A subgroup of patients with residual chemosensitive disease who attained complete response after high-dose therapy had an overall survival at 5 years of 69%. All patients with chemoresistant disease at the time of high-dose therapy died of relapsed or progressive disease (196). In an analysis of 35 patients treated with high-dose therapy and unpurged ABMT, overall survival at 5 years was 37% (197). Of the five patients older than 60 years of age, all died as the result of treatment-related complications, and other investigators have failed to note inferior outcomes for patients transplanted after histologic transformation. These studies suggest that autologous stem cell transplantation is a reasonable treatment option for selected patients after histologic transformation.

Allogeneic Transplantation for Follicular Lymphoma

A limited number of studies have been reported on the role of allogeneic bone marrow transplantation for patients with follicular lymphoma (Table 24.7). The concern over mortality from transplant-related complications and graft-versus-host disease has limited this approach to patients with disease refractory to chemotherapy and those with extensive bone marrow involvement. After allogeneic bone marrow transplantation, relapse-free and overall survival rates are quite similar, at approximately 80%, with exceedingly low relapse rates. However, treatment-related mortality remains high, approaching 30% (198).

The International Bone Marrow Transplant Registry has reported on allogeneic bone marrow transplantation in 113 patients with low-grade lymphoma, the majority of whom had chemosensitive disease at the time of transplantation (199). Kaplan-Meier estimates of relapse and overall survival at 3 years were 16% and 49%, respectively. Of 33 patients followed for longer than 2 years after allogeneic bone marrow transplantation, there was only one recurrence of lymphoma, suggesting a possible graft-versus-lymphoma effect.

In an attempt to decrease transplant-related morbidity and mortality, T-cell depletion as a means of graft-versus-host–disease prophylaxis was performed on allografts in 16 patients with indolent lymphoma at the Medical College of Wisconsin (200). At 5 years, disease-free survival was 62%, with a relapse rate of 13%. A very low treatment-related mortality after T-cell depletion has been observed at the

Dana-Farber Cancer Institute in patients with relapsed indolent lymphoma, with disease-free survival of 50% (201). Longer follow-up is needed to determine whether T-cell depletion in patients with lymphoma will interfere with a putative graft-versus-lymphoma effect.

Another strategy to decrease transplant-related mortality and foster a graft-versus-lymphoma effect involves the use of nonmyeloablative conditioning regimens. Twenty patients with indolent lymphoma were treated at the M.D. Anderson Cancer Center with fludarabine and cyclophosphamide, followed by allogeneic peripheral stem cell transplantation (202,203). Mixed chimerism was achieved in all patients, and the incidence of grade II to IV graft-versus-host disease was 20%. All patients achieved complete remission, and the probability of remission was 84% at 2 years, with no relapses seen. Studies are under way to define appropriate patients to consider for this approach.

UNIQUE COMPLICATIONS

The major unique complication of follicular lymphoma is histologic transformation. It is well recognized that an integral part of the natural history of indolent lymphoma is progression to a higher-grade histologic subtype, such as diffuse large B-cell lymphoma (31,77). However, the implications of histologic conversion for prognosis are controversial, because there are many associated variables, such as prior disease stage and treatment and length of survival before transformation, as well as the response of the transformed disease to more aggressive therapy. Armitage and colleagues compared the response of patients who had histologic conversion to diffuse large B-cell lymphoma with a similarly treated group of patients who developed diffuse large B-cell lymphoma de novo (82). They found no instances of prolonged complete remission in the former group, along with a significantly shorter median survival of 12 versus 40 months, respectively. The median survival of a large series of patients with follicular lymphoma undergoing histologic conversion was 11 months (84). An update from Stanford suggests that patients who were never treated had a better prognosis, as did patients with limited disease (78). Although the median survival for the entire group was only 22 months, patients who achieved a complete remission after histologic conversion had an actuarial survival of 75% at 5 years.

PROGNOSIS

The median survival from diagnosis for patients with follicular lymphoma is approximately 9 years. The median survival after relapse is 4.5 years (84). Weisdorf et al. reported that for patients younger than 60 years, the median survival after relapse was 5.9 years if the first complete remission was longer than 1.0 year, 4.2 years for patients whose first partial remission was longer than 1.0 year, and 2.4 years for patients whose initial remission was shorter than 1.0 year (204). The survival rates for patients who attained a second complete or partial remission were 53% and 28% at 10 years, respectively. The median survival for patients after histologic transformation ranged from 11 (84) to 22 (78) months. If patients attained a complete remission with combination therapy, the median survival was 81 months after transformation (84).

FUTURE DIRECTIONS

Improving Monoclonal Antibody Therapy

In an attempt to augment antibody-dependent cell-mediated cytotoxicity and improve the response rates and response duration of single-agent rituximab, several investigators have explored combination immunotherapy with rituximab and immunostimulants such as interleukin-2 (205), interleukin-12 (206), and interferon-α (207). These studies suggest that such combinations are safe and may prolong progression-free survival. Randomized studies are ongoing to further evaluate these rational combinations. Several other novel monoclonal antibodies with activity against B-cell lymphoma are also under development, including epratuzumab (anti-CD22, AMG412) and HU1D10 (anti-HLA-DR, Remitogen). In small studies, these antibodies have demonstrated efficacy and tolerability in patients with relapsed follicular lymphoma (208,209). Clinical trials are ongoing evaluating these antibodies as single agents and in combination with rituximab.

Antisense Therapy

The use of antisense therapy to "silence" genes involved in the malignant process is very attractive. One obvious target in lymphoma is the bcl-2 gene, which is overexpressed in more than 85% of patients with follicular lymphoma and t(14;18) (210). Currently, only phase I trials have been reported for such agents, although a limited number of responses have been obtained, even in the presence of advanced or relapsed disease. These agents are also under investigation in combination with rituximab.

Vaccines

Several approaches to vaccination have been used in clinical trials of patients with follicular lymphoma. The most frequent target of vaccination approaches is the idiotype (Id) (211). In two studies, anti-Id immune responses occurred after vaccination in approximately 50% of patients, and these patients had prolonged progression-free survival compared with historical controls (212,213). Currently, there is a randomized trial sponsored by the National Cancer Institute evaluating the role of Id vaccination after standard chemotherapy for follicular lymphoma. More recent studies have also used dendritic cells pulsed with Id as adoptive immunotherapy against follicular lymphoma (214). In one such study of 23 patients who completed the vaccination program, 15 (65%) mounted either a T-cell or humoral immune response. Six patients had disease progression after primary dendritic cell vaccination, and three of these patients responded to subsequent booster injections of Id-pulsed dendritic cells. Ongoing and future studies in these areas may provide novel alternatives and complement conventional therapy.

REFERENCES

1. Jaffe E, Harris N, Vardiman J. *Pathology and genetics: neoplasms of the hematopoietic and lymphoid tissues.* Lyon: IARC Press, 2001.
2. Glass AG, Karnell LH, Menck HR. The National Cancer Data Base report on non-Hodgkin's lymphoma. *Cancer* 1997;80:2311–2320.
3. A clinical evaluation of the International Lymphoma Study Group classification of non-Hodgkin's lymphoma. The Non-Hodgkin's Lymphoma Classification Project. *Blood* 1997;89:3909–3918.
4. Groves FD, Linet MS, Travis LB, et al. Cancer surveillance series: non-Hodgkin's lymphoma incidence by histologic subtype in the United States from 1978 through 1995. *J Natl Cancer Inst* 2000;92: 1240–1251.
5. Herrinton LJ, Goldoft M, Schwartz SM, et al. The incidence of non-Hodgkin's lymphoma and its histologic subtypes in Asian migrants to the United States and their descendants. *Cancer Causes Control* 1996;7:224–230.
6. Armitage J, Weisenburger D. New approach to classifying non-Hodgkin's lymphomas: clinical features of the major histologic subtypes. *J Clin Oncol* 1998;16:2780–2795.
7. National Cancer Institute–sponsored study of classification of non-Hodgkin's lymphomas: summary and description of a working formulation for clinical usage. The Non-Hodgkin's Lymphoma Pathologic Classification Project. *Cancer* 1982;49:2112–2135.
8. Herrinton LJ, Friedman GD. Cigarette smoking and risk of non-Hodgkin's lymphoma subtypes. *Cancer Epidemiol Biomarkers Prev* 1998;7:25–28.
9. Biagi JJ, Seymour JF. Insights into the molecular pathogenesis of follicular lymphoma arising from analysis of geographic variation. *Blood* 2002;99:4265–4275.
10. Nathwani BN, Anderson JR, Armitage JO, et al. Clinical significance of follicular lymphoma with monocytoid B cells. Non-Hodgkin's Lymphoma Classification Project. *Hum Pathol* 1999;30:263–268.
11. Mann RB, Berard CW. Criteria for the cytologic subclassification of follicular lymphomas: a proposed alternative method. *Hematol Oncol* 1983;1:187–192.
12. Harris NL, Jaffe ES, Diebold J, et al. World Health Organization classification of neoplastic diseases of the hematopoietic and lymphoid tissues: report of the Clinical Advisory Committee meeting-Airlie House, Virginia, November 1997. *J Clin Oncol* 1999;17:3835–3849.
13. Stein H, Gerdes J, Mason DY. The normal and malignant germinal centre. *Clin Haematol* 1982;11:531–559.
14. Anderson KC, Bates MP, Slaughenhoupt BL, et al. Expression of human B cell-associated antigens on leukemias and lymphomas: a model of human B cell differentiation. *Blood* 1984;63:1424–1433.
15. Cossman J, Neckers LM, Jones T, et al. Low grade lymphomas: expression of developmentally regulated B cell antigens. *Am J Pathol* 1984;115:117–124.
16. Jaffe ES, Shevach EM, Frank MM, et al. Nodular lymphoma—evidence for origin from follicular B lymphocytes. *N Engl J Med* 1974;290:814–819.
17. Harris NL, Nadler LM, Bhan AK. Immunologic characterization of two malignant lymphomas of germinal center type (centroblastic/centrocytic and centrocytic) with monoclonal antibodies. *Am J Pathol* 1984;117:262–272.
18. Flenghi L, Bigerna B, Fizzotti M, et al. Monoclonal antibodies PG-B6a and PG-B6p recognize, respectively, a highly conserved and a formol-resistant epitope on the human BCL-6 protein amino-terminal region. *Am J Pathol* 1996;148:1543–1555.
19. Pittaluga S, Ayoubi TA, Wlodarska I, et al. BCL-6 expression in reactive lymphoid tissue and in B-cell non-Hodgkin's lymphomas. *J Pathol* 1996;179:145–150.
20. Maio M, Pinto A, Carbone A, et al. Differential expression of CD54/intercellular adhesion molecule-1 in myeloid leukemias and in lymphoproliferative disorders. *Blood* 1990;76:783–790.
21. Picker LJ, Medeiros LJ, Weiss LM, et al. Expression of lymphocyte homing receptor antigen in non-Hodgkin's lymphoma. *Am J Pathol* 1988;130:496–504.
22. Cleary ML, Meeker TC, Levy S, et al. Clustering of extensive somatic mutations in the variable region of an immunoglobulin heavy chain gene from a human B cell lymphoma. *Cell* 1986;44:97–106.
23. Bahler DW, Campbell MJ, Hart S, et al. Ig VH gene expression among human follicular lymphomas. *Blood* 1991;78:1561–1568.
24. Bloomfield C, Arthur D, Frizzrera G, et al. Non-random chromosome abnormalities in lymphoma. *Cancer Res* 1983;43:2975.
25. Rowley J. Chromosome studies in non-Hodgkin's lymphomas: the role of the 14;18 translocation. *J Clin Oncol* 1988;6:919.
26. Cleary ML, Smith SD, Sklar J. Cloning and structural analysis of cDNAs for bcl-2 and a hybrid bcl-2/immunoglobulin transcript resulting from the t(14;18) translocation. *Cell* 1986;47:19–28.
27. Cleary ML, Galili N, Sklar J. Detection of a second t(14;18) breakpoint cluster region in human follicular lymphomas. *J Exp Med* 1986;164: 315–320.
28. Viardot A, Moller P, Hogel J, et al. Clinicopathologic correlations of genomic gains and losses in follicular lymphoma. *J Clin Oncol* 2002;20:4523–4530.
29. Gaidano G, Ballerini P, Gong JZ, et al. p53 mutations in human lymphoid malignancies: association with Burkitt lymphoma and chronic lymphocytic leukemia. *Proc Natl Acad Sci U S A* 1991;88:5413–5417.
30. Skinnider BF, Horsman DE, Dupuis B, et al. Bcl-6 and Bcl-2 protein expression in diffuse large B-cell lymphoma and follicular lymphoma: correlation with 3q27 and 18q21 chromosomal abnormalities. *Hum Pathol* 1999;30:803–808.
31. Longo D. What's the deal with follicular lymphomas? *J Clin Oncol* 1993;11:202–208
32. Elenitoba-Johnson K, Gascoyne R, Lim M, et al. Homozygous deletions at chromosome 9p21 involving p16 and p15 are associated with histologic progression in follicle center lymphoma. *Blood* 1998;91:4677–4685.
33. Lo Coco F, Gaidano G, Louie D, et al. p53 Mutations are associated with histologic transformation of follicular lymphoma. *Blood* 1993;82:2289–2295.
34. Tilly H, Rossi A, Stamatoullas A, et al. Prognostic value of chromosomal abnormalities in follicular lymphoma. *Blood* 1994;84:1043–1049.
35. Matolcsy A, Casali P, Warnke R, et al. Morphologic transformation of follicular lymphoma is associated with somatic mutation of the translocated bcl-2-gene. *Blood* 1996;88:3937–3944.
36. Lossos IS, Levy R. Higher-grade transformation of follicle center lymphoma is associated with somatic mutation of the 5′ noncoding regulatory region of the BCL-6 gene. *Blood* 2000;96:635–639.
37. Callanan MB, Le Baccon P, Mossuz P, et al. The IgG Fc receptor, FcgammaRIIB, is a target for deregulation by chromosomal translocation in malignant lymphoma. *Proc Natl Acad Sci U S A* 2000;97:309–314.
38. Graninger WB, Seto M, Boutain B, et al. Expression of Bcl-2 and Bcl-2-Ig fusion transcripts in normal and neoplastic cells. *J Clin Invest* 1987;80:1512–1515.
39. Ngan B, Chen-Levy Z, Weiss L, et al. Expression in non-Hodgkin's lymphoma of the bcl-2 protein associated with the t(14;18) chromosomal translocation. *N Engl J Med* 1988;318:1638.
40. Korsmeyer S. Bcl-2 initiates a new category of oncogenes: regulators of cell death. *Blood* 1992;80:879–886.
41. Nunez G, Hockenbery D, McDonnell TJ, et al. Bcl-2 maintains B cell memory. *Nature* 1991;353:71–73.
42. Boise L, Gonzalez-Garcia M, Postema C, et al. Bcl-x, a bcl-2 related gene that functions as a dominant regulator of apoptotic cell death. *Cell* 1993;74:597–608.
43. Oltvai Z, Milliman C, Korsmeyer S. Bcl-2 heterodimerizes *in vivo* with a conserved homolog, Bax, that accelerates programed cell death. *Cell* 1993;74:609–619.
44. Yin XM, Oltvai ZN, Korsmeyer SJ. BH1 and BH2 domains of Bcl-2 are required for inhibition of apoptosis and heterodimerization with Bax [see comments]. *Nature* 1994;369:321–323.
45. Zelenetz A, Chen T, Levy R. Clonal expansion in follicular lymphoma occurs subsequent to antigenic selection. *J Exp Med* 1992;176:1137–1148.
46. McDonnell TJ, Deane N, Platt FM, et al. bcl-2-immunoglobulin transgenic mice demonstrated extended B cell survival and follicular lymphoproliferation. *Cell* 1989;57:79–88.
47. McDonnell TJ, Korsmeyer SJ. Progression from lymphoid hyperplasia to high-grade malignant lymphoma in mice transgenic for the t(14:18). *Nature* 1991;349:254–256.

48. Liu Y, Hernandez A, Shibata D, et al. BCL-2 translocation frequency rises with age in humans. *Proc Natl Acad Sci U S A* 1994;91:8910–8914.
49. Summers KE, Goff LK, Wilson AG, et al. Frequency of the Bcl-2/IgH rearrangement in normal individuals: implications for the monitoring of disease in patients with follicular lymphoma. *J Clin Oncol* 2001;19:420–424.
50. Ji W, Qu GZ, Ye P, et al. Frequent detection of bcl-2/JH translocations in human blood and organ samples by a quantitative polymerase chain reaction assay. *Cancer Res* 1995;55:2876–2882.
51. Aster J, Kobayashi Y, Shiota M, et al. Detection of the t(14:18) at similar frequencies in hyperplastic lymphoid tissues from American and Japanese patients. *Am J Pathol* 1992;141:291–299.
52. Dolken G, Illerhaus G, Hirt C, et al. BCL-2/IgH rearrangements in circulating B cells of healthy blood donors and patients with nonmalignant diseases. *J Clin Oncol* 1996;14:1333–1344.
53. Alizadeh A, Eisen M, Davis R, et al. Distinct types of diffuse large B-cell lymphoma identified by gene expression profiling. *Nature* 2000;403:503–511.
54. Husson H, Carideo E, Neuberg D, et al. Gene expression profiling of follicular lymphoma and normal germinal center B cells using cDNA arrays. *Blood* 2002;99:282–289.
55. Velasquez WS, Jagannath S, Tucker SL, et al. Risk classification as the basis for clinical staging of diffuse large-cell lymphoma derived from 10-year survival data. *Blood* 1989;74:551–557.
56. Swan F Jr, Velasquez WS, Tucker S, et al. A new serologic staging system for large-cell lymphomas based on initial beta 2-microglobulin and lactate dehydrogenase levels. *J Clin Oncol* 1989;7:1518–1527.
57. Jerusalem G, Beguin Y, Najjar F, et al. Positron emission tomography (PET) with 18F-fluorodeoxyglucose (18F-FDG) for the staging of low-grade non-Hodgkin's lymphoma (NHL). *Ann Oncol* 2001;12:825–830.
58. Spaepen K, Stroobants S, Dupont P, et al. Prognostic value of positron emission tomography (PET) with fluorine-18 fluorodeoxyglucose ([18F]FDG) after first-line chemotherapy in non-Hodgkin's lymphoma: is [18F]FDG-PET a valid alternative to conventional diagnostic methods? *J Clin Oncol* 2001;19:414–419.
59. Anderson J, Vose J, Bierman P, et al. Clinical features and prognosis of follicular large-cell lymphoma: a report from the Nebraska Lymphoma Study Group. *J Clin Oncol* 1993;11:218–224.
60. Rodriguez J, McLaughlin P, Hagemeister F, et al. Follicular large cell lymphoma: an aggressive lymphoma that often presents with favorable prognostic features. *Blood* 1999;93:2202–2207.
61. Mirza I, Macpherson N, Paproski S, et al. Primary cutaneous follicular lymphoma: an assessment of clinical, histopathologic, immunophenotypic, and molecular features. *J Clin Oncol* 2002;20:647–655.
62. Cerroni L, Arzberger E, Putz B, et al. Primary cutaneous follicle center cell lymphoma with follicular growth pattern. *Blood* 2000;95:3922–3928.
63. Bekkenk MW, Postma TJ, Meijer CJ, et al. Frequency of central nervous system involvement in primary cutaneous B-cell lymphoma. *Cancer* 2000;89:913–919.
64. International Non-Hodgkin's Lymphoma Prognostic Factors Project: a predictive model for aggressive non-Hodgkin's lymphoma. *N Engl J Med* 1993;329:987.
65. Romaguera J, McLaughlin P, North L, et al. Multivariate analysis of prognostic factors in stage IV follicular low-grade lymphomas: a risk model. *J Clin Oncol* 1991;9:762–769.
66. Lopez-Guillermo A, Montserrat E, Bosch F, et al. Applicability of the International Index for aggressive lymphomas to patients with low-grade lymphomas. *J Clin Oncol* 1994;12:1343–1348.
67. Federico M, Vitolo U, Zinzani P, et al. Prognosis of follicular lymphoma: a predictive model based on a retrospective analysis of 987 cases. *Blood* 2000;95:783–789.
68. Decaudin D, Lepage E, Brousse N, et al. Low-grade stage III-IV follicular lymphoma: multivariate analysis of prognostic factors in 484 patients—a study of the Groupe d'Etude des Lymphomes de l'Adulte. *J Clin Oncol* 1999;17:2499–2505.
69. Kantarjian H, McLaughlin P, Fuller L, et al. Follicular large cell lymphoma: analysis and prognostic factors in 62 patients. *J Clin Oncol* 1984;2:811–819.
70. Rudders RA, Kaddis M, DeLellis RA, et al. Nodular non-Hodgkin's lymphoma (NHL): factors influencing prognosis and indications for aggressive treatment. *Cancer* 1979;43:1643–1651.
71. Warnke RA, Kim H, Fuks Z, et al. The coexistence of nodular and diffuse patterns in nodular non-Hodgkin's lymphomas: significance and clinicopathologic correlation. *Cancer* 1977;40:1229–1233.
72. Colby TV, Hoppe RT, Burke JS. Nodular lymphoma: clinicopathologic correlations of parafollicular small lymphocytes and degree of nodularity. *Cancer* 1980;45:2364–2367.
73. Glick J, McFadden E, Costello W, et al. Nodular histiocytic lymphoma: factors influencing prognosis and implications for aggressive chemotherapy. *Cancer* 1982;49:840.
74. Hu E, Weiss LM, Hoppe RT, et al. Follicular and diffuse mixed small-cleaved and large-cell lymphoma—a clinicopathologic study. *J Clin Oncol* 1985;3:1183–1187.
75. Ezdinli EZ, Costello WG, Kucuk O, et al. Effect of the degree of nodularity on the survival of patients with nodular lymphomas. *J Clin Oncol* 1987;5:413–418.
76. Hans CP, Weisenburger DD, Vose JM, et al. A significant diffuse component predicts for inferior survival in grade 3 follicular lymphoma, but cytological subtypes do not predict survival. *Blood* 2002;7:7.
77. Horning SJ, Rosenberg SA. The natural history of initially untreated low-grade non-Hodgkin's lymphoma. *N Engl J Med* 1984;311:1471–1508.
78. Yuen A, Kamel O, Halpern J, et al. Long-term survival after histologic transformation of low-grade follicular lymphoma. *J Clin Oncol* 1995;13:1726–1733.
79. Bastion Y, Sebban C, Berger F, et al. Incidence, predictive factors, and outcome of lymphoma transformation in follicular lymphoma patients. *J Clin Oncol* 1997;15:1587–1594.
80. Gallagher CJ, Gregory WM, Jones AE, et al. Follicular lymphoma: prognostic factors for response and survival. *J Clin Oncol* 1986;4:1470–1480.
81. Acker B, Hoppe RT, Colby TV, et al. Histologic conversion in the non-Hodgkin's lymphomas. *J Clin Oncol* 1983;1:11–16.
82. Armitage JO, Dick FR, Corder MP. Diffuse histiocytic lymphoma after histologic conversion: a poor prognostic variant. *Cancer Treat Rep* 1981;65:413–418.
83. Hubbard SM, Chabner BA, DeVita VT, et al. Histologic progression in non-Hodgkin's lymphoma. *Blood* 1982;59:258–264.
84. Johnson P, Rohatiner A, Whelan J, et al. Patterns of survival in patients with recurrent follicular lymphoma: a 20 year study from a single center. *J Clin Oncol* 1995;13:140–147.
85. Portlock CS, Rosenberg SA. No initial therapy for stage III and IV non-Hodgkin's lymphomas of favorable histologic types. *Ann Intern Med* 1979;90:10–13.
86. Anderson T, Chabner B, Young R, et al. Malignant lymphomas: the histology and staging of 473 patients at the National Cancer Institute. *Cancer* 1982;50:2699.
87. Gospodarowicz M, Lippuner T, Pintilie M, et al. Stage I and II follicular lymphoma: long-term outcome and pattern of failure following treatment with involved field radiation therapy alone. *Int J Radiat Oncol Biol Phys* 1999;45:217a.
88. Vaughan Hudson B, Vaughan Hudson G, MacLennan K, et al. Clinical stage 1 non-Hodgkin's lymphoma: long-term follow-up of patients treated by the British National Lymphoma Investigation with radiotherapy alone as initial therapy. *Br J Cancer* 1994;69:1088–1093.
89. MacManus M, Hoppe R. Is radiotherapy curative for stage I and II low-grade follicular lymphoma? Results of a long-term follow-up study of patients treated at Stanford University. *J Clin Oncol* 1996; 14:1282–1290.
90. Soubeyran S, Eghbali H, Bonichon F, et al. Localized follicular lymphomas: prognosis and survival of stages I and II in a retrospective series of 103 patients. *Radiother Oncol* 1988;13:91–98.
91. Wilder RB, Jones D, Tucker SL, et al. Long-term results with radiotherapy for Stage I-II follicular lymphomas. *Int J Radiat Oncol Biol Phys* 2001;51:1219–1227.
92. Taylor R, Allan S, McIntyre M, et al. Low grade stage I and II non-Hodgkin's lymphoma: results of treatment and relapse pattern following therapy. *Clin Radiol* 1988;39:287–290.
93. Lawrence T, Urba W, Steinberg S, et al. Retrospective analysis of stage I and II indolent lymphomas at the National Cancer Institute. *Int J Radiat Oncol Biol Phys* 1988;14:417–424.
94. Pendlebury S, el Awadi M, Ashley S, et al. Radiotherapy results in early stage low grade nodal non-Hodgkin's lymphoma. *Radiother Oncol* 1995;36:167–171.
94a. Monfardini S, Banfi A, Bonadonna G, et al. Improved five year survival after combined radio therapy-chemotherapy for stage I-II non-Hodgkin's lymphoma. *Int J Radat Oncol Biol Phys* 1980;6:125–134.
95. Landberg T, Hakansson L, Moller T, et al. CVP remission maintenance in stage I or II non-Hodgkin's lymphomas: preliminary results of a randomized study. *Cancer* 1979;44:831–838.
96. Toonkel LM, Fuller LM, Gamble JF, et al. Laparotomy staged I and II

non-Hodgkin's lymphomas: preliminary results of radiotherapy and adjunctive chemotherapy. *Cancer* 1980;45:249-260.

97. Kelsey S, Newland A, Hudson G, et al. A British National Lymphoma Investigation randomised trial of single agent chlorambucil plus radiotherapy versus radiotherapy alone in low grade, localised non-Hodgkin's lymphoma. *Med Oncol* 1994;11:19–25.

98. McLaughlin P, Fuller L, Redman J, et al. Stage I-II low-grade lymphomas: a prospective trial of combination chemotherapy and radiotherapy. *Ann Oncol* (suppl 2). 1991;2:137–140.

99. Seymour JF, McLaughlin P, Fuller LM, et al. High rate of prolonged remissions following combined modality therapy for patients with localized low-grade lymphoma. *Ann Oncol* 1996;7:157–163.

100. MacManus MP, Rainer Bowie CA, Hoppe RT. What is the prognosis for patients who relapse after primary radiation therapy for early-stage low-grade follicular lymphoma? *Int J Radiat Oncol Biol Phys* 1998;42:365–371.

101. Gattiker HH, Wiltshaw E, Galton DA. Spontaneous regression in non-Hodgkin's lymphoma. *Cancer* 1980;15:2627–2632.

102. Krikorian JG, Portlock CS, Cooney P, et al. Spontaneous regression of non-Hodgkin's lymphoma: a report of nine cases. *Cancer* 1980;46: 2093–2099.

103. Hoppe RT, Kushlan P, Kaplan HS, et al. The treatment of advanced stage favorable histology non-Hodgkin's lymphoma: a preliminary report of a randomized trial comparing single agent chemotherapy, and whole body irradiation. *Blood* 1981;58:592–598.

104. Ganem G, Lambin P, Socie G, et al. Potential role for low dose limited-field radiation therapy (2 × 2 Grays) in advanced low-grade non-Hodgkin's lymphomas. *Hematol Oncol* 1994;12:1–8.

105. Sawyer E, Timothy A. Low dose palliative radiotherapy in low grade non-Hodgkin's lymphoma. *Radiother Oncol* 1997;42:49–51.

106. Johnson RE, Canellos GP, Young RC, et al. Chemotherapy (cyclophosphamide, vincristine, and prednisone) versus radiotherapy (total-body irradiation) for stage III-IV poorly differentiated lymphocytic lymphoma. *Cancer Treat Rep* 1978;62:321–325.

107. Jacobs JP, Murray KJ, Schultz CJ, et al. Central lymphatic irradiation for stage III nodular malignant lymphoma: long-term results. *J Clin Oncol* 1993;11:233–238.

108. De Los Santos JF, Mendenhall NP, Lynch JW Jr. Is comprehensive lymphatic irradiation for low-grade non-Hodgkin's lymphoma curative therapy? Long-term experience at a single institution. *Int J Radiat Oncol Biol Phys* 1997;38:3–8.

109. Murtha AD, Knox SJ, Hoppe RT, et al. Long-term follow-up of patients with Stage III follicular lymphoma treated with primary radiotherapy at Stanford University. *Int J Radiat Oncol Biol Phys* 2001;49:3–15.

110. Ezdinli EZ, Costello WG, Icli F, et al. Nodular mixed lymphocytic-histiocytic lymphoma (NM): response and survival. Eastern Cooperative Oncology Group. *Cancer* 1980;45:261–267.

111. Glick JH, Barnes JM, Ezdinli EZ, et al. Nodular mixed lymphoma: results of a randomized trial failing to confirm prolonged disease-free survival with COPP chemotherapy. *Blood* 1981;58:920–925.

112. Jones SE, Grozea PN, Miller TP, et al. Chemotherapy with cyclophosphamide, doxorubicin, vincristine, and prednisone alone or with levamisole or with levamisole plus BCG for malignant lymphoma: a Southwest Oncology Group Study. *J Clin Oncol* 1985;3:1318–1324.

113. Young RC, Johnson RE, Canellos GP, et al. Advanced lymphocytic lymphoma: randomized comparisons of chemotherapy and radiotherapy, alone or in combination. *Cancer Treat Rep* 1977;61:1153–1159.

114. Anderson T, Ra B, Fisher RI, et al. Combination chemotherapy in non-Hodgkin's lymphoma: results of long-term followup. *Cancer Treat Rep* 1977;61:1057–1066.

115. Longo DL, Young RC, Hubbard SM, et al. Prolonged initial remission in patients with nodular mixed lymphoma. *Ann Intern Med* 1984;100:651–656.

116. Cabanillas F, Smith T, Bodey GP, et al. Nodular malignant lymphomas. Factors affecting complete response rate and survival. *Cancer* 1979;44:1983–1989.

117. Morrison V, Peterson B. Combination chemotherapy in the treatment of follicular low-grade lymphoma. *Leuk Lymphoma* 1993;10:29–33.

118. Ezdinli EZ, Anderson JR, Melvin F, et al. Moderate versus aggressive chemotherapy of nodular lymphocytic poorly differentiated lymphoma. *J Clin Oncol* 1985;3:769–775.

119. Jones SE, Grozea PN, Metz EN, et al. Superiority of adriamycin-containing combination chemotherapy in the treatment of diffuse lymphoma: a Southwest Oncology Group study. *Cancer* 1979;43:417–425.

120. Peterson BA, Petroni GR, Frizzera G, et al. Prolonged single-agent versus combination chemotherapy in indolent follicular lymphomas: a study of the Cancer And Leukemia Group B. *J Clin Oncol* 2003;21:5–15.

121. McLaughlin P, Fuller LM, Velasquez WS, et al. Stage III follicular lymphoma: durable remissions with a combined chemotherapy-radiotherapy regimen. *J Clin Oncol* 1987;5:867–874.

122. Travis LB, Weeks J, Curtis RE, et al. Leukemia following low-dose total-body irradiation and chemotherapy for non-Hodgkin's lymphoma. *J Clin Oncol* 1996;14:565–571.

123. Young RC, Longo DL, Glatstein E, et al. The treatment of indolent lymphomas: watchful waiting v aggressive combined modality treatment. *Semin Hematol* 1988;25:11–16.

124. Chun H, Leyland-Jones B, Cheson D. Fludarabine phosphate: a synthetic purine antimetabolite with significant activity against lymphoid malignancies. *J Clin Oncol* 1991;9:175–188.

125. Hochster H, Kim K, Green M, et al. Activity of fludarabine in previously treated non-Hodgkin's low-grade lymphoma: results of an Eastern Cooperative Oncology Group study. *J Clin Oncol* 1992;10:28–32.

126. Kay A, Saven A, Carrera C, et al. 2-Chlorodeoxyadenosine treatment of low-grade lymphomas. *J Clin Oncol* 1992;10:371–377.

127. Redman J, Cabanillas F, Velasquez W, et al. Phase II trial of fludarabine phosphate in lymphoma: an effective new agent in low-grade lymphoma. *J Clin Oncol* 1992;10:790–794.

128. Tefferi A, Witzig T, Reid J, et al. Phase I study of combined 2-chlorodeoxyadenosine and chlorambucil in chronic lymphoid leukemia and low-grade lymphoma. *J Clin Oncol* 1994;12:569–574.

129. Whelan J, Davis C, Rule S, et al. Fludarabine phosphate for the treatment of low grade lymphoid malignancy. *Br J Cancer* 1991;64:120–123.

130. Foran J, Rohatiner A, Coiffier B, et al. Multicenter phase II study of fludarabine phosphate for patients with newly diagnosed lymphoplasmacytoid lymphoma, Waldenstrom's macroglobulinemia, and mantle-cell lymphoma. *J Clin Oncol* 1999;17:546–553.

131. Solal-Celigny P, Brice P, Brousse N, et al. Phase II trial of fludarabine monophosphate as first-line treatment in patients with advanced follicular lymphoma: a multicenter study by the Groupe d'Etude des Lymphomes de l'Adulte. *J Clin Oncol* 1996;14:514–519.

132. Saven A, Emanuele S, Kosty M, et al. 2-Chlorodeoxyadenosine activity in patients with untreated, indolent non-Hodgkin's lymphoma. *Blood* 1995;86:1710–1716.

133. Hagenbeek A, Eghbali H, Monfardini S. Fludarabine compared with CVP chemotherapy in newly diagnosed patients with stages III and IV low grade malignant non-Hodgkin's lymphoma. Final analysis of a prospective randomized phase III Intergroup study of 381 patients. *Blood* 2001;98:843a.

134. Klasa R, Meyer R, Shustik C, et al. Fludarabine versus CVP in previously treated patients with progressive low grade non-Hodgkin's lymphomas. *Proc ASCO* 1999;18:9a.

135. Hochster HS, Oken MM, Winter JN, et al. Phase I study of fludarabine plus cyclophosphamide in patients with previously untreated low-grade lymphoma: results and long-term follow-up—a report from the Eastern Cooperative Oncology Group. *J Clin Oncol* 2000;18:987–994.

136. Flinn IW, Byrd JC, Morrison C, et al. Fludarabine and cyclophosphamide with filgrastim support in patients with previously untreated indolent lymphoid malignancies. *Blood* 2000;96:71–75.

137. Velasquez W, Lew D, Miller T, et al. SWOG 95-01: a phase II trial of a combination of fludarabine and mitoxantrone (FN) in untreated advanced low grade lymphoma. An effective, well tolerated therapy. *Proc Am Soc Clin Oncol* 1999;18:9a.

138. McLaughlin P, Hagemeister F, Swan F Jr, et al. Phase I study of the combination of fludarabine mitoxantrone, and dexamethasone in low-grade lymphoma. *J Clin Oncol* 1994;12:575–579.

139. Foon KA, Sherwin SA, Abrams PG, et al. Treatment of advanced non-Hodgkin's lymphoma with recombinant leukocyte A interferon. *N Engl J Med* 1984;311:1148–1152.

140. Rohatiner A, Radford J, Deakin D, et al. A randomized controlled trial to evaluate the role of interferon as initial and maintenance therapy in patients with follicular lymphoma. *Br J Cancer* 2001;85:29–35.

141. Smalley R, Andersen J, Hawkins M, et al. Interferon alfa combined with cytotoxic chemotherapy for patients with non-Hodgkin's lymphoma. *N Engl J Med* 1992;327:1336–1341.

142. Solal-Celigny P, Lepage E, Brousse N, et al. Recombinant interferon alfa-2b combined with a regimen containing doxorubicin in patients

with advanced follicular lymphoma. Groupe d'Etude des Lymphomes de l'Adulte. *N Engl J Med* 1993;329:1608–1614.

143. Arranz R, Garcia-Alfonso P, Sobrino P, et al. Role of interferon alfa-2b in the induction and maintenance treatment of low-grade non-Hodgkin's lymphoma: results from a prospective, multicenter trial with double randomization. *J Clin Oncol* 1998;16:1538–1546.

144. Hagenbeek A, Carde P, Meerwaldt J, et al. Maintenance of remission with human recombinant interferon alfa-2a in patients with stages III and IV low-grade malignant non-Hodgkin's lymphoma. *J Clin Oncol* 1998;16:41–47.

145. Solal-Celigny P, Lepage E, Brousse N, et al. Doxorubicin-containing regimen with or without interferon alfa-2b for advanced follicular lymphomas: final analysis of survival and toxicity in the Groupe d'Etude des Lymphomes Folliculaires 86 trial. *J Clin Oncol* 1998;16:2332–2338.

146. Aviles A, Duque G, Talavera A, et al. Interferon alpha 2b as maintenance therapy in low grade malignant lymphoma improves duration of remission and survival. *Leuk Lymphoma* 1996;20:495–499.

147. Fisher RI, Dana BW, LeBlanc M, et al. Interferon alpha consolidation after intensive chemotherapy does not prolong the progression-free survival of patients with low-grade non-Hodgkin's lymphoma: results of the Southwest Oncology Group randomized phase III study 8809. *J Clin Oncol* 2000;18:2010–2016.

148. McLaughlin P, Grillo-Lopez A, Link B, et al. Rituximab chimeric anti-CD20 monoclonal antibody therapy for relapsed indolent lymphoma: half of patients respond to a four-dose treatment program. *J Clin Oncol* 1998;16:2825–2833.

149. Foran JM, Gupta RK, Cunningham D, et al. A UK multicentre phase II study of rituximab (chimaeric anti-CD20 monoclonal antibody) in patients with follicular lymphoma, with PCR monitoring of molecular response. *Br J Haematol* 2000;109:81–88.

150. Piro LD, White CA, Grillo-Lopez AJ, et al. Extended Rituximab (anti-CD20 monoclonal antibody) therapy for relapsed or refractory low-grade or follicular non-Hodgkin's lymphoma. *Ann Oncol* 1999;10:655–661.

151. Davis TA, Grillo-Lopez AJ, White CA, et al. Rituximab anti-CD20 monoclonal antibody therapy in non-Hodgkin's lymphoma: safety and efficacy of re-treatment. *J Clin Oncol* 2000;18:3135–3143.

152. Hainsworth JD, Burris HA 3rd, Morrissey LH, et al. Rituximab monoclonal antibody as initial systemic therapy for patients with low-grade non-Hodgkin lymphoma. *Blood* 2000;95:3052–3056.

153. Colombat P, Salles G, Brousse N, et al. Rituximab (anti-CD20 monoclonal antibody) as single first-line therapy for patients with follicular lymphoma with a low tumor burden: clinical and molecular evaluation. *Blood* 2001;97:101–106.

154. Hainsworth JD, Litchy S, Burris HA 3rd, et al. Rituximab as first-line and maintenance therapy for patients with indolent non-Hodgkin's lymphoma. *J Clin Oncol* 2002;20:4261–4267.

155. Czuczman MS, Grillo-Lopez AJ, McLaughlin P, et al. Clearing of cells bearing the bcl-2 [t(14;18)] translocation from blood and marrow of patients treated with rituximab alone or in combination with CHOP chemotherapy. *Ann Oncol* 2001;12:109–114.

156. Czuczman M, Grillo-Lopez A, White C, et al. Treatment of patients with low-grade B-cell lymphoma with the combination of chimeric anti-CD20 monoclonal antibody and CHOP chemotherapy. *J Clin Oncol* 1999;17:268–276.

157. Czuczman M, Grillo-Lopez A, White C, et al. Progression free survival after six years (median) follow-up of the first clinical trial of rituximab/CHOP chemoimmunotherapy. *Blood* 2001;98:601(abstr.).

158. Maloney D, Press O, Braziel R, et al. A phase II trial of CHOP followed by rituximab chimeric monoclonal anti-CD20 antibody for treatment of newly diagnosed follicular non-Hodgkin's lymphoma: SWOG 9800. *Blood* 2001;98:843(abstr.).

159. Czuczman M, Fallon A, Mohr A, et al. Phase II study of rituximab plus fludarabine in patients with low-grade lymphoma: final report. *Blood* 2001;98:601(abstr.).

160. Hiddemann W, Forstpointner R, Fiedler F, et al. The addition of rituximab to combination chemotherapy with fludarabine, cyclophosphamide, mitoxantrone results in a significant increase of overall response as compared to FCM alone in patients with relapsed or refractory follicular and mantle cell lymphomas: results of a prospective randomized comparison of the German Low Grade Study group. *Blood* 2001;98:844(abstr.).

161. Zinzani P. A randomized trial of fludarabine and mitoxantrone plus rituximab versus CHOP plus rituximab as first-line treatment in patients with follicular lymphoma. *Blood* 2001;98:842(abstr.).

162. Multani P, Grossbard M. Monoclonal antibody-based therapies for hematologic malignancies. *J Clin Oncol* 1998;16:3691–3710.

163. Witzig TE, White CA, Wiseman GA, et al. Phase I/II trial of IDEC-Y2B8 radioimmunotherapy for treatment of relapsed or refractory CD20(+) B-cell non-Hodgkin's lymphoma. *J Clin Oncol* 1999;17:3793–3803.

164. Witzig TE, Gordon LI, Cabanillas F, et al. Randomized controlled trial of yttrium-90-labeled ibritumomab tiuxetan radioimmunotherapy versus rituximab immunotherapy for patients with relapsed or refractory low-grade, follicular, or transformed B-cell non-Hodgkin's lymphoma. *J Clin Oncol* 2002;20:2453–2463.

165. Kaminski MS, Estes J, Zasadny KR, et al. Radioimmunotherapy with iodine (131)I tositumomab for relapsed or refractory B-cell non-Hodgkin lymphoma: updated results and long-term follow-up of the University of Michigan experience. *Blood* 2000;96:1259–1266.

166. Press O, Unger J, Braziel R, et al. A phase II trial of CHOP followed by Bexxar (tositumomab and iodine-131-tositumomab) for treatment of newly diagnosed follicular non-Hodgkin's lymphomas. *Blood* 2001;98:843a.

167. Press OW, Eary JF, Gooley T, et al. A phase I/II trial of iodine-131-tositumomab (anti-CD20), etoposide, cyclophosphamide, and autologous stem cell transplantation for relapsed B-cell lymphomas. *Blood* 2000;96:2934–2942.

168. Vose JM, Wahl RL, Saleh M, et al. Multicenter phase II study of iodine-131 tositumomab for chemotherapy-relapsed/refractory low-grade and transformed low-grade B-cell non-Hodgkin's lymphomas. *J Clin Oncol* 2000;18:1316–1323.

169. Davis T, Kaminski M, Leonard J, et al. Results of a randomized study of Bexxar (tositumomab and Iodine-131 tositumomab) versus unlabelled tositumomab in patients with relapsed or refractory low-grade or transformed non-Hodgkin's lymphoma. *Blood* 2001;98:843a.

170. Bennett J, Zelenitz A, Press O, et al. Incidence of myelodysplastic syndromes and acute myeloid leukemia in patients with low-grade non-Hodgkin's lymphoma treated with Bexxar. *Blood* 2001;98:335a.

171. Schouten HC, Bierman PJ, Vaughan WP, et al. Autologous bone marrow transplantation in follicular non-Hodgkin's lymphoma before and after histologic transformation. *Blood* 1989;74:2579–2584.

172. Bierman P, Vose J, Anderson J, et al. High-dose therapy with autologous hematopoietic rescue for follicular low-grade non-Hodgkin's lymphoma. *J Clin Oncol* 1997;15:445–450.

173. Bastion Y, Brice P, Haioun C, et al. Intensive therapy with peripheral blood progenitor cell transplantation in 60 patients with poor-prognosis follicular lymphoma. *Blood* 1995;86:3257–3262.

174. Gazitt Y, Shaughnessy P, Liu Q. Differential mobilization of CD34+ cells and lymphoma cells in non-Hodgkin's lymphoma patients mobilized with different growth factors. *J Hematother Stem Cell Res* 2001;10:167–176.

175. Haas R, Moos M, Mohle R, et al. High-dose therapy with peripheral blood progenitor cell transplantation in low-grade non-Hodgkin's lymphoma. *Bone Marrow Transplant* 1996;17:149–155.

176. Tarella C, Corradini P, Astolfi M, et al. Negative immunomagnetic ex vivo purging combined with high-dose chemotherapy with peripheral blood progenitor cell autograft in follicular lymphoma patients: evidence for long-term clinical and molecular remissions. *Leukemia* 1999;13:1456–1462.

177. Freedman A, Neuberg D, Mauch P, et al. Long term followup of autologous bone marrow transplantation in patients with relapsed follicular lymphoma. *Blood* 1999;94:3325–3333.

178. Apostolidis J, Gupta RK, Grenzelias D, et al. High-dose therapy with autologous bone marrow support as consolidation of remission in follicular lymphoma: long-term clinical and molecular follow-up. *J Clin Oncol* 2000;18:527–536.

179. Rohatiner A, Johnson P, Price C, et al. Myeloablative therapy with autologous bone marrow transplantation as consolidation therapy for recurrent follicular lymphoma. *J Clin Oncol* 1994;12:1177–1184.

180. Brice P, Simon D, Bouabdallah R, et al. High-dose therapy with autologous stem-cell transplantation (ASCT) after first progression prolonged survival of follicular lymphoma patients included in the prospective GELF 86 protocol. *Ann Oncol* 2000;11:1585–1590.

181. Horning SJ, Negrin RS, Hoppe RT, et al. High-dose therapy and autologous bone marrow transplantation for follicular lymphoma in first complete or partial remission: results of a phase II clinical trial. *Blood* 2001;97:404–409.

182. Freedman AS, Ritz J, Neuberg D, et al. Autologous bone marrow transplantation in 69 patients with a history of low grade B cell non-Hodgkin's lymphoma. *Blood* 1991;77:2524–2529.

183. Colombat P, Donadio D, Fouillard L, et al. Value of autologous bone marrow transplantation in follicular lymphoma: a France Autogreffe retrospective study of 42 patients. *Bone Marrow Transplant* 1994; 13:157–162.

184. Cervantes F, Shu XO, McGlave PB, et al. Autologous bone marrow transplantation for non-transformed low-grade non-Hodgkin's lymphoma. *Bone Marrow Transplant* 1995;16:387–392.

185. Stein RS, Greer JP, Goodman S, et al. High-dose therapy with autologous or allogeneic transplantation as salvage therapy for small cleaved cell lymphoma of follicular center cell origin. *Bone Marrow Transplant* 1999;23:227–233.

186. Voso MT, Martin S, Hohaus S, et al. Prognostic factors for the clinical outcome of patients with follicular lymphoma following high-dose therapy and peripheral blood stem cell transplantation (PBSCT). *Bone Marrow Transplant* 2000;25:957–964.

187. Magni M, Di Nicola M, Devizzi L, et al. Successful *in vivo* purging of CD34-containing peripheral blood harvests in mantle cell and indolent lymphoma: evidence for a role of both chemotherapy and rituximab infusion. *Blood* 2000;96:864–869.

188. Moos M, Schulz R, Martin S, et al. The remission status before and the PCR status after high-dose therapy with peripheral blood stem cell support are prognostic factors for relapse-free survival in patients with follicular non-Hodgkin's lymphoma. *Leukemia* 1998;12:1971–1976.

189. Voso MT, Pantel G, Weis M, et al. *In vivo* depletion of B cells using a combination of high-dose cytosine arabinoside/mitoxantrone and rituximab for autografting in patients with non-Hodgkin's lymphoma. *Br J Haematol* 2000;109:729–735.

190. Freedman A, Gribben J, Neuberg D, et al. High dose therapy and autologous bone marrow transplantation in patients with follicular lymphoma during first remission. *Blood* 1996;88:2780–2786.

191. Freedman A, Neuberg D, Mauch P, et al. Cyclophosphamide, doxorubicin, vincristine, prednisone dose intensification with granulocyte colony-stimulating factor markedly depletes stem cell reserve for autologous bone marrow transplantation. *Blood* 1997;90:4996–5001.

192. Morel P, Laporte JP, Noel MP, et al. Autologous bone marrow transplantation as consolidation therapy may prolong remission in newly diagnosed high-risk follicular lymphoma: a pilot study of 34 cases. *Leukemia* 1995;9:576–582.

193. Seyfarth B, Kuse R, Sonnen R, et al. Autologous stem cell transplantation for follicular lymphoma: no benefit for early transplant? *Ann Hematol* 2001;80:398–405.

194. Foran J, Apostolidis J, Papamichael D, et al. High-dose therapy with autologous haematopoietic support in patients with transformed follicular lymphoma: a study of 27 patients from a single centre. *Ann Oncol* 1998;9:865–869.

195. Friedberg J, Neuberg D, Gribben J, et al. Autologous bone marrow transplantation following histologic transformation of indolent B cell malignancies. *Biol Blood Marrow Transplant* 1999;5:262–268.

196. Williams CD, Harrison CN, Lister TA, et al. High-dose therapy and autologous stem-cell support for chemosensitive transformed low-grade follicular non-Hodgkin's lymphoma: a case-matched study from the European Bone Marrow Transplant Registry. *J Clin Oncol* 2001;19:727–735.

197. Chen CI, Crump M, Tsang R, et al. Autotransplants for histologically transformed follicular non-Hodgkin's lymphoma. *Br J Haematol* 2001; 113:202–208.

198. Van Besien K, Khouri I, Giralt S, et al. Allogeneic bone marrow transplantation for refractory and recurrent low-grade lymphoma: the case for aggressive management. *J Clin Oncol* 1995;13:1096–1102.

199. van Besien K, Sobocinski K, Rowlings P, et al. Allogeneic bone marrow transplantation for low-grade lymphoma. *Blood* 1998;92:1832–1836.

200. Juckett M, Rowlings P, Hessner M, et al. T cell-depleted allogeneic bone marrow transplantation for high-risk non-Hodgkin's lymphoma: clinical and molecular follow-up. *Bone Marrow Transplant* 1998;21:893–899.

201. Soiffer R, Freedman A, Neuberg D, et al. CD6+ T-cell depleted allogeneic bone marrow transplantation for non-Hodgkin's lymphoma. *Bone Marrow Transplant* 1998;21:1177–1181.

202. Khouri I, Keating M, Korbling M, et al. Transplant-lite: induction of graft-versus-malignancy using fludarabine-based nonablative chemotherapy and allogeneic blood progenitor-cell transplantation as treatment for lymphoid malignancies. *J Clin Oncol* 1998;16:2817–2824.

203. Khouri IF, Saliba RM, Giralt SA, et al. Nonablative allogeneic hematopoietic transplantation as adoptive immunotherapy for indolent lymphoma: low incidence of toxicity, acute graft-versus-host disease, and treatment-related mortality. *Blood* 2001;98:3595–3599.

204. Weisdorf D, Andersen J, Glick J, et al. Survival after relapse of low-grade non-Hodgkin's lymphoma: implications for marrow transplantation. *J Clin Oncol* 1992;10:942–947.

205. Friedberg J, Neuberg D, Gribben J, et al. Combination immunotherapy with rituximab and interleukin-2 in patients with relapsed or refractory follicular non-Hodgkin's lymphoma. *Br J Haematol* 2002; 117:1–7.

206. Ansell SM, Witzig TE, Kurtin PJ, et al. Phase 1 study of interleukin-12 in combination with rituximab in patients with B-cell non-Hodgkin lymphoma. *Blood* 2002;99:67–74.

207. Davis TA, Maloney DG, Grillo-Lopez AJ, et al. Combination immunotherapy of relapsed or refractory low-grade or follicular non-Hodgkin's lymphoma with rituximab and interferon-alpha-2a. *Clin Cancer Res* 2000;6:2644–2652.

208. Link B, Kahl B, Czuczman M, et al. A phase II study of Remitogen (HU1D10), a humanized monoclonal antibody in patients with relapsed or refractory follicular, small lymphocytic or marginal zone/MALT lymphoma. *Blood* 2001;98:606(abstr.).

209. Leonard J, Coleman M, Matthews J, et al. Combination monoclonal antibody therapy for lymphoma: treatment with epratuzumab (anti-CD22) and rituximab (anti-CD20) is well tolerated. *Blood* 2001; 98:844(abstr.).

210. Waters JS, Webb A, Cunningham D, et al. Phase I clinical and pharmacokinetic study of bcl-2 antisense oligonucleotide therapy in patients with non-Hodgkin's lymphoma. *J Clin Oncol* 2000;18:1812–1823.

211. Bendandi M, Gocke CD, Kobrin CB, et al. Complete molecular remissions induced by patient-specific vaccination plus granulocyte-monocyte colony-stimulating factor against lymphoma. *Nat Med* 1999;5:1171–1177.

212. Hsu F, Caspar C, Czerwinski D, et al. Tumor-specific idiotype vaccines in the treatment of patients with B-cell lymphoma—long term-results of a clinical trial. *Blood* 1997;89:3129–3135.

213. Kwak L, Campbell M, Czerwinski D, et al. Induction of immune responses in patients with B-cell lymphoma against the surface-immunoglobulin idiotype expressed by their tumors. *N Engl J Med* 1992; 327:1209–1215.

214. Timmerman JM, Czerwinski DK, Davis TA, et al. Idiotype-pulsed dendritic cell vaccination for B-cell lymphoma: clinical and immune responses in 35 patients. *Blood* 2002;99:1517–1526.

CHAPTER 25

Anaplastic Large-Cell Lymphoma

Christian Gisselbrecht and Brunangelo Falini

The entity referred to as *anaplastic large-cell lymphoma* in the Revised European-American Lymphoma (REAL) (1) and World Health Organization (WHO) (2) classifications was first described by Stein et al. (3) in 1985 based on the anaplastic appearance of the tumor cells, their propensity to grow cohesively and to invade lymph node sinuses, and the consistent expression of the cytokine receptor CD30 (previously named *Ki-1*) (4) on neoplastic cells.

Further progress in the characterization of anaplastic large-cell lymphoma had to wait for the identification in a proportion of cases [sometimes mimicking "malignant histiocytosis" (5,6)] of a nonrandom t(2;5)(p23;q35) translocation (7–9) that in 1994 was shown to cause the fusion of the nucleophosmin (NPM) and anaplastic lymphoma kinase (ALK) genes (10). Since identification of the t(2;5)-associated NPM-ALK fusion gene, several methods have been developed to identify the genetic lesion by reverse transcriptase–polymerase chain reaction, fluorescent *in situ* hybridization, and immunohistochemistry (11). These techniques have been extensively applied to investigate the problem of morphologic and clinical heterogeneity of anaplastic large-cell lymphoma and that of the relationship between anaplastic large-cell lymphoma and Hodgkin's disease. Thanks to these studies, an entity has been identified within the heterogeneous group of anaplastic large-cell lymphomas—the so-called ALK[+] anaplastic large-cell lymphoma—which shows distinctive molecular, pathologic, and clinical features. This chapter provides an overview of the most important progress in this field.

MORPHOLOGY

Based on its architectural features (propensity of CD30[+] anaplastic large-cell lymphoma cells to grow cohesively and to invade lymph node sinuses), the wide cytologic spectrum of the tumor cells (ranging in size from small to large anaplastic), and the variable admixture of reactive elements, several morphologic forms of anaplastic large-cell lymphoma have been recognized (12).

The *common type* is the most frequent morphologic variant of anaplastic large-cell lymphoma (approximately 70% of cases).

It is characterized by large, pleomorphic tumor cells with an abundant, often vacuolated, cytoplasm (Color Plate 51A–C and Color Plate 52A) (1–3,12–14) and horseshoe- or kidney-shaped nuclei with evident, multiple basophilic nucleoli (Color Plate 51C and Color Plate 52A). Nuclear lobes sometimes surround the Golgi area, which appears as a clear or more eosinophilic zone. Cells with these cytologic features have been referred to as *hallmark cells* (Color Plate 52A) (15), because they can be detected in all morphologic variants of anaplastic large-cell lymphoma, including the small-cell and lymphohistiocytic types.

In the *small-cell variant* (5% to 10% of anaplastic large-cell lymphoma cases), a dominant population of small to medium-sized tumor cells with irregular, generally not cerebriform, nuclei (12,16) (Color Plate 52C) is admixed with large anaplastic elements that usually cluster around small vessels, as highlighted by immunostaining for CD30 (12) and ALK (15,17,18). Because of the predominance of the small-cell component, this variant was usually misdiagnosed in the past as pleomorphic T-cell lymphoma on conventional examination (12).

The *lymphohistiocytic variant* (1,13,19) (5% to 10% of anaplastic large-cell lymphoma cases) is closely related to the small-cell variant (2), as it often contains small neoplastic cells admixed with large anaplastic elements and a high number of pale reactive histiocytes (Color Plate 52E). The latter may be so abundant as to mask the tumor cell population, sometimes leading to a misdiagnosis of atypical inflammatory lesions, hemophagocytic syndrome, or malignant histiocytosis (12,19). Because of the small-sized tumor cell component, this variant was erroneously categorized as a *peripheral T-cell lymphoma* (20) in the Kiel Classification. The *small-cell* and *lymphohistiocytic* types are the only recognized variants in the new WHO Classification of the lymphoid neoplasms (2).

Although not regarded as distinctive variants, it is also important to recognize rare morphologic forms of anaplastic large-cell lymphoma [sarcomatoid (21,22), neutrophil-rich (23), hypocellular (24), and signet-ring (25)] (Color Plate 51B) that can be misdiagnosed as either atypical inflammatory lesions or malignant tumors other than anaplastic large-cell lymphoma. Some "anaplastic large-cell lymphomas" show a capsular thickening and a vaguely nodular fibrosis associated with the presence of a significant number of tumor cells resembling classic Hodgkin and Reed-Sternberg cells (26). It is now clear that these cases [previously assigned to the provisional category *Hodgkin's-like anaplastic large-cell lymphoma* in the REAL Classification (1)] mostly represent examples of Hodgkin's disease rich in tumor cells (e.g., anaplastic large-cell lymphoma–like Hodgkin's disease). For these reasons, the term *Hodgkin's-like anaplastic large-cell lymphoma* has been abandoned by the new WHO Classification of the lymphoid neoplasms (2).

IMMUNOPHENOTYPE

The hallmark of anaplastic large-cell lymphoma cells is the expression of the CD30 (Ki-1) molecule (3,13,27), a 120-kDa transmembrane cytokine receptor of the tumor necrosis factor receptor family (27,28), for which the corresponding ligand (CD30L) has been identified (29). CD30 is characteristically expressed on the cell membrane and in the Golgi area of tumor cells (Color Plates 51D,E). In the small-cell variant, only the large anaplastic cells (usually distributed around vessels) express CD30, whereas the small tumor cells are usually weakly positive or negative (12,16). The reproducibility of anaplastic large-cell lymphoma diagnosis on morphologic grounds is 46% but can be increased to 85% by immunostaining for CD30 (30). Epithelial membrane antigen positivity is also seen in most anaplastic large-cell lymphoma (31,32), although in some cases only a percentage of tumor cells express this molecule. Immunostaining for ALK is now recognized as one of the most specific diagnostic tools (Color Plates 51F and 52B,D,F) (13,15,17,18,33,34), and it is extensively discussed in the following sections. BCL2 expression has been reported in ALK[-] but not ALK[+] anaplastic large-cell lymphoma (35), thus suggesting that ALK expression may influence the apoptosis pathway in anaplastic large-cell lymphoma. Conversely, c-Myc nuclear expression has been observed in pediatric ALK[+] but not ALK[-] anaplastic large-cell lymphoma (36).

Primary systemic anaplastic large-cell lymphoma usually displays a T or null phenotype (3,37). Anaplastic large-cell lymphoma of the null-cell type is also likely to be derived from T cells, because the tumor cells usually express the cytotoxic molecules perforin, granzyme B, and TIA-1 (37,38) and harbor clonally rearranged T-cell antigen receptor genes (38).

The existence of a B-cell form of anaplastic large-cell lymphoma has been the subject of controversy. It was incorporated into the Kiel Classification as a separate entity (20), but the REAL (1) and WHO (2) classifications regard it as one morphologic extreme of the diffuse large B-cell–lymphoma spectrum. This view is supported by the following findings: (a) lack of ALK-protein expression (13,15,17,34,39), (b) evidence for transformation from follicular lymphomas (40); and (c) presence of somatic mutations of the immunoglobulin H–variable region genes (41).

MOLECULAR FEATURES OF ANAPLASTIC LARGE-CELL LYMPHOMA

Anaplastic large-cell lymphoma is associated with a t(2;5)(p23;q35) chromosome translocation (7–9) that causes the ALK gene on chromosome 2 to fuse with the NPM (also known as *B23* or *numatrin*) gene on chromosome 5 (10).

The NPM gene (42) encodes for a phylogenetically conserved and ubiquitously expressed 38-kDa acidic phosphoprotein that is mainly localized to nucleoli (43). NPM is a multifunctional protein engaged in cytoplasmic or nuclear trafficking (44) that also acts as a nuclear chaperone (45,46) and plays a key role in controlling centrosome duplication (47) and, therefore, successful M-phase entry and transit.

The ALK gene encodes for a glycosylated, 210-kDa transmembrane receptor tyrosine kinase that comprises a large extracellular domain, a lipophilic transmembrane segment, and a cytoplasmic tyrosine kinase domain (10,48,49). Recently, pleiotrophin has been proposed as the putative ligand for ALK (50). Under physiologic conditions, ALK is detectable only in the developing and mature central and peripheral nervous systems (34,49,51), but its function is unknown. In normal tissues and in tumors that express the native (full-length) protein (e.g., occasional cases of rhabdomyosarcomas), ALK is located on the surface membrane and in the cytoplasm.

The t(2;5) leads to the formation of the NPM-ALK fusion gene that encodes for an 80-kDa chimeric protein termed *NPM-ALK* (10) or *p80* (52). In the NPM-ALK fusion protein, the amino-terminal portion of NPM (amino acids 1 to 116) containing the oligomerization domain fuses to the entire cytoplasmic region of the ALK protein (the last 563 amino acids), which contains the tyrosine kinase domain (10) (Color Plate 53). Thus, the C-terminal domain of NPM (carrying the two nuclear localization signals) and the extracellular and transmembrane region of ALK are not retained in the NPM-ALK chimeric protein (10).

There are three important consequences of the t(2;5). First, it brings the ALK gene under the control of the strong NPM promoter, leading to the permanent high-level expression of the NPM-ALK fusion protein. Second, NPM-ALK can form homodimers (by cross-linking with other NPM-ALK molecules), which leads to the unregulated, constitutive activation of the tyrosine kinase catalytic domain of ALK (53), mimicking oligomerization of the receptor by the natural ligand. Third, NPM-ALK can form heterodimers (by cross-linking with the NPM wild-type protein encoded by the allele not involved in the translocation), which are responsible for the "aberrant" ALK nuclear-staining pattern revealed by immunohistochemistry in cases of anaplastic large-cell lymphoma with the t(2;5) (see the next section of this chapter).

A number of experimental data support the idea that NPM-ALK is the causative oncogene in ALK[+] anaplastic large-cell lymphoma. In fact, NPM-ALK displays strong transforming potential in both hematopoietic and fibroblast cell lines *in vitro* (54). Moreover, transplantation of NPM-ALK–transduced bone marrow cells into irradiated recipient mice can induce a lymphoma-like disease (55), and NPM-ALK transgenic mice spontaneously develop T-cell lymphomas and plasma cell tumors (56).

At least two signaling cascades involved in the control of proliferation and apoptosis appear to be activated by NPM-ALK *in vitro* (54) (Color Plate 54). NPM-ALK was found to recruit phospholipase C-gamma which is, in turn, responsible for the enhanced production of IP3 (57). The phospholipase C-gamma/IP3 pathway seems to be involved in the NPM-ALK–mediated mitogenicity (54). Moreover, NPM-ALK constitutively activates the antiapoptotic phosphatidylinositol-3 kinase/AKT pathway (58,59). This results in the phosphorylation and inactivation of the proapoptotic molecule BAD, which is, in turn, responsible for the apoptosis protection in NPM-ALK–bearing cells (54,58,59). NPM-ALK–mediated activation of STAT3 (60,61) and STAT5 (62) has also been suggested to play a role in lymphomagenesis (Color Plate 54).

ANAPLASTIC LARGE-CELL LYMPHOMA BEARING THE NUCLEOPHOSMIN-ANAPLASTIC LYMPHOMA KINASE FUSION PROTEIN

Detection of the NPM-ALK fusion gene/transcript or its chimeric product can be achieved using reverse transcriptase–polymerase chain reaction (11,63,64), *in situ* hybridization (65), two-color fluorescent *in situ* hybridization (66), or immunolabeling with specific antibodies directed against different portions of the NPM-ALK fusion protein (17,33,34,67,68). Because of its high specificity, simplicity, rapidity, and low cost, immunohistochemistry is, at present, the most useful and widely used technique. Additional advantages of this procedure are that it can be applied to archival paraffin-embedded material, provides information on the identity of labeled cells and their topographic distribution, and helps to identify molecular variants of anaplastic large-cell lymphoma (i.e., bearing fusion genes other than NPM-ALK) through demonstration of aberrant subcellular distribution of the ALK protein.

The ALK protein is not detectable by immunohistochemistry in normal tissues, with the exception of a few cells in neural tissues (34). Therefore, the finding of ALK positivity in tissues other than brain tissue can be taken as evidence of aberrant ALK expression, usually in the form of the t(2;5)-associated NPM-ALK fusion product (13,17,33,43,64,65,68).

In lymphomas, expression of the ALK protein is restricted to the approximately 60% of anaplastic large-cell lymphomas with T or null phenotype. Approximately 85% of the ALK+ anaplastic large-cell lymphomas bear the product of the t(2;5) translocation (e.g., the NPM-ALK fusion protein), as shown by the subcellular distribution of the ALK protein, which is characteristically seen not only in the cytoplasm (the expected location site of wild-type ALK), but also in the nucleus (13,43,68,69) (Color Plate 55). Transportation

of NPM-ALK into the nuclei of tumor cells through heterodimer formation with the wild-type NPM (70), which contains two nuclear localization signals (absent in the NPM portion of NPM-ALK), most likely accounts for this seemingly anomalous ALK nuclear-staining pattern (Color Plate 55). Anaplastic large-cell lymphoma with t(2;5) also shows a peculiar expression pattern of the N-terminus of NPM (retained in NPM-ALK). In fact, monoclonal antibodies directed against the N-terminus of NPM stain both the cytoplasm and the nucleus of tumor cells bearing the NPM-ALK fusion protein (14,43,68,69). In contrast, in tissues devoid of NPM-ALK, NPM positivity is restricted to the nucleus (43,68,69).

ANAPLASTIC LARGE-CELL LYMPHOMA BEARING ANAPLASTIC LYMPHOMA KINASE FUSION PROTEINS OTHER THAN NUCLEOPHOSMIN-ANAPLASTIC LYMPHOMA KINASE

In approximately 15% of cases of ALK+ anaplastic large-cell lymphoma, ALK fuses with a gene partner other than NPM to produce variant ALK fusion protein (15,17,34). These cases can be clearly distinguished from the most common NPM-ALK+ anaplastic large-cell lymphoma by immunohistochemistry, Western blotting, cytogenetics/ fluorescent *in situ* hybridization, and reverse transcriptase–polymerase chain reaction. At immunohistochemistry, they show a staining pattern different from that expected for the t(2;5), because they are characterized by cytoplasmic-restricted ALK expression (13,15,17,34,68,69) (Color Plate 56) and nucleus-restricted NPM (N-terminus) expression (69). Moreover, Western blotting with anti-ALK antibodies identifies fusion proteins with a molecular weight different from that expected for NPM-ALK (80 kDa) (71). When available, cytogenetic analysis of these cases has shown a variety of genetic abnormalities [e.g., the t(1;2)(q21;p23), the t(2;3)(p23;q21), and the inv(2)(p23;q35) (72–74)], strongly suggesting that the ALK gene at 2p23 fuses with partners other than NPM.

A number of genes involved in these chromosomal translocations have been now cloned (Color Plates 53 and 56) (13,68). The TPM3 (non-muscle tropomyosin)-ALK fusion gene, which encodes for a 104-kDa chimeric protein, is generated by the t(1;2)(q25;p23) translocation (75,76). Interestingly, fusion of TPM3 with ALK also occurs in a subset of myofibroblastic inflammatory tumors in children (77). Thus, TPM3-ALK is a remarkable example of an oncogenic fusion protein that can transform both lymphoid and mesenchymal human cells *in vivo* (77,78).

The TFG (tropomyosin receptor kinase–fused *gene*)-ALK fusion gene (79) may generate three chimeric proteins of different molecular weights [i.e., 83 kDa (short TFG-ALK), 97 kDa (large TFG-ALK), and 113 kDa (extra-large TFG-ALK)], which correspond to different breakpoints in the TFG

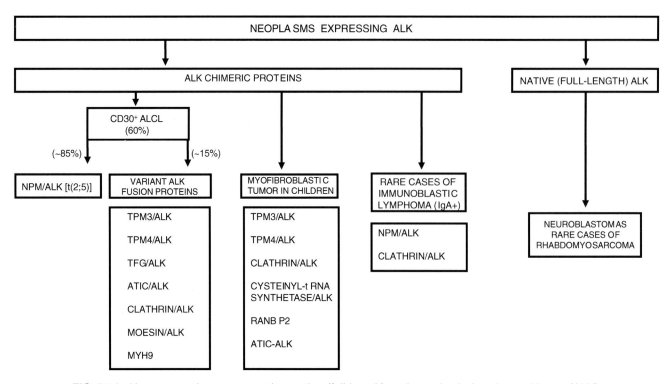

FIG. 25.1. Human neoplasms expressing native (full-length) and anaplastic lymphoma kinase (ALK) fusion proteins. ALCL, anaplastic large-cell lymphoma; NPM, nucleophosmin.

gene (79,80). At least the TFG-ALK 97-kDa chimeric product is known to be generated by the t(2;3)(p23;q21) (74).

The inv(2)(p23;q35) (73) leads to the creation of a fusion gene named *ATIC-ALK*, which encodes for a chimeric protein formed by the entire cytoplasmic portion of ALK and the amino-terminus of ATIC [5 Aminoimidazole-4-carboxamide-1-beta-D-ribonucleotide transfomylase/inosine monophosphate (IMP) cyclohydrolase] (81–83), a bifunctional homodimeric enzyme that catalyzes the penultimate and ultimate steps of *de novo* purine nucleotide biosynthesis (84). Finally, Meech et al. (85) have reported a case of childhood ALK⁺ anaplastic large-cell lymphoma with t(2;19)(p23;p13) in which ALK fuses to the TPM4 gene, which had been previously mapped to 19p13.1.

In some anaplastic large-cell lymphoma cases, the search for ALK gene partners alternative to NPM (usually prompted by the immunocytochemical finding of cytoplasmic-restricted ALK expression) has led to the identification of variant ALK fusion genes, for which the corresponding chromosomal translocation involving band 2p23 has been not yet identified. There are two such an examples: Touriol et al. (86) have reported the fusion of ALK with the CLTCL (clathrin heavy polypeptide-like) gene, which encodes for the main structural protein of coated vesicles (structures involved in the selective intracellular transport of molecules, such as hydrolytic enzymes). Because the CLTL gene is located on chromosome 22, the existence of an as yet unidentified t(2;22)(p23;q11.2) has been predicted. More recently, a case of anaplastic large-cell lymphoma bearing

a Moesin-ALK fusion gene encoding for a chimeric protein of 125 kDa has been reported (87). In this case, the ALK breakpoint differed from that consistently occurring in other translocations involving the ALK gene, being localized within the exonic sequence coding for the juxtamembrane portion of ALK (87). The Moesin-ALK fusion gene is predicted to be the result of an as yet unreported t(X;2)(q11;p23)(87).

The lack of nuclear localization signals in all identified ALK-variant fusion proteins accounts for their cytoplasmic-restricted expression. For some ALK-variant fusion proteins (CLTCL-ALK and Moesin-ALK), unique immunohistochemical staining patterns have been also recognized (Color Plate 57). Expression of CLTLC-ALK is associated with a typical cytoplasmic granular positivity (86) (Color Plate 57). This is due to the fact that the sequence responsible for clathrin heavy-chain assemblage is retained in the CLTCL-ALK fusion protein, which can, therefore, participate in the formation of the clathrin coat on the surface of the vesicles. In an anaplastic large-cell lymphoma case expressing Moesin-ALK, ALK expression was restricted to the surface membrane, reflecting the physiologic association of Moesin with cell membrane proteins (87) (Color Plate 57). Restriction of ALK positivity to the tumor cell surface has also been detected in occasional cases of rhabdomyosarcoma (17,88) and neuroblastoma (89). Surface/granular cytoplasmic expression of ALK also has been detected in a rare variant of large B-cell lymphoma (90) that is characterized by immunoblastic/plasmablastic (rather than anaplastic) morphology, cytoplasmic expression of immunoglobulin A, and absence of CD30. ALK positivity in these cases was initially thought to be the result of the expression of the 210-kDa full-length ALK protein (90). It is now clear that these cases bear ALK chimeric proteins, usually Clathrin-ALK (145–148). It is likely that the ALK⁺ lymphomas with B-cell phenotype recently reported by Gascoyne et al. (91) belong to this category. The spectrum of human neoplasms expressing ALK as a fusion protein or a native molecule is shown in Figure 25.1.

Although the contributions of the ALK-variant fusion proteins to lymphomagenesis *in vivo* remain to be established, a common theme is their ability to form homodimers (such as occurs with NPM-ALK) (13,14). Homodimer formation takes place through the dimerization sites present in the ALK-fusion partner (usually a molecule with strong and ubiquitous tissue expression). This event mimics ligand binding and leads to the activation of the ALK kinase catalytic domain (retained in all ALK-variant fusion proteins so far identified), which is in turn responsible for the oncogenic activity (53). The finding that TFG-ALK, TPM3-ALK, and Moesin-ALK fusion proteins are capable of autophosphorylation *in vitro* (75,79,87) further supports this view.

CORRELATION BETWEEN ANAPLASTIC LYMPHOMA KINASE EXPRESSION, MORPHOLOGY, AND PHENOTYPE IN HUMAN LYMPHOMAS

The term *ALK⁺ anaplastic large-cell lymphoma* has been proposed for anaplastic large-cell lymphoma expressing NPM-ALK or ALK-variant fusion proteins (15,17,18). On the contrary, the use of the term *ALKoma* should, in our opinion, be discouraged, because it may generate confusion with tumors other than anaplastic large-cell lymphoma that can express ALK either as fusion proteins (myofibroblastic tumors in children) or full-length proteins (rare rhabdomyosarcomas, neuroblastomas, rare B-cell immunoblastic tumors). At present, it is not clear whether the ALK⁻ anaplastic large-cell lymphoma is a separate entity or the end spectrum of peripheral T-cell lymphoma. Insights in this field can only derive from a better knowledge of the molecular mechanisms of tumorigenesis in these cases. For current clinical practice, the pathologist should diagnose anaplastic large-cell lymphoma according to the strict criteria outlined above but specify in each case whether it is ALK⁺ or ALK⁻, because this distinction apparently has a prognostic impact (see Prognostic and Predictive Factors later in this chapter).

ALK⁺ anaplastic large-cell lymphoma shows a broad morphologic spectrum ranging from the small-cell variant to the giant-cell–rich form of anaplastic large-cell lymphoma (13,15,17,68,92) (Color Plates 52B,D,E). The subcellular distribution of the ALK protein tends to correlate with the size of the neoplastic cells. In general, the large anaplastic tumor cells (the dominant population in the common and giant-cell types) show ALK positivity both in the cytoplasm and in the nucleus (Color Plate 55) or, less commonly, only in the cytoplasm (Color Plate 56). In contrast, the small tumor cells (the dominant population in the small-cell and lymphohistiocytic variants) exhibit a nuclear-restricted expression of the ALK protein (17) (Color Plates 52D,F). In the small-cell variant, a low percentage of large anaplastic cells that express ALK in the cytoplasm and nucleus is also found around vessels. Aberrant nuclear ALK expression (the immunohistochemical hallmark for the 2;5 translocation) in both small and large tumor cells strongly supports the view that they belong to the same neoplastic clone and excludes the notion that the large cells represent a subclone that has arisen in a (2;5)-translocation–negative low-grade (small-cell) lymphoma by acquiring the t(2;5) (93).

IMPACT OF IMMUNOHISTOCHEMISTRY IN THE DIAGNOSIS OF ANAPLASTIC LARGE-CELL LYMPHOMA

Immunohistochemistry plays a pivotal role in the differential diagnosis between anaplastic large-cell lymphoma and other reactive or malignant conditions.

Anaplastic Large-Cell Lymphoma versus Reactive Conditions

In the lymphohistiocytic variant of anaplastic large-cell lymphoma, the histiocytes may be so abundant as to mask the tumor-cell population (Color Plate 52E), thus leading to a misdiagnosis of atypical inflammatory lesions or hemophagocytic syndrome (12,19). Moreover, the neutrophil-rich (23) and hypocellular (24) forms of anaplastic large-cell lymphoma can be confused with an inflammatory process both in the lymph node (24) and in the skin (94,95). Immunostaining for CD30 and ALK usually allows a correct diagnosis.

Small-Cell Variant Anaplastic Large-Cell Lymphoma versus Peripheral T-Cell Lymphomas Not Otherwise Specified

The differential diagnosis between small-cell variant anaplastic large-cell lymphoma and peripheral T-cell lymphomas not otherwise specified is mainly based on the detection of nuclear ALK positivity on the small atypical cells (usually CD30⁻) (13,17) (Color Plate 52D). Such a distinction is clinically relevant, because ALK⁺ anaplastic large-cell lymphoma has a better prognosis than other peripheral T-cell lymphomas.

Anaplastic Large-Cell Lymphoma versus Hodgkin's Disease

Differential diagnosis between anaplastic large-cell lymphoma and Hodgkin's disease (usually in cases of lymphocyte depletion or nodular sclerosis with syncytial growth pattern) (12,13,26) is mainly based on the expression of the ALK and PAX5 molecules. The finding of ALK positivity excludes Hodgkin's disease. If the tumor turns out to have a null phenotype and to be ALK⁻, then PAX5 becomes the critical diagnostic tool. In fact, weak to moderate nuclear PAX5 expression (a specific B-cell marker) is typical of Hodgkin's disease (96). However, it is recognized that at least a percentage of cases at the interphase between anaplastic large-cell lymphoma and Hodgkin's disease still remain undiagnosed.

Anaplastic Large-Cell Lymphoma versus Extra-Hematopoietic Tumors

In the differential diagnosis between anaplastic large-cell lymphoma and undifferentiated carcinomas, cytokeratins (consistently negative in anaplastic large-cell lymphoma) are the discriminatory markers, because anaplastic large-cell lymphoma is frequently epithelial membrane antigen–positive, and CD30 can be expressed in some carcinomas (27). Immunohistochemistry easily distinguishes between anaplastic large-cell lymphoma and malignant fibrous histiocytoma, which consistently lacks CD30 and other lymphoid markers (21,27). The differential diagnosis between anaplastic large-cell lymphoma and the inflammatory myofibroblastic tumors that also express the ALK protein as a consequence of translocations involving the ALK and tropomyosin (TPM3 and TPM4) genes (77,97) is mainly based on CD30 and ALK immunostaining (98). In fact, neoplastic cells in anaplastic large-cell lymphoma are CD30⁺/ALK⁺, whereas inflammatory myofibroblastic tumors are CD30⁻/ALK⁺.

CLINICAL FEATURES: PRESENTATION, STAGING, AND UNUSUAL SYNDROMES

Primary systemic anaplastic large-cell lymphoma accounts for 2% to 8% of all lymphomas. Two distinct clinical forms of primary anaplastic large-cell lymphoma are now recognized: that limited to the skin (99) and systemic. However, rare cases of anaplastic large-cell lymphoma can occur in patients with a history of previous lymphoma and are considered secondary forms. The main clinical characteristics described in different series are reported in Table 25.1. Of particular interest are the comparisons within the same prospective study of treatment for lymphomas of patients with anaplastic large-cell lymphoma and those with other types of lymphomas, first irrespective of the immunophenotype, and then with peripheral T-cell lymphoma patients (100,101). In one report, 146 anaplastic large-cell lymphoma patients diagnosed based on morphology and CD30 expression were compared with 1,695 diffuse nonanaplastic large-cell lymphoma patients (100). Both subtypes predominantly affected males younger than

60 years of age. B symptoms were more frequent in anaplastic large-cell lymphoma, and a majority of anaplastic large-cell lymphoma patients had disseminated disease, with more skin and mediastinum lesions. Conversely, digestive tract involvement was less common in anaplastic large-cell lymphoma. According to that report, anaplastic large-cell lymphoma and nonanaplastic large-cell lymphoma had similar distributions in the different risk groups of the International Prognostic Index (IPI) (102), although a trend toward a lower risk category of the IPI presentation was found in the International Lymphoma Study Group (1). Anaplastic large-cell lymphoma with the T-cell phenotype (anaplastic large-cell lymphoma-T) had a higher rate of skin involvement, less disseminated disease, and lower lactate dehydrogenase level when compared with B- and null-cell anaplastic large-cell lymphoma. When compared with other nonanaplastic T-cell lymphomas, the same trend was found. In addition, anaplastic large-cell lymphoma-T had less frequent bone-marrow involvement or extranodal localizations leading to an IPI score distribution with 39% having zero factors and 24% with only one factor (101).

Clear clinicopathologic differences have been found between ALK⁺ and ALK⁻ subtypes in most studies (69,91,103,104) (Table 25.1). ALK⁺ patients were much younger, and anaplastic large-cell lymphoma occurred during the first three decades of life. B symptoms were observed in both groups, and ALK⁺ patients had significantly better performance status and fewer had above normal lactate dehydrogenase levels. Patients in both groups showed a nodal presentation, and more than 40% of children with disseminated disease had inguinal lymph node involvement. Mediastinal involvement was less common than in Hodgkin's lymphoma. An increased incidence of extranodal involvement was seen in the ALK⁻ group (104). Skin, bone, and soft tissues were commonly affected extranodal sites. Pelvic muscle involvement is not infrequent and can be mistaken for a soft tissue sarcoma. Central nervous system involvement seems rare, especially in children with ALK⁺ anaplastic large-cell lymphoma. Bone-marrow involvement is considered to be an uncommon event and can be difficult to detect on routine histologic examinations alone (18). In a series of 42 anaplastic large-cell lymphoma patients, 17% were bone marrow positive with conventional examination. However, after immunohistochemical analysis, occult malignant cells were detected in 23% of the patients with negative bone marrow biopsies on routine histology (105). The only way to detect these cells is by immunocytochemical labeling with anti-CD30 and anti-ALK antibodies (27,105,106). Prominent leukemic involvement in anaplastic large-cell lymphoma is uncommon and carries a poor prognosis (107–109). The ALK⁺ group was accorded lower IPI scores than was the ALK⁻ group. ALK expression is closely correlated with age and IPI. Clinical findings such as those described for ALK⁺ anaplastic large-cell lym-

TABLE 25.1. *Anaplastic large-cell lymphoma: clinical characteristics and comparison with nonanaplastic large-cell lymphoma or T-cell lymphoma*

Reference	Histology subtype	n	Age (%)	M/F (%)	Stage I–II/ III–IV (%)	PS >1 (%)	LDH >N (%)	B symptoms (%)	IPI 0–1 (%)	IPI ≥2 (%)	Skin involvement (%)	Bone involvement (%)	BM (%)	Med (%)
Tilly, 1997	ALCL CD30⁺	146	≤60 yr (73)	64/36	40/60	27	47	53	62	33	15	8	14	38
	Non ALCL B + T	1,695	≤60 yr (58)	54/46	42/58	25	52	40	57	36	6	8	16	—
Gisselbrecht, 1998	Non-ALCL-T	228	≤60 yr (76)	68/32	14/86	30	55	48	22	77	18	—	36	—
	ALCL-T	60	≤60 yr (75)	73/27	37/63	20	33	57	63	37	25	—	13	—
Suzuki, 2000	ALK⁺	83	≤30 yr (87)	63/37	34/66	19	41	54	78	22	21	12	11	6
	ALK⁻	60	≤30 yr (21)	75/25	31/69	33	60	55	57	40	32	5	20	12
Falini, 1999	ALK⁺	53	≤35 yr (88)	75/25	28/72	47	38	76	47	47	21	17	11	—
	ALK⁻	25	≤35 yr (60)	48/52	56/44	28	40	60	68	28	4	4	0	—
Gascoyne, 1999	ALK⁺	36	≤60 yr (51)		NA	28	36	—	—	—	—	—	—	—
	ALK⁻	34	≤60 yr (52)		NA	41	50	—	—	—	—	—	—	—
Seidemann, 2001	ALK⁺	35	≤17 yr (100)	68/32	31/69	—	91	57	NA	—	11	17	—	26
	ALK⁻	8	≤17 yr (100)	62/38	62/38	—	100	38	NA	—	13	13	—	25
Brugieres, 1998	ALK⁺ (93%)	82	≤17 yr (100)	56/44	34/66	—	16	68	NA	—	33	12	16	39

ALCL, anaplastic large-cell lymphoma; ALK, anaplastic lymphoma kinase; BM, bone marrow; IPI, International Prognostic Index; LDH, lactate dehydrogenase; Med, mediastinum; M/F, male/female; N, normal; NA, not available; PS, performance status.

phoma had been described in pediatric patients (110,111). In one report (110) on patients younger than 17 years of age, 93% of the patients were ALK⁺. Although not fully investigated in all series, ALK expression was high in young patients. Therefore, the entity—ALK⁺ anaplastic large-cell lymphoma—transcends the arbitrary boundaries of 15 or 20 years of age, so that there seems to be no good reason to divide this disease into two categories—pediatric and adults—to obtain a more accurate understanding of the disease.

True anaplastic large-cell lymphoma, especially the form bearing ALK proteins, is rare in posttransplant (112) and human immunodeficiency virus–infected patients (113,114). Most anaplastic large-cell lymphoma cases appear to be related to the anaplastic variant of diffuse large-cell B-cell lymphoma (113). Nevertheless, four out of eight cases of human immunodeficiency virus–associated anaplastic large-cell lymphoma reported in a New York series (115) had T-cell subtypes (no information about ALK expression is available). Their prognosis is determined by the immune status of the patient.

Secondary anaplastic large-cell lymphoma may arise in the progression of other lymphomas, most commonly during the course of mycosis fungoides, peripheral T-cell lymphomas, Hodgkin's lymphoma, or lymphomatoid papulosis (13) and has a poor prognosis (116).

PROGNOSTIC AND PREDICTIVE FACTORS

The complete-remission rate is generally higher for anaplastic large-cell lymphoma than for nonanaplastic large-cell lymphoma patients (100). In anaplastic large-cell lymphoma patients, survival is significantly longer than in nonanaplastic large-cell lymphoma patients. Multivariate analysis identified the anaplastic histology as an independent factor for survival. Moreover, patients with anaplastic large-cell lymphoma-T had significantly better survival than did those with nonanaplastic large-cell T-cell lymphoma (101,117) (Fig. 25.2). Event-free survival and overall survival of the anaplastic large-cell lymphoma-B patients were reported to be similar to those of the anaplastic large-cell lymphoma-T null cases (91,100). Initial investigations did not identify any IPI category as prognostic for anaplastic large-cell lymphoma (118), perhaps because of the small number of patients studied, but the results obtained with large populations recognized low IPI as having positive prognostic value (18,100,104). The value of histology type remains an independent parameter according to multivariate analysis integrating histology along with the other parameters. Shiota et al. (103) reported a significant prognostic difference between ALK⁺ and ALK⁻ anaplastic large-cell lymphoma, with the former having a far better 5-year survival rate (80%) than the latter (33%). This finding was subsequently confirmed by several other reports (18,91,104) (Fig. 25.3), except in

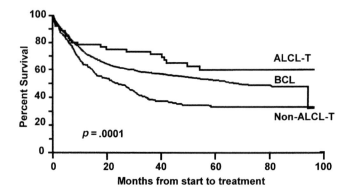

FIG. 25.2. Overall survival of 228 nonanaplastic T-cell lymphoma (non-ALCL-T) patients and 60 anaplastic T-cell lymphoma (ALCL-T) patients compared with 1,595 diffuse B-cell lymphoma (BCL) patients. ALCL, anaplastic T-cell lymphoma; ALK, anaplastic lymphoma kinase. (Adapted from Gisselbrecht C, et al. *Blood* 1998;92:76–82.)

children, because almost all of them are ALK⁺. These findings suggest that lymphomas expressing NPM-ALK can be considered as a single entity. Suzuki et al. (104) found CD56 expression to be a prognostic factor independent of IPI and ALK expression in multivariate analysis. In fact, in both ALK⁺ and ALK⁻ subgroups, CD56⁺ cases showed a poorer prognosis than did CD56⁻ cases. It is also possible that differences in expression of apoptosis-inhibiting proteins (119) might be responsible for the better prognosis of ALK⁺ as compared to ALK⁻ anaplastic large-cell lymphoma.

Several series of childhood and adult anaplastic large-cell lymphoma have been reported, but they are often difficult to compare because of the heterogeneity of the treatments or the lack of a common staging system. St. Jude's Hospital's classification has been used for children, whereas the Ann Arbor staging system and the IPI scoring are used for adults. Although ALK absence or presence is useful in association with the IPI score for adults to discriminate a patient's prognosis and to evaluate the impact of treatment, it is not applicable for children, as 90% of them have ALK⁺ disease (110). The European Intergroup Study of anaplastic large-cell lymphoma (120) compared the results and prognoses of 235 children enrolled in trials designed to treat childhood anaplastic large-cell lymphoma with short and intensive chemotherapy, similar to that used for B-cell lymphoma from the Berlin-Frankfurt-Munster group (93 patients), the French Society of Pediatric Oncology (82 patients), and the United Kingdom Childhood group (60 patients). Multivariate analysis adjusted for country has brought to light three prognostic factors: (a) mediastinal involvement; (b) visceral involvement defined as spleen, lung, or liver involvement; and (c) skin lesions. For the good-prognosis group with no factors, the 3-year event-free survival was 87%; for the poor-risk group with at least two factors, the expected 3-year overall survival was 61% (120).

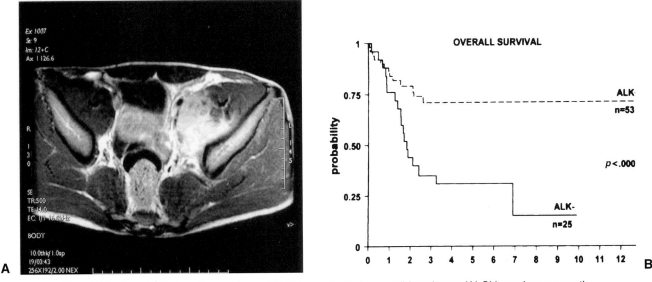

FIG. 25.3. Anaplastic lymphoma kinase (ALK)⁺ anaplastic large-cell lymphoma (ALCL): nuclear magnetic resonance image and survival curve. **A:** Involvement of the left obturator muscle in a 24-year-old patient with ALK⁺ ALCL. **B:** ALK⁺ ALCL shows better survival than ALK⁻ ALCL. (From Falini B, Pileri S, Zinzani PL, et al. ALK⁺ lymphoma: clinico-pathological findings and outcome. *Blood* 1999;93:2697–2706, with permission.)

TREATMENT

Anaplastic large-cell lymphoma accounts for only 10% to 15% of all childhood non-Hodgkin's lymphomas. In most European studies, anaplastic large-cell lymphoma is considered to be a separate entity and is treated with either a short and intensive chemotherapy regimen, as for B-cell lymphoma (111,121), or with more prolonged chemotherapy derived from T-cell lymphoma protocols (122,123). However, North Americans treated all large-cell lymphomas with the same chemotherapy regimen regardless of the histologic subgroup and immunophenotype (124,125). The opportunity to classify this disease into low- and high-risk cases according to IPI score and ALK positivity is highly relevant for the design of optimal therapeutic strategies. This concept is particularly applicable to children, whose treatment has mainly been based on the highly aggressive regimens used for lymphoblastic leukemia and lymphoma. The low frequency (less than 5%) of central nervous system involvement by ALK⁺ lymphomas also calls into question the general policy of intrathecal prophylaxis.

Due to the relatively high frequency of anaplastic large-cell lymphoma in childhood, prospective nonrandomized studies have been performed. Reports include generally successive protocols with stratification according to stage in Germany (Berlin-Frankfurt-Munster group) or the United States, whereas all patients received the same treatment regardless of stage in France (French Society of Pediatric Oncology). No randomized studies comparing different regimens have been reported so far. The main results obtained for children and adults are reported in Table 25.2. For the Berlin-Frankfurt-Munster group, after a cytoreductive prephase, treatment was stratified into three branches: nine patients in K1 (stage I and II resected) received

three 5-day cycles [methotrexate (MTX) 0.5 g/m², dexamethasone, oxazaphorins, etoposide, cytarabine, doxorubicin, and intrathecal therapy]; 65 patients in K2 (stage II nonresected and stage III) received six cycles without additional radiotherapy; 14 patients in K3 (stage IV or multifocal bone disease) received six intensified cycles, including MTX 5 g/m² and high-dose cytarabine/etoposide. K1, K2, and K3 had similar 5-year event-free survival rates at 76%, 73%, and 79% respectively (111). Therapy results of that study were similar to data previously obtained from 62 patients treated in earlier studies (121). Treatment lasted 2 months for localized resected stage I and II disease and 5 months for K3. After a cytoreductive prephase, French children (110) received two cycles of COPADM (MTX, cyclophosphamide, doxorubicin, vincristine, and prednisone) and 5 to 7 months of maintenance; radiotherapy was not used in localized stages. For all 82 children, the 3-year event-free–survival rate was 66%, with a 3-year event-free–survival rate of 47% for the 46 patients in the high-risk group differing significantly from the 95% rate for the 29 children at low risk. The 18 children treated at St. Jude's Hospital (124) with six cycles of CHOP [cyclophosphamide, hydroxydaunorubicin, Oncovin (vincristine), and prednisone]-like regimens achieved a 5-year event-free–survival rate of 75% for limited stages and 57% for extended stages. However, it must be kept in mind that those studies included small numbers of patients in each category, and no treatment was found superior to any other. Nevertheless, the impressive results obtained by the Berlin-Frankfurt-Munster group for each category with short-term administration and low cumulative doses of critical drugs, such as anthracyclines, warrant further study in randomized trials.

No large comparative studies of adults have been published. Most investigators reported that the anaplastic large-

TABLE 25.2. *Anaplastic large-cell lymphoma: evolution and treatments reported*

Authors	Histology subtype	No. of patients	Treatment	CR rate (%)	5-yr survival (%)	ALK+/ALK− survival (%)	Risk factor (IPI): 5-yr survival (%)			Prognostic factor (Cox model)
							0	1	2+	
Tilly, 1997	ALCL CD30+ T/B/Null	146	Dose-adjusted chemotherapy	75	66	Not done	82	78	50	IPI
	Non-ALCL B +T cells	1,695	CHOP/ACVB ASCT without RT	61	48	Not done	69	47	34	ALCL
Gisselbrecht, 1998	T-non ALCL	228	idem	49	35	Not done	64	56	34	IPI Non-ALCL
Zinzani, 1998	ALCL-HL	90	ABVD MACOP-B	73	60	Not available	—	—	—	Bulk/Stage B symptoms
Suzuki, 2000	ALCL ALK+, ALK−	139	CHOP-like regimen	72	Not precise	Significantly different	—	—	—	ALK
Gascoyne, 1999	ALK+, ALK−	70	CHOP-like ± RT	NA	65	79/46	85	69	37	IPI/ALK
Falini, 1999	ALK+, ALK−	96	CHOP-like ± RT	72	—	71/15	94 (0–1)	—	41 (2+)	IPI/ALK B symptoms
Seidemann, 2001	Pediatric	89	Dose duration	NA	76	NA	—	—	—	
Brugieres, 1998	Pediatric ALK+ 93%	82	COPADM	95 (EFS)	66	NA	NA	NA	NA	Mediastinum, ENS, LDH[a]

ABVD, Adriamycin (doxorubicin), bleomycin, vincristine, and dacarbazine; ACVB, Adriamycin (doxorubicin), cyclophosphamide, vindesine, bleomycin, and prednisone; ALCL, anaplastic large-cell lymphoma; ALK, anaplastic lymphoma kinase; ASCT, autologous stem cell transplantation; CHOP, cyclophosphamide, hydroxydaunorubicin, Oncovin (vincristine), and prednisone; COPADM, cyclophosphamide, vincristine, doxorubicin, prednisone, and methotrexate; CR, complete remission; EFS, event-free survival; ENS, extra-nodal sites; HL, Hodgkin's like; IPI, International Prognostic Index; LDH, lactate dehydrogenase; MACOP-B, methotrexate, Adriamycin (doxorubicin), cyclophosphamide, Oncovin (vincristine), prednisone, and bleomycin; NA, not available; RT, radiotherapy.
[a]IPI not used; replaced by prognostic factors mediastinum, ENS, and LDH. Absent = low risk, 1 present = high risk (5-yr survival: 95% for low-risk and 47% for high-risk groups).

cell lymphoma response rate to chemotherapy was good, ranging from 60% to 90%. Patients generally received the same treatment as that prescribed for diffuse large-cell lymphoma, according to the policy of the institution or in prospective trials. Due to the retrospective nature of the data, the same debate on whether CHOP is the standard of treatment for lymphoma can be reproduced. In one study, 40 cases of Hodgkin's-like anaplastic large-cell lymphoma were randomized to receive Hodgkin's-type chemotherapy [Adriamycin (doxorubicin), bleomycin, vinblastine, and dacarbazine (ABVD)] or lymphoma treatment [methotrexate, Adriamycin (doxorubicin), cyclophosphamide, Oncovin (vincristine), prednisone, and bleomycin (MACOP-B)], and it was concluded that the two regimens were equivalent (126). The overall survival of patients with localized stage without adverse IPI factors is known to exceed 90%. As in other adult studies—and in contrast to those in children—patients with more localized stages received radiotherapy. Patients with more advanced-stage disease frequently relapse, and their prognosis, in comparison to that of patients with other large-cell lymphomas, is controversial. Although a few studies have suggested that advanced-stage anaplastic large-cell lymphoma may have short disease-free survival and may require more intensive therapy (127–129), most investigators consider that anaplastic large-cell lymphomas generally behave like high-grade lymphomas (109,130). However, several comparative studies on diffuse large-cell lymphomas showed an association between CD30 expression and a favorable outcome (14, 30,100,131–133) when patients were treated with chemotherapy regimens similar to those used for other types of lymphomas (e.g., CHOP). According to the Groupe d'Etude des Lymphomes de l'Adulte study (100), which included T/null- and B-cell anaplastic large-cell lymphoma, the 5-year overall-survival rate for patients without adverse IPI factors was 82%, as compared to 78% for patients with one factor, 50% for the high-intermediate–risk group, and 25% for the high-risk group. Dose-intensive treatments have been used in this study, according to initial stratification based on prognostic factors. However, in that investigation, stratification according to ALK positivity had not been done, and results may also reflect the different percentage of ALK$^+$ lymphomas in adults. The age-adjusted IPI within the good-prognosis group of ALK$^+$ lymphomas showed that the 5-year overall-survival rate was 94% for patients with no or one factor versus 41% for those with two or more factors (18). Although ALK positivity is considered a marker of better prognosis, patients with two or more IPI factors still have a poor prognosis, and new approaches are needed. Systematic intensification of chemotherapy with the use of autologous stem cell support has been investigated in some institutions as part of a program designed for aggressive lymphoma (128,134,135). One study (128) described 16 consecutive anaplastic large-cell lymphoma cases, seven of which had an IPI score greater than or equal to 2, autografted in first-line therapy with impressive 100% disease-free and overall-survival rates at a median of 45 months. The other

publication (134) on 15 patients, six with an IPI score greater than or equal to 2 and seven ALK$^+$ patients, reported a 5-year overall-survival rate of 69%. In a retrospective study by the European Bone Marrow Transplantation group, the same authors reported on 64 patients with anaplastic large-cell lymphoma-T autografted during their treatment course, but the heterogeneity of patients and their therapeutic modalities prevented a clear appreciation of the role of autologous stem cell support (129). In addition, the number of patients with severe adverse factors was too small to extrapolate from these favorable results a set of recommendations differing from those advocated by the Consensus Conference on Aggressive Lymphoma (136). Only patients with at least two IPI adverse prognostic factors achieving complete remission after full treatment can be considered in a prospective study for consolidation with high-dose chemotherapy and autologous stem cell support.

Guidelines for the treatment of anaplastic large-cell lymphoma in the absence of large prospective studies in adults are not easy. Two factors should be taken in consideration: ALK positivity and adverse prognostic factors. Dose and duration of treatment without radiotherapy have been adjusted in children; 90% are ALK positive, according to their above-described prognostic factors. The same recommendations can be made for ALK$^+$ adult patients using the IPI as prognosis indicator, although the place of radiotherapy will remain controversial in localized stages (137,138). Comparison between CHOP and pediatric regimens could be of interest in the future.

Relapses occurred most frequently at the site of the primary tumor; however, involvement of new tumor sites distant from the initial manifestations was also observed frequently (110,111). Local recurrences of initial manifestations raise the question of additional local therapy with irradiation, as for other types of lymphomas. Questions not fully resolved by randomized studies include those of the potential late risks of radiotherapy and the fact that relapses may occur in new sites. As for other relapses, high-dose therapy with autologous stem cell support should be proposed to patients (128) chemosensitive to salvage chemotherapy. The role of allogeneic transplantation in relapsing patients is not yet determined as in other aggressive lymphomas but might be easier to investigate in this young population and has been performed in children (139).

It will also be important to look at the efficacy of innovative forms of therapy for ALK$^+$ anaplastic large-cell lymphoma with high IPI scores and for ALK$^-$ anaplastic large-cell lymphomas. Anti-CD30 monoclonal antibodies conjugated to toxins (140) or radioisotopes or vaccination strategies (141) may represent new tools. The use of drugs inhibiting NPM-ALK kinase activity (142) or interfering with the downstream signaling pathways (143) may also be expected to play a future role in the therapy of ALK$^+$ anaplastic large-cell lymphoma. The role of anti-CD20 should be explored in anaplastic large-cell lymphoma-B in combination with chemotherapy, as demonstrated with other large diffuse B-cell lymphomas (144).

REFERENCES

1. Harris NL, Jaffe ES, Stein H, et al. A revised European-American classification of lymphoid neoplasms: a proposal from the International Lymphoma Study Group. *Blood* 1994;84:1361–1392.
2. Jaffe ES, Harris NL, Stein H, et al., eds. *World Health Organization Classification of Tumours: Pathology and Genetics of Tumours of Haematopoietic and Lymphoid Tissues.* Lyon: IARC Press, 2001.
3. Stein H, Mason DY, Gerdes J, et al. The expression of the Hodgkin's disease associated antigen Ki-1 in reactive and neoplastic lymphoid tissue: evidence that Reed-Sternberg cells and histiocytic malignancies are derived from activated lymphoid cells. *Blood* 1985;66:848–858.
4. Schwab U, Stein H, Gerdes J, et al. Production of a monoclonal antibody specific for Hodgkin and Sternberg-Reed cells of Hodgkin's disease and a subset of normal lymphoid cells. *Nature* 1982;299:65–67.
5. Benz-Lemoine E, Brizard A, Huret JL, et al. Malignant histiocytosis: a specific t(2;5)(p23;q35) translocation? Review of the literature. *Blood* 1988;72:1045–1047.
6. Kaneko Y, Frizzera G, Edamura S, et al. A novel translocation, t(2;5)(p23;q35), in childhood phagocytic large T-cell lymphoma mimicking malignant histiocytosis. *Blood* 1989;73:806–813.
7. Rimokh R, Magaud JP, Berger F, et al. A translocation involving a specific breakpoint (q35) on chromosome 5 is characteristic of anaplastic large cell lymphoma ('Ki-1 lymphoma'). *Br J Haematol* 1989;71:31–36.
8. Bitter MA, Franklin WA, Larson RA, et al. Morphology in Ki-1(CD30)-positive non-Hodgkin's lymphoma is correlated with clinical features and the presence of a unique chromosomal abnormality, t(2;5)(p23;q35). *Am J Surg Pathol* 1990;14:305–316.
9. Mason DY, Bastard C, Rimokh R, et al. CD30-positive large cell lymphomas ('Ki-1 lymphoma') are associated with a chromosomal translocation involving 5q35. *Br J Haematol* 1990;74:161–168.
10. Morris SW, Kirstein MN, Valentine MB, et al. Fusion of a kinase gene, ALK, to a nucleolar protein gene, NPM, in non-Hodgkin's lymphoma. *Science* 1994;263:1281–1284.
11. Ladanyi M. The NPM/ALK gene fusion in the pathogenesis of anaplastic large cell lymphoma. *Cancer Surv* 1997;30:59–75.
12. Kadin ME. Anaplastic large cell lymphoma and its morphological variants. *Cancer Surv* 1997;30:77–86.
13. Stein H, Foss HD, Durkop H, et al. CD30(+) anaplastic large cell lymphoma: a review of its histopathologic, genetic, and clinical features. *Blood* 2000;96:3681–3695.
14. Falini B. Anaplastic large cell lymphoma: pathological, molecular and clinical features. *Br J Haematol* 2001;114:741–760.
15. Benharroch D, Meguerian-Bedoyan Z, Lamant L, et al. ALK-positive lymphoma: a single disease with a broad spectrum of morphology. *Blood* 1998;91:2076–2084.
16. Kinney MC, Collins RD, Greer JP, et al. A small-cell-predominant variant of primary Ki-1 (CD30)+ T-cell lymphoma. *Am J Surg Pathol* 1993;17:859–868.
17. Falini B, Bigerna B, Fizzotti M, et al. ALK expression defines a distinct group of T/null lymphomas ("ALK lymphomas") with a wide morphological spectrum. *Am J Pathol* 1998;153:875–886.
18. Falini B, Pileri S, Zinzani PL, et al. ALK+ lymphoma: clinico-pathological findings and outcome. *Blood* 1999;93:2697–2706.
19. Pileri S, Falini B, Delsol G, et al. Lymphohistiocytic T-cell lymphoma (anaplastic large cell lymphoma CD30+/Ki-1+ with a high content of reactive histiocytes). *Histopathology* 1990;16:383–391.
20. Lennert KF. *Histopathology of non-Hodgkin's lymphoma.* Berlin: Springer-Verlag, 1990.
21. Chan JK, Buchanan R, Fletcher CD. Sarcomatoid variant of anaplastic large-cell Ki-1 lymphoma. *Am J Surg Pathol* 1990;14:983–988.
22. Pereira EM, Maeda SA, Reis-Filho JS. Sarcomatoid variant of anaplastic large cell lymphoma mimicking a primary breast cancer: a challenging diagnosis. *Arch Pathol Lab Med* 2002;126:723–726.
23. Mann KP, Hall B, Kamino H, et al. Neutrophil-rich, Ki-1-positive anaplastic large-cell malignant lymphoma. *Am J Surg Pathol* 1995;19:407–416.
24. Cheuk W, Hill RW, Bacchi C, et al. Hypocellular anaplastic large cell lymphoma mimicking inflammatory lesions of lymph nodes. *Am J Surg Pathol* 2000;24:1537–1543.
25. Falini B, Liso A, Pasqualucci L, et al. CD30+ anaplastic large-cell lymphoma, null type, with signet-ring appearance. *Histopathology* 1997;30:90–92.
26. Chittal SM, Delsol G. The interface of Hodgkin's disease and anaplastic large cell lymphoma. *Cancer Surv* 1997;30:87–105.
27. Falini B, Pileri S, Pizzolo G, et al. CD30 (Ki-1) molecule: a new cytokine receptor of the tumor necrosis factor receptor superfamily as a tool for diagnosis and immunotherapy. *Blood* 1995;85:1–14.
28. Durkop H, Latza U, Hummel M, et al. Molecular cloning and expression of a new member of the nerve growth factor receptor family that is characteristic for Hodgkin's disease. *Cell* 1992;68:421–427.
29. Smith CA, Gruss HJ, Davis T, et al. CD30 antigen, a marker for Hodgkin's lymphoma, is a receptor whose ligand defines an emerging family of cytokines with homology to TNF. *Cell* 1993;73:1349–1360.
30. A clinical evaluation of the International Lymphoma Study Group classification of non-Hodgkin's lymphoma. The Non-Hodgkin's Lymphoma Classification Project. *Blood* 1997;89:3909–3918.
31. Delsol G, Al Saati T, Gatter KC, et al. Coexpression of epithelial membrane antigen (EMA), Ki-1, and interleukin-2 receptor by anaplastic large cell lymphomas. Diagnostic value in so-called malignant histiocytosis. *Am J Pathol* 1988;130:59–70.
32. ten Berge RL, Snijdewint FG, von Mensdorff-Pouilly S, et al. MUC1 (EMA) is preferentially expressed by ALK positive anaplastic large cell lymphoma, in the normally glycosylated or only partly hypoglycosylated form. *J Clin Pathol* 2001;54:933–939.
33. Shiota M, Fujimoto J, Takenaga M, et al. Diagnosis of t(2;5)(p23;q35)-associated Ki-1 lymphoma with immunohistochemistry. *Blood* 1994;84:3648–3652.
34. Pulford K, Lamant L, Morris SW, et al. Detection of anaplastic lymphoma kinase (ALK) and nucleolar protein nucleophosmin (NPM)-ALK proteins in normal and neoplastic cells with the monoclonal antibody ALK1. *Blood* 1997;89:1394–1404.
35. Rassidakis GZ, Medeiros, LJ, Herling M, et al. BCL-2 is expressed in ALK-negative but not ALK-positive anaplastic large cell lymphoma. *Blood* 2000;96.
36. Raetz EA, Perkins SL, Carlson MA, et al. The nucleophosmin-anaplastic lymphoma kinase fusion protein induces c-Myc expression in pediatric anaplastic large cell lymphomas. *Am J Pathol* 2002;161:875–883.
37. Krenacs L, Wellmann A, Sorbara L, et al. Cytotoxic cell antigen expression in anaplastic large cell lymphomas of T- and null-cell type and Hodgkin's disease: evidence for distinct cellular origin. *Blood* 1997;89:980–989.
38. Foss HD, Anagnostopoulos I, Araujo I, et al. Anaplastic large-cell lymphomas of T-cell and null-cell phenotype express cytotoxic molecules. *Blood* 1996;88:4005–4011.
39. Haralambieva E, Pulford KA, Lamant L, et al. Anaplastic large-cell lymphomas of B-cell phenotype are anaplastic lymphoma kinase (ALK) negative and belong to the spectrum of diffuse large B-cell lymphomas. *Br J Haematol* 2000;109:584–591.
40. Alsabeh R, Medeiros LJ, Glackin C, et al. Transformation of follicular lymphoma into CD30-large cell lymphoma with anaplastic cytologic features. *Am J Surg Pathol* 1997;21:528–536.
41. Kuze T, Nakamura N, Hashimoto Y, et al. Most of CD30+ anaplastic large cell lymphoma of B cell type show a somatic mutation in the IgH V region genes. *Leukemia* 1998;12:753–757.
42. Chan PK, Chan FY, Morris SW, et al. Isolation and characterization of the human nucleophosmin/B23 (NPM) gene: identification of the YY1 binding site at the 5' enhancer region. *Nucleic Acids Res* 1997;25:1225–1232.
43. Cordell JL, Pulford KA, Bigerna B, et al. Detection of normal and chimeric nucleophosmin in human cells. *Blood* 1999;93:632–642.
44. Borer RA, Lehner CF, Eppenberger HM, et al. Major nucleolar proteins shuttle between nucleus and cytoplasm. *Cell* 1989;56:379–390.
45. Okuwaki M, Matsumoto K, Tsujimoto M, et al. Function of nucleophosmin/B23, a nucleolar acidic protein, as a histone chaperone. *FEBS Lett* 2001;506:272–276.
46. Colombo E, Marine JC, Danovi D, et al. Nucleophosmin regulates the stability and transcriptional activity of p53. *Nat Cell Biol* 2002;4:529–533.
47. Okuda M. The role of nucleophosmin in centrosome duplication. *Oncogene* 2002;21:6170–6174.
48. Shiota M, Fujimoto J, Semba T, et al. Hyperphosphorylation of a novel 80 kDa protein-tyrosine kinase similar to Ltk in a human Ki-1 lymphoma cell line, AMS3. *Oncogene* 1994;9:1567–1574.
49. Morris SW, Naeve C, Mathew P, et al. ALK, the chromosome 2 gene locus altered by the t(2;5) in non-Hodgkin's lymphoma, encodes a novel neural receptor tyrosine kinase that is highly related to leukocyte tyrosine kinase (LTK). *Oncogene* 1997;14:2175–2188.

50. Powers C, Aigner A, Stoica GE, et al. Pleiotrophin signaling through anaplastic lymphoma kinase is rate-limiting for glioblastoma growth. *J Biol Chem* 2002;277:14153–14158.
51. Iwahara T, Fujimoto J, Wen D, et al. Molecular characterization of ALK, a receptor tyrosine kinase expressed specifically in the nervous system. *Oncogene* 1997;14:439–449.
52. Fujimoto J, Shiota M, Iwahara T, et al. Characterization of the transforming activity of p80, a hyperphosphorylated protein in a Ki-1 lymphoma cell line with chromosomal translocation t(2;5). *Proc Natl Acad Sci U S A* 1996;93:4181–4186.
53. Bischof D, Pulford K, Mason DY, et al. Role of the nucleophosmin (NPM) portion of the non-Hodgkin's lymphoma-associated NPM-anaplastic lymphoma kinase fusion protein in oncogenesis. *Mol Cell Biol* 1997;17:2312–2325.
54. Duyster J, Bai RY, Morris SW. Translocations involving anaplastic lymphoma kinase (ALK). *Oncogene* 2001;20:5623–5637.
55. Kuefer MU, Look AT, Pulford K, et al. Retrovirus-mediated gene transfer of NPM-ALK causes lymphoid malignancy in mice. *Blood* 1997;90:2901–2910.
56. Lange K, Uckert W, Blankenstein T, et al. Overexpression of NPM-ALK induces different types of malignant lymphomas in IL-9 transgenic mice. *Oncogene* 2003;22:517–527.
57. Bai RY, Dieter P, Peschel C, et al. Nucleophosmin-anaplastic lymphoma kinase of large-cell anaplastic lymphoma is a constitutively active tyrosine kinase that utilizes phospholipase C-gamma to mediate its mitogenicity. *Mol Cell Biol* 1998;18:6951–6961.
58. Slupianek A, Nieborowska-Skorska M, Hoser G, et al. Role of phosphatidylinositol 3-kinase-Akt pathway in nucleophosmin/anaplastic lymphoma kinase-mediated lymphomagenesis. *Cancer Res* 2001;61:2194–2199.
59. Bai RY, Ouyang T, Miething C, et al. Nucleophosmin-anaplastic lymphoma kinase associated with anaplastic large-cell lymphoma activates the phosphatidylinositol 3-kinase/Akt antiapoptotic signaling pathway. *Blood* 2000;96:4319–4327.
60. Zhang Q, Raghunath PN, Xue L, et al. Multilevel dysregulation of STAT3 activation in anaplastic lymphoma kinase-positive T/null-cell lymphoma. *J Immunol* 2002;168:466–474.
61. Zamo A, Chiarle R, Piva R, et al. Anaplastic lymphoma kinase (ALK) activates Stat3 and protects hematopoietic cells from cell death. *Oncogene* 2002;21:1038–1047.
62. Nieborowska-Skorska M, Slupianek A, Xue L, et al. Role of signal transducer and activator of transcription 5 in nucleophosmin/anaplastic lymphoma kinase-mediated malignant transformation of lymphoid cells. *Cancer Res* 2001;61:6517–6523.
63. Downing JR, Shurtleff SA, Zielenska M, et al. Molecular detection of the (2;5) translocation of non-Hodgkin's lymphoma by reverse transcriptase-polymerase chain reaction. *Blood* 1995;85:3416–3422.
64. Lamant L, Meggetto F, al Saati T, et al. High incidence of the t(2;5)(p23;q35) translocation in anaplastic large cell lymphoma and its lack of detection in Hodgkin's disease. Comparison of cytogenetic analysis, reverse transcriptase-polymerase chain reaction, and P-80 immunostaining. *Blood* 1996;87:284–291.
65. Herbst H, Anagnostopoulos J, Heinze B, et al. ALK gene products in anaplastic large cell lymphomas and Hodgkin's disease. *Blood* 1995;86:1694–1700.
66. Mathew P, Sanger WG, Weisenburger DD, et al. Detection of the t(2;5)(p23;q35) and NPM-ALK fusion in non-Hodgkin's lymphoma by two-color fluorescence in situ hybridization. *Blood* 1997;89:1678–1685.
67. Hutchison RE, Banki K, Shuster JJ, et al. Use of an anti-ALK antibody in the characterization of anaplastic large-cell lymphoma of childhood. *Ann Oncol* 1997;8:37–42.
68. Falini B, Mason DY. Proteins encoded by genes involved in chromosomal alterations in lymphoma and leukemia: clinical value of their detection by immunocytochemistry. *Blood* 2002;99:409–426.
69. Falini B, Pulford K, Pucciarini A, et al. Lymphomas expressing ALK fusion protein(s) other than NPM-ALK. *Blood* 1999;94:3509–3515.
70. Mason DY, Pulford KA, Bischof D, et al. Nucleolar localization of the nucleophosmin-anaplastic lymphoma kinase is not required for malignant transformation. *Cancer Res* 1998;58:1057–1062.
71. Pulford K, Falini B, Cordell J, et al. Biochemical detection of novel anaplastic lymphoma kinase proteins in tissue sections of anaplastic large cell lymphoma. *Am J Pathol* 1999;154:1657–1663.
72. Pittaluga S, Wiodarska I, Pulford K, et al. The monoclonal antibody ALK1 identifies a distinct morphological subtype of anaplastic large cell lymphoma associated with 2p23/ALK rearrangements. *Am J Pathol* 1997;151:343–351.
73. Wlodarska I, De Wolf-Peeters C, Falini B, et al. The cryptic inv(2)(p23q35) defines a new molecular genetic subtype of ALK-positive anaplastic large-cell lymphoma. *Blood* 1998;92:2688–2695.
74. Rosenwald A, Ott G, Pulford K, et al. t(1;2)(q21;p23) and t(2;3) (p23;q21): two novel variant translocations of the t(2;5)(p23;q35) in anaplastic large cell lymphoma. *Blood* 1999;94:362–364.
75. Lamant L, Dastugue N, Pulford K, et al. A new fusion gene TPM3-ALK in anaplastic large cell lymphoma created by a (1;2)(q25;p23) translocation. *Blood* 1999;93:3088–3095.
76. Siebert R, Gesk S, Harder L, et al. Complex variant translocation t(1;2) with TPM3-ALK fusion due to cryptic ALK gene rearrangement in anaplastic large-cell lymphoma. *Blood* 1999;94:3614–3617.
77. Lawrence B, Perez-Atayde A, Hibbard MK, et al. TPM3-ALK and TPM4-ALK oncogenes in inflammatory myofibroblastic tumors. *Am J Pathol* 2000;157:377–384.
78. Ladanyi M. Aberrant ALK tyrosine kinase signaling. Different cellular lineages, common oncogenic mechanisms. *Am J Pathol* 2000;157:341–345.
79. Hernandez L, Pinyol M, Hernandez S, et al. TRK-fused gene (TFG) is a new partner of ALK in anaplastic large cell lymphoma producing two structurally different TFG-ALK translocations. *Blood* 1999;94:3265–3268.
80. Hernandez L, Bea S, Bellosillo B, et al. Diversity of genomic breakpoints in TFG-ALK translocations in anaplastic large cell lymphomas: identification of a new TFG-ALK(XL) chimeric gene with transforming activity. *Am J Pathol* 2002;160:1487–1494.
81. Colleoni GW, Bridge JA, Garicochea B, et al. ATIC-ALK: a novel variant ALK gene fusion in anaplastic large cell lymphoma resulting from the recurrent cryptic chromosomal inversion, inv(2)(p23q35). *Am J Pathol* 2000;156:781–789.
82. Ma Z, Cools J, Marynen P, et al. Inv(2)(p23q35) in anaplastic large-cell lymphoma induces constitutive anaplastic lymphoma kinase (ALK) tyrosine kinase activation by fusion to ATIC, an enzyme involved in purine nucleotide biosynthesis. *Blood* 2000;95:2144–2149.
83. Trinei M, Lanfrancone L, Campo E, et al. A new variant anaplastic lymphoma kinase (ALK)-fusion protein (ATIC-ALK) in a case of ALK-positive anaplastic large cell lymphoma. *Cancer Res* 2000;60:793–798.
84. Beardsley GP, Rayl EA, Gunn K, et al. Structure and functional relationships in human pur H. *Adv Exp Med Biol* 1998;431:221–226.
85. Meech S, Grump J, McGavran L, et al. Tropomyosin 4 (TPM4) is fused to ALK by a t(2;19)(p23;p13) in an unusual childhood ALCL with the immunophenotype and functional properties of a natural killer cell malignancy. *Blood* 2000;92.
86. Touriol C, Greenland C, Lamant L, et al. Further demonstration of the diversity of chromosomal changes involving 2p23 in ALK-positive lymphoma: 2 cases expressing ALK kinase fused to CLTCL (clathrin chain polypeptide-like). *Blood* 2000;95:3204–3207.
87. Tort F, Pinyol M, Pulford K, et al. Molecular characterization of a new ALK translocation involving moesin (MSN-ALK) in anaplastic large cell lymphoma. *Lab Invest* 2001;81:419–426.
88. Pillay K, Govender D, Chetty R. ALK protein expression in rhabdomyosarcomas. *Histopathology* 2002;41:461–467.
89. Lamant L, Pulford K, Bischof D, et al. Expression of the ALK tyrosine kinase gene in neuroblastoma. *Am J Pathol* 2000;156:1711–1721.
90. Delsol G, Lamant L, Mariame B, et al. A new subtype of large B-cell lymphoma expressing the ALK kinase and lacking the 2;5 translocation. *Blood* 1997;89:1483–1490.
91. Gascoyne RD, Aoun P, Wu D, et al. Prognostic significance of anaplastic lymphoma kinase (ALK) protein expression in adults with anaplastic large cell lymphoma. *Blood* 1999;93:3913–3921.
92. Pileri SA, Pulford K, Mori S, et al. Frequent expression of the NPM-ALK chimeric fusion protein in anaplastic large-cell lymphoma, lympho-histiocytic type. *Am J Pathol* 1997;150:1207–1211.
93. Li G, Salhany KE, Rook AH, et al. The pathogenesis of large cell transformation in cutaneous T-cell lymphoma is not associated with t(2;5)(p23;q35) chromosomal translocation. *J Cutan Pathol* 1997;24:403–408.
94. Camisa C, Helm TN, Sexton C, et al. Ki-1-positive anaplastic large-cell lymphoma can mimic benign dermatoses. *J Am Acad Dermatol* 1993;29:696–700.

95. Simonart T, Kentos A, Renoirte C, et al. Cutaneous involvement by neutrophil-rich, CD30-positive anaplastic large cell lymphoma mimicking deep pustules. *Am J Surg Pathol* 1999;23:244–246.

96. Foss HD, Reusch R, Demel G, et al. Frequent expression of the B-cell-specific activator protein in Reed-Sternberg cells of classical Hodgkin's disease provides further evidence for its B-cell origin. *Blood* 1999;94:3108–3113.

97. Griffin CA, Hawkins AL, Dvorak C, et al. Recurrent involvement of 2p23 in inflammatory myofibroblastic tumors. *Cancer Res* 1999;59: 2776–2780.

98. Cessna MH, Zhou H, Sanger WG, et al. Expression of ALK1 and p80 in inflammatory myofibroblastic tumor and its mesenchymal mimics: a study of 135 cases. *Mod Pathol* 2002;15:931–938.

99. Harris NL, Jaffe ES, Diebold J, et al. World Heath Organization Classification of neoplastic diseases of the hematopoietic and lymphoid tissues: report of the Clinical Advisory Committee Meeting. Airlie House, Virginia, November 1997. *J Clin Oncol* 1999;17:3835–3849.

100. Tilly H, Gaulard P, Lepage E, et al. Primary anaplastic large-cell lymphoma in adults: clinical presentation, immunophenotype, and outcome. *Blood* 1997;90:3727–3734.

101. Gisselbrecht C, Gaulard P, Lepage E, et al. Prognostic significance of T-cell phenotype in aggressive non-Hodgkin's lymphomas. Groupe d'Etudes des Lymphomes de l'Adulte (GELA). *Blood* 1998;92:76–82.

102. Shipp M, Harrington DP, Anderson JR, et al. Development of a predictive model for aggressive lymphoma: the International Non-Hodgkins Lymphoma Prognostic Factors Project. *N Engl J Med* 1993;329:987–994.

103. Shiota M, Nakamura S, Ichinohasama R, et al. Anaplastic large cell lymphomas expressing the novel chimeric protein p80NPM/ALK: a distinct clinicopathologic entity. *Blood* 1995;86:1954–1960.

104. Suzuki R, Kagami Y, Takeuchi K, et al. Prognostic significance of CD56 expression for ALK-positive and ALK-negative anaplastic large-cell lymphoma of T/null cell phenotype. *Blood* 2000;96:2993–3000.

105. Fraga M, Brousset P, Schlaifer D, et al. Bone marrow involvement in anaplastic large cell lymphoma. Immunohistochemical detection of minimal disease and its prognostic significance. *Am J Clin Pathol* 1995;103:82–89.

106. Sadahira Y, Hata S, Sugihara T, et al. Bone marrow involvement in NPM-ALK-positive lymphoma: report of two cases. *Pathol Res Pract* 1999;195:657–661.

107. Bayle C, Charpentier A, Duchayne E, et al. Leukaemic presentation of small cell variant anaplastic large cell lymphoma: report of four cases. *Br J Haematol* 1999;104:680–688.

108. Chhanabhai M, Britten C, Klasa R, et al. t(2;5) positive lymphoma with peripheral blood involvement. *Leuk Lymphoma* 1998;28:415–422.

109. Greer JP, Kinney MC, Collins RD, et al. Clinical features of 31 patients with Ki-1 anaplastic large-cell lymphoma. *J Clin Oncol* 1991;9:539–547.

110. Brugieres L, Deley MC, Pacquement H, et al. CD30(+) anaplastic large-cell lymphoma in children: analysis of 82 patients enrolled in two consecutive studies of the French Society of Pediatric Oncology. *Blood* 1998;92:3591–3598.

111. Seidemann K, Tiemann M, Schrappe M, et al. Short-pulse B-non-Hodgkin lymphoma-type chemotherapy is efficacious treatment for pediatric anaplastic large cell lymphoma: a report of the Berlin-Frankfurt-Munster Group Trial NHL-BFM 90. *Blood* 2001;97:3699–3706.

112. Costes-Martineau V, Delfour C, Obled S, et al. Anaplastic lymphoma kinase (ALK) protein expressing lymphoma after liver transplantation: case report and literature review. *J Clin Pathol* 2002;55:868–871.

113. Tirelli U, Vaccher E, Zagonel V, et al. CD30 (Ki-1)-positive anaplastic large-cell lymphomas in 13 patients with and 27 patients without human immunodeficiency virus infection: the first comparative clinicopathologic study from a single institution that also includes 80 patients with other human immunodeficiency virus-related systemic lymphomas. *J Clin Oncol* 1995;13:373–380.

114. Gabarre J, Raphael M, Lepage E, et al. Human immunodeficiency virus-related lymphoma: relation between clinical features and histologic subtypes. *Am J Med* 2001;111:704–711.

115. Chadburn A, Cesarman E, Jagirdar J, et al. CD30 (Ki-1) positive anaplastic large cell lymphomas in individuals infected with the human immunodeficiency virus. *Cancer* 1993;72:3078–3090.

116. Salhany KE, Cousar JB, Greer JP, et al. Transformation of cutaneous T cell lymphoma to large cell lymphoma. A clinicopathologic and immunologic study. *Am J Pathol* 1988;132:265–277.

117. Lopez-Guillermo A, Cid J, Salar A, et al. Peripheral T-cell lymphomas: initial features, natural history, and prognostic factors in a series of 174 patients diagnosed according to the R.E.A.L. Classification. *Ann Oncol* 1998;9:849–855.

118. Shipp M. Prognostic factors in non-Hodgkin's lymphoma. *Curr Opin Oncol* 1992;4:856–862.

119. ten Berge RL, Meijer CJ, Dukers DF, et al. Expression levels of apoptosis-related proteins predict clinical outcome in anaplastic large cell lymphoma. *Blood* 2002;99:4540–4546.

120. Le Deley MC, Reiter A, Williams D, et al. Prognostic factors in childhood anaplastic large cell lymphoma: results of the European Intergroup Study. *Ann Oncol* 1999:10(Suppl 3).

121. Reiter A, Schrappe M, Tiemann M, et al. Successful treatment strategy for Ki-1 anaplastic large-cell lymphoma of childhood: a prospective analysis of 62 patients enrolled in three consecutive Berlin-Frankfurt-Munster group studies. *J Clin Oncol* 1994;12:899–908.

122. Vecchi V, Burnelli R, Pileri S, et al. Anaplastic large cell lymphoma (Ki-1+/CD30+) in childhood. *Med Pediatr Oncol* 1993;21:402–410.

123. Massimino M, Gasparini M, Giardini R. Ki-1 (CD30) anaplastic large-cell lymphoma in children. *Ann Oncol* 1995;6:915–920.

124. Sandlund JT, Pui CH, Santana VM, et al. Clinical features and treatment outcome for children with CD30+ large-cell non-Hodgkin's lymphoma. *J Clin Oncol* 1994;12:895–898.

125. Anderson JR, Jenkin RD, Wilson JF, et al. Long-term follow-up of patients treated with COMP or LSA2L2 therapy for childhood non-Hodgkin's lymphoma: a report of CCG-551 from the Childrens Cancer Group. *J Clin Oncol* 1993;11:1024–1032.

126. Zinzani PL, Martelli M, Magagnoli M, et al. Anaplastic large cell lymphoma Hodgkin's-like: a randomized trial of ABVD versus MACOP-B with and without radiation therapy. *Blood* 1998;92:790–794.

127. Shulman LN, Frisard B, Antin JH, et al. Primary Ki-1 anaplastic large-cell lymphoma in adults: clinical characteristics and therapeutic outcome. *J Clin Oncol* 1993;11:937–942.

128. Fanin R, Silvestri F, Geromin A, et al. Primary systemic CD30 (Ki-1)-positive anaplastic large cell lymphoma of the adult: sequential intensive treatment with the F-MACHOP regimen (+/– radiotherapy) and autologous bone marrow transplantation. *Blood* 1996;87:1243–1248.

129. Fanin R, Ruiz de Elvira MC, Sperotto A, et al. Autologous stem cell transplantation for T and null cell CD30-positive anaplastic large cell lymphoma: analysis of 64 adult and paediatric cases reported to the European Group for Blood and Marrow Transplantation (EBMT). *Bone Marrow Transplant* 1999;23:437–442.

130. Pileri S, Bocchia M, Baroni CD, et al. Anaplastic large cell lymphoma (CD30+/Ki-1+): results of a prospective clinico-pathological study of 69 cases. *Br J Haematol* 1994;86:513–523.

131. Romaguera JE, Garcia-Foncillas J, Cabanillas F. 16-year experience at M. D. Anderson Cancer Center with primary Ki-1 (CD30) antigen expression and anaplastic morphology in adult patients with diffuse large cell lymphoma. *Leuk Lymphoma* 1995;20:97–102.

132. Offit K, Ladanyi M, Gangi MD, et al. Ki-1 antigen expression defines a favorable clinical subset of non-B cell non-Hodgkin's lymphoma. *Leukemia* 1990;4:625–630.

133. Zinzani PL, Bendandi M, Martelli M, et al. Anaplastic large-cell lymphoma: clinical and prognostic evaluation of 90 adult patients. *J Clin Oncol* 1996;14:955–962.

134. Deconinck E, Lamy T, Foussard C, et al. Autologous stem cell transplantation for anaplastic large-cell lymphomas: results of a prospective trial. *Br J Haematol* 2000;109:736–742.

135. Haioun C, Lepage E, Gisselbrecht C, et al. Survival benefit of high-dose therapy in poor-risk aggressive non-Hodgkin's lymphoma: final analysis of the prospective LNH87-2 protocol—A Groupe d'Etude des Lymphomes de l'Adulte study. *J Clin Oncol* 2000;18:3025–3030.

136. Shipp MA, Abeloff MD, Antman KH, et al. International consensus conference on high-dose therapy with hematopoietic stem cell transplantation in aggressive non-Hodgkin's lymphomas: report of the jury [see comments]. *J Clin Oncol* 1999;17:423–429.

137. Miller TP, Dahlberg S, Cassady JR, et al. Chemotherapy alone compared with chemotherapy plus radiotherapy for localized intermediate- and high-grade non-Hodgkin's lymphoma. *N Engl J Med* 1998;339:21–26.

138. Reyes F, Lepage E, Munck JN, et al. Superiority of the ACVBP regimen over a combined treatment with three cycles of CHOP followed by involved field radiotherapy in patients (pts) with low risk localized aggressive non Hodgkin's lymphoma: results of the LNH93-1 study. *Blood* 2000;96(11).

139. Chakravarti V, Kamani NR, Bayever E, et al. Bone marrow transplantation for childhood Ki-1 lymphoma. *J Clin Oncol* 1990;8:657–660.

140. Falini B, Terenzi A, Liso A, et al. Targeted antibodies in the treatment of lymphomas. *Cancer Surv* 1997;30:295–309.

141. Passoni L, Scardino A, Bertazzoli C, et al. ALK as a novel lymphoma-associated tumor antigen: identification of 2 HLA-A2.1-restricted CD8+ T-cell epitopes. *Blood* 2002;99:2100–2106.

142. Turturro F, Arnold MD, Frist AY, et al. Model of inhibition of the NPM-ALK kinase activity by herbimycin A. *Clin Cancer Res* 2002;8:240–245.

143. Bonvini P, Gastaldi T, Falini B, et al. Nucleophosmin-anaplastic lymphoma kinase (NPM-ALK), a novel Hsp90-client tyrosine kinase: down-regulation of NPM-ALK expression and tyrosine phosphorylation in ALK(+) CD30(+) lymphoma cells by the Hsp90 antagonist 17-allylamino,17-demethoxygeldanamycin. *Cancer Res* 2002;62:1559–1566.

144. Coiffier B, Lepage E, Briere J, et al. CHOP chemotherapy plus rituximab compared with CHOP alone in elderly patients with diffuse large-B-cell lymphoma. *N Engl J Med* 2002;346:235–242.

145. Chikatsu N, Kojima H, Suzukawa K, et al. ALK+, CD30−, CD20− large B-cell lymphoma containing anaplastic lymphoma kinase (ALK) fused to clathrin heavy chain gene (CLTC). *Mod Pathol* 2003;16(8):828–832.

146. De Paepe P, Baens M, Van Krieken H, et al. ALK activation by the CTLC-ALK fusion is a recurrent event in large B-cell lymphoma. *Blood* 2003;May 15.

147. Gascoyne RD, Lamant L, Martin-Subero JI, et al. ALK-positive diffuse large B-cell lymphoma is associated with Clathrin-ALK rearrangements: report of six cases. *Blood* 2003;May 22.

148. Onciu M, Behm FG, Downing JR, et al. ALK-positive plasmablastic B-cell lymphoma with expression of the NPM-ALK fusion transcript: report of two cases. *Blood* 2003;Jun 19.

CHAPTER 26

Mature Nodal and Extranodal T-Cell and Non-Hodgkin–Cell Lymphomas (Peripheral T-Cell, Angioimmunoblastic, Nasal Natural Killer/T-Cell, Hepatosplenic T-Cell, Enteropathy-Type T-Cell, and Subcutaneous Panniculitis-Like T-Cell Lymphomas)

James O. Armitage, Raymond H. S. Liang, John W. Sweetenham, Félix Reyes, Elaine S. Jaffe, and Mark Raffeld

DEFINITION

The peripheral T-cell lymphomas are a subset of the non-Hodgkin's lymphomas that display T-cell or natural killer (NK)-cell immunophenotypes. In the broadest sense, any T-cell non-Hodgkin's lymphoma other than lymphoblastic lymphoma (i.e., the lymphoma that corresponds to T-cell acute lymphoblastic leukemia) is a peripheral T-cell lymphoma. However, by convention, anaplastic large T/null-cell lymphoma, mycosis fungoides, and adult T-cell lymphoma or leukemia are considered separately based on distinctive clinical features or pathogenesis. The remaining NK/T-cell lymphomas are lumped together under the name *peripheral T-cell lymphoma*. However, this is a heterogeneous group of disorders and includes peripheral T-cell lymphoma not otherwise specified (NOS) (i.e., those T-cell lymphomas not belonging to a defined entity) and several other less frequent disorders that represent distinctive clinical/pathologic syndromes. These include angioimmunoblastic T-cell lymphoma, subcutaneous panniculitis-like T-cell lymphoma, enteropathy-type T-cell lymphoma, nasal NK/T lymphoma, and hepatosplenic lymphoma.

FREQUENCY

The lymphomas lumped together under the title *peripheral T-cell lymphoma* represented 6% to 7% of non-Hodgkin's lymphomas in one large international study (1). In that study, peripheral T-cell lymphoma NOS represented approximately 4% of all non-Hodgkin's lymphomas; angioimmunoblastic T-cell lymphoma and angiocentric nasal NK/T-cell lymphoma each represented slightly more than 1% of all non-Hodgkin's lymphomas, and the other subtypes were rare. The exact frequency of the specific subtypes of peripheral T-cell lymphoma recognized in any particular study depends on the origin of the patients (2). Angioimmunoblastic T-cell lymphoma made up approximately 20% of all T-cell lymphomas in the Kiel Registry (3) and slightly less in a study from Italy (4). The extranodal NK/T-cell lymphoma of nasal type (sometimes called *angiocentric lymphoma*) has a striking geographic variation in frequency of occurrence and has been rarely observed in the United States and Europe but is seen frequently in Asia and in the native populations of Mexico and Central and South America (5). Enteropathy-type T-cell lymphoma has been most frequently recognized in patients with untreated gluten-sensitive enteropathy (6,7).

PATHOLOGY

Mature T-cell neoplasms are derived from mature or post-thymic T cells. Because NK cells are closely related and share some immunophenotypic and functional properties with T cells, these two classes of neoplasms are considered together (8).

T-cell lymphomas manifest the immunophenotypic features of postthymic T lymphocytes. There are two major classes of T-cells: αβ T cells and γδ T cells (9). This distinction is based on the structure of the T-cell receptor. The αβ and γδ chains are each composed of an external variable (V) and constant (C) portion. They both are associated with CD3, which is identical in both T-cell subsets. CD3 contains γ, δ, and ε chains. Although NK cells do not have a complete T-cell–receptor complex, NK cells usually express the ε chain of CD3 in the cytoplasm, which can be recognized by polyclonal antibodies to CD3.

γδ T cells are negative for both CD4 and CD8 and also usually negative for CD5. γδ T cells represent a more primitive type of immune response. They comprise less than 5% of all normal T cells and show a restricted distribution, being found mainly in the splenic red pulp, intestinal epithelium, and other epithelial sites. It is notable that these sites are more commonly affected by γδ T-cell lymphomas, which are relatively rare (10–12). γδ T cells have a restricted range of antigen recognition. They are not major histocompatibility complex restricted in their function and represent a first line of defense against bacterial peptides, such as heat shock proteins (9). They are often involved in responses to mycobacterial infections and mucosal immunity.

αβ T cells are divided into two major subtypes: CD4[+] and CD8[+]. In normal lymphoid tissues, CD4[+] cells exceed CD8[+] cells, and a similar ratio is seen among malignant diseases. CD4 T cells, or "helper T-cells," are mainly cytokine-secreting cells, whereas CD8 T cells are mainly involved in cytotoxic immune reactions. CD4 cells are divided into two major types based on their cytokine-secretion profiles: Th1 cells secrete interleukin (IL)-2 and interferon γ but not IL-4, -5, or -6. In contrast, Th2 cells secrete IL-4, -5, -6, and -10 (9). Th1 cells provide help mainly to other T cells and macrophages, whereas Th2 cells provide help mainly to B cells in their production of antibodies (13).

NK cells share some functions and markers with cytotoxic T cells. They can express CD2, CD7, CD8, CD56, and CD57, all of which can be seen in some T-cell subsets. As noted above, they also are often positive for the ε chain of CD3. However, they are usually positive for CD16, which is less often positive on T cells. Both NK cells and cytotoxic T cells express cytotoxic proteins, including perforin, granzyme B, and T-cell intracellular antigen (TIA)-1 (14). These antigens are also seen in cytotoxic T-cell and NK-cell malignancies (15).

The classification of T-cell and NK-cell neoplasms proposed by the World Health Organization (WHO) emphasizes a multiparameter approach, integrating morphologic, immunophenotypic, genetic, and clinical features (Table 26.1). Clinical features have particular importance in the subclassification of these tumors, in part due to the lack of specificity of other parameters. T-cell lymphomas show great morphologic diversity, and a spectrum of histologic appearances can

TABLE 26.1. *Mature T-cell and natural killer (NK)-cell neoplasms*

Leukemic or disseminated
  T-cell prolymphocytic leukemia
  T-cell granular lymphocytic leukemia
  Aggressive NK-cell leukemia
  Adult T-cell lymphoma/leukemia (human T-cell leukemia virus type I+)
Extranodal
  Extranodal NK/T-cell lymphoma, nasal type
  Enteropathy-type T-cell lymphoma
  Hepatosplenic T-cell lymphoma
  Subcutaneous panniculitis-like T-cell lymphoma
Cutaneous
  Blastic NK-cell lymphoma
  Mycosis fungoides/Sézary syndrome
  Anaplastic large-cell lymphoma, T/null-cell, primary cutaneous type
Nodal
  Peripheral T-cell lymphoma, not otherwise characterized
  Angioimmunoblastic T-cell lymphoma
  Anaplastic large-cell lymphoma, T/null-cell, primary systemic type

be seen within individual disease entities. The cellular composition can range from small cells with minimal atypia to large cells with anaplastic features. Moreover, there is morphologic overlap between disease entities. Many of the extranodal cytotoxic T-cell and NK-cell lymphomas share similar appearances, including prominent apoptosis, necrosis, and angioinvasion (Table 26.2) (16).

In contrast to B-cell lymphomas, specific immunophenotypic profiles are not associated with most T-cell–lymphoma subtypes. Although certain antigens are commonly associated with specific disease entities, these associations are not entirely disease specific. For example, CD30 is a universal feature of anaplastic large-cell lymphoma but can be expressed, usually to a lesser extent, in other T-cell and

TABLE 26.2. *Common features of extranodal T/natural killer–cell lymphomas*

Broad cytologic spectrum
Disease definition is heavily dependent on clinical features, not morphology
Infrequent lymph node involvement, even with recurrences
Frequent spread to other extranodal sites
Cytotoxic T-cell or natural killer–cell phenotype
Frequent apoptosis and/or necrosis, with or without angioinvasion
Increased incidence of hemophagocytic syndrome
Presence of Epstein-Barr virus correlates with both anatomic site and geographic factors

TABLE 26.3. *Extranodal natural killer (NK)/T-cell lymphomas*

Subtype	Epstein-Barr virus	CD3	TIA-1	GranB/Per	CD56	Major	Minor
SPTCL	–	+s	+	+	–/+	αβ	γδ
ETTL	–/+	+s	+	+	–/+	αβ	γδ/NK
Nasal	+	+c	+	+	+	NK	γδ/αβ
Hep/spl	–	+s	+	–	+	γδ	αβ

c, cytoplasmic CD3; ETTL, enteropathy-type T-cell lymphoma; GranB/Per, Granzyme B, perforin; Hep/spl, hepatosplenic T-cell lymphoma; Nasal, nasal NK/T-cell lymphoma; s, surface CD3; SPTCL, subcutaneous panniculitis-like T-cell lymphoma; TIA-1, T-cell intracellular antigen.

B-cell lymphomas. CD30 is, of course, also positive in Hodgkin's lymphoma. Similarly, although CD56 is a characteristic feature of nasal NK/T-cell lymphoma, it can be seen in other T-cell lymphomas and even malignant plasma cell neoplasms (17–19). Additionally, within a given disease entity, variation in the immunophenotypic features can be seen (Table 26.3). For example, hepatosplenic T-cell lymphomas are usually of γδ T-cell phenotype, but a minority of cases is of αβ derivation.

Finally, in contrast to B-cell lymphomas, there are no convenient immunophenotypic markers of monoclonality, although the presence of an aberrant immunophenotype may point toward a diagnosis of malignancy (20). Therefore, molecular studies, most commonly polymerase chain reaction studies for rearrangement of the T-cell–receptor genes, are generally required to evaluate the clonality of a T-cell proliferative process (21,22). Presently, specific genetic features have not been identified for many of the T-cell and NK-cell neoplasms. The molecular pathogenesis of most T-cell and NK-cell neoplasms remains to be defined. For the above reasons, clinical features at present play a major role in the subclassification of T-cell and NK-cell neoplasms. Several broad clinical groups are delineated: (a) leukemic or disseminated, (b) nodal, (c) extranodal, and (d) cutaneous. The diseases within these broad clinical groupings often share clinicopathologic and immunophenotypic features (16).

PATHOGENESIS OF THE PERIPHERAL T CELL

The peripheral T-cell and NK-cell lymphomas comprise an interesting group of neoplasms with regard to the relationship between their cellular origin and their pathology. These lymphomas show pathologic features that in many cases reflect their unique cellular origin and cytotoxic potential. For instance, the necrosis accompanying many of these lymphomas is most likely related to the presence of high concentrations of cytotoxic proteins, the granzymes and perforin that many of these lymphomas contain. The intraepithelial spread that is often seen in the enteropathy-type T-cell lymphomas most likely reflects their expression of CD103, a homing receptor unique to intraepithelial T

cells, and their derivative tumors (23). Abnormalities of the FAS death–signaling pathways and overexpression of cytotoxic protein inhibitors, reported to occur in extranodal NK/T-cell lymphoma, allow this cytotoxic lymphoma to escape from potential deleterious effects of their own cytotoxic machinery (24–26).

Unlike the mature B-cell lymphomas, for which the study of pathogenesis has been driven by the identification of tumor-specific translocations involving antigen-receptor genes, such as the t(14;18) in follicular lymphoma, the t(11;14) in mantle cell lymphoma, and the t(8;14) in Burkitt's lymphoma, there are no recurrent translocations characterizing the subtypes of peripheral T-cell lymphomas. Consequently, there is little information about the molecular pathogenesis of mature T-cell lymphomas. The one notable exception is anaplastic large-cell lymphoma, in which identification of the t(2;5) translocation led to the identification of the nucleophosmin/anaplastic lymphoma kinase fusion protein that results in the constitutive activation of the anaplastic lymphoma kinase and its downstream pathways (27). This T-cell lymphoma is covered in Chapter 25. The relative difficulty in obtaining cytogenetic data relates to the low incidence of the T- and NK-cell lymphomas, the polymorphous nature of many of these lymphomas, and the paucity of derivative cell lines. Recently, through the use of specialized cytogenetic technologies, such as comparative genomic hybridization and spectral karyotyping, some progress has been made in beginning to define the molecular lesions in the peripheral T-cell lymphomas.

The pathogenesis of peripheral T- and NK-cell lymphomas to date has been driven by an attempt to understand their clinical behavior and pathologic characteristics rather than through the identification of molecular cytogenetic abnormalities, as has been the case with the mature B-cell lymphomas. The molecular approach to pathogenesis has been stymied by the low incidence of these lymphomas, by their polymorphous histologies, and by a general lack of animal models and representative cell lines. Technical advances in cytogenetics, molecular biology, and protein chemistry are beginning to provide new insights into their pathogenesis, and it is only a matter of time before powerful genomic and proteomic technologies begin to shed more light on the enigmatic pathogenesis of these uncommon tumors.

Human γδ lymphocytes are a minor subset of normal postthymic T cells, with cytotoxic functions and preferential homing in restricted areas (28,29). There are two subsets of normal T cells, which differ by the structure of the T-cell receptor—αβ or γδ—the latter being expressed by less than 5% of normal T cells. γδ and αβ chains are each composed, like the chains of immunoglobulins in B cells, of V and C regions as a result of chronologically ordered events: γ and δ gene rearrangements first take place and, when not productive, are followed by α and β. Both αβ and γδ T-cell receptors are associated with the CD3 complex, which is identical in both T-cell subsets. αβ and γδ receptors can be detected at the cellular level—on cell suspensions or frozen tissue sections—by staining with the βF1 and δ T-cell antigen receptor (TCR)-1 monoclonal antibodies, which recognize a nonpolymorphic epitope of the β and δ chains, respectively. The CD3 complex can be detected at the cell surface and on frozen sections by the monoclonal Leu-4 antibody and also by both polyclonal and monoclonal antibodies recognizing its cytoplasmic ε chain in paraffin-embedded sections.

Thus, γδ cells express surface and cytoplasmic CD3, but unlike αβ cells, they usually have a double negative (CD4⁻ CD8⁻) phenotype (although some may express CD8) and are negative for CD5. Normal γδ T cells are preferentially located at extranodal sites, such as the splenic red pulp, intestinal epithelium, and skin (30,31). They have a limited range of antigen recognition in a non–major histocompatibility complex–restricted manner and are believed to act as a first line of defense against bacterial infections (28,29). Like a small subset of CD8⁻ αβ T cells, γδ T cells share with true (non-T) NK cells a cytotoxic potential, as revealed by the presence of cytoplasmic granules containing the cytotoxic TIA-1 protein and the expression of the CD56 marker (32). NK cells differ, however, in the absence of γδ/αβ T-cell–receptor rearrangements and protein and the lack of surface CD3, but in common with T cells, they exhibit the cytoplasmic ε chain of the TCR complex.

Based on clinical, pathologic, and phenotypic features, the recognition of the γδ T-cell hepatosplenic lymphoma subtype has been further supported by its association with the isochromosome 7q cytogenetic abnormality (33). More recently, cases of hepatosplenic lymphoma with an αβ T-cell–receptor phenotype have been reported (34–36) that are now considered in the WHO Classification as a phenotypic variant of the same disease entity (37).

SPECIFIC DISEASE ENTITIES

Peripheral T-Cell Lymphoma Not Otherwise Specified

There is a rapid change in our understanding of peripheral T-cell lymphomas currently under way. From a heterogeneous group of disorders, specific clinical-pathologic syndromes are steadily being split away. Many of those are dealt with later in this chapter. Those peripheral T-cell lymphomas that do not fit into a recognized clinical-pathologic entity are lumped together in the category *peripheral T-cell lymphoma NOS*. It is entirely possible that this category will dwindle as new insights are gained by clinical observations, new histologic observations, or, more likely, by ongoing genetic studies.

Many of the papers describing the clinical characteristics and treatment outcome in peripheral T-cell lymphomas were published before any of the currently recognized specific clinical-pathologic entities were described. Because of that, the data reviewed in this section sometimes include patients who would today be excluded. A recent international study of 1,378 cases of non-Hodgkin's lymphoma found that 7% of the cases represented peripheral T-cell lymphomas (1). Of these peripheral T-cell lymphomas, peripheral T-cell lymphoma NOS represented 55%, angiocentric nasal lymphomas 20%, angioimmunoblastic lymphomas 18%, intestinal T-cell lymphomas 5%, and only a single case of hepatosplenic T-cell lymphoma was identified (38). There were no cases of subcutaneous panniculitis–like T-cell lymphoma seen in that large series.

Peripheral T-cell lymphomas were not geographically evenly distributed in the previously mentioned international study (2). Peripheral T-cell or NK-cell lymphomas represented 2% of the cases studied in North America, 6% of the cases studied from Europe, 8% of the cases studied from southern Africa, and 18% of the cases studied from Hong Kong.

Pathology

The majority of peripheral T-cell lymphomas arising in lymph nodes fall into the unspecified category and are characterized by a heterogeneous cellular composition. There is usually a mixture of small and large atypical lymphoid cells. An inflammatory background is frequent, consisting of eosinophils, plasma cells, and histiocytes. If the epithelioid histiocytes are numerous and clustered, the case meets criteria for lymphoepithelioid-cell lymphoma, so-called Lennert's lymphoma (39). In the WHO Classification, lymphoepithelioid-cell lymphoma is considered a morphologic variant of peripheral T-cell lymphoma NOS and not a distinctive clinicopathologic entity. Peripheral T-cell lymphomas may show preferential involvement of the paracortical region of lymph nodes. In some cases, this architectural pattern is striking, with sparing of follicles. Such cases have been referred to as *T-zone lymphoma* (40,41), also considered a morphologic variant of peripheral T-cell lymphoma in the WHO Classification.

Thus far, immunophenotypic criteria have not been helpful in delineating subtypes. Most cases have a mature T-cell phenotype and express one of the major subset antigens: CD4 greater than CD8. These are not clonal markers, and antigen expression can change over time. Deletion of one of the pan T-cell antigens (CD3, CD5, CD2, or CD7) is seen in 75% of cases, with CD7 most frequently being absent (20).

Pathogenesis

Peripheral T-cell lymphomas NOS comprise the largest group within the general category of peripheral T-cell lymphoma. Nevertheless, our understanding of their pathogenesis is remarkably meager. The majority of cases show rearrangements of their T-cell–receptor genes and are phenotypically CD4+ αβ cells (42). Occasional CD8+ αβ-expressing nodal T-cell lymphomas have also been reported. These lymphomas do not appear to be a distinct clinicopathologic group but rather are likely to contain several entities, as is evidenced by their broad nonspecific phenotype and nonrecurrent complex chromosomal abnormalities (43,44). One intriguing preliminary report suggests a pathogenetic role for a novel putative oncogene called *human ral-GDS-related* (45). RalGDS-related was originally identified as one of the subunits of the RSC oncogene isolated from a rabbit squamous cell carcinoma. Truncated forms of both RSC and HRSc are able to transform NIH 3T3 cells (46). A preliminary screen of T- and B-cell lymphomas has shown high levels of truncated transcript in the majority of peripheral T-cell lymphomas (9 of 11 cases) and in a small percentage of mycoses fungoides cases (two of seven) and anaplastic large-cell lymphomas (two of five). Normal B and T cells and other forms of B- and T-cell lymphomas did not express the aberrant transcripts.

Clinical Features

Of 96 patients with peripheral T-cell lymphoma from a large international study of non-Hodgkin's lymphoma, 59 were felt to have peripheral T-cell lymphoma NOS (38). Of these, 44% were male, and 60% had stage IV disease. Forty-one percent of the patients had B symptoms. Nine percent of the patients had tumor masses larger than 10 cm. Seventy-two percent of the patients were ambulatory, and 28% had a reduced performance status. Forty percent of the patients had International Prognostic Index (IPI) scores of 0 to 2, and 60% had IPI scores of 3 to 5. The great majority of patients (i.e., 85%) had some site of extranodal involvement, but only 16% of the patients had the disease confined to extranodal sites. An elevated lactate dehydrogenase (LDH) was seen in 65%.

Chott et al. (47) described 75 patients with a variety of histologic subtypes of peripheral T-cell lymphoma. The median age of the patients was 54 years, with a slight female predominance. However, the comparatively young median age undoubtedly reflected the inclusion of anaplastic large-cell lymphomas in this series. Eighty percent of the patients presented primarily with lymphadenopathy and 20% with symptoms related to extranodal sites of disease. The most common sites of extranodal involvement were the skin, bone marrow, and upper aerodigestive track. Laboratory studies in these patients found 45% of the patients to be anemic and 75% to have an elevated LDH.

Lopez Guillermo et al. (48) described 184 patients with peripheral T-cell lymphoma and subdivided them based on the WHO Classification. Ninety-five patients had peripheral T-cell lymphoma NOS. Of these patients, 52% were older than 60 years of age, and 61% were male. Twenty-four percent had an Eastern Cooperative Oncology Group score of 2 or greater, and 57% of the patients had B symptoms. Some sign of extranodal disease was seen in 65% of the patients. Sixty-two percent had Ann Arbor stage IV disease, and 53% had a high LDH. A high β_2 microglobulin was seen in 62%. The IPI scores in these patients were 0 to 1 for 28%, 2 for 26%, 3 for 22%, and 4 or 5 for 24%. The most frequent sites of extranodal involvement were the bone marrow (41%), skin (12%), and liver (13%).

Armitage et al. (49) reported 134 cases of peripheral T-cell lymphoma. The median age of the patients was 57 years, and 59% of the patients were male. Sixty-seven percent of the patients had Ann Arbor stage IV disease, and 76% had B symptoms. An elevated LDH (measured in 113 patients) was seen in 87%. In this series, 27% of the patients had some preceding disorder of the immune system before the diagnosis of peripheral T-cell lymphoma. These diagnoses included a previous lymphoproliferative disorder (i.e., angioblastic lymphadenopathy, atypical dermatitis, mononucleosis, lymphomatoid papulosis, or lymphomatoid granulomatosis) in 11% of the patients; a different, usually B-cell, lymphoma in 8% of the patients; autoimmune arthritis in 4% of the cases; and a variety of other immune disorders in 3% of the patients.

Ansell et al. (50) reported 78 patients with peripheral T-cell lymphoma seen at the Mayo Clinic. Forty-two percent of the patients were older than 60 years of age, and 62% were male. Eighty-two percent had Ann Arbor stage III/IV disease. Fifty-three percent of the patients had B symptoms, and 54% percent of the patients had an Eastern Cooperative Oncology Group score of 2 or greater. Extranodal involvement was frequently seen, with the most commonly involved organs being the gastrointestinal tract (29%), bone marrow (28%), and liver (21%). An elevated LDH was seen in 42% of the patients. The findings in several series of patients with peripheral T-cell lymphoma NOS are presented in Table 26.4.

Prognostic Significance of B- versus T-Cell Immunophenotype

The prognostic significance of T-cell immunophenotype in aggressive non-Hodgkin's lymphomas has been a point for controversy. Although no series has found a better outcome in patients with peripheral T-cell lymphoma than in those with aggressive B-cell lymphomas, several have found no significant difference in outcome between T- and B-cell subgroups. Several of these are older studies in which assignment of immunophenotype may have been more imprecise due to technical limitation. For example, cases of T-cell–rich large B-cell lymphoma may have been included in the T-cell group.

Kwak et al. (51) studied 101 patients with diffuse large-cell lymphoma, of whom 21 had peripheral T-cell lymphomas. There was no significant difference in outcome between the B- and T-cell subgroups. Rudders et al. (52)

TABLE 26.4. *Clinical findings in patients with peripheral T-cell lymphoma not otherwise specified (PTCL-NOS)*

Reference	No. of patients	Type	Median age (yr)	Male (%)	B symptoms (%)	Ambulatory (%)	Any extranodal site (%)	Stage IV (%)	>10 cm mass (%)	Bone marrow involvement (%)	Skin involvement (%)	Liver involvement (%)	Increased lactate dehydrogenase (%)
38	53	PTCL-NOS	59	44	41	72	79	60	9	—	—	—	65
48	95	PTCL-NOS	52	61	57	76	65	62	—	41	12	13	53
4	78	PTCL-unspeci-fied	—	55	44	—	—	—	14	26	—	—	—

studied 130 patients with aggressive lymphomas and found no difference in survival between B- and T-cell subgroups. Cossman (53) cited 59 cases of diffuse aggressive lymphoma, of which 42% were peripheral T-cell lymphomas. There were no significant differences in treatment outcome between the B- and T-cell patients. Finally, Karakas et al. (54) studied 27 patients with peripheral T-cell lymphoma and 55 patients with aggressive B-cell lymphoma all treated with an aggressive chemotherapy regimen. There were no significant differences in outcome between the B- and T-cell patients. Liang et al. (55) studied 144 patients with peripheral T-cell lymphoma and 357 patients with aggressive B-cell lymphoma. Immunophenotype did not have a significant impact on survival.

In contrast, Coiffier (56) described 361 immunophenotyped patients with aggressive non-Hodgkin's lymphoma treated with one intensive chemotherapy regimen. Seventy percent were B-cell lymphomas, and 30% were peripheral T-cell lymphomas. There was no difference in response rate between the two groups, but patients with peripheral T-cell lymphoma were more likely to relapse (43% vs. 29%; $p < .001$). The overall survival was not significantly different. Lippman et al. (57) reported 103 patients with diffuse large-cell lymphoma who were successfully immunophenotyped. Twenty patients had peripheral T-cell lymphoma, and 83 patients had diffuse large B-cell lymphoma. Patients in each group were treated similarly. The median disease-free survival was 10.8 months for patients with peripheral T-cell lymphoma and 42.7 months for patients with diffuse large B-cell lymphoma ($p = .01$). The overall survival, although favoring B-cell patients, was not significantly different. Brown et al. (58) reported 51 cases with aggressive lymphoma that were successfully immunophenotyped. Forty-three were of B-cell and eight of T-cell immunophenotype. Even with these small numbers, the survival of the T-cell patients was significantly worse than that of their B-cell counterparts. Bloomfield et al. (59) reported 40 patients with diffuse aggressive lymphoma, of whom 23 had B-cell immunophenotype, five had T-cell immunophenotype, and 12 had null-cell immunophenotype. Patients with B-cell lymphoma had a significantly longer survival than did patients with T- or null-cell immunophenotype. Gisselbrecht et al. (60) reported 1,883 patients treated on the LNH-87 protocol by the Groupe d'Etude des Lymphomes de l'Adulte. Fifteen percent of the patients had peripheral T-cell lymphoma, and 85% had B-cell lymphoma. B-cell lymphoma patients were more likely to achieve a remission (63% vs. 54%; $p = .004$) and more likely to survive 5 years (53% vs. 41%; $p = .0004$). In a multivariate analysis, the immunophenotype had independent prognostic significance. Hutchison et al. (61) studied 69 children with aggressive lymphoma, of whom 25 had B-cell immunophenotype, 23 had T-cell immunophenotype, and 21 had indeterminate immunophenotype. B-cell patients had a significantly better survival than did the T-cell and indeterminate patients. Armitage et al. (62) studied 110 patients with diffuse aggressive lymphoma treated with a single combination chemotherapy regimen. Eighty-three percent of the patients had

B-cell lymphoma and 17% T-cell lymphoma. Patients with B-cell lymphoma overall did not have a significantly higher survival. However, patients with stage IV disease and peripheral T-cell lymphoma had a much worse complete-remission rate (67% vs. 0%; $p = .002$) and 3-year survival (44% vs. 0%; $p = .002$) than did stage IV patients with aggressive B-cell lymphoma. Shimizu et al. (63) studied 20 patients with peripheral T-cell lymphoma and 28 patients with diffuse aggressive B-cell lymphoma. Patients with T-cell lymphoma had a significantly worse outcome. Shimoyama (64) studied 541 patients, of whom 449 had aggressive B-cell lymphoma and 92 peripheral T-cell lymphoma (i.e., excluding adult T-cell leukemia/lymphoma). Patients with B-cell lymphoma had a significantly better overall survival than did the patients with peripheral T-cell lymphoma.

The balance of the data favors a poorer prognosis for patients with peripheral T-cell lymphoma than for those with diffuse large B-cell lymphoma. However, in most series, patients with peripheral T-cell lymphoma have a higher proportion of adverse risk factors. Although multivariate analyses in very large series have found peripheral T-cell lymphoma to be an independent adverse risk factor, patients with localized disease and low IPI scores can clearly have a good outcome.

Therapy

Patients with peripheral T-cell lymphoma have typically been treated with the same regimens used in diffuse large B-cell lymphoma. The tendency for poor survival in peripheral T-cell lymphoma patients suggests that the same regimens may not be equally efficacious in patients with B- and T-cell lymphoma. However, very little effort has been invested in finding the best regimen for patients with peripheral T-cell lymphoma.

Liang et al. (65) found an 84% complete-remission rate and a 60% overall survival at 18 months. In contrast, Greer et al. found a 24% complete-response rate in patients receiving combination chemotherapy regimens and only a 12% prolonged disease-free survival (66). Coiffier et al. (67) reported a 77% complete-remission rate in 39 patients treated with ACVPD [Adriamycin (doxorubicin), cyclophosphamide, vindesine, bleomycin, and prednisone], with a 23% relapse rate. Armitage et al. (49) described 80 patients treated for mucosa-associated lymphoid tissue (MALT) lymphoma with chemotherapy regimens having curative potential in diffuse large B-cell lymphoma. Fifty percent of the patients achieved a complete remission, and the actuarial 4-year survival was 45%. Rudiger et al. (38) reported 69 patients treated with Adriamycin (doxorubicin)-containing combination chemotherapy regimens, with only a 20% 5-year failure-free survival. The Nebraska Lymphoma Study Group reported 19 patients with peripheral T-cell lymphoma treated with CAP-BOP [cyclophosphamide, Adriamycin (doxorubicin), procarbazine, bleomycin, Oncovin (vincristine), and prednisone], with a 54% complete-remission rate and 41% 3-year overall survival. The Group d'Etude des Lymphomes de l'Adulte reported a study of 108 patients treated with ACVBP that found a 72% complete-remission rate and a 43% relapse rate.

Using regimens developed primarily for patients with diffuse large B-cell lymphoma, patients with peripheral T-cell lymphoma can also achieve complete remission and long-term disease-free survival. However, as noted above, both response rate and survival tend to be lower for patients with peripheral T-cell lymphoma. This undoubtedly reflects a lack of clinical trials aimed at developing regimens specifically for patients with peripheral T-cell lymphoma.

Three series have reported the results of bone marrow transplantation and compared the outcome in T- and B-cell lymphomas. Vose et al. (68) reported no difference in disease-free and overall survival in 17 patients with T-cell lymphoma and 24 patients with diffuse aggressive B-cell lymphoma. Rodriguez et al. (69) reported the results of transplantation in 36 patients with diffuse aggressive lymphoma who were immunophenotyped and found a 3-year survival of 37% that did not vary from what was seen in B-cell lymphomas. Blystad et al. (70) reported 27 patients with chemosensitive peripheral T-cell lymphoma who underwent autologous transplantation. Forty-four percent of these patients survived 4 years. All of these series suggest a comparable outcome with autologous transplantation in patients with diffuse aggressive B-cell lymphoma or peripheral T-cell lymphoma. These results might suggest the earlier use of high-dose therapy and autologous transplantation in patients with high-risk peripheral T-cell lymphomas. They also support the concept that patients with B- and T-cell lymphoma might not respond similarly to all regimens and that high-dose therapy with autotransplantation might overcome the treatment resistance seen with many standard chemotherapy regimens in treating peripheral T-cell lymphomas.

Multiple other salvage-chemotherapy regimens have been used in patients with peripheral T-cell lymphoma for whom primary therapy is unsuccessful. These include platinum-based and fludarabine-based combination-chemotherapy regimens, cyclosporin (71), pentostatin (72), cladribine (73), gemcitabine (74), retinoids (75), denileukin diftitox (76,77), interferon (78), Ara-G, and immunotoxins (79). All of these approaches have described some success. None has yet been advanced to frontline therapy.

Prognostic Factors

A large variety of prognostic factors have been described to be significantly associated with outcome in patients with peripheral T-cell lymphoma (4,38,48,49,55,56,60,65,67,80,81). These include response to treatment, high-stage disease, B symptoms, poor performance status, tumor bulk, extranodal disease, bone marrow infiltration, high serum LDH, high serum β_2 microglobulin level, liver involvement, and IPI score (1,38,50,82). At the present time, the most useful prognostic indicator is the IPI.

TABLE 26.5. *The International Prognostic Index (IPI) in patients with peripheral T-cell lymphoma*

Characteristic	IPI grouping				Reference
	0–1	2	3	4–5	
% of patients	19	27	26	28	50
	17	52		31	21,82
5-yr survival %	76	32	28	9	50
	36	28		15	21,82

The outcome of the IPI score in two series of patients with peripheral T-cell lymphoma is presented in Table 26.5. The survival of a series of patients with peripheral T-cell lymphoma by IPI score is presented in Figure 26.1.

Angioimmunoblastic T-Cell Lymphoma

Angioimmunoblastic lymphadenopathy with dysproteinemia was described by Frizzera et al. in 1974 (83). However, the same disorder had probably been reported by Flandrin in the French literature in 1972 (84). The patients characteristically presented with generalized lymphadenopathy, hepatosplenomegaly, fever, hypergammaglobulinemia, and frequently a positive Coombs test. A typical morphologic appearance involving proliferation of small arborizing vessels and a pleomorphic cellular infiltrate was described. Most patients had a short survival, although occasional patients seemed to have long-term benefit with prednisone therapy.

In 1987, Brice et al. described five patients with peripheral T-cell lymphoma that evolved from angioimmunoblastic lymphadenopathy (85). However, in 1979, Shimoyama et al. had proposed an entity that they called *immunoblastic lymphadenopathy–like T-cell lymphoma*, which was probably the same entity (86). Today, the accepted name for this lymphoma is *angioimmunoblastic T-cell lymphoma*. The angioimmunoblastic lymphadenopathy type of peripheral T-cell lymphoma has frequently been confused with lymphoepithelioid-cell lymphoma or Lennert's lymphoma (87). However, the Revised European-American Lymphoma Classification recognized angioimmunoblastic T-cell lymphoma as a separate entity (88), and this was confirmed in the WHO Classification (89).

Pathology

The nodal architecture is generally effaced, but peripheral sinuses are often open and even dilated. The abnormal infiltrate usually extends beyond the capsule into the surrounding adipose tissue. Hyperplastic germinal centers are usually, but not always, absent (90). However, there may be regressed follicles containing a proliferation of dendritic cells and blood vessels. These regressed follicles are referred to as *burned out*. At low power, there is usually a striking proliferation of postcapillary venules with prominent arborization. The cellularity of the

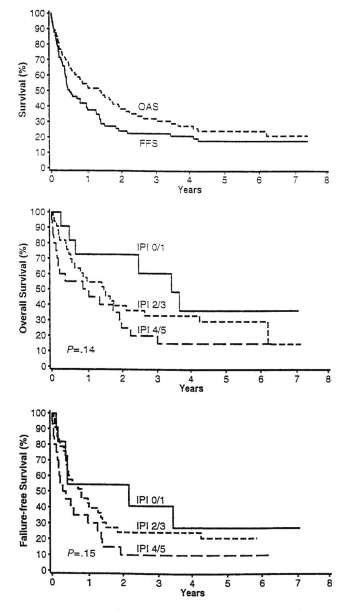

FIG. 26.1. Survival of a series of patients with peripheral T-cell lymphoma by International Prognostic Index (IPI) score. OAS, over-all survival; FFS, failure-free survival. (Reprinted from Armitage JO, Weisenburger DD. New approach to classifying non-Hodgkin's lymphomas: clinical features of the major histologic subtypes. Non-Hodgkin's Lymphoma Classification Project. *J Clin Oncol* 1998;16:2780–2795, with permission.)

lymph node usually appears reduced or depleted at low power. Clusters of lymphoid cells with clear cytoplasm may be seen. These are admixed with a polymorphous cellular background containing small normal-appearing lymphocytes, basophilic immunoblasts, plasma cells, and histiocytes, with or without eosinophils. The abnormal cells are usually CD4+ T cells, which can express both CD10 and bcl-6 (91). In paraffin sections, a helpful diagnostic feature is the presence of numerous CD21+ dendritic reticulum cells, which are especially prominent around postcapillary venules (87). Usually, scattered cells

positive for Epstein-Barr virus (EBV) are present (92). These are EBV+ B-cell blasts and not the neoplastic T cells. The expansion of EBV+ cells is felt to be secondary to the underlying immune deficiency of angioimmunoblastic T-cell lymphoma (93). The EBV+ cells may assume a Reed-Sternberg–like appearance, simulating Hodgkin's disease (94).

Pathogenesis

Angioimmunoblastic T-cell lymphomas comprise the second largest single group of peripheral T-cell lymphomas (peripheral T-cell lymphoma NOS being the largest) and are tumors of CD4+ αβ cells (95). TCR β and γ chain gene rearrangements can be seen in up to 75% of cases (96–98). Cytogenetic studies have shown that virtually all cases have abnormal karyotypes, with frequent trisomy 3, 5, and +X, and structural abnormalities at 1p32-33 (35,36). Schlegelberger et al. showed that the presence of multiple chromosomal abnormalities was associated with shortened survival (99).

The developmental pathogenesis of angioimmunoblastic T-cell lymphoma remains controversial. Initially, this disease was termed *angioimmunoblastic lymphadenopathy with dysproteinemia* (angioimmunoblastic lymphadenopathy) and was believed to be a systemic immunologic disease characterized by a variable clinical course, polyclonal gammopathy, a specific pattern of involvement of lymph nodes, and a predisposition for the development of T-cell lymphoma (100,101). With the development of improved methodologies to assess T-cell clonality and the identification of clonal T-cell populations in up to 75% of cases, the interpretation of this disease process has been shifting. The consensus opinion today is that this disease most likely represents a malignant T-cell lymphoma from its inception (hence the term *angioimmunoblastic T-cell lymphoma*) and that the associated immunologic abnormalities are secondary to the lymphoma (89). However, there is a significant minority viewpoint that this disease represents a continuum from reactive polyclonal T-cell proliferations to highly malignant T-cell lymphomas. This viewpoint is supported by the 25% of cases without identifiable clonal T-cell populations, even using sophisticated microdissection technologies (98), by the existence of cases in oligoclonal T-cell populations (102,103), and by reports of cases with transient T-cell clones (104).

Approximately 10% of cases show clonal immunoglobulin gene rearrangements (103,104). However, these have generally been attributed to clonal proliferations of EBV-infected B cells. EBV-infected B cells can be identified in a high proportion of angioimmunoblastic T-cell lymphomas and are believed to be a manifestation of the immune disturbance associated with this disease. In rare cases, overt B-cell lymphoma may supervene (105).

Clinical Features

Patients with angioimmunoblastic T-cell lymphoma typically present with generalized adenopathy, fever, weight loss, skin rash, polyclonal hypergammaglobulinemia, autoimmune manifestations that can include a positive Coombs test, and frequent infections. As with most other peripheral T-cell lymphomas, the patients have a median age of older than 65 years and a male predominance (106). In one series, 83% of the patients had stage IV disease; 65% had B symptoms and 65% an elevated LDH (38). Eighty-six percent had an IPI score of at least 3.

The most complicated factor in the care of patients in whom angioimmunoblastic-like T-cell lymphoma is considered is whether the patient has a "benign" condition mimicking T-cell lymphoma. Because some patients described with angioimmunoblastic lymphadenopathy and dysproteinemia seemed to have had long-term remissions induced by prednisone alone, this is an important issue. Although there are not characteristic cytogenetic abnormalities [however, trisomy 3, trisomy 5, and an additional X chromosome have been frequently described (99)], the presence of rearranged T-cell–receptor genes can be helpful in making the decision to treat for lymphoma.

Therapy

The optimal treatment for patients with angioimmunoblastic T-cell lymphoma remains uncertain. The results of several series of patients treated with regimens typically used in diffuse large B-cell lymphoma are presented in Table 26.6.

The complete-remission rates varied from 60% to 100%, with no obvious advantage to any particular treatment regimen. The complete-remission rate and the survival were not clearly lower than in other types of peripheral T-cell lymphoma (38).

An important study reported by Siegert et al. tested the relative merits of initial prednisone therapy versus initial treatment with an aggressive combination-chemotherapy regimen [i.e., COPBLAM/IMVP-16 (cyclophosphamide, Oncovin [vincristine], prednisone, bleomycin, Adriamycin [doxorubicin], and Matalane [procarbazine]/ifosfamide,

methotrexate, and etoposide)] (107). Patients in this study initially received prednisone, with the intention to give no further treatment if a complete remission were achieved. Patients with advanced disease were treated initially with chemotherapy. Twenty-eight patients received prednisone as their primary treatment. Eight patients (29%) achieved a complete remission, 16 patients achieved a partial remission, and four patients experienced early death. Of the eight patients achieving a complete remission with prednisone, five subsequently relapsed, and three remained in remission at the time of the report for 14 to 23 months. Eighteen patients who received initial prednisone subsequently were treated with aggressive chemotherapy. Ten, or 56%, of the patients achieved a complete remission, and six of these remissions were durable for 15 to 33 months. Eleven patients in the Siegert study received initial chemotherapy with COPBLAM/IMVP-16. Seven of these patients (64%) achieved a complete remission, and four remained in continuous remission for 3 to 50 months. The conclusion of the study was that patients with angioimmunoblastic lymphadenopathy–type T-cell lymphoma probably do better if treated initially with an effective combination-chemotherapy regimen.

Other treatments used for angioimmunoblastic T-cell lymphoma have included cyclosporin (108,109), low-dose oral methotrexate (110), interferon (111), and autologous transplantation (111).

Extranodal Natural Killer/T-Cell Lymphoma, Nasal Type

It is known that NK cells and T cells may have a common precursor. NK cells typically have abundant pale cytoplasm and azurophilic granules. Immunophenotypically, they express CD56 surface antigen. T-cell receptor and immunoglobulin gene rearrangements are uniformly absent. Functionally, NK cells are cytolytic cells targeting malignant or virally infected cells (112).

TABLE 26.6. *Response to primary chemotherapy for patients with angioimmunoblastic T-cell lymphoma*

Reference	No. of patients	Regimen	Complete remission (%)	Median survival (mo)
218	8	Doxorubicin-containing combinations	63	—
107	11	COPBLAM/IMVP-16	64	19
111	25	Variable (23/25 with anthracycline)	68	36
219	10	Doxorubicin-containing combination	60	>24
220	3	MOPP or COPP	100	—

COPBLAM/IMVP-16, cyclophosphamide, Oncovin (vincristine), prednisone, bleomycin Adriamycin (doxorubicin), and Matalane (procarbazine)/ifosfamide, methotrexate, and etoposide; COPP, cyclophosphamide, Oncovin (vincristine), procarbazine, and prednisone; MOPP, mechlorethamine, Oncovin (vincristine), procarbazine, and prednisone.

In the recent WHO Classification for hematopoietic and lymphoid tumors, NK cell malignancies are recognized as distinct clinicopathologic entities, and they include the extranodal NK/T-cell lymphoma, nasal type (113). Many other terms, including *polymorphic reticulosis*, *lethal midline granuloma*, *progressive lethal granulomatous ulceration*, *malignant granuloma*, *nonhealing granuloma*, and *midline malignant reticulosis*, have all been used in the past to describe this clinically malignant lesion involving midline facial structures (16,37,88,114–119). Because this lymphoma may present in sites other than the upper airway and nose, the term *nasal type* is used in the WHO Classification.

Epidemiology

Nasal NK/T-cell lymphoma is an uncommon tumor, and it shows great variations in incidence in different racial populations and geographic locations (120–122). In Asia, the tumor is seen mainly in southern China, Japan, and Korea. In our International Lymphoma Study, nasal NK/T-cell lymphoma comprised 8% of all the non-Hodgkin's lymphoma seen in Hong Kong. Nasal NK/T-cell lymphoma is also seen in patients of Native-American descent in Mexico and Central and South America, but it rarely affects whites. The tumor only accounts for less than 1% of all cases of non-Hodgkin's lymphoma seen in Europe and North America. It has, however, been sporadically reported in immunosuppressed and posttransplant patients.

Pathology

Extranodal NK/T-cell lymphoma is characterized by a broad cytologic spectrum. The atypical cells may be small or medium in size. Large atypical and hyperchromatic cells may be admixed or may predominate. If the small cells are in the majority, the disease may be difficult to distinguish from an inflammatory or infectious process. In early stages, there may also be a prominent admixture of inflammatory cells, further causing difficulty in diagnosis (123). Most cases of nasal NK/T-cell lymphoma have extensive tissue necrosis, often with vascular infiltration and necrosis. This feature led to the earlier description of this lymphoma type as *angiocentric lymphoma* (5,124). More recent studies have implicated chemokines and cytokines induced by EBV as mediating the vascular damage (125,126).

Because virtually all cases of nasal NK/T-cell lymphoma are positive for EBV, *in situ* hybridization studies with probes to EBV-encoded small nuclear ribonucleic acid (EBER 1/2) may be very helpful in diagnosis and can detect even small numbers of neoplastic cells (127,128). Although the cells express some T-cell–associated antigens, most commonly CD2, other T-cell markers, such as surface CD3, are usually absent (5). Cytoplasmic CD3 can be found in paraffin sections. However, cytoplasmic CD3 can be found in NK cells and is not specific for a T-cell lineage. In addition, molecular studies have not shown a clonal T-cell gene rearrangement,

despite clonality being shown by other methods (129–131). In favor of an NK-cell origin, the cells are nearly always CD56$^+$; however, CD16 and CD57 (other NK-cell antigens) are usually negative.

Pathogenesis

Extranodal NK/T-cell lymphomas, nasal type, are generally tumors of NK cells lacking rearranged T-cell receptors. By definition, all cases express cytotoxic proteins and contain EBV. Rare cases comprised of CD8$^+$ tumor cells possessing T-cell–receptor rearrangements that otherwise mimic cases with the NK phenotype have been described. There are few classical cytogenetic studies of these lymphomas, and among the abnormalities reported are trisomy 7, deletions of 6q, +X, trisomy 8, deletion of (13q), and deletion of (17p) (132). Comparative genomic hybridization and loss of heterozygosity studies have confirmed the high incidence of chromosomal loss at 6q (90% of cases) and 13q (approximately 70%), with lower frequencies of loss of heterozygosity observed at chromosomes 11q and 17p in approximately 30% of cases (133). Frequent chromosomal gains were also identified at 1p32-pter, 6p, 11q, 12q, 17q, 19p, 20q, and Xp. Recent studies using spectral karyotyping have identified the presence of cryptic translocations involving Xp21-pter and 8p23 (134). The genes involved are not known. These lymphomas show frequent overexpression of the p53 tumor-suppressor gene (122). This finding combined with reports of 17p deletions suggest that inactivation of p53 may be a common occurrence in NK/T-cell lymphomas; however, there is a lack of confirmatory mutational studies. Other tumor-suppressor loci have not been studied.

EBV is thought to play a prominent role in the pathogenesis of these tumors. EBV DNA sequences are found in 100% of tumors, and an EBV latency type II phenotype is usually seen (135). It is of interest that nearly all cases are infected with the EBV EBNA-1 p-ala variant sequence. This virus subtype is virtually never found in other types of EBV-associated neoplasms, although it is one of the major viral subtypes found in reactive conditions (136). Remarkably, Gutierrez et al. also identified ongoing mutations at a number of "hot spots" in the EBNA-1 sequence, although this finding is controversial (137). These observations raise interesting questions regarding the host–virus interaction and pathogenesis. Why are the other viral EBNA-1 subtypes not found in extranodal NK/T-cell lymphomas, nasal type, as they are in other EBV-associated cancers? Why is the p-ala EBNA-1 subtype selected specifically in NK cells? Are ongoing mutations an indication of genomic instability in these tumors?

Like their putative normal cellular progenitor, extranodal NK/T-cell lymphomas, nasal type, express several proteins capable of causing tissue destruction, including cytotoxic effectors, such as perforin and granzyme B and FAS ligand (FAS-L). Ng et al. demonstrated a correlation between the percentage of perforin-positive cells and the degree of zonal necrosis associated with the lesions (138). Although FAS-L is capable of initiating apoptotic death through activation of the FAS death pathway, the same investigators found no obvious correlation between the expression of FAS-L and zonal necrosis (139).

Cytotoxic NK cells and lymphomas of NK cells appear to have evolved elaborate mechanisms to control their potentially lethal activities. NK cells express a family of regulatory receptors termed *killer inhibitory receptors*, and they express FAS receptor (139,140). The killer inhibitory receptors are major histocompatibility complex class 1–specific NK-cell receptors that primarily function to inhibit the NK cytotoxic response. These receptors are comprised of two families: the immunoglobulin superfamily receptors (CD158a, CD158b, and NKB1) and the lectin-like receptors (CD94/NKG2A). Studies of killer inhibitory receptors in NK/T-cell lymphomas indicate that these receptors continue to be expressed in lymphomas, and it has been suggested that their presence may be important in modulating their potential antitumor activity to self (141,142).

It has been postulated that the expression of both FAS and FAS-L on NK cells may also play a role in preventing uncontrolled NK-cell activity and proliferation. Although one may have predicted downregulation of FAS on tumor cells, this is not the case. However, as many as one-half of all extranodal NK/T-cell lymphomas, nasal type, show potentially inactivating FAS coding–region mutations, including point mutations and frameshifts (24,25). Most of these mutations truncate the N-terminal death domain, leaving the C-terminal ligand-binding domain intact. Furthermore, when these mutations were modeled in mice, they were shown to confer resistance to FAS-mediated apoptosis. It has been suggested that these truncated FAS proteins behave in a dominant negative manner in the cell or, alternatively, result in a soluble ligand-binding domain that can block FAS-L activity. Thus, the presence of these FAS mutations should inactivate this potent death-signaling pathway and provide the tumor with a survival advantage.

Extranodal NK/T-cell lymphomas, nasal type, also express high levels of the serpin proteinase inhibitor 9 (26). This is the only known protein able to inhibit the proteolytic activity of granzyme B. It has been suggested that this is yet another mechanism by which tumor cells of extranodal NK/T-cell lymphomas, nasal type, can protect themselves from autologous granzyme B or enzyme directed from cytotoxic T cells and escape from immune surveillance.

Clinical Features

Nasal NK/T-cell lymphoma more commonly affects men, and the median age of the patients is approximately 50 years old (143–148). The tumor typically presents with nasal symptoms, including obstruction and bleeding, or a nasal mass. There may be local invasion into the orbit, nasal sinuses, nasopharynx, oropharynx, palate, and even larynx (Color Plate 58). Cranial nerves may also be involved, but meningeal involvement is not common (149,150). Systemic dissemination is often late but clinically very aggressive. Favorite metastatic sites include skin, gut, and testis, sites where CD56 is normally expressed. Patients may also present with a primary tumor in one of these sites. In a percentage of these patients, however, occult nasal disease may be present. Circulating lymphoma cells together with marrow involvement may be seen as a terminal event.

A high index of suspicion is essential for early diagnosis. Because of the anatomic location of the tumor, the size of the biopsy specimens from nasal endoscopy is often small. The presence of extensive necrosis, together with the marked presence of inflammatory cellular infiltrates, make this a big challenge for histopathologists. Multiple biopsies of adequate size are required before a definitive diagnosis can be made. For difficult cases, an opinion from an experienced histopathologist is beneficial, and the use of EBV markers may also provide additional clues.

A small subset of patients may have very aggressive disease at presentation. These patients have high fever, liver failure, and marrow failure. Features of hemophagocytosis may be observed. Studies have shown that this is usually associated with a high level of soluble FAS-L from the tumor (151).

Other than the usual staging investigations for non-Hodgkin's lymphoma, including computed tomographic scan of the thorax and abdomen and bone marrow biopsy, a computed tomographic scan or magnetic resonance imaging scan of the nasal region may give a better picture of the extent of local spread of the tumor (Fig. 26.2) (152,153).

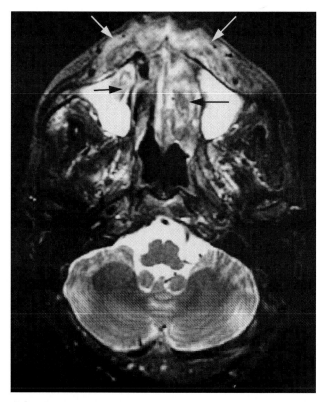

FIG. 26.2 Nuclear magnetic resonance scan showing natural killer–cell lymphoma in the midline nasal cavity.

Treatment and Monitoring

Local radiotherapy and chemotherapy are both effective treatments for primary nasal lymphoma. However, with radiotherapy or chemotherapy alone, treatment failure is still common (149,154,155). Local recurrences are usually followed by systemic relapse. Better clinical outcome has been obtained with the combined use of chemotherapy and local radiotherapy. For patients with localized disease at presentation, prolonged remission is achievable in approximately one-half of cases. For patients with disseminated disease at presentation or at disease progression, the disease is almost invariably fatal. The relatively poor clinical outcome may be explained by the ischemic nature of the tumor as well as the primary cellular drug resistance.

There is no consensus on the optimal chemotherapeutic regimen for this tumor. Because of the relative rarity of this disease, prospective clinical studies are not available. An anthracycline-containing regimen, such as CHOP [cyclophosphamide, hydroxydaunorubicin, Oncovin (vincristine), and prednisone], is commonly used. It remains uncertain that other more complicated regimens, such as ProMACE-CytaBOM [prednisone, methotrexate-leucovorin, Adriamycin (doxorubicin), cyclophosphamide, etoposide + cytarabine, bleomycin, Oncovin (vincristine), and methotrexate], are more effective.

After therapy, it is essential to monitor the patient closely with nasal endoscopy and biopsy. Random blind biopsy is recommended even if the nasal mucosa appears normal on endoscopy, as occult residual tumor cells may still persist. Interpretation of the biopsy specimens can be even more difficult at this stage. The use of EBV markers, such as Epstein-Barr early region staining, may sometimes be helpful (156). Further studies are ongoing to see whether molecular markers are even more useful.

The optimal timing of radiotherapy in relation to chemotherapy is also uncertain. The presence of residual tumor cells after 3 months of initial chemotherapy is usually indicative of inadequate response to therapy. A decision has to be made at that time to give local radiotherapy early and to switch to an alternative chemotherapy regime.

High-dose chemotherapy with autologous stem cell rescue may also have a role in the management of this tumor (157–159). The best result is seen when it is performed at the time of remission. There is very limited experience in the use of allogeneic transplants, including the nonmyeloablative approach, for this tumor.

Distant tumor dissemination appears to be the most important prognostic feature. It is well known that there is a wide variation in the cytologic appearance of the tumor. However, there is no evidence that the cytologic grade is useful in predicting prognosis.

Hepatosplenic T-Cell Lymphoma

Hepatosplenic lymphoma is an aggressive subtype of extranodal lymphoma accounting for less than 5% of all peripheral T-cell lymphomas. It has been previously recognized in the Revised European-American Lymphoma Classification as a provisional entity termed *hepatosplenic γδ T-cell lymphoma* (88,160). In 1990, a report of two patients with predominant infiltration of the spleen and liver led to a proposal that a new entity should be delineated within peripheral T-cell lymphomas on the basis of the clinical presentation, the pattern of histologic involvement showing a sinusal/sinusoidal tropism of neoplastic cells and the TCR-γδ phenotype of tumor cells (161). Subsequently, several reports, mostly of individual cases, have appeared, among which Cooke et al. (11) described a series of five cases of hepatosplenic T-cell lymphoma with a proven γδ phenotype. Finally, the characteristics of 45 published cases have been recently reviewed (162).

Pathology

The cells of hepatosplenic T-cell lymphoma are usually moderate in size, with a rim of pale cytoplasm. The nuclear chromatin is loosely condensed, with small, inconspicuous nucleoli. Usually, some irregularity of the nuclear contour can be seen. The liver and spleen show marked sinusoidal infiltration, with sparing of both portal triads and white pulp, respectively. In bone marrow biopsies, a similar sinusoidal infiltration is seen. The neoplastic cells have a phenotype that resembles that of normal γδ T cells. They are often negative for both CD4 and CD8, although CD8 may be expressed in some cases. Although they are positive for CD3, they are negative for antigens such as βF1, expressed on αβ cells, but positive for TCRδ. CD56 is also often positive (11,161). The neoplastic cells express markers associated with cytotoxic T cells, such as TIA-1. However, perforin is usually negative, suggesting that these cells are not functionally mature (11).

Pathogenesis

Hepatosplenic T-cell lymphomas are primarily tumors of nonactivated γδ-expressing T cells. (11,161,163). These rare lymphomas express the cytotoxic granule–associated protein TIA-1, (32,164) but do not express the effector cytotoxic proteins, the granzymes and perforin (32).

Clinical Presentation

Based on a series of 15 cases of γδ hepatosplenic lymphoma previously presented (160), as in the published literature (162), the disease occurs mainly in young men, presenting with splenomegaly and very often hepatomegaly but without peripheral lymphadenopathy. More than one half of the patients have B symptoms. Mild asymptomatic thrombocytopenia is a constant feature, associated with anemia and leucopenia in one-half of the patients. An overt leukemic picture with "atypical lymphoid cells" is uncommon at presentation, but after careful examination of blood smears, a minor population of such cells could be identified in one-half of our cases. The association with a hemophagocytic syndrome has been occasionally mentioned. Due to the constant bone marrow involvement and the frequency of an elevated serum LDH level or of an Eastern Cooperative Oncology Group index greater than 1, we found that 60% of patients had two to three adverse factors and, thus, belonged to the high-risk group of the age-adjusted IPI (165).

A number of cases have been reported in patients with immune manifestations or with a previous history of immune defect, especially in patients receiving long-term immunosuppressive therapy for solid-organ transplantation (160,166–168).

Genetics

As previously reported, DNA genotyping using the Southern blot technique performed in the first patients of our series demonstrated the clonality of the malignant cells and the presence of a biallelic rearrangement of the δ gene and occasionally of unproductive rearrangements of the TCR β gene (161). Subsequent analyses using polymerase chain reaction showed a clonal rearrangement of the TCR γ gene in all cases (169). In addition to the clonal rearrangement of γ chain, αβ hepatosplenic cases disclose a productive rearrangement of the TCR β chain.

Based on conventional cytogenetic and fluorescent *in situ* hybridization studies in approximately 30 published cases, most γδ hepatosplenic lymphoma cases have been characterized by the presence of an isochromosome 7q [i(7)(q10)], suggesting the primary role of this recurrent karyotypic abnormality in the pathogenesis of the disease (170–172). Trisomy 8 and loss of chromosome Y have occasionally been observed. It is noteworthy that an increased number of 7q signals has been found in progressive cases, indicating a tendency to multiply the i(7)(q10) chromosome during evolution of the disease (33). In hepatosplenic cases with αβ-phenotype (34–36), i(7)(q10) has also been found, thus providing further evidence that both γδ and αβ cases represent variants of the same entity.

Treatment and Outcome

Due to the rarity of the disease, information regarding therapeutic results has been obtained from single or sporadic reported cases with short follow-up at the time when they were published, resulting in a considerable heterogeneity of treatment modalities. As recently reviewed (162), treatment options have included—in addition to splenectomy performed for diagnostic purposes—steroids, alkylating agents, anthracycline-containing CHOP-like regimens, purine analogs, and autologous and allogeneic hematopoietic stem cell transplantation. From available reports, it appears that there are very few, if any, long-surviving patients. In a preliminary report (160), 70% of the patients responded to first-line treatment consisting of a CHOP-like regimen, but all relapsed early, despite consolidative high-dose therapy with stem cell transplantation in several cases. All of the patients have died, and median survival time was 12 months. Thus, therapeutic

strategies that have cured a significant proportion of other aggressive subtypes of lymphoma, such as diffuse large B-cell lymphoma, have failed in hepatosplenic T-cell lymphoma; efficient treatment modalities have yet to be defined.

Enteropathy-Type T-Cell Lymphoma

Enteropathy-type intestinal T-cell lymphoma is a rare type of non-Hodgkin's lymphoma comprising less than 1% of all non-Hodgkin's lymphomas in the recent reports from the International Lymphoma Study Group (1). Before the development of the WHO Classification of lymphoid tumors, enteropathy-type intestinal T-cell lymphoma was also known as *malignant histiocytosis of the intestine* (173) and *enteropathy-associated T-cell lymphoma* (174). It is a tumor of intraepithelial T lymphocytes most commonly occurring in the jejunum or ileum and is closely associated with celiac disease. The prognosis is poor, with reported 5-year survival rates of less than 30%. Optimal treatment strategies for enteropathy-type intestinal T-cell lymphoma are unclear.

Epidemiology, Etiology, and Relationship to Celiac Disease

Enteropathy-type intestinal T-cell lymphoma is a rare subtype of non-Hodgkin's lymphoma that is most common in those areas with a high incidence of celiac disease (175–178). In a study of 175 cases of gastrointestinal lymphoma from the British National Lymphoma Investigation, only 16 cases (9%) were enteropathy-type intestinal T-cell lymphoma (179). Patients with enteropathy-type intestinal T-cell lymphoma may have a history of celiac disease since childhood or a relatively brief history of adult-onset celiac disease before the development of lymphoma. It is thought that patients with adult-onset celiac disease may have occult clinical disease from early in life. In either case, a lack or loss of response of celiac disease to a gluten-free diet is often the first indication of the development of enteropathy-type intestinal T-cell lymphoma (180,181).

Most patients with enteropathy-type intestinal T-cell lymphoma have the HLA DQA1*0501, DQB1*0201 genotype, which is also associated with an increased risk of celiac disease [#1378;#1382]. However, additional HLA-DR/DQ-associated alleles that act independently may represent additional risk factors for enteropathy-type intestinal T-cell lymphoma but require further investigation (6).

Pathology

The small bowel usually shows ulceration, frequently with perforation. A mass may or may not be present. The infiltrate shows a varying cytologic composition with an admixture of small, medium, and larger atypical lymphoid cells. The adjacent small bowel may show villous atrophy associated with celiac disease (182). The neoplastic cells are CD3+, CD7+ T cells, which also express the homing receptor CD103 (HML-1) (183). The cells frequently express granzyme B, associated with cytotoxic T cells (184). Enteropathy-type T-cell lymphoma is usually EBV⁻, but some geographic differences have been seen (185,186). However, the possibility exists that these EBV⁺ cases are examples of extranodal NK/T-cell lymphoma presenting with intestinal disease.

Pathogenesis

Enteropathy-type T-cell lymphoma is a clonal T-cell proliferation, presumably originating from cytotoxic intraepithelial lymphocytes, in which the TCR β and γ genes are usually rearranged (187,188). Although the majority of these lymphomas express the αβ TCR, a minority express the γδ TCR receptor (189). Traditional cytogenetic studies that include cases of enteropathy-type T-cell lymphoma are rare. Recent studies using comparative genomic hybridization have demonstrated recurrent gains of chromosome 9q (58% of cases), 7q (24%), 5q (18%), and 1q (16%) and chromosomal losses of 8p (24%), 13q (24%), and 9p (18%) (190).

Like their nonneoplastic progenitors, enteropathy-type T-cell lymphoma cells express the homing and adhesion receptor CD103 (HML-1) (183,191). CD103 is a novel integrin composed of β7 and αE subunits, implicated in homing and adhesion properties of the intraepithelial lymphocytes (192). This receptor is expressed almost exclusively in enteropathy-type T-cell lymphoma, mycoses fungoides, and in hairy cell leukemia (23,193). The presence of this receptor may be responsible for the frequent intraepithelial spread of enteropathy-type T-cell lymphoma (188).

Enteropathy-type T-cell lymphomas often arise in patients with evidence of celiac disease, and nearly all cases are associated with the HLA DQA1*0501, DQB1*0201 genotype that is characteristic of celiac disease (6). Patients who progress and develop refractory sprue or ulcerative duodenitis frequently show intraepithelial lymphocytosis associated with clonal T-cell rearrangements (194,195). Furthermore, the intraepithelial lymphocytes of noninvolved intestinal mucosa in patients with enteropathy-type T-cell lymphoma frequently display T-cell receptor–gene rearrangements identical to those observed in their lymphoma (188). These observations suggest a stepwise progression from the polyclonal T-cell expansion seen in typical sprue to an early monoclonal T-cell expansion/low-grade lymphoma seen in refractory sprue and, finally, to a clinically evident overt T-cell lymphoma.

Sites of Involvement

Enteropathy-type intestinal T-cell lymphoma most commonly involves the jejunum or ileum, although involvement of other parts of the gastrointestinal tract, including the stomach, duodenum, and colon, has been reported. The typical macroscopic appearance is of circumferential ulceration of the bowel wall with marked edema of the adjacent small intestine (196). Enlargement of mesenteric lymph nodes in surgically resected specimens is observed in most cases, although only approximately 30% of these lymph nodes have evidence of infiltration by enteropathy-type intestinal T-cell lymphoma, with the remaining cases showing reactive changes only.

In addition to the histologic changes observed in the affected small bowel, most resected specimens show evidence of villous atrophy and crypt hyperplasia in the adjacent small bowel, with increased numbers of intraepithelial lymphocytes with a CD3⁺/CD8⁺ phenotype. These changes reflect those associated with the underlying celiac disease.

Clinical Features

In view of the rarity of enteropathy-type intestinal T-cell lymphoma, there are very few reports that specifically describe this entity. In the largest series, from Southampton, United Kingdom, the median age at onset of enteropathy-type intestinal T-cell lymphoma was 55 years (range, 20 to 80 years); 74% of patients were male and 26% female (196). Twelve of the patients in this series had a history of celiac disease, diagnosed between 3 months and 40 years before the diagnosis of enteropathy-type intestinal T-cell lymphoma. In a similar series from Ireland, where the prevalence of celiac disease is high, seven of 30 patients with enteropathy-type intestinal T-cell lymphoma had a previous diagnosis of celiac disease, from 12 to 252 months (median, 44 months) earlier (197). Other series have reported the onset of enteropathy-type intestinal T-cell lymphoma between 3 and 5 years after the diagnosis of celiac disease in adults, suggesting that close monitoring of patients with adult-onset celiac disease, especially in the first few years after diagnosis, is essential (198,199). Previous studies have demonstrated that between 5% and 10% of patients with adult-onset celiac disease may be at risk for enteropathy-type intestinal T-cell lymphoma (200,201).

The role of adherence to a gluten-free diet in the development of enteropathy-type intestinal T-cell lymphoma in patients with celiac disease is unclear, although Holmes et al. have reported that treatment of celiac disease with a gluten-free diet for longer than 5 years reduces the risk of lymphoma to that of the general population (202).

In the series for the United Kingdom (196), the most common presenting symptoms for enteropathy-type intestinal T-cell lymphoma were abdominal pain (84%), weight loss (81%), diarrhea (39%), and vomiting (29%). Small bowel perforation or small bowel obstruction were presenting features in 42%. In the series from Ireland, a similar proportion of patients without preceding celiac disease (60%) presented with intestinal obstruction or perforation (197). Night sweats and fevers are uncommon presenting symptoms in enteropathy-type intestinal T-cell lymphoma. Abdominal masses are uncommon (16%), and none of the patients in the UK series had peripheral lymphadenopathy at presentation.

The diagnosis of enteropathy-type intestinal T-cell lymphoma is most commonly made at laparotomy (80%), although in some patients, endoscopic biopsies from the proximal small bowel are diagnostic. In reported series, approximately two-thirds of patients have single-site disease in the small bowel, the remainder having multiple areas of involvement.

Most patients have clinical stage IE or IIE disease at presentation. Mesenteric lymph node involvement is relatively common, as is direct spread to the omentum or mesentery. Stage IV disease is uncommon, comprising only 20% of cases in the UK series.

Treatment and Complications

The optimal treatment strategy for patients with enteropathy-type intestinal T-cell lymphoma is unclear. In previous series, a small proportion of patients with stage IE disease has been managed with surgical resection alone. However, in one published series, of six patients managed with surgery alone, five subsequently relapsed (196), and it is now widely accepted that all patients presenting with enteropathy-type intestinal T-cell lymphoma should receive combination chemotherapy. The most commonly used regimen for patients with enteropathy-type intestinal T-cell lymphoma is CHOP (203). However, the use of combination chemotherapy in these patients is complicated, and less than 50% of patients in the Southampton series completed their planned courses of chemotherapy (196). In part, this may reflect the impaired nutritional status of this group of patients. Approximately 30% required parenteral or enteral nutrition during chemotherapy. Small bowel perforation is a well-documented complication of this treatment, most commonly after the first cycle of chemotherapy, when it is thought to be the result of tumor response in transmural disease. The risk of intestinal perforation in the UK series was four of 31 (13%). The risk of early treatment-related mortality in this group also appears to be high. In the same series, 21% of patients died of treatment-related complications (infection or gastrointestinal hemorrhage) after the first cycle of chemotherapy.

There have been no formal studies of other chemotherapy regimens in this disease, and CHOP is, therefore, generally considered the standard induction regimen.

Response and Survival

Response data are available from only one of the prior studies (196). Of 24 patients treated with combination chemotherapy, ten (41%) achieved a complete response and four (16%) a partial response. Five patients experienced treatment-related deaths, and the remaining patients either had no response or disease progression on chemotherapy.

Relapses occurred at a median of 6 months from the completion of initial therapy (range, 1 to 60 months), most commonly in the small intestine, although relapse at other sites, including the liver, spleen, and mesenteric lymph nodes, was documented. Central nervous system relapse has also been documented.

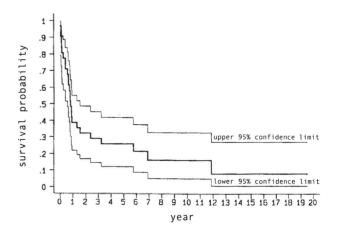

FIG. 26.3. Overall survival for 31 patients with enteropathy-type intestinal T-cell lymphoma. (Reprinted from Gale J, Simmonds PD, Mead GM, et al. Enteropathy-type intestinal T-cell lymphoma: clinical features and treatment of 31 patients in a single center. *J Clin Oncol* 2000;18:795, with permission.)

Results of salvage therapy have been poor, with very few patients achieving long-term disease-free survival after conventional dose salvage. Although anecdotal reports of long-term survival after high-dose therapy and autologous stem cell transplantation exist, there is no proven role for this approach.

Overall survival data from the UK series are shown in Figure 26.3. Twenty-six of the 31 patients died from disease progression or treatment-related complications. The actuarial 1-year and 5-year overall-survival rates were 39% and 20%, respectively. In the Irish study, of 23 patients who received chemotherapy, nine were alive and disease free with a median follow-up of 74 months (range, 10 to 196 months) (197). The latter series, however, included some patients in whom histologic review was not performed, and the outcome was not separately reported for the group who had undergone histologic review.

Subcutaneous Panniculitis-Like T-Cell Lymphoma

This entity represents the least well-defined and, perhaps, rarest of the subtypes of peripheral T-cell lymphoma. The first report is often ascribed to Gonzalez et al. (204), who reported eight cases of T-cell lymphoma primarily involving subcutaneous adipose tissue and stressed the resemblance of these tumors to panniculitis. Ashworth et al. (205) had previously described similar cases, as had Tanaka et al. (206). Wang et al., in 1996, described 23 patients seen at the Mayo Clinic (207). Many of the older cases were interpreted as an abnormal histiocytic proliferation, histiocytic cytophagic panniculitis. The total number of cases reported over the last decade is approximately 100.

Pathology

The cytologic composition of subcutaneous panniculitis-like T-cell lymphoma is extremely variable. The lesions may contain a predominance of small atypical lymphoid cells, often with clear cytoplasm, or larger atypical cells with hyperchromatic nuclei. Admixed reactive histiocytes are frequently present, particularly in areas of fat infiltration and destruction. The histiocytes are frequently vacuolated due to ingested lipid material. Vascular invasion may be seen in some cases, and necrosis and karyorrhexis are common.

The neoplastic cells invariably express a mature activated cytotoxic T-cell phenotype. Most cases are of αβ T-cell origin, although in approximately 25% of cases, a γδ T-cell phenotype can be seen. The γδ T-cell cases are clinically more aggressive and display more varied histologic features. For example, both dermal and epidermal involvement are often seen, in contrast to most cases of panniculitis-like T-cell lymphoma, which are generally confined to subcutaneous tissue.

Pathogenesis

Subcutaneous panniculitis-like T-cell lymphomas are exceedingly rare lymphomas that show an activated cytotoxic phenotype, with most cases expressing cytotoxic granule protein TIA-1 and the cytotoxic effector granzymes and perforin. The necrosis often associated with these lymphomas is likely to be related, at least in part, to their expression of these cytotoxic proteins. Most cases are derived from CD8$^+$ αβ T cells, whereas a minority are CD4$^-$CD8$^-$ and express the γδ T-cell receptor (19). All show clonal rearrangements of the T-cell receptor γ chain gene. The γδ cases exclusively use the Vδ2 gene, reflecting the predominant use of this variable-region gene in resident γδ cells of the skin (208). Cytogenetic and molecular genetic studies of these lymphomas are virtually nonexistent.

Clinical Features and Treatment Outcome

The clinical behavior of typical patients includes presentation with subcutaneous, sometimes painful nodules that can resemble lipomas. The lesions are typically first seen on the extremities and follow a several-year course of waxing and waning, but ultimately progressing. The nodules can sometimes ulcerate. Biopsies are frequently initially interpreted as showing panniculitis—particularly if not reviewed by an expert hematopathologist who is acquainted with this entity. When the diagnosis is made, it has been proposed that there is a distinction between those expressing αβ T-cell receptors and those expressing γδ T-cell receptors (209), with patients expressing γδ T-cell receptors being older, having a higher frequency of systemic symptoms, and having a shorter median survival. There is one case report of this lymphoma apparently being transmitted to the recipient of an allogeneic bone marrow transplant (210).

Although responses to standard combination-chemotherapy regimens are frequently seen (204,207,211–213), complete responses are not common, and the responses are rarely durable. Involved-field radiation has a high response rate, but the disease frequently relapses in unirradiated sites. Other treatments that have been used include platinum-based chemotherapy regimens (213,214), 13 cis-retinoid acid (215), cyclosporin (215), α-interferon, and zovudine (207,216), with success reported for each but no standard treatment being widely accepted.

The hemophagocytic syndrome is a well-described complication of subcutaneous panniculitis-like T-cell lymphoma (204,217). In cases reporting this association, it has been an often fatal complication. However, in many cases, the disease remains confined to the subcutaneous tissue, although any organ can be involved. It is likely that further evaluation of a large series of patients will better define this entity.

FUTURE DIRECTIONS

Peripheral T-cell lymphomas represent a wide variety of clinical/pathologic syndromes that are infrequent but share a poor prognosis. The explanation for a poor treatment outcome in patients with peripheral T-cell lymphoma in contrast to patients with aggressive B-cell lymphomas remains uncertain. However, one possibility is that the rarity of these disorders has made them difficult to study, and the results for patients with peripheral T-cell lymphoma in studies of the therapy of aggressive non-Hodgkin's lymphoma are "lost" because these patients represent such a small proportion of those being studied. The one thing that can be said with certainty is that what we currently consider optimal treatments for diffuse large B-cell lymphoma are not equally efficacious for patients with peripheral T-cell lymphoma.

Recognition of specific peripheral T-cell lymphomas as distinct entities should improve our ability to develop treatments for these disorders. A number of new agents, such as denileukin diftitox, alemtuzumab, Ara-G, α-interferon, purine analogs, and other new agents need to be studied in the treatment of patients with peripheral T-cell lymphoma. Improved understanding of the biology of the various peripheral T-cell lymphomas will, in all likelihood, offer new targets for developing specific treatments. There is every reason to believe that currently available treatments are not being optimally used in the treatment of patients with these disorders, and this is not likely to change until clinical trials focusing specifically on peripheral T-cell lymphomas are carried out.

REFERENCES

1. The Non-Hodgkin's Lymphoma Classification Project: a clinical evaluation of the International Lymphoma Study Group classification of non-Hodgkin's lymphoma. *Blood* 1997;89:3909–3918.
2. Anderson JR, Armitage JO, Weisenburger DD. Epidemiology of the non-Hodgkin's lymphomas: distributions of the major subtypes differ by geographic locations. Non-Hodgkin's Lymphoma Classification Project. *Ann Oncol* 1998;9:717–720.
3. Lennert K, Feller A. *Histopathology of non-Hodgkin's lymphomas.* New York: Springer-Verlag, 1992.
4. Ascani S, Zinzani PL, Gherlinzoni F, et al. Peripheral T-cell lymphomas. Clinico-pathologic study of 168 cases diagnosed according to the R.E.A.L. Classification. *Ann Oncol* 1997;8:583–592.
5. Jaffe ES, Chan JK, Su IJ, et al. Report of the Workshop on Nasal and Related Extranodal Angiocentric T/Natural Killer Cell Lymphomas.

Definitions, differential diagnosis, and epidemiology. *Am J Surg Pathol* 1996;20:103–111.

6. Howell WM, Leung ST, Jones DB, et al. HLA-DRB, -DQA, and -DQB polymorphism in celiac disease and enteropathy-associated T-cell lymphoma. Common features and additional risk factors for malignancy. *Hum Immunol* 1995;43:29–37.

7. Egan LJ, Stevens FM, McCarthy CF. Celiac disease and T-cell lymphoma [letter; comment]. *N Engl J Med* 1996;335:1611–1612.

8. Spits H, Blom B, Jaleco AC, et al. Early stages in the development of human T, natural killer and thymic dendritic cells. *Immunol Rev* 1998;165:75–86.

9. Delves PJ, Roitt IM. The immune system. First of two parts. *N Engl J Med* 2000;343:37–49.

10. Arnulf B, Copie-Bergman C, Delfau-Larue MH, et al. Non-hepatosplenic gammadelta T-cell lymphoma: a subset of cytotoxic lymphomas with mucosal or skin localization. *Blood* 1998;91:1723–1731.

11. Cooke CB, Krenacs L, Stetler-Stevenson M, et al. Hepatosplenic T-cell lymphoma: a distinct clinicopathologic entity of cytotoxic gamma delta T-cell origin [see comments]. *Blood* 1996;88:4265–4274.

12. Toro JR, Beaty M, Sorbara L, et al. Gamma delta T-cell lymphoma of the skin: a clinical, microscopic, and molecular study. *Arch Dermatol* 2000;136:1024–1032.

13. Delves PJ, Roitt IM. The immune system. Second of two parts. *N Engl J Med* 2000;343:108–117.

14. Jaffe ES, Krenacs L, Raffeld M. Classification of T-cell and NK-cell neoplasms based on the REAL classification. *Ann Oncol* 1997;8:17–24.

15. Jaffe ES. Classification of natural killer (NK) cell and NK-like T-cell malignancies. *Blood* 1996;87:1207–1210.

16. Jaffe ES, Krenacs L, Kumar S, et al. Extranodal peripheral T-cell and NK-cell neoplasms. *Am J Clin Pathol* 1999;111:S46–S55.

17. Van Camp B, Durie BG, Spier C, et al. Plasma cells in multiple myeloma express a natural killer cell-associated antigen: CD56 (NKH-1; Leu-19). *Blood* 1990;76:377–382.

18. Crouzier R, Martin T, Pasquali JL. Monoclonal IgM rheumatoid factor secreted by CD5-negative B cells during mixed cryoglobulinemia. Evidence for somatic mutations and intraclonal diversity of the expressed VH region gene. *J Immunol* 1995;154:413–421.

19. Kumar S, Krenacs L, Medeiros J, et al. Subcutaneous panniculitic T-cell lymphoma is a tumor of cytotoxic T lymphocytes. *Hum Pathol* 1998;29:397–403.

20. Picker LJ, Weiss LM, Medeiros LJ, et al. Immunophenotypic criteria for the diagnosis of non-Hodgkin's lymphoma. *Am J Pathol* 1987;128:181–201.

21. Greiner TC, Raffeld M, Lutz C, et al. Analysis of T cell receptor-gamma gene rearrangements by denaturing gradient gel electrophoresis of GC-clamped polymerase chain reaction products. Correlation with tumor-specific sequences. *Am J Pathol* 1995;146:46–55.

22. Krafft AE, Taubenberger JK, Sheng ZM, et al. Enhanced sensitivity with a novel TCRgamma PCR assay for clonality studies in 569 formalin-fixed, paraffin-embedded (FFPE) cases. *Mol Diagn* 1999;4:119–133.

23. Falini B, Flenghi L, Fagioli M, et al. Expression of the intestinal T-lymphocyte associated molecule HML-1: analysis of 75 non-Hodgkin's lymphomas and description of the first HML-1 positive T-lymphoblastic tumour. *Histopathology* 1991;18:421–426.

24. Shen L, Liang AC, Lu L, et al. Frequent deletion of Fas gene sequences encoding death and transmembrane domains in nasal natural killer/T-cell lymphoma. *Am J Pathol* 2002;161:2123–2131.

25. Takakuwa T, Dong Z, Nakatsuka S, et al. Frequent mutations of Fas gene in nasal NK/T cell lymphoma. *Oncogene* 2002;21:4702–4705.

26. Bladergroen BA, Meijer CJ, ten Berge RL, et al. Expression of the granzyme B inhibitor, protease inhibitor 9, by tumor cells in patients with non-Hodgkin and Hodgkin lymphoma: a novel protective mechanism for tumor cells to circumvent the immune system? *Blood* 2002;99:232–237.

27. Kutok JL, Aster JC. Molecular biology of anaplastic lymphoma kinase-positive anaplastic large-cell lymphoma. *J Clin Oncol* 2002;20:3691–3702.

28. Bluestone JA, Khattri R, Sciammas R, et al. TCR gamma delta cells: a specialized T-cell subset in the immune system. *Annu Rev Cell Dev Biol* 1995;11:307–353.

29. Haas W, Pereira P, Tonegawa S. Gamma/delta cells. *Annu Rev Immunol* 1993;11:637–685.

30. Bordessoule D, Gaulard P, Mason DY. Preferential localisation of human lymphocytes bearing gamma delta T cell receptors to the red pulp of the spleen. *J Clin Pathol* 1990;43:461–464.

31. Bucy RP, Chen CL, Cooper MD. Tissue localization and CD8 accessory molecule expression of T gamma delta cells in humans. *J Immunol* 1989;142:3045–3049.

32. Boulland ML, Kanavaros P, Wechsler J, et al. Cytotoxic protein expression in natural killer cell lymphomas and in alpha beta and gamma delta peripheral T-cell lymphomas. *J Pathol* 1997;183:432–439.

33. Wlodarska I, Martin-Garcia N, Achten R, et al. Fluorescence in situ hybridization study of chromosome 7 aberrations in hepatosplenic T-cell lymphoma: isochromosome 7q as a common abnormality accumulating in forms with features of cytologic progression. *Genes Chromosomes Cancer* 2002;33:243–251.

34. Lai R, Larratt LM, Etches W, et al. Hepatosplenic T-cell lymphoma of alphabeta lineage in a 16-year-old boy presenting with hemolytic anemia and thrombocytopenia. *Am J Surg Pathol* 2000;24:459–463.

35. Macon WR, Levy NB, Kurtin PJ, et al. Hepatosplenic alphabeta T-cell lymphomas: a report of 14 cases and comparison with hepatosplenic gammadelta T-cell lymphomas. *Am J Surg Pathol* 2001;25:285–296.

36. Suarez F, Wlodarska I, Rigal-Huguet F, et al. Hepatosplenic alpha-beta T-cell lymphoma: an unusual case with clinical, histologic, and cytogenetic features of gammadelta hepatosplenic T-cell lymphoma. *Am J Surg Pathol* 2000;24:1027–1032.

37. Harris NL, Jaffe ES, Diebold J, et al. World Health Organization classification of neoplastic diseases of the hematopoietic and lymphoid tissues: report of the Clinical Advisory Committee meeting-Airlie House, Virginia, November 1997. *J Clin Oncol* 1999;17:3835–3849.

38. Rudiger T, Weisenburger DD, Anderson JR, et al. Peripheral T-cell lymphoma (excluding anaplastic large-cell lymphoma): results from the Non-Hodgkin's Lymphoma Classification Project. *Ann Oncol* 2002;13:140–149.

39. Kim H, Jacobs C, Warnke RA, Dorfman RF. Malignant lymphoma with a high content of epithelioid histiocytes: a distinct clinicopathologic entity and a form of so-called "Lennert's lymphoma." *Cancer* 1978;41:620–635.

40. Suchi T, Lennert K, Tu LY, et al. Histopathology and immunohistochemistry of peripheral T cell lymphomas: a proposal for their classification. *J Clin Pathol* 1987;40:995–1015.

41. Rudiger T, Ichinohasama R, Ott MM, et al. Peripheral T-cell lymphoma with distinct perifollicular growth pattern: a distinct subtype of T-cell lymphoma? *Am J Surg Pathol* 2000;24:117–122.

42. Takagi N, Nakamura S, Ueda R, et al. A phenotypic and genotypic study of three node-based, low-grade peripheral T-cell lymphomas: angioimmunoblastic lymphoma, T-zone lymphoma, and lymphoepithelioid lymphoma. *Cancer* 1992;69:2571–2582.

43. Schlegelberger B, Himmler A, Godde E, et al. Cytogenetic findings in peripheral T-cell lymphomas as a basis for distinguishing low-grade and high-grade lymphomas. *Blood* 1994;83:505–511.

44. Lepretre S, Buchonnet G, Stamatoullas A, et al. Chromosome abnormalities in peripheral T-cell lymphoma. *Cancer Genet Cytogenet* 2000;117:71–79.

45. Leonardi P, Kassin E, Hernandez-Munoz I, et al. Human rgr: transforming activity and alteration in T-cell malignancies. *Oncogene* 2002;21:5108–5116.

46. D'Adamo DR, Novick S, Kahn JM, et al. rsc: a novel oncogene with structural and functional homology with the gene family of exchange factors for Ral. *Oncogene* 1997;14:1295–1305.

47. Chott A, Augustin I, Wrba F, et al. Peripheral T-cell lymphomas: a clinicopathologic study of 75 cases. *Hum Pathol* 1990;21:1117–1125.

48. Lopez-Guillermo A, Cid J, Salar A, et al. Peripheral T-cell lymphomas: initial features, natural history, and prognostic factors in a series of 174 patients diagnosed according to the R.E.A.L. Classification. *Ann Oncol* 1998;9:849–855.

49. Armitage JO, Greer JP, Levine AM, et al. Peripheral T-cell lymphoma. *Cancer* 1989;63:158–163.

50. Ansell SM, Habermann TM, Kurtin PJ, et al. Predictive capacity of the International Prognostic Factor Index in patients with peripheral T-cell lymphoma. *J Clin Oncol* 1997;15:2296–2301.

51. Kwak LW, Wilson M, Weiss LM, et al. Similar outcome of treatment of B-cell and T-cell diffuse large-cell lymphomas: the Stanford experience. *J Clin Oncol* 1991;9:1426–1431.

52. Rudders RA, DeLellis RA, Ahl ET Jr, et al. Adult non-Hodgkin's lymphoma. Correlation of cell surface marker phenotype with prog-

nosis, the new Working Formulation, and the Rappaport and Lukes-Collins histomorphologic schemes. *Cancer* 1983;52:2289–2299.

53. Cossman J, Jaffe ES, Fisher RI. Immunologic phenotypes of diffuse, aggressive, non-Hodgkin's lymphomas. Correlation with clinical features. *Cancer* 1984;54:1310–1317.

54. Karakas T, Bergmann L, Stutte HJ, et al. Peripheral T-cell lymphomas respond well to vincristine, adriamycin, cyclophosphamide, prednisone and etoposide (VACPE) and have a similar outcome as high-grade B-cell lymphomas. *Leuk Lymphoma* 1996;24:121–129.

55. Liang R, Todd D, Ho FC. Aggressive non-Hodgkin's lymphoma: T-cell versus B-cell. *Hematol Oncol* 1996;14:1–6.

56. Coiffier B, Brousse N, Peuchmaur M, et al. Peripheral T-cell lymphomas have a worse prognosis than B-cell lymphomas: a prospective study of 361 immunophenotyped patients treated with the LNH-84 regimen. The GELA (Groupe d'Etude des Lymphomes Agressives). *Ann Oncol* 1990;1:45–50.

57. Lippman SM, Miller TP, Spier CM, et al. The prognostic significance of the immunotype in diffuse large-cell lymphoma: a comparative study of the T-cell and B-cell phenotype. *Blood* 1988;72:436–441.

58. Brown DC, Heryet A, Gatter KC, et al. The prognostic significance of immunophenotype in high-grade non-Hodgkin's lymphoma. *Histopathology* 1989;14:621–627.

59. Bloomfield CD, Kersey JH, Brunning RD, et al. Prognostic significance of lymphocyte surface markers in adult non-Hodgkin's malignant lymphoma. *Lancet* 1976;2:1330–1333.

60. Gisselbrecht C, Gaulard P, Lepage E, et al. Prognostic significance of T-cell phenotype in aggressive non-Hodgkin's lymphomas. Groupe d'Etudes des Lymphomes de l'Adulte (GELA). *Blood* 1998;92:76–82.

61. Hutchison RE, Fairclough DL, Holt H, et al. Clinical significance of histology and immunophenotype in childhood diffuse large cell lymphoma. *Am J Clin Pathol* 1991;95:787–793.

62. Armitage JO, Vose JM, Linder J, et al. Clinical significance of immunophenotype in diffuse aggressive non-Hodgkin's lymphoma. *J Clin Oncol* 1989;7:1783–1790.

63. Shimizu K, Hamajima N, Ohnishi K, et al. T-cell phenotype is associated with decreased survival in non-Hodgkin's lymphoma. *Jpn J Cancer Res* 1989;80:720–726.

64. Shimoyama M, Oyama A, Tajima K, et al. Differences in clinicopathological characteristics and major prognostic factors between B-lymphoma and peripheral T-lymphoma excluding adult T-cell leukemia/lymphoma. *Leuk Lymphoma* 1993;10:335–342.

65. Liang R, Todd D, Chan TK, et al. Peripheral T cell lymphoma. *J Clin Oncol* 1987;5:750–755.

66. Greer JP, York JC, Cousar JB, et al. Peripheral T-cell lymphoma: a clinicopathologic study of 42 cases. *J Clin Oncol* 1984;2:788–798.

67. Coiffier B, Berger F, Bryon PA, et al. T-cell lymphomas: immunologic, histologic, clinical, and therapeutic analysis of 63 cases. *J Clin Oncol* 1988;6:1584–1589.

68. Vose JM, Peterson C, Bierman PJ, et al. Comparison of high-dose therapy and autologous bone marrow transplantation for T-cell and B-cell non-Hodgkin's lymphomas. *Blood* 1990;76:424–431.

69. Rodriguez J, Munsell M, Yazji S, et al. Impact of high-dose chemotherapy on peripheral T-cell lymphomas. *J Clin Oncol* 2001;19:3766–3770.

70. Blystad AK, Enblad G, Kvaloy S, et al. High-dose therapy with autologous stem cell transplantation in patients with peripheral T cell lymphomas. *Bone Marrow Transplant* 2001;27:711–716.

71. Cooper DL, Braverman IM, Sarris AH, et al. Cyclosporine treatment of refractory T-cell lymphomas. *Cancer* 1993;71:2335–2341.

72. Mercieca J, Matutes E, Dearden C, et al. The role of pentostatin in the treatment of T-cell malignancies: analysis of response rate in 145 patients according to disease subtype. *J Clin Oncol* 1994;12:2588–2593.

73. Saven A, Carrera CJ, Carson DA, et al. 2-Chlorodeoxyadenosine: an active agent in the treatment of cutaneous T-cell lymphoma. *Blood* 1992;80:587–592.

74. Zinzani PL, Baliva G, Magagnoli M, et al. Gemcitabine treatment in pretreated cutaneous T-cell lymphoma: experience in 44 patients. *J Clin Oncol* 2000;18:2603–2606.

75. Cheng AL, Su IJ, Chen CC, et al. Use of retinoic acids in the treatment of peripheral T-cell lymphoma: a pilot study. *J Clin Oncol* 1994;12:1185–1192.

76. Dang N, Hagemeister F, Fayad L, et al. Phase II study of denileukin diftitox (ONTAK) for relapsed/refractory B and T-cell non-Hodgkin's lymphoma. *Blood* 2002;100:154 [abstr 1405].

77. Mehta A, Hutchison R, Himpler B, et al. Treatment of T-cell anaplastic large cell lymphoma (ALCL) relapsing after autologous stem cell transplant (ASCT) with denileukin diftitox (Ontak). *Blood* 2002; 100:160–161 [abstract 4772].

78. Armitage JO, Coiffier B. Activity of interferon-alpha in relapsed patients with diffuse large B-cell and peripheral T-cell non-Hodgkin's lymphoma. *Ann Oncol* 2000;11:1–3.

79. Frankel AE, Laver JH, Willingham MC, et al. Therapy of patients with T-cell lymphomas and leukemias using an anti-CD7 monoclonal antibody-ricin A chain immunotoxin. *Leuk Lymphoma* 1997;26:287–298.

80. Liang R, Loke SL, Chan AC. The prognostic factors for peripheral T-cell lymphomas. *Hematol Oncol* 1992;10:135–140.

81. Haioun C, Gaulard P, Bourquelot P, et al. Clinical and biological analysis of peripheral T-cell lymphomas: a single institution study. *Leuk Lymphoma* 1992;7:449–455.

82. Armitage JO, Weisenburger DD. New approach to classifying non-Hodgkin's lymphoma: clinical features of the major histologic subtypes. Non-Hodgkin's Lymphoma Classification Project. *J Clin Oncol* 1998;16:2780–2795.

83. Frizzera G, Moran EM, Rappaport H. Angio-immunoblastic lymphadenopathy with dysproteinaemia. *Lancet* 1974;1:1070–1073.

84. Flandrin G, Daniel M, Yafi G, et al. Sarcomatoses ganglionnaires diffuses a differenciation plasmocytaire avec anemie hemolytique autoimmune. In: *Actualites Hematologiques.* Paris: Masson, 1972.

85. Brice P, Calvo F, d'Agay MF, et al. Peripheral T cell lymphoma following angioimmunoblastic lymphadenopathy. *Nouv Rev Fr Hematol* 1987;29:371–377.

86. Shimoyama M, Minato K, Saito H, et al. Immunoblastic lymphadenopathy (IBL)-like T-cell lymphoma. *Jpn J Clin Oncol* 1979;9:347.

87. Patsouris E, Noel H, Lennert K. Angioimmunoblastic lymphadenopathy—type of T-cell lymphoma with a high content of epithelioid cells. Histopathology and comparison with lymphoepithelioid cell lymphoma. *Am J Surg Pathol* 1989;13:262–275.

88. Harris NL, Jaffe ES, Stein H, et al. A revised European-American classification of lymphoid neoplasms: a proposal from the International Lymphoma Study Group [see comments]. *Blood* 1994;84:1361–1392.

89. Pathology and genetics of tumours of haematopoietic and lymphoid tissues. In: Jaffe E, Harris N, Stein H, Vardiman J, eds. *World Health Organization classification of tumors.* Lyon: IARC Press, 2001.

90. Ree HJ, Kadin ME, Kikuchi M, et al. Angioimmunoblastic lymphoma (AILD-type T-cell lymphoma) with hyperplastic germinal centers. *Am J Surg Pathol* 1998;22:643–655.

91. Attygalle A, Al-Jehani R, Diss TC, et al. Neoplastic T cells in angioimmunoblastic T-cell lymphoma express CD10. *Blood* 2002;99:627–633.

92. Weiss LM, Jaffe ES, Liu XF, et al. Detection and localization of Epstein-Barr viral genomes in angioimmunoblastic lymphadenopathy and angioimmunoblastic lymphadenopathy-like lymphoma. *Blood* 1992;79:1789–1795.

93. Jaffe ES. Angioimmunoblastic T-cell lymphoma: new insights, but the clinical challenge remains. *Ann Oncol* 1995;6:631–632.

94. Quintanilla-Martinez L, Fend F, Moguel LR, et al. Peripheral T-cell lymphoma with Reed-Sternberg-like cells of B-cell phenotype and genotype associated with Epstein-Barr virus infection. *Am J Surg Pathol* 1999;23:1233–1240.

95. Lee SS, Rudiger T, Odenwald T, et al. Angioimmunoblastic T cell lymphoma is derived from mature T-helper cells with varying expression and loss of detectable CD4. *Int J Cancer* 2003;103:12–20.

96. Weiss LM, Strickler JG, Dorfman RF, et al. Clonal T-cell populations in angioimmunoblastic lymphadenopathy and angioimmunoblastic lymphadenopathy-like lymphoma. *Am J Pathol* 1986;122:392–397.

97. Feller AC, Griesser H, Schilling CV, et al. Clonal gene rearrangement patterns correlate with immunophenotype and clinical parameters in patients with angioimmunoblastic lymphadenopathy. *Am J Pathol* 1988;133:549–556.

98. Willenbrock K, Roers A, Seidl C, et al. Analysis of T-cell subpopulations in T-cell non-Hodgkin's lymphoma of angioimmunoblastic lymphadenopathy with dysproteinemia type by single target gene amplification of T cell receptor-beta gene rearrangements. *Am J Pathol* 2001;158:1851–1857.

99. Schlegelberger B, Zwingers T, Hohenadel K, et al. Significance of cytogenetic findings for the clinical outcome in patients with T-cell

lymphoma of angioimmunoblastic lymphadenopathy type. *J Clin Oncol* 1996;14:593–599.

100. Frizzera G, Moran EM, Rappaport H. Angio-immunoblastic lymphadenopathy. Diagnosis and clinical course. *Am J Med* 1975;59:803–818.

101. Pangalis GA, Moran EM, Nathwani BN, et al. Angioimmunoblastic lymphadenopathy. Long-term follow-up study. *Cancer* 1983;52:318–321.

102. Hodges E, Quin CT, Wright DH, et al. Oligoclonal populations of T and B cells in a case of angioimmunoblastic T-cell lymphoma predominantly infiltrated by T cells of the VB5.1 family. *Mol Pathol* 1997;50:15–17.

103. Smith JL, Hodges E, Quin CT, et al. Frequent T and B cell oligoclones in histologically and immunophenotypically characterized angioimmunoblastic lymphadenopathy. *Am J Pathol* 2000;156:661–669.

104. Lipford EH, Smith HR, Pittaluga S, et al. Clonality of angioimmunoblastic lymphadenopathy and implications for its evolution to malignant lymphoma. *J Clin Invest* 1987;79:637–642.

105. Abruzzo LV, Schmidt K, Weiss LM, et al. B-cell lymphoma after angioimmunoblastic lymphadenopathy: a case with oligoclonal gene rearrangements associated with Epstein-Barr virus. *Blood* 1993;82:241–246.

106. Siegert W, Nerl C, Agthe A, et al. Angioimmunoblastic lymphadenopathy (AILD)-type T-cell lymphoma: prognostic impact of clinical observations and laboratory findings at presentation. The Kiel Lymphoma Study Group. *Ann Oncol* 1995;6:659–664.

107. Siegert W, Agthe A, Griesser H, et al. Treatment of angioimmunoblastic lymphadenopathy (AILD)-type T-cell lymphoma using prednisone with or without the COPBLAM/IMVP-16 regimen. A multicenter study. Kiel Lymphoma Study Group. *Ann Intern Med* 1992;117:364–370.

108. Advani R, Warnke R, Sikic BI, Horning S. Treatment of angioimmunoblastic T-cell lymphoma with cyclosporine. *Ann Oncol* 1997;8:601–603.

109. Takemori N, Kodaira J, Toyoshima N, et al. Successful treatment of immunoblastic lymphadenopathy-like T-cell lymphoma with cyclosporin A. *Leuk Lymphoma* 1999;35:389–395.

110. Quintini G, Iannitto E, Barbera V, et al. Response to low-dose oral methotrexate and prednisone in two patients with angio-immunoblastic lymphadenopathy-type T-cell lymphoma. *Hematol J* 2001;2:393–395.

111. Pautier P, Devidas A, Delmer A, et al. Angioimmunoblastic-like T-cell non Hodgkin's lymphoma: outcome after chemotherapy in 33 patients and review of the literature. *Leuk Lymphoma* 1999;32:545–552.

112. Kwong YL, Chan AC, Liang RH. Natural killer cell lymphoma/leukemia: pathology and treatment. *Hematol Oncol* 1997;15:71–79.

113. Chan J, Jaffe E, Ralfkiaer. Extranodal NK/T cell lymphoma, nasal type. In: Jaffe E, Harris N, Stein H, et al., eds. *Tumours of haematopoietic and lymphoid tissues, pathology and genetics. World Health Organization classification of tumours.* Lyon: IARC Press, 2001:204–207.

114. Ho FC, Choy D, Loke SL, et al. Polymorphic reticulosis and conventional lymphomas of the nose and upper aerodigestive tract: a clinicopathologic study of 70 cases, and immunophenotypic studies of 16 cases. *Hum Pathol* 1990;21:1041–1050.

115. Vidal RW, Devaney K, Ferlito A, et al. Sinonasal malignant lymphomas: a distinct clinicopathological category. *Ann Otol Rhinol Laryngol* 1999;108:411–419.

116. Liang R, Ng RP, Todd D, et al. Management of stage I-II diffuse aggressive non-Hodgkin's lymphoma of the Waldeyer's ring: combined modality therapy versus radiotherapy alone. *Hematol Oncol* 1987;5:223–230.

117. National Cancer Institute sponsored study of classifications of non-Hodgkin's lymphomas: summary and description of a working formulation for clinical usage. The Non-Hodgkin's Lymphoma Pathologic Classification Project. *Cancer* 1982;49:2112–2135.

118. Chan JK. Natural killer cell neoplasms. *Anat Pathol* 1998;3:77–145.

119. Chan JK. Peripheral T-cell and NK-cell neoplasms: an integrated approach to diagnosis. *Mod Pathol* 1999;12:177–199.

120. A clinical evaluation of the International Lymphoma Study Group classification of non-Hodgkin's lymphoma. The Non-Hodgkin's Lymphoma Classification Project. *Blood* 1997;89:3909–3918.

121. Liang R, Loke SL, Ho FC, et al. Histologic subtypes and survival of Chinese patients with non-Hodgkin's lymphomas. *Cancer* 1990;66:1850–1855.

122. Quintanilla-Martinez L, Franklin JL, Guerrero I, et al. Histological and immunophenotypic profile of nasal NK/T cell lymphomas from Peru: high prevalence of p53 overexpression. *Hum Pathol* 1999;30:849–855.

123. Lipford EH Jr, Margolick JB, Longo DL, et al. Angiocentric immunoproliferative lesions: a clinicopathologic spectrum of post-thymic T-cell proliferations. *Blood* 1988;72:1674–1681.

124. Chan JK, Ng CS, Ngan KC, et al. Angiocentric T-cell lymphoma of the skin. An aggressive lymphoma distinct from mycosis fungoides. *Am J Surg Pathol* 1988;12:861–876.

125. Teruya-Feldstein J, Jaffe ES, Burd PR, et al. The role of Mig, the monokine induced by interferon-gamma, and IP-10, the interferon-gamma-inducible protein-10, in tissue necrosis and vascular damage associated with Epstein-Barr virus-positive lymphoproliferative disease. *Blood* 1997;90:4099–4105.

126. Lay JD, Tsao CJ, Chen JY, et al. Upregulation of tumor necrosis factor-alpha gene by Epstein-Barr virus and activation of macrophages in Epstein-Barr virus-infected T cells in the pathogenesis of hemophagocytic syndrome. *J Clin Invest* 1997;100:1969–1979.

127. Dictor M, Cervin A, Kalm O, et al. Sinonasal T-cell lymphoma in the differential diagnosis of lethal midline granuloma using in situ hybridization for Epstein-Barr virus RNA. *Mod Pathol* 1996;9:7–14.

128. Tsang WY, Chan JK, Yip TT, et al. *In situ* localization of Epstein-Barr virus encoded RNA in non-nasal/nasopharyngeal CD56-positive and CD56-negative T-cell lymphomas. *Hum Pathol* 1994;25:758–765.

129. Medeiros LJ, Peiper SC, Elwood L, et al. Angiocentric immunoproliferative lesions: a molecular analysis of eight cases. *Hum Pathol* 1991;22:1150–1157.

130. Medeiros LJ, Jaffe ES, Chen YY, et al. Localization of Epstein-Barr viral genomes in angiocentric immunoproliferative lesions. *Am J Surg Pathol* 1992;16:439–447.

131. Ho FC, Srivastava G, Loke SL, et al. Presence of Epstein-Barr virus DNA in nasal lymphomas of B and 'T' cell type. *Hematol Oncol* 1990;8:271–281.

132. Wong KF, Zhang YM, Chan JK. Cytogenetic abnormalities in natural killer cell lymphoma/leukaemia—is there a consistent pattern? *Leuk Lymphoma* 1999;34:241–250.

133. Siu LL, Wong KF, Chan JK, et al. Comparative genomic hybridization analysis of natural killer cell lymphoma/leukemia. Recognition of consistent patterns of genetic alterations. *Am J Pathol* 1999;155:1419–1425.

134. Wong N, Wong KF, Chan JK, et al. Chromosomal translocations are common in natural killer-cell lymphoma/leukemia as shown by spectral karyotyping. *Hum Pathol* 2000;31:771–774.

135. Chiang AK, Tao Q, Srivastava G, et al. Nasal NK- and T-cell lymphomas share the same type of Epstein-Barr virus latency as nasopharyngeal carcinoma and Hodgkin's disease. *Int J Cancer* 1996;68:285–290.

136. Gutierrez MI, Spangler G, Kingma D, et al. Epstein-Barr virus in nasal lymphomas contains multiple ongoing mutations in the EBNA-1 gene. *Blood* 1998;92:600–606.

137. Gaal K, Weiss LM, Chen WG, et al. Epstein-Barr virus nuclear antigen (EBNA)-1 carboxy-terminal and EBNA-4 sequence polymorphisms in nasal natural killer/T-cell lymphoma in the United States. *Lab Invest* 2002;82:957–962.

138. Ng CS, Lo ST, Chan JK, et al. CD56+ putative natural killer cell lymphomas: production of cytolytic effectors and related proteins mediating tumor cell apoptosis? *Hum Pathol* 1997;28:1276–1282.

139. Ng CS, Lo ST, Chan JK. Peripheral T and putative natural killer cell lymphomas commonly coexpress CD95 and CD95 ligand. *Hum Pathol* 1999;30:48–53.

140. Binstadt BA, Brumbaugh KM, Leibson PJ. Signal transduction by human NK cell MHC-recognizing receptors. *Immunol Rev* 1997;155:197–203.

141. Haedicke W, Ho FC, Chott A, et al. Expression of CD94/NKG2A and killer immunoglobulin-like receptors in NK cells and a subset of extranodal cytotoxic T-cell lymphomas. *Blood* 2000;95:3628–3630.

142. Dukers DF, Vermeer MH, Jaspars LH, et al. Expression of killer cell inhibitory receptors is restricted to true NK cell lymphomas and a subset of intestinal enteropathy-type T cell lymphomas with a cytotoxic phenotype. *J Clin Pathol* 2001;54:224–228.

143. Chan JK, Sin VC, Wong KF, et al. Nonnasal lymphoma expressing the natural killer cell marker CD56: a clinicopathologic study of 49 cases of an uncommon aggressive neoplasm. *Blood* 1997;89:4501–4513.

144. Liang R, Todd D, Chan TK, et al. Nasal lymphoma. A retrospective analysis of 60 cases. *Cancer* 1990;66:2205–2209.

145. Yeh KH, Lien HC, Hsu SM, et al. Quiescent nasal T/NK cell lymphoma manifested as primary central nervous system lymphoma. *Am J Hematol* 1999;60:161–163.

146. Chim CS, Choy C, Liang R, et al. Isolated uterine relapse of nasal T/Nk cell lymphoma. *Leuk Lymphoma* 1999;34:629–632.

147. Kato N, Yasukawa K, Onozuka T, et al. Nasal and nasal-type T/NK-cell lymphoma with cutaneous involvement. *J Am Acad Dermatol* 1999;40:850–856.

148. Au WY, Chan AC, Kwong YL. Scrotal skin ulcer in a patient with a previous tonsillectomy because of natural killer cell lymphoma. *Am J Dermatopathol* 1998;20:582–585.

149. Liang R, Todd D, Chan TK, et al. Treatment outcome and prognostic factors for primary nasal lymphoma. *J Clin Oncol* 1995;13:666–670.

150. Kwong YL, Chan AC, Liang R, et al. CD56+ NK lymphomas: clinicopathological features and prognosis. *Br J Haematol* 1997;97:821–829.

151. Han JY, Seo EJ, Kwon HJ, et al. Nasal angiocentric lymphoma with hemophagocytic syndrome. *Korean J Intern Med* 1999;14:41–46.

152. Ooi GC, Chim CS, Liang R, et al. Nasal T-cell/natural killer cell lymphoma: CT and MR imaging features of a new clinicopathologic entity. *AJR Am J Roentgenol* 2000;174:1141–1145.

153. Chim CS, Ooi GC, Shek TW, et al. Lethal midline granuloma revisited: nasal T/Natural-killer cell lymphoma. *J Clin Oncol* 1999;17:1322–1325.

154. Kim GE, Cho JH, Yang WI, et al. Angiocentric lymphoma of the head and neck: patterns of systemic failure after radiation treatment. *J Clin Oncol* 2000;18:54–63.

155. Cheung MM, Chan JK, Lau WH, et al. Primary non-Hodgkin's lymphoma of the nose and nasopharynx: clinical features, tumor immunophenotype, and treatment outcome in 113 patients. *J Clin Oncol* 1998;16:70–77.

156. Lei KI, Chan LY, Chan WY, et al. Quantitative analysis of circulating cell-free Epstein-Barr virus (EBV) DNA levels in patients with EBV-associated lymphoid malignancies. *Br J Haematol* 2000;111:239–246.

157. Liang R, Chen F, Lee CK, et al. Autologous bone marrow transplantation for primary nasal T/NK cell lymphoma. *Bone Marrow Transplant* 1997;19:91–93.

158. Nawa Y, Takenaka K, Shinagawa K, et al. Successful treatment of advanced natural killer cell lymphoma with high-dose chemotherapy and syngeneic peripheral blood stem cell transplantation. *Bone Marrow Transplant* 1999;23:1321–1322.

159. Mukai HY, Kojima H, Suzukawa K, et al. High-dose chemotherapy with peripheral blood stem cell rescue in blastoid natural killer cell lymphoma. *Leuk Lymphoma* 1999;32:583–588.

160. Reyes F, Belhadj K, Tilly H, et al. Hepatosplenic gamma delta T-cell lymphoma: a recently recognized entity which is fatal. *Blood* 1997;90:338a [abstr].

161. Farcet JP, Gaulard P, Marolleau JP, et al. Hepatosplenic T-cell lymphoma: sinusal/sinusoidal localization of malignant cells expressing the T-cell receptor gamma delta. *Blood* 1990;75:2213–2219.

162. Weidmann E. Hepatosplenic T cell lymphoma. A review on 45 cases since the first report describing the disease as a distinct lymphoma entity in 1990. *Leukemia* 2000;14:991–997.

163. Wong KF, Chan JK, Matutes E, et al. Hepatosplenic gamma delta T-cell lymphoma. A distinctive aggressive lymphoma type [see comments]. *Am J Surg Pathol* 1995;19:718–726.

164. Felgar RE, Macon WR, Kinney MC, et al. TIA-1 expression in lymphoid neoplasms. Identification of subsets with cytotoxic T lymphocyte or natural killer cell differentiation. *Am J Pathol* 1997;150:1893–1900.

165. A predictive model for aggressive non-Hodgkin's lymphoma. The International Non-Hodgkin's Lymphoma Prognostic Factors Project [see comments]. *N Engl J Med* 1993;329:987–994.

166. Francois A, Lesesve JF, Stamatoullas A, et al. Hepatosplenic gamma/delta T-cell lymphoma: a report of two cases in immunocompromised patients, associated with isochromosome 7q. *Am J Surg Pathol* 1997;21:781–790.

167. Khan WA, Yu L, Eisenbrey AB, et al. Hepatosplenic gamma/delta T-cell lymphoma in immunocompromised patients. Report of two cases and review of literature. *Am J Clin Pathol* 2001;116:41–50.

168. Ross CW, Schnitzer B, Sheldon S, et al. Gamma/delta T-cell posttransplantation lymphoproliferative disorder primarily in the spleen. *Am J Clin Pathol* 1994;102:310–315.

169. Kanavaros P, Farcet JP, Gaulard P, et al. Recombinative events of the T cell antigen receptor delta gene in peripheral T cell lymphomas. *J Clin Invest* 1991;87:666–672.

170. Alonsozana EL, Stamberg J, Kumar D, et al. Isochromosome 7q: the primary cytogenetic abnormality in hepatosplenic gammadelta T cell lymphoma. *Leukemia* 1997;11:1367–1372.

171. Jonveaux P, Daniel MT, Martel V, et al. Isochromosome 7q and trisomy 8 are consistent primary, non-random chromosomal abnormalities associated with hepatosplenic T gamma/delta lymphoma. *Leukemia* 1996;10:1453–1455.

172. Wang CC, Tien HF, Lin MT, et al. Consistent presence of isochromosome 7q in hepatosplenic T gamma/delta lymphoma: a new cytogenetic-clinicopathologic entity. *Genes Chromosomes Cancer* 1995;12:161–164.

173. Mead GM, Whitehouse JM, Thompson J, et al. Clinical features and management of malignant histiocytosis of the intestine. *Cancer* 1987;60:2791–2796.

174. O'Farrelly C, Feighery C, O'Briain DS, et al. Humoral response to wheat protein in patients with coeliac disease and enteropathy associated T cell lymphoma. *BMJ (Clin Res Ed)* 1986;293:908–910.

175. Isaacson P, Wright DH. Intestinal lymphoma associated with malabsorption. *Lancet* 1978;1:67–70.

176. Isaacson P, Wright DH. Malignant histiocytosis of the intestine. Its relationship to malabsorption and ulcerative jejunitis. *Hum Pathol* 1978;9:661–677.

177. Whitehead R. Primary lymphadenopathy complicating idiopathic steatorrhoea. *Gut* 1968;9:569–575.

178. Gough K, Read A, Naish J. Intestinal reticulosis as a complication of idiopathic steatorrhoea. *Gut* 1962;3:232–239.

179. Morton JE, Leyland MJ, Vaughan Hudson G, et al. Primary gastrointestinal non-Hodgkin's lymphoma: a review of 175 British National Lymphoma Investigation cases. *Br J Cancer* 1993;67:776–782.

180. Trier JS. Celiac sprue. *N Engl J Med* 1991;325:1709–1719.

181. Weinstein W. Intractable celiac sprue. *Diff Dec Dig Dis* 1994:257-268.

182. Chott A, Dragosics B, Radaszkiewicz T. Peripheral T-cell lymphomas of the intestine. *Am J Pathol* 1992;141:1361–1371.

183. Spencer J, Cerf-Bensussan N, Jarry A, et al. Enteropathy-associated T cell lymphoma (malignant histiocytosis of the intestine) is recognized by a monoclonal antibody (HML-1) that defines a membrane molecule on human mucosal lymphocytes. *Am J Pathol* 1988;132:1–5.

184. de Bruin PC, Kummer JA, van der Valk P, et al. Granzyme B-expressing peripheral T-cell lymphomas: neoplastic equivalents of activated cytotoxic T cells with preference for mucosa-associated lymphoid tissue localization. *Blood* 1994;84:3785–3791.

185. de Bruin PC, Jiwa M, Oudejans JJ, et al. Presence of Epstein-Barr virus in extranodal T-cell lymphomas: differences in relation to site. *Blood* 1994;83:1612–1618.

186. Quintanilla-Martinez L, Lome-Maldonado C, Ott G, et al. Primary intestinal non-Hodgkin's lymphoma and Epstein-Barr virus: high frequency of EBV-infection in T-cell lymphomas of Mexican origin. *Leuk Lymphoma* 1998;30:111–121.

187. Isaacson PG, O'Connor NT, Spencer J, et al. Malignant histiocytosis of the intestine: a T-cell lymphoma. *Lancet* 1985;2:688–691.

188. Murray A, Cuevas EC, Jones DB, et al. Study of the immunohistochemistry and T cell clonality of enteropathy-associated T cell lymphoma. *Am J Pathol* 1995;146:509–519.

189. Katoh A, Ohshima K, Kanda M, et al. Gastrointestinal T cell lymphoma: predominant cytotoxic phenotypes, including alpha/beta, gamma/delta T cell and natural killer cells. *Leuk Lymphoma* 2000;39:97–111.

190. Zettl A, Ott G, Makulik A, et al. Chromosomal gains at 9q characterize enteropathy-type T-cell lymphoma. *Am J Pathol* 2002;161:1635–1645.

191. Stein H, Dienemann D, Sperling M, et al. Identification of a T cell lymphoma category derived from intestinal-mucosa-associated T cells. *Lancet* 1988;2:1053–1054.

192. Micklem KJ, Dong Y, Willis A, et al. HML-1 antigen on mucosa-associated T cells, activated cells, and hairy leukemic cells is a new integrin containing the beta 7 subunit. *Am J Pathol* 1991;139:1297–1301.

193. Simonitsch I, Volc-Platzer B, Mosberger I, et al. Expression of monoclonal antibody HML-1-defined alpha E beta 7 integrin in cutaneous T cell lymphoma. *Am J Pathol* 1994;145:1148–1158.

194. Cellier C, Delabesse E, Helmer C, et al. Refractory sprue, coeliac disease, and enteropathy-associated T-cell lymphoma. French Coeliac Disease Study Group. *Lancet* 2000;356:203–208.

195. Daum S, Weiss D, Hummel M, et al. Frequency of clonal intraepithelial T lymphocyte proliferations in enteropathy-type intestinal T cell lymphoma, coeliac disease, and refractory sprue. *Gut* 2001;49:804–812.

196. Gale J, Simmonds PD, Mead GM, et al. Enteropathy-type intestinal T-cell lymphoma: clinical features and treatment of 31 patients in a single center. *J Clin Oncol* 2000;18:795.

197. Egan LJ, Walsh SV, Stevens FM, et al. Celiac-associated lymphoma. A single institution experience of 30 cases in the combination chemotherapy era. *J Clin Gastroenterol* 1995;21:123–129.

198. Brandt L, Hagander B, Norden A, et al. Lymphoma of the small intestine in adult coeliac disease. *Acta Med Scand* 1978;204:467–470.

199. Cooper BT, Holmes GK, Ferguson R, et al. Celiac disease and malignancy. *Medicine (Baltimore)* 1980;59:249–261.

200. Cooper BT, Holmes GK, Cooke WT. Lymphoma risk in coeliac disease of later life. *Digestion* 1982;23:89–92.

201. Holmes GK, Stokes PL, McWalter R, et al. Proceedings: Coeliac disease, malignancy, and gluten-free diet. *Gut* 1974;15:339.

202. Holmes GK, Prior P, Lane MR, et al. Malignancy in coeliac disease—effect of a gluten-free diet. *Gut* 1989;30:333–338.

203. Armitage JO, Dick FR, Corder MP, et al. Predicting therapeutic outcome in patients with diffuse histiocytic lymphoma treated with cyclophosphamide, adriamycin, vincristine and prednisone (CHOP). *Cancer* 1982;50:1695–1702.

204. Gonzalez CL, Medeiros LJ, Braziel RM, et al. T-cell lymphoma involving subcutaneous tissue. A clinicopathologic entity commonly associated with hemophagocytic syndrome. *Am J Surg Pathol* 1991; 15:17–27.

205. Ashworth J, Coady AT, Guy R, et al. Brawny cutaneous induration and granulomatous panniculitis in large cell non-Hodgkin's (T suppressor/cytotoxic cell) lymphoma. *Br J Dermatol* 1989;120:563–569.

206. Tanaka K, Hagari Y, Sano Y, et al. A case of T-cell lymphoma associated with panniculitis, progressive pancytopenia and hyperbilirubinaemia. *Br J Dermatol* 1990;123:649–652.

207. Wang CY, Su WP, Kurtin PJ. Subcutaneous pannicultic T-cell lymphoma. *Int J Dermatol* 1996;35:1–8.

208. Przybylski GK, Wu H, Macon WR, et al. Hepatosplenic and subcutaneous panniculitis-like gamma/delta T cell lymphomas are derived from different Vdelta subsets of gamma/delta T lymphocytes. *J Mol Diagn* 2000;2:11–19.

209. Wang H, Medeiros LJ, Jones D. Subcutaneous panniculitis-like T-cell lymphoma. *Clin Lymphoma* 2002;3:181–183.

210. Berg KD, Brinster NK, Huhn KM, et al. Transmission of a T-cell lymphoma by allogeneic bone marrow transplantation. *N Engl J Med* 2001;345:1458–1463.

211. Perniciaro C, Zalla MJ, White JW Jr, et al. Subcutaneous T-cell lymphoma. Report of two additional cases and further observations. *Arch Dermatol* 1993;129:1171–1176.

212. Matsue K, Itoh M, Tsukuda K, et al. Successful treatment of cytophagic histiocytic panniculitis with modified CHOP-E. Cyclophosphamide, adriamycin, vincristine, prednisone, and etoposide. *Am J Clin Oncol* 1994;17:470–474.

213. Weenig RH, Ng CS, Perniciaro C. Subcutaneous panniculitis-like T-cell lymphoma: an elusive case presenting as lipomembranous panniculitis and a review of 72 cases in the literature. *Am J Dermatopathol* 2001; 23:206–215.

214. Abeloff M, Armitage J. *Journal of clinical oncology.* New York: Churchill Livingstone, 2000.

215. Papenfuss JS, Aoun P, Bierman PJ, et al. Subcutaneous panniculitis-like T-cell lymphoma: presentation of 2 cases and observations. *Clin Lymphoma* 2002;3:175–180.

216. Salhany KE, Macon WR, Choi JK, et al. Subcutaneous panniculitis-like T-cell lymphoma: clinicopathologic, immunophenotypic, and genotypic analysis of alpha/beta and gamma/delta subtypes. *Am J Surg Pathol* 1998;22:881–893.

217. Parisi M, McNutt N. Subcutaneous panniculitis-like T-cell lymphoma associated with a hemophagocytic syndrome in a patient with polycythemia vera and interferon-alpha therapy. *J Cutan Pathol* 1998;25.

218. Tobinai K, Minato K, Ohtsu T, et al. Clinicopathologic, immunophenotypic, and immunogenotypic analyses of immunoblastic lymphadenopathy-like T-cell lymphoma. *Blood* 1988;72:1000–1006.

219. Ohsaka A, Saito K, Sakai T, et al. Clinicopathologic and therapeutic aspects of angioimmunoblastic lymphadenopathy-related lesions. *Cancer* 1992;69:1259–1267.

220. Nathwani BN, Rappaport H, Moran EM, et al. Malignant lymphoma arising in angioimmunoblastic lymphadenopathy. *Cancer* 1978;41:578–606.

CHAPTER 27

Diffuse Large B-Cell Lymphoma

James O. Armitage, Peter M. Mauch, Nancy Lee Harris,
Riccardo Dalla-Favera, and Philip J. Bierman

DEFINITION

Diffuse large B-cell lymphoma, the most common non-Hodgkin's lymphoma, is a malignancy of large transformed B lymphocytes. Tumor cells can be predominately centroblastic, immunoblastic, anaplastic, or multilobated in appearance. Rare subtypes of diffuse large B-cell lymphoma can be difficult to diagnose because of a heavy infiltration of T-cells (i.e., T-cell–rich B-cell lymphoma) or obscured by other infiltrating cells (e.g., lymphomatoid granulomatosis, posttransplant lymphoproliferative disease). Diffuse large B-cell lymphoma can arise from small B-cell lymphoma, marginal zone lymphoma, or follicular lymphoma, a phenomenon that is often called a *transformed diffuse large B-cell lymphoma*. Diffuse large B-cell lymphomas can arise in nodal or extranodal sites. Diffuse large B-cell lymphomas that occur in sites where small-cell mucosa-associated lymphoid tissue (MALT) lymphomas are often found are best labeled as *diffuse large B-cell lymphoma* rather than *transformed* or *high-grade MALT lymphoma* to avoid confusion in therapeutic decisions.

It is certain that diffuse large B-cell lymphoma does not represent one clear-cut, clinical-pathologic entity. As is discussed below, clinical patterns of presentation and new studies of gene arrays are making it clear that all diffuse large B-cell lymphomas are not created equal. It may be that this subtype of lymphoma will be subdivided into more than one entity in the near future.

FREQUENCY AND ETIOLOGY

Diffuse large B-cell lymphoma is the most common non-Hodgkin's lymphoma, representing approximately one third of all non-Hodgkin's lymphomas worldwide (1). This is one type of non-Hodgkin's lymphoma in which the relative incidence does not seem to vary geographically (2). In almost all parts of the world, this is the most frequently occurring non-Hodgkin's lymphoma. The increasing incidence of non-Hodgkin's lymphoma seen in the latter half of the twentieth century was certainly due, at least in part, to an increase in the incidence of diffuse large B-cell lymphoma. Diffuse large B-cell lymphoma is most frequently seen in patients in the seventh decade of life and more frequently in men than women. However, it is also one of the more common non-Hodgkin's lymphomas of childhood.

When patients with immune deficiencies develop non-Hodgkin's lymphoma, diffuse large B-cell lymphoma and Burkitt's lymphoma are the most frequent subtypes. Patients with other immune disorders, such as rheumatoid arthritis, have been said to be at increased risk of developing non-Hodgkin's lymphoma (3,4). The most frequent subtype seen in this setting is diffuse large B-cell lymphoma.

Patients with immune deficiencies who develop non-Hodgkin's lymphoma often have the tumor associated with Epstein-Barr–virus infection. This is particularly true for patients with post–organ transplant lymphoma and central nervous system lymphomas developing in patients with autoimmune deficiency syndrome. Human herpes virus 8, or Kaposi's sarcoma–associated herpes virus, has been associated with diffuse large B-cell lymphoma developing in pleural effusions. The triggering factor for diffuse large B-cell lymphoma developing in preexisting small lymphocytic lymphoma, MALT lymphomas, or follicular lymphoma is unclear.

For more details regarding etiology and epidemiology, see Chapter 44.

PATHOLOGY

Diffuse large B-cell lymphoma is defined in the World Health Organization Classification as a lymphoma comprised of large neoplastic lymphoid cells similar in size to or larger than tissue macrophages and more than twice the size of normal lymphocytes, with a diffuse growth pattern. It is thought to be a heterogeneous category, but criteria for defining distinct subentities are, in general, lacking. Several clinically and morphologically distinct subtypes can be recognized at present and are described

TABLE 27.1. *Diffuse large B-cell lymphoma, variants and subtypes*

Diffuse large B-cell lymphoma, morphologic variants
  Centroblastic
  Immunoblastic
  Anaplastic large B-cell
  Plasmablastic
  Anaplastic lymphoma kinase–positive
Diffuse large B-cell lymphoma, subtypes
  Mediastinal (thymic) large B-cell lymphoma
  Intravascular large B-cell lymphoma
  T-cell/histiocyte-rich large B-cell lymphoma
  Lymphomatoid granulomatosis–type large B-cell lymphoma
  Primary effusion lymphoma

below and summarized in Table 27.1. Diffuse large B-cell lymphoma may also occur as a high-grade transformation of several low-grade B-cell lymphomas (small lymphocytic lymphoma/chronic lymphocytic leukemia, lymphoplasmacytic lymphoma, follicular lymphoma, MALT lymphoma, and splenic marginal zone lymphoma).

Morphology

Diffuse large B-cell lymphomas are a heterogeneous group of neoplasms. They are typically composed of large cells (three times the size of normal lymphocytes) that resemble either the proliferating cells of the germinal center (centroblasts/large noncleaved cells) or immunoblasts, most often with a mixture of the two (Color Plate 59). Several morphologic variants can be recognized, but their clinical significance is debated. The *centroblastic type* (80% of the cases) is composed of cells resembling centroblasts, with one to three peripheral nucleoli and a narrow rim of basophilic cytoplasm, often with a variable admixture of immunoblasts. Some cases have multilobated centroblasts. The *immunoblastic type* (10% of the cases) has more than 90% immunoblasts, with a prominent central nucleolus and abundant, basophilic cytoplasm, often with plasmacytoid differentiation. These cases are more common in immunosuppressed patients. In nonimmunosuppressed patients, they have been reported in some studies to have a worse prognosis, whereas others have failed to confirm this (5,6). In the *anaplastic type*, the cells are morphologically similar to those of T/null anaplastic large-cell lymphoma, with pleomorphic nuclei, abundant cytoplasm and sinusoidal growth pattern, and CD30 expression. Although these have been called *B-anaplastic large-cell lymphoma*, they do not have the same distinctive clinical or genetic features of T/null anaplastic large-cell lymphoma and are considered a morphologic variant of large B-cell lymphoma. Two other distinctive morphologic and immunophenotypic variants of diffuse large B-cell lymphomas are the *plasmablastic types* seen in human immunodeficiency virus–positive patients (7,8) and a rare

variant expressing the full-length anaplastic lymphoma kinase protein (9).

Bone marrow involvement in diffuse large B-cell lymphoma may take two forms. In approximately 10% of cases, there is large-cell lymphoma in the marrow. However, a slightly higher proportion may show so-called discordant marrow involvement—aggregates of small atypical lymphoid cells consistent with involvement of low-grade lymphoma, particularly follicular lymphoma. Several studies have shown that discordant marrow involvement is not associated with a worse prognosis than are cases without marrow involvement (10,11); however, these patients may be at risk for late relapses (12).

Immunophenotype and Genetic Features

Diffuse large B-cell lymphomas express one or more B cell–associated antigens (CD19, CD20, CD22, CD79a, PAX5), as well as CD45 and often surface immunoglobulin (Ig). They may coexpress CD5 or CD10 (13,14). Cases with plasmablastic morphology may lack CD20 and PAX5 and express only CD79a. Twenty-five percent to 80% of cases in various studies express bcl-2 protein, and this may be associated with a worse prognosis (15–19). Approximately 70% express bcl-6 protein, consistent with a germinal-center origin (18,19), independent of BCL-6 gene rearrangement.

Ig genes are rearranged, and most have somatic mutations in the variable-region genes (20,21). The BCL2 gene is rearranged in 15% to 30%; it is associated with disseminated nodal disease but not with either a worse prognosis or bcl-2 protein expression (15). The c-MYC gene is rearranged in 5% to 15% (22,23); the BCL6 gene is rearranged in 20% to 40% of cases (23,24) and shows mutations in the 5' noncoding region in 70% (25,26). Both the 5' noncoding mutations of the BCL-6 gene (27,28) and the Ig variable–region gene mutations are found in normal germinal center cells (29); their presence in diffuse large B-cell lymphoma is consistent with a germinal center or postgerminal center stage of differentiation.

The postulated normal counterpart is proliferating peripheral B cells—centroblasts or immunoblasts in most cases.

DIFFUSE LARGE B-CELL LYMPHOMA SUBTYPES

As mentioned, diffuse large B-cell lymphoma is believed to be a heterogeneous category for which we currently lack the tools to dissect into clinically relevant diseases. However, several distinctive subtypes of diffuse large B-cell lymphomas have been recognized; these are summarized in Table 27.1 and discussed briefly below.

Intravascular Large B-Cell Lymphoma

Rare cases of large-cell lymphoma, usually of the B-cell type, present with a disseminated intravascular proliferation of large lymphoid cells involving small blood vessels, without an obvious extravascular tumor mass or leukemia (30). This tumor has also been variously known as *intravascular lymphomatosis*, *angiotropic lymphoma*, and *malignant angioendotheliomatosis*. The neoplastic lymphoid cells are mainly lodged in the lumina of small vessels in many organs. The tumor cells may resemble centroblasts or immunoblasts and express B cell–associated antigens. Malignant cells are rarely seen in cerebrospinal fluid, blood, or bone marrow. The organs most commonly involved are the central nervous system, kidneys, lungs, and skin, but virtually any site may be involved. Patients present with a variety of symptoms related to organ dysfunction secondary to vascular occlusion. Because of this, the diagnosis is difficult, and many reported cases were diagnosed at autopsy. If a timely diagnosis is made and combination chemotherapy instituted, many patients achieve complete remission, and long-term survival appears to be possible (31).

T-Cell/Histiocyte–Rich Large B-Cell Lymphoma

Some cases of large B-cell lymphoma have a prominent background of reactive T cells and, often, histiocytes—so-called T-cell/histiocyte–rich large B-cell lymphoma. The tumors may resemble Hodgkin's lymphoma of lymphocyte predominance or mixed cellularity type (32,33). However, in contrast to either lymphocyte predominance or mixed cellularity Hodgkin's lymphoma, patients with T-cell/histiocyte–rich large B-cell lymphoma typically present with disseminated disease involving lymph nodes, liver, spleen, and bone marrow. They may respond to aggressive therapy for large-cell lymphoma. The relationship of this disease to lymphocyte-predominance or classical Hodgkin's lymphoma remains to be elucidated.

Large B-Cell Lymphoma, Lymphomatoid Granulomatosis Type

Recently, the entity described as *lymphomatoid granulomatosis* has been shown in most cases to be an Epstein-Barr virus–positive large B-cell lymphoma with a T-cell–rich background (34–37). Patients typically present with extranodal disease, most commonly involving lung, central nervous system, or kidneys. Evidence of past or present immunosuppression may be found. The infiltrates show extensive necrosis, often with only a few atypical large B cells in a background of small T lymphocytes; the infiltrate may be both angiocentric and angioinvasive. Although the infiltrates may resemble those of nasal-type natural killer/T-cell lymphoma, there is no biologic and little clinical overlap, because the latter is a natural killer/T-cell neoplasm that involves the upper airway and midfacial region, skin, and sometimes the gastrointestinal tract, but only rarely the lung or central nervous system. Lymphomatoid granulomatosis is graded according to the number of large B cells. The lower-grade cases are not typically treated as lymphoma; grade 3 cases fulfill the criteria for large B-cell lymphoma in a T-cell–rich background and may be clinically aggressive (38).

Primary Effusion Lymphoma

Primary effusion lymphoma is a recently recognized disease that occurs most often in immunosuppressed patients either with human immunodeficiency virus or in the posttransplant setting, but occasional cases in nonimmunosuppressed patients have been reported. Patients present with effusions in serous cavities: the pleura, pericardium, or peritoneum. Occasionally, infiltration of other tissues may be seen (39). The clinical course is usually very aggressive. The tumor cells are large, often pleomorphic, cells resembling either bizarre plasma cells or the cells of anaplastic large-cell lymphoma. They often lack B cell–associated antigens, such as CD20, and are bcl6− but may be CD79a+ and CD45+, sometimes contain cytoplasmic Ig, and often express CD30 and the plasma cell–associated antigen CD138 (40). Ig genes are clonally rearranged. They typically contain both Epstein-Barr virus and the recently-described Kaposi's sarcoma herpes virus/human herpes virus 8 (41).

PATHOGENESIS

Although biologically and clinically heterogeneous, all diffuse large B-cell lymphomas derive from germinal center B cells, as documented by the presence of somatic mutations in their Ig variable genes, by their expression of germinal center–related markers, and by the lack of expression of markers typical of plasma-cell differentiation. Recently, the genome-wide analysis of the pattern of expression of thousands of genes by DNA array technology has identified distinct subsets of diffuse large B-cell lymphomas that may correspond to distinct stages of germinal center development or to different mechanisms of malignant transformation (42,43). Taken together, these studies clearly indicate that diffuse large B-cell lymphomas comprise a heterogeneous group of tumors with distinct and still largely unknown biologic features.

The molecular pathogenesis of diffuse large B-cell lymphoma is complex and involves several mechanisms of genetic lesion: chromosomal translocations, the recently identified aberrant somatic hypermutation mechanism, and other mechanisms common to all malignancies, such as gene amplifications and deletions.

Chromosomal Translocations

Cytogenetic studies of non-Hodgkin's lymphoma have demonstrated that chromosomal alterations affecting band 3q27 are a frequent recurrent abnormality in B-lineage diffuse large-cell lymphoma (44,45). These alterations are represented by reciprocal translocations between the 3q27 region and several alternative partner chromosomes, including, although not restricted to, the sites of the Ig genes at 14q32 (Ig$_H$), 2p11 (Igκ), and 22q11 (Igλ) (44,45). The variability of the partner chromosomes juxtaposed to 3q27 in B-lineage diffuse large-cell lymphoma translocations suggests that these abnormalities belong to the group of "promiscuous" translocations, which involve a fixed chromosomal breakpoint on one side and, on the other side, different chromosomal partners in different cases. These translocations juxtapose heterologous promoters derived from different partner chromosomes to the coding region of the BCL6 gene, thereby leading to its deregulated expression by a mechanism called *promoter substitution* (46,47). The BCL6 gene encodes a transcription factor that binds the specific DNA sequences located in the promoter region of its target genes and represses their transcription (48). In the B-cell lineage, the bcl-6 protein is expressed only in germinal center cells but not in pregerminal center cells, for example the mantle zone cells, or postgerminal center cells, such as immunoblasts and plasma cells (49). Mice deficient for bcl-6 are not capable of forming germinal centers and show a complete lack of affinity maturation (50,51). Therefore, bcl-6 appears to be a pivotal regulator of germinal center development.

Chromosomal translocations involving the BCL6 gene can be detected in approximately 35% of diffuse large B-cell lymphomas and in a minority (5% to 10%) of follicular lymphomas (52). The majority of these translocations give rise to a fusion transcript in which exon1 and the promoter of BCL6 are replaced by the partner gene sequences (47). These fusion transcripts are initiated from the heterologous promoters, and they contain the intact coding exons of BCL6. Compared to the BCL6 promoter, these promoters demonstrate a broader spectrum of activity in B-cell development, including expression in the postgerminal center differentiation stage, such as immunoblasts and plasma cells (53). Consequently, they can prevent the normal downregulation of BCL6 expression that occurs during differentiation into postgerminal center cells. The constitutive expression of BCL6 is thought to contribute to lymphomagenesis by repressing the transcription of genes inducing cell-cycle arrest, apoptosis, and differentiation (54). *In vivo* studies in transgenic mice are necessary to confirm this hypothesis.

Besides promoter substitution, BCL6 gene can also be altered by somatic hypermutation of its 5' noncoding region. Hypermutation of BCL6 can be found in normal germinal center cells (27,55), and it is also found in many non-Hodgkin's lymphomas, most frequently in diffuse large B-cell lymphoma (73%) independent of BCL6 rearrangement (25,55). Functional analysis of BCL6 promoter–containing mutations indicates that some mutations associated with diffuse large B-cell lymphoma but not from normal germinal center cells may deregulate the basal level of BCL6 transcription by interfering with its physiologic mechanism of negative feedback regulation (56). Given the occurrence of BCL6 mutations in normal B cells and their frequency and heterogeneity, further studies are needed to identify the full spectrum of mutations, which have a pathogenetic significance.

In addition to translocations involving BCL6, diffuse large B-cell lymphoma displays a variety of other translocations, including those whose target gene has not yet been identified, as well as those involving the BCL2 gene. Based on the genetic configuration of BCL6 and BCL2, diffuse large B-cell lymphoma can be separated into three categories (22,26,57,58). The first one, accounting for approximately 40% of the cases, associates with rearrangement of BCL6 without other known genetic lesions. The second category contains BCL2 rearrangement with or without the presence of p53 alterations. This type probably presents diffuse large B-cell lymphoma evolving from clinical or subclinical follicular lymphoma. The third category contains germline BCL2 and BCL6 and, therefore, includes cases with mutated BCL6 as well as those with other types of translocations.

Aberrant Somatic Hypermutation

It has been recently shown that the process of somatic hypermutation, which normally engenders antibody diversity in germinal center B cells by mutating the variable region of Ig genes, malfunctions and aberrantly targets on-Ig genes in the majority of diffuse large B-cell lymphomas. As a consequence, the protooncogenes, PIM1, cMYC, PAX5 and RhoH/TTF, are hypermutated in more than 50% of diffuse large B-cell lymphomas (59). In the case of PIM1 and cMYC, the mutations affect nontranslated as well as coding regions, leading to amino acid changes, with potential functional consequences. This mechanism may represent a powerful mechanism of malignant transformation, because it may have an effect on multiple genes, with consequences in part analogous to DNA mismatch–repair defects in colon carcinogenesis. Although a comprehensive characterization of the potentially extensive genetic damage caused by aberrant somatic hypermutation is still lacking, this mechanism also provides a plausible explanation for the biologic and clinical heterogeneity of diffuse large B-cell lymphoma.

Methods of Presentation and Prognostic Factors

The most common presentation of patients with diffuse large B-cell lymphoma is rapidly enlarging lymphadenopathy. However, as many as 40% of patients can have presentation in extranodal sites, with gastrointestinal involvement being most common. Patients with primary nodal diffuse large B-cell lymphoma with disease in the chest or abdomen can present with symptoms related to those sites (e.g., shortness of breath with mediastinal nodes, pain with retroperitoneal nodes). Primary extranodal diffuse large B-cell lymphomas often present with symptoms related to dysfunction at the site of origin (e.g., neurologic symptoms with brain lymphomas, pain or digestive symptoms with stomach or bowel lymphomas, pain with bone lymphomas). Approximately one third of patients have B symptoms at the time of diagnosis.

Unusual presentations are seen with some uncommon subtypes of diffuse large B-cell lymphoma. Intravascular large B-cell lymphoma often presents with a bizarre system complex that reflects organ dysfunction secondary to vascular occlusion or systemic symptoms such as unexplained fever (31,60). Although the most common presentation is neurologic dysfunction, also reported are endocrine dysfunction, syndrome

TABLE 27.2. *Factors independently prognostic of overall survival in the International Prognostic Index*

All patients (n = 1,385)
  Age (≤60 yr vs. >60 yr)
  Serum LDH (≤1 × normal vs. >1 × normal)
  Performance status (0 or 1 vs. 2–4)
  Stage (I or II vs. III or IV)
  Extranodal involvement (≤1 site vs. >1 site)
Patients ≤60 yr old (n = 885)
  Stage (I or II vs. III or IV)
  Serum LDH (≤1 × normal vs. >1 × normal)
  Performance status (0 or 1 vs. 2–4)

From A predictive model for aggressive non-Hodgkin's lymphoma. The International Non-Hodgkin's Lymphoma Prognostic Factors Project [see comments]. *N Engl J Med* 1993;329:987–994, with permission.

of inappropriate secretion of antidiuretic hormone, disseminated intravascular coagulopathy, atypical skin lesions, anasarca, and thrombotic thrombocytopenic purpura.

Pleural cavity lymphoma has frequently been associated with tuberculosis and pyothorax but is also seen in human immunodeficiency virus–infected patients. Unless new symptoms in a patient with preexisting effusion are investigated aggressively or this unusual diagnosis is considered in an at-risk patient with a new effusion, the diagnosis will be missed.

Approximately 50% of patients with diffuse large B-cell lymphoma have disease that is stage I/II, and an equal proportion have stage III/IV disease. Approximately 25% of patients have truly localized, or stage I, disease. Very bulky (i.e., larger than 10 cm) tumor masses are not rare and are seen in one quarter to one third of patients. A reduced performance status is present in approximately one quarter of patients. The most common sites of extranodal disease are the gastrointestinal tract or bone marrow, although any site in the body can be involved. Bone marrow involvement is seen in approximately 15% of patients with diffuse large B-cell lymphoma. However, in many of these patients, bone marrow is infiltrated by smaller cells rather than large cells. Large-cell involvement of the marrow carries an ominous prognosis, but the same is not true for minimal involvement by small cleaved B lymphocytes (10,61).

Approximately 35% of patients with diffuse large B-cell lymphoma have an International Prognostic Index (IPI) score of 0 or 1. Forty-five percent have an IPI score of 2 to 3, and approximately 20% have an IPI score of 4 to 5. The IPI was developed by studying patients with diffuse large B-cell lymphoma and accurately predicts the survival of patients with this disease (62) (Tables 27.2 and 27.3) (Fig. 27.1). Other factors proposed to predict treatment outcome for patients with diffuse large B-cell lymphoma include large tumor masses, serum β_2-microglobulin level, tumor growth fraction, and genetics.

Physicians from the M.D. Anderson Cancer Center proposed an alternate prognostic index for patients with large-cell lymphomas using only the serum β_2-microglobulin level and serum lactate dehydrogenase level. Patients without an

TABLE 27.3. *Outcome according to risk group defined by the International Prognostic Index and the Age-Adjusted International Prognostic Index*

Index	Risk group	Number of risk factors	Distribution of patients (%)	Complete response rate (%)	2-yr relapse-free survival rate (%)	5-yr relapse-free survival rate (%)	2-yr survival rate (%)	5-yr survival rate (%)
International Index, all patients (n = 2,031)	Low	0 or 1	35	87	79	79	84	73
	Low intermediate	2	27	67	66	50	66	51
	High intermediate	3	22	55	59	49	54	43
	High	4 or 5	16	44	58	40	34	26
Age-adjusted Index, patients ≤60 yr (n = 1,274)	Low	0	22	92	88	86	90	83
	Low intermediate	1	3	78	74	66	79	69
	High intermediate	2	32	57	62	53	59	46
	High	3	14	46	61	58	37	32
Age-adjusted Index, patients >60 yr (n = 761)	Low	0	18	91	75	46	80	56
	Low intermediate	1	31	71	64	45	68	44
	High intermediate	2	35	56	60	41	48	37
	High	3	16	36	47	37	31	21

From A predictive model for aggressive non-Hodgkin's lymphoma. The International Non-Hodgkin's Lymphoma Prognostic Factors Project [see comments]. *N Engl J Med* 1993;329:987–994, with permission.

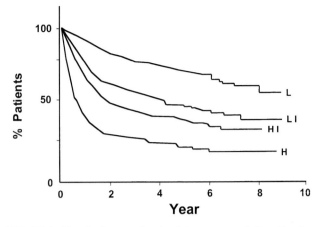

FIG. 27.1. Survival according to risk group as defined by the International Prognostic Index. [From A predictive model for aggressive non-Hodgkin's lymphoma. The International Non-Hodgkin's Lymphoma Prognostic Factors Project (see comments). *N Engl J Med* 1993;329:987–994, with permission.]

elevated lactate dehydrogenase or serum β_2-microgobulin were much more likely to survive therapy than were patients in whom both were elevated (81% vs. 26%) (63).

The rapidity of response to chemotherapy has been found to be prognostic in at least one study, in which patients achieving a complete remission in three cycles had a better chance for long-term disease-free survival than did patients who took longer to achieve a complete remission (64). Perhaps this was a reflection of chemotherapy sensitivity.

The importance of tumor proliferative rate has been studied on several occasions. Bauer et al. (65) and Wooldridge et al. (66) found that tumor proliferative rate predicted outcome in patients with diffuse large-cell lymphoma, with patients with a high proliferative rate having a poorer outlook. Those studies measured proliferation using flow cytometry, whereas Grogan et al. (67) measured Ki-67 expression and also found a high proliferative rate to be an independent prognostic factor predicting poor treatment outcome. In contrast, Wilson et al. (68) found that a low tumor proliferative rate was associated with a poor response to EPOCH (infusional etoposide, vincristine, and doxorubicin and bolus prednisone and cyclophosphamide).

The immune response of a diffuse large B-cell lymphoma has been studied as a prognostic factor. Patients with T-cell–rich B-cell lymphoma do not have a better survival than do patients with other subtypes of diffuse large B-cell lymphoma. However, a higher number of infiltrating CD4+ T cells in patients with diffuse large B-cell lymphoma was associated with an improved prognosis (69). The absence of expression of human leukocyte antigen-DR and β_2-microglobulin has been associated with a poor response to treatment (70,71).

A variety of cytokines or other endogenous protein expression have been studied for their prognostic impact in patients with diffuse aggressive lymphomas. Stasi et al. (72)

found that the combination of elevated soluble interleukin-2 receptors and interleukin-10 predicted a poor outcome in patients with diffuse aggressive non-Hodgkin's lymphoma. Seymour et al. (73) found that elevated interleukin-6 levels at diagnosis were associated with a poor treatment outcome. Ristamaki (74) found that elevated serum CD44 was associated with a poor treatment outcome in patients with diffuse large-cell lymphoma. Filipits et al. (75) found elevated levels of lung resistance protein, and multidrug resistance protein predicted a poor treatment outcome in patients with diffuse large B-cell lymphoma. Adida et al. (76) found that patients with diffuse large B-cell lymphoma treated with anthracycline-containing combination chemotherapy regimens had a poor survival rate with survivin expression. Finally, Salven et al. (77) found that a high pretreatment serum vascular endothelial growth–factor concentration predicted a poor treatment outcome in non-Hodgkin's lymphoma.

BCL 2 gene rearrangement and bcl-2 protein expression have been frequently studied in patients with diffuse large B-cell lymphoma. Gascoyne et al. (15) found that overexpression of bcl-2 protein, but not BCL 2 gene rearrangement, was associated with more frequent relapse in patients with diffuse large B-cell lymphoma. Yunis et al. (22) found BCL 2 gene rearrangement associated with a relatively poor prognosis. Hermine et al. (78) found that bcl-2 protein overexpression had an independent and adverse effect on disease-free survival in patients with diffuse large B-cell lymphoma treated with an anthracycline-containing chemotherapy regimen. Lossos (79) and Braaten et al. (80) both found that overexpression of the BCL 6 gene had a favorable impact on treatment outcome in patients with diffuse large B-cell lymphoma. Lossos et al. (81) described human germinal center–associated lymphoma, a novel interleukin-4–inducible gene associated with an improved survival in patients with diffuse large B-cell lymphoma. Leroy et al. (82) found that p53 gene mutations were associated with a low survival in low- and low-intermediate–risk patients with diffuse large B-cell lymphoma treated with an anthracycline-containing chemotherapy regimen. Filipits et al. (83) noted that cyclin D3 expression in patients with diffuse large B-cell lymphoma reduced the likelihood of achieving a complete remission.

Gene profiling has been shown to predict treatment outcome in patients with diffuse large B-cell lymphoma through the identification of specific patterns of gene expression (42,43,84,85). Using one system, patients can be divided into those with gene-expression patterns resembling normal germinal center B cells and those with gene-expression patterns similar to those seen in activated peripheral blood B lymphocytes. Another study, using an alternative algorithm to identify patterns of gene expression, also found patterns that predicted treatment outcomes, but no correlation was made to a normal cellular counterpart (43). Huang et al. (85) showed that the t(14;18)-containing diffuse large B-cell lymphomas were strongly associated with the germinal center B-cell gene-expression profile. Barrans et al. (86) showed that the germinal center immunophenotype as defined by expression of bcl-6 and CD10 predicted a favorable treatment outcome in patients with diffuse large B-cell lymphoma, whereas bcl-2 overexpression predicted a poor treatment outcome.

Therapy

Early-Stage Diffuse Large B-Cell Lymphoma

Radiation Therapy and Results of Early Clinical Trials

Before 1980, radiation therapy alone was often used as the primary treatment for patients with localized diffuse large-cell lymphoma. Approximately 50% of patients with stage I and 20% of patients with stage II disease were alive without recurrence 5 years after treatment (87,88). These results were even better in small series, in which selected stage I and II patients with a negative staging laparotomy were treated with extended-field irradiation alone. One series reported a 5-year survival of approximately 80% (89). Another study reported a 10-year actuarial relapse-free survival of 91% in stage I and 35% in stage II patients (90).

The relationship between radiation dose (and field size) and probability of tumor control has been the subject of numerous reports extending back to the early 1970s. A number of factors probably affect the relationship between dose and tumor control in diffuse large-cell lymphoma, including tumor size, use of chemotherapy before radiation therapy, and responsiveness to chemotherapy. However, there are no randomized trials evaluating the dose of radiation therapy in the management of lymphoma.

Two of the earliest retrospective papers on dose were published by Stanford University and the Princess Margaret Hospital in Toronto. Both series evaluated patients with early-stage diffuse large-cell lymphoma. In the 1973 Stanford study, Fuks and Kaplan reported that local control rates were 70% to 80% regardless of the dose of radiotherapy delivered (from 20 to 50 Gy) (91). In the Princess Margaret Hospital study, bulk of disease and patterns of relapse were evaluated (92,93). Patients with diffuse large-cell lymphoma had local or local-plus-distant recurrence rates of nearly 30%. Patients with medium- or large-bulk disease, defined as 2.5 to 5.0 cm in size and greater than 5 cm, respectively, had higher local or local-plus-distant recurrence rates (greater than 45%) than did patients with smaller-bulk disease (less than 20%). The dose–regional-control curve for diffuse large-cell lymphoma treated with radiation alone in patients with medium- or large-bulk disease showed 50% and 80% local-control rates with 25 and 40 Gy, respectively, with a plateau in the local-control curve after 40 Gy (92).

Several other retrospective studies using radiation therapy alone helped to establish early standards for the technical use of radiation therapy, including guidelines for dose and field size. These studies used a median dose of 50 Gy to the initial sites of involvement, and two of the retrospective studies treated extended fields to cover adjacent sites of disease (89,90,94,95).

Several randomized trials published from 1979 to 1982 helped to improve the outcome of patients with early-stage diffuse large-cell lymphoma. The trials compared radiation therapy alone to radiation therapy followed by CVP (cyclophosphamide, vincristine, and prednisone) or BACOP [bleomycin, Adriamycin (doxorubicin), cyclophosphamide, Oncovin (vincristine), and prednisone] chemotherapy (96–98). The addition of chemotherapy to radiation therapy resulted in a disease-free and overall survival advantage for combining the two regimens compared to radiation therapy alone. The trials somewhat reduced the dose of radiation therapy compared to previous reports without chemotherapy but continued to give prophylactic radiation therapy to uninvolved adjacent lymph node regions. In the Italian trial, 40 to 50 Gy was delivered to clinically involved areas, and proximal uninvolved lymph node–bearing areas received 35 to 45 Gy (96). Similar field sizes were used in the Danish trial, with the tumor receiving 37 to 43 Gy, with higher doses given for persistent disease (97). Data suggested that the addition of chemotherapy to radiation therapy not only reduced the incidence of distant relapse, but it also made the radiation therapy more effective for control of initial sites of involvement. In addition, approximately 10% of patients developed distant recurrences while on radiation therapy before chemotherapy was initiated. This suggested that the combination of the two modalities might be more effective with the chemotherapy given first. Results from these trials dramatically changed the treatment of localized large-cell lymphoma. Staging laparotomy and large-field radiation therapy became obsolete as combination chemotherapy with or without radiation therapy produced disease-free and overall survival rates equivalent to or better than those seen in even the most selective studies reporting results with radiation therapy alone.

Clinical Stage I and II Diffuse Large B-Cell Lymphoma Treated with Combined Adriamycin (Doxorubicin)- Based Chemotherapy and Radiation Therapy

With the use of the more effective doxorubicin-based regimens, a number of retrospective trials reported good data using smaller radiation fields limited to the initial regions of involvement and given at somewhat reduced doses in patients with diffuse large-cell lymphoma. Table 27.4 shows selected retrospective studies using doxorubicin-based chemotherapy regimens and radiation therapy (99–107). The first six series used six to eight cycles of chemotherapy (99,100,102–104,108); the last three series gave three to four cycles (105–107). Two of the three series using three to four cycles of chemotherapy excluded patients with bulky disease (greater than 10 cm). The median radiation doses range from 36 to 45 Gy in the first six studies and 35 to 40 Gy in the last three studies, except for some patients in the Rotterdam

TABLE 27.4. *Multiagent chemotherapy and local radiation therapy for stages I and II intermediate- or high-grade lymphomas: selected retrospective trials*

Institution (ref)	No. of patients	Stage	Median RT dose (Gy)	Type and median number of CT cycles	RT field size	MM/IF recur only	Freedom from recurrence (%)	Survival (%) (yr)
University of Florida (99)	121	I/II	NA	Nearly all ABR; ≥4 cycles	NA	5/121 (4%)	63 (10 yr)	44 (10)
Institute Gustave-Roussy (100)	96	I/II	45	CHVmP; NA	NA	7/95 (7%)	NA	77 (5)
Stanford University (101)	23	I	40	ABR (85%); 6 cycles	IF (86%)	6/94 (6%)	78	81 (5)
	71	II					70	72 (5)
Milan (102)	183	I/II	40-44	CHOP × 4 cycles (CR) or 6 cycles (PR)	IF (41%) REG (59%)	9/183 (3%)	—	83 (5)
The Netherlands Multicenter Trial (103)	94	I/IE	36 (6–8 cycles CT)	92% ABR; 3–8 cycles	IF (53%)	0/94, 3/94 local and distant	NA	70 (10)
			40 (3–4 cycles CT)		EF (47%)			
M.D. Anderson Cancer Center (104)	57	I	40 (CR)	CHOP-Bleo; 8 cycles	Gross disease + margin	5/147 (3%)	—	72 (10)
	90	II	50 (PR)				—	43 (10)
Rotterdam (105)	74	I/II	26 (CR)	CHOP; 4 cycles	IF	5/74 (7%)	69 (DFS)	76 (5)
	20		40 (CR)			1/20 (5%)	90	100 (5)
	34		40 (PR)			2/34 (6%)	75	75 (5)
British Columbia (106)	308	I/II	30/10 fx	ABR; 3 cycles	IF	7/308 (2%)	—	80 (5)
			35/20 fx					63 (10)
National Cancer Institute (107)	47	I	40	ProMACE-MOPP; 4 cycles	IF	2/47 (4%) 0/45 (CR)	96	94 (5)

ABR, Adriamycin-based regimens; Bleo, bleomycin; CHOP, cyclophosphamide, doxorubicin, Oncovin (vincristine), and prednisone; CHVmP, cyclophosphamide, doxorubicin, teniposide, and prednisone; CR, complete response; CT, chemotherapy; DFS, disease-free survival; EF, extended field; fx, fraction; IF, involved field; MM/IF recur only, recurrences limited to within or on the edge of the radiation field; NA, information not available; PR, partial response; REG, regional radiation, usually the involved region and immediately adjacent uninvolved regions; RT, radiation therapy.

study who received 26 Gy. In one study, a greater number of cycles of chemotherapy was used for patients not achieving a complete remission (102). The M.D. Anderson Cancer Center study used 40 Gy for patients in complete remission after chemotherapy and 50 Gy for a partial response or remission (104). Another study used a higher dose of radiation therapy (40 Gy) with three to four cycles of chemotherapy versus a lower dose (36 Gy) with six to eight cycles of chemotherapy. Most of the studies use involved-field irradiation; in two series, approximately one half of the patients were treated to larger fields (102,103). The majority of patients in the studies had diffuse large-cell lymphoma, although diffuse undifferentiated, follicular large-cell, and diffuse poorly differentiated small cleaved-cell lymphomas were included in many of the series. Recurrences within or on the edge of the radiation field as the only site of relapse were rare (0% to 7%). Although the range of median doses was small, no differences in local control were seen in the different studies within this dose range. Similarly, no differences in local control were seen in studies that used six to eight cycles of chemotherapy versus four cycles.

Four prospective randomized trials have further evaluated the role of radiation therapy in patients with early-stage diffuse large B-cell lymphoma (see Table 27.5). The Eastern Cooperative Oncology Group randomized 365 patients with bulky stage I (mediastinal or retroperitoneal

TABLE 27.5. *Chemotherapy versus combined modality therapy for stages I and II intermediate- or high-grade lymphoma: prospective randomized trials*

Reference	No. of evaluable patients	Stage	Chemotherapy	Radiation therapy dose (Gy)	CR or PR (%)	Failure-free survival (%)	Survival (%) (yr)
Eastern Cooperative Oncology Group (109)	345	CS I (B) and all CS II	CHOP × 8 (CR)	—	61% (CR)	58	70 (6)
			CHOP × 8 (CR)	30 (IF)		73[a]	84 (6)[a]
			CHOP × 8	40 (IF)	28% (PR)	60	64 (6)
Southwest Oncology Group (111)	401	CS I/IE (B/NB) and CS II (NB)	CHOP × 8	—	73	64	72 (5)
			CHOP × 3	40–55	75	77[b]	82 (5)[b]
Groupe d'Etude des Lymphomes de l'Adulte (112)	518	IPI 0, 1	CHOP × 4	—	—	69	78
		CS I-II	CHOP × 4	40	—	64	70
Groupe d'Etude des Lymphomes de l'Adulte (113)	631	CS I-II	ACVBP	—	—	83[c]	89[c]
		Low risk	CHOP × 3	30–40	—	74	80

ACVBP, Adriamycin (doxorubicin), cyclophosphamide, vindesine, bleomycin, and prednisone; B, bulky disease; CHOP, cyclophosphamide, doxorubicin, Oncovin (vincristine), and prednisone; CR, complete response; CS, clinical stage; IF, involved field; NB, no bulky disease; PR, partial response.
[a]Significant difference between radiation therapy and no radiation therapy.
[b]Borderline significant difference between radiation and no radiation therapy, *p* = .06.
[c]Significantly better result with ACVBP.

involvement or masses larger than 10 cm), stage IE, stage II, or stage IIE disease to eight cycles of CHOP [cyclophosphamide, doxorubicin, Oncovin (vincristine), and prednisone] chemotherapy with or without radiation therapy. Patients with no response or progression to chemotherapy were removed from the study. Patients in complete remission were randomized to 30 Gy involved-field radiation therapy (to sites of initial involvement) or no further treatment. Patients in partial remission received 40 Gy to the site or sites of pretreatment involvement plus radiation to contiguous uninvolved regions. In patients randomized after complete remission, the 5-year disease-free survival (73% vs. 58%; *p* = .03), freedom from recurrence (73% vs. 58%; *p* = .04), and survival (84% vs. 70%; *p* = .06) all favored the patients who received adjuvant involved-field irradiation (109). At 10 years, the disease-free survival continues to favor the addition of radiation therapy (57% vs. 46%; *p* = .04), but the survival differences no longer are statistically significant (110). In the patients who achieved a partial remission, 28% converted to a complete remission with the addition of 40 Gy of radiation therapy. Patients with a poor performance status or three or more sites of involvement at diagnosis were more likely to develop recurrent lymphoma. To date, the detailed results of this study have not been published.

The Southwest Oncology Group trial randomized 401 stage I and non-bulky stage II patients to receive either three cycles of CHOP and involved-field irradiation (40 Gy to 55 Gy) or eight cycles of CHOP alone. The 5-year progression-free survival (77% vs. 64%; *p* = .03) and overall survival

(82% vs. 72%, *p* = .02) favored the CHOP and involved-field radiation therapy treatment arm (111). A separate analysis of progression-free and overall survival was performed using a modified IPI. Patients with no or one risk factor had higher progression-free and overall survival rates compared to patients with two or three risk factors. As a result of these two trials, combination chemotherapy and adjuvant radiation therapy have become the standard care for patients with stage I or II diffuse large B-cell lymphoma. Patients with a higher modified IPI or poor prognostic pretreatment factors have a higher recurrence risk, suggesting that three cycles of CHOP (combined with radiation therapy) may not be enough chemotherapy for these patients.

The results of two European randomized trials were presented in abstract form at the 2002 American Society of Hematology meetings. Fillet el al. compared four cycles of CHOP with four cycles of CHOP followed by 40 Gy in 518 patients older than 60 years of age who all had an age-adjusted IPI score of 0 (112). Nine percent of the patients had bulky tumor masses larger than 10 cm in maximum diameter, and 8% had T-cell lymphoma, not diffuse large B-cell lymphoma. The 5-year event-free (CHOP, 69% vs. CHOP + radiation therapy, 64%) and overall (CHOP, 78% vs. CHOP + radiation therapy, 70%) survival did not differ between the two regimens. However, for patients older than 70 years, the overall survival was better in the group that received CHOP alone.

Reyes et al. compared three cycles of CHOP followed by 30 to 40 Gy involved-field radiotherapy with the chemotherapy regimen ACVBP [Adriamycin (doxorubicin), cyclophosphamide, vindesine, bleomycin, and prednisone] followed by consolidation chemotherapy using methotrexate, ifosfamide, etoposide, and cytarabine in 631 patients with low-risk, localized aggressive lymphoma (113). Bulky disease (i.e., a larger than 10-cm mass) was present in 10%, and 10% had T-cell lymphoma rather than diffuse large B-cell lymphoma. Event-free survival (CHOP + radiation therapy, 74% vs. ACVBP, 83%) and overall survival (CHOP + radiation therapy, 80% vs. ACVBP, 89%) were both significantly better in the chemotherapy-alone arm. Publication of these data and the Eastern Cooperative Oncology Group data in peer-reviewed journals would help in developing more precise treatment recommendations.

What can we conclude regarding the dose and field size of radiation therapy when combined with chemotherapy based on these retrospective and prospective trials? For diffuse large-cell lymphoma, radiation therapy alone is associated with a high distant-failure rate as well as a 20% infield recurrence rate despite doses of 45 Gy or higher. The infield recurrence rates appear to be higher for bulky disease than for patients with less bulky disease. In contrast, using doses of 35 to 45 Gy after a complete response to four to eight cycles of CHOP is associated with a low infield or margin of the field recurrence rate (0% to 7%, see Table 27.4). Furthermore, data do not appear to support the use of prophylactic adjacent nodal region irradiation. Similar local-control data are seen in patients in complete response after chemotherapy before radiation therapy compared to a partial response before involved-field irradiation (105). However, studies suggest somewhat lower recurrence-free and overall survival rates in the patients with a partial response to chemotherapy (102,105,109). Exactly what doses to recommend for patients with initial bulk disease is still unclear, but after a complete remission after CHOP, data suggest that doses of 36 Gy should be sufficient (114).

Based on all the above data, we recommend the following for diffuse large-cell lymphoma treated with combined modality therapy:

1. Use of involved fields
2. After a complete remission after six to eight cycles of CHOP: 36 Gy if initial bulky disease; 30 Gy for the remainder of patients
3. After three to four cycles of CHOP: 35 to 40 Gy
4. After a partial remission: 40 Gy

In the studies reported above, the definitions of *complete* or *partial remission* are not always consistent, especially because nuclear-medicine imaging was not available for the majority of patients in these reports. Residual masses are common on computed tomography after chemotherapy, especially in patients with bulky mediastinal or abdominal disease. We do not have data on the success of radiation therapy (or on the doses or field sizes needed) after a partial response based on a positive computed tomographic scan with a negative gallium or positron-emission tomography scan versus both positive computed tomography and positive

nuclear-medicine studies. The data that are available, using a variety of methods to define partial response, suggest that radiation therapy alone after a partial remission to chemotherapy can yield long-term survival (99,109,115).

In the Eastern Cooperative Oncology Group trial, patients with bulky or extranodal stage I and II intermediate-grade non-Hodgkin's lymphoma who achieved a complete response after eight cycles of CHOP were randomized to receive 30 Gy of radiation therapy versus no further treatment. All patients with a partial response to CHOP received radiation therapy to 40 Gy. Patients treated with radiation therapy after a partial remission had a 6-year disease-free survival rate of 54% and an overall survival rate of 64%. Another study from the M.D. Anderson Cancer Center also demonstrated the effectiveness of radiation therapy in achieving durable remission after a partial response to chemotherapy (116). The investigators reviewed 294 patients with large-cell lymphoma treated with CHOP-based chemotherapy. Computed tomography scans were obtained in every case to assess response to chemotherapy using the International Working Group guidelines. An unconfirmed complete response or partial response was documented in 44 patients. At a median follow-up of 43 months, compared with patients who received salvage chemotherapy, those who received salvage radiation therapy had a significantly better 4-year local-control rate (86% vs. 53%; $p = .009$) and 4-year progression-free survival (67% vs. 8%; $p < .0001$). Using historical controls, the authors also noted that the 6-year progression-free survival and overall survival rates of 61% and 70%, respectively, were comparable to results achieved by high-dose therapy with autologous stem cell rescue.

In a study by Zinzani et al. (115), 50 patients with primary mediastinal large B-cell lymphoma were prospectively treated with methotrexate, Adriamycin (doxorubicin), cyclophosphamide, Oncovin (vincristine), prednisone, and bleomycin (MACOP-B), followed by radiation therapy. Computed tomography and gallium-67-citrate single-photon emission scans (GaSPECT) were obtained at diagnosis, at the end of chemotherapy, and 3 months after radiation therapy. Three patients with progressive disease during chemotherapy were excluded from the analysis. After chemotherapy, 31 of 47 patients (66%) had a positive GaSPECT. Among these 31 patients, 22 became GaSPECT negative after radiation therapy. None of the patients with a negative GaSPECT posttreatment relapsed at a median follow-up of 39 months.

Disseminated Stage Diffuse Large B-Cell Lymphoma

The first convincing reports of the curability of diffuse large B-cell lymphoma with chemotherapy appeared in 1972 (117) and 1975 (118). In both of these reports, the majority of patients who achieved a complete remission documented at the end of the initial treatment did not relapse despite no further therapy. Subsequent to these reports, many combination-chemotherapy regimens were documented to be able to produce long-term disease-free survival in patients with this disorder. The most pop-

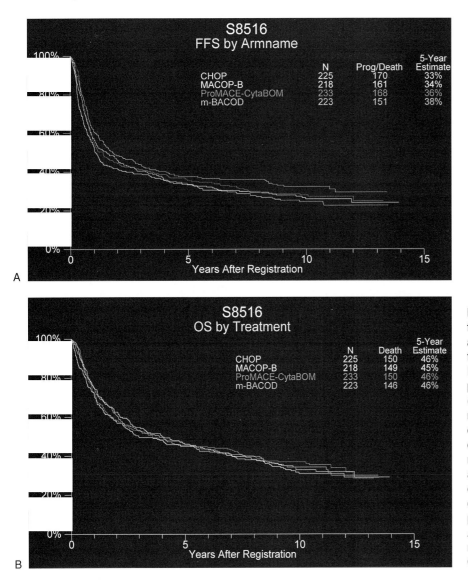

FIG. 27.2. Long-term follow-up of both failure-free survival (FFS) **(A)** and overall survival (OS) **(B)** by treatment arms for patients treated in the United States Intergroup trial (124). CHOP, cyclophosphamide, hydroxydaunorubicin, Oncovin (vincristine), and prednisone; MACOP-B, methotrexate, Adriamycin (doxorubicin), cyclophosphamide, Oncovin (vincristine), prednisone, and bleomycin; m-BACOD, [moderate-dose methotrexate, bleomycin, Adriamycin (doxorubicin), cyclophosphamide, and Oncovin dexamethasone; ProMACE-CytaBOM, prednisone, Matalane (procarbazine), Adriamycin (doxorubicin), cyclophosphamide, etoposide + cytarabine, bleomycin, Oncovin (vincristine), and methotrexate.

ular regimen in the United States has been CHOP. The most popular way to administer CHOP has been cyclophosphamide, 750 mg per m^2 intravenously (IV) on day 1; doxorubicin, 50 mg per m^2 IV on day 1; vincristine, 1.4 mg per m^2 IV on day 1, with a maximum dose of 2 mg; and prednisone, 100 mg orally daily for days 1 through 5 of each treatment cycle. The regimen is typically administered at 21-day intervals. When patients are documented to be in complete remission after four to six treatment cycles and two more cycles are subsequently given, the majority of complete responders appear to be cured (64,119). However, CHOP has been administered in a variety of different ways, including a day-1 and -8 schedule, and the prednisone doses have varied widely (120). Sometimes other drugs are added, and the regimen is referred to as a *CHOP-like* regimen.

With the design of a wide variety of new treatment regimens with documented curative potential in patients with diffuse large B-cell lymphoma, controversy developed over the relative merits of the new regimens in comparison to CHOP; a number of randomized clinical trials have been

performed to address these issues. Many of these studies are detailed in the subsequent paragraphs. However, apparent differences between CHOP and the other regimens seem to have frequently been based on patient selection. The treatment outcome for patients with diffuse large B-cell lymphoma varies considerably based on initial prognostic factors. The IPI (62) was developed in part to allow comparison of different treatment regimens and to ensure comparability of subgroups in clinical trials. Phase II trials of regimens such as m-BACOD [moderate-dose methotrexate, bleomycin, Adriamycin (doxorubicin), cyclophosphamide, and Oncovin dexamethasone], ProMACE/CytaBOM [prednisone, matalane (procarbazine), Adriamycin (doxorubicin), cyclophosphamide, etoposide + cytarabine, bleomycin, Oncovin (vincristine), and methotrexate], and MACOP-B seemed to show dramatic superiority over the CHOP regimen (121–123). However, in a landmark clinical trial (124), these regimens were found to be equivalent, with long-term disease-free survival in 35% to 40% of patients (Fig. 27.2).

The apparent discrepancy between the results of the phase II trials and the large randomized trial seemed to be explained by selection of patients with favorable IPI scores for participation in the phase II trials.

A variety of different approaches has been tried to improve treatment results in patients with diffuse large B-cell lymphoma. These include the incorporation of alternative chemotherapeutic agents, the addition of an immunotherapeutic approach, dose escalation supported by growth factors or hematopoietic stem cell transplantation, and infusion of one or more of the drugs in the regimen to prolong exposure of the tumor cells.

Many of these approaches have been tested in randomized trials.

The considerable number of randomized trials in which the majority or all of the patients had diffuse large B-cell lymphoma are presented in Tables 27.6, 27.7, and 27.8. The majority of these studies showed no advantage to one treatment over another.

Trials of Chemotherapy Including Younger Patients

Table 27.6 presents studies of predominantly younger patients with diffuse large B-cell lymphoma subdivided by

TABLE 27.6. *Trials of chemotherapy in disseminated diffuse large B-cell lymphoma including younger patients*

Clinical question	Reference	Comparison	No. of patients	Patient characteristics	Significant differences
The importance of including an anthracycline in the treatment regimen	125	CHOP vs. CVP	NA	Stage III–IV	Overall survival
	126	CHOP vs. BCOP	295	Stage II–IV	CR: CHOP 54%; BCOP 34%
	193	CHOP vs. MEV	141	Stage III–IV	CR: CHOP 61%; MEV 24% (*p* < .001)
					RFS: CHOP 34%; MEV 9% (*p* < .001)
	127	CHOP + Bleo vs. COP-Bleo			
The use of alternative anthracyclines or anthracine dions	194	CHOP vs. MEVP	57	Stage II–IV	None
	195	m-BACOD vs. m-BNCOD	70	Stage II–IV	None
	196	CHOP vs. CNOP	35	Stage II–IV	None
	129	CHOP vs. CIOP	103	Stage III–IV	None
	197	MACOP-B vs. MECOP-B	211	Stage I–IV	None
	198	CHOP vs. CNOP	89	Stage II–IV	None
	199	CHOP vs. CEOP-B	60	Stage I–IV	None
	131	CHOP vs. CNOP	325	Stage II–IV	None
Increased numbers of drugs or alternate combinations	200	CHOP vs. MACOP-B	236	Stage I–IV	5-yr failure-free survival: CHOP 30%; MACOP-B 42% (*p* = .04)
					5-yr overall survival: CHOP 41%; MACOP-B 54% (*p* = .03)
	134	CHOP vs. PACEBOM	459	Stage II–IV	Cause-specific survival in patients <50 yr of age: CHOP 55%; PACEBOM 78% (*p* = .004)
	135	CHVmP vs. CHVmP + VB (both arms received XRT to bulky or residual disease)	141	Stage III–IV	In diffuse large cell: CR: CHVmP 50%; CHVmP + VB 80% (*p* = .01)
					5-yr survival: CHVmP 29%; CHVmP + VB 53% (*p* = .002)
	124	CHOP vs. m-BACOD vs. Pro-MACE/CytaBOM vs. MACOP-B	899	Stage II–IV	None
	201	CHOP-B vs. ACOMLA	48	Stage III–IV	None

(continued)

TABLE 27.6. *Continued*

	Reference	Comparison	No. of patients	Patient characteristics	Significant differences
	202	CHOP-Mtx vs. CAPOME	281	Stage I–IV	None
	203	B-CHOP-M vs. PEEC/CHOP	325	Stage I–IV	None
	130	MACOP-B vs. ProMACE/ CytaBOM	210	Stage I–IV	None
	204	CHOP vs. m-BACOD	325	Stage III–IV	None
	205	MACOP-B vs. ProMACE/ MOPP	221	Stage II–IV	None
	133	CHOP vs. MACOP-B	374	Stage II–IV	None
	206	CHOEP vs. high-dose CHOP	146	Stage II–IV	None
	207	MACOP vs. F-MACHOP	286	Stage I–IV	None
	208	CHOEP + XRT vs. high-dose CHOP/IVEP + XRT	171	Stage II–IV	None
	132	CHOP vs. MACOP-B	236	Stage I–IV	None
	209	CHOP + high-dose Mtx vs. CHOP + low-dose Mtx vs. CHOP-B + high-dose Mtx vs. CHOP-B + low-dose Mtx	177	Stage III–IV	None
	210	m-BACOD vs. ACVBP	673	Stage I–IV	None
Continuous infusion	136	CHOP vs. EPOCH	78	Stage I–IV	4-yr overall survival: CHOP 71%; EPOCH 42% (p = .006)
Increasing dose or dose intensity	138	CHOP-14 vs. CHOP-21 vs. CHOEP-14 vs. CHOEP-21 (all arms received XRT to bulky sites)	762		Freedom from treatment failure: CHOP 63%; CHOEP 73% (p = .001)
	139	CEOP-B vs. high-dose CEOP-B	147	Stage I–IV	3-yr freedom from treatment failure: CEOP-B 37%; high-dose CEOP-B 76% (p < .01)
	137	CEOP vs. high-dose CEOP + filgrastim	250	Stage I–IV	None
Other approaches	211	CHOP vs. CHOP + α-interferon			None
	121	ProMACE/CytaBOM	193	Stage II–IV	CR Rate: P/C 85%; P/M 74% (p = .05)
		ProMACE/MOPP			Survival: P/C 67%; P/M 55% (p = .05)

ACOMLA, Adriamycin (doxorubicin), Cytoxan (cyclophosphamide), Oncovin (vincristine), methotrexate, cytarabine, leucovorin; ACVBP, Adriamycin (doxorubicin), cyclophosphamide, vindesine, bleomycin, and prednisone; BCOP, carmustine, cyclophosphamide, vincristine, and prednisone (B-BCNU); Bleo, bleomycin; CAPOME, cyclophosphamide, adriamycin, vincristine, prednisone methotrexate, and etoposide; CEOP-B, cyclophosphamide, Oncovin (vincristine), prednisone, and bleomycin; CHOEP, cyclophosphamide, doxorubicin, Oncovin (vincristine), etoposide, and prednisone; CHOP, cyclophosphamide, doxorubicin, Oncovin (vincristine), and prednisone; CHOP-B, CHOP + bleomycin; CHVmP, cyclophosphamide, doxorubicin, teniposide, and prednisone; CHVmP +VB, CHVmP + vincristine and bleomycin; CIOP, cyclophosphamide, idarubicin, vincristine, and prednisone; CNOP, Cytoxan (cyclophosphamide), Novantrone (mitoxantrone), Oncovin (vincristine), and prednisone; CR, complete remission; CVP, cyclophosphamide, vincristine, and prednisone; EPOCH, etoposide, prednisone, Oncovin (vincristine), Cytoxan (cyclophosphamide); F-MACHOP, fluorouracil, mthotrexate/leucovorin, cytarabine, cyclophosphamide, doxorubicin, vincristine, and prednisone; IVEP, ifosfamide, etoposide, vindesine, and prednisolone; MACOP-B, methotrexate, Adriamycin (doxorubicin), cyclophosphamide, Oncovin (vincristine), prednisone, and bleomycin; MECOP-B, methotrexate, epirubicin, cyclophosphamide, vincristine, prednisolone, and bleomycin; m-BACOD, moderate-dose methotrexate, bleomycin, Adriamycin (doxorubicin), cyclophosphamide, Oncovin (vincristine) dexamethasone; m-BNCOD, methotrexate, bleomycin, mitoxantrone, cyclophosphamide, vincristine, and dexamethasone; MEV, methotrexate, cyclophosphamide, and vincristine; MEVP, metoxantrone, etoposide, vindesine, and prednisolone; MOPP, mechlorethamine, Oncovin (vincristine), procarbazine, and prednisone; Mtx, methotrexate; PACEBOM, prednisolone, adriamycine, cyclophosphamide, etoposide, bleomycin, vincristine, and methotrexate; P/C, ProMACE/CytaBOM; P/M, PRoMACE/MOPP; PEEC, methylprednisolone, vindesine, etoposide, chlorambucil, and methotrexate; ProMACE/CytaBOM, prednisone, Matalane (procarbazine), Adriamycin (doxorubicin), cyclophosphamide, and etoposide + cytarabine, bleomycin, Oncovin (vincristine), methotrexate; RFS, relapse free survival; XRT, radiation therapy.

TABLE 27.7. *Randomized trials of autologous hematopoietic stem cell transplantation as part of initial therapy for diffuse large B-cell lymphoma*

Reference	Eligibility	Randomization	Treatment arms		Outcome		
			Standard	Transplant	Standard	Transplant	p
151	WF G, H + bulky stage I–II, or stage III or IV	All patients	MACOP-B ± XRT	Doxorubicin, vincristine, prednisone, methotrexate, etoposide, followed by FTBI + melphalan or mitoxantrone + melphalan, followed by ASCT ± XRT	49% 7-yr EFS	76% 7-yr EFS	.004
					55% 7-yr OS	81% 7-yr OS	.09
152	WF intermediate-high grade + bulky stage II, or stage III or IV	All patients	VACOP-B ± DHAP ± XRT	VACOP-B + ASCT ± XRT	48% 6-yr PFS[a]	60% 6-yr PFS[a]	.4
					65% 6-yr OS[a]	65% 6-yr OS[a]	.5
					37% 6-yr PFS[a]	65% 6-yr PFS[a]	.08
					55% 6-yr OS[a]	68% 6-yr OS[a]	.7
149	WF intermediate-high grade + PS 2-4, or ≥2 extranodal sites, or ≥10-cm bulk, or + BM or CNS, or Burkitt or lymphoblastic histology	Patients in CR after ACVB or NCVB	ACVB or NCVB + methotrexate, ifosfamide, L-asparaginase, cytarabine	ACVB or NCVB + methotrexate + ASCT	39% 8-yr DFS[a]	55% 8-yr DFS[a]	.02
					49% 8-yr OS[a]	64% 8-yr OS[a]	.04
153	WF F–H + aaIPI HI/H	After CHOP × 3	CHOP × 8 ± XRT	CHOP × 3 + ESHAP + ASCT ± XRT	15% 4-yr EFS	38% 4-yr EFS	.04
					30% 4-yr OS	51% 4-yr OS	.25
154	WF D–G, bulky stage I, or stage II–IV	If in PR or CR after CHVmP/BV × 3	CHVmP/BV × 8 ± XRT	CHVmP/BV × 6 + ASCT ± XRT	56% 5-yr PFS	61% 5-yr PFS	.712
					77% 5-yr OS	68% 5-yr OS	.336
155	Aggressive histology + stage II–IV + high LDH	All patients	CHOEP × 5 ± XRT	CHOEP × 3 + ASCT ± XRT	49% 3-yr EFS	59% 3-yr EFS	.22
					63% 3-yr OS	62% 3-yr OS	.68
150	Aggressive histology + aaIPI HI/H	All patients	ACVBP + methotrexate, etoposide, ifosfamide, cytarabine	CEOP × 1 + ECVBP × 2 + ASCT	51% 5-yr EFS	39% 5-yr EFS	.01
					60% 5-yr OS	46% 5-yr OS	.007
156	Aggressive histology + bulky stage I or stage II–IV, + aaIPI HI/H	All patients	MACOP-B × 12 wks ± XRT	MACOP-B × 8 wks + ASCT ± XRT	49% 5-yr PFS	61% 5-yr PFS	.21
					65% 5-yr OS	64% 5-yr OS	.95

aaIPI HI/H, age-adjusted International Prognostic Index high-intermediate/high-risk; ACVB, Adriamycin (doxorubicin), cyclophosphamide, vinblastine, and bleomycin; ACVBP, Adriamycin (doxorubicin), cyclophosphamide, vindesine, bleomycin, and prednisone; ASCT, autologous hematopoietic stem cell transplantation; CEOP, cyclophosphamide, epirubicin, Oncovin (vincristine), and prednisone; CHOEP, cyclophosphamide, doxorubicin, Oncovin (vincristine), etoposide, and prednisone; CHOP, cyclophosphamide, doxorubicin, Oncovin (vincristine), and prednisone; CHVmP/BV, cyclophosphamide, doxorubicin, teniposide, prednisone, bleomycin, and vincristine; DFS, disease-free survival; DHAP, dexamethasone, cytarabine, and Platinol (cisplatin); ECVBP, epirubicin, cyclophosphamide, vindesine, bleomycin, and prednisone; EFS, event free survival; ESHAP, etoposide, Solu-Medrol (methylprednisolone), cytarabine, and Platinol (cisplatin); FTBI, fractionated total-body irradiation; MACOP-B, methotrexate, Adriamycin (doxorubicin), cyclophosphamide, Oncovin (vincristine), prednisone, and bleomycin; NCVB, Novantrone (mitoxantrone), cyclophosphamide, vinblastine, and bleomycin; OS, overall survival; PFS, progression free survival; VACOP-B, VePesid (etoposide), Adriamycin (doxorubicin), cyclophosphamide, Oncovin (vincristine), prednisone, and bleomycin; WF, Working Formulation; XRT, radiation therapy.

[a]Applies to aaIPI high-intermediate/high-risk only.

TABLE 27.8. *Randomized therapeutic trials in elderly patients with diffuse large B-cell lymphoma*

Reference	Comparison	No. of patients	Patient characteristics	Significant differences
212	CHOP vs. CHOP + rituximab	399	Age 60–80 yr Stage II–IV All DLBC	CR: CHOP, 63%; CHOP-R, 76% (*p* = .005) 2-yr event-free survival: CHOP, 38%; CHOP-R, 57% (*p* = .001) 2-yr overall survival: CHOP, 57%; CHOP-R, 70% (*p* = .007)
213	CVP vs. CTVP	453	Age ≥70 yr Stage I–IV	CR: CVP, 32%; CTVP, 47% (*p* = .0001) 5-yr survival: CVP, 19%; CTVP, 26% (*p* = .05)
214	CHOP vs. ACVBP	635	Age 60–69 yr Age-adjusted IPI 1–3	Event-free survival: CHOP, 33%; ACVBP, 45% (*p* = .004)
215	ACVBP vs. alternating VIMMM/ACVBP	810	Age 55–69 yr Stage I–IV	CR: ACVBP, 58%; Alternating regimen, 48% (*p* = .003) 5-yr event-free survival: ACVBP, 33%; alternating regimen, 28% (*p* = .03)
161	CHOP vs. VMP	120	Age >70 yr Stage II–IV	Progression-free survival: CHOP, 55%; VMP, 30% (*p* =.004)
159	CHOP vs. CHOP + filgrastim vs. CNOP vs. CNOP + filgrastim	455	Age 60–86 yr Stage II–IV	CR: CHOP ± filgrastim, 60%; CNOP ± filgrastim, 43% (*p* < .001) 5-yr overall survival: CHOP ± filgrastim, 48%; CNOP ± filgrastim, 26% (*p* < .001)
160	CHOP vs. CNOP	148	Age ≥60 yr Stage II–IV	CR: CHOP, 49%; CNOP, 31% (*p* = .03) 3-yr overall survival: CHOP, 42%; CNOP, 26% (*p* = .03)
162	CHOP q 21 d vs. weekly CHOP	38	Age ≥65 yr Stage I–IV	None
163	VNCOP-B × 12 wk vs. VNCOP-B × 8 wk	306	Age ≥60 yr Stage II–IV	None

ACVBP, Adriamycin (doxorubicin), cyclophosphamide, vindesine, bleomycin, and prednisone; CHOP, cyclophosphamide, doxorubicin, vincristine, and prednisone; CHOP-R, cyclophosphamide, doxorubicin, vincristine, prednisone, and rituximab; CNOP, Cytoxan (cyclophosphamide), Novantrone (mitoxantrone), Oncovin (vincristine), and prednisone; CR, complete remission; CTVP, cyclophosphamide, pirarubicine (THP-doxorubicin), teniposide (VM-26), and prednisone; CVP, cyclophosphamide, teniposide (VM-26), and prednisone; DLBC, diffuse large B-cell lymphoma; IPI, International Prognostic Index; VIMMM, teniposide (VM-26), ifosfamide, mitroxantrone, methylgag, and methotrexate; VMP, VePesid (etoposide), mitoxantrone, prednimustine; VNCOP-B, VePesid (etoposide), Novantrone (mitoxantrone), cyclophosphamide, Oncovin (vincristine), prednisone, and bleomycin.

the types of clinical questions being tested. The value of incorporating an anthracycline into the treatment of patients with diffuse aggressive lymphoma—predominately diffuse large B-cell lymphoma—has been tested in four clinical trials. These studies tested CHOP versus COP [cyclophosphamide, Oncovin (vincristine), and prednisone] (125), CHOP versus COP plus bleomycin (126), CHOP plus bleomycin versus COP plus bleomycin, in which some patients also received Bacillus Calmette Guerin (BCG) (127), and CHOP versus methotrexate, etoposide, and vincristine (128). In each case, in patients with diffuse large-cell lymphoma, there was a treatment advantage for the anthracycline-containing regimen. One unequivocal statement about the treatment of patients with

diffuse large B-cell lymphoma is that the regimen should include an anthracycline if at all possible.

Eight randomized trials have tested the substitution of alternate anthracyclines or the substitution of an anthracenedione for doxorubicin in the treatment of younger patients with predominately diffuse large B-cell lymphoma. Most of these studies incorporated mitoxantrone at 12 mg per m² or 10 mg per m² rather than doxorubicin, but epirubicin and idarubicin have also been studied. Most of these studies were fairly small, with fewer than 100 patients in the trial, but three studies incorporated 103, 211, and 325 patients, respectively (129–131). In none of these studies was there an advantage for doxorubicin. This is in contrast to some studies performed in elderly patients that will be noted below. In young patients with diffuse large B-cell lymphoma, there is no evidence that an alternative anthracycline or an anthracendione leads to a poorer treatment outcome.

At least 17 studies have tested the value of the addition of extra drugs to those incorporated in CHOP or alternative drug combinations while still using an anthracycline. Fourteen of these studies have failed to show an advantage to the experimental arm. The most important of these negative studies, considering its impact on therapy, was a four-arm trial carried out in the United States comparing CHOP, m-BACOD, ProMACE/CytaBOM, and MACOP-B (124). As noted above, despite apparent differences in favor of the more complicated regimens seen in large phase II trials (121–123), the randomized trial incorporating 899 patients with bulky stage II, stage III, and stage IV diffuse large-cell lymphoma (i.e., predominantly diffuse large B-cell lymphoma) showed no superiority to any regimen, with approximately 35% to 40% of patients surviving disease free for extended periods. There were differences seen in toxicity, with CHOP being the easiest to administer and the least toxic regimen. This led to widespread incorporation of CHOP as the "standard" treatment for patients with diffuse large-cell lymphoma.

Three studies of alternative regimens in young patients with diffuse large-cell lymphoma did find a significant advantage to one treatment. Wolf et al. reported long follow-up on a comparative trial of CHOP versus MACOP-B in which 236 patients were studied. The initial report of this study was not positive (132). Long-term results showed an advantage to MACOP-B. Both the 5-year failure-free survival (42% vs. 30%; $p = .04$) and 5-year overall survival (54% and 41%; $p = .03$) favored MACOP-B. This is in contrast to the results from the large American study noted above and a Scandinavian trial (133). This result raises the important question of differences in short-term and long-term results of clinical trials and the possibility that studies initially either positive or negative might have the outcome change as the studies mature. Results such as this certainly complicate clinical decision making when studies are at one point negative and subsequently positive, and there are other, apparently similar, studies with conflicting results.

A large study of 459 patients from the United Kingdom studied the comparative merits of CHOP versus PACE-BOM [prednisolone, Adriamycin (doxorubicin), cyclophosphamide, etoposide, bleomycin, Oncovin (vincristine), methotrexate] (134). PACEBOM incorporates doxorubicin, cyclophosphamide, and etoposide IV on day 1 and bleomycin, vincristine, and methotrexate on day 8 of a 2-week cycle (i.e., alternating weekly IV therapy) plus oral prednisone. For patients younger than 50 years of age, cause-specific survival favored PACEBOM (78% vs. 55%; $p = .004$). This study raises the possibility of different regimens or treatment approaches working better in very young adults.

A European Organization for Research and Treatment of Cancer trial incorporating 141 patients substituted teniposide for vincristine in CHOP and compared that regimen to the same drugs plus vincristine and bleomycin (135). Patients in both arms received radiotherapy to bulky or residual disease at the completion of chemotherapy. Complete remissions were superior for the six-drug regimen (80% vs. 50%; $p = .01$), as was 5-year overall survival (53% vs. 49%, $p = .002$). The importance of the routine incorporation of radiotherapy in patients with bulky or residual disease in this study is in contrast to what is often done in the United States for patients with advanced diffuse large B-cell lymphoma. The impact of the radiation, although possibly important, remains uncertain.

One study tested the infusional regimen EPOCH compared to CHOP. This was a study of 78 patients reported by Khaled et al. (136). In contrast to the positive phase II results reported in the United States, this study found a superior 4-year overall survival for CHOP (71% vs. 42%, $p = .006$). The explanation for the striking difference between these results and phase II studies is unclear.

Three studies have tested the merits of increasing dose or dose intensity, or both, in treating patients with diffuse aggressive lymphoma (137–139). One study of 250 patients in which a CHOP-like regimen with epirubicin was substituted for doxorubicin was compared to the same regimen at higher doses supported by filgrastim (137). No significant advantage was seen for the higher doses. In contrast were the results found in a similar study of 147 patients who received a CHOP-like regimen with epirubicin substituted for doxorubicin with the addition of bleomycin in both arms. Patients in the high-dose arm received escalating doses of epirubicin, with the intended total dose being 420 mg per m^2 in the standard-dose arm and 710 mg per m^2 in the escalated-dose arm. Patients receiving the higher dose of epirubicin had a superior 3-year freedom from treatment failure (76% vs. 37%; $p = .01$). A complicated study from Germany recently reported in an abstract (138) compared CHOP at 14-day intervals to CHOP at 21-day intervals to CHOP plus etoposide at 14-day intervals to CHOP plus etoposide at 21-day intervals. In this study, all patients received radiotherapy to sites of bulky residual disease. In younger patients, the addition of etoposide to CHOP led to a superior freedom from treatment failure (73% vs. 63%; $p = .001$), whereas the increasing dose intensity of shorter regimens did not lead to a significant improvement of treatment outcome. This is in contrast to elderly patients from the same study, for whom CHOP at 14- rather than 21-day intervals did lead to a treatment advantage.

Two other studies deserve mention. Giles et al. performed a randomized trial testing the addition of interferon to the CHOP regimen (113). There was no significant advantage to incorporating interferon into the regimen. A study of 193 patients from the National Cancer Institute comparing ProMACE-CytaBOM to ProMACE-MOPP [Pro-

MACE + mechlorethamine, Oncovin (vincristine), procarbazine, and prednisone] found a significant advantage to ProMACE-CytaBOM (121). There were both a superior complete-remission rate (85% vs. 74%; $p = .05$) and superior overall survival (67% vs. 55%, $p = .05$). Although Pro-MACE-MOPP has not been a popular regimen for treating patients with advanced diffuse large B-cell lymphoma, this study suggests that cytarabine, bleomycin, and methotrexate are more effective than mechlorethamine and procarbazine for treating patients with diffuse large-cell lymphoma.

Given the very large number of randomized trials so far completed in patients with diffuse large B-cell lymphoma, it is somewhat discouraging that there is no general consensus on the best way to treat these patients. Although this demonstrates that randomized clinical trials are not a panacea for identifying the best treatment approach and, in fact, can yield conflicting results when apparently similar trials are conducted by two different groups, they remain the most powerful tool for answering important clinical questions. The trials reviewed here convincingly document the importance of incorporating an anthracycline or similar drug in the treatment for patients with diffuse large B-cell lymphoma. They certainly don't answer the question of the best treatment regimen and raise the question of the existence of specific subgroups based on clinical or biologic parameters in which there might be an advantage for one treatment regimen over the other. Our current ability to do genetic studies to look at activation of specific genes and, in the near future, the existence of over- or underexpression of specific proteins might eventually allow a choice of the specific treatment regimen most likely to benefit a patient with a specific lymphoma. However, this remains a goal for the future.

Trials of Bone Marrow Transplantation as Part of the Primary Therapy of Younger Patients

Another approach to improving the results of therapy for diffuse large B-cell lymphoma involves the incorporation of high-dose therapy and autologous hematopoietic stem cell transplantation into primary treatment. One of the earliest attempts at using "upfront" transplantation for non-Hodgkin's lymphoma was reported by investigators at Memorial Sloan-Kettering Cancer Center (140). Fourteen large-cell lymphoma patients with poor-prognosis characteristics were treated with autologous stem cell transplantation when in first complete or partial remission. The overall survival of this group was significantly better than that of a historical control group with similar characteristics and significantly better than that of a concurrent group of patients who refused early transplantation. After this, several phase II trials were reported describing the use of autologous stem cell transplantation as consolidation therapy for poor-prognosis non-Hodgkin's lymphoma patients in first remission after initial therapy (141–148). These tri-

als demonstrated that approximately 60% to 80% of these patients achieved long-term failure-free survival after autologous stem cell transplantation and that transplantation in this situation could frequently be performed with mortality rates below 5%. Despite these encouraging results, the value of upfront transplantation can only be demonstrated if survival of all poor-prognosis patients is reported from the time of diagnosis. However, most series only report outcomes for patients who undergo transplantation, and the "denominator" is rarely reported. Alternatively, benefits of early transplantation can be demonstrated through randomized trials.

Results of randomized trials examining the role of early autologous stem cell transplantation for poor-prognosis non-Hodgkin's lymphoma patients are displayed in Table 27.7. The trial designs in these studies are markedly different with respect to patient eligibility, time of randomization, and nature of treatment in the control arms.

In the LNH97-2 trial from the Groupe d'Etude des Lymphomes de l'Adulte (GELA), 541 patients in remission after an induction regimen were randomized to treatment with sequential conventional chemotherapy or to treatment with high-dose chemotherapy and autologous stem cell transplantation (149). No survival advantages were noted among patients who received autologous stem cell transplantation as consolidation therapy, although a retrospective analysis demonstrated significantly better disease-free survival and overall survival in the subset of patients in the high-intermediate– and high-risk groups identified with the age-adjusted IPI. The GELA group subsequently performed the LNH93-3 trial for patients with these same adverse prognostic characteristics (150). Patients were randomized to receive standard ACVBP chemotherapy or to receive treatment with a novel shortened initial chemotherapy regimen designed to increase the response rate and allow autologous stem cell transplantation by day 60. In this trial, event-free survival and overall survival rates were significantly higher in patients who were treated on the conventional treatment arm.

The Milan group used another approach to examine the role of upfront autologous stem cell transplantation (151). They randomized patients to receive the MACOP-B regimen or to receive a novel high-dose sequential regimen incorporating autologous stem cell transplantation. Patients for whom either treatment was unsuccessful were crossed over to the other treatment arm. The event-free survival was significantly better in the patients who received the high-dose sequential chemotherapy, and there was a trend toward improved overall survival.

Other trials have demonstrated improved progression-free survival or event-free survival in high-risk groups (152,153), although overall survival advantages have not been demonstrated in these trials or others (154–156).

There is considerable controversy regarding the role of upfront transplantation, although several conclusions can be drawn from these studies. Most important is the fact that early autologous stem cell transplantation is not warranted for all patients but is only beneficial for patients with adverse prognostic factors who are unlikely to do well with standard therapy. In addition, autologous stem cell transplantation consolidation does not appear to be beneficial for patients who receive abbreviated courses of conventional therapy before transplant. Benefits are most likely to be seen in patients who have maximal response after a full course of conventional chemotherapy. Ongoing trials in the United States, Europe, and Australia may clarify the role of early autologous stem cell transplantation for poor-prognosis diffuse large B-cell lymphoma.

Trials of Chemotherapy in Elderly Patients

Elderly patients present unique problems when they are diagnosed with diffuse large B-cell lymphoma. Although some elderly patients are at least as healthy as younger adults and can be treated with the same regimens, this is not always true. Older patients sometimes are less willing to accept very intensive and potentially more toxic regimens, even if they are apparently able to tolerate them. One trial noted above (138) suggested that regimens that might be optimal in younger patients would not be the same as those that would have optimal activity in elderly patients. In a large German trial reported as an abstract, elderly patients seemed to benefit more by shortening the treatment interval and increasing the dose intensity of CHOP, whereas younger patients benefited more from the addition of an extra drug to the CHOP regimen, with the drugs administered at 3-week intervals. A number of other randomized trials have been carried out specifically addressing the care of elderly patients with diffuse large-cell lymphoma in which most or all of the patients had diffuse large B-cell lymphoma. These trials are detailed in Table 27.8.

One of the most influential clinical trials ever carried out in the treatment of patients with lymphoma was a trial of CHOP versus CHOP plus the monoclonal anti-CD20 antibody rituximab in elderly patients (i.e., ages 60 to 80 years), all of whom had diffuse large B-cell lymphoma. This trial of 399 patients found a superior complete-remission rate (76% vs. 63%, $p = .005$), 2-year event-free survival (57% vs. 38%, $p = .001$), and 2-year overall survival (70% vs. 57%, $p = .007$), in each case favoring the combination of CHOP plus rituximab. In this trial, the rituximab was administered at a dose of 375 mg per m^2 on day 1 of each treatment cycle—the same day as the cyclophosphamide, Adriamycin, and vincristine were administered. Although this trial was restricted to elderly patients, this treatment approach has been broadly accepted in the United States, and currently, essentially all new patients with diffuse large B-cell lymphoma receive CHOP plus rituximab. However, there is an intergroup trial currently ongoing in the United States, albeit with a slightly different sequence of drug administration, that is testing this same point, and the results are expected soon. A recent report from the GELA investigators suggested that the advantage of adding rituximab to CHOP was confined to those patients with diffuse large B-cell lymphoma whose tumors overexpressed bcl-2 protein (157). Similar data regarding the particular efficacy of rituximab in patients with diffuse large B-cell lymphoma overexpressing bcl-2 protein had been reported in a single-arm study (158).

Another study from the same French group compared a regimen not containing an anthracycline (i.e., cyclophosphamide, teniposide, and prednisone) versus the same drugs plus the anthracycline pirarubicin in 453 patients with diffuse aggressive non-Hodgkin's lymphoma older than 70 years of age. Both the complete-remission rate (47% vs. 32%; $p = .0001$) and the 5-year survival (26% vs. 19%; $p = .05$) favored the anthracycline-containing regimen. This study supports the results in young patients indicating the importance of including an anthracycline or anthracenedione in the treatment of patients with diffuse large-cell lymphoma.

Two studies from the same French cooperative group compared the ACVBP regimen (doxorubicin, cyclophosphamide, vindesine, bleomycin, IV methylprednisolone, and intrathecal methotrexate followed by consolidative therapy with high-dose methotrexate, ifosfamide, etoposide, L-asparaginase, and cytarabine) to CHOP in one study and ACVBP without consolidation but alternating with VIMMM (mitoxantrone, ifosfamide, methylgag, teniposide, methotrexate, methylprednisolone, and intrathecal methotrexate) in another. The comparison of CHOP and ACVBP involved 635 patients aged 60 to 69 years. The event-free survival (45% vs. 33%; $p = .004$) favored ACVBP. The study of ACVBP versus ACVBP/VIMMM involved 810 patients aged 55 to 69 years. The complete-remission rate (58% vs. 48%; $p = .003$) and 5-year event-free survival (33% vs. 28%; $p = .03$) both favored ACVBP. When combined with the study in localized lymphoma showing an advantage of ACVBP over CHOP plus radiotherapy, the question is certainly raised as to whether this is a superior regimen for the treatment of patients with diffuse large B-cell lymphoma. However, one of the agents included in ACVBP (vindesine) is not available in the United States, and no studies have been undertaken in the United States using ACVBP.

Three studies in elderly patients have compared CHOP with alternate regimens incorporating the anthracenedione mitoxantrone rather than the anthracycline doxorubicin. The Scandinavian study compared CHOP plus or minus filgrastim to CNOP [Cytoxan (cyclophosphamide), Novantrone (mitoxantrone), Oncovin (vincristine), and prednisone] plus or minus filgrastim (159) in 455 patients aged 60 to 86 years. The dose of doxorubicin in this study was 50 mg per m^2 and the dose of mitoxantrone 10 mg per m^2. Both the complete-remission rate (60% vs. 43%; $p < .001$) and the 5-year survival (48% vs. 26%, $p < .001$) favored the CHOP regimens. In a Dutch study of 148 patients, CHOP was compared to CNOP (160); once again, the doxorubicin dose was 50 mg per m^2, and the mitoxantrone dose was 10 mg per m^2. In this study, both the complete-remission rate (49% vs. 31%; $p = .03$) and the 3-year overall survival (42% vs. 26%; $p = .03$) favored the CHOP regimen. Finally, the European Organization for Research and Treatment of Cancer studied 120 patients older than 70 years of age and compared CHOP with a regimen incorporating etoposide, mitoxantrone, and prednimustine (161). Once again, the doxorubicin dose was 50 mg per m^2, and the mitoxantrone dose 10 mg per m^2. The progression-free survival at 2 years (55% vs. 25%; $p = .002$) and the overall survival at 2 years (65% vs. 30%; $p = .004$) favored the CHOP regimen. Because the equitoxic dose of mitoxantrone to 50 mg per m^2 of doxorubicin is probably 12 mg per m^2, not 10 mg per m^2, these studies leave open the question of the results if the higher dose of mitoxantrone had been used. However, it would seem inappropriate to treat elderly patients with the mitoxantrone at a dose of 12 mg per m^2.

Two other randomized trials compared the frequency and duration of therapy in elderly patients. A Canadian study (162) compared traditional CHOP versus the same drugs administered at one-third–dose weekly to give the same total dose in 38 patients older than 65 years of age. This study found no treatment advantage to the weekly chemotherapy. An Italian study of 306 patients compared 8 versus 12 weeks of VNCOP-B (etoposide, mitoxantrone, cyclophosphamide, vincristine, prednisone, and bleomycin), in which the drugs were administered at weekly intervals supported by filgrastim (163). The patients in this study were all older than 60 years of age. There was no advantage to extending the treatment to 12 weeks.

Recurrent and Refractory Diffuse Large B-Cell Lymphoma

Conventional Treatment

At least 40% to 50% of patients with advanced-stage diffuse large B-cell lymphoma do not attain a remission with initial therapy or relapse after achieving a remission. Rare asymptomatic patients who are not candidates for curative therapy can sometimes be managed with a watch and wait approach. Selected patients may occasionally experience prolonged remissions with involved-field radiation therapy. However, the vast majority of patients require second-line (salvage) chemotherapy.

A variety of drugs have single-agent activity for patients with relapsed or refractory diffuse large B-cell lymphoma. The most commonly used agents include etoposide (164), cytarabine (165), cisplatin (166), mitoxantrone (167), and ifosfamide (168). Single-agent activity rates as high as 20% to 30% have been reported, although response durations are brief, and most patients are treated with combination-chemotherapy regimens. Results of several commonly used salvage-chemotherapy regimens are displayed in Table 27.9. Several of these regimens use infusional therapy as a means of overcoming drug resistance. It is difficult to compare results, because these series frequently contain patients who are heterogeneous with respect to prior therapy and other prognostic factors. In addition, patients with a variety of histologic subtypes may be included. Prognostic factors for patients treated with these salvage regimens are similar to the factors that are important for upfront treatment of newly diagnosed patients. These regimens are commonly used as short-duration treatments to reduce tumor burden before treatment with high-dose therapy and autologous hematopoietic stem cell transplantation. Because of this, it is frequently difficult to determine outcomes for patients who receive only these regimens. Although response rates exceeding 50% are commonly observed with these regimens, prior treatment frequently makes it difficult to administer repeated cycles of therapy, and few patients experience long-term disease-free survival with these regimens alone.

A number of newer agents, such as liposomal daunorubicin (169), gemcitabine (170,171), paclitaxel (172), docetaxel (173), and topotecan (174), and combinations of these agents (175,176) show promise. Some patients may

TABLE 27.9. Chemotherapy salvage regimens for diffuse large B-cell lymphoma

Regimen	Drugs	CR (%)	PR (%)	CR + PR (%)	Reference
IMVP-16	Ifosfamide, methotrexate, etoposide	37	25	62	216
DHAP	Dexamethasone, cytarabine, cisplatin	28	26	54	217
ESHAP	Etoposide, methylprednisolone, cytarabine, cisplatin	26	22	48	218
DICEP	Cyclophosphamide, etoposide, cisplatin	52	26	78	219
DICE	Dexamethasone, ifosfamide, cisplatin, etoposide	23	44	67	220
ICE	Ifosfamide, carboplatin, etoposide	—	—	66	221
I-CHOPE	Doxorubicin, vincristine, etoposide, cyclophosphamide, prednisone	17	31	48	222
EPOCH	Etoposide, vincristine, doxorubicin, cyclophosphamide, prednisone	36	34	70	223

CR, complete remission; PR, partial remission.

respond to therapy with interferon-α (177). Approximately one third of patients with relapsed or refractory diffuse large B-cell lymphomas respond to rituximab (178), and rituximab is commonly added to the regimens displayed in Table 27.9. There is relatively little experience with the use of radiolabeled antibodies for diffuse large B-cell lymphoma, although results appear to be poorer than those seen for low-grade and transformed lymphomas (179).

High-Dose Therapy

The poor results of treatment with conventional-dose salvage-chemotherapy regimens have led to the increasing use of high-dose therapy followed by autologous hematopoietic stem cell transplantation for patients with relapsed or refractory lymphoma. The first large series of autologous stem cell transplantation for aggressive lymphoma validated the observation that response to transplantation was related to chemotherapy sensitivity before transplant (180). Approximately 40% of patients who had relapsed after initial chemotherapy but responded to treatment with conventional salvage chemotherapy before receiving high-dose therapy (sensitive relapse) achieved long-term disease-free survival after autologous stem cell transplantation. The disease-free survival was approximately 15% for relapsed patients who did not respond to conventional salvage chemotherapy (resistant relapse). There were no long-term survivors among patients with primary refractory disease.

A large number of phase II trials of autologous stem cell transplantation for patients with relapsed or refractory aggressive lymphomas have subsequently been published (Table 27.10), and virtually all demonstrate the prognostic importance of chemotherapy sensitivity before transplantation. It is difficult to compare these results because of differences in patient-related prognostic factors and because of differences in the transplant procedures themselves. In addition, many of these series contain patients with histologic subtypes other than diffuse large B-cell lymphoma. Nevertheless, these trials demonstrate that substantial numbers of patients with relapsed or refractory disease can experience long-term disease-free survival after autologous stem cell transplantation. In addition, transplantation can be performed with low morbidity and mortality. Other prognostic factors usually associated with favorable outcomes after transplantation include good performance status, younger age, absence of tumor bulk, and absence of extensive prior therapy.

Despite the widespread use of autologous stem cell transplantation for aggressive lymphoma, the value of this approach was not validated until the results of the International PARMA trial were published (181). In this trial, patients with relapsed intermediate-grade or high-grade non-Hodgkin's lymphoma were treated with two cycles of DHAP [dexamethasone, high-dose ara-C, and Platinol

TABLE 27.10. *Selected series of autologous hematopoietic stem cell transplantation for aggressive non-Hodgkin's lymphoma*

Reference	No. of patients	Early mortality (%)	Outcome
180	100	21	19% actuarial 3-yr DFS
224	101	21	11% actuarial 5-yr EFS
225	158	NS	29% actuarial 3-yr FFS
226	107	7	35% actuarial 5-yr PFS
227	221	10	55% CCR (median 2.4 yr)
228	112	3	71% actuarial 3-yr DFS (for intermediate grade)
229	136	4.4	34% actuarial 5-yr EFS
230	94	10.6	33% actuarial 3-yr PFS
231	90	NS	40% actuarial 4-yr DFS

CCR, continuous complete remission; DFS, disease-free survival; EFS, event-free survival; FFS, failure-free survival; NS, not stated; PFS, progression-free survival.

(cisplatin)] salvage chemotherapy (Table 27.10). Sensitive patients were then randomized to treatment with four more cycles of DHAP or to treatment with high-dose chemotherapy followed by autologous stem cell transplantation. The 5-year event-free survival was 46% in patients randomized to transplant as compared with 12% for patients who received conventional salvage chemotherapy (p = .001). The 5-year overall survival rates were 53% and 32%, respectively (p = .038). A follow-up study demonstrated that patients with an IPI score of 0 at relapse did not benefit from transplantation, although overall survival was improved with transplantation for patients with an IPI score of 1 to 3 (182). Consensus panel recommendations indicate that high-dose therapy followed by autologous stem cell transplantation is now considered standard therapy for patients with chemotherapy-sensitive relapsed diffuse large B-cell lymphoma (183,184).

There is less agreement on the use of autologous stem cell transplantation for patients with resistant relapsed or refractory disease. However, two large series have investigated the role of autologous stem cell transplantation for patients with primary refractory disease and have demonstrated that 30% to 40% of these patients may experience long-term event-free survival after transplantation, especially if they have chemotherapy-sensitive disease (185,186). Patients with non-Hodgkin's lymphoma who respond slowly to initial therapy have a poor prognosis

(187). Two prospective randomized trials have evaluated the use of autologous stem cell transplantation performed after a partial course of chemotherapy for patients in partial remission (188,189). Neither trial showed survival advantages for transplanted patients. However, it is unknown whether completion of primary therapy followed by transplantation would be beneficial.

There is less experience with allogeneic hematopoietic stem cell transplantation for non-Hodgkin's lymphoma. When compared with autologous stem cell transplantation, this approach eliminates the possibility of infusing malignant cells and could be associated with a beneficial graft-versus-lymphoma effect. Comparative trials have demonstrated lower relapse rates after allogeneic transplantation, although overall survival advantages have not been seen because of the higher risk of transplant-related mortality (190–192). Transplant mortality may be decreased with the use of nonmyeloablative allogeneic transplantation, although there is limited experience using this approach for diffuse large B-cell lymphoma.

FUTURE DIRECTIONS

The subtype of non-Hodgkin's lymphoma that we refer to as *diffuse large B-cell lymphoma* is clearly a heterogeneous entity. We have known for many years that some patients could be cured with available therapies whereas others go on to die of their disease. The chances for a good survival have been found to be better with low stage, fewer symptoms, less bulky disease, low lactate dehydrogenase levels, no involvement of the liver or central nervous system, and other factors. Recently the use of gene arrays has demonstrated that patients with this disease can be subdivided based on gene-expression patterns. Patients with a gene-expression pattern that resembles normal germinal center B-cells have a better outcome than do those whose gene-expression pattern resembles activated peripheral blood lymphocytes. A third category with an outcome more like that for lymphomas whose gene-expression patterns resemble activated peripheral blood lymphocytes has more recently been identified. It is likely that further understanding of gene-expression and protein-expression patterns in diffuse large B-cell lymphomas will provide the biologic basis for the clinical prognostic factors that have been known for some time. These findings will provide the opportunity to divide patients with diffuse large B-cell lymphomas into subcategories based on gene and protein expression. If specific therapies are developed to target specific protein expression, these new subcategories will become key diagnostic features, and the disease we now call diffuse large B-cell lymphoma will be broken up into different diagnoses.

Thus, whether diffuse large B-cell lymphoma can be usefully further subdivided depends not only on our ability to find diagnostic tests to subcategorize the illness but also on

the development of specific therapies that make these subdivisions clinically important. It is likely that, to some degree, this will happen.

Diffuse large B-cell lymphoma is one of the chemotherapy-curable malignancies and can be cured in a significant portion of patients. Whether the prognosis for patients with this disorder improves will depend on the development of effective new therapies—probably targeted at specific proteins expressed in these lymphomas.

REFERENCES

1. A clinical evaluation of the International Lymphoma Study Group classification of non-Hodgkin's lymphoma. The Non-Hodgkin's Lymphoma Classification Project. *Blood* 1997;89:3909–3918.
2. Anderson JR, Armitage JO, Weisenburger DD. Epidemiology of the non-Hodgkin's lymphomas: distributions of the major subtypes differ by geographic locations. Non-Hodgkin's Lymphoma Classification Project. *Ann Oncol* 1998;9:717–720.
3. Kamel OW, Holly EA, van de Rijn M, et al. A population based, case control study of non-Hodgkin's lymphoma in patients with rheumatoid arthritis. *J Rheumatol* 1999;26:1676–1680.
4. Thomas E, Brewster DH, Black RJ, et al. Risk of malignancy among patients with rheumatic conditions. *Int J Cancer* 2000;88:497–502.
5. Engelhard M, Brittinger G, Huhn D, et al. Subclassification of diffuse large B-cell lymphomas according to the Kiel classification: distinction of centroblastic and immunoblastic lymphomas is a significant prognostic risk factor. *Blood* 1997;89:2291–2297.
6. Armitage JO, Weisenburger DD. New approach to classifying non-Hodgkin's lymphomas: clinical features of the major histologic subtypes. Non-Hodgkin's Lymphoma Classification Project. *J Clin Oncol* 1998;16:2780–2795.
7. Delecluse HJ, Anagnostopoulos I, Dallenbach F, et al. Plasmablastic lymphomas of the oral cavity: a new entity associated with the human immunodeficiency virus infection. *Blood* 1997;89:1413–1420.
8. Dupin N, Diss TL, Kellam P, et al. HHV-8 is associated with a plasmablastic variant of Castleman disease that is linked to HHV-8-positive plasmablastic lymphoma. *Blood* 2000;95:1406–1412.
9. Delsol G, Lamant L, Mariame B, et al. A new subtype of large B-cell lymphoma expressing the ALK kinase and lacking the 2;5 translocation. *Blood* 1997;89:1483–1490.
10. Fisher DE, Jacobson JO, Ault KA, et al. Diffuse large cell lymphoma with discordant bone marrow histology. Clinical features and biological implications. *Cancer* 1989;64:1879–1887.
11. Velasquez WS, Jagannath S, Tucker SL, et al. Risk classification as the basis for clinical staging of diffuse large-cell lymphoma derived from 10-year survival data. *Blood* 1989;74:551–557.
12. Cabanillas F, Velasquez WS, Hagemeister FB, et al. Clinical, biologic, and histologic features of late relapses in diffuse large cell lymphoma. *Blood* 1992;79:1024–1028.
13. Stein H, Lennert K, Feller AC, et al. Immunohistological analysis of human lymphoma: correlation of histological and immunological categories. *Adv Cancer Res* 1984;42:67–147.
14. Doggett RS, Wood GS, Horning S, et al. The immunologic characterization of 95 nodal and extranodal diffuse large cell lymphomas in 89 patients. *Am J Pathol* 1984;115:245–252.
15. Gascoyne RD, Adomat SA, Krajewski S, et al. Prognostic significance of Bcl-2 protein expression and Bcl-2 gene rearrangement in diffuse aggressive non-Hodgkin's lymphoma. *Blood* 1997;90:244–251.
16. Kramer MH, Hermans J, Parker J, et al. Clinical significance of bcl2 and p53 protein expression in diffuse large B-cell lymphoma: a population-based study. *J Clin Oncol* 1996;14:2131–2138.
17. Sanchez E, Chacon I, Plaza MM, et al. Clinical outcome in diffuse large B-cell lymphoma is dependent on the relationship between different cell-cycle regulator proteins. *J Clin Oncol* 1998;16:1931–1939.
18. Skinnider BF, Horsman DE, Dupuis B, et al. Bcl-6 and Bcl-2 protein expression in diffuse large B-cell lymphoma and follicular lym-

phoma: correlation with 3q27 and 18q21 chromosomal abnormalities. *Hum Pathol* 1999;30:803–808.

19. De Leval L, Shipp M, Neuberger D, et al. Diffuse large B-cell lymphomas are tumors of germinal center origin. *Blood* 1999:(in press).

20. Kuppers R, Rajewsky K, Hansmann ML. Diffuse large cell lymphomas are derived from mature B cells carrying V region genes with a high load of somatic mutation and evidence of selection for antibody expression. *Eur J Immunol* 1997;27:1398–1405.

21. Klein U, Goossens T, Fischer M, et al. Somatic hypermutation in normal and transformed human B cells. *Immunol Rev* 1998;162:261–280.

22. Yunis JJ, Mayer MG, Arnesen MA, et al. Bcl-2 and other genomic alterations in the prognosis of large-cell lymphoma [see comments]. *N Engl J Med* 1989;320:1047–1054.

23. Kramer MH, Hermans J, Wijburg E, et al. Clinical relevance of BCL2, BCL6, and MYC rearrangements in diffuse large B-cell lymphoma. *Blood* 1998;92:3152–3162.

24. Bastard C, Deweindt C, Kerckaert JP, et al. LAZ3 rearrangements in non-Hodgkin's lymphoma: correlation with histology, immunophenotype, karyotype, and clinical outcome in 217 patients. *Blood* 1994;83:2423–2427.

25. Migliazza A, Martinotti S, Chen W, et al. Frequent somatic hypermutation of the 5' noncoding region of the BCL6 gene in B-cell lymphoma. *Proc Natl Acad Sci U S A* 1995;92:12520–12524.

26. Vitolo U, Gaidano G, Botto B, et al. Rearrangements of bcl-6, bcl-2, c-myc and 6q deletion in B-diffuse large-cell lymphoma: clinical relevance in 71 patients. *Ann Oncol* 1998;9:55–61.

27. Shen HM, Peters A, Baron B, et al. Mutation of BCL-6 gene in normal B cells by the process of somatic hypermutation of Ig genes. *Science* 1998;280:1750–1752.

28. Peng HZ, Du MQ, Koulis A, et al. Nonimmunoglobulin gene hypermutation in germinal center B cells. *Blood* 1999;93:2167–2172.

29. Kuppers R, Zhao M, Hansmann ML, et al. Tracing B cell development in human germinal centres by molecular analysis of single cells picked from histological sections. *Embo J* 1993;12:4955–4967.

30. Ferry JA, Harris NL, Picker LJ, et al. Intravascular lymphomatosis (malignant angioendotheliomatosis). A B-cell neoplasm expressing surface homing receptors. *Mod Pathol* 1988;1:444–452.

31. DiGiuseppe JA, Nelson WG, Seifter EJ, et al. Intravascular lymphomatosis: a clinicopathologic study of 10 cases and assessment of response to chemotherapy. *J Clin Oncol* 1994;12:2573–2579.

32. Delabie J, Vandenberghe E, Kennes C, et al. Histiocyte-rich B-cell lymphoma. A distinct clinicopathologic entity possibly related to lymphocyte predominant Hodgkin's disease, paragranuloma subtype. *Am J Surg Pathol* 1992;16:37–48.

33. McBride JA, Rodriguez J, Luthra R, et al. T-cell-rich B large-cell lymphoma simulating lymphocyte-rich Hodgkin's disease [see comments]. *Am J Surg Pathol* 1996;20:193–201.

34. Guinee D Jr, Jaffe E, Kingma D, et al. Pulmonary lymphomatoid granulomatosis. Evidence for a proliferation of Epstein-Barr virus infected B-lymphocytes with a prominent T-cell component and vasculitis. *Am J Surg Pathol* 1994;18:753–764.

35. Haque AK, Myers JL, Hudnall SD, et al. Pulmonary lymphomatoid granulomatosis in acquired immunodeficiency syndrome: lesions with Epstein-Barr virus infection. *Mod Pathol* 1998;11:347–356.

36. Katzenstein AL, Peiper SC. Detection of Epstein-Barr virus genomes in lymphomatoid granulomatosis: analysis of 29 cases by the polymerase chain reaction technique. *Mod Pathol* 1990;3:435–441.

37. Myers JL, Kurtin PJ, Katzenstein AL, et al. Lymphomatoid granulomatosis. Evidence of immunophenotypic diversity and relationship to Epstein-Barr virus infection. *Am J Surg Pathol* 1995;19:1300–1312.

38. Wilson WH, Kingma DW, Raffeld M, et al. Association of lymphomatoid granulomatosis with Epstein-Barr viral infection of B lymphocytes and response to interferon-alpha 2b. *Blood* 1996;87:4531–4537.

39. Otsuki T, Kumar S, Ensoli B, et al. Detection of HHV-8/KSHV DNA sequences in AIDS-associated extranodal lymphoid malignancies. *Leukemia* 1996;10:1358–1362.

40. Carbone A, Gaidano G, Gloghini A, et al. Differential expression of BCL-6, CD138/syndecan-1, and Epstein-Barr virus-encoded latent membrane protein-1 identifies distinct histogenetic subsets of acquired immunodeficiency syndrome-related non-Hodgkin's lymphomas. *Blood* 1998;91:747–755.

41. Nador RG, Cesarman E, Chadburn A, et al. Primary effusion lymphoma: a distinct clinicopathologic entity associated with the Kaposi's sarcoma-associated herpes virus. *Blood* 1996;88:645–656.

42. Alizadeh AA, Eisen MB, Davis RE, et al. Distinct types of diffuse large B-cell lymphoma identified by gene expression profiling. *Nature* 2000;403:503–511.

43. Shipp MA, Ross KN, Tamayo P, et al. Diffuse large B-cell lymphoma outcome prediction by gene-expression profiling and supervised machine learning. *Nat Med* 2002;8:68–74.

44. Offit K, Jhanwar S, Ebrahim SA, et al. t(3;22)(q27;q11): a novel translocation associated with diffuse non-Hodgkin's lymphoma. *Blood* 1989;74:1876–1879.

45. Bastard C, Tilly H, Lenormand B, et al. Translocations involving band 3q27 and Ig gene regions in non-Hodgkin's lymphoma. *Blood* 1992;79:2527–2531.

46. Ye BH, Lista F, Lo Coco F, et al. Alterations of a zinc finger-encoding gene, BCL-6, in diffuse large-cell lymphoma. *Science* 1993;262:747–750.

47. Ye BH, Chaganti S, Chang CC, et al. Chromosomal translocations cause deregulated BCL6 expression by promoter substitution in B cell lymphoma. *Embo J* 1995;14:6209–6217.

48. Chang CC, Ye BH, Chaganti RS, et al. BCL-6, a POZ/zinc-finger protein, is a sequence-specific transcriptional repressor. *Proc Natl Acad Sci U S A* 1996;93:6947–6952.

49. Cattoretti G, Chang CC, Cechova K, et al. BCL-6 protein is expressed in germinal-center B cells. *Blood* 1995;86:45–53.

50. Dent AL, Shaffer AL, Yu X, et al. Control of inflammation, cytokine expression, and germinal center formation by BCL-6. *Science* 1997;276:589–592.

51. Ye BH, Cattoretti G, Shen Q, et al. The BCL-6 proto-oncogene controls germinal-centre formation and Th2-type inflammation. *Nat Genet* 1997;16:161–170.

52. Lo Coco F, Ye BH, Lista F, et al. Rearrangements of the BCL6 gene in diffuse large cell non-Hodgkin's lymphoma. *Blood* 1994;83:1757–1759.

53. Chen W, Iida S, Louie DC, et al. Heterologous promoters fused to BCL6 by chromosomal translocations affecting band 3q27 cause its deregulated expression during B-cell differentiation. *Blood* 1998;91:603–607.

54. Shaffer AL, Yu X, He Y, et al. BCL-6 represses genes that function in lymphocyte differentiation, inflammation, and cell cycle control. *Immunity* 2000;13:199–212.

55. Pasqualucci L, Migliazza A, Fracchiolla N, et al. BCL-6 mutations in normal germinal center B cells: evidence of somatic hypermutation acting outside Ig loci. *Proc Natl Acad Sci U S A* 1998;95:11816–11821.

56. Pasqualucci L, Migliazza A, Basso K, et al. Mutations of the BCL6 proto-oncogene disrupt its negative autoregulation in diffuse large B-cell lymphoma. *Blood* 2003;101:2914-2923.

57. Dalla-Favera R, Ye BH, Lo Coco F, et al. Identification of genetic lesions associated with diffuse large-cell lymphoma. *Ann Oncol* 1994;5:55–60.

58. Tang SC, Visser L, Hepperle B, et al. Clinical significance of bcl-2-MBR gene rearrangement and protein expression in diffuse large-cell non-Hodgkin's lymphoma: an analysis of 83 cases. *J Clin Oncol* 1994;12:149–154.

59. Pasqualucci L, Neumeister P, Goossens T, et al. Hypermutation of multiple proto-oncogenes in B-cell diffuse large-cell lymphomas. *Nature* 2001;412:341–346.

60. Fredericks RK, Walker FO, Elster A, et al. Angiotropic intravascular large-cell lymphoma (malignant angioendotheliomatosis): report of a case and review of the literature. *Surg Neurol* 1991;35:218–223.

61. Conlan MG, Bast M, Armitage JO, et al. Bone marrow involvement by non-Hodgkin's lymphoma: the clinical significance of morphologic discordance between the lymph node and bone marrow. Nebraska Lymphoma Study Group. *J Clin Oncol* 1990;8:1163–1172.

62. A predictive model for aggressive non-Hodgkin's lymphoma. The International Non-Hodgkin's Lymphoma Prognostic Factors Project [see comments]. *N Engl J Med* 1993;329:987–994.

63. Swan F Jr, Velasquez WS, Tucker S, et al. A new serologic staging system for large-cell lymphomas based on initial beta 2-microglobulin and lactate dehydrogenase levels. *J Clin Oncol* 1989;7:1518–1527.

64. Armitage JO, Weisenburger DD, Hutchins M, et al. Chemotherapy for diffuse large-cell lymphoma—rapidly responding patients have more durable remissions. *J Clin Oncol* 1986;4:160–164.

65. Bauer KD, Merkel DE, Winter JN, et al. Prognostic implications of ploidy and proliferative activity in diffuse large cell lymphomas. *Cancer Res* 1986;46:3173–3178.

66. Wooldridge TN, Grierson HL, Weisenburger DD, et al. Association of DNA content and proliferative activity with clinical outcome in patients with diffuse mixed cell and large cell non-Hodgkin's lymphoma. *Cancer Res* 1988;48:6608–6613.

67. Grogan TM, Lippman SM, Spier CM, et al. Independent prognostic significance of a nuclear proliferation antigen in diffuse large cell lymphomas as determined by the monoclonal antibody Ki-67. *Blood* 1988;71:1157–1160.

68. Wilson WH, Teruya-Feldstein J, Fest T, et al. Relationship of p53, bcl-2, and tumor proliferation to clinical drug resistance in non-Hodgkin's lymphomas. *Blood* 1997;89:601–609.

69. Ansell SM, Stenson M, Habermann TM, et al. Cd4+ T-cell immune response to large B-cell non-Hodgkin's lymphoma predicts patient outcome. *J Clin Oncol* 2001;19:720–726.

70. Miller TP, Lippman SM, Spier CM, et al. HLA-DR (Ia) immune phenotype predicts outcome for patients with diffuse large cell lymphoma. *J Clin Invest* 1988;82:370–372.

71. Swan F, Huh Y, Katz R, et al. Beta-2-microglobuin and HLA-DR cellular expression in relapsing large cell lymphomas (LCL): relationship to survival and serum beta-2-microglobulin levels. *Blood* 1990;76:375a [abstract].

72. Stasi R, Zinzani L, Galieni P, et al. Detection of soluble interleukin-2 receptor and interleukin-10 in the serum of patients with aggressive non-Hodgkin's lymphoma. Identification of a subset at high risk of treatment failure. *Cancer* 1994;74:1792–1800.

73. Seymour JF, Talpaz M, Cabanillas F, et al. Serum interleukin-6 levels correlate with prognosis in diffuse large-cell lymphoma. *J Clin Oncol* 1995;13:575–582.

74. Ristamaki R, Joensuu H, Lappalainen K, et al. Elevated serum CD44 level is associated with unfavorable outcome in non-Hodgkin's lymphoma. *Blood* 1997;90:4039–4045.

75. Filipits M, Jaeger U, Simonitsch I, et al. Clinical relevance of the lung resistance protein in diffuse large B-cell lymphomas. *Clin Cancer Res* 2000;6:3417–3423.

76. Adida C, Haioun C, Gaulard P, et al. Prognostic significance of survivin expression in diffuse large B-cell lymphomas. *Blood* 2000;96:1921–1925.

77. Salven P, Teerenhovi L, Joensuu H. A high pretreatment serum vascular endothelial growth factor concentration is associated with poor outcome in non-Hodgkin's lymphoma. *Blood* 1997;90:3167–3172.

78. Hermine O, Haioun C, Lepage E, et al. Prognostic significance of bcl-2 protein expression in aggressive non-Hodgkin's lymphoma. Groupe d'Etude des Lymphomes de l'Adulte (GELA). *Blood* 1996;87:265–272.

79. Lossos IS, Jones CD, Warnke R, et al. Expression of a single gene, BCL-6, strongly predicts survival in patients with diffuse large B-cell lymphoma. *Blood* 2001;98:945–951.

80. Braaten KM, Betensky RA, de Leval L, et al. BCL-6 expression predicts improved survival in patients with primary central nervous system lymphoma. *Clin Cancer Res* 2003;9:1063–1069.

81. Lossos IS, Alizadeh AA, Rajapaksa R, et al. HGAL is a novel interleukin-4-inducible gene that strongly predicts survival in diffuse large B-cell lymphoma. *Blood* 2003;101:433–440.

82. Leroy K, Haioun C, Lepage E, et al. p53 gene mutations are associated with poor survival in low and low-intermediate risk diffuse large B-cell lymphomas. *Ann Oncol* 2002;13:1108–1115.

83. Filipits M, Jaeger U, Pohl G, et al. Cyclin D3 is a predictive and prognostic factor in diffuse large B-cell lymphoma. *Clin Cancer Res* 2002;8:729–733.

84. Rosenwald A, Wright G, Chan WC, et al. The use of molecular profiling to predict survival after chemotherapy for diffuse large-B-cell lymphoma. *N Engl J Med* 2002;346:1937–1947.

85. Huang JZ, Sanger WG, Greiner TC, et al. The t(14;18) defines a unique subset of diffuse large B-cell lymphoma with a germinal center B-cell gene expression profile. *Blood* 2002;99:2285–2290.

86. Barrans SL, Carter I, Owen RG, et al. Germinal center phenotype and bcl-2 expression combined with the International Prognostic Index improves patient risk stratification in diffuse large B-cell lymphoma. *Blood* 2002;99:1136–1143.

87. Chen MG, Prosnitz LR, Gonzalez-Serva A, et al. Results of radiotherapy in control of stage I and II non-Hodgkin's lymphoma. *Cancer* 1979;43:1245–1254.

88. Reddy S, Saxena VS, Pellettiere EV, et al. Early nodal and extranodal non-Hodgkin's lymphomas. *Cancer* 1977;40:98–104.

89. Levitt SH, Lee CK, Bloomfield CD, et al. The role of radiation therapy in the treatment of early stage large cell lymphoma. *Hematol Oncol* 1985;3:33–37.

90. Hallahan DE, Farah R, Vokes EE, et al. The patterns of failure in patients with pathological stage I and II diffuse histiocytic lymphoma treated with radiation therapy alone. *Int J Radiat Oncol Biol Phys* 1989;17:767–771.

91. Fuks Z, Kaplan HS. Recurrence rates following radiation therapy of nodular and diffuse malignant lymphomas. *Radiology* 1973;108:675–684.

92. Bush R, Gospodarowicz M. The place of radiation therapy in the management of patients with localized non-Hodgkin's lymphoma. In: Rosenberg S, Kaplan HS, eds. *Malignant lymphomas: etiology, immunology, pathology, treatment*. Burlington, MA: Academic Press, 1982:485–502.

93. Gospodarowicz M, Bush R, et al. Role of radiation in treatment of patients with localized intermediate and high grade non-Hodgkin's lymphoma. *Proc Am Soc Clin Oncol* 1984;3:C–922 [abstract].

94. Mauch P, Leonard R, Skarin A, et al. Improved survival following combined radiation therapy and chemotherapy for unfavorable prognosis stage I-II non-Hodgkin's lymphomas. *J Clin Oncol* 1985;3:1301–1308.

95. Vokes EE, Ultmann JE, Golomb HM, et al. Long-term survival of patients with localized diffuse histiocytic lymphoma. *J Clin Oncol* 1985;3:1309–1317.

96. Monfardini S, Banfi A, Bonadonna G, et al. Improved five year survival after combined radiotherapy-chemotherapy for stage I-II non-Hodgkin's lymphoma. *Int J Radiat Oncol Biol Phys* 1980;6:125–134.

97. Nissen NI, Ersboll J, Hansen HS, et al. A randomized study of radiotherapy versus radiotherapy plus chemotherapy in stage I-II non-Hodgkin's lymphomas. *Cancer* 1983;52:1–7.

98. Landberg TG, Hakansson LG, Moller TR, et al. CVP-remission-maintenance in stage I or II non-Hodgkin's lymphomas: preliminary results of a randomized study. *Cancer* 1979;44:831–838.

99. Kamath SS, Marcus RB Jr, Lynch JW, et al. The impact of radiotherapy dose and other treatment-related and clinical factors on in-field control in stage I and II non-Hodgkin's lymphoma. *Int J Radiat Oncol Biol Phys* 1999;44:563–568.

100. Munck JN, Dhermain F, Koscielny S, et al. Alternating chemotherapy and radiotherapy for limited-stage intermediate and high-grade non-Hodgkin's lymphomas: long-term results for 96 patients with tumors > 5 cm. *Ann Oncol* 1996;7:925–931.

101. Prestidge BR, Horning SJ, Hoppe RT. Combined modality therapy for stage I-II large cell lymphoma. *Int J Radiat Oncol Biol Phys* 1988;15:633–639.

102. Tondini C, Giardini R, Bozzetti F, et al. Combined modality treatment for primary gastrointestinal non-Hodgkin's lymphoma: the Milan Cancer Institute experience [see comments]. *Ann Oncol* 1993;4:831–837.

103. van der Maazen RW, Noordijk EM, Thomas J, et al. Combined modality treatment is the treatment of choice for stage I/IE intermediate and high grade non-Hodgkin's lymphomas. *Radiother Oncol* 1998;49:1–7.

104. Velasquez WS, Fuller LM, Jagannath S, et al. Stages I and II diffuse large cell lymphomas: prognostic factors and long-term results with CHOP-bleo and radiotherapy. *Blood* 1991;77:942–947.

105. Krol AD, Berenschot HW, Doekharan D, et al. Cyclophosphamide, doxorubicin, vincristine and prednisone chemotherapy and radiotherapy for stage I intermediate or high grade non-Hodgkin's

lymphomas: results of a strategy that adapts radiotherapy dose to the response after chemotherapy. *Radiother Oncol* 2001;58:251–255.

106. Shenkier TN, Voss N, Fairey R, et al. Brief chemotherapy and involved-region irradiation for limited-stage diffuse large-cell lymphoma: an 18-year experience from the British Columbia Cancer Agency. *J Clin Oncol* 2002;20:197–204.

107. Longo DL, Glatstein E, Duffey PL, et al. Treatment of localized aggressive lymphomas with combination chemotherapy followed by involved-field radiation therapy. *J Clin Oncol* 1989;7:1295–1302.

108. Schlembach PJ, Wilder RB, Tucker SL, et al. Impact of involved field radiotherapy after CHOP-based chemotherapy on stage III-IV, intermediate grade and large-cell immunoblastic lymphomas. *Int J Radiat Oncol Biol Phys* 2000;48:1107–1110.

109. Glick J, Kim K, Earle J, et al. An ECOG randomized phase III trial of CHOP vs. CHOP + radiotherapy for intermediate grade early stage non-Hodgkin's lymphoma. *Proc Amer Soc Clin Oncol* 1995:391.

110. Horning S, Glick J, et al. Final report of E1484: CHOP v CHOP + radiotherapy for limited stage diffuse aggressive lymphoma. *Blood* 2001;98:724a [abstract].

111. Miller TP, Dahlberg S, Cassady JR, et al. Chemotherapy alone compared with chemotherapy plus radiotherapy for localized intermediate- and high-grade non-Hodgkin's lymphoma [see comments]. *N Engl J Med* 1998;339:21–26.

112. Fillet G, Bonnet C. Radiotherapy is unnecessary in elderly patients with localized aggressive non-Hodgkin's lymphoma: results of the GELA LNH 93-4 study. *Blood* 2002;100:92a [abstract 337].

113. Reyes F, Lepage E, et al. Superiority of chemotherapy alone with the ACVBP regimen over treatment with three cycles of CHOP plus radiotherapy in low risk localized aggressive lymphoma: the LNH93-1 GELA study. *Blood* 2002;100:93a [abstract].

114. Roy I, Yahalom J. Excellent local control with involved-field radiotherapy following CHOP chemotherapy: analysis of 145 patients with early-stage intermediate-grade non-Hodgkin's lymphoma. *Int J Radiat Oncol Biol Phys* 2001;51:362a–363a [abstract].

115. Zinzani PL, Martelli M, Magagnoli M, et al. Treatment and clinical management of primary mediastinal large B-cell lymphoma with sclerosis: MACOP-B regimen and mediastinal radiotherapy monitored by (67)Gallium scan in 50 patients. *Blood* 1999;94:3289–3293.

116. Wilder RB, Rodriguez MA, Tucker SL, et al. Radiation therapy after a partial response to CHOP chemotherapy for aggressive lymphomas. *Int J Radiat Oncol Biol Phys* 2001;50:743–749.

117. Levitt M, Marsh JC, DeConti RC, et al. Combination sequential chemotherapy in advanced reticulum cell sarcoma. *Cancer* 1972;29:630–636.

118. DeVita VT Jr, Canellos GP, Chabner B, et al. Advanced diffuse histiocytic lymphoma, a potentially curable disease. *Lancet* 1975;1:248–250.

119. Armitage JO, Fyfe MA, Lewis J. Long-term remission durability and functional status of patients treated for diffuse histiocytic lymphoma with the CHOP regimen. *J Clin Oncol* 1984;2:898–902.

120. Moreno A, Colon-Otero G, Solberg LA Jr. The prednisone dosage in the CHOP chemotherapy regimen for non-Hodgkin's lymphomas (NHL): is there a standard? *Oncologist* 2000;5:238–249.

121. Longo DL, DeVita VT Jr, Duffey PL, et al. Superiority of ProMACE-CytaBOM over ProMACE-MOPP in the treatment of advanced diffuse aggressive lymphoma: results of a prospective randomized trial [published erratum appears in *J Clin Oncol* 1991;9(4):710]. *J Clin Oncol* 1991;9:25–38.

122. Klimo P, Connors JM. MACOP-B chemotherapy for the treatment of diffuse large-cell lymphoma. *Ann Intern Med* 1985;102:596–602.

123. Shipp MA, Yeap BY, Harrington DP, et al. The m-BACOD combination chemotherapy regimen in large-cell lymphoma: analysis of the completed trial and comparison with the M-BACOD regimen. *J Clin Oncol* 1990;8:84–93.

124. Fisher RI, Gaynor ER, Dahlberg S, et al. Comparison of a standard regimen (CHOP) with three intensive chemotherapy regimens for advanced non-Hodgkin's lymphoma [see comments]. *N Engl J Med* 1993;328:1002–1006.

125. Bishop JF, Wiernik PH, Wesley MN, et al. A randomized trial of high dose cyclophosphamide, vincristine, and prednisone plus or minus doxorubicin (CVP versus CAVP) with long-term follow-up in advanced non-Hodgkin's lymphoma. *Leukemia* 1987;1:508–513.

126. Gams RA, Rainey M, Dandy M, et al. Phase III study of BCOP v CHOP in unfavorable categories of malignant lymphoma: a Southeastern Cancer Study Group trial. *J Clin Oncol* 1985;3:1188–1195.

127. Jones SE, Grozea PN, Metz EN, et al. Improved complete remission rates and survival for patients with large cell lymphoma treated with chemoimmunotherapy. A Southwest Oncology Group Study. *Cancer* 1983;51:1083–1090.

128. O'Connell M, Anderson J, Earle J, et al. Combined modality therapy of advanced unfavorable non-Hodgkin's lymphoma (NHL): an ECOG randomized clinical trial. *Proc Am Soc Clin Oncol* 1984:241 [abstract].

129. Zinzani PL, Martelli M, Storti S, et al. Phase III comparative trial using CHOP vs CIOP in the treatment of advanced intermediate-grade non-Hodgkin's lymphoma. *Leuk Lymphoma* 1995;19:329–335.

130. Silingardi V, Federico M, Cavanna L, et al. ProMECE-CytaBOM vs MACOP-B in advanced aggressive non-Hodgkin's lymphoma: long term results of a multicenter study of the Italian Lymphoma Study Group (GISL). *Leuk Lymphoma* 1995;17:313–320.

131. Bezwoda W, Rastogi RB, Erazo Valla A, et al. Long-term results of a multicentre randomised, comparative phase III trial of CHOP versus CNOP regimens in patients with intermediate- and high-grade non-Hodgkin's lymphomas. Novantrone International Study Group. *Eur J Cancer* 1995;31A:903–911.

132. Cooper IA, Wolf MM, Robertson TI, et al. Randomized comparison of MACOP-B with CHOP in patients with intermediate-grade non-Hodgkin's lymphoma. The Australian and New Zealand Lymphoma Group. *J Clin Oncol* 1994;12:769–778.

133. Jerkeman M, Anderson H, Cavallin-Stahl E, et al. CHOP versus MACOP-B in aggressive lymphoma—a Nordic Lymphoma Group randomised trial. *Ann Oncol* 1999;10:1079–1086.

134. Linch DC, Smith P, Hancock BW, et al. A randomized British National Lymphoma Investigation trial of CHOP vs. a weekly multi-agent regimen (PACEBOM) in patients with histologically aggressive non-Hodgkin's lymphoma. *Ann Oncol* 2000;11:87–90.

135. Carde P, Meerwaldt JH, van Glabbeke M, et al. Superiority of second over first generation chemotherapy in a randomized trial for stage III-IV intermediate and high-grade non-Hodgkin's lymphoma (NHL): the 1980-1985 EORTC trial. The EORTC Lymphoma Group. *Ann Oncol* 1991;2:431–435.

136. Khaled HM, Zekri ZK, Mokhtar N, et al. A randomized EPOCH vs. CHOP front-line therapy for aggressive non-Hodgkin's lymphoma patients: long-term results. *Ann Oncol* 1999;10:1489–1492.

137. Wolf M, Matthews J, Stone J, et al. Dose-intensification does not improve outcome in aggressive non-Hodgkin's lymphoma (NHL), report of a randomized trial by the Australasian Leukemia and Lymphoma Group. *Blood* 2000;96:832a.

138. Pfreundschuh M, Truemper L, Schmits R, et al. 2-weekly vs. 3 weekly CHOP with and without etoposide in young patients with low-risk (low LDH) aggressive non-Hodgkin's lymphoma: results of the completed NHL-B-1 trial of the DSHNHL. *Blood* 2002;100:92a.

139. Aviles A, Calva A, Diaz-Maqueo JC, et al. Dose escalation of epirubicin in the CEOP-BLEO regimen: a controlled clinical trial comparing standard doses for the treatment of diffuse large cell lymphoma. *Leuk Lymphoma* 1997;25:319–325.

140. Gulati SC, Shank B, Black P, et al. Autologous bone marrow transplantation for patients with poor-prognosis lymphoma. *J Clin Oncol* 1988;6:1303–1313.

141. Baro J, Richard C, Calavia J, et al. Autologous bone marrow transplantation as consolidation therapy for non-Hodgkin's lymphoma patients with poor prognostic features. *Bone Marrow Transplant* 1991;8:283–289.

142. Freedman AS, Takvorian T, Neuberg D, et al. Autologous bone marrow transplantation in poor-prognosis intermediate-grade and high-grade B-cell non-Hodgkin's lymphoma in first remission: a pilot study. *J Clin Oncol* 1993;11:931–936.

143. Pettengell R, Radford JA, Morgenstern GR, et al. Survival benefit from high-dose therapy with autologous blood progenitor-cell trans-

plantation in poor-prognosis non-Hodgkin's lymphoma. *J Clin Oncol* 1996;14:586–592.

144. Fanin R, Silvestri F, Geromin A, et al. Primary systemic CD30 (Ki-1)-positive anaplastic large cell lymphoma of the adult: sequential intensive treatment with the F-MACHOP regimen (+/- radiotherapy) and autologous bone marrow transplantation. *Blood* 1996;87:1243–1248.

145. Vitolo U, Cortellazzo S, Liberati AM, et al. Intensified and high-dose chemotherapy with granulocyte colony-stimulating factor and autologous stem-cell transplantation support as first-line therapy in high-risk diffuse large-cell lymphoma. *J Clin Oncol* 1997;15:491–498.

146. Schenkein DP, Roitman D, Miller KB, et al. A phase II multicenter trial of high-dose sequential chemotherapy and peripheral blood stem cell transplantation as initial therapy for patients with high-risk non-Hodgkin's lymphoma. *Biol Blood Marrow Transplant* 1997;3:210–216.

147. Nademanee A, Molina A, O'Donnell MR, et al. Results of high-dose therapy and autologous bone marrow/stem cell transplantation during remission in poor-risk intermediate- and high-grade lymphoma: international index high and high-intermediate risk group. *Blood* 1997;90:3844–3852.

148. Cortelazzo S, Rossi A, Bellavita P, et al. Clinical outcome after autologous transplantation in non-Hodgkin's lymphoma patients with high International Prognostic Index (IPI). *Ann Oncol* 1999;10:427–432.

149. Haioun C, Lepage E, Gisselbrecht C, et al. Survival benefit of high-dose therapy in poor-risk aggressive non-Hodgkin's lymphoma: final analysis of the prospective LNH87-2 protocol—a Groupe d'Etude des Lymphomes de l'Adulte study. *J Clin Oncol* 2000;18:3025–3030.

150. Gisselbrecht C, Lepage E, Molina T, et al. Shortened first-line high-dose chemotherapy for patients with poor-prognosis aggressive lymphoma. *J Clin Oncol* 2002;20:2472–2479.

151. Gianni AM, Bregni M, Siena S, et al. High-dose chemotherapy and autologous bone marrow transplantation compared with MACOP-B in aggressive B-cell lymphoma [see comments]. *N Engl J Med* 1997;336:1290–1297.

152. Santini G, Salvagno L, Leoni P, et al. VACOP-B versus VACOP-B plus autologous bone marrow transplantation for advanced diffuse non-Hodgkin's lymphoma: results of a prospective randomized trial by the Non-Hodgkin's Lymphoma Cooperative Study Group. *J Clin Oncol* 1998;16:2796–2802.

153. Intragumtornchai T, Prayoonwiwat W, Numbenjapon T, et al. CHOP versus CHOP plus ESHAP and high-dose therapy with autologous peripheral blood progenitor cell transplantation for high-intermediate-risk and high-risk aggressive non-Hodgkin's lymphoma. *Clin Lymphoma* 2000;1:219–225.

154. Kluin-Nelemans HC, Zagonel V, Anastasopoulou A, et al. Standard chemotherapy with or without high-dose chemotherapy for aggressive non-Hodgkin's lymphoma: randomized phase III EORTC study. *J Natl Cancer Inst* 2001;93:22–30.

155. Kaiser U, Uebelacker I, Abel U, et al. Randomized study to evaluate the use of high-dose therapy as part of primary treatment for "aggressive" lymphoma. *J Clin Oncol* 2002;20:4413–4419.

156. Martelli M, Gherlinzoni F, De Renzo A, et al. Early autologous stem-cell transplantation versus conventional chemotherapy as front-line therapy in high-risk, aggressive non-Hodgkin's lymphoma: an Italian Multicenter Randomized Trial. *J Clin Oncol* 2003;21:1255–1262.

157. Mounier N, Briere J, Gisselbrecht C, et al. Rituximab plus CHOP(R-CHOP) in the treatment of elderly patients with diffuse large B-cell lymphoma (DLBCL) overcomes Bcl2-asssociated chemotherapy resistance. *Blood* 2002;100:161a [abstract 603].

158. Wilson WH, Pittaluga S, O'Connor P, et al. Rituximab may overcome Bcl-2-associated chemotherapy resistance in untreated diffuse large B-cell lymphomas. *Blood* 2001;98:343a [abstract 1447].

159. Bjorkholm M, Osby E, Hagberg H, et al. Randomized trial of r-metHu granulocyte colony-stimulating factor (G-CSF) as adjunct to CHOP or CNOP treatment of elderly patients with aggressive non-Hodgkin's lymphoma. *Blood* 1999;94:599a.

160. Sonneveld P, de Ridder M, van der Lelie H, et al. Comparison of doxorubicin and mitoxantrone in the treatment of elderly patients with advanced diffuse non-Hodgkin's lymphoma using CHOP versus CNOP chemotherapy. *J Clin Oncol* 1995;13:2530–2539.

161. Tirelli U, Errante D, Van Glabbeke M, et al. CHOP is the standard regimen in patients > or = 70 years of age with intermediate-grade and high-grade non-Hodgkin's lymphoma: results of a randomized study of the European Organization for Research and Treatment of Cancer Lymphoma Cooperative Study Group. *J Clin Oncol* 1998;16:27–34.

162. Meyer RM, Browman GP, Samosh ML, et al. Randomized phase II comparison of standard CHOP with weekly CHOP in elderly patients with non-Hodgkin's lymphoma. *J Clin Oncol* 1995;13:2386–2393.

163. Zinzani PL, Gherlinzoni F, Storti S, et al. Randomized trial of 8-week versus 12-week VNCOP-B plus G-CSF regimens as front-line treatment in elderly aggressive non-Hodgkin's lymphoma patients. *Ann Oncol* 2002;13:1364–1369.

164. Schmoll H. Review of etoposide single-agent activity. *Cancer Treat Rev* 1982;9(Suppl):21–30.

165. Shipp MA, Takvorian RC, Canellos GP. High-dose cytosine arabinoside. Active agent in treatment of non-Hodgkin's lymphoma. *Am J Med* 1984;77:845–850.

166. Cavalli F, Jungi WF, Nissen NI, et al. Phase II trial of cis-dichlorodiammineplatinum (II) in advanced malignant lymphoma: a study of the Cancer and Acute Leukemia Group B. *Cancer* 1981;48:1927–1930.

167. Bajetta E, Buzzoni R, Valagussa P, et al. Mitoxantrone: an active agent in refractory non-Hodgkin's lymphomas. *Am J Clin Oncol* 1988;11:100–103.

168. Case DC Jr, Anderson J, Ervin TJ, et al. Phase II trial of ifosfamide and mesna in previously treated patients with non-Hodgkin's lymphoma: Cancer and Leukemia Group B study 8552. *Hematol Oncol* 1991;9:189–196.

169. Tulpule A, Rarick MU, Kolitz J, et al. Liposomal daunorubicin in the treatment of relapsed or refractory non-Hodgkin's lymphoma. *Ann Oncol* 2001;12:457–462.

170. Fossa A, Santoro A, Hiddemann W, et al. Gemcitabine as a single agent in the treatment of relapsed or refractory aggressive non-Hodgkin's lymphoma. *J Clin Oncol* 1999;17:3786–3792.

171. Savage DG, Rule SA, Tighe M, et al. Gemcitabine for relapsed or resistant lymphoma. *Ann Oncol* 2000;11:595–597.

172. Younes A, Sarris A, Melnyk A, et al. Three-hour paclitaxel infusion in patients with refractory and relapsed non-Hodgkin's lymphoma. *J Clin Oncol* 1995;13:583–587.

173. Budman DR, Petroni GR, Johnson JL, et al. Phase II trial of docetaxel in non-Hodgkin's lymphomas: a study of the Cancer and Leukemia Group B. *J Clin Oncol* 1997;15:3275–3279.

174. Kraut EH, Balcerzak SP, Young D, et al. A phase II study of topotecan in non-Hodgkin's lymphoma: an Ohio State University phase II research consortium study. *Cancer Invest* 2002;20:174–179.

175. Younes A, Preti HA, Hagemeister FB, et al. Paclitaxel plus topotecan treatment for patients with relapsed or refractory aggressive non-Hodgkin's lymphoma. *Ann Oncol* 2001;12:923–927.

176. Flinn IW, Goodman SN, Post L, et al. A dose-finding study of liposomal daunorubicin with CVP (COP-X) in advanced NHL. *Ann Oncol* 2000;11:691–695.

177. Armitage JO, Coiffier B. Activity of interferon-alpha in relapsed patients with diffuse large B-cell and peripheral T-cell non-Hodgkin's lymphoma. *Ann Oncol* 2000;11:1–3.

178. Coiffier B, Haioun C, Ketterer N, et al. Rituximab (anti-CD20 monoclonal antibody) for the treatment of patients with relapsing or refractory aggressive lymphoma: a multicenter phase II study. *Blood* 1998;92:1927–1932.

179. Kaminski MS, Estes J, Zasadny KR, et al. Radioimmunotherapy with iodine (131)I tositumomab for relapsed or refractory B-cell non-Hodgkin lymphoma: updated results and long-term follow-up of the University of Michigan experience. *Blood* 2000;96:1259–1266.

180. Philip T, Armitage JO, Spitzer G, et al. High-dose therapy and autologous bone marrow transplantation after failure of conventional chemotherapy in adults with intermediate-grade or high-grade non-Hodgkin's lymphoma. *N Engl J Med* 1987;316:1493–1498.

181. Philip T, Guglielmi C, Hagenbeek A, et al. Autologous bone marrow transplantation as compared with salvage chemotherapy in relapses of chemotherapy-sensitive non-Hodgkin's lymphoma [see comments]. *N Engl J Med* 1995;333:1540–1545.

182. Blay J, Gomez F, Sebban C, et al. The International Prognostic Index correlates to survival in patients with aggressive lymphoma in relapse: analysis of the PARMA trial. Parma Group. *Blood* 1998;92:3562–3568.

183. Shipp MA, Abeloff MD, Antman KH, et al. International Consensus Conference on High-Dose Therapy with Hematopoietic Stem Cell Transplantation in Aggressive Non-Hodgkin's Lymphomas: report of the jury. *J Clin Oncol* 1999;17:423–429.

184. Hahn T, Wolff SN, Czuczman M, et al. The role of cytotoxic therapy with hematopoietic stem cell transplantation in the therapy of diffuse large cell B-cell non-Hodgkin's lymphoma: an evidence-based review. *Biol Blood Marrow Transplant* 2001;7:308–331.

185. Vose J, Zhang M-J, Rowlings P, et al. Autologous transplantation for diffuse aggressive non-Hodgkin's lymphoma in patients never achieving remission: a report from the Autologous Blood and Marrow Transplant Registry. *J Clin Oncol* 2001;19:406–413.

186. Kewalramani T, Zelenetz AD, Hedrick EE, et al. High-dose chemoradiotherapy and autologous stem cell transplantation for patients with primary refractory aggressive non-Hodgkin lymphoma: an intention-to-treat analysis. *Blood* 2000;96:2399–2404.

187. Haw R, Sawka CA, Franssen E, et al. Significance of a partial or slow response to front-line chemotherapy in the management of intermediate-grade or high-grade non-Hodgkin's lymphoma: a literature review. *J Clin Oncol* 1994;12:1074–1084.

188. Verdonck LF, van Putten WL, Hagenbeek A, et al. Comparison of CHOP chemotherapy with autologous bone marrow transplantation for slowly responding patients with aggressive non-Hodgkin's lymphoma [see comments]. *N Engl J Med* 1995;332:1045–1051.

189. Martelli M, Vignetti M, Zinzani PL, et al. High-dose chemotherapy followed by autologous bone marrow transplantation versus dexamethasone, cisplatin, and cytarabine in aggressive non-Hodgkin's lymphoma with partial response to front-line chemotherapy: a prospective randomized Italian multicenter study. *J Clin Oncol* 1996;14:534–542.

190. Jones RJ, Ambinder RF, Piantadosi S, et al. Evidence of a graft-versus-lymphoma effect associated with allogeneic bone marrow transplantation. *Blood* 1991;77:649–653.

191. Ratanatharathorn V, Uberti J, Karanes C, et al. Prospective comparative trial of autologous versus allogeneic bone marrow transplantation in patients with non-Hodgkin's lymphoma. *Blood* 1994;84:1050–1055.

192. Schimmer AD, Jamal S, Messner H, et al. Allogeneic or autologous bone marrow transplantation (BMT) for non-Hodgkin's lymphoma (NHL): results of a provincial strategy. Ontario BMT Network, Canada. *Bone Marrow Transplant* 2000;26:859–864.

193. Hagberg H, Bjorkholm M, Glimelius B, et al. CHOP vs MEV for the treatment of non-Hodgkin's lymphoma of unfavourable histopathology: a randomized clinical trial. *Eur J Cancer Clin Oncol* 1985;21:175–179.

194. Takagi T, Sampi K, Sawada U, et al. A comparative study of CHOP versus MEVP (mitoxantrone, etoposide, vindesine, prednisolone) therapy for intermediate-grade and high-grade non-Hodgkin's lymphoma: a prospective randomized study. *Int J Hematol* 1993;57:67–71.

195. Gherlinzoni F, Guglielmi C, Mazza P, et al. Phase III comparative trial (m-BACOD v m-BNCOD) in the treatment of stage II to IV non-Hodgkin's lymphomas with intermediate- or high-grade histology. *Semin Oncol* 1990;17:3–8; discussion 8–9.

196. Brusamolino E, Bertini M, Guidi S, et al. CHOP versus CNOP (N = mitoxantrone) in non-Hodgkin's lymphoma: an interim report comparing efficacy and toxicity. *Haematologica* 1988;73:217–222.

197. Nair R, Ramakrishnan G, Nair NN, et al. A randomized comparison of the efficacy and toxicity of epirubicin and doxorubicin in the treatment of patients with non-Hodgkin's lymphoma. *Cancer* 1998;82:2282–2288.

198. Pavlovsky S, Santarelli MT, Erazo A, et al. Results of a randomized study of previously-untreated intermediate and high grade lymphoma using CHOP versus CNOP [see comments]. *Ann Oncol* 1992;3:205–209.

199. De Lena M, Maiello E, Lorusso V, et al. Comparison of CHOP-B vs CEOP-B in 'poor prognosis' non-Hodgkin's lymphomas. A randomized trial. *Med Oncol Tumor Pharmacother* 1989;6:163–169.

200. Wolf M, Matthews JP, Stone J, et al. Long-term survival advantage of MACOP-B over CHOP in intermediate-grade non-Hodgkin's lymphoma. The Australian and New Zealand Lymphoma Group. *Ann Oncol* 1997;8:71–75.

201. Todd M, Cadman E, Spiro P, et al. A follow-up of a randomized study comparing two chemotherapy treatments for advanced diffuse histiocytic lymphoma. *J Clin Oncol* 1984;2:986–993.

202. Bailey NP, Stuart NS, Bessell EM, et al. Five-year follow-up of a prospective randomised multi-centre trial of weekly chemotherapy (CAPOMEt) versus cyclical chemotherapy (CHOP-Mtx) in the treatment of aggressive non-Hodgkin's lymphoma. Central Lymphoma Group. *Ann Oncol* 1998;9:633–638.

203. Cameron DA, White JM, Proctor SJ, et al. CHOP-based chemotherapy is as effective as alternating PEEC/CHOP chemotherapy in a randomised trial in high-grade non-Hodgkin's lymphoma. Scotland and Newcastle Lymphoma Group. *Eur J Cancer* 1997;33:1195–1201.

204. Gordon LI, Harrington D, Andersen J, et al. Comparison of a second-generation combination chemotherapeutic regimen (m-BACOD) with a standard regimen (CHOP) for advanced diffuse non-Hodgkin's lymphoma [see comments]. *N Engl J Med* 1992;327:1342–1349.

205. Sertoli MR, Santini G, Chisesi T, et al. MACOP-B versus ProMACE-MOPP in the treatment of advanced diffuse non-Hodgkin's lymphoma: results of a prospective randomized trial by the non-Hodgkin's Lymphoma Cooperative Study Group. *J Clin Oncol* 1994;12:1366–1374.

206. Koppler H, Pfluger KH, Eschenbach I, et al. Sequential versus alternating chemotherapy for high grade non-Hodgkin's lymphomas: a randomized multicentre trial. *Hematol Oncol* 1991;9:217–223.

207. Mazza P, Zinzani PL, Martelli M, et al. MACOP-B vs F-MACHOP regimen in the treatment of high-grade non-Hodgkin's lymphomas. *Leuk Lymphoma* 1995;16:457–463.

208. Koppler H, Pfluger KH, Eschenbach I, et al. Randomised comparison of CHOEP versus alternating hCHOP/IVEP for high-grade non-Hodgkin's lymphomas: treatment results and prognostic factor analysis in a multi-centre trial. *Ann Oncol* 1994;5:49–55.

209. Gottlieb AJ, Anderson JR, Ginsberg SJ, et al. A randomized comparison of methotrexate dose and the addition of bleomycin to CHOP therapy for diffuse large cell lymphoma and other non-Hodgkin's lymphomas. Cancer and Leukemia Group B study 7851. *Cancer* 1990;66:1888–1896.

210. Tilly H, Mounier N, Lederlin P, et al. Randomized comparison of ACVBP and m-BACOD in the treatment of patients with low-risk aggressive lymphoma: the LNH87-1 study. Groupe d'Etudes des Lymphomes de l'Adulte. *J Clin Oncol* 2000;18:1309–1315.

211. Giles FJ, Shan J, Advani SH, et al. A prospective randomized study of CHOP versus CHOP plus alpha-2B interferon in patients with intermediate and high grade non-Hodgkin's lymphoma: the International Oncology Study Group NHL1 Study. *Leuk Lymphoma* 2000;40:95–103.

212. Coiffier B, Lepage E, Briere J, et al. CHOP chemotherapy plus rituximab compared with CHOP alone in elderly patients with diffuse large-B-cell lymphoma. *N Engl J Med* 2002;346:235–242.

213. Bastion Y, Blay JY, Divine M, et al. Elderly patients with aggressive non-Hodgkin's lymphoma: disease presentation, response to treatment, and survival—a Groupe d'Etude des Lymphomes de l'Adulte study on 453 patients older than 69 years. *J Clin Oncol* 1997;15:2945–2953.

214. Tilly H, Lepage E, Coiffier B, et al. A randomized comparison of ACVBP and CHOP in the treatment of advanced aggressive non-Hodgkin's lymphoma: The LNH93-5 study. *Blood* 2000;96:832a.

215. Bosly A, Lepage E, Coiffier B, et al. Outcome is not improved by the use of alternating chemotherapy in elderly patients with aggressive lymphoma. *Hematol J* 2001;2:279–285.

216. Cabanillas F. Ifosfamide combinations in lymphoma. *Semin Oncol* 1990;17:58–62.

217. Velasquez WS, Cabanillas F, Salvador P, et al. Effective salvage therapy for lymphoma with cisplatin in combination with high-dose Ara-C and dexamethasone (DHAP). *Blood* 1988;71:117–122.

218. Velasquez WS, McLaughlin P, Tucker S, et al. ESHAP—an effective chemotherapy regimen in refractory and relapsing lymphoma: a 4-year follow-up study. *J Clin Oncol* 1994;12:1169–1176.

219. Neidhart JA, Kubica R, Stidley C, et al. Multiple cycles of dose-intensive cyclophosphamide, etoposide, and cisplatinum (DICEP) produce durable responses in refractory non-Hodgkin's lymphoma. *Cancer Invest* 1994;12:1–11.

220. Goss P, Shepherd F, Scott JG, et al. DICE (dexamethasone, ifosfamide, cisplatin, etoposide) as salvage therapy in non-Hodgkin's lymphomas. *Leuk Lymphoma* 1995;18:123–129.

221. Moskowitz CH, Bertino JR, Glassman JR, et al. Ifosfamide, carboplatin, and etoposide: a highly effective cytoreduction and peripheral-blood progenitor-cell mobilization regimen for transplant-eligible patients with non-Hodgkin's lymphoma. *J Clin Oncol* 1999;17:3776–3785.

222. Lichtman SM, Niedzwiecki D, Barcos M, et al. Phase II study of infusional chemotherapy with doxorubicin, vincristine and etoposide plus cyclophosphamide and prednisone (I-CHOPE) in resistant diffuse aggressive non-Hodgkin's lymphoma: CALGB 9255. Cancer and Leukemia Group B. *Ann Oncol* 2000;11:1141–1146.

223. Gutierrez M, Chabner BA, Pearson D, et al. Role of a doxorubicin-containing regimen in relapsed and resistant lymphomas: an 8-year follow-up study of EPOCH. *J Clin Oncol* 2000;18:3633–3642.

224. Petersen FB, Appelbaum FR, Hill R, et al. Autologous marrow transplantation for malignant lymphoma: a report of 101 cases from Seattle. *J Clin Oncol* 1990;8:638–647.

225. Vose JM, Anderson JR, Kessinger A, et al. High-dose chemotherapy and autologous hematopoietic stem-cell transplantation for aggressive non-Hodgkin's lymphoma [see comments]. *J Clin Oncol* 1993;11:1846–1851.

226. Mills W, Chopra R, McMillan A, et al. BEAM chemotherapy and autologous bone marrow transplantation for patients with relapsed or refractory non-Hodgkin's lymphoma. *J Clin Oncol* 1995;13:588–595.

227. Stockerl-Goldstein KE, Horning SJ, Negrin RS, et al. Influence of preparatory regimen and source of hematopoietic cells on outcome of autotransplantation for non-Hodgkin's lymphoma. *Biol Blood Marrow Transplant* 1996;2:76–85.

228. Caballero MD, Rubio V, Rifon J, et al. BEAM chemotherapy followed by autologous stem cell support in lymphoma patients: analysis of efficacy, toxicity and prognostic factors. *Bone Marrow Transplant* 1997;20:451–458.

229. Rapoport AP, Lifton R, Constine LS, et al. Autotransplantation for relapsed or refractory non-Hodgkin's lymphoma (NHL): long-term follow-up and analysis of prognostic factors. *Bone Marrow Transplant* 1997;19:883–890.

230. Stiff PJ, Dahlberg S, Forman SJ, et al. Autologous bone marrow transplantation for patients with relapsed or refractory diffuse aggressive non-Hodgkin's lymphoma: value of augmented preparative regimens—a Southwest Oncology Group trial. *J Clin Oncol* 1998;16:48–55.

231. Popat U, Przepiork D, Champlin R, et al. High-dose chemotherapy for relapsed and refractory diffuse large B-cell lymphoma: mediastinal localization predicts for a favorable outcome. *J Clin Oncol* 1998;16:63–69.

CHAPTER 28

Primary Mediastinal Large B-Cell Lymphoma

Pier Luigi Zinzani, Riccardo Dalla-Favera, and Nancy Lee Harris

DEFINITION

Primary mediastinal large B-cell lymphoma was first described in the 1980s (1,2). It is an uncommon but not rare clinicopathologic entity with a worldwide distribution and was recently recognized in both the Revised European-American Lymphoma (REAL) and World Health Organization (WHO) classifications (3,4). This localized malignancy is characterized by aggressive and invasive behavior in an unusual site in a cohort of young adult females in whom large-cell lymphoma is infrequent. Although it resembles nodal large-cell lymphomas, it has distinct morphologic, immunophenotypic, and genetic features.

Primary mediastinal large B-cell lymphoma is a diffuse large B-cell lymphoma that arises in the thymus and is considered a peripheral B-cell neoplasm. Table 28.1 summarizes the clinical comparison of nodal diffuse large B-cell lymphoma and primary mediastinal large B-cell lymphoma.

EPIDEMIOLOGY

The precise frequency of this disease is difficult to discern with accuracy because of its relatively recent identification. Reports describing the same disease process have come from China, Japan, and the Middle East. In a review of 1,400 cases of non-Hodgkin's lymphomas from nine centers all over the world, primary mediastinal large B-cell lymphoma was found to account for 2% of all cases (5). It was the only tumor type for which clinical data were essential for its recognition (6). The disease is most common in young women, with a male to female ratio of 1:2 and a median age in the fourth decade (5–7). No risk factors have been clearly identified for the development of primary mediastinal large B-cell lymphoma.

DIAGNOSIS

Morphology

The tumor is composed of large cells with variable nuclear features, resembling centroblasts, large centrocytes, or mul-

tilobated cells, often with pale or "clear" cytoplasm. Less often, the tumor cells resemble immunoblasts. Reed-Sternberg–like cells may be present. Many cases have fine, compartmentalizing sclerosis (Color Plate 60).

Immunophenotype

The tumor cells are often immunoglobulin negative but express B cell–associated antigens (CD19, CD20, CD22, CD79a) and CD45 (8–10). Expression of CD10 and bcl6 is relatively common, and expression of late, plasma cell–associated antigens, such as CD138 and vs38c, is rare (11). Many cases express CD30, which can cause problems in differential diagnosis from Hodgkin's lymphoma.

Genetic Features

Immunoglobulin heavy and light chain genes are rearranged; the BCL2 gene is usually germline (12). BCL-6 and c-MYC gene rearrangements are uncommon (13). Amplification of the REL oncogene has been described in a minority of the cases (14).

Postulated Normal Counterpart

The postulated normal counterpart is the thymic medullary B cell.

Differential Diagnosis

This mediastinal lymphoma must be distinguished from other lymphomas that can present with anterior mediastinal masses, including Hodgkin's disease, nodal-type diffuse large B-cell lymphoma, anaplastic large T/null-cell lymphoma, and thymic mucosa-associated lymphoid tissue lymphoma. Knowledge of the clinical features, adequate tissue for morphologic analysis, complete immunophenotyping (T- and B-cell antigens, CD15, anaplastic lymphoma kinase-1), and assessment of proliferation fraction are all helpful in differential diagnosis.

TABLE 28.1. *Comparison of diffuse large B-cell lymphoma and primary mediastinal large B-cell lymphoma*

	Nodal diffuse large B-cell lymphoma	Primary mediastinal large B-cell lymphoma
Median age (yr)	55	35
Nodal/extranodal presentation (%)	65/35	0/100
Sex distribution (male:female)	1.2:1.0	1:2
Stage I–II/III–IV (%)	40/60	80/20
Bulky disease (%)	30	60–70

PATHOGENESIS

Primary mediastinal B-cell lymphoma displays clonal immunoglobulin gene rearrangements, immunoglobulin variable region and gene hypermutation, and frequently BCL6 hypermutation (14a). These observations, together with their specific immunophenotypic characteristics, suggest that these tumors derive from a mature germinal-center or postgerminal-center B cell (14a). These tumors seem to be associated with chromosomal translocations similar to those observed in other forms of diffuse large-cell lymphoma (14b,14c), suggesting a partially common pathogenesis. However, the genetic characterization of these tumors has been relatively limited.

CLINICAL FEATURES AND STAGING

Primary mediastinal large B-cell lymphoma is a distinct clinico-pathologic entity, characterized by a locally invasive anterior mediastinal mass that originates in the thymus and frequently compromises the airway, causing superior vena cava syndrome (2,15). In fact, 30% to 50% of patients have signs and symptoms of superior vena cava syndrome, thoracic and neck vein distension, facial edema, conjunctival swelling, and occasionally arm edema. At the time of diagnosis, the stage of disease is I or II in 80% of the patients. The mediastinal tumor is larger than 10 cm (bulky mass) in 60% to 70% of patients, infiltrating lung, chest wall, pleura, and pericardium (9,10). Figure 28.1 shows a chest x-ray illustrating a typical patient with this presentation. Pleural or pericardial effusions are present in one third of cases (16,17). The invasive neoplasm results in cough, chest pain, dyspnea, or complaints resulting from caval obstruction.

Despite the local invasiveness, distant spread is infrequent at the outset; even spread to the supraclavicular nodes is unusual at the time of presentation, although the upper border of the tumor can often be palpated at the base of the neck. The duration of symptoms oscillates between 6 weeks and 3 months. Systemic symptoms, mainly fever or weight loss, are present in fewer than 20% of cases.

Spread to peripheral lymph nodes is infrequent, and marrow or cerebrospinal fluid involvement is unusual. Distant relapses tend to be extranodal, including liver, gastrointestinal tract,

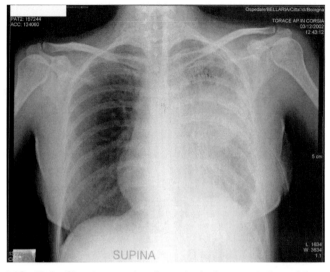

FIG. 28.1. Chest x-ray showing a typical presentation of the primary mediastinal large B-cell lymphoma.

kidneys, ovaries, adrenal glands, pancreas, and central nervous system (18–20). Moderate to high lactate dehydrogenase levels are observed in 70% to 80% of patients.

The complete staging work-up for primary mediastinal large B-cell lymphoma is the same as that routinely used for nodal lymphoma. It includes an accurate physical examination, complete hematologic and biochemical examinations, abdomen ultrasonography, total-body computerized tomography, and bone marrow biopsy. A diagnostic tissue sample is obtained by mediastinoscopy, biopsy of the tumor mass through the supraclavicular fossa, or anterior mediastinotomy or minithoracotomy. Formal thoracotomy is infrequently required, and total excision is rarely an option. Gallium-67 scanning ([67]GaSPECT) is a meaningful procedure for staging, response and relapse assessment, and follow-up. It is the most useful adjunctive test also to assess cure (17,21,22). [^{18}F]-2-fluoro-2-deoxy-D-glucose–positron-emission tomography (FDG-PET) has demonstrated an excellent usefulness in residual-mass assessment considering the elevated tracer uptake that characterizes this lymphoma, but a longer experience is necessary.

The standard staging system used for primary mediastinal large B-cell lymphoma is the same as that proposed for Hodgkin's disease at the Ann Arbor conference in 1971 (23). This system is currently used for all lymphomas, even if other staging systems are used in some extranodal lymphomas with particular biologic behavior. Concerning molecular analysis of minimal residual disease, no reliable molecular markers are available for monitoring minimal residual disease in primary mediastinal large B-cell lymphoma.

PROGNOSIS: NATURAL HISTORY AND PROGNOSTIC FACTORS

Recurrence is almost exclusively observed in the first 2 years of follow-up. Most early publications on primary mediastinal large B-cell lymphoma described an aggressive disease with poor prognosis (24,25). Further published series showed a 5-year survival of 65% with a CHOP [cyclophosphamide, hydroxydaunorubicin, Oncovin (vincristine), and prednisone] regimen followed by radiation therapy (15). Similar results have been obtained with third-generation regimens followed by radiation therapy, and some authors have suggested that the CHOP regimen is insufficient in patients with larger masses resulting from more aggressive lymphomas (19,26,27).

PROGNOSTIC FACTORS

Features associated with poor prognosis in primary mediastinal large B-cell lymphoma are poor performance status, pericardial effusion, bulky disease, and high serum lactate dehydrogenase. A compromised dose intensity of anthracycline and cyclophosphamide predicted a nonresponse to front-line chemotherapy, which is the major important predictor of survival in primary mediastinal large B-cell lymphoma (15,16,28). The age-adjusted International Prognostic Index did not provide a useful subdivision of primary mediastinal large B-cell lymphoma (16).

TREATMENT

Front-Line Therapy

The results of most series on primary mediastinal large B-cell lymphoma are reported in Table 28.2. Reported approaches to the treatment of this entity range from first-generation (15,18,28–35) to third-generation (5,9,16,19, 21,22,26,27,36,37) chemotherapy protocols. Early studies suggesting that primary mediastinal large B-cell lymphomas were unusually aggressive, with a poorer prognosis with respect to other large-cell lymphomas, have been contradicted by more recent reports. Complete-response rates of 53% to 80% have been reported after initial therapy, with a 50% to 65% overall survival rate at 5 years (5,15, 16,21,26,27,30,36). Regarding the use of different chemotherapeutic regimens (CHOP or CHOP-like vs. third-generation regimens), a report by Fisher et al. (38) showed that CHOP and intensive third-generation regimens produce equivalent results. This observation may limit discussion about the use of more aggressive protocols for primary mediastinal large B-cell lymphoma. Whereas the CHOP regimen has been used by American investigators, several European centers have suggested that

TABLE 28.2. *Studies on treatment and outcome of patients with primary mediastinal large B-cell lymphoma*

Author (reference)	No. of patients	Regimen (no. of patients)	Local radiation therapy	Partial remission (%)	Complete remission (%)	Failure-free survival (%)
Jacobson, 1988 (15)	30	CHOP/CHOP-like (22), C-MOPP (8)	Yes	—	80	59 (5-yr)
Haioun, 1989 (18)	20	CHOP (4) or variants (16)	Yes	55	45	40 (2-yr)
Todeschini, 1990 (27)	21	CHOP-B (6), MACOP-B (12), m-BACOD (3)	Yes	25	64	52 (3-yr)
Bertini, 1991 (26)	18	MACOP-B	Yes	6	89	73 (2-yr)
Kirn, 1993 (28)	57	M/m-BACOD (38), CHOP (10), other (9)	Yes	39	53	45 (5-yr)
Lazzarino, 1993 (19)	30	CHOP (14), MACOP-B or VACOP-B (16)	Yes	—	55	38 (3-yr)
Rodriguez, 1994 (30)	18	Doxorubicin regimens	Yes	12	67	45 (2-yr)
Falini, 1995 (9)	18	MACOP-B (7), F-MACHOP (11)	No	61	33	61 (2-yr)
Zinzani, 1996 (17)	22	MACOP-B (20), F-MACHOP (2)	Yes		95	86 (2-yr)
Cazals-Hatem, 1996 (5)	141	Intensive regimens	No	31	48	61 (3-yr)
Lazzarino, 1997 (16)	106	Doxorubicin regimens	Yes	42	23	50 (3-yr)
Martelli, 1998 (36)	37	F-MACHOP (10), MACOP-B (27)	No	90	10	70 (5-yr)
Abou Ellela, 1999 (31)	43	CAP-BOP and variants	NR		63	39 (5-yr)
Zinzani, 1999 (22)	50	MACOP-B	Yes		86	93 (8-yr)
Bieri, 1999 (34)	27	Doxorubicin regimens	Yes	15	55	44 (10-yr)
Nguyen, 2000 (35)	40	Doxorubicin regimens	Yes	41	41	67 (5-yr)
Zinzani, 2001 (37)	89	MACOP-B	Yes	4	88	91 (9-yr)

CAP-BOP, cyclophosphamide, Adriamycin (doxorubicin), procarbazine, bleomycin, Oncovin, and prednisone; CHOP, cyclophosphamide, hydroxydaunorubicin, Oncovin (vincristine), and prednisone; CHOP-B, CHOP and bleomycin; C-MOPP, cyclophosphamide, mechlorethamine, Oncovin (vincristine), procarbazine, and prednisone; F-MACHOP, 5-fluorouracil, methotrexate, cytosine arabinoside, cyclophosphamide, doxorubicin, Oncovin (vincristine), and prednisone; MACOP-B, methotrexate, Adriamycin (doxorubicin), cyclophosphamide, Oncovin (vincristine), prednisone, and bleomycin; m-BACOD, moderate-dose methotrexate, bleomycin, Adriamycin (doxorubicin), cyclophosphamide, Oncovin (vincristine) dexamethasone; NR, not reported; VACOP-B, VePesid (etoposide), Adriamycin (doxorubicin), cyclophosphamide, Oncovin (vincristine), prednisone, and bleomycin.

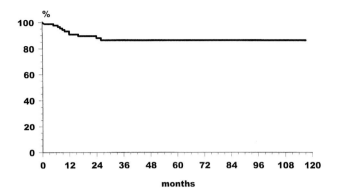

FIG. 28.2. Overall survival curve of 89 patients with primary mediastinal large B-cell lymphoma treated with MACOP-B [methotrexate, Adriamycin (doxorubicin), cyclophosphamide, Oncovin (vincristine), prednisone, and bleomycin] plus mediastinal radiation therapy. (From Zinzani PL, Martelli M, De Renzo A, et al. Primary mediastinal large B-cell lymphoma with sclerosis: a clinical study of 89 patients treated with MACOP-B chemotherapy and radiation therapy. *Haematologica* 2001;86:187–191, with permission.)

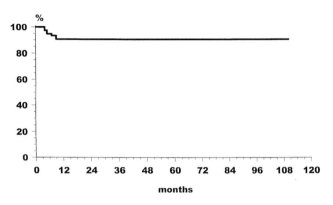

FIG. 28.3. Relapse-free survival curve of 78 complete-response patients treated with MACOP-B [methotrexate, Adriamycin (doxorubicin), cyclophosphamide, Oncovin (vincristine), prednisone, and bleomycin] plus mediastinal radiation therapy. (From Zinzani PL, Martelli M, De Renzo A, et al. Primary mediastinal large B-cell lymphoma with sclerosis: a clinical study of 89 patients treated with MACOP-B chemotherapy and radiation therapy. *Haematologica* 2001;86:187–191, with permission.)

the MACOP-B [methotrexate, Adriamycin (doxorubicin), cyclophosphamide, Oncovin (vincristine), prednisone, and bleomycin] regimen may be superior to CHOP (16,22, 26,27,37). However, the debate is still open, because it is difficult to compare the advantages of the different types of protocols, and it is also difficult to explain the rather different complete-response and survival rates reported by different institutions using similar regimens in phase II studies potentially influenced by patient-selection bias. Considering the published phase II data by centers that have used both first-generation chemotherapy regimens like CHOP and other more aggressive third-generation ones like MACOP-B, the results have clearly favored the latter. Todeschini et al. (27) used CHOP in six patients without achieving a single complete response; in the 15 patients treated with MACOP-B or F-MACHOP [5-fluorouracil, methotrexate, cytosine arabinoside, cyclophosphamide, doxorubicin, Oncovin (vincristine), and prednisone] (39) regimens, 87% achieved a complete response. Lazzarino et al. (19) treated 30 patients; the complete-response rate after CHOP was 36%, whereas that after MACOP-B or VACOP-B [VePesid (etoposide), Adriamycin (doxorubicin), cyclophosphamide, Oncovin (vincristine), prednisone, and bleomycin] was 73%. In a multicenter study of 106 patients, the 3-year relapse-free survival was 38% in the 47 patients treated with CHOP, whereas it was 58% in the 62 patients treated with MACOP-B or VACOP-B (16). In two previous studies (22,37), we used the MACOP-B regimen in 50 patients (a two-center prospective trial) and in 89 patients (an Italian multicenter prospective trial); the complete-response rates were 86% and 88%, respectively, whereas the 5-year relapse-free survival rates were 93% and 91%, respectively. Figures 28.2 and 28.3 show the overall and relapse-free survival curves of the Italian multicenter trial, respectively (37).

The role of high-dose approaches, including autologous stem cell transplantation and high-dose sequential treatment, needs to be confirmed, because the actual reported data do not prove the superiority of high-dose chemotherapy over conventional chemotherapy in phase II trials (40–42). The use of high-dose chemotherapy supported by stem cell transplantation to consolidate the initial response in high-risk patients is a matter of debate (40,43,44).

Radiation Therapy

The issue of adjuvant radiation therapy after chemotherapy also remains open, although it seems likely that it could play an important role in this locally aggressive disease, particularly in the presence of bulky disease. However, the excellent results obtained in the Groupe d'Etude des Lymphomes de l'Adulte study (5) without radiation therapy have called into question its necessity. The data from two recent publications of Italian studies (22,37) have indicated that the addition of radiation therapy after chemotherapy is of pivotal importance for the eradication of primary mediastinal large B-cell lymphoma in terms of increasing the complete-response rate or reinforcing existing complete responses after induction chemotherapy. In particular, in the first report (22), with the use of computed tomography (CT) scans, 70% of the patients had residual mediastinal tumor masses after chemotherapy (MACOP-B), and after radiation therapy, 44% of the patients had residual masses on CT scan. Regarding [67]GaSPECT, 66% of the patients showed persistent abnormal uptake after MACOP-B, whereas after radiation therapy, 19% of the patients were still [67]GaSPECT positive. In the second study (37), after the chemotherapy regimen (MACOP-B), 26% of the patients achieved a complete response, and 66% obtained a partial response, giving an overall-response rate of

92%. After radiation therapy, 93% of the patients who had already achieved a partial response obtained complete-response status. Thus, after the combined modality treatment, 88% of the patients achieved a complete response.

Gallium-67 Scanning

Concerning restaging, many patients with primary mediastinal large B-cell lymphoma have residual radiographic abnormalities in the mediastinum even after a complete clinical response, so chest x-ray and CT scans do not provide a valid basis for therapeutic decision making. [67]GaSPECT could be the best tool for selecting those patients who really require the addition of radiation therapy after chemotherapeutic induction. In our experience (22), after combined modality treatment, 60% of the patients with positive [67]GaSPECT and a negative CT scan relapsed, as opposed to no relapses with negative [67]GaSPECT and a negative CT scan. Twenty-one patients had a positive CT scan; of these, the four [67]GaSPECT positive patients all progressed, whereas there were no relapses among the 17 patients with negative [67]GaSPECT.

This restaging technique allows identification of a subset of patients with residual radiographic abnormalities who need no further therapy (negative [67]GaSPECT) and of poor-prognosis patients who do require further treatment.

Treatment of Recurrent Disease

Generally, patients with primary mediastinal large B-cell lymphoma who obtain a complete response lasting longer than 18 to 24 months after diagnosis are likely to be cured. In fact, most relapses occur within the first 12 months after the completion of the front-line treatment. A standard therapeutic option for patients with relapsed disease has not yet been identified. However, considering the young age of these patients and the pattern of relapse that spares the bone marrow, high-dose chemotherapy supported by autologous stem cell transplantation is suitable for individual clinical use (41,42). With this strategy, patients with relapsed mediastinal lymphoma seem to have a better prognosis than those with the other diffuse large-cell lymphomas, with 5-year disease-free survival rates of 55% and 35%, respectively (41,42). In contrast, patients treated with conventional second-line chemotherapy or with radiation therapy to the mediastinum (for patients who did not undergo radiation therapy after the front-line chemotherapy regimen) have a median survival after relapse of a few months.

FUTURE DIRECTIONS

Further improvements in the management of primary mediastinal large B-cell lymphoma depend on the design of prospective multicenter trials to assess the best chemotherapeutic regimen (first- vs. third-generation) to be combined with the radiation therapy, taking into account the pivotal role of the [67]GaSPECT (and FDG-PET) in posttreatment imaging

reevaluation. In addition, it will be important and interesting to add to the new therapeutic armamentarium of primary mediastinal large B-cell lymphoma the anti-CD20 monoclonal antibody alone or conjugated to radionuclides (radioimmunoconjugates) in an effort to increase the complete-response and survival rates.

REFERENCES

1. Lichtenstein AK, Levine A, Taylor CR, et al. Primary mediastinal lymphoma in adults. Am J Med 1980;68:509–514.
2. Levitt LJ, Aisenberg AC, Harris NL, et al. Primary non-Hodgkin's lymphoma of the mediastinum. Cancer 1982;50:2486–2492.
3. Harris NL, Jaffe ES, Stein H, et al. A revised European-American classification of lymphoid neoplasms: a proposal from the International Lymphoma Study Group [see comments]. Blood 1994;84:1361–1392.
4. Jaffe ES, Harris NL, Stein H, et al. Pathology and genetics of tumors of hematopoietic and lymphoid tissues. In: Kleihues P, Sobin L (eds), World Health Organization classification of tumours, vol. 3. Lyon: IARC Press, 2001.
5. Cazals-Hatem D, Lepage E, Brice P, et al. Primary mediastinal large B-cell lymphoma. A clinicopathologic study of 141 cases compared with 916 nonmediastinal large B-cell lymphomas, a GELA ("Groupe d'Etude des Lymphomes de l'Adulte") study. Am J Surg Pathol 1996;20:877–888.
6. A clinical evaluation of the International Lymphoma Study Group classification of non-Hodgkin's lymphoma. Blood 1997;89:3909–3918.
7. Armitage JO, Weisenburger DD. New approach to classifying non-Hodgkin's lymphomas: clinical features of the major histologic subtypes. J Clin Oncol 1998;16:2780–2795.
8. Lamarre L, Jacobson J, Aisenberg A, et al. Primary large cell lymphoma of the mediastinum. Am J Surg Pathol 1989;13:730–739.
9. Falini B, Venturi S, Martelli M, et al. Mediastinal large B-cell lymphoma: clinical and immunohistological findings in 18 patients treated with different third-generation regimens. Br J Haematol 1995; 89:780–789.
10. Moller P, Lammler B, Eberlein-Gonska M, et al. Primary mediastinal clear cell lymphoma of B-cell type. Virchows Arch A Pathol Anat Histopathol 1986;409:79–92.
11. de Leval L, Ferry JA, Falini B, et al. Expression of bcl-6 and CD10 in primary mediastinal large B-cell lymphoma: evidence for derivation from germinal center B cells? Am J Surg Pathol 2001;25:1277–1282.
12. Scarpa A, Bonetti F, Menestrina F. Mediastinal large cell lymphoma with sclerosis. Genotypic analysis establishes its B nature. Virchows Arch [A] 1987;412:17–21.
13. Tsang P, Cesarman E, Chadburn A, et al. Molecular characterization of primary mediastinal B cell lymphoma. Am J Pathol 1996;148:2017–2025.
14. Joos S, Otano-Joos MI, Ziegler S, et al. Primary mediastinal (thymic) B-cell lymphoma is characterized by gains of chromosomal material including 9p and amplification of the REL gene. Blood 1996;87:1571–1578.
14a. Pileri SA, Gaidano G, Zinzani PL, et al. Primary mediastinal B-cell lymphoma: high frequency of BCL-6 mutations and consistent expression of the transcription factors OCT-2, BOB.1, and PU.1 in the absence of immunoglobulins. Am J Pathol 2003;162(1):243–253.
14b. Tsang P, Cesarman E, Chadburn A, et al. Molecular characterization of primary mediastinal B cell lymphoma. Am J Pathol 1996;148(6):2017–2025.
14c. Joos S, Otano-Joos MI, Ziegler S, et al. Primary mediastinal (thymic) B-cell lymphoma is characterized by gains of chromosomal material including 9p and amplification of the REL gene. Blood 1996;87(4):1571.
15. Jacobson JO, Aisenberg AC, Lamarre L, et al. Mediastinal large cell lymphoma: an uncommon subset of adult lymphoma curable with combined modality therapy. Cancer 1988;62:1893–1898.
16. Lazzarino M, Orlandi E, Paulli M, et al. Treatment outcome and prognostic factors for primary mediastinal (thymic) B-cell lymphoma: A multicenter study of 106 patients. J Clin Oncol 1997;15:1646–1653.
17. Zinzani PL, Bendandi M, Frezza G, et al. Primary mediastinal B-cell lymphoma with sclerosis: clinical and therapeutic evaluation of 22 patients. Leuk Lymphoma 1996;21:311–316.
18. Haioun C, Gaulard P, Roudot-Thoraval F, et al. Mediastinal diffuse large B-cell lymphoma with sclerosis: a condition with a poor prognosis. Am J Clin Oncol 1989;12:425–429.

19. Lazzarino M, Orlandi E, Paulli M, et al. Primary mediastinal B-cell lymphoma with sclerosis: an aggressive tumor with distinctive clinical and pathological features. *J Clin Oncol* 1993;11:2306–2313.
20. Bishop P, Wilson W, Pearson D, et al. CNS involvement in primary mediastinal large B-cell lymphoma. *J Clin Oncol* 1999;17:2479–2485.
21. Abrahamsen AF, Lien HH, Aas M, et al. Magnetic resonance imaging and [67]gallium scan in mediastinal malignant lymphoma: a prospective pilot study. *Ann Oncol* 1994;5:433–436.
22. Zinzani PL, Martelli M, Magagnoli M, et al. Treatment and clinical management of primary mediastinal large B-cell lymphoma with sclerosis: MACOP-B regimen and mediastinal radiotherapy monitored by (67) gallium scan in 50 patients. *Blood* 1999;94:3289–3293.
23. Carbone PP, Kaplan HS, Musshoff K, et al. Report of the Committee on Hodgkin's Disease Staging Classification. *Cancer Res* 1971;31:1860–1861.
24. Lavabre-Bertrand T, Donadio D, Fegueux N, et al. A study of 15 cases of primary mediastinal lymphoma of B-cell type. *Cancer* 1992;69:2561–2566.
25. Rohatiner AZ, Whelan JS, Ganjoo RK, et al. Mediastinal large-cell lymphoma with sclerosis (MLCLS). *Br J Cancer* 1994;69:601–604.
26. Bertini M, Orsucci L, Vitolo U, et al. Stage II large B-cell lymphoma with sclerosis treated with MACOP-B. *Ann Oncol* 1991;2:733–737.
27. Todeschini G, Ambrosetti A, Meneghini V, et al. Mediastinal large-B-cell lymphoma with sclerosis: a clinical study of 21 patients. *J Clin Oncol* 1990;8:804–808.
28. Kirn D, Mauch P, Shaffer K, et al. Large-cell and immunoblastic lymphoma of the mediastinum: prognostic and pathologic features in 57 patients. *J Clin Oncol* 1993;11:1336–1343.
29. Aisenberg AC. Primary large-cell lymphoma of the mediastinum. *J Clin Oncol* 1993;11:2291–2298.
30. Rodriguez J, Pugh WC, Romaguera JE, et al. Primary mediastinal large cell lymphoma. *Haematol Oncology* 1994;12:175–184.
31. Abou-Elella AA, Weisenburger DD, Vose JM, et al. Primary mediastinal large B-cell lymphoma: a clinicopathologic study of 43 patients from the Nebraska Lymphoma Study Group. *J Clin Oncol* 1999;17:784–790.
32. Perrone T, Frizzera G, Rosai J. Mediastinal diffuse large-cell lymphoma with sclerosis. A clinicopathologic study of 60 cases. *Am J Clin Pathol* 1986;10:176–191.
33. Al-Sharabati M, Chittal S, Duga-Neulet I, et al. Primary anterior mediastinal B-cell lymphoma: a clinicopathological and immunohistochemical study of 16 cases. *Cancer* 1991;67:2579–2583.
34. Bieri S, Roggero E, Zucca E, et al. Primary mediastinal large B-cell lymphoma (PMLCL): the need for prospective controlled clinical trials. *Leuk Lymphoma* 1999;35:139–146.
35. Nguyen LN, Ha CS, Hess M, et al. The outcome of combined-modality treatments for stage I and II primary large B-cell lymphoma of the mediastinum. *Int J Radiat Oncol Biol Phys* 2000;47:1281–1285.
36. Martelli MP, Martelli M, Pescarmona E, et al. MACOP-B and involved field radiation therapy is an effective therapy for primary mediastinal large B-cell lymphoma with sclerosis. *Ann Oncol* 1998;9:1027–1029.
37. Zinzani PL, Martelli M, De Renzo A, et al. Primary mediastinal large B-cell lymphoma with sclerosis: a clinical study of 89 patients treated with MACOP-B chemotherapy and radiation therapy. *Haematologica* 2001;86:187–191.
38. Fisher RI, Gaynor ER, Dahlberg S, et al. Comparison of a standard regimen (CHOP) with three intensive chemotherapy regimens for advanced non-Hodgkin's lymphoma. *N Engl J Med* 1993;329:1002–1006.
39. Guglielmi C, Amadori S, Anselmo AP, et al. Sequential combination chemotherapy of high-grade non-Hodgkin's lymphoma with 5-fluorouracil, methotrexate, cytosine arabinoside, cyclophosphamide, doxorubicin, vincristine and prednisone (F-MACHOP). *Cancer Invest* 1987;5:159–169.
40. Nademanee A, Molina A, O'Donnell M, et al. Results of high-dose therapy and autologous bone marrow/stem cell transplantation during remission in poor-risk intermediate and high-grade lymphoma: international index high and high-intermediate risk group. *Blood* 1997;90:3844–3852.
41. Popat U, Przepiork D, Champlin R, et al. High-dose chemotherapy for relapsed and refractory diffuse large B-cell lymphoma: mediastinal localization predicts for a favorable outcome. *J Clin Oncol* 1998;16:63–69.
42. Sehn LH, Antin JH, Shulman LN, et al. Primary diffuse large B-cell lymphoma of the mediastinum. Outcome after high-dose chemotherapy and autologous hematopoietic cell transplantation. *Blood* 1998;91:717–723.
43. Aisenberg AC. Primary large cell lymphoma of the mediastinum. *Semin Oncol* 1999;26:251–258.
44. Van Besien K, Kelta M, Bahaguna P. Primary mediastinal B-cell lymphoma: a review of pathology and management. *J Clin Oncol* 2001;19:1855–1864.

CHAPTER 29

Mantle Cell Lymphoma

Wolfgang Hiddemann, Georg Lenz,
Dennis D. Weisenburger, and Martin H. Dreyling

DEFINITION

Mantle cell lymphoma is a subentity of malignant lymphoma which has only recently been generally accepted as a distinct disease (1,2). Twenty-five years ago, this entity was already described as *centrocytic lymphoma* in the Kiel Classification (3). In the Working Formulation (4), mantle cell lymphoma was not recognized as a separate entity and was grouped into different subtypes, including diffuse small cleaved-cell lymphoma, small lymphocytic lymphoma, follicular small cleaved-cell lymphoma, and diffuse mixed small- and large-cell lymphoma. It was not until the detection and functional characterization of the chromosomal translocation t(11; 14), which results in a juxtaposition of the BCL-1 gene locus to the immunoglobulin (Ig) heavy–chain promotor and the overexpression of the cell-cycle–regulator protein cyclin D1, that mantle cell lymphoma was considered as a distinct lymphoma entity (5).

Mantle cell lymphoma is derived from a subset of naive pregerminal center cells localized in primary follicles or in the mantle region of secondary follicles and is characterized by a nodular or diffuse growth pattern or a combination of the two (6–9).

EPIDEMIOLOGY AND ETIOLOGY

Mantle cell lymphoma represents approximately 5% of all lymphoma cases in North America (10) and 8% to 10% of all cases in Europe (11). The mean annual incidence of mantle cell lymphoma is approximately two to three cases per 100,000 per year, with a male predominance of 3:1 to 4:1. Patients with mantle cell lymphoma are usually elderly, with a median age of 65 to 70 years (12–15).

The molecular pathogenesis of mantle cell lymphoma is not yet fully elucidated. In the transgenic mouse model, the characteristic overexpression of cyclin D1 is not sufficient for generating a malignant phenotype (16).

PATHOLOGY

The pathology of mantle cell lymphoma has been refined, and the knowledge about the histologic spectrum of the dis-ease has been expanded in recent years through the use of immunologic, cytogenetic, and molecular techniques. A number of detailed descriptions of the pathology of mantle cell lymphoma have recently been published (10,17–22).

Lymph Nodes

The malignant lymphomas of mantle-cell type usually consist of atypical small lymphoid cells and have either a nodular or diffuse pattern of growth, or a combination of the two. Nodularity is present, at least focally, in approximately 40% of cases at the time of initial diagnosis. Early in the course of the disease, some or many of the nodules may consist of follicles with reactive germinal centers surrounded by broad mantles of small lymphoid cells (Fig. 29.1), the so-called *mantle-zone pattern*. In such cases, some neoplastic nodules without germinal centers, which mimic primary follicles, are also present. In other cases, these latter nodules may predominate or be present exclusively, and the process may be confused with a follicular center-cell lymphoma of the small cleaved-cell type. Later in the course of the disease, invasion and obliteration of the reactive germinal centers and interfollicular areas by neoplastic cells result in a diffuse pattern of growth and effacement of the nodal architecture. Residual vague nodularity may be seen in such cases, and naked germinal centers lacking a normal lymphocyte mantle are found.

Cytologically, mantle cell lymphoma usually consists of a monotonous population of atypical small lymphoid cells with irregular and indented nuclei, moderately coarse chromatin, inconspicuous nucleoli, and scant cytoplasm. Small, round lymphocytes, most of which are T cells, are admixed in variable numbers, and neoplastic cells with cleaved nuclei are often present as well. However, cases of mantle cell lymphoma with predominantly round nuclei or only slight nuclear irregularity and cases with markedly angulated and cleaved nuclei or even cerebriform nuclei do occur. Although the neoplastic lymphoid cells show a spectrum of nuclear irregularity from case to case, ranging from slight to marked, the cells usually show little variation within an individual neoplasm (Fig. 29.2). In some cases, the cells in focal

461

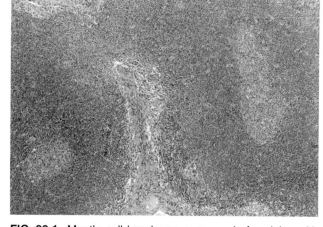

FIG. 29.1. Mantle cell lymphoma composed of nodules with reactive germinal centers surrounded by wide mantles of neoplastic small lymphoid cells (hematoxylin and eosin stain, 60× magnification).

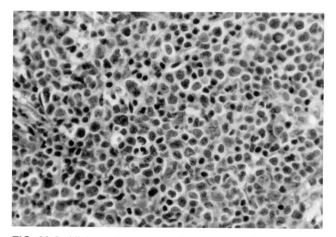

FIG. 29.3. High-grade mantle cell lymphoma of the pleomorphic type (hematoxylin and eosin stain, 200× magnification).

areas may have more abundant pale cytoplasm and resemble marginal-zone cells. In such cases, however, more typical areas are usually present, and it is unclear whether this finding is real or due to problems with fixation or processing.

In approximately 20% of cases of mantle cell lymphoma, the neoplastic cells are larger than usual and have more finely dispersed nuclear chromatin and small nucleoli. These high-grade variants have been referred to as *pleomorphic large-cell* or *blastic forms* of mantle cell lymphoma (10,17–23) and are associated with an aggressive clinical course. In some cases, a mixture of atypical small cells and larger cells with hyperchromatic nuclei and small nucleoli is present, imparting a pleomorphic cytologic picture (Fig. 29.3). In other cases, the cells are more blastic and quite monotonous, ranging from medium to large in size, with fine chromatin and multiple small nucleoli (Fig. 29.4). These high-grade variants of mantle cell lymphoma may occur *de novo* or as a

transformation during the course of more typical disease. Thus, the diversity of morphologies seen in different cases of mantle cell lymphoma is broad, ranging from small cells with round or slightly irregular nuclei at one end of the spectrum to large transformed cells with distinct nucleoli at the other end.

In general, large lymphoid cells with vesicular nuclei and multiple prominent nucleoli (large noncleaved cells or centroblasts) are not seen in the lymphocytic forms of mantle cell lymphoma, except in residual benign germinal centers. Plasma cells are usually absent or present in only small numbers and are polyclonal in nature. The mitotic rate is generally low (fewer than 20 mitoses per ten high-power fields) in the lymphocytic forms of mantle cell lymphoma, but an increased mitotic rate is usually seen in the high-grade variants and is often accompanied by admixed benign histiocytes. A high mitotic rate has been associated with shorter overall survival.

Histologic progression from a nodular pattern to a diffuse pattern of growth may be evident in a subsequent biopsy, and trans-

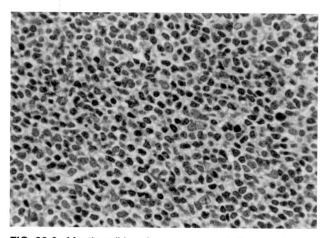

FIG. 29.2. Mantle cell lymphoma composed of a monotonous population of atypical small lymphoid cells with irregular nuclear contours (hematoxylin and eosin stain, 200× magnification).

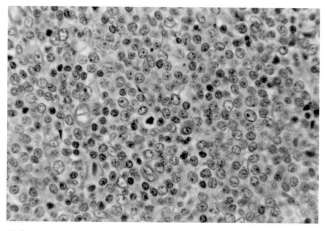

FIG. 29.4. High-grade mantle cell lymphoma seen of the blastic type (hematoxylin and eosin stain, 200× magnification).

formation from lymphocytic to high-grade cytology with a high mitotic rate is not uncommon. Norton and colleagues (24) noted histologic transformation to high-grade cytology on rebiopsy in 17% of their cases of mantle cell lymphoma and found evidence of transformation in 70% of their cases at autopsy. However, transformation of mantle cell lymphoma to the usual forms of diffuse large B-cell lymphoma is an uncommon event.

Cytology, Peripheral Blood, and Bone Marrow

In lymph node touch preparations and other cytologic specimens, the neoplastic cells are small to medium sized, with irregular, indented, and cleaved nuclear contours, moderately clumped (smudged) to more finely dispersed chromatin, one or more conspicuous nucleoli, and small to moderate amounts of cytoplasm (Fig. 29.5). Larger cells with round nuclei, fine chromatin, prominent nucleoli, and moderate amounts of basophilic cytoplasm are seen in the high-grade variants of mantle cell lymphoma. Smears of involved bone marrow and peripheral blood generally reflect the lymphoid population present in the lymph nodes (25,26). The neoplastic cells in the blood and bone marrow of a given patient may be quite heterogeneous in appearance (Fig. 29.6). In bone marrow sections, the neoplastic cells may infiltrate in either a focal, often paratrabecular, pattern or a diffuse pattern. However, one should not make a diagnosis of mantle cell lymphoma based on the examination of peripheral blood or bone marrow alone because of the lack of precise criteria for such a diagnosis. Immunologic analysis by flow cytometry (see Immunophenotype) may be very useful in the diagnosis of such specimens, but a lymph node biopsy is often necessary for definitive diagnosis.

Immunophenotype

The cells of mantle cell lymphoma have a characteristic phenotype. In frozen sections or by flow cytometry, the cells are

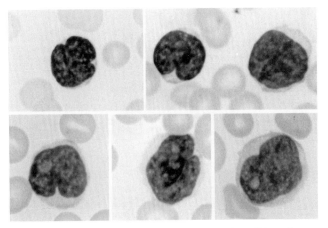

FIG. 29.6. Peripheral blood smear of mantle cell lymphoma showing a spectrum of lymphoma cells (Wright-Giemsa stain, 1,000× magnification).

monoclonal, almost always bearing surface IgM and often IgD. Surface IgG is expressed along with IgM in approximately 20% of cases. The κ to λ light ratio is reversed in mantle cell lymphoma, with approximately 60% of cases expressing monoclonal λ light chains, and the residual germinal centers are polyclonal. The neoplastic cells also stain for a variety of pan–B-cell antigens (CD19, CD20, CD22, and CD24) and human leukocyte antigen–DR antigen. The cells are usually negative for CD23 antigen, although weak expression may be detected by flow cytometry in some cases (27). Interestingly, the cells typically have the pan–T-cell antigen CD5 on the surface and are negative for CD10 antigen. The neoplastic cells may also bear the T-cell–associated antigens CD43 and Leu8, but fail to stain for other pan–T-cell antigens. Antibodies to dendritic reticulum cells reveal large aggregates of these cells in cases with a nodular or mantle-zone pattern, whereas a more sparse and irregular meshwork of dendritic cells is usually found in diffuse areas. Cases of high-grade mantle cell lymphoma are less likely to express IgD, CD5, and CD43 and may express CD10 antigen. The phenotype of mantle cell lymphoma is remarkably similar to that of small lymphocytic lymphoma and chronic lymphocytic leukemia, except for more intense surface Ig and CD20 staining and lack of CD23 expression. Studies of cellular proliferation in mantle cell lymphoma have generally found low rates in the lymphocytic forms and high rates in the high-grade variants, but with considerable overlap. Because the differential diagnosis of mantle cell lymphoma is complex and often difficult (8), immunophenotyping is usually necessary to confirm the diagnosis (Table 29.1).

Cytogenetics

The characteristic cytogenetic abnormality in mantle cell lymphoma is the t(11;14)(q13;q32), which is seen in approximately 60% of the cases (22). Variant translocations involving the 11q13 breakpoint have also been reported, but many

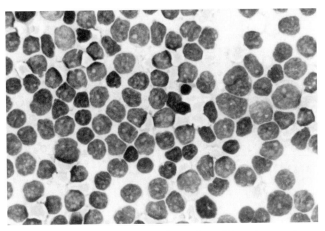

FIG. 29.5. Touch preparation of mantle cell lymphoma showing small- to medium-sized cells with irregular nuclear contours, moderately clumped chromatin, and scant cytoplasm (Wright-Giemsa stain, 400× magnification).

TABLE 29.1. *Phenotypes of the various B lymphocytic lymphomas*

Subtype	sIg	cIg	CD5	CD10	CD23	CD43
Mantle cell lymphoma	M ± D	−	+	−	−	+
Follicular lymphoma	G ± M	−	−	+/−	+/−	−
Small lymphocytic lymphoma/chronic lymphocytic leukemia	M ± D	−/+	+	−	+	+
Nodal marginal zone lymphoma	M	−/+	+	−	−/+	−
Mucosa-associated lymphoma	M	−/+	−	−	−	−/+
Lymphoplasmacytic lymphoma	M	+	−	−	−	−
Splenic marginal zone lymphoma	M ± D	−/+	−	−	−	−

cIg, cytoplasmic immunoglobulin; sIg, surface immunoglobulin; +, >80% positive; +/−, >50% positive; −/+, <50% positive; −, <20% positive.

cases are not informative, because the neoplastic cells do not proliferate in culture. Secondary abnormalities that appear to be nonrandom include the loss of chromosomes 13 and Y; deletions of chromosomes 1p, 6q, 11q22-23, 13q14, and 17p; and gains at chromosome 3q26-29, as well as trisomy 12 and various other abnormalities (28–31). The occurrence of deletions of chromosome 13q14 in 50% of cases suggests the presence of an important tumor-suppressor gene (28–32), whereas frequent deletions and mutations of the ATM gene on chromosome 11q22-23 may be a major event in the development of mantle cell lymphoma (33,34). Inactivation of the p53 gene on chromosome 17p by deletion or mutation also plays an important role in the evolution of mantle cell lymphoma and predicts for poor survival (23,35). The presence of a complex karyotype with hyperdiploidy has been associated with high-grade cytology and portends an aggressive clinical course (18,36). Similarly, secondary abnormalities involving the c-myc oncogene on chromosome 8q24 are associated with high-grade cytology and a short survival (37). Because the t(11;14)(q13;q32) also occurs, albeit quite infrequently, in other types of malignant lymphoma and lymphocytic leukemia and in multiple myeloma, positive cytogenetic findings need to be carefully correlated with the pathologic and immunologic features to confirm a diagnosis of mantle cell lymphoma.

The molecular counterpart of the t(11;14) involves an error in V-D-J joining during Ig heavy-chain gene rearrangement, resulting in the movement of a putative cellular oncogene adjacent to the BCL-1 (11q13) breakpoint into proximity of the enhancer region of the Ig heavy–chain gene (14q32). Breaks in the latter region are thought to occur during early B-cell development and to be mediated by the recombinase system (38). The breakpoints in the BCL-1 locus are not tightly clustered, although approximately 30% to 40% of cases of mantle cell lymphoma have breaks in the major translocation cluster region. However, using multiple probes,

including those for a number of minor breakpoint regions, investigators have detected clonal rearrangements in 50% to 70% of patients with mantle cell lymphoma. A polymerase chain reaction assay will detect most of the breaks in the major translocation cluster region and may be used on deoxyribonucleic acid extracted from paraffin-embedded tissues. Fluorescent *in situ* hybridization will detect the t(11;14) in interphase cells or in cells from paraffin tissue in nearly all cases tested, thus demonstrating the importance of this translocation in the pathogenesis and diagnosis of mantle cell lymphoma (39). The fluorescent *in situ* hybridization technique is also useful to detect minimal residual disease in mantle cell lymphoma.

The putative oncogene deregulated by the t(11;14) is located approximately 120 Kb telomeric from the major translocation cluster breakpoint and has been officially named *CCND1*. The gene encodes for cyclin D1 and is overexpressed in mantle cell lymphoma, whereas it is only rarely expressed in other forms of hematopoietic cancer. Because overexpression of this gene has been found in nearly all cases of mantle cell lymphoma, including those without detectable BCL-1 rearrangements, additional minor breakpoint sites outside of those detected by the available probes are involved in the translocation of chromosome 11q13. All of the known breakpoints leave the CCND1 coding region structurally intact and result in increased protein expression. Antibodies to cyclin D1, which stain formalin-fixed, paraffin-embedded tissue, have been shown to be highly sensitive and specific markers for mantle cell lymphoma and are very useful to confirm the diagnosis or elucidate the nature of diagnostically difficult cases (40). Nuclear staining is specific for cyclin D1, but only a subpopulation of the tumor cells may stain in mantle cell lymphoma (Fig. 29.7). Because cyclin D1 is quite labile and may be affected by poor fixation or harsh processing, positive staining of scattered internal

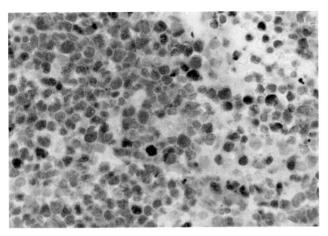

FIG. 29.7. Mantle cell lymphoma stained with antibody to cyclin D1. Note the nuclear positivity of variable intensity in most of the cells (immunoperoxidase stain, 200× magnification).

control cells, such as stromal or endothelial cells, should be observed before interpreting a case as negative. Cyclin D1–negative mantle cell lymphoma–like cases are best classified as *unclassifiable B-cell lymphoma*, because such cases appear to have a more indolent clinical course than does typical mantle cell lymphoma (41). Because a positive stain is not absolutely pathognomonic of mantle cell lymphoma due to the fact that other types of lymphocytic lymphoma or leukemia occasionally stain, careful correlation with the pathologic, immunologic, and cyto-

genetic features is necessary to confirm a diagnosis of mantle cell lymphoma. Detection of cyclin D1 overexpression by real-time, reverse transcriptase–mediated quantitative polymerase chain reaction analysis may also be useful for the diagnosis of mantle cell lymphoma or detection of minimal residual disease but requires fresh or snap-frozen tissue (42).

CLINICAL FEATURES

The clinical features of mantle cell lymphoma have been described in numerous studies (10,13,15,43–46). Mantle cell lymphoma patients have a median age of 60 to 65 years, with a predominance of the male gender (Table 29.2). The majority of cases are diagnosed at advanced Ann Arbor stages III or IV, usually with generalized lymphadenopathy. Extranodal involvement is found in approximately 90% of cases, including bone marrow infiltration (53% to 82%), liver (25%), and gastrointestinal tract (12% to 24%). A frequent extranodal presentation of mantle cell lymphoma is multiple lymphomatous polyposis of the intestine. However, this feature is frequently not diagnosed due to incomplete staging procedures (47). Less common extranodal sites are skin, lung, breast, and soft tissues. Central nervous system involvement is found in up to 4% to 22% of relapsed mantle cell lymphoma cases (48).

Mild anemia is not uncommon, and in approximately 50% of patients, a leukemic expression is found. Some

TABLE 29.2. *Features of presentation*

Authors (reference)	n	Median age (yr)	Stage IV (%)	Sex (male/female)	Bone marrow (%)	Leukemic expression (%)	Splenomegaly (%)	Gastrointestinal tract (%)
Berger et al., 1994 (111)	52	58% > 60	89 (III + IV)	NA	82	49	59	20
Zucca et al., 1995 (46)	65	64	72	2/1	58	20	35	15
Norton et al., 1995 (24)	66	62	82	3.7/1.0	80	NA	48	12
Fisher et al., 1995 (112)	36	55	NA	4/1	53	NA	NA	19
Teodorovic et al., 1995 (78)	64	58	NA	2.7/1.0	60	NA	33	NA
Pittaluga et al., 1995 (43)	55	68	62	6.8/1.0	66	NA	NA	NA
Hiddemann et al., 1996 (15)	573	63	75	2.5/1.0	69	NA	NA	NA
Velders et al., 1996 (13)	41	68	78	1.6/1.0	80	NA	NA	NA
Majlis et al., 1997 (56)	46	54	82 (III + IV)	1.7/1.0	69	NA	NA	24
Bosch et al., 1998 (44)	59	63	95 (III + IV)	3/1	81	58	44	17

n, number of patients; NA, not available.

patients present only with an elevated white blood count and massive splenomegaly. These leukemic mantle cell lymphoma patients seem to have a significantly worse outcome compared with the overall mantle cell lymphoma group (49). B-symptoms are described in less than 50% of cases.

PROGNOSTIC FACTORS IN MANTLE CELL LYMPHOMA

Mantle cell lymphoma is associated with poor prognosis and a median survival of 3 years, with virtually no long-term survivors due to the aggressive clinical course of the disease (Fig. 29.8). Several studies have analyzed prognostic factors in mantle cell lymphoma.

Clinical Prognostic Factors

In univariate analysis, the most important prognostic factors associated with a shorter time to treatment failure and a significantly poorer overall survival are age, poor performance status (46), advanced disease stages (III or IV) (44), a high serum level of lactate dehydrogenase (44,46), splenomegaly (50), and anemia (50). In the largest retrospective study presented so far, the parameters of the International Prognostic Index (IPI) were confirmed (Table 29.3) (15). In multivariate analyses, however, only age, poor performance status, leukemic generalization, and splenomegaly remained independent prognostic determinants (44,51).

The value of the IPI (52), which considers age (60 years or younger vs. older than 60 years), performance status (Eastern Cooperative Oncology Group 0 or 1 vs. 2 to 4), Ann Arbor stage (I or II vs. III or IV), extranodal involvement (fewer than two vs. two or more involved sites), and serum lactate dehydrogenase level (normal vs. high), is interpreted differently. Weissenburger et al. (20) reported a correlation between short-term survival and a high-risk

IPI classification. Bosch et al. (44) claimed that patients classified as high-risk IPI had lower response rates to chemotherapy. This was supported by a retrospective study of Zucca et al. (46) that demonstrated a benefit of anthracycline-containing chemotherapy regimens in patients with a favorable IPI score. In contrast, independent studies by Andersen et al. (50) and Samaha et al. (45) showed that the IPI has no impact on patients' survival. In the largest retrospective series published, the IPI identified different risk groups of patients. However, a significant overlap of survival curves in these groups was seen (15). Taken together, these studies suggest that the International Prognostic Index is of limited additional impact in predicting the clinical outcome of mantle cell lymphoma patients (Fig. 29.9).

A recent study of Pott et al. (53) investigated the value of molecular remission as a prognostic factor in mantle cell lymphoma patients after high-dose chemoradiotherapy and autologous stem cell transplantation. Similar to follicular lymphomas, molecular remission was a strong prognostic factor predicting progression-free survival in mantle cell lymphoma. Therefore, future studies may test response-dependent therapeutic concepts based on the molecular-remission status.

Biologic Prognostic Factors

Different studies analyzed the correlation between cytologic forms of mantle cell lymphoma and clinical outcome. In most studies, variant cytology, especially the blastoid variant, is associated with a worse prognosis than is classical mantle cell lymphoma. In the study by Bernard et al. (54), median overall survival for the blastoid variant was 14.5 months, compared to 53 months for patients with the common form of mantle cell lymphoma. This finding could be confirmed by the study by Bosch et al. (44), which showed a median survival of 50 months for patients with typical histology, whereas the median survival of patients with a blastic

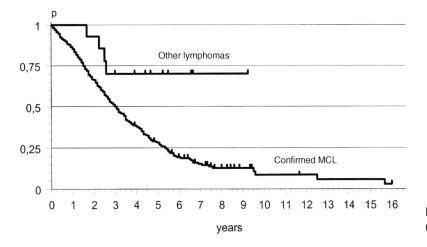

FIG. 29.8. European survey: clinical course of mantle cell lymphoma (MCL).

TABLE 29.3. *Prognostic determinants in mantle cell lymphoma*

Prognostic determinant	*p* value
Age (>60 yr)	< .0001
Performance status	< .0002
B symptoms	< .0018
Stage	< .0002
Extranodal involvement	< .0006
Elevated lactate dehydrogenase	< .0001

From Hiddemann W, Brittinger G, Tiemann M, et al. Presentation features and clinical course of mantle cell lymphomas—results of a European survey. *Ann Oncol* 1996;7:22, with permission.

variant was only 18 months. However, in the largest series published so far by Tiemann (55), cytology showed only borderline significance.

An additional prognostic feature investigated by different groups is the lymphoma growth pattern. Histopathologically, mantle cell lymphoma is characterized either by a diffuse, nodular, or so-called *mantle-zone* architecture. However, the results published so far differ, and the significance of the growth pattern remains unclear. Weisenburger (20) claimed a worse outcome for patients showing the diffuse growth pattern compared to those with nodular tumor architecture (16-month overall survival vs. 50 months). The study by Majlis et al. (56) demonstrated a poor treatment response and poor overall-survival rate in patients with a diffuse or nodular growth pattern compared to patients with a mantle-zone architecture. In contrast, Norton et al. (24) showed that growth pattern had no influence on the outcome.

Other groups determined the role of the p53 tumor-suppressor gene in mantle cell lymphoma. p53 gene mutations have been detected in other lymphoid malignancies, mainly in high-grade lymphomas and secondary transformation of follicular lymphoma. Analysis of the p53 gene in mantle cell lymphoma showed that mutations predict poor prognosis. Greiner et al. (23) found mutations of the p53 gene in 15% (eight out of 53) of mantle cell lymphoma cases and showed that median survival of cases with mutant p53 was only 1.3 years, compared to a median survival of 5.1 years of cases with germline p53. These findings could be confirmed by two other independent studies. Hernandez et al. (35) showed that patients with p53 mutations had a median survival of 18.3 months compared to a median survival of 49 months for patients with a nonmutated p53 gene. In addition, Zoldan et al. (57) could demonstrate the negative impact of p53 abnormalities on patients' survival. All studies confirmed the poor outcome of cases with mutated p53 gene.

The influence of the p16 gene on the pathogenesis of mantle cell lymphoma was determined by Pinyol et al. (58). Genetic alterations that led to loss of the normal protein expression were only detectable in 5% of the investigated cases. However, these cases followed an aggressive clinical course. In analogy to other investigated lymphoma subentities, in which p16 alterations led to aggressive tumor growth, Pinyol concluded that p16 genetic alterations are relatively infrequent in mantle cell lymphoma but are an indicator of a poor clinical outcome. In contrast, in another study, genomic alterations of the p16 region were the most frequently detected secondary aberration and closely related to cell proliferation (59).

Letestu et al. (60) investigated the prognostic influence of p27KIP1 expression in leukemic mantle cell lymphoma. This study showed that the downregulation of the cyclin-

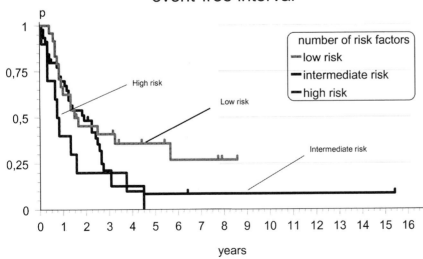

FIG. 29.9. European survey: prognostic value of the International Prognostic Index.

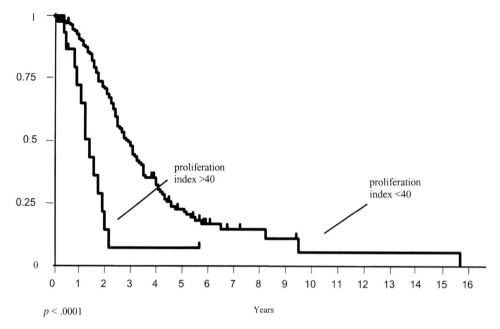

FIG. 29.10. Biologic risk factors: cell proliferation. Survival after diagnosis.

dependent kinase inhibitor p27KIP1 is associated with a shorter median survival in comparison to mantle cell lymphoma cases with p27KIP1 expression. However, further series have to be performed to confirm this finding.

In various studies, the most important biologic prognostic factor was the proliferation rate determined by the number of mitoses or the Ki67 staining index. Bosch et al. (44) showed that patients with more than 2.5 mitoses per high-power field had a median survival of 24 months, whereas those with 2.5 or fewer mitoses per high-power field had a median survival of 50 months, clearly indicating the prognostic value of this parameter. Furthermore, in a multivariant analysis, the proliferation rate was clearly superior to cytology and growth pattern as a prognostic factor (51) (Fig. 29.10).

Taken together, these studies suggest that the most prominent prognostic factor in mantle cell lymphoma is the proliferation rate, which might be closely regulated by distinct molecular aberrations (59). Important clinical prognostic factors are poor performance status, splenomegaly, anemia, and age, whereas the International Prognostic Index provides limited additional information. Therefore, future prognostic scores will combine clinical as well as biologic markers of mantle cell lymphoma to allow a risk-adapted therapy.

THERAPY

Mantle cell lymphoma has a clinically rapid and progressive course. In various epidemiologic studies, mantle cell lymphoma had the poorest long-term survival of all lymphoma subtypes. As a consequence, treatment should be applied as soon as possible, although at present, there is no evidence that any conventional chemotherapy is curative (11,43,46,61). Various conventional chemotherapeutic regimens induce overall-response rates of approximately 70% to 80%, with complete remissions in up to 20% to 50% of cases (Table 29.4). Splenectomy should only be performed in selected patients with prominent aplasia caused by hypersplenism (62).

Radiation Therapy

Due to the low incidence of mantle cell lymphoma and the fact that mantle cell lymphoma was not recognized as a distinct lymphoma entity until recently, only smaller trials have been reported. There are limited data suggesting that local-regional radiation therapy is curative in patients with stage I or II mantle cell lymphoma (63,64). Extrapolating from indolent lymphomas with a similar clinical presentation, doses of 30 to 36 Gy applied to modified involved or extended fields appear to be reasonable. In contrast, in advanced stage (III or IV), the benefit of radiation therapy in addition to chemotherapy is not proven. Thus, local radiation therapy should only be performed in cases with bulky disease not responsive to conventional therapy.

Chemotherapy

Anthracycline-Containing Regimens

Different studies investigated the use of anthracycline-containing regimens (Table 29.5). In the only prospective randomized study, Meusers et al. (65) compared COP

TABLE 29.4. *Therapy of mantle cell lymphoma with conventional chemotherapy*

Author (reference)	n	Complete remission (%)	Complete remission + partial response (%)	Overall survival (mo)
Pittaluga et al., 1995 (43)	55	NA	NA	32
Zucca et al., 1995 (46)	65	51	86	42
Vandenberghe et al., 1997 (61)	65	NA	NA	57

n, number of patients; NA, not available.

[cyclophosphamide, Oncovin (vincristine), and prednisone] and CHOP [cyclophosphamide, doxorubicin, Oncovin (vincristine), and prednisone]. The overall-response rate of complete and partial remissions was 84% after COP, as compared to 89% after CHOP. The median overall survival and relapse-free survival were not significantly different. In the COP group, overall survival was 32 months (relapse-free survival, 10 months) compared to 37 months in the patients who received the CHOP regimen (relapse-free survival, 7 months). In contrast, in a retrospective analysis of 65 mantle cell lymphoma patients, Zucca et al. (46) found anthracycline-containing regimens to be associated with superior complete-response rates, failure-free survival, and overall survival in the low-risk group of patients according to the International Prognostic Index. Another study by Zinzani et al. (66) compared the combination of fludarabine and idarubicin with fludarabine alone in patients with newly diagnosed mantle cell lymphoma. In terms of overall-response rates and toxicity, no differences could be observed. However, the fludarabine and idarubicin regimen seemed to confer a longer-lasting complete remission compared to fludarabine alone (Table 29.5). Unterhalt et al. (67) compared an anthrachinon-containing combination of prednimustine and mitoxantrone with the COP regimen. Overall-

response rates were similar (80%). However, prednimustine and mitoxantrone achieved a higher complete-response rate (Table 29.5). Thus, despite the contradicting study results published so far, most authors accept a CHOP-like regime as standard chemotherapy in mantle cell lymphoma.

Purine Analogs

The use of purine analogs in mantle cell lymphoma has been analyzed by different groups. Single-agent fludarabine phosphate (45,68,69), which has significant activity in follicular lymphoma, showed only moderate activity, with response rates of 32% to 41% (Table 29.6). However, various studies with a fludarabine-containing combination achieved high remission rates.

Cohen et al. (70) investigated the efficacy of cyclophosphamide and fludarabine in patients with newly diagnosed and relapsed or refractory mantle cell lymphoma. The overall-response rate was 63% (30% complete response and 33% partial response); the median failure-free survival and overall survival were 4.8 months and 17.5 months, respectively. The patients with newly diagnosed mantle cell lymphoma had especially high response rates (70% complete responses).

TABLE 29.5. *Anthracyclines in mantle cell lymphoma*

Authors (reference)	n	Regimen	Overall response/complete remission (%)
Meusers et al., 1989 (65)	37	COP	84/41
	26	CHOP	89/58
Unterhalt et al., 1996 (67)	20	COP: cyclophosphamide, 400 mg/m^2/d × 5; vincristine, 1.4 mg/m^2/d × 1; prednisone, 100 mg/m^2/d × 5	80/5
	19	PmM: prednimustine, 100 mg/m^2/d × 5; mitoxantrone, 8 mg/m^2/d × 2	80/27
Zinzani et al., 2000 (66)	11	Fludarabine, 25 mg/m^2/d × 5	72/27
	18	Fludarabine, 25 mg/m^2/d × 3; idarubicin, 12 mg/m^2/d × 1	61/33
Lefrere et al., 2002 (75)	28	CHOP followed by DHAP	89/82

CHOP, cyclophosphamide, doxorubicin, Oncovin (vincristine), and prednisone; DHAP, dexamethasone, high-dose ara-C, and Platinol (cisplatin); n, number of patients.

TABLE 29.6. *Purine analogs in mantle cell lymphoma*

Authors (reference)	n	Regimen	Overall response/ complete remission (%)
Samaha et al., 1998 (45)	12	Fludarabine (not specified)	33/25
Decaudin et al., 1998 (69)	15	Fludarabine, 25 mg/m^2/d × 5	33/0
Foran et al., 1999 (68)	17	Fludarabine, 25 mg/m^2/d × 5	41/29
Zinzani et al., 2000 (66)	11	Fludarabine, 25 mg/m^2/d × 5	72/27
	18	Fludarabine, 25 mg/m^2/d × 3; idarubicin 12 mg/m^2/d × 1	61/33
Cohen et al., 2001 (70)	30	Cyclophosphamide; fludarabine	63/30
Hiddemann et al., 2002 (71)	40	FCM: fludarabine, 25 mg/m^2/d × 3; cyclophosphamide 200 mg/m^2/d × 3; mitoxantrone 8 mg/m^2/d × 1	33/0
Rummel et al., 2002 (72)	18	Cladribine, 5 mg/m^2/d × 3; mitoxantrone, 8 mg/m^2/d × 2	100/44

n, number of patients.

In contrast, in a small, randomized, multicenter study, the combination of fludarabine and idarubicin did not show any difference concerning the complete-remission rate (66) compared to therapy with fludarabine alone. However, the combination achieved a longer-lasting progression-free survival.

In another study, the purine analog 2-CdA in combination with mitoxantrone achieved complete-response rates of 44% and overall-response rates of 100% (72), strongly suggesting a synergism of purine analogs and anthracycline or alkylating drugs.

Other promising response rates could be demonstrated for the combination of cisplatin, fludarabine, and cytarabine in patients with previously refractory mantle cell lymphoma (73).

Other Chemotherapy Schedules

The efficacy of the DHAP [dexamethasone, high-dose ara-C, and Platinol (cisplatin)] regimen in relapsed or refractory mantle cell lymphoma was investigated by Touati et al. (74). Overall-response rates of 67% were reported. A similar therapeutic approach is the sequential application of the CHOP regimen followed by the DHAP regimen, investigated by Lefrere et al. (75). After four cycles of CHOP, only 7% complete remissions were obtained. Patients who did not achieve a complete response received an additional four cycles of the DHAP regimen. In this group, 84% of the investigated patients obtained a complete response. Another attempt to improve prognosis by a more aggressive treatment strategy was published by Romaguera et al. (76). In a phase II study, an alternating regimen [hyper-CVAD (Cytoxan [cyclophosphamide], vincristine, Adriamycin [doxorubicin], and dexamethasone) and high doses of methotrexate and cytarabine] was investigated in previously untreated, elderly patients, who were ineligible for stem cell transplantation. Overall-response rates of 92% and complete-remission rates of 68% were remarkably high. Thus, the hyper-CVAD regimen with alternating high-doses of methotrexate and cytarabine seems to be a highly active and feasible regimen even in elderly patients with tolerable toxicity. These data strongly suggest a high efficacy of high-doses of cytarabine in mantle cell lymphoma. Prospective randomized trials are currently being performed to confirm the impact of high-dose cytarabine in mantle cell lymphoma.

A new approach in relapsed or refractory mantle cell lymphoma is the combination of gemcitabine, dexamethasone, and cisplatin. The overall-response rate in heavily pretreated patients was 50% (77). However, response duration was short (median duration of response, 5 months).

NEW THERAPEUTIC PERSPECTIVES

Interferon-α

A combined approach investigated by different study groups is the use of interferon-α as part of the induction or maintenance therapy. Interferon-α has been shown to extend progression-free survival in follicular lymphomas. The only studies published so far that investigated the effects of interferon-α in mantle cell lymphoma claimed a prolonged progression-free survival of patients receiving interferon-α maintenance therapy (12,78). However, the number of patients included in these studies is too low to allow definitive conclusions. Nevertheless, interferon may play a role in future approaches (e.g., in combination with rituximab).

Antilymphoma Antibodies

Over the past years, several studies have investigated the activity of the anti-CD20 antibody rituximab (Mabthera, Rit-

TABLE 29.7. *Anti-CD20 in mantle cell lymphoma*

Authors (reference)	n	Disease status	Overall response
Coiffier et al., 1998 (113)	12	Resistant/Relapse	4 (33%)
Nguyen et al., 1999 (82)	10	Resistant/Relapse	2 (20%)
Foran et al., 2000 (80)	34	Untreated	13 (38%)
	40	Relapsed	15 (37%)
Ghielmini et al., 2000 (81)	39	Relapsed	9 (23%)
Tobinai et al., 2002 (83)	13	Relapsed	6 (46%)

n, number of patients.

uxan) in mantle cell lymphoma. In numerous studies (Table 29.7), monotherapy with rituximab had only a limited efficacy, with partial-response rates of approximately 20% to 40% (79–83). The combination of chemotherapy and rituximab has been proposed to have some synergistic effect. In a phase II study, the combination of rituximab and the CHOP regimen achieved a complete response in 48% of cases and an overall-response rate of 96% (84). This better response in comparison to chemotherapy alone may potentially translate into a longer progression-free survival. However, Howard et al. (84) reported a median progression-free survival of just 16.6 months (Table 29.8).

In a prospective randomized study, Hiddemann et al. (71) compared immunochemotherapy with rituximab and a combination of fludarabine, mitoxantrone, and cyclophosphamide with chemotherapy (combination of fludarabine, mitoxantrone, and cyclophosphamide) alone in relapsed mantle cell lymphoma. Response rates were significantly higher in the group that included the anti-CD20 antibody (65% vs. 33%), indicating the superiority of a rituximab and chemotherapy combination in relapsed mantle cell lymphoma (Table 29.9).

TABLE 29.8. *Anti-CD20 and chemotherapy in mantle cell lymphoma*

Authors (reference)	n	Regimen	Complete remission/ overall response (%)
Hiddemann et al., 2002 (71)	17	R-FCM: rituximab, 375 mg m²/d × 1; fludarabine, 25 mg/m²/d × 3; cyclophosphamide, 200 mg/m²/d × 3; mitoxantrone, 8 mg/m²/d × 1	35/65
Howard et al., 2002 (84)	40	R-CHOP	48/96

n, number of patients; R-CHOP, rituximab, cyclophosphamide, Oncovin (vincristine), and prednisone.

TABLE 29.9. *Fludarabine, cyclophosphamide, and mitoxantrone (FCM) versus rituximab, fludarabine, cyclophosphamide, and mitoxantrone (R-FCM) in relapsed mantle cell lymphoma*

	FCM	R-FCM
Number of patients	18	17
Complete remission	0 (0%)	6 (35%)
Partial response	6 (33%)	5 (29%)
Complete remission + partial response	6 (33%)	11 (65%)
Progressive disease	9 (50%)	6 (35%)
Early death	3 (17%)	0 (0%)

From Hiddemann W, Dreyling MH, Unterhalt M, et al. Rituximab plus chemotherapy in follicular and mantle cell lymphomas. *Semin Oncol* 2003;30 N1, with permission.

The role of rituximab as maintenance therapy after conventional chemotherapy is currently being tested in several studies.

An alternative therapeutic setting in relapsed and refractory mantle cell lymphoma is the sequential rituximab consolidation after conventional or high-dose chemotherapy followed by peripheral blood stem transplantation. In a phase II trial by Horwitz et al. (85), patients with mantle cell lymphoma received a 4-week course of rituximab 40 days after transplant and a second course after 6 months. Overall-survival rates and freedom-from-progression rates after 2 years were higher than those observed after transplant therapy alone. Similar results were reported by Mangel et al. (86) in a small group of mantle cell lymphoma patients. However, the number of patients in these trials was too low, and further trials are needed to define the optimal sequence of rituximab and myeloablative chemotherapy.

Another innovative approach is the application of radioactive ^{131}Iodine- or ^{90}Yttrium-labeled anti-CD20 antibodies in a conventional or myeloablative regimen in mantle cell lymphoma. Different studies achieved remarkably long-lasting overall-survival rates (87,88). Therefore, the use of labeled antibodies in mantle cell lymphoma will be further investigated.

Autologous Stem Cell Transplantation

One of the recently established options in the treatment of mantle cell lymphoma is myeloablative chemotherapy followed by autologous stem cell transplantation. After the first report of Stewart et al. (89) in 1995, numerous clinical studies have been performed showing a wide range of clinical outcomes after transplantation (90–96) (Table 29.10). An analysis of the obtained results suggests that the different disease-free– and overall-survival rates are mainly due to the different time of transplantation (initial consolidation vs. relapse) and other patient-selection criteria. In addition, in a retrospective multivariate analysis, total-body irradiation was an independent prognostic marker (97).

TABLE 29.10. *High-dose chemotherapy and autologous stem cell transplantation*

Authors (reference)	Regimen	n	Disease status	Progression-free survival (%)	Overall survival
Stewart et al., 1995 (89)	Various	9	Relapsed	34	34% 2 yr
Haas et al., 1996 (93)	TBI	9	First CR or PR	76	92% 3 yr
	Cyclophosphamide	4	Relapsed		
Ketterer et al., 1997 (94)		6	First CR or PR	24	54% 2 yr
		10	Relapsed		16% 2 yr
Milpied et al., 1998 (97)	Various	10	First CR or PR	80	90% 4 yr
		8	Relapsed	18	66% 4 yr
Blay et al., 1998 (92)	Various	5	First CR or PR	75	91% 2 yr
		14	Relapsed		
Kröger et al., 1998 (91)	Various	7	First CR or PR	100	100% 2 yr
		2	Relapsed		
Freedman et al., 1998 (95)	TBI[a]	8	First CR or PR	31	62% 4 yr
		20	Relapsed	0	
Khouri et al., 1998 (96)	TBI	25	First CR or PR	72	92% 3 yr
	Cyclophosphamide	20	Relapsed	17	25% 3 yr
Decaudin et al., 2000 (90)	Various	9	First CR or PR	55	68% 3 yr
		15	Relapsed		
Vose et al., 2000 (114)	Various	40	Various	36	65% 2 yr
Hiddemann et al., 2001 (98)	TBI		Various		
	Cyclophosphamide				

CR, complete remission; n, number of patients; PR, partial response; TBI, total-body irradiation.
[a]Anti–B-cell antibody–purged autologous bone marrow transplantation.

In a randomized prospective study, the European Mantle Cell Lymphoma Intergroup compared high-dose radio-chemotherapy followed by autologous stem cell transplantation with the best conventional treatment (interferon maintenance) (98). The analysis of 109 patients showed a longer disease-free survival and a borderline improvement of overall survival in patients receiving myeloablative radio-chemotherapy and stem cell transplantation in first complete or partial remission, compared to interferon-α maintenance therapy (Fig. 29.11). Thus, patients who are treated in first remission with autologous stem cell transplantation benefit from this treatment. In contrast, the efficacy in heavily pre-treated patients seems to be limited (99). Consequently, high-dose consolidation in first remission may be accepted as the standard therapeutic approach in younger patients. However, the majority of patients will relapse. One explanation could be the contamination of the stem cells with circulating mantle cell lymphoma cells, as standard purging

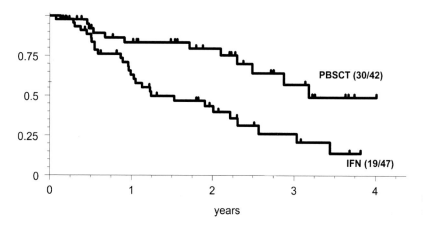

FIG. 29.11. Progression-free survival for patients in complete or partial remission. Peripheral blood stem cell transplant (PBSCT) versus interferon (IFN)-α in mantle cell lymphoma.

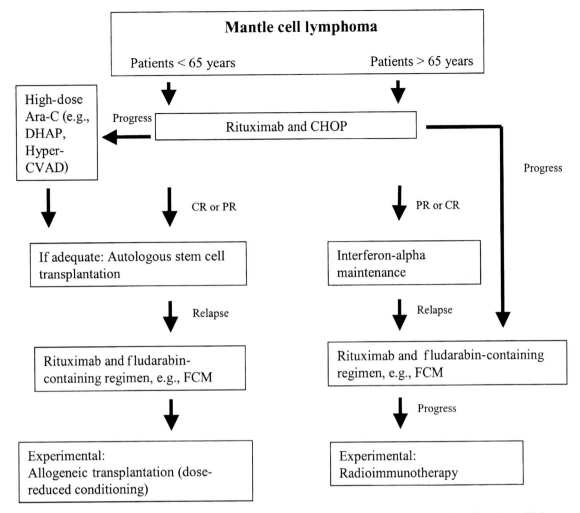

FIG. 29.12. Algorithm of management of mantle cell lymphoma. CHOP, cyclophosphamide, doxorubicin, Oncovin (vincristine), and prednisone; CR, complete response; FCM, fludarabine, cyclophosphamide, and mitoxantrone; DHAP, dexamethasone, high-dose ara-C, and Platinol (cisplatin); Hyper-CVAD, Cytoxan (cyclophosphamide), vincristine, Adriamycin (doxorubicin), and dexamethasone; PR, partial response.

procedures are not effective enough to avoid this problem (100). New antibody-based approaches with *in vivo* purging might overcome this dilemma (101).

Another new therapeutic approach is the combination of autologous stem cell transplantation and rituximab consolidation. The first promising results have been achieved in a multicenter phase II study published by Brugger et al. (102). At a median follow-up of 24 months, nine out of ten mantle cell lymphoma patients remained in clinical complete remission.

Allogeneic Transplantation

The only potentially curative therapy so far is allogeneic stem cell transplantation. Different studies showed that the induced graft-versus-lymphoma effect is able to achieve long-lasting complete remission even in patients with pretreated mantle cell lymphoma (103–107). However, trans-

plant-related toxicity is high, and especially, infectious complications are common. Alternatively, in patients who are ineligible for conventional myeloablative chemotherapy, human leukocyte antigen–identical stem cells can be transfused after a dose-reduced conditioning regimen. Khouri et al. (96) showed that allogeneic transplantation resulted in an overall survival and freedom from progression of 55% after 3 years. Molecular remission was achieved in five of seven patients within 7 months posttransplant. These data strongly support the role of a graft-versus-lymphoma effect in mantle cell lymphoma.

New Therapeutic Modalities

A new molecular-targeting agent in the treatment of mantle cell lymphoma is the specific inhibitor of cyclin D1 flavopiridol. Connors et al. (108) investigated the efficacy of flavopiridol given three times per week every 3 weeks. This application scheme showed only modest activity. Similarly, no remission could be achieved by a 72-hour continuous infusion in relapsed or refractory mantle cell lymphoma (109). However, cell-culture experiments suggest that flavopiridol might function as a "chemosensitizer" and might be investigated in combination with other chemotherapy.

Another approach in the treatment of mantle cell lymphoma is the proteasome inhibitor PS-341, which has been investigated in mantle cell lymphoma–derived cell lines and in a mantle cell lymphoma mouse model (110). PS-341 leads to a suppression of necrosis factor kB, an essential transcription factor that upregulates antiapoptotic genes, such as Bfl/A1 or c-IAP1. Different *in vitro* experiments could clearly demonstrate that PS-341 is capable of inhibiting cell growth and inducing apoptosis. Clinical studies to evaluate the efficacy of PS-341 are currently being performed.

FUTURE DIRECTIONS

In summary, mantle cell lymphoma remains a therapeutically resistant malignant lymphoma that is not curable using conventional chemotherapy. The clinical course is characterized by continuous progression, with a median survival of 3 years and only few long-term survivors. Due to the lack of prospective randomized multicenter trials, so far no standard chemotherapy has been established. However, recent prospective randomized studies confirmed the benefit of a combined immunochemotherapy with rituximab. In addition, in younger patients, high-dose chemotherapy followed by autologous stem cell transplantation improved the progression-free survival (Fig. 29.12). Nevertheless, the only curative approach to date is allogeneic bone marrow transplantation, indicating that new therapeutic strategies are necessary to further improve the clinical outcome of mantle cell lymphoma.

REFERENCES

1. Harris NL, Jaffe ES, Stein H, et al. A revised European-American classification of lymphoid neoplasms: a proposal from the International Lymphoma Study Group. *Blood* 1994;84:1361–1392.
2. Jaffe ES, Harris NL, Stein H, et al. *World Health Organisation classification of tumours: tumours of the haemopoietic and lymphoid tissues.* Lyon: IARC Press, 2001.
3. Lennert K, Stein H, Kaiserling E. Cytological and functional criteria for the classification of malignant lymphomata. *Br J Cancer* 1975;31[Suppl 2]:29–43.
4. Robb-Smith AH. U.S. National Cancer Institute working formulation of non-Hodgkin's lymphomas for clinical use. *Lancet* 1982;2:432–434.
5. Rimokh R, Berger F, Delsol G, et al. Rearrangement and overexpression of the BCL-1/PRAD-1 gene in intermediate lymphocytic lymphomas and in t(11q13)-bearing leukemias. *Blood* 1993;81:3063–3067.
6. Weisenburger DD, Kim H, Rappaport H. Mantle-zone lymphoma: a follicular variant of intermediate lymphocytic lymphoma. *Cancer* 1982;49:1429–1438.
7. Banks PM, Chan J, Cleary ML, et al. Mantle cell lymphoma. A proposal for unification of morphologic, immunologic, and molecular data. *Am J Surg Pathol* 1992;16:637–640.
8. Lardelli P, Bookman MA, Sundeen J, et al. Lymphocytic lymphoma of intermediate differentiation. Morphologic and immunophenotypic spectrum and clinical correlations. *Am J Surg Pathol* 1990;14:752–763.
9. Weisenburger DD, Armitage JO. Mantle cell lymphoma—an entity comes of age. *Blood* 1996;87:4483–4494.
10. Argatoff LH, Connors JM, Klasa RJ, et al. Mantle cell lymphoma: a clinicopathologic study of 80 cases. *Blood* 1997;89:2067–2078.
11. Meusers P, Hense J, Brittinger G. Mantle cell lymphoma: diagnostic criteria, clinical aspects and therapeutic problems. *Leukemia* 1997;11[Suppl 2]:S60–S64.
12. Hiddemann W, Unterhalt M, Herrmann R, et al. Mantle-cell lymphomas have more widespread disease and a slower response to chemotherapy compared with follicle-center lymphomas: results of a prospective comparative analysis of the German Low-Grade Lymphoma Study Group. *J Clin Oncol* 1998;16:1922–1930.
13. Velders GA, Kluin-Nelemans JC, De Boer CJ, et al. Mantle-cell lymphoma: a population-based clinical study. *J Clin Oncol* 1996;14:1269–1274.
14. Weisenburger DD, Nathwani BN, Diamond LW, et al. Malignant lymphoma, intermediate lymphocytic type: a clinicopathologic study of 42 cases. *Cancer* 1981;48:1415–1425.
15. Hiddemann W, Brittinger G, Tiemann M, et al. Presentation features and clinical course of mantle cell lymphomas—results of a European survey. *Ann Oncol* 1996;7:22.
16. Bodrug SE, Warner BJ, Bath ML, et al. Cyclin D1 transgene impedes lymphocyte maturation and collaborates in lymphomagenesis with the myc gene. *EMBO J* 1994;13:2124–2130.
17. Swerdlow SH, Zukerberg LR, Yang WI, et al. The morphologic spectrum of non-Hodgkin's lymphomas with BCL1/cyclin D1 gene rearrangements. *Am J Surg Pathol* 1996;20:627–640.
18. Ott G, Kalla J, Hanke A, et al. The cytomorphological spectrum of mantle cell lymphoma is reflected by distinct biological features. *Leuk Lymphoma* 1998;32:55–63.
19. Lai R, Medeiros LJ. Pathologic diagnosis of mantle cell lymphoma. *Clin Lymphoma* 2000;1:197–206; discussion, 198–207.
20. Weisenburger DD, Vose JM, Greiner TC, et al. Mantle cell lymphoma. A clinicopathologic study of 68 cases from the Nebraska Lymphoma Study Group. *Am J Hematol* 2000;64:190–196.
21. Yatabe Y, Suzuki R, Matsuno Y, et al. Morphological spectrum of cyclin D1-positive mantle cell lymphoma: study of 168 cases. *Pathol Int* 2001;51:747–761.
22. Swerdlow SH, Williams ME. From centrocytic to mantle cell lymphoma: a clinicopathologic and molecular review of 3 decades. *Hum Pathol* 2002;33:7–20.
23. Greiner TC, Moynihan MJ, Chan WC, et al. *p53* mutations in mantle cell lymphoma are associated with variant cytology and predict a poor prognosis. *Blood* 1996;87:4302–4310.
24. Norton AJ, Matthews J, Pappa V, et al. Mantle cell lymphoma: natural history defined in a serially biopsied population over a 20-year period. *Ann Oncol* 1995;6:249–256.
25. Wong KF, Chan JK, So JC, et al. Mantle cell lymphoma in leukemic phase: characterization of its broad cytologic spectrum with emphasis on the importance of distinction from other chronic lymphoproliferative disorders. *Cancer* 1999;86:850–857.
26. Schlette E, Lai R, Onciu M, et al. Leukemic mantle cell lymphoma: clinical and pathologic spectrum of twenty-three cases. *Mod Pathol* 2001;14:1133–1140.
27. Gong JZ, Lagoo AS, Peters D, et al. Value of CD23 determination by flow cytometry in differentiating mantle cell lymphoma from chronic lymphocytic leukemia/small lymphocytic lymphoma. *Am J Clin Pathol* 2001;116:893–897.
28. Cuneo A, Bigoni R, Rigolin GM, et al. Cytogenetic profile of lymphoma of follicle mantle lineage: correlation with clinicobiologic features. *Blood* 1999;93:1372–1380.
29. Bentz M, Plesch A, Bullinger L, et al. t(11;14)-positive mantle cell lymphomas exhibit complex karyotypes and share similarities with B-cell chronic lymphocytic leukemia. *Genes Chromosomes Cancer* 2000;27:285–294.
30. Bigoni R, Cuneo A, Milani R, et al. Secondary chromosome changes in mantle cell lymphoma: cytogenetic and fluorescence in situ hybridization studies. *Leuk Lymphoma* 2001;40:581–590.
31. Allen JE, Hough RE, Goepel JR, et al. Identification of novel regions of amplification and deletion within mantle cell lymphoma DNA by comparative genomic hybridization. *Br J Haematol* 2002;116:291–298.

32. Rosenwald A, Ott G, Krumdiek AK, et al. A biological role for deletions in chromosomal band 13q14 in mantle cell and peripheral T-cell lymphomas? *Genes Chromosomes Cancer* 1999;26:210–214.

33. Schaffner C, Idler I, Stilgenbauer S, et al. Mantle cell lymphoma is characterized by inactivation of the *ATM* gene. *Proc Natl Acad Sci U S A* 2000;97:2773–2778.

34. Camacho E, Hernandez L, Hernandez S, et al. *ATM* gene inactivation in mantle cell lymphoma mainly occurs by truncating mutations and missense mutations involving the phosphatidylinositol-3 kinase domain and is associated with increasing numbers of chromosomal imbalances. *Blood* 2002;99:238–244.

35. Hernandez L, Fest T, Cazorla M, et al. *p53* gene mutations and protein overexpression are associated with aggressive variants of mantle cell lymphomas. *Blood* 1996;87:3351–3359.

36. Bea S, Ribas M, Hernandez JM, et al. Increased number of chromosomal imbalances and high-level DNA amplifications in mantle cell lymphoma are associated with blastoid variants. *Blood* 1999;93:4365–4374.

37. Vaishampayan UN, Mohamed AN, Dugan MC, et al. Blastic mantle cell lymphoma associated with Burkitt-type translocation and hypodiploidy. *Br J Haematol* 2001;115:66–68.

38. Welzel N, Le T, Marculescu R, et al. Templated nucleotide addition and immunoglobulin JH-gene utilization in t(11;14) junctions: implications for the mechanism of translocation and the origin of mantle cell lymphoma. *Cancer Res* 2001;61:1629–1636.

39. Remstein ED, Kurtin PJ, Buno I, et al. Diagnostic utility of fluorescence in situ hybridization in mantle-cell lymphoma. *Br J Haematol* 2000;110:856–862.

40. Miranda RN, Briggs RC, Kinney MC, et al. Immunohistochemical detection of cyclin D1 using optimized conditions is highly specific for mantle cell lymphoma and hairy cell leukemia. *Mod Pathol* 2000;13:1308–1314.

41. Yatabe Y, Suzuki R, Tobinai K, et al. Significance of cyclin D1 overexpression for the diagnosis of mantle cell lymphoma: a clinicopathologic comparison of cyclin D1-positive MCL and cyclin D1-negative MCL-like B-cell lymphoma. *Blood* 2000;95:2253–2261.

42. Suzuki R, Takemura K, Tsutsumi M, et al. Detection of cyclin D1 overexpression by real-time reverse-transcriptase-mediated quantitative polymerase chain reaction for the diagnosis of mantle cell lymphoma. *Am J Pathol* 2001;159:425–429.

43. Pittaluga S, Wlodarska I, Stul MS, et al. Mantle cell lymphoma: a clinicopathological study of 55 cases. *Histopathology* 1995;26:17–24.

44. Bosch F, Lopez-Guillermo A, Campo E, et al. Mantle cell lymphoma: presenting features, response to therapy, and prognostic factors. *Cancer* 1998;82:567–575.

45. Samaha H, Dumontet C, Ketterer N, et al. Mantle cell lymphoma: a retrospective study of 121 cases. *Leukemia* 1998;12:1281–1287.

46. Zucca E, Roggero E, Pinotti G, et al. Patterns of survival in mantle cell lymphoma. *Ann Oncol* 1995;6:257–262.

47. Kadayifci A, Benekli M, Savas MC, et al. Multiple lymphomatous polyposis. *J Surg Oncol* 1997;64:336–340.

48. Oinonen R, Franssila K, Elonen E. Central nervous system involvement in patients with mantle cell lymphoma. *Ann Hematol* 1999;78:145–149.

49. Molina TJ, Delmer A, Cymbalista F, et al. Mantle cell lymphoma, in leukaemic phase with prominent splenomegaly. A report of eight cases with similar clinical presentation and aggressive outcome. *Virchows Arch* 2000;437:591–598.

50. Andersen NS, Jensen MK, de Nully Brown P, et al. A Danish population-based analysis of 105 mantle cell lymphoma patients. incidences, clinical features, response, survival and prognostic factors. *Eur J Cancer* 2002;38:401–408.

51. Dreyling MH. The increasing role of prognostic factors in the choice of treatment—mantle cell lymphoma. *Ann Oncol* 2002:13.

52. A predictive model for aggressive non-Hodgkin's lymphoma. The International Non-Hodgkin's Lymphoma Prognostic Factors Project. *N Engl J Med* 1993;329:987–994.

53. Pott C, Schrader C, Dermer N, Brüggemann M, et al. Molecular remission predicts progression-free survival in mantle cell lymphoma after peripheral blood stem cell transplantation. *Ann Oncol* 2002:69.

54. Bernard M, Gressin R, Lefrere F, et al. Blastic variant of mantle cell lymphoma: a rare but highly aggressive subtype. *Leukemia* 2001;15:1785–1791.

55. Tiemann M, Dreyling MH, et al. Pathology, proliferation indices and survival in 304 patients. *Ann Oncol* 1999:10.

56. Majlis A, Pugh WC, Rodriguez MA, et al. Mantle cell lymphoma: correlation of clinical outcome and biologic features with three histologic variants. *J Clin Oncol* 1997;15:1664–1671.

57. Zoldan MC, Inghirami G, Masuda Y, et al. Large-cell variants of mantle cell lymphoma: cytologic characteristics and *p53* anomalies may predict poor outcome. *Br J Haematol* 1996;93:475–486.

58. Pinyol M, Cobo F, Bea S, et al. p16(INK4a) gene inactivation by deletions, mutations, and hypermethylation is associated with transformed and aggressive variants of non-Hodgkin's lymphomas. *Blood* 1998;91:2977–2984.

59. Dreyling MH, Bullinger L, Ott G, et al. Alterations of the cyclin D1/p16-pRB pathway in mantle cell lymphoma. *Cancer Res* 1997;57:4608–4614.

60. Letestu R, Ugo V, Valensi F, et al. Prognostic impact of p27KIP1 expression in leukemic mantle cell lymphoma. *Blood* 2002;100:347a.

61. Vandenberghe E, De Wolf-Peeters C, Vaughan Hudson G, et al. The clinical outcome of 65 cases of mantle cell lymphoma initially treated with non-intensive therapy by the British National Lymphoma Investigation Group. *Br J Haematol* 1997;99:842–847.

62. Yoong Y, Kurtin PJ, Allmer C, et al. Efficacy of splenectomy for patients with mantle cell non-Hodgkin's lymphoma. *Leuk Lymphoma* 2001;42:1235–1241.

63. Stuschke M, Hoederath A, Sack H, et al. Extended field and total central lymphatic radiotherapy in the treatment of early stage lymph node centroblastic-centrocytic lymphomas: results of a prospective multicenter study. Study Group NHL-fruhe Stadien. *Cancer* 1997;80:2273–2284.

64. Zucca E, Fontana S, Roggero E, et al. Treatment and prognosis of centrocytic (mantle cell) lymphoma: a retrospective analysis of twenty-six patients treated in one institution. *Leuk Lymphoma* 1994;13:105–110.

65. Meusers P, Engelhard M, Bartels H, et al. Multicentre randomized therapeutic trial for advanced centrocytic lymphoma: anthracycline does not improve the prognosis. *Hematol Oncol* 1989;7:365–380.

66. Zinzani PL, Magagnoli M, Moretti L, et al. Randomized trial of fludarabine versus fludarabine and idarubicin as frontline treatment in patients with indolent or mantle-cell lymphoma. *J Clin Oncol* 2000;18:773–779.

67. Unterhalt M, Herrmann R, Tiemann M, et al. Prednimustine, mitoxantrone (PmM) vs cyclophosphamide, vincristine, prednisone (COP) for the treatment of advanced low-grade non-Hodgkin's lymphoma. German Low-Grade Lymphoma Study Group. *Leukemia* 1996;10:836–843.

68. Foran JM, Rohatiner AZ, Coiffier B, et al. Multicenter phase II study of fludarabine phosphate for patients with newly diagnosed lymphoplasmacytoid lymphoma, Waldenström's macroglobulinemia, and mantle-cell lymphoma. *J Clin Oncol* 1999;17:546–553.

69. Decaudin D, Bosq J, Tertian G, et al. Phase II trial of fludarabine monophosphate in patients with mantle-cell lymphomas. *J Clin Oncol* 1998;16:579–583.

70. Cohen BJ, Moskowitz C, Straus D, et al. Cyclophosphamide/fludarabine (CF) is active in the treatment of mantle cell lymphoma. *Leuk Lymphoma* 2001;42:1015–1022.

71. Hiddemann W, Dreyling MH, Unterhalt M, et al. Rituximab plus chemotherapy in follicular and mantle cell lymphomas. *Semin Oncol* 2003;30 N1.

72. Rummel M, Chow K, Karakas T, et al. Reduced-dose cladribine (2-CdA) plus mitoxantrone is effective in the treatment of mantle-cell and low-grade non-Hodgkin's lymphoma. *Eur J Cancer* 2002;38:1739.

73. Seymour JF, Grigg AP, Szer J, et al. Cisplatin, fludarabine, and cytarabine: a novel, pharmacologically designed salvage therapy for patients with refractory, histologically aggressive or mantle cell non-Hodgkin's lymphoma. *Cancer* 2002;94:585–593.

74. Touati M, Fitoussi O, Jaccard A, et al. DHAP regimen for relapsed or refractory low grade lymphomas: a study of 86 cases. *Blood* 2002;100:302b.

75. Lefrere F, Delmer A, Suzan F, et al. Sequential chemotherapy by CHOP and DHAP regimens followed by high-dose therapy with stem cell transplantation induces a high rate of complete response and improves event-free survival in mantle cell lymphoma: a prospective study. *Leukemia* 2002;16:587–593.

76. Romaguera JE, Khouri IF, Kantarjian HM, et al. Untreated aggressive mantle cell lymphoma: results with intensive chemotherapy without stem cell transplant in elderly patients. *Leuk Lymphoma* 2000;39:77–85.

77. Morschhauser F, Marit G, Jourdan E, et al. Gemcitabine with dexamethasone +/- cisplatin in patients with relapsing/refractory mantle cell lymphoma. Blood supplement, 44th annual meeting program and abstracts, 2002;100.

78. Teodorovic I, Pittaluga S, Kluin-Nelemans JC, et al. Efficacy of four different regimens in 64 mantle-cell lymphoma cases: clinicopathologic comparison with 498 other non-Hodgkin's lymphoma subtypes. European Organization for the Research and Treatment of Cancer Lymphoma Cooperative Group. *J Clin Oncol* 1995;13:2819–2826.

79. Foran JM, Cunningham D, Coiffier B, et al. Treatment of mantle-cell lymphoma with Rituximab (chimeric monoclonal anti-CD20 antibody): analysis of factors associated with response. *Ann Oncol* 2000;11:117–121.

80. Foran JM, Rohatiner AZ, Cunningham D, et al. European phase II study of rituximab (chimeric anti-CD20 monoclonal antibody) for patients with newly diagnosed mantle-cell lymphoma and previously treated mantle-cell lymphoma, immunocytoma, and small B-cell lymphocytic lymphoma. *J Clin Oncol* 2000;18:317–324.

81. Ghielmini M, Schmitz SF, Burki K, et al. The effect of Rituximab on patients with follicular and mantle-cell lymphoma. Swiss Group for Clinical Cancer Research (SAKK). *Ann Oncol* 2000;11:123–126.

82. Nguyen DT, Amess JA, Doughty H, et al. IDEC-C2B8 anti-CD20 (rituximab) immunotherapy in patients with low-grade non-Hodgkin's lymphoma and lymphoproliferative disorders: evaluation of response on 48 patients. *Eur J Haematol* 1999;62:76–82.

83. Tobinai K. Monoclonal antibody therapy for B-cell lymphoma: clinical trials of an anti-CD20 monoclonal antibody for B-cell lymphoma in Japan. *Int J Hematol* 2002;76:411–419.

84. Howard OM, Gribben JG, Neuberg DS, et al. Rituximab and CHOP induction therapy for newly diagnosed mantle-cell lymphoma: molecular complete responses are not predictive of progression-free survival. *J Clin Oncol* 2002;20:1288–1294.

85. Horwitz SM, Negrin RS, Stockerl-Goldstein KE, et al. Phase II trial of rituximab as adjuvant therapy to high-dose chemotherapy and peripheral blood stem cell transplantation for relapsed and refractory aggressive non-Hodgkin's lymphomas. *Blood* 2001;98:862a.

86. Mangel J, Buckstein R, Imrie K, et al. Immunotherapy with rituximab following high-dose therapy and autologous stem-cell transplantation for mantle cell lymphoma. *Semin Oncol* 2002;29:56–69.

87. Gopal AK, Rajendran JG, Petersdorf SH, et al. High-dose chemoradioimmunotherapy with autologous stem cell support for relapsed mantle cell lymphoma. *Blood* 2002;99:3158–3162.

88. Behr TM, Griesinger F, Riggert J, et al. High-dose myeloablative radioimmunotherapy of mantle cell non-Hodgkin lymphoma with the iodine-131-labeled chimeric anti-CD20 antibody C2B8 and autologous stem cell support. Results of a pilot study. *Cancer* 2002;94:1363–1372.

89. Stewart DA, Vose JM, Weisenburger DD, et al. The role of high-dose therapy and autologous hematopoietic stem cell transplantation for mantle cell lymphoma. *Ann Oncol* 1995;6:263–266.

90. Decaudin D, Brousse N, Brice P, et al. Efficacy of autologous stem cell transplantation in mantle cell lymphoma: a 3-year follow-up study. *Bone Marrow Transplant* 2000;25:251–256.

91. Kroger N, Hoffknecht M, Dreger P, et al. Long-term disease-free survival of patients with advanced mantle-cell lymphoma following high-dose chemotherapy. *Bone Marrow Transplant* 1998;21:55–57.

92. Blay JY, Sebban C, Surbiguet C, et al. High-dose chemotherapy with hematopoietic stem cell transplantation in patients with mantle cell or diffuse centrocytic non-Hodgkin's lymphomas: a single center experience on 18 patients. *Bone Marrow Transplant* 1998;21:51–54.

93. Haas R, Brittinger G, Meusers P, et al. Myeloablative therapy with blood stem cell transplantation is effective in mantle cell lymphoma. *Leukemia* 1996;10:1975–1979.

94. Ketterer N, Salles G, Espinouse D, et al. Intensive therapy with peripheral stem cell transplantation in 16 patients with mantle cell lymphoma. *Ann Oncol* 1997;8:701–704.

95. Freedman AS, Neuberg D, Gribben JG, et al. High-dose chemoradiotherapy and anti-B-cell monoclonal antibody-purged autologous bone marrow transplantation in mantle-cell lymphoma: no evidence for long-term remission. *J Clin Oncol* 1998;16:13–18.

96. Khouri IF, Lee MS, Romaguera J, et al. Allogeneic hematopoietic transplantation for mantle-cell lymphoma: molecular remissions and evidence of graft-versus-malignancy. *Ann Oncol* 1999;10:1293–1299.

97. Milpied N, Gaillard F, Moreau P, et al. High-dose therapy with stem cell transplantation for mantle cell lymphoma: results and prognostic factors, a single center experience. *Bone Marrow Transplant* 1998;22:645–650.

98. Hiddemann W, Dreyling MH, Pfreundschuh M, et al. Myeloablative radiochemotherapy followed by autologous blood stem cell transplantation leads to a significant prolongation of the event-free survival in patients with mantle cell lymphoma (MCL)—results of a prospective randomized European Intergroup study. *Blood* 2001;98.

99. Sweetenham JW. Stem cell transplantation for mantle cell lymphoma: should it ever be used outside clinical trials? *Bone Marrow Transplant* 2001;28:813–820.

100. Andersen NS, Donovan JW, Borus JS, et al. Failure of immunologic purging in mantle cell lymphoma assessed by polymerase chain reaction detection of minimal residual disease. *Blood* 1997;90:4212–4221.

101. Magni M, Di Nicola M, Devizzi L, et al. Successful in vivo purging of CD34-containing peripheral blood harvests in mantle cell and indolent lymphoma: evidence for a role of both chemotherapy and rituximab infusion. *Blood* 2000;96:864–869.

102. Brugger W, Hirsch J, Repp R, et al. Treatment of follicular and mantle cell lymphoma with rituximab after high-dose chemotherapy and autologous blood stem cell transplantation: a multicenter phase II study. *Blood* 2002;100:644a.

103. Kroger N, Hoffknecht M, Kruger W, et al. Allogeneic bone marrow transplantation for refractory mantle cell lymphoma. *Ann Hematol* 2000;79:578–580.

104. Adkins D, Brown R, Goodnough LT, et al. Treatment of resistant mantle cell lymphoma with allogeneic bone marrow transplantation. *Bone Marrow Transplant* 1998;21:97–99.

105. Berdeja JG, Jones RJ, Zahurak ML, et al. Allogeneic bone marrow transplantation in patients with sensitive low-grade lymphoma or mantle cell lymphoma. *Biol Blood Marrow Transplant* 2001;7:561–567.

106. Martinez C, Carreras E, Rovira M, et al. Patients with mantle-cell lymphoma relapsing after autologous stem cell transplantation may be rescued by allogeneic transplantation. *Bone Marrow Transplant* 2000;26:677–679.

107. Corradini P, Ladetto M, Astolfi M, et al. Clinical and molecular remission after allogeneic blood cell transplantation in a patient with mantle-cell lymphoma. *Br J Haematol* 1996;94:376–378.

108. Connors JM, Kouroukis C, Belch A, et al. Flavopiridol for mantle cell lymphoma: moderate activity and frequent disease stabilization. *Blood* 2001;98:807a.

109. Lin TS, Howard OM, Neuberg DS, et al. Seventy-two hour continuous infusion flavopiridol in relapsed and refractory mantle cell lymphoma. *Leuk Lymphoma* 2002;43:793–797.

110. Pham L, Tamayo A, Lo P, et al. Anti-tumor activity of the proteasome inhibitor ps-341 in mantle cell lymphoma B cells. *Blood* 2001;98:465b.

111. Berger F, Felman P, Sonet A, et al. Nonfollicular small B-cell lymphomas: a heterogeneous group of patients with distinct clinical features and outcome. *Blood* 1994;83:2829–2835.

112. Fisher RI, Dahlberg S, Nathwani BN, et al. A clinical analysis of two indolent lymphoma entities: mantle cell lymphoma and marginal zone lymphoma (including the mucosa-associated lymphoid tissue and monocytoid B-cell subcategories): a Southwest Oncology Group study. *Blood* 1995;85:1075–1082.

113. Coiffier B, Haioun C, Ketterer N, et al. Rituximab (anti-CD20 monoclonal antibody) for the treatment of patients with relapsing or refractory aggressive lymphoma: a multicenter phase II study. *Blood* 1998;92:1927–1932.

114. Vose JM, Bierman PJ, Weisenburger DD, et al. Autologous hematopoietic stem cell transplantation for mantle cell lymphoma. *Biol Blood Marrow Transplant* 2000;6:640–645.

CHAPTER 30

Burkitt's Lymphoma

Ian T. Magrath, Hemachandra Venkatesh, and Randy D. Gascoyne

Burkitt's lymphoma has sometimes been called a model tumor, for in spite of its low incidence throughout most of the world, its impact on the understanding and treatment of lymphomas, and doubtless on many other cancers, has been enormous. It was one of the first tumors shown to be curable by chemotherapy alone, thus providing critical support to pioneer chemotherapists. It was the first tumor to be shown to be associated with a virus (Epstein-Barr virus), an association that remains unexplained but that may eventually lead to highly specific targeted therapy. It was also one of the first tumors to be shown to be associated with a nonrandom chromosomal translocation, the first in which antigen receptor gene sequences were involved (now known to be a frequent occurrence in lymphoid neoplasia), and the first in which the consequences of the translocation are quite well understood, being the deregulation of an oncogene, c-myc. It remains possible that this finding, too, may eventually be relevant to targeted therapeutic approaches—indeed, experiments with antisense directed against the c-myc gene have provided at least "proof of principle" in this context. For now, however, the tumor can be cured in a high fraction of cases with intensive conventional chemotherapy—approximately 90% in children and possibly a similar fraction in adults, although more information is needed in the latter, particularly in elderly patients.

Burkitt's lymphoma, like all other lymphoma categories, is probably a family of tumors. It can be defined as a tumor of B-cell origin with a very high growth fraction, composed of uniform, medium-sized cells with a high nuclear to cytoplasmic ratio; relatively open chromatin; multiple nucleoli; basophilic cytoplasm, which usually contains lipid vacuoles; and the presence of a single translocation, which involves an immunoglobulin (Ig) gene locus and results in deregulation of the c-myc gene. Classical Burkitt's lymphoma does not, therefore, contain a 14;18 translocation or express Bcl-2. Morphologically, however, the tumor merges through atypical Burkitt's lymphoma and Burkitt-like lymphoma with diffuse large B-cell lymphoma and may arise *de novo* or in the context of a preexisting, less aggressive lymphoma. The tumor occurs at any age, although its peak incidence is in the first decade of life. It is almost unknown in children younger than the age of 2 years, and although usually considered a tumor of childhood, given that there are more decades of life in adults, the numbers of cases of adults and children are approximately equal at least in affluent countries. The incidence of the tumor varies quite markedly throughout the world, ranging from some one to three per million children in North America and Europe, to some five to ten per million in equatorial Africa. The tumor is sometimes associated with a herpes-type virus, Epstein-Barr virus (i.e., multiple viral genomes are present in the tumor cell nuclei), but the proportion of positive cases varies in different geographic regions and, doubtless, populations, to at least some degree in proportion to the incidence. Thus, in equatorial Africa, where the incidence is highest, quite probably because holoendemic malaria, which causes B-cell hyperplasia, is a co-factor, almost all cases are Epstein-Barr virus associated (a few percent are Epstein-Barr virus negative). In affluent countries, only 10% to 20% are Epstein-Barr virus positive. Burkitt's lymphoma also occurs in the context of human immunodeficiency virus infection, in which approximately 30% are Epstein-Barr virus associated. In addition, the tumor, in this circumstance, is most often associated with a phase of human immunodeficiency virus infection in which the immune system is relatively intact. In Africa, however, there does not appear to be an increased incidence of the disease in the context of human immunodeficiency virus infection. The reason for this remains unknown. Although Burkitt's lymphoma has been described as occurring in other immunodeficiency states, the majority of these tumors are atypical morphologically and, where tested, with respect to molecular characteristics. Thus, although the majority of cases can usually be precisely defined, the "margins" of the disease are, not surprisingly, blurred. It is, perhaps, most clearly defined when it occurs *de novo* in the absence of an underlying immunodeficiency syndrome or other lymphoma. Because it is likely that the spectrum of molecular abnormalities differs when the tumor is secondary to another lymphoma, its behavior and response to therapy may also be somewhat different in these circumstances, although given that the behavior of the disease varies, even when arising *de novo* (it can, for example, present clinically as relatively slow-growing, small-volume disease, or as explosive, widely disseminated tumor), distinction of subtypes on the basis of clinical characteristics in individual cases is difficult. Elucidation of these issues and, perhaps, a clearer definition of the entire family of tumors requires more extensive molecular studies, particularly, for example, microarray analysis of the expression of large numbers of genes from sufficient numbers of cases arising in different clinical or geographic settings.

DISCOVERY OF THE TUMOR

Burkitt's lymphoma was first recognized as a distinct clinicopathologic entity in Africa. The eponymous designation is probably well deserved, however, because Burkitt, a surgeon working in Kampala, Uganda, can certainly be said to have put the tumor "on the map" even though, as is so often the case, others, primarily pathologists, had made similar observations in Africa before Burkitt's classical 1958 paper (1). This tumor, which Burkitt referred to as a *sarcoma*, had a number of different clinical presentations, including jaw tumors and intraabdominal tumors (2–6), and it was the frequent association of the two that led Burkitt to propose that many children with isolated abdominal tumors had the same disease as those who presented with isolated jaw tumors. Unknown to Burkitt, O'Conor and Davies, pathologists also working at Mulago Hospital in Kampala, were at the same time undertaking a survey of the departmental collection of malignant tumors in children and were able to confirm Davies' earlier observation (3) that approximately one half of them were tumors of the "reticulo-endothelial system" (7). Thus, it soon became clear that the tumor recognized clinically by Burkitt was a lymphoma. Burkitt went on to recognize that the "African lymphoma," as it became known, had a high frequency in a broad band across equatorial Africa and that its distribution in Africa was climatically determined (8,9). Haddow, working in the Entebbe Virus Research Institute also in Uganda, found the distribution to be very similar to that of several viral diseases vectored by mosquitoes. This observation prompted Epstein, then working at the Middlesex Hospital in London, to search for virus particles in Burkitt's lymphoma tumor cells and, thus, led directly to the discovery of Epstein-Barr virus, although not in fresh tumor cells but in a tiny fraction of cells in cell lines derived from tumor samples (10). Subsequently, however, it has become clear, given the ubiquitous distribution of Epstein-Barr virus, that the climatic distribution in Africa is not due to the virus association. Most of the evidence supports the hypothesis, originally proposed by Dalldorf (11), that it is holoendemic malaria, which has a similar distribution to other insect-vectored diseases in equatorial Africa, that accounts for the geographic distribution on that continent. The distribution elsewhere has not been demonstrated to be climatically determined.

Subsequent to its discovery in Africa, pathologists who had worked there recognized that tumors with identical histology accounted for a fraction of the lymphomas occurring in children in other world regions (12–14). Initially, there was a general sense that patients with a leukemic presentation, almost unknown in Africa (although bone marrow involvement, in association with other disease sites, occurs in fewer than 10% of patients), had a different disease. However, through recognition that the molecular genetic abnormalities are identical to those with a more typical presentation and response to therapy is optimal with the same kinds of regimens, but not with regimens designed for acute lymphoblastic leukemia, it has become accepted that leukemic presentations [i.e., with bone marrow and peripheral blood involvement and frequently with lymphadenopathy, hepatosplenomegaly, or both of Burkitt's lymphoma (usually referred to as *acute B-cell leukemia* or *ALL-L3* by pediatric oncologists)] occur relatively frequently outside Africa. It has become conventional to refer to the disease as *acute B-cell leukemia* when the fraction of blast cells in the bone marrow is more than 25% (15–21).

DIAGNOSIS AND PATHOLOGY

Morphology

Classical Burkitt's Lymphoma

Virtually all cases of endemic Burkitt's lymphoma, the majority of sporadic Burkitt's lymphoma cases, and many cases of acquired immunodeficiency syndrome–related Burkitt's lymphoma have identical morphologic features described as *classical type* (20–25). The architecture is characteristically diffuse with a distinct starry-sky pattern evident at low-power magnification (Fig. 30.1). The latter feature imparts a "moth-eaten" appearance and is due to the presence of many benign phagocytic histiocytes engulfing the nuclear debris, which results from the apoptotic death of the Burkitt's lymphoma cells. Rare cases with a definite follicular pattern may be seen, but it is not

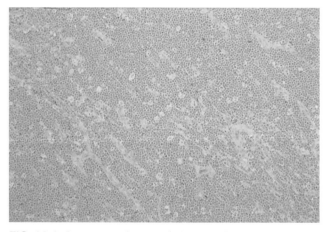

FIG. 30.1. Low-power image of classical Burkitt's lymphoma with prominent starry-sky appearance.

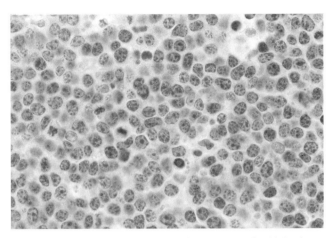

FIG. 30.2. High magnification of classical Burkitt's lymphoma showing the typical cytology of the neoplastic cells. Note the uniform appearance of the cells and the scattered mitotic figures.

possible to distinguish a true follicular growth pattern from colonization of residual benign lymphoid follicles in the majority of these cases (24). The cells are medium-sized with a monotonous and somewhat uniform appearance (Fig. 30.2). The cell size approximates the nuclear size of the macrophages in the same section. A so-called squaring-off of the cytoplasm may be encountered, as the cell borders appear to abut one another (Fig. 30.3) (26). This feature is particularly characteristic when using mercury-based fixatives, such as B5. The nuclear appearance is uniform with round to oval-shaped nuclei. The chromatin is clumped with relatively clear parachromatin and two to five centrally located small basophilic nucleoli. B5 fixation may enhance the visibility of cells with a single, central prominent nucleolus. There is a small amount of deeply basophilic cytoplasm that frequently contains lipid vacuoles (Color Plate 61).

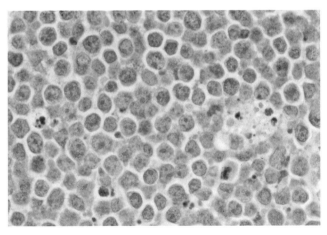

FIG. 30.3. Classical Burkitt's lymphoma at high magnification showing "squaring-off" of the cytoplasm. This feature is most easily seen in thin, formalin-fixed sections. Note the slight nuclear irregularity seen in classical Burkitt's lymphoma at increased magnification.

The latter feature is best seen in imprint preparations of lymph nodes or bone marrow aspirates and, although common, is not a universal finding (26). Multinucleated cells are quite uncommon. The classic diagnostic features of Burkitt's lymphoma are listed in Table 30.1 together with features that distinguish Burkitt's lymphoma from atypical Burkitt's lymphoma and Burkitt-like lymphoma.

Variant Burkitt's Lymphoma with Plasmacytoid Appearance

In the setting of human immunodeficiency virus infection, a variant form of Burkitt's lymphoma may be encountered that shares morphologic features with both classic Burkitt's lymphoma and diffuse large B-cell lymphoma (20–22,27–29). There is slight variation in cell size and shape, imparting a minimal degree of heterogeneity to the sections. The nuclei may be slightly eccentric, and the nucleoli are more often single and central, resembling small plasmacytoid immunoblasts. This appearance of Burkitt's lymphoma has been referred to as the *intermediate form* because it shares morphologic features intermediate between classic Burkitt's lymphoma and diffuse large B-cell lymphoma. Rarely, multinucleated cells may be present.

Atypical Burkitt's Lymphoma and Burkitt-Like Lymphoma

A diagnosis of *atypical Burkitt's lymphoma* is recommended for cases with a high proliferative fraction (Ki-67 or MIB-1 rate approximately 100%) and proven or presumptive evidence of an MYC translocation (19). This diagnosis implies that Burkitt's lymphoma is favored but recognizes the minimally atypical morphology that may occur in some cases (Fig. 30.4). Importantly, many of these atypical morphologic features may have no basis in biology but rather reflect minor artifacts introduced during tissue fixation and processing. These cases are otherwise typical of Burkitt's lymphoma, with expression of CD10, absence of Bcl-2 staining, and cytogenetic or molecular evidence of an MYC translocation without involvement of other common oncogenes (see below) (30). Most published reports that include karyotypic data have shown a diploid DNA content characterized by balanced translocations (31,32).

In the past and up to and including the recent World Health Organization Classification, the terms *atypical Burkitt's lymphoma* and *Burkitt-like lymphoma* have been used interchangeably (19). The term *Burkitt-like lymphoma* in particular has been the subject of much criticism, having been used to describe a heterogeneous group of neoplasms that morphologically resemble Burkitt's lymphoma (small, non-cleaved, non-Burkitt in the Working Formulation, or undifferentiated in the original Rappaport Classification) (25). Not surprisingly, this category of non-Hodgkin's lymphoma has lacked reproducibility and should now be distinguished from atypical Burkitt's lymphoma (33–34).

The term *Burkitt-like lymphoma* has most commonly been reserved for those gray-zone cases that appear to lie somewhere between classical Burkitt's lymphoma and diffuse

TABLE 30.1. *Diagnostic features distinguishing classical Burkitt's lymphoma from atypical Burkitt's lymphoma and Burkitt-like lymphoma*

Feature	Classical Burkitt's lymphoma	Atypical Burkitt's lymphoma	Burkitt-like lymphoma[a]
Architecture	Diffuse	Diffuse, rarely nodular	Diffuse, rarely nodular
Starry-sky pattern	Usually present	May be absent	May be absent
Mitoses	Many	Many	Many
Cytology	Monomorphic	Minimally pleomorphic	Pleomorphic with irregular nuclei
Nuclear shape	Round or oval	Some cells slightly irregular	Usually irregular
Nuclear size	Intermediate	Intermediate, some admixed larger cells	Intermediate, some admixed larger cells
Nucleoli	Multiple (two to five), basophilic	May be single and more prominent	May be single and more prominent
Cytoplasm	Basophilic and often vacuolated; squared-off appearance present	Basophilic; vacuoles may be absent and may lack squared-off appearance	Basophilic; vacuoles may be absent and usually lack squared-off appearance
CD10 expression	++	++	+/–
Bcl-6 expression	++	++	+/–
Bcl-2 expression	–	–	++/–
Cytogenetics	t(8;14) or variant t(2;8) or t(8;22)	t(8;14) or variant t(2;8) or t(8;22)	May lack MYC translocations or have both MYC and BCL2 translocations in the same metaphase
Molecular	MYC rearrangement	MYC rearrangement	+/– MYC; +/– BCL2

–, negative; +, postive.
[a]Burkitt-like lymphoma refers to those cases with overlapping features between classical Burkitt's lymphoma and diffuse large B-cell lymphoma.

large B-cell lymphoma (20,25). In contrast to atypical Burkitt's lymphoma, the traditional use of the category Burkitt-like lymphoma implies that the tumor differs from true Burmkitt's lymphoma. The results of immunophenotypic analyses and molecular cytogenetic studies are frequently different from classical Burkitt's lymphoma (Table 30.1). Typically, the infiltrate is diffuse, but rare cases with a follicular growth pattern are seen. Similar to classical Burkitt's lymphoma, a high mitotic rate and starry-sky pattern are often present. Some admixed large centroblasts are virtually always present, resulting in a morphologic overlap with diffuse large B-cell lymphoma. The cells vary slightly in size and shape and, thus, depart from the usual monotonous appearance of classical Burkitt's lymphoma (33,35). However, this feature is highly dependent on the quality of fixation and processing and, thus, is difficult to apply in routine practice. The Burkitt-like lymphoma variant is more common in adults than children (36). These cases reveal a lower proliferative rate as measured by MIB-1 stains, frequently express Bcl-2 protein, and less commonly express CD10, all of which contrast sharply with either classical or atypical Burkitt's lymphoma (37–39). Cautious interpretation of molecular and cytogenetic data is required, as rare cases of a lymphoma within the category of Burkitt-like lymphoma are characterized by the presence of both BCL2 and MYC translocations in the same cells (40–41). Clues to the correct diagnosis are provided by the recognition of the gray-zone morphology in addition to the immunophenotypic findings that include expression of Bcl-2 protein and a lower proliferative rate. The combination of these findings, molecular evidence for a BCL2 translocation, or both should discourage the pathologist from making a diagnosis of Burkitt's lymphoma.

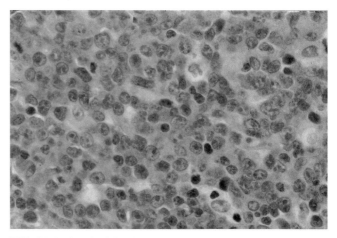

FIG. 30.4. Atypical Burkitt's lymphoma case with prominent starry-sky pattern. The cells have more nuclear irregularity and single central nucleoli than are normally seen in classical Burkitt's lymphoma.

Is MYC Translocation Specific to Burkitt's Lymphoma?

The role of dominant oncogenes can be primary or secondary. A primary role in pathogenesis is exemplified by the function of MYC in Burkitt's lymphoma. Secondary alterations are those that occur in the setting of clonal evolution and often herald a change to a more aggressive phenotype. A typical example is the significant role that the MYC gene plays in the downstream events that characterize clonal evolution in multiple myeloma (42–43). Thus, it is worth remembering that an MYC translocation, although characteristic of classical or atypical Burkitt's lymphoma, is by no means specific. The presence of an MYC translocation is well described in a small fraction of *de novo* diffuse large B-cell lymphoma cases (44–49). In these cases, MYC is believed to be a primary event in pathogenesis. A recent report describes immunophenotypic features that distinguish such cases from Burkitt's lymphoma, including a lower proliferative fraction, expression of Bcl-2 protein, and less frequent coexpression of CD10 (48).

High-grade transformation of follicular lymphoma may involve the acquisition of an MYC translocation as a secondary cytogenetic alteration on a background of t(14;18) (40). The resultant morphology is highly variable, including diffuse large B-cell lymphoma, Burkitt-like lymphoma, and terminal deoxynucleotidyl transferase–positive lymphoblastic lymphoma (50–59). The morphology, immunophenotypic findings, and molecular alterations usually allow distinction from classical/atypical Burkitt's lymphoma. These tumors are usually aggressive and have in the past been included within the rubric of Burkitt-like lymphoma. This category is probably best avoided when referring to cases that result from histologic transformation of preexisting low-grade lymphoma. Perhaps "high-grade transformation of follicular lymphomas, unclassifiable" is a better term. The concomitant presence of the t(14;18) in such cases precludes a diagnosis of classical Burkitt's lymphoma in any setting. Rarely, such cases may present as acute leukemia, typically in adults (60–68). It is important to note that one-half of the patients with dual translocations of BCL2 and MYC may present *de novo*, presumably due to both the t(14;18) and t(8;14) or variant occurring in rapid succession and, therefore, are not associated with a clinically apparent follicular lymphoma (40). In this setting, classification of the tumor may be difficult. Typically, the morphology is not that of classical Burkitt's lymphoma. The cells usually show a moderate to marked degree of nuclear irregularity, and admixed centroblasts are often present. The immunophenotype is not typical of Burkitt's lymphoma as the cells are usually Bcl-2+, may fail to express CD10, and often display a lower proliferation rate (less than 95% Ki-67 or MIB-1 immunostains) (40,48). The cases do not harbor latent Epstein-Barr virus. Molecular studies need to be carefully coordinated to search for the presence of both BCL2 and MYC alterations. Moreover, standard cytogenetic or locus-specific fluorescent *in situ* hybridization techniques may be required, as fully half of these dual-translocation cases have variant MYC translocations that would normally be missed by Southern blot or polymerase chain reaction analysis (69). MYC alterations occurring as secondary events have also been described in mantle cell lymphoma, splenic marginal zone lymphoma, and myeloma (43,70,71).

Immunophenotype

The tumor cells in classical Burkitt's lymphoma and atypical Burkitt's lymphoma variants are mature B cells and, thus, express CD19, CD20, CD22, and CD79a. Usually, the cells express membrane Ig M with light chain restriction (19–22,26,72,73). The cells are frequently positive for both CD10 and Bcl-6, which helps to define Burkitt's lymphoma as a germinal-center cell lymphoma (see Color Plate 62) (74). Burkitt's lymphoma cells are negative for CD5, CD23, cyclin D1, and terminal deoxynucleotidyl transferase. Bcl-2 is characteristically negative, although rare, weakly positive cases may be seen (75). CD21, which represents the receptor for both the C3d component of human complement and Epstein-Barr virus, is commonly expressed on the cell surface of endemic Burkitt's lymphoma. Sporadic Burkitt's lymphoma is typically CD21−, a finding in keeping with the lower incidence of latent Epstein-Barr virus infection in these cases. Cases of human immunodeficiency virus–associated Burkitt's lymphoma with the "intermediate" morphology may be shown to express monotypic intracytoplasmic immunoglobulin (29). Moreover, Burkitt's lymphoma cases in the setting of acquired immunodeficiency syndrome are phenotypically distinct from both diffuse large B-cell lymphoma and immunoblastic lymphomas in human immunodeficiency virus–infected patients (76). Burkitt's lymphoma cases are Bcl-6+ and lack expression of MUM1/IRF4 and CD138 (syndecan). Although they are uniformly LMP-1−, they harbor latent Epstein-Barr virus, as evidenced by postive *in situ* hybridization for Epstein-Barr early region in approximately 30% of cases (29,77).

Atypical Burkitt's lymphoma shares immunophenotypic features with otherwise classical Burkitt's lymphoma, in particular the lack of Bcl-2 expression (19). The less well-defined variant of Burkitt-like lymphoma is more phenotypically heterogeneous. Depending on the series, tumors diagnosed as Burkitt-like lymphoma often express Bcl-2 protein (40,48). They are much more frequently CD10+ and p53+ in comparison to *de novo* diffuse large B-cell lymphoma. They may lack expression of cell adhesion molecules, including CD44 (36), and the proliferative fraction may be lower than in classical Burkitt's lymphoma, as measured by MIB-1 staining. The frequency of expression of many of these markers is affected by the inclusion of cases of Burkitt-like lymphoma with antecedent follicular lymphoma, particularly those cases with dual translocation of both BCL2 and MYC oncogenes (described above).

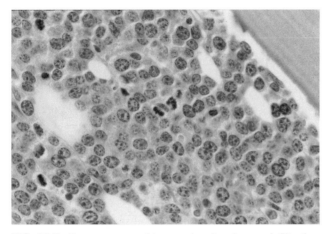

FIG. 30.5. Bone marrow biopsy showing heavy infiltration with Burkitt's lymphoma. The packed bone marrow led to a diagnosis of L3 acute lymphoblastic leukemia.

When Burkitt's lymphoma presents in leukemic form (L3 acute lymphoblastic leukemia), the blast cells nearly always have a mature immunophenotype (there are rare exceptions) and, thus, differ significantly from classic precursor B-cell acute lymphoblastic leukemia (Fig. 30.5) (17–18). The CD45 expression is brighter than typical acute lymphoblastic leukemia; the cells express monotypic immunoglobulin and lack expression of nuclear terminal deoxyribonucleotide transferase.

Burkitt's lymphoma in equatorial Africa (endemic Burkitt's lymphoma) differs from both sporadic Burkitt's lymphoma and acquired immunodeficiency syndrome–related lymphoma with respect to the frequency of latent Epstein-Barr virus infection. Endemic Burkitt's lymphoma demonstrates Epstein-Barr virus with a latency type I pattern—that is, expression of only one of the Epstein-Barr virus nuclear antigens, Epstein-Barr nuclear antigen 1, and none of the latent proteins, known as LMP-1 and -2, in more than 90% of cases (78). Sporadic Burkitt's lymphoma, on the other hand, is Epstein-Barr virus positive in only 5% to 30% of cases (19). Burkitt's lymphoma in most developing countries is Epstein-Barr virus associated (50% to 90% of cases), whereas acquired immunodeficiency syndrome–associated Burkitt's lymphoma reveals the presence of latent Epstein-Barr virus in approximately 25% to 40% of cases (29,77).

Molecular Genetics

That Burkitt's lymphoma cells have a germinal-center cell phenotype is supported not only by its immunophenotype but also by the finding of somatic mutations within the variable-regions of immunoglobulin genes (72,79,80). Similarly, mutations in the 5' noncoding region of the BCL6 gene serve as a molecular marker of transit through the germinal center. These are found in all types of Burkitt's lymphoma, occurring in approximately 37% of cases (81–83). This does not necessarily indicate that the classical chromosomal translocations arise in the germinal

center. Indeed, the latter may arise in immature B lymphoid cells (which are occasionally found in germinal centers). However, it certainly appears that potential Burkitt's lymphoma cells must transit a germinal center or at least undergo programmed expression of set of genes characteristic of germinal-center B cells to become fully transformed.

In 1972, Manolov and Manolova identified a marker chromosome 14, which was subsequently shown by Zech and coworkers (1976) to be a balanced reciprocal translocation between chromosomes 8q24 and 14q32 (84,85). Thus, Burkitt's lymphoma represents the first lymphoma for which a recurrent chromosomal aberration was described. Classical Burkitt's lymphoma demonstrates translocation t(8;14)(q24;q32) in approximately 75% to 80% of the cases or, less frequently, one of its variants, t(8;22)(q24;q11) or t(2;8)(p12;q24) (86,87). Thus, the diagnosis of Burkitt's lymphoma in a case having a clonal karyotype should reveal the presence of one of these MYC translocations; otherwise, an alternative diagnosis should be sought. However, the opposite is not true, as MYC translocations or other alterations involving the MYC locus are seen in a number of different lymphomas, including follicular lymphomas, transformed follicular lymphomas, mantle cell lymphomas, multiple myeloma, diffuse large B-cell lymphoma, and others (described above) (40,43,44,46,70,88,89). In these malignancies, the t(8;14) and variants frequently constitute secondary chromosomal changes, distinguishing them from classical Burkitt's lymphoma in which MYC alterations are considered primary events. Of the published cases of Burkitt-like lymphoma with a clonal karyotype, between 60% and 80% have been shown to carry translocations with breakpoints in 8q24 (36,40). These series, however, contain cases that other pathologists designate as atypical Burkitt's lymphoma. Burkitt-like lymphoma cases defined using more stringent criteria often fail to show evidence of molecular abnormalities in MYC (35) but do show the presence of BCL2 translocations, either alone or with an MYC translocation. Clearly, morphologic criteria alone are unsatisfactory for making the subtle distinctions between atypical Burkitt's lymphoma and Burkitt-like lymphoma. When MYC alterations are present in Burkitt-like lymphoma, they are similar to those in classical Burkitt's lymphoma; the translocation partners involve the usual immunoglobulin locus sites, including 14q32, 2p12, and 22q11. However, increasing numbers of reports of variant translocations and cryptic alterations of MYC highlight the complexity of mechanisms that affect the MYC locus (90–92). Moreover, the growing awareness of the role of MYC alterations in the clonal evolution of multiple myeloma has expanded the role of this dominant oncogene (42,43). Being a critical gene in the regulation of cell replication, survival, and viability, this broader role is perhaps not surprising, nor are the observations that additional mechanisms of MYC deregulation have recently been described and that the spectrum of diseases associated with this molecular alteration is continuing to expand.

At the molecular level, the t(8;14) and variants juxtapose the MYC gene located at chromosome region 8q24 next to one of the Ig gene loci, namely the Ig heavy chain (IgH) locus at

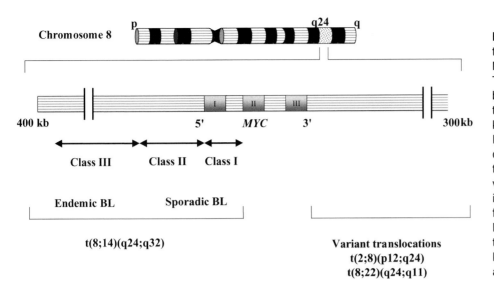

FIG. 30.6. The schematic shows the molecular structure of the MYC locus on chromosome 8q24. The location of class I, II, and III breakpoints and their relationship to either sporadic or endemic Burkitt's lymphoma is depicted. Class III breakpoints can occur at some distance from the coding exons of the MYC gene. The location of the variant translocation breakpoints is also shown, emphasizing that for both t(2;8) and t(8;22), the MYC gene remains on the derivative chromosome 8, with either kappa or lambda sequences lying adjacent.

chromosome region 14q32, the Ig κ (IgK) locus in 2p12 or the Ig λ (IgL) locus in 22q11. As a result of these translocations involving the immunoglobulin loci, the normal control mechanisms of MYC expression are disrupted, leading to constitutive expression of the protein throughout the cell cycle. MYC encodes a transcription factor that can function both as transcriptional activator and transcriptional repressor capable of inducing apoptosis as well as proliferation (86,87,93).

The molecular breakpoints within the MYC locus at 8q24 depend on the translocation partners and show considerable interindividual variation (94–96) (Fig. 30.6). In the case of classical t(8;14), the breakpoints in 8q24 typically lie within the centromeric (5') part of the MYC locus (Table 30.2). These have been classified according to the position of the chromosomal breakpoints relative to the MYC gene. Translocations with breakpoints in the first (5') exon or intron of MYC (but not disruptive of the protein coding region) have been designated as class I, those with breakpoints immediately upstream of the gene as class II, and those with distant breakpoints as class III. In sporadic and immunodeficiency-associated Burkitt's lym-

phoma, class I (and II) translocations predominate, whereas in endemic (African) Burkitt's lymphoma cases, class III translocations with breakpoints dispersed over approximately 300 kb upstream of the gene are most frequent (86,87,97–99). The t(8;14), thus, leads to activation of MYC on the der(14) chromosome containing the intact coding region of the gene. The breakpoints in the IgH locus at 14q32 more often occur 5' of the intron enhancer in a joining (J) or diversity (D) segment in Burkitt's lymphoma, but breakpoints 3' of the intron enhancer in the switch μ region, which are rare in endemic Burkitt's lymphoma, occur more often in sporadic and human immunodeficiency virus–associated Burkitt's lymphoma. The breakpoints suggest that these translocations occur during an aberrant variable-diversity-joining (VDJ) or class-switch recombination process, respectively (86,87,97). There is also evidence that Burkitt translocations might be the result of a misdirected somatic mutation (100). Somatic and, in part, ongoing V_H mutations have been observed in some cases of Burkitt's lymphoma. Similarly, mutations of the MYC gene are very frequent, particularly in endemic Burkitt's lymphoma carrying t(8;14),

TABLE 30.2. *Characteristic genetic features of Burkitt's lymphoma (BL)*

Feature	Endemic BL	Sporadic BL	Acquired immunodeficiency syndrome–associated BL
Usual class of MYC breakpoint	Class III	Classes I and II	Class I
Predominant MYC breakpoint site	Centromeric (5') of MYC	Within the first exon or intron of MYC, or centromeric of MYC (class II)	Within the first exon or intron of MYC
Predominant IGH breakpoint in t(8;14)(q24;q32)	VDJ region, 80%; switch region, 20%	VDJ, 70%; switch region, 30%	Switch region
Somatic IGH mutations	Yes	Yes	Yes
BCL6 mutations	Yes	Yes	Yes

IGH, immunoglobulin heavy chain; VDJ, variable-diversity-joining.

presumably due to somatic hypermutation driven by the immunoglobulin sequences juxtaposed to the MYC locus on the derivative chromosome 14 (100–105). Such mutations can alter MYC transcription or influence phosphorylation, stability, and activity of the protein (87–89). They frequently cluster near the 3' boundary of the first MYC exon. A surrogate marker for the presence of these mutations is the status of the hypermutable PvuII site in the first exon of the MYC gene (89,104,106).

In contrast to the classical Burkitt translocation t(8;14), both variant translocations t(2;8) and t(8;22) lead to deregulation of MYC on the derivative chromosome 8 caused by juxtaposition of the translocated IgK and IgL genes, respectively. The chromosome 8 breakpoints of these variants are located 3' of MYC and can be dispersed over a region up to 300 kb telomeric of the MYC gene (96). The breaks on chromosomes 2 and 22 usually occur 5' of the IgK and IgL gene constant region segments, respectively (86,87).

To establish a confident diagnosis of a Burkitt's lymphoma, the detection of a Burkitt translocation should be sought. Conventional cytogenetic analysis using chromosomal banding techniques still has to be considered the gold standard for the analysis of Burkitt's lymphoma. In addition to the detection of the diagnostic translocations, cytogenetic analyses can identify variant MYC translocations involving non-Ig-loci as well as other characteristic primary chromosomal aberrations that may indicate an aggressive transformation of a variety of different underlying low-grade non-Hodgkin's lymphomas. Chromosomal banding analysis and spectral karyotyping are the only techniques that provide a complete genomic overview of balanced and unbalanced secondary changes (31,32). Molecular methods, such as the Southern blot or polymerase chain reaction–based approaches, have been used for the diagnosis of Burkitt-associated MYC alterations but suffer from the requirement for fresh or cryopreserved material as well as from the widely dispersed breakpoints over several hundred kilobases for both MYC and Ig loci. For example, alterations of MYC occurring as secondary events in follicular lymphomas often involve the light chain gene. Such alterations are more difficult to detect using the Southern blot or, polymerase chain reaction approach. (50,69). This molecular variability requires the application of multiple probes or sequence-specific primers that render Southern blot and polymerase chain reaction analysis time-consuming and expensive. Nevertheless, long-distance polymerase chain reaction techniques using various sets of primers have been described to reliably detect Ig-MYC junctions in classical and variant Burkitt translocations (91). Perhaps the best technique currently available for the routine detection of the Burkitt translocation is interphase fluorescent *in situ* hybridization, which can be applied to virtually every type of tissue (108–116). In principle, two different types of fluorescent *in situ* hybridization assays have been developed for use in Burkitt's lymphoma, including break-apart and colocalization assays. Break-apart assays are, on the whole, more robust and are likely to become the new gold standard for the molecular analysis of most oncogene alterations. It is important to note that interphase fluorescent *in situ* hybridization approaches can now be combined in assays that detect the immunophenotype, referred to as *multicolor-FICTION* (114,115). These will undoubtedly prove to be powerful techniques for the *in situ* analyses of genetic alterations in single cells.

Pathogenetic Mechanisms

The hallmark translocations involving MYC and immunoglobulin genes, coupled to experimental data indicating that c-Myc expression can be induced by juxtaposed enhancer elements from immunoglobulin loci (117,118), leave no doubt that the translocations are a central element of Burkitt's lymphoma pathogenesis. However, because abnormal expression of c-Myc normally results in diversion of the cell to an apoptotic pathway, it appears that the translocations need to be associated with lesions that simultaneously inhibit apoptosis. Such lesions have been described in Burkitt's lymphoma, in which the Fas pathway is frequently abrogated, and mutations in the proapoptotic protein bax have been described (119,120) [although it must be pointed out that abrogation of specific pathways does not prevent the induction of apoptosis via others (119)—which may be relevant to treatment]. In addition to lesions in EBV-associated apoptotic genes, however, another potential means whereby Burkitt's lymphoma cells may avoid apoptosis is through the expression of viral genes. In this respect, recent reports that the Epstein-Barr virus Epstein-Barr early region small-molecular-weight RNA, highly expressed in Epstein-Barr virus–associated Burkitt's lymphoma, can protect against apoptosis are of considerable interest, although it also remains possible that this molecule may be relevant to pathogenesis in other ways (121–123). Although the pattern of Epstein-Barr virus protein expression is restricted in Burkitt's lymphoma, it is possible that before full malignant transformation, other viral proteins are expressed that inhibit apoptosis (either directly or via upregulation of Bcl2), as occurs when B cells are transformed by Epstein-Barr virus when the full range of Epstein-Barr nuclear antigens and latent membrane proteins are expressed (a so-called latency III pattern). These proteins, with the exception of Epstein-Barr nuclear antigen 1, are highly immunogenic, and their expression in Burkitt's lymphoma would lead to an immune reaction against the tumor cells. It is likely that they are expressed *in vivo* only in privileged sites, such as germinal centers where cytotoxic T cells are essentially absent. Recently, evidence supporting the possibility that Burkitt's lymphoma evolves from Epstein-Barr virus–transformed cells expressing a latency III pattern has been provided by the observation of Burkitt's lymphomas in which Epstein-Barr nuclear antigen 2 has been deleted. Such cells also fail to express the latent membrane proteins that are regulated by Epstein-Barr nuclear antigen 2 (124). It is interesting to note that the expression of Epstein-Barr nuclear antigen 2, although necessary for the transformation of B cells, antagonizes c-Myc and appears to have a negative impact on the growth of Burkitt's lymphoma cells (125,126). This may be because Epstein-Barr nuclear antigen 2 inhibits c-Myc expression via its ability to inhibit the immunoglobulin μ gene, which, by virtue of the t(8;14), regulates MYC in Burkitt's lymphoma (127). But Burkitt's lymphoma cells lack immunogenicity for other reasons; in particular, the peptide transporters are inactive, and there is reduced HLA class I protein expression such that there is an inability to present endogenously expressed Epstein-Barr virus–latent proteins to cytotoxic T cells. Although Epstein-Barr nuclear antigen 1 is not immunogenic, a small number of additional proteins expressed in latency I are, such that this mechanism of reducing immunogenicity from virally derived proteins is critically important to the survival of Burkitt's lymphoma cells. It is interesting to note that all of these characteristics can be produced in lymphoblastoid cell lines transformed by Epstein-Barr virus simply by over-expressing c-Myc (128), suggesting that the oncogene does more than simply drive cell proliferation.

The mechanism whereby the latency switch (type III to type I)—if, indeed, it does occur—is accomplished as cells undergo progressive transformation remains unknown. It is not due to over-expression of c-Myc (129) but could, instead, result from a mechanism operative when normal B cells infected by Epstein-Barr virus leave the germinal center; peripheral memory cells that contain Epstein-Barr virus express a latency I pattern, suggesting the existence of such a mechanism. A latency switching mechanism may be critical to Epstein-Barr virus's survival strategy in the host, because cells expressing the highly immunogenic latency III pattern of viral proteins are immediately eliminated by Epstein-Barr virus antigen-specific cytotoxic T cells (without this mechanism, Epstein-Barr virus infection might always result, eventually, in massive B-cell proliferation and death of the host). Although c-Myc cannot induce a latency I pattern, it is able to replace the growth-stimulating effects of Epstein-Barr nuclear antigen 2 (130) such that the Burkitt's lymphoma cells are independent of the need for expression of Epstein-Barr nuclear antigen 2 and the latent membrane proteins.

In the normal germinal center, the drive to proliferation is antigen. Recent gene expression profiling data suggest that the naive B cells become centroblasts through a proliferation program that does not include c-Myc expression (131). Such cells are primed to undergo apoptosis in the absence of antigen stimulation. Thus, if the transcriptional data reflect the protein data (which remains open to question) (132), even modest levels of c-Myc expression induced by the MYC translocation are clearly abnormal for germinal center cells, and c-Myc alone may not be sufficient to rescue them from apoptosis—in fact, its abnormal expression is more likely to drive the cell into an apoptotic pathway. Epstein-Barr virus, through its ability to mimic antigen stimulation and CD40 binding (through the latent membrane proteins) is able to prevent apoptosis and presumably permit the cell to exit the germinal center and become a memory cell, thus ensuring its own survival in the host.

Taken together, these findings suggest that EBV+ Burkitt's lymphoma arises from a B cell that has been transformed by Epstein-Barr virus and that first expresses a latency III pattern, perhaps in the context of a germinal center. Because the latency III pattern is incompatible with the survival of Burkitt's lymphoma cells in an immunologically normal host (such proteins

often are expressed in Epstein-Barr virus–containing lymphomas in immunodeficient hosts), the c-Myc expression, brought about by the MYC chromosomal translocations, is necessary before exit from the germinal center, both to replace the normal transforming but immunogenic Epstein-Barr virus proteins, thereby ensuring continued proliferation, and to reduce the immunogenicity of the tumor cells. A latency I pattern further contributes to the reduced immunogenicity and also avoids inhibition of expression of the translocated c-Myc gene by Epstein-Barr nuclear antigen 2. The recent demonstration that c-Myc can enhance the expression of the potentially antiapoptotic Epstein-Barr early region RNAs (133) supports, if indirectly, the notion that Epstein-Barr early region expression is relevant to Burkitt's lymphoma transformation.

Given the probable cooperation between Epstein-Barr virus and the MYC translocation in the pathogenesis of Burkitt's lymphoma, it seems likely that individuals carrying more Epstein-Barr virus–transformed lymphocytes and perhaps releasing more virus capable of transforming other cells would be at greater risk of developing Burkitt's lymphoma. This is entirely consistent with the observation of Geser and de Thé that individuals with higher antiviral capsid antigen in Africa are at higher risk for the development of Burkitt's lymphoma (134) and with the finding that acute malaria is associated with an increased number of circulating Epstein-Barr virus–containing cells (as is human immunodeficiency virus infection) (135). Malaria may also increase the risk of the development of Burkitt's lymphoma in Africa through its ability to cause B-cell hyperplasia and potentially, therefore, increase the likelihood that a chromosomal translocation will occur.

This hypothesis, constructed on the basis of available information, is also entirely consistent with the markedly increased incidence of Burkitt's lymphoma in equatorial Africa, where Epstein-Barr virus infection occurs at a very early age, and malaria is holoendemic. Epstein-Barr virus–negative Burkitt's lymphoma may well use similar pathways but is much less likely to occur, because the role played by Epstein-Barr virus must be subserved by, presumably, a series of genetic events. It is not known whether the differences in clinical behavior between endemic Burkitt's lymphoma and Burkitt's lymphoma in other world regions (see below) are a consequence of differences in the molecular abnormalities present in the tumor, differences in the host, or both.

CLINICAL FEATURES

The clinical features of Burkitt's lymphoma overlap throughout the world, but differences, particularly with respect to the frequency of involvement of various sites in equatorial African cases versus cases elsewhere, can be readily discerned. Thus, jaw tumors are present in perhaps 50% to 70% of patients in equatorial Africa, and most patients have multiple-quadrant involvement. Jaw tumors in African patients are age associated; whereas almost all young children of 3 years of age have jaw or orbital tumor, or both, only 25% of patients older than the age of 16 years have jaw tumors. In the endemic region of Africa itself, the percentage of patients with jaw tumors appears to be inversely proportional to the incidence of the disease. In addition, the median age of patients tends to be higher in lower incidence areas, such as highlands or arid regions (136). Jaw involvement in sporadic Burkitt's lymphoma, in contrast to endemic Burkitt's lymphoma, occurs in a small percentage of patients at presentation (less than 10% in most series) and is not age related (137). Such patients frequently have involvement of other bony sites or of the bone marrow, suggesting that jaw involvement arises for quite different pathobiologic reasons than in African patients (138). A higher percentage of patients with jaw tumors than is the case in the United States and Europe has been reported in some Asian countries, South Africa (where both whites and nonwhites appear to have as high a frequency of jaw tumors as in the endemic form of the disease), Turkey, Japan, and equatorial Brazil (15,139–144).

Between 50% and 90% of patients with Burkitt's lymphoma throughout the world present with abdominal tumor, which gives rise to abdominal pain or swelling, sometimes with a symptom complex caused by intussusception, a change in bowel habits, nausea and vomiting, evidence of gastrointestinal bleeding, or, rarely, intestinal perforation (15,144–149). Presentation with a right iliac fossa mass is quite frequent outside Africa, occurring in perhaps 25% of patients (150), and can be confused with an inflammatory appendiceal mass. Such presentations are uncommon, however, in the endemic form of disease. Frequently at surgery, there are multiple enlarged mesenteric lymph nodes that may or may not contain microscopically visible tumor, and multiple peritoneal plaques of tumor may be observed. Involvement of retroperitoneal structures, including kidneys and pancreas, is second only to bowel and mesentery involvement, whereas liver and particularly splenic involvement are seen somewhat less frequently. Ovarian involvement is frequent in females. Pleural effusions and ascites, which nearly always contain Burkitt's lymphoma cells, and bone involvement, not infrequently multiple, are common, and pharyngeal or nasopharyngeal sites of disease, as well as paranasal sinus involvement, are all occasionally seen. Thyroid and salivary gland involvement are not common in endemic patients although occasionally observed, appear to be less common outside Africa. Adrenal gland involvement is occasionally seen. Isolated lymphadenopathy, tonsillar (or any form of pharyngeal tumor), splenic and testicular involvement are all rare in African Burkitt's lymphoma and somewhat more common in other world regions. Breast involvement, regardless of geography, occurs almost exclusively in pubertal girls or lactating women (151–154). Unusual presentations of Burkitt's lymphoma include isolated tonsillar (uni- or bilateral) involvement, sometimes only recognized after tonsillectomy for presumptive tonsillitis, and isolated cervical adenopathy.

Bone marrow involvement is perhaps more common in sporadic Burkitt's lymphoma than had previously been believed. At presentation, marrow involvement occurs in some 20% of patients (155). As already mentioned, some patients present with a clinical syndrome consistent with leukemia without any solid lymphomatous masses apart from lymphadenopathy and hepatosplenomegaly. Interestingly, bone marrow involvement often appears to occur with lower frequency in several series from outside the United States or Europe, as is the case in equatorial Africa (156–158). It is not clear whether this is truly because of the low frequency of bone marrow involvement in these geographic regions or because some patients with bone marrow involvement (e.g., those with a leukemic blood picture) were excluded from these series.

Central nervous system disease, either cerebrospinal fluid pleocytosis or cranial nerve palsies, is much more frequently observed in endemic Burkitt's lymphoma than in the sporadic variety, occurring in approximately one third of patients at presentation in one Ugandan series. Any cranial nerve can be involved, but the ophthalmic nerves and the facial nerve are more often affected (142,159). Very rarely, cranial nerve involvement and cerebrospinal fluid pleocytosis have been the sole sites of disease (160), and peripheral neuropathy is occasionally seen (161). Also rare, even in the presence of other cranial neuropathies, the optic nerve may be infiltrated, giving rise to blindness. In Uganda, approximately 15% of patients present with isolated epidural lymphoma and paraplegia, requiring laminectomy for diagnosis (142,159). Intracerebral disease has been described but is usually diagnosed only at recurrence (162). In sporadic patients, intracranial disease is not infrequently extradural (163). When central nervous system disease occurs in sporadic patients, it is usually associated with bone marrow involvement (approximately two thirds of patients with marrow disease have central nervous system disease) or with multiple other bony sites of disease. It may consist of cerebrospinal fluid pleocytosis or cranial nerve palsies. Compression of the inferior alveolar nerve as it passes through the mandible with numbness of the lip and chin occurs quite frequently in patients with widespread bone marrow disease, and this, as with compression of cranial nerves by orbital tumor, is not a sign of central nervous system involvement, although such

TABLE 30.3. *Disease sites at presentation in endemic and sporadic Burkitt's lymphoma*

Site	Patients with involvement (%)	
	Endemic	Sporadic
Abdomen	58	91
Pleural effusion	3	19
Bone marrow	7	20
Peripheral nodes	9	13
Bone	8	9
Central nervous system	19	14
Paraspinal	17	2
Testis	2	6
Pharynx	0	10
Jaw	58	7
Orbit	11	1

patients are at high risk to develop central nervous system disease. Occasionally, it can be the sole presenting sign (165).

A comparison of sites of disease at presentation in endemic (Ugandan) and sporadic (U.S.) Burkitt's lymphoma is shown in Table 30.3. In addition to the differences in jaw involvement, there are striking differences in the frequency of involvement of the bone marrow (higher in sporadic); central nervous system, including spinal epidural disease (higher in endemic); and other sites including, it is interesting to note, those involved in mucosa-associated lymphoid tissue lymphomas, such as the thyroid and salivary glands.

STAGING

Staging provides a short-hand categorization of patients into different risk groups defined largely on the basis of extent of disease. Lactate dehydrogenase levels correlate well with stage (as do anti–Epstein-Barr virus early antigen titers in equatorial African patients) (164). The most widely used staging system in children and young adults, the St. Jude system, is shown in Table 30.4. This staging system works perfectly well for adults, but the more usual system is the Ann Arbor system. This suffers from the fact that it was originally used for staging patients with Hodgkin's disease, which is primarily a nodal lymphoma. Burkitt's lymphoma is largely extranodal (Burkitt-like lymphoma tends to more often involve nodes but is also frequently extrano-

TABLE 30.4. *St. Jude staging system for childhood non-Hodgkin's lymphoma*

Stage	Definition
I	Single tumor (extranodal), excluding mediastinum or abdomen
	Single anatomic area (nodal)
II	Single tumor (extranodal) with regional node involvement
	Primary gastrointestinal tumor with or without involvement of associated mesenteric nodes only, grossly completely resected
	On same side of diaphragm
	a. Two or more nodal areas
	b. Two single (extranodal) tumors with or without regional node involvement
III	On both sides of the diaphragm
	a. Two single tumors (extranodal)
	b. Two or more nodal areas
	All primary intrathoracic tumors (mediastinal, pleural thymic)
	All extensive primary intraabdominal disease
	All primary paraspinal or epidural tumors regardless of other sites
IV[a]	Any of the above with initial central nervous system or bone marrow involvement

[a]Patients with more than 25% of tumor cells in the bone marrow are generally referred to as having acute B-cell leukemia.

dal) such that this staging scheme does not work well in dividing patients into risk groups.

GENERAL PRINCIPLES OF CHEMOTHERAPY OF BURKITT'S LYMPHOMA AND BURKITT-LIKE LYMPHOMA

Progress in the treatment of Burkitt's lymphoma and Burkitt-like lymphoma in both children and adults in the last three decades has been dramatic, with long-term remission rates having improved from approximately 25% to 80% to 90% (with the most effective protocols) since the 1960s. This success was accomplished through a series of improvements in the multi-agent chemotherapy regimens used in children and by adopting similar approaches in adults (at least up to the age of 60 years). Independent, simultaneous efforts were made by Berlin-Frankfurt-Münster (BFM), Societé Française d'Oncologie Pediatrique (SFOP), the U.S. National Cancer Institute (NCI), and cooperative group investigators (166–179) who improved on the initial successes achieved in African patients in the 1960s (142,180–185). Clinical trials at the NCI in the last three decades have shown that it is possible to achieve the same degree of success in children and adult patients with Burkitt's lymphoma and Burkitt-like lymphoma by using identical regimens (167–169). Applying the same chemotherapy regimens to the treatment of children with diffuse large B-cell lymphoma has been so successful that most pediatric oncologists use the same regimen to treat all aggressive B-cell lymphomas in children. However, in adult patients with diffuse large B-cell lymphoma the same regimens that have been successfully used in Burkitt's and Burkitt-like lymphoma have not been adequately tested. Although it is probable that diffuse large B-cell lymphoma in children represents a somewhat different spectrum of diseases than diffuse large B-cell lymphoma in adults, it still seems worth applying the principles learned in children with B-cell lymphomas to adults because at least a subfraction, perhaps identifiable with modern gene expression studies or even simply Ki-67 or MIB1 expression (high expression of which is associated with a poor prognosis in diffuse large B-cell lymphoma in adults), may do as well or almost as well as children. This approach is being adopted by the United Kingdom Lymphoma Group, which achieved very good results in adults with Burkitt's lymphoma using an NCI protocol and is now exploring the value of this regimen in diffuse large B-cell lymphoma with high Ki-67 expression (186).

An analysis of the Burkitt's lymphoma regimens tested in the last 30 years shows that the following strategies played a crucial role in improving the long-term outlook for these patients: (a) dose intensity; (b) the addition of high-dose methotrexate and high-dose Ara-C, which are both active in central nervous system and systemic disease; (c) the inclusion of additional agents, such as etoposide and possibly ifosfamide; (d) central nervous system prophylactic therapy and central nervous system–directed therapy; (e) risk stratification and risk-adapted therapy; (f) exclusion of radiotherapy; (g) short-duration regimens; and (h) prompt initiation of successful treatment cycles as soon as the bone marrow recovers (neutrophil count, 500 to 1,000 per mm^3; platelet count, 50,000 per mm^3 or more).

Dose Intensity

Maintaining an appropriate dose intensity based on the risk category is an important component of effective therapy. Most of the modern chemotherapy regimens are dose intensive and of short duration. Several studies have clearly shown that there is no benefit to long-duration treatment regimens (168,169,175,177–179). This remains true for patients with high-risk or extensive disease, including patients with leukemic presentation.

High-Dose Methotrexate and High-Dose Ara-C

The BFM, SFOP, and NCI regimens have been very effective in Burkitt's lymphoma, and all three regimens have given significant emphasis to high-dose methotrexate and high-dose Ara-C, which were first evaluated in patients with recurrent disease (187–189). In BFM trials, simply increasing the dose of methotrexate from 500 to 5,000 mg/m^2 for patients with stage III abdominal disease and lactate dehydrogenase levels greater than 500 resulted in an increase in event-free survival from 43% to 81%, whereas for patients with leukemic presentation, event-free survival improved from 50% to 78% (179). High-dose Ara-C is an important component of all these protocols for high-risk patients. At the NCI, addition of high-dose Ara-C along with etoposide and ifosfamide improved the survival rate in high-risk patients from less than 20% to approximately 80% (169).

Additional Agents

Good responses to ifosfamide and etoposide have been shown in relapse and refractory settings, even in patients previously treated with high cumulative doses of cyclophosphamide (190,191). The incorporation of these two drugs, along with Ara-C, into early primary treatment at the NCI resulted in two major gains. First, there was a dramatic improvement in the survival of high-risk patients; second, the number of cycles of chemotherapy for these patients was reduced from 15 to 4 with an improved outcome (168,169). Alternating noncross-resistant regimens appear, therefore, able to prevent the emergence of drug-resistant clones, which is crucial to a successful outcome. Although there is no direct information that can be brought to bear on the issue, it may also be critical to use these drugs early in treatment rather than later as consolidation therapy because resistant clones might, by then, have already emerged.

Central Nervous System Prophylaxis and Therapy

Central nervous system involvement in Burkitt's lymphoma is a poor prognostic feature; survival for patients with central nervous system involvement in the United States and Europe was extremely poor when only intrathecal chemotherapy and radiation were used to treat central nervous system disease (174,175).

The addition of high-dose methotrexate and Ara-C along with intrathecal chemotherapy has improved the results from approximately 20% to 75% to 80%. High-dose methotrexate and Ara-C, being active in both systemic and central nervous system disease, are likely to play a major role in improving the outcome of patients with central nervous system involvement or of patients who have a high risk for central nervous system relapse.

Risk Stratification and Risk-Adapted Therapy

The dramatically different survival rates of children with limited and advanced disease were most obvious when therapy was still relatively unintensive (150,167,170). Thus, patients with more limited disease have continued to receive less intensive therapy, which is sufficient to produce a high survival rate in this group of patients (171,172,178), whereas patients with more advanced disease, in successive trials, received progressively increasing intensity of therapy (169,175,177,178). Today, stratification by risk permits patients to be separated into different prognostic categories so that each group of patients can receive the appropriate dose and combination of drugs (168,174,179). This strategy has been a very important part of all pediatric studies. BFM protocols now recognize four different risk categories, and the treatment is tailored to each of these risk groups so that treatment toxicity is minimized for low-risk patients and more toxic and efficacious therapy used only in patients with higher-risk disease. Appropriate risk stratification must take into consideration various prognostic features in addition to stage of disease. For example, in BFM protocols, patients with stage III abdominal disease are divided into two subgroups based on lactate dehydrogenase levels of more than or less than 500. The BFM group has clearly shown that these two groups of stage III patients have a big difference in their outcome when treated with a low-dose methotrexate regimen (179). Risk stratification has not been used in many of the adult protocols, except for those in which a regimen developed in childhood Burkitt's lymphoma has been used without modification (17,167,168). Risk stratification must clearly be a component of any effective modern chemotherapy regimen.

The results of NCI, SFOP, and BFM protocols in which the principle of risk stratification is used to demonstrate that excellent results can be achieved regardless of the extent of disease, although the intensity of therapy varies for patients in different groups (Tables 30.5 through 30.10). In particular, the SFOP's LMB 89 and the German BFM 90 protocols have been used in more than 1,000 patients with event-free survival rates ranging from 76% in patients with the most extensive disease (leukemic patients) treated on BFM 90 to 98% for stage II patients treated on this same protocol. However there are no statistically significant differences in event-free survival among any of the groups, with an average event-free survival at several years of approximately 90% (172,178) (Table 30.11). More recent protocols from these groups are producing similar, if not better, results. Comparable results have been obtained by the NCI protocol 89-C-41 (Table 30.11), but the number of patients accrued is much smaller (168,169). In these protocols, the significance of prog-

TABLE 30.5. *Definitions of therapy arms for Burkitt's lymphoma and large B-cell lymphoma in Berlin-Frankfurt-Münster protocol NHL-BFM 95*

Risk group	Definition
1	Complete surgical resection
2	Incomplete surgical resection
	Stages I and II
	Stage III and LDH <500 U/L
3	Incomplete surgical resection
	Stage III and LDH 500–999 U/L
	Stage IV or B-cell leukemia and LDH <1000 U/L; CNS negative
4	Incomplete surgical resection
	Stage III and LDH >999 U/L
	Stage IV or B-cell leukemia and LDH >999 U/L ± CNS

CNS, central nervous system; LDH, lactate dehydrogenase.

nostic factors has largely been lost. Even patients with stage IV disease (bone marrow disease, central nervous system disease, or both) do not have a significantly worse prognosis, although central nervous system disease in some studies, although now not connoting a poor prognosis, may be associated with a worse outcome (173). Thus, at this point, the major questions to be asked in the treatment of these diseases are whether equally good results can be achieved with less toxicity and whether further improvements in risk stratification can be made. In addition to the potential to further limit therapy when this can be accomplished without detriment, there is also the possibility that further therapeutic modifications in the regimens for patients at exceptionally high risk may increase survival rates.

Exclusion of Local Radiotherapy

Although radiation has been used in the past, at least by some investigators, for central nervous system prophylaxis, central nervous system therapy, consolidation treatment at sites of bulk disease, or in spinal cord compression, in the last three decades it has become clear that radiation has essentially no role in the

TABLE 30.6. *Definitions of therapy groups in French-American-British protocol LMB 96 for B-cell lymphomas*

Therapy group	Definition
A	Complete surgical resection stage I or abdominal stage II
B	All patients not eligible for Group A or C
C	Any central nervous system[a] involvement or bone marrow involvement ≥25% blasts

[a]Central nervous system involvement is defined as any blasts in cerebrospinal fluid; cranial nerve palsies not explained by extracranial tumor; clinical spinal cord compression; isolated intracerebral mass; parameningeal extension, cranial or spinal.

TABLE 30.7. *Definitions of therapy groups in NCI protocol 89-C-41 for B-cell lymphomas*

Therapy group	Definition
Low-risk patients	Stage I or II and lactate dehydrogenase <150% of normal
High-risk patients	All other patients

therapy of Burkitt's lymphoma. Indeed, early studies in Africa with standard fractions of radiation demonstrated the poor response of irradiated tumors (192). A randomized clinical trial has shown that there is no benefit to adding radiation therapy in limited-stage disease (193), and although not formally studied, patients with central nervous system disease, bulky sites, and even testicular disease no longer receive radiation without detriment (169,173,179,194,195). On the other hand, combined modality therapy causes more acute, as well as long-term, complications, including acute and late neurologic toxicity from central nervous system radiation (in combination with intrathecal therapy) and, potentially, second malignancies (196). As the majority of patients with Burkitt's lymphoma are cured, particular attention needs to be paid to late complications.

Surgery, also once considered a useful therapeutic modality if almost all tumor could be removed (197), has become of limited value in the era of highly effective chemotherapy. At the present time, surgery is limited to obtaining a diagnostic sample (which may entail complete resection of a small abdominal mass) or to the management of complications such as an acute abdomen (198–200).

Short-Duration, Dose-Intensive Therapy

The experience with Burkitt's lymphoma in Africa during the 1960s and 1970s demonstrated that short-duration therapy of

TABLE 30.8. *Outline of therapy in protocol BFM-NHL 90 for B-cell lymphomas[a]*

Risk group	Therapy
1	Cycles A and B (no prephase and vincristine is omitted)
2	Prephase followed by 4 cycles: A-B-A-B
3	Prephase followed by 5 cycles: AA-BB-CC-AA-BB
4	Prephase followed by 6 cycles: AA-BB-CC-AA-BB-CC

A cycles consist of dexamethasone, VePesid, Ara-C, intermediate-dose methotrexate, ifosfamide, and triple intrathecal therapy; B cycles consist of dexamethasone, adriamycin, intermediate-dose methotrexate, cyclophosphamide, and triple intrathecal therapy. In AA and BB cycles, high-dose methotrexate is given instead of intermediate-dose methotrexate, and vincristine is added to the regimen. CC cycles consist of dexamethasone, vindesine, high-dose Ara-C, VePesid, and triple intrathecal therapy.

TABLE 30.9. *Outline of therapy in protocol French-American-British LMB 96[a]*

Therapy group	Therapy
A	Two cycles of COPAD
B	COP
	COPADM 1
	COPADM 2
	COPADM 2 (reduced cyclophosphamide)
	CYM 1 and 2
	COPADM 3
C[b]	COP
	COPADM 1
	COPADM 2
	CYVE 1 and 2
	Mini-CYVE 1 and 2
	CYVE and intrathecal therapy and high-dose methotrexate
	Mini-CYVE and intrathecal therapy and high-dose methotrexate
	Maintenance 1
	Maintenance 2–4
	COPADM 3

AD, doxorubicin; C, cyclophosphamide; CY, cytarabine (Ara-C); M, methotrexate with leucovorin rescue; O, vincristine; P, prednis(ol)one; VE, etoposide.

[a]Intrathecal therapy is administered in all cycles except COPAD, CYVE, mini-CYVE, and maintenance courses 2–4, except when indicated.

[b]Patients with central nervous system disease receive additional high-dose methotrexate after CYVE 1 or mini-CYVE 1 and additional intrathecal drugs at the beginning of CYVE or mini-CYVE.

even one or a few doses of a single agent could cure Burkitt's lymphoma; in fact a high fraction of patients with limited disease (perhaps 70% to 80%) were curable with a single agent (180–185). This experience has been recently repeated (201). In the 1970s, given the success of the treatment of acute lymphoblastic leukemia and the notion, at that time, that lymphomas were a variant form of leukemia and should be treated as such (205), the question whether long-duration leukemia-like therapy (i.e., with multiple, different treatment cycles, including induction, consolidation, and maintenance) is superior to short-duration regimens with repeated cycles of the same drug

TABLE 30.10. *Outline of therapy in NCI protocol 89-C-41 for B-cell lymphomas[a]*

Therapy group	Therapy
Low-risk patients	Three A cycles
High-risk patients	Four cycles: A-B-A-B

[a]A cycles consist of cyclophosphamide, Adriamycin, vincristine, and high-dose methotrexate (given on day 10). B cycles consist of ifosfamide, etoposide, and high-dose Ara-C.

TABLE 30.11. *Results of French (LMB 89), German-Austrian (BFM 90), and NCI (89-C-41) protocols in the treatment of B-cell lymphomas*

Protocol	No. of patients	Event-free survival at 3 yr (%)
LMB 89		
Stage I and II	122	96 ± 4
Stage III	280	93 ± 3
Stage IV	97	95 ± 4
Leukemic patients	67	79 ± 8
BFM 90		
Stage I	49	95 ± 5
Stage II	114	98 ± 1
Stage III	171	86 ± 3
Stage IV	23	83 ± 8
Leukemic patients	56	76 ± 8
NCI 89-C-41		
Low risk	18	100
High risk	66	85

combinations was considered of primary importance. In 1977, the Children's Cancer Study Group initiated a study in which children with non-Hodgkin's lymphoma were randomized to a regimen based on therapy for acute lymphoblastic leukemia, LSA_2-L_2, or to the COMP [cyclophosphamide, Oncovin (vincristine), methotrexate, prednisone] regimen. The duration of therapy for both regimens was 18 months, and radiation was given to sites of bulk disease. The results were better with COMP for advanced-stage Burkitt's lymphoma, whereas patients with lymphoblastic lymphoma had a better outcome with LSA_2-L_2 (170). In a subsequent study, the Children's Cancer Study Group compared 6 months of COMP with 18 months of COMP for patients with localized Burkitt's lymphoma and showed that 6 months is as good as 18 months (171). Protocol NCI 7704, a regimen consisting of Cytoxan (cyclophosphamide), Oncovin (vincristine), doxorubicin (Adriamycin), and prednisone alternating with high-dose methotrexate (CODOX-M), was used to treat both adult and pediatric patients with Burkitt's lymphoma and Burkitt-like lymphoma; patients with "high-risk" disease received 15 cycles of therapy. Overall, between 50% and 60% of patients achieved long-term survival (167). A subsequent NCI regimen, 89-C-41, consisted of only four cycles of alternating CODOX-M therapy, with a combination of ifosfamide, (VePesid) etoposide, and high-dose Ara-C (IVAC) shown to be effective in patients with recurrent disease after cyclophosphamide-containing regimens (168,169). Despite the drastic reduction in the number of cycles, this short-duration therapy resulted in a markedly superior outcome for both low-risk and high-risk patients. A study from the Pediatric Oncology Group in pediatric patients with limited-stage nonlymphoblastic lymphoma showed that 9 weeks of chemotherapy is as efficacious as 8 months of chemotherapy whether or not radiation is used (193). Recently, cure of a high fraction of patients with Burkitt's lymphoma with an intensive regimen of only 45 days has been reported (202). These studies clearly support the concept that short-duration therapy with an effective regimen is sufficient to cure Burkitt's lymphoma/Burkitt-like lymphoma and that long-duration therapies have no advantage. In fact, long-duration regimens containing fewer drugs are clearly inferior in terms of their curative potential, especially in high-risk patients.

In light of the efficacy of these approaches, which, although intensive, do not require stem cell rescue, there appears to be no routine role of stem cell transplantation in Burkitt's lymphoma or Burkitt-like lymphoma. Although induction of remission followed by transplantation has been used by some in an attempt to improve survival rates, particularly in adults, there seems to be no advantage to this approach; in fact, there is a potential disadvantage because the number of agents that can be used in such therapies is limited, and using the patients' own stem cells risks reinfusion of some tumor cells. Because it appears that one of the reasons for improved survival rates is the addition of additional agents at high, but conventional, dosage, it appears retrogressive to use a small number of agents at very high dosage. Indeed, such approaches, anecdotally, yield worse results (17,203). Even when used only for patients who achieve a complete response, which is unlikely to be more than 60% with conventional regimens used, the overall event-free survival rate is necessarily considerably lower than that achieved with modern, intensive, multidrug protocols (203,204). This is because not all patients are able to receive transplantation, and even those who do are unlikely to achieve a survival rate of more than 70% (giving a "best-case" scenario of cure of some 40% to 45% of patients). If high-intensity regimens are used to ensure a high complete response rate, then there is clearly no need for regimens that require stem cell rescue.

Prompt Initiation of Successive Cycles of Chemotherapy

Burkitt's lymphoma and Burkitt-like lymphoma both have a very high proliferative index and very short tumor doubling time. This is perhaps one of the reasons that these tumors are particularly responsive to chemotherapy, but it also has implications for the therapeutic strategy. Successful treatment regimens for Burkitt's lymphoma or Burkitt-like lymphoma allow as little delay between therapy cycles as possible—subsequent chemotherapy cycles are started as soon as there are signs of bone marrow recovery (usually based on the neutrophil count). Waiting for a fixed period of time between cycles, as may be reasonable for much more slowly growing solid tumors, may be detrimental; it is not unusual to see progressive growth before the next cycle of therapy when the tumor is resistant to chemotherapy. Because of the urgency of commencing the next cycle of therapy, it is considered inappropriate to wait for full marrow recovery. The required neutrophil count varies among different protocols. In BFM 95, it is 200 per mm^3 in early cycles and 500 per mm^3 in later cycles, with a platelet count of 50,000 per mm^3 or more. For NCI 89-C-41, a neutrophil count of 1,000 per mm^3

or more and a platelet count of 50,000 per mm^3 were used, whereas in SFOP trials, a neutrophil count of 1,500 per mm^3 or more and platelet count of 100,000 per mm^3 or more are required. Because all of these protocols are equally successful (although not necessarily equitoxic), it appears that once marrow recovery has begun, it is safe to proceed with the next therapy cycle and also that there is a relatively short interval between the achievement of a count of 200 or 500 per mm^3 and, for example, 1,000 per mm^3. Nonetheless, the principle of initiating therapy as soon as possible is common to all three protocols.

These general principles apply to both pediatric and adult patients with Burkitt's lymphoma/Burkitt-like lymphoma; application of these principles to the treatment of adult patients (up to age 60 years) has shown great success in improving the results (which, at least in published studies, appear to be similar to those achieved in children), although there is some evidence that medical oncologists or adult patients are less tolerant of the degree of toxicity encountered; in one multicenter study in which patients were treated with a slightly modified 89-C-41 protocol, only 43% of patients received the treatment as planned (186). In contrast, standard chemotherapy regimens used for aggressive B-cell lymphomas, primarily diffuse large B-cell lymphoma, give poor results (206,207) in Burkitt's lymphoma/Burkitt-like lymphoma, or the results are based on very few patients (208). Indeed, it was for this reason (survival rates of 20% to 25%) that patients with these diseases were originally included in a "high-grade" category in the Working Formulation for Clinical Usage (24). In adult patients with significant comorbidities and in patients who are very elderly, the application of the therapeutic principles described may not be possible. In this group of patients, significant modifications in the doses may be required, and newer strategies may be necessary (e.g., combining chemotherapy with B-cell antibodies against CD20, CD22, and use of radiolabeled antibodies).

CHEMOTHERAPY REGIMENS AND RESULTS OF TREATMENT

Limited-Stage Disease

Patients with limited disease, that is, localized or completely resected intraabdominal disease (stages I and II, St. Jude), have an excellent prognosis, with cure rates between 90% and 100%. The definition of limited-stage or low-risk patients varies among the different protocols. The NCI protocol has only two risk groups, SFOP protocols have three risk groups, and BFM has four risk groups (Tables 30.5, 30.6, and 30.7). Patients with limited disease are treated with only two or three cycles of chemotherapy (without radiation), which is also less intensive than the therapy used for patients with extensive disease; yet recently published NCI, BFM, and SFOP trials have all reported 100% cure rates in these patients (168,173,178). A randomized study from Pediatric Oncology Group has shown no benefit of combined chemoradiation when compared with chemotherapy alone in patients with limited disease (193).

The importance of not undertreating patients with a limited tumor burden is underscored by the recent Pediatric Oncology Group results reported at a meeting but not yet published. This group demonstrated that patients with completely resected gastrointestinal disease enjoyed an excellent prognosis of some 95% long-term survival when treated with a CHOP [cyclophosphamide, hydroxydaunomycin, Oncovin (vincristine), prednisone] regimen for 9 weeks. However, the other side of this coin is that other "low-risk" patients treated with this same regimen achieved a survival rate of only just over 80%. Thus, even within the low-risk patient group, a very low-risk group—that in which a small gastrointestinal tumor is completely resected—can be identified and separated from the remaining slightly higher-risk patients who presumably should be treated with somewhat more intensive therapy. This observation also emphasizes the potential disadvantages of stage as a means of stratifying patients because those with completely resected gastrointestinal disease—that is, the best-risk patients—are included in stage II in the St. Jude system. Occasional patients with stage I disease have quite an extensive tumor (e.g., a localized mass of more than 10 cm). Although there are insufficient published data from which to draw firm conclusions, it seems that such patients ought to be included in a higher risk category than would be the case if stage alone were the determinant of therapy. These patients may also be anticipated to have elevated serum lactate dehydrogenase levels. If this were included as a marker of risk, they would receive more intensive therapy. Risk stratification should not, therefore, be based exclusively on clinical stage (not, at least, as determined by the existing staging systems).

Extensive-Stage Disease

Patients had a very poor prognosis in the 1970s, especially patients with bone marrow involvement, central nervous system involvement, or both. The newer, more intensive short-duration regimens, which consisted of seven to nine drugs instead of the four to five drug regimens used in the 1970s for 1 year to 18 months, have dramatically improved overall survival. These regimens also demonstrated that chemotherapy alone is sufficient to treat sites of bulky disease, treat central nervous system disease (including paraplegia), prevent central nervous system disease, and even treat disease in so-called sanctuary sites, such as testicular disease—all of which were previously treated with radiation therapy.

For patients with extensive disease, the basic cyclophosphamide, vincristine, and methotrexate (with or without prednisone) has been supplemented with higher dose methotrexate (5–8 g per m^2) and frequently high-dose Ara-C, in addition to other drugs, such as etoposide and sometimes ifosfamide (169, 174,178,209), shown to be active in patients with recurrent disease (17,187–191). Of considerable significance is the observation that in spite of the shorter number of cycles, the survival rate for patients with marrow or central nervous system involvement improved from 20% to 80%. High-dose Ara-C and etoposide are used in NCI, BFM, and SFOP regimens for high-risk patients. In the NCI and BFM regimens, ifosfamide replaces

Cytoxan (cyclophosphamide) in every other cycle. Although designed independently, it is clear that these three regimens (NCI, BFM, and SFOP) have more similarities than differences. Moreover, in children at least, they have also improved the outcome of patients with diffuse large B-cell lymphoma. Although adult patients with Burkitt's lymphoma/Burkitt-like lymphoma comprise less than 2% of lymphomas, they have had major survival benefit (from approximately 25% to 30% cure rates to 65% to 90% cure rates) from these newer regimens (17,186,210–213). Other intensive therapy approaches that use some of the strategies used in these protocols are effective but not as effective (214). These results contrast with poor survival rates (40% to 50% cure rates with currently used regimens) seen in adult diffuse large B-cell lymphoma (which constitutes approximately 30% to 33% of all adult lymphomas). In view of the success in children with diffuse large B-cell lymphoma, it might be legitimately concluded that these regimens, or at least the principles learned from these regimens, ought to be formally tested in adult patients with diffuse large B-cell lymphoma.

Variations in individual and cumulative drug doses, timing, and total treatment duration exist among the several protocols in use, and it is probable that emphasis in the immediate future will be on "fine tuning" (i.e., refining drug dosage and administration and reducing toxicity). For example, the optimal duration of methotrexate infusions (4 hours vs. 24 hours) is a major study question in the present BFM trial for B-cell lymphomas, whereas the present French-American-British protocol for B-cell lymphomas, based on protocol LMB 89 of the SFOP (which is longer in duration and more complicated than the other protocols) is designed to determine whether reduction in dosage and in the total duration of therapy for specific patient subgroups can be accomplished without detracting from the excellent results it achieves. Although the evidence suggests that more than four or five active drugs are necessary to achieve excellent results, it is difficult to determine the relative value of each drug in any given regimen. In this respect, it is of interest that corticosteroids are not included in one effective protocol (168,169), whereas anthracyclines have been shown, in a yet unpublished, randomized study conducted by the Children's Cancer Study Group, to add no therapeutic value to the four-drug regimen COMP. Because anthracyclines have the potential for acute or late cardiac toxicity and certainly add to the acute toxicity of combination regimens (particularly with respect to myelosuppression and stomatitis), further studies of their use in the present-day six-to-eight-drug regimens may be warranted.

Treatment and Prevention of Central Nervous System Disease

Patients with central nervous system disease have for long been considered to have a particularly poor prognosis. There are several possible explanations for this. Such patients could have biologically different disease, which is more resistant to the particular chemotherapy in use; central nervous system disease may be associated with particularly extensive systemic disease; or the chemotherapy used may be less effective because of maldistribution to the central nervous system. Of interest in this context is the observation that African patients with Burkitt's lymphoma and central nervous system disease do not appear to have a worse prognosis than other patients. Indeed, even with the therapy delivered in the 1960s and 1970s, often single-agent therapy, 50% of patients could be expected to achieve long-term survival (182,215). This is probably related to the fact that in endemic Burkitt's lymphoma, central nervous system disease is frequently associated with rather small tumor burdens. In contrast, in sporadic Burkitt's lymphoma it is associated with extensive systemic disease, frequently including bone marrow involvement (194). Thus, the probability is that central nervous system disease in sporadic Burkitt's lymphoma previously had a poor prognosis because of its association with a high tumor burden, perhaps coupled to the inadequate therapeutic approach to central nervous system disease.

The use of high-dose S-phase agents [i.e., methotrexate and Ara-C, both of which are highly active in Burkitt's lymphoma (187,189–191) and provide effective drug levels in the spinal fluid and central nervous system parenchyma] has dramatically improved the results of therapy in patients with central nervous system disease (175). Before this, intrathecal therapy and radiation were the only therapeutic modalities used specifically against the central nervous system. However, the potential role of better systemic therapy in improving the results in patients with central nervous system disease must also be considered. Both high-dose methotrexate and high-dose Ara-C are also effective, of course, against systemic disease. High-dose Ara-C and high-dose methotrexate are potential neurotoxins, and this must be taken into consideration in protocol design because neurotoxicity may be considerably increased if other potential neurotoxins are used (216). The risk of enhancing the neurotoxicity of these drugs with radiation is another reason to avoid central nervous system irradiation.

In adults as well as children with Burkitt's lymphoma/Burkitt-like lymphoma, prophylaxis against the spread of tumor to the central nervous system is an essential component of therapy for the majority of patients. At the present time, the only patient groups that do not routinely receive prophylaxis against central nervous system disease are those with minimal disease, such as patients with intraabdominal disease that is completely resected or patients with stage I disease that is not in proximity to the central nervous system (i.e., not in the head and neck region or epidural) in whom central nervous system spread is extremely rare. Although there are risks to such treatment, the potential for harm appears to be greatly outweighed by the risk of the development of central nervous system recurrence if such therapy is not given. Intrathecal therapy with methotrexate alone or methotrexate and Ara-C is usually the mainstay of central nervous system prophylactic therapy, but in patients with extensive disease, high-dose intravenous infusions of the S-phase specific agents, methotrexate and Ara-C, are administered in most effective protocols and clearly play a role in preventing central nervous system spread or dealing with occult central nervous system involvement.

Radiation of the cranium or craniospinal axis is generally not considered to have an advantage over chemotherapeutic central nervous system prophylactic therapy in children with lymphoma, and in some studies in patients with B-cell lymphomas, it has been shown to be ineffective (217,218). Moreover, prophylactic cranial irradiation in acute lymphoblastic leukemia, in which there is considerably more experience with this approach, has been associated with significant toxicity, including impaired growth, intellectual impairment, and secondary brain tumors (219,220).

TREATMENT OF ELDERLY PATIENTS WITH BURKITT'S LYMPHOMA/ BURKITT-LIKE LYMPHOMA

Despite the fact that most modern Burkitt's lymphoma regimens can cure 80% to 90% of pediatric and adult patients, the treatment of elderly patients is a challenge. Most adults treated on intensive protocols designed for Burkitt's lymphoma have been 60 years of age or younger. Elderly patients (patients older than 65 or 70 years of age) have a high incidence of comorbid conditions that may include cardiac problems, renal insufficiency, pulmonary problems, neurologic problems, and poor performance status. These factors can make it impossible to treat these patients with unmodified short-duration, dose-intensive regimens, which, in elderly patients, have a high likelihood of being associated with increased morbidity and mortality from toxicity. Such patients need regimens that are individually tailored to minimize toxicity while still maintaining reasonable efficacy. However, there is very limited published information available, largely because it is difficult to conduct clinical trials in this age group given the rarity of Burkitt's lymphoma/Burkitt-like lymphoma and the frequent presence of significant comorbidities. These patients may be worthy of particular consideration for the use of unlabeled antibodies against CD20, CD22, and CD52 in concert with modified chemotherapy. There is good evidence from in vitro experiments in Burkitt's lymphoma cell lines and animal studies using Burkitt's lymphoma cell-line xenografts that CD20 antibody has antitumor activity by itself and also enhances the efficacy of chemotherapy or radiation (221). A randomized study in elderly patients with diffuse large B-cell lymphoma has demonstrated a superior outcome for the chemotherapy plus Rituxan group when compared with the group that received chemotherapy alone (222). However, because this effect appears to be due to overcoming bcl-2 resistance, it may not apply to Burkitt's lymphoma, which does not express bcl-2. Elderly patients may tolerate radioimmunotherapy more easily than intensive chemotherapy, and the possibility of using radioimmunoconjugates, such as Yttrium and ^{131}I tagged to CD20 antibody, which presumably act independently of any effect on bcl-2, should be considered (223). The addition of radioconjugates could allow a decrease in the dose intensity or the number of cycles of chemotherapy, making, in either event, therapy more tolerable for the elderly, but a negative note in this regard is the limited—if any—contribution made by radiation to therapy in Burkitt's lymphoma and Burkitt-like lymphoma. Nonetheless, given the very different considerations in the case of radioimmunotherapy (e.g., it homes to tumor anywhere in the body and exposes tumor cells constantly to radiation), it should not be assumed that it will not be of value. Radioimmunotherapy overcomes some of these drawbacks of traditional external-beam radiation therapy, which presumably can make this slightly more effective than external-beam radiation. Potential side effects might include an increased incidence of myelodysplasia and secondary acute myelogenous leukemia. This may be of less concern in very elderly patients who may still be able to enjoy several years of remission from Burkitt's lymphoma.

Treatment of Elderly Patients with Limited Disease

Elderly patients with localized non-bulky disease or with completely resected intraabdominal disease may tolerate therapy as well as younger patients because it is less intensive and shorter. If a regimen with methotrexate is preferred, then an intermediate dose of methotrexate, such as 500 to 1,000 mg/m^2, is preferable. Based on the studies in elderly patients with diffuse large B-cell lymphoma, it may be reasonable to use Rituxan along with chemotherapy because this may increase the efficacy of treatment. Cure rates for elderly patients with limited disease are likely to be as good, or only slightly worse, as in younger patients. The need for intrathecal prophylaxis is presumably similar to younger patients, although there are no data in this regard.

Treatment of Elderly Patients with Extensive Disease

Treatment of this group of patients is extremely challenging, as the risks and benefits of therapy have to be delicately weighed in the balance. Extreme care should be given to postchemotherapy supportive care, as the treatment-related morbidity and mortality can be significant. Treatment regimen may have to be individualized to each patient, depending on extent of disease, renal function, cardiac status, and overall health. Elderly patients (older than 70 years of age) may have particular problems in handling high-dose methotrexate; in patients older than 70 years of age and in patients with significant associated medical problems, it may be safer to limit the dose of methotrexate to 1 to 3 g per m^2 or less. In some patients (especially those with renal insufficiency), it may not be possible to give any methotrexate. Comments regarding the use of anti-CD20 or other antibodies apply as discussed above.

If an NCI 89-C-41 regimen is used, then doses of CODOX [Cytoxan (cyclophosphamide), Oncovin (vincristine), doxorubicin (Adriamycin)] may also have to be modified (based on patients' total disease burden and the ability to tolerate the toxicity of therapy). In patients who have high disease burden, are at particular risk for central nervous system involvement, or who already have central nervous system involvement, the highest tolerated dose of methotrexate should be given. Patients who are in good physical condition and who have normal renal function may tolerate full doses of methotrexate without serious complications (if extreme care is taken to facilitate elimination of methotrexate by hyperhydration and alkalinization). Cyclophosphamide and ifosfamide as well as Ara-C may need dose reduction, but Adriamycin and vincristine may not in the absence of cardiac or neurologic problems, respectively. Similarly, individualized dose and schedule modification of BFM or SFOP regimens may be required in patients older than 70 years of age. In making such modifications, it must be recognized that there is likely to be an associated reduction in the chance for a good outcome. The use of prophylactic antibiotics, antiviral and antifungal medication, high-dose growth factor support, and very close follow-up until complete recovery from the treatment toxicity are particularly important in the elderly. In the near future, with advances in biologic therapies and targeted therapies directed to specific molecular lesions, treatment may become less toxic and more efficacious—perhaps equally effective and minimally toxic in elderly patients too.

SUPPORTIVE CARE

The success of treatment in Burkitt's lymphoma/Burkitt-like lymphoma is equally dependent on (a) the effectiveness of the regimen, and (b) the efficacy of supportive care. Because of the intensive nature of most of the effective regimens, patients demand very intensive postchemotherapy supportive care. Effective and careful management of treatment-related toxicity and complications is very critical to a successful outcome. Important aspects of postchemotherapy care include (a) prevention and management of tumor lysis syndrome; (b) pre– and post–high-dose methotrexate hyperhydration and alkalinization to maintain a good urine output (greater than 100 to 150 mL/hour) and an alkaline urine pH (pH greater than 7.0); (c) intensive growth factor support; (d) prophylactic antibiotics, antifungals, and antivirals; and (e) close follow-up care as an inpatient or outpatient (almost daily visits to the clinic or physician's office).

Prevention and Management of Uric Acid Nephropathy and Tumor Lysis Syndrome

In patients with a large tumor burden, pretreatment uricosemia is likely to be present, perhaps associated with renal failure from uric acid nephropathy. This syndrome can be compounded by obstruction to the renal outflow tract, and such patients are at heightened risk for the development of a tumor lysis syndrome (224–226). Management includes the use of alkaline hyperhydration and allopurinol or, probably more effective, a urate oxidase. In extreme circumstances, or in cases in which treatment must be begun urgently, management includes hemodialysis or filtration. In general, it is wise not to commence therapy until the serum uric acid level is normal or close to normal and the patient has an excellent urine output because such patients are at particular risk to develop a tumor lysis syndrome. In the first few days of therapy, continuation of the above measures, with the exception of alkalinization (because hyperphosphatemia occurs post-therapy, and phosphates are less soluble in an alkaline urine), is essential, the most important component being hydration because all oxypurines can be dissolved in a sufficiently large volume of urine. Patients must be monitored carefully, particularly with respect to fluid intake and output, such that additional measures (diuretics, dialysis, filtration) may be taken if necessary. It is advisable to avoid intravenous potassium or calcium in these patients because potassium levels tend to rise rapidly within hours of therapy, whereas elevated phosphorus can lead to deposition of calcium in soft tissues. In general, because of the significant risks and close monitoring required, most patients at risk for a tumor lysis syndrome (i.e., with a significant tumor burden) should be cared for in a critical care unit.

Pre– and Post–High-Dose Methotrexate Hydration and Alkalinization

Most of the effective Burkitt's lymphoma regimens include high-dose methotrexate as an important component of the regimen. Among all the other drugs used in these regimens, high-dose methotrexate administration demands utmost care; this component of these regimens also discourages many oncologists from using these highly effective regimens. Despite the fact that high-dose methotrexate is potentially very toxic or even fatal if care is not taken to facilitate its timely elimination, it can be administered safely by following a number of simple principles. For patients younger than 70 years of age, these include the following:

1. Premethotrexate hydration and alkalinization.
2. Monitoring urine pH.
3. Strict monitoring of serum methotrexate levels and, of course, input and output, as well as renal and hepatic function.
4. Prompt initiation of leucovorin rescue. Carboxypeptidase, which cleaves methotrexate, can be used if levels remain high, particularly in the presence of renal failure.
5. Temporary discontinuation of all potentially nephrotoxic drugs and drugs that compete with methotrexate for renal excretion (including nonsteroidal antiinflammatories, aminoglycosides, and acyclovir) before, during, and until complete clearance of methotrexate. It is very important to make sure the patient's renal function is normal or adequate (creatinine clearance of 50 to 60) before high-dose methotrexate administration; if renal function is suboptimal secondary to lymphoma or tumor lysis, then methotrexate should be withheld until renal function is satisfactory to meet the guidelines.
6. Patients with localized fluid accumulation (e.g., pleural effusion, ascites) may accumulate methotrexate in the fluid with resultant delayed elimination and toxicity. In such cases, drainage of the fluid or very careful monitoring of methotrexate excretion may be necessary.

Intensive Growth Factor Support

Many of the serious complications related to intensive chemotherapy are secondary to severe pancytopenia. All of the effective regimens used in Burkitt's lymphoma cause prolonged severe neutropenia, which invariably leads to neutropenic infections (in most, if not all, patients) without prophylactic antibiotics. Granulocyte colony-stimulating factor or granulocyte-macrophage colony-stimulating factor can reduce the number of days of neutropenia and shorten the time for neutrophil recovery. By reducing the number of days of severe neutropenia, the risks of infection are lessened. Neutrophil recovery also increases the likelihood of, and potentially speeds, recovery from an existing infection. The use of growth factors should result in patients being treated in a timely fashion and maintaining the dose intensity of these highly effective regimens. In practice, although the kinetics of neutrophil recovery can be clearly demonstrated (169), the impact on rate of infection and number of days in the hospital has not been clearly documented and may depend on dose, patient age group, and many other factors. Anecdotal experience does suggest that the use of high-dose growth factors has minimized treatment delays and has decreased morbidity from neutropenic infections. They may be particularly useful in combination with prophylactic antibiotics.

Prophylactic Antibiotics, and Antifungal and Antiviral Medications

Because most patients invariably develop neutropenic infections because of the depth and duration of neutropenia from these regimens, the use of antibiotics during periods of neutropenia may help to reduce infection (in protocol 89-C-41, for example, 80% to 90% of cycles are associated with febrile neutropenia in the absence of prophylactic antibiotics, such that patients are at very high risk). Antifungal and antiviral prophylaxis may also be valuable when given before the onset of neutropenia until recovery from neutropenia. Antiviral prophylaxis should not be given during high-dose methotrexate administration.

Close Follow-Up

Effective but intensive Burkitt's lymphoma regimens demand close physician follow-up for a successful outcome. Follow-up care should be similar to that for transplant and acute myelogenous leukemia patients. If close, detailed follow-up care cannot be provided, these patients should be referred to an institution where such care is available. In most instances, patients need inpatient care, but in places where outpatient transplant and leukemia therapy is given, it is possible to treat at least some patients on an outpatient basis, usually seeing them every day.

TREATMENT OF RELAPSE

When the highly effective, short-duration, high-intensity therapies described above are used in primary therapy, the few patients who relapse tend to have highly resistant disease. It is also highly unlikely that these patients who relapse after intensive therapy will be salvaged by additional intensive therapy (e.g., accompanied by autologous stem cell rescue). In this situation, salvage therapy accompanied by allogeneic transplantation appears to be a reasonable approach, which at least has the theoretical benefit of a potential graft-versus-tumor effect (231). Combinations containing platinum compounds [e.g., ICE (ifosfamide, carboplatin, etoposide)] are frequently chosen, particularly in patients who have not already been treated with ifosfamide and etoposide.

FUTURE DIRECTIONS

Although patients with Burkitt's lymphoma or Burkitt-like lymphoma treated with modern intensive regimens have a high cure rate, this is not without toxic cost—usually related to neutropenia during chemotherapy and occasionally from a nonhematologic toxicity, such as neuropathy. Late effects are likely to be relatively minor, perhaps in part because relatively low cumulative doses of drugs are given because of the short duration of therapy. Even in earlier protocols, late toxicity appeared mainly due to combined modality therapy or to Adriamycin cardiotoxicity (196). Lower cumulative doses of Adriamycin and no radiotherapy are given in more recent protocols, and it is clear that fertility, even if somewhat impaired, is frequently maintained (186,197). Thus, maintaining excellent survival rates while further reducing toxicity is the primary goal. It may also be reasonable to attempt to identify (e.g., through gene expression studies using microarrays) the small number of patients at high risk not to achieve complete response or to relapse. Such patients may then be assigned to more experimental approaches. There can be no doubt that highly targeted therapy, directed at the molecular lesions or their consequences, will be the therapy of the twenty-first century, not only for Burkitt's lymphoma and Burkitt-like lymphoma but for perhaps all cancers. Such approaches have the advantage of being much more tumor specific, such that toxicity should be more tolerable. Therapeutic targets in Burkitt's lymphoma include the deregulated c-Myc gene (227) and, where Epstein-Barr virus is present, the virus itself. In the latter case, induction of the viral protein, zebra, induces production of virus particles, which results in cell death. This system can be made highly tumor specific by ensuring that zebra induction occurs only in cells that contain Epstein-Barr virus in a latent phase (228). Although the demonstration of the effectiveness of targeted therapy *in vitro* has been conducted in these systems through the use of antisense and a DNA construct, respectively, it seems likely that a similar effect could be achieved through use of small-molecular-weight drugs. It is already known, for example, that various butyrates, such as arginine butyrate, can induce the virus lytic cycle (229,230). Analysis of gene expression patterns may also lead to new leads with respect to the identification of additional therapeutic targets, and it is entirely possible that therapy tailored to the particular set of molecular abnormalities in the patient—that is, consisting of a combination of drugs targeted at the several molecular lesions present in the tumor—may be in use in the course of the present century.

REFERENCES

1. Burkitt D. A sarcoma involving the jaws in African children. *Br J Surg* 1958;46:218–223.
2. Smith EC, Elmes BGT. Malignant disease in natives of Nigeria. *Ann Trop Med Parasitol* 1934;28;461–512.
3. Davies JNP. Reticuloendothelial tumours. *East Afr Med J* 1948;25:117.
4. Edington GM. Malignant disease in the Gold Coast. *Br J Cancer* 1956; 10;41–54.
5. Thijs A. Considérations sur les tumeurs malignes des indigénes du Congo belge et du Ruanda-Urundi. A propos de 2,536 cas. *Ann Soc Belge Med Trop* 1957;37:483–514.
6. De Smet MP. Observations cliniques de tumeurs malignes des tissus réticuloendothéliaux et des tissus hémolymphopoiétiques au Congo. *Ann Soc Belge Med Trop* 1956;36:53–70.
7. O'Conor GT, Davies JNP. Malignant tumors in African children with special reference to malignant lymphomas. *J Pediat* 1960;56: 526–535.
8. Burkitt D. Determining the climatic limitations of a children's cancer common in Africa. *BMJ* 1962;2:1019–1026.
9. Burkitt D. A children's cancer dependent on climatic factors. *Nature* 1962;194:232–234.
10. Epstein MA, Achong BG, Barr YM. Viral particles in cultured lymphoblasts from Burkitt's lymphoma. *Lancet* 1964;1:702–703.
11. Dalldorf G, Linsell CA, Marnhart FE, et al. An epidemiological approach to the lymphomas of African children and Burkitt's sarcoma of the jaws. *Perspect Biol Med* 1964;7:435–449.
12. O'Conor G, Rappaport H, Smith EB. Childhood lymphoma resembling Burkitt's tumor in the United States. *Cancer* 1965;18:411–417.
13. Dorfman RF. Childhood lymphosarcoma in St. Louis, Missouri, clinically and histologically resembling Burkitt's tumor. *Cancer* 1965;18:418–130.
14. Wright DH. Burkitt's tumour in England. A comparison with childhood lymphosarcoma. *Int J Cancer* 1966;1:503–514.
15. Magrath IT, Sariban E. Clinical features of Burkitt's lymphoma in the USA. *IARC Sci Publ* 1985:119–127.
16. Preudhomme C, Dervite I, Wattel E, et al. Clinical significance of p53 mutations in newly diagnosed Burkitt's lymphoma and acute lymphoblastic leukemia: a report of 48 cases. *J Clin Oncol* 1995;13:812–820.
17. Soussain C, Patte C, Ostronoff M, et al. Small noncleaved cell lymphoma and leukemia in adults. A retrospective study of 65 adults treated with the LMB pediatric protocols. *Blood* 1995;85:664–674.
18. van der Burg M, Barendregt BH, van Wering ER, et al. The presence of somatic mutations in immunoglobulin genes of B cell acute lymphoblastic leukemia (ALL-L3) supports assignment as Burkitt's leukemia-lymphoma rather than B-lineage ALL. *Leukemia* 2001;15:1141–1143.
19. Jaffe ES, Harris NL, Stein H, Vardiman JW. *World Health Organization classification of tumours. pathology & genetics: tumours of haematopoietic and lymphoid tissues.* Lyon, France: IARC Press, 2001.
20. Harris NL, Jaffe ES, Stein H, et al. A revised European-American classification of lymphoid neoplasms: a proposal from the International Lymphoma Study Group. *Blood* 1994;84:1361–1392.

21. Harris NL, Jaffe ES, Diebold J, et al. World Health Organization classification of neoplastic diseases of the hematopoietic and lymphoid tissues: report of the Clinical Advisory Committee meeting-Airlie House, Virginia, November 1997. *J Clin Oncol* 1999;17:3835–3849.

22. Hui PK, Feller AC, Lennert K. High-grade non-Hodgkin's lymphoma of B-cell type. I. Histopathology. *Histopathology* 1988;12:127–143.

23. Anonymous. Histopathological definition of Burkitt's tumour. *Bull World Health Organ* 1969;40:601–607.

24. Anonymous. National Cancer Institute sponsored study of classifications of non-Hodgkin's lymphomas: summary and description of a working formulation for clinical usage. The Non-Hodgkin's Lymphoma Pathologic Classification Project. *Cancer* 1982;49:2112–2135.

25. Wright DH. What is Burkitt's lymphoma? *J Pathol* 1997;182:125–127.

26. Warnke RA, Weiss LM, Chan JKC, et al. *Tumors of the lymph nodes and spleen*, 3rd ed. Washington, DC: Armed Forces Institute Of Pathology, 1994.

27. Carbone A, Gloghini A, Gaidano G, et al. AIDS-related Burkitt's lymphoma. Morphologic and immunophenotypic study of biopsy specimens. *Am J Clin Pathol* 1995;103:561–567.

28. Raphael M, Gentilhomme O, Tulliez M, et al. Histopathologic features of high-grade non-Hodgkin's lymphomas in acquired immunodeficiency syndrome. The French Study Group of Pathology for Human Immunodeficiency Virus-Associated Tumors. *Arch Pathol Lab Med* 1991;115:15–20.

29. Carbone A. AIDS-related non-Hodgkin's lymphomas: from pathology and molecular pathogenesis to treatment. *Hum Pathol* 2002;33:392–404.

30. Spina D, Leoncini L, Megha T, et al. Cellular kinetic and phenotypic heterogeneity in and among Burkitt's and Burkitt-like lymphomas. *J Pathol* 1997;182:145–150.

31. Schlegelberger B, Zwingers T, Harder L, et al. Clinicopathogenetic significance of chromosomal abnormalities in patients with blastic peripheral B-cell lymphoma. Kiel-Wien-Lymphoma Study Group. *Blood* 1999;94:3114–3120.

32. Johansson B, Mertens F, Mitelman F. Cytogenetic evolution patterns in non-Hodgkin's lymphoma. *Blood* 1995;86:3905–3914.

33. Grogan TM, Warnke RA, Kaplan HS. A comparative study of Burkitt's and non-Burkitt's "undifferentiated" malignant lymphoma: immunologic, cytochemical, ultrastructural, cytologic, histopathologic, clinical and cell culture features. *Cancer* 1982;49:1817–1828.

34. Anonymous. A clinical evaluation of the International Lymphoma Study Group classification of non-Hodgkin's lymphoma. *Blood* 1997;89:3909–3918.

35. Yano T, van Krieken JH, Magrath IT, et al. Histogenetic correlations between subcategories of small noncleaved cell lymphomas. *Blood* 1992;79:1282–1290.

36. Braziel RM, Arber DA, Slovak ML, et al. The Burkitt-like lymphomas: a Southwest Oncology Group study delineating phenotypic, genotypic, and clinical features. *Blood* 2001;97:3713–3720.

37. Akasaka T, Akasaka H, Ueda C, et al. Molecular and clinical features of non-Burkitt's, diffuse large-cell lymphoma of B-cell type associated with the c-MYC/immunoglobulin heavy-chain fusion gene. *J Clin Oncol* 2000;18:510–518.

38. Gaulard P, Delsol G, Callat MP, et al. Cytogenetic and clinicopathologic features of B-cell lymphomas associated with the Burkitt translocation t(8;14)(q24;q32) or its variants. *Ann Oncol* 2002;13[Suppl 2]:33.

39. Hutchison RE, Finch C, Kepner J, et al. Burkitt lymphoma is immunophenotypically different from Burkitt-like lymphoma in young persons. *Ann Oncol* 2000;11[Suppl 1]:35–38.

40. Macpherson N, Lesack D, Klasa R, et al. Small noncleaved, non-Burkitt's (Burkitt-like) lymphoma: cytogenetics predict outcome and reflect clinical presentation. *J Clin Oncol* 1999;17:1558–1567.

41. Mintzer DM, Andreeff M, Filippa DA, et al. Progression of nodular poorly differentiated lymphocytic lymphoma to Burkitt's-like lymphoma. *Blood* 1984;64:415–421.

42. Shou Y, Martelli ML, Gabrea A, et al. Diverse karyotypic abnormalities of the c-myc locus associated with c-myc dysregulation and tumor progression in multiple myeloma. *Proc Natl Acad Sci U S A* 2000;97:228–233.

43. Avet-Loiseau H, Gerson F, Magrangeas F, et al. Rearrangements of the c-myc oncogene are present in 15% of primary human multiple myeloma tumors. *Blood* 2001;98:3082–3086.

44. Sigaux F, Berger R, Bernheim A, et al. Malignant lymphomas with band 8q24 chromosome abnormality: a morphologic continuum extending from Burkitt's to immunoblastic lymphoma. *Br J Haematol* 1984;57:393–405.

45. Vitolo U, Gaidano G, Botto B, et al. Rearrangements of bcl-6, bcl-2, c-myc and 6q deletion in B-diffuse large-cell lymphoma: clinical relevance in 71 patients. *Ann Oncol* 1998;9:55–61.

46. Ladanyi M, Offit K, Jhanwar SC, et al. MYC rearrangement and translocations involving band 8q24 in diffuse large cell lymphomas. *Blood* 1991;77:1057–1063.

47. Kramer MH, Hermans J, Wijburg E, et al. Clinical relevance of BCL2, BCL6, and MYC rearrangements in diffuse large B-cell lymphoma. *Blood* 1998;92:3152–3162.

48. Nakamura N, Nakamine H, Tamaru J, et al. The distinction between Burkitt lymphoma and diffuse large B-cell lymphoma with c-myc rearrangement. *Mod Pathol* 2002;15:771–776.

49. Cigudosa JC, Parsa NZ, Louie DC, et al. Cytogenetic analysis of 363 consecutively ascertained diffuse large B-cell lymphomas. *Genes Chromosomes Cancer* 1999;25:123–133.

50. Thangavelu M, Olopade O, Beckman E, et al. Clinical, morphologic, and cytogenetic characteristics of patients with lymphoid malignancies characterized by both t(14;18)(q32;q21) and t(8;14)(q24;q32) or t(8;22)(q24;q11). *Genes Chromosomes Cancer* 1990;2:147–158.

51. Kroft SH, Domiati-Saad R, Finn WG, et al. Precursor B-lymphoblastic transformation of grade I follicle center lymphoma. *Am J Clin Pathol* 2000;113:411–418.

52. De Jong D, Voetdijk BM, Beverstock GC, et al. Activation of the c-myc oncogene in a precursor-B-cell blast crisis of follicular lymphoma, presenting as composite lymphoma. *N Engl J Med* 1988;318:1373–1378.

53. Donti E, Falini B, Giuseppe Pelicci P, et al. Immunological and molecular studies in a case of follicular lymphoma with an extra chromosome 12 and t(2;8) translocation. *Leukemia* 1988;2:41–44.

54. Lee JT, Innes DJ Jr, Williams ME. Sequential bcl-2 and c-myc oncogene rearrangements associated with the clinical transformation of non-Hodgkin's lymphoma. *J Clin Invest* 1989;84:1454–1459.

55. Wlodarska I, Mecucci C, De Wolf-Peeters C, et al. Two translocations: a follicular variant 2;18 and a Burkitt 8;14 in a small non cleaved non Hodgkin's lymphoma. *Leuk Lymphoma* 1991;5:65–69.

56. Aventin A, Mecucci C, Guanyabens C, et al. Variant t(2;18) translocation in a Burkitt conversion of follicular lymphoma. *Br J Haematol* 1990;74:367–369.

57. Carli MG, Cuneo A, Piva N, et al. Lymphoblastic lymphoma with primary splenic involvement and the classic 14;18 translocation. *Cancer Genet Cytogenet* 1991;57:47–51.

58. Gauwerky CE, Haluska FG, Tsujimoto Y, et al. Evolution of B-cell malignancy: pre-B-cell leukemia resulting from MYC activation in a B-cell neoplasm with a rearranged BCL2 gene. *Proc Natl Acad Sci U S A* 1988;85:8548–8552.

59. Gauwerky CE, Hoxie J, Nowell PC, Croce CM. Pre-B-cell leukemia with a t(8; 14) and a t(14; 18) translocation is preceded by follicular lymphoma. *Oncogene* 1988;2:431–435.

60. Hammami A, Chan WC, Michels SD, Nassar VH. Mature B-cell acute leukemia: a clinical, morphological, immunological, and cytogenetic study of nine cases. *Hematol Pathol* 1991;5:109–118.

61. Smith SR, Bown N, Wallis JP. Acute lymphoblastic leukemia of Burkitt type (L3) with a t(14;18) and an atypical (8;22) translocation. *Cancer Genet Cytogenet* 1992;62:197–199.

62. Gluck WL, Bigner SH, Borowitz MJ, Brenckman WD Jr. Acute lymphoblastic leukemia of Burkitt's type (L3 ALL) with 8;22 and 14;18 translocations and absent surface immunoglobulins. *Am J Clin Pathol* 1986;85:636–640.

63. Kramer MH, Raghoebier S, Beverstock GC, et al. De novo acute B-cell leukemia with translocation t(14;18): an entity with a poor prognosis. *Leukemia* 1991;5:473–478.

64. Brito-Babapulle V, Crawford A, Khokhar T, et al. Translocations t(14;18) and t(8;14) with rearranged bcl-2 and c-myc in a case presenting as B-ALL (L3). *Leukemia* 1991;5:83–87.

65. Marosi C, Bettelheim P, Chott A, et al. Simultaneous occurrence of t(14;18) and t(8;22) common acute lymphoblastic leukemia. *Ann Hematol* 1992;64:101–104.

66. Fiedler W, Weh HJ, Zeller W, et al. Translocation (14; 18) and (8; 22) in three patients with acute leukemia/lymphoma following centrocytic/centroblastic non-Hodgkin's lymphoma. *Ann Hematol* 1991;63:282–287.

67. Mufti GJ, Hamblin TJ, Oscier DG, Johnson S. Common ALL with pre-B-cell features showing (8;14) and (14;18) chromosome translocations. *Blood* 1983;62:1142–1146.

68. Stamatoullas A, Buchonnet G, Lepretre S, et al. De novo acute B cell leukemia/lymphoma with t(14;18). *Leukemia* 2000;14:1960–1966.

69. Karsan A, Gascoyne RD, Coupland RW, et al. Combination of t(14;18) and a Burkitt's type translocation in B-cell malignancies. *Leuk Lymphoma* 1993;10:433–441.

70. Au WY, Horsman DE, Viswanatha DS, et al. 8q24 translocations in blastic transformation of mantle cell lymphoma. *Haematologica* 2000;85:1225–1227.

71. Batanian JR, Dunphy CH, Richart JM, et al. Simultaneous presence of t(2;8)(p12;q24) and t(14;18)(q32;q21) in a B-cell lymphoproliferative disorder with features suggestive of an aggressive variant of splenic marginal-zone lymphoma. *Cancer Genet Cytogenet* 2000;120:136–140.

72. Klein U, Klein G, Ehlin-Henriksson B, et al. Burkitt's lymphoma is a malignancy of mature B cells expressing somatically mutated V region genes. *Mol Med* 1995;1:495–505.

73. Mann RB, Jaffe ES, Braylan RC, et al. Non-endemic Burkitts's lymphoma. A B-cell tumor related to germinal centers. *N Engl J Med* 1976;295:685–691.

74. Dogan A, Bagdi E, Munson P, Isaacson PG. CD10 and BCL-6 expression in paraffin sections of normal lymphoid tissue and B-cell lymphomas. *Am J Surg Pathol* 2000;24:846–852.

75. Lai R, Arber DA, Chang KL, et al. Frequency of bcl-2 expression in non-Hodgkin's lymphoma: a study of 778 cases with comparison of marginal zone lymphoma and monocytoid B-cell hyperplasia. *Mod Pathol* 1998;11:864–869.

76. Carbone A, Gaidano G, Gloghini A, et al. Differential expression of BCL-6, CD138/syndecan-1, and Epstein-Barr virus-encoded latent membrane protein-1 identifies distinct histogenetic subsets of acquired immunodeficiency syndrome-related non-Hodgkin's lymphomas. *Blood* 1998;91:747–755.

77. Carbone A, Gloghini A, Larocca LM, et al. Expression profile of MUM1/IRF4, BCL-6, and CD138/syndecan-1 defines novel histogenetic subsets of human immunodeficiency virus-related lymphomas. *Blood* 2001;97:744–751.

78. Tao Q, Robertson KD, Manns A, et al. Epstein-Barr virus (EBV) in endemic Burkitt's lymphoma: molecular analysis of primary tumor tissue. *Blood* 1998;91:1373–1381.

79. Chapman CJ, Mockridge CI, Rowe M, et al. Analysis of VH genes used by neoplastic B cells in endemic Burkitt's lymphoma shows somatic hypermutation and intraclonal heterogeneity. *Blood* 1995;85:2176–2181.

80. Tamaru J, Hummel M, Marafioti T, et al. Burkitt's lymphomas express VH genes with a moderate number of antigen-selected somatic mutations. *Am J Pathol* 1995;147:1398–1407.

81. Capello D, Vitolo U, Pasqualucci L, et al. Distribution and pattern of BCL-6 mutations throughout the spectrum of B-cell neoplasia. *Blood* 2000;95:651–659.

82. Gaidano G, Pastore C, Capello D, et al. Involvement of the bcl-6 gene in AIDS-related lymphomas. *Ann Oncol* 1997;8[Suppl 2]:105–108.

83. Gaidano G, Carbone A, Pastore C, et al. Frequent mutation of the 5' noncoding region of the BCL-6 gene in acquired immunodeficiency syndrome-related non-Hodgkin's lymphomas. *Blood* 1997;89:3755–3762.

84. Manolov G, Manolova Y. Marker band in one chromosome 14 from Burkitt lymphomas. *Nature* 1972;237:33–34.

85. Zech L, Haglund U, Nilsson K, Klein G. Characteristic chromosomal abnormalities in biopsies and lymphoid-cell lines from patients with Burkitt and non-Burkitt lymphomas. *Int J Cancer* 1976;17:47–56.

86. Hecht JL, Aster JC. Molecular biology of Burkitt's lymphoma. *J Clin Oncol* 2000;18:3707–3721.

87. Boxer LM, Dang CV. Translocations involving c-myc and c-myc function. *Oncogene* 2001;20:5595–5610.

88. Ladanyi M, Offit K, Parsa NZ, et al. Follicular lymphoma with t(8;14)(q24;q32): a distinct clinical and molecular subset of t(8;14)-bearing lymphomas. *Blood* 1992;79:2124–2130.

89. Yano T, Jaffe ES, Longo DL, Raffeld M. MYC rearrangements in histologically progressed follicular lymphomas. *Blood* 1992;80:758–767.

90. Nacheva E, Dyer MJ, Fischer P, et al. C-MYC translocations in de novo B-cell lineage acute leukemias with t(14;18)(cell lines Karpas 231 and 353). *Blood* 1993;82:231–240.

91. Denyssevych T, Lestou VS, Knesevich S, et al. Establishment and comprehensive analysis of a new human transformed follicular lymphoma B cell line, Tat-1. *Leukemia* 2002;16:276–283.

92. Sonoki T, Siebert R, Taniguchi I, et al. Activation of myc by cytogenetically cryptic chromosomal translocation t(8;17)(q24;q22). *Ann Oncol* 2002;13[Suppl 2]:50.

93. Willis TG, Dyer MJ. The role of immunoglobulin translocations in the pathogenesis of B-cell malignancies. *Blood* 2000;96:808–822.

94. Joos S, Falk MH, Lichter P, et al. Variable breakpoints in Burkitt lymphoma cells with chromosomal t(8;14) translocation separate c-myc and the IgH locus up to several hundred kb. *Hum Mol Genet* 1992;1:625–632.

95. Joos S, Haluska FG, Falk MH, et al. Mapping chromosomal breakpoints of Burkitt's t(8;14) translocations far upstream of c-myc. *Cancer Res* 1992;52:6547–6552.

96. Zeidler R, Joos S, Delecluse HJ, et al. Breakpoints of Burkitt's lymphoma t(8;22) translocations map within a distance of 300 kb downstream of MYC. *Genes Chromosomes Cancer* 1994;9:282–287.

97. Bower M. Acquired immunodeficiency syndrome-related systemic non-Hodgkin's lymphoma. *Br J Haematol* 2001;112:863–873.

98. Gutierrez M, Bhatia K, Barriga R, et al. Molecular epidemiology of Burkitt's lymphoma from South America: differences in breakpoint locations and EBV association from tumors in other world regions. *Blood* 1992;79:3261–3266.

99. Gutierrez MI, Hamdy N, Bhatia K, et al. Geographic variation in t (8;14) chromosomal breakpoint locations and EBV association in Burkitt's lymphoma. *Int J Pediatr Hematol Oncol* 1999;6:161–168.

100. Kuppers R, Dalla-Favera R. Mechanisms of chromosomal translocations in B cell lymphomas. *Oncogene* 2001;20:5580–5594.

101. Pasqualucci L, Neumeister P, Goossens T, et al. Hypermutation of multiple proto-oncogenes in B-cell diffuse large-cell lymphomas. *Nature* 2001;412:341–346.

102. Cesarman E, Dalla-Favera R, Bentley D, Groudine M. Mutations in the first exon are associated with altered transcription of c-myc in Burkitt lymphoma. *Science* 1987;238:1272–1275.

103. Gu W, Bhatia K, Magrath IT, et al. Binding and suppression of the Myc transcriptional activation domain by p107. *Science* 1994;264:251–254.

104. Raffeld M, Yano T, Hoang AT, et al. Clustered mutations in the transcriptional activation domain of Myc in 8q24 translocated lymphomas and their functional consequences. *Curr Top Microbiol Immunol* 1995;194:265–272.

105. Bemark M, Neuberger MS. The c-MYC allele that is translocated into the IgH locus undergoes constitutive hypermutation in a Burkitt's lymphoma line. *Oncogene* 2000;19:3404–3410.

106. Pelicci PG, Knowles DM 2nd, Magrath I, Dalla-Favera R. Chromosomal breakpoints and structural alterations of the c-myc locus differ in endemic and sporadic forms of Burkitt lymphoma. *Proc Natl Acad Sci U S A* 1986;83:2984–2988.

107. Akasaka T, Muramatsu M, Ohno H, et al. Application of long-distance polymerase chain reaction to detection of junctional sequences created by chromosomal translocation in mature B-cell neoplasms. *Blood* 1996;88:985–994.

108. Siebert R, Matthiesen P, Harder S, et al. Application of interphase fluorescence in situ hybridization for the detection of the Burkitt translocation t(8;14)(q24;q32) in B-cell lymphomas. *Blood* 1998;91:984–990.

109. Taniwaki M, Matsuda F, Jauch A, et al. Detection of 14q32 translocations in B-cell malignancies by in situ hybridization with yeast artificial chromosome clones containing the human IgH gene locus. *Blood* 1994;83:2962–2969.

110. Veronese ML, Ohta M, Finan J, et al. Detection of myc translocations in lymphoma cells by fluorescence in situ hybridization with yeast artificial chromosomes. *Blood* 1995;85:2132–2138.

111. Rack KA, Delabesse E, Radford-Weiss I, et al. Simultaneous detection of MYC, BVR1, and PVT1 translocations in lymphoid malignancies by fluorescence in situ hybridization. *Genes Chromosomes Cancer* 1998;23:220–226.

112. Tamura A, Miura I, Iida S, et al. Interphase detection of immunoglobulin heavy chain gene translocations with specific oncogene loci in 173 patients with B-cell lymphoma. *Cancer Genet Cytogenet* 2001;129:1–9.

113. Martin-Subero JI, Harder L, Gesk S, et al. Interphase FISH assays for the detection of translocations with breakpoints in immunoglobulin light chain loci. *Int J Cancer* 2002;98:470–474.

114. Martin-Subero JI, Chudoba I, Harder L, et al. Multicolor-FICTION: expanding the possibilities of combined morphologic, immunophenotypic, and genetic single cell analyses. *Am J Pathol* 2002;161:413–420.

115. Martin-Subero JI, Chudoba I, Harder L, et al. Multi-color-fluorescence immunophenotyping and interphase cytogenetics as a tool for the investigation of neoplasms; expanding possibilities of combined morphologic, immunophenotypic and genetic single cell analyses. *Am J Pathol* 2002;161:413–420.

116. Haralambieva E, Kleiverda K, Mason DY, et al. Detection of three common translocation breakpoints in non-Hodgkin's lymphomas by fluorescence in situ hybridization on routine paraffin-embedded tissue sections. *J Pathol* 2002;198:163–170.

117. Kanda K, Hu HM, Zhang L, et al. NF-kappa B activity is required for the deregulation of c-myc expression by the immunoglobulin heavy chain enhancer. *J Biol Chem* 2000;275:32338–32346.

118. Hu HM, Arcinas M, Boxer LM. A Myc-associated zinc finger protein-related factor binding site is required for the deregulation of c-myc expression by the immunoglobulin heavy chain gene enhancers in Burkitt's lymphoma. *J Biol Chem* 2002;277:9819–9824.

119. Hussain A, Doucet JP, Gutierrez M, et al. Tumor necrosis factor-related apoptosis-inducing ligand (TRAIL) and Fas apoptosis in Burkitt's lymphomas with loss of multiple pro-apoptotic proteins. *Haematologica* 2003;88:167–175.

120. Gutierrez MI, Cherney B, Hussain A, et al. Bax is frequently compromised in Burkitt's lymphomas with irreversible resistance to Fas-induced apoptosis. *Cancer Res* 1999;59:696–703.

121. Nanbo A, Takada K. The role of Epstein-Barr virus-encoded small RNAs (EBERs) in oncogenesis. *Rev Med Virol* 2002;12:321–326.

122. Nanbo A, Inoue K, Adachi-Takasawa K, Takada K. Epstein-Barr virus RNA confers resistance to interferon-alpha-induced apoptosis in Burkitt's lymphoma. *EMBO J* 2002;21:954–965.

123. Takada K, Nanbo A. The role of EBERs in oncogenesis. *Semin Cancer Biol* 2001;11:461–467.

124. Kelly G, Bell A, Rickinson A. Epstein-Barr virus-associated Burkitt lymphomagenesis selects for downregulation of the nuclear antigen EBNA2. *Nat Med* 2002;8:1098–1104.

125. Pajic A, Staege MS, Dudziak D, et al. Antagonistic effects of c-myc and Epstein-Barr virus latent genes on the phenotype of human B cells. *Int J Cancer* 2001;93:810–816.

126. Kempkes B, Zimber-Strobl U, Eissner G, et al. Epstein-Barr virus nuclear antigen 2 (EBNA2)-oestrogen receptor fusion proteins complement the EBNA2-deficient Epstein-Barr virus strain P3HR1 in transformation of primary B cells but suppress growth of human B cell lymphoma lines. *J Gen Virol* 1996;77:227–237.

127. Jochner N, Eick D, Zimber-Strobl U, et al. Epstein-Barr virus nuclear antigen 2 is a transcriptional suppressor of the immunoglobulin mu gene: implications for the expression of the translocated c-myc gene in Burkitt's lymphoma cells. *EMBO J* 1996;15:375–382.

128. Staege MS, Lee SP, Frisan T, et al. MYC overexpression imposes a nonimmunogenic phenotype on Epstein-Barr virus-infected B cells. *Proc Natl Acad Sci U S A* 2002;99:4550–4555.

129. Pajic A, Polack A, Staege MS, et al. Elevated expression of c-myc in lymphoblastoid cells does not support an Epstein-Barr virus latency III-to-I switch. *J Gen Virol* 2001;82:3051–3055.

130. Polack A, Hortnagel K, Pajic A, et al. c-myc activation renders proliferation of Epstein-Barr virus (EBV)-transformed cells independent of EBV nuclear antigen 2 and latent membrane protein 1. *Proc Natl Acad Sci U S A* 1996;93:10411–10416.

131. Klein U, Tu Y, Stolovitzky GA, et al. Transcriptional analysis of the B cell germinal center reaction. *Proc Natl Acad Sci U S A* 2003;25.

132. Cutrona G, Dono M, Pastorino S, et al. The propensity to apoptosis of centrocytes and centroblasts correlates with elevated levels of intracellular myc protein. *Eur J Immunol* 1997;27:234–238.

133. Niller HH, Salamon D, Ilg K, et al. The in vivo binding site for oncoprotein c-Myc in the promoter for Epstein-Barr virus (EBV) encoding RNA (EBER) 1 suggests a specific role for EBV in lymphomagenesis. *Med Sci Monit* 2003;9:HY1–HY9.

134. Geser A, de Thé G, Lenoir G, et al. Final case reporting from the Ugandan prospective study of the relationship between EBV and Burkitt's lymphoma. *Int J Cancer* 1982;29:397–400.

135. Whittle HC, Brown J, Marsh K, et al. T-cell control of Epstein-Barr virus infected B-cells is lost during *P. falciparum* malaria. *Nature* 1984;312:449–450.

136. Kitinya JN, Lauren PA. Burkitt's lymphoma on Mount Kilimanjaro and in the inland regions of North Tanzania. *East Afr Med J* 1982;59:256–260.

137. Sariban E, Donahue A, Magrath IT. Jaw involvement in American Burkitt's lymphoma. *Cancer* 1984;53:141–146.

138. Haddy T, Jaffe E, Keenan A, Magrath IT. Bone involvement in young patients with non-Hodgkin's lymphoma: efficacy of chemotherapy without local radiotherapy. *Blood* 1988;72:1141–1147.

139. Sabbah RS, Ali MA, Lewall DB, Aur RJ. Burkitt's lymphoma in Saudi Arabia: clinical, pathological, and epidemiological analyses of 16 cases. *King Faisal Spec Hosp Med J* 1982;2:77–83.

140. Suvatte V, Mahasandana C, Tanphaichitr VS, et al. Burkitt's lymphoma in Thai children: an analysis of 25 cases. *Southeast Asian J Trop Med Public Health* 1983;14:385–393.

141. Wood RE, Nortje CJ, Hesseling P, Mouton S. Involvement of the maxillofacial region in African Burkitt's lymphoma in the Cape Province and Namibia. *Dentomaxillofac Radiol* 1988;17:57–60.

142. Magrath IT. African Burkitt's lymphoma. *Am J Ped Hematol Oncol* 1991;13:222–246.

143. Cavdar AO, Yavuz G, Babacan E, et al. Burkitt's lymphoma in Turkish children: clinical, viral [EBV] and molecular studies. *Leuk Lymphoma* 1994;14:323–330.

144. Ertem U, Duru F, Pamir A, et al. Burkitt's lymphoma in 63 Turkish children diagnosed over a 10 year period. *Pediatr Hematol Oncol* 1996;13:123–134.

145. Sandlund JT, Fonseca T, Leimig T, et al. Predominance and characteristics of Burkitt lymphoma among children with non-Hodgkin lymphoma in northeastern Brazil. *Leukemia* 1997;11:743–746.

146. Madanat FF, Amr SS, Tarawneh MS, et al. Burkitt's lymphoma in Jordanian children: epidemiological and clinical study. *J Trop Med Hyg* 1986;89;189–191.

147. Amr SS, Tarawneh MS, Jitawi SA, Oran LW. Malignant neoplasms in Jordanian children. *Ann Trop Paediatr* 1986;6:161–166.

148. Hathirat P, Isarangkura P, Nitiyanant P, et al. Lymphoma in children: study of 100 cases. *Southeast Asian J Trop Med Public Health* 1986;17:135–137.

149. Thomas OA, Abdelaal MA, Ayoub DA, et al. Childhood lymphoma in Saudi Arabia: experience at the King Khalid National Guard Hospital. *East Afr Med J* 1996;73:343–345.

150. Janus C, Edwards BK, Sariban E, Magrath IT. Surgical resection and limited chemotherapy for abdominal undifferentiated lymphomas. *Cancer Treat Rep* 1984;68:599–605.

151. Shepherd JJ, Wright DH. Burkitt's tumour presenting as bilateral swelling of the breast in women of child-bearing age. *Br J Surg* 1967;54:776–780.

152. Durodola JI. Burkitt's lymphoma presenting during lactation. *Int J Gynaecol Obstet* 1976;14:225–231.

153. Plantaz D, Bachelot C, Dyon JF, et al. [Massive breast involvement in Burkitt's lymphoma]. *Arch Fr Pediatr* 1987;44:199–200.

154. Hugh JC, Jackson FI, Hanson J, Poppema S. Primary breast lymphoma. An immunohistologic study of 20 new cases. *Cancer* 1990;66:2602–2611.

155. Magrath IT, Ziegler JL. Bone marrow involvement in Burkitt's lymphoma and its relationship to acute B-cell leukemia. *Leukemia Res* 1980;4;33–59.

156. Advani S, Pai S, Adde M, et al. Preliminary report of an intensified, short duration chemotherapy protocol for the treatment of pediatric non-Hodgkin's lymphoma in India. *Ann Oncol* 1997;8:893–897.

157. Chantada GL, Felice MS, Zubizarreta PA, et al. Results of a BFM-based protocol for the treatment of childhood B-non-Hodgkin's lymphoma and B-acute lymphoblastic leukemia in Argentina. *Med Pediatr Oncol* 1997;28:333–341.

158. Gad-el-Mawla N, Hamza MR, Abdel-Hadi S, et al. Prolonged disease-free survival in pediatric non-Hodgkin's lymphoma using ifosfamide-containing combination chemotherapy. *Hematol Oncol* 1991;9:281–286.

159. Ziegler JL, Magrath IT. Burkitt's lymphoma. In: Ioachim HL, ed. *Pathobiology annual*. New York: Appleton Century Croft, 1974:129–142.

160. Osuntokun BO, Osuntokun O, Adeloye A, et al. Primary neuro-ophthalmological presentation of Burkitt's lymphoma. *Afr J Med Sci* 1973;4:111–117.

161. Nkrumah FK, Perkins IV. Neurological manifestations of Burkitt's lymphoma in Ghana. *Afr J Med Sci* 1973;4:209–214.

162. Magrath IT, Mugerwa J, Bailey I, et al. Intracerebral Burkitt's lymphoma: pathology clinical features and treatment. *Q J Med* 1974;43;489–508.

163. Sanchez Pina C, Pascual-Castroviejo I, Martinez Fernandez V, et al. Burkitt's lymphoma presenting as Tolosa-Hunt syndrome. *Pediatr Neurol* 1993;9:157–158.

164. Magrath IT, Lee YJ, Anderson T, et al. Prognostic factors in Burkitt's lymphoma: Importance of total tumor burden. *Cancer* 1980;45:l507–1515.

165. Landesberg R, Yee H, Datikashvili M, Ahmed AN. Unilateral mandibular lip anesthesia as the sole presenting symptom of Burkitt's lymphoma: case report and review of literature. *J Oral Maxillofac Surg* 2001;59:322–326.

166. Ziegler JL. Treatment results of 54 American patients with Burkitt's lymphoma are similar to the African experience. *N Engl J Med* 1977;297:75.

167. Magrath IT, Janus C, Edwards B, et al. An effective therapy for both undifferentiated (including Burkitt's) lymphomas and lymphoblastic lymphomas in children and young adults. *Blood* 1984;63:1102–1111.

168. Magrath I, Adde M, Shad A, et al. Adults and children with small non-cleaved-cell lymphoma have a similar excellent outcome when treated with the same chemotherapy regimen. *J Clin Oncol* 1996;14:925–934.

169. Adde M, Shad A, Venzon D, et al. Additional chemotherapy agents improve treatment outcome for children and adults with advanced B-cell lymphomas. *Semin Oncol* 1998;2[Suppl 4]:33–39.

170. Anderson JR, Jenkin RD, Wilson JF, et al. Long-term follow-up of patients treated with COMP or LSA2L2 therapy for childhood non-Hodgkin's lymphoma: a report of CCG-551 for the Children's Cancer Group. *J Clin Oncol* 1993;13:1024–1032.

171. Meadows AT, Sposto R, Jenkin RD, et al. Similar efficacy of 6 and 18 months of therapy with four drugs (COMP) for localized non-Hodgkin's lymphoma of children: a report from the Childrens Cancer Study Group. *J Clin Oncol* 1989;7:92–99.

172. Link MP, Shuster JJ, Donaldson SS, et al. Treatment of children and young adults with early-stage non-Hodgkin's lymphoma. *N Engl J Med* 1997;337:1259–1266.

173. Patte C, Auperin A, Michon J, et al. The Société Française d'Oncologie Pediatrique LMB89 protocol: highly effective multiagent chemotherapy tailored to the tumor burden and initial response in 561 unselected children with B-cell lymphomas and L3 leukemia. *Blood* 2001;97:3370–3379.

174. Patte C, Michon J, Frappaz D, et al. Therapy of Burkitt and other B-cell acute lymphoblastic leukaemia and lymphoma: experience with the LMB protocols of the SFOP (French Paediatric Oncology Society) in children and adults. *Baillieres Clin Haematol* 1994;2:339–348.

175. Patte C, Philip T, Rodary C, et al. High survival rate in advanced stage B cell lymphomas and leukemias without CNS involvement with a short intensive polychemotherapy: results from the French Pediatric Oncology Society of a randomized trial of 216 children. *J Clin Oncol* 1991;9:123–132.

176. Patte C. Treatment of mature B-ALL and high grade B-NHL in children. *Best Pract Res Clin Haematol* 2002;15:695–711.

177. Reiter A, Schrappe M, Ludwig WD, et al. Favorable outcome of B-cell acute lymphoblastic leukemia in childhood: a report of three consecutive studies of the BFM group. *Blood* 1992;80:2471–2478.

178. Reiter A, Schrappe M, Parwaresch R, et al. Non-Hodgkin's lymphomas of childhood and adolescence: results of a treatment stratified for biologic subtypes and stage—a report of the Berlin-Frankfurt-Munster Group. *J Clin Oncol* 1995;13:359–372.

179. Reiter A, Schrappe M, Tiemann M, et al. Improved treatment results in childhood B-cell neoplasms with tailored intensification of therapy: a report of the Berlin-Frankfurt-Munster Group Trial NHL-BFM 90. *Blood* 1999;94:3294–3306.

180. Burkitt D. Long term remissions following one and two dose chemotherapy for African lymphoma. *Cancer* 1967;20;756–759.

181. Clifford P. Long term survival of patients with Burkitt's lymphoma. An assessment of treatment and other factors which may relate to survival. *Cancer Res* 1967;27:2578.

182. Ziegler J, Magrath IT, Olweny CLM. Cure of Burkitt's lymphoma: 10 year follow-up of 157 Ugandan patients. *Lancet* 1979;2;936–938.

183. Ziegler JL, Morrow RH Jr, Fass L, et al. Treatment of Burkitt's tumor with cyclophosphamide. *Cancer* 1970;26:474–484.

184. Olweny CLM, Katongole-Mbidde E, Kaddu-Mukasa A, et al. Treatment of Burkitt's lymphoma: randomized clinical trials of single-agent versus combination chemotherapy. *Int J Cancer* 1976;17:436–440.

185. Olweny CLM, Katongole-Mbidde E, Otim D, et al. Long term experience with Burkitt's lymphoma in Uganda. *Int J Cancer* 1980;26:261–266.

186. Mead GM, Sydes MR, Walewski J, et al. An international evaluation of CODOX-M and CODOX-M alternating with IVAC in adult Burkitt's lymphoma: results of the United Kingdom Lymphoma Group LY06 study. *Ann Oncol* 2002;13:1264–1274.

187. Djerassie I, Kim JS. Methotrexate and citrovorum factor rescue in the management of childhood lymphosarcoma and reticulum cell sarcoma (non-Hodgkin's lymphomas). Prolonged unmaintained remissions. *Cancer* 1976;38:1043–1051.

188. Jones GR, Ettinger LJ. Continuous infusion of high-dose cytosine arabinoside for treatment of childhood acute leukemia and non-Hodgkin's lymphoma in relapse. *Semin Oncol* 1985;12[Suppl 3]:150.

189. Patte C, Bernard A, Hartmann O, et al. High-dose methotrexate and continuous infusion Ara-C in children's non-Hodgkin's lymphoma: phase II studies and their use in further protocols. *Pediatr Hematol Oncol* 1986;3:11–18.

190. Gentet JC, Patte C, Quintana E. Phase II study of cytarabine and etoposide in children with refractory or relapsed non-Hodgkin's lymphoma: a study of the French Society of Pediatric Oncology. *J Clin Oncol* 1990;8:661–665.

191. Magrath I, Adde M, Sandlund J, and Jain V. Ifosfamide in the treatment of high-grade recurrent non-Hodgkin's lymphomas. *Hematol Oncol* 1991;9:267–274.

192. Norin T, Clifford P, Einhorn J, et al. Radiotherapy in Burkitt's lymphoma. Conventional or superfractionated radiation therapy in Burkitt's lymphoma. *Acta Radiol Ther Phys Biol* 1971;10:545.

193. Link MP, Donaldson SS, Berard CW, et al. Results of treatment of childhood localized non-Hodgkin's lymphoma with combination chemotherapy with or without radiotherapy. *N Engl J Med* 1990;322;1169–1174.

194. Magrath IT, Adde M, Haddy T. Treatment of patients with high grade non-Hodgkin's lymphomas and central nervous system involvement: is radiation an essential component of therapy? *Leuk Lymphoma* 1996;21:99–105.

195. Kellie SJ, Pui CH, Murphy SB. Childhood non-Hodgkin's lymphoma involving the testis: clinical features and treatment outcome. *J Clin Oncol* 1989;7:1066–1070.

196. Haddy T, Adde M, McCalla J, et al. Late effects in long-term survivors of high-grade non-Hodgkin's lymphomas. *J Clin Oncol* 1998;16:2070.

197. Magrath IT, Lwanga S, Carswell W, et al. Surgical reduction of tumour bulk in management of abdominal Burkitt's lymphoma. *Br Med J* 1974;2;308.

198. Attarbaschi A, Mann G, Dworzak M, et al. The role of surgery in the treatment of pediatric B-cell non-Hodgkin's lymphoma. *J Pediatr Surg* 2002;37:1470–1475.

199. LaQuaglia MP, Stolar CHJ, Krailo M, et al. The role of surgery in abdominal non-Hodgkin's lymphoma: experience from the Children's Cancer Study Group. *J Pediatr Surg* 1992;27:230–235.

200. Reiter A, Zimmermann W, Zimmermann M, et al. The role of initial laparotomy and second-look surgery in the treatment of abdominal B-cell non-Hodgkin's lymphoma of childhood. A report of the BFM Group. *Eur J Pediatr Surg* 1994;4:74–81.

201. Kazembe P, Hesseling PB, Griffin BE, et al. Long term survival of children with Burkitt lymphoma in Malawi after cyclophosphamide monotherapy. *Med Pediatr Oncol* 2003;40:23–25.

202. Spreafico F, Massimino M, Luksch R, et al. Intensive, very short-term chemotherapy for advanced Burkitt's lymphoma in children. *J Clin Oncol* 2002;20:2783–2788.

203. Jost LM, Jacky E, Dommann-Scherrer C, et al. Short-term weekly chemotherapy followed by high-dose therapy with autologous bone marrow transplantation for lymphoblastic and Burkitt's lymphomas in adult patients. *Ann Oncol* 1995;6:445–451.

204. Sweetenham JW, Pearce R, Taghipour G, et al. Related adult Burkitt's and Burkitt-like non-Hodgkin's lymphoma—outcome for patients treated with high-dose therapy and autologous stem-cell transplantation in first remission or at relapse: results from the European Group for Blood and Marrow Transplantation. *J Clin Oncol* 1996;14:2465–2472.

205. Arseneau JC, Canellos GP, Banks PM, et al. American Burkitt's lymphoma—a clinicopathological study of 30 cases. I. Clinical factors relating to long term survival. *Am J Med* 1975;58:314–321.

206. Waits TM, Greco FA, Greer JP, Hainsworth JD. Treatment of poor prognosis non-Hodgkin's lymphoma with intensive, inpatient combi-

nation chemotherapy of brief duration: long-term followup. *Leuk Lymphoma* 1993;10:453–459.

207. Shipp MA, Harrington DP, Anderson JR, et al. A predictive model for aggressive non-Hodgkin's lymphoma. *N Engl J Med* 1993;329:987–994.

208. Longo DL, Duffey PL, Jaffe ES, et al. Diffuse small noncleaved-cell, non-Burkitt's lymphoma in adults: a high-grade lymphoma responsive to ProMACE-based combination chemotherapy. *J Clin Oncol* 1994;12:2153–2159.

209. Brecher ML, Schwenn MR, Coppes MJ, et al. Fractionated cyclophosphamide and back to back high dose methotrexate and cytosine arabinoside improves outcome in patients with stage III high grade small non-cleaved cell lymphomas (SNCCL): a randomized trial of the Pediatric Oncology Group. *Med Pediatr Oncol* 1997;6:526–533.

210. Holte H, Smeland S, Blystad AK, et al. [Intensive chemotherapy in Burkitt's lymphoma and aggressive non-Hodgkin's lymphoma]. *Tidsskr Nor Laegeforen* 2002;122:364–369.

211. Pees HW, Radtke H, Schwamborn J, Graf N. The BFM-protocol for HIV-negative Burkitt's lymphomas and L3 ALL in adult patients: a high chance for cure. *Ann Hematol* 1992; 65:201–205(abst).

212. Todeschini G, Tecchio C, Degani D, et al. Eighty-one percent event-free survival in advanced Burkitt's lymphoma/leukemia: no differences in outcome between pediatric and adult patients treated with the same intensive pediatric protocol. *Ann Oncol* 1997;8[Suppl 1]: 77–81.

213. Evens AM, Gordon LI. Burkitt's and Burkitt-like lymphoma. *Curr Treat Options Oncol* 2002;3:291–305.

214. Thomas DA, Cortes J, O'Brien S, et al. Hyper-CVAD program in Burkitt's-type adult acute lymphoblastic leukemia. *J Clin Oncol* 1999;17:2461–2470.

215. Ziegler JL, Bluming AZ, Morrow RH, et al. Central nervous system involvement in Burkitt's lymphoma. *Blood* 1970;36:718–728.

216. Macdonald DR. Neurologic complications of chemotherapy. *Neurol Clin* 1991;9:955–967.

217. Olweny CLM, Atime I, Kaddu-Mukasa A, et al. Cerebrospinal irradiation of Burkitt's lymphoma. *Acta Radiol* 1977;12:225–231.

218. Gasparini M, Lombardi F, Bellani FF, et al. Childhood non-Hodgkin's lymphoma: long-term results of an intensive chemotherapy regimen. *Cancer* 1981;48;1508–1512.

219. Smibert E, Anderson V, Godber T, Ekert H. Risk factors for intellectual and educational sequelae of cranial irradiation in childhood acute lymphoblastic leukaemia. *Br J Cancer* 1996;73:825–830.

220. Walter AW, Hancock ML, Pui CH, et al. Secondary brain tumors in children treated for acute lymphoblastic leukemia at St. Jude Children's Research Hospital. *J Clin Oncol* 1998;16:3761–3767.

221. Chow KU, Sommerlad WD, Boehrer S, et al. Anti-CD20 antibody (IDEC-C2B8, rituximab) enhances efficacy of cytotoxic drugs on neoplastic lymphocytes in vitro: role of cytokines, complement, and caspases. *Haematologica* 2002;87:33–43.

222. Coiffier B. Rituximab in combination with CHOP improves survival in elderly patients with aggressive non-Hodgkin's lymphoma. *Semin Oncol* 2002;29[2 Suppl 6]:18–22.

223. Pagel JM, Hedin N, Subbiah K, et al. Comparison of anti-CD20 and anti-CD45 antibodies for conventional and pretargeted radioimmunotherapy of B-cell lymphomas. *Blood* 2003;101:2340–2348.

224. Cohen LF, Balow JE, Magrath IT. Acute tumor lysis syndrome: a review of 37 patients with Burkitt's lymphoma. *Am J Med* 1980;68; 486–491.

225. Cabanillas F. Metabolic abnormalities in lymphoma. *Clin Lymphoma* 2002;3[Suppl 1]:S32–S36.

226. Cairo MS. Prevention and treatment of hyperuricemia in hematological malignancies. *Clin Lymphoma* 2002;3[Suppl 1]:S26–S31.

227. McManaway ME, Neckers LM, Loke SL, et al. Tumor-specific inhibition of lymphoma growth by an antisense oligodeoxynucleotide. *Lancet* 1990;335:808–811.

228. Gutierrez MI, Judde JG, Magrath IT, Bhatia KG. Switching viral latency to viral lysis: a novel therapeutic approach for Epstein-Barr virus-associated neoplasia. *Cancer Res* 1996;56;969–972.

229. Oertel SH, Riess H. Antiviral treatment of Epstein-Barr virus-associated lymphoproliferations. *Recent Results Cancer Res* 2002;159:89–95.

230. Mentzer SJ, Perrine SP, Faller DV. Epstein-Barr virus post-transplant lymphoproliferative disease and virus-specific therapy: pharmacological re-activation of viral target genes with arginine butyrate. *Transpl Infect Dis* 2001;3:177–185.

231. Grigg AP, Seymour JF. Graft versus Burkitt's lymphoma effect after allogeneic marrow transplantation. *Leuk Lymphoma* 2002;43:889–892.

CHAPTER 31

Precursor B- and T-Cell Lymphoblastic Lymphoma

John W. Sweetenham and Michael J. Borowitz

DEFINITION

Precursor B-cell and T-cell lymphoblastic leukemias/lymphoblastic lymphomas are neoplasms of lymphoblasts. The designation of *lymphoblastic lymphoma* has been used previously to describe precursor B- and T-cell tumors with predominantly lymph node–based disease (most commonly affecting the anterior mediastinum). As a consequence, the entity of lymphoblastic lymphoma has been recognized by most classifications of lymphoid neoplasms, including the Kiel and Working Formulation systems. However, the clinical distinction between lymphoblastic lymphoma and lymphoblastic leukemia has been arbitrary and has varied among different studies and different institutions.

Because it is now recognized that acute lymphoblastic leukemias and lymphoblastic lymphomas represent the same disease entity at the morphologic, immunophenotypic, and genotypic level, the World Health Organization Classification has unified these entities as precursor B- or T-cell lymphoblastic leukemia/lymphoma.

Although it is now acknowledged that the distinction between lymphoblastic leukemia and lymphoma has no biologic basis, the clinical literature describing these entities has been distinct until very recently. Consequently, the treatment approach to lymphoblastic lymphoma, particularly in the adult population, has developed separately from the approach used in acute lymphoblastic leukemia. Therefore, although the biology of all lymphoblastic disease is discussed in detail in this chapter, the clinical aspects are confined to the entity previously designated as lymphoblastic lymphoma.

FREQUENCY

Lymphoblastic lymphoma is a rare disease that accounts for approximately 2% of all non-Hodgkin's lymphomas (1). Approximately 85% to 90% of adult cases are of T-cell phenotype and occur most frequently in adolescent and young adult males (2–5). B-cell lymphoblastic lymphoma com-

prises approximately 10% of adult cases of this disease (6). The reported median age for patients with lymphoblastic lymphoma is approximately 20 years, with most series reporting male predominance. There has been no clear evidence for a change in the incidence of lymphoblastic lymphoma in recent years, although in view of the variability in the definition between lymphoblastic lymphoma and acute lymphoblastic leukemia, incidence trends may have been obscured.

DIAGNOSIS

The histopathologic and immunophenotypic features of lymphoblastic lymphoma are distinctive, so that diagnosis, if properly approached, is rarely a problem. In many cases, a tissue diagnosis of lymphoblastic lymphoma may be inferred if only peripheral blood, bone marrow, or, in the case of a patient with a mediastinal mass, pleural fluid can be shown to contain lymphoblasts with characteristic immunophenotypic properties. However, the majority of cases of lymphoblastic lymphoma are still diagnosed by tissue examination, coupled with flow cytometric or immunophenotypic analysis.

Histopathologic Findings

Morphologically, lymphoblastic lymphoma is composed of medium-sized cells with finely dispersed chromatin and scant cytoplasm (3) (Color Plate 63). Nucleoli are inconspicuous. The cells may have round nuclei or highly convoluted ones, although this is of no clinical significance. Because it is a high-grade malignancy, mitotic features are invariably present, and there are often numerous apoptotic bodies. These may be phagocytosed by macrophages, thereby imparting a "starry-sky" pattern to the tissue. Although this pattern is often thought of as a characteristic of Burkitt's lymphoma, it may be seen in other high-grade lymphomas as well. Morphologic distinction between lymphoblastic and Burkitt's lymphoma is easy to accomplish in many cases because the latter tumor has a distinct rim of cytoplasm and multiple nucleoli. However, some caveats are in order. First, the classically described histopathologic findings of lymphoblastic lymphoma correspond to L1 acute lymphoblastic leukemia in the French-American-British Classification of acute lymphoblastic leukemia. L2 acute lymphoblastic leukemia, by contrast, has more cytoplasm and more prominent nucleoli and, thus, can in some cases more closely resemble Burkitt's lymphoma in tissue sections (7).

The other concern is that finding the histologic features of lymphoblastic lymphoma is very dependent on optimal tissue fixation and processing. Over-stained material can resemble tumors of more mature lymphocytes, whereas the cells of poorly fixed lymphoblastic lymphoma may greatly enlarge and resemble diffuse large-cell lymphoma.

Differential diagnostic considerations also include cases of lymphocyte-rich thymoma and, in children, other small round-cell tumors. The latter are readily separated by immunophenotyping studies, particularly if one realizes that CD99, the antigen characteristically present on Ewing's sarcoma and peripheral neuroectodermal tumor, is also present in lymphoblastic malignancies (8). Distinction from thymoma is sometimes made more complicated by the fact that lymphoid cells in both tumors have a thymic T-cell phenotype, but the cytology of the cells is generally different, and the characteristic epithelial distribution of thymoma is not present in lymphomas.

Immunophenotypic Analysis

Immunophenotypic analysis almost always allows a diagnosis of lymphoblastic lymphoma to be made with certainty. The great majority of lymphoblastic lymphomas are tumors of precursor T lymphocytes (7,9,10), and finding such a phenotype is essentially pathognomonic of such an entity, although there is no single phenotype associated with precursor T lymphoblastic lymphoma. CD7, CD5, and CD2 are most commonly expressed, whereas CD3 is often present in the cytoplasm but not on the surface (11). Immunohistochemical staining generally does not allow this distinction. Thus, by immunocytochemistry, most cases are CD3+, whereas the sCD3−/cCD3+ phenotype is best demonstrated by flow cytometry. CD4 and CD8 can be expressed in any combination: one alone, neither, or both together. The best means of distinguishing a T lymphoblastic lymphoma from a peripheral T-cell lymphoma is by the expression of non–lineage-specific immature markers, such as terminal deoxynucleotidyl transferase or CD99, or in some cases, CD34 (8,12,13). Cytoplasmic CD3 without surface expression is also a relatively specific finding. CD1a, when positive, is also a relatively specific feature. Although coexpression of CD4 and CD8 is a characteristic of normal thymocytes, there is some controversy about the specificity of this expression for lymphoblastic lymphoma, as it has also been described in T-cell prolymphocytic leukemia.

The less common precursor B lymphoblastic lymphomas also generally express immature markers, such as CD99,

CD34, and terminal deoxynucleotidyl transferase. They are positive for early-expressed pan B markers, including CD79a and CD19, but often lack or show only patchy expression of CD20. CD45 is often negative. By definition, precursor B tumors are surface immunoglobulin negative, but in practice, this is not often the best way to identify them. If only fixed tissue is available, surface immunoglobulin determinations are not reliably done in paraffin sections, and in addition, some lymphomas of mature B cells also lack surface immunoglobulin. In children, precursor B lymphoblastic lymphomas often present as cutaneous disease (14).

Molecular Diagnostics

The great majority of T lymphoblastic lymphomas show clonal rearrangements of T-cell receptor genes, with T-cell receptor δ being the most sensitive (15), but this is not a lineage-specific finding, as many B—or even blastic myeloid—tumors may show this as well (16). Thus, gene rearrangement studies play little role in the diagnosis of this disease. Many precursor T-cell lymphoblastic lymphomas have translocations involving the T-cell receptor gene (17), and although these are important for an understanding of the pathogenesis of the disease (see Pathogenesis), such studies are not particularly important diagnostically or prognostically. Compared with acute lymphoblastic leukemia, there is relatively little literature on the role of cytogenetics or molecular analysis of particular translocations. The rare case of precursor B lymphoblastic lymphoma should probably be screened for the presence of the bcr-abl translocation because of the poor prognosis associated with that abnormality, although specific examples of bcr-abl+ B lymphoblastic lymphoma have not been described.

PATHOGENESIS

Understanding of the pathogenesis and molecular basis of precursor T-cell lymphoblastic disease has mainly arisen from studies of recurrent chromosomal translocations and chromosomal rearrangements in this disease. Approximately one third of patients have translocations involving the α and δ T-cell receptor loci at 14q11.2, the β locus at 7q35, and the γ locus at 7p14-15 (46). The typical result of these translocations is to juxtapose promoter and enhancer elements producing high levels of T-cell receptor gene expression with transcription factor genes, such as HOX11/TLX1, TAL1/SCL, TAL 2, and LYL 1, resulting in aberrant expression of these genes in the developing thymocyte (47–49).

Recent microarray studies have demonstrated molecular subtypes of precursor T-cell lymphoblastic disease that characterize different stages in thymocyte maturation and may identify prognostic subgroups (50). For example, patients with HOX11 expression show a pattern of gene expression corresponding to the early cortical thymocyte. This subgroup appears to have a more favorable clinical outcome, possibly related to the lower frequency of expression of the antiapoptotic BCL-2 gene. These cells are apparently developmentally arrested at a stage at which they are particularly sensitive to drug-induced apoptosis.

In contrast, those samples with gene expression profiles associated with TAL1 or LYL1 expression resemble late cortical and early pro-T thymocytes, respectively, and show more drug resistance and correspondingly higher levels of *bcl-2*.

METHODS OF PRESENTATION

Characteristic clinical features of lymphoblastic lymphoma include male predominance and peak incidence in the second and third decades. Mediastinal involvement at presentation is common, occurring in 60% to 70% of patients, reflecting the thymic origin of the malignant cells in lymphoblastic lymphoma. Mediastinal masses are uncommon in patients with B-cell lymphoblastic lymphoma. Pleural effusions are also a common presenting feature, and pericardial effusions, with resulting cardiac tamponade, may also occur. In addition, symptoms and signs of superior vena caval obstruction may be present.

Peripheral lymph node involvement is present in 60% to 80% of patients at diagnosis, most commonly in cervical, supraclavicular, and axillary regions.

Lymphoblastic lymphoma has a propensity for dissemination to the bone marrow and central nervous system. The frequency of bone marrow involvement at presentation is very difficult to determine from published series in view of the arbitrary and variable distinction between lymphoblastic lymphoma and acute lymphoblastic leukemia. In a recent prospective study from Europe, 21% of adult patients with lymphoblastic lymphoma had bone marrow involvement at presentation (18). Leukemic overspill is also common, but again, the frequency is obscured by inconsistencies in distinction between lymphoblastic lymphoma and acute lymphoblastic leukemia.

Central nervous system involvement is uncommon at presentation, occurring in approximately 5% to 10% of patients. Several reports suggest that it is more common in patients with bone marrow involvement at presentation. Typical manifestations of central nervous system involvement include meningeal involvement with a pleocytosis in the cerebrospinal fluid or cranial nerve involvement, characteristically involving ophthalmic or facial nerves. Although central nervous system involvement at presentation is uncommon, it is a frequent site of relapse in the absence of adequate prophylaxis. In one series from Stanford University, central nervous system relapse was reported in 31% of patients (19).

Other less common sites of involvement include the liver, spleen, and subdiaphragmatic lymph nodes, as well as bone, skin, and testes. Presentation in the pharynx and in the skin is especially typical of precursor B-cell lymphoblastic lymphoma/leukemia in children (20).

UNIQUE ASPECTS OF STAGING

Some centers have adopted the Murphy staging system for lymphoblastic lymphoma in view of the fact that it was devised specifically to address staging of children with non-Hodgkin's lymphoma, in whom disseminated, noncontiguous involvement of nodal and extranodal sites is common. In most children with non-Hodgkin's lymphoma, the Murphy staging system has been shown to provide more useful prognostic information (4). However, in a comparison of the Ann Arbor and Murphy staging systems in adult lymphoblastic lymphoma, the Ann Arbor system was shown to predict survival more accurately and is, therefore, now used in most centers (19).

The applicability of the International Prognostic Index for aggressive non-Hodgkin's lymphomas has now been investigated in three studies. A study from the Non-Hodgkin's Lymphoma Classification Project included a retrospective analysis of a small sample of 26 patients with a median age of 28 years (range, 4 to 65 years) with lymphoblastic lymphoma (21). For the entire group, the 5-year overall and failure-free survival rates were approximately 20%. The number of International Prognostic Index risk factors was not shown to be predictive of overall or failure-free survival in this series. A retrospective series of 62 patients from France also concluded that the International Prognostic Index did not have prognostic significance in adults with lymphoblastic lymphoma (22). The predictive value of the International Prognostic Index was also explored in the context of a European randomized trial in adults with lymphoblastic lymphoma (18). Sixty patients had complete data. The number of International Prognostic Index risk factors was shown to be predictive of overall survival, but this reached significance only for the group with three adverse factors, according to the age-adjusted International Prognostic Index. Larger patient samples are needed to determine whether the International Prognostic Index proves to be a suitable staging and prognostic system for lymphoblastic lymphoma. At present, the Ann Arbor system is still in most widespread use, although because all patients with lymphoblastic lymphoma require intensive systemic therapy (see Treatment below), its relevance is doubtful.

PROGNOSTIC AND PREDICTIVE FACTORS

Identification of prognostic factors in lymphoblastic lymphoma has been variable and inconsistent partly because of the variable criteria used for the distinction between lymphoblastic lymphoma and acute lymphoblastic leukemia and for the distinction between adult and pediatric cases. However, some consistent data, particularly with respect to "biologic" predictors of outcome, have emerged.

"Biologic" Predictive Factors

Various studies have identified phenotypic and genotypic predictors of prognosis. There have been inconsistent reports with respect to the role of B-cell versus T-cell immunophenotype as a prognostic factor. Although there have been reports suggesting a worse outcome for adult lymphoblastic lymphoma patients with precursor B-cell phenotype, more recent retrospective studies have failed to confirm this, possibly because the number of patients with B-cell immunophenotype is very small.

For patients with T-cell precursor lymphoblastic disease, although genetic abnormalities have been described in approximately 30% of cases, particularly involving α and δ T-cell receptor loci, or deletion of 9p, none of these abnormalities has been shown to have prognostic significance (23). In adult patients with acute lymphoblastic leukemia, expression of T-cell antigens, including CD1, CD2, CD4, and CD5, has been associated with a more favorable prognosis. In the Cancer and Leukemia Group B 8364 study, overall and disease-free survival were shown to correlate with the number of T-cell antigens expressed (24). Similar studies have not been performed in patients with lymphoblastic lymphoma.

For patients with precursor B-cell disease, most prognostic information has been derived from patients classified with acute lymphoblastic leukemia. For example, in childhood B acute lymphoblastic leukemia, translocations involving the MLL gene at 11q23 are associated with adverse prognosis (25), as are those involving the t(9;22)(q34;q11.2). Features associated with good prognosis in children include hyperdiploid karyotype, particularly as it is associated with trisomy 4, 10, and 17, and t(12;21)(p13;q22) (26). As in children, adults with B acute lymphoblastic leukemia with 11q23 abnormalities or the t(9;22)(q34;q11.2) translocation have a poor prognosis, although specific studies of these abnormalities as prognostic factors have not been performed in B lymphoblastic lymphoma.

Clinical Predictive Factors

Before the description of the International Prognostic Index, multiple, small retrospective series of patients with lymphoblastic lymphoma identified adverse clinical prognostic factors for overall and disease-free survival (27–29). These have varied in different series, reflecting the small patient numbers and the variable criteria for categorizing acute lymphoblastic leukemia and lymphoblastic lymphoma. Some of the more commonly identified factors are summarized in Table 31.1. Few of these have been consistent across different retrospective series.

Until the description of the International Prognostic Index, the most widely accepted prognostic factors for lymphoblastic lymphoma were those described by Coleman et al. from Stanford University (19). Patients with Ann Arbor stage less than IV or Ann Arbor stage IV, but without bone marrow or central nervous system involvement, with a serum lactate dehydrogenase level less than 300 IU/L (normal = 200 IU/L) were considered good risk. This group had a 5-year freedom-from-relapse rate of 94%. All other patients were considered poor risk. The 5-year freedom from relapse in the poor-risk group was only 19%.

TABLE 31.1. *Clinical prognostic factors in adult lymphoblastic lymphoma*

Adverse factor	Reference
Advanced age	17
Ann Arbor stage	8,16
Bone marrow involvement	8
Central nervous system involvement	8
Leukemic overspill	15
Serum lactate dehydrogenase	8,17
B symptoms	8,17
Time to attainment of complete response	15
International Prognostic Index risk group	7

As mentioned previously, the predictive value of the International Prognostic Index has been assessed in three previous studies. Although the numbers of patients in all series are small, the study from Europe represents the only prospectively collected data set in a relatively unselected population of adult patients with lymphoblastic lymphoma (18). This study demonstrated a statistically significant trend for lower overall survival with an increasing number of adverse factors according to the age-adjusted International Prognostic Index ($p = .016$). However, although there was a clearly inferior survival in patients with three adverse factors, there was little distinction between those with zero, one, or two factors, and the value of the International Prognostic Index as a prognostic model remains unclear.

Although prognostic factors for acute lymphoblastic leukemia have been reasonably well-defined in large prospective studies, there are no consistent data for lymphoblastic lymphoma, and therefore, no clear rationale exists for designing different treatment strategies according to risk group for these patients at present.

TREATMENT

Early studies of the treatment of lymphoblastic lymphoma were conducted in combined populations of children and adults during the 1970s (3,4,30). These and many of the more recent studies are difficult to interpret because patient numbers in most have been small, and variable criteria have been used to assign patients to protocols for acute lymphoblastic leukemia or lymphoblastic lymphoma.

Initial trials in lymphoblastic lymphoma used first- and second-generation chemotherapy regimens initially developed for the treatment of other, less aggressive, types of non-Hodgkin's lymphoma (3,4,31–33). Results with these regimens were poor. Nathwani et al. reported results in 95 adult and pediatric patients with lymphoblastic lymphoma treated on a variety of collaborative group protocols, none of which included central nervous system prophylaxis (3). This series included some patients with leukemic involvement. The complete response rate was only 24%, and for the 87 patients on whom survival information was available, the median survival was only 17 months, with less than 10% of patients alive and disease free at 5 years. Similar results were reported for other low-intensity chemotherapy regimens.

The introduction of intensive chemotherapy and radiation therapy protocols in childhood lymphoblastic lymphoma produced marked improvements in outcome. Protocols such as the LSA$_2$-L$_2$ regimen combined intensive chemotherapy, comparable to that used in childhood acute lymphoblastic leukemia, with central nervous system irradiation (34). Long-term disease-free survival rates between 60% and 80% were reported for children treated with this and similar regimens. A subsequent randomized trial comparing the LSA$_2$-L$_2$ regimen with COMP [cyclophosphamide, Oncovin (vincristine), methotrexate, prednisone] demonstrated a 2-year actuarial failure-free survival of 76% for children with lymphoblastic lymphoma receiving LSA$_2$-L$_2$, compared with only 26% for those receiving COMP (p = .0002) (35).

Subsequently, chemotherapy/radiotherapy regimens similar in design to LSA$_2$-L$_2$ adapted from those in adult acute lymphoblastic leukemia have been applied to adult patients with lymphoblastic lymphoma (19,27,28,36–39). Most of these regimens are characterized by intensive remission-induction chemotherapy, central nervous system prophylaxis, a phase of consolidation chemotherapy, and a prolonged maintenance phase, often lasting for 12 to 18 months. Results from some of these regimens are summarized in Table 31.2.

TABLE 31.2. *Results of intensive combination chemotherapy regimens in adults with lymphoblastic lymphoma*

First author (reference)	Regimen	No. of patients	Response rate	Failure-free survival (FFS)/ relapse-free survival (RFS)	Overall survival (OS)	Comments
Levine (36)	Modified LSA$_2$-L$_2$	15	73% CR; 27% PR	5-yr actuarial FFS = 35%	5-yr actuarial OS = 40%	Median age = 25 yr.
Weinstein (37)	APO	21	95% CR	3-yr actuarial FFS = 58%	5-yr actuarial OS = 69%	Median age = 13 yr.
Slater (27)	Various ALL protocols	51	80% CR for "non-leukemic"; 77% CR for leukemic	N/A	5-yr actuarial OS = 45%	Median age = 22 yr. Four successive ALL regimens used. No difference in outcome according to regimen.
Morel (29)	CHOP plus various ALL protocols	80	82% CR	46% at 30 mo FFS	51% at 30 mo	Median age = 33.7 yr. No difference in outcome according to induction protocol.
Bernasconi (28)	Various ALL protocols	31	77% OR	3-yr RFS = 45%	3-yr OS = 59%	Median age = 25 yr.
Coleman (19)	Two ALL-type protocols with intensified CNS prophylaxis in the second	44	100%	3-yr FFS = 56%	—	—
Hoelzer (38)	Two ALL-type protocols, both including CNS and mediastinal irradiation	45	93% CR	7-yr actuarial DFS = 62%	7-yr actuarial OS = 51%	Median age = 25 yr. All patients had T lymphoblastic lymphoma. No benefit for mediastinal radiotherapy for DFS, OS, or incidence of mediastinal relapse. No prognostic factors identified. Age-adjusted IPI was not predictive of survival.

ALL, acute lymphoblastic leukemia; APO, Adriamycin (doxorubicin), prednisone, Oncovin (vincristine); CHOP, cyclophosphamide, hydroxydaunomycin, Oncovin (vincristine), prednisone; CNS, central nervous system; CR, complete response; DFS, disease free survival; IPI, International Prognostic Index; N/A, not available; OR, overall response; PR, partial response.

Most of these studies report long-term disease-free survival rates between 40% and 60%. Because all of these patient series are relatively small, the apparent minor differences in reported outcomes according to treatment regimens are unlikely to be significant. Results from the unselected patient series reported by the Non-Hodgkin's Lymphoma Classification Project are inferior to this, with a reported 5-year actuarial overall survival of only approximately 20% (21). This may reflect selection bias in the clinical series.

AUTOLOGOUS STEM CELL TRANSPLANTATION IN FIRST REMISSION

Despite the high remission rates reported for first-line therapy in lymphoblastic lymphoma, relapse rates are also relatively high. This has provided a rationale for investigation of the role of high-dose therapy with autologous or allogeneic stem cell transplantation in first remission in an attempt to reduce the incidence of relapse after induction therapy. Most studies to date have explored the role of autologous transplantation in this setting, although some series have also included small numbers of patients receiving sibling-matched allogeneic stem cell transplants (22,39–41).

The results of this approach have appeared superior to those achieved with conventional-dose consolidation and maintenance chemotherapy, and these are summarized in Table 31.3. Long-term disease-free survival in most of these

series has been between 60% and 80%, although many of these series are not analyzed according to intention to treat. The patient populations included in many of these reports represent patients already in complete or partial remission at the time of inclusion in the study, and they are, therefore, a relatively favorable group.

The study reported by Jost et al. is one of the few to include a true intent-to-treat analysis, with follow-up on all patients from diagnosis. In this study, adult patients with lymphoblastic lymphoma received initial induction chemotherapy with MACOP-B [methotrexate, Adriamycin (doxorubicin), cyclophosphamide, Oncovin (vincristine), prednisone, bleomycin] or VACOP-B [VePesid (etoposide), Adriamycin (doxorubicin), cyclophosphamide, Oncovin (vincristine), prednisone, bleomycin] followed by high-dose therapy and autologous stem cell transplantation. The 3-year actuarial overall and event-free survival rates were 48% and 31%, respectively (40). These results do not appear superior to those reported for conventional-dose first-line therapy.

A single, small randomized trial conducted by the European Group for Blood and Marrow Transplantation and the United Kingdom Lymphoma Group has compared the use of high-dose therapy and autologous stem cell transplantation with conventional-dose consolidation and maintenance therapy in adult patients with lymphoblastic lymphoma (18).

This study included 119 adult patients who were treated with intensive acute lymphoblastic leukemia–type induction chemotherapy, of whom 111 were assessable for

TABLE 31.3. *Results of first remission stem cell transplantation in adults with lymphoblastic lymphoma*

First author (reference)	Induction therapy/high-dose regimen/stem cell source	No. of patients	Failure-free survival/relapse-free survival	Overall survival (OS)	Comments
Verdonck (39)	CHOP- or ALL-like induction/ high-dose cyclophosphamide and TBI/autologous bone marrow	9	6/9 in long-term remission	6/9 long-term survivors	Median age = 22 yr.
Jost (40)	MACOP-B or VACOP-B induction/high-dose cyclophosphamide and TBI or CBV/ autologous bone marrow	20	3-yr EFS = 31%	3-yr OS = 48%	Median age = 27 yr. Intent-to-treat analysis with survival calculated from start of induction therapy.
Sweetenham (41)	Multiple-induction and high-dose regimens/ autologous bone marrow	105	6-yr PFS = 63%	6-yr OS = 64%	Median age = 25.8 yr. Registry-based study.
Bouabdallah (22)	Various ALL-type induction regimens/high-dose cyclophosphamide and TBI/12 allogeneic BMT and 18 autologous BMT	62 (30 received BMT in first complete remission)	5-yr EFS = 58%	5-yr OS = 60%	Apparent advantage to allogeneic vs. autologous transplant.

ALL, acute lymphoblastic leukemia; BMT, bone marrow transplant; CBV, Cytoxan, BCNU, VP-16; CHOP, cyclophosphamide, hydroxydaunomycin, Oncovin (vincristine), prednisone; EFS, event free survival; MACOP-B, methotrexate, Adriamycin (doxorubicin), cyclophosphamide, Oncovin (vincristine), prednisone, bleomycin; PFS, progression-free survival; TBI, total-body irradiation; VACOP-B, VePesid (etoposide), Adriamycin (doxorubicin), cyclophosphamide, Oncovin (vincristine), prednisone, bleomycin.

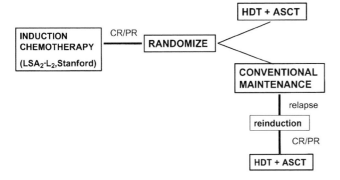

FIG. 31.1. Study design for United Kingdom Lymphoma Group/European Group for Blood and Marrow Transplantation randomized trial of first-remission stem cell transplant for adult patients with lymphoblastic lymphoma. ASCT, autologous stem cell transplant; CR, complete response; HDT, high-dose therapy; PR, partial response.

response to induction therapy. The study design is summarized in Figure 31.1. The overall-response rate to induction chemotherapy was comparable to other series at 82%. However, of 98 patients eligible for randomization, only 65 were actually randomized. Reasons for failure to randomize included patient refusal, early disease progression before transplantation, and elective allogeneic transplantation in patients with human leukocyte antigen (HLA)-matched sibling donors.

Results from this small study are summarized in Figure 31.2. The 3-year actuarial relapse-free survival rate was 24% for patients receiving conventional consolidation and maintenance therapy, compared with 55% for those receiving high-dose therapy and autologous stem cell transplan-

tation (p = .065). The corresponding values for overall survival were 45% and 56% (p = .71). The fact that there was a nonsignificant trend for improved relapse-free survival in the transplant arm but no difference in overall survival may be due to the fact that some patients who relapsed after conventional-dose consolidation therapy were "rescued" by high-dose therapy in second remission. On the basis of the above data, many centers now use high-dose therapy and autologous stem cell transplantation in first remission as standard therapy for adults with lymphoblastic lymphoma. However, the use of conventional-dose consolidation and maintenance therapy, with high-dose strategies being reserved for relapsing patients, is an alternative approach that appears to be associated with an equivalent overall survival.

Although no direct comparisons have been reported, there is no clear evidence that any high-dose regimen is superior to another before autologous transplantation. Similarly, there is no evidence to suggest that the source of hematopoietic stem cells (peripheral blood vs. bone marrow) has an influence on outcome, and for most centers, peripheral blood progenitors are regarded as the preferred stem cell source.

AUTOLOGOUS STEM CELL TRANSPLANTATION FOR RELAPSED OR REFRACTORY DISEASE

Results of salvage therapy for adult patients with lymphoblastic lymphoma with relapsed or refractory disease are very poor. The use of second-line conventional-dose regimens in this situation produces response rates of less than 10%, and median overall survival in these series is only

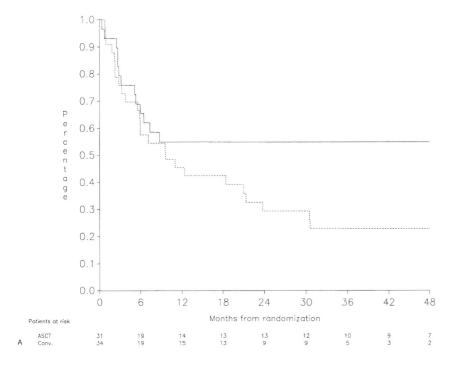

FIG. 31.2. Results from the United Kingdom Lymphoma Group/European Group for Blood and Marrow Transplantation randomized trial of high-dose therapy and stem cell transplant versus conventional consolidation therapy in adult lymphoblastic lymphoma. Relapse-free survival **(A)**. *(continued)*

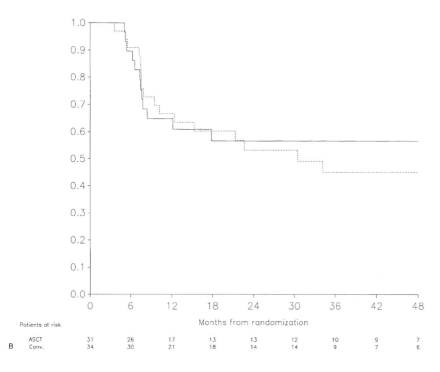

Patients at risk

ASCT	31	26	17	13	13	12	10	9	7
B Conv.	34	30	21	18	14	14	9	7	6

FIG. 31.2. Continued. Overall survival **(B)**. ASCT, autologous stem cell transplant; Conv., conventional. (Reproduced from Sweetenham JW, Santini G, Qian W, et al. High-dose therapy and autologous stem-cell transplantation versus conventional-dose consolidation/maintenance therapy as post-remission therapy for adult patients with lymphoblastic lymphoma: results of a randomized trial of the European Group for Blood and Marrow Transplantation and the United Kingdom Lymphoma Group. *J Clin Oncol* 2001;19: 2927–2936, with permission.)

approximately 9 months (19,27–29). High-dose therapy with autologous stem cell rescue has been used increasingly in this situation, either as a component of second-line remission-induction therapy or to consolidate remission after a conventional-dose second-line regimen.

Very few published studies have specifically addressed the role of autologous stem cell transplantation in this situation. In a retrospective study from Morel et al., of 37 patients with adult lymphoblastic lymphoma who required salvage therapy, 14 achieved a second complete remission with conventional- dose reinduction (29). Seven of these patients underwent consolidation with autologous stem cell transplantation, of whom three achieved long-term disease-free survival.

In a retrospective study from the European Group for Blood and Marrow Transplantation, 41 patients underwent high-dose therapy and autologous stem cell transplantation in second complete remission (41). The 3-year actuarial progression-free survival and overall survival for this group were 30% and 31%, respectively (Fig. 31.3). This series also included patients in whom high-dose therapy was used before the attainment of second complete remission. As with other types of non-Hodgkin's lymphoma, the responsiveness of the disease to conventional-dose therapy given before the transplant was predictive of outcome. The 5-year actuarial overall survival for those with chemosensitive relapse was 31%, compared with 18% for those with chemorefractory disease (Fig. 31.4).

Because patients in chemosensitive relapse have a superior outcome to those with chemorefractory relapse, all relapsing patients should receive conventional-dose salvage therapy in an attempt to induce a second remission before

high-dose therapy. However, even in those patients with refractory disease, the reported long-term disease-free survival of 18% is superior to that achieved with conventional-dose salvage, and these patients should also be offered high-dose therapy.

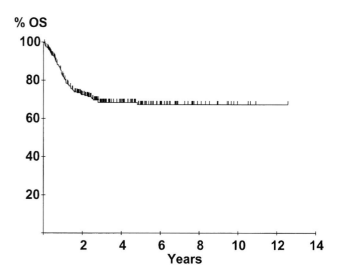

FIG. 31.3. Results of high-dose therapy and autologous stem cell transplant in adult patients with lymphoblastic lymphoma transplanted in second complete remission. OS, overall survival. (Reproduced from Sweetenham JW, Santini G, Pearce R, et al. High-dose therapy and autologous bone marrow transplantation for adult patients with lymphoblastic lymphoma: results from the European Group for Bone Marrow Transplantation. *J Clin Oncol* 1994;12:1358–1365, with permission.)

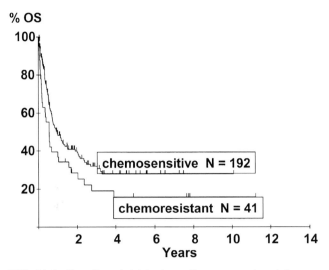

FIG. 31.4. Results of high-dose therapy and autologous stem cell transplant in adult patients with lymphoblastic lymphoma transplanted in chemosensitive or chemoresistant relapse. OS, overall survival. (Reproduced from Sweetenham JW, Santini G, Pearce R, et al. High-dose therapy and autologous bone marrow transplantation for adult patients with lymphoblastic lymphoma: results from the European Group for Bone Marrow Transplantation. *J Clin Oncol* 1994;12:1358–1365, with permission.)

ALLOGENEIC STEM CELL TRANSPLANTATION

The role of allogeneic stem cell transplantation in adults with lymphoblastic lymphoma is unclear. In view of the relatively young age of adult patients with lymphoblastic lymphoma, it is anticipated that their regimen-related mortality after allogeneic transplantation is likely to be relatively low. If a graft-versus-lymphoma effect exists in this disease, then the low relapse rate observed in patients who survive allogeneic transplantation might result in improved overall survival, compared with autologous transplantation. A retrospective, case-controlled analysis from the European Group for Blood and Marrow Transplantation comparing autologous with allogeneic stem cell transplantation reported a lower relapse rate for patients receiving allogeneic compared with autologous stem cell transplantation (2% vs. 48%, respectively; $p = .035$) (42). However, progression-free survival for both groups was equivalent because of the higher procedure-related mortality in the allogeneic group. Although one other series has reported a superior outcome for patients receiving HLA-matched allogeneic transplants, this was also a small retrospective series (22). Patients proceeding to allogeneic transplant are likely to be favorable in terms of age, performance status, and time in remission before transplant—all factors that might bias for improved survival.

The only prospectively collected data on the role of allogeneic transplantation were reported in the context of the European randomized trial (18). In this study, a small series of 12 patients with HLA-identical sibling donors were treated with allogeneic transplantation in first remission. The 3-year actu-arial overall survival of 58% for this group is comparable to results in patients receiving autologous transplants.

There are currently no convincing data to suggest that allogeneic stem cells are a better stem cell source or that a clinically significant graft-versus-lymphoma effect is active in this disease. Autologous stem cells should still be regarded as the preferred source of hematopoietic rescue in these patients.

UNIQUE COMPLICATIONS

Central Nervous System Relapse

The central nervous system is a frequent site of relapse in lymphoblastic lymphoma when treated with first- and second-generation non-Hodgkin's lymphoma regimens (2–4,30–33). Most of these protocols did not include specific central nervous system prophylaxis. The effectiveness of central nervous system prophylaxis in lymphoblastic lymphoma was demonstrated in two sequential studies from Stanford University (19). The first protocol described by this group included intrathecal and moderate-dose systemic methotrexate. The second protocol introduced the central nervous system prophylaxis phase earlier and used intrathecal methotrexate with cranial irradiation. The incidence of central nervous system relapse in these two relatively small patient groups was reduced from 31% in the first protocol to 3% in the second. Although the effectiveness of this specific protocol in controlling central nervous system disease has been questioned in one series (43), the reported incidence of central nervous system relapse with most acute lymphoblastic leukemia–like chemotherapy regimens has been low. The use of first remission stem cell transplantation has also been associated with a very low subsequent incidence of central nervous system recurrence in most reported series.

Acute Tumor Lysis Syndrome

Lymphoblastic lymphoma is an extremely chemosensitive disease. All patients with active disease, and especially those with a large tumor burden, are at risk of developing acute tumor lysis after the initiation of chemotherapy. Appropriate prophylactic measures should therefore be taken in all patients before chemotherapy.

PROGNOSIS AND MEDIAN SURVIVAL

As summarized in Tables 31.2 and 31.3, for most published series that include adult patients treated with intensive combination chemotherapy protocols with or without the use of stem cell transplantation to consolidate first remission, 5-year overall survival rates of 50% to 65% are typical, with no obvious benefit from stem cell transplantation. Although the International Prognostic Index may provide some prognostic information, there are inadequate data to suggest that patients should have treatment strategies modified according to risk group.

After relapse after first-line chemotherapy, subsequent prognosis is poor, with typical reported median survival rates of 6 to 9 months when conventional chemotherapy is used, although for relapsed and primary refractory patients, long-term survival rates of approximately 30% and 20%, respectively, are reported after stem cell transplantation.

FUTURE DIRECTIONS

Dose-intensive, multiagent, induction chemotherapy, similar to that used in acute lymphoblastic leukemia, has increased response rates and overall survival for adult patients with lymphoblastic lymphoma, compared with standard non-Hodgkin's lymphoma–type regimens. Whether further enhancement of dose intensity will improve response rates more is unclear. The use of very intensive induction therapy, such as hyper-CVAD [Cytoxan (cyclophosphamide), vincristine, Adriamycin (doxorubicin), and dexamethasone] has been reported to produce high overall-response rates in acute lymphoblastic leukemia and some subtypes of non-Hodgkin's lymphoma. Regimens such as this may have similar activity in patients with lymphoblastic lymphoma (44).

Reports of the use of relatively T-cell–specific agents, such as 506U78, suggest that such agents may have useful activity in this disease (45).

Stem cell transplant strategies also require further evaluation. In particular, nonmyeloablative stem cell transplantation may offer an opportunity to exploit the reported graft-versus-tumor effect in this disease, with lower risk of regimen-related mortality.

REFERENCES

1. The Non-Hodgkin's Lymphoma Classification Project: a clinical evaluation of the International Lymphoma Study Group classification of non-Hodgkin's lymphomas. *Blood* 1997;89:3909–3918.
2. Rosen PJ, Feinstein DI, Pattengale PK, et al. Convoluted lymphocytic lymphoma in adults: a clinicopathological entity. *Ann Intern Med* 1978;89:319–324.
3. Nathwani BN, Diamond LW, Winberg CD, et al. Lymphoblastic lymphoma: a clinicopathologic study of 95 patients. *Cancer* 1978;48:2347–2357.
4. Murphy SB. Management of childhood non-Hodgkin's lymphoma. *Cancer Treat Rep* 1977;61:1161–1173.
5. Warnke RA, Weiss LM, Chan JKC, et al. Tumors of the lymph nodes and spleen. In: *Atlas of tumor pathology.* Washington, DC: Armed Forces Institute of Pathology, 1995.
6. Borowitz MJ, Crocker BP, Metzgar RS. Lymphoblastic lymphoma with the phenotype of common acute lymphoblastic leukemia. *Am J Clin Pathol* 1983;79:387–391.
7. Griffith RC, Kelly DR, Nathwani BN, et al. A morphologic study of childhood lymphoma of the lymphoblastic type: the Pediatric Oncology Group experience. *Cancer* 1987;59:1126–1131.
8. Riopel M, Dickman PS, Link MP, et al. MIC analysis in pediatric lymphoma and leukemia. *Hum Pathol* 1994;25:396–399.
9. Cossman J, Chused TM, Fisher RI, et al. Diversity of immunologic phenotypes of lymphoblastic lymphoma. *Cancer Res* 1983;43:4486–4490.
10. Sheibani K, Nathwani BN, Winberg CD, et al. Antigenically defined subgroups of lymphoblastic lymphoma: relationship to clinical presentation and biological behavior. *Cancer* 1987;60:183–190.
11. Link MP, Stewart SJ, Warnke RA, et al. Discordance between surface and cytoplasmic expression of the Leu-4(T3) antigen I thymocytes and in blast cells from childhood T lymphoblastic malignancies. *J Clin Invest* 1985;76:248–253.
12. Chilosi M, Pizzolog G. Review of terminal deoxynucleotidyl transferase: biological aspects, methods of detection, and selected diagnostic applications. *Appl Immunohistochem* 1995;3:209–221.
13. Borowitz MJ. Immunologic markers in childhood acute lymphoblastic leukemia. *Hematol Oncol Clin North Am* 1990;4:743–765.
14. Bernard A, Murphy SM, Melvin S, et al. Non-T, non-B lymphomas are rare in childhood and are associated with cutaneous tumor. *Blood* 1982;59:549–554.
15. Knowles DM. Immunophenotypic and antigen receptor gene rearrangement analysis in T cell neoplasia. *Am J Pathol* 1989;134:761–785.
16. Pilozzi E, Muller-Hermelink HK, Falini B, et al. Gene rearrangements in T cell lymphoblastic lymphoma. *J Pathol* 1999;188:267–270.
17. Kaneko Y, Frizzera G, Shikano T, et al. Chromosomal and immunophenotypic patterns in T cell acute lymphoblastic leukemia and lymphoblastic lymphoma. *Leukemia* 1989;3:886–892.
18. Sweetenham JW, Santini G, Qian W, et al. High-dose therapy and autologous stem-cell transplantation versus conventional dose consolidation/maintenance therapy as post-remission therapy for adult patients with lymphoblastic lymphoma: results of a randomized trial of the European Group for Blood and Marrow Transplantation and the United Kingdom Lymphoma Group. *J Clin Oncol* 2001;19:2927–2936.
19. Coleman CN, Picozzi VJ, Cox RS, et al. Treatment of lymphoblastic lymphoma in adults. *J Clin Oncol* 1986;4:1626–1637.
20. Murphy SB, Fairclough DL, Hutchison RE, et al. Non-Hodgkin's lymphomas of childhood: an analysis of the histology, staging and response to treatment of 338 cases at a single institution. *J Clin Oncol* 1989;7:186–193.
21. Armitage JO, Weisenberger DD. New approach to classifying non-Hodgkin's lymphomas: clinical features of the major histologic subtypes. *J Clin Oncol* 1998;16:2780–2795.
22. Bouabdallah R, Xerri L, Bardou V-J, et al. Role of induction chemotherapy and bone marrow transplantation in adult lymphoblastic lymphoma: a report on 62 patients from a single center. *Ann Oncol* 1998;9:619–625.
23. Okuda T, Fisher R, Downing JR. Molecular diagnostics in pediatric acute lymphoblastic leukemia. *Mol Diag* 1996;1:139–151.
24. Czuczman MS, Dodge RK, Stewart CC, et al. Value of immunophenotype in intensively treated adult acute lymphoblastic leukemia: Cancer and Leukemia Group B study 8364. *Blood* 1999;93:3931–3939.
25. Secker-Walker LM, Moorman AV, Bain BJ, et al. Secondary acute leukemia and myelodysplastic syndrome with 11q23 abnormalities. EU Concerted Action 11q23 Workshop. *Leukemia* 1998;12:840–844.
26. Raimondi SC. Current status of cytogenetic research in childhood acute lymphoblastic leukemia. *Blood* 1993;81:2237–2251.
27. Slater DE, Mertelsmann R, Koriner B, et al. Lymphoblastic lymphoma in adults. *J Clin Oncol* 1986;4:57–67.
28. Bernasconi C, Brusamolino E, Lazzarino M, et al. Lymphoblastic lymphoma in adult patients; clinicopathological features and response to intensive multi-agent chemotherapy analogous to that used in acute lymphoblastic leukemia. *Ann Oncol* 1990;1:141–160.
29. Morel P, Lepage E, Brice P, et al. Prognosis and treatment of lymphoblastic lymphoma in adults: a report on 80 patients. *J Clin Oncol* 1992;10:1078–1085.
30. Murphy SB. Childhood non-Hodgkin's lymphoma. *N Engl J Med* 1977;299:1446–1448.
31. Voakes JB, Jones SE, McKelvey EM. The chemotherapy of lymphoblastic lymphoma. *Blood* 1981;57:186–188.
32. Colgan JP, Anderson J, Habermann TM, et al. Long-term follow-up of a CHOP-based regimen with maintenance chemotherapy and central nervous system prophylaxis in lymphoblastic non-Hodgkin's lymphoma. *Leuk Lymphoma* 1994;15:291–296.
33. Kaiser U, Uebelacker I, Havemann K. Non-Hodgkin's lymphoma protocols in the treatment of patients with Burkitt's lymphoma and lymphoblastic lymphoma: a report on 58 patients. *Leuk Lymphoma* 1999;36:101–108.
34. Woolner N, Burchenal JH, Liberman PH, et al. Non-Hodgkin's lymphoma in children. A progress report on the original patient treated with the LSA$_2$-L$_2$ protocol. *Cancer* 1979;44:1990–1999.
35. Anderson JR, Wilson JF, Jenkin RDT, et al. Childhood non-Hodgkin's lymphoma. The results of a randomized therapeutic trial comparing a 4-drug regimen (COMP) with a 10-drug regimen (LSA$_2$-L$_2$). *N Engl J Med* 1983;308:559–565.
36. Levine AM, Forman SJ, Meyer PR, et al. Successful therapy of convoluted T-lymphoblastic lymphoma in the adult. *Blood* 1983;61:92–99.

37. Weinstein HJ, Cassady JR, Levey R. Long-term results of the APO protocol (vincristine, doxorubicin [adriamycin] and prednisone) for the treatment of mediastinal lymphoblastic lymphoma. *J Clin Oncol* 1983;1:537–541.

38. Hoelzer D, Gokbuget N, Digel W, et al. Outcome of adult patients with T-lymphoblastic lymphoma treated according to protocols for acute lymphoblastic leukemia. *Blood* 2002;99:4379–4385.

39. Verdonck LF, Dekker AW, deGast GC, et al. Autologous bone marrow transplantation for adult poor risk lymphoblastic lymphoma in first remission. *J Clin Oncol* 1992;4:644–646.

40. Jost LM, Jacky E, Dommann-Scherrer C, et al. Short-term weekly chemotherapy followed by high dose therapy with autologous bone marrow transplantation for lymphoblastic and Burkitt's lymphomas in adult patients. *Ann Oncol* 1995;6:445–451.

41. Sweetenham JW, Santini G, Pearce R, et al. High-dose therapy and autologous bone marrow transplantation for adult patients with lymphoblastic lymphoma: results from the European Group for Bone Marrow Transplantation. *J Clin Oncol* 1994;12:1358–1365.

42. Chopra R, Goldstone AH, Pearce R, et al. Autologous versus allogeneic bone marrow transplantation for non-Hodgkin's lymphoma: a case controlled analysis of the European Bone Marrow Transplant Group registry data. *J Clin Oncol* 1992;10:1690–1695.

43. Sweetenham JW, Mead GM, Whitehouse JMA. Adult lymphoblastic lymphoma: high incidence of central nervous system relapse in patients treated with the Stanford University protocol. *Ann Oncol* 1992;3:839–841.

44. Thomas D, Kantarjian H, O'Brien S, et al. Outcome with the hyper-CVAD regimen in lymphoblastic lymphoma. *Proc Am Soc Clin Oncol* 1999;18:38a.

45. Kurtzberg J, Keating M, Moore JO, et al. 2-Amino-9-B-D-arabinosyl-6-methoxy-9H-guanine (GW506U; compound 506U) is highly active in patients with T-cell malignancies: results of a phase I trial in pediatric and adult patients with refractory hematological malignancies. *Blood* 1996;88:2666a.

46. Okuda T, Fisher R, Downing JR. Molecular diagnostics in pediatric acute lymphoblastic leukemia. *Mol Diag* 1996;1:139–151.

47. Finger LR, Kagan J, Christopher G, et al. Involvement of the TCL5 gene on human chromosome 1 in T-cell leukemia and melanoma. *Proc Natl Acad Sci U S A* 1989;86:5039–5043.

48. Mellentin JD, Smith SD, Cleary ML. Lyl-1, A novel gene altered by chromosomal translocation in T-cell leukemia, codes for a protein with helix-loop-helix DNA binding motif. *Cell* 1989;58:77–83.

49. Xia Y, Brown L, Yang CY, et al. TAL2, a helix-loop-helix gene activated by the t(7;9)(q34;q32) translocation in human T-cell leukemia. *Proc Natl Acad Sci U S A* 1989;88:11416–11420.

50. Ferrando AA, Neuberg D, Staunton J, et al. Gene expression signatures define novel oncogenic pathways in T cell acute lymphoblastic leukemia. *Cancer Cell* 2002;1:75–87.

CHAPTER 32

Plasma Cell Neoplasms: Multiple Myeloma and Plasmacytoma

Noopur Raje, Carl J. O'Hara, Richard W. Tsang, and Kenneth C. Anderson

Multiple myeloma is a plasma cell dyscrasia characterized by a clonal proliferation of lymphoid B cells and infiltration of the bone marrow by plasma cells. The presence of a monoclonal immunoglobulin in the serum or urine is characteristic of this disease (1,2). It is the second most common hematologic malignancy and is responsible for at least 2% of cancer-related deaths (3). It accounted for 14,600 new cancer cases in the United States in 2002. Despite our understanding of its biology and the use of aggressive treatment strategies, including transplantation, myeloma remains incurable.

EPIDEMIOLOGY

Contrary to the dogma that myeloma is a disease of the elderly, a significant proportion of patients are younger than 70 years of age and can tolerate aggressive therapeutic approaches. In a large Mayo Clinic series, the mean age was 62 years for men and 61 years for women (2). Although the majority of myeloma patients were 40 years of age or older, 35% of men and 41% of women were younger than 60 years of age. There was a slight male predominance in this series. The incidence rates are highest among African Americans and Pacific Islanders. Whites have intermediate rates, whereas generally low rates have been reported among Asians (4). Exposure to radiation and petroleum products is a potential risk factor for the development of myeloma (5). A genetic predisposition has also been suggested (6).

BIOLOGY AND PATHOGENESIS

Normal B-cell differentiation is characterized by a process of immunoglobulin variable diversity joint rearrangement, somatic mutation, and immunoglobulin class switching. Some evidence suggests that pre-B and naïve B cells migrate from the bone marrow to the lymph node where antigen recognition, selection, and somatic hypermutation occur. The memory B-cell compartment is believed to contain the cyto-

plasmic μ-positive precursor cell of myeloma, which then undergoes immunoglobulin class switching in the lymph node (7). Immunoglobulin variable (VH) gene sequence analysis has shown myeloma tumor cells to be post-follicular (8), and VH gene analysis of immunoglobulin M myeloma indicates an origin from a memory cell undergoing isotype switch events (9). Translocations involving switch regions (10) indicate that the final oncogenic molecular event in myeloma occurs late in B-cell ontogeny.

Karyotypic abnormalities are detected at a frequency of 30% to 50% by conventional cytogenetic analysis (Table 32.1) (11–13). Recent fluorescent *in situ* hybridization studies have shown that immunoglobulin H gene rearrangements are present in 73% of multiple myeloma patients (14), and spectral karyotyping identifies even higher frequencies of gene rearrangements. Translocations involving 14q32 are seen in 30% of myeloma patients. The partner chromosomal locus identified is 11q13 (bcl-1, cyclin D1), and transcriptional activation of cyclin D1 has been confirmed in some primary tumors (15,16), as has cyclin D3 activation associated with t(6;14(p21;q32) translocation (17). The t(4;14) translocation regulates FGFR3 and MMSET, resulting in immunoglobulin H/MMSET hybrid transcripts (18). FGFR3 promotes multiple myeloma cell proliferation and prevents apoptosis (19), and its oncogenic potential has been tested in a murine model confirming its capacity to transform hematopoietic cells (20). Other recurrent partner loci have been identified infrequently, including 8q24(c-myc) in less than 5%, 18q21(bcl-2), 11q23(MLL-1), and 6p21.1. Chromosome 13 deletions are present in more than 50% of multiple myeloma cases and are associated with poor prognosis (16,21–23). However, these deletions are also associated with monoclonal gammopathy of undetermined significance (16,24,25), and their role in transformation to multiple myeloma is at present undefined. There is evidence to suggest that RAS, p16, and p53 mutations play a role in disease biology and progression (1). Gene expression profiling studies are ongoing and help better define disease

515

TABLE 32.1. *Chromosomal abnormalities in multiple myeloma*

Chromosome	Incidence (%)	Genes	Function
11q13	30	Cyclin D1	Growth factor
4q16	25	FGFR3, MMSET	Growth factor
8q24	5	c-myc	Growth/apoptosis
16q23	1	c-maf	Transcription factor

biology, highlight prognostic factors, identify potential targets for novel therapies (15,19), and identify mechanisms of drug resistance (26,27).

ROLE OF THE BONE MARROW MICROENVIRONMENT IN MULTIPLE MYELOMA PATHOGENESIS

Adhesion molecules on multiple myeloma cells as well as bone marrow stromal cells play a key role in the homing of tumor cells to the bone marrow microenvironment and are crucial to the growth, survival, and development of drug resistance of multiple myeloma cells within the bone marrow milieu (Fig. 32.1). Our previous studies have identified adhesion molecules mediating multiple myeloma cell binding to fibronectin and bone marrow stromal cells. A growth and survival advantage is conferred on the tumor cells by this binding (28–31). Furthermore, secretion of cytokines, such as interleukin-6 (1) and insulin growth factor-1 (32), is upregulated by this binding, and it augments cell growth, survival, and drug resistance of multiple myeloma cells in the bone marrow milieu. Adhesion of multiple myeloma cells to bone marrow stromal cells also triggers the paracrine NF-κB–dependent transcription and secretion of interleukin-6 in bone marrow stromal cells (29,33). In addition, vascular endothelial growth factor is secreted by both multiple myeloma cells and bone marrow stromal cells, and its secretion is similarly upregulated by the binding of multiple myeloma cells to bone marrow stromal cells (34). Although tumor necrosis factor α does not directly alter multiple myeloma cell growth and survival, it induces NF-κB–dependent upregulation in cell surface expression of adhesion molecules on both multiple myeloma cells and bone marrow stromal cells. This results in increased binding and related

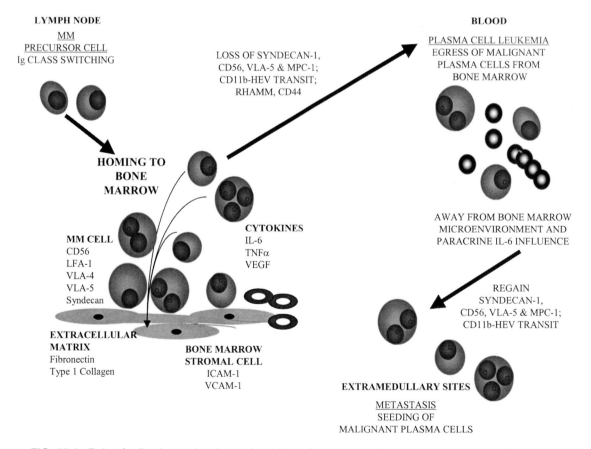

FIG. 32.1. Role of adhesion molecules and cytokines in myeloma disease pathogenesis and progression. ICAM-1, intercellular adhesion molecule-1; Ig, immunoglobulin; IL, interleukin; MM, multiple myeloma; TNFα, tumor necrosis factor α; VCAM-1, vascular cell adhesion molecule-1; VEGF, vascular endothelial growth factor.

induction of interleukin-6 transcription and secretion in bone marrow stromal cells (35). Multiple myeloma cell adhesion to fibronectin confers conventional drug resistance with induction of p27 and G1 growth arrest (36), and we have demonstrated that adhesion of multiple myeloma cells to paraformaldehyde-fixed bone marrow stromal cells triggers mitogen-activated protein kinase activation and proliferation in multiple myeloma cells (37) independent of cytokine induction in bone marrow stromal cells. Homing and localization of the multiple myeloma cell in the bone marrow milieu therefore promotes tumor cell growth, survival, migration, and drug resistance, supporting our focus to target multiple myeloma cell-host bone marrow stromal cells' interactions and their sequelae in novel therapeutics. Recent studies show that mitogen-activated protein kinase activation and proliferation of multiple myeloma cells triggered by adherence to paraformaldehyde-fixed bone marrow stromal cells are completely abrogated by novel agents, such as PS 341 (37), validating this approach.

ROLE OF CYTOKINES IN MULTIPLE MYELOMA PATHOGENESIS

Interleukin-6

Interleukin-6 plays a key role in the growth and survival of myeloma cells (38). Multiple reports support an autocrine interleukin-6–mediated growth mechanism in myeloma (39,40). Autocrine interleukin-6 production is associated with a highly malignant phenotype, with a high proliferative index and resistance to drug-induced apoptosis (41). An interleukin-6–mediated paracrine growth mechanism has also been postulated based on studies of the bone marrow microenvironment and multiple myeloma cell/bone marrow stromal cell adhesion as previously described (29,33,42).

Interleukin-6 mediates growth of myeloma cells via activation of the mitogen-activated protein kinase and phosphatidylinositol-3 kinase/Akt kinase signaling cascades, and blockade of these pathways abrogates the proliferative response. Interleukin-6 is not only a growth factor but also a survival factor in multiple myeloma (43,44). Recent studies have begun to identify cascades mediating dexamethasone-induced multiple myeloma cell death as well as resistance to apoptosis conferred by interleukin-6. Dexamethasone-induced apoptosis in multiple myeloma cells is associated with tyrosine phosphorylation and kinase activity of related adhesion focal tyrosine kinase, also known as *proline-rich tyrosine kinase 2* (45). Interleukin-6 blocks both dexamethasone-induced proline-rich tyrosine kinase 2 tyrosine phosphorylation and apoptosis via activation of Src homology protein tyrosine phosphatase 2 (SHP2), which modulates proline-rich tyrosine kinase 2 tyrosine kinase activity (46). We have further identified that dexamethasone-induced apoptosis is mediated by downstream activation of caspase-9 (26,47) and resultant caspase-3 cleavage by the release of second mitochondrial activator caspase (48). Interleukin-6,

via its triggering of phosphatidylinositol-3 kinase/Akt kinase signaling (47) and its association with Src homology protein tyrosine phosphatase 2, inactivates caspase-9 and protects against dexamethasone-induced apoptosis. These studies therefore identify signals triggering dexamethasone-induced multiple myeloma cell death as well as the protective effects of interleukin-6 against apoptosis. Characterization of these pathways may suggest novel treatment strategies based on triggering of apoptosis in tumor cells or inhibiting survival signals. For example, it appears that myeloma cells selected for resistance to Fas-mediated apoptosis are not cross-resistant to cytotoxic drugs, providing evidence for independent mechanisms of caspase activation (49).

Elevated interleukin-6 serum levels in some studies correlate with poor prognosis and higher tumor cell mass (50,51). Interleukin-6 is an important osteoclast activating factor in myeloma bone disease (52), and anti–interleukin-6 monoclonal antibody therapy can transiently reverse disease manifestations in patients with myeloma (53). Several studies suggest potential therapeutic usefulness of inhibiting interleukin-6 in myeloma; anti-humanized interleukin-6R and gp130 antibodies inhibit the growth of interleukin-6–dependent plasmacytoma cells *in vivo* (54). Interleukin-6 receptor superantagonists, which bind interleukin-6 but do not trigger via gp130, block interleukin-6–dependent myeloma cell growth (55–57). Dexamethasone has been shown to inhibit interleukin-6 and interleukin-6 receptor gene expression (58), as have bisphosphonates (56). Because the Kaposi's sarcoma herpesvirus genome encodes a homolog of the human interleukin-6 gene, a causal association with Kaposi's sarcoma herpesvirus was postulated (59). This association remains controversial (60), and to date, we have been unable to identify biologically relevant Kaposi's sarcoma herpesvirus gene products in myeloma (61).

Tumor Necrosis Factor α

Cytokines, such as tumor necrosis factor α, play an important role in bone resorption and myeloma bone disease (62). Although it induces only modest proliferation and activation of mitogen-activated protein kinase/extracellular signal-regulated protein kinase in multiple myeloma cells, tumor necrosis factor α upregulates certain adhesion molecules on multiple myeloma cells (CD11a, CD54, CD106, CD49d, and MUC-1) as well as on bone marrow stromal cells (CD54 and CD106), thereby increasing binding and triggering enhanced interleukin-6 secretion in bone marrow stromal cells (33,35). Blockade of NF-κB activation, on the other hand, has been shown to inhibit these sequelae.

Vascular Endothelial Growth Factor

Myeloma cells secrete vascular endothelial growth factor, which augments interleukin-6 secretion in stroma, and interleukin-6, in turn, augments vascular endothelial growth factor secretion from tumor cells (63,64). The presence of Flt-1 on some myeloma cells also suggests autocrine vascular endothelial growth factor–mediated myeloma cell growth (65). We have shown that vascular endothelial growth factor induces proliferation and triggers migration of multiple myeloma cells via activation of the Raf-1-MEK–extracellular signal-regulated protein kinase pathway and the protein kinase C–dependent cascade, respectively (34,66).

Other Cytokines

Similarly, other growth factors, including transforming growth factor β (67), interleukin-1α (68), interleukin-1β (69), lymphotoxin (70), interleukin-4 (71), oncostatin M, leukemia inhibitory factor, ciliary neurotropic factor (72), granulocyte-macrophage colony-stimulating factor (73), interleukin-11 (74,75), and interleukin-10 (76), have been shown to support myeloma cell growth directly or indirectly. Recently, insulin growth factor-1 has been shown to augment myeloma cell growth, survival, and drug resistance (32). Macrophage inflammatory protein-1α is a potential osteoclast stimulatory factor in multiple myeloma (77). These are discussed in the section Bone Disease and Hypercalcemia. Autocrine growth mediated by interleukin-15 (78), and most recently interleukin-21 (79), has been demonstrated in both myeloma cell lines and patient cells.

ROLE OF ANGIOGENESIS IN MULTIPLE MYELOMA PATHOGENESIS

Recent evidence suggests that angiogenesis may be important in the context of hematologic malignancies such as leukemia and multiple myeloma (80,81). Bone marrow neovascularization, plasma cell angiogenic potential, and matrix metalloproteinase-2 secretion have paralleled disease progression (82). Specifically, microvessel density is increased in patients with active myeloma, compared with patients with asymptomatic myeloma and monoclonal gammopathy of undetermined significance. Culture supernatants from patients with active myeloma have demonstrated increased angiogenic activity *in vitro*. Bone marrow plasma cells from patients with active myeloma express more matrix metalloproteinase-2 messenger RNA and protein than those with inactive myeloma or monoclonal gammopathy of undetermined significance (83). Progressive increase in bone marrow angiogenesis has been noted across the spectrum of plasma cell dyscrasias from monoclonal gammopathy of undetermined significance to advanced myeloma. The relevance of increased angiogenesis remains to be determined because despite targeted antiangiogenic therapy, such as thalidomide, clinical responses have not been associated with decreased marrow angiogenesis (84,85).

DIAGNOSTIC CRITERIA

The diagnosis of myeloma is based on the presence of major and minor criteria, which have been defined (Table 32.2)

TABLE 32.2. *Durie and Salmon criteria for diagnosis of myeloma*

Major criteria
1. Plasmacytomas on tissue biopsy.
2. BM plasmacytosis (>30% plasma cells).
3. Monoclonal Ig spike on serum or urine electrophoresis: IgG >3.5 g/dL or IgA >2.0 g/dL; kappa or lambda light chain urinary excretion >1.0 g/d.

Minor criteria
a. BM plasmacytosis (10–30% plasma cells).
b. Monoclonal Ig spike present but at a lower magnitude than above.
c. Lytic bone lesions.
d. Normal IgM >500 mg/L, IgA >1 g/L, or IgG >6 g/L.

The diagnosis of myeloma requires a minimum of one major and one minor criterion, although *1 + a* is not sufficient, or three minor criteria that must include *a* and *b*.

Patients with the above criteria and associated with the following are categorized as those with indolent myeloma and do not require immediate therapy:

Absent or limited bone lesions (≤ 3 lytic lesions), no compression fractures.

Stable paraprotein levels: IgG <70 g/L, IgA <50 g/L.

No symptoms and associated disease features, including Karnofsky performance status >70%, hemoglobin >10 g/L, normal serum calcium, serum creatinine <2 mg/dL, and no infections.

Plasma cell labeling index ≤0.5%.

BM, bone marrow; Ig, immunoglobulin.

(86). These include the presence of excess monotypic bone marrow plasma cells, monoclonal immunoglobulin in serum or urine, decreased normal serum immunoglobulin levels, and lytic bone disease. These criteria help to distinguish myeloma from other plasma cell dyscrasias and B-cell malignancies, which produce a paraprotein.

CLINICAL AND LABORATORY FEATURES

Myeloma is often regarded as a disease of older age, but, as previously described, a significant proportion of patients are younger than 60 years of age. A slight male preponderance has been described. Symptoms of bone pain and anemia remain the most common presenting features. Other features include renal insufficiency, hypercalcemia, and symptoms associated with infection and hyperviscosity (2). Laboratory evaluation identifies a monoclonal immunoglobulin in serum or urine in the majority of cases. In most series, 50% to 60% of patients with myeloma have both serum and urinary monoclonal protein; 20% to 30% of patients have serum without urinary protein; 15% to 20% of patients have monoclonal protein in urine only; and only 1% to 2% of patients do not secrete monoclonal protein in blood or urine. Immunoglobulin G or immunoglobulin A monoclonal proteins are most common, and immunoglobulin D or immunoglobulin E are rare. A biclonal process is much more common than previously appreciated, often only documented by immunofixation techniques (87). The natural history of myeloma is a progressive increase in tumor growth. The M protein doubling time, which is reflective of the myeloma growth rate, shortens with each relapse. Eventually, marrow failure develops, with sideroblastic anemia, leukopenia, and thrombocytopenia. The median interval from marrow failure to death is 3 (range, 1 to 9) months (88). Infection and renal failure account for 52% and 21% of deaths, respectively, in patients with myeloma (89).

BONE MARROW EXAMINATION IN MULTIPLE MYELOMA

One of the major criteria required to make a diagnosis of multiple myeloma is the presence of bone marrow plasmacytosis (90). In full-blown cases, plasma cells comprise more than 30% of the marrow cellularity. These plasma cells can be assessed by two separate yet complementary modalities: the core biopsy and the Wright-Giemsa–stained aspirate smears. The core biopsy offers the unique advantage of capturing plasma cells in their *in situ* environment, which in turn allows a more accurate assessment of proportional marrow involvement as well as demonstrates the propensity of malignant plasma cells to occur in sheets, clusters, and aggregates. This ability of neoplastic plasma cells to form cohesive tumoral masses contrasts with reactive plasmacytosis in which plasma cells are more likely to occur singly or in small clusters typically surrounding blood vessels. Recognition of these growth patterns may be very important, as these are reactive conditions (acquired immunodeficiency syndrome, rheumatoid arthritis) in which bone marrow plasmacytosis may exceed 30% of the cellularity (91). The bone marrow aspirate smear offers a greater appraisal of the morphologic spectrum of plasma cells. The typical plasma cell is quite distinctive and readily identified in Wright-Giemsa–stained smears with its eccentric nucleus, clumped nuclear chromatin, blue cytoplasm, and paranuclear halo. In multiple myeloma, plasma cells may range from being mature (indistinguishable from normal reactive plasma cells), to immature (slightly larger cells with central nuclei, dispersed chromatin, and nucleoli), to anaplastic (large cells with vesicular nuclei, prominent eosinophilic nucleoli, and abundant cytoplasm). These latter cells may be difficult to distinguish from immunoblasts. Not infrequently, binucleated and trinucleated plasma cells may be encountered, however, multinucleation in and of itself is not indicative of malignancy; such cells may be seen in reactive processes. Similarly, plasma cells may exhibit distinctive cytoplasmic inclusions (Russell's bodies, Mott cells), representing inspissated cytoplasmic immunoglobulin or, rarely, crystalline inclusions. These inclusions however are not particularly indicative of malignancy, as they may be seen in reactive plasma cells (92). Color Plate 64 demonstrates typical findings on bone marrow examination.

Although the morphologic findings in the core biopsy and aspirate smears may be sufficient to make a diagnosis of multiple myeloma, the demonstration of plasma cell monoclonality by immunohistochemical stains for light-chain immunoglobulins can be an extremely useful adjunct, especially in cases in which the degree of plasmacytosis is relatively low and overlaps with reactive plasmacytosis. The expression of kappa and lambda light-chain immunoglobulins by plasma cells in the core biopsy can be readily demonstrated by immunohistochemistry. An important technical point to emphasize is the far superior results obtained in this regard when biopsies are fixed in Zenker's fixative, compared with the more universally used formalin fixative. In kappa-positive myeloma, kappa-positive plasma cells exceed the normal kappa to lambda ratio of 3:1. In lambda-positive cases, inversion of the kappa to lambda ratio is by itself indicative of monoclonality. In addition to immunoglobulins, plasma cells can express the surface antigens CD38 and CD138. Typically, plasma cells do not express the B-cell antigen CD20, but they are positive for another pan-B–cell antigen, CD79a. Normal plasma cells express CD19 and lack CD56/CD58, whereas malignant plasma cells are believed to lack CD19 and are positive for CD56/CD58 (93). These latter antigens are more readily detected by flow cytometry than by immunohistochemistry.

BONE DISEASE AND HYPERCALCEMIA

Eighty percent of patients with myeloma present with bone pain and radiologic evidence of bone disease in the way of isolated, discrete lytic abnormalities or diffuse osteopenia. Skeletal surveys are routinely performed, but magnetic resonance imaging is becoming more frequently used and is more sensitive. Bone resorption leads to increased calcium in extracellular fluid. Although patients with normal renal function can increase urinary calcium excretion, those with renal failure develop hypercalcemia. Therefore, hypercalcemia is more likely to occur in the setting of Bence Jones proteinuria, myeloma kidney, chronic infection, or uric acid nephropathy. Overall, hypercalcemia occurs in 20% to 40% of patients with myeloma (94). Osteosclerosis occurs in less than 1% of patients.

Osteoclast activating factors, such as lymphotoxin, tumor necrosis factor α, hepatocyte growth factor, interleukin-6, interleukin-1, metalloproteinases (matrix metalloproteinase 1, matrix metalloproteinase 2, matrix metalloproteinase 9), RANKL, MIP-Iα, and insulin growth factor-4, are produced by multiple myeloma cell in the bone marrow and are responsible for bone resorption (69,70,77,94–98). The levels of RANKL/osteoprotegerin ligand, an osteoclast-like activation and differentiation factor, and of osteoprotegerin, which is a decoy receptor for osteoprotegerin ligand, modulate osteoclast formation, and an imbalance favoring osteoclast activation has been seen in multiple myeloma patients (99–101). Although osteoprotegerin levels are decreased in multiple myeloma patients with osteolytic lesions, the levels do not correlate with clinical stage or survival. Osteoprotegerin, which neutralizes osteoprotegerin ligand, may have therapeutic application in multiple myeloma bone disease (97). The use of osteoprotegerin to inhibit osteolytic bone disease has been demonstrated in an *in vivo* model by Croucher et al. (102). Another antagonist of osteoprotegerin ligand is the RANK-Fc molecule, a fusion of the Fc portion of immunoglobulin to a soluble form of the RANK receptor. RANK-Fc alone or in combination with bisphosphonates has been evaluated using *in vivo* models and also blocks bone destruction (103,104).

Pamidronate has been shown in a prospective randomized trial to reduce skeletal-related events, including pathologic fractures, need for radiation therapy, and spinal cord compression in patients with Durie-Salmon stage III myeloma and more than one lytic bone lesion (105). This benefit was maintained until 21 months in a follow-up study (106), and it is now recommended that myeloma patients remain on intravenous bisphosphonates indefinitely to reduce skeletal events and pain, regardless of their response to chemotherapy (107). More recently, the anti-myeloma activity of bisphosphonates via downregulation of interleukin-6 and direct apoptosis of osteoclasts and tumor cells has been studied (56,108,109). Pamidronate has been studied in patients with indolent myeloma (110), and although bone turnover was reduced in treated patients, no significant antitumor activity was noted. More potent bisphosphonates, such as zoledronate, are undergoing clinical evaluation and offer the benefit of shorter infusion times, compared with pamidronate (111–113). Ibandronate, a third-generation bisphosphonate, on the other hand, has failed to enhance survival or reduce morbidity from bone disease in patients with stage II or III multiple myeloma (114).

RENAL FAILURE

The causes of renal failure in myeloma are often multifactorial and include hypercalcemia, myeloma kidney, hyperuricemia, toxicity from intravenous urography, dehydration, plasma cell infiltration, pyelonephritis, and amyloidosis. The most important predisposing factor is dehydration; aggressive hydration is therefore crucial to avoid irreversible renal dysfunction. Combination chemotherapy should be used in patients with renal failure due to the more rapid response than is observed with melphalan and prednisone.

PROGNOSTIC FACTORS

Based on clinical and laboratory parameters, various staging systems have been identified (115–118). Of the many staging systems, the Durie-Salmon system is most commonly used and is of prognostic relevance (116). Tumor-cell mass correlates with stage, and survival duration is 61.2, 54.5, 30.1, and 14.7 months for patients with stage IA, stage IB+ IIA+ IIB, stage IIIA, and stage IIIB disease, respectively. Besides staging, serum β_2-microglobulin has been found to be a powerful prognostic indicator, with serum albumin being the only other variable adding to this significantly (115). These two variables were noted to be better than any staging systems. Many additional single parameters have been examined, including plasma cell morphology, plasma cell labeling index, tumor cell karyotype, cell surface phenotype, and percentage of circulating peripheral plasma cells.

SOLITARY PLASMACYTOMA

Solitary plasmacytomas account for less than 10% of plasma cell neoplasms (119–125). Although there has been variation of diagnostic criteria in the literature, the minimum requirements include the following: a histologically confirmed single lesion, normal bone marrow biopsy (less than 10% plasma cells), negative skeletal survey, no anemia, and normal calcium and renal function (119). A serum paraprotein (M protein) is present in 30% to 70% of cases, usually minimally elevated (120). The disease can present in bone or in extramedullary sites such as soft tissues or lymph nodes. Patients have a median age of 50 to 55 years, which on average is 5 to 10 years younger than those diagnosed with multiple myeloma (median age, 60 years) (119,121). A bony presentation is more common, and in such cases, it really represents early multiple myeloma.

Solitary Plasmacytoma of Bone

Patients with bone involvement often present with pain, neurologic compromise, and occasionally pathologic fracture. A lytic lesion is typical, with or without adjacent soft-tissue infiltration. The most common location is the vertebra. Rarely, a patient may present with demyelinating polyneuropathy (126). Detailed staging investigations, including the use of magnetic resonance imaging of the spine, have been shown to demonstrate disease in a significant proportion (4/ 12 patients, 33%) of patients who otherwise would be diagnosed with a solitary bone plasmacytoma (127,128). Although patients often progress to multiple myeloma despite initial successful local treatment with surgery and radiation therapy (119,121,123,125,128–134), a significant proportion (approximately 20% to 30%) have durable control of disease and would die of unrelated illness without development of myeloma. Early use of systemic therapy has not been shown to reduce the risk of progression to myeloma; therefore, radiation therapy remains the standard treatment (134). For patients treated with gross tumor excision, radiation therapy is still indicated for presumed or proven microscopic residual disease. The whole bone is usually included in the radiation portals. A review of the literature (Table 32.3) indicated a high local control rate with radiation therapy, yet a modest disease-free survival of approximately 50% at 8 years. As shown in Table 32.3, more than 50% of patients with osseous tumors progressed to myeloma (119,121,129,135) at a median of 2 to 3 years after treatment. The median survival is 7 to 11 years (121,125,128–130). Age is a significant factor affecting the risk of progression to myeloma in some series (119,129) but not in others (123,131,132,135). The presence of M protein preradiation was not associated with a higher risk of progression to multiple myeloma (129), but the persistence of M protein after radiation is ominous for subsequent systemic failure

TABLE 32.3. *Solitary plasmacytoma of bone: representative treatment results from the literature*

First author, yr (reference)	Institution	No. of patients (median follow-up)	Local control (%)	Progression to myeloma (10-yr rate %)	Overall survival (10-yr rate %)
Bataille, 1981 (119)	Hopital St. Eloi, France	114 (>10 yr)	88	58	68[a]
Knowling, 1983 (121)	Princess Margaret Hospital, Canada	25 (45 mo)	91	86	50
Chak, 1987 (129)	Stanford[b]	65[b] (87 mo)	95	77	52
Frassica, 1989 (130)	Mayo Clinic	46 (90 mo)	89	54[a]	45
Mayr, 1990 (123)	University of Iowa	17 (12 yr)	88	53[a]	47[a] (at 5 yr)
Holland, 1992 (131)	Mallinckrodt	32 (66 mo)	94	53[a]	—
Shih, 1995 (132)	Chang Gung Memorial Hospital, Taiwan	22 (48 mo)	91	32[a]	68 (5-yr rate)
Bolek, 1996 (135)	University of Florida	27 (N/A)	96	54	55
Jyothirmayi, 1997 (133)	Royal Marsden, United Kingdom	23 (64 mo)	100	39[a]	33
Tsang, 2001 (125)	Princess Margaret Hospital, Canada	32 (95 mo)	87	64 (8-yr rate)	65 (8-yr rate)
Wilder, 2002 (137)	M.D. Anderson Cancer Center	60 (94 mo)	90	62	59

N/A, not available.
[a]Crude rate.
[b]Combined results of four institutions.

(128,136,137). Radiation therapy treatment details are discussed in Radiation Therapy Dose Prescription.

As for local control, data from Princess Margaret Hospital showed that tumor size assessed preradiation is important because all the local failures were in bulky tumors greater than or equal to 5 cm (125). After radiotherapy, persistent residual abnormalities are often found; therefore, the majority of authors in the literature define *local control* as the absence of disease progression in the local irradiated site. In the long term, local control of disease is reflected by absence of symptoms and follow-up imaging showing stability, with the lytic bone lesion developing sclerosis, with no or minimal surrounding soft-tissue mass.

Although it is recognized that some patients recur with plasmacytoma(s) of bone or soft tissues without bone marrow involvement (119,121,131), this occurrence is infrequent, and the subsequent development of multiple myeloma is high—75% according to one series (119).

Solitary Extramedullary Plasmacytoma

Nonosseous tumors often present with a mass, and approximately 80% are located in the upper aerodigestive passages (138) and produce local compressive symptoms. The histologic diagnosis of extramedullary plasmacytoma can be difficult, with the differential diagnosis being non-Hodgkin's lymphoma, particularly of the mucosa-associated lymphoid tissue type, in which there can be extensive infiltration by plasmacytoid cells (139). Although complete surgical excision may be curative for small lesions (138), most patients with larger lesions or location

not amenable to complete excision should receive local radiation therapy. Additionally, postoperative radiation therapy is indicated for patients treated with incomplete local excision. Based on an extensive review of the literature, the incidence of regional nodal involvement is low, 7.6% for upper aerodigestive locations, and even lower for other sites (138). Therefore, routine nodal treatment is unnecessary, and significant regional nodal failure was not observed with radiation treatment plans that did not include first echelon lymph nodes (122,125,140,141).

In contrast to solitary plasmacytoma of bone, a review of the literature showed that extramedullary plasmacytomas are frequently cured with local radiation (Table 32.4), with a lower rate of progression to myeloma, ranging from 8% to 41% (121–123,131,132,135,138,140–147). Therefore, definitive local radiotherapy is the treatment of choice for extramedullary plasmacytoma.

Radiation Therapy Dose Prescription

The optimal radiation dose is controversial, and recommendations vary from 35 Gy (148) to 40 Gy (135,146,149) or higher (120,130,131,141,144,150,151). Although some authors reported no dose-response relationship in radiation therapy for plasmacytomas (131,148), others indicated that 45 to 50 Gy is required for a high local control rate (123,124,128,130), particularly for extramedullary plasmacytomas (122) or a nonvertebral bone lesion (120). The recommendation of a minimum dose of 40 Gy originated from a dose-response analysis by Mendenhall et al. reported in 1980 based on a review of the lit-

TABLE 32.4. *Solitary extramedullary plasmacytoma: representative treatment results from the literature*

First author, yr (reference)	Institution/location	No. of patients (median follow-up)	Local control (%)	Progression to myeloma (10-yr rate %)	Overall survival (10-yr rate %)
Wiltshaw, 1976 (142)	Royal Marsden, United Kingdom	44	70	41[a]	40
Bush, 1981 (144)	Stanford	10 (4.5 yr)	80	20[a]	70[a]
Kapadia, 1982 (143)	University of Pittsburgh	17 (62 mo)	85	31[a]	31[a] (5-yr rate)
Knowling, 1983 (121)	Princess Margaret Hospital, Canada	25 (71 mo)	88	28	43
Brinch, 1990 (146)	Oslo, Norway	18	—	—	90
Mayr, 1990 (123)	University of Iowa	13 (12 yr)	92	23[a]	58[a] (5-yr rate)
Soeson, 1991 (145)	Padua, Italy	25 (44 mo)	88	—	~50
Holland, 1992 (131)	Mallinckrodt	14 (66 mo)	93	36[a]	—
Shih, 1995 (132)	Chang Gung Memorial Hospital, Taiwan	10 (48 mo)	70	20[a]	100
Bolek, 1996 (135)	University of Florida	10	100	11	80
Susnerwala, 1997 (140)	Christie Hospital, United Kingdom	25 (73 mo)	79	8[a]	59 (5-yr rate)
Liebross, 1999 (122)	M.D. Anderson Cancer Center	22	95	44 (5-yr rate)	50
Galieni, 2000 (147)	Siena, Italy	46 (118 mo)	92	15	78 (15 yr)
Strojan, 2002 (141)	Slovenia Cancer Registry	26 (61 mo)	90	8	61

[a]Crude rate.

erature including 81 patients (149). A total dose of 40 Gy or more resulted in a local failure rate of 6% versus 31% for lower doses (149). Retrospective analyses are always confounded by important factors that affect tumor control such as tumor size. A recent series indicated that smaller tumors (less than 5 cm) have a high control rate with a total dose of less than or equal to 35 Gy (125), similar to that reported by Harwood et al. (148), who recommended 35 Gy in 15 fractions. However, for extensive, bulky plasmacytomas, it is important to optimize local control with a higher total dose of 45 to 50 Gy (141). Despite higher doses, local control is not guaranteed, as local failure has been documented even after doses as high as 60 to 67 Gy (144,152). The dose per fraction should be kept at 2 Gy or less to minimize the long-term side effects of radiation.

Role of Combined Modality Therapy

The addition of chemotherapy for bulky solitary plasmacytomas is theoretically advantageous, both in enhancing local control and potentially eradicating subclinical disease to delay or prevent the development of myeloma. Mayr et al. (123) reported a lower rate of progression to myeloma with chemotherapy (combined modality therapy, 0 of 5 patients progressed; radiation therapy alone, 9 of 12 patients progressed) (123), although other studies did not document a similar effect (131,132). One randomized trial suggested benefit with adjuvant melphalan and prednisone given for 3 years after radiotherapy (153). After a median follow-up of 8.9 years, 15 of 28 patients in the radiation therapy arm progressed to myeloma (54%), whereas only 3 of 25 patients in the combined modality arm developed myeloma (12%) (153). This study is limited by the small sample size and the obvious concerns about prolonged use of alkylating agents in this setting. In using chemotherapy with fewer long-term consequences, such as VAD [vincristine, Adriamycin (doxorubicin), dexamethasone] (154), or novel agents, such as thalidomide (84), a combined modality approach (drug plus radiation therapy) is worthy of further investigation, particularly for bulky solitary plasmacytomas.

TREATMENT OF MULTIPLE MYELOMA

Chemotherapy with alkylating agents is established therapy for symptomatic myeloma. Response to therapy can be monitored because of the presence of the paraprotein in serum. The most commonly used response criteria are the Southwest Oncology Group criteria (155). An objective response by these criteria was defined as a reduction of at least 75% of the calculated serum paraprotein or a decrease of at least 90% in urinary light chains sustained for a period of 2 months. More recently, the European Group for Blood and Marrow Transplant, the International Bone Marrow Transplant Registry, and the Autologous Blood and Marrow Transplant Registry (156) have defined criteria for response and disease progression. These criteria include a more sensitive and rigorous definition of complete response, including absence of paraprotein assayed by immunofixation, and exclude transient responses.

CONVENTIONAL THERAPY

Melphalan and Prednisone

Oral administration of MP (melphalan, prednisone) has been used for more than three decades and produces objective response in up to 50% to 60% of patients (157,158). The dosage of melphalan, due to the variability of absorption, should be modified if necessary so that some reduction in leukocytes and platelets occurs 3 to 4 weeks after the beginning of each cycle. Unless there is disease progression, MP should be given for at least 1 year until the monoclonal immunoglobulin levels in the serum or urine have been stable for at least 6 months (plateau state) and then discontinued if the patient has no other evidence of active disease. Typical dosages of melphalan are 0.15 mg per kg daily for 7 days (8 to 10 mg/day) and 20 mg of prednisone three times daily for the same period. Melphalan must be given before meals because food reduces absorption. It is important to remember that the natural course of multiple myeloma is one of progression, so that alleviation of pain and lack of progressive disease may be beneficial, even in the absence of an objective response.

Combination Chemotherapy

Combination chemotherapy has been used in the treatment of myeloma, and although improved responses are seen, these may not translate into prolonged survival (159). Various combinations have been tried, including VMCP (vincristine, melphalan, cyclophosphamide, prednisone) alternating with VBAP [vincristine, BCNU, Adriamycin (doxorubicin), prednisone]. One study demonstrated a 54% response rate and a 48-month survival in those receiving VMCP/VBAP (160). Initial combination therapy with VAD produced a high response rate (84%), with 28% of all patients achieving a complete response; however, duration of response was only 18 months (161). Initial therapy with high-dose dexamethasone achieved response rates approximately 15% less than those seen with VAD and similar to those with MP (162). VAD chemotherapy was, however, associated with increased toxicity, and survival was similar. The inclusion of high doses of corticosteroids increased the frequency of response to chemotherapy and was noted to prolong survival (163). In a recent Southwest Oncology Group study, alternate-day prednisone at a dose of 50 mg was noted to improve overall survival and event free survival after induction treatment with a VAD-like induction regimen (164). The M2 protocol, which includes VBMCP [vincristine, BCNU (carmustine), melphalan, prednisone, and cyclophosphamide], was evaluated in an Eastern Cooperative Oncology Group study in which 220 evaluable patients were randomized to VBMCP and 221 to MP. The objective response was 72% for VBMCP and 51% for MP, but the median survival was not different at 30 versus 28 months, respectively (165). Table 32.5 represents some of the commonly used combination chemotherapies with the regimen.

TABLE 32.5. *Representative combination chemotherapy for myeloma*

Regimen (reference)	Drugs	Dosages	Treatment schedule
M2 (165)	Vincristine	1.2 mg/m^2 i.v. on d 1	Cycle is repeated every 35 d.
	Carmustine (BCNU)	20 mg/m^2 i.v. on d 1	
	Cyclophosphamide	400 mg/m^2 i.v. on d 1	
	Melphalan	8 mg/m^2 p.o. on d 1–4	
	Prednisone	40 mg/m^2 p.o. on d 1–7 and 20 mg/m^2 on d 8–14 for cycles 1–3 only	
VMCP (160)	Vincristine	1 mg/m^2 i.v. on d 1 (1.5 mg maximum)	Alternating cycles of VMCP and VBAP are given at 3-wk intervals.
	Melphalan	6 mg/m^2 p.o. on d 1–4	
	Cyclophosphamide	125 mg/m^2 p.o. on d 1–4	
	Prednisone	60 mg/m^2 p.o. on d 1–4	
VBAP (160)	Vincristine	1 mg/m^2 i.v. on d 1 (1.5 mg maximum)	Cycles are repeated at 21-d intervals, depending on the extent of myelosuppression.
	BCNU (carmustine)	30 mg/m^2 i.v. on d 1	
	Adriamycin (doxorubicin)	30 mg/m^2 i.v. on d 1	
	Prednisone	60 mg/m^2 p.o. on d 1–4	
VAD (161)	Vincristine	0.4 mg/d by continuous i.v. infusion on d 1–4	Cycles are repeated at 21-d intervals, depending on the extent of myelosuppression.
	Adriamycin (doxorubicin)	9 mg/m^2/ by continuous i.v. infusion on d 1–4	
	Dexamethasone	40 mg p.o., q.d. on d 1–4, 9–12, and 17–20	

TABLE 32.6. *Conventional treatment of myeloma*

Therapy	Response (%)	Median survival (yr)
MP	50–60	3
VBMCP	72	≅3
VMCP/VBAP	54	4
VAD	84	≅3

MP, melphalan and prednisone; VAD, vincristine, Adriamycin (doxorubicin), dexamethasone; VBAP, vincristine, BCNU (carmustine), Adriamycin (doxorubicin), prednisone; VBMCP, vincristine, BCNU (carmustine), melphalan, prednisone, (Cytoxan) cyclophosphamide; VMCP, vincristine, melphalan, cyclophosphamide, prednisone.
From Myeloma Trialists' Collaborative Group. Combination chemotherapy versus melphalan plus prednisone as treatment for multiple myeloma: an overview of 6633 patients from 27 randomized trials. *J Clin Oncol* 1998;16:3832, with permission.

In a metaanalysis performed by Gregory et al., 18 randomized, controlled trials comparing MP with combination therapy in the primary treatment of 3,814 patients were studied (166). The overall results showed no difference in efficacy between these treatment modalities. A subgroup analysis showed that MP is superior for patients with an intrinsically good prognosis and inferior for those patients with a poor prognosis. A second overview of 6,633 patients from 27 randomized trials of combination therapy versus MP confirmed higher response rates to combination therapy but equivalent mortality and survival (167). In patients who are potential candidates for high-dose therapies, prolonged use of alkylating agents, such as melphalan, should be avoided. Table 32.6 shows the response and median survival with conventional treatment in that overview.

ALPHA-2B INTERFERON THERAPY

Several prospective randomized trials have examined the usefulness of combined interferon-α and chemotherapy for induction therapy. The duration of the plateau phase was prolonged by 5 to 6 months without a statistically significant increase in median survival (168–171). A metaanalysis of 16 randomized trials involving 2,286 patients receiving combined interferon-α chemotherapy for induction treatment yielded higher response rates (complete response or partial response) in the interferon-α arms, but the average gain was only approximately 10% (169).

The role of interferon-α as maintenance therapy was studied by Mandelli et al. in a randomized trial in patients who had achieved complete response, partial response, or stable disease after MP or VMCP/VBAP (172). Although the duration of response and survival were superior with interferon-α, subsequent studies had variable results. The remission duration was always longer in the interferon-α arm (163,169,173–175), but the observed differences reached statistical significance in only a few studies (169,174,175) and were minimal in others (163,176). Substantial increases in survival times were also observed only in some trials (169,174,175). Metaanalysis of eight trials of 929 patients receiving maintenance interferon-α

revealed that both remission duration and survival were significantly longer in the interferon-α arm than in the control arm, but median gains were only 6 and 5 months, respectively (169). Interferon-α maintenance treatment therefore appears to benefit a subset of patients who have achieved low tumor burden, and its marginal benefit needs to be balanced against side effects in this patient group.

HIGH-DOSE TREATMENT OF MULTIPLE MYELOMA

The rationale for the administration of alkylating agents in myeloablative doses with or without total-body irradiation followed by transplantation of syngeneic, allogeneic, or autologous bone marrow or peripheral-blood progenitor cells stems from the fact that dose response has been noted in multiple myeloma. More important, documented complete responses have been associated with high-dose therapy.

Autologous Stem Cell Transplantation

High-dose chemoradiotherapy followed by transplantation of autologous bone marrow or peripheral-blood progenitor cells has resulted in high (40%) complete response rates; however, the median duration of these responses has only been 24 to 36 months (177,178). Patients with sensitive disease and those who are less heavily pretreated have the most favorable outcomes. In a landmark national French trial of 200 patients with myeloma, patients were randomized after two courses of VMCP alternating with VBAP to receive either conventional chemotherapy (eight additional courses of VMCP/VBAP) or high-dose therapy (melphalan and total-body irradiation) followed by autologous bone marrow transplantation. Significantly higher response rates, event-free survival, and overall survival for those patients treated with high-dose therapy, compared with those receiving conventional therapy, were noted (179). Response rates in the high-dose and conventional arms were 81% versus 57%, respectively. The 5-year probabilities of event-free survival and overall survival were 28% and 52%, respectively, in recipients of high-dose therapy and only 10% and 12%, respectively, in patients treated with conventional therapy. Prognostic factors, such as age and renal failure, have been evaluated in several studies in the setting of high-dose treatment. Although high-dose therapy is feasible, increased toxicity is noted (180–183). A second randomized trial in myeloma examined the relative merits of high-dose therapy early or late as salvage therapy for relapse after conventional therapy (184). The overall survival was 64 months in both groups, but the quality-adjusted time without symptoms and toxicity strongly favored the early transplant arm. The use of high-dose melphalan at 200 mg per m² versus melphalan at 140 mg per m² plus total-body irradiation as ablative therapies has also been studied, and melphalan-alone conditioning proved to be more efficacious with improved survival and decreased toxicity (185). More recently, a population-based Scandinavian study demonstrated prolonged survival for patients with

TABLE 32.7. *Comparison of high-dose therapy (HDT) versus conventional chemotherapy (CCT) for newly diagnosed myeloma*

Study (reference)	Therapy	Complete response (%)	Median event-free survival (mo)	Overall survival
Barlogie et al. (271)	CCT	—	22	48 mo (median)
	HDT	40	49	62 mo (median)
Lenhoff et al. (186)	CCT	—	—	44 mo (median)
	HDT	41	32	61% at 4 yr
Attal et al. (179)	CCT	5	18	37 mo (median)
	HDT	22	27	52% at 5 yr
Blade et al. (*unpublished data*)	CCT	83	34	66.6 mo (median)
	HDT	81	42.5	67.4 mo (median)

myeloma younger than 60 years of age treated with intensive therapy, compared with historical controls who received conventional therapy (186). We have compared 228 patients undergoing transplantation over a 10-year period, including 166 patients who underwent autografting and 66 patients who were allografted (187). The outcomes were similar in the two groups, with high relapses in the autografting group versus increased toxicity in the allograft recipients. Therefore, relapse remains the major problem with autografting, likely due to a contaminated graft or the persistence of minimal residual disease. Table 32.7 compares the outcome of patients treated with high-dose therapy with conventional chemotherapy. Table 32.8 demonstrates the role of early versus late transplants.

A strategy to decrease relapse and improve the outcome of autografting includes the use of depletion of tumor cells in the graft (188,189) or positive selection of normal hematopoietic progenitor cells by virtue of CD34 expression (190). Despite a median of 3.1 log reduction in myeloma cells within the CD34+-selected autografts (191), there was no impact on survival at 2 years (192). A second trial showed that CD34+ selection also had no impact on the outcome of single or tandem high-dose chemotherapy (193).

Alternate approaches include the use of multiple high-dose therapies and stem cell transplantation (194–196). Response rates are higher relative to historically matched controls, but the impact on long-term disease-free survival requires further follow-up. A French randomized trial has compared a single versus double transplant in the autologous setting. In this study, 403 patients were randomized to receive a single or a double autotransplant, the first prepared with melphalan and the second prepared with melphalan and total-body irradiation. Out of 199 patients assigned to the single autograft arm, 177 (85%) received the planned transplant, and there were three toxic deaths. Out of 200 patients randomized to the double transplant, 156 (78%) actually received two transplants, and there were five toxic deaths. There was no significant difference in the complete remission rate between the single and double transplantation arms, and event-free survival and overall survival curves separated only after 3 years (197). Table 32.9 demonstrates results of single versus double transplantation for myeloma. Strategies to stimulate autologous immunity to

myeloma cells to treat minimal residual disease post autografting have been studied and hold promise (198,199). Hsu and coworkers have vaccinated patients using autologous dendritic cells pulsed *ex vivo* with tumor-specific idiotypic protein to stimulate host antitumor immunity and demonstrated T-cell–mediated antiidiotype and anti–keyhole limpet hemocyanin proliferative responses specific for the immunizing immunoglobulin in some patients (200).

Allogeneic Stem Cell Transplant

Syngeneic or allogeneic bone marrow transplantation has also been associated with a dramatic reduction in tumor mass in some cases, with complete-response rates commonly in the 40% range and a similar number of partial responses (177,201). Syngeneic bone marrow transplantation has been done infrequently, but some patients reported from Seattle (202) and in the European Group for Blood and Marrow Transplant (203) remain progression free at long intervals post bone marrow transplantation. The European Group for Blood and Marrow Transplant allografting data in myeloma (204–206) demonstrate an actuarial overall survival of 32% at 4 years and 28% at 7 years for the 72 patients (44%) who achieved complete response after bone marrow transplantation. However,

TABLE 32.8. *Early versus late stem cell transplantation for myeloma*

End point	Early peripheral-blood stem cell transplant (mo)	Late peripheral-blood stem cell transplant (mo)
Median overall survival	64.6	64
Median event-free survival	39	13
Time without symptoms and toxicity	27.8	22.3

From Fermand J-P, Ravaud P, Chevret S, et al. High-dose therapy and autologous peripheral blood stem cell transplantation in multiple myeloma: up-front or rescue treatment? Results of a multicenter sequential randomized clinical trial. *Blood* 1998;92:3131, with permission.

TABLE 32.9. *Single versus double transplantation for myeloma*

Study (reference)	Therapy (n)	Complete response (%)	Event-free survival	Overall survival
Attal et al. (197)	Single (88)	50	20% at 60 mo	40% at 60 mo
	Double (92)	61	35% at 60 mo	60% at 60 mo
Cavo et al. (unpublished)	Single (81)	34	21.5 mo median	71% at 48 mo
	Double (97)	41	29.5 mo median	74% at 48 mo

overall progression-free survival was 34% at 6 years, and few patients remain in continuing complete response at more than 4 years post allograft. Favorable pretransplantation prognostic factors for both response and survival after bone marrow transplantation were female sex, immunoglobulin A myeloma, low serum β_2-microglobulin, stage I disease at diagnosis, one line of previous treatment, and being in complete response before bone marrow transplantation. The Seattle data demonstrate actuarial probabilities of overall survival and event-free survival for the 36% of patients achieving complete response to be 0.50 ± 0.21 and 0.43 ± 0.17, respectively, at 4.5 years. Adverse prognostic factors include transplantation more than 1 year from diagnosis; serum β_2-microglobulin more than 2.5 mg per dL at transplant; female patients transplanted from male donors; having received more than eight cycles of chemotherapy; and Durie-Salmon stage III disease at presentation. Again, toxicity was common, with 35 patients (44%) dying of transplant-related causes within 100 days of bone marrow transplantation (207). A major concern is the 40% transplant-related mortality associated with allografting seen in most series. Nonetheless, molecular remissions are noted in allogeneic bone marrow transplantation (208), due in part to a graft-versus-myeloma effect (209–211), and the emphasis now is to develop strategies to achieve and maintain high remission rates

TABLE 32.10. *Allogeneic transplantation for myeloma*

Study	Complete response (%)	TRM (%)	Overall survival	Event-free survival
EBMTR	44	41	28% at 7 yr	45% at 5 yr
Seattle	36	44	20% at 4.6 yr	24% at 4.6 yr
DFCI	28	5	40% at 3 yr	20% at 3 yr

DFCI, Dana-Farber Cancer Institute; EBMTR, European Group for Blood and Marrow Transplant Registry; TRM, transplant-related mortality.

while avoiding transplant-related morbidity and mortality. Results of allografting are depicted in Table 32.10.

An approach to improve transplant results is to offer transplant earlier in the course of disease. The European Group for Blood and Marrow Transplant registry data demonstrate improved survival with low transplant-related mortality in patients transplanted between 1994 and 1998 because of better patient selection, early transplantation, and less pretransplant treatment (212). We have carried out T-cell (CD6)–depleted allografting using histocompatible sibling donors in 61 patients with myeloma whose disease remained sensitive to conventional chemotherapy (189,213–215). Although transplant related mortality was markedly reduced (5%), disease relapse adversely affected survival. To overcome the problem of relapse, we have demonstrated that the graft-verus-myeloma effect of donor lymphocyte infusions can be preserved, and graft-versus-host disease can be abrogated, by using CD8-depleted (CD4$^+$) donor lymphocyte infusions (211). Overall, only 8 of 32 patients (25%) evaluable for toxicity developed acute or chronic graft-versus-host disease. Although feasible, only 58% of patients were able to receive donor lymphocyte infusions despite T-cell–depleted bone marrow transplantation (216), underlying the need for less toxic transplantation strategies. Our laboratory data have confirmed that prophylactic infusion of CD4$^+$ donor lymphocyte infusions, besides enhancing reconstitution of donor T cells, also helps reconstitute donor hematopoiesis and promotes antitumor immunity (217–219). Ongoing studies are addressing the role of nonmyeloablative transplantation to preserve graft-versus-myeloma effect while avoiding the toxicity of allografting (220,221).

TOTAL-BODY IRRADIATION IN HIGH-DOSE THERAPY PROTOCOLS

In light of the radiation sensitivity of myeloma cells and the successful use of total-body irradiation in leukemia transplant protocols, many high-dose protocols for multiple myeloma incorporate total-body irradiation into the conditioning regimen. A phase III study conducted by the Intergroupe Francophone du Myelome (IFM 90) showed that autologous stem cell transplant (melphalan, 140 mg per m^2, plus total-body irradiation, 8 Gy in four daily fractions) gave superior 5-year event-free survival rates (28%), compared with conventional chemotherapy (10%) ($p = .01$) (179,222). However, there was no plateau on the event-free survival curve, suggesting that autologous stem cell transplant is not curative. Because of toxicity concerns (mucosal and hematologic) with total-body irradiation, another IFM trial (#9502) studied a higher dose of melphalan, 200 mg per m^2, versus total-body irradiation (8 Gy in 4 fractions) plus melphalan, 140 mg per m^2 (185). Patients in the total-body irradiation–containing arm suffered more grade 3–4 mucosal toxicity (51% vs. 30%), a heavier transfusion requirement, and a longer median hospitalization stay (23 days vs. 19 days) and had a higher toxic death rate (3.6% vs. 0%) than patients who did not get total-body irradiation. Although event-free survival was no different between the two treatment arms, the 45-month overall survival favored the melphalan, 200 mg per m², arm with borderline statistical significance [65.8% vs. 45.5% (p = .05)] (185). Similarly, another IFM protocol tested total-body irradiation in the tandem transplant setting by intensifying the conditioning regimen for the second transplant to melphalan, 200 mg per m², without total-body irradiation and comparing it with the standard tandem regimen (melphalan, 140 mg per m², for the first; melphalan, 140 mg per m², plus total-body irradiation for the second). There was no benefit with total-body irradiation, and increased toxicity was again observed. Therefore, all subsequent IFM trials abandoned the use of total-body irradiation (223). Another study from the Spanish bone marrow transplant registry compared melphalan, 140 mg per m², plus total-body irradiation with three other chemotherapy conditioning regimens (melphalan, 200 mg per m²; melphalan and busulfan; busulfan and cyclophosphamide) (224). There were no significant differences in the hospitalization duration, hematologic recovery, event-free survival, and overall survival among the four regimens, although the melphalan-busulfan regimen had the highest rate of complete response. The authors concluded that no one regimen was clearly superior to another (224).

The Toronto protocol with intensification of the conditioning regimen to melphalan, 140 mg per m², etoposide, 60 mg per kg, and fractionated total-body irradiation (12 Gy in six fractions over 3 days with a high dose rate) was used in 100 patients. The main toxicity was interstitial pneumonitis (28% of patients); seven patients died (225), leading to discontinuation of the total-body irradiation in the subsequent protocol. Presently, the use of total-body irradiation is based on institutional experience and the specific drug regimen used for conditioning. The tandem transplant programs at the University of Arkansas (194,196,226) and Memorial Hospital (New York City) (124) continue to use total-body irradiation in their autologous stem cell transplant programs for specific indications.

RADIOIMMUNOTHERAPY

Innovative therapy with bone-seeking radiopharmaceuticals, which target the bone marrow, has been studied as an alternative to total-body irradiation. Typically, a β-emitting isotope is conjugated to a phosphonate complex such as ^{153}Samarium-ethylene diamine tetramethylene phosphonate (samarium lexidronam). The isotope also emits a γ ray, therefore permitting scanning of the patient to locate areas of uptake. This agent has been used successfully for palliation of bone metastasis (227). Hogan et al. reported its use as part of the conditioning regimen before autologous stem cell transplantation for a patient with POEMS syndrome (228), and the feasibility of this approach in myeloma patients was also reported from Australia in a pilot study of 20 patients treated with stem cell transplantation (228a). The chemotherapy conditioning regimens consisted of

melphalan, 200 mg per m², in 14 patients with autologous transplant and cyclophosphamide, 50 mg per m², for 4 days in six patients treated with allogeneic transplant. Because of preferential uptake in the axial skeleton, the protocol required administration of external-beam radiation boosts to the long bones. Another bone-seeking pharmaceutical is ^{166}Holmium–1,4,7,10-tetraazacyclododecane-1,4,7,10-tetramethylene-phosphonic acid, with a higher energy β emission than ^{153}Samarium (maximum energy, 1.85 MeV) and a shorter half-life of 26.8 hours. It also has a γ emission (81 keV) suitable for imaging. A phase I/II study incorporating ^{166}Holmium–1,4,7,10-tetraazacyclododecane-1,4,7,10-tetramethylene-phosphonic acid into a transplant regimen has been performed at the M.D. Anderson Cancer Center with encouraging results (229,230). With the ability to deliver much higher doses to the bone marrow than total-body irradiation, in the range of 30 to 60 Gy, yet sparing the dose-limiting normal tissues such as lung, mucosa, and kidneys, the concept of applying targeted radiation therapy is tantalizing. However, there remains a problem of heterogeneity of uptake in the skeleton, and the dosimetric variation may be even larger at a microscopic level due to the limited range of the β particle and, hence, lead to significant underdosage of tumor cells.

Whether targeted bone/bone marrow radiotherapy has a more favorable therapeutic ratio than standard conditioning regimens with chemotherapy alone or chemotherapy plus total-body irradiation in the autologous transplantation setting awaits larger scale phase II and phase III trials.

TREATMENT OF REFRACTORY DISEASE

Despite aggressive upfront treatment for multiple myeloma, all patients with multiple myeloma ultimately relapse. Patients who progress with initial therapy have a 40% response to high-dose or pulsed corticosteroid therapy (231). Patients who relapse during therapy or within 6 months of stopping initial treatment have a 75% response rate to VAD chemotherapy (231–233). Patients who relapse more than 6 months after stopping therapy have a 60% to 70% response rate when initial therapy is reinstituted (158); if no response is achieved, then VAD or alternate regimens can be used. Treatment for refractory myeloma consisting of EDAP [etoposide, dexamethasone, Ara-C (cytarabine), Platinol (cisplatin)] led to a 40% response in patients resistant to MP, VAD, and high-dose melphalan. However, median survival after EDAP was only 4.5 months (234). Chemosensitizers, such as verapamil, tamoxifen, cyclosporine, and PSC 833, have been evaluated for reversing multidrug resistance in refractory/resistant disease both *in vitro* and in clinical trials (235–237).

A major advance in the treatment of resistant myeloma has been the emergence of thalidomide as an effective therapy (84). The University of Arkansas Cancer Center has evaluated thalidomide as a sole therapeutic agent for advanced and refractory myeloma (84). Before receiving thalidomide, 85% of subjects in this open-label experience underwent at least one cycle of graft-supported high-dose therapy, and 66% had disease relapse/progression after two transplants. The majority of these patients had poor prognostic factors, including immunoglobulin A subclass and adverse cytogenetic changes. A 32% response rate by Southwest Oncology Group criteria was noted. In a follow-up study, these authors have identified prognostic factors in 169 multiple myeloma patients with advanced or refractory multiple myeloma treated with single-agent thalidomide (85). An overall response rate of 37% was noted; low plasma cell labeling index and normal cytogenetics were associated with higher response rates. The 2-year event-free survival and overall survival were 20% and 48%, respectively; low plasma cell labeling index, normal cytogenetics, and a β_2-microglobulin of less than 3 mg per L were good prognostic factors for survival. Based on the impressive results of single-agent thalidomide in refractory or relapsed multiple myeloma and *in vitro* data suggesting its synergy with dexamethasone, thalidomide has been coupled with dexamethasone to treat patients with disease refractory to either agent alone; even in this setting, half of patients treated respond (238). Thalidomide has also been combined with chemotherapy and bisphosphonates in the treatment of refractory multiple myeloma (239,240) and is now under evaluation to treat patients earlier in their disease course.

PALLIATIVE RADIATION THERAPY FOR MULTIPLE MYELOMA

The indications for local radiation therapy are palliation of bone pain and the compression of the spinal cord (241,242), cranial nerves, or peripheral nerves. The role of radiation therapy in preventing impending pathologic fracture is unclear. In general, lesions at high risk for pathologic fracture should be referred for surgical stabilization, and radiation therapy can be administered after surgery for control of residual disease at the local site (243). When radiation therapy is given for pain due to disease involving a long bone, a generous local field suffices, and it is unnecessary to treat the entire bone (244). Doses of 10 to 20 Gy (in 5 to 10 fractions) are effective, although the pain relief is often partial (151). With an average dose of 25 Gy given to 306 sites in 101 patients, Leigh et al. found that 97% of symptomatic patients responded (complete pain relief in 26% and partial relief in 71%) (245). There was no dose-response relationship down to 10 Gy. Recurrence of symptoms requiring further treatment was seen in 6% of sites after a median of 16 months (245). In contrast, Adamietz et al. reported a higher rate of response with higher radiation dose and with the use of ongoing chemotherapy (response rate, 80% with chemotherapy and 40% without) (246). An important adjunctive treatment is bisphosphonate drugs (e.g., pamidronate), which have been shown to reduce skeletal complications and pain in patients with multiple myeloma (247,248).

HEMIBODY RADIATION

Diffuse bone pain involving wide areas of the skeleton can be effectively palliated by half-body radiation with single doses of 5 to 8 Gy (249,250). The bone marrow in the unirradiated half body serve as hematologic reserve and slowly repopulates the irradiated marrow after treatment. The dose for upper half-body radiation is limited by lung tolerance and should not exceed 8 Gy (251). The main toxicity is myelosuppression, and the use of hemibody radiation must be carefully considered, particularly in patients heavily pretreated with chemotherapy. Growth factor support may be helpful to reduce the risk of febrile neutropenia, whereas transfusions of packed red cells and platelets should be given as needed. For diffuse pain involving both the upper and lower half body, sequential half-body radiation can be used, usually separated by 4 to 8 weeks to allow general and hematologic recovery. The sequential hemibody radiation technique has been used in phase II (252,253) and phase III trials as "systemic" treatment to control multiple myeloma in patients with or without skeletal pain. A phase III trial by Southwest Oncology Group included newly diagnosed patients treated with chemotherapy; complete responders were randomized to sequential hemibody radiation (7.5 Gy in 5 fractions, upper hemibody, followed 6 weeks later by lower hemibody) or further chemotherapy (254). Survival was significantly poorer with radiation, compared with chemotherapy (254). At present, there is no standard role for planned sequential hemibody radiation as systemic treatment for multiple myeloma outside of a clinical trial.

FUTURE DIRECTIONS: NOVEL TARGETED THERAPIES

Novel targeted therapies are currently under evaluation in the treatment of multiple myeloma. These therapies are aimed at targeting not only the tumor cell but also its microenvironment, which has been shown to play a central role in disease progression and development of resistance (Fig. 32.2) (255). Increased angiogenesis in multiple myeloma bone marrow, coupled with the known antiangiogenesis activity of thalidomide, provided the rationale for its use in refractory multiple myeloma. We, and others (84,256), have shown remarkable responses even in multiple myeloma refractory to all other known therapies. It is important to note that our studies to date demonstrate that thalidomide and immunomodulatory derivatives not only act to inhibit angiogenesis, but also act directly to induce apoptosis or G1 growth arrest in multiple myeloma cells, including those refractory to standard chemotherapy agents (256). Thalidomide also abrogates the adhesion of multiple myeloma cells to bone marrow stromal cells and related protection against apoptosis (64). It blocks the increased secretion of multiple myeloma growth, survival, and migratory factors (interleukin-6, vascular endothelial growth factor) triggered by binding of multiple myeloma cells to bone marrow stromal cells (64). Finally, it expands

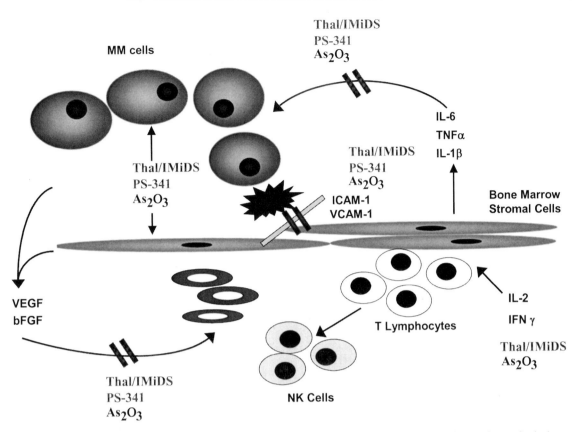

FIG. 32.2. Potential targets and mechanisms of action of novel therapeutic agents in myeloma, including thalidomide (Thal) and analogs, PS-341, and arsenic trioxide (As₂O₃). bFGF, basic fibroblast growth factor; IFN γ, interferon γ; IL, interleukin; IMiDS, immunomodulatory derivatives; MM, multiple myeloma; NK, natural killer; TNFα, tumor necrosis factor α; VEGF, vascular endothelial growth factor.

patients' natural killer cell number and function against human multiple myeloma cells (257) and downregulates protectin expression in multiple myeloma cells (258), thereby enhancing their susceptibility to antibody-dependent cellular cytotoxicity. Using our severe combined immunodeficiency model, we have shown that thalidomide/immunomodulatory derivatives mediate both anti–multiple myeloma activity and antiangiogenesis *in vivo* (259). Based on these promising preclinical data, we have recently carried out a phase I immunomodulatory derivative (CC-5013) dose escalation (5 mg/day, 10 mg/day, 25 mg/day, and 50 mg/day) study in 27 patients (median age, 57; range, 40 to 71 years) with relapsed or refractory relapsed multiple myeloma (260). Best responses of more than 25% reduction in paraprotein occurred in 17 of 24 patients (71%), including 11 patients (46%) who had received prior thalidomide. Stable disease (less than 25% reduction in paraprotein) was observed in an additional two patients (8%). This study, therefore, provides the basis for the evaluation of CC-5013, either alone or in combination, to treat patients with multiple myeloma at earlier stages of disease. Studies already ongoing or to begin soon in multiple myeloma include CC-5013 as initial therapy, treatment for first relapse, and as maintenance post high-dose therapy and stem cell transplantation.

Proteasome inhibitors represent a second class of therapeutics targeting the multiple myeloma cell in its bone marrow microenvironment. Specifically, based on our prior finding that interleukin-6 is the major growth and survival factor for human multiple myeloma cells (1) and our observation that multiple myeloma cell adhesion to bone marrow stromal cells triggers the transcription and secretion of interleukin-6 in bone marrow stromal cells via an NF-κB–dependent mechanism (33), we postulate that blockade of NF-κB using the proteasome inhibitor PS-341 may mediate anti–multiple myeloma activity by inhibiting paracrine interleukin-6 production in bone marrow stromal cells. Our studies demonstrate that PS-341 acts directly on multiple myeloma cells to induce apoptosis of cells resistant to known conventional therapies, overcomes the protective effects of interleukin-6, and adds to the anti–multiple myeloma effects of dexamethasone (37). Importantly, it acts in the bone marrow microenvironment to inhibit the binding of multiple myeloma cells to bone marrow stromal cells, the transcription and secretion of interleukin-6 triggered by multiple myeloma to bone marrow stromal cell adhesion, and bone marrow angiogenesis. Our recent gene microarray profiling studies demonstrate that PS-341 induces transcriptional downregulation of growth/survival signaling pathways as well as upregulation of apoptotic cascades, ubiquitin/proteasome pathways, and heat-shock proteins (27). These preclinical studies, coupled with phase I studies of PS-341 demonstrating clinical promise in patients with refractory multiple myeloma, provided the strong rationale for a recently completed multicenter phase II trial of PS-341 in multiple myeloma (261). Two hundred two patients with relapsed or refractory multiple myeloma were treated, and analysis of the first cohort of 78 patients is currently available. Patients had received a mean of five (2 to 13) prior therapies, including thalidomide (74%) and stem cell transplant (54%). Twenty-five percent or more decreases in multiple myeloma paraprotein were noted in 47% of patients, and no change in protein in an additional 30% of patients. Excitingly, greater than 90% decreases in multiple myeloma paraprotein were observed in 20% of patients, including some complete responses. At a follow-up of 6.2 months, the median duration of response has not been reached. Based on preclinical studies showing additive anti–multiple myeloma activity of dexamethasone and PS-341 (37), dexamethasone was added to those 25 patients who progressed or achieved only stabilization of disease on PS-341 alone; all but one patient achieved additional anti–multiple myeloma response. The drug was well tolerated, with nausea, fatigue, diarrhea, peripheral neuropathy, and thrombocytopenia as the most common adverse events. Importantly, neuropathy and thrombocytopenia were rare unless present before PS-341 therapy. Based on this clinical promise, a phase III, international, randomized trial of PS-341 versus dexamethasone in relapsed multiple myeloma, and trials of PS-341 in newly diagnosed multiple myeloma patients, are ongoing.

Recent studies in our laboratory have also identified arsenic (As_2O_3) as a third agent targeting both the multiple myeloma and the bone marrow microenvironment. Arsenic at clinically achievable levels induces apoptosis of drug-resistant multiple myeloma cell lines and patient cells via caspase-9 activation, adds to dexamethasone-induced apoptosis, and can overcome the antiapoptotic effects of interleukin-6 (262). It also decreases multiple myeloma cell binding to bone marrow stromal cells, inhibits interleukin-6 and vascular endothelial growth factor secretion in bone marrow stromal cells induced by multiple myeloma cell adhesion, and blocks proliferation even of those multiple myeloma cells adherent to bone marrow stromal cells.

We are also attempting to generate and expand anti–myeloma-specific autologous T cells ex vivo for adoptive immunotherapy of minimal residual disease in the patient post-autotransplant (263–266). Immunologic responses are being tested to enhance the immunogenicity of the whole tumor cell. Specifically, CD40 activation of myeloma cells upregulates class I and II human leukocyte antigen, costimulatory, GRP94, and other molecules, and these CD40–activated myeloma cells also trigger a brisk autologous T-cell response (267). Although T cells can be harvested from myeloma patients before autografting, expanded ex vivo using CD40–activated autologous myeloma cells as a stimulus, and then given as adoptive immunotherapy to treat minimal residual disease posttransplant, this is logistically complex. Therefore, we and others are developing and examining the clinical usefulness of a variety of myeloma vaccines, including autologous CD40–activated tumor cells, recombinant vaccinia virus containing the Muc-1 gene, autologous dendritic cells transduced using adenoviral vectors with Muc-1, and myeloma dendritic cell fusion vaccines. In a syngeneic murine myeloma model, vaccinations with myeloma cell–dendritic cells fusions, but not with either myeloma cells or dendritic cells alone, demonstrate both protective and therapeutic efficacy (268). Most important, we have shown that patient myeloma cells can be fused to autologous dendritic cells, which are readily isolated from either patient bone marrow or peripheral blood (269), and that autologous myeloma cell–dendritic cell fusions can trigger specific cytolytic autologous T-cell responses in vitro (270). Combining these targeted therapies with conventional strategies with or without transplantation will translate into more durable remissions and ultimately a cure in multiple myeloma.

REFERENCES

1. Hallek M, Bergsagel PL, Anderson KC. Multiple myeloma: increasing evidence for a multistep transformation process. Blood 1998;91:3.
2. Kyle RA. Multiple myeloma: review of 869 cases. Mayo Clin Proc 1975;50:29.
3. Greenlee R, Hill-Harmon M, Murray T, et al. Cancer statistics, 2001. CA Cancer J Clin 2000;51:15.
4. Herrinton LJ, Weiss NS, Olshan AF. Epidemiology of myeloma. In: Malpas JS, Bergsagel DE, Kyle R, Anderson K, eds. Myeloma: biology and management. Oxford, UK: Oxford Medical Publications, 1997:150.
5. Bergsagel DE, Wong O, Bergsagel PL, et al. Benzene and multiple myeloma: appraisal of the scientific evidence. Blood 1999;94:1174.
6. Bourguet CC, Grufferman S, Delzell E, et al. Multiple myeloma and family history of cancer. Cancer 1985;56:2133.
7. Bakkus MHC, Heirman C, van Riet I, et al. Evidence that multiple myeloma Ig heavy chain VDJ genes contain somatic mutations but show no intraclonal variation. Blood 1992;80:2326.
8. Vescio RA, Cao J, Hong CH, et al. Myeloma Ig heavy chain V region sequences reveal prior antigenic selection and marked somatic mutation but no intraclonal diversity. J Immunol 1995;155:2487.
9. Sahota SS, Garand R, Mahroof R, et al. VH gene analysis of IgM-secreting myeloma indicates an origin from a memory cell undergoing isotype switch events. Blood 1999;94:1070.
10. Bergsagel PL, Chesi M, Nardini E, et al. Promiscuous translocations into immunoglobulin heavy chains with regions in multiple myeloma. Proceedings of the National Academy of Sciences of the United States of America 1996;93.
11. Dewald GW, Kyle RA, Hicks GA, et al. The clinical significance of cytogenetic studies in 100 patients with multiple myeloma, plasma cell leukemia, or amyloidosis. Blood 1985;66:380.
12. Gould J, Alexanian R, Goodacre A, et al. Plasma cell karyotype in multiple myeloma. Blood 1988;71:453.
13. Sawyer JR, Waldron JA, Jagannath S, et al. Cytogenic findings in 200 patients with multiple myeloma. Cancer Genet Cytogenet 1995;82:41.
14. Avet-Loiseau H, Daviet A, Brigaudeau C, et al. Cytogenetic, interphase, and multicolor fluorescence in situ hybridization analyses in primary plasma cell leukemia: a study of 40 patients at diagnosis, on behalf of the Intergroupe Francophone du Myelome and the Groupe Français de Cytogenetique Hematologique. Blood 2001;97:822.
15. Zhan F, Hardin J, Kordsmeier B, et al. Global gene expression profiling of multiple myeloma, monoclonal gammopathy of undetermined significance, and normal bone marrow plasma cells. Blood 2002;99:1745.

16. Fonseca R, Bailey RJ, Ahmann GJ, et al. Genomic abnormalities in monoclonal gammopathy of undetermined significance. *Blood* 2002;100: 1417.

17. Shaughnessy J Jr, Gabrea A, Qi Y, et al. Cyclin D3 at 6p21 is dysregulated by recurrent chromosomal translocations to immunoglobulin loci in multiple myeloma. *Blood* 2001;98:217.

18. Chesi M, Nardini E, Lim RSC, et al. The t(4;14) translocation in myeloma dysregulates both FGFR3 and a novel gene, MMSET, resulting in IgH/MMSET hybrid transcripts. *Blood* 1998;92:3025.

19. Plowright EE, Li Z, Bergsagel PL, et al. Ectopic expression of fibroblast growth factor receptor 3 promotes myeloma cell proliferation and prevents apoptosis. *Blood* 2000;95:992.

20. Li Z, Zhu YX, Plowright EE, et al. The myeloma-associated oncogene fibroblast growth factor receptor 3 is transforming in hematopoietic cells. *Blood* 2001;97:2413.

21. Tricot G, Barlogie B, Jagannath S, et al. Poor prognosis in multiple myeloma is associated only with partial or complete deletions of Chr 13 or abnormalities involving 11q and not with other karyotype abnormalities. *Blood* 1995;86:4250.

22. Tricot G, Spencer T, Sawyer J, et al. Predicting long-term (> or = 5 years) event-free survival in multiple myeloma patients following planned tandem autotransplants. *Br J Haematol* 2002;116:211.

23. Facon T, Avet-Loiseau H, Guillerm G, et al. Chromosome 13 abnormalities identified by FISH analysis and serum beta2-microglobulin produce a powerful myeloma staging system for patients receiving high-dose therapy. *Blood* 2001;97:1566.

24. Konigsberg R, Zojer N, Ackermann J, et al. Predictive role of interphase cytogenetics for survival of patients with multiple myeloma. *J Clin Oncol* 2000.

25. Avet-Loiseau H, Li JY, Morineau N, et al. Monosomy 13 is associated with the transition of monoclonal gammopathy of undetermined significance to multiple myeloma. Intergroupe Francophone du Myelome. *Blood* 1999;94:2583.

26. Chauhan D, Auclair D, Robinson EK, et al. Identification of genes regulated by dexamethasone in multiple myeloma cells using oligonucleotide arrays. *Oncogene* 2002;21:1346.

27. Mitsiades N, Mitsiades C, Poulaki V, et al. Molecular sequelae of proteasome inhibition in human multiple myeloma cells. *Proc Natl Acad Sci U S A* 2002;99(22):14374.

28. Uchiyama H, Barut BA, Chauhan D, et al. Characterization of adhesion molecules on human myeloma cell lines. *Blood* 1992;80:2306.

29. Uchiyama H, Barut BA, Mohrbacher AF, et al. Adhesion of human myeloma-derived cell lines to bone marrow stromal cells stimulates IL-6 secretion. *Blood* 1993;82:3712.

30. Uchiyama H, Anderson KC. Cellular adhesion molecules. *Transfus Med Rev* 1994;8:84.

31. Teoh G, Anderson KC. Interaction of tumor and host cells with adhesion and extracellular matrix molecules in the development of multiple myeloma. *Hematol Oncol Clin North Am* 1997;11:27.

32. Mitsiades C, Mitsiades N, Poulaki V, et al. IGF-1 induced activation of NF-kB and upregulation of intracellular anti-apoptotic proteins in human multiple myeloma cells: therapeutic implications. *Oncogene* (in press).

33. Chauhan D, Uchiyama H, Akbarali Y, et al. Multiple myeloma cell adhesion-induced interleukin-6 expression in bone marrow stromal cells involves activation of NF-kB. *Blood* 1996;87:1104.

34. Podar, K, Tai YT, Davies FE, et al. Vascular endothelial growth factor triggers signaling cascades mediating multiple myeloma cell growth and migration. *Blood* 2001;98:428.

35. Hideshima T, Chauhan D, Schlossman RL, et al. Role of TNF-alpha in the pathophysiology of human multiple myeloma: therapeutic applications. *Oncogene* 2001;20:4519.

36. Damiano JS, Cress AE, Hazlehurst LA, et al. Cell adhesion mediated drug resistance (CAM-DR): role of integrins and resistance to apoptosis in human myeloma cell lines. *Blood* 1999;93:1658.

37. Hideshima T, Richardson P, Chauhan D, et al. The proteosome inhibitor PS341inhibits growth, induces apoptosis, and overcomes drug resistance in human multiple myeloma cells. *Cancer Res* 2001;61: 3071.

38. Klein B, Lu Y, Gaillard JP, et al. Inhibiting IL-6 in human multiple myeloma. *Curr Top Microbiol Immunol* 1992;182:236.

39. Kawano MM, Hirano T, Matsuda T, et al. Autocrine generation and requirement of BSF-2/IL-6 for human multiple myeloma. *Nature* 1988;332:83.

40. Urashima M, Chauhan D, Uchiyama H, et al. CD40 ligand triggered interleukin-6 secretion in multiple myeloma. *Blood* 1995;85:1903.

41. Frassanito MA, Cusmai A, Iodice G, et al. Autocrine interleukin-6 production and highly malignant multiple myeloma: relation with resistance to drug-induced apoptosis. *Blood* 2001;97:483.

42. Lokhorst HM, Lamme T, de Smet M, et al. Primary tumor cells of myeloma patients induce interleukin-6 secretion in long-term marrow cultures. *Blood* 1994;84:2269.

43. Chauhan D, Kharbanda S, Ogata A, et al. Interleukin-6 inhibits Fas-induced apoptosis and stress-activated protein kinase activation in multiple myeloma cells. *Blood* 1997;89:227.

44. Chauhan D, Pandey P, Ogata A, et al. Dexamethasone induces apoptosis of multiple myeloma cells in a JNK/SAP kinase independent mechanism. *Oncogene* 1997;15:837.

45. Chauhan D, Hideshima T, Pandey P, et al. RAFTK/PYK2-dependent and independent apoptosis in multiple myeloma cells. *Oncogene* 1999; 18:6733.

46. Chauhan D, Anderson KC. Apoptosis in multiple myeloma: therapeutic implications. *Apoptosis* 2001;6(1–2):47.

47. Hideshima T, Nakamura N, Chauhan D, et al. Biologic sequelae of interleukin-6 induced PI3-K/Akt signaling in multiple myeloma. *Oncogene* 2001;20:5991.

48. Chauhan D, Hideshima T, Rosen S, et al. Apaf-1/cytochrome c independent and Smac dependent induction of apoptosis in multiple myeloma cells. *J Biol Chem* 2001;276:24453.

49. Landowski TH, Shain KH, Oshiro MM, et al. Myeloma cells selected for resistance to CD95-mediated apoptosis are not cross-resistant to cytotoxic drugs: evidence for independent mechanisms of caspase activation. *Blood* 1999;94:265.

50. Bataille R, Jourdan M, Zhang XG, et al. Serum levels of interleukin-6, a potent myeloma cell growth factor, as a reflection of disease severity in plasma cell dyscrasias. *J Clin Invest* 1989;84:2008.

51. Ludwig H, Nachbaur DM, Fritz E, et al. Interleukin-6 is a prognostic factor in multiple myeloma. *Blood* 1991;77:2794.

52. Barille S, Collette M, Bataille R, et al. Myeloma cells upregulate IL-6 but downregulate osteocalcin production by osteoblastic cells through cell to cell contact. *Blood* 1995;86:3151.

53. Bataille R, Barlogie B, Yang Z, et al. Biologic effects of anti-interleukin-6 murine monoclonal antibody in advanced multiple myeloma. *Blood*1995; 86:685.

54. Ogata A, Nishimoto N, Shima Y, et al. Inhibitory effect of All-trans retinoic acid on the growth of freshly isolated myeloma cells via interference with interleukin-6 signal transduction. *Blood* 1994;84:3040.

55. Ehlers M, de Hon FD, Klasse Bos H, et al. Combining two mutations of human interleukin-6 that affect gp130 activation results in a potent interleukin-6 receptor antagonist on human myeloma cells. *J Biol Chem* 1995;270:8158.

56. Savage AD, Belson DJ, Vescio RA, et al. Pamidronate reduces IL-6 production by bone marrow stroma from multiple myeloma patients. *Blood* 1996;88:105a.

57. Sporeno E, Savino R, Ciapponi L, et al. Human interleukin-6 receptor super antagonists with high potency and wide spectrum on multiple myeloma cells. *Blood* 1996;87:4510.

58. Klein B, Zhang XG, Lu XY, et al. Interleukin-6 in human multiple myeloma. *Blood* 1995;85:863.

59. Rettig MB, Ma HJ, Vescio RA, et al. Kaposi's sarcoma-associated herpesvirus infection of bone marrow dendritic cells from multiple myeloma patients. *Science* 1997;276:1851.

60. Tarte K, Chang Y, Klein B. Kaposi's sarcoma-associated herpesvirus and multiple myeloma: lack of criteria for causality. *Blood* 1999;93: 3159.

61. Brander C, Raje N, O'Connor PG, et al. Absence of biologically important Kaposi sarcoma-associated herpesvirus gene products and virus-specific cellular immune responses in multiple myeloma. *Blood* 2002;100:698.

62. Davies FE, Rollinson SJ, Rawstron AC, et al. High-producer haplotypes of tumor necrosis factor alpha and lymphotoxin alpha are associated with an increased risk of myeloma and have an improved progression-free survival after treatment. *J Clin Oncol* 2000;18:2843.

63. Dankar B, Padro T, Leo R, et al. Vascular endothelial growth factor and interleukin-6 in paracrine tumor-stromal cell interactions in multiple myeloma. *Blood* 2000;95:2630.

64. Gupta D, Treon SP, Shima Y, et al. Adherence of multiple myeloma cells to bone marrow stromal cells upregulates vascular endothelial

growth factor secretion: therapeutic applications. *Leukemia* 2001;15:1950.

65. Bellamy W, Richter L, Frutiger Y, et al. Expression of vascular endothelial growth factor and its receptor in hematological malignancies. *Cancer Res* 1999;59:728.

66. Podar K, Tai YT, Lin BK, et al. Vascular endothelial growth factor-induced migration of multiple myeloma cells is associated with beta 1 integrin- and phosphatidylinositol 3-kinase-dependent PKC alpha activation. *J Biol Chem* 2002;277:7875.

67. Urashima M, Ogata A, Chauhan D, et al. Transforming growth factor b1: differential effects on multiple myeloma versus normal B cells. *Blood* 1996;87:1928.

68. Kawano M, Tanaka H, Ishikawa H, et al. Interleukin-1 accelerates autocrine growth of myeloma cells through interleukin-6 in human myeloma. *Blood* 1989;73:2145.

69. Cozzolino F, Torcia M, Aldinucci D, et al. Production of interleukin-1 by bone marrow myeloma cells: its role in the pathogenesis of lytic bone lesions. *Blood* 1989;74:380.

70. Garrett IR, Durie BGM, Nedwin GE, et al. Production of lymphotoxin, a bone resorbing cytokine, by cultured human myeloma cells. *N Engl J Med* 1987;317:526.

71. Hermann F, Andreff M, Gruss J, et al. Interleukin 4 inhibits growth of multiple myeloma by suppressing interleukin 6 expression. *Blood* 1991;78:2070.

72. Chauhan D, Kharbanda S, Ogata A, et al. Oncostatin M induces association of Grb2 with Janus Kinase JAK2 in multiple myeloma cells. *J Exp Med* 1995;182:1801.

73. Zhang XG, Bataille R, Jourdan M, et al. Granulocyte-macrophage colony-stimulating factor synergizes with interleukin-6 in supporting the proliferation of human myeloma cells. *Blood* 1990;76:2599.

74. Anderson KC, Morimoto C, Paul SR, et al. Interleukin-11 promotes accessory cell dependent B cell differentiation in man. *Blood* 1992;80:2797.

75. Paul SD, Barut BA, Cochran MA, et al. Lack of a role of interleukin-11 in the growth of multiple myeloma. *Leuk Res* 1992;16:247.

76. Lu ZY, Zhang XG, Rodriguez C, et al. Interleukin-10 is a proliferation factor but not a differentiation factor for human myeloma cells. *Blood* 1995;85:2521.

77. Choi SJ, Cruz JC, Craig F, et al. Macrophage inflammatory protein 1-alpha is a potential osteoclast stimulatory factor in multiple myeloma. *Blood* 2000;96:671.

78. Tinhofer I, Marschitz I, Henn T, et al. Expression of functional interleukin-15 receptor and autocrine production of interleukin-15 as mechanisms of tumor propagation in multiple myeloma. *Blood* 2000;95:610.

79. Brenne AT, Baade Ro T, Waage A, et al. Interleukin-21 is a growth and survival factor for human myeloma cells. *Blood* 2002;99:3756.

80. Munshi N, Wilson CC, Penn MJ. Angiogenesis in newly diagnosed multiple myeloma: poor prognosis with increased microvessel density in bone marrow biopsies. *Blood* 1998;92[Suppl]:98a.

81. Rajkumar SV, Fonseca R, Witzig TE, et al. Bone marrow angiogenesis in patients achieving complete response after stem cell transplantation for multiple myeloma. *Leukemia* 1999;13:469.

82. Ribatti D, Vacca A, Nico B, et al. Bone marrow angiogenesis and mast cell density increase simultaneously with progression of human multiple myeloma. *Br J Cancer* 1999;79:451.

83. Vacca A, Ribatti D, Presta M, et al. Bone marrow neovascularization, plasma cell angiogenic potential, and matrix metalloproteinase-2 secretion parallel progression of human multiple myeloma. *Blood* 1999;93:3064.

84. Singhal S, Mehta J, Desikan R, et al. Anti-tumor activity of thalidomide in refractory multiple myeloma. *N Engl J Med* 1999;341:1565.

85. Barlogie B, Desikan R, Eddlemon P, et al. Extended survival in advanced and refractory multiple myeloma after single-agent thalidomide: identification of prognostic factors in a phase 2 study of 169 patients. *Blood* 2001;98:492.

86. Durie BGM. Staging and kinetics of multiple myeloma. *Semin Oncol* 1986;13:300.

87. Blade J, Lust JA, Kyle RA. Immunoglobulin D multiple myeloma: presenting features, response to therapy, and survival in a series of 53 cases. *J Clin Oncol* 1994;12:2398.

88. Bergsagel DE. Acute leukemia and multiple myeloma: natural history or iatrogenic disease? *Drug Ther* 1996;8.

89. Kapadia SB. Multiple myeloma: a clinicopathologic study of 62 consecutively autopsied cases. *Medicine* 1980;59:380.

90. Jaffe ES, Harris NL, Stein H, et al. WHO classification of tumours: tumours of haematopoietic and lymphoid tissues. *Plasma Cell Neoplasms* 2001:144.

91. Bartl R, Frisch B, Burkhardt R, et al. Bone marrow histology in myeloma. *Br J Haematol* 1982;51:361.

92. Zucker-Franklin D. The pathology of multiple myeloma and related disorders. In: Wiernick P, Canellos GP, Kyle R, eds. *Neoplastic diseases of the blood.* New York: Churchill Livingstone, 1985:462.

93. Van Camp B, Durie BG, Spier C, et al. Plasma cells in multiple myeloma express natural killer cell-associated antigen: CD56 (NKH-1; Leu-19). *Blood* 1990;76:377.

94. Mundy GR, Bertolini DR. Bone destruction and hypercalcemia in plasma cell myeloma. *Semin Oncol* 1986;13:291.

95. Barille S, Bataille R, Rapp MJ, et al. Production of metalloproteinase-7 (matrilysin) by human myeloma cells and its potential involvement in metalloproteinase-2 activation. *J Immunol* 1999;163:5723.

96. Hjertner O, Torgersen ML, Seidel C, et al. Hepatocyte growth factor (HGF) induces interleukin-11 secretion from osteoblasts: a possible role for HGF in myeloma-associated osteolytic bone disease. *Blood* 1999;94:3883.

97. Lacey DL, Timms E, Tan H-L, et al. Osteoprotegerin ligand is a cytokine that regulates osteoclast differentiation and activation. *Cell* 1998;93:165.

98. Han JH, Choi SJ, Kurihara N, et al. Macrophage inflammatory protein-1alpha is an osteoclastogenic factor in myeloma that is independent of receptor activator of nuclear factor kappaB ligand. *Blood* 2001;97:3349.

99. Giuliani N, Bataille R, Mancini C, et al. Myeloma cells induce imbalance in the osteoprotegerin/osteoprotegerin ligand system in the human bone marrow environment. *Blood* 2001;98:3527.

100. Pearse RN, Sordillo EM, Yaccoby S, et al. Multiple myeloma disrupts the TRANCE/osteoprotegerin cytokine axis to trigger bone destruction and promote tumor progression. *Proc Natl Acad Sci U S A* 2001;98:11581.

101. Seidel C, Hjertner O, Abildgaard N, et al. Serum osteoprotegerin levels are reduced in patients with multiple myeloma with lytic bone disease. *Blood* 2001;98:2269.

102. Croucher PI, Shipman CM, Lippitt J, et al. Osteoprotegerin inhibits the development of osteolytic bone disease in multiple myeloma. *Blood* 2001;98:3534.

103. Oyajobi BO, Anderson DM, Traianedes K, et al. Therapeutic efficacy of a soluble receptor activator of nuclear factor kappaB-IgG Fc fusion protein in suppressing bone resorption and hypercalcemia in a model of humoral hypercalcemia of malignancy. *Cancer Res* 2001;61:2572.

104. Yaccoby S, Barlogie B, Epstein J. Primary myeloma cells growing in SCID-hu mice: a model for studying the biology and treatment of myeloma and its manifestations. *Blood* 1998;92:2908.

105. Berenson J, Lichtenstein A, Porter L, et al. Pamidronate disodium reduces the occurrence of skeletal events in patients with advanced multiple myeloma. *N Engl J Med* 1996;334:488.

106. Berenson JR, Lichtenstein A, Porter L, et al. Long-term pamidronate treatment of advanced multiple myeloma patients reduces skeletal events. *J Clin Oncol* 1998;16:593.

107. Bloomfield DJ. Should bisphosphonates be part of the standard therapy of patients with multiple myeloma or bone metastases from other cancers? An evidence-based review. *J Clin Oncol* 1998;16:1218.

108. Dhodapkar MV, Singh J, Mehta J, et al. Anti-myeloma activity of pamidronate in vivo. *Br J Haematol* 1998;103:530.

109. Hughes DE, Wright KR, Uy HL. Bisphosphonates promote apoptosis in murine osteoclasts *in vitro* and *in vivo*. *J Bone Miner Res* 1995;10:1478.

110. Martin A, Garcia-Sanz R, Hernandez J, et al. Pamidronate induces bone formation in patients with smouldering or indolent myeloma, with no significant anti-tumour effect. *Br J Haematol* 2002;118:239.

111. Berenson JR, et al. Phase-1 clinical study of a new bisphosphonate, zoledronate (CGP-42446), in patients with osteolytic bone metastases. *Blood* 1996;88(Suppl 1):586a.

112. Lipton A, et al. Phase 11 study of the bisphosphonate, zoledronate in patients with osteolytic lesions. Abstract #48, Secondary International Conference: Cancer-Induced Bone Diseases. Davos, Switzerland, March 27–29, 1999.

113. Lipton A, et al. The effects of the bisphosphonate, zoledronic acid, when administered as a short intravenous infusion in patients with bone metastases: a phase-1 study. Abstract #848, American Society of Clinical Oncology Annual Meeting, Denver, CO, May 17–20, 1997.

114. Menssen HD, Sakalova A, Fontana A, et al. Effects of long-term intravenous ibandronate therapy on skeletal-related events, survival, and bone resorption markers in patients with advanced multiple myeloma. *J Clin Oncol* 2002;20:2353.
115. Bataille R, Durie BGM, Grenier J, et al. Prognostic factors and staging in multiple myeloma: a reappraisal. *J Clin Oncol* 1986;4:80.
116. Durie BGM, Salmon SE. A clinical staging system for multiple myeloma. Correlation of measured cell mass with presenting clinical features, response to treatment and survival. *Cancer* 1975;36:842.
117. Gassmann W, Pralle H, Haferlach T, et al. Staging systems for multiple myeloma: a comparison. *Br J Haematol* 1985;59:703.
118. Greipp PR. Prognosis in myeloma. *Mayo Clin Proc* 1994;69:895.
119. Bataille R, Sany J. Solitary myeloma: clinical and prognostic features of a review of 114 cases. *Cancer* 1981;48:845.
120. Dimopoulos MA, Moulopoulos LA, Maniatis A, et al. Solitary plasmacytoma of bone and asymptomatic multiple myeloma. *Blood* 2000;96:2037.
121. Knowling MA, Harwood AR, Bergsagel DE. Comparison of extramedullary plasmacytomas with solitary and multiple plasma cell tumors of bone. *J Clin Oncol* 1983;1:255.
122. Liebross RH, Ha CS, Cox JD, et al. Clinical course of solitary extramedullary plasmacytoma. *Radiother Oncol* 1999;52:245.
123. Mayr NA, Wen BC, Hussey DH, et al. The role of radiation therapy in the treatment of solitary plasmacytomas. *Radiother Oncol* 1990;17:293.
124. Hu K, Yahalom J. Radiotherapy in the management of plasma cell tumors. *Oncology* 2000;14:101.
125. Tsang RW, Gospodarowicz MK, Pintilie M, et al. Solitary plasmacytoma treated with radiotherapy: impact of tumor size on outcome. *Int J Radiat Oncol Biol Phys* 2001;50:113.
126. Schindler OS, Briggs TW, Gillies SA. Bilateral demyelinating neuropathy in a solitary lytic and sclerotic myeloma of the proximal humerus: a case report. *Int Orthop* 1997;21:59.
127. Moulopoulos LA, Dimopoulos MA, Weber D, et al. Magnetic resonance imaging in the staging of solitary plasmacytoma of bone. *J Clin Oncol* 1993;11:1311.
128. Liebross RH, Ha CS, Cox JD, et al. Solitary bone plasmacytoma: outcome and prognostic factors following radiotherapy. *Int J Radiat Oncol Biol Phys* 1998;41:1063.
129. Chak LY, Cox RS, Bostwick DG, et al. Solitary plasmacytoma of bone: treatment, progression, and survival. *J Clin Oncol* 1997;5:1811.
130. Frassica DA, Frassica FJ, Schray MF, et al. Solitary plasmacytoma of bone: Mayo Clinic experience. *Int J Radiat Oncol Biol Phys* 1989;16:43.
131. Holland J, Trenkner DA, Wasserman TH, et al. Plasmacytoma. Treatment results and conversion to myeloma. *Cancer* 1992;9:1513.
132. Shih LY, Dunn P, Leung WM, et al. Localised plasmacytomas in Taiwan: comparison between extramedullary plasmacytoma and solitary plasmacytoma of bone. *Br J Cancer* 1995;71:128.
133. Jyothirmayi R, Gangadharan VP, Nair MK, et al. Radiotherapy in the treatment of solitary plasmacytoma. *Br J Radiol* 1997;70:511.
134. Dimopoulos MA, Moulopoulos LA, Maniatis A, et al. Solitary plasmacytoma of bone and asymptomatic multiple myeloma. *Blood* 2000;96:2037.
135. Bolek TW, Marcus RB, Mendenhall NP. Solitary plasmacytoma of bone and soft tissue. *Int J Radiat Oncol Biol Phys* 1996;36:329.
136. Dimopoulos MA, Goldstein J, Fuller L, et al. Curability of solitary bone plasmacytoma. *J Clin Oncol* 1992;10:587.
137. Wilder RB, Ha CS, Cox JD, et al. Persistence of myeloma protein for more than one year after radiotherapy is an adverse prognostic factor in solitary plasmacytoma of bone. *Cancer* 2002;94:1532.
138. Alexiou C, Kau RJ, Dietzfelbinger H, et al. Extramedullary plasmacytoma: tumor occurrence and therapeutic concepts. *Cancer* 1999;85:2305.
139. Hussong JW, Perkins SL, Schnitzer B, et al. Extramedullary plasmacytoma. A form of marginal zone cell lymphoma? *Am J Clin Pathol* 1999;111:111.
140. Susnerwala SS, Shanks JH, Banerjee SS, et al. Extramedullary plasmacytoma of the head and neck region: clinicopathological correlation in 25 cases. *Br J Cancer* 1997;75:921.
141. Strojan P, Soba E, Lamovec J, et al. Extramedullary plasmacytoma: clinical and histopathologic study. *Int J Radiat Oncol Biol Phys* 2002;53:692.
142. Wiltshaw E. The natural history of extramedullary plasmacytoma and its relation to solitary myeloma of bone and myelomatosis. *Medicine* 1976;55:217.
143. Kapadia SB, Desai U, Cheng VS. Extramedullary plasmacytoma of the head and neck. *Medicine* 1982;61:317.
144. Bush SE, Goffinet DR, Bagshaw MA. Extramedullary plasmacytoma of the head and neck. *Radiology* 1981;140:801.
145. Soesan M, Paccagnella A, Chiarion-Sileni V, et al. Extramedullary plasmacytoma: clinical behavior and response to treatment. *Ann Oncol* 1992;3:51.
146. Brinch L, Hannisdal E, Abrahamsen AF, et al. Extramedullary plasmacytomas and solitary myeloma cell tumours of bone. *Eur J Haematol* 1990;44:131.
147. Galieni P, Cavo M, Pulsoni A, et al. Clinical outcome of extramedullary plasmacytoma. *Haematologica* 2000;85:47.
148. Harwood AR, Knowling MA, Bergsagel DE. Radiotherapy of extramedullary plasmacytoma of the head and neck. *Clin Radiol* 1981;32:31.
149. Mendenhall CM, Thar TL, Million RR. Solitary plasmacytoma of bone and soft tissue. *Int J Radiat Oncol Biol Phys* 1980;6:1497.
150. Corwin J, Lindberg RD. Solitary plasmacytoma of bone vs. extramedullary plasmacytoma and their relationship to multiple myeloma. *Cancer* 1979;43:1007.
151. Mill WB, Griffith R. The role of radiation therapy in the management of plasma cell tumors. *Cancer* 1980;45:647.
152. Petrovich Z, Fishkin B, Hittle RE, et al. Extramedullary plasmacytoma of the upper respiratory passages. *Int J Radiat Oncol Biol Phys* 1977;2:723.
153. Aviles A, Huerta-Guzman J, Delgado S, et al. Improved outcome in solitary bone plasmacytomata with combined therapy. *Hematol Oncol* 1996;14:111.
154. Alexanian R, Barlogie B, Tucker S. VAD-based regimens as primary treatment for multiple myeloma. *Am J Hematol* 1990;33:86.
155. Salmon SE, Haut A, Bonnet JD, et al. Alternating combination chemotherapy and levamisole improves survival in multiple myeloma: a Southwest Oncology Group Study. *J Clin Oncol* 1983;1:453.
156. Blade J, Samson D, Reece D, et al. Criteria for evaluating disease response and progression in patients with multiple myeloma treated by high-dose therapy and haemopoietic stem cell transplantation. Myeloma Subcommittee of the EBMT. European Group for Blood and Marrow Transplant. *Br J Haematol* 1998;102:1115.
157. Alexanian R, Dimopoulos M. The treatment of multiple myeloma. *N Engl J Med* 1994;330:484.
158. Kyle RA. Newer approaches to the therapy of multiple myeloma. *Blood* 1990;76:1678.
159. Blade J, San Miguel JF, Alcala A. Alternating combination VCMP/VBAP chemotherapy versus melphalan/prednisone in the treatment of multiple myeloma: a randomized multicentric study of 487 patients. *J Clin Oncol* 1993;11:1165.
160. Durie BGM, Dixon DO, Carter S, et al. Improved survival duration with combination chemotherapy induction for multiple myeloma: a Southwest Oncology Group Study. *J Clin Oncol* 1996;4:1227.
161. Samson D, Gaminara E, Newland A, et al. Infusion of vincristine and doxorubicin with oral dexamethasone as first-line therapy for multiple myeloma. *Lancet* 1989;2:882.
162. Alexanian R, Dimopoulos MA, Delasalle K, et al. Primary dexamethasone treatment of multiple myeloma. *Blood* 1992;80:887.
163. Salmon SE, Crowley JJ, Grogan TM, et al. Combination chemotherapy, glucocorticoids, and interferon alpha in the treatment of multiple myeloma: a Southwest Oncology Group Study. *J Clin Oncol* 1994;12:2405.
164. Berenson JR, Crowley JJ, Grogan TM, et al. Maintenance therapy with alternate-day prednisone improves survival in multiple myeloma patients. *Blood* 2002;99:3163.
165. Oken MM, Harrington DP, Abramson N, et al. Comparison of melphalan and prednisone with vincristine, carmustine, melphalan, cyclophosphamide, and prednisone in the treatment of multiple myeloma—results of Eastern Cooperative Oncology Group Study E2479. *Cancer* 1997;79:1561.
166. Gregory WM, Richards MA, Malpas JS. Combination chemotherapy versus melphalan and prednisolone in the treatment of multiple myeloma: an overview of published trials. *J Clin Oncol* 1992;10:334.
167. Myeloma Trialists' Collaborative Group. Combination chemotherapy versus melphalan plus prednisone as treatment for multiple myeloma: an overview of 6633 patients from 27 randomized trials. *J Clin Oncol* 1998;16:3832.
168. The Nordic Myeloma Study Group. Interferon-alpha 2b added to melphalan-prednisone for initial and maintenance therapy in multiple myeloma. A randomized, controlled trial. *Ann Intern Med* 1996;124:212.

169. Ludwig H, Cohen AM, Polliack A, et al. Interferon-alpha for induction and maintenance in multiple myeloma: results of two multicenter randomized trials and summary of other studies. *Ann Oncol* 1995:467.

170. Montuoro A, De Rosa L, De Blasio A, et al. Alpha-2a-interferon/melphalan/prednisone versus melphalan/prednisone in previously untreated patients with multiple myeloma. *Br J Haematol* 1990;76:365.

171. Osterborg A, Bjorkholm M, Bjoreman M, et al. Natural interferon-a in combination with melphalan/prednisone versus melphalan/prednisone in the treatment of multiple myeloma stages II and III: a randomized study from the Myeloma Group of Central Sweden. *Blood* 1993;81:1428.

172. Mandelli F, Avvisati G, Amadori S, et al. Maintenance treatment with recombinant interferon alpha-2b in patients with multiple myeloma responding to conventional induction chemotherapy. *N Engl J Med* 1990;322:1430.

173. Browman GP, Bergsagel DP, Sicheri D, et al. Randomized trial of interferon maintenance in multiple myeloma: a study of the National Cancer Institute of Canada Clinical Trials Group. *J Clin Oncol* 1995;13:2354.

174. Cunningham D, Powles R, Malpas J, et al. A randomized trial of maintenance therapy with Intron-A following high-dose chemotherapy in multiple myeloma—long-term follow-up results. *Br J Haematol* 1998;102:495.

175. Westin J. Interferon therapy during the plateau phase of multiple myeloma: an update of a Swedish Multicenter Study. *Semin Oncol* 1991;18:37.

176. Peest D, Deicher H, Coldeway R, et al. Melphalan and prednisone versus vincristine, BCNU, adriamycin, melphalan and dexamethasone induction chemotherapy and interferon maintenance treatment in multiple myeloma: current results of a multicenter trial. *Onkologie* 1990;13:458.

177. Anderson KC. Who benefits from high dose therapy for multiple myeloma? *J Clin Oncol* 1995;13:1291.

178. Harousseau J-L, Attal M. The role of autologous hematopoietic stem cell transplantation in multiple myeloma. *Semin Hematol* 1997;34:61.

179. Attal M, Harousseau JL, Stoppa AM, et al. Autologous bone marrow transplantation versus conventional chemotherapy in multiple myeloma: a prospective, randomized trial. *N Engl J Med* 1996;335:91.

180. Siegel DS, Desikan KR, Mehta J, et al. Age is not a prognostic variable with autotransplants for multiple myeloma. *Blood* 1999; 93:51.

181. Badros A, Barlogie B, Siegel E, et al. Autologous stem cell transplantation in elderly multiple myeloma patients over the age of 70 years. *Br J Haematol* 2001;114:600.

182. Palumbo A, Triolo S, Argentino C, et al. Dose-intensive melphalan with stem cell support (MEL100) is superior to standard treatment in elderly myeloma patients. *Blood* 1999;94:1248.

183. Badros A, Barlogie B, Siegel E, et al. Results of autologous stem cell transplant in multiple myeloma patients with renal failure. *Br J Haematol* 2001;114:822.

184. Fermand J-P, Ravaud P, Chevret S, et al. High-dose therapy and autologous peripheral blood stem cell transplantation in multiple myeloma: up-front or rescue treatment? Results of a multicenter sequential randomized clinical trial. *Blood* 1998;92:3131.

185. Moreau P, Facon T, Attal M, et al. Comparison of 200 mg/m(2) melphalan and 8 Gy total body irradiation plus 140 mg/m(2) melphalan as conditioning regimens for peripheral blood stem cell transplantation in patients with newly diagnosed multiple myeloma: final analysis of the Intergroupe Francophone du Myeloma 9502 randomized trial. *Blood* 2002;99:731.

186. Lenhoff S, Hjorth M, Holmberg E, et al. Impact on survival of high-dose therapy with autologous stem cell support in patients younger than 60 years with newly diagnosed multiple myeloma: a population-based study. *Blood* 2000;95:7.

187. Alyea E, Weller E, Schlossman R, et al. Outcome after autologous and allogeneic stem cell transplantation for patients with multiple myeloma: impact of graft versus myeloma effect. *Bone Marrow Transplant (in press)*

188. Anderson KC, Anderson J, Soiffer R, et al. Monoclonal antibody-purged bone marrow transplantation therapy for multiple myeloma. *Blood* 1993;82:2568.

189. Seiden M, Schlossman R, Andersen J, et al. Monoclonal antibody-purged bone marrow transplantation therapy for multiple myeloma. *Leuk Lymphoma* 1995;17:87.

190. Schiller G, Vescio R, Freytes C, et al. Transplantation of CD34 positive peripheral blood progenitor cells following high dose chemotherapy for patients with advanced multiple myeloma. *Blood* 1995;86:390.

191. Vescio R, Schiller GJ, Stewart AK, et al. Multicenter phase III trial to evaluate CD34+ selected versus unselected autologous peripheral blood progenitor cell transplantation in multiple myeloma. *Blood* 1999;93:1858.

192. Stewart AK, Vescio R, Schiller G, et al. Purging of autologous peripheral blood stem cells from multiple myeloma patients using CD34+ selection does not improve overall or progression free survival following high-dose chemotherapy: results of a multicenter randomized controlled trial. *J Clin Oncol* 2001;19(17):3771.

193. Lemoli RM, Martinelli G, Zamagni E, et al. Engraftment, clinical, and molecular follow-up of patients with multiple myeloma who were reinfused with highly purified CD34+ cells to support single or tandem high-dose chemotherapy. *Blood* 2000;95:2234.

194. Barlogie B, Jagannath S, Desikan KR, et al. Total therapy with tandem transplants for newly diagnosed multiple myeloma. *Blood* 1999;93:55.

195. Vesole DH, Tricot G, Jagannath S, et al. Autotransplants in multiple myeloma: what have we learned? *Blood* 1996;88:838.

196. Desikan R, Barlogie B, Sawyer J, et al. Results of high-dose therapy for 1000 patients with multiple myeloma: durable complete remissions and superior survival in the absence of chromosome 13 abnormalities. *Blood* 2000;95:4008.

197. Attal M, Harousseau J-I, Facon T, et al. Double autologous transplantation improves survival of multiple myeloma patients: final analysis of a prospective randomized study of the Intergroupe Francophone du Myeloma (IFM 94). *Blood* 2002;100(11):5a (abstr).

198. Qing Y, Osterborg A. Idiotype-specific T cells in multiple myeloma: targets for an immunotherapeutic intervention? *Med Oncol* 1996;13:1.

199. Bergenbrant S, Yiu Q, Osterborg A, et al. Modulation of antiidiotypic immune response by immunization with the autologous M component protein multiple myeloma patients. *Br J Haematol* 1996;92:840.

200. Hsu FJ, Benike C, Fagnoni F, et al. Vaccination of patients with B-cell lymphoma using autologous antigen-pulsed dendritic cells. *Nat Med* 1996;2:52.

201. Kovasics TJ, Delay A. Intensive treatment strategies in multiple myeloma. *Semin Hematol* 1997;34:49.

202. Bensinger WI, Demirer T, Buckner CD, et al. Syngeneic marrow transplantation in patients with multiple myeloma. *Bone Marrow Transplant* 1996;18:527.

203. Gahrton G, Svensson H, Bjorkstrand B, et al. Syngeneic transplantation in multiple myeloma-a case-matched comparison with autologous and allogeneic transplantation. *Bone Marrow Transplant* 1999;7:741.

204. Gahrton G, Tura S, Ljungman P, et al. Allogeneic bone marrow transplantation in multiple myeloma. *N Engl J Med* 1991;325:1267.

205. Gahrton G, Tura S, Ljungman P, et al. Prognostic factors in allogeneic bone marrow transplantation for multiple myeloma. *J Clin Oncol* 1995;13:1312.

206. Gahrton G, Anderson K, Bensinger W. *Allogeneic transplantation in myeloma.* Totowa, NJ: The Humana Press, 1999.

207. Bensinger WI, Buchner CD, Anasetti C, et al. Allogeneic marrow transplantation for multiple myeloma: an analysis of risk factors on outcome. *Blood* 1996;88:2787.

208. Corradini P, Voena C, Tarella C, et al. Molecular and clinical remissions in multiple myeloma: role of autologous and allogeneic transplantation of hematopoietic cells. *J Clin Oncol* 1999;17:208.

209. Tricot G, Vesole DH, Jagannath S, et al. Graft-versus myeloma effect: proof of principle. *Blood* 1996;87:1196.

210. Verdonck LF, Lokhorst HM, Dekker AW, et al. Graft-versus-myeloma effect in two cases. *Lancet* 1996;347:800.

211. Alyea EP, Soiffer RJ, Canning C, et al. Toxicity and efficacy of defined doses of CD4+ donor lymphocytes for treatment of relapse after allogeneic bone marrow transplant. *Blood* 1998;91:3671.

212. Gahrton G, Svensson H, Cavo M, et al. Progress in allogeneic bone marrow and peripheral blood stem cell transplantation for multiple myeloma: a comparison between transplants performed 1983–93 and 1994–8 at European Group for Blood and Marrow centers. *Br J Haematol* 2001;113:209.

213. Schlossman SF, Alyea E, Orsini E, et al. Immune based strategies to improve hematopoietic stem cell transplantation in multiple myeloma. In: Dicke KA, Keating A, eds. *Autologous marrow and blood transplantation.* Charlottesville, VA: Carden, Jennings Publishing Co., Ltd., 1999:207.

214. Schlossman SF, Anderson KC. Bone marrow transplantation in multiple myeloma. In: Jones R, ed. *Current opinion in oncology* (vol. 11). Philadelphia: Lippincott Williams & Wilkins, 1999:102.

215. Soiffer RJ, Murray C, Mauch P, et al. Prevention of graft-versus-host disease by selective depletion of CD6-positive T lymphocytes from donor bone marrow. *J Clin Oncol* 1992;10:1191.

216. Alyea E, Weller E, Schlossman R, et al. T-cell–depleted allogeneic bone marrow transplantation followed by donor lymphocyte infusion in patients with multiple myeloma: induction of graft-versus-myeloma effect. *Blood* 2001;98:934.

217. Orsini E, Alyea EP, Schlossman R, et al. Changes in T cell receptor repertoire associated with graft-versus-tumor effect and graft-versus host disease in patients with relapsed multiple myeloma receiving donor lymphocyte infusions. *Bone Marrow Transplant* 2000;25(6):623.

218. Orsini E, Alyea EP, Chillemi A, et al. Conversion to full donor chimerism following donor lymphocyte infusion is associated with disease response in patients with multiple myeloma. *Biol Blood Marrow Transplant* 2000;6(4):375.

219. Bellucci R, Alyea EP, Weller E, et al. Immunologic effects of prophylactic donor lymphocyte infusion after allogeneic marrow transplantation for multiple myeloma. *Blood* 2002;99:4610.

220. Badros A, Barlogie B, Morris C, et al. High response rate in refractory and poor-risk multiple myeloma after allotransplantation using a nonmyeloablative conditioning regimen and donor lymphocyte infusions. *Blood* 2001;97:2574.

221. Kroger N, Schwerdtfeger R, Kiehl M, et al. Autologous stem cell transplantation followed by a dose-reduced allograft induces high complete remission rate in multiple myeloma. *Blood* 2002;100:755.

222. Attal M, Harousseau JL, Stoppa AM, et al. A prospective, randomized trial of autologous bone marrow transplantation and chemotherapy in multiple myeloma. *N Engl J Med* 1996;335:91.

223. Harousseau JL, Attal M. Autologous stem cell transplantation in multiple myeloma: the IFM experience. Dallas: Proceedings of the Tenth International Symposium on Autologous Blood and Marrow Transplantation, 2000.

224. Lahuerta JJ, Grande C, Blade J, et al. Myeloablative treatments for multiple myeloma: update of a comparative study of different regimens used in patients from the Spanish registry for transplantation in multiple myeloma. *Leuk Lymphoma* 2002;43:67.

225. Abraham R, Chen C, Tsang R, et al. Intensification of the stem cell transplant induction regimen results in increased treatment-related mortality without improved outcome in multiple myeloma. *Bone Marrow Transplant* 1999;24:1291.

226. Barlogie B, Jagannath S, Vesole DH, et al. Superiority of tandem autologous transplantation over standard therapy for previously untreated multiple myeloma. *Blood* 1997;89:789.

227. Anderson PM, Wiseman GA, Dispenzieri A, et al. High-dose samarium-153 ethylene diamine tetramethylene phosphonate: low toxicity of skeletal irradiation in patients with osteosarcoma and bone metastases. *J Clin Oncol* 2002;20:189.

228. Hogan WJ, Lacy MQ, Wiseman GA, et al. Successful treatment of POEMS syndrome with autologous hematopoietic progenitor cell transplantation. *Bone Marrow Transplant* 2001;28:305.

228a. Durrant STS, Irving IM, Morton J, et al. 5m-153 Lexidronam, limb irradiation and stem-cell transplantation for the treatment of multiple myeloma. *Blood* 2001;98(11):778a (abstr.).

229. Bayouth JE, Macey DJ, Boyer AL, et al. Radiation dose distribution within the bone marrow of patients receiving holmium-166-labeled-phosphonate for marrow ablation. *Med Phys* 1995;22:743.

230. Bayouth JE, Macey DJ, Kasi LP, et al. Pharmacokinetics, dosimetry and toxicity of holmium-166-DOTMP for bone marrow ablation in multiple myeloma. *J Nucl Med* 1995;36:730.

231. Barlogie B, Smith L, Alexanian R. Effective treatment of advanced multiple myeloma refractory to alkylating agents. *N Engl J Med* 1984; 310:1353.

232. Monconduit M, Le Loet X, Bernard JF, et al. Combination chemotherapy with vincristine, doxorubicin, dexamethasone for refractory or relapsing multiple myeloma. *Br J Haematol* 1986;63:599.

233. Sheehan T, Judge M, Parker AC. The efficacy and toxicity of VAD in the treatment of myeloma and related disorders. *Scand J Haematol* 1986;37:425.

234. Barlogie B, Valasquez WS, Alexanian R, et al. Etoposide, dexamethasone, cytarabine, and cisplatin in vincristine, doxorubicin and dexamethasone-refractory myeloma. *J Clin Oncol* 1989;7:1514.

235. Salmon SE, Dalton WS, Grogan TM, et al. Multidrug-resistant myeloma: laboratory and clinical effects of verapamil as a chemosensitizer. *Blood* 1991;78:44.

236. Sonneveld P, Schoester M, de Leeuw K. Clinical modulation of multidrug resistance in multiple myeloma: effects of cyclosporine on resistant tumor cells. *J Clin Oncol* 1994;12:1584.

237. Sonneveld P. Drug resistance in myeloma. In: *VI international workshop on multiple myeloma.* Boston, 1997.

238. Weber DM, Gavino M, Delasalle K, et al. Thalidomide alone or with dexamethasone for multiple myeloma. *Blood Suppl* 1999;94:604a.

239. Moehler TM, Neben K, Benner A, et al. Salvage therapy for multiple myeloma with thalidomide and CED chemotherapy. *Blood* 2001; 98:3846.

240. Garcia-Sanz R, Gonzalez-Fraile MI, Sierra M, et al. The combination of thalidomide, cyclophosphamide and dexamethasone (ThaCyDex) is feasible and can be an option for relapsed/refractory multiple myeloma. *Hematol J* 2002;3:43.

241. Ampil FL, Chin HW. Radiotherapy alone for extradural compression by spinal myeloma. *Radiat Med* 1995;13:129.

242. Wallington M, Mendis S, Premawardhana U, et al. Local control and survival in spinal cord compression from lymphoma and myeloma. *Radiother Oncol* 1997;42:43.

243. Chang SA, Lee SS, Ueng SW, et al. Surgical treatment for pathological long bone fracture in patients with multiple myeloma: a retrospective analysis of 22 cases. *Chang Gung Med J* 2001;24:300.

244. Catell D, Kogen Z, Donahue B, et al. Multiple myeloma of an extremity: must the entire bone be treated? *Int J Radiat Oncol Biol Phys* 1998;40:117.

245. Leigh BR, Kurtts TA, Mack CF, et al. Radiation therapy for the palliation of multiple myeloma. *Int J Radiat Oncol Biol Phys* 1993;25: 801.

246. Adamietz IA, Schober C, Schulte RW, et al. Palliative radiotherapy in plasma cell myeloma. *Radiother Oncol* 1991;20:111.

247. Berenson J, Crowley J, Barlogie B, et al. Alternate day oral prednisone maintenance therapy improves progression-free survival and overall survival in multiple myeloma patients. *Blood* 1998;92[Suppl 1]:318a.

248. Djulbegovic B, Wheatley K, Ross J, et al. Bisphosphonates in multiple myeloma (Cochrane review). *Cochrane Database Syst Rev* 2002:CD003188.

249. McSweeney EN, Tobias JS, Blackman G, et al. Double hemibody irradiation (DHBI) in the management of relapsed and primary chemoresistant multiple myeloma. *Clin Oncol (R Coll Radiol)* 1993;5:378.

250. Tobias JS, Richards JD, Blackman GM, et al. Hemibody irradiation in multiple myeloma. *Radiother Oncol* 1985;3:11.

251. van Dyk J, Keane TJ, Kan S, et al. Radiation pneumonitis following large single dose irradiation: a re-evaluation based on absolute dose to lung. *Int J Radiat Oncol Biol Phys* 1981;7:461.

252. Rowland CG, Garrett MJ, Crowley FA. Half body radiation in plasma cell myeloma. *Clin Radiol* 1983;34:507.

253. Singer CR, Tobias JS, Giles F, et al. Hemibody irradiation. An effective second-line therapy in drug-resistance multiple myeloma. *Cancer* 1989;63:2446.

254. Salmon SE, Tesh D, Crowley J, et al. Chemotherapy is superior to sequential hemibody irradiation for remission consolidation in multiple myeloma: a Southwest Oncology Group study. *J Clin Oncol* 1990;8:1575.

255. Anderson KC. Targeted therapy for multiple myeloma. *Semin Hematol* 2001;38:286.

256. Hideshima T, Chauhan D, Shima Y, et al. Thalidomide and its analogues overcome drug resistance of human multiple myeloma cells to conventional therapy. *Blood* 2000;96(9):2943.

257. Davies FE, Raje N, Hideshima T, et al. Thalidomide and immunomodulatory derivatives augment natural killer cell cytotoxicity in multiple myeloma. *Blood* 2001;98:210.

258. Treon SP, Mitsiades C, Mitsiades N, et al. Tumor cell expression of CD59 is associated with resistance to CD20 serotherapy in patients with B-cell malignancies. *J Immunother* 2001;24:263.

259. Lentzsch S, LeBlanc R, Podar K, et al. Immunomodulatory analogs of thalidomide inhibit growth of HS Sultan cells and angiogenesis *in vivo*. *Leukemia* 2003;17:41.

260. Richardson P, Schlossman R, Weller E, et al. The IMiD CC 5013 overcomes drug resistance and is well tolerated in patients with relapsed multiple myeloma. *Blood* 2002;100:3063.

261. Richardson P, Berenson J, Irwin D, et al. Phase II trial of pS-341, a novel proteasome inhibitor, alone or in combination with dexamethasone, in patients with multiple myeloma who have relapsed following front-line therapy and are refractory to their most recent therapy. *Blood* 2001;98:774a.

262. Hayashi T, Hideshima T, Akiyama M, et al. Arsenic trioxide inhibits growth of human multiple myeloma cells in the bone marrow microenvironment. *Mol Cancer Ther* 2002;1:851.

263. Trojan A, Schultze JL, Witzens M, et al. Immunoglobulin framework-derived peptides function as cytotoxic T-cell epitopes commonly expressed in B-cell malignancies. *Nat Med* 2000;6:667.

264. Vonderheide RH, Hahn WC, Schultze JL, et al. The telomerase catalytic subunit is a widely expressed tumor-associated antigen recognized by cytotoxic T lymphocytes. *Immunity* 1999;10:673.

265. Treon SP, Mollick JA, Urashima M, et al. Muc-1 core protein is expressed on multiple myeloma cells and is induced by dexamethasone. *Blood* 1999;93:1287.

266. Maecker B, Sherr DH, Shen C, et al. Targeting universal tumor antigens with cytotoxic T cells: potential of CYP1B1 for broadly applicable antigen-specific immunotherapy. *Blood* 1999;94[Suppl]:438a.

267. Schultze JL, Anderson KC, Gilleece MH, et al. Autologous adoptive T cell transfer for a patient with plasma cell leukemia: results of a pilot phase I trial. *Br J Haematol* 2001;113:455–460.

268. Gong J, Koido S, Chen D, et al. Immunization against murine multiple myeloma with fusions of dendritic and plasmacytoma cells is potentiated by interleukin 12. *Blood* 2002;99:2512.

269. Raje N, Gong J, Chauhan D, et al. Bone marrow and peripheral blood dendritic cells from patients with multiple myeloma are phenotypically and functionally normal. *Blood* 1999;93:1487.

270. Raje N, Hideshima T, Avigan D, et al. Tumor cell/dendritic cell fusions as a vaccination strategy for multiple myeloma. *Blood (in press)*.

271. Barlogie B, Jagannath S, Vesole DH, et al. Superiority of tandem autologous transplantation over standard therapy for previously untreated multiple myeloma. *Blood* 1997;89:789.

SECTION V

Late Effects

CHAPTER 33

Second Cancers

Lois B. Travis and Flora E. van Leeuwen

Survival rates for patients with lymphoma have improved dramatically in the last few decades, due largely to the introduction of effective treatment regimens. Five-year and 10-year relative survival rates are currently 58% and 46%, respectively (1). Now that considerable numbers of lymphoma patients have such a favorable prognosis, it becomes increasingly important to assess the long-term sequelae of treatment. Results of studies conducted over the past few decades have clearly shown that some of the modalities used to treat cancer are associated with late complications, including the development of second primary malignancies (2). Second cancers are generally considered to be one of the most significant complications of treatment and can be associated with substantial morbidity and mortality (3). Other influences, however, should be considered in the development of second cancers and include shared etiologic factors, underlying host susceptibility, and the effects of chance, particularly in an aging population in which the underlying cancer incidence is increasing. Thus, critical to any assessment of second cancers is an evaluation of whether their occurrence exceeds expectation; if second tumors are indeed shown to occur in excess, the influence of other risk factors must be ruled out before increased risks can be attributed to treatment. A number of measures have been introduced to quantify risk, as described below.

METHODS TO ASSESS SECOND-CANCER RISK

Cohort Studies

The epidemiologic study designs generally used for the assessment of second-cancer risk are the cohort and case-control studies. Although the pursuit of case reports can hardly be considered a sound research strategy, it is irrefutable that some associations between treatment and second cancers (i.e., acute myelogenous leukemia after alkylating-agent chemotherapy) (4) have been recognized relatively early through the publication of case series by astute clinicians. In a cohort study, large numbers of patients with a first malignancy (the cohort) who meet well-defined criteria are followed for a number of years to determine the incidence of second cancers. To evaluate whether second-cancer risk in the cohort is increased compared with cancer risk in the general population, the observed number of second malignant neoplasms in the cohort is compared with the number expected on the basis of age-, sex- and calendar year–specific cancer incidence rates in the general population. This analytic approach takes into account the observation period of individual patients (person-years) (5). The relative risk of developing a second cancer is estimated by comparing the ratio of the observed number of second cancers in the cohort with the number expected based on population rates. When the relative risk is increased, the question of whether the excesses are due to therapy then arises. This issue can be evaluated by comparing risks between treatment groups, preferably within specified follow-up intervals and, when possible, with a reference group of patients not treated with radiotherapy and chemotherapy. The temporal trend of the relative risk of second cancers may also provide an important clue to etiology, for example, the risk of solid tumors after radiotherapy for lymphoma is generally not increased in the first 5 years of follow-up but continues to increase thereafter with time since exposure (6). Such a pattern demonstrates that the excess solid-tumor risk is not due solely to host susceptibility or common risk factors but rather points to a role of treatment.

Cumulative Risk

Second-cancer risk in the cohort can also be measured in terms of the cumulative (actuarial estimated) risk (7), which yields the proportion of patients alive at time t (e.g., 10 years from diagnosis) who can be expected to develop a second malignancy. When the cohort's death rate due to causes other than second malignancy is high, the assumptions underlying the actuarial method may not be valid, and competing risk techniques should be considered to estimate cumulative risk (8,9). Because many treatment-related cancers are rare in the general population (e.g., leukemia, sarcoma), a high relative risk (compared with the population) may still translate into a rather low cumulative risk. Absolute excess risk, which estimates the excess number of second malignancies per 10,000 patients per year, perhaps best reflects the additional cancer burden in a cohort. This risk measure is also the most appropriate one by which to identify those second malignancies that contribute the most to increased risks.

Examples

The authors illustrate an application of the above approaches with an example from an international study of 6,171 2-year survivors of lymphoma (6). In this cohort, 14 cases of acute nonlymphocytic leukemia were observed during a mean follow-up period of 7.4 years, whereas only 2.9 cases were expected on the basis of age-, sex-, and calendar period–specific incidence rates of leukemia in the general population. Hence, the observed to expected ratio (also denoted as relative risk or standardized incidence ratio) is 4.8 (95% confidence interval, 2.6 to 8.1). In the same study, 39 cases of bladder cancer were observed against 22 expected cases, resulting in an observed to expected ratio of 1.8 (95% confidence interval, 1.3 to 2.4). The absolute excess risk [i.e., the excess number of second cancer cases (beyond the background incidence) per 10,000 patients per year] can be easily derived by subtracting the expected number from the observed number and dividing by person-years at risk. In the above example, the number of person-years at risk was 45,794 (6,171 people multiplied by an average follow-up time of 7.4 years). The absolute excess risk for leukemia is [(14 − 2.9)/45,794] × 10,000 = 2.4 per 10,000 person-years. The absolute excess risk for bladder cancer is [(39 − 22)/ 45,794 × 10,000 = 3.7 per 10,000 person-years, demonstrating that bladder cancer contributes more to the absolute excess risk of second malignancies than leukemia, although the relative risk for bladder cancer is lower. Although cumulative risk measures were not provided in the above study, it can be predicted that the 20-year cumulative risk of developing leukemia is considerably smaller than for bladder cancer, given the lower background incidence of the former.

Cohort studies that provide estimates of second-cancer risk can be based on patient data derived from several sources, including population-based cancer registries, hospital-based cancer registries, or clinical trial series (10). Each of the data sources used to construct cohorts has inherent advantages and disadvantages.

Population-Based Cancer Registries

Population-based cancer registries frequently have large numbers of patients available, which allows the detection of even small increases in the site-specific risk of second cancers (11); an additional advantage is that the observed and expected numbers of cancers derive from the same reference population. Disadvantages of population-based cancer registries include the limited availability of treatment data, possible underreporting of second cancers (12,13), and differing diagnostic criteria for second cancers. Population-based registries vary greatly in these aspects and, hence, in their usefulness for second-cancer studies. When treatment data are not available, it is impossible to determine whether excess second cancers might be related to prior therapy, shared etiologic factors with the first cancer, other influences, or a combination of factors. Despite the disadvantages of population-based registries, they are particularly conducive to the global evaluation of site-specific cancer risk after a broad spectrum of first primary malignancies. These resources also serve as a valuable starting point for case-control studies that evaluate treatment effects in detail (see below).

Clinical Trial Databases

A major strength of clinical trial databases is that detailed treatment data on all patients are available. Comparison of second-cancer risk between the treatment arms of the trial adjusts for any intrinsic risk for a second malignancy associated with the first cancer. Limitations of most trials, however, include small numbers of patients and the frequent lack of data on subsequent therapy. The dearth of large numbers becomes especially critical when the second cancer of interest has a low background incidence (e.g., leukemia). Further, the endpoints of interest in the majority of clinical trials include only treatment response and survival, not the development of second cancers. Therefore, many clinical trials do not routinely collect information on second malignancies, and some do not compile any data beyond 5 years. Routine reporting and assessment of second-malignancy risk should become an integral part of clinical trial research (14).

Hospital-Based Cancer Registries

Many large cancer treatment centers maintain registries of all admitted patients. Most of these registries have been in existence for decades and collect extensive data on treatment and follow-up. As compared with clinical trial data, hospital registries provide larger patient numbers and a wider variety of treatments and dose levels, which may yield important information on drug and radiation carcinogenesis. For example, most studies of second-cancer risk after Hodgkin's disease, a related lymphoma, have been based on data accrued from hospital registries (15–17). Complete patient follow-up and confirmation of second malignancies through careful review of pathology reports constitute critical methodologic features in second-cancer research. Overestimation of second-malignancy risk occurs when follow-up in the original treatment center is more complete for survivors who developed a second tumor than for those who remain healthy. This bias is likely to result when patients who remain healthy lose contact with the original treatment center, whereas those with late complications return for clinical follow-up. In view of this potential bias, it is critical that investigators obtain recent information on medical status for all patients lost to follow-up in the original treatment center. This can be accomplished by a variety of procedures, including contact of treating physicians in other hospitals or

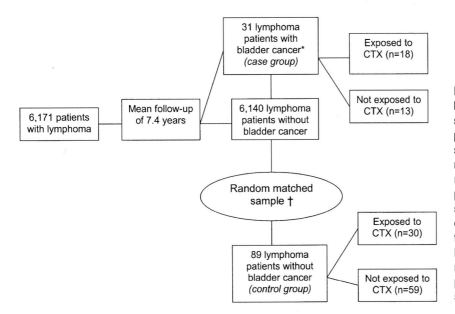

FIG. 33.1. Nested case-control design of bladder cancer in a cohort of 6,171 2-year survivors of lymphoma. CTX, cyclophosphamide; *, pathologically confirmed transitional cell carcinomas of the bladder; †, matched on cancer registry, gender, age, race, calendar year of diagnosis of lymphoma, and interval between the case subject's diagnosis of lymphoma and bladder cancer. (Adapted from Travis LB, Curtis RE, Holowaty EJ, et al. Bladder and kidney cancer following cyclophosphamide therapy for non-Hodgkin's lymphoma. *J Natl Cancer Inst* 1995;87:524–530, with permission of Oxford University.)

general practitioners. However, completeness of follow-up is rarely reported in second cancer studies. Pathologic confirmation of second primary cancers is important to ensure that the second tumor is not a metastasis of the first one.

Nested Case-Control Studies

The cohort study is not an efficient design when examining the role of detailed treatment factors (e.g., cumulative dose of alkylating agents, radiation dose) in relation to second-cancer risk. Most cohorts are fairly large (to yield reliable estimates of second-cancer risk), rendering the collection of detailed treatment data for all patients prohibitively expensive and time-consuming. In such instances, the case-control study nested within an existing cohort is the preferred approach. The case group consists of all patients identified with the second cancer of interest, whereas the controls are a matched sample of all patients in the cohort who did not develop the cancer of interest, although they experienced the same amount of follow-up time. Matching factors typically include age, sex, and calendar year of diagnosis of the first cancer. The use of the above matching criteria adjusts for several potentially confounding factors between treatment and second-cancer risk.

Example

The nested case-control design is illustrated in Figure 33.1 using data from a study of bladder cancer (18) conducted in the international cohort of 6,171 2-year survivors of lymphoma described above (6). In this well-defined cohort, 31 cases of pathologically confirmed transitional cell carcinoma of the bladder were identified. Risk factors for bladder cancer were examined in a case-control study in which the complete treatment histories (with an emphasis on the use of cyclophosphamide) for the 31 case subjects were compared with those of 89 matched controls in whom bladder cancer was not diag-

nosed. A major advantage of a case-control study nested within a cohort is that it is necessary to collect detailed treatment information for only a small proportion of the entire population. Even in the above example, in which the control group is three times as large as the case group, detailed data had to be obtained for only 2% of the underlying cohort. The marked efficiency of this design stems from the fact that the outcome of interest in many late effects studies is relatively rare.

Methodologic Issues

In the case-control investigation, it is critical to the validity of the study that the controls are truly representative of all patients who did not develop the second cancer of interest. Bias in the selection of the control group can lead to spurious associations or obscure a true association. The advantage of case-control studies nested in a cohort, as compared with traditional case-control studies, is that both case subjects and controls are identified from the same well-defined population (the cohort), thus minimizing selection bias. However, selection bias in nested case-control studies may still arise when the medical records of controls who were initially selected cannot be traced. A patient's medical chart may be untraceable for various reasons, some of which may be related to the intensity of treatment or directly to the risk of second-cancer development (e.g., a record stored in a private file cabinet), whereas other factors may be unrelated to patient outcome (e.g., misfiling of charts). In the former case, bias may arise when control subjects with untraceable records are replaced by patients with obtainable charts.

In the analysis of case-control studies, treatment factors are compared between cases and controls, and the risk associated with specific therapies is estimated relative to the risk in patients who received other treatments. The ideal reference group in second-cancer studies consists of patients treated with surgery only; however, such a group is not available when studying the risk of second neoplasms after lymphoma.

The cumulative risk of developing a second malignancy cannot be derived from a case-control study. Treatment-specific absolute excess risks can be estimated, however, when the case-control study follows a cohort analysis in which basic treatment data were available. Numerous landmark studies (18–26) have demonstrated the strengths of the case-control approach when evaluating second-cancer risk.

INCIDENCE AND RISK FACTORS OF SELECTED SECOND CANCERS

Estimates of the risk of second malignancies after lymphoma have been provided by several population-based studies (6,27–29). In the largest published investigation to date, the incidence of second cancers was estimated in 29,153 patients diagnosed with lymphoma between 1973 and 1987 and reported to population-based cancer registries that participate in the National Cancer Institute's Surveillance, Epidemiology, and End Results (SEER) Program (27). Compared with the general population, significant excesses were observed for all second cancers taken together (observed to expected ratio, 1.2; observed, 1,231; absolute excess risk, 20.2 excess cancers per 10,000 lymphoma patients per year). Risk increased with time to reach 1.8 in 10-year survivors (p trend < .05). These findings were confirmed in an international study of 6,171 2-year survivors of lymphoma, which showed that significant excesses of second cancers persisted for two decades (6). An update of the SEER Program data (1973 to 1998) includes more than 66,000 2-month survivors of lymphoma, with 22,755, 9,812, 3,843, and 1,200 patients surviving 5, 10, 15, and 20 years, respectively (30). Overall, 4,600 subsequent cancers were diagnosed, representing a significantly elevated risk (observed to expected ratio, 1.1; absolute excess risk, 19.3) (Table 33.1). Significant excesses were

TABLE 33.1. *Relative and absolute site-specific risks of selected second malignant neoplasms among 66,171 2-month survivors of lymphoma reported to the SEER Program (1973 to 1998)[a]*

Cancer site	Observed	Observed to expected ratio	95% confidence interval	Absolute excess risk[b]
All sites	4,638	1.1[c]	1.1–1.2	19.3
Buccal cavity and pharynx	147	1.4[c]	1.2–1.6	1.4
Esophagus	37	0.9	0.6–1.2	−0.2
Stomach	107	1.2	1.0–1.4	0.5
Colon	471	1.1	1.0–1.2	1.3
Rectum	111	1.1	0.9–1.2	0.2
Liver, gallbladder, bile ducts	55	0.9	0.7–1.1	−0.3
Pancreas	95	0.8	0.7–1.0	−0.6
Lung	876	1.3[c]	1.3–1.4	7.4
Female breast	393	0.8[c]	0.7–0.9	−7.1
Cervix	13	0.6[c]	0.3–0.9	−0.7
Uterine corpus	103	0.9	0.8–1.1	−0.6
Ovary	60	0.9	0.7–1.2	−0.4
Prostate	669	0.9[c]	0.8–0.96	−5.3
Testis	5	0.9	0.3–2.2	0
Urinary bladder	295	1.3[c]	1.2–1.5	2.4
Kidney	137	1.7[c]	1.4–2.0	1.9
Melanomas of skin	158	1.6[c]	1.4–1.9	2.1
Brain, central nervous system	46	1.1	0.8–1.4	0.1
Thyroid	38	1.6[c]	1.1–2.2	0.5
Bone and joints	14	3.6[b]	2.0–6.1	0.3
Soft tissue	26	1.6[c]	1.01–2.30	0.3
Kaposi's sarcoma	106	13.0[c]	10.6–15.7	3.3
Hodgkin's disease	49	4.5[c]	3.3–5.9	1.3
Multiple myeloma	34	0.6[c]	0.4–0.9	−0.6
Acute myelogenous leukemia	89	3.4[c]	2.7–4.1	2.9

SEER, Surveillance, Epidemiology, and End Results.
[a]Excludes second diagnoses of non-Hodgkin's lymphoma.
[b]Number of excess second cancers per 10,000 lymphoma patients per year.
[c]p < .05.

observed for malignant melanoma, Kaposi's sarcoma, acute myelogenous leukemia, and cancers of buccal cavity and pharynx, lung, bladder, kidney, thyroid, bone and joint, and soft tissue. The largest absolute excess risk was observed for lung cancer. The risk of all solid tumors (n = 4,195) increased with time to reach 1.6 (95% confidence interval, 1.2 to 2.0; absolute excess risk, 84.2; p trend < .0001) among 20-year survivors of lymphoma, who experienced significantly elevated threefold site-specific risks for cancers of colon, rectum, and bladder. In contrast, significant excesses of acute myelogenous leukemia were restricted to the first 15 years after lymphoma diagnosis, with risks (observed to expected ratio) of 2.6, 3.2, 4.7, and 2.3 in the latency intervals of 2 months to 1 year, 1 to 4 years, 5 to 9 years, and 10 to 14 years, respectively. Analytic studies to examine increased risks for second cancers in relation to lymphoma treatment have been conducted only for genitourinary cancers (18,31) and acute myelogenous leukemia (32–38).

Genitourinary Cancer

The largest investigation (18) of secondary bladder cancer was conducted in a cohort of more than 6,100 2-year survivors of lymphoma who were first diagnosed between 1965 and 1980 (6). This case-control study included 31 patients with transitional cell carcinoma of the bladder and 17 patients with kidney cancer. For each patient with a secondary genitourinary cancer, three controls were selected from the defined cohort by means of stratified random sampling. Matching factors included cancer registry, sex, age, calendar year of lymphoma diagnosis, and survival at least as long as the time between the case's diagnosis of lymphoma and subsequent genitourinary cancer. For all cases and controls, data on drug dose and duration of administration were collected for all alkylating agents, including cyclophosphamide. Radiation dose to the bladder or kidney was estimated using detailed radiotherapy records for each patient. Sources of treatment information included hospitals, clinics, and radiotherapy facilities and offices of physicians. For approximately 95% of patients, data on cumulative dose of cyclophosphamide were available from all abstracted sources. A significant 4.5-fold increased risk of bladder cancer followed therapy with cyclophosphamide, with risk strongly dependent on cumulative dose (Table 33.2).

The risks of bladder cancer after a total dose of less than 20 g, 20 to 49 g, or 50 g or more of cyclophosphamide were 2.4-, 6.3-, and 14.5-fold, respectively (p trend for dose = .004). Radiotherapy without cyclophosphamide was associated with a nonsignificant 2.8-fold risk of bladder cancer, compared with subjects whose treatment included neither treatment modality. Excess bladder-cancer risk after treatment with both cyclophosphamide and radiotherapy was as expected if individual risks were summed. Based on the above findings taken together with results of the underlying cohort survey (6), the absolute risk of bladder cancer for lymphoma patients given between 20 and 49 g of cyclophosphamide and followed for 15 years was three excess cancers per 100 patients. At cumulative doses of 50 g or more, the excess risk increased to approximately seven bladder cancers per 100 lymphoma patients. For patients included in this case-control study, it is unlikely that procedures now known to ameliorate cyclophosphamide-related bladder toxicity, such as the administration of sodium 2-mercaptoethane-sulfonate (39) or intensive

TABLE 33.2. *Risk of bladder cancer according to cumulative dose and duration of cyclophosphamide therapy for lymphoma*

Cyclophosphamide	Median dose or duration[a]	No. of cases	No. of controls	Matched relative risk[b]	95% confidence interval
Cumulative dose					
<20 g[c]	10.0 g	8	22	2.4	0.7–8.4
20–49 g	34.0 g	5	6	6.3[d]	1.3–29.0
≥50 g	87.7 g	5	2	14.5[d,e]	2.3–94.0
Duration of therapy					
<1 yr	6 mo	8	20	2.5	0.7–9.0
1–2 yr	18 mo	3	6	3.7	0.6–22.0
≥2 yr	51 mo	7	4	11.8[d,e]	2.3–61.0

[a]Median cumulative dose of cyclophosphamide or median duration of therapy among all patients within the specified category.
[b]The referent group consists of six case subjects and 42 control subjects who did not meet study exposure criteria.
[c]The minimum cumulative dose of cyclophosphamide in this group was 2.1 g.
[d]p < .05.
[e]p for trend < .005.
From Travis LB, Curtis RE, Holowaty EJ, et al. Bladder and kidney cancer following cyclophosphamide therapy for non-Hodgkin's lymphoma. *J Natl Cancer Inst* 1995;87:524–530, with permission of Oxford University Press.

TABLE 33.3. *Overview of analytic studies of secondary acute nonlymphocytic leukemia (ANLL) after lymphoma*

First author, yr	No. of lymphoma patients	Type of treatment for lymphoma	No. of ANLL	Risk (95% confidence interval or *p* value)
Gomez et al., 1982	41	Total-lymphoid irradiation	1	O/E, 162 (n/a)
	40	Total-lymphoid irradiation, carmustine, mechlorethamine, cyclophosphamide, vincristine	4	O/E, 1,082 (n/a)
	81	All treatments	5	O/E, 341 (*p* <.001)
Greene et al., 1983	517	Varied: involved or extended-field radiotherapy, total-nodal irradiation, total-body irradiation, or hemi-body irradiation, chemotherapy (frequently cyclophosphamide)	9	O/E, 105 (48–199)
Pedersen-Bjergaard et al., 1985	498	Alkylating agents, usually long-term cyclophosphamide	9	O/E, 76 (n/a)
Lavey et al., 1990	322	Chemotherapy	5	RR, 10.6 (3.4–24.8)
	72	Radiotherapy	0	RR, 0 (0–183)
	292	Combined modality therapy	4	RR ,11.9 (3.2–30.6)
Lishner et al., 1991	3,021	Varied: radiotherapy, chemotherapy, or both	8	RR, 6.9 (2.9–13.1)
Travis et al., 1994[a]	11,386	Prednimustine	4	RR, 13.4 (1.1–156)
		Mechlorethamine/procarbazine	4	RR, 12.6 (2.0–79)
		Cyclophosphamide	11	RR, 1.8 (0.7–4.9)
		Chlorambucil	6	RR, 2.4 (0.7–8.6)
		Radiotherapy, high-dose	6	RR, 3.1 (0.7–13.7)

n/a, not available; O/E, observed to expected ratio; RR, relative risk.

[a]Case-control study: referent group for calculation of relative risks associated with alkylating agents consisted of patients not given these drugs. Referent group for high-dose radiotherapy group (defined by median cumulative dose to bone marrow or 6.35 Gy) consisted of patients who received no radiation or low-dose radiation (<6.35 Gy).

From Travis LB, Weeks J, Curtis RE, et al. Leukemia following total body irradiation and chemotherapy for non-Hodgkin's lymphoma. *J Clin Oncol* 1996;14:565–571, with permission of Lippincott Williams & Wilkins.

hydration, were undertaken. Although lymphoma patients today are unlikely to receive the high cumulative doses of cyclophosphamide administered from the mid-1960s to early 1980s, the large spectrum of doses in the above investigation permitted an evaluation of the risk of bladder cancer across a wide range of amounts. The strong dose-response relation and high absolute risk of bladder cancer show that it is important to restrict the total amount of cyclophosphamide to that which is necessary to reach therapeutic endpoints, especially for patients with nonneoplastic conditions who may receive total amounts of more than 200 g during long-term therapy (40). Bladder cancer is known to be induced by radiation with a dose-dependent response (41), and the magnitude of the risk after radiotherapy for lymphoma is consistent with excesses reported in other populations exposed to comparable doses. Neither radiotherapy nor cyclophosphamide-based chemotherapy was associated with excess renal cancers in the above investigation (18), and the kidney is generally not regarded as a radiogenic site (41). In a separate study of archived bladder cancer tissue derived from the above investigation, Khan and colleagues (42) showed that the TP53 mutational spectrum of cyclophosphamide-associated tumors appeared to differ significantly from patterns reported for sporadic, smoking-related, and schistosomiasis-linked bladder cancers but not arylamine-associated cancers (43).

Therapy-Related Acute Leukemia

Treatment-related acute myelogenous leukemia represents one of the most feared complications of cancer therapy, given the extraordinarily poor survival associated with this diagnosis (44). A number of studies have provided global estimates of the risk of leukemia after lymphoma, with relative risks ranging from 1 to 1,000 based on small numbers of patients (32,35,36). Few series have quantified the risk of acute myelogenous leukemia in relation to specific lymphoma treatments (33,34,37). Major analytic studies of acute myelogenous leukemia after lymphoma are summarized in Table 33.3; in view of the possible misclassification between leukemic progressions of lymphoma and acute myelogenous leukemia, histopathologic confirmation of leukemia diagnosis has comprised an integral part of most series.

In the largest analytic study to date (37), 35 cases of acute myelogenous leukemia or myelodysplastic syndrome were identified among a cohort of 11,386 2-year survivors of lymphoma (1965 to 1989). For all reported cases, an independent evaluation of all available peripheral blood smears, bone marrow aspirates and biopsies, or accompanying reports was undertaken to ensure that the disorders did not represent leukemic progressions of lymphoma. For all confirmed leukemia cases and matched controls, detailed information on all chemotherapeutic drugs and radiotherapy was collected. Cyclophosphamide-based regimens (median cumulative dose, 12.5 g) were associated with a nonsignificant 1.8-fold risk of acute myelogenous leukemia, compared with treatments that did not include alkylating agents. Increasing cumulative dose or duration of treatment with cyclophosphamide was not associated with increasing risk of acute myelogenous leukemia (p trend = .57 and .33, respectively). Substantially larger risks (relative risk, 105 and 76, respectively) of secondary leukemia were reported in other investigations of lymphoma patients based on small numbers (nine cases each) (33,34). The weak association between small cumulative doses of cyclophosphamide and acute myelogenous leukemia (37) is consistent with the results of other studies (12,24,45) and is reassuring, given the frequent use of this alkylating agent in current treatment regimens for lymphoma. In terms of absolute risk, Travis et al. (37) estimated that among 10,000 lymphoma patients treated for 6 months with chemotherapy regimens containing low cumulative doses of cyclophosphamide and followed for 10 years, an excess of four cases of acute myelogenous leukemias might occur.

For lymphoma patients treated with chlorambucil in the above study (37), elevated risks of leukemia were limited to those who received cumulative doses greater than 1,300 mg (relative risk = 6.5) or who were treated for more than 13 months (relative risk = 8.3). Significantly increased risks of leukemia also followed treatment with prednimustine (relative risk = 13.4), the prednisolone ester of chlorambucil. Risk increased with increasing cumulative dose or increasing duration of therapy of prednimustine (p trend for each < .05); a 23-fold risk of leukemia was evident among patients who received the highest doses. Combination chemotherapy regimens that included mechlorethamine and procarbazine were also associated with significantly increased 13-fold risks of leukemia. Overall, leukemia excesses after alkylating-agent therapy did not differ significantly by age at lymphoma diagnosis when assessed by multivariate statistical methods; risks for patients aged 60 years or older, 50 to 59 years, or younger than 50 years were 3.6, 1.8, and 2.7, respectively. Risk of leukemia after alkylating-agent therapy did not differ by sex or stage of lymphoma. Treatment with epipodophyllotoxins (ten patients), doxorubicin (37 patients), or bleomycin (ten patients) was not associated with increased leukemia risk when the effects of alkylating agents were taken into account. These chemotherapeutic drugs, however, were typically not administered without alkylating agents.

The risk of leukemia among patients treated for lymphoma with radiotherapy without alkylating agents was calculated by classifying subjects into two categories based on the median radiation dose received by active bone marrow among controls. The risk of leukemia among patients who received a radiation dose of 6.35 Gy or more to active bone marrow (6 cases, 22 controls) was 3.1 (p = .13), compared with patients receiving lower doses or no radiation (three cases, 41 controls). The extent of irradiation (i.e., percentage of exposed bone marrow) did not affect leukemia risk when

adjusted for radiation dose. Excesses of leukemia after combined modality therapy were similar to risks observed among patients treated with alkylating agents alone when adjusted for drug dose and type.

Although low-dose total-body irradiation was used in past therapeutic approaches to lymphoma, few studies have evaluated the associated risk of second cancers (38,46). In this unique treatment modality, low individual total-body irradiation fraction sizes (most commonly 10 to 15 cGy) were administered several times a week until a total dose of approximately 150 cGy was given (38). Larger cumulative doses of total-body irradiation (e.g., 1,000 cGy) are used in some conditioning regimens before bone marrow transplantation (9). In a collaborative study between the National Cancer Institute and the Harvard Joint Center for Radiation Therapy (38), a cohort of 61 2-year lymphoma survivors who were given low-dose total-body irradiation as primary therapy was identified. Patients were followed for an average of 9.7 years (median, 8.6; range, 2.0 to 21.7 years) after lymphoma diagnosis. Subsequent courses of therapy included radiotherapy (12 patients), alkylating agents (six patients), or both (35 patients). Eight patients were subsequently diagnosed with solid tumors (observed to expected ratio = 2.0; 95% confidence interval, 0.9 to 4.0). Acute myelogenous leukemia developed in four patients at a median of 9.1 years after lymphoma diagnosis (range, 2.6 to 13.1 years; observed to expected ratio = 117, compared with population rates; 95% confidence interval, 31.5 to 300). Myelodysplastic syndrome developed in a fifth patient. All lymphoma patients in whom secondary myelodysplastic syndrome/acute myelogenous leukemia were diagnosed had received salvage treatment with alkylating-agent chemotherapy, either alone or in combination with radiotherapy. The cumulative risks for secondary acute myelogenous leukemia or all second cancers taken together were 17% and 37%, respectively, 15 years after initial treatment. The authors observed that the risk of acute myelogenous leukemia after primary therapy for lymphoma with low-dose total-body irradiation was considerably larger than risks observed in an international investigation of lymphoma patients (37), although comparable chemotherapy regimens were administered. High-dose, extended-field radiotherapy in combination with alkylating-agent chemotherapy for lymphoma has also been followed by exceptionally high risks (100- to 1,000-fold) of acute myelogenous leukemia (32,33). Results of preclinical investigations suggest that low-dose total-body irradiation may increase the number of bone marrow stem cells susceptible to potential transformation by alkylating agents (47). Thus, it is likely that salvage alkylating-agent chemotherapy for lymphoma contributed to the exceptionally high risks of leukemia after low-dose total-body irradiation through a direct carcinogenic influence or by potentiating the effect of radiotherapy.

The results of numerous investigations indicate that autologous bone marrow transplantation for lymphoma is followed by increased risks of secondary myelodysplastic syndrome/acute myelogenous leukemia (9,48–53). Based on follow-up of a large cohort, Friedberg et al. (54) reported that the actuarial risk of myelodysplastic syndrome/acute myelogenous leukemia at 10 years was approximately 20%, with no evidence of a plateau. Differentiation of the influence of previous treatments for lymphoma from the contribution of the preparative regimen for transplantation in the development of leukemia is difficult because most patients tend to be intensively treated before autologous bone marrow transplantation (48,49). Moreover, many of these treatments are known to confer an increased risk of leukemia (37), and several investigators have found chromosomal abnormalities associated with myelodysplastic syndrome/acute myelogenous leukemia in pretransplant specimens (55–57). Traweek et al. (58) pointed out that although prior therapy for lymphoma may play a pivotal role in the development of secondary leukemia, an additional role for the transplantation procedure cannot be discounted.

Radioimmunotherapy is an effective treatment modality for selected B-cell lymphomas (59), with iodine-131 (^{131}I) and yttrium-90 the most commonly used isotopes. In one series of 60 lymphoma patients treated with ^{131}I tositumomab, four secondary myelodysplastic syndromes were reported (median latency, 35.5 months) (60). Because all patients had previously been intensively treated with chemotherapy, it was not possible to attribute the development of the myelodysplastic syndrome to any particular therapeutic modality; the major acute toxicity of ^{131}I tositumomab in this study, however, was hematologic. It is of interest that van Leeuwen and colleagues (61) previously showed that the degree of thrombocytopenia after alkylating-agent chemotherapy for Hodgkin's disease was a significant predictor of secondary leukemia risk, even when adjusted for cumulative dose of mechlorethamine, the administration of other alkylating agents, and the number of chemotherapy episodes. Thus, in some settings, acute organ toxicity might be a predictor of late effects. Clearly, further follow-up of lymphoma patients treated with radioimmunotherapy is required to accurately assess the incidence of any late complications.

Lung Cancer

According to some reports (27,37), but not others (28,29), patients with lymphoma experience significantly increased risks of lung cancer. To our knowledge, analytic studies in which excess lung cancers are examined in relation to prior treatment for lymphoma have not been conducted, in contrast to several such investigations of Hodgkin's disease patients (26,62–64). Given the overlap in treatment regimens for Hodgkin's disease and lymphoma, it is noteworthy that in the most recent investigation (26), alkylating-agent chemotherapy for Hodgkin's disease was associated with a significantly increased 4.2-fold risk of lung cancer. Risk after 1 to 4, 5 to 8, or 9 or more cycles was 4.0, 6.2 and 13.0, respectively (p trend < .001). After treatment that included

MOPP [mechlorethamine, Oncovin (vincristine), procarbazine, prednisone], lung cancer risk increased with increasing cumulative dose of mechlorethamine and procarbazine (p < .001) when assessed separately. Treatment with other alkylating agents (i.e., non-MOPP) was associated with significantly increased sixfold risks of lung cancer (relative risk, 6.3; 95% confidence interval, 2.5 to 17.7). A large number of Hodgkin's disease patients had also received mantle radiotherapy, which can also be used to treat lymphoma. Radiotherapy that resulted in a dose of at least 5 Gy to the area of the lung in which cancer subsequently developed was associated with a 5.9-fold risk (95% confidence interval, 2.7 to 13.5) of lung cancer that increased with increasing dose (p trend < .001). The risk of lung cancer after therapy with both alkylating agents and radiotherapy was as expected if individual excess relative risks were added together (relative risk = 8.0; 95% confidence interval, 3.6 to 18.5). Smoking was associated with a 20-fold risk of lung cancer and appeared to multiply treatment-associated risks. Whether findings in patients with Hodgkin's disease, however, can be applied to lymphoma patients is not clear, given the specific immune defects associated with Hodgkin's disease (65) and the high prevalence of tobacco use in the aforementioned investigation (26). Studies in laboratory animals indicate that mechlorethamine and procarbazine cause lung cancer (66), and mechlorethamine is structurally similar to sulfur mustard, a known human lung carcinogen (67). It is noteworthy that increased risks for lung cancer have also been observed after treatment for chronic lymphocytic leukemia (68).

Other Sites

Elevated risks for malignant melanoma have been observed in patients with lymphoma (6,27,28) as well as in those with other lymphopoietic malignancies, such as Hodgkin's disease (16,17) and chronic lymphocytic leukemia (68). A significantly increased reciprocal risk (1.3-fold) of lymphoma is also evident among malignant melanoma patients reported to the SEER Program (1973 to 1988) (30), an observation that is consistent with a role of shared etiologic influences. Subsequent excesses of malignant melanoma are likely related to the immunologic defects associated with various lymphopoietic cancers, including lymphoma (see Chapter 45), although diagnostic surveillance may also play a role.

Significantly elevated risks of Hodgkin's disease after non-Hodgkin's lymphoma have been reported in several investigations (6,27,29), but not others (28). Because diagnostic misclassification may influence risk, in one population-based survey (27), all pathologic materials were requested for 14 patients in whom Hodgkin's disease was reported after non-Hodgkin's lymphoma. For 11 of 12 cases, archived material for both sets of diagnoses was available; independent pathologic review confirmed diagnoses of both non-Hodgkin's lymphoma and subsequent Hodgkin's disease in nine patients (observed to expected ratio = 2.68; 95% confidence interval, 1.22 to 5.09) (69). In a separate study, Zarate-Osorno et al. (70) provided clinicopathologic descriptions of nine patients with Hodgkin's disease after non-Hodgkin's lymphoma. The relation between non-Hodgkin's lymphoma and Hodgkin's disease is discussed in Chapter 6.

CLINICAL IMPLICATIONS (RECOMMENDATIONS FOR SCREENING/TREATMENT)

Although lymphoma patients experience significantly elevated risks for therapy-related leukemia and several solid tumors, the second-cancer burden is substantially less than for patients with Hodgkin's disease. Increased risks for acute myelogenous leukemia and bladder cancer have been related to treatment for lymphoma, although analytic studies have not yet examined the association of other excess cancers with prior therapies. The findings summarized in this chapter have numerous clinical implications, including the need for close surveillance of lymphoma patients and recommendations directed at avoidance of other carcinogenic exposures, especially smoking and ultraviolet light. Second cancers are frequently viewed as a problem of success (71); thus, the issue of treatment-induced cancers must always be considered in relation to the marked improvements in survival rates for lymphoma patients. Clinical trials should continue to develop therapeutic regimens that have less carcinogenic potential and also should follow patients long term so that treatment efficacy can be accurately weighed against late effects. In the interim, arbitrary modification of highly successful lymphoma treatments to decrease second-cancer risk is unwarranted. For newer therapies to treat lymphoma (59), late sequelae have not yet been fully characterized, and patients should continue to be followed for long periods. Whenever feasible, future investigations of second-cancer risk should include studies at the molecular level (72–77). Data derived from laboratory analyses may help elucidate the effect of genetic susceptibility on therapy-related second-cancer risk and advance our knowledge of the underlying mechanisms of drug- and radiation-related carcinogenesis.

REFERENCES

1. Ries LAG, Eisner MP, Kosary CL, et al. SEER cancer statistics review, 1973–1997. NIH Pub. No. 00-2789. Bethesda, MD: National Cancer Institute, 2000.
2. Van Leeuwen FE, Travis LB. "Second cancers." In: Devita VT, et al., eds. Cancer: principles and practice of oncology, 6th ed. Philadelphia: Lippincott Williams & Wilkins, 2001:2939–2964.
3. Hoppe RT. Hodgkin's disease: complications of therapy and excess mortality. Ann Oncol 1997;8:115–118.
4. Kyle RA, Pierre RV, Bayrd ED. Multiple myeloma and acute myelomonocytic leukemia. N Engl J Med 1970;283:1121–1125.
5. Makuch R, Simon R. Recommendations for the analysis of the effect of treatment on the development of second malignancies. Cancer 1979;44:250–253.
6. Travis LB, Curtis RE, Glimelius B, et al. Second cancer among long-term survivors of non-Hodgkin's lymphoma. J Natl Cancer Inst 1993;85:1932–1937.
7. Kaplan EL, Meier P. Non-parametric estimation from incomplete observations. J Am Stat Assoc 1958;53:457–481.
8. Pepe MS, Mori M. Kaplan-Meier, marginal or conditional probability curves in summarizing competing risks failure time data? Stat Med 1993;12:737–751.
9. Darrington DL, Vose JM, Anderson JR, et al. Incidence and characterization of secondary myelodysplastic syndrome and acute myelogenous leukemia following high-dose chemoradiotherapy and autologous stem-cell transplantation for lymphoid malignancies. J Clin Oncol 1994;12:2527–2534.
10. Kaldor JM, Day NE, Shiboski S. Epidemiological studies of anticancer drug carcinogenicity. IARC Sci Publ 1986;78:189–201.
11. Boice JD Jr, Day NE, Andersen A, et al. Second cancers following radiation treatment for cervical cancer. An international collaboration among cancer registries. J Natl Cancer Inst 1985;74:955–975.
12. Kaldor JM, Day NE, Pettersson F, et al. Leukemia following chemotherapy for ovarian cancer. N Engl J Med 1990;322:1–6.
13. Storm HH, Prener A. Second cancer following lymphatic and hematopoietic cancers in Denmark, 1943–80. Natl Cancer Inst Monogr 1985;68:389–409.
14. Greene MH. Is cisplatin a human carcinogen? [Review]. J Natl Cancer Inst 1992;84:306–312.
15. Coleman CN, Williams CJ, Flint A, et al. Hematologic neoplasia in patients treated for Hodgkin's disease. N Engl J Med 1977;297:1249–1252.
16. Tucker MA, Coleman CN, Cox RS, et al. Risk of second cancers after treatment for Hodgkin's disease. N Engl J Med 1988;318:76–81.
17. Van Leeuwen FE, Klokman WJ, Hagenbeek A, et al. Second cancer risk following Hodgkin's disease: a 20-year follow-up study. J Clin Oncol 1994;12:312–325.
18. Travis LB, Curtis RE, Holowaty EJ, et al. Bladder and kidney cancer following cyclophosphamide therapy for non-Hodgkin's lymphoma. J Natl Cancer Inst 1995;87:524–530.
19. Boice JD Jr, Blettner M, Kleinerman RA, et al. Radiation dose and leukemia risk in patients treated for cancer of the cervix. J Natl Cancer Inst 1987;79:1295–1311.
20. Tucker MA, D'Angio GJ, Boice JD Jr, et al. Bone sarcomas linked to radiotherapy and chemotherapy in children. N Engl J Med 1987;317:588–593.
21. Tucker MA, Meadows AT, Boice JD Jr, et al. Leukemia after therapy with alkylating agents for childhood cancer. J Natl Cancer Inst 1987;78:459–464.
22. Kaldor JM, Day NE, Clarke EA, et al. Leukemia following Hodgkin's disease [see comments]. N Engl J Med 1990;322:7–13.
23. Boice JD Jr, Harvey EB, Blettner M, et al. Cancer in the contralateral breast after radiotherapy for breast cancer. N Engl J Med 1992;326:781–785.
24. Curtis RE, Boice JD Jr, Stovall M, et al. Risk of leukemia after chemotherapy and radiation treatment for breast cancer. N Engl J Med 1992;326:1745–1751.
25. Travis LB, Holowaty E, Hall P, et al. Risk of leukemia following platinum-based chemotherapy for ovarian cancer. N Engl J Med 1999;340:351–357.
26. Travis LB, Gospodarowicz M, Curtis RE, et al. Lung cancer following chemotherapy and radiotherapy for Hodgkin's disease. J Natl Cancer Inst 2002;94:182–192.
27. Travis LB, Curtis RE, Boice JD Jr, et al. Second cancers following non-Hodgkin's lymphoma. Cancer 1991;67:2002–2009.
28. Brennan P, Coates M, Armstrong B, et al. Second primary neoplasms following non-Hodgkin's lymphoma in New South Wales, Australia. Br J Cancer 2000;82:1344–1347.
29. Dong C, Hemminki K. Second primary neoplasms among 53,159 haematolymphoproliferative malignancy patients in Sweden, 1958–1996: a search for common mechanisms. Br J Cancer 2001;85:997–1005.
30. Dores G, Cote T, Travis L. Second cancers following Hodgkin's disease, non-Hodgkin's lymphoma, and multiple myeloma (in preparation).
31. Pedersen-Bjergaard J, Ersboll J, Hansen VL, et al. Carcinoma of the urinary bladder after treatment with cyclophosphamide for non-Hodgkin's lymphoma. N Engl J Med 1988;318:1028–1032.
32. Gomez GA, Aggarwal KK, Han T. Post-therapeutic acute malignant myeloproliferative syndrome and acute nonlymphocytic leukemia in non-Hodgkin's lymphoma. Cancer 1982;50:2285–2288.

33. Greene MH, Young RC, Merrill JM, DeVita VT. Evidence of a treatment dose response in acute nonlymphocytic leukemias which occur after therapy of non-Hodgkin's lymphoma. *Cancer Res* 1983;43:1891–1898.

34. Pedersen-Bjergaard J, Ersboll J, Sorensen HM, et al. Risk of acute nonlymphocytic leukemia and preleukemia in patients treated with cyclophosphamide for non-Hodgkin's lymphomas. Comparison with results obtained in patients treated for Hodgkin's disease and ovarian carcinoma with other alkylating agents. *Ann Intern Med* 1985;103:195–200.

35. Lavey RS, Eby NL, Prosnitz LR. Impact on second malignancy risk of the combined use of radiation and chemotherapy for lymphomas. *Cancer* 1990;66:80–88.

36. Lishner M, Slingerland J, Barr J, et al. Second malignant neoplasms in patients with non Hodgkin's lymphoma. *Hematol Oncol* 1991;9:169–179.

37. Travis LB, Curtis RE, Stovall M, et al. Risk of leukemia following treatment for non-Hodgkin's lymphoma. *J Natl Cancer Inst* 1994;86:1450–1457.

38. Travis LB, Weeks J, Curtis RE, et al. Leukemia following low-dose total body irradiation and chemotherapy for non-Hodgkin's lymphoma. *J Clin Oncol* 1996;14:565–571.

39. DeVries CR, Freiha FS. Hemorrhagic cystitis; a review. *J Urol* 1990;143:1–7.

40. Hoffman GS, Kerr GS, Leavitt RY, et al. Wegener granulomatosis: an analysis of 158 patients. *Ann Intern Med* 1992;116:488–498.

41. United Nations Scientific Committee on the Effects of Atomic Radiation. Report to General Assembly, with Scientific Annexes, Sources and Effects of Ionizing Radiation. UNSCEAR. New York: United Nations, 2000.

42. Khan MA, Travis LB, Lynch CF, et al. P53 mutations in cyclophosphamide-associated bladder cancer. *Cancer Epidemiol Biomarkers Prev* 1998;7:397–403.

43. Taylor JA, Li Y, He M, et al. p53 mutations in bladder tumors from arylamine-exposed workers. *Cancer Res* 1996;56:294–298.

44. Neugut AI, Robinson E, Nieves J, et al. Poor survival of treatment-related acute nonlymphocytic leukemia. *JAMA* 1990;264:1006–1008.

45. Greene MH, Harris EL, Gershenson DM, et al. Melphalan may be a more potent leukemogen than cyclophosphamide. *Ann Intern Med* 1986;105:360–367.

46. Mendenhall NP, Noyes WD, Million RR. Total body irradiation for stage II-IV non-Hodgkin's lymphoma: ten-year follow-up. *J Clin Oncol* 1989;7:67–74.

47. Rubin P, Constine LS 3rd, Scarantino CW. The paradoxes in patterns and mechanism of bone marrow regeneration after irradiation. 2. Total body irradiation. *Radiother Oncol* 1984;2:227–233.

48. Miller JS, Arthur DC, Litz CE, et al. Myelodysplastic syndrome after autologous bone marrow transplantation: an additional late complication of curative cancer therapy. *Blood* 1994;83:3780–3786.

49. Stone RM, Neuberg D, Soiffer R, et al. Myelodysplastic syndrome as a late complication following autologous bone marrow transplantation for non-Hodgkin's lymphoma. *J Clin Oncol* 1994;12:2535–2542.

50. Pedersen-Bjergaard J, Pedersen M, Myhre J, et al. High risk of therapy-related leukemia after BEAM chemotherapy and autologous stem cell transplantation for previously treated lymphomas is mainly related to primary chemotherapy and not to the BEAM-transplantation procedure. *Leukemia* 1997;11:1654–1660.

51. Milligan DW, Ruiz De Elvira MC, Kolb HJ, et al. Secondary leukaemia and myelodysplasia after autografting for lymphoma: results from the EBMT (European Group for Blood and Marrow Transplantation). *Br J Haematol* 1999;106:1020–1026.

52. Micallef INM, Lillington DM, Apostolidis J, et al. Therapy-related myelodysplasia and secondary acute myelogenous leukemia after high-dose therapy with autologous hematopoietic progenitor-cell support for lymphoid malignancies. *J Clin Oncol* 2000;18:947–955.

53. Krishnan A, Bhatia S, Slovak ML, et al. Predictors of therapy-related leukemia and myelodysplasia following autologous transplantation for lymphoma: an assessment of risk factors. *Blood* 2000;95:1588–1593.

54. Friedberg JW, Neuberg D, Stone RM, et al. Outcome in patients with myelodysplastic syndrome after autologous bone marrow transplantation for non-Hodgkin's lymphoma. *J Clin Oncol* 1999;17:3128–3135.

55. Mach-Pascual S, Legare RD, Lu D, et al. Predictive value of clonality assays in patients with non-Hodgkin's lymphoma undergoing autologous bone marrow transplant: a single-institution study. *Blood* 1998;91:4496–4503.

56. Abruzzese E, Radford JE, Miller JS, et al. Detection of abnormal pretransplant clones in progenitor cells of patients who developed myelodysplasia after autologous transplantation. *Blood* 1999;94:1814–1819.

57. Lillington DM, Micallef INM, Carpenter E, et al. Detection of chromosome abnormalities pre-high-dose treatment in patients developing therapy-related myelodysplasia and second acute myelogenous leukemia after treatment for non-Hodgkin's lymphoma. *J Clin Oncol* 2001;19:2472–2481.

58. Traweek ST, Slovak ML, Nademanee AP, et al. Myelodysplasia and acute myeloid leukemia occurring after autologous bone marrow transplantation for lymphoma [Review]. *Leuk Lymphoma* 1996;20:365–372.

59. Press OW, Rasey J. Principles of radioimmunotherapy for hematologists and oncologists. *Semin Oncol* 2000;27:62–73.

60. Kaminski MS, Zelenetz AD, Press OW, et al. Pivotal study of iodine I 131 tositumomab for chemotherapy-refractory low-grade or transformed low-grade B-cell non-Hodgkin's lymphomas. *J Clin Oncol* 2001;19:3918–3928.

61. van Leeuwen FE, Chorus AMJ, van den Belt-Dusebout AW, et al. Leukemia risk following Hodgkin's disease: relation to cumulative dose of alkylating agents, treatment with teniposide combinations, number of episodes of chemotherapy, and bone marrow damage. *J Clin Oncol* 1994;12:1063–1073.

62. Kaldor JM, Day NE, Bell J, et al. Lung cancer following Hodgkin's disease: a case-control study. *Int J Cancer* 1992;52:677–682.

63. Van Leeuwen FE, Klokman WJ, Stovall M, et al. Roles of radiotherapy and smoking in lung cancer following Hodgkin's disease. *J Natl Cancer Inst* 1995;87:1530–1537.

64. Swerdlow AJ, Schoemaker MJ, Allerton R, et al. Lung cancer after Hodgkin's disease: a nested case-control study of the relation to treatment. *J Clin Oncol* 2001;19:1610–1618.

65. Mauch PM, Armitage JO, Diehl V, et al, eds. *Hodgkin's disease*. Philadelphia: Lippincott Williams & Wilkins, 1999.

66. World Health Organization, International Agency for Research on Cancer. *IARC monographs on the evaluation of carcinogenic risks to humans, overall evaluation of carcinogenicity: an updating of IARC monographs* (vol. 1–42). Lyon, France, 1987.

67. Blair A, Kazerouni N. Reactive chemicals and cancer. *Cancer Causes Control* 1997;8:473–490.

68. Travis LB, Curtis RE, Hankey BF, et al. Second cancers in patients with chronic lymphocytic leukemia. *J Natl Cancer Inst* 1992;84:1422–1427.

69. Travis LB, Gonzalez CL, Hankey BF, Jaffe ES. Hodgkin's disease following non-Hodgkin's lymphoma. *Cancer* 1992;69:2337–2342.

70. Zarate-Osorno A, Medeiros LJ, Kingma DW, et al. Hodgkin's disease following non-Hodgkin's lymphoma. A clinicopathologic and immunophenotypic study of nine cases. *Am J Surg Pathol* 1993;17:123–132.

71. Boice JD Jr, Travis LB. Late effects of cancer therapy (editorial). *J Natl Cancer Inst* 1995;87:705–706.

72. Felix CA. Chemotherapy-related second cancers. In: Neugut AI, Meadows AT, Robinson E, eds. *Multiple primary cancers*. Philadelphia: Lippincott Williams & Wilkins, 1999.

73. Berwick M, Vineis P. Markers of DNA repair and susceptibility to cancer in humans: an epidemiologic review. *J Natl Cancer Inst* 2000;92:874–897.

74. Liotta L, Petricoin E. Molecular profiling of human cancer. *Nat Rev Genet* 2000;1:48–56.

75. Daly MJ, Rioux JD, Schaffner SE, et al. High-resolution haplotype structure in the human genome. *Nature Genet* 2001;29:229–232.

76. Liotta LA, Kohn EC, Petricoin EF. Clinical proteomics. Personalized molecular medicine. *J Am Med Assoc* 2001;286:2211–2214.

77. Patil N, Berno AJ, Hinds DA, et al. Blocks of limited haplotype diversity revealed by high-resolution scanning of human chromosome 21. *Science* 2001;249:1719–1723.

CHAPTER 34

Late Effects of Treatment after Lymphoma

Marc P. E. André

Because of the increasing incidence of non-Hodgkin's lymphoma over the past two decades and improvements in curing this disease, long-term survivors should be observed for late toxicities. The relative contribution of the treatment modalities to the development of these toxicities may be approached in an attempt to improve the quality of life of long-term survivors. Second cancer is the most devastating toxicity of treatments and is reviewed in the previous section of this book. This chapter is dedicated to nonneoplastic toxicities. Late effects that are reviewed in this section include toxicities that occurred after treatment was completed, as well as toxicities that occurred during therapy and continued after therapy was completed.

CARDIAC TOXICITY

For frequently used chemotherapy, such as anthracyclines, the risk of acute cardiovascular toxicity has been extensively evaluated and is well known (Table 34.1) (1). Long-term effects on survivors of childhood cancer treated with anthracycline-based chemotherapy regimens or of Hodgkin's disease treated with radiotherapy (2) have made oncologists aware that cardiovascular damage can manifest many years after the end of treatment (3). Today, the evaluation of long-term cardiovascular complications is of growing importance for adults and also for elderly patients who might expect cure with the currently available treatments. The study of long-term cardiac complications in the population between 40 and 60 years of age is more complicated, because the risk of cardiovascular disease increases above the age of 50 years. Therefore, it is more difficult to establish whether the cardiovascular morbidity occurring during the follow-up period is the result of chemotherapy or the consequence of aging. Compared to the multitude of studies on long-term consequences of treatments in the Hodgkin's disease survivor, the literature on non-Hodgkin's lymphoma is limited.

Radiation-Associated Cardiac Toxicity

Most of the data in the literature on radiotherapy late effects come from observation of Hodgkin's disease survivors, most

of whom received mediastinal irradiation. Pericarditis was an important complication in the 1960s and 1970s, but this complication has virtually vanished with new treatment approaches.

An association between coronary artery disease and irradiation was first reported in the late 1960s (4). The association between age at treatment and dose of radiotherapy in relation to risk remains uncertain, and conflicting results are reported in the literature (5,6) depending on treatment techniques, use of chemotherapy, and duration of observation.

So far, there is no evidence of a synergy between radiotherapy and chemotherapy—the combination increases neither the coronary risk associated with radiotherapy, nor the chronic heart failure associated with chemotherapy.

Chemotherapy-Associated Cardiac Toxicity

For patients with advanced intermediate-grade or high-grade lymphoma, the cyclophosphamide, doxorubicin, vincristine, and prednisone regimen (CHOP) is considered the standard treatment and has been recently shown to improve the cure rate when combined with rituximab (7,8). However, various other standard or high-dose chemotherapy regimens are used after relapse or progression and might contain drugs with potential cardiac toxic effects, such as high-dose ifosfamide, paclitaxel, or vinca alkaloids.

Acute Cardiovascular Toxicity

Myocardial Toxicity

Although the initial anthracycline-induced damage to the myocyte occurs shortly after its administration, overt heart failure presents weeks, months, or years after chemotherapy. Acute cardiotoxic effects that can occur during or shortly (i.e., within hours) after administration of anthracyclines include electrocardiographic changes and rhythm disturbances (9). These changes appear to be of minor clinical relevance, as they rarely happen with current treatment regimens and do not predict chronic cardiac toxicity (10).

TABLE 34.1. *Cardiac toxicities associated with the treatment of lymphoma*

Type of treatment	Effects	References
Radiotherapy	Increases coronary risk	4
Chemotherapy	Acute	
	Myocardiotoxicity (anthracycline)	13–16,18,19
	Cardiovascular (vinca alkaloids)	20,21
	Other vascular effects (bleomycin)	22
	Late	
	Myocardiotoxicity	25–27
	Coronary vasculature	28,29
	Pulmonary vasculature	30
Interferon	Hypotension, arrhythmia, myocardial infarction, congestive cardiomyopathy	31–35
High-dose chemotherapy	Acute cardiomyopathy related to cyclophosphamide	36–37
	Late cardiomyopathy: infrequent	27

The other agent that can cause acute cardiotoxicity is cyclophosphamide, which is mainly cardiotoxic at higher doses, such as those used before stem cell transplantation. The reported cardiotoxicity ranges from transient electrocardiographic changes to more severe cardiotoxicity, such as exudative pericardial effusion, ventricular hypertrophy, and fatal myocardial necrosis (11,12). The onset of the latter type of cardiac toxicity is acute, with death within 15 days. The cardiotoxic effect of cyclophosphamide may be potentiated by anthracycline administration (13). In 2000, Brockstein et al. evaluated the risk factors in patients receiving high-dose cyclophosphamide before stem cell transplantation. In this series of 138 patients, they showed in a multivariate analysis that lymphoma (as opposed to breast cancer) and older age were the risk factors associated with cardiac toxicity. History of an abnormal ejection fraction and higher doses of anthracyclines before high-dose chemotherapy may also contribute to the cardiac toxicity (14). The authors concluded that patients who are seemingly poor cardiac risks may fare well with high-dose chemotherapy if carefully selected with the aid of a thorough cardiac evaluation.

Another agent that can cause cardiac toxicity is high-dose ifosfamide. In one study, cardiac arrhythmias were observed (15). In another study by Quezado et al. in 1993, high-dose ifosfamide was associated with severe but usually reversible myocardial depression and malignant arrhythmias (16). Given the close chemical resemblance between cyclophosphamide and ifosfamide, it is possible that they induce myocardial depression through a similar mechanism, even if no histopathologic evidence of hemorrhagic myocarditis, the

hallmark of cyclophosphamide cardiomyopathy, could be found (17).

Although high-dose cyclophosphamide or ifosfamide is often used in the setting of autologous stem cell transplantation, cardiac toxicity is infrequent. Hertenstein et al. reported an occurrence of less than 2%. Occurrence of cardiac toxicity was correlated with an echographic reduction in ejection fraction before bone marrow transplantation, but life-threatening cardiac toxicity could not be predicted in individual patients (18).

Other drugs, such as paclitaxel, may be associated with cardiac toxicity. One study of 60 patients treated with a 3-hour infusion of 200 mg per m² did not show any significant cardiac toxicity (19).

Cardiovascular Events

Although rare, patients have been described who developed acute myocardial infarction during or after chemotherapy for lymphomas (20,21). In these reports, the cause of these events was attributed to the administration of vinca alkaloids. The mechanism by which chemotherapy, specifically vinca alkaloids, could cause myocardial infarction remains speculative (21).

Other Vascular Events

There are at least two manifestations of acute vascular toxicity associated with chemotherapy for lymphomas. Bleomycin-containing regimens may induce pneumonitis, which is thought to be a result of damage to endothelium of the lung vasculature. Another manifestation of acute vascular toxicity may be the thromboembolic events that occur during chemotherapy. Clarke et al. evaluated 85 non-Hodgkin's lymphoma patients and found thromboembolic events in 4 of 11 patients who received weekly chemotherapy; this was not the case in patients treated with a less-intensive schedule (22).

Late Cardiovascular Toxicity

Myocardial Toxicity

Of the agents used in the treatment for non-Hodgkin's lymphoma, anthracyclines are the most important in causing direct injury to the heart. The exact mechanism of how anthracyclines affect the myocardium is not fully elucidated, but the formation of free radicals and calcium overload in the myocytes play an important role (23). These processes lead to patchy myocyte damage, leading to intramyocyte vacuolization and eventually myocyte death. As a consequence, cardiomyopathy develops, which can result in congestive heart failure (24). However, because the heart has considerable compensatory reserves, a long time elapses before heart failure manifests, if it does at all. The majority of chronic heart failure occurs within 1 year, and cardiotoxicity increases with the cumulative dose given; however, wide interindividual susceptibility exists. In childhood cancer survivors, incidences of subclinical cardiotoxicity have been reported to increase with the extent of follow-up duration. These figures cannot be reliably extrapolated to adults, but they illustrate that the risk of chronic heart failure continues long after the completion of treatment.

In the study by Miller et al. in 1998, left ventricular dysfunction was found in 7 of 201 patients treated with eight cycles of CHOP (cumulative dose of doxorubicin, 400 mg/m^2), whereas in the group treated with three cycles combined with radiotherapy, none of 200 patients developed left ventricular dysfunction (25). Seven patients treated with eight cycles of CHOP and only two patients treated with three cycles of CHOP and radiotherapy subsequently died of heart disease. In the study by Haddy et al. in 1998, 103 young long-term survivors were observed up to 20 years with a median time to cardiac evaluation of 9.9 years. Left ventricular dysfunction was detected in 8 (14%) of 57 patients who had received cumulative doses of doxorubicin of 200 to 560 mg per m^2. Four were symptomatic, of whom two needed cardiac medication, and four were asymptomatic. Cardiac toxicity was the predominant major late effect observed in this series (26).

Although high-dose cyclophosphamide can cause acute cardiotoxicity, late toxicity in the first year after stem cell transplantation seems exceptional, as was recently described by Ghielmini et al. (27). However, longer follow-up is needed to exclude long-term cardiotoxicity with certainty.

Coronary Vasculature

Mediastinal irradiation is known to affect coronary arteries, but different large series were unable to find an association between chemotherapy and death from myocardial infarction, suggesting that chemotherapy alone was not directly affecting coronary artery disease (28,29). However, because cardiac death was not an end point in these trials, risk of coronary artery disease might be underestimated and therefore not detected.

Pulmonary Vasculature

Several cases of pulmonary veno-occlusive disease have been described after chemotherapy for lymphoma. Although the number of cases is limited in the literature, this might be due to the failure to recognize this complication (30).

Interferon-Associated Cardiac Toxicity

In clinical trials, interferon has demonstrated activity in the treatment of several tumors, including follicular lymphoma (31). Adverse cardiovascular effects due to interferon have been reported infrequently and consist mainly of transient hypotension and tachyarrhythmias that are commonly associated with the initial febrile reaction. More severe adverse cardiac events, including arrhythmia and myocardial infarction, have been reported (32,33). The etiologic role of inter-

feron-α in the development of these adverse cardiac events, however, cannot be firmly established due to the presence of preexisting heart disease or significant previous doxorubicin exposure. The development of congestive cardiomyopathy has also been infrequently described in patients receiving interferon-α (34,35). The cardiomyopathy occurred while receiving interferon and subsequently improved on discontinuation of interferon. The mechanism for the development of this cardiomyopathy remains unclear. In a randomized trial comparing an anthracycline-based chemotherapy with and without interferon, Solal-Celigny did not report any significant increase in cardiac toxicity among follicular lymphoma patients (31).

High-Dose Chemotherapy–Associated Cardiac Toxicity

Cardiac toxicity associated with high-dose chemotherapy and stem cell transplantation has been reported in different series (36–38). In two series, 12% of patients died of cardiac or pulmonary toxicities. Cardiac toxicity is clearly related to the high dose of cyclophosphamide as used in the BEAC regimen [carmustine (BCNU), 300 mg/m^2; VP16, 800 mg/m^2; cytarabine, 800 mg/m^2; and cyclophosphamide, 140 mg/kg] and has not been reported to be significant when cyclophosphamide is replaced by melphalan, such as in the BEAM regimen (BCNU, 300 mg/m^2; VP16, 800 mg/m^2; cytarabine, 800 mg/m^2; melphalan, 140 mg/m^2). In Rapoport's series in 1993 (37), toxicity appeared to be related to the bulk of disease at time of transplant, but for van Besien in 1995 (36), cyclophosphamide-associated cardiac toxicity was unpredictable. It was not related to pretreatment left ventricular ejection fraction or any other pretreatment factors. Cardiac toxicity has been reported most frequently when cyclophosphamide was combined either with BCNU or cytarabine. Carmustine can lead to intracellular glutathione depletion and therefore enhance cardiac toxicity (39). In addition, high-dose nitrosoureas can cause myocardial ischemia, hypotension, tachycardia, myocardial infarction, and even non–Q-wave infarction (40). It is also possible that high-dose cytarabine contributes to the cardiac toxicity of BEAC, as suggested by the absence of cardiac toxicity in cyclophosphamide, BCNU, and etoposide (CBV)-treated Hodgkin's disease patients. Twenty-nine relapsed B-cell lymphoma patients treated with iodine-131–labelled anti-CD20 antibody and autologous stem cell rescue did not show any significant late cardiopulmonary toxicities (41).

Reducing the Risk

Studies evaluating the extent of cardiac toxicity have used various combinations of rest and exercise echocardiography and radionuclide scintigraphy scanning. However, it has become evident that chemotherapy-induced left ventricular dysfunction often occurs without symptoms and that new tools to identify higher-risk patients needing close monitoring or cardiologic treatment are needed. In 2000, Cardinale et al. reported a series of 204 patients treated with high-dose chemotherapy for various tumors, including 46 lymphomas (42). Cardiac troponin, a new specific marker of minor myocardial damage, was measured shortly after high-dose chemotherapy. In the troponin-negative group, left ventricular ejection fraction progressively decreased after the treatment, but this was transient and no longer detectable after later follow-up. In the troponin-positive group, left ventricular ejection depression was more marked and still evident at the end of follow-up. In this group, a close relationship between the short-term troponin increment and the greatest left ventricular ejection fraction reduction was found. All three patients developing symptoms of heart failure and needing treatment were in this group.

In general, efforts should be aimed at reducing all risk factors after treatments of lymphoma patients to reduce potentially fatal cardiac complications. Cessation of cigarette smoking and optimal management of hypertension, lipids, and diabetes are absolutely mandatory.

PULMONARY TOXICITY

Development of pulmonary complications in lymphoma patients is frequent and nonspecific (Table 34.2). Patients with lung damage frequently receive empirical antibiotics and frequently invasive diagnostic procedures to rule out infection before lung toxicity is suspected. Both radiotherapy, including total-body irradiation used before autologous stem cell transplantation, and chemotherapeutic agents (mainly bleomycin, methotrexate, and cyclophosphamide) may induce short- and long-term pulmonary toxicity. Because most patients receive combination chemotherapy, additional or synergistic effects may overlap and make the relative contribution of each different toxic effect difficult to evaluate. The toxic effects of both radiotherapy and mainly bleomycin have been the subject of many publications on Hodgkin's disease because of the use of the ABVD regimen (doxorubicin, bleomycin, vinblastine, and

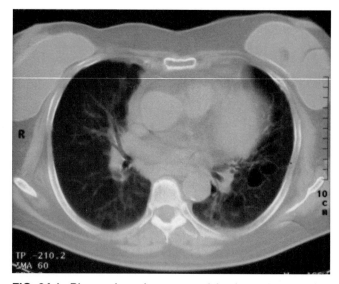

FIG. 34.1. Bleomycin pulmonary toxicity in a 62-year-old patient treated with bleomycin-containing chemotherapy for lymphoma.

dacarbazine) and long-term follow-up of many survivors (43–45). Although not demonstrated, it can be speculated that most of the information obtained in Hodgkin's disease might be translated to non-Hodgkin's lymphoma.

Radiotherapy

Two successive phases of lung damage may occur after radiation therapy of the chest. The first phase is a radiation pneumonitis developing usually within the first 6 months of the radiotherapy and responsible for radiologic changes. The second phase is the progressive development of fibrosis that occurs in the field of radiation therapy. Recent data suggest an activation of inflammatory reaction; mainly, transforming growth factor-β and interleukin-1α, leading to the expression of a cytokine cascade and an overexpression of collagen genes (46). Actually, combination chemotherapy with or without radiotherapy is used because of reported inferior results with radiation alone in clinically staged patients (47,48). In 1996, Lee and Levitt reported a small series of stage I large-cell non-Hodgkin's lymphoma patients treated exclusively with radiotherapy and did not report any significant lung toxicity (49). However, this treatment modality remains infrequently used, and most lung toxicity occurs after combination therapy, leading to difficulty in estimating the contribution of radiotherapy to this toxic effect.

Chemotherapy Toxicity

It is quite well recognized that at a cumulative doses of approximately 400 to 450 mg of bleomycin, the incidence of pulmonary toxicity (e.g., interstitial chronic fibrosis) increases dramatically, reaching approximately 13%. However, the relationship between dose and toxicity is unclear, and severe interstitial pulmonary fibrosis (Fig. 34.1) has been shown to

TABLE 34.2. *Pulmonary toxicities associated with the treatment of lymphoma*

Type of treatment	Effects	References
Radiotherapy	Radiation pneumonitis	46–49
	Progressive fibrosis	
Chemotherapy	Bleomycin toxicity	50
	Methotrexate toxicity	51–52
	Granulocyte colony-stimulating factor: poor evidence of association	53–59
High-dose chemotherapy	BCNU toxicity	63–64
	BCNU + cyclophosphamide toxicity	65–68

BCNU, carmustine.

develop with cumulative doses of less than 50 mg in sensitive patients. Most patients with acute pulmonary damage associated with bleomycin responded favorably to steroids (50).

Methotrexate pneumonitis was described in patients with hematologic and solid tumors. The pathogenesis of the pulmonary injury related to methotrexate is not identified, although some features, such as peripheral eosinophilia, suggest an immune-mediated hypersensitivity mechanism. It is interesting to note that MACOP-B (methotrexate-leucovorin, doxorubicin, cyclophosphamide, vincristine, prednisone, and bleomycin), which contains the same component drugs as m-BACOD (methotrexate, bleomycin, doxorubicin, cyclophosphamide, vincristine, and dexamethasone), has no reported pulmonary toxicity (51). These regimens differ in several ways, including the dosage and schedule of the component drugs and the use of steroids. High doses of steroids are administered throughout the MACOP-B treatment course, and the immunosuppressive and antiinflammatory properties of steroids may suppress methotrexate pneumonitis; short intermittent courses of steroids, such as in m-BACOD, may promote its development. Shapiro et al. compared three different chemotherapy regimens [m-BACOD, m-ACOD (methotrexate, calcium, leucovorin, doxorubicin, cyclophosphamide, vincristine, and dexamethasone), and CHOP] containing the same drugs but differing primarily in the addition of bleomycin and methotrexate. Pulmonary toxicity occurred in 24 of 134 (18%) of the m-BACOD–treated patients and in 6 of 43 (14%) of the m-ACOD–treated patients (p = not significant). None of the CHOP-treated patients had pulmonary toxicity. This suggested that methotrexate may play an important role in the pathogenesis of pulmonary toxicity (52).

Some patients have developed pulmonary toxicity after receiving chemotherapy and granulocyte colony-stimulating factor (G-CSF) (53–56). The G-CSF increases the number and functional properties, such as superoxide production and expression of adhesion-related molecules, of neutrophils. Therefore, it might be speculated that G-CSF has a causal association with the pulmonary toxicity. However, there is no full consensus that G-CSF is involved in the development of pulmonary toxicity (57,58). In one series, Yokose in 1998 retrospectively compared CHOP and CHOP with G-CSF. He reported six patients with pulmonary toxicity out of 52 patients (11.5%) in the G-CSF group and none in the CHOP-alone group (59). The mean peak leukocyte count with each therapy cycle was associated with development of this toxicity. Because the toxicity was associated with a high mean peak leukocyte count and did not recur in readministration of G-CSF, an idiosyncratic reaction to G-CSF is unlikely to be the pathogenesis of this phenomenon. Early use of steroids and lowering the dose of G-CSF seem to be useful in the management of this toxicity. However, the probability of an increase of bleomycin-induced toxicity by G-CSF remains controversial and questionable. Two randomized GELA (Groupe d'Etude des Lymphomes de l'Adulte) trials comparing placebo versus G-CSF after bleomycin-containing chemotherapy did not observe any increase in pulmonary toxicity in 278 patients (57).

High-Dose Chemotherapy–Associated Pulmonary Toxicity

The major risk factor for serious pulmonary toxicity is previous radiation therapy or prior treatment with bleomycin, as indicated by different studies (36,37,59–62). Mild delayed drug toxicity related to carmustine, cyclophosphamide, or previous radiotherapy might be responsive to treatment with steroids.

Drug-induced lung injury has been associated with the use of several alkylating agent–based high-dose chemotherapy regimens but is particularly problematic when high-dose BCNU is administered in combination with multiple alkylating agents. In the dose-finding series of Wheeler et al. in 1990, it was reported that a BCNU dose escalation to 600 mg per m^2 was associated with a significant increase in the incidence of interstitial pneumonitis (63). In another study by Kalaycioglu et al. in 1995, 30 of 59 patients required steroids for a decline in the diffusing capacity of the lung for carbon monoxide (DL$_{CO}$) after high-dose chemotherapy combining BCNU at a dose of 600 mg per m^2 with etoposide and cyclophosphamide (64).

Pulmonary toxicity appears to be enhanced when BCNU is combined with high-dose cyclophosphamide (65,66). It has been suggested that cyclophosphamide and BCNU act synergistically by depleting reduced glutathione and impairing antioxidant defenses (67,68). Seiden et al. in 1992 retrospectively evaluated the incidence of pulmonary toxicity after six high-dose chemotherapy cycles. Eighteen of 178 patients had fatal or life-threatening toxicity (66). A significant decrease in DL$_{CO}$ and forced expiratory volume in 1 second values was observed in patients treated with a regimen containing cyclophosphamide and BCNU, respectively. In another study by Jones et al. in 1993 (65), 20 of 38 patients treated with high-dose cyclophosphamide, cisplatin, and BCNU at a dose of 600 mg/m^2 developed pulmonary toxicity. Thirteen of 20 patients were treated with steroids for shortness of breath, and the majority of patients were diagnosed 1 to 3 months' posttransplantation.

GONADAL TOXICITY

Because the annual incidence of lymphoma is increasing, especially among men younger than 55 years (69), and the cure rate is increasing, the detrimental effect of treatment on fertility and its psychological consequences are of growing interest to physicians.

Several reports have described severe gonadal toxicity in patients with Hodgkin's disease (ranging from 40 to 90%), particularly ovarian failure in women and infertility in men, after chemotherapy such as MOPP (mechlorethamine, vincristine, procarbazine, and prednisone) (70) or COPP (cyclophosphamide, vincristine, procarbazine, and prednisone)/ABVD (Table 34.3) (71). However, recent randomized trials have demonstrated that ABVD achieves comparable or better results than MOPP and alternating regimens (72). Because ABVD has been associated with 30% azoospermia

TABLE 34.3. *Gonadal toxicities associated with the treatment of lymphoma*

Type of treatment	Effects	References
Radiotherapy	Women: ovarian castration if >5 Gy	74–75
	Men: sterility at 1–2 Gy	
Chemotherapy	Women: low effect	73,77,78
	Men: sterility with chlorambucil, cyclophosphamide, busulfan	75
High-dose chemotherapy	Female: increased preterm labor and delivery, increase of low-birth-weight infants	77,82–85

and 100% recovery, it has become the standard treatment, and it seems that cyclophosphamide and procarbazine, as components of COPP, are mainly responsible for the occurrence of gonadal toxicity. The comparison of gonadal toxicity between patients with Hodgkin's disease and non-Hodgkin lymphoma is complicated by the facts that different drugs are used and more radiotherapy is used for Hodgkin's disease. However, patients with non-Hodgkin's lymphoma have a lower incidence of long-term gonadal damage after therapy (73). In lymphoma, chemotherapy—mainly cyclophosphamide—and radiation may contribute to gonadal damage. Fever, the general state of the patient, and psychological factors were all suggested as other possible causes.

Ovary

Injury to the ovary can cause sterility and suppressed hormone production. The assessment of gonadal function after treatment of lymphoma in women is difficult because the ova and ovary are not easily accessible for study. Therefore, the surrogate markers of a woman's fertility are regular menses, estrogen levels greater than 20 pmol per L, and the ability to become pregnant.

The dose of radiation that ablates ovarian function depends on whether the dose is fractionated and the age at the time of radiation. The ovary has a smaller number of cells that undergo meiotic activity than the testis and therefore is sensitive to radiation at a higher dosage than the testis. Subsequent to radiation, a woman may have months of amenorrhea followed by the return of normal menses, because cessation of menses does not imply permanent sterility. However, in general, women older than 25 years who receive an ovarian dose greater than 5 Gy tend to undergo ovarian castration (74). However, even after total-body irradiation, pregnancies have been reported (75). If pelvis radiotherapy is planned in a patient who still desires pregnancy, oophoropexy may be performed. Shielding of the gonads is performed but is less successful in preserving the fertility of

a woman than it is for a man. For chemotherapy, cyclophosphamide, age, dosage, and combination with pelvic radiation are risk factors for ovarian injury. The basic ovarian lesions after chemotherapy are fibrosis and follicle destruction (74). Protection of gonad function with hormonal manipulation has shown encouraging preliminary data but is still an area of investigation (76), and, unfortunately, storage of oocytes is not readily available because of technical difficulties. Bokemeyer et al. in 1994 reported on 10 women with lymphoma treated with CHOP plus radiotherapy. One of the women showed an elevated level of serum gonadotropins and decreased estradiol as an indicator of gonadal toxicity, with abnormalities of the menstrual cycle (73). In the series of Müller and Stahel in 1993, one of seven women was found to have gonadal dysfunction after MACOP-B or VACOP-B (doxorubicin, cyclophosphamide, etoposide, vincristine, prednisone, and bleomycin) (77). After autologous transplantation, all patients became menopausal immediately after the procedure in the Schimmer et al. series in 1998 (78). Twenty-nine percent recovered ovarian function, and younger age at transplantation predicted ovarian recovery, whereas use of total-body irradiation had a borderline negative impact. Pregnancies have been reported, essentially for women younger than 26 years of age. Brice et al. found that a small number of normal pregnancies can be achieved in women treated with chemotherapy for non-Hodgkin's lymphoma regardless of whether high-dose therapy with autologous stem cell transplantation is included. The pregnancy rate did not seem to have been impaired in the group treated with high-dose chemotherapy. On the other hand, these pregnancies occurred in the youngest patients, and no pregnancy was observed in women older than 29 years at non-Hodgkin's lymphoma diagnosis in this group (79). The question of pregnancy complications or birth defects after stem cell transplantation is difficult. Sanders et al. reported in 1996 that women who received high doses of alkylating agents with total-body irradiation were at increased risk for spontaneous abortion, and women who were treated with high-dose alkylating agents had an increased incidence of preterm labor and delivery as well as an increased incidence of low-birth-weight infants (75).

Testes

Chemotherapy and radiotherapy affect gonadal function primarily by progressive, dose-related injury to the germinal epithelium of the seminiferous tubules. This damage can lead to oligospermia or aspermia that may be reversible. After therapy, the Leydig cells remain at normal values, whereas follicle-stimulating hormone increases secondary to the germinal aplasia. Drugs commonly associated with germinal aplasia include chlorambucil, cyclophosphamide, and busulfan. However, semen anomalies, which are reflected by low sperm count ($<20 \times 10^6$/mL) and reduced sperm motility, are well documented in the range of 20 to 67% at diagnosis and before treatment (80,81). These anomalies were attributed to emotional stress, elevated body temperature, and immunologic influences (82). Spermatogonia are very sensitive to radiation therapy, and small doses can produce damage. Multiple small fractions of radiation are more toxic to spermatogenesis than are large, single fractions. Semen cryopreservation and testicular shielding are used to preserve gonadal function after treatment.

In a 2000 series of 33 Hodgkin's disease and non-Hodgkin's lymphoma patients, Tal et al. found that stage III and IV patients had a greater probability of long-lasting sperm anomalies after treatment, but that B symptoms had no predictive value (83). The overall incidence of long-term gonadal toxicity was 21% among men, but all of them received COP (cyclophosphamide, vincristine, and prednisone) maintenance therapy with cumulative doses of cyclophosphamide between 12 and 43 g. Similarly, in the series of Pryzant et al. in 1993, cumulative cyclophosphamide doses of greater than 9.5 g per m^2 were associated with a high risk of permanent sterility in lymphoma patients treated with the CHOP-bleomycin regimen; other drugs from this combination might increase the risk associated with cyclophosphamide alone. The fractions of patients whose sperm counts recovered were 83% and 47% for those who received less than 9.5 g per m^2 and greater than 9.5 g per m^2, respectively. As expected, pelvic radiation therapy also had an increased risk of sterility, and all patients were azoospermic during treatment (84). Normal follicle-stimulating hormone values and spermatogenesis were found in 70% to 80% of the patients after treatments with COPP or the LNH-80 regimen (85,86). In the series of Müller in 1993, all patients had normal testosterone, luteinizing hormone, and follicle-stimulating hormone values after conventional treatment with MACOP-B or VACOP-B (77). In contrast, three out of seven patients undergoing autologous stem cell transplantation showed abnormal values. Haddy et al. showed that, among 18 lymphoma patients who elected to have a semen analysis performed after completion of radiotherapy, all showed azoospermia or oligospermia. Nine of the 18 patients later fathered children. Of the nine patients who did not father children, six were shown to have azoospermia or oligospermia 10 to 14 years later, and the others were not tested (26).

NEUROLOGIC TOXICITIES

Primary Central Nervous System Lymphoma

Late leukoencephalopathy is a common complication in patients treated with high-dose methotrexate and cranial radiation for primary central nervous system lymphoma (87,88). However, the exact incidence of this devastating neurologic dysfunction is not very well-known and has been reported to be between 4% and 36% in different series (89,90). In the series of Blay et al. in 1998, it was found to be 19% at 5 years and correlated with the dose administered to the brain (>50 Gy) and with the use of postradiation chemotherapy (91). Haddy et al. in 1998 reported a pediatric

series of 103 young survivors. Two patients who received 3,000 cGy of cranial irradiation subsequently developed seizures and required continuous anticonvulsant therapy; both had leukomalacia shown by magnetic resonance imaging. One of them required a special education class at school. Two others who received 900 and 1,200 cGy of cranial irradiation did not develop neurologic deficits. Three patients who did not receive cranial irradiation developed seizures during or after chemotherapy. One of them required tutoring in school due to short-term memory loss. This late neurologic toxicity also contributes to the poor social outcome of primary central nervous system lymphoma patients. In one series, only 6% of patients returned to work. In the study of Sandor et al. (87), the incidence of late neurologic effects (3 out of 14, 21%) does not seem to be dramatically decreased by the use of chemotherapy alone and case reports of fatal leukoencephalopathy after CHOP chemotherapy without radiotherapy have been reported (92).

Vincristine

Vincristine, a common agent in treating lymphoma, is associated with peripheral, central, and autonomic neuropathies. In the series of Haim et al. in 1994, mild to moderately severe neuropathy was seen in 92% of the lymphoma patients exposed to the drug at full dose, without capping at a total of 2 mg (93). After discontinuation of vincristine, the median time to recovery was 3 months for paresthesia and motor weakness and 5 months for muscle cramps. Residual minor abnormalities have, in some cases, persisted for years. Relapsed or refractory patients may be treated with ifosfamide and cisplatin, both known to cause central and peripheral neurotoxicity. Fludarabine, used in indolent lymphomas, induces mild and reversible central nervous system toxicity in 15% of treated patients; however, delayed and severe encephalopathy have been reported (94).

ENDOCRINE TOXICITIES

The thyroid is likely to produce clinically significant abnormalities after external radiotherapy. Functional clinical changes after direct radiation exceeding 30 Gy are essentially related to hypothyroidism, which may be clinically overt or subclinical with normal serum free thyroxine levels and high thyrotropin concentrations (95). In the series by Hancock et al. in 1991, 512 out of 1,677 irradiated Hodgkin's disease patients presented with hypothyroidism, and 486 patients received thyroxine therapy; the 20-year actuarial risk among irradiated patients was 43%. The risk of hyperthyroidism (95), silent thyroiditis, and Hashimoto's disease (96) is also increased after radiation therapy. Secondary hypothyroidism related to the irradiation of the hypothalamus and pituitary gland may arise with doses higher than 40 to 50 Gy. After total-body irradiation, subclinical thyroid dysfunction was seen in 39% of patients. No evidence of direct damage to the hypothalamic-pituitary axis was found in one series (97).

Thyroid dysfunction has been the most common late complication after myeloablative radioimmunotherapy with iodine-131–labelled anti-CD20 antibody. Seventeen of 29 patients developed abnormal elevations of thyroid-stimulating hormone during follow-up. The estimated cumulative probability of hypothyroidism is 62%. All patients who developed hypothyroidism have done so within the first year, and the median time to development of an elevated thyroid-stimulating hormone has been 6 months. No patient developed symptomatic hypothyroidism, as thyroid replacement therapy was initiated as soon as monitoring showed elevated thyroid-stimulating hormone levels (41).

As the number of young patients surviving lymphoma increases, the growth impairment resulting from radiotherapy, especially from cranial radiation greater than 24 Gy, or from aggressive chemotherapy has become a matter of concern. Growth hormone deficiency is of primary importance among the various potential alterations in hypothalamic and pituitary function associated with radiotherapy or chemotherapy, and the hypothalamus appears to be the main site of damage (98). Normal spontaneous growth hormone secretion during sleep but failure to show the normal growth hormone response to arginine, growth hormone-releasing factor, and glucagon-propanolol test suggest hypothalamic dysfunction and secondary pituitary atrophy as demonstrated in central nervous system relapsing patients (99). Age at initial diagnosis and at central nervous system relapse seems to be the best predictive factor of the severity of the subsequent growth impairment. Children younger than 2 years may be particularly sensitive to the radiation and systemic or intrathecal chemotherapy and therefore experience more severe growth impairment.

MISCELLANEOUS

Bone Damage

Ionizing radiation may induce an impairment of growing bone. This fact is of particular importance in children and represents the most important dose-limiting factor in the radiotherapeutic management of children with malignant disease. Scoliosis, epiphyseal slippage, avascular necrosis, and abnormalities of craniofacial growth may be observed after radiation. The child's age at the time of treatment, the location of irradiated bone, and irradiation characteristics may influence the radiation-related observed effects (100). There is no evidence that chemotherapy may affect bone growth in lymphoma patients, as is suggested for medulloblastoma (101). In adults, pathologic analysis of mature bone after ionizing radiation exposure is rare, suggesting that it is difficult to draw a clear picture of the action of radiation on the bone. Osteoporosis, medullary fibrosis, and cytotoxicity on bone cells can lead to fracture or necrosis. Various factors can influence bone tolerance to radiation, such as bone involvement or infection, which is frequent in mandibular osteonecrosis. Technical improvements in radiation techniques have also decreased radio-induced bone complication. The most common effect of chemotherapy is skeletal demineralization (osteoporosis) leading to fractures after use of corticosteroids.

Avascular necrosis of bone (AVNB) is a well-known but rare complication of chemotherapy for lymphoma, with a reported incidence ranging from 1 to 10%. Early diagnosis is essential for optimal therapeutic management. Using magnetic resonance imaging, the most sensitive means of detecting the earlier stages of AVNB, 100 patients treated with standard chemotherapy for lymphoma were assessed. Fifteen patients were found to have changes of AVNB, ten with early changes, but five with advanced segmental collapse of the femoral head. None of the patients with AVNB had more than the standard course of corticosteroids. Almost one fourth of the study group complained of joint pain during or after their treatment, one third of whom were found to have AVNB—a strong indicator to screen all those with pain. However, 40% of those with AVNB were asymptomatic. The clinical significance of the "silent hip" has yet to be elucidated (102).

Muscle

There are few data regarding the adverse effects of chemotherapy or radiotherapy on skeletal muscle. This tissue is considered to be radioresistant, and the most common effect on muscle is hypoplasia, but the effects on strength are not pronounced. Therefore, the effect is more cosmetic than functional.

Skin

The skin response to ionizing radiation is characterized by an acute reaction during and after the treatment and a chronic effect, subcutaneous fibrosis, resulting from a continuous and self-maintained local process, possibly sensitive to therapeutic intervention (103). At the present time, late skin effects should rarely be observed if appropriate dose, fractionation, and beam energy are used. Alopecia generally occurs in radiation field with doses of 25 to 40 Gy, and regrowth is generally seen within 3 months.

Cutaneous hyperpigmentation is observed after administration of doxorubicin and bleomycin, often at the sites of skin trauma. Nail changes are also commonly observed as radiation recall reactions and photosensitivity.

Immune System

The different treatment modalities used in non-Hodgkin's lymphoma may cause more or less pronounced immunodeficiency. Deficiencies in the humoral system, even using anti-CD20, an antigen present on every B cell, are generally not long-lasting and not very clinically significant (8). However, T-cell reconstitution may be more affected by therapy. After autologous stem cell transplantation, T-cell CD3$^+$ repopulation typically occurs by 2 to 4 months, low CD4$^+$/CD8$^+$ ratios

TABLE 34.4. *Recommendations of the European Bone Marrow Transplantation Registry for vaccination after stem cell transplantation*

Vaccine	Allograft	Autograft	Delay after transplant
Tetanus	Recommended for all patients	Recommended for all patients	6–12 mo
Diphtheria	Recommended for all patients	Recommended for all patients	6–12 mo
Poliomyelitis (inactivated)	Recommended for all patients	Recommended for all patients	6–12 mo
Streptococcus pneumoniae (Pneumo 23)	Recommended for all patients (low efficacy)	Recommended for all patients (low efficacy)	6–12 mo
Haemophilus influenzae	Recommended for all patients	Recommended for children and patients with respiratory deficiency	4–5 mo
Flu	Recommended for all patients	Recommended for all patients	>6 mo and 1/yr for at least 2 yr
Hepatitis B	According to epidemiology	According to epidemiology	6–12 mo

may exist during the first 6 to 12 months, and T-cell function, as measured by mitogen studies, returns to baseline by 1 year (104). The introduction of CD34$^+$ selection technique to reduce tumor contamination does not greatly influence long-term immunologic reconstitution. However, unusual viral infections, progressive multifocal leukoencephalopathy, and cytomegalovirus have recently been reported with concomitant use of CD34$^+$ selection and peritransplant rituximab (105). Recommendations for vaccination after stem cell transplantation have been proposed by the European Bone Marrow Transplantation Registry and U.S. Centers for Disease Control and Prevention (106) (Table 34.4).

REFERENCES

1. Singal PK, Iliskovic N. Doxorubicin-induced cardiomyopathy. *N Engl J Med* 1998;339:900–905.
2. Pohjola-Sintonen S, Totterman KJ, Salmo M, et al. Late cardiac effects of mediastinal radiotherapy in patients with Hodgkin's disease. *Cancer* 1987;60:31–37.
3. Lipshultz SE, Colan SD, Gelber RD, et al. Late cardiac effects of doxorubicin therapy for acute lymphoblastic leukemia in childhood. *N Engl J Med* 1991;324:808–815.
4. Cohn KE, Stewart JR, Fajardo LF, et al. Heart disease following radiation. *Medicine (Baltimore)* 1967;46:281–298.
5. Hancock SL, Tucker MA, Hoppe RT. Factors affecting late mortality from heart disease after treatment of Hodgkin's disease. *JAMA* 1993;270:1949–1955.
6. Boivin JF, Hutchison GB, Lubin JH, et al. Coronary artery disease mortality in patients treated for Hodgkin's disease. *Cancer* 1992;69:1241–1247.
7. Fisher RI, Gaynor ER, Dahlberg S, et al. Comparison of a standard regimen (CHOP) with three intensive chemotherapy regimens for advanced non-Hodgkin's lymphoma. *N Engl J Med* 1993;328:1002–1006.
8. Coiffier B, Lepage E, Briere J, et al. CHOP chemotherapy plus rituximab compared with CHOP alone in elderly patients with diffuse large-B-cell lymphoma. *N Engl J Med* 2002;346:235–242.
9. Bristow MR, Billingham ME, Mason JW, et al. Clinical spectrum of anthracycline antibiotic cardiotoxicity. *Cancer Treat Rep* 1978;62:873–879.
10. Shan K, Lincoff AM, Young JB. Anthracycline-induced cardiotoxicity. *Ann Intern Med* 1996;125:47–58.
11. Laufman LR, Jones JJ, Morrice B, et al. Case report of a lethal cardiac toxic effect following high-dose cyclophosphamide. *J Natl Cancer Inst* 1995;87:539–540.
12. Tulleken JE, Kooiman CG, van der Werf TS, et al. Constrictive pericarditis after high-dose chemotherapy. *Lancet* 1997;350:1601.
13. Isberg B, Paul C, Jonsson L, et al. Myocardial toxicity of high-dose cyclophosphamide in rabbits treated with daunorubicin. *Cancer Chemother Pharmacol* 1991;28:171–180.
14. Brockstein BE, Smiley C, Al-Sadir J, et al. Cardiac and pulmonary toxicity in patients undergoing high-dose chemotherapy for lymphoma and breast cancer: prognostic factors. *Bone Marrow Transplant* 2000;25:885–894.
15. Kandylis K, Vassilomanolakis M, Tsoussis S, et al. Ifosfamide cardiotoxicity in humans. *Cancer Chemother Pharmacol* 1989;24:395–396.
16. Quezado ZM, Wilson WH, Cunnion RE, et al. High-dose ifosfamide is associated with severe, reversible cardiac dysfunction. *Ann Intern Med* 1993;118:31–36.
17. Gottdiener JS, Appelbaum FR, Ferrans VJ, et al. Cardiotoxicity associated with high-dose cyclophosphamide therapy. *Arch Intern Med* 1981;141:758–763.
18. Hertenstein B, Stefanic M, Schmeiser T, et al. Cardiac toxicity of bone marrow transplantation: predictive value of cardiologic evaluation before transplant. *J Clin Oncol* 1994;12:998–1004.
19. Younes A, Sarris A, Melnyk A, et al. Three-hour paclitaxel infusion in patients with refractory and relapsed non-Hodgkin's lymphoma. *J Clin Oncol* 1995;13:583–587.
20. House KW, Simon SR, Pugh RP. Chemotherapy-induced myocardial infarction in a young man with Hodgkin's disease. *Clin Cardiol* 1992;15:122–125.
21. Scholz KH, Herrmann C, Tebbe U, et al. Myocardial infarction in young patients with Hodgkin's disease—potential pathogenic role of radiotherapy, chemotherapy, and splenectomy. *Clin Investig* 1993;71:57–64.
22. Clarke CS, Otridge BW, Carney DN. Thromboembolism. A complication of weekly chemotherapy in the treatment of non-Hodgkin's lymphoma. *Cancer* 1990;66:2027–2030.
23. Klencke B, Kaplan L. Advances and future challenges in non-Hodgkin's lymphoma. *Curr Opin Oncol* 1998;10:422–427.
24. Shan K, Lincoff AM, Young JB. Anthracycline-induced cardiotoxicity. *Ann Intern Med* 1996;125:47–58.
25. Miller TP, Dahlberg S, Cassady JR, et al. Chemotherapy alone compared with chemotherapy plus radiotherapy for localized intermediate- and high-grade non-Hodgkin's lymphoma. *N Engl J Med* 1998;339:21–26.
26. Haddy TB, Adde MA, McCalla J, et al. Late effects in long-term survivors of high-grade non-Hodgkin's lymphomas. *J Clin Oncol* 1998;16:2070–2079.
27. Ghielmini M, Zappa F, Menafoglio A, et al. The high-dose sequential (Milan) chemotherapy/PBSC transplantation regimen for patients with lymphoma is not cardiotoxic. *Ann Oncol* 1999;10:533–537.
28. Hancock SL, Tucker MA, Hoppe RT. Factors affecting late mortality from heart disease after treatment of Hodgkin's disease. *JAMA* 1993;270:1949–1955.

29. Henry-Amar M, Hayat M, Meerwaldt JH, et al. Causes of death after therapy for early stage Hodgkin's disease entered on EORTC protocols. EORTC Lymphoma Cooperative Group. *Int J Radiat Oncol Biol Phys* 1990;19:1155–1157.

30. Rose AG. Pulmonary veno-occlusive disease due to bleomycin therapy for lymphoma. Case reports. *S Afr Med J* 1983;64:636–638.

31. Solal-Celigny P, Lepage E, Brousse N, et al. Recombinant interferon alfa-2b combined with a regimen containing doxorubicin in patients with advanced follicular lymphoma. Groupe d'Etude des Lymphomes de l'Adulte. *N Engl J Med* 1993;329:1608–1614.

32. Dickson D. Deaths halt interferon trials in France. *Science* 1982;218:772.

33. Grunberg SM, Kempf RA, Itri LM, et al. Phase II study of recombinant alpha interferon in the treatment of advanced non-small cell lung carcinoma. *Cancer Treat Rep* 1985;69:1031–1032.

34. Deyton LR, Walker RE, Kovacs JA, et al. Reversible cardiac dysfunction associated with interferon alfa therapy in AIDS patients with Kaposi's sarcoma. *N Engl J Med* 1989;321:1246–1249.

35. Zimmerman S, Adkins D, Graham M, et al. Irreversible, severe congestive cardiomyopathy occurring in association with interferon alpha therapy. *Cancer Biother* 1994;9:291–299.

36. van Besien K, Tabocoff J, Rodriguez M, et al. High-dose chemotherapy with BEAC regimen and autologous bone marrow transplantation for intermediate grade and immunoblastic lymphoma: durable complete remissions, but a high rate of regimen-related toxicity. *Bone Marrow Transplant* 1995;15:549–555.

37. Rapoport AP, Rowe JM, Kouides PA, et al. One hundred autotransplants for relapsed or refractory Hodgkin's disease and lymphoma: value of pretransplant disease status for predicting outcome. *J Clin Oncol* 1993;11:2351–2361.

38. Salloum E, Jillella AP, Nadkarni R, et al. Assessment of pulmonary and cardiac function after high dose chemotherapy with BEAM and peripheral blood progenitor cell transplantation. *Cancer* 1998;82:1506–1512.

39. Friedman HS, Colvin OM, Aisaka K, et al. Glutathione protects cardiac and skeletal muscle from cyclophosphamide-induced toxicity. *Cancer Res* 1990;50:2455–2462.

40. Kanj SS, Sharara AI, Shpall EJ, et al. Myocardial ischemia associated with high-dose carmustine infusion. *Cancer* 1991;68:1910–1912.

41. Liu SY, Eary JF, Petersdorf SH, et al. Follow-up of relapsed B-cell lymphoma patients treated with iodine-131-labeled anti-CD20 antibody and autologous stem-cell rescue. *J Clin Oncol* 1998;16:3270–3278.

42. Cardinale D, Sandri MT, Martinoni A, et al. Left ventricular dysfunction predicted by early troponin I release after high-dose chemotherapy. *J Am Coll Cardiol* 2000;36:517–522.

43. Villani F, De Maria P, Bonfante V, et al. Late pulmonary toxicity after treatment for Hodgkin's disease. *Anticancer Res* 1997;17:4739–4742.

44. Horning SJ, Adhikari A, Rizk N, et al. Effect of treatment for Hodgkin's disease on pulmonary function: results of a prospective study. *J Clin Oncol* 1994;12:297–305.

45. Hirsch A, Vander Els N, Straus DJ, et al. Effect of ABVD chemotherapy with and without mantle or mediastinal irradiation on pulmonary function and symptoms in early-stage Hodgkin's disease. *J Clin Oncol* 1996;14:1297–1305.

46. Rubin P, Johnston CJ, Williams JP, et al. A perpetual cascade of cytokines postirradiation leads to pulmonary fibrosis. *Int J Radiat Oncol Biol Phys* 1995;33:99–109.

47. Nissen NI, Ersboll J, Hansen HS, et al. A randomized study of radiotherapy versus radiotherapy plus chemotherapy in stage I-II non-Hodgkin's lymphomas. *Cancer* 1983;52:1–7.

48. Sutcliffe SB, Gospodarowicz MK, Bush RS, et al. Role of radiation therapy in localized non-Hodgkin's lymphoma. *Radiother Oncol* 1985;4:211–223.

49. Lee CK, Levitt SH. Long-term follow-up of pathologic stage I large cell non-Hodgkin's lymphoma patients after primary radiotherapy. *Am J Clin Oncol* 1996;19:93–98.

50. Kreisman H, Wolkove N. Pulmonary toxicity of antineoplastic therapy. *Semin Oncol* 1992;19:508–520.

51. Klimo P, Connors JM. MACOP-B chemotherapy for the treatment of diffuse large-cell lymphoma. *Ann Intern Med* 1985;102:596–602.

52. Shapiro CL, Yeap BY, Godleski J, et al. Drug-related pulmonary toxicity in non-Hodgkin's lymphoma. Comparative results with three different treatment regimens. *Cancer* 1991;68:699–705.

53. Iki S, Yoshinaga K, Ohbayashi Y, et al. Cytotoxic drug-induced pneumonia and possible augmentation by G-CSF—clinical attention. *Ann Hematol* 1993;66:217–218.

54. Matthews JH. Pulmonary toxicity of ABVD chemotherapy and G-CSF in Hodgkin's disease: possible synergy. *Lancet* 1993;342:988.

55. Lei KI, Leung WT, Johnson PJ. Serious pulmonary complications in patients receiving recombinant granulocyte colony-stimulating factor during BACOP chemotherapy for aggressive non-Hodgkin's lymphoma. *Br J Cancer* 1994;70:1009–1013.

56. Couderc LJ, Stelianides S, Frachon I, et al. Pulmonary toxicity of chemotherapy and G/GM-CSF: a report of five cases. *Respir Med* 1999;93:65–68.

57. Bastion Y, Reyes F, Bosly A, et al. Possible toxicity with the association of G-CSF and bleomycin. *Lancet* 1994;343:1221–1222.

58. Bastion Y, Coiffier B. Pulmonary toxicity of bleomycin: is G-CSF a risk factor? *Lancet* 1994;344:474.

59. Yokose N, Ogata K, Tamura H, et al. Pulmonary toxicity after granulocyte colony-stimulating factor-combined chemotherapy for non-Hodgkin's lymphoma. *Br J Cancer* 1998;77:2286–2290.

60. Petersen FB, Appelbaum FR, Hill R, et al. Autologous marrow transplantation for malignant lymphoma: a report of 101 cases from Seattle. *J Clin Oncol* 1990;8:638–647.

61. Gingrich RD, Ginder GD, Burns LJ, et al. BVAC ablative chemotherapy followed by autologous bone marrow transplantation for patients with advanced lymphoma. *Blood* 1990;75:2276–2281.

62. Ghalie R, Szidon JP, Thompson L, et al. Evaluation of pulmonary complications after bone marrow transplantation: the role of pretransplant pulmonary function tests. *Bone Marrow Transplant* 1992;10:359–365.

63. Wheeler C, Antin JH, Churchill WH, et al. Cyclophosphamide, carmustine, and etoposide with autologous bone marrow transplantation in refractory Hodgkin's disease and non-Hodgkin's lymphoma: a dose-finding study. *J Clin Oncol* 1990;8:648–656.

64. Kalaycioglu M, Kavuru M, Tuason L, et al. Empiric prednisone therapy for pulmonary toxic reaction after high-dose chemotherapy containing carmustine (BCNU). *Chest* 1995;107:482–487.

65. Jones RB, Matthes S, Shpall EJ, et al. Acute lung injury following treatment with high-dose cyclophosphamide, cisplatin, and carmustine: pharmacodynamic evaluation of carmustine. *J Natl Cancer Inst* 1993;85:640–647.

66. Seiden MV, Elias A, Ayash L, et al. Pulmonary toxicity associated with high dose chemotherapy in the treatment of solid tumors with autologous marrow transplant: an analysis of four chemotherapy regimens. *Bone Marrow Transplant* 1992;10:57–63.

67. Babson JR, Reed DJ. Inactivation of glutathione reductase by 2-chloroethyl nitrosourea-derived isocyanates. *Biochem Biophys Res Commun* 1978;82:754–762.

68. Friedman HS, Colvin OM, Aisaka K, et al. Glutathione protects cardiac and skeletal muscle from cyclophosphamide-induced toxicity. *Cancer Res* 1990;50:2455–2462.

69. Wingo PA, Ries LA, Rosenberg HM, et al. Cancer incidence and mortality, 1973-1995: a report card for the U.S. *Cancer* 1998;82:1197–1207.

70. Schilsky RL, Sherins RJ, Hubbard SM, et al. Long-term follow up of ovarian function in women treated with MOPP chemotherapy for Hodgkin's disease. *Am J Med* 1981;71:552–556.

71. Kreuser ED, Felsenberg D, Behles C, et al. Long-term gonadal dysfunction and its impact on bone mineralization in patients following COPP/ABVD chemotherapy for Hodgkin's disease. *Ann Oncol* 1992; 3(Suppl 4):105–110.

72. Canellos GP, Anderson JR, Propert KJ, et al. Chemotherapy of advanced Hodgkin's disease with MOPP, ABVD, or MOPP alternating with ABVD. *N Engl J Med* 1992;327:1478–1484.

73. Bokemeyer C, Schmoll HJ, van Rhee J, et al. Long-term gonadal toxicity after therapy for Hodgkin's and non-Hodgkin's lymphoma. *Ann Hematol* 1994;68:105–110.

74. Chapman RM, Sutcliffe SB, Malpas JS. Cytotoxic-induced ovarian failure in women with Hodgkin's disease. I. Hormone function. *JAMA* 1979;242:1877–1881.

75. Sanders JE, Hawley J, Levy W, et al. Pregnancies following highdose cyclophosphamide with or without high-dose busulfan or totalbody irradiation and bone marrow transplantation. *Blood* 1996;87: 3045–3052.

76. Whitehead E, Shalet SM, Blackledge G, et al. The effect of combination chemotherapy on ovarian function in women treated for Hodgkin's disease. *Cancer* 1983;52:988–993.

77. Müller U, Stahel RA. Gonadal function after MACOP-B or VACOP-B with or without dose intensification and ABMT in young patients with aggressive non-Hodgkin's lymphoma. *Ann Oncol* 1993;4:399–402.

78. Schimmer AD, Quatermain M, Imrie K, et al. Ovarian function after autologous bone marrow transplantation. *J Clin Oncol* 1998;16:2359–2363.

79. Brice P, Haioun C, André M, et al. Pregnancies after high-dose chemotherapy and autologous stem cell transplantation in aggressive lymphomas. *Blood* 2002;100:736.

80. Marmor D, Elefant E, Dauchez C, et al. Semen analysis in Hodgkin's disease before the onset of treatment. *Cancer* 1986;57:1986–1987.

81. Viviani S, Ragni G, Santoro A, et al. Testicular dysfunction in Hodgkin's disease before and after treatment. *Eur J Cancer* 1991;27:1389–1392.

82. Barr RD, Clark DA, Booth JD. Dyspermia in men with localized Hodgkin's disease. A potentially reversible, immune-mediated disorder. *Med Hypotheses* 1993;40:165–168.

83. Tal R, Botchan A, Hauser R, et al. Follow-up of sperm concentration and motility in patients with lymphoma. *Hum Reprod* 2000;15:1985–1988.

84. Pryzant RM, Meistrich ML, Wilson G, et al. Long-term reduction in sperm count after chemotherapy with and without radiation therapy for non-Hodgkin's lymphomas. *J Clin Oncol* 1993;11:239–247.

85. Dumontet C, Bastion Y, Felman P, et al. Long-term outcome and sequelae in aggressive lymphoma patients treated with the LNH-80 regimen. *Ann Oncol* 1992;3:639–644.

86. Roeser HP, Stocks AE, Smith AJ. Testicular damage due to cytotoxic drugs and recovery after cessation of therapy. *Aust N Z J Med* 1978;8:250–254.

87. Sandor V, Stark-Vancs V, Pearson D, et al. Phase II trial of chemotherapy alone for primary central nervous system and intraocular lymphoma. *J Clin Oncol* 1998;16:3000–3006.

88. Bessell EM, Graus F, Punt JA, et al. Primary non-Hodgkin's lymphoma of the CNS treated with BVAM or CHOD/BVAM chemotherapy before radiotherapy. *J Clin Oncol* 1996;14:945–954.

89. Glass J, Gruber ML, Cher L, et al. Preirradiation methotrexate chemotherapy of primary central nervous system lymphoma: long-term outcome. *J Neurosurg* 1994;81:188–195.

90. Abrey LE, DeAngelis LM, Yahalom J. Long-term survival in primary CNS lymphoma. *J Clin Oncol* 1998;16:859–863.

91. Blay JY, Conroy T, Chevreau C, et al. High-dose methotrexate for the treatment of primary cerebral lymphomas: analysis of survival and late neurologic toxicity in a retrospective series. *J Clin Oncol* 1998;16:864–871.

92. Cain MS, Burton GV, Holcombe RF. Fatal leukoencephalopathy in a patient with non-Hodgkin's lymphoma treated with CHOP chemotherapy and high-dose steroids. *Am J Med Sci* 1998;315:202–207.

93. Haim N, Epelbaum R, Ben-Shahar M, et al. Full dose vincristine (without 2-mg dose limit) in the treatment of lymphomas. *Cancer* 1994;73:2515–2519.

94. Johnson PW, Fearnley J, Domizio P, et al. Neurological illness following treatment with fludarabine. *Br J Cancer* 1994;70:966–968.

95. Hancock SL, Cox RS, McDougall IR. Thyroid diseases after treatment of Hodgkin's disease. *N Engl J Med* 1991;325:599–605.

96. Tamura K, Shimaoka K, Friedman M. Thyroid abnormalities associated with treatment of malignant lymphoma. *Cancer* 1981;47:2704–2711.

97. Littley MD, Shalet SM, Morgenstern GR, et al. Endocrine and reproductive dysfunction following fractionated total body irradiation in adults. *Q J Med* 1991;78:265–274.

98. Shalet SM, Clayton PE, Price DA. Growth and pituitary function in children treated for brain tumours or acute lymphoblastic leukaemia. *Horm Res* 1988;30:53–61.

99. Yamada S, Ishii E, Okabe Y, et al. Growth retardation in childhood leukemia and lymphoma. Special reference to patients with CNS relapse. *Am J Pediatr Hematol Oncol* 1992;14:236–240.

100. Willman KY, Cox RS, Donaldson SS. Radiation induced height impairment in pediatric Hodgkin's disease. *Int J Radiat Oncol Biol Phys* 1994;28:85–92.

101. Olshan JS, Gubernick J, Packer RJ, et al. The effects of adjuvant chemotherapy on growth in children with medulloblastoma. *Cancer* 1992;70:2013–2017.

102. Ratcliffe MA, Gilbert FJ, Dawson AA, et al. Diagnosis of avascular necrosis of the femoral head in patients treated for lymphoma. *Hematol Oncol* 1995;13:131–137.

103. Lefaix JL, Delanian S, Leplat JJ, et al. Successful treatment of radiation-induced fibrosis using Cu/Zn-SOD and Mn-SOD: an experimental study. *Int J Radiat Oncol Biol Phys* 1996;35:305–312.

104. Steingrimsdottir H, Gruber A, Bjorkholm M, et al. Immune reconstitution after autologous hematopoietic stem cell transplantation in relation to underlying disease, type of high-dose therapy and infectious complications. *Haematologica* 2000;85:832–838.

105. Goldberg SL, Pecora AL, Alter RS, et al. Unusual viral infections (progressive multifocal leukoencephalopathy and cytomegalovirus disease) after high-dose chemotherapy with autologous blood stem cell rescue and peritransplantation rituximab. *Blood* 2002;99:1486–1488.

106. Ljungman P. Immunization of transplant recipients. *Bone Marrow Transplant* 1999;23:635–636.

CHAPTER 35

Assessing Quality of Life in Patients with Lymphoma

Andrea K. Ng and Michel Henry-Amar

BACKGROUND

In 1948, the World Health Organization defined *health* as the presence of physical, mental, and social well-being and not merely the absence of disease or infirmity (1). Over the years, and especially in the last two decades, there has been increasing effort to incorporate quality-of-life assessment in clinical research and practice. Quality-of-life consideration is of special interest in the field of oncology, given the toxicity associated with many cancer treatments. In addition, with the growing therapeutic successes, the evaluation of cancer survivors in terms of their physical, functional, emotional, and social health is important. Listed in Table 35.1 are commonly used generic quality-of-life instruments in oncology (2–14).

Quality-of-life research and publications related to non-Hodgkin's lymphoma, however, are still relatively scarce, in part because it is a heterogeneous disease, and the relevance of quality-of-life consideration varies greatly among the different subtypes of lymphoma, each of which has different presentation, natural courses, treatment, and prognosis. To date, no validated lymphoma-specific quality-of-life instrument has been developed. In this chapter, we provide an overview of quality-of-life assessment in oncologic clinical research, with an emphasis on available quality-of-life data in patients with non-Hodgkin's lymphoma.

WHY IS QUALITY-OF-LIFE ASSESSMENT IMPORTANT IN ONCOLOGY?

Disease response, disease control, and survival have been the traditional endpoints in measuring the effectiveness of interventions in oncology. More aggressive and intensive treatment may improve disease-specific and overall survival but at the expense of increased toxicities. The impact of the treatment on patients' quality of life needs to be taken into account in assessing the overall benefits of an intervention. In addition

to curative treatment, palliative care is another important component of oncologic management. Although palliative treatments often do not prolong survival, they can improve patients' quality of life by offering symptomatic relief and providing assurance as an intervention is being made against the cancer. Finally, as cancer treatment continues to improve and as the number of cancer survivors accumulate, examining the quality of life of patients with a history of cancer, including aspects of long-term physical and psychological morbidity and social adaptation, can help facilitate the management of these patients. Exploring the effect of a cancer diagnosis and its treatment on interpersonal relationships, family dynamics, work environment, and insurance coverage may also help bring closer attention to the psychosocial needs and legal rights of cancer survivors.

Quality-of-life measurement serves a number of important purposes in the practice of oncology. In situations in which multiple treatment options exist with similar survival outcome or if a new therapeutic strategy needs to be evaluated, the inclusion of quality of life as an endpoint can provide additional data and help in clinical decision making. Furthermore, information on quality of life has been shown to be of prognostic value in the treatment outcome of specific cancers and may help in guiding treatment selection. Quality-of-life assessment also allows the description of the overall well-being of the patient population. It helps in the understanding of the nature and extent of functional and psychosocial impairment patients encounter during their cancer therapy as well as after treatment completion. Understanding the risk factors for dysfunction can help identify high-risk patients who can be targeted for counseling and medical and psychosocial intervention. In addition, the incorporation of quality of life in clinical trials and the performance of cost-utility analysis can help in the allocation of limited resources. Finally, quality-of-life assessment provides clinicians, researchers, and administrators a means to measure, monitor, and improve quality of care.

TABLE 35.1. *Generic measures commonly used in oncology quality-of-ife research*

Measures	Reference
European Organization for Research and Treatment of Cancer Quality of Life Questionnaire-C30 (EORTC QLQ-C30)	4
Functional Assessment of Cancer Therapy-General Version (FACT-G)	5
Medical Outcomes Study 36-Item Short-Form (SF-36) Health Survey	7
Cancer Rehabilitation Evaluation System (CARES)	8
Edmonton Symptom Assessment System (ESAS) (Palliative Care)	9
Functional Living Index for Cancer (FLIC)	11
Spitzer Quality of Life Index (QLI)	12
Quality-adjusted Time Without Symptoms and Toxicity (Q-TWiST)	13
Memorial Symptom Assessment Scale (MSAS)	15
Quality-Quantity Questionnaire (QQ-q)	16
Quality of Life Scale-Cancer (QOL-CA)	17

INSTRUMENTS FOR QUALITY-OF-LIFE ASSESSMENT

Dimensions of Quality of Life

Health-related quality of life is a multifaceted construct and should be measured with multidimensional instruments. Karnofsky performance status is one of the earlier tools widely used for measuring quality of life in cancer patients (15). However, it is limited by the fact that it is a unidimensional tool, allowing assessment of only the functional status domain. Many other studies also reported on treatment toxicities using toxicity scales. However, again, such measurements are only unidimensional. By current standards, most consider such reports insufficient measures of quality of life. The key domains that are considered in most instruments include physical and role functioning, emotional well-being, and social functioning. Examples of other dimensions that may be pertinent to specific patient population, cancer sites, and treatment include sexuality, body image, fertility, pain, cognition, and financial impact.

Attributes of a Good Quality-of-Life Instrument

According to the Scientific Advisory Committee of the Medical Outcomes Trust (16), the key properties to be considered in reviewing a health-related quality-of-life instrument include the following: conceptual and measurement model, reliability, validity, responsiveness, interpretability, respondent and administrative burden, alternative forms, and cultural and language adaptations. *Reliability* is the degree to which an instrument is free from random error. Internal consistency is the most frequently used estimate in reliability testing, measured by Cronbach's alpha coefficient, a statistic that reflects the homogeneity of the scale. Other estimates used in estimating reliability include test-retest and inter-rater reliability, measured by the kappa coefficients. Kappa coefficients exceeding 0.7 are considered good to excellent. *Validity* refers to the degree to which an instrument measures what it purports to measure. The three approaches in establishing an instrument's validity are construct validity (the extent to which the measure performs in the expected direction and the ability to distinguish between groups), content validity (the ability of the instrument to measure the appropriate entity), and criterion validity (correlation of the measure with a gold standard).

Quality-of-Life Instruments in Oncology

For cancer patients, the two most widely used cancer-specific instruments for assessing overall quality of life are the European Organization for Research and Treatment of Cancer Quality of Life Questionnaire-C30 (EORTC QLQ-C30) (2) and the Functional Assessment of Cancer Therapy-General Version (FACT-G) (3). The former is a 33-item instrument developed by the EORTC that covers the domains of physical functioning, social functioning, emotional functioning, cognitive functioning, role functioning, symptoms, and financial impact. In addition to the generic core questionnaire, the EORTC Quality of Life Group has adopted a modular approach for disease-specific treatment measurements (17). The FACT-G may be considered the U.S. counterpart of the EORTC instrument. It is a 29-item questionnaire that covers the domains of physical, social and family, emotional, and functional well-being. Modules specific to disease site, treatment modality, symptoms, and condition are also available. Commonly used generic measures in the field of oncology are listed in Table 35.1 (2–14). As an example, Figure 35.1 illustrates the content of the EORTC QLQ-C30 questionnaire.

STUDY DESIGNS IN QUALITY-OF-LIFE RESEARCH

Quality-of-life measurements can be broadly divided into two main categories: health profile and preference based. The former approach uses questionnaires with sound psychometric properties designed to yield scores reflecting multiple domains of health-related quality of life. A commonly used study design using such health profile measurements is a cross-sectional longitudinal study. This approach involves a large patient population with a wide range of states of health, with the goal being identification of predictors of various aspects of quality of life. Another study design is a prospective trial in which measurements of health profile are performed prospectively at various time points. In trials in which patients are being randomized to different arms, the results allow direct comparisons of quality-of-life outcomes of different clinical interventions over time and yield addi-

EORTC QLQ-C30 (version 3)

We are interested in some things about you and your health. Please answer all of the questions yourself by circling the number that best applies to you. There are no "right" or "wrong" answers. The information that you provide will remain strictly confidential.

Please fill in your initials:
Your birthdate (Day, Month, Year):
Today's date (Day, Month, Year):

	Not at all	A little	Quite a bit	Very much
1. Do you have any trouble doing strenuous activities, like carrying a heavy shopping bag or a suitcase?	1	2	3	4
2. Do you have any trouble taking a long walk?	1	2	3	4
3. Do you have any trouble taking a short walk outside of the house?	1	2	3	4
4. Do you need to stay in bed or a chair during the day?	1	2	3	4
5. Do you need help with eating, dressing, washing yourself or using the toilet?	1	2	3	4

During the past week:	Not at All	A little	Quite a bit	Very much
6. Were you limited in doing either your work or other daily activities?	1	2	3	4
7. Were you limited in pursuing your hobbies or other leisure time activities?	1	2	3	4
8. Were you short of breath?	1	2	3	4
9. Have you had pain?	1	2	3	4
10. Did you need to rest?	1	2	3	4
11. Have you had trouble sleeping?	1	2	3	4
12. Have you felt weak?	1	2	3	4
13. Have you lacked appetite?	1	2	3	4
14. Have you felt nauseated?	1	2	3	4
15. Have you vomited?	1	2	3	4
16. Have you been constipated?	1	2	3	4

Please go on to the next page

During the past week:	Not at all	A little	Quite a bit	Very much
17. Have you had diarrhea?	1	2	3	4
18. Were you tired?	1	2	3	4
19. Did pain interfere with your daily activities?	1	2	3	4
20. Have you had difficulty in concentrating on things, like reading a newspaper or watching television?	1	2	3	4
21. Did you feel tense?	1	2	3	4
22. Did you worry?	1	2	3	4
23. Did you feel irritable?	1	2	3	4
24. Did you feel depressed?	1	2	3	4
25. Have you had difficulty remembering things?	1	2	3	4
26. Has your physical condition or medical treatment interfered with your family life?	1	2	3	4
27. Has your physical condition or medical treatment interfered with your social activities?	1	2	3	4
28. Has your physical condition or medical treatment caused you financial difficulties?	1	2	3	4

For the following questions please circle the number between 1 and 7 that best applies to you

29. How would you rate your overall health during the past week?

1	2	3	4	5	6	7
Very poor						Excellent

30. How would you rate your overall quality of life during the past week?

1	2	3	4	5	6	7
Very poor						Excellent

SPECIMEN

FIG. 35.1. The European Organization for Research and Treatment of Cancer Quality of Life Questionnaire-C30 (version 3), a 33-item instrument covering the domains of physical functioning, social functioning, emotional functioning, cognitive functioning, role functioning, symptoms, and financial impact. (From Aaronson NK, Ahmedzai S, Bergman B, et al. The European Organization for Research and Treatment of Cancer QLQ-C30: a quality-of-life instrument for use in international clinical trials in oncology. *J Natl Cancer Inst* 1993;85:365–376, with permission.)

tional useful information beyond the traditional endpoints of clinical trials.

Preference-based measures, unlike health profile measures, are designed to produce a single score, known as a *utility*, that summarizes the different aspects of health-related quality of life. A utility score reflects one's preference for a specific health state, typically in reference to health states of death and perfect health, represented by scores of 0 and 1, respectively. Commonly used elicitation methods include visual analog scales, time tradeoff, and standard gamble. Another way to elicit utilities is through the use of health index models, such as the Quality of Well-Being (18), EuroQoL (19), and Health Utility Index (20), in which previously obtained utilities are mapped onto the index scores. Utilities are used to estimate quality-adjusted survival and, through modeling techniques, can be applied in cost-effectiveness or cost-utility analyses. The development of the quality-adjusted time without symptoms and toxicity (Q-TWiST) of treatment also allows the estimation of quality-adjusted survival using actual survival data from clinical trials (10). In the analysis, the average time spent in each of a number of health states is estimated from clinical trial data. Each health state is assigned a utility, or quality-of-life weight, and the results are combined to produce an estimate of quality-adjusted survival.

RELEVANT QUALITY-OF-LIFE CONCERNS IN PATIENTS WITH NON-HODGKIN'S LYMPHOMA

Non-Hodgkin's lymphoma is a heterogeneous disease. Over the years, a number of different classification systems have been adopted to distinguish the various subtypes of non-Hodgkin's lymphoma. In the Revised European-American Lymphoma Classification of lymphoid neoplasms (21), the most recently developed and proposed system, in addition to distinctive morphologic and immunophenotypic features, each subtype of lymphoma also has its unique clinical characteristics. Different subtypes affect different patient populations and have different disease presentation and clinical course. In addition, treatment intent, management approaches, treatment toxicity, responses to therapy, and overall prognosis may vary. As such, aspects of quality of life that are relevant can differ, depending on the subtype of non-Hodgkin's lymphoma and the clinical situation under consideration.

Indolent Lymphoma

Among indolent lymphomas, the most common subtype is follicular lymphoma, accounting for 22% of all cases of non-Hodgkin's lymphoma (22). The natural history of follicular lymphoma is typified by a prolonged clinical course with slow disease progression. Despite the indolent nature of the disease, it is generally considered to be incurable. Treatment options, including chemotherapy, immunotherapy, local radiation therapy, and radioimmunotherapy, are available. However, the treatments frequently can only induce a temporary response. Although treatments can provide palliation, such as pain control, relieving obstruction, improving cosmesis, or alleviating neurologic damage, they also carry toxicity and costs. Common side effects of treatment include hair loss, nausea, vomiting, loss of appetite, and fatigue, which in turn may influence patients' ability to carry out normal daily activities as well as affect their emotional status. The strategy of watchful waiting is sometimes adopted in follicular lymphoma, particularly in patients who are clinically asymptomatic. However, despite the lack of symptoms, these patients may bear substantial emotional burden and are faced with the stigma and psychosocial consequences of carrying a diagnosis of an essentially incurable cancer. In weighing the benefits against the drawbacks of the available management options for indolent lymphoma, quality-of-life data can be of considerable value, especially in the absence of clear survival differences among the various approaches.

Aggressive Lymphoma

Aggressive lymphoma tends to be associated with a more rapid clinical course and can potentially be fatal within a relatively short time frame. Paradoxically, however, unlike indolent lymphoma, aggressive lymphoma is curable in 30% to 40% of the cases. Diffuse large B-cell lymphoma is the most common of the aggressive non-Hodgkin's lymphomas. The introduction of CHOP [cyclophosphamide, hydroxydaunomycin, Oncovin (vincristine), prednisone] in 1975 has resulted in long-term survival rates of close to 50% (22). In the 1980s, phase II trials evaluating more intensive combination chemotherapy showed initial promising results with high remission and survival rates (23–28). However, a subsequent large, prospective, randomized trial did not demonstrate a survival benefit of the second and third generation regimens (29). In the absence of survival differences, quality-of-life consideration is

of particular interest. Investigators are continuing to seek other treatment strategies that may further improve the survival outcome of aggressive lymphoma. More recently, a randomized study demonstrated a survival benefit with the addition of rituximab to CHOP in elderly patients with diffuse large B-cell lymphoma (30). In these trials, toxicity profile was evaluated, but formal quality-of-life assessment was typically not performed or reported. Incorporation of quality of life as one of the endpoints in future trials evaluating novel, more intensive, and potentially more toxic regimens as curative treatments for aggressive lymphoma may provide further insights into the important tradeoffs of the alternative regimens.

High-Dose Therapy with Hematopoietic Stem Cell Rescue

High-dose therapy with hematopoietic stem cell rescue has been shown to improve survival in patients with relapsed/refractory non-Hodgkin's lymphoma (31), although its role as consolidation in patients with aggressive lymphoma in first remission is less conclusive (32–34). It is a one-time, high-risk treatment that offers the potential of cure for patients who are otherwise largely incurable. However, it is also associated with numerous acute and chronic morbidities that may have profound effects on multiple aspects of quality of life. It begins with the demanding schedule in preparation for the procedure, along with the anxiety and anticipation; then come the hospitalization, receiving the conditioning regimen, and experiencing the side effects while being in isolation and awaiting engraftment. After discharge from the hospital, patients continue to experience the lingering side effects and remain in precautions due to the immunosuppression, while at the same time attempting to return to the structures of their lives before their illness. Patients undergoing high-dose therapy with hematopoietic stem cell rescue are one group of patients with hematologic malignancies in whom considerable amounts of quality-of-life data are available, both during and in the immediate period after the high-dose therapy as well as after long-term remission has been achieved.

Long-Term Survivors of Non-Hodgkin's Lymphoma

Lymphoma and its treatment may leave many survivors with a wide range of physical and psychological problems. Although there are numerous reports in the literature on health-related quality of life of long-term survivors of Hodgkin's disease (35–45), similar data are not as readily available for patients with history of non-Hodgkin's lymphoma. This is because unlike Hodgkin's disease, which is a highly curable malignancy, the overall cure rate of non-Hodgkin's disease is lower. In addition, on average, patients with non-Hodgkin's lymphoma tend to be older at the time of presentation. Most information on the long-term physical and psychosocial functioning in survivors of non-Hodgkin's lymphoma is included in quality-of-life studies on patients who had undergone high-dose therapy with hematopoietic stem cell or bone marrow support.

QUALITY-OF-LIFE STUDIES IN NON-HODGKIN'S LYMPHOMA

A review of the literature shows that publications on quality-of-life assessment in non-Hodgkin's lymphoma are relatively scarce. The majority of the available data has been reported in the last 5 to 10 years, as the topic gained in popularity in recent years. To illustrate the types of quality-of-life studies available and the commonly used instruments and methodology, existing studies are summarized below in which quality of life of patients with non-Hodgkin's lymphoma is evaluated.

Prospective Quality-of-Life Evaluations

A number of prospective trials on treatment of non-Hodgkin's lymphoma formally assessed quality of life, which was reported as one of the endpoints. The focus is typically on the immediate effect of the disease and its treatment on patients' quality of life. The available studies are summarized in Table 35.2 (46–53).

In a phase III study reported by Aviles et al. (46), the efficacy and toxicity of interferon alfa-2b as maintenance therapy were evaluated in patients with low-grade non-Hodgkin's lymphoma. In this study, 98 patients were randomized to a year of interferon alfa-2b versus no further treatment after a complete remission had been achieved with conventional induction chemotherapy. The Medical Outcomes Study 36-Item Short Form (SF-36) Health Survey (4), a well-validated and widely accepted generic quality-of-life instrument, was applied to patients at 6 months during the maintenance therapy and 6 months after the patient completed the study. Whereas a significantly longer duration of response was found in the interferon alfa-2b maintenance therapy arm, significant differences in the mean scored values of the SF-36 scales were not detected between the two arms. The results led to the authors'

conclusions that interferon should be considered as good maintenance therapy that improves the duration of remission without compromising quality of life.

The Groupe d'Etude des Lymphomes Folliculaires used a different approach in incorporating quality of life as an endpoint in their randomized study (47). In this trial, patients with advanced-stage follicular lymphoma were randomized to CHVP [cyclophosphamide, hydroxydaunomycin (doxorubicin), VM-26 (teniposide), prednisone] alone versus CHVP and interferon alfa-2b. Using collected data on the type and grade of adverse events in each 3-month period as a surrogate for the duration of toxicity, a Q-TWiST analysis was applied (10). Even with adjustment for quality of life, taking into account the toxicities of treatment, the analysis showed that the clinical benefit of concomitant interferon alfa-2b persisted. Sensitivity analysis was also performed, demonstrating how changes in utility values of different health states affected the magnitude of the benefit, the results of which can serve as a useful aid in clinical decision making for individual patients.

The Q-TWiST analysis was also used on the results of a randomized trial conducted by the Groupe d'Etude des Lymphomes de l'Adulte comparing high-dose therapy with autologous bone marrow transplantation versus chemotherapy for patients with aggressive lymphoma in first remission (48). Patients were divided into low-, intermediate-, and high-risk groups based on their serum lactate dehydrogenase and disease stage. The quality-adjusted survival was found to be significantly higher with high-dose therapy in high-risk patients but not in low-risk patients. Diagrams were also provided, illustrating changes in differences of quality-adjusted survival between the two groups as the utilities for the treatment toxicity and relapse health state changed, allowing clinicians to determine optimal treatment based on patients' risk group and relative preferences regarding toxicity and relapse.

TABLE 35.2. *Prospective quality-of-life studies*

Author, yr (reference)	Disease	Design	Instruments (references)
Aviles, 1996 (46)	Low-grade lymphoma	Phase III	SF-36 (7)
Cole, 1998 (47)	Follicular lymphoma	Phase III	Q-TWiST (13)
Mounier, 2000 (48)	Aggressive lymphoma	Phase III	Q-TWiST (13)
Gordon, 2002 (49)	Relapsed/refractory follicular lymphoma	Phase III	FACT-G (5)
Jerkeman, 1999 (50)	Aggressive lymphoma	Phase III	EORTC QLQ-C30 (4)
Remick, 2001 (51)	Acquired immunodeficiency syndrome–related non-Hodgkin's lymphoma	Comparison of two prospective phase II studies	FLIC and BSI (12,11)
Olsen, 2001 (52)	Cutaneous T-cell lymphoma	Phase III	FACT-G (5)
Duvic, 2001 (53)	Cutaneous T-cell lymphoma	Multiinstitutional phase II-III trial results	Spitzer QLI; "cutaneous T-cell lymphma–specific" instrument (12)

BSI, Brief Symptom Inventory; EORTC QLQ-C30, European Organization for Research and Treatment of Cancer Quality of Life Questionnaire-C30; FACT-G, Functional Assessment of Cancer Therapy-General Version; FLIC, Functional Living Index for Cancer; QLI, Quality of Life Index; Q-TWiST, Quality-adjusted Time Without Symptoms and Toxicity; SF-36, the Medical Outcomes Study 36-Item Short Form Health Survey.

Recent studies have shown promising results in the use of immunotherapy and radioimmunotherapy on patients with non-Hodgkin's lymphoma. Quality of life was included as a secondary endpoint in the pivotal phase III trial comparing ibritumomab tiuxetan (Zevalin) with rituximab (Rituxan) in 143 patients with relapsed or refractory low-grade non-Hodgkin's lymphoma (49). Patients on each arm were asked to complete the FACT-G questionnaire at baseline and at various time points after completion of treatment. It was found that quality-of-life scores improved for patients in both arms. The difference between the FACT-G scores at baseline and at 3 months, however, was significant only for the ibritumomab tiuxetan group. The results suggested that ibritumomab tiuxetan, a more aggressive treatment with a higher response rate, is also well tolerated and significantly improves patients' quality of life.

The only available randomized trial that incorporated quality-of-life assessment in comparing CHOP chemotherapy with a second or third generation regimen was conducted by the Nordic Lymphoma Group (50). In this study, patients with aggressive lymphoma were randomized to CHOP versus MACOP-B [methotrexate, Adriamycin (doxorubicin), cyclophosphamide, Oncovin (vincristine), prednisone, bleomycin]. The EORTC QLQ-C30 was administered to a subset of patients' pretreatment and at nine subsequent time points 6 to 56 weeks after study entry. As has been found in other earlier studies, no significant differences in overall or failure-free survival were detected between the two arms. However, patients who received MACOP-B had a significantly lower global quality-of-life and physical function scores after 12 weeks, although the differences disappeared after 56 weeks. The results confirmed the role of CHOP chemotherapy as standard therapy for patients with aggressive lymphoma.

Remick et al. reported the efficacy and toxicity profile of an oral combination chemotherapy regimen in patients with acquired immunodeficiency syndrome–related non-Hodgkin's lymphoma (51). In the earlier part of the study, 18 patients were enrolled in the study, receiving five cycles of lomustine, etoposide, cyclophosphamide, and procarbazine. Subsequently, an additional 20 patients received a shortened duration of chemotherapy, with granulocyte colony-stimulating factor added to lessen myelosuppression. The Functional Living Index for Cancer (FLIC) (8), which assesses the functional status of daily living activities, and the Brief Symptom Inventory (54), which evaluates for psychological distress, were administered at baseline and on completion of treatment. The results showed that this novel chemotherapy regimen yielded response rates and median survival duration that compared favorably to other regimens for patients with acquired immunodeficiency syndrome–related lymphoma. Furthermore, with the addition of granulocyte colony-stimulating factor, the number of hospitalizations for febrile neutropenia was reduced by half. This translated to an effect on quality of life, as noted by the significant deterioration of the FLIC scores in patients who developed febrile neutropenia.

In the study of cutaneous lymphoma, quality-of-life considerations are of particular importance. Because of the nature of the disease and its treatment, patients are often plagued by pain and itching. Their physical appearance, role, and social functioning are also frequently adversely affected. In a prospective trial, the efficacy, safety, and pharmacokinetics of denileukin diftitox (52), a novel recombination fusion protein that has been shown to have antitumor effects in patients with cutaneous T-cell lymphoma that expresses interleukin-2R, was evaluated. Two dose levels were compared in a randomized fashion. In addition to reporting objective responses, patients were asked to independently assess subjective response and to assess the severity of pruritus using a visual analog scale. Furthermore, general quality of life was measured using the FACT-G questionnaire. Among patients who responded to treatment, more favorable pruritus scores, as well as quality-of-life composite scores, were observed.

A phase I–II trial evaluating another novel agent for cutaneous T-cell lymphoma was reported by the Bexarotene Worldwide Study Group (53). Ninety-four patients with advanced-stage cutaneous T-cell lymphoma were treated with bexarotene, an orally administered retinoid, at varying doses. The primary endpoint of the study was clinical response rate, but also included in the trial were quality-of-life parameters. The Spitzer Quality of Life Index (QLI) (9), which measures general status, and a nonvalidated cutaneous T-cell lymphoma–specific questionnaire were administered to patients on a monthly basis. Results showed that the Spitzer QLI did not change substantially over the course of the treatment, with the scores generally remaining high for both responders and nonresponders. The cutaneous T-cell lymphoma–specific questionnaire, however, did show an improvement from baseline to week 16 after treatment in both the level of pruritus and satisfaction with level of physical appearance.

Longitudinal Cross-Sectional Surveys

In cross-sectional quality-of-life studies, patients are typically at different time points in their clinical course. Therefore, unlike in prospective evaluation of quality of life as part of a clinical trial, it may be difficult to compare among patients within the study and to assess changes over time. However, this type of study design allows a one-time glimpse of patients' quality of life during or after treatment. The focus is generally on the long-term effect of the cancer diagnosis and treatment on patients' quality of life, and comparisons are often made with a normative population. A number of cross-sectional surveys have been conducted in survivors of Hodgkin's disease and other childhood malignancies evaluating various aspects of quality of life. Similar studies for non-Hodgkin's lymphoma are much more limited and of smaller scale, and they are summarized in Table 35.3 (55–58).

Wallwork et al. conducted a study interviewing a convenience sample of ten adult lymphoma patients at a minimum of 18 months after the completion of successful treatments (55). The Cancer Survivorship Questionnaire was used, which covered questions on abilities to perform daily activities, body function, health habits, self-image, relationships and support, work, social activities, spiritual issues, and

TABLE 35.3. *Longitudinal quality-of-life studies*

Author, yr (reference)	Disease	Design	Instruments
Wallwork, 1994 (55)	Lymphoma	Cross-sectional; recorded interview	Cancer survivorship question-naire
Dumontet, 1992 (56)	Aggressive lymphoma	Cross-sectional; self-administered questionnaire	Ad hoc survey evaluating work, sexual function, fertility, and other long-term sequelae
Guha-Thakurta, 1999 (57)	Primary central nervous system lymphoma	Cross-sectional; self-administered questionnaire	FACT-BR, SQ, SAS-SR, PSI
Wang, 2002 (58)	Hematologic malignancies (54% non-Hodgkin's lymphoma)	Cross-sectional; self-administered questionnaire	Brief Fatigue Inventory

FACT-BR, Functional Assessment of Cancer Therapy-Brain; PSI, Problem Solving Inventory; SAS-SR, Social Adjustment Scale Self-Report; SQ, Symptom Questionnaire.

health service contact. In this descriptive study, significant changes in patients' lives after treatment were noted, but most patients were accepting of the changes and were able to successfully adjust to their new lives.

In a study by Dumontet et al. (56), 100 patients with aggressive lymphoma were treated with a regimen consisting of three intensive courses of Adriamycin, cyclophosphamide, vindesine, and bleomycin, followed by consolidation and final intensification. The long-term sequelae of treatment were evaluated in 52 survivors at a median of 9.1 years after treatment. A questionnaire that covered job situations, sexual function, fertility, and other adverse physical and emotional effects was used. It was found that a large majority of patients were able to resume work and have children and overall reported an acceptable quality of life. The results led to the authors' conclusions that the dose intensity applied in the regimen offers satisfactory response without significantly compromising patients' long-term quality of life.

The quality of life of 11 patients with primary central nervous system lymphoma treated with high-dose methotrexate without radiation therapy was reported as part of a study by Guha-Thakurta et al. (57). All 11 patients had been in complete remission for a median duration of 16 months. Four self-administered questionnaires assessing different aspects of quality of life were used, including a modified FACT-Brain (FACT-BR), Symptom Questionnaire (SQ), Social Adjustment Scale Self-Report (SAS-SR), and Problem Solving Inventory (PSI). The mean total score on the modified FACT-BR was found to be significantly higher in the study population, compared with 26 pretreatment glioma patients. Compared with the normal population, however, survivors of primary central nervous system lymphoma had higher scores for depression and anxiety based on the SQ scores. Also, results from the SAS-SR and PSI showed that compared with the normal population, the study group had similar work, social/leisure, family interactions, marital functions, problem solving abilities, and stress coping abilities. Based on these results, it was concluded that patients with primary central nervous system lymphoma treated with high-dose systemic methotrexate maintain high levels of psychosocial adjustment and well-being.

Fatigue, which can significantly impair health-related quality of life, has been shown to be a prevalent problem among cancer survivors. In a cross-sectional study by Wang et al. (58), 228 patients with the diagnosis of a hematologic malignancy were asked to complete a demographic data sheet and the Brief Fatigue Inventory, a validated fatigue assessment instrument. Among the 122 patients with non-Hodgkin's lymphoma, 46% reported their fatigue as "severe." In these patients, the severe fatigue significantly interfered with their general activity, mood, walking ability, work, relationships with others, and enjoyment of life. On multivariate analysis, the presence of nausea and low albumin levels were significant predictors of fatigue. These results illustrate the substantial burden of cancer-related fatigue on patients, provide information on those who are more likely to experience the problem, and allow better understanding of the potential underlying mechanisms.

QUALITY-OF-LIFE STUDIES OF PATIENTS WITH BONE MARROW/STEM CELL TRANSPLANTATION

Many patients with various hematologic diseases that were previously considered fatal are now able to achieve long-term cure through high-dose therapy with bone marrow or hematopoietic stem cell rescue. Over the years, the efficacy and safety of high-dose therapy have improved, and its usefulness has expanded to include broader patient groups, leading to an increasing number of survivors of the procedure. Quality-of-life issues of these patients have become a topic of interest among researchers. Considerable data with varying focuses are available on the quality of life of patients who are undergoing or have undergone high-dose therapy with bone marrow or peripheral stem cell support.

Recovery in the Posttransplantation Period

A number of studies prospectively followed and assessed the quality of life of patients after high-dose therapy with bone marrow or stem cell transplantation. At Stanford University, the quality of life of 58 patients was evaluated every 90 days posttransplant until 1 year after the autologous bone marrow transplantation (59). Twenty-three of the 58 patients had non-Hodgkin's lymphoma, and the remaining patients had Hodgkin's disease or leukemia. A "home-grown" telephone questionnaire that addressed physical concerns, sleep patterns, colds, occupational functioning, sexual functioning, body image, and global quality of life was administered. Results at 90 days and 1 year were reported, but pretransplant quality-of-life data were not available. It was found that the quality-of-life ratings of patients with non-Hodgkin's lymphoma were the highest, compared with other patient groups. The overall quality of life improved significantly from 90 days to 1 year posttransplant. By the end of 1 year of follow-up, most ratings had increased, and the differences between groups had disappeared.

Similar findings were reported in another prospective quality-of-life study in which patients who underwent allogeneic versus autologous stem cell transplantation were evaluated (60). The EORTC QLQ-C30 was given to patients pretransplant and at several time points until 1 year after the transplantation. As noted in the previous study, the majority of patients recovered reasonably well 1 year posttransplant, especially in the physical function domain.

Investigators have also attempted to identify ways to improve the physical and psychological well-being of patients undergoing bone marrow or stem cell transplantation. Courneya et al. conducted a study designed to examine the relationship between physical exercise and quality of life of 25 patients undergoing autologous bone marrow transplantation (61). Patients were asked to recall their exercise levels before the diagnosis and before the transplantation. During the course of hospitalization, patients were asked to prospectively record their exercise patterns. Quality-of-life assessments were made on a weekly basis after the baseline assessment until discharge. The FACT-Bone Marrow Transplant Scale, which also included a Fatigue Scale, was used to assess quality of life. In addition, the Affect Balance Scale, measuring psychological well-being; the Satisfaction with Life Scale; Center for Epidemiological Studies Depression Scale; and State-Trait Anxiety Inventory were administered. A significant correlation was found between exercise and physical and psychological well-being. Level of exercise also correlated negatively with depression and anxiety. The results suggested a potential role of exercise in the rehabilitation of bone marrow or stem cell transplantation patients.

Psychosocial Consequences

The psychosocial consequences of bone marrow transplantation appear to persist longer over time. In a study by Broers et al., the psychological functioning and quality of life of patients were prospectively evaluated from baseline to 3 years posttransplant (62). In this study, six self-reported instruments were used, including the Functional Limitations Battery, the General Health Questionnaire, the revised Symptom Checklist-90 (SCL-90), the Health Locus of Control Scale, Rosenberg's Self-Esteem Scale, and a two-item general quality-of-life instrument. It was found that up to one fourth of patients had persistent psychological distress based on the SCL-90 scores,

especially in depression and anxiety. The main predictor of long-term psychological problems was patients' baseline psychological functioning, suggesting that increased attention should be paid to patients with underlying psychological distress before the transplantation.

Baker et al. reported results of 84 bone marrow transplantation patients who completed interviews regarding quality of life and psychosocial adaptation before, at 6 months, and at 1 year after transplantation (63). The three main areas of concern addressed by the interview included physical, psychological, and community reintegration. Fear about the future was a psychological problem identified by more than one third of the patients at 6 months, and the fear persisted in one fourth of the patients at 1 year. Patients also reported problems in returning to former social roles, dealing with stigmatization, and financial and employment difficulties. The results suggest the need to prepare patients and families for life after the transplantation. Patients deemed to be at high risk for psychosocial maladaptation may benefit from problem-solving training and psychosocial rehabilitation programs.

Andrykowski et al. attempted to identify predictors of psychosocial concerns in 110 patients at a mean of 17 months after stem cell transplantation (64). A nonvalidated Stem Cell Transplant Concerns Questionnaire was used, which consisted of 30 items, each identifying a specific area of potential concern to stem cell transplant recipients. Women, younger patients, and patients with low performance status reported more current or past concerns on the questionnaire, whereas education level, income, type of stem cell transplantation, and type of malignant diagnosis were not predictive.

Fatigue

A number of somatic and psychiatric conditions may contribute to fatigue, but its pathophysiology and optimal management remain largely unclear. The prevalence of fatigue and the health-related quality of life of 85 patients with malignant lymphoma more than 3 years after autologous bone marrow transplantation were evaluated by Knobel et al. (65). In this cross-sectional study, the Fatigue Questionnaire, which measures both physical and mental fatigue, and the EORTC QLQ-C30 were used. Physical fatigue was found to be significantly more prevalent in the patient group, compared with the general population. Women reported significantly more total and physical fatigue, compared with men and with the general population. Similar findings were noted in the study by Baker et al. (63), in which fatigue was the most common physical symptom experienced by the survivors. It was reported by half of the patients at 6 months, and it persisted in 40% of patients at 1 year.

Factors Predicting for Impaired Quality of Life Posttransplantation

The relationship between treatment and patient factors and health-related quality of life after transplantation has been addressed in a number of studies. Researchers have shown that quality of life differs between patients who undergo allogeneic transplants and those who undergo autologous transplantation. In the study by Hjermstad et al., at baseline before the transplantation, the allogeneic stem cell transplantation group had consistently higher functional scores and less symptomatology than the autologous stem cell transplantation group (60). After 1 year, however, the scores of patients who underwent allogeneic stem cell transplantation remained relatively unchanged, whereas the scores of those who underwent autologous stem cell transplantation improved significantly, with the greatest differences found in social function, role function, fatigue, constipation, and appetite. The differences were attributed to the different underlying malignancies in the two groups, and the fact that patients in the allogeneic transplantation group, who all had leukemia, were more heavily pretreated and had multiple relapses or refractory disease at the time of transplantation. The two types of transplantation were also compared in a cross-sectional study by Andrykowski et al. (66). In this study, the quality of life of patients who were more than 1 year posttransplantation was assessed. Among several factors evaluated, allogeneic bone marrow transplantation was found to be a significant predictor of inferior quality of life.

The source of transplantation has also been shown to influence quality of life. A study from Japan used the FLIC to evaluate the quality of life of 282 survivors at a median of 35 months after stem cell transplantation (67). Patients who underwent unrelated allogeneic transplantation had significantly lower ratings on relief from pain, stability in weight, and confidence in dealing with daily life, compared with patients who underwent related allogeneic transplantation. Vellenga et al. conducted a phase III study comparing autologous peripheral blood stem cell transplantation with bone marrow transplantation in patients with relapsed or refractory non-Hodgkin's lymphoma (68). Quality-of-life assessment was performed using the EuroQoL, SF-36, and Rotterdam Symptom Checklist (RSCL) at baseline, and 14 days and 3 months posttransplantation. At 14 days, the RSCL physical and activity domain scores were significantly better in the peripheral stem cell transplantation arm, and the more favorable activity domain scores persisted at 3 months.

Factors other than treatment type for predicting quality of life have also been evaluated. In the study from Stanford University, the global quality of life 90 days posttransplantation was found to be significantly influenced by employment status, appetite, sleep patterns, and body image (59). Hjermstad et al. found that 1 year after transplantation, patients who relapsed had significantly inferior global quality of life and physical and social function and more fatigue, dyspnea, and sleep disturbances (60). Older patients and patients who were living alone also had significantly lower global quality of life. Among 200 patients who were more than 1 year posttransplantation, Andrykowski et al. reported that lower education level, allogeneic transplantation, advanced-stage disease, shorter time since transplantation, and older age at treatment significantly predicted for poorer quality-of-life

status (66). In addition, patients with chronic graft-versus-host disease reported more concerns regarding decreases in attractiveness. The cross-sectional study from Japan on survivors of transplantation also found that time since transplantation and diagnosis of chronic graft-versus-host disease were significantly associated with reduced total current functioning score on the FLIC (67).

SUMMARY

As in many other disease sites, information on quality of life of patients with non-Hodgkin's lymphoma is accumulating. To capture the impact of the cancer and its treatment on health-related quality of life, the report of toxicity data as part of a clinical trial is no longer considered adequate. Quality-of-life data should be assessed by well-validated instruments rather than ad hoc surveys and administered at baseline as well as over time. In addition, effort should also be put into improving the compliance rate and response rate in quality-of-life studies. Future directions in the field include the development of multidimensional, lymphoma-specific quality-of-life instruments and exploring strategies that enhance posttreatment quality of life in specific patient groups. As quality-of-life studies on lymphoma patients increase in number and improve in quality, the results may provide important insights into the treatment design, counseling, and follow-up of patients with various types of non-Hodgkin's lymphoma.

REFERENCES

1. Constitution of the World Health Organization. *World Health Organization. Handbook of basic documents,* 5th ed. Geneva, Switzerland, 1952:3–20.
2. Aaronson NK, Ahmedzai S, Bergman B, et al. The European Organization for Research and Treatment of Cancer QLQ-C30: a quality-of-life instrument for use in international clinical trials in oncology. *J Natl Cancer Inst* 1993;85:365–376.
3. Cella DF, Tulsky DS, Gray G, et al. The Functional Assessment of Cancer Therapy scale: development and validation of the general measure. *J Clin Oncol* 1993;11:570–579.
4. Stewart A, Sherbourne C, Hays R, et al. Summary and discussion of MOS measures. In: Stewart AL, Ware JE, eds. *Measuring functioning and well-being: the Medical Outcomes Study approach.* Durham, NC: Duke University Press 1992:345–371.
5. Ganz PA, Schag CA, Lee JJ, et al. The CARES: a generic measure of health-related quality of life for patients with cancer. *Qual Life Res* 1992;1:19–29.
6. Bruera E, Kuehn N, Miller MJ, et al. The Edmonton Symptom Assessment System (ESAS): a simple method for the assessment of palliative care patients. *J Palliat Care* 1991;7:6–9.
7. Cella DF, Tulsky DS, Gray G, et al. The Functional Assessment of Cancer Therapy scale: development and validation of the general measure. *J Clin Oncol* 1993;11:570–579.
8. Schipper H, Clinch J, McMurray A, et al. Measuring the quality of life of cancer patients: the Functional Living Index-Cancer: development and validation. *J Clin Oncol* 1984;2:472–483.
9. Spitzer WO, Dobson AJ, Hall J, et al. Measuring the quality of life of cancer patients: a concise QL-index for use by physicians. *J Chronic Dis* 1981;34:585–597.
10. Gelber RD, Goldhirsch A, Cole BF. Evaluation of effectiveness: Q-TWiST. The International Breast Cancer Study Group. *Cancer Treat Rev* 1993;19:73–84.
11. Chang VT, Hwang SS, Feuerman M. Validation of the Edmonton Symptom Assessment Scale. *Cancer* 2000;88:2164–2171.

12. Portenoy RK, Thaler HT, Kornblith AB, et al. The Memorial Symptom Assessment Scale: an instrument for the evaluation of symptom prevalence, characteristics and distress. *Eur J Cancer* 1994;9:1326–1336.

13. Stiggelbout AM, de Haes JC, Kiebert GM, et al. Tradeoffs between quality and quantity of life: development of the QQ Questionnaire for Cancer Patient Attitudes. *Med Decis Making* 1996;16:184–192.

14. Padilla GV, Presant C, Grant MM, et al. Quality of life index for patients with cancer. *Res Nurs Health* 1983;6:117–126.

15. Karnofsky D, Burchenal J. The clinical evaluation of chemotherapeutic agents in cancer. In: Macleod CM, ed. *Evaluation of chemotherapeutic agents*. New York: Columbia University Press, 1949:199–205.

16. Lohr KN, Aaronson NK, Alonso J, et al. Evaluating quality-of-life and health status instruments: development of scientific review criteria. *Clin Ther* 1996;18:979–992.

17. Sprangers MA, Cull A, Groenvold M, et al. The European Organization for Research and Treatment of Cancer approach to developing questionnaire modules: an update and overview. EORTC Quality of Life Study Group. *Qual Life Res* 1998;7:291–300.

18. Anderson JP, Kaplan RM, Berry CC, et al. Interday reliability of function assessment for a health status measure. The Quality of Well-Being scale. *Med Care* 1989;27:1076–1083.

19. EuroQoL Group. EuroQoL: a new facility for the measurement of health-related quality of life. *Health Policy* 1990;16:199–208.

20. Torrance GW, Furlong W, Feeny D, et al. Multi-attribute preference functions. Health Utilities Index. *Pharmacoeconomics* 1995;7:503–520.

21. Harris NL, Jaffe ES, Stein H, et al. A revised European-American classification of lymphoid neoplasms: a proposal from the International Lymphoma Study Group. *Blood* 1994;84:1361–1392.

22. Armitage JO, Weisenburger DD. New approach to classifying non-Hodgkin's lymphomas: clinical features of the major histologic subtypes. Non-Hodgkin's Lymphoma Classification Project. *J Clin Oncol* 1998;16:2780–2795.

23. Klimo P, Connors JM. MACOP-B chemotherapy for the treatment of diffuse large-cell lymphoma. *Ann Intern Med* 1985;102:596–602.

24. Coiffier B, Bryon PA, Berger F, et al. Intensive and sequential combination chemotherapy for aggressive malignant lymphomas (protocol LNH-80). *J Clin Oncol* 1986;4:147–153.

25. Lee R, Cabanillas F, Bodey GP, et al. A 10-year update of CHOP-bleo in the treatment of diffuse large-cell lymphoma. *J Clin Oncol* 1986;4:1455–1461.

26. Boyd DB, Coleman M, Papish SW, et al. COPBLAM III: infusional combination chemotherapy for diffuse large-cell lymphoma. *J Clin Oncol* 1988;6:425–433.

27. Shipp MA, Yeap BY, Harrington DP, et al. The m-BACOD combination chemotherapy regimen in large-cell lymphoma: analysis of the completed trial and comparison with the M-BACOD regimen. *J Clin Oncol* 1990;8:84–93.

28. Longo DL, DeVita VT Jr, Duffey PL, et al. Superiority of ProMACE-CytaBOM over ProMACE-MOPP in the treatment of advanced diffuse aggressive lymphoma: results of a prospective randomized trial. *J Clin Oncol* 1991;9:25–38.

29. Fisher RI, Gaynor ER, Dahlberg S, et al. Comparison of a standard regimen (CHOP) with three intensive chemotherapy regimens for advanced non-Hodgkin's lymphoma. *N Engl J Med* 1993;328:1002–1006.

30. Coiffier B, Lepage E, Briere J, et al. CHOP chemotherapy plus rituximab compared with CHOP alone in elderly patients with diffuse large-B-cell lymphoma. *N Engl J Med* 2002;346:235–242.

31. Philip T, Guglielmi C, Hagenbeek A, et al. Autologous bone marrow transplantation as compared with salvage chemotherapy in relapses of chemotherapy-sensitive non-Hodgkin's lymphoma. *N Engl J Med* 1995;333:1540–1545.

32. Gianni AM, Bregni M, Siena S, et al. High-dose chemotherapy and autologous bone marrow transplantation compared with MACOP-B in aggressive B-cell lymphoma. *N Engl J Med* 1997;336:1290–1297.

33. Santini G, Salvagno L, Leoni P, et al. VACOP-B versus VACOP-B plus autologous bone marrow transplantation for advanced diffuse non-Hodgkin's lymphoma: results of a prospective randomized trial by the non-Hodgkin's Lymphoma Cooperative Study Group. *J Clin Oncol* 1998;16:2796–2802.

34. Haioun C, Lepage E, Gisselbrecht C, et al. Survival benefit of high-dose therapy in poor-risk aggressive non-Hodgkin's lymphoma: final analysis of the prospective LNH87-2 protocol—a Groupe d'Etude des Lymphomes de l'Adulte study. *J Clin Oncol* 2000;18:3025–3030.

35. Fobair P, Hoppe RT, Bloom J, et al. Psychosocial problems among survivors of Hodgkin's disease. *J Clin Oncol* 1986;4:805–814.

36. Cella DF, Tross S. Psychological adjustment to survival from Hodgkin's disease. *J Consult Clin Psychol* 1986;54:616–622.

37. Siegel K, Christ G. *Psychosocial consequences in Hodgkin's disease: the consequences of survival*. Philadelphia: Lea & Febiger, 1990:383-399.

38. Kornblith AB, Anderson J, Cella DF, et al. Hodgkin disease survivors at increased risk for problems in psychosocial adaptation. The Cancer and Leukemia Group B. *Cancer* 1992;70:2214–2224.

39. van Tulder MW, Aaronson NK, Bruning PF. The quality of life of long-term survivors of Hodgkin's disease. *Ann Oncol* 1994;5:153–158.

40. Joly F, Henry-Amar M, Arveux P, et al. Late psychosocial sequelae in Hodgkin's disease survivors: a French population-based case-control study. *J Clin Oncol* 1996;14:2444–2453.

41. Loge JH, Abrahamsen AF, Ekeberg O, et al. Psychological distress after cancer cure: a survey of 459 Hodgkin's disease survivors. *Br J Cancer* 1997;76:791–796.

42. Flechtner H, Ruffer JU, Henry-Amar M, et al. Quality of life assessment in Hodgkin's disease: a new comprehensive approach. First experiences from the EORTC/GELA and GHSG trials. EORTC Lymphoma Cooperative Group. Groupe D'Etude des Lymphomes de l'Adulte and German Hodgkin Study Group. *Ann Oncol* 1998;9:S147–S154.

43. Loge JH, Abrahamsen AF, Ekeberg O, et al. Hodgkin's disease survivors more fatigued than the general population. *J Clin Oncol* 1999;17:253–261.

44. Loge JH, Abrahamsen AF, Ekeberg O, et al. Reduced health-related quality of life among Hodgkin's disease survivors: a comparative study with general population norms. *Ann Oncol* 1999;10:71–77.

45. Loge JH, Abrahamsen AF, Ekeberg O, et al. Fatigue and psychiatric morbidity among Hodgkin's disease survivors. *J Pain Symptom Manage* 2000;19:91–99.

46. Aviles A, Duque G, Talavera A, et al. Interferon alpha 2b as maintenance therapy in low grade malignant lymphoma improves duration of remission and survival. *Leuk Lymphoma* 1996;20:495–499.

47. Cole BF, Solal-Celigny P, Gelber RD, et al. Quality-of-life-adjusted survival analysis of interferon alfa-2b treatment for advanced follicular lymphoma: an aid to clinical decision making. *J Clin Oncol* 1998;16:2339–2344.

48. Mounier N, Haioun C, Cole BF, et al. Quality of life-adjusted survival analysis of high-dose therapy with autologous bone marrow transplantation versus sequential chemotherapy for patients with aggressive lymphoma in first complete remission. Groupe d'Etude des Lymphomes de l'Adulte (GELA). *Blood* 2000;95:3687–3692.

49. Gordon LI, Witzig TE, Wiseman GA, et al. Yttrium 90 ibritumomab tiuxetan radioimmunotherapy for relapsed or refractory low-grade non-Hodgkin's lymphoma. *Semin Oncol* 2002;29:87–92.

50. Jerkeman M, Anderson H, Cavallin-Stahl E, et al. CHOP versus MACOP-B in aggressive lymphoma—a Nordic Lymphoma Group randomised trial. *Ann Oncol* 1999;10:1079–1086.

51. Remick SC, Sedransk N, Haase RF, et al. Oral combination chemotherapy in conjunction with filgrastim (G-CSF) in the treatment of AIDS-related non-Hodgkin's lymphoma: evaluation of the role of G-CSF; quality-of-life analysis and long-term follow-up. *Am J Hematol* 2001;66:178–188.

52. Olsen E, Duvic M, Frankel A, et al. Pivotal phase III trial of two dose levels of denileukin diftitox for the treatment of cutaneous T-cell lymphoma. *J Clin Oncol* 2001;19:376–388.

53. Duvic M, Hymes K, Heald P, et al. Bexarotene is effective and safe for treatment of refractory advanced-stage cutaneous T-cell lymphoma: multinational phase II-III trial results. *J Clin Oncol* 2001;19: 2456–2471.

54. Derogatis LR, Melisaratos N. The Brief Symptom Inventory: an introductory report. *Psychol Med* 1983;13:595–605.

55. Wallwork L, Richardson A. Beyond cancer: changes, problems and needs expressed by adult lymphoma survivors attending an out-patients clinic. *Eur J Cancer Care (Engl)* 1994;3:122–132.

56. Dumontet C, Bastion Y, Felman P, et al. Long-term outcome and sequelae in aggressive lymphoma patients treated with the LNH-80 regimen. *Ann Oncol* 1992;3:639–644.

57. Guha-Thakurta N, Damek D, Pollack C, et al. Intravenous methotrexate as initial treatment for primary central nervous system lymphoma: response to therapy and quality of life of patients. *J Neurooncol* 1999; 43:259–268.

58. Wang X, Giralt S, Mendoza T, et al. Clinical factors associated with cancer-related fatigue in patients being treated for leukemia and non-Hodgkin's lymphoma. *J Clin Oncol* 2002;20:1319–1328.

59. Chao NJ, Tierney DK, Bloom JR, et al. Dynamic assessment of quality of life after autologous bone marrow transplantation. *Blood* 1992;80:825–830.

60. Hjermstad MJ, Evensen SA, Kvaloy SO, et al. Health-related quality of life 1 year after allogeneic or autologous stem-cell transplantation: a prospective study. *J Clin Oncol* 1999;17:706–718.

61. Courneya KS, Keats MR, Turner AR. Physical exercise and quality of life in cancer patients following high dose chemotherapy and autologous bone marrow transplantation. *Psychooncology* 2000;9:127–136.

62. Broers S, Kaptein AA, Le Cessie S, et al. Psychological functioning and quality of life following bone marrow transplantation: a 3-year follow-up study. *J Psychosom Res* 2000;48:11–21.

63. Baker F, Zabora J, Polland A, et al. Reintegration after bone marrow transplantation. *Cancer Pract* 1999;7:190–197.

64. Andrykowski MA, Cordova MJ, Hann DM, et al. Patients' psychosocial concerns following stem cell transplantation. *Bone Marrow Transplant* 1999;24:1121–1129.

65. Knobel H, Loge JH, Nordoy T, et al. High level of fatigue in lymphoma patients treated with high dose therapy. *J Pain Symptom Manage* 2000;19:446–456.

66. Andrykowski MA, Greiner CB, Altmaier EM, et al. Quality of life following bone marrow transplantation: findings from a multicentre study. *Br J Cancer* 1995;71:1322–1329.

67. Yano K, Kanie T, Okamoto S, et al. Quality of life in adult patients after stem cell transplantation. *Int J Hematol* 2000;71:283–289.

68. Vellenga E, van Agthoven M, Croockewit AJ, et al. Autologous peripheral blood stem cell transplantation in patients with relapsed lymphoma results in accelerated haematopoietic reconstitution, improved quality of life and cost reduction compared with bone marrow transplantation: the Hovon 22 study. *Br J Haematol* 2001;114:319–326.

SECTION VI

Special Topics

CHAPTER 36

Management of Lymphoma in Children

John T. Sandlund, Karen J. Marcus, and Frederick G. Behm

The malignant lymphomas, which include both Hodgkin's disease and non-Hodgkin's lymphoma, are the third most common malignancies of childhood; only acute lymphoblastic leukemia and brain tumors are more common (1–8). Among children younger than 15 years, approximately 60% of cases are non-Hodgkin's lymphoma; however, among children younger than 18 years, there is a slight predominance of Hodgkin's disease (4,5,8).

There are significant differences between the non-Hodgkin's lymphomas that occur in children and in adults. The pediatric non-Hodgkin's lymphomas are primarily aggressive tumors, whereas in adults, indolent low-grade lymphomas are more common (9,10). Children with non-Hodgkin's lymphomas often present with diffuse extranodal disease, whereas adults more frequently present with primary nodal disease. These differences in histologic subtype likely reflect age-related differences in the immune system and associated susceptibility to malignant transformation (2,10).

Dramatic improvements have been made in our understanding of these diseases with respect to pathogenesis, diagnosis, and treatment. As survival rates have improved, efforts to refine therapy have in part focused on reducing or eliminating the risk of treatment-related late effects such as cardiotoxicity, infertility, and second malignancy. This chapter reviews these advances and discusses future directions.

EPIDEMIOLOGY

Approximately 500 new cases of pediatric non-Hodgkin's lymphoma are diagnosed each year in the United States (5–8). The median age at the time of diagnosis is approximately 10 years (3). Although non-Hodgkin's lymphoma can occur at any age, it is less common in children younger than 3 years (3,11). Unlike Hodgkin's disease, which has a bimodal age distribution, non-Hodgkin's lymphoma continues to increase in frequency with advancing age. For reasons that have yet to be elucidated, non-Hodgkin's lymphoma is more common in the white than in the black population and is two to three times more common in males than in females (2,3).

There are specific populations of children who are at increased risk of non-Hodgkin's lymphoma (1–3). These groups include children with congenital immunodeficiency disorders such as Wiskott-Aldrich syndrome, ataxia-telangiectasia (12), and X-linked lymphoproliferative syndrome. It is important that these underlying conditions be recognized so that an appropriate management plan can be designed. For example, in children with ataxia-telangiectasia, electron beam irradiation and use of radiomimetics such as bleomycin should be avoided, and judicious use of diagnostic x-rays is recommended. Additionally, patients with ataxia-telangiectasia are at a much higher risk of hemorrhagic cystitis when treated with cyclophosphamide or ifosfamide; thus, vigorous hydration and mesna uroprotection should be implemented, even when low doses of these chemotherapeutic agents are used. Boys with X-linked lymphoproliferative syndrome are at risk of both fatal infectious mononucleosis and B-cell lymphoma. Because allogeneic bone marrow transplantation may be a treatment option for children with X-linked lymphoproliferative syndrome, the diagnosis should be considered in any male patient who presents with a B-cell lymphoma and whose brother has had either fatal infectious mononucleosis or B-cell lymphoma, or in any male who has two primary B-cell lymphomas. Children with acquired immunodeficiency conditions are also at increased risk for non-Hodgkin's lymphoma (13–18). This group comprises children who are recipients of bone marrow or organ transplants and those who have the acquired immunodeficiency syndrome.

CLASSIFICATION

There are three major subtypes of non-Hodgkin's lymphoma in children: Burkitt's, lymphoblastic, and large-cell lymphoma. These groupings are recognized in the National Cancer Institute's Working Formulation (9), the Revised European-American Lymphoma (REAL) Classification (19), and the World Health Organization (WHO) Classification of Tumors of Haematopoietic and Lymphoid Tissues (20). Table 36.1 summarizes the different classification terms used by these three schemes for the three major pediatric lymphoma subtypes. According to the National Cancer Institute's Working Formula-

TABLE 36.1. *Comparison of the updated REAL/WHO lymphoma classifications with the NCI Working Formulation for pediatric lymphomas*

Updated REAL and WHO classifications	NCI Working Formulation
Common pediatric lymphomas	
B-cell lymphomas	
Precursor B-lymphoblastic lymphoma/leukemia	Lymphoblastic
Burkitt's lymphoma	Small noncleaved cell, Burkitt's or non-Burkitt's
Diffuse large B-cell lymphoma	Diffuse large-cell/large-cell immunoblastic
Mediastinal (thymic) large B-cell lymphoma	Diffuse large cell/large-cell immunoblastic
T-cell lymphomas	
Precursor T-lymphoblastic lymphoma/leukemia	Lymphoblastic
Anaplastic large-cell lymphoma	Diffuse large-cell, immunoblastic
Peripheral T-cell lymphoma	Diffuse, mixed small- and large-cell/large-cell immunoblastic
Uncommon pediatric lymphomas	
Follicular lymphoma (grade 1, 2, or 3)	Follicular, small cleaved, mixed small and large, or large-cell
Hepatosplenic T-cell lymphoma	Not recognized

NCI, National Cancer Institute; REAL, Revised European-American Lymphoma; WHO, World Health Organization.

Adapted from National Cancer Institute sponsored study of classification of non-Hodgkin's lymphoma. Summary and description of a working formulation for clinical usage. *Cancer* 1982;49:2112–2135; Harris NL, Jaffe ES, Stein H, et al. A revised European-American classification of lymphoid neoplasms: a proposal from the International Lymphoma Study Group. *Blood* 1994;84;1361–1392; and Jaffe ES, Harris NL, Stein H, et al., eds. *World Health Organization classification of tumors. Pathology and genetics of tumors of haematopoietic and lymphoid tissues.* Lyon, France: IARC Press, 2001.

tion, which incorporates both morphologic features and clinical aggressiveness, the majority of pediatric lymphomas are high-grade lesions. The more recent REAL and WHO systems incorporate additional histopathologic and genetic features. Table 36.2 summarizes the clinical and biologic features of each main subtype. For the classification of pediatric lymphoma, the REAL and WHO classifications are comparable, and both are significant improvements over the older Working Formulation that did not recognize anaplastic large-cell lymphoma and mediastinal B-cell large-cell lymphoma.

Burkitt's Lymphoma

Burkitt's lymphoma is the designation for lymphomas classified as "small noncleaved cell lymphoma" in the Lukes-Collins Classification and the National Cancer Institute Working Formulation (9,21) (Table 36.1). Lukes and Collins coined the term "small noncleaved cell lymphomas" because of the morphologic and biologic resemblance of the malignant lymphoid cells to similar cells in the normal lymph node germinal center. The intent of the authors of these systems was to separate this neoplastic process from large-cell lymphomas with large noncleaved cells. Large noncleaved cell lymphomas were also thought to resemble another type of germinal center cell. However, the cells of small noncleaved cell lymphoma are larger than those of small lymphocytic lymphoma and most lymphoblastic lymphomas. The size of the cells in small noncleaved cell lymphoma may even approach that of some larger-cell lymphomas. In the updated REAL and new WHO classifications, "small noncleaved cell lymphoma" is replaced by Burkitt's lymphoma (19,20). The REAL and WHO classifications also combine the L3-acute lymphoblastic leukemia of the French-American-British classification of acute leukemia with Burkitt's lymphoma. Indeed, most, but not all, L3-acute lymphoblastic leukemia appears to be the leukemic phase of Burkitt's lymphoma (22). Biologic differences between Burkitt's lymphoma and primary Burkitt's leukemia have not been reported.

Classical Burkitt's lymphoma consists of a diffuse infiltrative pattern of uniform, medium-sized cells with moderate amounts of basophilic cytoplasm (19,20). The cells have round nuclei, clumped or condensed chromatin with clear parachromatin, and 1 to 3 nucleoli. The malignant cells characteristically have multiple, small, clear, cytoplasmic vacuoles. A "starry-sky" appearance imparted by interspersed tingible body macrophages is usually present. Frequent mitotic and apoptotic cells are present and reflect this lymphoma's high proliferative rate and apoptotic index, respectively.

The WHO Classification also recognizes two morphologic variants: Burkitt's lymphoma with plasmacytoid differentiation and atypical Burkitt's or Burkitt-like lymphoma (20). In the former variant, many of the tumor cells have eccentrically placed nuclei with a single central nucleolus, which are features of plasma cells (19,20). This variant is not uncommon in children and is frequently found in immunodeficiency-related Burkitt's lymphomas (23). No prognostic significance in children has been described for this variant.

The cells of the other variant, atypical Burkitt's or Burkitt-like lymphoma, display greater pleomorphism in nuclear size and shape and fewer but larger nucleoli. These morphologic features can make this variant difficult to differentiate from large B-cell lymphoma. To be considered a variant of Burkitt's lymphoma, these lymphomas should have evidence of a MYC translocation such as the t(8;14), t(8;22), or t(2;8). However, MYC translocations may also be present in some large B-cell lymphomas. In classical Burkitt's lymphoma, MYC deregulation causes almost 100% of the tumor cells to be in cell cycle. This proliferative activity can be detected with anti-Ki-67 antibodies, and almost all of the Burkitt's lymphoma cells will express Ki-67. The WHO committee suggests that a "Burkitt-like" lymphoma diagnosis should be

TABLE 36.2. *Clinical and biologic characteristics of non-Hodgkin's lymphoma in children*

Subtype	Proportion of cases (%)[a]	Phenotype	Primary site	Translocation	Affected genes
Burkitt's	39	B-cell	Abdomen or head and neck	t(8;14)(q24;q32)	IgH-MYC
				t(2;8)(p11;q24)	Igκ-MYC
				t(8;22)(q24;q11)	Igλ-MYC
Lymphoblastic	28	T-cell[b]	Mediastinum or head and neck	t(1;14)(p32;q11)	TCRαδ-TAL1
				t(11;14)(p13;q11)	TCRαδ-RHOMB2
				t(11;14)(p15;q11)	TCRαδ-RHOMB1
				t(10;14)(q24;q11)	TCRαδ-HOX11
				t(7;19)(q35;p13)	TCRβ-LYL1
				t(8;14)(q24;q11)	TCRαδ-MYC
				t(1;7)(p34;q34)	TCRβ-LCK
Large cell	26	B-cell, T-cell[c], indeterminate[c]	Mediastinum, abdomen, head and neck, or skin[c]	t(2;5)(p23;q35)[c]	NPM-ALK

Ig, immunoglobulin; TCR, T-cell receptor.
[a]Proportion at St. Jude Children's Research Hospital; other histotypes account for approximately 7%.
[b]B-cell progenitor variants have also been described.
[c]Associated with anaplastic large-cell lymphoma subtype: approximately 10% of childhood non-Hodgkin's lymphoma.
Adapted from Sandlund JT, Downing JR, Crist WM. Non-Hodgkin's lymphoma in children. *N Engl J Med* 1996;334:1238–1248.

made for tumors with morphologic features intermediate between Burkitt's lymphoma and diffuse large B-cell lymphoma in which the Ki-67 fraction of viable cells is at least 99% or a MYC translocation is present (24). Lymphomas with features typical of large-cell lymphoma plus a MYC translocation or a very high Ki-67–positive fraction and Burkitt-like lymphomas with a low Ki-67 index should be classified as diffuse large B-cell lymphomas (24). It is not known whether large-cell lymphomas with a MYC translocation and high proliferative rate will respond to the therapy used for Burkitt's lymphoma. The atypical Burkitt's variant is more common in adults than in children, and its clinical significance in children remains controversial (25).

Burkitt's lymphoma and its variants have a characteristic immunophenotypic profile: CD19+, strongly CD20+, CD22+, CD79α+, and Ki-67+ with moderately strong expression of surface immunoglobulin M or, less commonly, immunoglobulin A or immunoglobulin G, with light chain κ or λ restriction (26). Nuclear bcl-6 is present without evidence of BCL6 rearrangement (27). Markers CD5, CD34, bcl-2, and terminal deoxynucleotidyl transferase (Tdt) are negative. CD10 is expressed in almost half of cases and is often cited as evidence of a germinal center origin. CD21, the receptor for complement fragment Cd3 and the Epstein-Barr virus (EBV), is more frequently detected in the endemic than sporadic form. A small percentage of Burkitt's lymphomas have cytoplasmic immunoglobulin μ with no detectable surface immunoglobulin and a rare case may have neither (28,29). These unusual Burkitt's lymphomas, unlike B-lymphoblastic lymphomas, do not express CD34 or Tdt, strongly express CD20, and have a MYC translocation.

Translocations of MYC on chromosome 8 at band q24 to the immunoglobulin heavy-chain locus on chromosome band

14 q32, the lambda immunoglobulin light chain loci on 2q11, or 22q11 are found in all cases of Burkitt's lymphoma. The t(8;14)(q24;q32) occurs in approximately 80% of Burkitt's lymphomas (30). The breakpoint on chromosome 14 in endemic Burkitt's lymphoma involves the heavy chain joining region. Sporadic cases demonstrate a translocation of MYC to the immunoglobulin switch region. As a result of these translocations, MYC comes under the influence of the promoter region of the immunoglobulin genes, resulting in constitutive expression of MYC (31). The deregulation of MYC drives cells through the cell cycle and activates genes involved in apoptosis. As noted above, MYC translocations are not entirely specific for Burkitt's lymphoma, having been reported in large B-cell lymphomas, follicular lymphomas, and precursor B-lymphoblastic transformation of follicular lymphoma. MYC translocations are relatively easily detected by classic cytogenetic methods and more recently by fluorescence *in situ* hybridization of interphase nuclei (32).

Epidemiology

The incidence and distribution of histologic subtypes of non-Hodgkin's lymphoma in children differ geographically (4,33–37). Although non-Hodgkin's lymphoma is very rare in Japan, it is very common in equatorial Africa (36). The Burkitt's subtype is the most common childhood malignancy in equatorial Africa and is the most common histologic subtype of non-Hodgkin's lymphoma in northeastern Brazil and areas of the Middle East (35). In contrast, the predominant histologic subtype in Southern India is lymphoblastic lymphoma (35).

Burkitt's lymphoma is of particular interest with respect to the geographic variation of clinical and biologic features

(36). The endemic subtype, which occurs in equatorial Africa, is characterized clinically by younger age at diagnosis and by frequent involvement of the jaw, abdomen, orbit, and paraspinal area (35–37). In contrast, the sporadic subtype (which occurs in the United States and Western Europe) is characterized by an older median age at diagnosis and frequent involvement of the abdomen, nasopharynx, and bone marrow (35–37). There are also geographic differences with respect to location of the MYC breakpoint in Burkitt's lymphoma cells. Among sporadic cases, the breakpoint tends to occur within the MYC gene, whereas it tends to occur upstream of the MYC gene in endemic cases (36).

The association of EBV with Burkitt's lymphoma has also been shown to vary with geographic location (36,37). The overlap of the Burkitt's lymphoma belt and the malaria belt in equatorial Africa first suggested the involvement of an infectious agent in Burkitt's lymphoma pathogenesis. This hypothesis led to the discovery that EBV is associated with the endemic (African) subtype. Although there is little direct evidence of its role in pathogenesis, the circumstantial evidence is provocative. EBV, a B-cell mitogen, is hypothesized to expand the target pool of cells susceptible to malignant transformation (36,37). This hypothesis is supported by studies demonstrating that expression of the recombination activating gene can be induced by EBV, theoretically increasing the chance of a chromosomal translocation during immunoglobulin gene rearrangement (38). The observation that lymphomas develop in transgenic mice expressing EBNA-1 is also compelling (39). A more direct role of EBV in pathogenesis was suggested by a recent finding that the EBV-positive cell line Akata loses its malignant phenotype with spontaneous loss of EBV but regains the malignant phenotype upon reinfection with EBV (40). EBV is associated with approximately 85% of cases of endemic Burkitt's lymphoma but with only 15% of sporadic cases (36). An intermediate degree of EBV association has been identified in other parts of the world (33).

Treatment

Two of the most successful early treatment regimens for the management of pediatric non-Hodgkin's lymphoma were the cyclophosphamide-based COMP regimen (cyclophosphamide, vincristine, methotrexate, and prednisone) (41) and the multiagent anti–acute lymphoblastic leukemia regimen LSA$_2$-L$_2$ (41–43). The Children's Cancer Group performed a randomized trial of these two regimens (41). The outcomes of children with limited-stage disease were excellent regardless of histologic subtype, whereas the outcomes of patients with advanced-stage disease depended on histologic subtype. Specifically, treatment with the COMP regimen was more effective for children with Burkitt's lymphoma, whereas the LSA$_2$-L$_2$ regimen produced a superior outcome in children with lymphoblastic lymphoma. Subsequent trials build on these observations (44–79).

For children with limited-stage disease, the primary focus of clinical trials has been to reduce treatment-related acute and late effects without compromising the excellent outcome (48,49). Therefore, trials investigated the reduction of the dose intensity and the duration of therapy. The Pediatric Oncology Group demonstrated in the first of two sequential trials that involved field irradiation could be safely eliminated when three cycles of CHOP (cyclophosphamide, doxorubicin, vincristine, and prednisone) are followed by a 24-week maintenance phase of 6-mercaptopurine and methotrexate (49). The second trial demonstrated that the 24-week maintenance phase could be eliminated without compromising outcome, except in the case of lymphoblastic disease (49).

For children with advanced-stage disease, improvements in outcome have been achieved in part through refinement of risk-adapted histology-directed and immunophenotype-directed approaches. Treatment of Burkitt's lymphoma was first improved by adding cytarabine or high-dose methotrexate or both to the cyclophosphamide-based COMP regimen (47,50–52,54,57,58). For example, the Total B regimen featured courses of fractionated cyclophosphamide, vincristine, and doxorubicin given in alternation with courses of high-dose methotrexate and cytarabine (47). The results were excellent for children with stage III disease (2-year event-free survival estimate of 80%). However, patients who had bone marrow or central nervous system involvement had a 2-year event-free survival estimate of only approximately 20%. Over the last decade, further improvement in outcome has been achieved by dose intensification of cyclophosphamide, methotrexate, and cytarabine and by the inclusion of new active agents such as etoposide (Table 36.3) (46,54,56,69,72,75). One of the most successful regimens to date is the LMB-89 regimen designed by Patte et al. (French Society of Pediatric Oncology) (46). In this strategy, patients are grouped on the basis of disease extent and degree of resection (Fig. 36.1). Group A comprises those with completely resected limited-stage disease. Group C comprises those with central nervous system involvement or greater than 70% replacement of the bone marrow by lymphoma cells, and group B comprises the remainder of patients (i.e., those with incompletely resected limited-stage disease, stage III disease, or less than 70% replacement of the bone marrow). Eighty-five percent of children with advanced-stage disease are long-term event-free survivors with this regimen. This approach has also been very effective for adults with Burkitt's lymphoma (80).

The largest current clinical trial for children with Burkitt's lymphoma is an international collaboration between institutions in France, the United States, and the United Kingdom. This randomized trial is designed to determine whether the duration and dose intensity of therapy of the highly successful French LMB-89 protocol can be reduced without compromising outcome (46). Immunotherapeutic approaches may ultimately permit additional reduction in the intensity of cytotoxic therapy. In this regard, the Children's Oncology Group has designed a pilot study that incorporates rituximab (i.e., anti-CD20) into the LMB-89 regimen. If this approach is feasible, subsequent studies may focus on further reduction of cytotoxic dose intensity.

TABLE 36.3. *Treatment outcome for advanced-stage small noncleaved cell non-Hodgkin's lymphoma*

Protocol	Stage	No. of patients	EFS rate (%)	Reference
POG 8617	IV	34	79 ± 9 (4-yr)	51
	B-ALL	47	65 ± 8 (4-yr)	
LMB-89[a]	III	278	91 (95% CI, 87–94%) (5-yr)	46
	IV	62	87 (95% CI, 77–93%) (5-yr)	
	B-ALL	102	87 (95% CI, 79–92%) (5-yr)	
BFM 90	III	169	86 ± 3 (6-yr)	72
	IV	24	73 ± 10 (6-yr)	
	B-ALL	56	74 ± 6 (6-yr)	
Randomized Children's Cancer Group[a]:				
Orange vs. LMB-86	III/IV/B-ALL	43	83 (12-mo)	56
	III/IV/B-ALL	42	84 (12-mo)	

B-ALL, B-cell acute lymphoblastic leukemia; BFM, Berlin-Frankfurt-Münster; EFS, event-free survival; POG, Pediatric Oncology Group.

[a]Includes patients with B-cell large-cell non-Hodgkin's lymphoma.

Lymphoblastic Lymphoma (Precursor B- or T-cell Lymphoblastic Lymphoma/Leukemia)

Lymphoblastic lymphomas are neoplasms of either B- or T-lineage lymphoblasts (Tables 36.2 and 36.4). Acute lymphoblastic leukemia and lymphoblastic lymphoma have overlapping morphologic, immunophenotypic, and cytogenetic features, and, thus, the distinction between these two processes is considered by many to be largely arbitrary (81–83). The International Lymphoma Study Group and the WHO have designated these malignancies *precursor B- and T-lymphoblastic leukemia/lymphoma* in the updated REAL and WHO classifications (19,20). However, subtle immunophenotypic, molecular, and cytogenetic differences suggest that primary acute lymphoblastic leukemia and lymphoblastic lymphomas are fundamentally biologically different. Patients may present with lymphoblastic lymphoma confined to a lymphoid tissue or an extranodal site, but molecular studies usually reveal the involvement of bone marrow and blood. When disease is confined to an extramedullary site, a diagnosis of lymphoblastic lymphoma is rendered. Whereas the St. Jude criteria define acute lymphoblastic leukemia by a proportion of lymphoblasts in the bone marrow greater than 25%, others require only 10% lymphoblasts in the marrow (61,84,85). However, it is often difficult to distinguish between a leukemic phase of lymphoblastic lymphoma and extramedullary involvement by acute lymphoblastic leukemia. Common presentation sites of precursor T-lymphoblastic lymphoma are the mediastinum, lymph nodes, skin, bone, and soft tissues. Rarely, the presenting site may be the kidney, lung, or orbit. By contrast, B-lymphoblastic lymphoma more often presents in the skin, lymph nodes, bone, soft tissues, or breast, and mediastinal involvement is very uncommon (87–89). The most frequent location of skin lesions in children is the head (90). With aggressive chemotherapy, patients with precursor B-lymphoblastic lymphoma have a better prognosis than those with T-lymphoblastic lymphoma and may also fare better than precursor B-lymphoblastic leukemia patients (87–89).

Typically, lymphoblastic lymphomas and acute lymphoblastic leukemia show a diffuse pattern of tissue involvement by a uniform population of small to medium-sized blastic cells. Partially involved lymphoid tissues may show residual normal follicles and germinal centers. Large phagocytically active histiocytes interspersed among the malignant lymphoblasts may impart a "starry-sky" microscopic appearance in some cases. This pattern is a characteristic feature of Burkitt's lymphoma, but the unique biologic features of Burkitt's lymphoma can distinguish it from lymphoblastic lymphoma. The malignant lymphoblasts characteristically have scant to moderate amounts of basophilic cytoplasm and finely dispersed chromatin with small, indistinct nucleoli. The nuclei of either B or T types may be markedly irregular or convoluted, although this feature is more common in T-lymphoblastic lymphomas. Mitotic cells are particularly frequent in T-lymphoblastic lymphoma.

Immunophenotypic studies have revealed only minor differences in antigen expression between B- and T-lymphoblastic lymphomas and their acute lymphoblastic leukemia counterparts. Approximately 90% of lymphoblastic lymphomas are of T lineage, and the remaining 10% are of B lineage (91–95). Rarely, lymphoblastic lymphoma is derived from a natural killer cell of origin (94,96,97). Lymphoblastic lymphomas are usually Tdt positive, a marker that distinguishes them from all other types of lymphoma (98–102). Previously, Tdt-positive cells were thought to be confined to the bone marrow and thymus, which are sites of normal B- and T-cell development, respectively. The presence of Tdt-positive cells in the peripheral blood or lymph nodes was considered evidence of lymphoblastic malignancy in these tissues. However, improved immunohistochemical and flow cytometric analysis now allows the detection of small numbers of benign immature Tdt-positive lymphocytes in blood and lymph nodes (103). In addition to Tdt, CD34 and CD99 (MIC2) are also expressed by the majority of lymphoblastic lymphomas and prove useful in distinguishing these malignancies from Burkitt's lymphoma tumor biopsies embedded in paraffin (104). B- (and many T-) lympho-

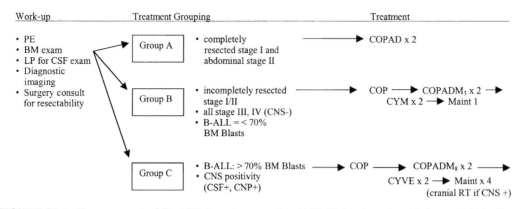

Work-up   Treatment Grouping   Treatment

FIGURE 36.1. Management of Burkitt's lymphoma using LMB-89 treatment guidelines. B-ALL, B-cell acute lymphoblastic leukemia; BM, bone marrow; CNP, cranial nerve palsy; CNS, central nervous system; COP, cyclophosphamide, vincristine, prednisone; COPADM$_3$, cyclophosphamide, vincristine, prednisone doxorubicin, methotrexate (3 g vs. 8 g); CSF, cerebrospinal fluid; CYM, cytarabine, methotrexate; CYVE, cytarabine, etoposide; LP, lumbar puncture; Maint, maintenance courses; PE, physical examination; RT, radiation therapy. (From Patte C, Auperin A, Michon J, et al. The Société Française d'Oncologie Pédiatrique LMB89 protocol: highly effective multiagent chemotherapy tailored to the tumor burden and initial response in 561 unselected children with B-cell lymphomas and L3 leukemia. *Blood* 2001;97:3370–3379, with permission.)

blastic lymphomas express CD10 or the common acute lymphoblastic leukemia antigen. A favorable clinical outcome is associated with CD10$^+$ T-cell acute lymphoblastic leukemias, but a similar association has not been described in T-cell lymphoblastic lymphoma (94,105).

The lymphoblastic lymphomas may be subclassified by their apparent stage of bone marrow or intrathymic maturation in a manner analogous to acute lymphoblastic leukemia classification (Table 36.4). In general, lymphoblastic lymphomas have antigen expression profiles consistent with a more mature stage of intrathymic T-cell development than does T-cell acute lymphoblastic leukemia (91–94,106–109). However, attempts at separating lymphoblastic lymphoma from acute lymphoblastic leukemia by immunophenotypic

features and the identification of clinically significant immunologic subtypes have been largely unsuccessful. In our and others' experience, B-lymphoblastic lymphomas may correspond to any of the four subtypes listed in Table 36.4. A pre-B stage of maturation (i.e., cytoplasmic mu heavy-chain expression without detectable kappa or lambda immunoglobulin light chains) appears more frequently in lymphoblastic lymphoma than in B-lineage acute lymphoblastic leukemia (93,110,111). Rare cases of B-lymphoblastic lymphoma may express surface immunoglobulin without detectable Tdt and should not be confused with Burkitt's lymphoma (112). T-lymphoblastic malignancies can also be subdivided according to corresponding stages of normal intrathymic T cell maturation: early thymic stage (CD7$^+$,

TABLE 36.4. *Immunophenotypic features of precursor B- and T-lymphoblastic lymphomas*

Subtype	CD45	CD34	Tdt	CD3[a]	CD5	CD7	CD19	CD20	CD22	CD79α[a]	CD10	Immunoglobulin expression
Early pre-B	+[b]	+	+	–	–	–	+	±	+	+	+[c]	clgμ$^-$, slgμ$^-$, κ$^-$, λ$^-$
Pre-B	+	±	+	–	–	–	+	±	+	+	+	clgμ$^+$, slgμ$^-$, κ$^-$, λ$^-$
Late pre-B[c]	+	±	±	–	–	–	+	±	+	+	+	clgμ$^+$, slgμ$^+$, κ$^-$, λ$^-$
Mature B[d]	+	±	±	–	–	–	+	±	+	+	+	clgμ$^+$, slgμ$^+$, κ$^±$, λ$^±$
T[e]	+	±	±	+	±	+	–	–	–	±	–	—

clgμ, cytoplasmic immunoglobulin μ; slgμ, surface immunoglobulin μ; Tdt, terminal deoxynucleotidyl transferase; κ, immunoglobulin light chain κ; λ, immunoglobulin light chain λ.
[a]Cytoplasmic antigen expression.
[b]10% of cases may have very weak to no detectable CD45 antigen.
[c]Also termed *transitional-pre-B*.
[d]Rare subtype not to be confused with Burkitt's lymphoma.
[e]May be subclassified into early thymic stage (CD7$^+$, cytoplasmic CD3$^+$, CD5$^±$, CD2$^±$, CD1a$^-$, CD4$^-$, CD8$^-$), midthymic stage (CD7$^+$, CD5$^+$, CD2$^+$, cytoplasmic CD3$^+$, surface CD3$^±$, CD1a$^±$, CD4$^±$, CD8$^±$), and late thymic stage (CD7$^+$, CD5$^+$, CD2$^+$, surface CD3$^+$, CD1a$^-$, CD4$^+$ or CD8$^+$).

cytoplasmic CD3⁺, CD5±, CD2±, CD1a⁻, CD4⁻, CD8⁻), mid-thymic stage (CD7⁺, CD5⁺, CD2⁺, cytoplasmic CD3⁺, surface CD3±, CD1a±, CD4±, CD8±), and late thymic stage (CD7⁺, CD5⁺, CD2⁺, surface CD3⁺, CD1a⁻, CD4⁺or CD8⁺). The majority of T-lymphoblastic lymphomas correspond to the late stage of intrathymic T-cell maturation (98–102). Most lymphoblastic lymphomas retain the expression of pan-T-cell antigens—for example, CD7, CD2, CD5, and CD6—whereas one or more of these are often undetectable in T large-cell lymphomas. A more frequent expression of T-cell receptor αβ than of γδ has been reported in T-lymphoblastic lymphoma as compared to T-cell acute lymphoblastic leukemia (113).

Aberrant expression of myeloid-associated antigen, a feature of some B- and T-lineage acute lymphoblastic leukemias, can occur in lymphoblastic lymphomas (92,114,115). Some investigators have suggested that the expression of CD56 is more common in T-lymphoblastic lymphoma than in its leukemic counterpart. Interestingly, a small number of T-lymphoblastic lymphomas may undergo a phenotypic switch to acute myeloid leukemia (116,117). Although some of these lineage switches may occur secondary to treatment, we have seen examples of T-lymphoblastic malignancies that contain a very small blast cell population with committed myeloid maturation features. Treatment directed at lymphoblasts induced a clinical remission, but there was a subsequent outgrowth of the myeloblastic cell population.

Reported cytogenetic studies of lymphoblastic lymphomas have been fewer than those for acute lymphoblastic leukemia and include small numbers of patients (118–120). Additionally, many reports describing molecular and cytogenetic findings of lymphoblastic lymphoma include cases of acute lymphoblastic leukemia and vice-versa. Thus, an accurate summary of cytogenetic abnormalities in lymphoblastic lymphoma devoid of the influence of acute lymphoblastic leukemia remains elusive. T-lymphoblastic lymphoma and T-cell acute lymphoblastic leukemia demonstrate similar chromosomal abnormalities for the most part. Chromosome abnormalities involving the T-cell receptor are relatively common and include abnormalities at bands 7q34-36, 7p15, and 14q11 (119,120). The t(9;17) translocation appears more commonly in T-lymphoblastic lymphoma than in T-cell acute lymphoblastic leukemia (119,121). Patients with this translocation often present with a mediastinal mass and have an aggressive disease course. The t(8;13)(p11;q11-14) has been described in rare cases of T-lymphoblastic lymphoma that present with myeloid hyperplasia and eosinophilia (122–124). The t(10;11)(p13-14;q14-21) is an uncommon but recurring translocation associated with acute lymphoblastic leukemia, acute myelogenous leukemia, and lymphoblastic lymphoma (125,126). Unlike the case in acute lymphoblastic leukemia, cytogenetic abnormalities have not been shown to be of prognostic significance in lymphoblastic lymphoma. Gene expression profile (microarray) studies have demonstrated possible clinically relevant subgroups of T-cell acute lymphoblastic leukemia, but similar studies of lymphoblastic lymphoma have yet to be reported at the time of this writing (127,128).

Treatment

For children with lymphoblastic lymphoma, various strategies have been implemented to further improve the treatment outcome achieved with LSA₂-L₂ (Table 36.5) (60,67,70,73,76). The French Society of Pediatric Oncology incorporated courses of high-dose methotrexate into an LSA₂-L₂ backbone with excellent results (67). Other groups have also obtained successful outcomes with the inclusion of high-dose methotrexate (76). Of these, the German Berlin-Frankfurt-Münster group has reported results among the best (i.e., 5-year event-free survival of 90%) with a regimen whose consolidation phase includes four courses of high-dose methotrexate (5 g/m² given every 2 weeks; Fig. 36.2) (76). This improvement in outcome may be the result of higher intracellular levels of methotrexate polyglutamates achieved with a higher dose of methotrexate (129). Other refinements in therapy that are thought to contribute to improved treatment outcome include the incorporation of a reinduction (i.e., reintensification) phase, as well as the incorporation of L-asparaginase and new active agents (60,73,76).

In the United States, the Children's Oncology Group is currently performing a randomized trial to determine whether

TABLE 36.5. *Treatment outcome for advanced-stage lymphoblastic non-Hodgkin's lymphoma*

Protocol	Stage	No. of patients	EFS/DFS rate (%)	Reference
POG 8704 (no extra L-asp)	III/IV	83	4-yr CCR = 64 ± 6	73
POG 8704 (extra L-asp)	III/IV	84	4-yr CCR = 78± 5	
LSA₂-L₂ (modified); CCG-551	III/IV	124	5-yr EFS = 64	41
BFM 90	III	82	5-yr EFS = 90 ± 3	76
	IV	19	5-yr EFS = 95 ± 5	
X-H SJCRH	III/IV	22	4-yr DFS = 73	60
APO (Dana Farber)	III/IV	21	3-yr DFS = 58 ± 23	61
ACOP + (POG)	III	33	3-yr DFS = 54 ± 9	62

ACOP, doxorubicin (Adriamycin), cyclophosphamide, vincristine, and prednisone; APO, Adriamycin, prednisone, and vincristine; BFM, Berlin-Frankfurt-Münster; CCG, Children's Cancer Group; CCR, continuous complete remission; DFS, disease-free survival; EFS, event-free survival; L-asp, L-asparaginase; POG, Pediatric Oncology Group.

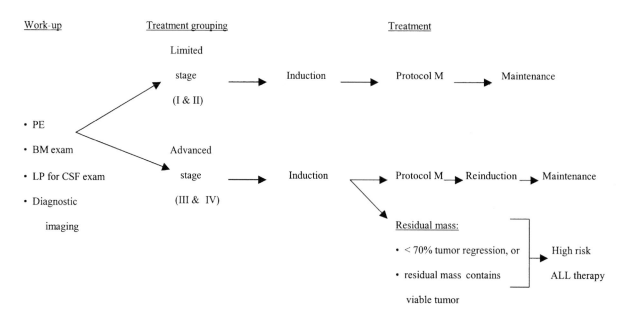

FIGURE 36.2. Management of lymphoblastic lymphoma using BFM-90 (Berlin-Frankfurt-Münster) treatment guidelines. BM, bone marrow; induction, prednisone, vincristine, L-asparaginase, cyclophosphamide, high-dose methotrexate; LP, lumbar puncture; PE, physical examination; reinduction, dexamethasone, vincristine, doxorubicin, L-asparaginase, cyclophosphamide, cytarabine, 6-thioguanine, methotrexate. (From Reiter A, Schrappe M, Ludwig W-D, et al. Intensive ALL-type therapy without local radiotherapy provides a 90% event-free survival for children with T-cell lymphoblastic lymphoma: a BFM group report. *Blood* 2000;95:416–421, with permission.)

extended intrathecal-administration of methotrexate can be safely used as a substitute for high-dose methotrexate in the context of the very successful Berlin-Frankfurt-Münster regimen (76), which includes a consolidation phase featuring four doses of high-dose methotrexate (at 5 g/m^2) given every other week. Data from a Pediatric Oncology Group study suggested that high-dose methotrexate may not be necessary, in the context of a regimen based on anthracycline and L-asparaginase, for children with advanced-stage lymphoblastic lymphoma (130), even though it was necessary for T-cell leukemia. The Children's Oncology Group's current trial is also testing the benefit of an intensification phase of cyclophosphamide and an anthracycline. Early response, as measured by diagnostic imaging and minimal residual disease studies, will also be evaluated.

In the Pediatric Oncology Group limited-stage non-Hodgkin's lymphoma trial, which featured three courses of CHOP followed by a 24-week maintenance phase of 6-mercaptopurine and methotrexate, one third of children with lymphoblastic lymphoma experienced relapse even with the maintenance phase; however, the majority were successfully salvaged, and their overall survival did not differ from that of children with other histologic subtypes (49). Some groups, such as the French Society of Pediatric Oncology, take a more aggressive initial approach to avoid the need to retreat (67).

In an attempt to reduce the 30% rate of relapse observed with the Pediatric Oncology Group approach (49) (three cycles of CHOP followed by a 24-week maintenance phase of 6-mercaptopurine and methotrexate) without exposing patients to the toxicity of therapy for high-risk T-cell acute

lymphoblastic leukemia, the Children's Oncology Group is currently studying a regimen similar in design to a treatment plan for low-risk acute lymphoblastic leukemia.

Large-Cell Lymphoma

Large-cell lymphoma, as the name implies, is composed of large lymphoid cells that are larger than the diameter of a histiocytic nucleus or two to three times the width of small inactive-appearing lymphocytes. These lymphomas are of B- or T-cell origin (Table 36.6) (275). The term *non-B, non-T, or null-cell large-cell lymphoma* usually indicates incomplete laboratory characterization of the cell of origin and not a true nonlineage neoplasm. Large-cell neoplasms of true monocytic/histiocytic or dendritic phenotype should not be considered lymphomas, as their clinical course and treatment differ. The revised REAL (19) and recent WHO (20) classifications recognize multiple types of large-cell lymphoma, including diffuse large B-cell, mediastinal (thymic) B-cell, intravascular large B-cell, peripheral T-cell unspecified, angioimmunoblastic T-cell, and anaplastic large-cell lymphomas. Other lymphomas, including adult T-cell leukemia/lymphoma, extranodal nasal natural killer T-cell lymphoma, enteropathy-type T-cell lymphoma, subcutaneous panniculitis-like T-cell lymphoma, and primary cutaneous CD30+ T-cell disorders, may have a prominent large-cell component but are defined by other biologic or clinical features. Anaplastic large-cell, diffuse large B-cell, and, to a markedly lesser degree, peripheral T-cell lymphomas compose the vast majority of pediatric large-cell lymphomas, although rare exam-

TABLE 36.6. *Tissue markers of large-cell lymphomas of children*

	CD20	CD79	Ig	CD5	CD3	CD30	CD15	ALK	CA	bcl-2	bcl-6
ALCL[a]	–	–	–	±	±	+	±	+	+	–	±
PTL	–	–	–	±	±	±	–	–	±	–	±
MBCLCL	+	+	±	–	–	±	–	–	–	–	–
DLBCL	+	+	±	±	–	–	–	–	–	±	±

ALCL, anaplastic large-cell lymphoma; CA, cytotoxic antigen (perforin, TIA-1); DLBCL, diffuse large B-cell lymphoma; Ig, immunoglobulin; MBCLCL, mediastinal B-cell large-cell lymphoma; PTL, peripheral T-cell lymphoma.

[a]Marker features are for ALCL with ALK gene rearrangements. Rare ALCL without ALK rearrangements are ALK-negative and may express bcl-2 protein.

From Falini B, Mason DY. Proteins encoded by genes involved in chromosomal alterations in lymphoma and leukemia: clinical value of their detection by immunocytochemistry. *Blood* 2002;99:409–426.

ples of other types of large-cell lymphomas in children have been reported. In the St. Jude Children's Research Hospital experience, T-cell anaplastic large-cell lymphomas account for 40% to 50% of pediatric large-cell lymphomas, diffuse large B-cell lymphomas comprise another 30% to 40%, and the remainder consists of nonanaplastic peripheral T-cell lymphomas. Investigations have revealed few morphologic and immunophenotypic differences between the large-cell lymphomas of adults and children. However, strikingly few investigations of the laboratory and biologic features of pediatric large-cell lymphomas other than the anaplastic large-cell type have been reported.

The treatment of large-cell lymphoma has historically been selected on the basis of histology in the United States and on the basis of immunophenotype in Europe (131). Most of the regimens in the United States have been CHOP-based (Table 36.7) (41,44,45,55,56,131–133). With these approaches, approximately 60% to 70% of patients are long-term event-free survivors. In a randomized trial performed by the Children's Oncology Group comparing doxorubicin (Adriamycin), prednisone, and vincristine (APO) with Adriamycin, cyclophosphamide, vincristine, and prednisone (ACOP⁺), patients with a B-cell immunophenotype appeared to have a survival advantage, although the number of immunophenotyped cases was relatively small (45). In Europe, children with T-cell large-cell lymphoma are treated on regimens used for T-cell lymphoblastic lymphoma, and children with B-cell large-cell lymphoma are treated with regimens used for Burkitt's lymphoma. With the French LMB-89 regimen, children with B-cell large-cell lymphoma had results comparable to those of children with Burkitt's lymphoma (77).

Current trials in the United States are moving toward an immunophenotype-directed approach, which has been used in Europe for many years. Children with B-cell large-cell lymphoma will be treated on regimens designed for children with Burkitt's lymphoma.

Anaplastic Large-Cell Lymphoma

Anaplastic large-cell lymphoma is rare in very young children but has a peak incidence in adolescence. In children, anaplastic large-cell lymphoma tends to involve lymph nodes and extranodal sites, including skin, soft tissues, lungs, and bones (134,135). Approximately 20% to 25% of patients have bone marrow involvement at diagnosis that may not be obvious without special studies (136).

Anaplastic large-cell lymphoma is usually composed of variable numbers of small, medium-size, and large neoplastic cells. The hallmark cells of anaplastic large-cell lymphoma are large cells with eccentrically placed, monocytoid or horse-shoe-shaped nuclei and an eosinophilic patch near the nucleus. Often, these cells are mutinucleated, with the nuclei forming a wreath-like appearance. The large cells may be mistaken for Reed-Sternberg cells. The lymphoma cells commonly proliferate within the sinuses of lymphoid tissues, resulting in a cohesive appearance that mimics metastatic tumor. The smaller cells usually have smaller amounts of cytoplasm and lack the nuclear characteristics of the large cells.

Several morphologic variants of anaplastic large-cell lymphoma are recognized, including the common, lymphohistiocytic, and small cell (28,137). The common variant accounts for more than 70% of cases and features the hall-

TABLE 36.7. *Treatment outcome for advanced-stage large-cell non-Hodgkin's lymphoma*

Protocol	Stage	No. of patients	EFS rate (%)	Reference
CHOP	III/IV	21	62 ± 11 (3-yr)	44
MACOP-B	III/IV	11	55 ± 16 (3-yr)	65
Randomized				
COMP vs.	III/IV	42	52 (5-yr)	41
LSA₂-L₂	III/IV	18	43 (5-yr)	
APO vs.	III/IV	62	72 ± 6 (3-yr)	133
ACOP+	III/IV	58	62 ± 7 (4-yr)	

ACOP, doxorubicin (Adriamycin), cyclophosphamide, vincristine, and prednisone; APO, Adriamycin, prednisone, and vincristine; CHOP, cyclophosphamide, doxorubicin, vincristine, and prednisone; COMP, cyclophosphamide, vincristine, methotrexate, and prednisone; EFS, event-free survival; MACOP-B, methotrexate, doxorubicin, cyclophosphamide, vincristine, prednisone, and bleomycin.

mark large anaplastic tumor cells. Varying numbers of small and medium lymphoid cells may also be present. Erythrophagocytosis by histiocytes can also be found in some cases. The lymphohistiocytic variant accounts for less than 20% of anaplastic large-cell lymphoma in children and consists of a mixture of small and larger lymphoid cells and many histiocytes (138). The histiocytes may be so numerous as to partially obscure the lymphoid cells. Not infrequently, there is evidence of active histiocytic erythrophagocytosis simulating hemophagocytic syndrome (139,140). Neutrophils and sometimes eosinophils may also be present. When neutrophils are particularly numerous, sometimes with associated necrosis, the lymphoma is referred to as *neutrophil-rich form of anaplastic large cell lymphoma* (141–143). The small-cell variant accounts for less than 10% of cases and may not be recognized if the hallmark cells are scarce and immunophenotyping and cytogenetic studies are not performed (144). In the past, this variant in children and adults was often called *peripheral T-cell lymphoma*. Other rare forms of anaplastic large-cell lymphoma not recognized as a variant in the WHO Classification include sarcomatoid, signet ring, and granulomatous forms (145–147). Rare examples of children and adults who present with a leukemic process or who develop a leukemic phase during the course of their disease have recently been described (148–153). Patients who initially present with a leukemic process may not have adenopathy or extranodal masses. The circulating lymphoma cells are usually small to medium in size and are atypical appearing without the features of lymphoblasts. White blood cell counts may be more than 100×10^9 per L. Tissue masses, when present, may show the more typical morphologic features of common anaplastic large-cell lymphoma, but most cases reported to date resemble the small-cell variant. The bone marrow may have infiltrates resembling the peripheral blood cells or may have a component of large cells with anaplastic features. The circulating cells have a T-cell phenotype profile but usually have atypical patterns of T-cell antigen expression. In contrast to T-cell acute lymphoblastic leukemia, CD1a, CD34, or Tdt are negative. Anaplastic lymphoma kinase and epithelial membrane antigen-expressing cells may be detected in the bone marrow. Cytogenetic or molecular studies for ALK translocations are necessary to confirm a primary diagnosis. A t(2;5)(p23;q35) is demonstrable in most cases. A novel t(2;19)(p23;p13) was found in an 18-month-old boy who presented with a leukemic process and hepatosplenomegaly but no overt bone marrow involvement, adenopathy, or other extranodal masses (152). Studies revealed an unusual immunophenotype: cells were positive for CD45, CD13, CD30, CD33, CD16/56, perforin, and granzyme B, and negative for CD3, CD34, Tdt, and myeloperoxidase. The neoplastic cells also stained strongly with antibodies to anaplastic lymphoma kinase and epithelial membrane antigen. The phenotype of this leukemia was suggestive of a natural killer cell of origin, raising the possibility that some cases of null anaplastic large-cell lymphoma may likewise arise from this cell lineage (152).

Membrane and Golgi expression of CD30 is characteristic of the neoplastic cells of anaplastic large-cell lymphoma (154). The most intense reactivity to anti-CD30 antibodies is seen in the large cells, whereas the smaller cells are weakly positive or, more often, negative. Most anaplastic large-cell lymphomas are positive for the epithelial membrane antigen, in a manner analogous to CD30 (155). Most anaplastic large-cell lymphomas express one or more T-cell–associated antigens, including CD2, CD3, CD4, CD7, or CD45RO. T-cell antigens CD5 and CD8 are usually negative. Some cases lack demonstrable T-cell antigens but have evidence of T-cell receptor gene rearrangement. These cases are similar to T-cell antigen–positive cases in every other way and may be referred to as *null/T anaplastic large-cell lymphoma* (20). Most anaplastic large-cell lymphomas express the cytoplasmic cytotoxic cell–associated proteins TIA-1, granzyme B, or perforin. Myeloid-associated CD15 may be weakly expressed by some neoplastic cells in a minority of cases. Some antibodies to the monocytic/histiocytic-associated CD68 may react with the lymphoma cells. B-cell–associated antigens CD19, CD20, CD22, and CD79a are not expressed except in rare, controversial cases of B-lineage anaplastic large-cell lymphoma.

A t(2;5)(p23;q35) translocation is demonstrable in more than 75% of anaplastic large-cell lymphomas (156,157). Several other translocations of ALK have been described, including t(1;2)(q25;p23), t(2;3)(p23;q21), inv(2)(p23;q35), t(2;22), t(2;17)(p23;q11), and t(2;19)(p23;p13) (158–160). With the t(2;5), NPM (nucleophosmin) on chromosome 5q35 is fused with ALK (anaplastic lymphoma kinase) on chromosome 2p23, resulting in expression of a chimeric npm-Alk protein (161). Alk protein is a transmembrane protein normally expressed by some cells of the brain but not by lymphoid or hematopoietic elements. The result of ALK translocations is upregulation of ALK with resultant aberrant expression of a chimeric alk protein in the lymphoma cells. The lymphoma cells in more than 85% of anaplastic large-cell lymphoma cases express alk proteins detectable with the p80 or ALK1 antibodies (161–163). Thus, tumor cell expression of ALK is specific for anaplastic large-cell lymphoma except for rare examples of large B-cell lymphomas with plasmacytoid features and immunoglobulin A expression, rhabdomyosarcoma, neuroblastoma, and some examples of inflammatory myofibroblastic tumor (164–167). Anaplastic large-cell lymphomas with the t(2;5) display a cytoplasmic plus nuclear alk expression pattern, whereas other ALK translocations display only a cytoplasmic pattern (159,168). Rare cases of anaplastic large-cell lymphoma with the t(2;17)(q23;q11) display granular cytoplasmic staining with anti-alk antibodies (169). Approximately 10% of anaplastic large-cell lymphomas do not have a detectable ALK translocation or express alk (138). Conversely, rare lymphomas with a t(2;5) do not have the morphologic features of anaplastic large-cell lymphoma (135). Lymphomas that have anaplastic large-cell leukemia morphology and immunophenotype but that are negative for a detectable ALK translocation and expression should be regarded as phenotypic variants of anaplastic large-cell lymphoma or a different entity, because alk positivity may have prognostic utility (20).

In adults, alk protein expression in anaplastic large-cell lymphoma is a favorable prognostic factor (170–172). Treatment responses in adults are similar for patients with the t(2;5) or its variant translocations (173). A similar favorable outcome is found in children with immunochemically documented alk-positive anaplastic large-cell lymphoma (66,135,138). In a multivariate analysis of childhood anaplastic large-cell lymphoma, mediastinal, visceral (lung, liver, spleen), and skin involvement were poor prognostic factors (175,176).

The optimal treatment approach for anaplastic large-cell lymphomas has yet to be elucidated (131,132). Although the treatment strategies studied thus far have been quite varied, the estimated 3-year event-free survival rates for children with advanced-stage disease are approximately 60% to 70% (131). A Pediatric Oncology Group randomized study of APO versus ACOP⁺ showed no significant difference in outcome between the two arms ($p = .90$) (45). One of the best results to date was that reported by the Berlin-Frankfurt-Münster, who used their B-cell lymphoma protocol to treat children with anaplastic large-cell lymphoma, which typically has a non–B-cell immunophenotype. They achieved an 80% probability of 3-year event-free survival with this approach (66).

There are currently two major initiatives worldwide for the anaplastic large-cell lymphomas. Both of these build on the results of a French study showing that patients with recurrent anaplastic large-cell lymphoma could be successfully treated with single-agent vinblastine (177). In Europe, a multinational trial is using the very successful Berlin-Frankfurt-Münster regimen (66) for B-cell lymphoma, with randomization to a vinblastine maintenance phase. In the United States, the Children's Oncology Group is planning a study that builds on the successful results of the APO regimen (61), which comprises primarily Adriamycin, prednisone, and vincristine (APO). In this study, the substitution of vinblastine for vincristine will be studied in a randomized fashion.

Diffuse Large B-Cell Lymphomas

Diffuse large B-cell lymphomas are postulated to be of germinal or postgerminal-center B-cell origin. In children and adults, these lymphomas can be divided into morphologic variants, including centroblastic, immunoblastic, T-cell/histiocytic–rich, anaplastic, and mediastinal large B-cell lymphomas (20). Unfortunately, the intraobserver reproducibility of these designations is relatively poor and not useful for clinical studies. A particular problem in pediatric lymphomas is distinguishing among Burkitt's, Burkitt-like, and diffuse large B-cell lymphomas. In a recent study, consensus for identifying Burkitt's and diffuse large B-cell lymphoma were 88% and 80%, respectively, and 42% for Burkitt-like lymphoma (178).

One or more pan-B–associated markers—CD19, CD20, CD22, and CD79a—are expressed by diffuse large B-cell lymphoma. Surface or cytoplasmic immunoglobulins are expressed by 50% or more cases. Some cases may express CD5, CD10, bcl-2, or bcl-6. Most B-cell anaplastic large-cell lymphomas and some nonanaplastic cases express CD30. In adults, alk protein may be detected in a rare subtype of diffuse large B-cell lymphoma that has plasmacytoid features but no rearrangement of the ALK gene (164). The proliferative index, as measured by nuclear Ki-67 expression, may be high in some diffuse large B-cell lymphomas but less than that observed in Burkitt's lymphoma.

Investigations of adult diffuse large B-cell lymphoma show that approximately 30% express bcl-2 or have a t(14;18) translocation, indicative of germinal center origin. Another 30% of cases may have abnormalities of the chromosome 3 band q27, the locus of BCL6. A small number of cases may have a t(8;14) translocation. Only scanty information is available on the incidence of genetic lesions in childhood diffuse large B-cell lymphoma. In a recent small study of pediatric diffuse large B-cell lymphoma, expression of bcl-6, c-myc, and bcl-2 were detected in 66%, 100%, and 50% of cases, respectively (179). Recent gene expression profiling studies of adult diffuse large B-cell lymphoma have identified two genotype patterns consistent with different stages of peripheral B-cell development: germinal center B cells and activated peripheral blood B cells (180,181). Gene profiling studies of pediatric large-cell lymphomas have not been reported.

Mediastinal Large B-Cell Lymphoma

Mediastinal large B-cell lymphoma is an uncommon subtype of diffuse large B-cell lymphoma but recognized as a unique B-cell lymphoma by the WHO Classification (20,182–187). Mediastinal large B-cell lymphoma accounts for less than 10% of all large-cell lymphomas in children. Although it is more prevalent in female adults, this lymphoma may occur slightly more frequently in male children and adolescents. Other names for this lymphoma include *mediastinal diffuse large-cell lymphoma with sclerosis* and *mediastinal clear-cell lymphoma of B-cell type*. These neoplasms are of thymic origin with features analogous to those of noncirculating thymic medullary B cells (188). Patients present with signs and symptoms of a large mediastinal mass, frequently with extension into adjacent structures, including lung, pericardium, chest wall, and superior vena cava. Extrathoracic extension at diagnosis is uncommon but with disease progression can involve kidneys, brain, soft tissue, skin, and adrenal glands.

Biopsy of mediastinal large B-cell lymphoma typically shows thin to thick, dense fibrotic bands that divide the neoplastic cells into small clusters. The clustering effect can mimic the lobules of metastatic undifferentiated carcinoma. Remnant thymic epithelial cells expressing cytokeratin may also be present and, in small biopsies, may be confused with an epithelial tumor. Not infrequently, intense fibrosis can obscure the neoplastic cells. The lymphoma may comprise a mixture of small, medium, or large lymphoid cells or consist primarily of large cells with ample amounts of clear and, less commonly, acidophilic or weakly basophilic cytoplasm (189). Not infrequently, small benign-appearing lymphocytes and eosinophils are dispersed among the tumor cells, mimicking Hodgkin's disease. The tumor cells express the common leukocyte antigen CD45 and B-cell–associated antigens CD19, CD20, CD22, and CD79, but not CD21. Expression of bcl-6 and CD10 by these lymphomas suggests a possible derivation from germinal center B cells (190). Immunoglobulin expression may be weak but often is not detectable (191). Unlike lymphoblastic lymphoma, these tumors do not express Tdt or CD34. The CD30 antigen, a marker common to anaplastic large-cell lymphoma and classical Hodgkin's disease, may be weakly to strongly expressed by a few or sometimes by the majority of lymphoma cells (192). In contrast to other aggressive B lymphomas, patients with mediastinal large B-cell lymphoma exhibit low serum levels of β_2-microglobulin due to absence or weak expression of major histocompatibility complex class I antigens by tumor cells (193,194).

Molecular studies uniformly reveal clonal immunoglobulin gene rearrangements even when immunoglobulins are not demonstrable by immunologic techniques. Studies reveal that the tumor cells harbor mutated immunoglobulin V region genes consistent with antigen-experienced or postgerminal-center B cells (195). Uncommonly, evidence of clonal EBV genome may be present in the tumor cells. Few cytogenetic studies have been reported, but those available show aneuploid tumor cells, often with gains of chromosome 9p or Xq (196–198). The t(14;18) chromosomal translocation and its variants, which are common to adult large-cell follicular lymphomas, are rare (198). The tumor cells may overexpress REL or MAL in a minority of cases (199). BCL6, p53, and p16[INK4] alterations and MYC rearrangements may be present (196–198,200).

Despite previous designations of mediastinal large B-cell lymphoma as an aggressive neoplasm, current treatment regimens in children and adults with localized disease induce remissions with greater than 80% overall survivals (183,185). Pediatric patients presenting with extrathoracic disease fare less well (185). Rebiopsy of residual posttreatment masses are necessary to distinguish between residual tumor and persistent fibrosis and necrosis.

Uncommon Pediatric Lymphomas

Pediatric Follicular Lymphoma

Follicular lymphoma is a neoplasm of follicular-center B cells that retains a follicular or nodular growth pattern. The WHO Classification recognizes three morphologic grades of follicular lymphoma based on ratios of centroblasts or centrocytes (noncleaved and cleaved follicular center cells, respectively) (20). Follicular lymphomas comprise approximately 35% of adult non-Hodgkin's lymphomas and in this age group usually present in lymph nodes, spleen, and bone marrow (20). More than two thirds of adult patients have disseminated disease at diagnosis and are not cured with chemotherapy. In contrast,

follicular lymphoma accounts for less than 3% of all pediatric lymphomas (201–206). Furthermore, in children, these lymphomas usually present with disease localized to tonsillar, cervical, and inguinal lymphoid tissues. Localized testicular follicular large-cell lymphomas in children have also been reported (206–210). Transformation to higher-grade diffuse lymphoma or leukemic phase is distinctly uncommon in children, unlike adults, and most children have prolonged remissions with or without therapy. The actuarial 5-year event-free survival was 94% in a series reported by Ribeiro (204). In another study, six of seven children were in complete remission, including three who had no chemotherapy (205). In a recent study of 23 pediatric patients, 15 of 19 patients had stage I disease, and 11 of 13 with sufficient follow-up achieved a durable clinical remission (206).

Despite good morphologic criteria for follicular lymphoma, the rarity of this disease in children requires additional immunophenotypic and molecular studies to confirm a lymphoma diagnosis and to clearly separate it from the more frequent finding of benign follicular hyperplasia. Although no morphologic differences between adult and pediatric follicular lymphomas have been identified, recent studies show biologic differences between these tumors. Studies of pediatric testicular follicular lymphomas show that these neoplasms express bcl-6 or have BCL6 rearrangements but lack t(14;18)(q32;q21) chromosomal translocations and BCL2 and p53 abnormalities (207–210). By contrast, more than three fourths of adult follicular lymphomas express bcl-2, have a t(14;18) that involves rearrangement of BCL2, and will have disease progression despite chemotherapy (20). Bcl-2 is a mitochondrial protein that plays a central role in resistance to apoptosis. Bcl-2 is normally expressed by T cells and mantle zone B cells but not by germinal center cells. Aberrant expression of bcl-2 by follicular lymphomas appears to be a primary etiologic factor in most cases of adult follicular lymphomas and may influence the response to therapy. In two other separate investigations of pediatric nontesticular follicular lymphomas, bcl-2 expression was detected in only 6 of 20 patients and BCL2 rearrangements by polymerase chain reaction in 2 of 16 patients (205,206). Furthermore, in one of these studies, all four patients with lymphomas expressing bcl-2 either presented with advanced disease or had disease refractory to therapy, whereas children with bcl-2–negative tumors had stage I disease, achieved complete remission, and had no relapses (206). Thus, bcl-2 expression does not appear to contribute to the pathogenesis of most pediatric follicular lymphomas. However, it does identify a subset of pediatric patients in whom the lymphoma is often disseminated and is more refractory to chemotherapy.

Hepatosplenic T-Cell Lymphoma

Hepatosplenic T-cell lymphoma is an aggressive extranodal malignancy of cytotoxic T-cells, usually of $\gamma\delta$ and less commonly $\alpha\beta$ T-cell receptor type (28,211–213). This systemic lymphoma is rare in children and adults, with the peak incidence in adolescents and young adults (20,212). Males are more frequently afflicted than females, although a female predisposition is reported for αβ hepatosplenic lymphomas (214,215). Patients typically present with enlarged spleens and livers, with no appreciable lymphadenopathy (216). Thrombocytopenia is common, as is anemia. Circulating lymphoma cells are commonly present at diagnosis but may be difficult to distinguish from atypical lymphocytes. A more obvious leukemic phase may develop as the disease progresses (214,215). Cases of αβ hepatosplenic lymphoma are histologically, cytogenetically, and clinically similar to the γδ form (215). A relatively high percentage of cases after solid-organ transplant suggests that an underlying immune problem predisposes to this neoplasm (217–220). The neoplastic cells are medium-sized with scant to moderate amounts of cytoplasm. Azurophilic cytoplasmic granules have been described in a minority of cases. The nuclei may be round or convoluted, with condensed chromatin and inconspicuous nucleoli. Mitotic cells are infrequent. With disease progression, a blast-cell transformation may occur, with cells having prominent nucleoli (217,221,222). The lymphoma cells may be difficult to appreciate in bone marrow aspirates, but bone marrow needle biopsy frequently shows the presence of a characteristic sinusoidal infiltrate (215,216,222). The spleen and liver also show marked sinusoidal infiltration by the neoplastic cells (215,216). Erythrophagocytosis may be evident in splenic and bone marrow sinusoids (215,216,223,224). The lymphoma cells have a fairly consistent immunophenotypic expression pattern (CD2$^+$, CD3$^+$, CD4$^-$, CD8$^\pm$, CD5$^-$, CD7$^+$, CD16$^+$, and CD56$^\pm$) (20,224), although exceptions to this phenotype are not uncommon. The αβ hepatosplenic lymphomas have a similar immunophenotype except for a slightly more frequent expression of CD57 (215). T-cell receptor γδ or, less commonly, T-cell receptor αβ proteins can be detected by flow cytometric analysis (211,216). Cytotoxic granular protein TIA-1 is detected in most cases, whereas granzyme B or perforin is detected in only a minority of cases (214,215,223,225,226). An isochromosome 7q, often with trisomy 8 and other random chromosomal abnormalities, is found in the majority of reported cases (215,219,221,222,227–230). T-cell receptor γ- and β-chain gene rearrangement studies show reciprocal findings between αβ and γδ types of hepatosplenic lymphomas and should not be used as a distinguishing test (215,216). Investigators have reported preferential expression of the Vδ 1 gene by γδ hepatosplenic lymphomas (214,231). The majority of γδ cytotoxic T cells in the sinuses of normal spleens also preferentially utilize Vδ 1, which has been cited as evidence that this splenic cell is the origin of hepatosplenic T cell lymphoma. T-cell receptor rearrangement studies can be used for monitoring the response to treatment (232). EBV genome may be present in the neoplastic cells of some cases, but there does not appear to be any causative relationship (215,233).

Hepatosplenic T-cell lymphoma has only recently been recognized and in children may have been previously confused with a T-cell lymphoblastic malignancy or other forms of peripheral T-cell lymphomas. Reports of pediatric cases are limited to case discussions or inclusions in adult investigations (211,214,215,228,230,232). Children with αβ hepatosplenic lymphoma tend to be younger than those with the γδ form of lymphoma (215). As in adults, the clinical course in children is aggressive. Initial responses to chemotherapy are followed rapidly by relapse and death in the majority of patients. Bone marrow transplantation with subsequent relapse has been mentioned in one report (215).

Rare Pediatric Lymphomas

Rare lymphomas of children and adolescents include mycosis fungoides, panniculitis T-cell lymphoma, mucosa-associated lymphoid tissue lymphoma, human T-lymphotropic virus-1–associated leukemia/lymphoma, and natural killer lymphoma (234–249). For the most part, the clinical and biologic features of these lymphomas in children resemble their adult counterparts. However, because of their rarity in children, clinical and biologic features of these lymphomas can be gleaned only from compilations of case reports. The diagnosis of these rare lymphomas in children is often delayed or initially interpreted as a reactive process or as one of the more common pediatric lymphomas.

CLINICAL FEATURES

The signs and symptoms of presentation seen in children with non-Hodgkin's lymphoma are in large part determined by the sites of tumor involvement. There is a striking relationship between the primary site of disease at presentation and the lymphoblastic and Burkitt's lymphoma histologic subtypes (3). Children with Burkitt's lymphoma typically present with primary involvement of the abdomen or head and neck region but not of the mediastinum, whereas children with lymphoblastic lymphoma usually present with primary involvement of the head and neck area or mediastinum, but not of the abdomen. In contrast, children with large-cell lymphoma may present with primary involvement at almost any location.

Children who have a mediastinal mass (e.g., those who have lymphoblastic lymphoma) may present with a spectrum of respiratory symptoms ranging from slight cough to severe respiratory distress (2). An associated pleural effusion may contribute to worsening respiratory status. A mediastinal mass may also compromise venous return, resulting in a superior vena cava syndrome (2). This syndrome is characterized by prominent venous vasculature and swelling in the shoulder and neck region—a condition that may favor the development of deep venous thrombosis. An abdominal mass with or without associated ascites is a common finding in children with advanced-stage Burkitt's lymphoma. The tumor often arises from the terminal ileum and may result in intussusception and nausea, vomiting, and abdominal pain. Extension of the mass into the pelvis may result in compression of the ureter and secondary hydronephrosis.

The extent of disease ranges from isolated peripheral node involvement with an otherwise normal physical examination to a leukemic picture with associated pallor and increased bruising. Involvement of the central nervous system may result in headache and vision changes or in the finding of cranial nerve palsy on physical examination. Bony invasion by tumor may result in local pain or limping. Skin lesions may be present in as many as 4% of children with non-Hodgkin's lymphoma and are usually associated with CD30+ anaplastic large-cell lymphoma (250,251).

DIAGNOSIS

The diagnosis is best established by examination of tissue obtained by an open biopsy of the involved site. Sufficient tissue should be resected for histologic, cytochemical, flow cytometric, cytogenetic, and molecular pathologic studies. However, all patients should undergo bilateral iliac crest bone marrow aspiration and biopsy before open biopsy, because the diagnosis may be established by studies of these specimens without the need for more invasive procedures. Some patients, such as those with a large mediastinal mass, may not be good candidates for general anesthesia. In those cases, the diagnosis may be established by examination of pleural fluid obtained by thoracentesis. If there is no pleural fluid, the diagnosis may be established in some cases by a parasternal core biopsy of the mass obtained under local anesthesia (252).

TABLE 36.8. *Stages of non-Hodgkin's lymphoma*

Stage I

A single tumor (extranodal) or involvement of a single anatomic area (nodal), with the exclusion of the mediastinum and abdomen.

Stage II

A single tumor (extranodal) with regional node involvement.

Two or more nodal areas on the same side of the diaphragm.

Two single (extranodal) tumors, with or without regional node involvement, on the same side of the diaphragm.

A primary gastrointestinal tract tumor (usually in the ileocecal area), with or without involvement of associated mesenteric nodes, that is completely resectable.

Stage III

Two single tumors (extranodal) on opposite sides of the diaphragm.

Two or more nodal areas above and below the diaphragm.

Any primary intrathoracic tumor (mediastinal, pleural, or thymic).

Extensive primary intraabdominal disease.

Any paraspinal or epidural tumor, whether or not other sites are involved.

Stage IV

Any of the above findings with initial involvement of the central nevous system, bone marrow, or both.

Based on the classification proposed by Murphy SB. Classification, staging and end results of treatment of childhood non-Hodgkin's lymphomas: dissimilarities from lymphoma in adults. *Semin Oncol* 1980;7:332–339.

STAGING WORK-UP

The treatment of children with non-Hodgkin's lymphoma depends on both histologic subtype and disease stage. Therefore, after a diagnosis is established, an expeditious and comprehensive staging work-up must be performed. Such a work-up generally includes computed tomography of the neck, chest, abdomen and pelvis; nuclear imaging (i.e., gallium scan and bone scan); bilateral iliac crest bone marrow aspiration and biopsy; and lumbar puncture for examination of cerebrospinal fluid (1,3). Positron emission tomography is commonly used in the staging work-up of adults with malignant lymphoma, but it is not routinely used in children (253). Studies are currently being designed to compare positron emission tomography to other nuclear imaging approaches in children. After completion of the staging work-up, patients are generally classified according to the St. Jude staging system described by Murphy (Table 36.8) (10). A stage I or II classification is considered to denote limited-stage disease, whereas stage III or IV is considered to denote advanced-stage disease.

INITIAL MANAGEMENT

The lymphomas of childhood are very rapidly growing malignancies; therefore, pathologic confirmation of the diagnosis, completion of staging work-up, and initiation of chemotherapy should be expeditious. Before chemotherapy is started, various issues must be considered. A complete blood count and chemistry panel should be obtained. Children who are at high risk of tumor lysis syndrome, such as those who have advanced-stage Burkitt's lymphoma and a high serum lactate dehydrogenase value, require excellent intravenous access, vigorous hydration, and management of hyperuricemia. Historically, hyperuricemia has been managed in the United States with hyperhydration, alkalinization, and administration of allopurinol. In France, the use of uricolytic agents such as uricozyme has proven to be very effective. More recently, the recombinant form of this drug (i.e., SR29142) has become available and has been studied in the United States (254). This agent directly cleaves uric acid, converting it to allantoin, which is readily excreted; uric acid is often undetectable in the serum within several hours of administration of the drug. In a recent study of recombinant uricozyme, renal function was preserved, and there were no significant problems with hyperphosphatemia or hyperkalemia (254). When SR29142 is administered, patients at risk of tumor lysis syndrome require hyperhydration but not alkalinization or administration of allopurinol.

RELAPSE

Although there has been significant progress in the treatment of childhood lymphoma, approximately 25% to 30% of children with these diseases experience treatment failure and have refractory or recurrent disease (1). The prognosis for these children is generally considered to be poor; therefore, most investigators consider high-dose chemotherapy followed by an intensification phase with either autologous or allogeneic hematopoietic stem cell transplantation. However, such strategies remain somewhat controversial, and a recent publication has questioned their benefit (255).

Although there are relatively few reports on the role of hematopoietic stem cell transplantation in childhood lymphoma, a number of studies have suggested that some children with refractory or recurrent lymphoma benefit from this treatment approach (256–265). For example, European cooperative group trials have demonstrated successful salvage of children with Burkitt's lymphoma who have a poor early response to initial therapy while using high-dose multiagent chemotherapy followed by autologous hematopoietic stem cell rescue (256,259,261,262,264). The French Pediatric Oncology Society reported that 8 of 24 children who had hematopoietic stem cell transplantation for refractory or recurrent non-Hodgkin's lymphoma are long-term disease-free survivors (262). The Spanish Working Party for Bone Marrow Transplantation reported that of 46 children who underwent hematopoietic stem cell transplantation for refractory or recurrent non-Hodgkin's lymphoma or high-risk non-Hodgkin's lymphoma in first complete remission, 58% were event-free survivors after transplantation (261). In a St. Jude report of 20 children with refractory or recurrent non-Hodgkin's lymphoma, approximately 45% were alive and free of disease after hematopoietic stem cell transplantation (266). The available reports vary with regard to the type of hematopoietic stem cell transplantation (allogeneic vs. autologous), histologic subtype of non-Hodgkin's lymphoma, salvage therapy, and preparative regimen used; therefore, these trials must be compared with caution.

Histologic subtype does appear to be an important factor in determining the appropriate type of transplant (i.e., autologous vs. allogeneic) for children with recurrent non-Hodgkin's lymphoma. Some of the earliest studies of the use of autologous hematopoietic stem cell transplantation for non-Hodgkin's lymphoma demonstrated its efficacy in children with Burkitt's lymphoma who were poor early responders (i.e., induction failure) (257). These observations have been validated by subsequent studies (256,262). However, it is less clear whether allogeneic or autologous hematopoietic stem cell transplantation is optimal for children with Burkitt's lymphoma who develop widespread recurrent disease involving the bone marrow. Allogeneic hematopoietic stem cell transplantation from a matched sibling donor is favored by many investigators, although more data are clearly needed. For children with recurrent large-cell lymphoma, various studies have shown that autologous hematopoietic stem cell transplantation is a very effective salvage approach (260,266). In contrast, the results of autologous hematopoietic stem cell transplantation for recurrent or refractory lymphoblastic lymphoma have been less encouraging (255).

Various preparative regimens have proved to be effective in hematopoietic stem cell transplantation strategies for children with recurrent or refractory lymphoma (Table 36.9) (256–266). Carmustine, cytarabine, cyclophosphamide, and

TABLE 36.9. *Hematopoietic stem cell transplantation preparative regimens for non-Hodgkin's lymphoma in children*

Regimen or group	Components	Reference
BACT	Carmustine, cytarabine, cyclophosphamide, thioguanine	257,258
BEAM	Carmustine, etoposide, cytarabine, melphalan	257,258
Spanish Working Party	Cyclophosphamide, TBI	261
French Society of Pediatric Oncology	Busulfan, cyclophosphamide, melphalan	262
Nebraska	Thiotepa, etoposide, TBI	260

BACT, carmustine, cytarabine, cyclophosphamide, and thioguanine; BEAM, carmustine, etoposide, cytarabine, and melphalan; TBI, total-body irradiation.

thioguanine (BACT) and carmustine, etoposide, cytarabine, and melphalan (BEAM) are two of the earliest multiagent drug combinations used successfully (257,258,265). A report by the French Pediatric Oncology Society attributed their successful salvage of children with refractory or recurrent B-cell lymphomas to the inclusion of high-dose busulfan in the preparative regimen (262). In another study, excellent results for children with peripheral T-cell lymphoma were obtained by using a regimen that featured thiotepa; however, oral mucositis was reported as a significant toxicity in some children (260).

Currently, many investigators consider autologous hematopoietic stem cell transplantation for children with Burkitt's lymphoma who have a poor early response and for those with large-cell lymphoma who have chemosensitive recurrent disease. An allogeneic hematopoietic stem cell transplantation is often considered for children with systemic, chemosensitive recurrent lymphoblastic or Burkitt's lymphoma. There is clearly a need, however, for additional prospective clinical trials examining hematopoietic stem cell transplantation strategies for children with refractory or recurrent lymphoma of all histologies and relapse patterns. One report suggested that a potential graft-versus-lymphoma effect be studied in those who experience relapse, because of the very intensive initial therapy that children with lymphoma now receive (264).

RADIATION THERAPY

The role of local radiation therapy in the management of childhood non-Hodgkin's lymphoma has been changing as the survival of children with non-Hodgkin's lymphoma has been increasing with more effective chemotherapy regimens. The improved outcomes with chemotherapy have allowed trials to evaluate the need for local radiation therapy. Pediatric Oncology Group carried out a prospective randomized trial from 1987 to 1991 comparing 8 months of chemotherapy with radiotherapy to 8 months of chemotherapy without radiotherapy in children with early-stage lymphoma (49). The radiation therapy was administered during induction chemotherapy and consisted of 27 Gy in 18 fractions. Chemotherapy consisted of three cycles of CHOP followed by a 24-week maintenance phase that included 6-mercaptopurine and methotrexate. At 5 years, the rates of continuous complete remission were 88% for those receiving radiotherapy and 86% for those treated without radiotherapy. A second trial built on the results of the first and compared 8 months of chemotherapy to 9 weeks of chemotherapy (49). No patient received radiotherapy in the second trial, with projected 5-year continuous complete remission rates of 89% and 86% for the patients treated with 9 weeks of chemotherapy and for those given 8 months of chemotherapy, respectively.

The management of localized lymphoma of bone has traditionally included radiation therapy. In the initial Pediatric Oncology Group trial, the subset of children with primary lymphoma of bone was not randomized on the first trial and was nonrandomly treated with 37.5 Gy of radiotherapy. The results of three consecutive Pediatric Oncology Group trials that included 31 patients with localized lymphoma of bone were reported; seven had received chemotherapy and radiotherapy and 24 were treated with chemotherapy without the addition of radiation therapy (267). All patients achieved complete remission; one child with lymphoblastic lymphoma relapsed in the testicle 1 year after completion of therapy. There were no local relapses. Based on these results, the current management of localized lymphoma of bone involves chemotherapy without consolidative radiation therapy.

Children with advanced lymphoma do not benefit from the addition of involved-field radiation therapy as demonstrated in a randomized trial from St. Jude Children's Research Hospital (268).

Cranial irradiation has been eliminated as part of central nervous system prophylaxis in childhood lymphoma, although some institutions continue to include cranial irradiation for the treatment of advanced lymphoblastic lymphoma. Radiation therapy is used in patients with relapsed or refractory disease and in the palliation of symptomatic end-stage lymphoma. Children with persistent disease after chemotherapy or with relapsed or refractory disease may be considered for high-dose chemotherapy protocols with stem cell rescue if they have chemoresponsive disease. In such patients, radiation therapy can be used to consolidate residual disease either pre– or post–high-dose therapy, although no prospective randomized trials in pediatrics have been done to determine the benefit of the addition of radiation therapy. Radiation therapy can be useful in the palliation of symptomatic incurable disease. Hyperfractionation or accelerated fractionation can be useful to obtain responses in rapidly growing tumors. The elimination of radiation therapy in the management of childhood lymphoma can help to decrease the long-term sequelae in survivors. The late effects include musculoskeletal deformities, secondary malignan-

cies, and hypothyroidism, as well as cardiac and pulmonary sequelae (268).

LATE EFFECTS

As the cure rates for children with lymphoma have improved, many studies have focused on reducing the risk of treatment-related late effects. Three of the most serious treatment-related late effects are infertility, cardiotoxicity, and second malignancies. Various trials have explored the possibility of eliminating involved-field radiation, whereas others have attempted to eliminate or reduce the intensity of certain chemotherapeutic agents that are highly associated with specific sequelae, without compromising treatment outcome.

Chemotherapy with alkylating agents, such as cyclophosphamide, results in a dose-related depletion of germinal cells and tends to be more gonadotoxic in males than females. Recovery of spermatogenesis after cyclophosphamide-induced azoospermia is related to the total cumulative dose received (269). The results of previous trials suggest that sterility is likely at cumulative doses higher than 7.5 g per m^2, whereas fertility is usually maintained at doses less than 4 g per m^2 (269). The Pediatric Oncology Group has published the results of a randomized trial of APO versus ACOP$^+$, showing that cyclophosphamide can be eliminated altogether if a relatively anthracycline-rich chemotherapy regimen is used (133). Other trials are examining reduction of the dose of cyclophosphamide; these include a current international trial for Burkitt's lymphoma and B-cell acute lymphoblastic leukemia.

The desire to avoid anthracycline-induced cardiac toxicity has also strongly influenced protocol development for children with lymphoma. Although some adults are reported to tolerate a cumulative dose of doxorubicin of 550 mg per m^2 relatively well, children with acute lymphoblastic leukemia who were treated with lower cumulative doses of doxorubicin have shown troubling abnormalities in ventricular afterload and contractility (270). Various factors have been identified as predictive of cardiac dysfunction, including higher anthracycline dose intensity, cumulative anthracycline dose, younger age at the time of therapy, female sex, time interval since completion of therapy, and combined-modality therapy with mediastinal irradiation (271,272). A randomized trial by the Children's Cancer Group demonstrated that the addition of Adriamycin did not improve the outcome achieved with COMP alone (55). Nevertheless, anthracyclines remain an important class of agents in lymphoma treatment; one example is the use of Adriamycin in the APO regimen for large-cell non-Hodgkin's lymphoma. Therefore, investigations of cardioprotectants, such as the Pediatric Oncology Group Zinecard study, are indicated.

FUTURE DIRECTIONS

Significant progress has been made in the treatment of children with non-Hodgkin's lymphoma; however, 25% to 30% of children with newly diagnosed non-Hodgkin's lymphoma have recurrent or refractory disease despite having received aggressive modern therapy. The development of serious treatment-related late effects is of additional concern. Therefore, the goal of the pediatric oncologist is to improve the treatment result for children with non-Hodgkin's lymphoma while minimizing or eliminating the risk of therapy-induced seque-lae. The achievement of this goal requires further refinement of our current risk-adapted therapeutic approach. As additional clinical and biologic prognostic factors are identified, children with a poorer prognosis can be targeted with more aggressive or novel therapeutic approaches, whereas those with an excellent prognosis can be targeted with less intensive therapy, thus protecting them from undesirable treatment-related late effects.

The outcome of treatment for non-Hodgkin's lymphoma may be improved in a number of ways: the development of new active agents, the study of novel ways to give presently used agents, and the investigation of new drug combinations. Novel immunotherapeutic approaches may also hold promise. For example, rituximab has been shown to be active against certain adult CD20+ B-cell lymphomas (273,274). This agent is currently under investigation in children, and a study of a radiolabeled form of this monoclonal antibody is planned. Small molecule inhibitors, which have been shown to be active against adult chronic myelogenous leukemia, may also benefit children with certain non-Hodgkin's lymphoma sub-types, such as the alk+ anaplastic large-cell lymphoma.

The molecular characterization of the chromosomal abnormalities in pediatric non-Hodgkin's lymphoma has proven to be valuable in disease classification, confirmation of diagnosis, and evaluation of response to therapy (i.e., in cases such as anaplastic large-cell lymphoma in which mini-mal residual disease can be assessed by polymerase chain reaction). As mechanisms of molecular pathogenesis are more completely elucidated, insights into novel tumor-specific therapeutic approaches should emerge.

REFERENCES

1. Sandlund JT, Downing JR, Crist WM. Non-Hodgkin's lymphoma in childhood. *N Engl J Med* 1996;334:1238–1248.
2. Magrath IT. Malignant non-Hodgkin's lymphomas in children. In: Pizzo PA, Poplack DG, eds. *Principles and practice of pediatric oncology*, 2nd ed. Philadelphia: JB Lippincott Co, 1993:537–575.
3. Murphy S, Fairclough DL, Hutchison RE, et al. Non-Hodgkin's lymphomas of childhood: an analysis of the histology, staging, and response to treatment of 338 cases at a single institution. *J Clin Oncol* 1989;7:186–193.
4. Robison LL. General principles of the epidemiology of childhood cancer. In: Pizzo PA, Poplack DG, eds. *Principles and practice of pediatric oncology*, 2nd ed. Philadelphia: JB Lippincott Co, 1993:3–10.
5. Young JL Jr., Ries LG, Silverberg E, et al. Cancer incidence, survival and mortality for children younger than age 15 years. *Cancer* 1986; 58:598–602.
6. Bleyer WA. The impact of childhood cancer on the United States and the world. *CA Cancer J Clin* 1990;40:355–366.
7. Parker SL, Tong T, Bolden S, et al. Cancer statistics, 1996. *CA Cancer J Clin* 1996;65:5–27.
8. Ries LAG, Miller BA, Hankey BF, et al. *SEER cancer statistics review, 1973-1991.* Bethesda, Maryland: National Institutes of Health, 1994.
9. National Cancer Institute sponsored study of classifications of non-Hodgkin's lymphoma. Summary and description of a working formulation for clinical usage. *Cancer* 1982;49:2112–2135.
10. Murphy SB. Classification, staging and end results of treatment of childhood non-Hodgkin's lymphomas: Dissimilarities from lymphoma in adults. *Semin Oncol* 1980;7:332–339.
11. Hutchison RE, et al. Non-Hodgkin's lymphoma in children younger than three years. *Cancer* 1988;62:1371.
12. Taylor AMR, Metcalfe JA, Thick J, et al. Leukemia and lymphoma in ataxia telangiectasia. *Blood* 1996;87:423–438.
13. Ellaurie M. Lymphoma in pediatric HIV infection. *Pediatr Res* 1989;25:884(abst).
14. Murphy SB, Jenson HB, McClain KL, et al. AIDS related tumors. *Med Ped Oncol* 1997;29:381.
15. McClain KL, Joshi VV, Murphy SB. Cancers in children with HIV infection. *Hematol Oncol Clin North Am* 1996;10:1189.
16. Pluda JM, Yarchoan R, Jaffe ES, et al. Development of non-Hodgkin lymphoma in a cohort of patients with severe human immunodeficiency virus (HIV) infection on long-term antiretroviral therapy. *Ann Intern Med* 1990;113:276.
17. Filipovich AH, Heinitz KJ, Robison LL, et al. The immunodeficiency cancer registry. A research resource. *Am J Pediat Hematol Oncol* 1987;9:183–184.
18. Gatti RA, Good RA. Occurrence of malignancy in immunodeficiency disease. A literature review. *Cancer* 1971;28:89–98.
19. Harris NL, Jaffe ES, Stein H, et al. A revised European-American classification of lymphoid neoplasms: a proposal from the International Lymphoma Study Group. *Blood* 1994;84:1361–1392.
20. Jaffe ES, Harris NL, Stein H, et al., eds. *World Health Organization classification of tumours. Pathology and genetics of tumours of haematopoietic and lymphoid tissues.* Lyon, France: IARC Press, 2001.
21. Lukes R, Collins R. Immunologic characterization of human malignant lymphomas. *Cancer* 1974;34:1488.
22. Bennett JM, Catovsky D, Daniel M-T, et al. The morphologic classification of acute lymphoblastic leukemia: Concordance among observers and clinical correlations. *Br J Haematol* 1981;41:553.
23. Raphael M, Gentilhomme O, Tulliez M, et al. Histopathological features of high-grade non-Hodgkin's lymphoma in acquired immunodeficiency syndrome. The French Study Group of Pathology for Human Immunodeficiency Virus-Associated Tumors. *Arch Pathol Lab Med* 1991;115:15–20.
24. Harris NL, Jaffe ES, Diebold J, et al. The World Health Organization Classification of Hematologic Malignancies: report of the Clinical Advisory Committee meeting. *J Clin Oncol* 1999;17:3835–3849.
25. Hutchison RE, Murphy SB, Fairclough DL, et al. Diffuse small non-cleaved cell lymphoma in children. Burkitt's versus non-Burkitt's types. Results from the Pediatric Oncology Group and St. Jude Children's Research Hospital. *Cancer* 1988;64:23–28.
26. Behm FG, Campana D. Immunophenotyping. In: Pui C-H, ed. *Childhood leukemias.* New York: Cambridge University Press, 1999:111–141.
27. Falini B, Fizzotti M, Pileri S, et al. Bcl-6 protein expression in normal and neoplastic lymphoid tissue. *Ann Oncol* 1997;8[Suppl 2]:101–104.
28. Navid F, Mosijczuk AD, Head DR, et al. Acute lymphoblastic leukemia with the (8;14)(q24;q32) translocation and FAB L3 morphology associated with a B-precursor immunophenotype: the Pediatric Oncology Group experience. *Leukemia* 1999;13:135–141.
29. Loh ML, Samson Y, Motte E, et al. Translocation (2;8)(p12;q24) associated with a cryptic t(12;21)(p13;q22) TEL/AML1 gene rearrangement in a child with acute lymphoblastic leukemia. *Cancer Genet Cytogenet* 2000;122:70–82.
30. Kornblau SM, Goodacre A, Cabanillas F. Chromosomal abnormalities in adult non-endemic Burkitt's lymphoma and leukemia: 22 new reports and a review of 148 cases from the literature. *Hematol Oncol* 1991;9:63–78.
31. Krolewski JJ, Dalla-Favera R. Molecular genetic approaches in the diagnosis and classification of lymphoid malignancies. *Hematol Pathol* 1989;3:45–61.
32. Nishida K, Ritterbach J, Repp R, et al. Characterization of chromosome 8 abnormalities by fluorescence in situ hybridization in childhood B-acute lymphoblastic leukemia/non-Hodgkin lymphoma. *Cancer Genet Cytogenet* 1995;79:8–14.
33. Sandlund J, Fonseca T, Leimig T, et al. Predominance and characteristics of Burkitt's lymphoma among children with non-Hodgkin lymphoma (NHL) in northeast Brazil. *Leukemia* 1997;11:743–746.
34. Madanat FF, Amr SS, Tarawneh MS, et al. Burkitt's lymphoma in Jordanian children: epidemiological and clinical study. *Trop Med Hyg* 1986;89:189–191.

35. Shad A, Magrath I. Non-Hodgkin's lymphoma. *Pediatr Clin North Am* 1997;44:863.
36. Magrath IT, Bhatia K. Pathogenesis of small noncleaved cell lymphomas (Burkitt's lymphoma). In: Magrath IT, ed. *The non-Hodgkin's lymphomas*. London: Arnold, 1997:385–409.
37. Gutierrez MI, Bhatia K, Barriga F, et al. Molecular epidemiology of Burkitt's lymphoma from South America: differences in breakpoint location and Epstein-Barr virus association from tumors in other world regions. *Blood* 1992;79:3261–3266.
38. Kuhn-Hallek I, Sage DR, Stein L, et al. Expression of recombination activating genes (RAG-1 and RAG-2) in Epstein-Barr virus-bearing B-cells. *Blood* 1995;85:1289–1299.
39. Wilson JB, Levine AJ. The oncogenic potential of Epstein-Barr virus nuclear antigen 1 in transgenic mice. *Curr Top Microbiol Immunol* 1992;182:375–385.
40. Ruf IK, Rhyne PW, Yang H, et al. Epstein-Barr virus regulates c-MYC, apoptosis, and tumorigenicity in Burkitt lymphoma. *Mol Cell Biol* 1999;19(3):1651–1660.
41. Anderson JR, Jenkin RDT, Wilson JF, et al. Long-term follow-up of patients treated with COMP or LSA$_2$-L$_2$ therapy for childhood non-Hodgkin's lymphoma: A report of CCG-551 from the Children's Cancer Group. *J Clin Oncol* 1993;11:1024–1032.
42. Wollner N, Burchenal JH, Liebermann PH. Non-Hodgkin's lymphoma in children: a comparative study of two modalities of therapy. *Cancer* 1976;37:123.
43. Sullivan MP, Boyett J, Pullen J, et al. Pediatric Oncology Group experience with modified LSA$_2$-L$_2$ therapy in 107 children with non-Hodgkin's lymphoma (Burkitt's lymphoma excluded). *Cancer* 1985;55:323–336.
44. Sandlund JT, Santana V, Abromowitch M, et al. Large cell non-Hodgkin lymphoma of childhood: Clinical characteristics and outcome. *Leukemia* 1994;8:30–34.
45. Hutchison RE, Berard CW, Shuster JJ, et al. B-cell lineage confers a favorable outcome among children and adolescents with large-cell lymphoma: A Pediatric Oncology Group Study. *J Clin Oncol* 1995;13:2023–2032.
46. Patte C, Auperin A, Michon J, et al. The Société Française d'Oncologie Pédiatrique LMB89 protocol: highly effective multiagent chemotherapy tailored to the tumor burden and initial response in 561 unselected children with B-cell lymphomas and L3 leukemia. *Blood* 2001;97:3370–3379.
47. Murphy SB, Bowman WP, Abromowitch M, et al. Results of treatment of advanced-stage Burkitt's lymphoma and B cell (SIg+) acute lymphoblastic leukemia with high-dose fractionated cyclophosphamide and coordinated high-dose methotrexate and cytarabine. *J Clin Oncol* 1986;4:1732–1739.
48. Murphy SB, Hustu HO, Rivera G, et al. End results of treating children with localized non-Hodgkin's lymphomas with a combined modality approach of lessened intensity. *J Clin Oncol* 1983;1:326–330.
49. Link MP, Shuster JJ, Donaldson SS, et al. Treatment of children and young adults with early-stage non-Hodgkin's lymphoma. *N Engl J Med* 1997;337:1259–1266.
50. Brecher M, Schwenn MR, Coppes MJ, et al. Fractionated cyclophosphamide and back to back high dose methotrexate and cytosine arabinoside improves outcome in patients with stage III high grade small non-cleaved cell lymphomas (SNCCL): a randomized trial of the Pediatric Oncology Group. *Med Pediatr Oncol* 1997;29:526–533.
51. Bowman WP, Shuster J, Cook B, et al. Improved survival for children with B-cell acute lymphoblastic leukemia and stage IV small non-cleaved cell lymphoma: a Pediatric Oncology Group study. *J Clin Oncol* 1996;14:1252–1261.
52. Patte C, Philip T, Rodary C, et al. High survival rate in advanced-stage B-cell lymphomas and leukemias without CNS involvement with a short intensive polychemotherapy: results from the French Pediatric Oncology Society of a randomized trial of 216 children. *J Clin Oncol* 1991;9:123–132.
53. Patte C, Leverger G, Perel Y, et al. Updated results of the LMB86 protocol of the French Pediatric Oncology Society (SFOP) for B-cell non-Hodgkin's lymphomas (B-NHL) with CNS involvement (CNS+) and B-ALL. *Med Ped Oncol* 1990;18:397.
54. Reiter A, Schrappe M, Ludwig W. Favorable outcome of B-cell acute lymphoblastic leukemia in childhood: a report of three consecutive studies of the BFM Group. *Blood* 1992;80:2471.
55. Sposto R, Meadows AT, Chilcote RR, et al. Comparison of long-term outcome of children and adolescents with disseminated non-lymphoblastic non-Hodgkin lymphoma treated with COMP or daunomycin-COMP: A report from the Children's Cancer Group. *Med Pediatr Oncol* 2001;37:432–441.
56. Cairo MS, Krailo M, Hutchinson R, et al. Results of a phase II trial of "French" (F) (LMB-86) or "orange" (O) (CCG-hybrid) in children with advanced non-lymphoblastic non-Hodgkin's lymphoma: an improvement in survival. *Proc Am Soc Clin Oncol* 1994;13:392(abst).
57. Magrath IT, Janus C, Edwards BK, et al. An effective therapy for both undifferentiated (including Burkitt's) lymphomas and lymphoblastic lymphomas in children and young adults. *Blood* 1984;63:1102–1111.
58. Schwenn MR, Blattner SR, Lynch E, et al. HiC-COM: A 2-month intensive chemotherapy regimen for children with stage III and IV Burkitt's lymphoma and B-cell acute lymphoblastic leukemia. *J Clin Oncol* 1991;9:133–138.
59. Muller-Weihrich S, Henze G, Odenwald E. BFM trials for childhood non-Hodgkin's lymphomas. In: Cavalli F, Bonadonna G, Rozencweig M, eds. *Malignant lymphomas and Hodgkin's disease: experimental and therapeutic advances*. Boston: Martinus Nijhoff, 1985:633.
60. Dahl GV. A novel treatment of childhood lymphoblastic non-Hodgkin's lymphoma: early and intermittent use of teniposide plus cytarabine. *Blood* 1985;66:1110–1114.
61. Weinstein HJ, Cassady JR, Levey R. Long-term results of the APO protocol [vincristine, doxorubicin (Adriamycin) and prednisone] for treatment of mediastinal lymphoblastic lymphoma. *J Clin Oncol* 1983;1:537–541.
62. Hvizdala E. Lymphoblastic lymphoma in children—a randomized trial comparing LSA$_2$L$_2$ with the A-COP therapeutic regimen: a POG study. *J Clin Oncol* 1988;6:26–33.
63. Weinstein HJ, Lack EE, Cassady JR. APO therapy for malignant lymphoma of large cell histiocytic type of childhood: analysis of treatment results for 29 patients. *Blood* 1984;64:422–426.
64. Hvizdala EV, Berard C, Callihan T. Nonlymphoblastic lymphoma in children: histology and stage-related response to therapy: a POG study. *J Clin Oncol* 1991;9:1189–1195.
65. Santana VM, Abromowitch M, Sandlund JT, et al. MACOP-B treatment in children and adolescents with advanced diffuse large-cell non-Hodgkin's lymphoma. *Leukemia* 1993;7:187–191.
66. Reiter A, Schrappe M, Tiemann M, et al. Successful treatment strategy for Ki-1 anaplastic large-cell lymphoma of childhood: a prospective analysis of 62 patients enrolled in three consecutive Berlin-Frankfurt-Munster group studies. *J Clin Oncol* 1994;12:899–908.
67. Patte C, Kalifa C, Flamant F, et al. Results of the LMT81 protocol, a modified LSA$_2$L$_2$ protocol with high dose methotrexate, in 84 children with non-B-cell (lymphoblastic) lymphoma. *Med Ped Oncol* 1992;20:105–113.
68. Meadows A, Sposto R, Jenkin R, et al. Similar efficacy of 6 and 18 months of therapy with four drugs (COMP) for localized non-Hodgkin's lymphoma of children: a report from the children's cancer study group. *J Clin Oncol* 1989;7:92–99.
69. Patte C, Philip T, Rodary C, et al. Improved survival rate in children with stage III and IV B cell non-Hodgkin's lymphoma and leukemia using multi-agent chemotherapy: results of a study of 114 children from the French Pediatric Oncology Society. *J Clin Oncol* 1986;4:1219–1226.
70. Tubergen DG, Krailo MD, Meadows AT, et al. Comparison of treatment regimens for pediatric lymphoblastic non-Hodgkin's lymphoma: a Children's Cancer Group study. *J Clin Oncol* 1995;13:1368–1376.
71. Reiter A, Schrappe M, Parwaresch R, et al. Non-Hodgkin's lymphomas of childhood and adolescence: results of a treatment stratified for biologic subtypes and stage. A report of the Berlin-Frankfurt-Munster Group. *J Clin Oncol* 1995;13:359–372.
72. Reiter A, Schrappe M, Tiemann M, et al. Improved treatment results in childhood B-cell neoplasms with tailored intensification of therapy: A report of the Berlin-Frankfurt-Munster Group Trial NHL-BFM 90. *Blood* 1999;94:3294–3306.
73. Amylon MD, Shuster J, Pullen J, et al. Intensive high-dose asparaginase consolidation improves survival for pediatric patients with T cell acute lymphoblastic leukemia and advanced stage lymphoblastic lymphoma: a Pediatric Oncology Group Study. *Leukemia* 1999;13:335–342.
74. Magrath I, Adde M, Shad A, et al. Adult and children with small non-cleaved cell lymphoma have a similar excellent outcome when

treated with the same chemotherapy regimen. *J Clin Oncol* 1996; 14:925–934.

75. Magrath I, Adde M, Venzon D, et al. Additional chemotherapy agents improve treatment outcome for children and young adults with B-cell lymphomas. SIOP XXIX. *Med Pediat Oncol* 1997;29:358.

76. Reiter A, Schrappe M, Ludwig W-D, et al. Intensive ALL-type therapy without local radiotherapy provides a 90% event-free survival for children with T-cell lymphoblastic lymphoma: a BFM group report. *Blood* 2000;95:416–421.

77. Patte C, Michon J, Behrendt H, et al. B-cell large cell lymphoma in children, description and outcome when treated with the same regimen as Burkitt. SFOP experience with the LMB 89 protocol. *Ann Oncol* 1996;7:(abst 092).

78. Mann G, Yakisan E, Schrappe M, et al. Diffuse large B-cell lymphomas in childhood and adolescence: favorable outcome with a Burkitt's lymphoma directed therapy in trial NHL-BFM 90. A report of the BFM group. SIOP XXIX. *Med Pediatr Oncol* 1997; 29:358.

79. Patte C. Non-Hodgkin's lymphoma. *Eur J Cancer* 1998;34:359–363.

80. Soussain C, Patte C, Ostronoff M, et al. Small noncleaved cell lymphoma and leukemia in adults. A retrospective study of 65 adults treated with the LMB pediatric protocols. *Blood* 1995;85: 664–674.

81. Williams AH, Taylor CR, Higgins GR, et al. Childhood lymphoma-leukemia: I. Correlation of morphology and immunological studies. *Cancer* 1978;42:171–181.

82. Mitchell CD, Gordon I, Chessells JM. Clinical, haematological and radiological features in T-cell lymphoblastic malignancy in childhood. *Clin Radiol* 1986;37:257–261.

83. Head DR, Behm FG. Acute lymphoblastic leukemia and the lymphoblastic lymphoma of childhood. *Semin Diagn Pathol* 1995;12:325–334.

84. Murphy SB. Classification, staging, and end results of treatment of childhood non-Hodgkin's lymphomas: Dissimilarities from lymphomas in adults. *Semin Oncol* 1980;7:332.

85. Murphy SB. Childhood non-Hodgkin's lymphoma. *N Engl J Med* 1978;299:1446.

86. Reference deleted.

87. Maitra A, McKenna RW, Weinberg AG, et al. Precursor B-cell lymphoblastic lymphoma. A study of nine cases lacking blood and bone marrow involvement and review of the literature. *Am J Clin Pathol* 2001;115:868–875.

88. Lin P, Jones D, Dorfman DM, et al. Precursor B-cell lymphoblastic lymphoma: a predominantly extranodal tumor with low propensity for leukemic involvement. *Am J Surg Pathol* 2000;24:1480–1490.

89. Neth O, Seidemann K, Jansen P, et al. Precursor B-cell lymphoblastic lymphoma in childhood and adolescence: clinical features, treatment, and results in trials NHL-BFM 86 and 90. *Med Pediatr Oncol* 2000; 35:20–27.

90. Millot F, Robert A, Bertrand Y, et al. Cutaneous involvement in children with acute lymphoblastic leukemia or lymphoblastic lymphoma. The Children's Leukemia Cooperative Group of the European Organization of Research and Treatment of Cancer (EORTC). *Pediatrics* 1997;100:60–64.

91. Bernard A, Boumsell L, Reinherz EL, et al. Cell surface characterization of malignant T cells from lymphoblastic lymphoma using monoclonal antibodies: Evidence for phenotypic differences between malignant T cells from patients with acute lymphoblastic leukemia and lymphoblastic lymphoma. *Blood* 1981;57:1105.

92. Weiss LM, Bindl JM, Picozzi VJ, et al: Lymphoblastic lymphoma: An immunophenotypic study of 26 cases in comparison with T-cell acute lymphoblastic leukemia. *Blood* 1986;67:464.

93. Cossman J, Chused T, Fisher R, et al. Diversity of immunologic phenotypes of lymphoblastic lymphoma. *Cancer Res* 1983;43:4486.

94. Sheibani K, Nathwani BN, Winberg CD, et al. Antigenically defined subgroups of lymphoblastic lymphoma: Relationship to clinical presentation and biologic behavior. *Cancer* 1987;60:183.

95. Grogan T, Spier C, Wirt DP, et al: Immunologic complexity of lymphoblastic lymphoma. *Diagn Immunol* 1986;4:81.

96. Swerdlow SH, Habeshaw JA, Richards MA, et al. T lymphoblastic lymphoma with Leu-7 positive phenotype and unusual clinical course: A multiparameter study. *Leuk Res* 1985;9:167.

97. Sheibani K, Winberg CD, Burke JS, et al. Lymphoblastic lymphoma expressing natural killer cell-associated antigens: A clinicopathologic study of six cases. *Leuk Res* 1987;11:371.

98. Braziel RM, Keneklis T, Donlan JA, et al. Terminal deoxynucleotide transferase in non-Hodgkin's lymphomas. *Am J Clin Pathol* 1983;80: 655.

99. Kung PC, Long JC, McCaffrey RP, et al. Terminal deoxynucleotidyl transferase in the diagnosis of leukemia and malignant lymphoma. *Am J Med* 1978;64:788.

100. Murphy S, Jaffe ES. Terminal transferase activity and lymphoblastic neoplasm. *N Engl J Med* 1984;311:1373.

101. Bearman RM, Winberg CD, Maslow WC, et al. Terminal deoxynucleotidyl transferase activity in neoplastic and non-neoplastic hematopoietic cells. *Am J Clin Pathol* 1981;75:794.

102. McCaffrey R, Smoler DF, Baltimore D. Terminal deoxynucleotidyl transferase in a case of childhood acute lymphoblastic leukemia. *Proc Natl Acad Sci U S A* 1973;70:521.

103. Onciu M, Lorsbach RB, Henry C, et al. Terminal deoxynucleotidyl transferase (TdT)-positive cells in reactive lymph nodes from children with malignant tumors. *Am J Clin Pathol* 2002;118:248–254.

104. Soslow RA, Bhargave V, Warnke RA. MIC2, Tdt, bcl-2, and CD34 expression in paraffin-embedded high-grade lymphoma/acute lymphoblastic leukemia distinguishes between distinct clinicopathologic entities. *Hum Pathol* 1997;28:1158–1165.

105. Pui C-H, Rivera GK, Hancock ML, et al. Clinical significance of CD10 expression in childhood acute lymphoblastic leukemia. *Leukemia* 1993;7:35–40.

106. Pui C-H, Behm FG, Crist WM. Clinical and biological relevance of immunologic marker studies in childhood acute lymphoblastic leukemia. *Blood* 1993;82:343–362.

107. Roper M, Crist WM, Metzgar R, et al. Monoclonal antibody characterization of surface antigens in childhood T-cell lymphoid malignancies. *Blood* 1983;61:830–837.

108. Magrath IT. Malignant non-Hodgkin's lymphomas in children. *Hematol Oncol Clin North Am* 1987;1:577–602.

109. Crist WM, Shuster JJ, Falletta J, et al. Clinical features and outcome in childhood T-cell leukemia-lymphoma according to stage of thymocyte differentiation: a Pediatric Oncology Study Group study. *Blood* 1988;72:1891–1897.

110. Link MP, Roper M, Dorfman RF, et al: Cutaneous lymphoblastic lymphoma with pre-B markers. *Blood* 1983;61:838.

111. Borowitz MJ, Croker BP, Metzgar RS. Lymphoblastic lymphoma with the phenotype of common acute lymphoblastic leukemia. *Am J Clin Pathol* 1983;79:387.

112. Stroup R, Sheibani K, Misset JL, et al. Surface immunoglobulin positive lymphoblastic lymphoma: a report of three cases. *Cancer* 1990; 65:2559–2563.

113. Gouttefangeas C, Bensussan A, Boumsell L. Study of the CD3-associated T-cell receptors reveals further differences between T-cell acute lymphoblastic lymphoma and leukemia. *Blood* 1990;75:931.

114. Childs CC, Chrystal CS, Strauchen JA, et al. Biphenotypic lymphoblastic lymphoma: An unusual tumor with lymphocytic and granulocytic differentiation. *Cancer* 1986;57:1019.

115. Somers GR, Slater H, Rockman S, et al. Coexistent T-cell lymphoblastic lymphoma and an atypical myeloproliferative disorder associated with t(8;13)(p21;q14). *Pediatr Pathol Lab Med* 1997;17(1):141–158.

116. Thandla S, Alashari M, Green DM, et al. Therapy-related T cell lymphoblastic lymphoma with t(11;19)(q23;p13) and MLL gene rearrangement. *Leukemia* 1999;12(12):2116–2118.

117. Nagano M, Kimura N, Akiyoshi T, et al. T-stem cell leukemia/lymphoma with both myeloid lineage conversion and T-specific delta recombination. *Leuk Res* 1997;21(8):763–773.

118. Thomas DA, Kantarjian HM. Lymphoblastic lymphoma. *Hematol Oncol Clin North Am* 2001;15(1):51–95, vi.

119. Shikano T, Ishikawa Y, Naito H, et al. Cytogenetic characteristics of childhood non-Hodgkin lymphoma. *Cancer* 1992;70(3):714–719.

120. Kaneko Y, Frizzera G, Shikano T, et al. Chromosomal and immunophenotypic patterns in T-cell acute lymphoblastic leukemia and lymphoblastic lymphoma. *Leukemia* 1989;3:886.

121. Kaneko Y, Frizzera G, Maseki N, et al. A novel translocation, t(9;17)(q34;q23), in aggressive childhood lymphoblastic lymphoma. *Leukemia* 1988;2:745.

122. Naeem R, Singer S, Fletcher JA. Translocation t(8;13)(p11;q11-12) in stem cell leukemia/lymphoma of T-cell and myeloid changes. *Genes Chromosomes Cancer* 1995;12(2):148–150.

123. Inhorn RC, Aster JC, Roach SA, et al. A syndrome of lymphoblastic lymphoma, eosinophilia, and myeloid hyperplasia/malignancy asso-

ciated with t(8;13)(p11;q11): description of a distinctive clinico-pathologic entity. *Blood* 1995;85:1881–1887.

124. Xiao S, Nalabolu SR, Aster JC, et al. FGFR1 is fused with a novel zinc-finer gene, ZNF198, in the t(8;13) leukemia/lymphoma syndrome. *Nat Genet* 1998;18:84–87.

125. Narita M, Shimizu K, Hayashi Y, et al. Consistent detection of CALM-AF10 chimaeric transcripts in haematological malignancies with t(10;11)(p13;q14) and identification of novel transcripts. *Br J Haematol* 1999;105:928–937.

126. Bohlander SK, Muschinsky V, Schrader K, et al. Molecular analysis of the CALM/AF10 fusion: identical rearrangement in acute myeloid leukemia, acute lymphoblastic leukemia and malignant lymphoma patients. *Leukemia* 2000;14(1):93–99.

127. Yeoh E-J, Ross MB, Shurtleff S, et al. Classification, subtype discovery and prediction of outcome in pediatric acute lymphoblastic leukemia by gene expression profiling. *Cancer Cell* 2002;1:133–143.

128. Ferrando AA, Neuberg DS, Staunton J, et al. Gene expression signatures define novel oncogenic pathways in T-cell acute lymphoblastic leukemia. *Cancer Cell* 2002;1:75–87.

129. Synold TW, Relling MV, Boyett JM, et al. Blast cell methotrexate-poly-glutamate accumulation in vivo differs by lineage, ploidy, and methotrexate dose in acute lymphoblastic leukemia. *J Clin Invest* 1994;94:1996–2001.

130. Asselin B, Shuster J, Amylon M, et al. Improved event-free survival (EFS) with high dose methotrexate (HDM) in T-cell lymphoblastic leukemia (T-All) and advanced lymphoblastic lymphoma (T-NHL): a Pediatric Oncology Group (POG) study. *Ped Oncol* 2001;1464:367a.

131. Murphy SB. Pediatric lymphomas: recent advances and commentary on Ki-1-positive anaplastic large-cell lymphomas of childhood. *Ann Oncology* 1994;5[Suppl 1]:S31–S33.

132. Brugieres L, Le Deley MC, Pacquement H, et al. Anaplastic large cell lymphoma in children: analysis of 63 patients enrolled in two consecutive studies of the SFOP. SIOP XXIX. *Med Pediat Oncol* 1997;29:357.

133. Laver JH, Mahmoud H, Pick TE, et al. Results of a randomized phase III trial in children and adolescents with advanced stage diffuse large cell non-Hodgkin's lymphoma: a Pediatric Oncology Group study. *Leuk Lymphoma* 2002;43:105–109.

134. Rubie H, Gladieff L, Robert A, et al. Childhood anaplastic large cell lymphoma Ki-1/CD30: clinicopathologic features of 19 cases. *Med Pediatr Oncol* 1994;22:155–161.

135. Sandlund J, Pui C, Santana V, et al. Clinical features and treatment outcome for children with CD30+ large-cell non-Hodgkin's lymphoma. *J Clin Oncol* 1994;12:895–898.

136. Fraga M, Brousset P, Schlaifer D, et al. Bone marrow involvement in anaplastic large cell lymphoma. Immunohistochemical detection of minimal disease and its prognostic significance. *Am J Clin Pathol* 1995;103:82–89.

137. Benharroch D, Meguerian-Bedoyan Z, Lamant L, et al. ALK-positive lymphoma: a single disease with a broad spectrum of morphology. *Blood* 1998;91:2076–2084.

138. Brugieres L, Le Deley MC, Pacquement H, et al. CD30⁺ anaplastic large-cell lymphoma in children: analysis of 82 patients enrolled in two consecutive studies of the French Society of Pediatric Oncology. *Blood* 1998;92:3591–3598.

139. Sandlund JT, Roberts WM, Pui C-H, et al. Systemic hemophagocytosis masking the diagnosis of large cell non-Hodgkin lymphoma. *Med Pediatr Oncol* 1997;29:167–169.

140. Blatt J, Weston B, Belhorn T, et al. Childhood non-Hodgkin lymphoma presenting as hemophagocytic syndrome. *Pediatr Hematol Oncol* 2002;19:45–49.

141. Mann KP, Hall B, Kamino H, et al. Neutrophil-rich, Ki-1-positive anaplastic large-cell malignant lymphoma. *Am J Surg Pathol* 1995;19:407–416.

142. McCluggage WG, Walsh MY, Bharucha H. Anaplastic large cell malignant lymphoma with extensive eosinophilic or neutrophilic infiltration. *Histopathology* 1998;32:110–115.

143. Simonart T, Kentos A, Renoirte C, et al. Cutaneous involvement by neutrophil-rich, CD30-positive anaplastic large cell lymphoma mimicking deep pustules. *Am J Surg Pathol* 1999;23:244–266.

144. Kinney MC, Collins RD, Greer JP, et al. A small-cell-predominant variant of primary Ki-1 CD30+ T-cell lymphoma. *Am J Surg Pathol* 1993;17:859–868.

145. Chan JK, Buchanan R, Fletcher CD. Sarcomatoid variant of anaplastic large-cell Ki-1 lymphoma. *Am J Surg Pathol* 1990;14:983–988.

146. Falini B, Liso A, Pasqualucci L, et al. CD30+ anaplastic large cell lymphoma, null type, with signet-ring appearance. *Histopathology* 1997;30:90–92.

147. Piccaluga PP, Ascani S, Fraternali Orcioni G, et al. ALK expression as a marker of malignancy. Application to a case of anaplastic large cell lymphoma with high granulomatous reaction. *Haematologica* 2000;85:978–981.

148. van den Berg H, Noorduyn A, van Kullenburg ABP, et al. Leukemic expression of anaplastic large cell lymphoma with 46,XX,ins(2;5)(p23;q15q36) in a child with dihydropyrimidine dehydrogenase deficiency. *Leukemia* 2000;14:769–770.

149. Anderson MM, Ross CW, Singleton TP, et al. Ki-1 anaplastic large cell lymphoma with a prominent leukemic phase. *Hum Pathol* 1996;27:1093–1095.

150. Villamor N, Rozman M, Esteve J, et al. Anaplastic large-cell lymphoma with rapid evolution to leukemic phase. *Ann Hematol* 1999;78:478–482.

151. Bayle C, Charpentier A, Duchayne E, et al. Leukaemic presentation of small cell variant anaplastic large cell lymphoma: report of four cases. *Br J Haematol* 1999;104:680–688.

152. Meech SJ, McGavaran L, Odom LF, et al. Unusual childhood extramedullary hematologic malignancy with natural killer cell properties that contains tropomyosin 4-anaplastic lymphoma kinase gene fusion. *Blood* 2001;98:1209–1216.

153. Chhanabhai M, Britten C, Klasa R, et al. t(2;5) positive lymphoma with peripheral blood involvement. *Leukemia Lymphoma* 1998;28;415–422.

154. Stein H, Foss HD, Durkop H, et al. CD30-positive anaplastic large cell lymphoma: a review of its histopathological, genetic, and clinical features. *Blood* 2000;96:3681–3695.

155. Delsol GA, Al Saati T, Gatter KC, et al. Coexpression of epithelial membrane antigen (EMA), Ki-1, and interleukin-2 receptor by anaplastic large cell lymphoma. Diagnostic value in so-called malignant histiocytosis. *Am J Pathol* 1988;130:59–70.

156. Kaneko Y, Frizzera G, Edamura S, et al. A novel translocation, t(2;5)(p23;q35), in childhood phagocytic large T-cell lymphoma mimicking malignant histiocytosis. *Blood* 1989;73:806.

157. Mason DY, Bastard C, Rimokh R, et al. CD30-positive large cell lymphomas ('Ki-1 lymphoma') are associated with a chromosomal translocation involving 5q35. *Br J Haematol* 1990;74:161–168.

158. Lamant L, Dastugue N, Pullford K, et al. A new fusion gene TPM3-ALK in anaplastic large cell lymphoma created by a (1;2)(q25;p23) translocation. *Blood* 1999;93:3088–3095.

159. Rosenwald A, Ott G, Pullford K, et al. t(1;2)(q21;p23) and t(2;3)(p23;q21): two novel variant translocations of the t(2;5)(p23;q35) in anaplastic large cell lymphoma. *Blood* 1999;94:362–364.

160. Colleoni GW, Bridge JA, Garicochea B, et al. ATIC-ALK: a novel variant ALK gene fusion in anaplastic large cell lymphoma resulting form the recurrent cryptic chromosome inversion, inv(2)(p23q35). *Am J Pathol* 2000;156:781–789.

161. Morris SW, Kirstein MN, Valentine MB, et al. fusion of a kinase gene, ALK, to a nucleolar protein gene, NPM, in non-Hodgkin's lymphoma. *Science* 1994;263:1281–1284.

162. Lamant L, Meggetto F, Al Saati TA, et al. High incidence of the t(2;5)(p23;q35) translocation in anaplastic large cell lymphoma and its lack of detection in Hodgkin's disease: comparison of cytogenetic analysis, reverse transcriptase-polymerase chain reaction, and P-80 immunostaining. *Blood* 1996;87:284–291.

163. Pulford K, Lamant L, Morris SW, et al. Detection of anaplastic lymphoma kinase (ALK) and nucleolar protein (NPM)-ALK proteins in normal and neoplastic cells with the monoclonal antibody ALK1. *Blood* 1997;89:1394–1404.

164. Delsol G, Lamant L, Mariame B, et al. A new subtype of large B-cell lymphoma expressing the ALK kinase and lacking the 2;5 translocation. *Blood* 1997;89:1483–1490.

165. Falini B, Bigerna B, Pizzotti M, et al. ALK expression defines a distinct group of t/null lymphomas ('ALK lymphomas') with a wide morphologic spectrum. *Am J Pathol* 1998;153:875–886.

166. Lawrence B, Perez-Atayde A, Hibbard MK, et al. TPM3-ALK and TPM4-ALK oncogenes in inflammatory myofibroblastic tumors. *Am J Pathol* 2000;157:377–384.

167. Lamant L, Pullford K, Bischof D, et al. Expression of the ALK tyrosine kinase gene in neuroblastoma. *Am J Pathol* 2000;156:1711–1721.

168. Falini B. Anaplastic large cell lymphoma: pathological, molecular and clinical features. *Br J Haematol* 2001;114:741–760.

169. Touriol C, Greenland C, Lamant L, et al. Further demonstration of the diversity of chromosomal changes involving 2p23 in ALK-positive lymphoma: 2 cases expressing ALK kinase fused to CLTCL (clathrin chain polypeptide-like). *Blood* 2000;95:3204–3207.

170. Shiota M, Nakamura S, Ichinohasama R, et al. Anaplastic large cell lymphoma expressing the novel chimeric protein p80NPM/ALK: a distinct clinicopathologic entity. *Blood* 1995;86(5):1954–1960.

171. Falini B, Pileri S, Zinzani PL, et al. ALK+ lymphoma: clinico-pathological findings and outcome. *Blood* 1999;03(8):2697–2700.

172. Gascoyne RD, Aoun P, Wu D, et al. Prognostic significance of anaplastic lymphoma kinase (ALK) protein expression in adults with anaplastic large cell lymphoma. *Blood* 1999;93:3913–3921.

173. Falini B, Pulford K, Pucciarini A, et al. Lymphomas expressing ALK fusion protein(s) other than NPM-ALK. *Blood* 1999;94(10):3509–3515.

174. Reference deleted.

175. Le Deley MC, Reiter A, Williams D, et al. Prognostic factors in childhood anaplastic large cell lymphoma: results of the European Intergroup Study. *Ann Oncol* 1999;10[Suppl 3]:28.

176. Williams DM, Hobson R, Imeson J, et al. Anaplastic large cell lymphoma in childhood: analysis of 72 patients treated on The United Kingdom Children's Cancer Study Group chemotherapy regimens. *Br J Haematol* 2002;117:812–820.

177. Brugieres L, Quartier P, LeDeley MC, et al. Relapses of childhood anaplastic large cell lymphoma: treatment results in a series of 41 children—a report from the French Society of Pediatric Oncology. *Ann Oncol* 200;11:53–58.

178. Lones MA, Auperin A, Raphael M, et al. Mature B-cell lymphoma/leukemia in children and adolescents: intergroup pathologist consensus with the Revised European-American Lymphoma Classification. *Ann Oncol* 2000;11:47–51.

179. Hutchison RE, Finch C, Kepner J, et al. Burkitt lymphoma is immunophenotypically different from Burkitt-like lymphoma in young persons. *Ann Oncol* 2000;11[Suppl 1]:35–38.

180. Alizadeh AA, Eisen MB, Davis RE, et al. Distinct types of diffuse large B-cell lymphoma identified by gene expression proofing. *Nature* 2000;403:503–511.

181. Davis RE, Staudt LM. Molecular diagnosis of lymphoid malignancies by gene expression profiling. *Curr Opin Hematol* 2002;9:333–338.

182. Lazzarino M, Orlandi E, Paulli M, et al. Treatment outcome and prognostic factors for primary mediastinal (thymic) B-cell lymphoma: a multicenter study of 106 patients. *J Clin Oncol* 1997;15:1646–1653.

183. Zanzani PL, Bendandi M, Frezza G, et al. Primary mediastinal B-cell lymphoma with sclerosis: clinical and therapeutic evaluation of 22 patients. Leuk Lymphoma 1996;21:311–316.

184. Pauli M, Lazzarino M, Gianelli U, et al. Primary mediastinal B-cell lymphoma: update of its clinicopathologic features. *Leukemia Lymphoma* 1997;26:115–123.

185. Lones MA, Perkins SL, Sposto R, et al. Large-cell lymphoma arising in the mediastinum of children and adolescents is associated with an excellent outcome: a Children's Cancer Group report. *J Clin Oncol* 2000;18:3845–3853.

186. van Besien K, Kelta M, Bahaguna. Primary mediastinal B-cell lymphoma: a review of pathology and management. *J Clin Oncol* 2001;19:1855–1864.

187. Abou-Ellela AA, Weinburger DD, Vose JM, et al. Primary mediastinal large B-cell lymphoma: a clinicopathologic study of 43 patients from the Nebraska Lymphoma Study Group. *J Clin Oncol* 1999;17:784–790.

188. Kanavaros P, Gaulard P, Charlotte F, et al. Discordant expression of immunoglobulin and its associated molecular mb-1/CD79a is frequently found in mediastinal large B cell lymphomas. *Am J Pathol* 1995;146:735–741.

189. Pauli M, Strater J, Gianelli U, et al. Mediastinal B-cell lymphoma: a study of its histomorphologic spectrum based on 109 cases. *Human Pathol* 1999;30:178–187.

190. de Leval L, Ferry JA, Falini B, et al. Expression of bcl-6 and CD10 in primary mediastinal large B-cell lymphoma: evidence for derivation from germinal center B cells? *Am J Surg Pathol* 2001;25:1277–1282.

191. Lamarre L, Jacobson JO, Aisenberg AC, et al. Primary large cell lymphoma of the mediastinum: a histologic and immunophenotype study of 29 cases. *Am J Surg Pathol* 1989;13:730–739.

192. Higgins JP, Warnke RA. CD30 expression is common in mediastinal large B-cell lymphoma. *Am J Clin Pathol* 1999;112:241–247.

193. Lazzarino M, Orlandi E, Astori C, et al. A low pretreatment serum level β2-microglobulin level despite bulky tumor is a characteristic feature of primary mediastinal large B-cell lymphoma: implications for serologic staging. *Eur J Haematol* 1996;57:331–333.

194. Moller P, Herrman B, Moldenhauer G, et al. Defective expression of MHC class I antigens is frequent in B-cell lymphomas of high-grade malignancy. *Int J Cancer* 1987;40:32–39.

195. Kuppers R, Rajewsky K, Hansmann ML. Diffuse large cell lymphomas are derived from mature B cells carrying V region genes with a high load of somatic mutation and evidence of selection for antibody expression. *Eur J Immunol* 1997;27:1398–1405.

196. Scarpa A, Moore PS, Riguad G, et al. Molecular features of primary mediastinal B-cell lymphoma: involvement of p16INK4A, p53, and c-myc. *Br J Haematol* 1999;107:106–113.

197. Bentz M, Barth TF, Bruderlein S, et al. Gain of chromosome arm 9p is characteristic of primary mediastinal B-cell lymphoma (MBL): comprehensive molecular cytogenetic analysis and presentation of a novel MBL cell line. *Genes Chromosomes Cancer* 2001;30:393–401.

198. Palanisamy N, Abou-Elella AA, Chaganti SR, et al. Similar patterns of genomic alteration characterize primary mediastinal large-B-cell lymphoma and diffuse large-B-cell lymphoma. *Genes Chromosomes Cancer* 2002;33:114–122.

199. Joos S, Otano-Joos MI, Ziegler S, et al. Primary mediastinal (thymic) B-cell lymphoma is characterized by gains of chromosome material including 9p and amplification of the REL gene. *Blood* 1996;87:1571–1578.

200. Tsang P, Cesarman E, Chadburn A, et al. Molecular characterization of primary mediastinal B cell lymphoma. *Am J Pathol* 1996;148:2017–2025.

201. Frizzera G, Murphy SB. Follicular (nodular) lymphoma in childhood: a rare clinical-pathological entity, report of eight cases from four cancer centers. *Cancer* 1979;44:2218–2235.

202. Murphy SB, Fairclough DL, Hutchison RE, et al. Non-Hodgkin's lymphomas of childhood: an analysis of the histology, staging, and response to treatment of 338 cases at a single institution. *J Clin Oncol* 1989;7:186–193.

203. Pinto A, Hutchison RE, Grant LH, et al. Follicular lymphomas in pediatric patients. *Mod Pathol* 1990;3:308–313.

204. Ribeiro RC, Pui CH, Murphy SB, et al. Childhood malignant non-Hodgkin's lymphomas of uncommon histology. *Leukemia* 1992;6:761–765.

205. Atra A, Meller ST, Stevens RS, et al. Conservative management of follicular non-Hodgkin's lymphoma in childhood. *Br J Haematol* 1998;103:320–323.

206. Lorsbach RB, Shay-Seymour D, Moore J, et al. Clinicopathologic analysis of follicular lymphoma occurring in children. *Blood* 2002;99:1959–1964.

207. Moertel CL, Watterson J, McCormick SR, et al. Follicular large cell lymphoma of the testis in a child. *Cancer* 1995;75:1182–1186.

208. Finn LS, Viswanatha DS, Belasco JB, et al. Primary follicular lymphoma of the testis in childhood. *Cancer* 1999;85:1626–1635.

209. Lu D, Medeiros LJ, Eskenazi AE, et al. Primary follicular large cell lymphoma of the testis in a child. *Arch Pathol Lab Med* 2001;125:551–554.

210. Pakzad K, MacLennan GT, Elder JS, et al. Follicular large cell lymphoma localized to the testis in children. *J Urol* 2002;168:225–228.

211. Lai R, Larratt LM, Etches W, et al. Hepatosplenic T-cell lymphoma of alphabeta lineage in a 16-year-old boy presenting with hemolytic anemia and thrombocytopenia. *Am J Surg Pathol* 2000;24:459–463.

212. Weidmann E. Hepatosplenic T cell lymphoma. A review on 45 cases since the first report describing the disease as a distinct lymphoma entity in 1990. *Leukemia* 2000;14:991–997.

213. Suarez F, Wlodarska I, Rigal-Huguet F, et al. Hepatosplenic alpha-beta T-cell lymphoma: an unusual case with clinical, histologic, and cytogenetic features of gammadelta hepatosplenic T-cell lymphoma. *Am J Surg Pathol* 2000;24:1027–1032.

214. Cooke CB, Krenacs L, Stetler-Stevenson M, et al. Hepatosplenic T-cell lymphoma: a distinct clinicopathologic entity of cytotoxic gamma delta T-cell origin. *Blood* 1996;88:4265–4274.

215. Macon WR, Levy NB, Kurtin PJ, et al. Hepatosplenic αβ T-cell lymphomas. *Am J Surg Pathol* 2001;25:285–296.

216. Farcet J, Gaulard P, Marolleau J, et al. Hepatosplenic T-cell lymphoma: sinusal/sinusoidal localization of malignant cells expressing the T-cell receptor αβ. *Blood* 1990;75:2213–2219.

217. Francois A, Lesesve J-F, Stamatoullas A, et al. Hepatosplenic gamma/delta T-cell lymphoma: a report of two cases in immunocompromised patients associated with isochromosome 7q. *Am J Surg Pathol* 1997;21:781–790.

218. Ross CW, Schnitzer B, Sheldon S, et al. γδ T cell posttransplantation lymphoproliferative disorder primarily in the spleen. *Am J Clin Pathol* 1994;102:310–315.

219. Khan WA, Yu L, Eisenbrey AB, et al. Hepatosplenic gamma/delta T-cell lymphoma in immunocompromised patients. Report of two cases and review of literature. *Am J Clin Pathol* 2001;116:41–50.

220. Steurer M, Stauder R, Grunewald K, et al. Hepatosplenic gamma-delta-T-cell lymphoma with leukemic course after renal transplant. *Hum Pathol* 2002;33:253–258.

221. Wang CC, Tien HF, Lin MT, et al. Consistent presence of isochromosome 7q in hepatosplenic T gamma/delta lymphoma: a new cytogenetic-clinicopathologic entity. *Genes Chromosomes Cancer* 1995;12:161–164.

222. Vega F, Medeiros LJ, Bueso-Ramos C, et al. Hepatosplenic lymphoma in bone marrow. A sinusoidal neoplasm with blastic cytologic features. *Am J Clin Pathol* 2001;116:410–419.

223. Salhany KE, Feldman M, Kahn MJ, et al. Hepatosplenic gamma/delta T-cell lymphoma: ultrastructural, immunophenotypic, and functional evidence for cytotoxic T lymphocyte differentiation. *Hum Pathol* 1997;28:674–685.

224. Nosari A, Oreste PL, Biondi A, et al. Hepato-splenic gamma/delta T-cell lymphoma: a rare entity mimicking the hemophagocytic syndrome. *Am J Hematol* 1999;60:61–65.

225. Felger RE, Macon WR, Kinney MC, et al. TIA-1 expression in lymphoid neoplasms. Identification of subsets with cytotoxic T lymphocyte or natural killer cell differentiation. *Am J Pathol* 1997;150:1893–1900.

226. Boulland ML, Kanavaros P, Wechsler J, et al. Cytotoxic protein expression in natural killer cell lymphomas and in alpha beta and gamma delta peripheral T-cell lymphomas. *J Pathol* 1997;183:432–439.

227. Joneaux P, Daniel MT, Martel V, et al. Isochromosome 7q and trisomy 8 are consistent primary, non-random chromosomal abnormalities associated with hepatosplenic T gamma/delta lymphoma. *Leukemia* 1996;10:1453–1455.

228. Coventry S, Punnett HH, Tomczak EZ, et al. Consistency of isochromosome 7q and trisomy 8 in hepatosplenic gammadelta T-cell lymphoma: detection by fluorescence in situ hybridization of a splenic touch-preparation from a pediatric patient. *Pediatr Dev Pathol* 1999;2:478–483.

229. Wlodarska I, Martin-Garcia N, Achten R, et al. Fluorescence in situ hybridization study of chromosome 7 aberrations in hepatosplenic T-cell lymphoma: isochromosome 7q as a common abnormality accumulating in forms with features of cytologic progression. *Genes Chromosomes Cancer* 2002;33:243–251.

230. Rossbach HC, Chamizo W, Dumont DP, et al. Hepatosplenic gamma/delta T-cell lymphoma with isochromosome 7q, translocation t(7;21), and tetrasomy 8 in a 9-year-old girl. *J Pediatric Hematol* 2002;24:154–157.

231. Przybylski GK, Wu H, Macon WR, et al. Hepatosplenic and subcutaneous panniculitis-like gamma-delta T cell lymphomas are derived from different delta subsets of gamma/delta T lymphocytes. *J Mol Diagn* 2000;2:11–19.

232. Garcia-Sanchez F, Menarguez J, Cristobal E, et al. Hepatosplenic gamma-delta T-cell malignant lymphoma: report of the first case in childhood, including molecular minimal residual disease follow-up. Br J Haematol 1995;90:943–946.

233. Ohshima K, Haraoka S, Harada N, et al. Hepatosplenic gammadelta T-cell lymphoma: relation to Epstein-Barr virus and activated cytotoxic molecules. *Histopathol* 2000;36:127–135.

234. Agnarrsson BA, Kadin ME. Peripheral T-cell lymphomas in children. *Semin Diagn Pathol* 1995;12:314–324.

235. El-Hoshy K, Hashimoto K. Adolescence mycosis fungoides: an unusual presentation with hypopigmentation. *J Dermatol* 1995;22:424–427.

236. Grunwald MH, Amichai B. Localized hypopigmented mycosis fungoides in a 12-year-old Caucasian boy. *J Dermatol* 1999;26:70–71.

237. Schmid H, Dummer R, Kempf W, et al. Mycosis fungoides with mucinous follicularis in childhood. *Dermatology* 1999;198:284–287.

238. Garzon MC. Cutaneous T cell lymphoma in children. *Semin Cutan Med Surg* 1999;18:226–232.

239. Tan E, Tay YK, Giam YC. Profile and outcome of childhood mycosis fungoides in Singapore. *Pediatr Dermatol* 2000;17:352–356.

240. Neuhaus IM, Ramos-Caro FA, Hassanein AM. Hypopigmented mycosis fungoides in childhood and adolescence. *Pediatr Dermatol* 2000;17:403–406.

241. Whittam LR, Calonje E, Orchard G, et al. CD8-positive juvenile onset mycosis fungoides: an immunohistochemical and genotypic analysis of six cases. *Br J Dermatol* 2000;143:199–204.

242. Gold BD. New approaches to *Helicobacter pylori* infection in children. *Curr Gastroenterol Rep* 201;3:235–247.

243. Sen F, Rassidakis GZ, Jones D, et al. Apoptosis and proliferation in subcutaneous panniculitis-like T-cell lymphoma. *Mod Pathol* 2002;15:625–631.

244. Thomson AB, McKenzie KJ, Jackson R, et al. Subcutaneous panniculitic T-cell lymphoma in childhood: successful response to chemotherapy. *Med Pediatr Oncol* 2001;37:549–552.

245. Lewis JM, Vasef MA, Seabury Stone M. HTLV-1-associated granulomatous T-cell lymphoma in a child. *J Am Acad Dermatol* 2001;44:525–529.

246. Broniscer A, Ribeiro RC, Srinivas RV, et al. An adolescent with HTLV-I-associated adult T-cell leukemia treated with interferon-alpha and zidovudine. *Leukemia* 1996;10:1244–1254.

247. Miyazaki M, Lin Y-W, Okiada M, et al. Childhood cutaneous natural killer/T-cell lymphoma successfully treated with only one course of chemotherapy and incomplete tumor resection. *Haematologica* 2001;86:883–884.

248. Ohnuma K, Toyada Y, Nishihira H, et al. Aggressive natural killer (NK) cell lymphoma: report of a pediatric case and review of the literature. *Leuk Lymphoma* 1997;25:387–392.

249. Shaw PH, Cohn SL, Morgan ER, et al. Natural killer cell lymphoma: report of two pediatric cases, therapeutic options, and review of the literature. *Cancer* 2001;91:642–646.

250. Kadin ME. Ki-1-positive anaplastic large-cell lymphoma: A clinicopathologic entity? *J Clin Oncol* 1991;9:533–536.

251. Kadin ME. Ki-1/CD30+ (anaplastic) large-cell lymphoma: maturation of a clinicopathologic entity with prospects of effective therapy. *J Clin Oncol* 1994;12:884–887.

252. Garrett KM, Hoffer FA, Behm FG, et al. Interventional radiology techniques for the diagnosis of lymphoma or leukemia. *Pediatr Radiol* 2002;32:653–662.

253. Naumann R, Vaic A, Beuthien-Baumann B, et al. Prognostic value of positron emission tomography in the evaluation of post-treatment residual mass in patients with Hodgkin's disease and non-Hodgkin's lymphoma. *Br J Haematol* 2001;115:793–800.

254. Pui C-H, Mahmoud HH, Wiley JM, et al. Recombinant urate oxidase for the prophylaxis or treatment of hyperuricemia in patients with leukemia or lymphoma. *J Clin Oncol* 2001;19:697–704.

255. Korinsky NL, Sposto R, Shah NR, et al. Outcomes of treatment of children and adolescents with recurrent non-Hodgkin's lymphoma and Hodgkin's disease with dexamethasone, etoposide, cisplatin, cytarabine, and L-asparaginase, maintenance chemotherapy, and transplantation: Children's Cancer Group Study CCG-5912. *J Clin Oncol* 2001;19:2390–2396.

256. Reiter A, Schrappe M, Tiemann M, et al. Improved treatment results in childhood B-cell neoplasm with tailored intensification of therapy: a report of the Berlin-Frankfurt-Münster Group Trial NHL-BFM 90. *Blood* 1999;94:3294–3306.

257. Philip T, Biron P, Philip I, et al. Massive therapy and autologous bone marrow transplantation in pediatric and young adults Burkitt's lymphoma (30 courses on 28 patients: a 5-year experience). *Eur J Cancer Clin Oncol* 1986;22:1015–1027.

258. Philip T, Armitage JO, Spitzer G, et al. High-dose therapy and autologous bone marrow transplantation after failure of conventional chemotherapy in adults with intermediate-grade or high-grade non-Hodgkin's lymphoma. *N Engl J Med* 1987;316:1493–1498.

259. Philip T, Hartmann O, Biron P, et al. High-dose therapy and autologous bone marrow transplantation in partial remission after first-line induction therapy for diffuse non-Hodgkin's lymphoma. *J Clin Oncol* 1988;6:1118–1124.

260. Gordon BG, Warkentin PI, Weisenburger DD, et al. Bone marrow transplantation for peripheral T-cell lymphoma in children and adolescents. *Blood* 1992;80:2938–2942.

261. Bureo E, Ortega JJ, Muñoz A, et al. Bone marrow transplantation in

46 pediatric patients with non-Hodgkin's lymphoma. *Bone Marrow Transplant* 1995;15:353–359.

262. Avet Loiseau H, Hartmann O, Valteau D, et al. High-dose chemotherapy containing busulfan followed by bone marrow transplantation in 24 children with refractory or relapsed non-Hodgkin's lymphoma. *Bone Marrow Transplant* 1991;8:465–472.

263. O'Leary M, Ramsay NKC, Nesbit ME, et al. Bone marrow transplantation for non-Hodgkin's lymphoma in children and young adults. *Am J Med* 1983;74:497.

264. Ladenstein R, Pearce R, Hartmann O, et al. High-dose chemotherapy with autologous bone marrow rescue in children with poor-risk Burkitt's lymphoma: a report from the European Lymphoma Bone Marrow Transplantation Registry. *Blood* 1997;90:2921–2930.

265. Appelbaum FR, Deisseroth AB, Graw RG, et al. Prolonged complete remission following high-dose chemotherapy of Burkitt's lymphoma in relapse. *Cancer* 1978;41:1059–1063.

266. Sandlund JT, Bowman L, Heslop HE, et al. Intensive chemotherapy with hematopoietic stem-cell support for children with recurrent or refractory NHL. *Cytotherapy* 2002;4:253–258.

267. Suryanarayan K, Shuster JJ, Donaldson SS, et al. Treatment of localized primary non-Hodgkin's lymphoma of bone in children: a Pediatric Oncology Group study. *J Clin Oncol* 1999;17:456–459.

268. Murphy SB, Hustu HO. A randomized trial of combined modality therapy of childhood non-Hodgkin's lymphoma. *Cancer* 1980;45:630–637.

269. Meistrich ML, Wilson G, Brown BW, et al. Impact of cyclophosphamide on long-term reduction in sperm count in men treated with combination chemotherapy for Ewing and soft tissue sarcomas. *Cancer* 1992;70:2703–2712.

270. Lipshultz SE, Colan SD, Gelber RD, et al. Late cardiac effects of doxorubicin therapy for acute lymphoblastic leukemia in childhood. *N Engl J Med* 1991;324:808–815.

271. Sorensen K, Levitt G, Bull C, et al. Anthracycline dose in childhood acute lymphoblastic leukemia: Issues of early survival versus late cardiotoxicity. *J Clin Oncol* 1997;15:61–68.

272. Nysom K, Holm K, Lipsitz SR, et al. Relationship between cumulative anthracycline dose and late cardiotoxicity in childhood acute lymphoblastic leukemia. *J Clin Oncol* 1998;16:545–550.

273. Colombat P, Salles G, Brousse N, et al. Rituximab (anti-CD20 monoclonal antibody) as single first-line therapy for patients with follicular lymphoma with a low tumor burden: clinical and molecular evaluation. *Blood* 2001;97:101–106.

274. Coiffier B, Haioun C, Ketterer N, et al. Rituximab (anti-CD20 monoclonal antibody) for the treatment of patients with relapsing or refractory aggressive lymphoma: a multicenter phase II study. *Blood* 1998;92:1927–1932.

275. Falini B, Mason DY. Proteins encoded by genes involved in chromosomal alterations in lymphoma and leukemia: clinical value of their detection by immunocytochemistry. *Blood* 2002;99:409–426.

CHAPTER 37

Management of Lymphoma in the Elderly

Bertrand Coiffier

Lymphomas in elderly patients need special attention because elderly patients represent one half of the cases (the median age for all lymphomas is approximately 60 years) and because these patients usually require different management than younger patients. Indeed, most of these patients had one or several other diseases before the lymphoma that may alter the capacity to tolerate the treatment of the lymphoma (1). Moreover, the incidence of lymphoma in elderly patients has increased in recent years, probably more than it has in young patients (2), although recent results show a trend toward stabilization during the 1990s (3). Very few differences have been described for morphology and clinical presentation between young and elderly patients with lymphoma (4). However, outcome for elderly patients with lymphoma is worse, particularly for those with aggressive subtypes, because of the difficulties encountered during treatment, difficulties related to the presence of other diseases, diminished organ function, and altered drug metabolism (1,5). A recent study concludes that the best way to improve the survival of elderly patients with lymphoma is to have the intention to treat them correctly, that is with an optimal chemotherapy regimen (6).

HIGH INCIDENCE OF LYMPHOMA IN THE ELDERLY

The prolonged human life expectancy has naturally resulted in an increase in the number of elderly patients; current estimates indicate that the percentage of people older than 65 years of age will rise from 12% to 20% over the next 25 years (7). An increase in the incidence of lymphomas has been documented in Europe and the United States, particularly among elderly patients (3,8–10). For the last 25 years, lymphoma incidence has increased by more than 50% and even more in patients older than 60 years of age; now it is 15 to 16 new cases a year for each 100,000 inhabitants in the United States (11). One half of all newly diagnosed patients with lymphoma are older than 60 years of age (Fig. 37.1). All lymphoma subtypes increased, but diffuse large B-cell lymphoma was the one with the most important increase in elderly patients (12).

LYMPHOMA SUBTYPES IN THE ELDERLY

All lymphoma subtypes may be observed in elderly patients but with some differences when compared with those encountered in younger patients (4,13). Most of the large epidemiologic studies have been done with the Working Formulation for Clinical Usage (14) and found a higher percentage of aggressive lymphoma among the elderly (3,8,9,11,15). Recent studies use the Revised European-American Classification of Lymphoid Neoplasms (16), not too different from the World Health Organization Classification (13), and allow more precise definition of the subtypes. Only one large study has defined the differences between young and elderly patients, but it is not an epidemiologic study (4,17). All cases included in this study were reviewed by five expert pathologists. This study shows that, in the eight referral centers worldwide, there are some differences; elderly patients more frequently have lymphocytic/lymphoplasmacytoid lymphoma, diffuse large B-cell lymphoma, and peripheral T-cell lymphoma and less frequently have anaplastic large cell lymphoma, lymphoblastic lymphoma, and Burkitt's lymphoma (Table 37.1). In all studies, the two most frequent subtypes are diffuse large B-cell lymphoma and follicular lymphoma, accounting for 40% and 20% of all cases, respectively.

No specific chromosomal or genetic abnormalities have been described in elderly patients, but very few studies have looked at them.

SPECIAL PROBLEMS FOR STAGING IN THE ELDERLY

As in young patients, the Ann Arbor staging system for Hodgkin's lymphoma has proved inappropriate in the elderly, and since 1993, prognosis has been better described by the International Prognostic Index than the stage (18). The International Prognostic Index includes age (younger or older than 60 years), disease stage (localized or disseminated), performance status (good, 0 to 1; or poor, less than 1), lactate dehydrogenase (LDH) levels (normal or above normal), and

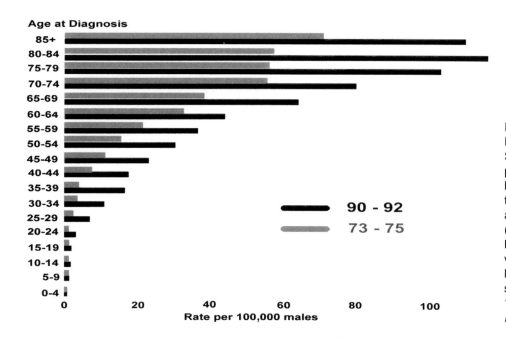

Age at Diagnosis

FIG. 37.1. Incidence of non-Hodgkin's lymphoma in the United States according to age of the patient at diagnosis. Data collected by the National Cancer Institute in the Surveillance, Epidemiology and End Results (SEER) Program. (Adapted from Groves FD, Linet MS, Travis LB, et al. Cancer surveillance series: non-Hodgkin's lymphoma incidence by histologic subtype in the United States from 1978 through 1995. *J Natl Cancer Inst* 2000;92:1240–1251.)

number of extranodal disease sites (0 to 1 or more than 1) to classify patients into four risk categories, ranging from low risk to high risk. For patients older than 60 years of age, a simplified index, the age-adjusted International Prognostic Index, only uses stage, performance status, and LDH level to estimate the risk of failure or death. Otherwise, staging is comparable to young patients, with clinical examination, computed tomographic scanning of the body, other examination if there are clinical symptoms, blood counts, bone marrow biopsy,

LDH and β_2-microglobulin measurements, human immunodeficiency virus status, and hepatitis B and C virus serology.

In assessing treatment options for elderly patients, a great deal of attention must be paid to age-related factors. Presence of other diseases (19), diminished organ function, and health problems resulting from long-term use or abuse of tobacco, alcohol, and medications are factors that can compromise the ability of elderly patients to tolerate therapy. Furthermore, older patients typically have reduced emotional or physio-

TABLE 37.1. *Frequency of different lymphomas reported in the Revised European-American Lymphoma Classification in 1,283 patients according to age*

Lymphoma subtypes	No. of patients	Percentages of patients by age				
		<35 yr	35–49 yr	50–59 yr	60–69 yr	≥70 yr
Small lymphocytic/lymphoplasmacytoid lymphoma	98	1	14	18	33	34
Mucosa-associated lymphoid tissue lymphoma	108	9	14	24	26	27
Marginal zone lymphoma (splenic and nodal)	32	6	22	22	34	16
Follicular lymphoma	317	8	22	22	26	22
Mantle cell lymphoma	72	—	11	31	33	25
Diffuse large B-cell lymphoma	448	16	15	16	21	32
Peripheral T-cell lymphomas	93	11	18	17	26	28
Anaplastic large T/null-cell lymphoma	32	53	19	6	13	9
Burkitt's lymphoma	9	78	—	11	11	—
Lymphoblastic lymphoma	28	68	14	14	4	—
Unclassified	46	6	22	20	22	30
All patients	1283	13	17	19	24	27

Adapted from Coiffier B. The Non-hodgkin's Lymphoma Classification Project. Effect of age on the characteristics and clinical behavior of non-Hodgkin's lymphoma patients. *Ann Oncol* 1997;8:973–978.

logic tolerance to invasive and toxic procedures. Elderly patients often have alterations in the absorption, distribution, activation, detoxification, metabolism, and clearance of drugs, which modify the pharmacodynamics of therapeutic drugs (20). Decreases in the glomerular filtration rate and tubular reabsorption delay drug excretion, such that doses may have to be tailored to creatinine clearance (21). Because of decreased liver function, the metabolism of certain drugs, such as cyclophosphamide or anthracyclines, may be altered. However, the adjustment of the drug based on hepatic function is not associated with a better tolerance (22). Hematopoietic reserve capacity may be altered as well and myelotoxicity increased with standard doses (23). However, decreasing dosage because of a putative increased toxicity has proved to be associated with poorer therapeutic results (24).

In a recently reported study with 577 patients treated in community and academic hospitals, patients older than 65 years of age had more heart disease and comorbid conditions, were planned for lower average dose intensity, and received fewer cycles than younger patients (25). Even with this less intensive treatment, they had more hospitalizations for febrile neutropenia (28%, compared with 16% in younger patients). None of these patients received granulocyte colony-stimulating factor, and such a preventive treatment must be considered for elderly patients, particularly those with poor performance status or comorbid conditions. Such early use was associated with a decrease in repeated hospitalizations and a shorter length of stay in hospital in another study (26).

AGE AS A PROGNOSTIC FACTOR

Several studies reported that older age correlated with shorter disease-free and overall survivals. A retrospective analysis of 312 diffuse large B-cell lymphoma patients shows that age older than 60 years was the only prognostic factor affecting survival (27). In a study of 307 patients treated with CHOP [cyclophosphamide, hydroxydoxorubicin, Oncovin (vincristine), prednisone], the disease-free survival rates decreased from 65% at 96 months for subjects younger than 40 years of age to 50% at 36 months for those older than 65 years of age (24). Although comparable complete-response rates are observed in patients younger than 60 years or older than 60 years of age who are treated with the CAP-BOP [cyclophosphamide, Adriamycin (doxorubicin), procarbazine, bleomycin, Oncovin (vincristine), prednisone] regimen, the survival rate is significantly lower for older patients (34% vs. 62%; $p = .001$) (28). Likewise, age older than 50 years versus younger than 50 years was a major factor predicting outcome in an English study of 459 patients treated with two dissimilar regimens (29). A Scottish study demonstrated that stage and histology are comparable in patients younger than and older than 60 years of age, although the elderly have a significantly

TABLE 37.2. *Response to treatment and survival according to patient age at diagnosis*

Treatment outcome	No. of patients	Percentages of patients by age				
		<35 yr	35–49 yr	50–59 yr	60–69 yr	≥70 yr
Response to treatment						
Complete response	686	68	64	64	56	45
Partial response	313	21	18	27	32	30
No response	119	8	12	6	9	13
Not precise	65	3	6	3	3	12
Progression at time of analysis						
Yes	595	38	49	49	51	43
No	688	62	51	51	49	57
Relapse from complete remission	253	20	41	40	42	36
Event-free survival						
3-yr	—	59	54	55	50	47
5-yr	—	59	48	44	43	41
Median	—	NR	4.0	3.9	3.4	2.4
Overall survival						
3-yr	—	65	70	70	61	44
5-yr	—	61	66	62	51	34
Median	—	NR	NR	7.9	5.5	2.2

NR, not reached.
Adapted from Coiffier. The non-Hodgkin's lymphoma classification project. Effect of age on the characteristics and clinical behavior of non-Hodgkin's lymphoma patients. *Ann Oncol* 1997;8:973–978.

poorer survival (30). Advancing age has also been associated with increased treatment-related death rates. In patients with advanced-stage diffuse large B-cell lymphoma treated with VAPEC-B [vincristine, Adriamycin (doxorubicin), predniso-lone, etoposide, cyclophosphamide, bleomycin], the treatment-related death rate was higher in subjects older than 60 years of age, compared with younger patients (31). In Peru, patients older than 60 years treated with CHOP plus granulo-cyte-macrophage colony-stimulating factor had a good response rate and a 50% 4-year disease-free survival, although toxicity was greater in those older than 70 years of age (32).

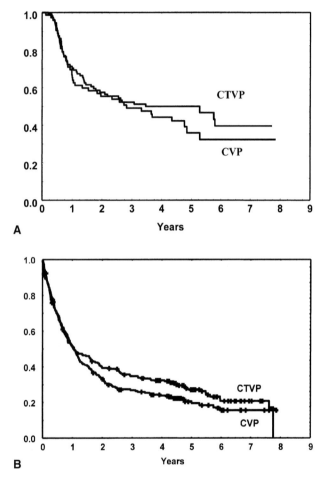

FIG. 37.2. Disease-free survival **(A)** and overall survival **(B)** in elderly patients treated with CVP (cyclophosphamide, vin-cristine, prednisone) or a CHOP [cyclophosphamide, hydroxy-daunomycin, Oncovin (vincristine), and prednisone]–like regimen. Disease-free survival is very good and not different between the two treatment arms, underscoring the fact that a complete remission must be the first goal of treatment. Over-all survival was not good because few of the patients reached a complete remission, and all others progressed and died from the disease or the toxicity of the treatment. (Adapted from Bastion Y, Blay JY, Divine M, et al. Elderly patients with aggressive non-Hodgkin's lymphoma: disease presentation, response to treatment, and survival—a Groupe d'Etude des Lymphomes de l'Adulte study on 453 patients older than 69 years. *J Clin Oncol* 1997;15:2945–2953.)

It was recently demonstrated that elderly patients usually have more severe disease than young and middle-aged patients; complete remission rates decline steadily with age, from 68% in the young to 45% in the elderly (4). Median event-free and overall survivals also decline with age (Table 37.2) (4). All published studies show shorter survival in the elderly, compared with younger patients matched for lymphoma and clinical characteristics (4,9). This difference persists after correction for non-lymphoma–related deaths (Fig. 37.1). The shorter survival has been ascribed to two main causes: a tendency by physicians to administer weaker, "better tolerated" (hence, less effective) treatment in the elderly (24); and poor drug tolerance in the elderly, largely due to the presence of concomitant disease (28). In the absence of concomitant disease, survival is no shorter in those older than 70 years of age, compared with those 70 years of age or younger (33). As in young patients, therapy in the elderly must be based on the type of lymphoma and the presence or absence of adverse prognostic factors.

Several studies have demonstrated that elderly patients treated with the appropriate therapy and effective management of putative toxicities may have a survival comparable to that observed in younger patients (34–36). Once a complete response has been obtained, disease-free survival in elderly patients may be comparable to that of younger patients, even if the initial chemotherapy regimen was less aggressive (33). However, in one study this did not result in an identical survival because the complete-response rate was inferior to that observed in younger patients (Fig. 37.2). The major difficulty for physicians treating elderly lymphoma patients is, thus, to successfully administer the chemotherapy required by the lymphoma without adverse toxicities and to reach a high complete-remission rate.

THERAPEUTIC STRATEGIES FOR DIFFUSE LARGE B-CELL LYMPHOMAS

Given their age and the presence of concomitant disease, the elderly have sometimes been considered ineligible for treatment with regimens that are potentially curative in the young. Thus, two approaches have been proposed: The first prioritizes the possibility of cure and uses the same treatments as in the young, provided there is no severe concomitant disease contraindicating their use; the second prioritizes quality of life and uses specific treatment regimens tailored to the elderly, which are reputedly less toxic but also less effective. The debate has essentially centered on the treatment of diffuse large B-cell lymphoma because it is potentially curable with proper treatment, CHOP being the reference therapy (37). When CHOP is used at lower doses in the elderly, the remission rate declines and survival shortens, compared with results in patients younger than 60 years of age (24). The standard CHOP regimen, on the other hand, achieves progression-free survival similar to that in younger patients but carries a much higher risk of severe toxicity or death: 15% to 30% in different retrospective series. Several recent randomized studies have compared results obtained with standard CHOP

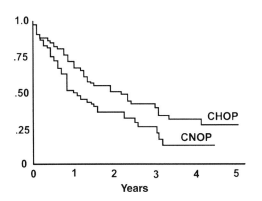

FIG. 37.3. Overall survival for CHOP [cyclophosphamide, hydroxydaunomycin, Oncovin (vincristine), and prednisone] versus CNOP [Cytoxan (cyclophosphamide), Novantrone (mitoxantrone), Oncovin (vincristine), prednisone] in patients older than 60 years of age with aggressive lymphoma. This study demonstrates that a so-called better tolerated chemotherapy regimen (CNOP) is not associated with a longer survival than that obtained with classic CHOP. The difference was statistically significant ($p < .05$). (Adapted from Zinzani PL, Storti S, Zaccaria A, et al. Elderly aggressive-histology non-Hodgkin's lymphoma: first-line VNCOP-B regimen experience on 350 patients. *Blood* 1999;94:33–38.)

with those obtained using less intensive therapy in elderly patients with diffuse large B-cell lymphoma. Sonneveld showed that CHOP was well tolerated in patients older than 60 years of age; toxicity did not differ from that of a reputedly less toxic regimen, CNOP [Cytoxan (cyclophosphamide), Novantrone (mitoxantrone), Oncovin (vincristine), prednisone], in which mitoxantrone replaced doxorubicin. The complete-remission rate was also higher, and survival was longer with the CHOP regimen (Fig. 37.3) (38). In another study, CHOP was compared with "chop" using the same drugs at the same overall doses but in three weekly injections instead of a single injection every 3 weeks, leading to decreased drug toxicity (39). In this study, survival at 2 years was longer in patients receiving standard CHOP than in those receiving chop. In a similar study, the Central Lymphoma Group in the United Kingdom reported the failure of CAPOMEt (CHOP with methotrexate and etoposide), a weekly regimen based on CHOP drugs plus etoposide, to increase survival over that reached with the CHOP regimen and reported an increase in neurologic toxicity (40). Finally, CHOP was compared with VMP [VePesid (etoposide), mitoxantrone, prednimustine] in an Italian study and was found superior to this previously used regimen in the European Organization for the Research and Treatment of Cancer group (41). These data confirm the similarity of response rates in elderly and younger patients and also the high correlation between complete response and long-term survival, irrespective of patient age (Fig. 37.2) (33).

The only comparative study that has shown a regimen to be superior to anthracycline-based regimens for elderly patients

compared PAdriaCEBO with PMitCEBO and used a low dose of doxorubicin (35 mg/m^2) versus mitoxantrone (7 mg/m^2) with each drug combined with cyclophosphamide (300 mg/m^2), etoposide, vincristine, and bleomycin (42). In this study, complete-remission rates were 60% and 52% and 4-year survival rates were 50% and 28% for PMitCEBO and PAdriaCEBO, respectively. This does not signify that PMitCEBO may be superior to CHOP, as the previously reported comparative studies have shown inferior results with CNOP (38).

A recent German trial, not yet completely reported, shows that therapeutic results may be improved if the dose intensity of the CHOP regimen is increased—that is, CHOP given every 2 weeks (CHOP-14) rather than the classic 3 weeks (CHOP-21) in patients older than 60 years of age (43). This increase in dose intensity is not associated with an increase in severe complications. However, the median age of the patients included in this study is only 65 years, and only 20% of the patients are older than 70 years of age. So, the conclusion of all these trials is that CHOP should be recommended for the treatment of elderly patients with diffuse large B-cell lymphoma, except for patients with a known cardiac contraindication to doxorubicin.

Recently, the combination of rituximab plus CHOP (R-CHOP) for eight cycles was demonstrated as being superior to CHOP alone in elderly patients (44). In this prospective randomized study, patients aged 60 to 80 years with untreated diffuse large B-cell lymphoma were included (Table 37.3). The complete response rate was 15% higher in patients treated with the R-CHOP combination. Event-free, disease-free, and

TABLE 37.3. Outcome of elderly patients included in the randomized study comparing CHOP to R-CHOP[a]

Treatment outcome	CHOP	R-CHOP
Number of patients	197	202
Complete-response rate (CR + CRu)	63%	75%
Number of events at 2 yr	61%	46%
Progression during treatment	22%	9%
Relapse after CR	25%	14%
Event-free survival at 2 yr	38%	57%
Median event-free survival (mo)	13	NR
Overall survival at 2 yr	57%	70%
Median overall survival	NR	NR

CHOP, cyclophosphamide, hydroxydaunomycin, Oncovin (vincristine), and prednisone; CR, complete remission; CRu, unconfirmed/uncertain complete remission; NR, not reached; R-CHOP, CHOP plus rituximab.
[a]All endpoints were statistically significant in favor of the R-CHOP arm.
Adapted from Coiffier B, Lepage E, Brière J, et al. CHOP chemotherapy plus rituximab compared with CHOP alone in elderly patients with diffuse large B-cell lymphoma. *N Engl J Med* 2002;346:235–242.

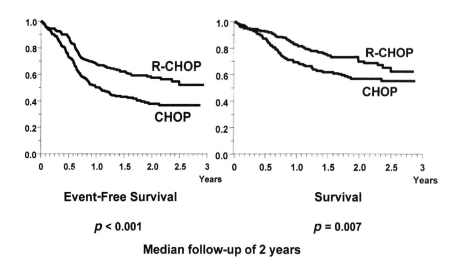

Event-Free Survival

p < 0.001

Survival

p = 0.007

Median follow-up of 2 years

FIG. 37.4. Event-free survival and overall survival in patients included in the Groupe d'Etude des Lymphomes de l'Adulte (GELA) trial, comparing CHOP [cyclophosphamide, hydroxydaunomycin, Oncovin (vincristine), and prednisone] and R-CHOP (CHOP plus rituximab) in previously untreated elderly patients with diffuse large B-cell lymphoma. (Adapted from Coiffier B, Lepage E, Brière J, et al. CHOP chemotherapy plus rituximab compared with CHOP alone in elderly patients with diffuse large B-cell lymphoma. *N Engl J Med* 2002;346:235–242.)

overall survivals were significantly longer with a 2-year median follow-up (Fig. 37.4). Because of the magnitude of the difference between CHOP and R-CHOP and the very good safety ratio, these data have established R-CHOP as the new standard for the treatment of previously untreated elderly patients with diffuse large B-cell lymphoma. Questions that remain to be settled are: How many cycles of CHOP and infusions of rituximab? Is there any indication for prolonged treatment with rituximab to decrease the relapse rate? Might increasing the dose intensity by giving R-CHOP every 2 weeks increase the efficacy without increasing the toxicity? Currently, no randomized study has shown that six cycles of CHOP do the same as the classic eight cycles. As the toxicity of this regimen is essentially observed for the first cycles (45), there is not any reason not to do eight cycles. Moreover, with the use of granulocyte colony-stimulating factor, all studies have shown that full-dose CHOP can be safely administered to elderly patients (46,47). Decreasing the number of rituximab infusions may decrease the cost of this regimen but may also decrease the efficacy. Only a randomized study may respond to this point, but the current ideas of increasing the duration of the treatment with rituximab maintenance after reaching a complete response are against this hypothesis (48).

REGIMENS IN PATIENTS WITH CONTRAINDICATION TO ANTHRACYCLINES

Patients with altered cardiac function and a decrease in ventricular ejection rates are not able to tolerate doxorubicin or other anthracyclines, or even mitoxantrone. The use of cisplatin-containing regimens, such as DHAP [dexamethasone, high-dose Ara-C, Platinol (cisplatin)] or ESHAP [etoposide, Solu-Medrol (methylprednisone), high-dose Ara-C, Platinol (cisplatin)], is also frequently contraindicated because of the hydration necessary to avoid renal toxicity or because of the altered renal function associated with cardiac disease. Protocols with good efficacy but less cardiac toxicity have been designed for these patients; however, they never have been

compared to CHOP. Comparison of these trials is impeded by differences in the inclusion criteria (age limits, clinical features at diagnosis) and length of follow-up that may well explain the dissimilarities in their results. Overall survival rates in these phase II trials, for example, ranged from 34% to 64% (49,50).

The first question to ask when treating an elderly patient is: Is there really any contraindication to using CHOP? A recent study in the Netherlands showed that patients not treated with CHOP had a worse survival and a much higher death rate from lymphoma, 77% compared with 53% for those treated with CHOP (6,51). The addition of granulocyte colony-stimulating factor allowed more patients to receive the correct chemotherapy regimen without decreasing the results. The conclusion of the authors was that the outcome of elderly patients with diffuse large B-cell lymphoma may be good if the physicians in charge make the good decision to treat them as they would younger patients with CHOP and granulocyte colony-stimulating factor, if necessary (6).

THERAPEUTIC STRATEGIES FOR OTHER LYMPHOMA SUBTYPES

Although the therapeutic strategies have begun to be settled for the treatment of elderly patients with diffuse large B-cell lymphoma, very few proposals have been made for the treatment of other lymphoma subtypes. Burkitt's lymphoma is a problem because of the worse results obtained with classical CHOP and the near impossibility of increasing the dose intensity, except in "younger" elderly patients—that is, those between the ages of 60 and 65 or 68 years. R-CHOP is recommended, and if the patient relapses, palliative treatment is certainly the best strategy.

For patients with indolent lymphomas, there are not any data that show that the conclusions drawn for diffuse large B-cell lymphoma may not be applied—that is, to treat them as younger patients. Mantle cell lymphoma and peripheral T-cell lymphoma are the only two difficulties because no standard has been defined for young patients, and the currently recommended treatments use high-dose therapy with autologous stem cell transplantation (52). This high-dose therapy certainly has to be reserved for a small subgroup of elderly patients (see High-Dose Therapy with Autologous Stem Cell Transplantation), and other patients have to be treated with standard chemotherapy approaches. The best treatment known for mantle cell lymphoma, even if it only cures a small percentage of patients, is the combination of CHOP plus rituximab (53). There is not any better regimen recommended for patients with peripheral T-cell lymphoma.

HIGH-DOSE THERAPY WITH AUTOLOGOUS STEM CELL TRANSPLANTATION

High-dose chemotherapy with autologous stem cell transplantation is an established procedure in the treatment of poor-prognosis lymphoma (54), and advances in supportive care have allowed consideration of its extension to older patients who are otherwise medically fit (55,56). Collection of a sufficient number of CD34+ stem cells does not seem to be an obstacle in these patients. This combination can thus be regarded as an up-front therapy for a well-defined and restricted group of patients with high-risk lymphoma or at the time of relapse.

TREATMENT FOR PATIENTS OLDER THAN 80 YEARS OF AGE

Currently, patients older than 80 years of age are not rare and always pose a difficult problem because of the presence of minor or major dysfunction in every body organ. However, very few, if any, studies report data on these patients. They may have a lymphoma while their performance status is still good, their dependence on others for help is low, and their intellectual function is near normal. For these patients, except for those with indolent disease, the solution of not treating is not considered satisfactory, at least by the patient. On the other hand, the clinical status may deteriorate rapidly because of the lymphoma, other diseases, or the hospitalization, in which case palliative treatment with an appropriate chemotherapy regimen is the best solution (57). An appropriate chemotherapy regimen may be defined as a regimen associated with efficacy, which is a disappearance of the lymphoma symptoms, and a low toxicity. No such marvel has been described, and every physician may have his or her recipe. In this setting, the combination of ifosfamide, 1,000 mg per m^2, and etoposide, 300 mg per m^2, given every 2 or 3 weeks is used. This regimen is nearly devoid of hematologic toxicity and may decrease the tumor volume. This usually gives the patient a few more weeks to arrange his or her affairs.

CONCLUSION

Age has been described as an adverse prognostic factor for survival of patients with diffuse large B-cell lymphoma, especially when other diseases are also present. These poorer results in the elderly may reflect, at least partially, the use of lower doses of chemotherapeutic agents. However, once a complete remission is reached, the disease-free survival of elderly patients does not differ from that of younger patients, emphasizing the importance of achieving complete remission (8,33). As R-CHOP is a very well-tolerated regimen, it must be recommended for the treatment of these patients, and decreasing dosage in the hope of having better tolerance only decreases the benefit associated with chemotherapy. Such an attitude must formally be reserved for patients having a contraindication to doxorubicin. Inclusion of growth factors in the therapeutic protocol can offset the risk of neutropenia, neutropenic infection, and a higher treatment-related death rate, and these must certainly be used in the management of these elderly patients, particularly for patients with a poor performance status at diagnosis, for whom the risk of treatment-related death is the highest (45,46).

REFERENCES

1. Armitage JO, Potter JF. Aggressive chemotherapy for diffuse histiocytic lymphoma in the elderly: increased complications with advancing age. *J Am Geriatr Soc* 1984;32:269–273.
2. Devesa SS, Blot WJ, Stone BJ, et al. Recent cancer trends in the United States. *J Nat Cancer Inst* 1995;87:175–182.
3. Howe HL, Wingo PA, Thun MJ, et al. Annual report to the nation on the status of cancer (1973 through 1998), featuring cancers with recent increasing trends. *J Natl Cancer Inst* 2001;93:824–842.
4. The Non-Hodgkin's Lymphoma Classification Project. Effect of age on the characteristics and clinical behavior of non-Hodgkin's lymphoma patients. *Ann Oncol* 1997;8:973–978.
5. Balducci L, Ballester OF. Non-Hodgkin's lymphoma in the elderly. *Cancer Control* 1996;3:5–14.
6. Peters FPJ, Lalisang RI, Fickers MMF, et al. Treatment of elderly patients with intermediate- and high-grade non-Hodgkin's lymphoma: a retrospective population-based study. *Ann Hematol* 2001;80:155–159.
7. Kennedy BJ. Aging and cancer. *J Clin Oncol* 1988;6:1903–1911.
8. Maartense E, Hermans J, Kluin-Nelemans JC, et al. Elderly patients with non-Hodgkin's lymphoma: population-based results in The Netherlands. *Ann Oncol* 1998;9:1219–1227.
9. d'Amore F, Brincker H, Christensen BE, et al. Non-Hodgkin's lymphoma in the elderly. A study of 602 patients aged 70 or older from a Danish population-based registry. The Danish LYFO-Study Group. *Ann Oncol* 1992;3:379–386.
10. Carbone A, Tirelli U, Volpe R, et al. Non-Hodgkin's lymphoma in the elderly. A retrospective clinicopathologic study of 50 patients. *Cancer* 1986;57:2185–2189.
11. Greiner TC, Medeiros LJ, Jaffe ES. Non-Hodgkin's lymphoma. *Cancer* 1995;75:370–380.
12. Groves FD, Linet MS, Travis LB, Devesa SS. Cancer surveillance series: non-Hodgkin's lymphoma incidence by histologic subtype in the United States from 1978 through 1995. *J Natl Cancer Inst* 2000;92:1240–1251.
13. Jaffe ES, Harris NL, Stein H, Vardiman JW. *World Health Organization classification of tumours: pathology and genetics of tumours of haematopoietic and lymphoid tissues.* Lyon, France: IARC, 2001.
14. The Non-Hodgkin's Lymphoma Pathologic Classification Project. National Cancer Institute sponsored study of classifications of non-Hodgkin's lymphomas. Summary and description of a working formulation for clinical usage. *Cancer* 1982;49:2112–2135.
15. Carbone A, Volpe R, Gloghini A, et al. Non-Hodgkin's lymphoma in the elderly. I. Pathologic features at presentation. *Cancer* 1990;66:1991–1994.
16. Harris NL, Jaffe ES, Stein H, et al. A revised European-American classification of lymphoid neoplasms. A proposal from the International Lymphoma Study Group. *Blood* 1994;84:1361–1392.

17. The Non-Hodgkin's Lymphoma Classification Project. A clinical trial of the International Lymphoma Study Group classification of non-Hodgkin's lymphoma. *Blood* 1997;89:3909–3918.

18. The International Non-Hodgkin's Lymphoma Prognostic Factors Project. A predictive model for aggressive non-Hodgkin's lymphoma. *N Engl J Med* 1993;329:987–994.

19. Balducci L. Cancer in the elderly: tailoring treatment. *Hosp Pract (Off Ed)* 2000;35:73–79; discussion, 79–80; quiz, 135.

20. Balducci L, Parker M, Sexton W, et al. Pharmacology of antineoplastic agents in the elderly patient. *Semin Oncol* 1989;16:76–84.

21. Lindeman RD, Tobin J, Shock NW. Longitudinal studies on the rate of decline in renal function with age. *J Am Geriatr Soc* 1986;33:278–285.

22. Durnas C, Loi CM, Cusack BJ. Hepatic drug metabolism and aging. *Clin Pharmacokinet* 1990;19:359–380.

23. Lipschitz DA. Age-related declines in hematopoietic reserve capacity. *Semin Hematol* 1995;22[Suppl 1]:3–5.

24. Dixon DO, Neilan B, Jones SE, et al. Effect of age on therapeutic outcome in advanced diffuse histiocytic lymphoma: the Southwest Oncology Group experience. *J Clin Oncol* 1986;4:295–305.

25. Morrison VA, Picozzi V, Scott S, et al. The impact of age on delivered dose intensity and hospitalizations for febrile neutropenia in patients with intermediate-grade non-Hodgkin's lymphoma receiving initial CHOP chemotherapy: a risk factor analysis. *Clin Lymphoma* 2001;2:47–56.

26. Chrischilles E, Delgado DJ, Stolshek BS, et al. Impact of age and colony-stimulating factor use on hospital length of stay for febrile neutropenia in CHOP-treated non-Hodgkin's lymphoma. *Cancer Control* 2002;9:203–211.

27. Simon R, Durrleman S, Hoppe RT, et al. The Non-Hodgkin Lymphoma Pathologic Classification Project. Long-term follow-up of 1153 patients with non-Hodgkin lymphomas. *Ann Intern Med* 1988;109:939–945.

28. Vose JM, Armitage JO, Weisenburger DD, et al. The importance of age in survival of patients treated with chemotherapy for aggressive non-Hodgkin's lymphoma. *J Clin Oncol* 1988;6:1838–1844.

29. Linch DC, Vaughn Hudson B, Hancock BW, et al. A randomised comparison of a third-generation regimen (PACEBOM) with a standard regimen (CHOP) in patients with histologically aggressive non-Hodgkin's lymphoma: a British National Lymphoma Investigation report. *Br J Cancer* 1996;74:318–322.

30. Neilly IJ, Ogston M, Bennett B, Dawson AA. High grade non-Hodgkin's lymphoma in the elderly:12-year experience in the Grampian Region of Scotland. *Hematol Oncol* 1995;13:99–106.

31. Radford JA, Whelan JS, Rohatiner AZS, et al. Weekly VAPEC-B chemotherapy for high grade non-Hodgkin's lymphoma: results of treatment in 184 patients. *Ann Oncol* 1994;5:147–151.

32. Gomez H, Mas L, Casanova L, et al. Elderly patients with aggressive non-Hodgkin's lymphoma treated with CHOP chemotherapy plus granulocyte-macrophage colony-stimulating factor: identification of two age subgroups with differing hematologic toxicity. *J Clin Oncol* 1998;16:2352–2358.

33. Bastion Y, Blay JY, Divine M, et al. Elderly patients with aggressive non-Hodgkin's lymphoma: disease presentation, response to treatment, and survival—a Groupe d'Etude des Lymphomes de l'Adulte study on 453 patients older than 69 years. *J Clin Oncol* 1997;15:2945–2953.

34. Zinzani PL, Storti S, Zaccaria A, et al. Elderly aggressive-histology non-Hodgkin's lymphoma: first-line VNCOP-B regimen experience on 350 patients. *Blood* 1999;94:33–38.

35. Tirelli U, Carbone A, Monfardini S, Zagonel V. A 20-year experience on malignant lymphomas in patients aged 70 and older at a single institute. *Crit Rev Oncol Hematol* 2001;37:153–158.

36. Miller TP, Dahlberg S, Cassady JR, et al. Chemotherapy alone compared with chemotherapy plus radiotherapy for localized intermediate- and high-grade non-Hodgkin's lymphoma. *N Engl J Med* 1998;339:21–26.

37. Fisher RI, Gaynor ER, Dahlberg S, et al. Comparison of a standard regimen (CHOP) with three intensive chemotherapy regimens for advanced non-Hodgkin's lymphoma. *N Engl J Med* 1993;328:1002–1006.

38. Sonneveld P, de Ridder M, van der Lelie H, et al. Comparison of doxorubicin and mitoxantrone in the treatment of elderly patients with advanced diffuse non-Hodgkin's lymphoma using CHOP versus CNOP chemotherapy. *J Clin Oncol* 1995;13:2530–2539.

39. Meyer RM, Browman GP, Samosh ML, et al. Randomized phase II comparison of standard CHOP with weekly CHOP in elderly patients with non-Hodgkin's lymphoma. *J Clin Oncol* 1995;13:2386–2393.

40. Bailey NP, Stuart NSA, Bessell EM, et al. Five-year follow-up of a prospective randomised multi-centre trial of weekly chemotherapy (Capomet) versus cyclical chemotherapy (Chop-Mtx) in the treatment of aggressive non-Hodgkin's-lymphoma. *Ann Oncol* 1998;9:633–638.

41. Tirelli U, Errante D, Vanglabbeke M, et al. CHOP is the standard regimen in patients greater than or equal to 70 years of age with intermediate-grade and high-grade non-Hodgkin's lymphoma. Results of a randomized study of the European Organization for Research and Treatment of Cancer Lymphoma Cooperative Study Group. *J Clin Oncol* 1998;16:27–34.

42. Mainwaring PN, Cunningham D, Gregory W, et al. Mitoxantrone is superior to doxorubicin in a multiagent weekly regimen for patients older than 60 with high-grade lymphoma: results of a BNLI randomized trial of PAdriaCEBO versus PMitCEBO. *Blood* 2001;97:2991–2997.

43. Pfreundschuh M, Trümper L, Kloess M, et al. 2-weekly CHOP (CHOP-14): the new standard regimen for patients with aggressive non-Hodgkin's lymphoma >60 years of age. *Hematol J* 2001;1[Suppl 1]:194.

44. Coiffier B, Lepage E, Brière J, et al. CHOP chemotherapy plus rituximab compared with CHOP alone in elderly patients with diffuse large B-cell lymphoma. *N Engl J Med* 2002;346:235–242.

45. Gomez H, Hidalgo M, Casanova L, et al. Risk factors for treatment-related death in elderly patients with aggressive non-Hodgkin's lymphoma: results of a multivariate analysis. *J Clin Oncol* 1998;16:2065–2069.

46. Guerci A, Lederlin P, Reyes F, et al. Effect of granulocyte colony-stimulating factor administration in elderly patients with aggressive non-Hodgkin's lymphoma treated with a pirarubicin-combination chemotherapy regimen. Groupe d'Etudes des Lymphomes de l'Adulte. *Ann Oncol* 1996;7:966–969.

47. Jacobson JO, Grossbard M, Shulman LN, Neuberg D. CHOP chemotherapy with preemptive granulocyte colony-stimulating factor in elderly patients with aggressive non-Hodgkin's lymphoma: a dose-intensity analysis. *Clin Lymphoma* 2000;1:211–217; discussion, 218.

48. Hainsworth JD. Rituximab as first-line and maintenance therapy for patients with indolent non-Hodgkin's lymphoma: interim follow-up of a multicenter phase II trial. *Semin Oncol* 2002;29:25–29.

49. Coiffier B. What treatment for elderly patients with aggressive lymphoma? *Ann Oncol* 1994;5:873–875.

50. Bertini M, Boccomini C, Calvi R. The influence of advanced age on the treatment and prognosis of diffuse large-cell lymphoma (DLCL). *Clin Lymphoma* 2001;1:278–284.

51. Peters FP, Fickers MM, Erdkamp FL, et al. The effect of optimal treatment on elderly patients with aggressive non-Hodgkin's lymphoma: more patients treated with unaffected response rates. *Ann Hematol* 2001;80:406–410.

52. Lazzarino M, Arcaini L, Bernasconi P, et al. A sequence of immunochemotherapy with Rituximab, mobilization of *in vivo* purged stem cells, high-dose chemotherapy and autotransplant is an effective and non-toxic treatment for advanced follicular and mantle cell lymphoma. *Br J Haematol* 2002;116:229–235.

53. Howard OM, Gribben JG, Neuberg DS, et al. Rituximab and CHOP induction therapy for newly diagnosed mantle-cell lymphoma: molecular complete responses are not predictive of progression-free survival. *J Clin Oncol* 2002;20:1288–1294.

54. Haioun C, Lepage E, Gisselbrecht C, et al. Survival benefit of high-dose therapy in poor-risk aggressive non-Hodgkin's lymphoma: final analysis of the prospective LNH87-2 protocol—A Groupe d'Etude des Lymphomes de l'Adulte Study. *J Clin Oncol* 2000;18:3025–3030.

55. Gopal AK, Gooley TA, Golden JB, et al. Efficacy of high-dose therapy and autologous hematopoietic stem cell transplantation for non-Hodgkin's lymphoma in adults 60 years of age and older. *Bone Marrow Transplant* 2001;27:593–599.

56. Jantunen E, Mahlamaki E, Nousiainen T. Feasibility and toxicity of high-dose chemotherapy supported by peripheral blood stem cell transplantation in elderly patients (>/=60 years) with non-Hodgkin's lymphoma: comparison with patients <60 years treated within the same protocol. *Bone Marrow Transplant* 2000;26:737–741.

57. Fiorentino MV. Lymphomas in the elderly. *Leukemia* 1991;5[Suppl 1]:79–85.

CHAPTER 38

Management of Lymphoma during Pregnancy

Thomas M. Habermann and Thomas E. Witzig

The synchronous presentation of non-Hodgkin's lymphoma and pregnancy is rare. This presentation leads to a complex set of management decisions throughout the pregnancy and the immediate postpartum period.

The management of the pregnant patient with non-Hodgkin's lymphoma requires a team with a broad-based knowledge of many factors, including high-risk pregnancy, the natural history of the histologic type of lymphoma the patient has, pharmacology of chemotherapeutic agents, side effects of radiation (diagnostic and therapeutic) to the fetus, and psychosocial and ethical issues. The management team needs to be cognizant that decisions have potential implications that may affect both the patient and the fetus.

Management has evolved over time and depends on the histology at the time of the diagnosis of lymphoma, the trimester of the pregnancy, and other factors. This chapter focuses on the reported experiences in the literature and recommends an approach to this complex clinical situation.

HISTOLOGY

It is important to obtain an adequate biopsy to establish a definitive diagnosis and classification of the lymphoma. This determines the prognosis, potential for curability, and type of treatment. One hundred twenty-two cases of non-Hodgkin's lymphoma in pregnancy are reported in the English literature (1–59). Cross-translation from earlier lymphoma histologic classifications into current classification schemes is not always feasible. The most common histologic subtypes in these pregnant patients are diffuse large B-cell, lymphoblastic, and Burkitt's lymphomas. Specifically, 31 patients had histologically high-grade disease (9,12,14,16–18,21,26,27,29,33, 35,38,39,41,52); 36 had diffuse large-cell non-Hodgkin's lymphoma (19,20,22,23,32,34,35,40–42,44,45,52,56,58). There were individual cases of composite lymphoma [follicular lymphoma and nodular sclerosing Hodgkin's lymphoma (56)] natural killer–cell lymphoma (55), anaplastic large-cell lymphoma (54), and two patients were reported with undifferentiated non-Hodgkin's lymphoma (31,35).

Follicular histologic disease was rare (52,53,56). Four cases of immunophenotypically confirmed T-cell non-Hodgkin's lymphoma at initial diagnosis have been reported (25, 31,56,59). One case of adult T-cell leukemia/lymphoma has been reported (59).

SITE OF DISEASE

Non-Hodgkin's lymphoma in pregnancy commonly involves nodal sites. Primary and secondary extranodal disease presentations have been reported in a diverse group of patients. Eight cases involving the breast have been reported. Four of these cases were African Burkitt's lymphoma (9,12,16,18,27,40). Three cases have involved the gastrointestinal tract (13,35). Gynecologic presentations have included two cervical cases (8,23,53), one perineal (7), and one uterine (9). Uterine involvement resulted in an abruptio placentae in one case (35) and was diagnosed 3 weeks after normal delivery in another patient. Placental involvement has been reported (41,47–49,55). The cervix may be pathologically involved (54). Central nervous system involvement may be parenchymal or meningeal (9,52,56). The bone marrow may be involved (51,55,56,59). One patient presented with acute spontaneous tumor lysis syndrome (57).

TRIMESTER AT THE TIME OF PRESENTATION

The diagnosis of the lymphoma can occur at anytime during the pregnancy but is more likely in the second and third trimesters (Tables 38.1 through 38.3). Among 79 patients for whom adequate information was available, lymphoma appeared in the first trimester in 18 (23%) (8,12,18,26,33,41,43,56), in the second trimester in 29 (37%) (7,16,17,25,31,33,41,44,47,51, 52,53,55–58), and in the third trimester in 32 (40%) (6,12–15,20,21,28,30,34,35,37,38,41,42,45–47,51–53,55). In addition, 21 of the reported cases of non-Hodgkin's lymphoma were histologically documented in the immediate postpartum period (4,10,12,13,23,33,35,38,40,47–49,55).

It has been suggested that hormonal or immunologic changes in pregnancy may influence the course and progres-

TABLE 38.1. *Strategy by trimester*

First trimester

 When possible, avoid therapy during the first 12 wk of gestation

Second trimester

 Diffuse large B-cell lymphoma

  CHOP chemotherapy

  If radiation therapy is incorporated, then lead apron abdominal/pelvis shielding is indicated

  No data are available in pregnancy for monoclonal antibody therapy

 Variant Burkitt's lymphoma

  Intensive combination chemotherapy regimens

Third trimester

 If close to delivery, consider delivery before therapeutic intervention if fetal maturity has been established

Postpartum

 Treatment should reflect the standard of care for histology

 Breast-feeding is contraindicated

CHOP, cyclophosphamide, doxorubicin, Oncovin (vincristine), prednisone.

sion of disease (33). In support of this possibility, Steiner-Salz et al. (35) reported that disease progressed in two patients after delivery, suggesting that pregnancy has a lymphoma-mediated suppressing effect. In contrast, others have suggested no effect (52,60–62) or even a protective effect (33,63).

TABLE 38.2. *Specific issues in diagnosis, treatment, and management*

Histology

 Diffuse large B-cell lymphoma is the most common

 Lymphoblastic and non-Burkitt's do occur and likely because of the age of the patients

 Follicular histology is uncommon

Trimester of pregnancy/postpartum

 The incidence is essentially equal in these four categories

 The therapeutic intervention strategies differ

Psychosocial and religious issues

Stage

 Nodal versus extranodal

 Bulky versus localized

Fetal maturity

Radiation exposure to the fetus: lead apron shielding of the abdomen for chest X-ray

 Magnetic resonance imaging

 Contraindicated scans: gallium, positron emission tomography, bone

 Relatively contraindicated scans: computed axial tomography scan abdomen/pelvis

TABLE 38.3. *General issues*

Outcome by trimester
Outcome by histology
Potential risk to fetus by trimester
Strategies by trimester

OUTCOME OF THE PREGNANCY

Information on the course of the pregnancy is known for 86 patients (7–9,12–21,23,25–27,30–35,38–40,42,44–47,51–56, 58,59). Therapeutic abortion was induced in four (17,33,52) and performed at the time of abdominal exploration in two (16,18). Of the remaining 82 pregnancies intended to continue to term, three resulted in miscarriages (27,31,56), one of which occurred after a radiation dose of 9 Gy and administration of doxorubicin, vincristine, and prednisone (31). Three additional patients died before delivery (12,25,33). Thirty-one patients delivered before any treatment; 14 had a cesarean section (7,8,13,23,35,52–56,58,59), and 19 had a vaginal delivery (9,12,20,33,35,38, 40,46,52,56). Twenty-eight patients had a vaginal delivery after initial treatment (14,19,21,26,30,32–34,41,42,45,51,56). Sixty-six fetuses (80%) were reported to be alive, and 16 did not survive.

OUTCOME OF THE NON-HODGKIN'S LYMPHOMA

Ortega (19) first reported on the use of chemotherapy in pregnant patients with non-Hodgkin's lymphoma. Since that time, additional patients with intermediate- and high-grade lymphoma have been treated with chemotherapy during pregnancy. The largest single reported series is by Avilés et al., who treated 19 patients and reported the results in 16 patients (41). Fifteen patients received a regimen that contained doxorubicin. Eight patients were alive and disease free at 4 to 9 years after delivery. In the Stanford experience, many women deferred therapy until after delivery or spontaneous/therapeutic abortion (52). This group reported that four patients were alive with no evidence of disease, three were alive with disease, and four had died of lymphoma. In the Mayo series (56), which included diffuse large B-cell lymphoma or peripheral T-cell lymphoma patients, all five patients who were treated with anthracycline-based chemotherapy (one during pregnancy, four after delivery, and two received radiation therapy during the pregnancy) achieved a complete remission, and four are alive and disease free, with a median follow-up of 13.5 years.

There have been multiple case reports using various chemotherapy regimens. CPOB [cyclophosphamide, prednisone, Oncovin (vincristine), bleomycin] was used in a patient in the second trimester with complete remission at 2 years (19); CHOP [cyclophosphamide, doxorubicin, Oncovin (vincristine), prednisone] in the third trimester with complete remission at 28 and 36 months (34,42); CHOP-BLEO (CHOP plus bleomycin) in the second trimester (44); procarbazine and prednisone (32); teniposide (29); CVP (cyclophosphamide, vincristine, prednisone) and intrathecal methotrexate in the third trimester with maternal death in 21 days (30); and CHOP-BLEO in the second trimester (44). Two spontaneous abortions have been reported after chemotherapy (25,31). Four cycles of rituximab (anti-CD20 monoclonal antibody) and CHOP were administered in the second trimester followed by two more cycles and mediastinal radiation therapy after a cesarean section (58). The child was found to have a normal B-cell population at 4 months.

Two patients with Burkitt's lymphoma who received cyclophosphamide died at 4.5 months and 5.0 months (14,18). One patient with lymphoblastic lymphoma was treated with 41 Gy to the mediastinum in the second trimester (33). The patient eventually had a relapse and died 3 years later (33). Other treatments included cyclophosphamide in the third trimester in a mother who died 23 days after giving birth (23), dexamethasone in the third trimester (28), and teniposide (29). CHOP was administered in a case of adult T-cell leukemia/lymphoma (59). On the eighth day, a healthy fetus was delivered. The mother subsequently died of septicemia after the first cycle.

TERATOGENIC EFFECTS OF THERAPEUTIC INTERVENTION

The patient with potentially curable malignant disease in pregnancy who requires chemotherapy presents a therapeutic dilemma. In contrast to findings in laboratory animals, data on teratogenicity and mutagenicity of chemotherapeutic agents are incomplete. The critical teratogenic period for chemotherapeutic agents is in the first trimester. Drugs implicated as having adverse effects on the fetus include cyclophosphamide (64,65), methotrexate (66), and chlorambucil (67). Cyclophosphamide administered in the first trimester in two patients with Hodgkin's disease was associated with absent toes and a single coronary artery (64,65). Congenital anomalies with folic acid antagonists, such as methotrexate, administered in the first trimester for indications other than non-Hodgkin's lymphoma have been reported to be associated with multiple cranial ossification defects, abnormal facies, digital anomalies, and other defects (66). Chlorambucil has been implicated in causing renal agenesis and hypoplasia (67). Radiotherapy has been reported to be teratogenic in animals and humans (68,69). Anthracyclines have been incorporated in the treatment of malignant disease in pregnancy. Karp et al. (31), in a report on a patient with undifferentiated lymphoma of T-cell origin who received doxorubicin during pregnancy, measured drug levels in fetal and placental material. After miscarriage, no doxorubicin was detectable in any tissue. In a recent review of anthracycline agents in pregnancy with long-term follow-up, Turchi and Villasis (70) found that 28 pregnancies had resulted in 24 normal infants. Effects on offspring have been reported (71–73). Avilés has subsequently reported on a

series of 84 patients with hematologic malignancies and found no congenital abnormalities at a median follow-up of 18.7 years (74). No secondary malignancies were reported in the children in this large series.

MANAGEMENT RECOMMENDATIONS FOR NON-HODGKIN'S LYMPHOMA IN PREGNANCY

Recommendations regarding the management of pregnant patients with lymphoma are based on current concepts of lymphoma management in the nonpregnant patient and the results from the case reports reviewed above. Therapeutic intervention depends on histologic type, stage of disease, extranodal presentation of disease, and trimester in which lymphoma is detected. Early and accurate tissue diagnosis is essential.

Staging

A careful history should be conducted to elicit symptoms of disease such as fatigue out of proportion to that usually experienced with pregnancy, weight loss, fever, and drenching night sweats. Staging procedures are necessary to assess extent of disease and determine if normal organs, such as liver and kidney, are involved or threatened by bulky lymphoma. Recommended staging studies in the pregnant patient with non-Hodgkin's lymphoma include physical examination; blood chemistries (electrolytes, lactate dehydrogenase, aspartate aminotransferase, bilirubin, alkaline phosphatase, uric acid, and creatinine); single-view chest radiograph with adequate abdominal shielding; magnetic resonance imaging of the chest, abdomen, and pelvis; pelvic ultrasound; and bone marrow aspiration and biopsy. Cerebral spinal fluid analysis is suggested in patients with lymphoblastic, Burkitt's, and non-Burkitt's lymphomas. Gallium scans, positron emission tomography scans, and bone scans are contraindicated because the radioisotopes used may cause harm to the fetus. Computed axial tomography should also be avoided because of the radiation exposure to the fetus, and other alternative imaging procedures (magnetic resonance imaging, ultrasound) are available.

Pregnancy Management

The patient should be evaluated by an obstetrician experienced in the management of high-risk pregnancies, and a fetal ultrasound is recommended to determine fetal age and health.

Termination of the pregnancy is rarely medically indicated in patients with an initial presentation of non-Hodgkin's lymphoma. The risk of transplacental transmission is rare. One case of transfer to the fetus of a rare natural killer–cell lymphoma with fatal consequences to the fetus in a 15-year-old girl who presented at 33 weeks has been reported (55). The delivery must be coordinated with the obstetrician and the team involved in the treatment. When possible, the fetus should be carried to term. Placental blood should be stored (68). Breast-feeding is not recommended during staging and treatment.

The issue of therapeutic abortion is one with complex religious, psychological, cultural, and social implications. The published cases in the literature with maternal and fetal outcomes support an approach that maintains the pregnancy. Ongoing management of the lymphoma is feasible. Different authors have supported the approach of therapeutic abortion. It is likely that therapeutic abortions have been underreported in the literature in patients with a synchronous presentation of pregnancy and non-Hodgkin's lymphoma.

Treatment

After staging of the patient is complete and an assessment of fetal health completed, a decision as to the therapeutic approach and timing of treatment is required. The following principles should be followed:

Whenever possible, all therapy should be avoided during the first 12 weeks of gestation. This is the most critical period of development of the fetus and the period when the use of antimetabolites is the most damaging.

Patients with localized disease above the diaphragm may be treated with radiation therapy with abdominal shielding, with a low risk to the fetus.

Patients with advanced-stage, low-grade lymphoma who are asymptomatic can usually be observed without treatment during pregnancy.

Corticosteroids may be used at any time during the pregnancy, with low risk to the fetus. This treatment can relieve symptoms and shrink lymphomatous masses and delay the need for cytotoxic drugs until after delivery or at least until the third trimester, when the risk of teratogenic effects on the fetus is less.

Treatment of patients in the second trimester depends on the bulk of disease, symptoms, stage of disease, and fetal gestation. If the patient has a curable lymphoma, such as a diffuse large-cell, then chemotherapy should proceed with a CHOP-based regimen. Chemotherapy is not contraindicated in the second and third trimester, and successful results have been reported. In the second and third trimesters, chemotherapy is associated with a low risk of fetal malformations—1.3% of 150 patients (69). However, long-term delayed effects remain a concern (70). Methotrexate should be avoided. If the disease is determined to be of low bulk, the patient asymptomatic, and the pace of disease is determined to be stable or slow, then careful observation until delivery or the third trimester is reasonable.

Treatment of patients in the third trimester is less problematic. As mentioned above, chemotherapy at this stage has a low risk of fetal malformations. On the other hand, if the fetus is determined to be mature enough to survive after delivery, elective induction can proceed, and chemotherapy

can be initiated after delivery. The hematologist/oncologist should work in close collaboration with an obstetrician to time delivery and chemotherapy. Amniocentesis to assess fetal lung maturity can be helpful in choosing the optimal time of delivery.

Lymphoblastic and Burkitt's lymphomas require an early and aggressive approach.

Treatment postdelivery should reflect the standard of care for the particular histology and stage.

Non-Hodgkin's lymphoma during pregnancy is rare. Adequate long-term follow-up information is not available on children exposed to chemotherapy for malignant disease. A multidisciplinary approach can result in long-term survival for both mother and fetus. More information needs to be accumulated on the long-term outcome of the fetus exposed to radiation or chemotherapeutic agents. The objective of the management and treatment in non-Hodgkin's lymphoma and pregnancy is to ensure that both the mother and the fetus achieve the optimal outcome.

REFERENCES

1. Issacs R. Lymphosarcoma cell leukemia. *Ann Intern Med* 1937;11:657–662.
2. Moracci E. Insopetta linfosarcomatosi di Kundrat gravidanze. *Arch Obstet Gynecol* 1942;6:15.
3. Hesseltine HC, Loth MF. Malignant diseases associated with pregnancy. *West J Surg Obstet Gynecol* 1956;64:529–535.
4. Goodman M. Reticulum cell sarcoma in pregnancy. *J Obstet Gynecol Br Empire* 1958;65:641–643.
5. Rosenberg SA, Diamond HD, Jaslowitz B, Craver LF. Lymphosarcoma: a review of 1269 cases. *Medicine* 1961;40:31–84.
6. Bulska M. A case of reticulosarcoma appearing as a thrombosis of the femoral vein in a pregnant woman. *Ginekol Pol* 1962;33:373–378.
7. Lysyj M, Bergquist JR. Pregnancy complicated by sarcoma: report of two cases. *Obstet Gynecol* 1963;21:506–509.
8. Vieaux JW, McGuire DE. Reticulum cell sarcoma of the cervix. *Am J Obstet Gynecol* 1964;89:134–135.
9. Bannerman RHO. Burkitt's tumor in pregnancy [Letter]. *BMJ* 1966;2:1136–1137.
10. Leeks SR. Lymphosarcoma complicating pregnancy. *N Z Med J* 1966;65:467–468.
11. Mehta A, Vakil RM. Use of Endoxan in case of lymphosarcoma with pregnancy during the third trimester (a case report). *Indian J Cancer* 1966;3:198–202.
12. Sheperd JJ, Wright DH. Burkitt's tumour presenting as bilateral swelling of the breast in women of child-bearing age. *Br J Surg* 1967;54:776–780.
13. Henderson M, Paterson WG. Perforation of jejunum by reticulum cell sarcoma in pregnancy. *Am J Surg* 1968;115:385–389.
14. Hardin JA. Cyclophosphamide treatment of lymphoma during third trimester of pregnancy. *Obstet Gynecol* 1972;39:850–851.
15. Inoue Y, Masuda, H, Shiojima Y. Pregnancy complicated by sarcoma. *Acta Obstet Gynaecol Jpn* 1972;19:222–225.
16. Finkle HI, Goldman RL. Burkitt's lymphoma—gynecologic considerations. *Obstet Gynecol* 1974;43:281–284.
17. Armon PJ. Burkitt's lymphoma of the ovary in association with pregnancy: two case reports. *Br J Obstet Gynaecol* 1976;83:169–172.
18. Armitage JO, Feagler JR, Skoog DP. Burkitt lymphoma during pregnancy with bilateral breast involvement. *JAMA* 1977;237:151.
19. Ortega J. Multiple agent chemotherapy including bleomycin of non-Hodgkin's lymphoma during pregnancy. *Cancer* 1977;40:2829–2835.
20. VillaSanta U, Attar S, Jiji R. Malignant histiocytic lymphoma (reticulum cell sarcoma) in pregnancy. *Gynecol Oncol* 1978;6:383–390.
21. Newman RA, Gallagher JG, Clements JP, Krakoff IH. Demonstration of Ga-67 localization in human placenta. *J Nucl Med* 1978;19:504–506.

22. Durodola JI. Administration of cyclophosphamide during late pregnancy and early lactation: a case report. *J Natl Med Assoc* 1979;71:165–166.
23. Tunca JC, Reddi PR, Shah SH, Slack ST. Malignant non-Hodgkin's type lymphoma of the cervix uteri occurring during pregnancy. *Gynecol Oncol* 1979;7:385–393.
24. Bornkamm GW, Kaduk B, Kachel G, et al. Epstein-Barr virus-positive Burkitt's lymphoma in a German woman during pregnancy. *Blut* 1980;40:167–177.
25. Case BW, Benaroya S. Dyspnea in a pregnant young woman. *Can Med Assoc J* 1980;122:890–896.
26. Falkson HC, Simson IW, Falkson G. Non-Hodgkin's lymphoma in pregnancy. *Cancer* 1980;45:1679–1682.
27. Jones DED, d'Avignon MB, Lawrence R, et al. Burkitt's lymphoma: obstetric and gynecologic aspects. *Obstet Gynecol* 1980;56:533–536.
28. Cheson BD, Johnston JL, Junco GD. Cytologic evidence for disseminated immunoblastic lymphoma. *Am J Clin Pathol* 1981;75:621–625.
29. Lowenthal RM, Funnel CF, Hope DM, et al. Normal infant after combination chemotherapy including teniposide for Burkitt's lymphoma in pregnancy. *Med Pediatr Oncol* 1982;10:165–169.
30. Berrebi A, Schattner A, Mogilner BM. Disseminated Burkitt's lymphoma during pregnancy. *Acta Haematol* 1983;70:139–140.
31. Karp GI, van Oeyen P, Valone F, et al. Doxorubicin in pregnancy: possible transplacental passage. *Cancer Treat Rep* 1983;67:773–777.
32. Schapira DV, Chudley AE. Successful pregnancy following continuous treatment with combination chemotherapy before conception and throughout pregnancy. *Cancer* 1984;54:800–803.
33. Ioachim HL. Non-Hodgkin's lymphoma in pregnancy: three cases and review of the literature. *Arch Pathol Lab Med* 1985;109:803–809.
34. Garg A, Kochupillai V. Non-Hodgkin's lymphoma in pregnancy. *South Med J* 1985;78:1263–1264.
35. Steiner-Salz S, Yahalom J, Samuelov A, et al. Non-Hodgkin's lymphoma associated with pregnancy: a report of six cases, with a review of the literature. *Cancer* 1985;56:2087–2091.
36. Mulvihill JJ, McKeen EA, Rosner F, et al. Pregnancy outcome in cancer patients: experience in a large cooperative group. *Cancer* 1987;60:1143–1150.
37. Trombley BA, Marcus CS, Koci T. Unexpected demonstration of superior vena caval obstruction in third trimester lung imaging. *Clin Nucl Med* 1988;13:407–409.
38. Giovannini M, Saccucci P, Cannone D, et al. Can pregnancy aggravate the course of non-Hodgkin's lymphoma? *Eur J Gynaecol Oncol* 1989;10:287–289.
39. Natel S, Parboosingh J, Poon MC. Treatment of an aggressive non-Hodgkin's lymphoma during pregnancy with MACOP-B chemotherapy. *Med Pediatr Oncol* 1990;18:143–145.
40. Roumen FJME, de Leeuw JW, Van der Linden PJQ, et al. Non-Hodgkin's lymphoma of the puerperal uterus. *Obstet Gynecol* 1990;75:527–529.
41. Avilés A, Díaz-Maqueo JC, Torras V, et al. Non-Hodgkin's lymphomas and pregnancy: presentation of 16 cases. *Gynecol Oncol* 1990;37:335–337.
42. Toko H, Okabe K, Kamei H, et al. Successful chemotherapy on a pregnant non-Hodgkin's lymphoma patient. *Acta Med Okayama* 1990;44:321–323.
43. Ba-Thike K, Oo N. Non-Hodgkin's lymphoma in pregnancy. *Asia Oceania J Obstet Gynaecol* 1990;16:229–232.
44. Lambert J, Wijermans PW, Dekker GA, et al. Chemotherapy in non-Hodgkin's lymphoma during pregnancy. *Neth J Med* 1991;38:80–85.
45. Spitzer M, Citron M, Ilardi CF, et al. Non-Hodgkin's lymphoma during pregnancy. *Gynecol Oncol* 1991;43:309–312.
46. Valemzuela PL, Montalban C, Matorras R, et al. Pregnancy and relapse of peripheral T cell lymphoma: a case report. *Gynecol Obstet Invest* 1991;32:59–61.
47. Kurtin PJ, Gaffey TA, Habermann TM. Peripheral T-cell lymphoma involving the placenta. *Cancer* 1992;70:2963–2968.
48. Tsujimura T, Matsumoto K, Aozasa K. Placental involvement by maternal non-Hodgkin's lymphoma. *Arch Pathol Lab Med* 1993;117:325–327.
49. Pollack RN, Sklarin NT, Rao S, et al. Metastatic placental lymphoma associated with maternal human immunodeficiency virus infection. *Obstet Gynecol* 1993;81:856–857.
50. Lishner M, Zemlickis D, Sutcliffe SB, et al. Non-Hodgkin's lymphoma and pregnancy. *Leuk Lymphoma* 1994;14:411–413.
51. Imai A, Kawabata I, Tamaya T. Case report—primary brain malignant lymphoma newly diagnosed during pregnancy. *J Med* 1995;26:333–336.
52. Gelb AB, van de Rijn M, Warnke RA, et al. Pregnancy-associated lymphomas, a clinicopathologic study. *Cancer* 1996;78:304–309.
53. Wang PH, Chao KC, Lin G, et al. Primary malignant lymphoma of the cervix in pregnancy, a case report. *J Reprod Med* 1999;53:630–632.
54. Meguerian-Bedoyan Z, Lamant L, Hopfner C, et al. Anaplastic large cell lymphoma of maternal origin involving the placenta: case report and literature survey. *Am J Surg Pathol* 1997;21:1236–1241.
55. Catlin EA, Roberts JD Jr, Erana R, et al. Brief report: transplacental transmission of natural-killer-cell lymphoma. *N Engl J Med* 1999;341:85–91.
56. Habermann TM, Kurtin PJ, Johansen KL, et al. The synchronous presentation of non-Hodgkin's lymphoma and pregnancy: a greater than ten-year follow-up. *Blood* 2000;96:224a(abst).
57. El-Sonbaty MR, Bitar Z, Abdulrazak AA. Acute spontaneous tumor-lysis syndrome. *Int J Hematol* 2001;73:386–389.
58. Herold M, Schnohr S, Bittrich H. Efficacy and safety of a combined rituximab chemotherapy during pregnancy. *J Clin Oncol* 2001;19:3439.
59. Safdar A, Johnson N, Gonzalez F, et al. Adult T-cell leukemia-lymphoma during pregnancy. *N Engl J Med* 2002;346:2014–2015.
60. Sutcliffe SB, Chapman RM. Lymphomas and leukemias. In: Allen HH, Nisker JA eds. *Cancer in pregnancy*. Mt. Kisco, NY: Futura Publishing Co., 1986:135–198.
61. Zuazu J, Julia A, Sierra J, et al. Pregnancy outcome in hematologic malignancies. *Cancer* 1991;67:703–709.
62. Rodriguez JM, Haggag M. VACOP-B chemotherapy for high-grade non-Hodgkin's lymphoma in pregnancy. *Clin Oncol* 1995;7:337–338.
63. Banks PM. Pregnancy and lymphoma. *Arch Pathol Lab Med* 1985;109:182.
64. Greenberg LH, Tanaka KR. Congenital anomalies probably induced by cyclophosphamide. *JAMA* 1964;188:423–426.
65. Toledo TM, Harper RC, Moser RH. Fetal effects during cyclophosphamide and irradiation therapy. *Ann Intern Med* 1971;74:87–91.
66. Milunsky A, Graef JW, Gaynor MF Jr. Methotrexate-induced congenital malformations: with review of the literature. *J Pediatr* 1968;72:790–795.
67. Shotton D, Monie IW. Possible teratogenic effect of chlorambucil on a human fetus. *JAMA* 1963;186:74–75.
68. Sweet DW Jr, Kinzie J. Consequences of radiotherapy and antineoplastic therapy for the fetus. *J Reprod Med* 1976;17:241–246.
69. Shepart T. *Catalog of teratogenic agents*, 3rd ed. Baltimore: Johns Hopkins University Press, 1980.
70. Turchi JJ, Villasis V. Anthracyclines in the treatment of malignancy in pregnancy. *Cancer* 1988;61:435–440.
71. Varadi G, Elchalal U, Shushan A, et al. Umbilical and cord blood for use in transplantation. *Obstet Gynecol Surv* 1995;50:611.
72. Byrne J, Rasmussen SA, Steinhorn SC, et al. Genetic disease in offspring of childhood and adolescent cancer survivors. *N Engl J Med* 1998;338:1339–1344.
73. Doll DC, Ringenberg QS, Yarbro JW. Antineoplastic agents and pregnancy. *Semin Oncol* 1989;16:337–346.
74. Avilés A, Neri N. Hematological malignancies and pregnancy: a final report of 84 children who received chemotherapy *in utero*. *Clin Lymphoma* 2001;2:1723–1727.

CHAPTER 39

Management of Acquired Immunodeficiency Syndrome–Related Lymphoma

Alexandra M. Levine and Jonathan W. Said

EPIDEMIOLOGY OF ACQUIRED IMMUNODEFICIENCY SYNDROME–RELATED LYMPHOMA

Epidemiology of Acquired Immunodeficiency Syndrome in the United States

Human immunodeficiency virus (HIV)/acquired immunodeficiency syndrome (AIDS) is now the fourth leading cause of death in the world, accounting for 4.8% of all mortality (1). Approximately 42 million people are living with AIDS, of whom 25 million live in sub-Saharan Africa. Cumulative deaths due to AIDS now approach 22 million people worldwide (1).

The peak of the AIDS epidemic in the United States occurred in 1993, a year in which new infections continued unabated and additional patients were added on the basis of an expanded case definition (2). New clinical AIDS-defining conditions were added at that time, including development of cervical cancer, recurrent bacterial pneumonia, or tuberculosis in HIV-infected people. Further, a new category termed *immunologic AIDS* was added to the case definition of AIDS, characterized not by the development of a clinical illness, but by the presence of very low CD4 cells (less than 200/mm^3 CD4$^+$ lymphocytes) in the peripheral blood (2). In sharp contrast to the initial dramatic increases in the incidence of AIDS in the United States in the 1980s and early 1990s, a decline in the incidence of new AIDS cases was first documented in 1995, clearly as a result of the widespread use of highly active antiretroviral therapy (HAART) (3). This antiretroviral therapy, modeled after the concepts of multiagent chemotherapy for malignant disease, usually consists of three or more antiretroviral agents, each of which comes from a different chemical class, with differing mechanisms of action and differing toxicities (4). The widespread use of HAART in the United States and Europe has resulted in a remarkable 73% decrease in the development of new AIDS cases among HIV-infected people (3,5) and in an equally remarkable approximately 75% decline in mortality among patients with AIDS (3,6). Nonetheless, the prevalence of HIV continues to increase in the United States, driven by a stable number of new infections each year along with prolongation in survival of previously infected individuals. It is thus apparent that increasing numbers of HIV-infected individuals will require care in the decades ahead.

Epidemiology of AIDS–Related Lymphoma

Lymphoma has traditionally been considered a late manifestation of HIV infection, more likely to occur in the setting of significant immune suppression (7), with CD4 cells less than 200/mm^3 and history of an AIDS-defining illness. Thus, after an earlier diagnosis of AIDS, the relative risk of immunoblastic lymphoma is approximately 627-fold increased, whereas that of diffuse large-cell lymphoma is 145-fold increased over that expected in the general population (8,9). Of interest, when linking cancer and AIDS registries, even low-grade lymphoma is found to be increased 14-fold over that expected in individuals who had already been diagnosed with an AIDS-defining illness (8,9), while the incidence of T-cell lymphoma has also increased among patients with AIDS (10).

Although HAART therapy has been associated with a significant decrease in the incidence of various opportunistic infections and Kaposi's sarcoma (3,11), such a major and significant decrease has not yet been uniformly described in terms of systemic AIDS lymphoma. In a cohort of 6,636 HIV-infected individuals from Switzerland, reflecting more than 18,000 person-years of follow-up, no decrease in lymphoma was seen, when comparing the period 1992 to 1994 (before the widespread use of HAART) with the period from July 1997 to June 1998 (11). A recent report of more than 7,300 HIV-infected patients from 52 European countries compared data on AIDS-defining illnesses diagnosed during 1994, before the HAART era, with those diagnosed in 1998, after widespread use of HAART in these regions (12). The incidence of AIDS-defining conditions declined from 30.7 per 100 patient-years in 1994 to 2.5 per 100 patient-years during 1998 ($p < .0001$). However, whereas the proportion of new AIDS cases due to various opportunistic infections decreased, the proportion of new AIDS cases secondary to lymphoma increased significantly, with lymphoma representing less than 4% of all AIDS cases diagnosed in 1994 and 16% of all AIDS cases diagnosed in 1998 ($p < .0001$). In contrast, there was no evidence for an increase in the proportion of AIDS diagnoses due to primary central nervous system lymphoma (12). Matthews and colleagues from England have also documented a statistically significant increase in lymphoma as the initial AIDS-defining condition among a large group of HIV-infected individuals (13).

An international collaborative study, including cancer incidence data from 23 prospective studies that included 47,936 HIV-seropositive individuals from North America, Europe, and Australia, sought to determine the adjusted incidence rates of various AIDS-defining conditions since the advent of HAART (14). In terms of lymphoma incidence, the rate ratio showed a significant reduction when cases diagnosed in 1992 to 1996 were compared with those from 1997 through 1999. Of interest, however, the rate ratio for immunoblastic lymphoma and primary central nervous system lymphoma decreased significantly during these two time intervals, whereas that of Burkitt's lymphoma and Hodgkin's disease showed no such decrease (14).

Multiple additional studies have been conducted recently that seek to determine if the incidence of HIV lymphoma has decreased in the era of HAART. Some of these studies indicate no significant decrease (13,15), whereas others have documented highly significant decreases in the incidence of HIV lymphoma in recent years (12,16,17). The true situation may, perhaps, best be understood within the context of the immune

status of the population being evaluated. Thus, Besson and colleagues from France evaluated the incidence of HIV lymphoma in terms of the strata or level of CD4 cells (17). As the number of CD4 cells in a given group of patients decreased, the incidence of HIV lymphoma increased, as shown in Table 39.1. The same inverse relationship between decreased CD4 levels and increased risk of HIV lymphoma was apparent both in the time frame before institution of HAART and after the availability of HAART. Thus, if HAART is available in a given population and has been used effectively, with resultant decrease in HIV-1 viral load (16) and increase in CD4 cells (17), one would expect a significant decline in the incidence of HIV lymphoma. However, in populations that do not have access to HAART or in those in whom HAART has been ineffective, no decrease in the incidence of HIV lymphoma is observed.

Taken together, the current population-based data would suggest that the incidence of primary central nervous system and systemic lymphoma has decreased since the widespread use of HAART. However, the decline in lymphoma is far less impressive than that observed for opportunistic infections or Kaposi's sarcoma, resulting in a proportionate increase in lymphoma as an initial AIDS-defining illness. Furthermore, although initial controlled clinical trials have indicated that approximately 80% of treated subjects achieve a nondetectable HIV viral load after HAART, only approximately 40% achieve this endpoint in "real world" conditions (18). The effect of HAART on the incidence of AIDS lymphoma will clearly be dependent on the long-term efficacy of combination antiretroviral therapy when assessed at the population level. Issues of access, compliance, drug resistance, and underlying host and environmental factors will all likely be operative. Additional time is thus required to elucidate the full impact of HAART on the incidence of AIDS-related systemic and primary central nervous system lymphoma.

TABLE 39.1. *Incidence of acquired immunodeficiency syndrome lymphoma since highly active antiretroviral therapy stratified by CD4 cells[a]*

| | Systemic | | | | | Primary central nervous system | | | | |
| | 1993–1994 | | 1997–1998 | | | 1993–1994 | | 1997–1999 | | |
CD4	Cases (n)	Incidence	Cases (n)	Incidence	p Value	Cases (n)	Incidence	Cases (n)	Incidence	p Value
≥350	15	15.6	37	15.9	NS	2	2.0	3	1.3	NS
200–349	25	34.8	45	33.6	NS	5	6.8	6	4.4	NS
100–199	40	76.8	53	73.3	NS	5	9.2	6	8.1	NS
50–99	34	103.8	40	164.7	.053	10	29.6	7	28.0	NS
<50	202	253.8	50	223.2	NS	77	93.9	25	107.5	NS
All	415	86.0	285	42.9	$<10^{-30}$	135	27.8	65	9.7	$<10^{-11}$

NS, not significant.
[a]Rate/100,000 person-years.
From Besson C, Goubar A, Gabarre J, et al. Changes in AIDS-related lymphoma since the era of highly active antiretroviral therapy. *Blood* 2001;98:2339–2344, with permission.

Genetic Epidemiology of AIDS–Related Lymphoma

In distinction to Kaposi's sarcoma, which occurs primarily in men who have sex with men, lymphoma is seen in all population groups at risk for HIV (19). Similar to *de novo* lymphoma occurring in HIV-negative individuals (20,21), AIDS lymphoma is more common in men than in women. All age groups are affected, and lymphoma is the most common malignancy in HIV-infected children (22). Epidemiologic studies have failed to identify major environmental factors associated with AIDS lymphoma among HIV-infected individuals (23–25). However, host genetic factors may be operative. Thus, HIV-infected patients who are heterozygotes for the CCR5Δ32 deletion are statistically less likely to develop lymphoma (26), whereas those with SDF-1 mutations (3'A) are statistically more likely to develop lymphoma (27).

Changing Characteristics of Patients with AIDS-Related Lymphoma in the Era of Highly Active Antiretroviral Therapy

At this time, there is some inconsistency regarding potential changes in the clinical or pathologic characteristics of patients with AIDS lymphoma since the widespread use of HAART. These inconsistencies may be related to differing patient populations, access to HAART, or other unknown factors. Levine and colleagues reviewed records of 369 patients diagnosed with AIDS lymphoma at a single institution from 1982 through 1998 and compared these data to population-based information from the County of Los Angeles (15). Significant changes in the demographic characteristics of AIDS lymphoma occurred in both populations, with the latter period characterized by statistically significant increases among women, those of nonwhite ethnicity (Latino/Hispanic individuals), and those who acquired HIV heterosexually. The median CD4+ lymphocyte count at the time of lymphoma diagnosis decreased significantly over the years, with a median count of 177 per mm^3 in the earliest time period and 53 per mm^3 in the latest. A decrease in small noncleaved (Burkitt's or Burkitt-like) lymphomas occurred over time, whereas the prevalence of diffuse large-cell lymphoma increased. In the large EuroSIDA study of AIDS lymphoma (16), similar changes were seen in terms of both pathologic and certain clinical characteristics of disease. Thus, the incidence of Burkitt's lymphoma decreased from the pre-HAART to the post-HAART eras, whereas that of diffuse large-cell/immunoblastic lymphoma increased. In the post-HAART era, a statistically decreased incidence of HIV lymphoma was seen among homosexuals and whites, with an increase among those who acquired HIV by heterosexual contact (16). The median age of affected patients increased from 38 years in the pre-HAART era to 42 years in the post-HAART time frame (16). Similarly, Matthews and colleagues, reporting on experience in London with 7,840 HIV-positive

patients, noted a statistically significant increase in median age of patients diagnosed with HIV lymphoma in the post-HAART era (13). On multivariate analysis, characteristics statistically associated with development of AIDS lymphoma included lower CD4 lymphocyte count (both at baseline and at nadir), older age, and lack of HAART (13). In a study of HIV-infected patients followed in Paris, the incidence of AIDS lymphoma decreased since the advent of HAART, and the median CD4 cell count at lymphoma diagnosis increased significantly, from 63 per mm^3 in the earliest to 191 per mm^3 in the latest time interval (17). Although not statistically significant, trends similar to those identified in Los Angeles and London were observed, with an increase of HIV lymphoma among women (from 6.3% in the pre-HAART to 11.9% in the post-HAART era) and heterosexuals (from 11.1% to 14.3%) and a decrease among those who acquired HIV by homosexual contact.

These changes indicate that the demographic profile of patients with HIV/AIDS is similar to that in patients with AIDS lymphoma as well.

PATHOGENESIS AND PATHOLOGY OF AIDS–RELATED LYMPHOMA

Immunosuppression and Epstein-Barr Virus Infection

Studies of HIV lymphoma offer a paradigm for the development of lymphoid malignancy in the setting of profound immunosuppression (28). One of the factors that contributes to lymphomagenesis is chronic antigenic stimulation, driven by HIV, multiple coinfecting agents, and B-cell expansion, which is frequently poly- or oligoclonal (7).

The Epstein-Barr virus also plays a pivotal role in this process, with Epstein-Barr virus demonstrated in approximately 40% of cases (29–34). Lymphomas associated with HIV are associated with both A and B types of Epstein-Barr virus, which differ from lymphomas associated with transplantation (35–39). Viral infection may be associated with production of cytokines, including interleukin (IL)-6, IL-10, and IL-13, which also support proliferation of neoplastic lymphoid cells (40,41). Table 39.2 demonstrates the relative prevalence of Epstein-Barr virus in various subtypes of AIDS lymphoma.

TABLE 39.2. *Relative prevalence of Epstein-Barr virus (EBV) in various subtypes of acquired immunodeficiency syndrome (AIDS) lymphoma*

Subtype of AIDS lymphoma	Percentage positive for EBV
Burkitt's lymphoma	30–50
Diffuse large B-cell lymphoma	20
Immunoblastic lymphoma	80
Immunoblastic lymphoma of the central nervous system	100

Gene Rearrangements and Clonality

Monoclonal rearrangements of the immunoglobulin (Ig) genes depicting a single dominant clone can be detected in almost all B-cell HIV lymphomas, regardless of subtype. This may be confirmed by clonal presence of Epstein-Barr virus as well as clonal cytogenetic abnormalities. A rare exception (see below) occurs in posttransplant lymphoproliferative disorder–like polymorphous lymphomas (42).

Many of the key oncogenic events associated with the pathogenesis of HIV lymphoma have been linked to known oncogenes, including MYC, p53, RAS, and TCL-1 (43,44). Molecular events in AIDS-related lymphoma are often multiple and complex and are still poorly understood. New molecular techniques, such as gene expression profiling, are being applied to AIDS-related lymphoma and will likely uncover further genetic abnormalities. Molecular pathogenesis of specific disease entities is discussed below.

Classification of AIDS–Related Lymphomas

HIV lymphomas have been classified by the World Health Organization into three groups: those occurring specifically in HIV-positive patients, those also occurring in other immunodeficiency states, and those that also arise in immunocompetent patients. These are depicted in Table 39.3 (45,46).

Pathology and Pathogenesis of Burkitt's Lymphomas (30% of AIDS Lymphomas)

Patients with Burkitt's lymphomas may present with nodal disease but more often present with mass lesions in extranodal sites, such as the bowel, or leukemia-like infiltration in the bone marrow in a pattern resembling acute lymphoblastic leukemia. Histologically, there are sheets of intermediate-sized lymphoid cells with regular round or oval nuclear outlines or slight nuclear irregularities. The cells have one or more distinct nucleoli and amphophilic, often vacuolated, cytoplasm. Mitoses are frequent, and there are characteristically scattered phagocytic or tingible body macrophages imparting a "starry-sky" appearance. AIDS-related Burkitt's lymphomas usually have atypical features, including greater nuclear pleomorphism than endemic cases (atypical Burkitt's or Burkitt-like), and some cases have more amphophilic cytoplasm or a plasmacytoid appearance (45,47–50). The cells often have a cohesive or clustered appearance in tissue sections, and all variations share an extremely high mitotic rate and a Ki67 or mib-1 score approaching 100%.

Molecular findings in Burkitt's lymphoma characteristically involve translocations of the MYC gene on chromosome 8, with the heavy-chain gene on chromosome 14 or the kappa- and lambda-light chain genes in chromosomes 2 and 22, respectively. In addition, dysregulation of C-MYC may arise from point mutations in the first intron-first exon regulatory regions and amino acid substitution in the second exon (51). The molecular characteristics of C-MYC activation

TABLE 39.3. *World Health Organization Classification of acquired immunodeficiency syndrome–related lymphomas*

A. Lymphomas also occurring in immunocompetent patients
1. Burkitt's lymphoma
   Classical
   With plasmacytoid differentiation
   Atypical
2. Diffuse large B-cell lymphoma
   Centroblastic
   Immunoblastic
3. Extranodal marginal zone B-cell lymphoma of mucosa-associated lymphoid tissue
4. Peripheral T-cell lymphoma
5. Classical Hodgkin's lymphoma
B. Lymphomas occurring more specifically in human immunodeficiency virus–positive patients
1. Primary effusion lymphoma
2. Plasmablastic lymphoma of the oral cavity
C. Lymphomas also occurring in other immunodeficiency states
   Polymorphic lymphoma (posttransplant lymphoproliferative disorder–like)

resemble sporadic rather than endemic Burkitt's lymphoma. The second most common molecular alteration in Burkitt's lymphomas is point mutations in the tumor suppressor gene p53, which occurs in up to 60% of cases (52).

In terms of Epstein-Barr virus, only approximately 40% of tumors are positive, a prevalence that resembles sporadic rather than endemic Burkitt's lymphoma. Also of interest are patterns of viral latency in HIV-related Burkitt's lymphomas that resemble endemic Burkitt's lymphomas in expressing latent Epstein-Barr virus nuclear antigen 1 transcripts 1 but differ in that they also express transcripts for Epstein-Barr virus latent membrane protein-1.

Diffuse Large B-Cell Lymphomas (30% of AIDS-Related Lymphomas)

Diffuse large B-cell lymphomas are a heterologous group, and HIV is associated with an increased incidence of specific subtypes. Although common in the general population, diffuse large B-cell lymphoma of follicular or centroblastic type accounts for only approximately 20% of AIDS lymphoma. This group of lymphomas may present with nodal or extranodal disease and consists of diffuse sheets of large lymphoid cells with round or oval nuclei and prominent nucleoli. These malignant cells are monoclonal for Ig gene rearrangements. Not surprisingly, and in keeping with their likely pathogenesis from centroblasts, cases of diffuse large B-cell lymphoma are often associated with expression of BCL-6 (53,54,55). BCL-6 amplification can be demonstrated with immunohistochemistry in tissue sections. Epstein-Barr virus is found in approximately 20% of cases. The frequency of latent membrane protein-1 deletion variants and of Epstein-Barr virus type 1 and type 2 strains in AIDS diffuse large B-cell lymphomas overlaps those in the general population and is not specific for HIV (39). The proliferation rate is usually high but not at the levels characteristically seen with small noncleaved cell or Burkitt's lymphomas.

The immunoblastic subtype of AIDS lymphoma (approximately 20% of cases) is more characteristic of AIDS infection and usually occurs at extranodal sites, particularly the central nervous system. The cells are large with a single prominent, often central, nucleolus and plasmacytoid cytoplasm. In some cases, Reed-Sternberg–like cells may be found, but the background proliferation does not resemble Hodgkin's lymphoma. Mitoses are frequent. In the central nervous system, there is often clustering around blood vessels, and the lesions may be multiple (56). The incidence of Epstein-Barr virus infection is highest in central nervous system lymphomas in which it approaches 100%, whereas the central nervous system AIDS lymphomas are uniformly negative for C-MYC (57).

Plasmablastic Lymphomas

Plasmablastic lymphomas were first described in the oral cavity but may occur at other sites (58,59). These distinctive lymphomas are characterized by a diffuse proliferation consisting almost entirely of large lymphoid cells with a marked plasmablastic appearance (Fig. 39.1). The cells have blast-like nuclei with prominent central nucleolus and plasmacytoid cytoplasm. These cells are usually positive for Epstein-Barr virus but invariably negative for the Kaposi's sarcoma-associated herpesvirus (human herpesvirus type 8). Most are positive for Epstein-Barr early region by in situ hybridization, variably positive for Epstein-Barr virus latent membrane protein-1, and negative for Epstein-Barr virus nuclear antigen 2. As suggested by their morphologic appearance, they resemble plas-

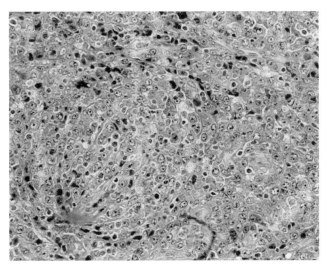

FIG. 39.1. Plasmablastic lymphoma of the oral cavity revealing sheets of plasmablasts infiltrating soft tissues of the jaw. Hematoxylin and eosin, original ×250.

mablasts rather than centroblasts in their phenotype, usually negative for CD45 and CD20 but expressing cytoplasmic IgG and plasma cell–related epitopes, such as VS38c and CD138.

Salivary Gland Lymphoid Hyperplasias and Extranodal Marginal Zone Lymphomas (Mucosa-Associated Lymphoid Tissue Lymphomas)

Symptoms and mass lesions relating to the salivary glands and related lymph nodes are common in patients infected with HIV. The most common abnormality is hyperplasia of salivary lymphoid tissue causing ductal obstruction and salivary duct cysts. There is frequently a proliferation of myoepithelial cells forming lymphoepithelial lesions analogous to those encountered in Sjögren's syndrome. Other features of sicca syndrome, including rheumatoid arthritis, are not encountered. The lesions usually involve the parotid gland, but other salivary glands may also be affected.

The lymphoid hyperplasia resembles that seen in the generalized, persistent lymphadenopathy syndrome, and the ductal lesions are almost always cystic (60,61). The lymphoid proliferation is polyclonal and not associated with lymphoma in adults, but in the pediatric HIV-infected population, salivary lymphoid infiltrates have similarities with lymphocytic interstitial pneumonitis and cystic hyperplasia of the thymus (62). In HIV-infected children, mucosa-associated lymphoid tissue (MALT) lymphomas, similar to those occurring in the general population, have been described in the salivary glands and also at other sites, including the lung and stomach. The relationship of pulmonary MALT lymphoma to lymphocytic interstitial pneumonitis suggests that an infectious agent may be causally related, including exposure to Epstein-Barr virus (63). Morphologically, these are indistinguishable from MALT lymphomas in the general population and are defined by nodules of centrocyte-like cells with slightly irregular nuclei and monocytoid cytoplasm, with a tendency to infiltrate epithelium, forming lymphoepithelial lesions.

Polymorphic B-Cell Lymphoma (Posttransplant Lymphoproliferative Disorder–Like)

Unlike in the iatrogenically immunosuppressed transplant population, polymorphic B-cell lymphoma, for unexplained reasons, is only occasionally encountered in the setting of HIV (42). Posttransplant lymphoproliferative disorder–like lymphomas in HIV-positive patients closely resemble posttransplant lymphomas in their association with Epstein-Barr virus and their polymorphous appearance, which includes small lymphocytes, plasma cells, and plasmacytoid immunoblasts (Fig. 39.2). In the higher-grade lesions, large cells are more prominent, and there may be tumor necrosis. This lesion is not associated with specific HIV risk factors and occurs in men, women, and children with AIDS. Disease may be encountered at nodal or extranodal sites, including salivary glands, lung, and skin, and must be distinguished from benign forms of HIV-related lymphoid hyper-

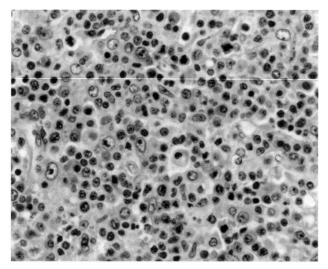

FIG. 39.2. Polymorphic lymphoid proliferation resembling posttransplant-associated lymphoproliferative disease showing a mixture of lymphoid cells, plasma cells, and immunoblasts. Hematoxylin and eosin, original ×160.

plasia (64). Although they are usually monoclonal with regard to Ig gene rearrangements, occasional cases may be polyclonal or exhibit only a small clonal rearranged band in a polyclonal background (42).

Other Low-Grade Lymphomas, Including Small Lymphocytic Lymphoma, Follicular Lymphoma, and Marginal Zone Lymphoma

Although indolent lymphomas, including small lymphocytic and marginal zone lymphoma, are increasingly encountered in the HIV-infected population (8,9), it is not clear at this point if there is a causal relationship to AIDS. HIV-positive patients with low-grade lymphomas tend to be less immunosuppressed and have higher CD4 counts, compared with patients with aggressive lymphomas, and demonstrate prolonged survival despite a high incidence of bone marrow infiltration and advanced stage disease at presentation (65).

Myeloma, Plasmacytoma, Plasma Cell Leukemia, and Monoclonal Gammopathy of Undetermined Significance

The relationship of HIV to plasma cell dyscrasias is of particular interest because polyclonal hypergammaglobulinemia and oligoclonal B-cell expansion are commonly encountered in patients with HIV. AIDS is associated with an increased risk for myeloma, and patients with myeloma tend to have aggressive disease with an anaplastic or blastic morphology and frequent involvement of body fluids (66,67).

Lymphomatoid Granulomatosis

Lymphomatoid granulomatosis is a rare Epstein-Barr virus–related disorder in which immunodeficiency is a contributory

factor. This lesion has been described in the oral cavity and gingival areas in patients with HIV (68). The lymphomatous infiltrates are characteristically associated with angioinvasion and extensive necrosis. Numerous Epstein-Barr early region 1–containing lymphoid cells can be found clustered about affected vessels.

Peripheral T/Natural Killer–Cell and Anaplastic Large-Cell Lymphomas

Although AIDS-related lymphomas are usually of B-cell type, peripheral T-cell lymphomas are occasionally associated with AIDS (69,70), and T-cell lymphomas are statistically increased among patients with a prior diagnosis of AIDS (10). These occur most frequently in the skin and subcutaneous tissues where they present with tumor-like masses, frequently associated with vascular invasion and necrosis. Unlike mycosis fungoides, they usually lack epidermotropism. Morphologically, they resemble peripheral T-cell lymphomas with a spectrum of pleomorphic neoplastic T cells.

T/natural killer–cell anaplastic large-cell lymphomas usually present at extranodal sites, including the gastrointestinal tract, skin, and nasal sinuses (69,70). These consist of large anaplastic lymphoid cells with the characteristic "hallmark" cells with markedly deformed nuclei most common around blood vessels. Because of the unusual presentation and anaplastic morphology, they may be confused with carcinoma. Some of these cases may be positive for Epstein-Barr virus. Cases in the skin are usually negative for ALK protein. Neutrophil-rich anaplastic large-cell lymphoma has also been described in association with HIV (71). In addition, the Epstein-Barr virus–associated nasal type T/natural killer–cell lymphoma has been described in the setting of HIV, although this appears quite rare (72).

Mycosis Fungoides

There appears to be an increased incidence of mycosis fungoides in the HIV-infected population (69,70). The lesions resemble mycosis fungoides in the general population and may present on the buttocks among other cutaneous sites. Histologically, there are characteristically cerebriform lymphoid cells infiltrating the epidermis and forming Pautrier-like intraepidermal clusters. Although mycosis cells are almost invariably CD4$^+$ in the general population, in HIV patients with CD4 cell depletion, there may be cutaneous eruptions and infiltration of CD8$^+$ mycosis cells. These cells may also infiltrate regional lymph nodes and the bone marrow and are associated with a poor prognosis (73). Mycosis fungoides lesions must be distinguished from atypical lymphoid infiltrates in the skin, which are common in HIV and often related to drug reactions.

Human Herpesvirus 8–Associated Lymphomas

In addition to causing multicentric Castleman's disease in patients infected with HIV, human herpesvirus 8 infection is also associated with characteristic lymphoproliferative disorders, which include primary effusion lymphomas, extracavitary lymphomas not associated with effusions, and plasmablastic lymphomas (not to be confused with plasmablastic lymphomas of the oral cavity).

Primary Effusion Lymphomas

Primary effusion lymphoma is a distinct clinicopathologic entity occurring usually, but not exclusively, in the setting of HIV infection (74–78). Patients with HIV and primary effusion lymphoma tend to be older males with homosexuality as a risk factor, late-stage disease, and severe immunosuppression, with CD4 counts less than 100 per mm^3. Approximately one third of patients with primary effusion lymphoma also have Kaposi's sarcoma (79). Although rare, this lymphoma is of interest because of the causal relationship with the Kaposi's sarcoma-associated herpesvirus, also known as *human herpesvirus 8*. Kaposi's sarcoma-associated herpesvirus/human herpesvirus 8 was the first human gamma-2 herpes virus identified and has been shown to be the cause of Kaposi's sarcoma, from which it was first isolated (80,81). Kaposi's sarcoma-associated herpesvirus sequences are, in fact, present in much higher copy numbers in primary effusion lymphoma tissues when compared with tissues of Kaposi's sarcoma (82).

Patients with primary effusion lymphoma present with symptoms of an effusion (pleural, pericardial, or ascitic) in the absence of a tumor mass. In some cases, although the disease is predominantly in body cavities, there may be extension to adjacent structures, such as the chest wall, pleura, or peritoneum (83). Examination of the fluid reveals large pleomorphic lymphoma cells with cytologic features that range between immunoblastic, plasmablastic, and anaplastic large-cell lymphoma (Fig. 39.3). The cells may be multinucleated and resemble Reed-Sternberg cells but are negative for CD15. The malignant cells also have a distinctive phenotype, staining for leukocyte common antigen CD45 and various activation antigens (HLA-DR, EMA, CD30, CD38, CD77), but are usually negative for other B- and T-cell markers, including CD20, CD19, and CD79a. Rare cases may coexpress both B- and T-cell antigens despite a B-cell genotype (84,85). The B-cell nature can be demonstrated by the presence of Ig gene rearrangements in Southern blots or polymerase chain reaction (86). Presence of human herpesvirus type 8 is demonstrable by polymerase chain reaction for various transcripts or by immunohistochemistry using antibodies to the latent nuclear antigen. There is active viral replication in the nuclei of the malignant cells, and viral particles are packaged in the cytoplasm to be shed from the cell surface (87). Virus can be found in saliva and the gastrointestinal tract of infected individuals.

Primary effusion lymphoma appears to derive from a late differentiated (postfollicular) B cell because there are clonal rearrangements and somatic mutations of the Ig genes. The pathogenesis of primary effusion lymphoma is of interest because the Kaposi's sarcoma-associated herpesvirus is a herpes virus with a number of oncogenic sequences, including a

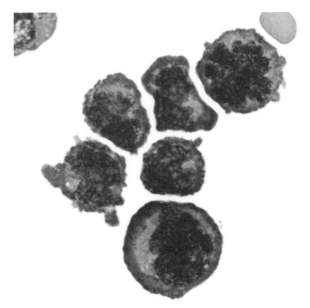

FIG. 39.3. Primary effusion lymphoma showing large anaplastic malignant cells from a pleural effusion. Hematoxylin and eosin, original ×400.

bcl-2–like sequence, a G-coupled receptor, and a type D cyclin similar to PRAD1 (88). Cytogenetic studies suggest multiple complex abnormalities (89), but most known oncogenes, including BCL6, MYC, RAS, TCL-1, and p53, do not appear to be implicated (43). The virus also produces cytokines, such as viral IL-6, capable of contributing to angiogenesis and tumor cell growth (90). Although there is invariably coinfection with Epstein-Barr virus in the setting of HIV, Kaposi's sarcoma-associated herpesvirus is capable of producing lymphomas in the absence of Epstein-Barr virus. Primary effusion lymphoma may also occur in Kaposi's sarcoma-associated herpesvirus–infected individuals in the absence of HIV and may be seen in both men and women (78,91).

Extracavitary Human Herpesvirus 8–Associated Lymphoma

Rare cases of lymphoma are associated with human herpesvirus type 8 in patients who do not develop effusions at presentation or during the course of the disease (92). These usually occur at extranodal sites and have similar morphologic and phenotypic findings to primary effusion lymphoma, frequently taking on an anaplastic appearance (93).

Human Herpesvirus 8–Positive Lymphomas Associated with Multicentric Castleman's Disease

Human herpesvirus 8–positive lymphoma occurs in association with Kaposi's sarcoma-associated herpesvirus–related multicentric Castleman's disease (94,95). The disease usually presents in the spleen where there are aggregates of plasmablasts forming clusters termed *microlymphomas* or in

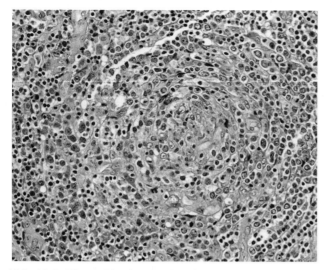

FIG. 39.4. Plasmablastic microlymphoma in a spleen from a patient with multicentric Castleman's disease showing clusters of plasmablasts. Hematoxylin and eosin, ×250.

some cases mass lesions. Morphologically, these resemble immunoblasts or plasmablasts but differ from plasmablastic lymphomas of the oral cavity, which are not associated with Kaposi's sarcoma-associated herpesvirus (Fig. 39.4). The plasmablasts are monotypic for IgM λ and are infected with Kaposi's sarcoma-associated herpesvirus, which can be demonstrated by immunohistochemical staining for latent nuclear antigen. These cells do not harbor somatic mutations in the rearranged Ig genes and appear to originate from naïve B cells in the follicular mantle (94).

CLINICAL ASPECTS OF AIDS-RELATED LYMPHOMA

Clinical Presentation

Systemic "B" Symptoms

Most patients with AIDS lymphoma present with systemic "B" symptoms, including unexplained fever, drenching night sweats, or weight loss in excess of 10% of normal body weight (19,96,97). These symptoms may also be seen in various opportunistic infections or in Hodgkin's disease or Kaposi's sarcoma. Nonetheless, after careful evaluation to exclude these other causes of systemic symptoms, the possibility of lymphoma should be considered.

Bone Marrow Involvement

Bone marrow involvement is diagnosed in approximately 20% of patients at initial presentation, with Burkitt's lymphoma the most common in this setting (98). The median hemoglobin level in patients with marrow involvement is 10.6 g per dL, whereas approximately one third of patients present with platelet counts less than 100,000. Marrow involvement is statistically associated with leptomeningeal

involvement. More than 50% marrow involvement is associated with decreased survival in these patients (98).

Gastrointestinal Tract Lymphoma

The gastrointestinal tract is involved by lymphoma in approximately one fourth of reported patients, who may present with abdominal pain, anorexia, nausea and vomiting, or a change in bowel habits. Abdominal distention or an abdominal mass may be noted. Involvement of the rectum is not unusual, presenting as a rectal mass or pain on defecation. Lymphoma within the liver is also relatively common, occurring in approximately 10% to 25% of reported series (19,96,97). These patients may present with jaundice, systemic "B" symptoms, abdominal pain, or anorexia.

Involvement of the Cerebrospinal Fluid

Leptomeningeal involvement by lymphoma occurs in approximately 10% to 20% of patients with newly diagnosed systemic AIDS lymphoma. These patients may be entirely asymptomatic in terms of the central nervous system. When symptoms do occur, the most common include altered mental status, cranial nerve palsies, or headache. Numbness of the chin may also be seen in patients with leptomeningeal lymphoma (99). Presence of Epstein-Barr virus within the cerebrospinal fluid, with Epstein-Barr virus nuclear antigen 1 detected by polymerase chain reaction, may also be used to diagnose lymphomatous meningitis in patients with systemic AIDS lymphoma (100). Leptomeningeal lymphoma is associated with higher CD4 cell counts than seen in patients with primary central nervous system lymphoma. Intrathecal cytosine arabinoside or methotrexate has been used successfully, both to treat known leptomeningeal lymphoma and to prevent its occurrence in patients at risk.

Other Sites

Any site may be involved by lymphoma in patients with underlying HIV infection. Unusual sites include the lung, oral cavity, adrenal gland, kidney, heart, and others. Lymphoma within the gallbladder has been described as well as involvement of the earlobe and multiple other unusual sites of lymphomatous disease (19,96).

Staging Evaluation in Patients with AIDS Lymphoma

The specific evaluation and management of patients with newly diagnosed AIDS lymphoma are presented in Table 39.4.

Routine Blood Work

Routine blood work is often abnormal at the time of diagnosis, with anemia expected in the majority, even in the

TABLE 39.4. *Staging and management of systemic acquired immunodeficiency syndrome lymphoma*

History.

Physical examination.

Blood tests: complete blood cell count, lactate dehydrogenase, uric acid, chemistries.

CAT scan: chest, abdomen, pelvis.

CAT or magnetic resonance imaging scan: brain.

Gallium-67 scan or fluorodeoxyglucose positron emission tomography scan of body.

Bone-marrow aspirate and biopsy.

Lumbar puncture with evaluation of cerebrospinal fluid for lymphoma.

Systemic chemotherapy is used for all stages of disease.

HAART is recommended in combination with chemotherapy.

Restage patient after two or four cycles of chemotherapy.

Give two cycles of chemotherapy beyond complete remission.

CAT, computed axial tomography; HAART, highly active antiretroviral therapy.

absence of marrow involvement (98). Although thrombocytopenia or leukopenia may also be observed, these abnormalities may occur secondary to HIV itself or to various commonly used medications or opportunistic infections.

The level of lactate dehydrogenase is often elevated and should always be checked because an increased lactate dehydrogenase level has prognostic implications associated with decreased survival (101).

Uric acid levels may also be increased at diagnosis. Allopurinol is indicated before institution of chemotherapy to prevent hyperuricemia associated with tumor lysis. Serum calcium levels may also be elevated at diagnosis.

Computed Axial Tomography Scan of Chest, Abdomen, and Pelvis

Generalized or localized lymphadenopathy is commonly seen on computed axial tomography scans of patients with AIDS lymphoma. Special attention should be given to the retroperitoneal and mesenteric nodes as well as to lymph node areas adjacent to sites of extranodal disease.

In the presence of gastrointestinal involvement, abdominal computed axial tomography scan reveals evidence of focal lymphomatous involvement, documented in 58 of 59 such patients described by Radin and colleagues (102). Focal hepatic lesions are expected with liver involvement, varying from solitary to innumerable and ranging from relatively small 1-cm nodules to large masses greater than 15 cm in diameter. Lesions are typically less dense than the adjacent liver parenchyma. Larger masses are often heterogeneous in density, with areas of necrosis. Isolated hepatomegaly alone, without focal mass lesions, is quite unusual (102).

With lymphoma in the lung, interstitial infiltrates, pulmonary nodules, or alveolar lung disease have all been described, with pleural effusions also commonly encountered (103).

Gallium-67 Scan

Gallium-67 scanning can be particularly useful in patients with AIDS lymphoma and may differentiate malignant lymphoma from reactive lymphadenopathy (104). High- and intermediate-grade lymphomas are almost always gallium avid, and the gallium scan may be useful in identifying lesions that have not yet caused specific organ or nodal enlargement on computed axial tomography scan. Aside from its known sensitivity and specificity in lymphoma, gallium-67 scanning may be particularly useful in the assessment of residual, stable masses after the completion of chemotherapy. These residual masses may occur in as many as 40% of patients with lymphoma who have been successfully treated. The residual masses in these instances represent fibrosis and are gallium negative. In the presence of a residual mass that remains gallium avid at the conclusion of chemotherapy, the clinician can assume that remaining active lymphomatous disease is still present and that further therapy is required.

Fluorodeoxyglucose Positron Emission Tomography

Although formal studies of fluorodeoxyglucose positron emission tomography (FDG-PET) scanning have not yet been accomplished in patients with AIDS-related systemic lymphoma, the usefulness of these scans has been confirmed in patients with *de novo* lymphoma, with sensitivity rates of 89% and specificity of 100% in a group of 18 such patients (105). By comparison, sensitivity of computed axial tomography scanning on detection of lymphoma in these patients was 86%, and specificity was 67%. FDG-PET has also been useful in the detection of residual active lymphomatous disease after completion of chemotherapy (106). Further, early response to chemotherapy, as detected by FDG-PET scan, may be useful as an indicator of subsequent prognosis (107).

Lumbar Puncture

Although not routine in patients with *de novo* lymphoma, patients with systemic AIDS lymphoma should undergo diagnostic lumbar puncture at the time of initial staging evaluation. As many as 20% of patients may have lymphoma within the spinal fluid in the absence of any specific symptom or clinical sign of such involvement (108). In the presence of lymphomatous meningitis, the cell count may be normal or high, with presence of abnormal cells cytologically. The median cell count is usually only minimally elevated, at 12 per mm^3 (109). The glucose level may be low or normal, whereas the protein in the cerebrospinal fluid may be elevated or normal (109). The presence of Epstein-Barr virus nuclear antigen 1 by polymerase chain reaction is associated with lymphomatous involvement of the cerebrospinal fluid and may also predict eventual lymphomatous meningitis (100).

Bone Marrow Aspirate and Biopsy

Bone marrow aspirate and biopsy are also indicated during the initial staging evaluation of a patient with AIDS lymphoma, with marrow involvement in approximately 20% of patients (19,98). Lymphomatous involvement of marrow is statistically associated with lymphoma in the cerebrospinal fluid and in bones (98).

Prognostic Factors in Patients with Systemic AIDS–Related Lymphoma

The factors associated with shorter survival of patients with AIDS-related lymphoma include CD4 cells less than 100 per mm^3, stage III or IV disease, age older than 35 years, history of injection drug use, and elevated lactate dehydrogenase (101,110,111). The International Prognostic Index for aggressive lymphoma has also been validated in patients with AIDS lymphoma (112). Recently, the use of HAART has been associated with significant prolongation in survival among HIV-infected patients with lymphoma (17,113).

Therapy of Patients with Systemic AIDS–Related Lymphoma: Standard versus Low-Dose Chemotherapy

Before the advent of HAART, patients with AIDS-related lymphoma were highly immunocompromised, with low CD4 cells and increased proclivity for developing serious opportunistic infections, from which they often died (19). The propensity for developing serious infectious complications was augmented by the use of multiagent chemotherapy, which in itself is associated with development of opportunistic infections, even in the absence of underlying HIV infection (19). In an attempt to ascertain the potential value of low-dose chemotherapy in this setting, Levine and her colleagues developed a low-dose modification of m-BACOD [moderate-dose methotrexate, bleomycin, Adriamycin (doxorubicin), cyclophosphamide, Oncovin (vincristine), dexamethasone], which was associated with a complete remission rate of approximately 50% and a median survival of approximately 6 months (108). The AIDS Clinical Trials Group in the United States evaluated the use of standard-versus low-dose m-BACOD chemotherapy in patients with newly diagnosed AIDS lymphoma (108,114). Although standard-dose therapy was associated with a statistically greater likelihood of severe hematologic toxicity, neither response rates nor overall or disease-free survival was influenced by dose intensity. It is important to note that this study was conducted before the widespread use of HAART. It is certainly possible that toxicity may have been ameliorated and survival prolonged if HAART had been available and if

patients had initiated chemotherapy at higher CD4 lymphocyte counts.

Use of Concomitant Highly Active Antiretroviral Therapy Plus Chemotherapy

The use of dose-reduced and standard-dose CHOP [cyclophosphamide, doxorubicin, Oncovin (vincristine), prednisone] was studied by the National Cancer Institute–sponsored AIDS Malignancy Consortium, with chemotherapy administered along with HAART in a cohort of 65 patients with newly diagnosed AIDS lymphoma (115). In this study, HAART consisted of indinavir, stavudine, and lamivudine. Grade 3 or 4 neutropenia was more common among patients receiving full-dose CHOP (25% vs. 12%), but there were similar numbers of patients who experienced other toxicities. Doxorubicin clearance and indinavir concentration curves were comparable in patients on this study when compared with historical controls. Of interest, although cyclophosphamide clearance was decreased 1.5-fold when compared with controls, no clinical consequence of this change was apparent. With complete remission rates of 30% in the low-dose CHOP group and 48% among those who received standard-dose CHOP in this nonrandomized phase II trial, the authors concluded that either regimen, when delivered with HAART, was effective and tolerable (115). Despite these results, however, caution should be used when employing chemotherapy together with zidovudine, which may cause significant bone marrow compromise in itself and should be avoided in this setting (116).

Relationship between Response to Highly Active Antiretroviral Therapy and Response to Chemotherapy in Patients with AIDS-Related Lymphoma

The use of HAART has been associated with an approximate 75% decline in the development of new AIDS-defining conditions among HIV-infected people and a similar decline in mortality among those with full-blown AIDS (3). It would thus appear reasonable to assume that HAART would also be associated with an increase in survival among patients with AIDS-related lymphoma. Although this relationship has been demonstrated in several recent studies (17,113), other studies have not yet confirmed an increase in overall median survival among AIDS lymphoma patients treated in the era of HAART (13,15,16). Differences in the actual use of HAART among the cohorts may provide one explanation. Furthermore, although HAART may be used in a given patient or patient population, this does not necessarily imply that the antiretroviral regimen was actually effective in reducing the HIV-1 viral load or increasing the CD4 cells or overall state of immune function. To address this question, Antinori and colleagues from Italy recently evaluated the relationship between effective HAART use and outcome in 44 patients with newly diagnosed AIDS lymphoma (113). Of importance, complete response to chemo-

TABLE 39.5. *Infusional CDE regimen*

Cyclophosphamide, 200 mg/m^2/d × 4 d

Doxorubicin, 12.5 mg/m^2/d × 4 d

Etoposide, 60 mg/m^2/d × 4 d

Intrathecal prophylaxis in patients with marrow involvement or small noncleaved (Burkitt's or Burkitt-like) histology

Prophylaxis against opportunistic infections (cotrimoxazole, fluconazole)

CDE, cyclophosphamide, doxorubicin, etoposide.

TABLE 39.6. *EPOCH regimen of infusional chemotherapy*

Etoposide, 50 mg/m^2/d × 4 d

Vincristine, 0.4 mg/m^2/d × 4 d

Doxorubicin, 10 mg/m^2/d × 4 d

Cyclophosphamide, 187 mg/m^2 IV on d 5 for CD4$^+$ <100 cells/ mm^3 or 375 mg/m^2 IV on d 5 for CD4$^+$ ≥100 cells/mm^3

Prednisone, 60 mg/m^2 orally, d 1–5

Granulocyte colony-stimulating factor: start on d 6

Repeat on d 22 times six cycles

EPOCH, etoposide, prednisone, Oncovin (vincristine), cyclophosphamide, hydroxydaunomycin (doxorubicin).

therapy was statistically related to virologic response to HAART, and, on multivariate analysis, the virologic response to HAART was the only factor associated with attainment of complete remission status. Furthermore, a higher relative dose intensity of chemotherapy could be safely administered to patients who attained a virologic response to HAART, and, in this setting, receipt of higher-dose chemotherapy was advantageous, in terms of attainment of complete remission status and in terms of longer overall survival. On multivariate analysis, an immunologic response to HAART (development of higher CD4 cell count), receipt of higher relative dose intensity of chemotherapy, and attainment of complete remission to chemotherapy were all associated with longer survival (113). These data imply a major advantage to the combined use of HAART with chemotherapy not only in terms of overall survival, but in terms of the ability to achieve complete-remission status as well.

Infusional Cyclophosphamide, Doxorubicin, and Etoposide

Sparano and colleagues have developed and tested the CDE (cyclophosphamide, doxorubicin, etoposide) regimen (117, 118) in patients with newly diagnosed AIDS lymphoma, as shown in Table 39.5. In a large, multiinstitutional Eastern Cooperative Oncology Group trial, 107 patients received the 4-day infusion, including 48 patients who received concomitant antiretroviral therapy with didanosine, and 59 received HAART regimens (117,118). For the group as a whole, the rate of complete remission was 44%, with partial responses in 11%. Although there was no difference in complete remission rates among patients who received HAART versus didanosine, the median overall survival was longer in those patients who received combination antiretroviral therapy. This series of trials indicates that although response rates to infusional CDE appear similar to those achieved with either low-dose or standard-dose m-BACOD, survival appears superior in those patients who receive concomitant HAART.

Infusional Risk-Adjusted Etoposide, Prednisone, Oncovin (Vincristine), Cyclophosphamide, Hydroxydaunomycin Regimen

Wilson and his group at the National Cancer Institute have developed the EPOCH [etoposide, prednisone, Oncovin (vin-

cristine), cyclophosphamide, hydroxydaunomycin (doxorubicin)] regimen (Table 39.6), consisting of a 4-day infusion of etoposide, vincristine, and doxorubicin, with risk-adjusted bolus dosing of cyclophosphamide on day 5 and prednisone given orally on days 1 through 5 of each 22-day cycle (119). Granulocyte colony-stimulating factor is used uniformly, beginning at day 6, and all antiretroviral therapy is withheld until day 6 of the last cycle of chemotherapy. With a total of 39 patients reported thus far, a complete remission rate of 74% was achieved, including 56% in those with CD4 lymphocyte counts less than 100 per mm^3 and 87% among patients with CD4 lymphocyte counts greater than 100 per mm^3. A total of 60% of the group as a whole remains alive at 33 months, and, notably, only three patients have yet experienced relapse of lymphoma. The HIV viral load rose by 1,000-fold by cycle 4 of therapy but returned to pretreatment levels within 3 months of restarting antiretroviral therapy. Likewise, although CD4 lymphocyte counts decreased during chemotherapy, they returned to baseline values by 12 to 24 months post EPOCH. No increase in opportunistic infections was noted, despite the fact that antiretroviral therapy was withheld during the 6 months of chemotherapy. This study implies that concomitant use of HAART may not be necessary in patients with AIDS lymphoma, provided that this therapy is begun very quickly after discontinuation of multiagent chemotherapy. Nonetheless, these data have not yet been confirmed in settings outside of the National Cancer Institute in the United States, and the bulk of current data suggests an advantage to the use of combined HAART and chemotherapy (17,113,115,118).

Current Questions Regarding Optimal Therapy of Systemic AIDS-Related Lymphoma

The studies discussed above leave several important questions unanswered. First, the relative importance of HAART used together with combination chemotherapy in patients with newly diagnosed AIDS lymphoma remains unanswered. The value of dose-reduced versus standard-dose–intensity chemotherapy remains unknown in the current era of HAART, when patients have higher median CD4 lymphocyte counts and may be more able to tolerate dose-intensive therapy. The optimal regimen of chemotherapy remains uncertain, as does the value of rituximab when added to standard chemotherapy regimens such as CHOP. All of these questions are being addressed within the context of ongoing clinical trials, and results are awaited with great interest. Table 39.7 summarizes results of current regimens for patients with systemic AIDS lymphoma.

Therapy of Patients with Relapsed or Primary Resistant AIDS-Related Lymphoma

Treatment options for patients with relapsed or refractory AIDS–related lymphoma are extremely limited. The infusional CDE regimen has been associated with a complete-remission rate of 10% in a group of 40 patients with relapsed/refractory disease and a partial-remission rate of 18% (121). The median duration of complete remission was 6 months, whereas that for the partial responder patients was 5 months. The overall median survival of these 40 patients was 4 months (range, less than 1 to 33 months), and the median survival for responding patients was 10 months (121). A regimen consisting of etoposide, prednimustine, and mitoxantrone resulted in complete response in 8 of 21 patients (38%) but a median survival of only 2 months (122). Although associated with uniform grade 4 neutropenia, the ESHAP [etoposide, Solu-Medrol (methylprednisolone), high-dose ara-C, Platinol (cisplatin)] regimen, when given to 13 patients with relapsed or refractory AIDS lymphoma, led to complete remission in 31%, overall response in 54%, and median survival of 7.1 months from the time of ESHAP (123). Clearly, additional work is required to ascertain the optimal therapy for patients who show no response to first-line therapy for AIDS lymphoma or relapse after initial response.

PRIMARY CENTRAL NERVOUS SYSTEM AIDS-RELATED LYMPHOMA

Patients with AIDS-related primary central nervous system lymphoma tend to present with extremely advanced HIV disease, with median CD4 cell counts less than 50 per mm^3 and history of previous AIDS-defining clinical illnesses in approximately 75% (19,124,125). Recent large series have confirmed a major, highly significant decrease in primary central nervous system lymphoma since the advent of HAART (12,14,16,17).

Patients with AIDS lymphoma primary to the brain usually seek medical attention because of altered mental status, seizures, or focal neurologic abnormalities (124–126). Systemic "B" symptoms are seen in 80% to 90%. Imaging studies of the brain reveal mass lesion(s) within brain parenchyma, which may be found at any site. Computed tomographic scans or magnetic resonance imaging scans are relatively nonspecific in terms of identifying a lesion as lymphoma, whereas thallium single-positron emission tomography scan (127) or FDG-PET scan (128) may be more helpful in terms of differentiating primary central nervous system lymphoma from other AIDS-related disease entities. Because AIDS-related primary central nervous system lymphoma is uniformly associated with Epstein-Barr virus (129), when combined with Epstein-Barr virus testing of cerebrospinal fluid, FDG-PET scanning yields even more specific results (127).

TABLE 39.7. *Results of therapy in patients with systemic acquired immunodeficiency syndrome lymphoma*

Regimen (reference)	Patients (n)	Antiretroviral therapy	Complete remission (%)	Overall median survival	Comments
Low-dose m-BACOD (114)	98	Optional; no HAART	41	8.75 mo	No significant differences in response or survival between low-dose m-BACOD and standard-dose m-BACOD
Standard-dose m-BACOD	94	Optional; no HAART	52	7.75 mo	—
CDE (117)	48	Didanosine	46	8.2 mo	—
CDE (118)	59	HAART	42	17.8 mo	—
CHOP (120)	80	None	36	7 mo	Retrospective review of patients treated with CHOP or CHOP-like regimens
CHOP (120)	24	HAART	50	Not reached at median follow-up of 8.5 mo	—
EPOCH (119)	33	HAART began at completion of EPOCH	79	73% survival at 33 mo	—

CDE, cyclophosphamide, doxorubicin, etoposide; CHOP, cyclophosphamide, hydroxydaunomycin (doxorubicin), Oncovin (vincristine), prednisone; EPOCH, etoposide, prednisone, Oncovin (vincristine), cyclophosphamide, hydroxydaunomycin (doxorubicin); HAART, highly active antiretroviral therapy; m-BACOD, moderate-dose methotrexate, bleomycin, Adriamycin (doxorubicin), cyclophosphamide, Oncovin (vincristine), dexamethasone.

The optimal therapy for patients with AIDS-related primary central nervous system lymphoma remains problematic. Median survival is in the range of 2 to 4 months in the setting of either radiation therapy or no treatment at all (126). Nonetheless, whole-brain radiation has been associated with improved quality of survival and is advocated on this basis (126). Antiretroviral therapy (zidovudine) along with ganciclovir and IL-2 has been explored, with some evidence of efficacy in small numbers of patients (130). Hydroxyurea, in an attempt to suppress Epstein-Barr virus infection, was recently used in two patients, with excellent objective responses (131). Additional work is required to define effective modalities of therapy in affected individuals.

REFERENCES

1. Quinn TC. The global HIV/AIDS pandemic. Program and abstracts of the 5th International AIDS Malignancy Conference; April 23–25, 2001. Bethesda, MD, S23(abst).
2. Buehler JW, Ward JW. A new definition for AIDS surveillance. *Ann Intern Med* 1993;118:390–391.
3. Palella FJ Jr, Delaney KM, Moorman AC, et al. Declining morbidity and mortality among patients with advanced human immunodeficiency virus infection. *N Engl J Med* 1998;338:853–860.
4. Carpenter CCJ, Cooper DA, Fischel MA, et al. Antiretroviral therapy in adults: updated recommendations of the International AIDS Society-USC Panel. *JAMA* 2000;283:381–390.
5. Ledergerber B, Egger M, Erard V, et al. AIDS related opportunistic illnesses occurring after initiation of potent antiretroviral therapy: The Swiss HIV Cohort Study. *JAMA* 1999;282:2220–2226.
6. Lee LM, Karon JM, Selik R, et al. Survival after AIDS diagnosis in adolescents and adults during the treatment era, United States, 1984–1997. *JAMA* 2001;285:1308–1315.
7. Grulich AE, Wan X, Law MG, et al. B cell stimulation and prolonged immune deficiency are risk factors for non-Hodgkin's lymphoma in people with AIDS. *AIDS* 2000;14:144.
8. Cote TR, Biggar RJ, Rosenberg PS, et al. Non-Hodgkin's lymphoma among people with AIDS: incidence, presentation and public health burden. *Int J Cancer* 1997;73:645–650.
9. Biggar RJ, Rosenberg PS, Cote T: Kaposi's sarcoma and non-Hodgkin's lymphoma following the diagnosis of AIDS. *Int J Cancer* 1996;68:754–758.
10. Biggar RJ, Engels EA, Frisch M, Goedert JJ. Risk of T cell lymphomas in persons with AIDS. *J AIDS* 2001;26:371–376.
11. Ledergerber B, Telenti A, Effer M. Risk of HIV related Kaposi's sarcoma and non-Hodgkin's lymphoma with potent antiretroviral therapy: prospective cohort study. *Br Med J* 1999;319:23–24.
12. Mocroft A, Katama C, Johnson AM, et al. AIDS across Europe, 1994–1998: the EuroSIDA study. *Lancet* 2000;356:291–296.
13. Matthews GV, Bower M, Mandalia S, et al. Changes in acquired immunodeficiency syndrome-related lymphoma since the introduction of highly active anti-retroviral therapy. *Blood* 2000;96:2730–2734.
14. International Collaboration on HIV and Cancer. Highly active antiretroviral therapy and incidence of cancer in human immunodeficiency virus infected adults. *J NCI* 2000;92:1823–1830.
15. Levine AM, Seneviratne L, Espina BM, et al. Evolving characteristics of AIDS-related lymphoma. *Blood* 2000;96:4084–4090.
16. Kirk O, Pedersen C, Cozzi-Lepri A, et al. Non-Hodgkin lymphoma in HIV-infected patients in the era of highly active antiretroviral therapy. *Blood* 2001;98:3406–3412.
17. Besson C, Goubar A, Gabarre J, et al. Changes in AIDS-related lymphoma since the era of highly active antiretroviral therapy. *Blood* 2001;98:2339–2344.
18. Lucas GM, Chaisson RE, Moore RD. Highly active anti-retroviral therapy in a large urban clinic: risk factors for virologic failure and adverse drug reactions. *Ann Intern Med* 1999;130:81–87.
19. Levine AM. AIDS related lymphoma (review). *Blood* 1992;80:8–20.
20. Hartge P, Devesa SS, Fraumeni JF Jr. Hodgkin's and non-Hodgkin's lymphomas. *Cancer Surv* 1994;20:423–453.
21. Nelson RA, Levine AM, Bernstein L. Reproductive factors and risk of intermediate or high grade B cell non-Hodgkin's lymphoma in women. *J Clin Oncol* 2001;19:1381–1387.
22. Granovsky MO, Mueller BU, Nicholson HS, et al. Cancer in human immunodeficiency virus infected children: a case series from the Children's Cancer Group and the National Cancer Institute. *J Clin Oncol* 1998;16:1729–1735.
23. Holly EA, Lele C. Non-Hodgkin's lymphoma in HIV positive and HIV negative homosexual men in the San Francisco Bay area: allergies, prior medication use, and sexual practice. *J AIDS* 1997;15:211–222.
24. Holly EA, Lele C, Bracci P. Non-Hodgkin's lymphoma in homosexual men in the San Francisco Bay area: occupational, chemical and environmental exposures. *J AIDS* 1997;15:223–231.
25. Armenian H, Hoover DR, Rubb S, et al. Risk factors for non-Hodgkin's lymphomas in AIDS. *Am J Epidemiol* 1996;143:374–379.
26. Dean M, Jacobson LP, McFarlane G, et al. Reduced risk of AIDS lymphoma in individuals heterozygous for the CCR5-delta32 mutation. *Cancer Res* 1999;59:3561–3564.
27. Rabkin CS, Yang Q, Goedert JJ, et al. Chemokine and chemokine receptor gene variants and risk of non-Hodgkin's lymphoma in human immunodeficiency virus-1 infected individuals. *Blood* 1999;93:1838–1842.
28. Pluda JM, Yarchoan R, Jaffe ES, et al. Development of non-Hodgkin lymphoma in a cohort of patients with severe human immunodeficiency virus (HIV) infection on long-term antiretroviral therapy. *Ann Intern Med* 1990;113:276–282.
29. Shibata D, Weiss LM, Hernandez AM, et al. Epstein-Barr virus-associated non-Hodgkin's lymphoma in patients infected with the human immunodeficiency virus. *Blood* 1993;81:2102–2109.
30. Shibata D, Weiss LM, Nathwani BN, et al. Epstein-Barr virus in benign lymph node biopsies from individuals infected with the human immunodeficiency virus is associated with concurrent or subsequent development of non-Hodgkin's lymphoma. *Blood* 1991;77:1527–1533.
31. Neri A, Barriga F, Inghirami G, et al. Epstein-Barr virus infection precedes clonal expansion in Burkitt's and acquired immunodeficiency syndrome-associated lymphoma. *Blood* 1991;77:1092–1095.
32. Subar M, Neri A, Inghirami G, et al. Frequent c-myc oncogene activation and infrequent presence of Epstein-Barr virus genome in AIDS-associated lymphoma. *Blood* 1988;72:667–671.
33. Ballerini P, Gaidano G, Gong J, et al. Molecular pathogenesis of HIV-associated lymphomas. *AIDS Res Hum Retroviruses* 1992;8:731–735.
34. Ballerini P, Gaidano G, Gong JZ, et al. Multiple genetic lesions in acquired immunodeficiency syndrome-related non-Hodgkin's lymphoma. *Blood* 1993;81:166–176.
35. Boyle MJ, Sculley TB, Cooper DA, et al. Epstein-Barr virus and HIV play no direct role in persistent generalized lymphadenopathy syndrome. *Clin Exp Immunol* 1992;87:357–361.
36. Boyle MJ, Sewell WA, Milliken ST, et al. HIV and malignancy. *J Acquir Immune Defic Syndr* 1993;6[Suppl 1]:S5–S9.
37. Boyle MJ, Sewell WA, Sculley TB, et al. Subtypes of Epstein-Barr virus in human immunodeficiency virus-associated non-Hodgkin's lymphoma. *Blood* 1991;78:3004–3011.
38. Boyle MJ, Swanson CE, Turner JJ, et al. Definition of two distinct types of AIDS-associated non-Hodgkin lymphoma. *Br J Haematol* 1990;76:506–512.
39. Fassone L, Cingolani A, Martini M, et al. Characterization of Epstein-Barr virus genotype in AIDS-related non-Hodgkin's lymphoma. *AIDS Res Hum Retroviruses* 2002;18:19–26.
40. Knowles DM, Chamulak GA, Subar M, et al. Lymphoid neoplasia associated with the acquired immunodeficiency syndrome (AIDS). The New York University Medical Center experience with 105 patients (1981–1986). *Ann Intern Med* 1988;108:744–753.
41. Emilie D, Zou W, Fior R, et al. Production and roles of IL-6, IL-10, and IL-13 in B-lymphocyte malignancies and in B-lymphocyte hyperactivity of HIV infection and autoimmunity. *Methods* 1997;11:133–142.
42. Nador R, Chadburn A, Cesarman E, et al. AIDS-related polymorphic lymphoproliferative disorders. *J Acquir Immune Defic Syndr Hum Retroviol* 1997;14:45a.
43. Said JW, Hoyer KK, French SW, et al. TCL1 oncogene expression in B cell subsets from lymphoid hyperplasia and distinct classes of B cell lymphoma. *Lab Invest* 2001;81:555–564.

44. Weinberg RA. Oncogenes, antioncogenes, and the molecular bases of multistep carcinogenesis. *Cancer Res* 1989;49:3713–3721.

45. Raphael M, Borisch B, Jaffe ES. Lymphomas associated with infection by the human immunodeficiency virus (HIV). In: Jaffe ES, Harris NL, Stein H, Vardiman JW, eds. *World Health Organization classification of tumours.* Lyon, France: IARC Press, 2001:260–263.

46. Jaffe ES, Harris NL, Stein H, Vardiman JW. *Pathology & genetics. Tumours of haematopoietic and lymphoid tissues. World Health Organization classification of tumors.* Lyon, France: IARC Press, 2001.

47. Raphael M, Gentilhomme O, Tulliez M, et al. Histopathologic features of high-grade non-Hodgkin's lymphomas in acquired immunodeficiency syndrome. The French Study Group of Pathology for Human Immunodeficiency Virus-Associated Tumors. *Arch Pathol Lab Med* 1991;115:15–20.

48. Carbone A, Gloghini A, Gaidano G, et al. AIDS-related Burkitt's lymphoma. Morphologic and immunophenotypic study of biopsy specimens. *Am J Clin Pathol* 1995;103:561–567.

49. Davi F, Delecluse HJ, Guiet P, et al. Burkitt-like lymphomas in AIDS patients: characterization within a series of 103 human immunodeficiency virus-associated non-Hodgkin's lymphomas. Burkitt's Lymphoma Study Group. *J Clin Pathol* 1998;16:3788–3795.

50. Delecluse HJ, Raphael M, Magaud JP, et al. Variable morphology of human immunodeficiency virus-associated lymphomas with c-myc rearrangements. The French Study Group of Pathology for Human Immunodeficiency Virus-Associated Tumors, I. *Blood* 1993;82:552–563.

51. Bhatia K, Spangler G, Gaidano G, et al. Mutations in the coding region of c-myc occur frequently in acquired immunodeficiency syndrome-associated lymphomas. *Blood* 1994;84:883–888.

52. Nakamura H, Said JW, Miller CW, Koeffler HP. Mutation and protein expression of p53 in acquired immunodeficiency syndrome-related lymphomas. *Blood* 1993;82:920–926.

53. Gaidano G, Carbone A, Pastore C, et al. Frequent mutation of the 5' noncoding region of the BCL-6 gene in acquired immunodeficiency syndrome-related non-Hodgkin's lymphomas. *Blood* 1997;89:3755–3762.

54. Gaidano G, Lo Coco F, Ye BH, et al. Rearrangements of the BCL-6 gene in acquired immunodeficiency syndrome-associated non-Hodgkin's lymphoma: association with diffuse large-cell subtype. *Blood* 1994;84:397–402.

55. Carbone A, Gaidano G, Gloghini A, et al. BCL-6 protein expression in AIDS-related non-Hodgkin's lymphomas: inverse relationship with Epstein-Barr virus-encoded latent membrane protein-1 expression. *Am J Pathol* 1997;150:155–165.

56. Camilleri-Broet S, Davi F, Feuillard J, et al. AIDS-related primary brain lymphomas: histopathologic and immunohistochemical study of 51 cases. The French Study Group for HIV-Associated Tumors. *Hum Pathol* 1997;28:367–374.

57. Meeker TC, Shiramizu B, Kaplan L, et al. Evidence for molecular subtypes of HIV-associated lymphoma: division into peripheral monoclonal, polyclonal and central nervous system lymphoma. *AIDS* 1991;5:669–674.

58. Delecluse HJ, Anagnostopoulos I, Dallenbach F, et al. Plasmablastic lymphomas of the oral cavity: a new entity associated with the human immunodeficiency virus infection. *Blood* 1997;89:1413–1420.

59. Flaitz CM, Nichols CM, Walling DM, Hicks MJ. Plasmablastic lymphoma: an HIV-associated entity with primary oral manifestations. *Oral Oncol* 2002;38:96–102.

60. Ihrler S, Zietz C, Riederer A, et al. HIV-related parotid lymphoepithelial cysts. Immunohistochemistry and 3-D reconstruction of surgical and autopsy material with special reference to formal pathogenesis. *Virchows Arch* 1996;429:139–147.

61. Ihrler S, Zietz C, Sendelhofert A, et al. Lymphoepithelial duct lesions in Sjogren-type sialadenitis. *Virchows Arch* 1999;434:315–323.

62. Mishalani SH, Lones MA, Said JW. Multilocular thymic cyst. A novel thymic lesion associated with human immunodeficiency virus infection. *Arch Pathol Lab Med* 1995;119:467–470.

63. Teruya-Feldstein J, Temeck BK, Sloas MM, et al. Pulmonary malignant lymphoma of mucosa-associated lymphoid tissue (MALT) arising in a pediatric HIV-positive patient. *Am J Surg Pathol* 1995;19:357–363.

64. Tao J, Valderrama E. Epstein-Barr virus-associated polymorphic B-cell lymphoproliferative disorders in the lungs of children with AIDS: a report of two cases. *Am J Surg Pathol* 1999;23:560–566.

65. Levine AM, Sadeghi S, Espina B, et al. Characteristics of indolent non-Hodgkin lymphoma in patients with type 1 human immunodeficiency virus infection. *Cancer* 2002;94:1500–1506.

66. Goedert JJ, Cote TR, Virgo P, et al. Spectrum of AIDS-associated malignant disorders. *Lancet* 1998;351:1833–1839.

67. Kumar S, Kumar D, Schnadig VJ, et al. Plasma cell myeloma in patients who are HIV-positive. *Am J Clin Pathol* 1994;102:633–639.

68. Jaffe ES. Lymphoid lesions of the head and neck: a model of lymphocyte homing and lymphomagenesis. *Mod Pathol* 2002;15:255–263.

69. Beylot-Barry M, Vergier B, Masquelier B, et al. The spectrum of cutaneous lymphomas in HIV infection: a study of 21 cases. *Am J Surg Pathol* 1999;23:1208–1216.

70. Gonzalez-Clemente JM, Ribera JM, Campo E, et al. Ki-1+ anaplastic large-cell lymphoma of T-cell origin in an HIV-infected patient. *AIDS* 1991;5:751–755.

71. Jhala DN, Medeiros LJ, Lopez-Terrada D, et al. Neutrophil-rich anaplastic large cell lymphoma of T-cell lineage. A report of two cases arising in HIV-positive patients. *Am J Clin Pathol* 2000;114:478–482.

72. Canioni D, Arnulf B, Asso-Bonnet M, et al. Nasal natural killer lymphoma associated with Epstein-Barr virus in a patient infected with human immunodeficiency virus. *Arch Pathol Lab Med* 2001;125:660–662.

73. Guitart J, Variakojis D, Kuzel T, Rosen S. Cutaneous CD8 T cell infiltrates in advanced HIV infection. *J Am Acad Dermatol* 1999;41:722–727.

74. Nador RG, Cesarman E, Knowles DM, Said JW. Herpes-like DNA sequences in a body-cavity-based lymphoma in an HIV-negative patient. *N Engl J Med* 1995;333:943.

75. Green I, Espiritu E, Ladanyi M, et al. Primary lymphomatous effusions in AIDS: a morphological, immunophenotypic, and molecular study. *Mod Pathol* 1995;8:39–45.

76. Ansari MQ, Dawson DB, Nador R, et al. Primary body cavity-based AIDS-related lymphomas. *Am J Clin Pathol* 1996;105:221–229.

77. Cobo F, Hernandez S, Hernandez L, et al. Expression of potentially oncogenic HHV-8 genes in an EBV-negative primary effusion lymphoma occurring in an HIV-seronegative patient. *J Pathol* 1999;189:288–293.

78. Said JW, Tasaka T, Takeuchi S, et al. Primary effusion lymphoma in women: report of two cases of Kaposi's sarcoma herpes virus-associated effusion-based lymphoma in human immunodeficiency virus-negative women. *Blood* 1996;88:3124–3128.

79. Nador RG, Cesarman E, Chadburn A, et al. Primary effusion lymphoma: a distinct clinicopathologic entity associated with the Kaposi's sarcoma-associated herpes virus. *Blood* 1996;88:645–656.

80. Chang Y, Cesarman E, Pessin MS, et al. Identification of herpesvirus-like DNA sequences in AIDS-associated Kaposi's sarcoma. *Science* 1994;266:1865–1869.

81. Moore PS, Chang Y. Kaposi's sarcoma findings. *Science* 1995;270:15.

82. Cesarman E, Chang Y, Moore PS, et al. Kaposi's sarcoma-associated herpesvirus-like DNA sequences in AIDS-related body-cavity-based lymphomas. *N Engl J Med* 1995;332:1186–1191.

83. Mbulaiteye SM, Biggar RJ, Goedert JJ, Engels EA. Pleural and peritoneal lymphoma among people with AIDS in the United States. *J Acquir Immune Defic Syndr* 2002;29:418–421.

84. Said JW, Shintaku IP, Asou H, et al. Herpesvirus 8 inclusions in primary effusion lymphoma: report of a unique case with T-cell phenotype. *Arch Pathol Lab Med* 1999;123:257–260.

85. Beaty MW, Kumar S, Sorbara L, et al. A biphenotypic human herpesvirus 8-associated primary bowel lymphoma. *Am J Surg Pathol* 1999;23:992–994.

86. Walts AE, Shintaku IP, Said JW. Diagnosis of malignant lymphoma in effusions from patients with AIDS by gene rearrangement. *Am J Clin Pathol* 1990;94:170–175.

87. Said JW, Chien K, Tasaka T, Koeffler HP. Ultrastructural characterization of human herpesvirus 8 (Kaposi's sarcoma-associated herpesvirus) in Kaposi's sarcoma lesions: electron microscopy permits distinction from cytomegalovirus (CMV). *J Pathol* 1997;182:273–281.

88. Cesarman E, Mesri EA, Gershengorn MC. Viral G protein-coupled receptor and Kaposi's sarcoma: a model of paracrine neoplasia? *J Exp Med* 2000;191:417–422.

89. Wilson KS, McKenna RW, Kroft SH, et al. Primary effusion lymphomas exhibit complex and recurrent cytogenetic abnormalities. *Br J Haematol* 2002;116:113–121.

90. Aoki Y, Jaffe ES, Chang Y, et al. Angiogenesis and hematopoiesis induced by Kaposi's sarcoma-associated herpesvirus-encoded interleukin-6. *Blood* 1999;93:4034–4043.

91. Teruya-Feldstein J, Zauber P, Setsuda JE, et al. Expression of human herpesvirus-8 oncogene and cytokine homologues in an HIV-seronegative patient with multicentric Castleman's disease and primary effusion lymphoma. *Lab Invest* 1998;78:1637–1642.

92. Chadburn A, Cesarman E, Hyjek E, et al. Kaposi's sarcoma-associated herpesvirus positive extra-cavitary lymphomas in HIV-positive patients: part of the spectrum of primary effusion lymphoma. *Mod Pathol* 2002 (*in press*).

93. Katano H, Suda T, Morishita Y, et al. Human herpesvirus 8-associated solid lymphomas that occur in AIDS patients take anaplastic large cell morphology. *Mod Pathol* 2000;13:77–85.

94. Du MQ, Liu H, Diss TC, et al. Kaposi sarcoma-associated herpesvirus infects monotypic (IgM lambda) but polyclonal naive B cells in Castleman disease and associated lymphoproliferative disorders. *Blood* 2001;97:2130–2136.

95. Dupin N, Diss TL, Kellam P, et al. HHV-8 is associated with a plasmablastic variant of Castleman disease that is linked to HHV-8-positive plasmablastic lymphoma. *Blood* 2000;95:1406–1412.

96. Ziegler JL, Beckstead JA, Volberding PA, et al. Non-Hodgkin's lymphoma in 90 homosexual men: relation to generalized lymphadenopathy the acquired immunodeficiency syndrome. *N Engl J Med* 1984;311:565–570.

97. Kaplan LD, Abrams DI, Feigal E, et al. AIDS associated non-Hodgkin's lymphoma in San Francisco. *JAMA* 1989;261:719–724.

98. Seneviratne LC, Tulpule A, Espina BM, et al. Clinical, immunologic and pathologic correlates of bone marrow involvement in 291 patients with AIDS-related lymphoma. *Blood* 2001;98:2358–2363.

99. Lossos A, Siegal T. Numb chin syndrome in cancer: etiology, response to treatment, and prognostic significance. *Neurology* 1992;42:1181–1184.

100. Cingolani A, De Luca A, Larocca LM, et al. Minimally invasive diagnosis of acquired immunodeficiency syndrome-related primary central nervous system lymphoma. *J Natl Cancer Inst* 1998;90:364–370.

101. Vaccher E, Tirelli U, Spina M, et al. Age and serum LDH level are independent prognostic factors in HIV related non-Hodgkin's lymphoma: a single institution study of 96 patients. *J Clin Oncol* 1996;14:2217–2223.

102. Radin DR, Esplin J, Levine AM, Ralls PW. AIDS-related non-Hodgkin's lymphoma: abdominal CT findings in 112 patients. *AJR Am J Roentgenol* 1993;160:1133–1139.

103. Sider L, Weiss AJ, Smith MD, et al. Varied appearance of AIDS-related lymphoma in the chest. *Radiology* 1989;171:629–632.

104. Podzamczer D, Ricat I, Bolao F, et al. Gallium-67 scan for distinguishing follicular hyperplasia from other AIDS associated disease in lymph nodes. *AIDS* 1990;4:683–685.

105. Stumpe KD, Urbinelli M, Steinert HC, et al. Whole body positron emission tomography using fluorodeoxyglucose for staging of lymphoma: effectiveness and comparison with computed tomography. *Eur J Nucl Med* 1998;25:721–728.

106. DeWit M, Bumann D, Beyer W, et al. Whole body positron emission tomography (PET) for diagnosis of residual mass in patients with lymphoma. *Ann Oncol* 1997;8:[Suppl 1]:57–60.

107. Romer W, Hanauske AR, Ziegler S, et al. Positron emission tomography in non-Hodgkin's lymphoma: assessment of chemotherapy with fluorodeoxyglucose. *Blood* 1998;91:4464–4471.

108. Levine AM, Wernz JC, Kaplan L, et al. Low dose chemotherapy with central nervous system prophylaxis and zidovudine maintenance in AIDS-related lymphoma: a prospective multi-institutional trial. *JAMA* 1991;266:84–88.

109. Mummaneni M, Tulpule A, Palmer M, et al. Leptomeningeal involvement in AIDS-lymphoma: clinical, immunologic and pathologic features. *Proc ASCO* 1998;17:41A(abst 160).

110. Levine AM, Sullivan-Halley J, Pike MC, et al. HIV-related lymphoma: prognostic factors predictive of survival. *Cancer* 1991;68:2466–2472.

111. Straus, DJ, Juang J, Testa MA, et al. Prognostic factors in the treatment of HIV associated non-Hodgkin's lymphoma: analysis of AIDS Clinical Trials Group protocol 142: low dose versus standard dose m-BACOD plus GM-CSF. *J Clin Oncol* 1998;16:3601–3606.

112. Rossi G, Donisi A, Casari S, et al. The International Prognostic Index can be used as a guide to treatment decisions regarding patients with HIV related systemic non-Hodgkin's lymphoma. *Cancer* 1999;86:2391–2397.

113. Antinori A, Cingolani A, Alba L, et al. Better response to chemotherapy and prolonged survival in AIDS-related lymphomas responding to highly active antiretroviral therapy. *AIDS* 2001;15:1483–1491.

114. Kaplan LD, Straus DJ, Testa MA, et al. Randomized trial of standard-dose versus low dose mBACOD chemotherapy for HIV-associated non-Hodgkin's lymphoma. *N Engl J Med* 1997;336:1641–1648.

115. Ratner L, Lee J, Tang S, et al. Chemotherapy for HIV-associated non-Hodgkin's lymphoma in combination with highly active anti-retroviral therapy. *J Clin Oncol* 2001;19:2171–2178.

116. Gill PS, Rarick MU, Brynes RL, et al. Azidothymidine and bone marrow failure in AIDS. *Ann Intern Med* 1987;107:502–505.

117. Sparano JA, Wiernik PH, Hu X, et al. Pilot trial of infusional cyclophosphamide, doxorubicin and etoposide plus didanosine and filgrastim in patients with HIV associated non-Hodgkin's lymphoma. *J Clin Oncol* 1996;14:3026–3035.

118. Sparano JA, Lee S, Henry DH, et al. Infusional cyclophosphamide, doxorubicin and etoposide in HIV associated non-Hodgkin's lymphoma: a review of the Einstein, Aviano, and ECOG experience in 182 patients. Abstracts of the 4th International AIDS Malignancy Conference; May 16–18, 2000; Bethesda, MD. *J Acquir Immune Defic Syndr* 2000;23:A11(abst S15).

119. Little RF, Pittaluga S, Grant N, et al. Highly effective treatment of acquired immunodeficiency syndrome-related lymphoma with dose-adjusted EPOCH: impact of antiretroviral therapy suspension and tumor biology. *Blood* 2003;101:4653–4659.

120. Vaccher E, Spina M, di Gennaro R, et al. Concomitant cyclophosphamide, doxorubicin, vincristine and prednisone chemotherapy plus highly active antiretroviral therapy in patients with human immunodeficiency virus-related non-Hodgkin's lymphoma. *Cancer* 2001;91:155–163.

121. Spina M, Vaccher E, Juzbasic S, et al. Human immunodeficiency virus related non-Hodgkin lymphoma: activity of infusional cyclophosphamide, doxorubicin, and etoposide as second line chemotherapy in 40 patients. *Cancer* 2001;92:200–206.

122. Tirelli U, Errante D, Spina M, et al. Second line chemotherapy in HIV related non-Hodgkin's lymphoma. *Cancer* 1996;77:2127–2131.

123. Bi J, Espina BM, Tulpule A, et al. High dose cytosine arabinoside and cisplatin regimens as salvage therapy for refractory or relapsed AIDS-related non Hodgkin's lymphoma. *J AIDS* 2001;28:416–421.

124. Gill PS, Levine AM, Meyer RP, et al. Primary central nervous system lymphoma in homosexual men. Clinical, immunologic, and pathologic features. *Am J Med* 1985;78:742–748.

125. So YT, Beckstead JH, Davis RL. Primary central nervous system lymphoma in AIDS: a clinical and pathological study. *Ann Neurol* 1986;20:566–572.

126. Baumgartner JE, Rachlin JR, Beckstead JH, et al. Primary central nervous system lymphomas: natural history and response to radiation therapy in 55 patients with AIDS. *J Neurosurg* 1990;73:206–211.

127. Antinori A, De Rossi G, Ammassari A, et al. Value of combined approach with thallium-201 single photon emission computed tomography and Epstein-Barr virus DNA polymerase chain reaction in CSF for the diagnosis of AIDS related primary CNS lymphoma. *J Clin Oncol* 1999;17:554–560.

128. Hoffman JM, Waskin HA, Schifter T, et al. FDG-PET in differentiating lymphoma from non-malignant central nervous system lesions in patients with AIDS. *J Nucl Med* 1993;34:567–575.

129. MacMahon EME, Glass JD, Hayward SCD, et al. Epstein Barr virus in AIDS related primary central nervous system lymphoma. *Lancet* 1991;338:969–973.

130. Raez L, Cabral L, Cai J-P, et al. Antivirals induce apoptosis and tumor regression in AIDS related primary central nervous system lymphoma. Third AIDS Malignancy Conference, Bethesda, MD, 1999. *J AIDS* 1999;21:A31(abst 87).

131. Slobod KS, Taylor GH, Sandlund JT, et al. Epstein-Barr virus-targeted therapy for AIDS-related primary lymphoma of the central nervous system. *Lancet* 2000;356:1493–1494.

CHAPTER 40

Diagnosis and Management of Posttransplant and Other Iatrogenic Immune Deficiency Lymphoproliferative Disorders

Lode J. Swinnen and Steven H. Swerdlow

Initially recognized as a complication of iatrogenic immunosuppression after organ transplantation, immunodeficiency-related lymphoma has now been described in a number of iatrogenic, congenital, and acquired immunodeficiency states. The disease comprises a spectrum of clinical, pathologic, and molecular findings that are unique to the setting of immunodeficiency. Although the majority of proliferations are of B-cell origin and are associated with the Epstein-Barr virus, T-cell and Epstein-Barr virus–negative tumors have recently been recognized, usually after many years of immunodeficiency. The increasing number of organ and bone marrow recipients, longer patient survival, increasing use of transplantation in the pediatric age group, and the use of highly immunosuppressive drugs in new settings all contribute to the increasing prevalence of iatrogenic immunodeficiency-related lymphoproliferation. The disease presents significant diagnostic and therapeutic challenges. Despite progress in recent years and the curability of a proportion of patients, mortality remains high.

INCIDENCE AND PREDISPOSING FACTORS

Posttransplant lymphoproliferative disorder after solid-organ or allogeneic bone marrow transplantation has been studied much more extensively than lymphoproliferations in other settings of iatrogenic immunodeficiency. The type of transplant, the specific immunosuppressives used, and the proportion of patients who are Epstein-Barr virus seronegative at the time of transplant all influence the risk for posttransplant lymphoproliferative disorder. Incidence estimates from retrospective single-institution series correspond well with more recent large population-based registry data (Tables 40.1 and 40.2). A single-institution incidence of 3.4% after heart transplantation and 7.9% after lung transplantation was reported from the University of Pittsburgh (1). The multicenter European and North American Collaborative Transplant Study analyzing 14,284 heart recipients and 72,360 kidney recipients reported a cumulative posttransplant lymphoproliferative disorder incidence of 5% by 7 years of follow-up in heart recipients and 1% by 10 years of follow-up in renal recipients. Again in keeping with observations from smaller series, incidence was highest in the first posttransplant year. During that first year, 0.2% of renal and 1.2% of cardiac recipients developed posttransplant lymphoproliferative disorder, rates that were calculated to be 20 and 120 times higher than those seen in the general population. The incidence of posttransplant lymphoproliferative disorder in subsequent years was approximately 0.04% per year in renal and 0.30% per year in cardiac recipients (2–4). The incidence of posttransplant lymphoproliferative disorder after allogeneic bone marrow transplantation is typically low, on the order of 1%, in the absence of T-cell depletion or graft mismatching. An analysis of data reported to the International Bone Marrow Transplant Registry for 18,014 allogeneic bone marrow transplant recipients showed a cumulative posttransplant lymphoproliferative disorder incidence of 1.0% ± 0.3% at 10 years of follow-up. Incidence was highest in the first 5 months after transplantation (120 cases per 10,000 patient-years), with a marked and stable decrease in incidence to a very low level (5 cases per 10,000 patient-years) after 1 year posttransplant (5). That observation is at odds with the continued increase in cumulative incidence seen after solid-organ transplantation and is likely due to the fact that immunosuppressives are usually discontinued at approximately 1 year after bone marrow transplantation but are maintained lifelong in most organ recipients.

The risk of developing posttransplant lymphoproliferative disorder is influenced by several factors, including the immunosuppressive regimen (Table 40.3). A posttransplant

TABLE 40.1. *Incidence of posttransplant lymphoproliferative disorder in organ transplant*

Organ (reference)	Incidence (%)
Kidney (2–4)	1.0 (10-yr cumulative incidence)
Liver (84)	2.2 (single institution)
Heart (2–4)	5.0 (7-yr cumulative incidence)
Lung (1,84)	7.9 (single institution)

TABLE 40.3. *Predisposing factors for posttransplant lymphoproliferative disorder (reference)*

Type of organ transplant (1–4,84)
Epstein-Barr virus seronegativity at time of transplant (13–16)
Pediatric age group (13)
Use of monoclonal anti-CD3 antibodies (5,10–12)
Mismatched bone marrow transplant (5)
T-cell depleted bone marrow transplant (5)

lymphoproliferative disorder incidence on the order of 12% was noted after the introduction of cyclosporine (6), which diminished with blood level monitoring (7). The incidence of posttransplant lymphoproliferative disorder under FK506 immunosuppression appears to be comparable to what has been seen with cyclosporine (8,9). Posttransplant lymphoproliferative disorder incidence has consistently been higher in nonrenal than in renal transplants, possibly because of the greater intensity of immunosuppression in vital organ recipients. The immunosuppressive antibody OKT3, a potent anti–T-cell agent, has been shown to result in a ninefold higher incidence of posttransplant lymphoproliferative disorder in cardiac transplant recipients receiving induction immunotherapy, with an incidence of 35.7% in patients who had received two courses of the drug (10). A number of other observations underscore the fact that the intensity of immunosuppression, and particularly the use of selective anti–T-cell therapy, constitutes a major risk factor for the development of posttransplant lymphoproliferative disorder (11,12). Analysis of the International Bone Marrow Transplant Registry data showed that the risk of posttransplant lymphoproliferative disorder after allogeneic bone marrow transplant was strongly associated with donor-recipient mismatch (relative

risk, 4.1), T-cell depletion of the allograft (relative risk, 12.7), the prophylactic use of polyclonal antithymocyte globulin (relative risk, 6.4), or anti-CD3 monoclonal antibodies (relative risk, 43.2). Patients with two of these risk factors had a posttransplant lymphoproliferative disorder incidence of 8%, whereas those with three or more risk factors had a 22% incidence. Methods selectively targeting T cells were associated with a much higher risk than were approaches that remove both T and B cells, such as Campath-1 monoclonal antibody or elutriation (5).

Pretransplant Epstein-Barr virus seronegativity is a major risk factor for posttransplant lymphoproliferative disorder. Virtually all seronegative recipients seroconvert shortly after transplantation. Ninety percent or more of adults are Epstein-Barr virus seropositive. The majority of seronegatives are therefore children, with the likelihood of seronegativity being determined by age and by social and geographic factors (13,14). Data regarding the incidence of posttransplant lymphoproliferative disorder in such seroconverters exist only from institutional series, so the exact level of risk is difficult to determine (13,15,16). In a series from Mayo Clinic, the risk of posttransplant lymphoproliferative disorder in Epstein-Barr virus–seronegative recipients was determined to be 76 times higher than in seropositive recipients (14). In a study of adult cardiac recipients, a much higher proportion of patients who went on to develop posttransplant lymphoproliferative disorder were Epstein-Barr virus seronegative before transplantation than were patients who did not develop the disease (30% vs. 5%) (10), and similar findings have been reported in pediatric liver recipients (16). A series from the University of Pittsburgh identified a four times higher risk of posttransplant lymphoproliferative disorder for pediatric transplant recipients than for adult transplant recipients (13). Primary Epstein-Barr virus infection in an immunodeficient host therefore appears to carry a particularly high risk of posttransplant lymphoproliferative disorder and represents a significant problem among pediatric transplant recipients.

TABLE 40.2. *Incidence of posttransplant lymphoproliferative disorder in allogeneic bone marrow transplant*

ABMT	Incidence
Overall	1.0% ± 0.3% (10-yr cumulative incidence)
Mismatched	Relative risk, 4.1
T-cell depletion of graft	Relative risk, 12.7
Use of polyclonal antithymocyte globulin	Relative risk, 6.4
Use of anti-CD3 monoclonal antibodies	Relative risk, 43.2
Two risk factors	8%
Three or more risk factors	22%

ABMT, allogenic bone marrow transplant.
From Curtis RE, Travis LB, Rowlings PA, et al. Risk of lymphoproliferative disorders after bone marrow transplantation: a multiinstitutional study. *Blood* 1999;94:2208–2216, with permission.

Pathology of Posttransplant Lymphoproliferative Disorder

The posttransplant lymphoproliferative disorders are a heterogeneous group of frequently Epstein-Barr virus–

associated lymphoid or plasmacytic proliferations with varied morphologic, phenotypic, and genotypic features. They form a spectrum from polyclonal lesions to monoclonal proliferations indistinguishable from a lymphoma of non-Hodgkin's or Hodkin's type. Posttransplant lymphoproliferative disorders after solid-organ transplantation are usually of recipient origin, whereas those after bone marrow transplantation usually are of donor origin (17–20). Posttransplant lymphoproliferative disorders arising in allografts, however, are more frequently of donor origin (21). Other iatrogenic immunodeficiency-associated lymphoproliferative disorders include those associated with methotrexate and seen most frequently in patients with rheumatoid arthritis (22), fludarabine-associated lymphoproliferative disorders in patients treated for B-cell chronic lymphocytic leukemia, and others (23).

As with other lymphoid proliferations, posttransplant lymphoproliferative disorder is best characterized by handling biopsy and resection specimens using a standard protocol such as that used for evaluating potential lymphomas (Table 40.4). Although much information can be gained from fine-needle aspiration biopsies, when possible, larger tissue biopsies are recommended for potential posttransplant lymphoproliferative disorder because of the marked heterogeneity that can be seen even in single lesions and the need sometimes for a variety of ancillary studies (24).

Pathologic classifications of posttransplant lymphoproliferative disorder have evolved over the last two decades (25–29), with the most recent being that of the World Health Organization (Table 40.5) (30).

TABLE 40.4. *Pathologic work-up for suspected immune deficiency–associated lymphoproliferative disorders*

Histopathology to evaluate architectural and cytologic features.

Immunophenotype to assess cell lineage, B-cell clonality, "aberrant" markers, B- or T-cell subset markers associated with specific types of lymphoma. Flow cytometric immunophenotypic studies are the most sensitive method for detecting surface light chain class restriction (B-cell clonality) and the easiest way to identify antigenic coexpression. Paraffin section immunostains, however, can provide a large amount of information that is sufficient for a diagnosis in the vast majority of cases.

Detection of EBV small RNAs (Epstein-Barr early region 1) using *in situ* hybridization. Although not essential, diagnostically useful, especially in allografts and to identify EBV⁻ cases.

Genotypic/cytogenetic studies. Although not usually required for minimal diagnostic purposes, these studies can be used to identify clonality and lineage when morphologic and immunophenotypic studies are problematic and to look for secondary changes that may be useful for detailed classification and prognostication. In addition, EBV terminal repeat analysis can be used to document the presence of even very small clonal EBV⁺ populations.

EBV, Epstein-Barr virus.

TABLE 40.5. *World Health Organization Classification of posttransplant lymphoproliferative disorder (PTLD)*

Early lesions
  Reactive plasmacytic hyperplasia
  Infectious mononucleosis–like
Polymorphic PTLD
Monomorphic PTLD (classify according to lymphoma classification)
  B-cell neoplasms
    Diffuse large B-cell lymphoma (immunoblastic, centroblastic, anaplastic)
    Burkitt's/Burkitt-like lymphoma
    Plasma cell myeloma
    Plasmacytoma-like lesions
  T-cell neoplasms
    Peripheral T-cell lymphoma, not otherwise specified
    Other types
Hodgkin's lymphoma and Hodgkin's lymphoma–like PTLD

From Harris NL, Swerdlow SH, Frizzera G, et al. Post-transplant lymphoproliferative disorders. In: Jaffe E, Harris NL, Stein H, Vardiam JW, eds. *Pathology and genetics of tumours of haematopoietic and lymphoid tissues.* World Health Organization classification of tumours. Lyon, France: IARC Press, 2001:264–269, with permission.

The pathology of the other iatrogenic immunodeficiency–related lymphoproliferative disorders bears many similarities to that of posttransplant lymphoproliferative disorder, and they are often categorized in a similar fashion. The pathologic criteria for the different types of posttransplant lymphoproliferative disorder, including immunophenotypic and genotypic features, are described below. As discussed, there are a number of problematic gray zones, and patients can have one or more posttransplant lymphoproliferative disorder lesions with varied histologic patterns, different B-cell clones, and even both B- and T-cell clones (31–33). Posttransplant lymphoproliferative disorder can also show histologic progression over time (34).

"Early" and "late" clinicopathologic disease patterns have consistently been described. The terms refer more to the time after transplantation than necessarily to an evolution of the disease over time, which has not been described with any frequency.

The "early" lesions include *plasmacytic hyperplasia* and *infectious mononucleosis–like posttransplant lymphoproliferative disorder.* "Early" in this setting denotes early in the posttransplant course, typically less than 1 year. In both cases, underlying architectural features are retained, even if partially obscured, with these diagnoses most often rendered in lymph node biopsies and tonsillectomies. Plasmacytic hyperplasia demonstrates mostly small lymphocytes and plasma cells and, especially if Epstein-Barr virus–positive cells are absent or not very numerous, cannot be distinguished from a completely nonspecific hyperplasia, which can occur in transplant patients. Some do not consider these

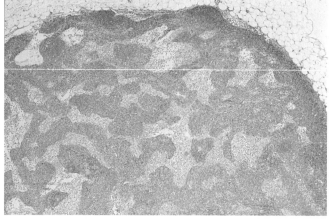

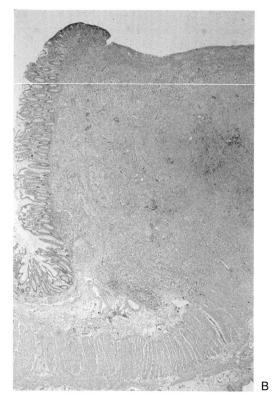

FIG. 40.1. Posttransplant lymphoproliferative disorder with distinct infectious mononucleosis–like and monomorphic diffuse large B-cell lymphoma lesions in a 44-year-old woman post lung transplant. **A:** This abdominal lymph node shows an intact architecture with intact sinuses. **B:** This patient, however, also demonstrated large mass lesions in the colon. (See also Color Plate 65.)

as posttransplant lymphoproliferative disorder. The plasma cells are polyclonal when immunostains are used, with only a minority of these cases showing a very small clonal lymphoid population or a clonal population of Epstein-Barr virus–infected cells (26). Infectious mononucleosis–like posttransplant lymphoproliferative disorder resembles infectious mononucleosis in the normal host and is diagnosed as such by some. In addition to plasma cells and small lymphocytes, variable numbers of immunoblasts are present, and there may be necrosis and Reed-Sternberg–like cells. Immunophenotypic studies are not expected to demonstrate clonal B-cell populations; however, in some cases, genotypic studies do, due to their ability to detect even very small clonal expansions. Caution is advised, as some patients may have early lesions at one site and more overt posttransplant lymphoproliferative disorder at adjacent or more distant sites (Fig. 40.1 and Color Plate 65). Partial nodal involvement by a monomorphic posttransplant lymphoproliferative disorder also must be excluded in these circumstances. Distinction from polymorphic posttransplant lymphoproliferative disorder in tonsils is in part a matter of definition.

Polymorphic posttransplant lymphoproliferative disorders demonstrate effacement of the underlying tissues by a heterogeneous population of variably sized and shaped lymphocytes admixed with plasma cells, immunoblasts, and sometimes histiocytes (Fig. 40.2 and Color Plate 66). As with other posttransplant lymphoproliferative disorders, necrosis, atypical immunoblasts or Reed-Sternberg–like cells, and marked angioinvasion may be seen. The presence of necrosis and atypical immunoblasts was used in the past to distinguish polymor-

phic B-cell hyperplasia from polymorphic B-cell lymphoma; however, that distinction is no longer made. A higher proportion of immunoblasts is often seen adjacent to areas of necrosis, sometimes making pathologic distinction from a monomorphic posttransplant lymphoproliferative disorder difficult (see below). Immunophenotypic studies may demonstrate clonal B cells, with genotypic studies demonstrating variably sized B-cell clones in almost all cases. Individual patients with posttransplant lymphoproliferative disorder can have more than one clone or both monoclonal and polyclonal

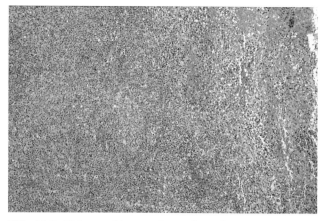

FIG. 40.2. Polymorphic posttransplant lymphoproliferative disorder (Epstein-Barr virus positive) in lymph node from a man post liver transplant. There is diffuse architectural effacement in this epitrochlear lymph node. Note the geographic necrosis on the right side. (See also Color Plate 66.)

or oligoclonal lesions. With the exception of BCL-6 mutations, seen in somewhat less than half of the cases, additional genotypic abnormalities are not expected (26,35).

Monomorphic posttransplant lymphoproliferative disorders are destructive infiltrative proliferations that fulfill the criteria for one of the conventional non-Hodgkin's lymphomas or plasma cell neoplasms. This does not mean that the biology or clinical behavior of such lesions is the same as for the histologically equivalent lesion seen in the general population. It should be recognized that nodal involvement may be focal, and, in some instances, involvement at extranodal sites can be very patchy. The most common monomorphic posttransplant lymphoproliferative disorders fulfill the criteria for one of the types of diffuse large B-cell lymphoma, being composed predominantly of large transformed B cells that may resemble centroblasts of follicular centers, immunoblasts, or very anaplastic cells. These cases may not appear completely monotonous, as the cells may be pleomorphic, and there can be admixed smaller lymphoid cells or differentiation to plasma cells. Immunophenotypic studies are critical in demonstrating the B-cell nature of the large cells, often with CD20 expression. The latter is important to know if rituximab therapy is being contemplated. In some circumstances in which the diagnosis is not readily apparent, immunophenotypic documentation of B-cell clonality can be very helpful. Immunophenotypic studies also illustrate the heterogeneity of the diffuse large B-cell lymphoma type of monomorphic posttransplant lymphoproliferative disorders that range from some cases having phenotype-like follicular center cells (CD10$^+$, BCL6$^+$, MUM-1$^-$, CD138$^-$) to others that are clearly postfollicular (CD10$^-$, BCL6$^-$, MUM-1$^+$, CD138$^+$). Genotypic studies are expected to demonstrate significant B-cell clones in these cases. Some patients will have different clones at different posttransplant lymphoproliferative disorder sites, especially those with multiple gastrointestinal tract lesions (33). BCL6 mutations are very common in monomorphic posttransplant lymphoproliferative disorders (35), and at least a proportion have other genotypic abnormalities, including C-MYC rearrangements, N-RAS mutations, and p53 mutations (26). Other monomorphic posttransplant lymphoproliferative disorders resemble Burkitt's or Burkitt-like lymphomas and have a similar phenotype and genotype, including C-MYC rearrangements (Color Plate 67). In some monomorphic posttransplant lymphoproliferative disorders, there is a proliferation of numerous plasma cells with the clinicopathologic picture of multiple myeloma or, more commonly, an extramedullary plasmacytoma. These plasma cells should be monoclonal, and at least the myeloma cases can have secondary genotypic abnormalities, such as N-RAS mutations (26). Data regarding cytogenetic abnormalities in posttransplant lymphoproliferative disorders are limited. Abnormalities have been identified, usually in tumors with monomorphic histology, but no characteristic abnormality has been found. In a series of 28 patients, no clonal cytogenetic abnormalities were identified among ten polymorphic tumors, all of which were polyclonal or oligoclonal. Analysis of 12 monomorphic cases revealed a variety of abnormalities in ten cases: chromosome 8 translocations involving the MYC gene, trisomy 9, trisomy 11, and 11q27 (36). Gastric and salivary gland Epstein-Barr virus–negatuve extranodal marginal zone B-cell lymphomas of mucosa-associated lymphoid tissue type have also been described in the posttransplant setting (37,38). However, these are best separately designated and not grouped together with the other monomorphic posttransplant lymphoproliferative disorders.

Although the descriptions of the above posttransplant lymphoproliferative disorders have concentrated on the nature of the B cells and plasma cells present, all contain variable numbers of admixed T cells. Cases of infectious mononucleosis–like posttransplant lymphoproliferative disorder and polymorphic posttransplant lymphoproliferative disorder especially can have greater than 50% T cells, with some monomorphic posttransplant lymphoproliferative disorders also reported to be T-cell rich (39,40). The nature of the T cells present appears to be variable, with some cases showing a predominance of CD8$^+$ cells and others predominantly CD4$^+$ cells (40,41). Cytokine profiles are complex; however, posttransplant lymphoproliferative disorders are believed to be associated with a TH2 cytokine environment that promotes B-cell growth (42).

Monomorphic posttransplant lymphoproliferative disorder of T-cell origin may be more difficult to distinguish from polymorphic posttransplant lymphoproliferative disorders because they are morphologically heterogeneous and can include many small- to intermediate-sized lymphoid cells (Fig. 40.3 and Color Plate 68). These cases should fulfill the criteria for one of the standard T-cell lymphomas. Many of the

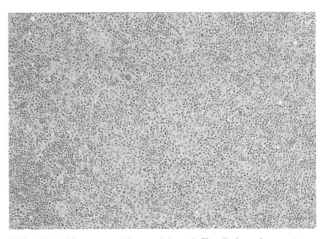

FIG. 40.3. Monomorphic peripheral T-cell lymphoma–type posttransplant lymphoproliferative disorder (Epstein-Barr virus positive) in a child 5 years post heart–lung transplant who presented with fever, sore throat, and cervical adenopathy. Large areas of this lymph node show diffuse architectural effacement. The larger cells have an aberrant T-cell phenotype, and a T-cell clone is documented by genotypic studies. The lesion responded to decreased immunosuppression. (See also Color Plate 68.)

cases resemble a peripheral T-cell lymphoma, unspecified type, with a significant proportion of extranodal cytotoxic T-cell lymphomas (43,44). In fact, 15% of all hepatosplenic lymphomas reportedly arise posttransplantation (45). Occasional cases of other specific types of T-cell or natural killer–cell neoplasms are also reported, such as anaplastic large-cell lymphoma or extranodal natural killer/T-cell lymphoma of nasal type (43,46). At least some of the reported lymphoblastic cases may relate to the patients' underlying disorders. Another subset of cases that are probably best separately designated are those of large granular lymphocyte type (47). Identification of all of these T-cell posttransplant lymphoproliferative disorders requires at least morphologic and immunophenotypic studies. Genotypic proof of clonality and T-cell lineage is also useful in some circumstances. A detailed description of these entities is included in other chapters.

Hodgkin's lymphoma or *Hodgkin's lymphoma–like posttransplant lymphoproliferative disorders* are diagnosed in cases that fulfill the morphologic and phenotypic criteria for classical Hodgkin's lymphoma in the normal host (Color Plate 69). In brief, these cases require the presence of Reed-Sternberg cells and variants in an appropriate background of lymphocytes and variable numbers of other inflammatory cells. Immunophenotypic studies are critical because many posttransplant lymphoproliferative disorders have Reed-Sternberg–like cells, and some also have numerous admixed inflammatory cells. In the most definite cases, the Reed-Sternberg cells should be $CD45^-$, $CD15^+$, and $CD30^+$, with negative or variable CD20 expression. Cases with less typical phenotypes should be interpreted with great caution, with the term Hodgkin's lymphoma–like posttransplant lymphoproliferative disorder then sometimes used. Hodgkin's lymphoma–type posttransplant lymphoproliferative disorder should be distinguished from infectious mononucleosis–like posttransplant lymphoproliferative disorder, polymorphic posttransplant lymphoproliferative disorder, and monomorphic posttransplant lymphoproliferative disorder of diffuse large B-cell lymphoma type, all of which are rich in T cells.

Bone marrow involvement is not common in most types of posttransplant lymphoproliferative disorders. When present, there may be large overt lesions or only small focal lesions (25,48). Nonspecific lymphoplasmacytic lesions of uncertain significance may also be found (48).

Differential Diagnosis

Not all lymphoid or plasmacytic infiltrates in posttransplant patients represent posttransplant lymphoproliferative disorders. Inflammatory and infectious disorders must always be considered and worked up appropriately. Posttransplant lymphoproliferative disorders not uncommonly occur in the allografts, so that rejection is another critical differential diagnosis with often completely opposite therapeutic implications. Sometimes both processes are present. Some pathologic features favoring the diagnosis of a posttransplant lymphoproliferative disorder include lymphoid mass lesions, numerous

transformed cells, numerous plasma cells, extensive serpiginous necrosis, a very B-cell–rich infiltrate, and numerous Epstein-Barr virus–positive cells (49–52). Scattered Epstein-Barr virus–positive cells may be seen in non–posttransplant lymphoproliferative disorder lesions (53).

Epstein-Barr Virus

The majority of posttransplant lymphoproliferative disorders are Epstein-Barr virus-associated. Tumor-associated Epstein-Barr virus is clonal, and the pattern of viral clones corresponds to B-cell clonality. Lesions consisting of polyclonal or multiclonal B-cell proliferations contain multiple Epstein-Barr virus clones, whereas monoclonal proliferations show evidence of a single infectious event (54,55). The virus is usually of type A (type 1) (56). In most cases, the infected cells have a latency type III pattern similar to what is seen in lymphoblastoid cell lines; however, cases with a latency type II pattern, as seen in Hodgkin's lymphoma, or type I pattern, as seen in Burkitt's lymphoma, are reported (57–61). Some evidence of lytic activity has been reported (58,62,63). Although some require the presence of Epstein-Barr virus before diagnosing a posttransplant lymphoproliferative disorder, approximately 15% to 30% of posttransplant lymphoproliferative disorders do not demonstrate evidence of Epstein-Barr virus, even when the very sensitive Epstein-Barr early region *in situ* hybridization stain is performed (64–66). Use of the latent membrane protein-1 immunostain is less sensitive than the Epstein-Barr early region *in situ* hybridization stain but is less likely to be positive in non–posttransplant lymphoproliferative disorder lesions. Epstein-Barr virus–negative posttransplant lymphoproliferative disorders are more likely to be of monomorphic type than Epstein-Barr virus–positive cases and are more likely to occur later after transplantation (65,66). Epstein-Barr virus negativity is also reported to be an adverse prognostic indicator (65). Certain types of posttransplant lymphoproliferative disorders are more likely to be Epstein-Barr virus negative, such as those of myeloma type, whereas Hodgkin's-type cases are generally positive. Only up to approximately one third of T-cell posttransplant lymphoproliferative disorders are Epstein-Barr virus positive (43,67). Whether some other specific stimulus, such as another virus, is responsible for these Epstein-Barr virus–negative posttransplant lymphoproliferative disorders or whether they have a pathogenesis similar to non-Hodgkin's lymphomas in nonimmunosuppressed hosts is uncertain. Only rare cases have been associated with human herpesvirus-8 (68–70).

Prognostic Implications of Pathologic Classification and Other Ancillary Studies

The lack of sufficient data from well-controlled studies that take into account the many variables that affect the occurrence and behavior of posttransplant lymphoproliferative disorder; contradictory conclusions from the studies that do exist; varied criteria used for the different types of posttransplant lymphoproliferative disorders; subjective elements in applying the criteria, even when agreed on; and the variability between lesions that can occur in a given patient all complicate using the pathologic classification or the additional ancillary findings discussed above in making therapeutic decisions or assessing prognosis. Nevertheless, there are some conclusions that can be rendered. Cases diagnosed as plasmacytic hyperplasia are the most likely to regress with decreased immunosuppression (71), perhaps in part because some are nonspecific hyperplasias. Cases of infectious mononucleosis–like posttransplant lymphoproliferative disorder have not been extensively studied. Although some cases may be fatal, posttransplant patients are recognized who have a disease very much like infectious mononucleosis in a normal host (72). In view of this uncertainty, caution should be used in applying high-risk treatments to what may be a self-limited process. A question that has long been controversial is whether polymorphic posttransplant lymphoproliferative disorder behaves differently from the more monomorphic types. This matter is complicated further by the fact that monomorphic posttransplant lymphoproliferative disorder is not a homogeneous category. Some studies suggest that polymorphic or benign-appearing posttransplant lymphoproliferative disorder is more likely to respond to reduction in immunosuppression than is monomorphic posttransplant lymphoproliferative disorder (71,73–76); however, others have reported no correlation between histology and clinical behavior (77,78). Of the plasma cell–rich posttransplant lymphoproliferative disorders, patients with the clinicopathologic features of an extramedullary plasmacytoma have a more variable outcome than those resembling systemic myeloma, who are considered to have a more aggressive disorder (79). Among the B-cell posttransplant lymphoproliferative disorders, BCL-6 mutations have been reported to predict refractoriness to decreased immunosuppression and to be an adverse prognostic indicator (35). The number of patients studied was, however, small; the clinical correlations were retrospective and subject to many variables; and no confirmatory studies have been reported. The finding of a C-MYC rearrangement or other secondary genotypic abnormality has also been found to correlate with clinical behavior that more closely resembles that of malignancies seen in immunocompetent patients, although the numbers studied are again small (26,80). With the increasing therapeutic use of the anti-CD20 antibody rituximab, it is important not to underestimate CD20 positivity, as many of the cells in a posttransplant lymphoproliferative disorder may be infiltrating benign T cells. Monomorphic posttransplant lymphoproliferative disorders of T-cell type are considered to be clinically aggressive. Clinical data remain limited; although some apparently do respond to decreased immunosuppression, most do not, and results with chemotherapy have been generally poor (43,45,81,82). There are certain types of T-cell posttransplant lymphoproliferative disorders that have behaved in a more uniformly aggressive fashion such as the late-occurring cases composed of large cells often with cytoplasmic granules (81) and those of hepatosplenic type (45,82). In contrast, the posttransplant large granular lymphocyte disorders are indolent processes (47).

Methotrexate-Associated Lymphoproliferative Disorders

The methotrexate-associated lymphoproliferative disorders have a spectrum similar to the posttransplant lymphoproliferative disorders; however, the relative distribution of cases differs, and only approximately one half of the cases are reported to be Epstein-Barr virus positive (22). The most common histopathologic types of methotrexate-associated lymphoproliferative disorder are those that resemble diffuse large B-cell lymphomas, with a much smaller proportion resembling Burkitt's lymphomas. Many of the former cases are CD30 (Ki-1) positive. P53 mutations are described in approximately one half of the cases. Very few T-cell methotrexate-associated lymphoproliferative disorders or polymorphic cases are reported. Approximately 25% of the cases are of classical Hodgkin's type (22). A variety of small B-cell lymphoid neoplasms, such as follicular lymphomas, have also been reported in patients after methotrexate therapy.

Other Iatrogenic Immune Deficiency–Associated Lymphoproliferative Disorders

Other iatrogenic immune deficiency–associated lymphoproliferative disorders have been described in a variety of different circumstances, often as case reports. One group of cases recently highlighted are those following fludarabine therapy for B-cell chronic lymphocytic leukemia (23). Although more difficult to diagnose because they are arising in patients who already have a clonal B-cell disorder, the most definitive cases are those that are clonally distinct from the underlying B-cell chronic lymphocytic leukemia. The fludarabine-associated cases are Epstein-Barr virus positive and can resemble polymorphic, monomorphic, or Hodgkin's lymphoma–like posttransplant lymphoproliferative disorders. As with some posttransplant lymphoproliferative disorders, they may also resemble lymphomatoid granulomatosis.

CLINICAL PRESENTATION

One of the most striking features of posttransplant lymphoproliferative disorder is its clinical variability. This heterogeneity makes it difficult to generalize and likely accounts for the frequently variant results reported in small series of patients. Nonetheless, some general patterns are recognizable. A presentation with marked constitutional symptoms and rapid enlargement of the tonsils and cervical nodes is often the case for posttransplant lymphoproliferative disorder presenting early after transplantation—within less than approximately 1 year from the time of transplant (83). Highly immunosuppressed patients may present with rapidly progressive, widespread disease; diffusely infiltrative multiorgan involvement; and systemic sepsis, sometimes within weeks of transplantation. The diagnosis can be difficult to distinguish from sepsis alone, as fever is frequent, the disease is typically extranodal, and mass lesions may not be evident. Multiorgan failure is often the outcome, and the diagnosis may not be evident until autopsy (84,85).

Posttransplant lymphoproliferative disorder presenting later than approximately 1 year after transplantation is likely to be more circumscribed anatomically, manifest fewer systemic symptoms, and progress less rapidly. Extranodal disease and visceral nodal involvement, often in the absence of superficial nodal involvement, are common, which makes the establishment of a histologic diagnosis more difficult. Gastrointestinal involvement is frequent; approximately 25% of patients in one series presented with gastrointestinal disease manifesting as acute abdominal pain, obstruction, or hemorrhage (84). The transplanted organ itself may be affected in up to 20% of cases and may be the only site of disease. Histologic confusion between rejection and posttransplant lymphoproliferative disorder is a significant concern in such cases. Central nervous system involvement is mainly seen as part of very extensive disease but may occur in isolation. Unlike classic systemic non-Hodgkin's lymphomas, parenchymal central nervous system involvement is not rare. Multiple pulmonary nodules have been commonly described and must be differentiated from infectious etiologies in an immunocompromised host (85,86).

One large retrospective series of 61 patients was analyzed for factors prognostic of outcome. Epstein-Barr virus negativity in the tumor or T-cell phenotype was a negative prognostic factor. The International Prognostic Index, as used in immunocompetent patients, was less predictive in posttransplant lymphoproliferative disorder than was a specific index using two risk factors: performance status 0 or 1 versus 2 or more and number of involved sites (1 versus greater than 1) (87).

TREATMENT

There is at present no uniform approach to the treatment of posttransplant lymphoproliferative disorder. The literature consists of small series and anecdotal reports (Table 40.6). Certain observations can, however, be generalized. Unlike

TABLE 40.6. *Treatment options for posttransplant lymphoproliferative disorder (PTLD) (reference)*

Reduction in immunosuppressives (84)

Surgical resection or limited-field irradiation (84)

Monoclonal anti–B-cell antibodies

   Anti-CD21/CD24 (not commercially available) (96,97)

   Anti-CD20 (rituximab) (98,99)

Chemotherapy (88,100)

Donor leukocyte infusion (101) (for PTLD after T-cell–depleted allogeneic BMT)

Epstein-Barr virus–specific adoptive T-cell therapy (102–104) (for PTLD after allogeneic BMT)

BMT, bone marrow transplant.

non-Hodgkin's lymphoma in general, posttransplant lymphoproliferative disorder can be cured in some cases by surgical resection or by irradiation of unresectable, strictly localized lesions (84). Reduction in immunosuppression can result in partial or complete regression of some posttransplant lymphoproliferative disorders, with permanent resolution of a proportion of those (1,84). Resection of a limited number of residual lesions after a partial response to reduced immunosuppression has been achieved has also been reported (1,84).

Reduction in Immunosuppression

The probability of a response to reduction in immunosuppression appears to correlate with the interval since transplantation, perhaps because that interval also shows a degree of correlation with the morphology and clonality of lymphoproliferations. In a retrospective series of patients from the University of Pittsburgh, more than 80% of patients presenting at less than 1 year after transplantation responded to reduction in immunosuppression, whereas none presenting at more than 1 year did so (1). More variable results with reduced immunosuppression have been reported in other series: lower response rates and greater variability in terms of the interval since transplantation (88,89). Attempts at formulating a clinicopathologic classification based on clinical features, histology, clonality, and the presence of oncogene alterations capable of predicting disease behavior have been limited by the considerable overlap in categories, and the course of an individual patient remains difficult to predict (25,26,77,83). The presence of mutations in the BCL-6 protooncogene has been reported to be predictive of response to reduced immunosuppression; the assay is, however, not feasible within a clinically relevant time frame, the study involved small numbers, and the retrospective clinical correlations impart significant uncertainty to that analysis (35). It is, however, true that tumors classified as immunoblastic lymphoma or multiple myeloma by the Knowles-Frizzera classification system and tumors arising very late after transplantation or having a T-cell phenotype or showing no Epstein-Barr virus association are much more likely to be refractory to reduced immunosuppression. A trial of reduced immunosuppressives therefore still appears justified as the initial approach to all cases occurring within the first year after transplantation but becomes more problematic in the face of the above-mentioned factors predictive of a low likelihood of success. Rapid disease progression, rejection of a vital organ and the loss of a renal allograft complicating subsequent management are all valid concerns. The extent and duration of a reduction in immunosuppression for recipients of a vital organ remain poorly defined and highly subjective. Furthermore, since the advent of rituximab as a less toxic next therapeutic step than chemotherapy, the motivation to apply a trial of reduced immunosuppressives in all cases has likely waned. After a trial of immunosuppressive reduction, immunosuppressives need to be reinstituted before the onset of rejection. Nonvital organ recipients who have achieved a complete remission should probably be an exception to this. Based on the model of posttransplant lymphoproliferative disorder as a disease of over-immunosuppression, immunosuppressive agents have often been reinstituted at moderately reduced dosage. Data regarding the level of subsequent immunosuppressives required remain anecdotal.

Antiviral Drugs

Although regression of lymphoproliferations has been described after the use of high-dose acyclovir in a small number of cases, the therapeutic value of acyclovir remains very unclear (86,90). Acyclovir and ganciclovir have furthermore proved to be ineffective as prophylaxis for posttransplant lymphoproliferative disorders in animals and in humans (91–93). It is not known whether other drugs, such as foscarnet, are of any greater efficacy. A course of full-dose intravenous acyclovir is viewed as relatively nontoxic and has often been given simultaneously with reduction in immunosuppressives as initial management of posttransplant lymphoproliferative disorder.

Interferon-α

Durable complete responses have been achieved with low-dose interferon α-2b. Neither the response rate nor the mechanism of action is defined at this point. The drug might exert an antiviral or an antitumor effect; both early polyclonal proliferations and late-presenting monoclonal lesions have been reported to respond (91,94,95). Larger scale studies are needed to fully define the toxicity and the efficacy of interferon-α as treatment for posttransplant lymphoproliferative disorder.

Anti–B-Cell Monoclonal Antibodies

Two anti–B-cell monoclonal antibody preparations have shown significant activity with minimal toxicity in the treatment of posttransplant lymphoproliferative disorder. In 1991, the therapeutic use of a mixture of anti-CD21 and anti-CD24 anti–B-cell monoclonal antibodies was reported to be effective in patients with polyclonal or oligoclonal disease in a European multicenter trial involving both organ and bone marrow transplant recipients with posttransplant lymphoproliferative disorder (96), with long-term follow-up reported 7 years later (97). Fifty-eight patients with posttransplant lymphoproliferative disorder (27 after bone marrow and 31 after organ transplantation) were treated. The overall complete response rate was 61%. The relapse rate was low at 8%. The long-term overall survival was 46% (high-dose chemotherapy and hematopoietic stem cell rescue, 35%; organ transplant, 55%) at a median follow-up of 61 months. Complete remission was achieved in 46% of monoclonal and in 80% of oligoclonal cases (p = .05). Multivisceral disease, central nervous system involvement, and late-onset posttransplant

lymphoproliferative disorder (more than 1 year posttransplant) were identified as predictive for poorer response on multivariate analysis. Only 29% of patients with central nervous system involvement and 22% of patients presenting later than 1 year posttransplant achieved complete remission. Toxicity was mild, consisting of transient fever, hypotension, and neutropenia. The antibodies used are not currently clinically available.

The commercially available anti-CD20 antibody rituximab has shown efficacy in posttransplant lymphoproliferative disorder and has come to be widely used as treatment for the disease. Several anecdotes and very small series and a retrospective study of 32 patients with posttransplant lymphoproliferative disorder have been reported (98). Immunosuppressives had been modified in 27 patients in a variable fashion. Among 26 evaluable patients, 54% complete response and 15% partial response were reported. Median duration of follow-up at that time was 5 months. Two relapses were seen at approximately 9 months. Early data on a prospective multicenter study of rituximab for posttransplant lymphoproliferative disorder after solid-organ or bone marrow transplantation are reported. Fifty-five patients (19 renal, 11 cardiac, 7 lung or heart–lung, 7 liver, 11 hematopoietic stem cell transplant recipients) were recruited from 19 centers. Rituximab was given as four weekly doses of 375 mg per m^2; solid-organ transplant recipients had not responded to prior tapering of immunosuppressives. The median interval from transplant was 2.4 years (0.4 months to 17 years). Twenty-five patients (45.5%) responded (15 complete response, 3 unconfirmed/uncertain complete remission, 7 partial response); 2 had stable disease; 19 progressed; and 9 died (99).

Rituximab therefore has significant efficacy against B-cell posttransplant lymphoproliferative disorder. Toxicity as reported to date is usually minor and does not appear to differ from that seen with this drug in the immunocompetent population. The long-term follow-up data from the earlier study using anti-CD21/CD24 antibodies suggest that complete responses after antibody therapy can be durable in many patients. However, a significant proportion of patients—approximately one half—do not achieve complete remission and require other therapy.

Cytotoxic Chemotherapy

Chemotherapy has traditionally been viewed as a treatment of last resort for posttransplant lymphoproliferative disorder refractory to a reduction in immunosuppression, often in patients with disease presenting more than 1 year after transplantation. A mortality of 70% has been reported for such patients (1,86). Sepsis and other complications of chemotherapy have been the major problem in some centers, whereas others have found refractory disease to be common (1,86,89). Poor results have been obtained with a variety of regimens usually used for aggressive non-Hodgkin's lymphomas in the immunocompetent population. More encouraging results have been achieved in two series: one using very aggressive multiagent chemotherapy and one using low-dose single-agent treatment. In a series of adult cardiac recipients refractory to reduction or discontinuation of immunosuppressives and treated predominantly with Pro-MACE-CytaBOM [prednisone, Adriamycin (doxorubicin), cyclophosphamide, etoposide + cytarabine, bleomycin, Oncovin (vincristine), high-dose methotrexate and leuco-vorin], 75% durable complete remission was achieved with a median follow-up of 64 months (85). The advent of better supportive care measures, granulocyte colony-stimulating factor, and preventive antibiotics may further reduce the toxicity of intensive chemotherapy in this patient population. On the other hand, favorable preliminary data have been reported from a series of pediatric organ transplant recipients treated with low-dose chemotherapy. Thirty-six patients (17 liver, 6 liver/bowel/pancreas, 5 renal, 3 heart, 3 bowel, 2 lung recipients) were treated with cyclophosphamide, 600 mg per m^2 intravenously on day 1, and prednisone, 2 mg per kg on days 1 to 5, repeated every 3 weeks for a total of six cycles. All patients had failed prior modification of immunosuppressives; immunosuppressives were not reescalated during chemotherapy. Median age was 4.9 years; median time from transplant was 5.3 months. The overall response rate was 86% (77% complete remission, 9% partial remission). Four patients (11%) experienced progressive disease; two died of treatment-related causes. Median follow-up was 32 months; only five patients have relapsed (100).

Both the treatment regimens and the patient population in these two studies were very different from each other. A large proportion of patients in the pediatric study are likely to have had posttransplant lymphoproliferative disorder after primary Epstein-Barr virus infection early after transplant; histopathologic data are not available, but polymorphic, polyclonal, or oligoclonal proliferations, with few structural genetic abnormalities, are expected in that setting. The treatment may have controlled Epstein-Barr virus–driven lymphoproliferation long enough for Epstein-Barr virus–specific immunocompetence to develop. Although this study represents an excellent result in a pediatric population, it is unclear how well low-dose therapy would work in adult patients against tumors presenting late after transplant in the face of established Epstein-Barr virus–specific immunity and with malignant histologic and biochemical features.

T-Cell Therapy

Clinical posttransplant lymphoproliferative disorder is most clearly the result of insufficient host immune control at that particular moment in patients who develop the disease as part of primary Epstein-Barr virus infection or in T-cell–depleted allogeneic bone marrow recipients. Whether late-presenting posttransplant lymphoproliferative disorder is still amenable to immune control is much less clear.

It has been shown that Epstein-Barr virus–specific immunocompetence can rapidly be restored in T-cell–depleted allogeneic bone marrow recipients by the infusion of a lim-

ited number of peripheral blood leukocytes from the donor. Posttransplant lymphoproliferative disorder could be controlled in these cases without incurring graft-versus-host disease, probably because of the high frequency of Epstein-Barr virus–specific effector cells in the relatively small number of leukocytes transfused (101). More selective adoptive transfer of T-cell immunity has been achieved using *in vitro* expanded Epstein-Barr virus–specific cytotoxic T cells as treatment and prophylaxis for posttransplant lymphoproliferative disorder in bone marrow transplant recipients (102,103). Polyclonal T-cell lines containing both CD4 and CD8 cells were used, as it is not presently clear which antigens expressed by Epstein-Barr virus–infected cells are important in generating an effector response. Adoptive transfer of Epstein-Barr virus–specific T-cell immunity in solid-organ recipients is constrained by the MHC-restricted nature of the T-cell response and the fact that the majority of posttransplant lymphoproliferative disorders arise from recipient rather than donor lymphocytes in the organ transplant setting. Encouraging preliminary data using autologous Epstein-Barr virus–specific T cells expanded *in vitro* have been reported for pediatric liver recipients (104).

Several challenges remain, most notably the elaboration of suitable cytotoxic T cells for patients experiencing primary Epstein-Barr virus infection posttransplant, a particular problem in pediatric recipients, and demonstration of efficacy in patients with malignant, monomorphic histologies, tumors that usually do not respond to reduction in immunosuppressives and may or may not be amenable to Epstein-Barr virus–specific immune control.

Early Diagnosis and Screening

Early diagnosis of posttransplant lymphoproliferative disorder is clearly attractive, in view of the negative prognostic significance of extensive disease and poor performance status. Reliable tests for subclinical lymphoproliferation might allow identification of over-immunosuppression or early preemptive treatment. There are extensive data supporting such a subclinical phase to the disease. Analysis of prior liver biopsy specimens in liver transplant recipients has shown the presence of Epstein-Barr virus, as determined by polymerase chain reaction or by *in situ* immunohistochemical staining for Epstein-Barr early region–expressing cells, in 70% of patients who subsequently developed posttransplant lymphoproliferative disorder. Only 10% of patients who did not go on to develop the disease had such findings (105). A preclinical phase for posttransplant lymphoproliferative disorder is also suggested by observations that circulating viral load, as determined in peripheral blood mononuclear cells or in serum, increases before the appearance of clinically detected disease—increases that resolve after eradication of the posttransplant lymphoproliferative disorder. It is not clear when such increases in Epstein-Barr virus load are indicative of Epstein-Barr virus–driven neoplasia and when they only reflect the degree of immunodeficiency at the time. Obstacles to an effective screening test are determination of the best compartment (peripheral blood mononuclear cells, serum, or whole blood) to sample, methodologies for detection, and the determination of sensitivity and specificity parameters. Current data are generally from small series with, at times, conflicting results (106–114).

REFERENCES

1. Armitage JM, Kormos RL, Stuart RS, et al. Posttransplant lymphoproliferative disease in thoracic organ transplant patients: ten years of cyclosporine-based immunosuppression. *J Heart Lung Transplant* 1991;10:877–886.
2. Opelz G, Henderson R. Incidence of non-Hodgkin lymphoma in kidney and heart transplant recipients. *Lancet* 1993;342:1514–1516.
3. Opelz G. Collaborative transplant study—10-year report. *Transplant Proc* 1992;24:2342–2355.
4. Opelz G. Are post-transplant lymphomas inevitable? *Nephrol Dial Transplant* 1996;11:1952–1955.
5. Curtis RE, Travis LB, Rowlings PA, et al. Risk of lymphoproliferative disorders after bone marrow transplantation: a multiinstitutional study. *Blood* 1999;94:2208–2216.
6. Starzl TE, Nalesnik MA, Porter KA, et al. Reversibility of lymphomas and lymphoproliferative lesions developing under cyclosporin-steroid therapy. *Lancet* 1984;1:583–587.
7. Beveridge T, Krupp P, McKibbin C. Lymphomas and lymphoproliferative lesions developing under cyclosporin therapy [Letter]. *Lancet* 1984;1:788.
8. Armitage JM, Fricker FJ, del Nido P, et al. A decade (1982 to 1992) of pediatric cardiac transplantation and the impact of FK 506 immunosuppression. *J Thorac Cardiovasc Surg* 1993;105:464–472.
9. Cacciarelli TV, Reyes J, Jaffe R, et al. Primary tacrolimus (FK506) therapy and the long-term risk of post-transplant lymphoproliferative disease in pediatric liver transplant recipients. *Pediatr Transplant* 2001;5:359–364.
10. Swinnen LJ, Costanzo-Nordin MR, Fisher SG, et al. Increased incidence of lymphoproliferative disorder after immunosuppression with the monoclonal antibody OKT3 in cardiac-transplant recipients. *N Engl J Med* 1990;323:1723–1728.
11. Penn I. The changing pattern of posttransplant malignancies. *Transplant Proc* 1991;23:1101–1103.
12. Witherspoon RP, Fisher LD, Schoch G, et al. Secondary cancers after bone marrow transplantation for leukemia or aplastic anemia. *N Engl J Med* 1989;321:784–789.
13. Ho M, Jaffe R, Miller G, et al. The frequency of Epstein-Barr virus infection and associated lymphoproliferative syndrome after transplantation and its manifestations in children. *Transplantation* 1988;45:719–727.
14. Walker RC, Paya CV, Marshall WF, et al. Pretransplantation seronegative Epstein-Barr virus status is the primary risk factor for posttransplantation lymphoproliferative disorder in adult heart, lung, and other solid organ transplantations. *J Heart Lung Transplant* 1995;14:214–221.
15. Cacciarelli TV, Esquivel CO, Moore DH, et al. Factors affecting survival after orthotopic liver transplantation in infants. *Transplantation* 1997;64:242–248.
16. Newell KA, Alonso EM, Whitington PF, et al. Posttransplant lymphoproliferative disease in pediatric liver transplantation. Interplay between primary Epstein-Barr virus infection and immunosuppression. *Transplantation* 1996;62:370–375.
17. Shapiro RS, McClain K, Frizzera G, et al. Epstein-Barr virus associated B cell lymphoproliferative disorders following bone marrow transplantation. *Blood* 1988;71:1234–1243.
18. Larson RS, Scott MA, McCurley TL, et al. Microsatellite analysis of posttransplant lymphoproliferative disorders: determination of donor/recipient origin and identification of putative lymphomagenic mechanism. *Cancer Res* 1996;56:4378–4381.
19. Weissmann DJ, Ferry JA, Harris NL, et al. Posttransplantation lymphoproliferative disorders in solid organ recipients are predominantly aggressive tumors of host origin. *Am J Clin Pathol* 1995;103:748–755.
20. Chadburn A, Suciu-Foca N, Cesarman E, et al. Post-transplantation lymphoproliferative disorders arising in solid organ transplant recipients are usually of recipient origin. *Am J Pathol* 1995;147:1862–1870.
21. Nuckols JD, Baron PW, Stenzel TT, et al. The pathology of liver-localized post-transplant lymphoproliferative disease: a report of three cases and a review of the literature. *Am J Surg Pathol* 2000;24:733–741.
22. Harris NL, Swerdlow SH. Methotrexate-associated lymphoproliferative disorders. In: Jaffe E, Harris NL, Stein H, Vardiman JW, eds. *Pathology and genetics of tumours of haematopoietic and lymphoid tissues*. World Health Organization classification of tumours. Lyon, France: IARC Press, 2001:270–271.
23. Abruzzo LV, Rosales CM, Medeiros LJ, et al. Epstein-Barr virus-positive B-cell lymphoproliferative disorders arising in immunodeficient patients previously treated with fludarabine for low-grade B-cell neoplasms. *Am J Surg Pathol* 2002;26:630–636.
24. Paya CV, Fung JJ, Nalesnik MA, et al. Epstein-Barr virus-induced posttransplant lymphoproliferative disorders. ASTS/ASTP EBV-PTLD Task Force and The Mayo Clinic Organized International Consensus Development Meeting. *Transplantation* 1999;68:1517–1525.
25. Frizzera G, Hanto DW, Gajl-Peczalska KJ, et al. Polymorphic diffuse B-cell hyperplasias and lymphomas in renal transplant recipients. *Cancer Res* 1981;41:4262–4279.
26. Knowles DM, Cesarman E, Chadburn A, et al. Correlative morphologic and molecular genetic analysis demonstrates three distinct categories of posttransplantation lymphoproliferative disorders. *Blood* 1995;85:552–565.
27. Nalesnik MA, Jaffe R, Starzl TE, et al. The pathology of posttransplant lymphoproliferative disorders occurring in the setting of cyclosporine A-prednisone immunosuppression. *Am J Pathol* 1988;133:173–192.
28. Swerdlow SH. Classification of the posttransplant lymphoproliferative disorders: from the past to the present. *Semin Diagn Pathol* 1997;14:2–7.
29. Harris NL, Ferry JA, Swerdlow SH. Posttransplant lymphoproliferative disorders: summary of Society for Hematopathology Workshop. *Semin Diagn Pathol* 1997;14:8–14.
30. Harris NL, Swerdlow SH, Frizzera G, et al. Post-transplant lymphoproliferative disorders. In: Jaffe E, Harris NL, Stein H, Vardiman JW, eds. *Pathology and genetics of tumours of haematopoietic and lymphoid tissues. World Health Organization classification of tumours*. Lyon, France: IARC Press, 2001:264–269.
31. Nelson BP, Locker J, Nalesnik MA, et al. Clonal and morphological variation in a posttransplant lymphoproliferative disorder: evolution from clonal T-cell to clonal B-cell predominance. *Hum Pathol* 1998;29:416–421.
32. Swerdlow SH. Post-transplant lymphoproliferative disorders: a morphologic, phenotypic and genotypic spectrum of disease. *Histopathology* 1992;20:373–385.
33. Chadburn A, Cesarman E, Liu YF, et al. Molecular genetic analysis demonstrates that multiple posttransplantation lymphoproliferative disorders occurring in one anatomic site in a single patient represent distinct primary lymphoid neoplasms. *Cancer* 1995;75:2747–2756.
34. Wu TT, Swerdlow SH, Locker J, et al. Recurrent Epstein-Barr virus-associated lesions in organ transplant recipients. *Hum Pathol* 1996;27:157–164.
35. Cesarman E, Chadburn A, Liu YF, et al. BCL-6 gene mutations in posttransplantation lymphoproliferative disorders predict response to therapy and clinical outcome. *Blood* 1998;92:2294–2302.
36. Liebowitz D. Epstein-Barr virus and a cellular signaling pathway in lymphomas from immunosuppressed patients. *N Engl J Med* 1998;338:1413–1421.
37. Hsi ED, Singleton TP, Swinnen L, et al. Mucosa-associated lymphoid tissue-type lymphomas occurring in post-transplantation patients. *Am J Surg Pathol* 2000;24:100–106.
38. Wotherspoon AC, Diss TC, Pan L, et al. Low grade gastric B-cell lymphoma of mucosa associated lymphoid tissue in immunocompromised patients. *Histopathology* 1996;28:129–134.
39. Minervini MI, Swerdlow SH, Nalesnik MA. Polymorphism and T-cell infiltration in posttransplant lymphoproliferative disorders. *Transplant Proc* 1999;31:1270.
40. Kowal-Vern A, Swinnen L, Pyle J, et al. Characterization of postcardiac transplant lymphomas. Histology, immunophenotyping, immunohistochemistry, and gene rearrangement. *Arch Pathol Lab Med* 1996;120:41–48.

41. Perera SM, Thomas JA, Burke M, et al. Analysis of the T-cell micro-environment in Epstein-Barr virus-related post-transplantation B lymphoproliferative disease. *J Pathol* 1998;184:177–184.
42. Nalesnik MA, Zeevi A, Randhawa PS, et al. Cytokine mRNA profiles in Epstein-Barr virus-associated post-transplant lymphoproliferative disorders. *Clin Transplant* 1999;13:39–44.
43. Van Gorp J, Doornewaard H, Verdonck LF, et al. Posttransplant T-cell lymphoma. Report of three cases and a review of the literature. [Review]. *Cancer* 1994;73:3064–3072.
44. Kluin PM, Feller A, Gaulard P, et al. Peripheral T/NK-cell lymphoma: a report of the IXth Workshop of the European Association for Haematopathology. *Histopathology* 2001;38:250–270.
45. Steurer M, Stauder R, Grunewald K, et al. Hepatosplenic gamma delta-T-cell lymphoma with leukemic course after renal transplantation. *Hum Pathol* 2002;33:253–258.
46. Mukai HY, Kojima H, Suzukawa K, et al. Nasal natural killer cell lymphoma in a post-renal transplant patient. *Transplantation* 2000; 69:1501–1503.
47. Gentile TC, Hadlock KG, Uner AH, et al. Large granular lymphocyte leukaemia occurring after renal transplantation. *Br J Haematol* 1998;101:507–512.
48. Koeppen H, Newell K, Baunoch DA, et al. Morphologic bone marrow changes in patients with posttransplantation lymphoproliferative disorders. *Am J Surg Pathol* 1998;22:208–214.
49. Rizkalla KS, Asfar SK, McLean CA, et al. Key features distinguishing post-transplantation lymphoproliferative disorders and acute liver rejection. *Mod Pathol* 1997;10:708–715.
50. Rosendale B, Yousem SA. Discrimination of Epstein-Barr virus-related posttransplant lymphoproliferations from acute rejection in lung allograft recipients. *Arch Pathol Lab Med* 1995;119:418–423.
51. Randhawa PS, Magnone M, Jordan M, et al. Renal allograft involvement by Epstein-Barr virus associated post-transplant lymphoproliferative disease. *Am J Surg Pathol* 1996;20:563–571.
52. Drachenberg CB, Abruzzo LV, Klassen DK, et al. Epstein-Barr virus-related posttransplantation lymphoproliferative disorder involving pancreas allografts: histological differential diagnosis from acute allograft rejection. *Hum Pathol* 1998;29:569–577.
53. Hubscher SG, Williams A, Davison SM, et al. Epstein-Barr virus in inflammatory diseases of the liver and liver allografts: an *in situ* hybridization study. *Hepatology* 1994;20:899–907.
54. Cleary ML, Nalesnik MA, Shearer WT, et al. Clonal analysis of transplant-associated lymphoproliferations based on the structure of the genomic termini of the Epstein-Barr virus. *Blood* 1988;72:349–352.
55. Kaplan MA, Ferry JA, Harris NL, et al. Clonal analysis of posttransplant lymphoproliferative disorders, using both episomal Epstein-Barr virus and immunoglobulin genes as markers. *Am J Clin Pathol* 1994;101:590–596.
56. Frank D, Cesarman E, Liu YF, et al. Posttransplantation lymphoproliferative disorders frequently contain type A and not type B Epstein-Barr virus. *Blood* 1995;85:1396–1403.
57. Delecluse HJ, Kremmer E, Rouault JP, et al. The expression of Epstein-Barr virus latent proteins is related to the pathological features of post-transplant lymphoproliferative disorders. *Am J Pathol* 1995;146:1113–1120.
58. Oudejans JJ, Jiwa M, van den Brule AJ, et al. Detection of heterogeneous Epstein-Barr virus gene expression patterns within individual post-transplantation lymphoproliferative disorders. *Am J Pathol* 1995; 147:923–933.
59. Rea D, Fourcade C, Leblond V, et al. Patterns of Epstein-Barr virus latent and replicative gene expression in Epstein-Barr virus B cell lymphoproliferative disorders after organ transplantation. *Transplantation* 1994;58:317–324.
60. Garnier JL, Lebranchu Y, Dantal J, et al. Hodgkin's disease after transplantation. *Transplantation* 1996;61:71–76.
61. Rooney CM, Smith CA, Heslop HE. Control of virus-induced lymphoproliferation: Epstein-Barr virus-induced lymphoproliferation and host immunity. [Review]. *Mol Med Today* 1997;3:24–30.
62. Murray PG, Swinnen LJ, Constandinou CM, et al. BCL-2 but not its Epstein-Barr virus-encoded homologue, BHRF1, is commonly expressed in posttransplantation lymphoproliferative disorders. *Blood* 1996;87:706–711.
63. Montone KT, Hodinka RL, Salhany KE, et al. Identification of Epstein-Barr virus lytic activity in post-transplantation lymphoproliferative disease. *Mod Pathol* 1996;9:621–630.
64. Muti G, De Gasperi A, Cantoni S, et al. Incidence and clinical characteristics of posttransplant lymphoproliferative disorders: report from a single center. *Transplant Int* 2000;13[Suppl 1]:S382–S387.
65. Leblond V, Davi F, Charlotte F, et al. Posttransplant lymphoproliferative disorders not associated with Epstein-Barr virus: a distinct entity? *J Clin Oncol* 1998;16:2052–2059.
66. Nelson BP, Nalesnik MA, Locker JD. EBV negative post-transplant lymphoproliferative disorders: a distinct entity? *Lab Invest* 1996;74:118 (abst).
67. Dockrell DH, Strickler JG, Paya CV. Epstein-Barr virus-induced T cell lymphoma in solid organ transplant recipients. *Clin Infect Dis* 1998;26:180–182.
68. Kapelushnik J, Ariad S, Benharroch D, et al. Post renal transplantation human herpesvirus 8-associated lymphoproliferative disorder and Kaposi's sarcoma. *Br J Haematol* 2001;113:425–428.
69. Matsushima AY, Strauchen JA, Lee G, et al. Posttransplantation plasmacytic proliferations related to Kaposi's sarcoma-associated herpesvirus. *Am J Surg Pathol* 1999;23:1393–1400.
70. Dotti G, Fiocchi R, Motta T, et al. Primary effusion lymphoma after heart transplantation: a new entity associated with human herpesvirus-8. *Leukemia* 1999;13:664–670.
71. Chadburn A, Chen JM, Hsu DT, et al. The morphologic and molecular genetic categories of posttransplantation lymphoproliferative disorders are clinically relevant. *Cancer* 1998;82:1978–1987.
72. Billiar TR, Hanto DW, Simmons RL. Inclusion of uncomplicated infectious mononucleosis in the spectrum of Epstein-Barr virus infections in transplant recipients. *Transplantation* 1988;46:159–161.
73. Miller WT Jr, Siegel SG, Montone KT. Posttransplantation lymphoproliferative disorder: changing manifestations of disease in a renal transplant population. *Crit Rev Diagn Imaging* 1997;38:569–585.
74. Hanto DW. Classification of Epstein-Barr virus-associated posttransplant lymphoproliferative diseases: implications for understanding their pathogenesis and developing rational treatment strategies. *Ann Rev Med* 1995;46:381–394.
75. Hayashi RJ, Kraus MD, Patel AL, et al. Posttransplant lymphoproliferative disease in children: correlation of histology to clinical behavior. *J Pediatr Hematol Oncol* 2001;23:14–18.
76. Cohen JI. Epstein-Barr virus lymphoproliferative disease associated with acquired immunodeficiency. *Medicine (Baltimore)* 1991;70:137–160.
77. Green M, Michaels M, Weber S. Predicting outcome from post-transplant lymphoproliferative disease: a risky business. *Pediatr Transplant* 2001;5:235–238.
78. Nalesnik MA. Involvement of the gastrointestinal tract by Epstein-Barr virus—associated posttransplant lymphoproliferative disorders. *Am J Surg Pathol* 1990;14[Suppl 1]:92–100.
79. Joseph G, Barker RL, Yuan B, et al. Posttransplantation plasma cell dyscrasias. *Cancer* 1994;74:1959–1964.
80. Locker J, Nalesnik M. Molecular genetic analysis of lymphoid tumors arising after organ transplantation. *Am J Pathol* 1989;135:977–987.
81. Hanson MN, Morrison VA, Peterson BA, et al. Posttransplant T-cell lymphoproliferative disorders—an aggressive, late complication of solid-organ transplantation. *Blood* 1996;88:3626–3633.
82. Wu H, Wasik MA, Przybylski G, et al. Hepatosplenic gamma-delta T-cell lymphoma as a late-onset posttransplant lymphoproliferative disorder in renal transplant recipients. *Am J Clin Pathol* 2000;113:487–496.
83. Hanto DW, Birkenbach M, Frizzera G, et al. Confirmation of the heterogeneity of posttransplant Epstein-Barr virus-associated B cell proliferations by immunoglobulin gene rearrangement analyses. *Transplantation* 1989;47:458–464.
84. Nalesnik MA, Makowka L, Starzl TE. The diagnosis and treatment of posttransplant lymphoproliferative disorders. *Curr Probl Surg* 1988;25: 367–472.
85. Swinnen LJ, Mullen GM, Carr TJ, et al. Aggressive treatment for postcardiac transplant lymphoproliferation. *Blood* 1995;86:3333–3340.
86. Morrison VA, Dunn DL, Manivel JC, et al. Clinical characteristics of post-transplant lymphoproliferative disorders. *Am J Med* 1994;97:14–24.
87. Leblond V, Dhedin N, Mamzer Bruneel MF, et al. Identification of prognostic factors in 61 patients with posttransplantation lymphoproliferative disorders. *J Clin Oncol* 2001;19:772–778.
88. Swinnen LJ, Mullen GM, Carr TJ, et al. Aggressive treatment for postcardiac transplant lymphoproliferation. *Blood* 1995;86:3333–3340.

89. Leblond V, Sutton L, Dorent R, et al. Lymphoproliferative disorders after organ transplantation: a report of 24 cases observed in a single center. *J Clin Oncol* 1995;13:961–968.

90. Hanto DW, Frizzera G, Gajl-Peczalska KJ, et al. Epstein-Barr virus-induced B-cell lymphoma after renal transplantation: acyclovir therapy and transition from polyclonal to monoclonal B-cell proliferation. *N Engl J Med* 1982;306:913–918.

91. Filipovich AH, Mathur A, Kamat D, et al. Lymphoproliferative disorders and other tumors complicating immunodeficiencies [Review]. *Immunodeficiency* 1994;5:91–112.

92. McDiarmid SV, Jordan S, Lee GS, et al. Prevention and preemptive therapy of posttransplant lymphoproliferative disease in pediatric liver recipients. *Transplantation* 1998;66:1604–1611.

93. Green M, Kaufmann M, Wilson J, et al. Comparison of intravenous ganciclovir followed by oral acyclovir with intravenous ganciclovir alone for prevention of cytomegalovirus and Epstein-Barr virus disease after liver transplantation in children. *Clin Infect Dis* 1997;25:1344–1349.

94. Shapiro RS, Chauvenet A, McGuire W, et al. Treatment of B-cell lymphoproliferative disorders with interferon alfa and intravenous gamma globulin [Letter]. *N Engl J Med* 1988;318:1334.

95. Liebowitz D, Anastasi J, Hagos F, et al. Post-transplant lymphoproliferative disorders (PTLD): clinicopathologic characterization and response to immunomodulatory therapy with interferon-alpha. *Ann Oncol* 1996;7:28(abst).

96. Fischer A, Blanche S, Le Bidois J, et al. Anti-B-cell monoclonal antibodies in the treatment of severe B-cell lymphoproliferative syndrome following bone marrow and organ transplantation. *N Engl J Med* 1991;324:1451–1456.

97. Benkerrou M, Jais JP, Leblond V, et al. Anti-B-cell monoclonal antibody treatment of severe posttransplant B-lymphoproliferative disorder: prognostic factors and long-term outcome. *Blood* 1998;92:3137–3147.

98. Milpied N, Antoine C, Garnier JL, et al. Humanized anti-CD20 monoclonal antibody (rituximab) in B post-transplant lymphoproliferative disorders (B PTLDs): a retrospective analysis of 32 patients. *Ann Oncol* 1999;10:5(abst).

99. Choquet S, Herbrecht R, Socie G, et al. Efficacy and safety of rituximab in B-cell post-transplantation lymphoproliferative disorders (B-PTLD): preliminary results of a multicenter, open label, phase II trial (M9037 trial). *Blood* 2002;100:1811(abst).

100. Gross TG, Park J, Bucuvalas J, et al. Low-dose chemotherapy for refractory EBV associated post transplant lymphoproliferative disease (PTLD) following solid organ transplant in children. *Blood* 2002;100:598(abst).

101. Papadopoulos EB, Ladanyi M, Emanuel D, et al. Infusions of donor leukocytes to treat Epstein-Barr virus-associated lymphoproliferative disorders after allogeneic bone marrow transplantation. *N Engl J Med* 1994;330:1185–1191.

102. Rooney CM, Smith CA, Ng CY, et al. Use of gene-modified virus-specific T lymphocytes to control Epstein-Barr-virus-related lymphoproliferation. *Lancet* 1995;345:9–13.

103. O'Reilly RJ, Small TN, Papadopoulos E, et al. Biology and adoptive cell therapy of Epstein-Barr virus-associated lymphoproliferative disorders in recipients of marrow allografts [Review]. *Immunol Rev* 1997;157:195–216.

104. Savoldo B, Huls HM, Lopez T, et al. Autologous EBV-specific cytotoxic T lymphocyte (CTL) infusions as early intervention for liver transplant recipients with lymphoproliferative disease. *Blood* 2002;1001407(abst).

105. Randhawa PS, Jaffe R, Demetris AJ, et al. Expression of Epstein-Barr virus-encoded small RNA (by the EBER-1 gene) in liver specimens from transplant recipients with post-transplantation lymphoproliferative disease. *N Engl J Med* 1992;327:1710–1714.

106. Riddler SA, Breinig MC, McKnight JL. Increased levels of circulating Epstein-Barr virus (EBV)-infected lymphocytes and decreased EBV nuclear antigen antibody responses are associated with the development of posttransplant lymphoproliferative disease in solid-organ transplant recipients. *Blood* 1994;84:972–984.

107. Rooney CM, Loftin SK, Holladay MS, et al. Early identification of Epstein-Barr virus-associated post-transplantation lymphoproliferative disease. *Br J Haematol* 1995;89:98–103.

108. Swinnen LJ, Gulley ML, Hamilton E, Schichman SA. EBV DNA quantitation in serum is highly correlated with the development and regression of post-transplant lymphoproliferative disorder in solid organ transplant recipients. *Blood* 1998;92:1291(abst).

109. Lucas KG, Burton RL, Zimmerman SE, et al. Semiquantitative Epstein-Barr virus (EBV) polymerase chain reaction for the determination of patients at risk for EBV-induced lymphoproliferative disease after stem cell transplantation. *Blood* 1998;91:3654–3661.

110. Rose C, Green M, Webber S, et al. Detection of Epstein-Barr virus genomes in peripheral blood B cells from solid-organ transplant recipients by fluorescence *in situ* hybridization. *J Clin Microbiol* 2002;40:2533–2544.

111. Rowe DT, Qu L, Reyes J, et al. Use of quantitative competitive PCR to measure Epstein-Barr virus genome load in the peripheral blood of pediatric transplant patients with lymphoproliferative disorders. *J Clin Microbiol* 1997;35:1612–1615.

112. Wagner HJ, Wessel M, Jabs W, et al. Patients at risk for development of posttransplant lymphoproliferative disorder: plasma versus peripheral blood mononuclear cells as material for quantification of Epstein-Barr viral load by using real-time quantitative polymerase chain reaction. *Transplantation* 2001;72:1012–1019.

113. Smets F, Latinne D, Bazin H, et al. Ratio between Epstein-Barr viral load and anti-Epstein-Barr virus specific T-cell response as a predictive marker of posttransplant lymphoproliferative disease. *Transplantation* 2002;73:1603–1610.

114. Stevens SJ, Verschuuren EA, Pronk I, et al. Frequent monitoring of Epstein-Barr virus DNA load in unfractionated whole blood is essential for early detection of posttransplant lymphoproliferative disease in high-risk patients. *Blood* 2001;97:1165–1171.

CHAPTER 41

Management of Central Nervous System Lymphoma

Sumul N. Raval, Joachim Yahalom, and Lisa M. DeAngelis

Malignant lymphoma can involve the nervous system, most commonly from metastasis from systemic non-Hodgkin's lymphoma. Lymphoma rarely metastasizes to the brain, but it can spread to the leptomeninges in as many as 10% of patients. In approximately 3% to 5% of patients, it can indirectly affect the central nervous system by causing epidural spinal cord compression. Lymphoma can also arise within the central nervous system as primary central nervous system lymphoma that typically involves the brain and, to a lesser extent, the eyes, leptomeninges, and spinal cord. Primary central nervous system lymphoma has been diagnosed with greater frequency in the past 25 years, and survival has significantly improved with the use of chemotherapy as part of the initial treatment. Primary central nervous system lymphoma has a predilection to affect immunosuppressed patients, especially those with acquired immune deficiency syndrome (AIDS). However, the introduction of highly active antiretroviral therapy has resulted in a significant decline of primary central nervous system lymphoma in this population (1,2).

EPIDEMIOLOGY

In 1929, Bailey first described primary central nervous system lymphoma as a perithelial sarcoma (3). Through the decades, it became known by other names, including *microglioma* (because microglia was the presumed cell of origin), *reticulum cell sarcoma* (because of the reticulum deposition around blood vessels), and *lymphosarcoma* (4,5). In 1974, Henry et al. described these tumors as primary malignant lymphomas of the central nervous system because their morphologic characteristics were similar to systemic malignant lymphomas (6). Current advances in immunohistochemical techniques confirmed the lymphoid nature of primary central nervous system lymphoma (7–10).

Formerly, primary central nervous system lymphoma accounted for approximately 1% of all primary brain tumors and 1% to 2% of all lymphomas (11,12). In the past three

decades, the incidence of primary central nervous system lymphoma in immunocompetent patients increased to 3% to 4% of all brain tumors (13). The reason for this increase is unclear, although it is part of a general trend in the United States of an increase in all extranodal lymphomas. Analysis of the National Cancer Institute Surveillance, Epidemiology, and End Results data shows a tenfold increase in primary central nervous system lymphoma from two to five cases per 10 million people in 1973 to 30 cases per 10 million in 1992. This increased incidence was not observed worldwide. Reports from Germany, Scotland, and Canada do not show an increased incidence of primary central nervous system lymphoma in immunocompetent patients (14–16), raising the question of an environmental contribution to tumor formation.

Isolated ocular lymphoma is being seen with increased frequency as well. There are three reasons to consider ocular lymphoma as part of the spectrum of primary central nervous system lymphoma: (a) Ocular involvement is a common feature of primary central nervous system lymphoma; (b) the central nervous system is the primary site of tumor progression or relapse in patients who present with isolated ocular lymphoma; and (c) embryologically and anatomically, the eye is part of the nervous system.

Primary central nervous system lymphoma has a special predilection for immunocompromised patients, including those with congenital or acquired immunodeficiencies (Table 41.1) (17–24). AIDS is the most common immunocompromised state that predisposes to primary central nervous system lymphoma, and AIDS patients have a 10% lifetime risk of developing primary central nervous system lymphoma; however, 4% to 7% of organ transplant recipients also develop primary central nervous system lymphoma (25). A variety of congenital immunodeficiency states (Wiskott-Aldrich syndrome, ataxia-telangiectasia) have also been associated with primary central nervous system lymphoma. Primary central nervous system lymphoma occurs when cellular immunity is markedly depressed; in AIDS

643

TABLE 41.1. *Immunodeficiency conditions associated with primary central nervous system lymphoma*

Congenital
1. Wiskott-Aldrich syndrome
2. Ataxia-telangiectasia
3. Severe combined immunodeficiency
4. X-linked immunoproliferative disorder

Other rare conditions
1. Sjögren's syndrome
2. Rheumatoid arthritis
3. Systemic lupus erythematosus

Acquired
1. Acquired immunodeficiency syndrome
2. Organ transplant patients

patients, it develops late in the disease when CD4 counts are less than 100 to 200 per mm³. Recently, the incidence of AIDS–related primary central nervous system lymphoma has declined secondary to better human immunodeficiency virus control with highly active antiretroviral therapy (1,2), but there is concern that the incidence could increase if human immunodeficiency virus resistance develops to current antiretroviral therapy.

Primary central nervous system lymphoma may represent a second malignancy in some patients. Approximately 17% of primary central nervous system lymphoma patients had a prior systemic cancer, such as colon, thyroid, breast, non-Hodgkin's lymphoma, or Hodgkin's lymphoma. The primary central nervous system lymphoma frequently occurs many years or decades after the initial systemic cancer (26). There is no uniform treatment-related factor that may explain primary central nervous system lymphoma in these patients; in fact, many had their primary cancer treated with surgery alone, and they never received chemotherapy or radiotherapy. There may be diagnostic confusion in these patients because new brain lesions are often presumed to be brain metastases from their original cancer. However, biopsy of cerebral lesions should always be considered in patients whose systemic cancer is remote and inactive.

Primary central nervous system lymphoma affects patients of all ages, with a peak incidence in the sixth and seventh decades of life. The median age is 55 years in immunocompetent patients (27,28). There is a slight male predominance in immunocompetent patients, approximately 1.5:1.0, but more than 90% of primary central nervous system lymphoma patients are male, which reflects the sex distribution of human immunodeficiency virus in the United States (29). When reported in children, primary central nervous system lymphoma is almost always associated with inherited or acquired immunodeficiency (30–33.) In immunosuppressed patients, median age of primary central nervous system lymphoma is lowest in

patients with inherited immunodeficiency syndromes (10 years), followed by acquired immunodeficiency states, such as AIDS (31 years), and by organ allograft transplantation (37 years) (34,35).

ETIOLOGY

In immunocompromised patients, primary central nervous system lymphoma always arises from B lymphocytes infected with the Epstein-Barr virus (1,36). After primary Epstein-Barr virus infection, which usually occurs early in life, a small population of B cells remains latently infected and resides for life within the individual. These B cells are immortalized but not transformed, and their proliferation is controlled by suppressor T cells. Any immunosuppressive process that disturbs T-cell function leads to uncontrolled proliferation of the latently infected B-cell population, eventually leading to development of a neoplasm. Epstein-Barr virus–driven lymphomas have a propensity to develop in the central nervous system because there is limited normal immune surveillance in the nervous system, and, therefore, these cells are further protected from any functioning immune system. Epstein-Barr virus can be detected in the cerebrospinal fluid or in tumor tissue of almost all immunocompromised patients with primary central nervous system lymphoma (37,38).

Neither Epstein-Barr virus nor any of the human herpesviruses have been identified as etiologic factors in immunocompetent patients, and the pathogenesis of primary central nervous system lymphoma in these patients is unknown. There are no lymph nodes or lymphatics in the nervous system to serve as a reservoir for lymphoid tissue. There are three possible origins of this tumor: (a) A clone of lymphocytes transforms systemically, enters the nervous system, and grows there; the malignant clone is eradicated systemically by an intact immune system but grows in the immunoprivileged central nervous system; (b) normal lymphocytes passing through the central nervous system become transformed during passage and remain sequestered there and grow; and (c) there is an antigenic stimulus in the central nervous system that attracts B cells where they develop into a neoplasm. There are no convincing data to support or disprove any of these three potential mechanisms.

PATHOLOGY

The Revised European-American Lymphoma Classification system differentiates lymphoma as either B cell, T cell, or Hodgkin's disease (39). Primary central nervous system lymphoma is a B-cell tumor in almost all cases; less than 1% to 2% of primary central nervous system lymphomas are of T-cell origin (Color Plate 70) (40). The majority of primary central nervous system lymphomas are large-cell or large-cell immunoblastic subtypes, although low-grade subtypes are occasionally seen. Primary central nervous system lymphoma involves the brain parenchyma in more than 90% of patients and most commonly affects the frontal lobes, corpus callosum, basal ganglia, and cerebellum. It typically grows in periventricular regions and commonly comes in contact with the ventricles or the subarachnoid space (41). Primary central nervous system lymphoma rarely involves the leptomeninges or spinal cord in the absence of a brain lesion (42).

Macroscopically, primary central nervous system lymphoma lesions are fleshy and usually discrete from normal brain. Microscopically, they are composed of high-grade neoplastic cells that grow in a characteristic perivascular pattern in concentric rings around blood vessel walls without invasion of the lumen (Color Plate 70) (43). Autopsy typically shows extensive brain invasion with microscopic tumor growing in areas remote from bulky lesions seen on imaging studies (44). Reactive T lymphocytes may infiltrate these B-cell tumors, causing diagnostic difficulty, particularly in patients treated with corticosteroids before sampling. Steroids may cause lysis of the malignant B cells, leaving the reactive T cells behind, leading to misdiagnosis of an inflammatory reaction (45,46). Primary central nervous system lymphoma does not have the degree of vascular proliferation commonly seen in high-grade gliomas; necrosis and hemorrhage are uncommon. In immunocompromised patients, however, necrosis and hemorrhage are frequent (43).

Cytogenetic studies showed abnormalities of chromosomes 1 (1q21), 6 (6q15, 6q21), 7 (7q15), and 14 (14q24, 14q32) (47). A genomic imbalance was confirmed in 95% of patients with primary central nervous system lymphoma by comparative genomic hybridization; the most common were losses of 6q (47% with common deletion of 6q21-q22) and gains of 12q (63%), 18q (37%), and 22q (37%). Weber et al. reported gains involving 1q, 9q, 11q, 12p, 16p, and 17p (48). Conflicting data were reported for p53 as being overexpressed, mutated, or absent in different studies (49–52). Bcl-2 and bcl-6 were overexpressed in 20% to 50% of primary central nervous system lymphomas (49,51,52), but they were absent in p53-expressing tumors (49). It appears that one of several central pathways involved in apoptosis is affected in primary central nervous system lymphoma. Sixty-six percent of primary central nervous system lymphomas contained less than or equal to 10% apoptotic cells detectable by terminal deoxynucleotidyl transferase–mediated uradine triphosphatase nick end labeling assay (51). Other evidence indicates an abnormal G_1-S phase of the cell cycle in primary central nervous system lymphoma. In one report of immunocompetent patients with primary central nervous system lymphoma, approximately 50% showed deletion of p15 and p16 or 5' CpG island methylation of the p16 gene (52,53). In another report, further testing for p16 expression by reverse transcriptase–mediated polymerase chain reaction revealed that messenger RNA expression was absent in 63% and weakly present in 36% (52). Immunohistochemistry indicated that p16 was absent or restricted to single tumor cells intermingled among negative tumor cells. P16 binds and inhibits the cyclin D–regulated CDK4 and 6 kinases that control transition into the late G_1 phase of the cell cycle.

Deletion of p16 may relieve this block, and cells would progress into S phase. Primary central nervous system lymphomas were also reported to be MIB-1 positive; 53% showed high proliferative activity with more than 20% MIB-1–positive cells (51).

CLINICAL PRESENTATIONS

Primary central nervous system lymphoma presents as a fast-growing brain tumor, and patients usually have only a few weeks of symptoms (54). Signs and symptoms depend on the size and location of the tumor.

The frontal lobes are involved in 30% to 40% of patients, causing cognitive deficit or personality changes in 24% to 70% of patients (Table 41.2) (54,55). Focal neurologic deficits (e.g., hemiparesis and ataxia) and signs of increased intracranial pressure (e.g., headache and nausea) are common (55). Because these tumors are located deep in white matter, seizures are less common than with other primary brain tumors. Primary central nervous system lymphoma presenting as isolated leptomeningeal disease is rare, but involvement of the leptomeninges occurs in approximately 42% of patients at diagnosis and approximately 41% at recurrence (56). However, patients rarely have symptoms suggestive of leptomeningeal spread, such as cranial neuropathies, hydrocephalus, or spinal radiculopathy (57).

Primary involvement of the spinal cord is extremely rare and usually occurs at the thoracic level. Patients present with a painless, progressive myelopathy (58). Primary central nervous system lymphoma involving the eye is common and can be the sole site of disease. Fifty percent to 80% of patients with isolated ocular lymphoma eventually develop cerebral lymphoma at a mean of approximately 23 months after ocular diagnosis (59). In contrast, ocular involvement is reported in 20% to 25% of primary central nervous system lymphoma

TABLE 41.2. *Presenting signs and symptoms of primary central nervous system lymphoma*

Symptoms and signs	Percentage range
Common	
Changes in mental status	24–73
Focal neurologic signs (hemiparesis, aphasia)	40–50
Increased intracranial pressure (headache, nausea)	15–60
Ataxia	15–40
Visual blurring, floaters	8–10
Less common	
Seizures	2–33
Nuchal rigidity	0–36
Cranial neuropathy	5–31
Spinal radiculopathy	1–2
Bladder or bowel dysfunction	1–2

patients at diagnosis, and only one half of those have visual symptoms (60). The symptoms of ocular lymphoma include floaters, visual blurring, or segmental visual loss secondary to retinal detachment from subretinal deposits of lymphoma. In patients with isolated ocular lymphoma, the diagnosis may be delayed because these nonspecific symptoms and the accompanying cellular infiltrate of the vitreous are similar to those occurring in common inflammatory eye conditions, such as uveitis, chorioretinitis, or vitreitis.

DIAGNOSIS AND STAGING

The initial evaluation for the diagnosis and staging of primary central nervous system lymphoma includes cranial magnetic resonance imaging; cerebrospinal fluid studies; ophthalmologic examination; computed tomography scan of chest, abdomen, and pelvis; bone marrow biopsy; and human immunodeficiency virus test (Table 41.3). Magnetic resonance imaging is the optimal technique for neuroimaging, but occasionally computed tomographic scanning must be used in patients who cannot undergo magnetic resonance imaging, such as those with a pacemaker. On computed tomographic scanning, primary central nervous system lymphomas usually appear as iso- or hyperdense lesions, and on magnetic resonance imaging, the lesions are iso- to hypointense on T1-weighted images. Homogeneous contrast enhancement is seen in more than 90% of cases (Fig. 41.1) (61). The lesions usually have irregular borders; the amount of surrounding edema is variable, compared with the reliably prominent edema usually seen with metastatic tumors or gliomas. The lesions occur in the subcortical white matter, often adjacent to the ventricles, and are soli-

TABLE 41.3. *Initial work-up and staging for primary central nervous system lymphoma*

Immunocompetent patients
  Cranial MRI with and without contrast (if contraindicated, CT)
  Lumbar puncture
    CSF markers: β_2-microglobulin, soluble CD27, CD20 cytology
  Ophthalmologic evaluation including slit-lamp examination
  Human immunodeficiency virus test
  CT chest, abdomen, pelvis
  Possible bone marrow biopsy
  MRI of spine with contrast if indicated
Immunocompromised patients
  As above and additional tests
  Lumbar puncture
    CSF for Epstein-Barr virus DNA
  Cranial positron emission tomography or single-photon emission CT scan

CSF, cerebrospinal fluid; CT, computed tomography; MRI, magnetic resonance imaging.

tary in 60% to 70% of cases and multifocal in 30% to 40% of cases. In immunocompromised patients, primary central nervous system lymphoma typically appears as a ring-enhancing lesion on magnetic resonance imaging or computed tomographic scanning. The central necrosis seen radiographically correlates with the necrosis identified pathologically in these patients. It is impossible in AIDS patients to differentiate radiographically primary central nervous system lymphoma from an infectious process, such as toxoplasmosis (62). Positron emission tomography or single-photon emission computed tomography can be helpful in distinguishing primary central nervous system lymphoma, which is hypermetabolic, from infection, which is typically hypometabolic (63,64). Nonenhancing tumors have also been reported in approximately 10% of mainly immunosuppressed patients with primary central nervous system lymphoma (Fig. 41.2) (65).

Stereotactic biopsy is the diagnostic test for immunocompetent and immunocompromised patients. Resection is not performed because most lesions are deep, many are multifocal, and resection does not improve survival over biopsy alone. Occasionally, resection is necessary to decompress a rapidly expanding mass in herniating patients. In these patients, resection is life-saving and restores neurologic function so that medical therapy can follow. In AIDS patients, the combination of a hypermetabolic positron emission tomography or single-photon emission computed tomography scan and a positive cerebrospinal fluid test for Epstein-Barr virus DNA is 100% specific for primary central nervous system lymphoma; therefore, biopsy can be avoided in these cases (66). Stereotactic biopsy is associated with an 11.5% incidence of intracranial hemorrhage in AIDS patients, in contrast to a 1% incidence in non AIDS patients (67,68). Thus, biopsy for AIDS patients should be reserved for those suspected of primary central nervous system lymphoma in whom noninvasive tests are nondiagnostic.

Even though stereotactic biopsy in immunocompetent patients is the definitive surgical approach to diagnose primary central nervous system lymphoma (69), the diagnosis may become difficult when the patient is treated preoperatively with corticosteroids (70). Primary central nervous system lymphoma may shrink or disappear after steroid administration (45,46). The steroids have a direct cytotoxic effect on malignant lymphocytes, which is mediated by a cytoplasmic steroid receptor that translocates to the nucleus and induces apoptosis (70). Not all primary central nervous system lymphoma lesions respond to steroids; thus, the absence of tumor regression after steroids does not preclude the diagnosis of primary central nervous system lymphoma (71). However, when primary central nervous system lymphoma is suspected on imaging, steroids should be withheld until a biopsy has been performed. It is safe to defer steroid use for most patients.

Lumbar puncture for cerebrospinal fluid analysis is essential for neurologic staging. It is safe in the majority of

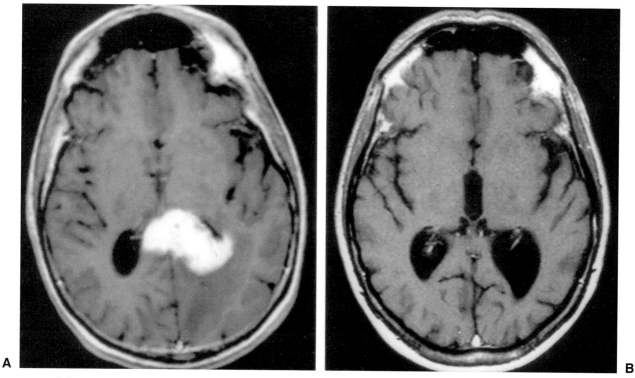

A

B

FIG. 41.1. Gadolinium-enhanced magnetic resonance scans showing complete response of primary central nervous system lymphoma to high-dose methotrexate, procarbazine, and vincristine.

patients and must be avoided only in those with large posterior fossa lesions. Eighty percent to 90% of patients have elevation of cerebrospinal fluid protein, usually less than 100 mg/dL. Positive cytology is reported in 0% to 50% of patients. Identification of malignant cells may be difficult when cell counts are low, reactive lymphocytes are present, or steroids have been administered (72). Because most primary central nervous system lymphomas are B-cell tumors,

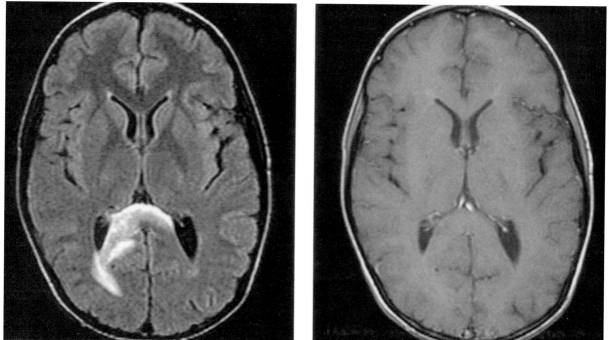

A

B

FIG. 41.2. Non-enhancing Epstein-Barr virus–positive cerebral lymphoma in an immunocompromised patient after allogeneic T-cell–depleted bone marrow transplant acute lymphocytic leukemia.

demonstration of a monoclonal B-cell population by immunocytochemistry or immunoglobulin gene rearrangement may facilitate diagnosis (73).

Soluble CD27 in the cerebrospinal fluid has been reported as a useful marker for primary central nervous system lymphoma. A CD27 level greater than 15 units/mL was associated with primary central nervous system lymphoma but was not found in the cerebrospinal fluid of patients with glial tumors or inflammatory neurologic conditions (74,75). In AIDS patients, cerebrospinal fluid analysis for both cytology and Epstein-Barr virus DNA using polymerase chain reaction analysis can establish the diagnosis. Cerebrospinal fluid studies can also exclude other processes, such as progressive multifocal leukoencephalopathy, by testing for JC virus by polymerase chain reaction (76,77). Gleissner et al. recently demonstrated the usefulness of molecular genetic testing for primary central nervous system lymphoma in the cerebrospinal fluid (78). Polymerase chain reaction analysis of the complementary determining region III identified a monoclonal population of lymphoma cells in the cerebrospinal fluid of patients with primary and secondary central nervous system lymphoma. This may be an important new technique, but its sensitivity and specificity remain to be established.

Complete ophthalmologic work-up, including slit-lamp, is an essential part of the initial staging evaluation. Ocular lymphoma can appear as choroidal scleral thickening, widening of the optic nerve, or vitreous debris (58). These findings may be nonspecific, but in a patient with known primary central nervous system lymphoma, they confirm the presence of ocular lymphoma. Biopsy of the vitreous, or an anterior chamber tap, can be confirmatory in patients with isolated ocular lymphoma or ocular relapse (79). Patients treated with steroids can have a false-negative vitrectomy if the tumor has regressed (80). Alternatively, vitreitis that initially responds but then becomes refractory to corticosteroids suggests ocular lymphoma.

A systemic evaluation reveals another site of disease in approximately 3% to 4% of immunocompetent patients who present with typical primary central nervous system lymphoma (81). Consequently, systemic staging has a low yield and, in the absence of a clinical trial, probably adds little to the evaluation and care of a patient with primary central nervous system lymphoma.

DIFFERENTIAL DIAGNOSIS

The differential diagnosis for primary central nervous system lymphoma differs for immunocompetent and immunodeficient patients (Table 41.4). In the immunocompetent patient, brain metastases and primary brain tumors are the most common diagnostic concerns; demyelinating disease and inflammatory processes, such as neurosarcoidosis, may also be considered in some patients. Acute exacerbation of multiple sclerosis can resemble a periventricular enhancing lesion that improves or disappears after steroid administration (82). However, recurrent stereotypic symptoms reflect-

TABLE 41.4. *Most common differential diagnoses of primary central nervous system lymphoma*

Immunocompetent patients
  Glioma
  Metastasis
  Multiple sclerosis
  Sarcoid
Immunocompromised patients
  Infections
    Toxoplasmosis
    Fungal
    Viral (progressive multifocal leukoencephalopathy)
  Human immunodeficiency virus encephalopathy
  Abscess
  Glioma
  Metastasis

ing a single neurologic location and associated with a single recurrent enhancing lesion are suspicious for primary central nervous system lymphoma. Sarcoidosis may have a similar appearance to primary central nervous system lymphoma and responds to steroids (83,84), but it usually involves the hypothalamus and is frequently associated with pulmonary involvement. The diffuse enhancement pattern on magnetic resonance imaging often differentiates primary central nervous system lymphoma from glial tumors or metastases, which typically have areas of central necrosis. In addition, the deep location of most primary central nervous system lymphoma lesions is unusual for metastatic disease (85–90).

The main differential diagnoses for primary central nervous system lymphoma in the AIDS patient are toxoplasmosis and progressive multifocal leukoencephalopathy. Other opportunistic infections, human immunodeficiency virus encephalopathy, and other brain tumors should also be considered. To further complicate the situation, these processes may coexist with primary central nervous system lymphoma in the AIDS patient. In addition, systemic lymphoma in an AIDS patient is frequently extranodal with spread to the central nervous system. Therefore, an AIDS patient with primary central nervous system lymphoma should undergo a complete evaluation for systemic lymphoma to exclude a central nervous system presentation of systemic disease. In AIDS–related primary central nervous system lymphoma, the incidence of ocular involvement is unknown, but the high incidence of cytomegalovirus retinitis in AIDS patients can make the diagnosis difficult.

TREATMENT

Immunocompetent Patients

Early diagnosis and treatment are critical because primary central nervous system lymphoma is a highly aggressive tumor and, if not treated, is fatal. The median survival is approximately 2 to 3 months for untreated patients (Table 41.5) (91,92). Surgical resection alone gives a median survival of only 4 to 5 months, and resection may worsen the patient's neurologic deficit because of the deep location of most lesions (93). Therefore, the appropriate surgical approach for patients with primary central nervous system lymphoma is a stereotactic needle biopsy for diagnosis. Surgical resection should be reserved only for patients acutely deteriorating due to herniation from a large tumor mass.

A complete response to radiation treatment has been reported in up to 80% of patients with primary central nervous system lymphoma (94). Whole-brain radiation therapy was the standard treatment for primary central nervous system lymphoma and increased median survival to 12 to 18 months (71). Whole-brain radiation therapy is necessary because of the widespread, infiltrative nature of primary central nervous system lymphoma, even in a patient with only a single lesion on magnetic resonance imaging. Even though radiotherapy is highly effective at producing remission, recurrence is common within 1 year, and 5-year survival is only 3% to 4% (92,95–97). Different authors observed a threshold dose of 30 to 50 Gy, but no clear dose response could be documented. In a Radiation Therapy Oncology Group prospective study, patients were given 40 Gy whole-brain radiation therapy with a 20 Gy boost to the tumor site. The focal increase in the dose to 60 Gy did not improve local control; relapse was as frequent within the boosted field as outside of it. Patients older than 60 years of age had a median survival of 7.6 months, whereas those younger than 60 years of age had a median survival of 23.1 months (98). A similar observation was made regarding Karnofsky performance score. Patients with a Karnofsky performance score greater than or equal to 70 had a median survival of 21.1 months, whereas the median survival was 5.6 months for patients with a Karnofsky performance score of 40 to 60. In other studies, the importance of age and Karnofsky performance score was seen repeatedly (99).

Currently, when using whole-brain radiation therapy, a dose of 45 Gy is considered effective and sufficient; a boost

TABLE 41.5. *Median survival in months with different treatments*

Treatments	Months
Untreated	2–3
Surgery alone	4–5
CHOP + WBRT	9.5–16
WBRT	12–18
High-dose methotrexate ± WBRT	40–60

CHOP, cyclophosphamide, doxorubicin, Oncovin (vincristine), prednisone; WBRT, whole-brain radiation therapy.

is avoided. If ocular lymphoma is present, the eyes are included in the radiation port in addition to whole-brain radiation therapy. Radiation therapy can effectively control ocular lymphoma; however, relapse may occur after radiation therapy. The dose for ocular radiation therapy is 36 to 40 Gy to minimize any risk of permanent ocular toxicity. This dose usually causes accelerated cataract formation, which often requires repair several years after completion of radiation therapy. Because occult involvement of the leptomeninges is common in primary central nervous system lymphoma, craniospinal radiation therapy (24 to 40 Gy) was used in a group of patients; however, survival was not improved (100). In addition, neuraxis radiation therapy compromises subsequent chemotherapy administration by irradiating a large volume of bone marrow.

Chemotherapy is currently the initial treatment of choice for primary central nervous system lymphoma. In all chemotherapy-based studies, age and performance status were critical prognostic factors (99). Due to the histologic similarities between primary central nervous system lymphoma and systemic lymphoma, standard chemotherapy regimens for systemic lymphoma were used. Three trials used CHOP [cyclophosphamide, doxorubicin, Oncovin (vincristine), prednisone] combined with whole-brain radiation therapy, and all had a median survival identical to whole-brain radiation therapy alone (9.5 to 16 months) (101–103). Furthermore, patients incurred significant chemotherapy-related toxicity (101). These patients frequently developed leptomeningeal disease and brain recurrence, typically in areas remote from the primary site (103). The initial lesion(s) seen on imaging often responded to the first few cycles of CHOP because the drugs could penetrate the disrupted blood–brain barrier associated with bulky disease and reach the tumor. However, the microscopic tumor residing behind an intact blood–brain barrier and, therefore, not visualized on magnetic resonance imaging continued to grow, resulting in early recurrence (104). A successful chemotherapy regimen for primary central nervous system lymphoma requires drugs that penetrate the blood–brain barrier either because they can be delivered in high doses (e.g., methotrexate) or because they are intrinsically lipophilic (e.g., thiotepa).

Methotrexate administered in a standard dose does not cross the blood–brain barrier in a sufficient amount to treat tumor, but higher doses can reach a therapeutic concentration in the central nervous system. In multiple studies, high-dose methotrexate with leucovorin rescue emerged as the most effective drug for the treatment of primary central nervous system lymphoma (105–109). A wide range of doses has been used (1 to 8 g/m^2) without a clear dose-response relationship. Systemic high-dose methotrexate plus intra-Ommaya methotrexate, followed by whole-brain radiation therapy and high-dose cytarabine as initial therapy of primary central nervous system lymphoma gave a median survival of 42 months with a 22% 5-year survival. However, significant neurotoxicity was observed, especially in patients older than age 60 years at diagnosis (110). These patients developed progressive dementia, ataxia, and urinary incontinence. Some patients benefitted temporarily from a ventriculoperitoneal shunt, but the syndrome was irreversible (111).

More recently, preradiation methotrexate at 3.5 g per m² combined with procarbazine and vincristine was used to treat primary central nervous system lymphoma (Fig. 41.1). Chemotherapy was followed by whole-brain radiation therapy and high-dose cytarabine. The median survival was 60 months, giving a 50% 5-year survival. In an effort to reduce neurotoxicity, whole-brain radiation therapy was eliminated in patients older than 60 years of age; survival was identical in those who did or did not receive radiotherapy, and neurotoxicity was significantly decreased in those treated with chemotherapy alone. However, relapse was more common in those treated with only chemotherapy, and these patients died of recurrent primary central nervous system lymphoma, whereas those treated with chemotherapy and radiation therapy died of neurotoxicity. Despite these limitations, the quality of life was far superior when radiation therapy was not administered. In addition, some authors have reported that the use of single-agent high-dose methotrexate given in a prolonged regimen produced a high response rate, whereas others reported a poor outcome (112). Thus, every effort should be made to withhold whole-brain radiation therapy in patients older than 60 years of age who attain a complete response to chemotherapy; younger patients should receive whole-brain radiation therapy as part of the treatment regimen to minimize the risk of relapse. The standard dose of whole-brain radiation therapy administered in most combined modality studies is 45 Gy. Lower radiation doses may still be effective and potentially less toxic in patients who have attained a complete response after a high-dose methotrexate program. Yet, radiation dose reduction remains investigational because one study showed that radiation dose reduction from 45.0 to 30.6 Gy in patients younger than 60 years of age resulted in a significantly inferior 3-year survival (113).

An alternative approach is the use of intraarterial methotrexate after blood–brain disruption, with intraarterial mannitol plus systemic cyclophosphamide and procarbazine (114). This regimen is delivered monthly and rotated to all three arterial distributions; whole-brain radiation therapy is reserved for recurrence. The median survival is 40 months, and the authors report no delayed neurotoxicity (114–117). However, some patients develop procedure-related toxicity, including seizures, strokes, arterial dissection and cerebral swelling, pulmonary embolism, and renal toxicity (111,114). In addition, intraarterial chemotherapy markedly increases the drug exposure of normal brain, which may be associated with leukoencephalopathy (114,118).

High-dose systemic chemotherapy followed by autologous peripheral stem cell transplant has had some success for refractory or recurrent disease, but response was disappointing when used as the initial treatment (119,120). Different transplant regimens may have partially accounted for the disparate results. There is a single case report of remission of recurrent primary central nervous system lymphoma by a graft-versus-lymphoma reaction after allogeneic peripheral-blood stem cell transplantation (121). Despite all aggressive measures, 20% to 30% of patients do not respond to chemotherapy, and the median survival of these patients is 6 to 10 months (106). Alternately, approximately 50% of patients have a second remission with salvage treatment; 25% survive many years after reinduction.

Systemic high-dose methotrexate or cytarabine can also treat ocular lymphoma, as therapeutic drug levels can be achieved in the vitreous (122,123). If ocular disease is present at diagnosis, initial treatment with chemotherapy is often effective for both ocular and cerebral involvement. Ocular radiation therapy can follow chemotherapy to consolidate treatment of the eye disease. Intravitreal methotrexate has been used successfully for recurrent ocular lymphoma (124).

Immunocompromised Patients

Patients with AIDS have a median survival of 1 to 2 months when treated symptomatically. Even when treated with steroids and whole-brain radiation therapy, the median survival is only 2 to 5 months (125,126). Because primary central nervous system lymphoma occurs late in the course of human immunodeficiency virus infection, many patients die from opportunistic infections and not from primary central nervous system lymphoma. A few selected patients can tolerate chemotherapy and survive a median of approximately 1 year (127,128).

The institution of highly active antiretroviral therapy and antiviral therapy directed against Epstein-Barr virus can induce prolonged remission in some patients with AIDS–related primary central nervous system lymphoma (129,130). Tumor regression due to reconstitution of the immune system may explain the occasional AIDS patient with spontaneous remission of primary central nervous system lymphoma (131–134).

CENTRAL NERVOUS SYSTEM METASTATIC COMPLICATIONS OF SYSTEMIC NON-HODGKIN'S LYMPHOMA

Leptomeningeal Metastasis

Leptomeningeal metastasis develops in approximately 5% to 15% of patients with systemic non-Hodgkin's lymphoma, particularly in patients with a lymphoblastic or diffuse undifferentiated histology. Gururangan et al. reported a series of 362 children with central nervous system metastasis, 49 of whom had central nervous system disease at diagnosis (135). The median interval between the diagnosis of systemic non-Hodgkin's lymphoma and central nervous system involvement was 6 to 9 months in the 362 patients.

In another large series of 2,561 adult patients with lymphoma, 140 had central nervous system involvement from systemic lymphoma, and 67% of these 140 patients had leptomeningeal involvement (136). Leptomeningeal metastasis involves all levels of the neuraxis, leading to multifocal symptoms and signs, including headache, ataxia, cranial nerve palsies, back pain, radiculopathy, and sensory symptoms. The diagnosis is established by cerebrospinal fluid cytology or enhanced magnetic resonance imaging, showing definitive evidence of subarachnoid tumor such as enhancing nodules on the cauda equina or infiltration of cranial nerves.

Focal radiotherapy in a dose of approximately 30 Gy provides effective palliation to symptomatic sites such as the lumbosacral spine for cauda equina symptoms or the brain for cranial neuropathies. Neuraxis radiation therapy is avoided because of its high morbidity and limited efficacy. Radiation therapy is sometimes administered to areas of bulky disease seen on neuroimaging, even if they are not yet symptomatic, to prevent the development of additional neurologic disability, or to open potential sites of cerebrospinal fluid obstruction to facilitate subsequent intrathecal chemotherapy. This must be decided within the context of the patient's overall condition and therapeutic plan.

Intrathecal chemotherapy with methotrexate or cytarabine usually supplements radiotherapy of the involved neuraxis to treat the entire subarachnoid space. Intrathecal methotrexate (12 mg) or cytarabine (50 mg) is administered every 3 to 4 days for the first 3 weeks, with subsequent doses decreasing in frequency depending on the patient's response. The intrathecal drug is given as a fixed dose and not calculated according to the body surface area because the cerebrospinal fluid volume is approximately 150 cc in all adults regardless of size. Several reports suggest improved median survival when intrathecal chemotherapy is delivered through an Ommaya reservoir, compared with lumbar puncture (137–139). An Ommaya reservoir is also easier for the patient (and physician) for repeated drug instillation, and the physician can be assured that drug is actually delivered into the subarachnoid space, whereas some injections by lumbar puncture can lead to drug pooling in the epidural space. Furthermore, drug can also be given to patients via an Ommaya reservoir even when the patient is thrombocytopenic (≥20,000/mm³), whereas lumbar puncture is associated with a risk of epidural hematoma in this setting. Therefore, an Ommaya reservoir should be used in all patients with leptomeningeal metastasis in whom intrathecal chemotherapy is a planned component of treatment.

Intrathecal chemotherapy is distributed by bulk flow through the subarachnoid space and requires normal cerebrospinal fluid dynamics. Cerebrospinal fluid flow can be assessed by cerebrospinal fluid studies with radiolabeled indium. Intrathecal chemotherapy must be avoided in patients with obstruction of cerebrospinal fluid flow because drug delivery is impaired and can cause neurotoxicity. When drug is instilled into the ventricular system and does not egress properly, it can leak into the subependymal tissue, leading to leukoencephalopathy. Impaired cerebrospinal fluid flow is present when hydrocephalus is evident on imaging, there is increased intracranial pressure, or there are large subarachnoid tumor nodules. Occasionally, cerebrospinal fluid flow is abnormal even in the setting of normal

neuroimaging. Alternative treatment in the form of radiotherapy or systemic chemotherapy may be used until cerebrospinal fluid flow can be restored.

In patients with leptomeningeal lymphoma, high-dose methotrexate or cytarabine are alternatives to intrathecal chemotherapy. Response is comparable to intrathecal treatment, and systemic drugs can penetrate into areas of bulky disease that intrathecal chemotherapy does not treat well; however, there are more systemic side effects (137,140–142). In addition, systemic drug can be given in the presence of impaired cerebrospinal fluid flow.

Central nervous system prophylaxis with radiation therapy and chemotherapy has been effective in patients with non-Hodgkin's lymphoma (143,144). Usually, intrathecal or intraventricular chemotherapy is administered concurrently, with chemotherapy targeted against the systemic disease (145,146). Central nervous system prophylaxis is recommended for patients with stage IV disease, Waldeyer's ring involvement, and lymphoblastic undifferentiated, diffuse histocytic lymphoma, or small cell–type histologies (137,147). Haddy et al. demonstrated that prophylactic intrathecal chemotherapy effectively prevented spread to the central nervous system in patients without initial central nervous system involvement; 28% of patients who did not receive prophylaxis had a central nervous system relapse, compared with 8% who received intrathecal drug (147). In ocular adnexal lymphoma, central nervous system prophylaxis with radiotherapy or chemotherapy did not reduce central nervous system relapse (148).

Epidural Tumors

Symptomatic spinal cord compression was due to lymphoma in 10% of 583 patients with malignant cord compression (149). In another series of 265 patients with epidural spinal metastasis from various systemic cancers, 6.8% had lymphoma (149). Epidural metastasis from systemic lymphoma usually involves the thoracic spine and is associated with extensive retroperitoneal disease; less commonly, the lumbosacral and cervical spine can also be involved (150). Diffuse large-cell is the most common histology, although all histologic subtypes of lymphoma have been described causing epidural metastasis (136,151,152).

The most common signs and symptoms of epidural tumor are back pain, weakness, sensory loss, autonomic dysfunction, and ataxia. Pain is the earliest and most frequent presenting symptom of cord compression. Pain can be local, radicular, referred, or funicular in nature. Pain from epidural metastasis is generally mild at onset, but if not diagnosed and treated in a timely fashion, it progresses with increasing severity. More than one half of patients with thoracic epidural metastasis and cord compression have a radiating, tight, band-like pain around the chest or abdomen. In cervical and lumbosacral spine epidural disease, pain generally radiates to the arms or leg. Weakness is the second most common symptom resulting from root compression or corticospinal tract involvement (153,154). Motor signs may include bilateral leg weakness, spasticity, hyperactive deep tendon reflexes, and a Babinski's sign. Cauda equina involvement is manifest as unilateral or asymmetric leg weakness, hypotonia, decreased reflexes, and early sphincter disturbance. Sensory symptoms may include numbness and paresthesias that usually begin in the legs and ascend to the level of cord compression.

Diagnosis is established by spinal magnetic resonance imaging. Contrast is not necessary, and the entire spine must be imaged, even in patients with a single focus of pain, because multilevel epidural tumor can be found in approximately 10% of patients. Plain films and bone scan can miss epidural tumor, particularly in lymphoma patients, because disease can extend directly into the epidural space from paravertebral tumor without destroying the bony elements of the spine. Thus, any lymphoma patient with back pain should undergo magnetic resonance imaging of the spine.

Once diagnosed, patients with epidural metastasis should be treated with high-dose corticosteroids, which rapidly relieve pain and may improve neurologic function. For a patient with a confirmed systemic lymphoma and newly diagnosed epidural metastasis, local radiation therapy using 30 to 40 Gy is the treatment of choice (155,156). If the diagnosis is not confirmed or the patient has relapsed, surgical decompression may become necessary for diagnosis or treatment. Initial surgery followed by radiation therapy does not improve survival or functional outcome, as compared with radiation therapy alone. Systemic chemotherapy is an alternative for patients with spinal epidural disease, and minimal or no symptoms or signs, who need to receive chemotherapy for their systemic tumor. Such patients need to be followed closely, and if they do not experience a rapid response or there is progression of the epidural disease, then focal radiation therapy needs to be administered promptly (157).

Brain Metastasis

Brain metastasis develops in less than 1% of patients with lymphomas. Patients with cerebral metastasis can be symptomatically treated with high-dose steroids. If the diagnosis is not confirmed, steroids should be withheld until biopsy. These patients may be treated with the same high-dose methotrexate regimens as primary central nervous system lymphoma patients, because regular systemic chemotherapy for non-Hodgkin's lymphoma does not penetrate the blood–brain barrier effectively. If the patient's medical condition does not permit high-dose chemotherapy or in patients with advanced systemic disease, palliative whole-brain radiation therapy can be effective. Patients with intracerebral disease frequently have leptomeningeal involvement and should be treated with intrathecal chemotherapy as well.

REFERENCES

1. Forsyth PA, DeAngelis LM. Biology and management of AIDS associated primary CNS lymphoma. *Hematol Oncol Clin North Am* 1996; 10:1125–1134.
2. Lutz J-M, Coleman MP. Trends in primary cerebral lymphoma. *Br J Cancer* 1994;70:716–718.
3. Bailey P. Intracranial sarcomatous tumors of leptomeningeal origin. *Arch Surg* 1929;18:1359–1402.
4. Schaumburg HH, Plank CR, Adams RD. The reticulum cell sarcoma—microglioma group of brain tumors. A consideration of their clinical features and therapy. *Brain* 1972;95:199–212.
5. Yulie CL. Case of primary reticulum cell sarcoma of the brain. Relationship of microglial cells to histiocytes. *Arch Path* 1938;26:1037–1044.
6. Henry JM, Heffner RR Jr, Dillard SH, et al. Primary malignant lymphomas of the central nervous system. *Cancer* 1974;34:1293–1302.
7. Hochberg FH, Miller DC. Primary central nervous lymphoma. *J Neurosurg* 1988;68:835–853.
8. Nakhleh RE, Manivel JC, Hurd D, et al. Central nervous system lymphoma immunohistochemical and immunopathologic study of 26 autopsy cases. *Arch Pathol Lab Med* 1989;113:1050–1056.
9. Taylor CR, Russel R, Lukes RJ, et al. An immunohistological study of immunoglobulin content of primary central nervous system lymphoma. *Cancer* 1978;41:2197–2205.
10. Tomlinson FH, Kurtin PJ, Suman VJ, et al. Primary intracerebral lymphoma: a clinicopathological study of 89 patients. *J Neuro surg* 1995;82:558–566.
11. Jellinger KA, Radaskiewicz TH, Slowik F. Primary malignant lymphomas of the central nervous system in man. *Acta Neuro Pathol* 1975;6:95–102.
12. Zimmerman HM. Malignant lymphomas of the nervous system. *Acta Neuropathol* 1975;6:69–74.
13. Eby NL, Grufferman S, Flannelly CM, et al. Increasing incidence of primary brain lymphoma in the U.S. *Cancer* 1988;62:461–465.
14. Krogh-Jensen M, D'Amore FD, Jensen MK, et al. Clinicopathological features, survival, and prognostic factors of primary central nervous system lymphoma: trends in incidence of primary central nervous system lymphoma and primary malignant brain tumors in a well-defined geographic area. *Leuk Lymph* 1995;19:223–233.
15. Yau Y, O'Sullivan M, Signorini D, et al. Primary lymphoma of the central nervous system in immunocompetent patients in south-east Scotland. *Lancet* 1996;348:890.
16. Hao D, DiFrancesco LM, Brasher P, et al. Is the incidence of primary CNS lymphoma increasing? A population based study of incidence, clinicopathological features, and outcomes in Alberta from 1975 to 1996. *Ann Neurol* 1997;42:537.
17. Raizer JR, DeAngelis LM. Primary central nervous system lymphoma. In: Raghaven D, Brecher ML, Johnson DH, eds. *Textbook of uncommon cancer*, 2nd ed. Sussex, UK: John Wiley and Sons, 1999:323.
18. Lehrich JR, Richardson EP Jr. Malignant lymphoma with Sjögren's syndrome. Case records of the Massachusetts General Hospital. *N Engl J Med* 1978;299:1349–1359.
19. Good AE, Russo RH, Schnitzer B, et al. Intracranial histiocytic lymphoma with rheumatoid arthritis. *J Rheumatol* 1978;5:75–78.
20. Lipsmeyer EA. Development of malignant cerebral lymphoma in a patient with systemic lupus erythematous treated with immunosuppression. *Arthritis Rheum* 1972;15:183–186.
21. Diette KM, Caro WA, Roenigk HH Jr. Malignant lymphoma presenting with cutaneous granulomas. *J Am Acad Dermatol* 1984;10:896–902.
22. Jellinger K, Slowik, F, Sluga E. Primary intracranial malignant lymphomas. A fine structure, cytochemical and CSF immunological study. *Clin Neurol Neurosurg* 1979;81:173–184.
23. Varadachari C, Palutke M, Climie AR, et al. Immunoblastic sarcoma (histiocytic lymphoma) of the brain with B cell markers. *J Neurosurg* 1978;49:887–892.
24. Neault RW, Van Scoy RE, Okazaki H, et al. Uveitis associated with isolated reticulum cell sarcoma of the brain. *Am J Ophthalmol* 1972;73:431–436.
25. Schabet M. Epidemiology of primary CNS lymphoma. *J Neurooncol* 1999;43:199–201.
26. DeAngelis LM. Primary central nervous system lymphoma as a secondary malignancy. *Cancer* 1991;67:431–435.
27. Hochberg FH, Miller DC. Primary central nervous system lymphoma. *J Neurosurg* 1988;68:835–853.
28. Fine HA, Mayer RJ. Primary central nervous system lymphoma. *Ann Int Med* 1993;119:1093–1104.
29. Remick SC, Diamond C, Migliozzi JA, et al. Primary central nervous system lymphoma in patients with and without the acquired immunodeficiency syndrome. A retrospective analysis and review of the literature. *Medicine* 1990;69:345–360.
30. Epstein LG, Dicarlo FJ Jr, Joshi VV, et al. Primary lymphoma of the central nervous system with acquired immunodeficiency syndrome. *Pediatrics* 1988;82:355–363.

31. Andiman WA, Eastman R, Martin K, et al. Opportunistic lymphoproliferations associated with Epstein-Barr viral DNA in infants and children with AIDS. *Lancet* 1985:2:1390–1393.
32. Belman AL, Diamond G, Dickson D, et al. Pediatric acquired immunodeficiency syndrome: neurologic syndromes. *Am J Dis Child* 1988; 142:29–35.
33. Del Mistro A, Laverda A, Calabrese F, et al. Primary lymphoma of the central nervous system in 2 children with acquired immune deficiency syndrome. *Am J Clin Pathol* 1990;94:722–728.
34. Filipovich AH, Heinitz KJ, Robison LL, et al. The immunodeficiency cancer registry. A research resource. *Am J Pediatr Hematol Oncol* 1987;9:183–184.
35. Penn I, Porat G. Central nervous system lymphomas in organ allograft recipients. *Transplantation* 1995;59:240–244.
36. Bashir RM, Harris NL, Hochberg FH, et al. Detection of Epstein-Barr virus in CNS lymphoma by in-situ hybridization. *Neurology* 1989; 39:813–817.
37. Cingolani A, Gastaldi R, Fassone L, et al. Epstein-Barr virus infection is predictive of CNS involvement in systemic AIDS-related non-Hodgkin's lymphomas. *J Clin Oncol* 200;18:3325–3330.
38. Cinque P, Brytting M, Vago L, et al. Epstein-Barr virus DNA in cerebrospinal fluid from patients with AIDS-related primary lymphoma of the central nervous system. *Lancet* 1993;342:398–401.
39. Morgello S. Pathogenesis and classification of primary central nervous system lymphoma: an update. *Brain Pathol* 1995;5:383–393.
40. Gijtenbeek JMM, Rosenblum M, DeAngelis LM. Primary central nervous system T-cell lymphoma. *Neurology* 2001;57:716–718.
41. Shibata S. Sites of origin of primary intracerebral malignant lymphoma. *Neurosurgery* 1989;25:14–19.
42. Miller DC, Hochberg FH, Harris NL, et al. Pathology with clinical correlations of primary central nervous system non-Hodgkin's lymphoma. The Massachusetts General Hospital experience 1958–1989. *Cancer* 1994;74:1383–1397.
43. Burger PC, Scheithauer BW. *Atlas of tumor pathology. Tumors of the central nervous system*, 3rd series. Washington, DC: Armed Forces Institute of Pathology, 1994.
44. Nakhleh RE, Manivel JC, Hurd D, et al. Central nervous system lymphomas. Immunohistochemical and clinicopathologic study of 26 autopsy cases. *Arch Pathol Lab Med* 1989;113:1050–1056.
45. Singh A, Strobos RJ, Singh BM, et al. Steroid-induced remissions in CNS lymphoma. *Neurology* 1982;32:1267–1271.
46. Van den Bent MJ, Vanneste JA, Ansink BJ. Prolonged remission of primary central nervous system lymphoma after discontinuation of steroid therapy. *J Neurooncol* 1992;13:257–259.
47. Itoyama T, Sadamori N, Tsutsumi K, et al. Primary central nervous system lymphomas. Immunophenotypic, virologic, and cytogenetic findings of three patients without immune defects. *Cancer* 1994;73:455–463.
48. Weber T, Weber RG, Kaulich K, et al. Characteristic chromosomal imbalances in primary central nervous system lymphomas of the diffuse large B-cell type. *Brain Pathol* 2000;10:73–84.
49. Nozaki M, Tada M, Mizugaki Y. Expression of oncogenic molecules in primary central nervous system lymphomas in immunocompetent patients. *Acta Neuropathol* 1998;95:505–510.
50. Koga H, Zhang S, Ichikawa T. Primary malignant lymphoma of the brain: demonstration of the p53 gene mutations by PCR-SSCP analysis and immunohistochemistry. *Noshuyo Byori* 1994;11:151–155.
51. Deckert-Schlüter M, Rang A, Wiestler OD. Apoptosis and apoptosis-related gene products in primary non-Hodgkin's lymphoma of the central nervous system. *Acta Neuropathol* 1998;96:157–162.
52. Cobbers JM, Wolter M, Reifenberger J, et al. Frequent inactivation of CDKN2A and rare mutation of TP53 in PCNSL. *Brain Pathol* 1999; 8:263–276.
53. Zhang SJ, Endo S, Ichikawa T, et al. Frequent deletion and 5' CpG island methylation of the p16 gene in primary malignant lymphoma of the brain. *Cancer Res* 1998;58:1231–1237.
54. DeAngelis LM. Primary central nervous system lymphoma. *Curr Opin Neurol* 1999;112:687–691.
55. Herrlinger U, Schabet M, Bitzer M, et al. Primary central nervous system lymphoma: from clinical presentation to diagnosis. *J Neurooncol* 1999;3:219–226.
56. Balmaceda C, Gaynor JJ, Sun M, et al. Leptomeningeal tumor in primary central nervous system lymphoma: recognition, significance, and implications. *Ann Neurol* 1995;38:202–209.
57. Chamberlain M. Leptomeningeal metastases. In: Levin V, ed. *Cancer in the nervous system*. New York: Churchill Livingstone, 1996:282.
58. Schild SE, Wharen RE Jr, Menke DM, et al. Primary lymphoma of the spinal cord. *Mayo Clin Proc* 1995;70:256–260.
59. Ursea R, Heinemann MH, Silverman RH, et al. Ophthalmic, ultrasonographic findings in primary central nervous system lymphoma with ocular involvement. *Retina* 1997;17:118–123.
60. Peterson K, Gordon KB, Heinemann MH, et al. The clinical spectrum of ocular lymphoma. *Cancer* 1993;72:843–849.
61. Buhring U, Herrlinger U, Krings T, et al. MRI features of primary central nervous system lymphomas at presentation. *Neurology* 2001;57:393–396.
62. Ciricillo SF, Rosenblum ML. Use of CT and MR imaging to distinguish intracranial lesions and to define the need for biopsy in AIDS patients. *J Neurosurg* 1990;73:720–724.
63. Kosuda S, Aoki S, Suzuki K, et al. Primary malignant lymphoma of the central nervous system by Ga-67 and TI-201 brain SPECT. *Clin Nucl Med* 1992;17:961–964.
64. Akiyama Y, Moritake K, Yamasaki T, et al. The diagnostic value of 123I-IMP SPECT in non-Hodgkin's lymphoma of the central nervous system. *J Nucl Med* 2000;41:1777–1783.
65. DeAngelis LM. Cerebral lymphoma presenting as a non-enhancing lesion on computed tomographic/magnetic resonance scan. *Ann Neurol* 1993;33:308–311.
66. Antinori A, De Rossi G, Ammassari A, et al. Value of combined approach with thallium-201 single-photon emission computed tomography and Epstein-Barr virus DNA polymerase chain reaction in CSF for the diagnosis of AIDS-related primary CNS lymphoma. *J Clin Oncol* 1999;17:554–560.
67. Luzzati R, Ferrari S, Nicolato A, et al. Stereotactic brain biopsy in human immunodeficiency virus-infected patients. *Arch Intern Med* 1996;156:565–568.
68. Apuzzo ML, Chandrasoma PT, Cohen D, et al. Computed imaging stereotaxy: experience and perspective related to 500 procedures applied to brain masses. *Neurosurgery* 1987;20:930–937.
69. Boiardi A, Silvani A. Primary cerebral non-Hodgkin's lymphoma (PCNSL): a review of new trends in management. *Ital J Neurol Sci* 1997;18:1–7.
70. Weller M. Glucocorticoid treatment of primary CNS lymphoma. *J Neurooncol* 1999;43:237–239.
71. DeAngelis LM. Current management of primary central nervous system lymphoma. *Oncology* 1995;9:63–71.
72. Ferreri AJ, Reni M, Villa E. Therapeutic management of primary central nervous system lymphoma: lessons from prospective trials. *Ann Oncol* 2000;11:927–937.
73. Hochberg FH, Miller DC. Primary central nervous system lymphoma. *J Neurosurg* 1988;68:835–853.
74. Murase S, Saio M, Takenata K, et al. Increased level of CSF soluble CD 27 in patients with primary central nervous lymphoma. *Cancer Lett* 1998;132:181–186.
75. Murase S, Saio M, Andoh H, et al. Diagnostic utility of CSF soluble CD27 for primary central nervous system lymphoma in immunocompetent patients. *Neurol Res* 2000;22:434–442.
76. Fedele CG, Avellon A, Ciardi M, et al. Quantitation of polyomavirus DNA by a competitive nested polymerase chain reaction. *J Virol Methods* 2000;88:51–61.
77. Samorei IW, Schmid M, Pawlita M, et al. High sensitivity detection of JC-virus DNA in postmortem brain tissue by *in situ* PCR. *J Neurovirol* 2000;6:61–74.
78. Gleissner B, Siehl J, Korfel A, et al. CSF evaluation in primary CNS lymphoma patients by PCR of the CDR III IgH genes. *Neurology* 2002;58:390–396.
79. Akpek EK, Ahmed I, Hochberg FH, et al. Intraocular-central nervous system lymphoma: clinical features, diagnosis, and outcomes. *Ophthalmology* 1999;106:1805–1810.
80. Peterson K, Gordon KB, Heinemann MH, et al. The clinical spectrum of ocular lymphoma. *Cancer* 1993;72:843–849.
81. O'Neill BP, Dinapoli RP, Kurtin PJ, et al. Occult systemic non-Hodgkin's lymphoma (NHL) in patients initially diagnosed as primary central nervous system lymphoma (PCNSL): how much staging is enough? *J Neurooncol* 1995;25:67–71.
82. DeAngelis LM. Primary central nervous system lymphoma imitates multiple sclerosis. *J Neurooncol* 1990;9:177–181.

83. Lexa FJ, Grossman RI. MR of sarcoidosis in the head and spine: spectrum of manifestations and radiographic responses to steroid therapy. *AJNR Am J Neuroradiol* 1994;15:973–982.

84. Pickuth D, Spielmann RP, Heywang-Kobrunner SH. Role of radiology in the diagnosis of neurosarcoidosis. *Eur Radiol* 2000;10:941–944.

85. Vecht CJ. Clinical management of brain metastasis. *J Neurol* 1998;245:127–131.

86. Davey P. Brain metastases. *Curr Prob Cancer* 1999;23:59–98.

87. Wen PY, Loeffler JS. Management of brain metastases. *Oncology* 1999:941–954, 957–961.

88. Chidel MA, Suh JH, Barnett GH. Brain metastases: presentation, evaluation, and management. *Cleve Clin J Med* 2000;67:120–127.

89. Bentson JR, Steckel RJ, Kagan AR. Diagnostic imaging in clinical cancer management: brain metastases. *Invest Radiol* 1988;23:335–341.

90. Patchell RA. Brain metastases. *Neurol Clin* 1991;9:817–824.

91. Henry JM, Heffner RR Jr, Dillard SH, et al. Primary malignant lymphomas of the central nervous system. *Cancer* 1974;34:1293–1302.

92. Reni M, Ferreri AJ, Garancini MP, et al. Therapeutic management of primary central nervous system lymphoma in immunocompetent patients: results of a critical review of the literature. *Ann Oncol* 1997; 8:227–234.

93. Murray K, Kun L, Cox J. Primary malignant lymphoma of the central nervous system. Results of treatment of 11 cases and review of the literature. *J Neurosurg* 1986;65:600–607.

94. Corn BW, Dolinskas C, Scott C, et al. Strong correlation between imaging response and survival among patients with primary central system lymphoma: a secondary analysis of RTOG studies 83-15 and 88-06. *Int J Radiat Oncol Biol Phys* 2000;47:299–303.

95. Phan TG, O'Neill BP, Kurtin PJ. Post-transplant primary CNS lymphoma. *J Neurooncol* 2000;2:229–238.

96. Sagerman RH, Cassady JR, Chang CH. Radiation therapy for intracranial lymphoma. *Radiology* 1967;88:552–554.

97. Pollack IF, Lunsford LD, Flickinger JC, et al. Prognostic factors in the diagnosis and treatment of primary central nervous system lymphoma. *Cancer* 1989;63:939–947.

98. Nelson DF, Martz KL, Bonner H, et al. Non-Hodgkin's lymphoma of the brain: can high dose, large volume radiation therapy improve survival? Report on a prospective trial by the Radiation Therapy Oncology Group (RTOG): RTOG 8315. *Int J Radiat Oncol Biol Phys* 1992;23:9–17.

99. Correy J, Smith JG, Wirth A, et al. Primary central nervous lymphoma: age and performance status are more important than treatment modality. *Int J Radiat Oncol Biol Phys* 1998;41:615–620.

100. Brada M, Dearnaley D, Horwich A, et al. Management of primary cerebral lymphoma with initial chemotherapy: preliminary results and comparison with patients treated with radiotherapy alone. *Int J Radiat Oncol Biol Phys* 1990;18:787–792.

101. Schultz C, Scott C, Sherman W, et al. Pre-irradiation chemotherapy with cyclophosphamide, doxorubicin, vincristine, and dexamethasone for primary CNS lymphomas: initial report of radiation therapy oncology group protocol 88-06. *J Clin Oncol* 1996;2:556–564.

102. O'Neill BP, Wang CH, O'Fallon JR, et al. Primary central nervous system non-Hodgkin's lymphoma (PCNSL): survival advantages with combined initial therapy? A final report of the North Central Cancer Treatment Group (NCCTG) Study 86-72-52. *Int J Radiat Oncol Biol Phys* 1999;43:559–563.

103. Lachance DH, Brizel DM, Gockerman JP, et al. Cyclophosphamide, doxorubicin, vincristine, and prednisone for primary central nervous system lymphoma: short-duration response and multifocal intracerebral recurrence preceding radiotherapy. *Neurology* 1994;9:44:1721–1727.

104. Ott RJ, Brada M, Flower MA, et al. Measurements of blood-brain barrier permeability in patients undergoing radiotherapy and chemotherapy for primary cerebral lymphoma. *Eur J Cancer* 1991;27:1356–1361.

105 Blay JY, Conroy T, Chevreau C, et al. High-dose methotrexate for the treatment of primary cerebral lymphoma: analysis of survival and late neurologic toxicity in a retrospective series. *J Clin Oncol* 1998;16:864–871.

106. DeAngelis LM, Yahalom J, Thaler HT, et al. Combined modality therapy for primary CNS lymphoma. *J Clin Oncol* 1992;10:635–643.

107. DeAngelis LM. Primary CNS lymphoma: treatment with combined chemotherapy and radiotherapy. *J Neurooncol* 1999;43:249–257.

108. DeAngelis LM, Yahalom J, Heinemann MH, et al. Primary CNS lymphoma: combined treatment with chemotherapy and radiotherapy. *Neurology* 1990;40:80–86.

109. Blay JY, Bouhour D, Carrie C, et al. The C5R protocol: a regimen of high-dose chemotherapy and radiotherapy in primary cerebral non-Hodgkin's lymphoma of patients with no known cause of immunosuppression. *Blood* 1995;86:2922–2929.

110. Schlegel U, Pels H, Oehring R. Neurologic sequelae of treatment of primary CNS lymphoma. *J Neurooncol* 1999;43:277–286.

111. McAllister LD, Doolittle ND, Guastadisegni PE, et al. Cognitive outcomes and long-term follow-up results after enhanced chemotherapy delivery for primary central nervous system lymphoma. *Neurosurgery* 2000;46:51–60.

112. Herrlinger U, Schaber M, Brugger W, et al. German Cancer Society Neuro-Oncology Working Group NOA-03 multicenter trial of single-agent high dose methotrexate for primary central nervous system lymphoma. *Ann Neurol* 2002;51:247–252.

113. Bessell EM, Lopez-Guillermo A, Villa S, et al. Importance of radiotherapy in the outcome of patients with primary CNS lymphoma: an analysis of the CHOD/BVAM regimen followed by two different radiotherapy treatments. *J Clin Oncol* 2001;20:231–236.

114. Doolittle ND, Miner ME, Hall WA, et al. Safety and efficacy of a multicenter study using intraarterial chemotherapy in conjunction with osmotic opening of the blood-brain barrier for the treatment of patients with malignant brain tumors. *Cancer* 2000;88:637–647.

115. Neuwelt EA, Pagel M, Barnett P, et al. Pharmacology and toxicity of intracarotid adriamycin administration following osmotic blood-brain barrier modification. *Cancer Res* 1981;41:4466–4470.

116. Rosenblum MK, Delattre JY, Walker RW, et al. Fatal necrotizing encephalopathy complicating treatment of malignant gliomas with intra-arterial BCNU and irradiation: a pathological study. *J Neurooncol* 1989;7:269–281.

117. Dahlborg SA, Henner WD, Crossen JR, et al. Non-AIDS primary CNS lymphoma: first example of a durable response in a primary brain tumor using enhanced chemotherapy delivery without cognitive loss and without radiotherapy. *Cancer J Sci Am* 1996;2:166.

118. Gelman M, Chakeres DN, Newton HB. Brain tumors: complications of cerebral angiography accompanied by intraarterial chemotherapy. *Radiology* 1999;10:135–140.

119. Abrey LE, Rosenblum MK, Papadopoulos E, et al. High-dose chemotherapy with autologous stem cell rescue in adults with malignant primary brain tumors. *J Neurooncol* 1999;9:147–153.

120. Soussain C, Suzan F, Hoang-Xuan K, et al. Results of intensive chemotherapy followed by hematopoietic stem-cell rescue in patients with refractory or recurrent primary CNS lymphoma or intraocular lymphoma. *J Clin Oncol* 2001;19:742–749.

121. Varadi G, Or R, Kapelushnik J, et al. Graft-versus-lymphoma effect after allogeneic peripheral blood stem cell transplantation for primary central nervous system lymphoma. *Leuk Lymphoma* 1999;34:185–190.

122. De Smet MD, Stark-Vancs V, Kohler DR. Intraocular level of methotrexate after intravenous administration. *Am J Ophthalmol* 1996;121:442–444.

123. Strauchen JA, Dalton J, Friedman AH. Chemotherapy in the management of intraocular lymphoma. *Cancer* 1989;63:1918–1921.

124. De Smet MD, Stark-Vanes V, Kohler D, et al. Intravitreal chemotherapy for the treatment of recurrent intraocular lymphoma. *Br J Ophthalmol* 1999;83:448–451.

125. Kaufmann T, Nisce LZ, Coleman M. A comparison of survival of patients treated for AIDS-related central nervous system lymphoma with and without tissue diagnosis. *Int J Radiat Oncol Biol Phys* 1996;36:429–432.

126. Ling SM, Roach A, Larson DA, et al. Radiotherapy of primary CNS lymphoma in patients with and without HIV. *Cancer* 1994;73:2570–2582.

127. Forsyth PA, Yahalom J, DeAngelis LM. Combined-modality therapy in the treatment of primary central nervous system lymphoma in AIDS. *Neurology* 1994;44:1473–1479.

128. Chamberlain MC, Kormanik PA. AIDS-related central nervous system lymphomas. *J Neurooncol* 1999;43:269–276.

129. Hoffmann C, Tabrizian S, Wolf E, et al. Survival of AIDS patients with primary central nervous system lymphoma is dramatically improved by HAART-induced immune recovery. *AIDS* 2001;15:2119–2127.

130. Chow KU, Mitrou PS, Geduldig K, et al. Changing incidence and survival in patients with AIDS-related non-Hodgkin's lymphomas in the era of highly active antiretroviral therapy (HAART). *Leuk Lymphoma* 2001;41:105–116.

131. Sugita Y, Shigemori M, Yuge T, et al. Spontaneous regression of primary malignant intracranial lymphoma. *Surg Neurol* 1988;30:148–152.

132. Heinzlef O, Poisson M, Delattre JY. Spontaneous regression of primary cerebral lymphoma. *Rev Neurol* 1996;152:135–138.

133. Al-Yamany M, Lozano A, Nag S, et al. Spontaneous remission of pri-

mary central nervous system lymphoma: report of 3 cases and discussion of pathophysiology. *J Neurooncol* 1999;42:151–159.

134. Daniels D, Lowdell CP, Glaser MG. The spontaneous regression of lymphoma in AIDS. *Clin Oncol* 1992;4:196–197.

135. Gururangan S, Sposto R, Cairo MS, et al . Outcome of CNS disease at diagnosis in disseminated small noncleaved-cell lymphoma and B-cell leukemia: a Children's Cancer Group study. *J Clin Oncol* 2000;18:2017–2025.

136. Hollender A, Kvaloy S, Lote K, et al. Prognostic factors in 140 adult patients with non-Hodgkin's lymphoma with systemic central nervous system (CNS) involvement. A single centre analysis. *Eur J Cancer* 2000;36:1762–1768.

137. Mackintosh FR, Colby TV, Podolsky, et al. Central nervous system involvement in non-Hodgkin's lymphoma: an analysis of 105 cases. *Cancer* 1982;49:586–595.

138. Raz I, Siegal T, Polliack A. CNS involvement by non-Hodgkin's lymphoma. *Arch Neurol* 1984;41:1167–1171.

139. Recht L, Straus DJ, Cirrincione C, et al. Central nervous system metastases from non-Hodgkin's lymphoma: treatment and prophylaxis. *Am J Med* 1988;84:425–435.

140. Skarin AT, Zuckermann KS, Pitman SW, et al. High dose methotrexate with folinic acid in the treatment of advanced non-Hodgkin lymphoma including CNS involvement. *Blood* 1977;50:1039–1047.

141. Amadori S, Papa G, Avvisati G, et al. Sequential combination of systemic high-dose ara-C and asparaginase for the treatment of central nervous system leukemia and lymphoma. *J Clin Oncol* 1984;2:98–101.

142. Morra E, Lazzarino M, Brusamolino E, et al. The role of systemic high-dose cytarabine in the treatment of central nervous system leukemia. *Cancer* 1993;72:439–445.

143. Duque-Hammershaimb L, Wollner N, Miller DR. LSA2-L2 protocol treatment of stage IV non-Hodgkin's lymphoma in children with partial and extensive bone marrow involvement. *Cancer* 1983;52:39–43.

144. Tomita N, Kodama F, Sakai R, et al. Predictive factors for central nervous system involvement in non-Hodgkin's lymphoma: significance of very high serum LDH concentrations. *Leuk Lymphoma* 2000;38:335–343.

145. Recht L, Straus DJ, Cirrincione C, et al. Central nervous system metastasis from non-Hodgkin's lymphoma: treatment and prophylaxis. *Am J Med* 1988;84:425–435.

146. Cortes J, O'Brien SM, Pierce S, et al. The value of high-dose systemic chemotherapy and intrathecal therapy for central nervous system prophylaxis in different risk groups of adult acute lymphoblastic leukemia. *Blood* 1995;86:2091–2097.

147. Haddy TB, Adde MA, Magrath IT. CNS involvement in small noncleaved-cell lymphoma: is CNS disease per se a poor diagnostic sign? *J Clin Oncol* 1991;9:1973–1982.

148. Restrepo A, Raez LE, Byrne GE Jr. Is central nervous system prophylaxis necessary in ocular adnexal lymphoma? *Crit Rev Oncol* 1998;9:269–273.

149. Posner JB. *Neurologic complications of cancer*. Philadelphia: F.A. Davis, 1995.

150. Levitt LJ, Dawson DM, Rosenthal DS, et al. CNS involvement in non-Hodgkin's lymphoma. *Cancer* 1980;45:545–552.

151. Jellinger K, Radaszkiewicz T, Slowik F. Primary malignant lymphomas of the central nervous system in man. *Acta Neuropathologica* 1975;6:95–102.

152. Herman TS, Hammond N, Jones SE, et al. Involvement of the central nervous system by non-Hodgkin's lymphoma. *Cancer* 1979;43:390–397.

153. Gilbert RW, Kim J-H, Posner JB. Epidural spinal cord compression from metastatic tumor: diagnosis and treatment. *Ann Neurol* 1978;3:40–51.

154. Greenberg HS, Kim J-H, Posner JB. Epidural spinal cord compression from metastatic tumor: results with a new treatment protocol. *Ann Neurol* 1980;8:361–366.

155. Haddad P, Thaell JF, Kiely JM, et al. Lymphoma of the spinal extradural space. *Cancer* 1976;38:1862–1966.

156. Mead GM, Kennedy P, Smith JL, et al. Involvement of the central nervous system by non-Hodgkin's lymphoma in adults: a review of 36 cases. *Q J Med* 1986;60:699–714.

157. Wong ET, Portlock CS, O'Brien JP, et al. Chemosensitive epidural spinal cord disease in non-Hodgkin's lymphoma. *Neurology* 1996;46:1543–1547.

CHAPTER 42

Diagnosis and Management of Other Lymphoproliferative Disorders

Andre H. Goy, Hesham M. Amin, Fernando Cabanillas, and L. Jeffrey Medeiros

A wide variety of conditions can be associated with lymphadenopathy and mimic bona fide malignant lymphomas. These lymphoproliferative disorders are a heterogeneous group on the basis of their clinical presentation, pathogenesis, and outcome. In this chapter, we describe the diagnosis and management of a subset of these diseases, which have not been discussed comprehensively in other chapters.

CASTLEMAN'S DISEASE

Castleman's disease, also known as *angiofollicular lymph node hyperplasia*, was initially described as a mediastinal mass (1). This disorder is now recognized as a heterogeneous group of diseases with variable morphology and clinical presentation. Two main types are recognized: the hyaline vascular and the plasma cell variants. A mixed form of the disease has also been described. However, most of these cases, in our opinion, fit within the spectrum of the plasma cell variant. The hyaline vascular form of Castleman's disease is a well-defined entity. By contrast, the plasma cell variant is a heterogeneous entity.

Clinical Features

Hyaline Vascular Variant

The hyaline vascular variant of Castleman's disease almost always presents as a localized mass, most often involving the mediastinum (1–3), but other anatomic sites may be involved, including neck (4,5), the paraspinal region with spinal cord compression (6), retroperitoneal or abdominal masses (7,8), or even as an isolated pulmonary nodule (9). Typically, patients present with symptoms related to the mass, or the mass is identified incidentally. Patients rarely present with systemic (B type) symptoms.

Plasma Cell Variant

Patients with the plasma cell variant of Castleman's disease may present with localized or multicentric disease. Most

patients are adults in the sixth decade (median age, 55.5 years), and men are affected more often than women (1.4:1.0). Only rare cases have been reported in children, mostly in the context of primary immunodeficiency (10). The disease may be detected incidentally, usually in patients with localized disease. However, patients may present with systemic illness and B symptoms, particularly patients with multicentric disease.

The clinical characteristics of patients with multicentric plasma cell variant Castleman's disease have been defined in several series (11–13) and are summarized in Table 42.1. These patients can develop deep-seated lymphadenopathy, hepatosplenomegaly, rash, and skin lesions (14,15). Neurologic manifestations are uncommon but can occur, including seizures, central nervous system involvement, and occasionally leptomeningeal disease (16) or neuropathy (17). Demyelinating disease also has been reported (18). Other rare findings include blood-vessel compression leading to esophageal varices (19), destructive polyarthritis (20), glomerulonephritis (21), and connective-tissue diseases (22).

Pathogenesis

Human Herpesvirus-8

Human herpesvirus-8, originally described as *Kaposi's sarcoma herpesvirus*, is found in approximately 50% of cases of plasma cell variant Castleman's disease, a subset of localized cases, and most cases that are multicentric. Human herpesvirus-8 infects both B cells and T cells in Castleman's disease, and viral load has been shown to correlate with the aggressiveness of disease (23,24).

Human herpesvirus-8 carries at least 11 open reading frames that encode for homologs to cellular proteins involved in signal transduction (viral analogs of the interferon regulatory factors), cell cycle regulation proteins, inhibition of apoptosis proteins, and immune modulation proteins. Therefore, human herpesvirus-8 has the genetic machinery of an oncogenic virus (25–27).

Human herpesvirus-8 encodes for a homolog of the human interleukin (IL)-6, viral (v) IL-6, that is believed to play an

TABLE 42.1. *Clinical findings in multicentric Castleman's disease*

Finding	Percent
Clinical	
Lymphadenopathy	100
Peripheral	100
Abdominal	33
Mediastinal	10
B symptoms	98
Splenomegaly	69
Hepatomegaly	54
Edema/effusions	23
Rash	20
Neurologic changes	11
Laboratory	
Elevated sedimentation rate	90
Anemia	88
Hypergammaglobulinemia	82
Hypoalbuminemia	67
Thrombocytopenia	63
Proteinuria	16

important role in pathogenesis (described below) (27). Although v-IL-6 induces the same changes *in vitro* as does human IL-6, human herpesvirus-8 in plasma cell variant Castleman's disease may play a role in pathogenesis via other viral proteins, such as v-cyclin D1 and v-bcl-2, or indirectly through deregulation of the production of human cytokines (28,29).

Other Viruses

Plasma cell variant Castleman's disease, particularly the multicentric form, is relatively more frequent in the context of human immunodeficiency virus infection, in which the disease is typically florid (30,31). Most, but not all, cases of human immunodeficiency virus–associated Castleman's disease also show infection by human herpesvirus-8 (31). Epstein-Barr virus is only rarely detected in Castleman's disease of hyaline vascular or plasma cell type, as shown using a variety of molecular methods (32,33). This suggests that Epstein-Barr virus does not have a direct role in the pathogenesis of Castleman's disease, although Epstein-Barr virus may be involved in progression of disease.

Interleukin-6

The role of IL-6 in the plasma cell variant of Castleman's disease, either the localized or multicentric type, is well documented (34–37). Cells from lymph nodes involved by plasma cell variant Castleman's disease have been shown to produce high levels of IL-6. Human IL-6–positive cells also

can be identified by *in situ* hybridization or other techniques within biopsy specimens of patients with plasma cell variant Castleman's disease (36). v-IL-6 has been found in many cases that are associated with human herpesvirus-8 (38,39). In addition, B cells from Castleman's disease patients have been shown to overexpress IL-6 receptor (CD126) (40); therefore, both autocrine and paracrine mechanisms exist secondary to high IL-6 production by B cells.

IL-6 is a pleiotropic lymphokine produced by a variety of cells, including B and T lymphocytes, monocytes/macrophages, fibroblasts, endothelial cells, epidermal keratinocytes, and mesangial cells (34,41). IL-6 is an important B-cell growth factor involved in the terminal differentiation of activated B cells to plasma cells (42). IL-6 also stimulates plasma cells and hematopoiesis, regulates T cells, is an endogenous pyrogen, and stimulates the production of acute-phase reactants (C-reactive protein, fibrinogen, haptoglobin) from hepatocytes but inhibits albumin synthesis (43). Overproduction of IL-6 in plasma cell variant Castleman's disease patients may explain a number of phenomena that occur in these patients, including B symptoms, B-cell hyperreactivity and elevated sedimentation rate acute-phase reactants, hypergammaglobulinemia and hypoalbuminemia. The identification of many IL-6–positive cells in biopsy specimens of Castleman's disease correlates with the presence of B symptoms. Mice injected with bone marrow cells genetically engineered to overexpress IL-6 develop a syndrome similar to multicentric plasma cell variant Castleman's disease (44), and mice lacking a negative transcriptional regulator for IL-6 also develop abnormalities similar to multicentric plasma cell variant Castleman's disease. The "primary" defect that leads to overexpression of IL-6 in Castleman's disease, except for those cases associated with human herpesvirus-8 infection, is still poorly understood. Other cytokines are likely to be involved (45). The role of IL-6 in the hyaline vascular variant of Castleman's disease is not conclusive, and the results of studies that have assessed IL-6 expression in these lesions have been contradictory (36).

Immune Dysfunction

Frequent autoimmune phenomena or immune defects are associated with plasma cell variant Castleman's disease and cannot be explained only by the factors mentioned above. One theory is that the overexpression of IL-6 in the germinal centers affects the elimination of B cells that have undergone inappropriate gene mutations, thereby favoring the emergence of autoreactive clones (46). B cells in plasma cell variant Castleman's disease frequently coexpress CD5 and may correspond to the long-lived memory B cells that commonly produce autoantibodies (47). In this scenario, plasma cell variant Castleman's disease is a lymphoproliferation of autoantibody-producing cells, driven by IL-6, resulting in accumulation of plasma cells, bridging somewhat the overlap between Castleman's disease and autoimmune diseases. Others have suggested a primary immune defect in germinal center cell formation (25,48,49), leading to poor control and suppression of the humoral response, which participates in the accumulation of autoreactive cells (25).

Pathologic Features

Hyaline Vascular Variant

Hyaline vascular variant represents 80% to 90% of all cases of Castleman's disease and usually presents as a mass (that can be quite large) involving lymph node. The nodal architecture is preserved or partially effaced (50–52). Sclerosis is commonly present in the periphery of the lymph node, around the venules, and as bands traversing the nodal parenchyma. The subcapsular sinus is commonly obliterated. Lymphoid follicles can be small or large and often contain more than one small germinal center, so-called twinning (Fig. 42.1). Characteristically, the germinal centers are depleted of lymphocytes, have prominent follicle dendritic cells, and are penetrated by radial small blood vessels with hyalinized walls, forming so-called lollipop lesions (Fig. 42.2) (50–52). The mantle zones surrounding affected germinal centers are broad and often are composed of concentric rings of small lymphocytes referred to as an *onion skin–like pattern* (Fig. 42.3). In some cases, the follicle dendritic cells can be large and bizarre with dysplastic features (53). The interfollicular regions are rich in sclerotic blood vessels (high endothelial venules), and clusters of plasmacytoid monocytes (more recently designated as DC2 cells) are sometimes identified. Sheets of plasma cells are absent.

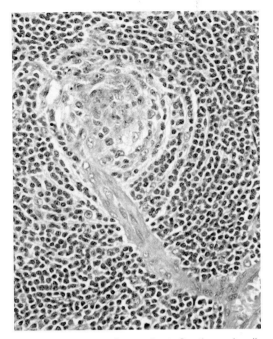

FIG. 42.2. Hyaline vascular variant Castleman's disease. Lymphoid follicle showing lymphocyte depletion and the characteristic "lollipop vascular lesion" (hematoxylin-eosin).

Immunophenotypic studies in hyaline vascular Castleman's disease, using flow cytometry or immunohistochemistry, show that the B cells are polytypic and the T cells have no evidence of an aberrant immunophenotype. In the lymphocyte-

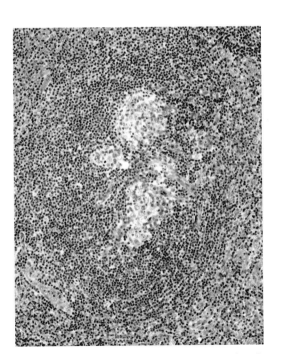

FIG. 42.1. Hyaline vascular variant Castleman's disease. Large lymphoid follicle that contains more than one lymphocyte-depleted germinal center, so-called twinning (hematoxylin-eosin).

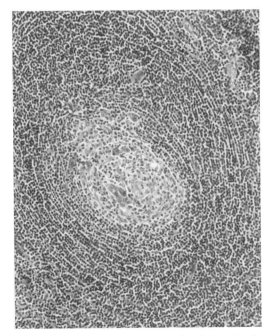

FIG. 42.3. Hyaline vascular variant Castleman's disease. Large lymphoid follicle showing lymphocyte depletion of the germinal center and surrounded by a broad mantle zone that forms the "onion skin–like" pattern (hematoxylin-eosin).

depleted germinal centers, the follicle dendritic cells often are present in tight clusters and are positive for CD21 (C3d receptor), CD23 [FcIgE receptor], and CD35 (C3b receptor). B cells in the expanded mantle zones have the immunophenotype of normal mantle-zone B cells [immunoglobulin (Ig) M and IgD positive] but are less well organized than in normal mantle zones. T cells are decreased within the interfollicular areas, with more CD4$^+$ than CD8$^+$ cells. The interfollicular blood vessels are positive for vascular markers, such as factor VIII and CD34. The interfollicular plasmacytoid monocytes are positive for CD68 and other markers of DC2 lineage.

Molecular studies of antigen receptor genes, most often the Ig heavy-chain (IgH) and T-cell receptor β-chain genes, usually have not shown evidence of gene rearrangements in hyaline vascular Castleman's disease. Conventional cytogenetic studies have been performed only rarely on these lesions. One case of hyaline vascular Castleman's disease reported had cytogenetic abnormalities after short-term cell culture (53), and the cells had the following karyotype: 46,XX,t(1;16)(p11;p11), del(7)(q21q22),del(8)(q12q22).

The differential diagnosis of the hyaline vascular variant of Castleman's disease includes non-Hodgkin's lymphomas, such as mantle cell lymphoma and follicular lymphoma. The germinal centers in mantle cell lymphoma and follicular lymphoma are usually not depleted of lymphocytes nor do they show hyaline vascular changes. Furthermore, the interfollicular areas are not hypervascular in lymphomas. Plasmacytoid monocytes are generally absent in lymphomas. The prominent mantle zones in hyaline vascular Castleman's disease can mimic the mantle-zone pattern of mantle cell lymphoma but are unusual in follicular lymphoma. Immunophenotypic and molecular studies are very helpful in difficult cases, as both mantle cell and follicular lymphomas show evidence of a monoclonal B-cell population.

Plasma Cell Variant

Plasma cell variant represents 10% to 20% of cases of Castleman's disease and may be localized or multicentric. Histologic features are similar in localized and multicentric plasma cell Castleman's disease (11,12,51,54). The lymphoid follicles are hyperplastic or normal in size, and usually at least a few follicles have hyaline vascular features. Characteristically, sheets of plasma cells are seen in the interfollicular zones. It has become clear that plasma cell variant Castleman's disease can be subdivided into two groups: cases associated with human herpesvirus-8 infection and those without human herpesvirus-8 infection (54,55). Virtually all cases of multicentric and a subset of localized plasma cell variant Castleman's disease are positive for human herpesvirus-8. Distinct histologic differences exist between the human herpesvirus-8–positive and human herpesvirus-8–negative cases (54).

The most prominent histologic feature in human herpesvirus-8–positive cases is blurring or obliteration of the boundaries between the mantle zones and the interfollicular areas (Fig. 42.4) (54). Another feature is the presence of increased

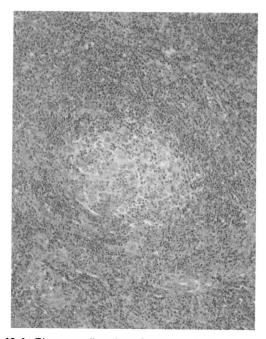

FIG. 42.4. Plasma cell variant Castleman's disease, human herpesvirus-8 positive. Lymph node showing obliteration of the boundaries between the mantle zone and the interfollicular areas (hematoxylin-eosin).

numbers of plasma cells and atypical plasmablasts/immunoblasts in the mantle zones (Fig. 42.5). Marked interfollicular vascularity (increased high endothelial venules) is also observed in most human herpesvirus-8–positive cases.

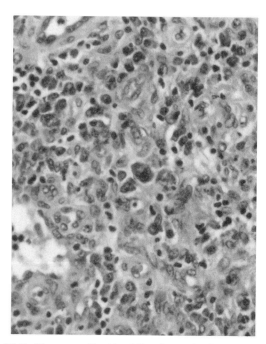

FIG. 42.5. Plasma cell variant Castleman's disease, human herpesvirus-8 positive. Increased atypical plasma cells in the mantle zone of a lymphoid follicle (hematoxylin-eosin).

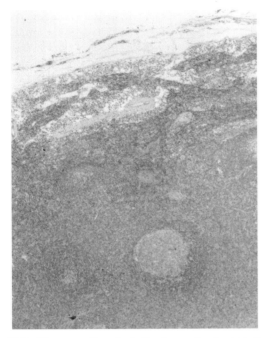

FIG. 42.6. Plasma cell variant Castleman's disease, human herpesvirus-8 negative. Lymph node at low power showing expansion of the interfollicular areas. The subcortical sinuses are dilated (hematoxylin-eosin).

In contrast, in human herpesvirus-8–negative cases of plasma cell variant Castleman's disease, the plasma cells are restricted to their normal location in interfollicular and medullary regions (Fig. 42.6). Compared with human herpesvi-

rus-8–positive cases, usually there are numerous intact hyperplastic follicles with modestly expanded mantle zones that are sharply demarcated from the surrounding interfollicular areas (Fig. 42.7). Interfollicular vascularity is generally less prominent in these lesions (54).

Immunophenotypically, there are distinct differences between the human herpesvirus-8–positive and human herpesvirus-8–negative cases of plasma cell variant Castleman's disease. Human herpesvirus-8 latent proteins ORF73/LNA-1 are detected in immunoblasts and small lymphocytes, largely present within the mantle zone of the lymphoid follicles (Fig. 42.8) (54,56). Human herpesvirus-8 lytic proteins K8, K10, K11, ORF59, and ORF65 are also expressed in these cells (57). Human herpesvirus-8 v-IL-6 is detectable in lymphoid cells surrounding the lymphoid follicles as well as in follicular dendritic cells (58,59). Vascular endothelial growth factor is expressed in the interfollicular plasma cells (60). The plasma cells in human herpesvirus-8–positive cases may express cytoplasmic monotypic Ig lambda light chain in approximately 40% of the cases (11,55). These findings suggest that human herpesvirus-8–positive Castleman's disease probably represents a lymphoproliferative disease (55). In human herpesvirus-8–negative Castleman's disease, by definition, viral proteins are absent, and the plasma cells are almost always polytypic.

Molecular studies have shown IgH gene rearrangements in 25% to 35% of cases of plasma cell variant Castleman's disease (61,62). Although the human herpesvirus-8 status of these cases was not known in many of these studies, gene rearrangements were most common in cases with human immunodeficiency

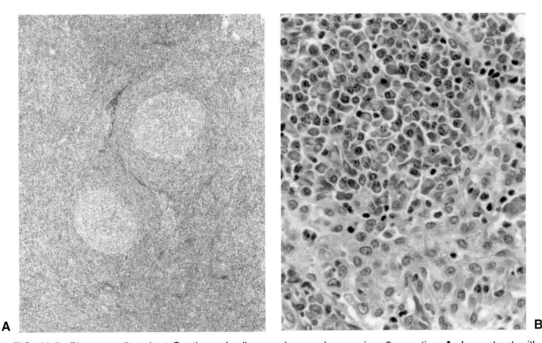

FIG. 42.7. Plasma cell variant Castleman's disease, human herpesvirus-8 negative. **A:** In contrast with human herpesvirus-8–positive cases (see Fig. 42.5), the reactive germinal centers are well defined. **B:** The plasma cells in human herpesvirus-8–negative cases also show typical morphologic features and are restricted to the interfollicular and medullary regions (hematoxylin-eosin).

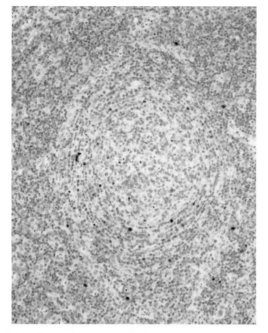

FIG. 42.8. Plasma cell variant Castleman's disease, human herpesvirus-8 positive. Immunostain for human herpesvirus-8 showing positive cells predominantly localized in the mantle zone of a lymphoid follicle (immunoperoxidase).

virus or Epstein-Barr virus infection, both being much more common in human herpesvirus-8–positive cases. In some cases, a predominant clone with an oligoclonal background has been described, similar to what is observed in immunodeficient patients such as those who have undergone organ transplantation (62). Rarely, T-cell receptor β-chain gene rearrangements have been reported in plasma cell variant Castleman's disease, usually in conjunction with IgH gene rearrangements, and may be examples of lineage infidelity that is known to occur in lymphoid neoplasms (63). The prognostic significance of these rearrangements is not clear nor is their presence considered unequivocal evidence of transformation to lymphoma.

Cytogenetic abnormalities have been detected infrequently in plasma cell variant Castleman's disease (64). One case of multicentric plasma cell variant Castleman's disease with the t(7;14)(p22;q22) involving the IL-6 gene locus was observed in a patient who had high serum levels of IL-6 (65).

The differential diagnosis of plasma cell variant Castleman's disease includes hyaline vascular variant Castleman's disease, other types of reactive lymphadenopathy with follicular hyperplasia and plasmacytosis, and malignant lymphomas. In most cases, the distinction between hyaline vascular and plasma cell variant Castleman's disease is obvious. However, many cases of the plasma cell variant can also have a few hyaline-vascular follicles. Others have designated these cases as being of mixed type (11). These mixed lesions, in most ways, resemble plasma cell variant Castleman's disease cases without hyaline-vascular follicles; thus, most pathologists now include these cases within the plasma cell variant category.

The distinction of plasma cell variant Castleman's disease from other types of reactive lymphadenopathy can be problematic. Syphilitic lymphadenopathy is one example in which prominent follicular hyperplasia and plasmacytosis can resemble, in part, plasma cell variant Castleman's disease. Unlike Castleman's disease, syphilis generally involves inguinal lymph nodes, and histologically, spirochetes are identified, and granulomas are frequently seen, particularly in cases of primary syphilis. Infection with human immunodeficiency virus also may show increased plasma cells, prominent vascularity in the interfollicular regions, and follicular hyperplasia in early-stage lesions that can resemble plasma cell variant Castleman's disease. Usually, the histologic findings are not as prominent as those observed in plasma cell variant Castleman's disease, and the clinical history is very helpful.

The plasma cell variant of Castleman's disease can also resemble malignant lymphoproliferative diseases involving lymph nodes, such as lymphoplasmacytic lymphoma and plasmacytoma. In lymphoplasmacytic lymphoma, reactive follicles are usually absent, the neoplastic cells usually have lymphoplasmacytoid cytologic features, and the tumor replaces architecture, unlike Castleman's disease. In addition, lymphoplasmacytic lymphoma usually expresses monotypic IgM and does not preferentially express Ig lambda. Usually, plasmacytoma shows diffuse replacement of the architecture, and the neoplastic plasma cells are cytologically atypical with prominent nucleoli, unlike Castleman's disease. Plasmacytomas more commonly are positive for monotypic Ig kappa, unusual in plasma cell variant Castleman's disease.

Castleman-Like Changes in Lymph Nodes of Patients with Malignant Lymphomas

Not uncommonly, lymph nodes involved by either Hodgkin's disease or non-Hodgkin's lymphoma or lymph nodes in proximity to affected lymph nodes can have many of the histologic changes of Castleman's disease, either the hyaline vascular or plasma cell variant. However, often the entire constellation of histologic findings that define either variant of Castleman's disease is absent, and patients do not have symptoms attributable to Castleman's disease. (The cases with symptoms attributable to plasma cell variant Castleman's disease are described below.) In the literature, lymph nodes with these changes have been referred to as having Castleman-like changes or being involved by Castleman's disease itself (50,66). Most likely, the histologic changes in these lymph nodes are nonspecific and may be caused by secretion of IL-6 or other cytokines related to the presence of the neoplasm. Underlying immune dysregulation associated with the neoplasm also may explain these Castleman-like changes.

Cancers Associated with Castleman's Disease

Patients with Castleman's disease are prone to developing a variety of neoplasms, in part dependent on the type of Castleman's disease. These may occur within the affected lymph node(s) or may occur subsequently, long after the diagnosis of Castleman's disease is established.

Tumors That Occur Simultaneously with Castleman's Disease

Follicle dendritic cell sarcomas may occur in lymph nodes involved by hyaline vascular Castleman's disease (53,67). In addition, in a subset of hyaline vascular Castleman's disease cases, dysplastic changes can be identified in follicle dendritic cells, suggesting that these are precursor lesions (53). Vascular neoplasms, but rarely Kaposi's sarcoma, also have been rarely described in hyaline vascular Castleman's disease (68).

Kaposi's sarcoma may arise in lymph nodes involved by plasma cell variant Castleman's disease and is particularly common in multicentric cases and those that occur in patients with human immunodeficiency virus infection (11,58). Lymphomas also can be associated with plasma cell variant Castleman's disease, in the same lymph node, or in nearby anatomic locations. The mixed cellularity type of Hodgkin's disease, often the interfollicular variant, is the most common type of Hodgkin's disease associated with plasma cell variant Castleman's disease (65,69). A number of non-Hodgkin's lymphomas have been reported to be associated with plasma cell variant Castleman's disease. In studies in which human herpesvirus-8 status was negative or unknown, mantle cell lymphoma, diffuse large B-cell lymphoma, and peripheral T-cell lymphoma were common (70). In patients with human herpesvirus-8 infection, as expected, there is an increased risk of human herpesvirus-8–positive lymphomas, including primary effusion lymphoma and plasmablastic lymphoma (71–73).

Solid tumors also have been reported to be associated with Castleman's disease of hyaline vascular or plasma cell type, usually as isolated case reports, including rectal carcinoma, pheochromocytoma, renal carcinoma, and thyroid carcinoma (74–78).

Tumors That Arise Subsequent to Castleman's Disease

Hodgkin's disease, non-Hodgkin's lymphomas, and plasma cell disorders have been reported to occur in patients subsequent to the diagnosis of plasma cell variant Castleman's disease. The risk of each lymphoma type correlates with presence or absence of human herpesvirus-8 infection. A recent review (70) described a relatively large group of human immunodeficiency virus–negative patients who had Castleman's disease and lymphoma. Human herpesvirus-8 status was not known for many of these patients. This group included 23 cases of non-Hodgkin's lymphoma and 27 cases of Hodgkin's disease. The non-Hodgkin's lymphomas occurred more often in patients with multicentric Castleman's disease and commonly arose within 2 years. Diffuse large B-cell lymphoma, with or without immunoblastic features, was the most common type. Hodgkin's disease, most often mixed cellularity type, more

often occurred in patients with localized Castleman's disease. As stated above, there is an increased risk of primary effusion lymphoma and plasmablastic lymphoma in human herpesvirus-8–positive patients (71–73).

Other Diseases Associated with Castleman's Disease

Pathologic features suggestive of Castleman's disease also can be seen in other nonneoplastic diseases, such as lymphoid interstitial pneumonia, pulmonary hyalinizing granuloma, myasthenia gravis, amyloidosis, and benign liver lesions (79–83). Castleman's disease plasma cell variant also occurs as a part of POEMS (polyneuropathy, organomegaly, endocrinopathy, M protein, and skin changes) syndrome as described below (84).

Management and Outcome

Hyaline Vascular Variant

Hyaline vascular Castleman's disease is usually localized; thus, it can be treated locally with surgical resection. In some cases in which resection might be impossible or incomplete, radiation has been used with good results (85,86). Hyaline vascular Castleman's disease recurs rarely, and the outcome is favorable.

Plasma Cell Variant

The treatment of plasma cell Castleman's disease is much more difficult and depends on the context. In the presence of human herpesvirus-8 infection, often associated with human immunodeficiency virus infection and multicentric disease, the prognosis is poor, with survival usually ranging from 9 to 12 months (31). Survival may also be poor if Castleman's disease is associated with aggressive malignant neoplasms such as diffuse large B-cell lymphoma or Kaposi's sarcoma. There are some reports of improvement of constitutional symptoms by using interferon-α, with prolonged remissions in some cases (87–89). Retinoids have been used in some patients (90). Nonspecific and temporary improvement occurs with steroids, but long-term toxicity obviously prevents prolonged use. Although conceptually appealing, reports of attempts to block IL-6–induced symptoms by monoclonal anti–IL-6 antibody remain anecdotal (91). Use of immunomodulators (e.g., suramin) in the authors' experience has resulted in improvement in a few cases. Conventional chemotherapy also has been used. Single agents, such as etoposide (30), or combination chemotherapy regimens identical to the ones used in aggressive lymphomas have been tried. At the authors' institution (92) and at others (93), intensive combination chemotherapy has resulted in complete remission in some patients. Surgical excision alone for patients with symptomatic plasma cell variant Castleman's disease is often inadequate, and patients die of the disease (92).

POEMS SYNDROME

POEMS syndrome also has been designated as *Crow-Fukase* (94), *PEP* (*p*lasma cell dyscrasia, *e*ndocrinopathy, and *p*oly-neuropathy), or *Takatsuki syndrome* (95) in the literature. The acronym POEMS, coined by Bardwick and colleagues in 1980 (84), captures a constellation of findings that are common in this syndrome, including polyneuropathy, organomegaly, endocrinopathy, M protein, and skin changes.

Clinical Features

A number of large case series and reviews of POEMS syndrome have been reported in the literature (84,94–98), the most recent being a series of 99 cases from the Mayo Clinic (98). Affected patients are usually adults in the sixth decade of life, and men are affected more often than women. The authors of the Mayo Clinic study suggest that the diagnosis of POEMS syndrome is best made by a combination of findings, which they divide into major and minor criteria as shown in Table 42.2.

Peripheral neuropathy is an almost constant finding in patients with POEMS syndrome. The neuropathy is usually symmetrical, ascending, and affects both sensory and muscular functions. When sural nerve biopsy is performed, in most cases demyelinization and edema are observed. Organomegaly includes hepatomegaly, splenomegaly, and lymphadenopathy. Lymph node biopsy, if performed, commonly shows plasma

TABLE 42.2. *Criteria for the diagnosis of POEMS syndrome*[a]

Major criteria
  Polyneuropathy
  Monoclonal plasmaproliferative disorder
Minor criteria
  Sclerotic bone lesions
  Castleman's disease
  Organomegaly (splenomegaly, hepatomegaly, or lymphadenopathy)
  Edema (edema, pleural effusion, or ascites)
  Endocrinopathy (adrenal, thyroid, pituitary, gonadal, parathyroid, pancreatic)
  Skin changes (hyperpigmentation, hypertrichosis, plethora, hemangiomata, white nails)
  Papilledema
Known associations
  Clubbing
  Weight loss
  Thrombocytosis
  Polycythemia
  Hyperhidrosis

POEMS, polyneuropathy, organomegaly, endocrinopathy, M protein, skin changes.
[a]Two major criteria and at least one minor criterion required for diagnosis (98).

cell variant Castleman's disease. In the Mayo Clinic study, 26% of patients had lymphadenopathy, but biopsy was performed in only 15; 11 patients had plasma cell variant Castleman's disease, and four patients had reactive but nonspecific lymph node findings (98). Endocrinopathy includes hypogonadism (most common), hypothyroidism, adrenal pituitary axis dysfunction, and diabetes mellitus. A monoclonal plasma cell dyscrasia is another virtually constant finding. Most patients have a monoclonal paraprotein in serum or urine. Skin changes can be variable and include hyperpigmentation (most common), hypertrichosis, acrocyanosis and plethora, and skin thickening.

Although not captured by the acronym POEMS, a number of other findings occur in this syndrome, including sclerotic or mixed lytic and sclerotic bone lesions that may be single or multiple, extravascular volume overload (peripheral edema or body-cavity effusions), papilledema, thrombocytosis, polycythemia, fatigue, renal failure, pulmonary hypertension, thrombotic events, and congestive heart failure (94–98).

Pathogenesis

The pathogenesis of POEMS syndrome is believed to be cytokine related, probably an imbalance of proinflammatory cytokines. IL-1, IL-6, vascular endothelial growth factor, and tumor necrosis factor-α are usually increased in the serum of patients with POEMS syndrome (99–104). An autoimmune disorder induced by a monoclonal gammopathy also has been suggested (105).

Pathologic Features

Monoclonal gammopathy is virtually always present in POEMS syndrome patients, more commonly in serum than in urine and most often composed of Ig lambda and either IgA or IgG (94,96–98). Nevertheless, iliac-crest bone marrow aspiration and biopsy usually show only a mild plasmacytosis. In the Mayo Clinic study, only 14% of patients had a plasmacytosis of more than 10%, and less than 5% of patients had more than 20% plasma cells (98). The plasma cells are commonly monotypic. In a subset of biopsy specimens, lymphoid aggregates are present that may contain lymphocyte-depleted germinal centers as are seen in Castleman's disease (106).

Bone lesions are commonly involved by osteosclerotic myeloma. These lesions resemble plasmacytoma, and bone marrow trabeculae are thickened by peritrabecular fibrosis. In these patients, bone marrow apart from the lesions, such as the iliac crests (mentioned above), usually shows only slight plasmacytosis (98).

As mentioned above, enlarged lymph nodes in POEMS syndrome patients are usually involved by plasma cell variant Castleman's disease, although some specimens may only show nonspecific reactive changes (97,98). The histologic features are similar to other cases of plasma cell variant Castleman's disease arising in other settings, as described previously. The frequency of Castleman's disease in POEMS syndrome is underestimated in the literature, as many patients do not undergo lymph node biopsy. Some of these cases have been associated with human herpesvirus-8 (107), but other studies have failed to demonstrate human herpesvirus-8 (108). In some cases of plasma cell variant Castleman's disease associated with POEMS syndrome, the affected lymph nodes also have had nodules or a diffuse infiltrate of monotypic plasma cells arising within a background of polytypic plasma cells, raising the differential diagnosis with plasmacytoma.

Management and Outcome

In the recent Mayo Clinic study, the median survival for patients with POEMS syndrome was 165 months (98). This survival is substantially better than that reported in other studies in which median survival has ranged from 12 to 33 months (94–97). The explanation for this discrepancy is uncertain. The number of aspects of the syndrome present in an individual patient do not correlate with prognosis, perhaps because patients continue to acquire different aspects of the syndrome during the course of the disease. Certain findings, however, do correlate with poorer prognosis, such as extravascular volume overload (98). Polyneuropathy and cachexia are the main causes of death.

Patients have been treated with some success using a variety of therapeutic modalities, including radiation therapy (109–111), chemotherapy (111–113), and high-dose chemotherapy with stem cell support (114,115). Radiation therapy is best used for patients with a single bone lesion or patients who have multiple bone lesions with one dominant lesion. Chemotherapy regimens used with some success include melphalan and prednisone or alkylator agents. There appears to be little role for plasmapheresis, cyclosporine, azathioprine, or intravenous Ig.

KIKUCHI-FUJIMOTO DISEASE

This disorder was first described independently by Kikuchi (116) and Fujimoto and colleagues (117) in Japan in 1972. *Kikuchi-Fujimoto disease*, also known as *necrotizing histiocytic lymphadenitis*, is a self-limited disorder that most often affects cervical lymph nodes in young Asian women. However, any nodal or extranodal site can be involved, and the disease has a worldwide distribution.

Clinical Features

Patients with Kikuchi-Fujimoto disease usually present with cervical lymphadenopathy and are often asymptomatic (118–120). However, Kikuchi-Fujimoto disease may be associated with fever of unknown origin, neutropenia, atypical lymphocytes in the peripheral blood, an elevated erythrocyte sedimentation rate, myalgias, or skin rash (118,120,121). Splenomegaly also has been reported in a small subset of patients. Extranodal presentations can occur but are unusual (122,123). Rare cases of Kikuchi-Fujimoto disease with skin involvement (124,125),

aseptic meningitis (126), polymyositis (127), brachial plexus neuritis (128), thyroiditis (129), or panuveitis also have been reported (130). The clinical course of patients with Kikuchi-Fujimoto disease is almost invariably benign, and the disease usually resolves spontaneously within a few months. Recurrence is rare (121,131). Multisystem involvement (132,133) also has been reported. In this circumstance, outcome may be poor, particularly in patients who have undergone organ transplantation (133). Although clinical presentation and radiologic studies can be suggestive of Kikuchi-Fujimoto disease, the final diagnosis requires tissue biopsy.

Laboratory studies show that approximately 25% to 50% of the patients have a decreased peripheral blood leukocyte count with neutropenia. Two percent to 5% of patients present with leukocytosis (120). Approximately one third of patients have atypical lymphocytes in their peripheral blood smears. Thrombocytopenia has been reported rarely in Kikuchi-Fujimoto disease patients (118). Some patients have an elevated erythrocyte sedimentation rate and C-reactive protein level. Autoimmune antibody studies, including rheumatoid factor, lupus erythematosus preparations, and antinuclear antibodies, are negative.

Pathogenesis

Little is known about the etiology and pathogenesis of Kikuchi-Fujimoto disease. Genetic susceptibility is likely to be involved. For example, certain human leukocyte antigen (HLA) class II alleles (e.g., DPBI *0202) are more common in Asians, perhaps explaining the higher frequency of Kikuchi-Fujimoto disease in Asia (134). The disease also has been reported in two sisters who were HLA identical, although they were not twins (135). In some cases, Kikuchi-Fujimoto disease has been associated with systemic diseases, such as systemic lupus erythematosus (136,137), adult Still's disease (138), and scleroderma (139). These associations further suggest a genetic component.

Kikuchi-Fujimoto disease may be the result of local hyperimmune stimulation after viral, bacterial, or parasitic infection. A variety of viruses have been identified in a subset of Kikuchi-Fujimoto disease cases using various techniques. These viruses include adenovirus, parvovirus (140), and members of the herpes virus family, including cytomegalovirus (141), Epstein-Barr virus (142–144), and human herpesvirus-6 (141,145). More recently, human herpesvirus-8 has been implicated, but this is controversial (146). Rare cases of Kikuchi-Fujimoto disease have been reported to be associated with human immunodeficiency virus (147) or human T-cell leukemia virus type I (148). Bacterial infections reportedly associated with Kikuchi-Fujimoto disease include *Yersinia enterocolitica* (149) and *Brucella* (150).

Whatever the etiology of Kikuchi-Fujimoto disease, apoptotic mechanisms are involved in pathogenesis. Histologic examination shows numerous cells with morphologic features of apoptosis, including nuclear pyknosis and fragmentation, but acute inflammation is absent (151,152). This has been confirmed using methods to assess apoptosis, such as terminal

FIG. 42.9. Kikuchi-Fujimoto disease. Lymph node showing extensive fibrinoid necrosis (upper right of field) located predominantly in the paracortical areas (hematoxylin-eosin).

deoxynucleotidal transferase (TdT) mediated dUTP nick end labeling (TUNEL) assay. The presence of CD8+ T cells positive for cytotoxic proteins in Kikuchi-Fujimoto disease also suggests that cytolytic T cells are involved and may mediate apoptosis (151).

Pathologic Features

Grossly, lymph nodes involved by Kikuchi-Fujimoto disease are typically less than 3 cm in greatest dimension, although there have been reports of much larger lymph nodes up to 6 to 7 cm in size.

Lymph nodes affected by Kikuchi-Fujimoto disease have a characteristic histologic appearance that is attributable to a number of features, including (a) patchy lymph node involvement predominantly located in the paracortical areas; (b) fibrinoid necrosis, present in all cases except very early lesions (Fig. 42.9); (c) a mixture of benign histiocytes (so-called crescentic or C shaped), immunoblasts, plasmacytoid monocytes, and small lymphocytes surrounding necrotic areas; (d) absence of granulocytes; (e) absence or paucity of plasma cells; and (f) abundant, predominantly extracellular apoptotic debris (Fig. 42.10) (116–120). The uninvolved lymph node has a mottled appearance at low power due to paracortical hyperplasia, with scattered immunoblasts in a sea of lymphocytes (118,153). A variable number of reactive follicles with secondary germinal centers may be present, but these are relatively less conspicuous. The lymph node capsule is usually intact and may show partial thickening in the areas overlying necrotic areas. Whereas partial involvement and confinement to the lymph node are most common, occasional cases may show extensive replacement of lymph node with extension into the perinodal soft tissue, evoking the differential diagnosis with malignant lymphoma (153). All of these findings describe the so-called mature or classical lesion.

Other lymph nodes involved by Kikuchi-Fujimoto disease can have a different appearance, believed to be related to the "age" of the lesion. These include an early proliferative lesion with a predominance of histiocytes (Fig. 42.11), a slightly later

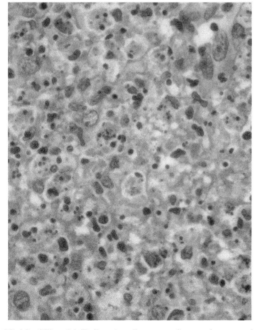

FIG. 42.10. Kikuchi-Fujimoto disease. Area of necrosis with extracellular apoptotic debris as well as residual cellular elements, including small lymphocytes, plasmacytoid monocytes, and histiocytes (hematoxylin-eosin).

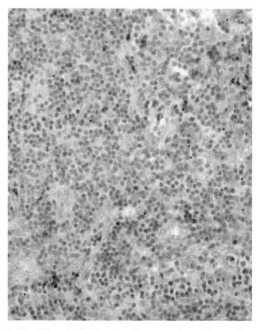

FIG. 42.11. Kikuchi-Fujimoto disease. Lymph node showing early proliferative stage of this disease. Sheets of histiocytes with minimal necrosis are present (hematoxylin-eosin).

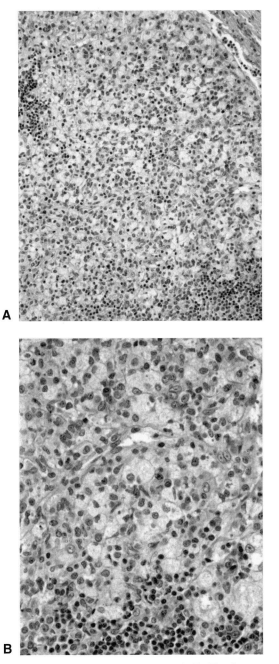

FIG. 42.12. Kikuchi-Fujimoto disease. **A, B:** The late postnecrotic xanthomatous lesion in a lymph node. Numerous lipid-laden "foamy" histiocytes are seen in the interfollicular areas (hematoxylin-eosin). (Figure courtesy of Mihaela Onciu, M.D., St. Jude Children's Research Hospital, Memphis, TN.)

prenecrotizing phagocytic lesion lacking necrosis, and a late postnecrotic xanthomatous lesion with numerous lipid-laden or foamy histiocytes (Fig. 42.12) (116,118,120). All of these morphologic variations appear to represent stages of an evolving process, supported by occasional case reports that multiple histologic variants can occur sequentially in a single patient (154).

Kikuchi-Fujimoto disease also has been reported in extranodal locations, including skin (120,124,125,155), bone marrow (155), and viscera. In the skin, the dermis and subcutaneous adipose tissue is infiltrated by a dense, perivascular, and interstitial inflammatory infiltrate similar to that seen in lymph nodes. This includes a mixture of lymphocytes and histiocytes associated with karyorrhectic debris. In some cases, rare eosinophils and focal interstitial mucin accumulation may be present. Associated changes include vacuolar change at the dermal-epidermal junction and variable degrees of papillary edema, ranging from mild to severe, the latter associated with intraepidermal and subepidermal vesiculation (120,124,125).

Rarely, bone marrow is involved by Kikuchi-Fujimoto disease, invariably in the context of extranodal dissemination (155). The bone marrow is infiltrated by a population of lymphohistiocytic cells with phagocytosis of nuclear debris. Hemophagocytosis may be present.

Very limited information is available regarding the histologic features of Kikuchi-Fujimoto disease involving the viscera of patients with widespread dissemination. In two transplant patients who underwent autopsy, multiple organs, including the grafts, were infiltrated by a lymphohistiocytic cell population associated with karyorrhexis and necrosis. In these cases, granulocytes and plasma cells were absent (156). In another case report, lymph nodes showed typical features of Kikuchi-Fujimoto disease, whereas many viscera, including lung, liver, spleen, and thymus, were infiltrated by lymphocytes and histiocytes (157).

The immunophenotypic findings of Kikuchi-Fujimoto disease are distinctive (118,120,124,151,158,159). The lymphoid component consists predominantly of mature T cells with variable members of T-suppressor (CD8+) and T-helper (CD4+) cells. In most cases, the CD8+ T cells express cytotoxic markers, such as TIA-1 and granzyme B, and usually outnumber the CD4+ lymphocytes (151,160). The latter appear to correlate with the stage of the lesion (120)—fewer in earlier lesions, most numerous at 1 to 3 months, and then declining in number at later stages. Immunoblasts are positive for CD30 and CD45 and are usually of T-cell lineage. Few B cells are present.

The histiocytes of Kikuchi-Fujimoto disease express many monocyte/histiocyte-associated antigens, such as CD11b, CD11c, CD14, CD68, Mac387, Ki-MP1, and lysozyme (118,120,158). In addition, as recently reported by Pileri and colleagues (160), the histiocytes of Kikuchi-Fujimoto disease express myeloperoxidase, a feature characteristic of the histiocytes in Kikuchi-Fujimoto disease and systemic lupus erythematosus. Plasmacytoid monocytes share monocytic markers with the histiocytic population, are positive for CD10, and are negative for myeloperoxidase (159,160). Staining for S-100 protein highlights increased numbers of interdigitating reticulum cells in the uninvolved paracortical areas (159). Proliferation markers, such as Ki-67, are positive in the lymphoid population and predominantly negative within histiocytes and plasmacytoid monocytes.

The differential diagnosis of Kikuchi-Fujimoto disease includes a variety of other disorders, including non-Hodgkin's lymphoma, Hodgkin's disease, and nonneoplastic disorders associated with necrotizing lymphadenitis, such as autoimmune diseases and infectious lymphadenitis.

Non-Hodgkin's lymphoma and Hodgkin's disease enter the differential diagnosis, particularly in cases with extensive lymph node involvement, extranodal extension, and early lesions with a predominance of atypical mononuclear cells, including immunoblasts and plasmacytoid monocytes without extensive necrosis (153,154). Features that help with this distinction in Kikuchi-Fujimoto disease include presence of cytologically bland histiocytes; presence of predominantly extracellular apoptotic debris or "nuclear dust"; absence of neutrophils, eosinophils, and plasma cells in areas of necrosis; and a predominance of T immunoblasts, with only rare B immunoblasts. The presence of Reed-Sternberg–like cells has not been described in Kikuchi-Fujimoto disease. In most cases of Kikuchi-Fujimoto disease, the lymph node biopsy specimen includes small uninvolved areas that show the characteristic paracortical hyperplasia with "mottling" by histiocytes and transformed lymphoid cells (153). Immunohistochemical studies are also helpful when needed. An immunostain for CD68 highlights the crescentic histiocytes and plasmacytoid monocytes, unlike non-Hodgkin's lymphomas in which sheets of B cells or T cells are present. Unlike classical Hodgkin's disease, immunoblasts are negative for CD15 and positive for LCA (CD45).

The finding of numerous crescent-shaped histiocytes and sometimes signet ring histiocytes may suggest the possibility of metastatic adenocarcinoma. However, the histiocytes of Kikuchi-Fujimoto disease are not cytologically atypical nor are they cohesive, unlike metastatic carcinoma. Patients with Kikuchi-Fujimoto disease are also relatively young, unusual for patients with carcinoma. Immunohistochemical studies are very helpful for this distinction; histiocytes of Kikuchi-Fujimoto disease are positive for histiocyte-associated markers and are negative for keratin.

The histologic features of systemic lupus erythematosus lymphadenopathy (described below) overlap significantly with those seen in Kikuchi-Fujimoto disease to the extent that these entities may not be distinguishable on the basis of morphologic and immunophenotypic findings (118,161). Thus, patients with Kikuchi-Fujimoto disease should be evaluated for evidence of connective-tissue diseases. Hematoxylin bodies, when present, support systemic lupus erythematosus, although these bodies are found in only a small subset of systemic lupus erythematosus cases. Histologic features that favor systemic lupus erythematosus include the presence of numerous plasma cells, DNA deposition on blood-vessel walls, and extensive areas of acellular coagulative necrosis devoid of karyorrhectic debris (161).

In Kawasaki's disease, areas of patchy necrosis are present, reminiscent of Kikuchi-Fujimoto disease. In Kawasaki's disease, however, the necrosis is associated with neutrophils and thrombosis of small vessels (162). These histologic features and the associated characteristic mucocutaneous manifestations help to establish the diagnosis.

Infectious agents that can cause necrotizing lymphadenitis also are part of the differential diagnosis, including *Y. enterocolitica*, *Bartonella henselae* (cat-scratch disease), Epstein-Barr virus, and cytomegalovirus.

Y. enterocolitica lymphadenitis is usually located in mesenteric lymph nodes. Histologically, features present in *Yersinia* lymphadenitis but not Kikuchi-Fujimoto disease include microabscesses that contain granulocytes, frequently involving germinal centers, as well as aggregates of epithelioid histiocytes (163).

In cat-scratch disease, stellate microabscesses containing numerous granulocytes are characteristic, often surrounded by palisading histiocytes (Fig. 42.13) (162,163). These abscesses

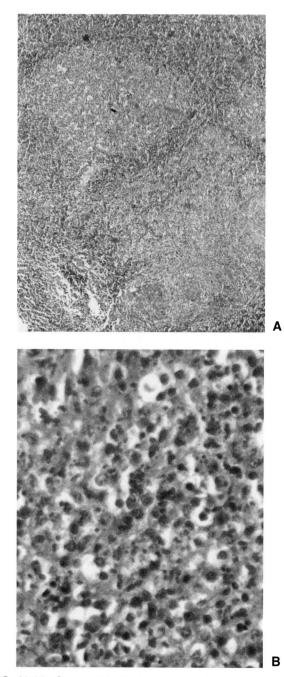

FIG. 42.13. Cat-scratch disease. **A:** A microabscess (lower right of field) surrounded by palisading histiocytes in lymph node. A reactive germinal center is at the upper left. **B:** Higher magnification of the microabscess showing necrotic cells, nuclear debris, and neutrophils (hematoxylin-eosin).

may be associated with thickening and plasma-cell infiltration of the overlying capsule. A Warthin-Starry stain can be helpful in highlighting the characteristic microorganisms located in capillary walls, in macrophages, or adjacent to germinal centers and microabscesses (164). Serologic testing is also a helpful tool for establishing the diagnosis (165).

Viral lymphadenitis, most notoriously observed in infectious mononucleosis secondary to Epstein-Barr virus infection, may raise the possibility of Kikuchi-Fujimoto disease due to the prominent immunoblastic proliferation and patchy necrosis that are often associated with these cases. However, some features of Epstein-Barr virus–associated lymphadenitis are distinctive (162). Such cases usually show prominent follicular hyperplasia and a florid immunoblastic proliferation associated with plasma cells and granulocytes in the interfollicular areas. Reed-Sternberg–like cells are also common in Epstein-Barr virus–infected lymph nodes. Immunophenotypically, most of the proliferating cells in infectious mononucleosis are B immunoblasts (positive for CD30) that express Epstein-Barr virus proteins (166). Lymphadenitis associated with cytomegalovirus infection shows similar features. In addition, characteristic nuclear ("owl eye") and cytoplasmic inclusions of cytomegalovirus are present in endothelial cells and T-lymphoid cells associated with areas of necrosis (161).

Cases of Kikuchi-Fujimoto disease with extensive and confluent areas of necrosis need to be distinguished from lymph node infarction. The latter entity, often associated with malignant lymphoma, usually presents with a thickened lymph node capsule. The areas of necrosis are surrounded by granulation tissue rather than the cell population seen in Kikuchi-Fujimoto disease (167). The infarcted areas also often contain eosinophilic cell "ghosts" rather than the amorphous fibrinoid material seen in Kikuchi-Fujimoto disease. There may be prominent vascular thrombosis. Such findings should prompt a careful search for viable areas of malignant lymphoma, often found external to the lymph node capsule. Immunohistochemical studies show that the cell ghosts are of B-cell or T-cell lineage, if the cells retain their antigenicity, supporting necrotic lymphoma (167).

Management and Outcome

In most patients, Kikuchi-Fujimoto disease is a self-limited disorder that resolves spontaneously (116–120), generally within 1 to 4 months, although in rare cases lymphadenopathy may persist for up to 1 year after diagnosis (168). There are no disease-specific therapies. In patients with significant systemic manifestations, steroids or nonsteroidal antiinflammatory agents have been administered. In cases associated with hemophagocytic syndrome, immunosuppressive therapy, including steroids and etoposide, has yielded excellent results (169,170).

Approximately 1% to 3% of the patients may experience relapse of Kikuchi-Fujimoto disease, usually manifested as recurrent lymphadenopathy at the site of initial presentation or, less commonly, at another distant site. These recurrent episodes may develop anywhere between 4 months and 8 to 9 years from the time of initial diagnosis (118,120,168). These relapses often resolve spontaneously.

A small number of fatal cases of Kikuchi-Fujimoto disease has been reported. One Kikuchi-Fujimoto disease patient reported by Wong et al. (170) developed a fatal pulmonary hemorrhage. Four patients described by Tsai and colleagues (156) were organ-transplant recipients who developed acute febrile illness and graft failure within 1 month after transplantation. All of these patients had widespread organ-system involvement and died rapidly. It appears that most fatalities associated with Kikuchi-Fujimoto disease occur in cases with widespread involvement in the setting of a compromised immune system. It is also possible that these fatal cases do not truly belong to the clinicopathologic spectrum of Kikuchi-Fujimoto disease.

A small number of patients initially diagnosed as Kikuchi-Fujimoto disease go on to develop the characteristic clinical and laboratory features of systemic lupus erythematosus (118,120). Such cases most likely represent examples of systemic lupus erythematosus presenting with isolated lymphadenopathy, rather than transformation from Kikuchi-Fujimoto disease. However, it has been suggested that Kikuchi-Fujimoto disease may be a *forme fruste* of systemic lupus erythematosus in some patients (118).

To date, patients who have recovered from Kikuchi-Fujimoto disease have not subsequently developed lymphoma, either non-Hodgkin's lymphoma or Hodgkin's disease. However, Kikuchi-Fujimoto disease has been reported in two patients who previously had diffuse large B-cell lymphoma (171).

LYMPHADENOPATHY ASSOCIATED WITH SYSTEMIC LUPUS ERYTHEMATOSUS

Clinical Features

The diagnosis of systemic lupus erythematosus is based on well-defined clinical and serologic criteria that have been reviewed elsewhere (172). Patients with systemic lupus erythematosus are usually young, with onset in the second to fourth decades, and the male to female ratio is approximately 1:3 (173). Lymphadenopathy is common in systemic lupus erythematosus patients, occurring in 50% to 60% of patients (173,174). Cervical lymph nodes are most commonly affected, but all lymph node groups may be involved. In approximately 10% of patients, lymphadenopathy may be generalized, which can develop gradually or suddenly (173,174). Thus, lymphoma may be considered in some clinical settings.

Pathogenesis

Systemic lupus erythematosus is a complex, multifactorial, autoimmune disease (175). Genetic factors may also contribute to its pathogenesis, especially through association with certain major histocompatibility class II alleles, complement deficiencies, polymorphisms of Fc γ receptor genes (a complement-related gene), and cytokine genes. During the past several years, linkage analyses using systemic lupus erythematosus families have provided many chromosomal regions for further exploration of susceptibility genes. Six of these regions exhibit significant linkage to systemic lupus erythematosus and are promising loci for candidate genes (176).

Pathologic Features

In the era of effective diagnosis and therapy, the need for biopsy in the management of systemic lupus erythematosus patients has been reduced, and autopsy is rarely performed on patients with untreated disease. The pathologic findings of systemic lupus erythematosus also have been modified by therapy. The reader is referred to older studies that describe the pathologic findings of acute systemic lupus erythematosus in the era before effective therapy (177). Relevant to this chapter is a discussion of lymphadenopathy in systemic lupus erythematosus.

Lymph nodes in systemic lupus erythematosus patients are often enlarged but are typically less than 2 to 3 cm in greatest dimension. Histologically, lymph nodes can show a variety of appearances that may correlate with the stage of the disease or the therapy received by the patient (161,173,178–180).

The classic findings in systemic lupus erythematosus lymphadenopathy, also known as *lupus lymphadenitis*, occur in patients with acute illness. Necrosis, either focal or extensive, is present in the paracortex and is surrounded by lymphocytes, plasma cells, histiocytes, and immunoblasts (Fig. 42.14) (161,173,178,179). Neutrophils and eosinophils are absent. In the residual cortex, reactive follicular hyperplasia

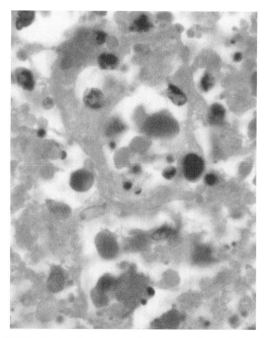

FIG. 42.15. Systemic lupus erythematosus (lupus lymphadenitis). Extracellular clumps of amorphous, necrotic material, known as *hematoxylin bodies*, are characteristic when present. These bodies are composed of DNA, mucopolysaccharides, and immunoglobulins (hematoxylin-eosin).

is present. The lymph nodes are also usually edematous with distension of the subcapsular sinuses. Although identified in only a subset of cases, hematoxylin bodies (Fig. 42.15) are the most specific finding for systemic lupus erythematosus lymphadenopathy (61,173). Hematoxylin bodies are extracellular clumps of amorphous, necrotic material that are composed of DNA, mucopolysaccharides, and Igs (181). Hematoxylin bodies, as stated in the name, are highlighted by hematoxylin in the routine hematoxylin-eosin stain and are also positive for the periodic acid-Schiff reaction. Extracellular DNA may also surround and highlight the walls of blood vessels (the so-called Azzopardi phenomenon) in systemic lupus erythematosus lymph nodes (161,173). Granulomas and fibrosis are consistently absent.

Immunophenotypic studies have been reported in very few cases of lupus lymphadenitis and are not helpful diagnostically (161). The lymphocytes that surround areas of necrosis are predominantly CD8+ T cells. Histiocytes surrounding areas of necrosis express histiocyte-associated antigens. B cells are confined to the cortex in areas of follicular hyperplasia. Molecular studies to assess clonality in systemic lupus erythematosus lymph node biopsy specimens have not been reported.

The true frequency of the classic lesion in systemic lupus erythematosus lymph nodes (i.e., lupus lymphadenitis) is unknown in the era of steroid therapy and other immunosuppressive therapeutic agents. Other histologic findings also have been reported in lymph node biopsy specimens from systemic lupus erythematosus patients. Kojima and col-

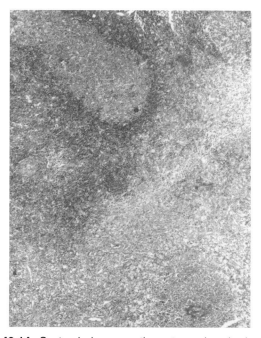

FIG. 42.14. Systemic lupus erythematosus lymphadenopathy (lupus lymphadenitis). Extensive paracortical necrosis in lower right of field. A reactive lymphoid follicle is present at the upper left (hematoxylin-eosin).

leagues (180) described 21 Japanese patients with active systemic lupus erythematosus who underwent lymph node biopsy and divided the cases into three groups on the basis of the histologic findings. One third of patients had nonspecific reactive follicular hyperplasia, one third of patients had follicular hyperplasia with prominent arborizing blood vessels in the paracortex, and six patients had Castleman's disease (CD). In the latter group, two patients had hyaline vascular Castleman's disease, and four patients had Castleman's disease with mixed features of both the hyaline vascular and plasma cell variants. It is of interest that no specimens in their study had the classic morphologic findings described in systemic lupus erythematosus lymph nodes. Because most of the patients in their study were being treated for active disease, perhaps therapy administered to these patients modified the histologic findings in the lymph node biopsy specimens.

The differential diagnosis of lupus lymphadenitis includes a number of diseases characterized by necrosis in lymph nodes, including Kikuchi-Fujimoto disease, cat-scratch disease, lymphogranuloma venereum, syphilitic lymphadenitis, infectious mononucleosis, and lymph node infarct.

With the exception of hematoxylin bodies in systemic lupus erythematosus, the histologic findings in Kikuchi-Fujimoto disease and lupus lymphadenitis are virtually identical (118–120). Thus, clinical history and laboratory findings are mandatory in making this distinction. Some investigators have reported an association between systemic lupus erythematosus and Kikuchi-Fujimoto disease (136,137), and rarely patients with Kikuchi-Fujimoto disease have gone on to develop systemic lupus erythematosus, further suggesting a pathogenetic relationship (182).

Both cat-scratch disease and lymphogranuloma venereum are characterized by stellate microabscesses composed of numerous neutrophils (162,164). In cat-scratch disease, Warthin-Starry stain can identify the bacilli of *B. henselae* in some cases. In syphilitic lymphadenitis, plasma cells are numerous, vasculitis and epithelioid granulomas are common, and Warthin-Starry stain may identify spirochetes (162).

Unlike lymph node infarct, in lupus lymphadenitis the areas of necrosis are not surrounded by granulation tissue nor are eosinophilic cell ghosts present within the necrosis (167). Because most infarcts in lymph node represent infarcted lymphoma, immunohistochemical studies are useful in distinguishing systemic lupus erythematosus lymphadenopathy from lymph node infarct.

Management and Outcome

Therapy directed toward the activity of systemic lupus erythematosus is the best approach for treating acute onset of localized or generalized lymphadenopathy. Patients with systemic lupus erythematosus are also known to be at increased risk for developing lymphoma, both non-Hodgkin's lymphomas and Hodgkin's disease (183–185). In a recent study of 5,175 hospitalized patients with systemic lupus erythemato-

sus followed from 1964 to 1995 in Sweden, 32 patients developed non-Hodgkin's lymphomas, and six patients developed Hodgkin's disease (183). This corresponded with a threefold and fourfold increased risk over normal individuals, respectively, of these neoplasms. The specific histologic types of non-Hodgkin's lymphoma and Hodgkin's disease were not specified in this study.

ROSAI-DORFMAN DISEASE

Rosai-Dorfman disease, first described in the English literature by Rosai and Dorfman in 1969 (186), was initially designated as *sinus histiocytosis with massive lymphadenopathy*; this term is still used. This disease can involve a variety of extranodal sites, however, and, in this circumstance, the term sinus histiocytosis with massive lymphadenopathy is less applicable. Thus, the name *Rosai-Dorfman disease* is becoming more popular. Rosai-Dorfman disease is a rare disorder of unknown etiology that occurs worldwide, affecting all ages, races, and socioeconomic groups (186–188).

Clinical Features

Rosai-Dorfman disease most commonly affects patients in the second and third decades, and the male to female ratio is approximately 1.5:1.0 (188). Rare cases have occurred in siblings (189,190), including identical twins (191), suggesting a genetic predisposition to this disease. Most patients are asymptomatic, but approximately 25% of patients have fever, weight loss, or night sweats.

Patients with Rosai-Dorfman disease most often present with painless, often bulky, lymphadenopathy. The cervical regions, either unilateral or bilateral, are most commonly affected. Axillary, inguinal, and mediastinal lymph nodes are also affected. Depending on the series reported, approximately 25% to 40% of patients with Rosai-Dorfman disease have extranodal involvement, alone or associated with lymph node involvement. All anatomic sites may be involved, but skin (192), soft tissue (193), and the head and neck region (including sinuses and ocular adnexa) (194, 195) are most commonly involved. Other sites involved at moderate frequency include the gastrointestinal tract (196), bone (197), respiratory tract (198), breast (199), and central nervous system (200). The lesions of Rosai-Dorfman disease in the central nervous system are more often dural (200) and less frequently involve the parenchyma (201).

Abnormal laboratory findings in Rosai-Dorfman disease patients include anemia (usually of chronic disease; less frequently hemolytic), neutrophilia, a moderately elevated erythrocyte sedimentation rate, and polyclonal hypergammaglobulinemia (188).

Pathogenesis

The etiology of Rosai-Dorfman disease is unknown. A viral etiology has been considered, and human herpesvirus-6 DNA sequences and proteins have been identified in a subset of cases (202,203). Serologic or molecular studies for other viruses have been generally negative (188). Patients with Rosai-Dorfman disease often have evidence of underlying immunologic dysfunction (204) that may be involved in etiology or pathogenesis. An interesting *in vitro* model suggests that macrophages can suppress lymphocyte function via phagocytosis (205).

As expected in a histiocytic disorder, molecular studies to assess clonality of B and T lymphocytes have shown that the lymphocytes are polyclonal. Studies using an assay to assess the human androgen receptor locus have also shown that the histiocytes of Rosai-Dorfman disease are also polyclonal (206).

Pathologic Features

Grossly, affected lymph nodes are usually substantially enlarged. The cut surface of these lymph nodes is yellow-white and nodular, and the nodules may be surrounded by fibrous bands.

Histologically, in lymph nodes, the most prominent finding is massive dilatation of the sinuses by histiocytes with abundant pale cytoplasm and centrally located vesicular nuclei with or without small nucleoli (Fig. 42.16-42.18) (186–188). The cytoplasm often contains engulfed lymphocytes (emperipolesis). In residual lymph node between the sinuses, reactive follicular hyperplasia and plasmacytosis are present. The

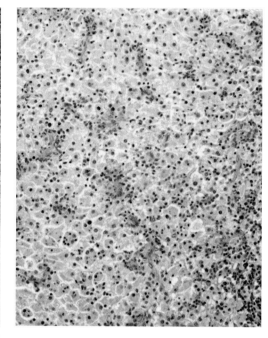

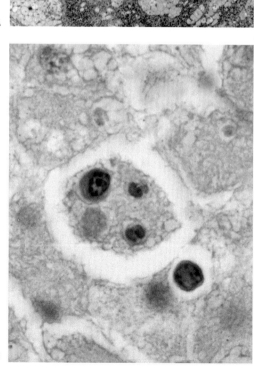

FIG. 42.16. Rosai-Dorfman disease. **A:** Lymph node showing marked dilation of the lymph node sinuses by sheets of histiocytes with abundant pale cytoplasm. **B:** Higher power view showing histiocytes with centrally located nuclei. **C:** One histiocyte contains engulfed lymphocytes and a plasma cell (hematoxylin-eosin).

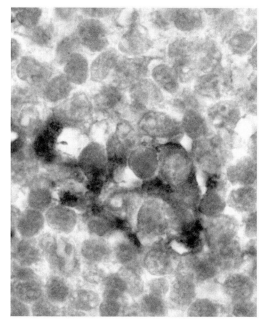

FIG. 42.17. Rosai-Dorfman disease. Immunostain for S-100 protein highlights positive histiocyte nucleus and cytoplasm, the latter surrounding negative lymphocytes engulfed by the histiocyte (immunoperoxidase).

lymph node capsule is often fibrotic. Necrosis and granulocytes are unusual in Rosai-Dorfman disease involving lymph nodes. In general, extranodal lesions of Rosai-Dorfman disease are more difficult to recognize histologically. Fibrosis is commonly present, superimposed acute inflammation may be present, and emperipolesis is less prominent or absent (188,192,194).

Immunohistochemical studies are extremely helpful for establishing the diagnosis of Rosai-Dorfman disease. The histiocytes are strongly positive for S-100 protein, with a nuclear and cytoplasmic pattern of staining (Fig. 42.17) (207). S-100 immunostaining also outlines negative lymphocytes within the histiocyte cytoplasm. The histiocytes of Rosai-Dorfman disease are also positive for CD31, placental alkaline phosphatase and histiocyte-associated antigens (e.g., CD11b, CD14, CD62) but are negative for CD1a and B- and T-cell markers (206). Human herpesvirus-6 antigens have been detected within histiocytes and follicle dendritic cells in a subset of cases (203).

The differential diagnosis of Rosai-Dorfman disease in lymph nodes includes Langerhans' cell histiocytosis; common sinus histiocytosis; and metastatic tumors, such as melanoma or carcinoma.

Langerhan's cell histiocytosis (also known as *eosinophilic granuloma*, *histiocytosis X*, and *Langerhan's cell granulomatosis*) may involve a variety of anatomic sites, most commonly bone, lung, lymph nodes, and rarely viscera (208,209). In lymph nodes, Langerhan's cell histiocytosis is primarily situated in sinuses, such as Rosai-Dorfman disease, but is associated with necrosis and eosinophilia. Cytologically, Langerhan's cells are easily distinguished from the histiocytes of Rosai-Dorfman disease. Langerhan's cells have elongated and twisted nuclei

(resembling a twisted towel) with linear grooves. Immunohistochemically, Langerhan's cells are positive for S-100 protein, as are the histiocytes of Rosai-Dorfman disease (208,209). However, unlike Rosai-Dorfman disease histiocytes, Langerhan's cells are also positive for CD1a. Electron microscopy studies show Birbeck granules within the cytoplasm of Langerhan's cells, a feature unique to these cells (209).

Sinus histiocytosis is a common reaction pattern in lymph nodes, particularly in lymph nodes excised as a part of the staging work-up for various types of tumors (e.g., breast carcinoma). In sinus histiocytosis, the lymph nodes are of nor-

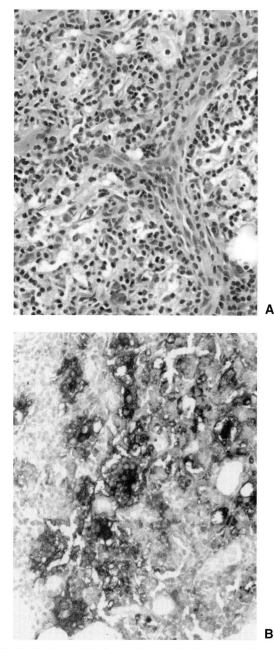

FIG. 42.18. Rosai-Dorfman disease. **A:** A case involving the breast showing an infiltrate of lymphocytes and pale histiocytes (hematoxylin-eosin). **B:** Staining for S-100 is strongly positive in these histiocytes (immunoperoxidase).

mal size or are slightly enlarged, and the sinuses are moderately expanded by morphologically typical histiocytes. Emperipolesis is absent and plasmacytosis is unusual. The histiocytes of sinus histiocytosis are negative or weakly positive for S-100 protein and strongly express histiocyte-associated markers.

Rosai-Dorfman disease may be mistaken for metastatic tumor, less likely in lymph node than in extranodal sites. Although individual histiocytes of Rosai-Dorfman disease can resemble tumor cells because of their abundant cytoplasm, Rosai-Dorfman disease histiocytes are not cytologically atypical nor are they cohesive. Immunohistochemical positivity for S-100 protein in Rosai-Dorfman disease may further raise the possibility of metastatic melanoma, but Rosai-Dorfman disease histiocytes are negative for other melanoma-associated antigens, such as HMB-45 and Melan A (MART-1). The histiocytes of Rosai-Dorfman disease are also negative for keratin, unlike metastatic carcinoma.

Focal Rosai-Dorfman Disease Associated with Lymphoma

Rarely, Rosai-Dorfman disease may occur in lymph nodes involved by Hodgkin's disease or non-Hodgkin's lymphomas. In a recent study, eight cases of this occurrence were described or collected from the literature (210). Both nodular lymphocyte predominant and mixed cellularity types of Hodgkin's disease have been reported to be associated with Rosai-Dorfman disease. Follicular lymphoma is the most common type of non-Hodgkin's lymphoma associated with Rosai-Dorfman disease.

In cases of lymphoma associated with Rosai-Dorfman disease, the latter is focal, less than 1 cm in size, and is discovered incidentally (210). In the cases that have been reported, patients did not have evidence of Rosai-Dorfman disease elsewhere, and the detection of focal Rosai-Dorfman disease did not influence patient management (210).

Autopsy Findings in Patients with Rosai-Dorfman Disease

Only a small number of patients with Rosai-Dorfman disease have died, with a subset of these studied by autopsy. In 1984, Foucar and colleagues (211) reviewed 215 patients in their Rosai-Dorfman disease patient registry, 14 of whom had died. Eight of these patients were studied by autopsy. Two patients died from Rosai-Dorfman disease infiltrating vital organs. The other patients had persistent Rosai-Dorfman disease but died of immunologic abnormalities or infection (211). No patient had malignant tumors at time of autopsy.

Management and Outcome

Patients with Rosai-Dorfman disease usually have a prolonged clinical course with occasional exacerbation and remission phases. However, this disease commonly resolves spontaneously without specific therapy. In a recent literature review of cases with clinical information reported between 1969 and 2000, 80% of patients had spontaneous resolution (212). Uncommonly, patients require systemic or local therapy for extranodal disease, visceral compression, or systemic involvement (212–214). Various therapeutic strategies have been tried in this clinical context, including local therapy with radiation and surgery, chemotherapy (213), interferon-α (214), and steroids (215). Radiotherapy alone has yielded conflicting results: Complete remissions were obtained in 3 of 9 patients treated with this approach (212). Surgical debulking, when required because of vital organ compression, was effective for 8 of 9 patients. Chemotherapy generally has not been effective, and interferon-α has only been of anecdotal benefit. Thus, clinical observation without treatment is advised, if at all possible. Patients with Rosai-Dorfman disease do not appear to be at increased risk of developing lymphoma or other neoplastic diseases (211).

PROGRESSIVE TRANSFORMATION OF GERMINAL CENTERS

Progressive transformation of germinal centers, initially described by Lennert and Muller-Hermelink (216), is a nonspecific but histologically distinctive reaction pattern that can occur in lymph nodes and extranodal lymphoid tissues. In one large study, progressive transformation of germinal centers was identified in 3.5% of reactive lymph node biopsy specimens (217). Progressive transformation of germinal centers is also detected in up to 30% to 40% of patients with nodular lymphocyte predominant Hodgkin's disease (218,219). In these patients, progressive transformation of germinal centers is more often detected simultaneously with nodular lymphocyte predominant Hodgkin's disease or subsequent to its diagnosis, and progressive transformation of germinal centers less often precedes nodular lymphocyte predominant Hodgkin's disease. Progressive transformation of germinal centers has been reported much less frequently in biopsy specimens of patients with a variety of other lymphoma types, including 2% of patients with mixed cellularity or nodular sclerosis Hodgkin's disease (217), follicular lymphoma, and rarely other types of B- and T-cell lymphoma and plasma cell myeloma (218,219).

Clinical Features

The clinical features of patients with progressive transformation of germinal centers were recently reviewed by Hicks and Flaitz (220). Patients with progressive transformation of germinal centers may be children or adults. The youngest patient reported in the literature with progressive transformation of germinal centers was 4 years of age, but most affected children are adolescents. The oldest adult reported in the literature with progressive transformation of germinal centers was 82 years of age, but most affected adults are in their third or fourth decade. This disorder is more common in boys or men, with a male to female ratio of 3:1. Peripheral lymph nodes are usually involved, most commonly the cervical region; abdominal lymph nodes are uncommonly involved.

Patients with progressive transformation of germinal centers are usually asymptomatic and seek medical attention because of lymphadenopathy. Uncommonly, patients present with widespread lymphadenopathy involved by florid progressive transformation of germinal centers (221). More commonly, patients present with localized lymphadenopathy, and progressive transformation of germinal centers often focally involves the lymph node (217,218). Lymphadenopathy in most patients eventually resolves, but in a subset of patients, lymphadenopathy can persist for a number of years, more often in children than adults (220). Progressive transformation of germinal centers does not undergo transformation to malignant lymphoma.

Pathogenesis

The pathogenesis of progressive transformation of germinal centers is unknown. The clinical syndrome of systemic, florid progressive transformation of germinal centers suggests the possibility of a viral infection or another infectious agent.

At one time, the association between progressive transformation of germinal centers and nodular lymphocyte predominant Hodgkin's disease led to the hypothesis that progressive transformation of germinal centers was a precursor lesion of nodular lymphocyte predominant Hodgkin's disease; however, this is now not believed to be the case. The majority of patients with progressive transformation of germinal centers do not have evidence of lymphoma at the time of diagnosis and only rarely do they develop nodular lymphocyte predominant Hodgkin's disease with prolonged clinical follow-up (218, 222,223). Furthermore, progressive transformation of germinal centers is a polyclonal process, unlike nodular lymphocyte predominant Hodgkin's disease (224). The explanation for the association between progressive transformation of germinal centers and nodular lymphocyte predominant Hodgkin's disease is unknown.

Recently, a familial syndrome known as *autoimmune lymphoproliferative syndrome* has been described (225). The lymph nodes in these patients show florid follicular hyperplasia that is often associated with progressive transformation of germinal centers. FAS gene mutations have been identified in these cases, associated with defects in apoptosis. These findings raise the possibility that abnormalities of the FAS gene may also be associated with florid progressive transformation of germinal centers.

Pathologic Features

A spectrum of histologic findings are present in lymph nodes involved by progressive transformation of germinal centers. At its early stage, progressive transformation of germinal centers is characterized by large lymphoid follicles that contain more than one germinal center (Fig. 42.19). In its more fully developed stage, follicles involved by progressive transformation of germinal centers are two to four times the size of normal follicles, and germinal centers are infiltrated

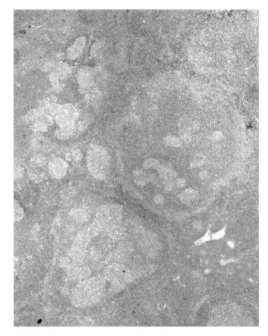

FIG. 42.19. Progressive transformation of germinal centers. Early stage showing large lymphoid follicles that contain more than one germinal center (hematoxylin-eosin).

by small lymphocytes from the mantle zones. As a result, the germinal centers have irregular borders, and the boundary between germinal centers and mantle zones is blurred. At its late stages, germinal centers within progressive transformed follicles are extensively infiltrated by small mantle zone lymphocytes, leaving single and small groups of germinal center cells (Fig. 42.20).

Immunohistochemical studies of progressive transformation of germinal centers have shown that the small lymphocytes that infiltrate germinal centers are mantle-zone B cells, positive for IgM and IgD (224,226). The germinal center cells express CD10, bcl-6, and other antigens of germinal center lineage. T cells are present in progressive transformation of germinal centers, with CD4+ cells outnumbering CD8+ cells, but these T cells are less well organized than those in typical reactive lymphoid follicles with secondary germinal centers. CD57+ T cells are present in progressive transformation of germinal centers, as they are in normal follicles. In a small subset of cases of florid progressive transformation of germinal centers, T cells form rosettes around germinal-center B cells (226). However, T-cell rosetting is absent or rare in most progressive transformation of germinal centers cases. Molecular studies of progressive transformation of germinal centers have shown that the mantle-zone and germinal-center B cells are polyclonal (224).

The differential diagnosis of progressive transformation of germinal centers includes nodular lymphocyte predominant Hodgkin's disease (225,226) and follicular lymphoma (227). Unlike progressive transformation of germinal centers, the nodules of nodular lymphocyte predominant Hodgkin's disease contain neoplastic lymphocytic and histi-

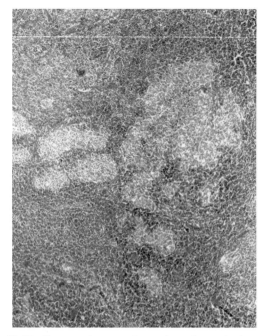

FIG. 42.20. Progressive transformation of germinal centers. A later stage in which the follicles are invaded by small mantle zone lymphocytes, leaving small groups of germinal-center cells (hematoxylin-eosin).

ocytic, (L&H) cells. These large cells, also known as *popcorn cells*, have distinctive clear nuclei and multilobated nuclear contours resembling popped kernels of corn. Furthermore, the nodules of nodular lymphocyte predominant Hodgkin's disease are more vague and replace lymph node architecture, unlike progressive transformation of germinal centers. Immunohistochemical studies can be helpful in distinguishing progressive transformation of germinal centers from nodular lymphocyte predominant Hodgkin's disease. In the latter, the nodules have an irregular broken-up pattern when stained for CD20, and (L&H) cells are often surrounded by rosettes of T cells that may be positive for CD57. These features are less common in progressive transformation of germinal centers. Single-cell polymerase chain reaction studies have shown that the (L&H) cells in nodular lymphocyte predominant Hodgkin's disease are monoclonal, unlike the germinal-center B cells of progressive transformation of germinal centers.

In follicular lymphoma, the neoplastic follicles are back-to-back, replace architecture, and often extend into perinodal adipose tissue. In addition, the neoplastic follicles of follicular lymphoma have relatively round outlines. In contrast, the nodules of progressive transformation of germinal centers do not replace the architecture or extend outside the lymph node capsule, and the nodules have irregular outlines. However, one type of follicular lymphoma, the so-called floral variant, is composed of neoplastic follicles with irregular outlines and superficially resembles florid progressive transformation of germinal centers at low power (227). In these cases, attention to the

cellular composition of the follicles is helpful. In follicular lymphoma, the nodules are composed of a mixture of small-cleaved, large-cleaved, and large-noncleaved cells in varying proportions. In contrast, the follicles of progressive transformation of germinal centers are relatively more heterogeneous, being composed of small round lymphocytes, histiocytes, and germinal center B cells. Flow cytometry immunophenotypic and molecular studies are useful for distinguishing progressive transformation of germinal centers from follicular lymphoma in the small subset of morphologically difficult cases. The finding of a monoclonal B-cell population or the t(14;18)(q32;q21) supports the diagnosis of follicular lymphoma.

Management and Outcome

There is no specific therapy for patients with progressive transformation of germinal centers. Therapy aimed at providing relief of symptoms may be needed for patients with systemic, florid progressive transformation of germinal centers. No specific therapy is required for focal involvement of lymph nodes involved by other processes.

DRUG-RELATED LYMPHADENOPATHY

Patients receiving a variety of drugs may develop lymphadenopathy, either generalized or local, that clinically may resemble malignant lymphoma (Table 42.3). Of these, phenytoin and carbamazepine are best known and are models for the following discussion.

Clinical Features

Patients affected by drug-induced lymphadenopathy can be of any age, and there is no sex preference (228–231). Most commonly, lymphadenopathy develops relatively shortly after initiation of drug therapy, in days to weeks, suggesting a drug hypersensitivity reaction. However, some patients develop lymphadenopathy years after onset of drug therapy. In the latter group of patients, lymph node enlargement may

TABLE 42.3. *Medications associated with lymphadenopathy*

Phenytoin (Dilantin)	Tetracycline
Carbamazepine (Tegretol)	Sulfasalazine
Propylthiouracil	Phenylbutazone
Methimazole (Tapazole)	Halothane
Abacavir (Ziagen)	Allopurinol
Ivermectin (Stromectol)	Aspirin
Potassium iodide	Antithymocyte globulin
Indomethacin	Iron dextran
Sulfonamides	Gold
Penicillins	Bacillus Calmette-Guerin (BCG)
Gentamicin	Methyldopa

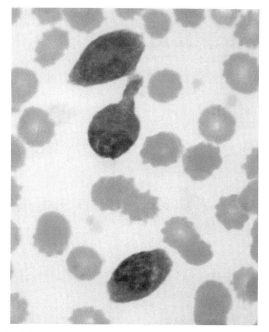

FIG. 42.21. Drug reaction peripheral blood smear shows atypical lymphoid cells with basophilic cytoplasm, so called immunocytes, that should not be interpreted as lymphoma cells (Wright-Giemsa).

be either a manifestation of a hypersensitivity reaction or coincidental (229). Lymphadenopathy is generalized in approximately 25% to 50% of patients.

Patients with lymphadenopathy attributable to drug hypersensitivity also may have a constellation of other findings, including fever, skin rash, nausea, facial edema, and hepatosplenomegaly (229,231). Laboratory abnormalities are also common and may include eosinophilia, leukocytosis or leukopenia, atypical lymphocytosis (Fig. 42.21), and either hypo- or hypergammaglobulinemia.

In most patients, lymphadenopathy regresses with discontinuation of the drug. In a small subset of patients, lymphadenopathy may persist or subsequently recur. Bona fide cases of malignant lymphoma also have been reported in patients being treated with drugs, particularly phenytoin and carbamazepine (229,231). In one study, two patients with clinically and histologically documented phenytoin-associated lymphadenopathy underwent subsequent biopsy for recurrent lymphadenopathy involved by malignant lymphoma (229).

Pathogenesis

The cause of lymphadenopathy in response to drug therapy is unknown. Long-term phenytoin administration to mice causes a similar syndrome (232). Three hypotheses have been proposed. One possibility, most likely for lymphadenopathy associated with a hypersensitivity syndrome, is a hapten-like interaction between the drug and an unknown host antigen (229,231). Other possibilities include an illness analogous to serum sickness or drug-induced chronic immunosuppression

or immunodysregulation allowing emergence of B- or T-cell clones (233,234). This latter possibility may be applicable for cases of true lymphoma that arise in patients treated chronically with drug. A genetic predisposition to drug-associated lymphadenopathy also may be involved as hypersensitivity to phenytoin occurs in families (235).

Pathologic Features

The histologic findings in lymphadenopathy secondary to phenytoin are well described and are probably representative of other drug-related lymphadenopathies (229,231). Thus, phenytoin-associated lymphadenopathy is discussed here in detail.

In lymph nodes that become enlarged shortly after drug exposure, corresponding to a hypersensitivity syndrome, there is marked paracortical hyperplasia. The paracortical regions are expanded by numerous immunoblasts, often associated with vascular proliferation, foci of necrosis, histiocyte clusters, eosinophilia, and, in a smaller subset of cases, vasculitis (Fig. 42.22). Follicular hyperplasia is also present in these lymph nodes. In lymph nodes that become enlarged one to several years after onset of drug therapy, paracortical hyperplasia with an immunoblastic proliferation is also often observed, but follicles are atrophic or absent. In these cases, foci of necrosis and vasculitis are less frequent.

Drug-associated lymphoproliferations also can arise in a number of extranodal sites, including skin, liver, spleen, and bone marrow. Lesions in the skin may be reminiscent of mycosis fungoides (Fig. 42.23) or cutaneous anaplastic large-cell lymphoma (236,237).

Immunophenotypic studies of lymph nodes that become enlarged as part of a drug reaction show no evidence of monoclonality. Immunoblasts are most often of B-cell lineage and usually express the CD30 antigen. Numerous small T cells and histiocytes are also often present. Molecular studies of occasional cases reported in the literature have shown no evidence of antigen receptor gene rearrangements, as assessed by Southern blot analysis (238).

The differential diagnosis of drug-induced lymphadenopathy includes viral lymphadenitis, such as infectious mononucleosis, and malignant lymphomas. In cases of infectious mononucleosis, lymphoid follicles are very prominent, and the paracortical regions show plasmacytosis and Reed-Sternberg–like cells. In tissues involved by infectious mononucleosis, numerous cells are positive for Epstein-Barr virus, as shown by *in situ* hybridization. Eosinophils are relatively less numerous in infectious mononucleosis than in drug-associated lymphadenopathy; in the latter, Epstein-Barr virus is absent or is detected in relatively few cells.

Lymphomas that may be confused with drug-associated lymphadenopathy include angioimmunoblastic T-cell lymphoma, diffuse large B-cell lymphoma, and mixed cellularity Hodgkin's disease. The distinction between angioimmunoblastic T-cell lymphoma and drug-reaction lymphadenopathy may not be possible using histologic criteria alone. Prolonged follow-up showing regression without specific therapy sup-

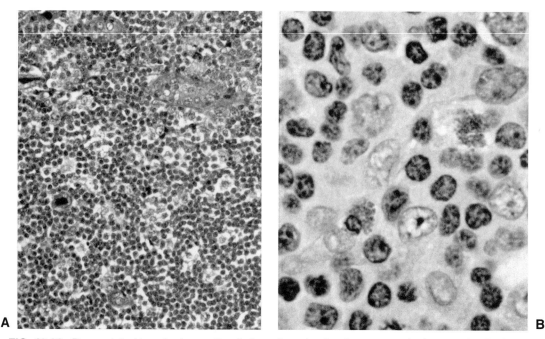

FIG. 42.22. Drug-related lymphadenopathy. **A:** Lymph node showing paracortical expansion by immunoblasts, small lymphocytes, and vascular proliferation. **B:** At higher magnification, a heterogeneous group of immunoblasts, small lymphocytes, histiocytes, and eosinophils is present (hematoxylin-eosin).

ports a drug reaction (231). Detection of clonal abnormalities by conventional cytogenetics or a monoclonal population shown by molecular techniques supports lymphoma. In diffuse large B-cell lymphomas, large cells are relatively more monotonous and form sheets replacing architecture. In contrast, the immunoblastic proliferation of drug-induced lymphadenopathy tends to be confined to the paracortical regions and is often associated with eosinophils, histiocytes, and focal necrosis. Similar to drug-associated lymphadenopathy, mixed cellularity Hodgkin's disease is composed of a heterogeneous mixture of cells with many eosinophils. However, the Reed-Sternberg cells and mononuclear (Hodgkin's) cells of Hodgkin's disease are not observed in drug-associated lymphadenopathy. Furthermore, Epstein-Barr virus is often present within the neoplastic cells of mixed cellularity Hodgkin's disease and is usually absent, or observed in only a few cells, in drug-related lymphadenopathy.

Lymphomas Associated with Drug Therapy

A variety of lymphomas have been reported in patients treated with phenytoin (229) or carbamazepine (231), with non-Hodgkin's lymphomas being at least twice as common as Hodgkin's disease (229). A number of types of non-Hodgkin's lymphomas have been reported, including angioimmunoblastic T-cell lymphoma, follicular lymphoma, small lymphocytic lymphoma/chronic lymphocytic leukemia, and diffuse large B-cell lymphoma (229,231).

Cases in the literature diagnosed as angioimmunoblastic lymphadenopathy with dysproteinemia or immunoblastic lymphadenopathy, old names for angioimmunoblastic T-cell

lymphoma, need to be reviewed critically. In many of these cases, the lesions regressed once drug therapy was discontinued; thus, these lesions were probably not truly lymphoma (231). Furthermore, these lesions were not studied molecularly. The percentage of cases in the literature that are truly

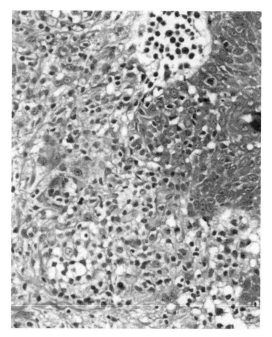

FIG. 42.23. Drug-related skin reaction. A skin biopsy specimen showing a lymphoid infiltrate at the dermal-epidermal junction with epidermotropism reminiscent of mycosis fungoides (hematoxylin-eosin).

angioimmunoblastic T-cell lymphoma is uncertain, but these tumors do occur.

Cases of Hodgkin's disease also have been reported after phenytoin therapy, including nodular sclerosis, mixed cellularity, and nodular lymphocyte predominant types.

Management and Outcome

Discontinuation of the offending drug, without specific therapy, results in resolution of lymphadenopathy in patients with a hypersensitivity-type reaction. In patients who develop lymphoma, therapy specific for the type of lymphoma is required.

REFERENCES

1. Castleman B, Iverson L, Menendez V. Localized mediastinal lymph node resembling thymoma. *Cancer* 1956;9:822–830.
2. Cioffi U, De Simone M, Nosotti M, et al. Hyaline vascular Castleman's disease of the mediastinum. *Int Surg* 1999;84:115–117.
3. Iyoda A, Yusa T, Hiroshima K, et al. Castleman's disease in the posterior mediastinum: report of a case. *Surg Today* 2000;30:473–476.
4. Kooper DP, Tiwari RM, van der Valk P. Castleman's disease as an uncommon cause of a neck mass. *Eur Arch Otorhinolaryngol* 1994; 251:370–372.
5. Frank DK, Charney D, Kashani A. Plasma cell variant of Castleman's disease occurring concurrently with Hodgkin's disease in the neck. *Head Neck* 2001;23:166–169.
6. Kachur E, Ang LC, Megyesi JF. Castleman's disease and spinal cord compression: case report. *Neurosurgery* 2002;50:399–402.
7. Kim TJ, Han JK, Kim YH, et al. Castleman disease of the abdomen: imaging spectrum and clinicopathologic correlations. *J Comput Assist Tomogr* 2001;25:207–214.
8. Gonzalez Sanchez FJ, Landeras Alvaro RM, Encinas Gaspar MB, et al. [Castleman's disease: isolated retroperitoneal mass. Report of a case]. *Arch Esp Urol* 1999;52:282–285.
9. Spedini C, Lombardi C, Lanzani G, et al. Castleman's disease presenting as an asymptomatic solitary pulmonary nodule. *Monaldi Arch Chest Dis* 1995;50:363–365.
10. Parez N, Bader-Meunier B, Roy CC, Dommergues JP. Paediatric Castleman disease: report of seven cases and review of the literature. *Eur J Pediatr* 1999;158:631–637.
11. Frizzera G. Castleman's disease and related disorders. *Semin Diagn Pathol* 1988;5:346–364.
12. Frizzera G, Peterson BA, Bayrd ED, Goldman A. A systemic lymphoproliferative disorder with morphologic features of Castleman's disease: clinical findings and clinicopathologic correlations in 15 patients. *J Clin Oncol* 1985;3:1202–1216.
13. Weisenburger DD, Nathwani BN, Winberg CD, Rappaport H. Multicentric angiofollicular lymph node hyperplasia: a clinicopathologic study of 16 cases. *Hum Pathol* 1985;16:162–172.
14. Sherman D, Ramsay B, Theodorou NA, et al. Reversible plane xanthoma, vasculitis, and peliosis hepatis in giant lymph node hyperplasia (Castleman's disease): a case report and review of the cutaneous manifestations of giant lymph node hyperplasia. *J Am Acad Dermatol* 1992;26:105–109.
15. Hsiao CJ, Hsu MM, Lee JY, et al. Paraneoplastic pemphigus in association with a retroperitoneal Castleman's disease presenting with a lichen planus pemphigoides-like eruption. A case report and review of literature. *Br J Dermatol* 2001;144:372–376.
16. Cummings TJ, Gong JZ, Friedman AH, McLendon RE. Castleman's disease confined to the leptomeninges. *Ann Clin Lab Sci* 2000;30: 278–282.
17. Vingerhoets F, Kuntzer T, Delacretaz, et al. Chronic relapsing neuropathy associated with Castleman's disease (angiofollicular lymph node hyperplasia). *Eur Neurol* 1995;35:336–340.
18. Fernandez-Torre JL, Polo JM, Calleja J, Berciano J. Castleman's disease associated with chronic inflammatory demyelinating polyradiculoneuropathy: a clinical and electrophysiological follow-up study. *Clin Neurophysiol* 1999;110:1133–1138.

19. Serin E, Ozer B, Gumurdulu Y, et al. A case of Castleman's disease with "downhill" varices in the absence of superior vena cava obstruction. *Endoscopy* 2002;34:160–162.
20. Carpentier-Planchon V, Bouillanne O, Cabane J, et al. [A unique case of destructive polyarthritis associated with multicentric Castleman's disease]. *Ann Med Interne (Paris)* 2001;152:139–144.
21. Lui SL, Chan KW, Li FK, et al. Castleman's disease and mesangial proliferative glomerulonephritis: the role of interleukin-6. *Nephron* 1998;78:323–327.
22. Gohlke F, Marker-Hermann E, Kanzler S, et al. Autoimmune findings resembling connective tissue disease in a patient with Castleman's disease. *Clin Rheumatol* 1997;16:87–92.
23. Kikuta H, Itakura O, Ariga T, Kobayashi K. Detection of human herpesvirus 8 DNA sequences in peripheral blood mononuclear cells of children. *J Med Virol* 1997;53:81–84.
24. Grandadam M, Dupin N, Calvez V, et al. Exacerbations of clinical symptoms in human immunodeficiency virus type 1-infected patients with multicentric Castleman's disease are associated with a high increase in Kaposi's sarcoma herpesvirus DNA load in peripheral blood mononuclear cells. *J Infect Dis* 1997;175:1198–1201.
25. Palestro G, Turrini F, Pagano M, Chiusa L. Castleman's disease. *Adv Clin Path* 1999;3:11–22.
26. Hengge UR, Ruzicka T, Tyring SK, et al. Update on Kaposi's sarcoma and other HHV8 associated diseases. Part 2: pathogenesis, Castleman's disease, and pleural effusion lymphoma. *Lancet Infect Dis* 2002;2:344–352.
27. Boshoff C, Chang Y. Kaposi's sarcoma-associated herpesvirus: a new DNA tumor virus. *Annu Rev Med* 2001;52:453–470.
28. Luppi M, Barozzi P, Maiorana A, et al. Expression of cell-homologous genes of human herpesvirus-8 in human immunodeficiency virus-negative lymphoproliferative diseases. *Blood* 1999;94:2931–2933.
29. Foussat A, Fior R, Girard T, et al. Involvement of human interleukin-6 in systemic manifestations of human herpesvirus type 8-associated multicentric Castleman's disease. *AIDS* 1999;13:150–152.
30. Scott D, Cabral L, Harrington WJ Jr. Treatment of HIV-associated multicentric Castleman's disease with oral etoposide. *Am J Hematol* 2001;66:148–150.
31. Oksenhendler E, Duarte M, Soulier J, et al. Multicentric Castleman's disease in HIV infection: a clinical and pathological study of 20 patients. *AIDS* 1996;10:61–67.
32. Ohyashiki JH, Ohyashiki K, Kawakubo K, et al. Molecular genetic, cytogenetic, and immunophenotypic analyses in Castleman's disease of the plasma cell type. *Am J Clin Pathol* 1994;101:290–295.
33. Murray PG, Deacon E, Young LS, et al. Localization of Epstein-Barr virus in Castleman's disease by in situ hybridization and immunohistochemistry. *Hematol Pathol* 1995;9:17–26.
34. Yoshizaki K, Kuritani T, Kishimoto T. Interleukin-6 in autoimmune disorders. *Semin Immunol* 1992;4:155–166.
35. Ishiyama T, Nakamura S, Akimoto Y, et al. Immunodeficiency and IL-6 production by peripheral blood monocytes in multicentric Castleman's disease. *Br J Haematol* 1994;86:483–489.
36. Hsu SM, Waldron JA, Xie SS, Barlogie B. Expression of interleukin-6 in Castleman's disease. *Hum Pathol* 1993;24:833–839.
37. Leger-Ravet MB, Peuchmaur M, Devergne O, et al. Interleukin-6 gene expression in Castleman's disease. *Blood* 1991;78:2923–2930.
38. Cannon JS, Nicholas J, Orenstein JM, et al. Heterogeneity of viral IL-6 expression in HHV-8-associated diseases. *J Infect Dis* 1999;180:824–828.
39. Staskus KA, Sun R, Miller G, et al. Cellular tropism and viral interleukin-6 expression distinguish human herpesvirus 8 involvement in Kaposi's sarcoma, primary effusion lymphoma, and multicentric Castleman's disease. *J Virol* 1999;73:4181–4187.
40. Ishiyama T, Koike M, Nakamura S, et al. Interleukin-6 receptor expression in the peripheral B cells of patients with multicentric Castleman's disease. *Ann Hematol* 1996;73:179–182.
41. Akira S, Taga T, Kishimoto T. Interleukin-6 in biology and medicine. *Adv Immunol* 1993;54:1–78.
42. Kawano MM, Mihara K, Huang N, et al. Differentiation of early plasma cells on bone marrow stromal cells requires interleukin-6 for escaping from apoptosis. *Blood* 1995;85:487–494.
43. Ramadori G, Christ B. Cytokines and the hepatic acute-phase response. *Semin Liver Dis* 1999;19:141–155.
44. Brandt SJ, Bodine DM, Dunbar CE, Nienhuis AW. Dysregulated interleukin 6 expression produces a syndrome resembling Castleman's disease in mice. *J Clin Invest* 1990;86:592–599.

45. Winter SS, Howard TA, Ritchey AK, et al. Elevated levels of tumor necrosis factor-beta, gamma-interferon, and IL-6 mRNA in Castleman's disease. *Med Pediatr Oncol* 1996;26:48–53.
46. Emilie D, Zou W, Fior R, et al. Production and roles of IL-6, IL-10, and IL-13 in B-lymphocyte malignancies and in B-lymphocyte hyperactivity of HIV infection and autoimmunity. *Methods* 1997;11:133–142.
47. Hall PA, Donaghy M, Cotter FE, et al. An immunohistological and genotypic study of the plasma cell form of Castleman's disease. *Histopathology* 1989;14:333–346; discussion 429–432.
48. Danon AD, Krishnan J, Frizzera G. Morpho-immunophenotypic diversity of Castleman's disease, hyaline-vascular type: with emphasis on a stroma-rich variant and a new pathogenetic hypothesis. *Virchows Arch A Pathol Anat Histopathol* 1993;423:369–382.
49. Ruco LP, Gearing AJ, Pigott R, et al. Expression of ICAM-1, VCAM-1 and ELAM-1 in angiofollicular lymph node hyperplasia (Castleman's disease): evidence for dysplasia of follicular dendritic reticulum cells. *Histopathology* 1991;19:523–528.
50. Keller AR, Hochholzer L, Castleman B. Hyaline-vascular and plasma-cell types of giant lymph node hyperplasia of the mediastinum and other locations. *Cancer* 1972;29:670–683.
51. Menke DM, Camoriano JK, Banks PM. Angiofollicular lymph node hyperplasia: a comparison of unicentric, multicentric, hyaline vascular, and plasma cell types of disease by morphometric and clinical analysis. *Mod Pathol* 1992;5:525–530.
52. McCarty MJ, Vukelja SJ, Banks PM, Weiss RB. Angiofollicular lymph node hyperplasia (Castleman's disease). *Cancer Treat Rev* 1995;21:291–310.
53. Pauwels P, Dal Cin P, Vlasveld LT, et al. A chromosomal abnormality in hyaline vascular Castleman's disease: evidence for clonal proliferation of dysplastic stromal cells. *Am J Surg Pathol* 2000;24:882–888.
54. Amin HM, Medeiros LJ, Manning JT, Jones D. Dissolution of the lymphoid follicle is a feature of the HHV8+ variant of plasma cell Castleman's disease. *Am J Surg Pathol* 2003;27:91–100.
55. Dupin N, Diss TL, Kellam P, et al. HHV-8 is associated with a plasmablastic variant of Castleman disease that is linked to HHV-8-positive plasmablastic lymphoma. *Blood* 2000;95:1406–1412.
56. Dupin N, Fisher C, Kellam P, et al. Distribution of human herpesvirus-8 latently infected cells in Kaposi's sarcoma, multicentric Castleman's disease, and primary effusion lymphoma. *Proc Natl Acad Sci U S A* 1999;96:4546–4551.
57. Katano H, Sato Y, Kurata T, et al. Expression and localization of human herpesvirus 8-encoded proteins in primary effusion lymphoma, Kaposi's sarcoma, and multicentric Castleman's disease. *Virology* 2000;269:335–344.
58. Brousset P, Cesarman E, Meggetto F, et al. Colocalization of the viral interleukin-6 with latent nuclear antigen-1 of human herpesvirus-8 in endothelial cells spindle cells of Kaposi's sarcoma and lymphoid cells of multicentric Castleman's disease. *Hum Pathol* 2001;32:95–100.
59. Menke DM, Chadbum A, Cesarman E, et al. Analysis of human herpesvirus 8 (HHV-8) genome and HHV-8 vIL-6 expression in archival cases of Castleman disease at low risk for HIV infection. *Am J Clin Pathol* 2002;117:268–275.
60. Nishi J, Maruyama I. Increased expression of vascular endothelial growth factor (VEGF) in Castleman's disease: proposed pathomechanism of vascular proliferation in the affected lymph node. *Leuk Lymphoma* 2000;38:387–394.
61. Hanson CA, Frizzera G, Patton DF, et al. Clonal rearrangement for immunoglobulin and T-cell receptor genes in systemic Castleman's disease. Association with Epstein-Barr virus. *Am J Pathol* 1988;131:84–91.
62. Soulier J, Grollet L, Oksenhendler E, et al. Molecular analysis of clonality in Castleman's disease. *Blood* 1995;86:1131–1138.
63. Klein A, Zemer R, Manor Y, et al. Lymphoma with multi gene rearrangement on the level of immunoglobulin heavy chain, light chains, and T-cell receptor beta chain. *Am J Hematol* 1997;56:219–223.
64. Menke DM, DeWald GW. Lack of cytogenetic abnormalities in Castleman's disease. *South Med J* 2001;94:472–474.
65. Nakamura H, Nakaseko C, Ishii A, et al. [Chromosomal abnormalities in Castleman's disease with high levels of serum interleukin-6]. *Rinsho Ketsueki* 1993;34:212–217.
66. Zarate-Osorno A, Medeiros LJ, Danon AD, Neiman RS. Hodgkin's disease with coexistent Castleman-like histologic features. A report of three cases. *Arch Pathol Lab Med* 1994;118:270–274.
67. Chan AC, Chan KW, Chan JK, et al. Development of follicular dendritic cell sarcoma in hyaline-vascular Castleman's disease of the

nasopharynx: tracing its evolution by sequential biopsies. *Histopathology* 2001;38:510–518.
68. Gerald W, Kostianovsky M, Rosai J. Development of vascular neoplasia in Castleman's disease. Report of seven cases. *Am J Surg Pathol* 1990;14:603–614.
69. Maheswaran PR, Ramsay AD, Norton AJ, et al. Hodgkin's disease presenting with the histological features of Castleman's disease. *Histopathology* 1991;18:249–253.
70. Larroche C, Cacoub P, Soulier J, et al. Castleman's disease and lymphoma: report of eight cases in HIV-negative patients and literature review. *Am J Hematol* 2002;69:119–126.
71. Oksenhendler E, Boulanger E, Galacier L, et al. High incidence of Kaposi sarcoma-associated herpesvirus-related non-Hodgkin lymphoma in patients with HIV infection and multicentric Castleman disease. *Blood* 2002;99:2331–2336.
72. Ascoli V, Signoretti S, Onetti-Muda A, et al. Primary effusion lymphoma in HIV-infected patients with multicentric Castleman's disease. *J Pathol* 2001;193:200–209.
73. Dupin N, Diss TL, Kellam P, et al. HHV-8 is associated with a plasmablastic variant of Castleman disease that is linked to HHV-8-positive plasmablastic lymphoma. *Blood* 2000;95:1406–1412.
74. Wengrower D, Libson E, Okon E, Goldin E. Gastrointestinal manifestations in Castleman's disease. *Am J Gastroenterol* 1990;85:1179–1181.
75. Stelfox HT, Stewart AK, Bailey D, et al. Castleman's disease in a 44-year-old male with neurofibromatosis and pheochromocytoma. *Leuk Lymphoma* 1997;27:551–556.
76. Tissier F, de Pinieux G, Thiounn N, et al. [Castleman's disease and chromophobe carcinoma of the kidney. An incidental association?]. *Ann Pathol* 1998;18:429–431.
77. Mizutani N, Okada S, Tanaka J, et al. Multicentric giant lymph node hyperplasia with ascites and double cancers, an autopsy case. *Tohoku J Exp Med* 1989;158:1–7.
78. Baker WJ, Vukelja SJ, Weiss RB, Dich N. Multicentric angiofollicular lymph node hyperplasia and associated carcinoma. *Med Pediatr Oncol* 1994;22:384–388.
79. Torii K, Ogawa K, Kawabata Y, et al. Lymphoid interstitial pneumonia as a pulmonary lesion of idiopathic plasmacytic lymphadenopathy with hyperimmunoglobulinemia. *Intern Med* 1994;33:237–241.
80. Atagi S, Sakatani M, Akira M, et al. Pulmonary hyalinizing granuloma with Castleman's disease. *Intern Med* 1994;33:689–691.
81. Pasaoglu I, Dogan R, Topcu M, Gungen Y. Multicentric angiofollicular lymph-node hyperplasia associated with myasthenia gravis. *Thorac Cardiovasc Surg* 1994;42:253–256.
82. West KP, Morgan DR, Lauder I. Angiofollicular lymph node hyperplasia with amyloidosis. *Postgrad Med J* 1989;65:108–111.
83. Molina T, Delmer A, Le Tourneau A, et al. Hepatic lesions of vascular origin in multicentric Castleman's disease, plasma cell type: report of one case with peliosis hepatis and another with perisinusoidal fibrosis and nodular regenerative hyperplasia. *Pathol Res Pract* 1995;191:1159–1164.
84. Bardwick PA, Zvaifler NJ, Gill GN, et al. Plasma cell dyscrasia with polyneuropathy, organomegaly, endocrinopathy, M protein, and skin changes: the POEMS syndrome. Report on two cases and a review of the literature. *Medicine (Baltimore)* 1980;59:311–322.
85. Latz D, Mende U, Schraube P, Rieden K. [The radiotherapy of Castleman's lymphoma]. *Strahlenther Onkol* 1992;168:297–299.
86. Cioffi U, DeSimone M, Nosotti M, et al. Hyaline vascular Castleman's disease of the mediastinum. *Int Surg* 1999;84:115–117.
87. Pavlidis NA, Briassoulis E, Klouvas G, et al. Is interferon-α an active agent in Castleman's disease? *Ann Oncol* 1992;3:85–86.
88. Andres E, Maloisel F. Interferon-alpha as first-line therapy for treatment of multicentric Castleman's disease. *Ann Oncol* 2000;11:1613–1614.
89. Tamayo M, Gonzalez C, Majado MJ, et al. Long-term complete remission after interferon treatment in a case of multicentric Castleman's disease. *Am J Hematol* 1995;49:359–360.
90. Rieu P, Droz D, Gessain A, et al. Retinoic acid for treatment of multicentric Castleman's disease. *Lancet* 1999;354:1262–1263.
91. Beck JT, Hsu SM, Wijdenes J, et al. Brief report: alleviation of systemic manifestations of Castleman's disease by monoclonal anti-interleukin-6 antibody. *N Engl J Med* 1994;330:602–605.
92. Herrada J, Cabanillas F, Rice L, et al. The clinical behavior of localized and multicentric Castleman disease. *Ann Intern Med* 1998;128:657–662.
93. Repetto L, Jaiprakash MP, Selby PJ, et al. Aggressive angiofollicular lymph node hyperplasia (Castleman's disease) treated with high dose

melphalan and autologous bone marrow transplantation. *Hematol Oncol* 1986;4:213–217.

94. Nakanishi T, Sobue I, Toyokura Y, et al. The Crow-Fukase syndrome: a study of 102 cases in Japan. *Neurology* 1984;34:712–720.

95. Pruzanski W. Takatsuki syndrome: a reversible multisystem plasma cell dyscrasia. *Arthritis Rheum* 1986;29:1534–1535.

96. Driedger H, Pruzanski W. Plasma cell neoplasia with peripheral polyneuropathy: a study of five cases and a review of the literature. *Medicine (Baltimore)* 1980;59:301–310.

97. Miralles GD, O'Fallon JR, Talley NJ. Plasma-cell dyscrasia with polyneuropathy. The spectrum of POEMS syndrome. *N Engl J Med* 1992;327:1919–1923.

98. Dispenzieri A, Kyle RA, Lacy MQ, et al. POEMS syndrome: a retrospective review. *Blood* 2003;101:2496–2506.

99. Bova G, Pasqui AL, Saletti M, et al. POEMS syndrome with vascular lesions: a role for interleukin-1 beta and interleukin-6 increase—a case report. *Angiology* 1998;149:937–940.

100. Watanabe O, Maruyama I, Arimura K, et al. Overproduction of vascular endothelial growth factor/vascular permeability factor is causative in Crow-Fukase (POEMS) syndrome. *Muscle Nerve* 1998;21:1390–1397.

101. Rose C, Zandecki M, Copin MC, et al. POEMS syndrome: report on six patients with unusual clinical signs, elevated levels of cytokines, macrophage involvement and chromosomal aberrations of bone marrow plasma cells. *Leukemia* 1997;11:1318–1323.

102. Atsumi T, Kato K, Kurosawa S, et al. A case of Crow-Fukase syndrome with elevated soluble interleukin-6 receptor in cerebrospinal fluid. Response to double-filtration plasmapheresis and corticosteroids. *Acta Haematol* 1995;94:90–94.

103. Gherardi RK, Authier FJ, Belec L. [Pro-inflammatory cytokines: a pathogenic key of POEMS syndrome]. *Rev Neurol (Paris)* 1996;152:409–412.

104. Nakazawa K, Itoh N, Shigematu H, Koh CS. An autopsy case of Crow-Fukase (POEMS) syndrome with a high level of IL-6 in the ascites: special reference to glomerular lesions. *Acta Pathol Jpn* 1992;42:651–656.

105. Farhangi M, Merlini G. The clinical implications of monoclonal immunoglobulins. *Semin Oncol* 1986;13:366–379.

106. Menke DM, Horny HP, Dispenzieri A. Bone marrow pathology of POEMS syndrome. *Mod Pathol* 2003;16:244A.

107. Belec L, Mohamed AS, Authier FJ, et al. Human herpesvirus 8 infection in patients with POEMS syndrome-associated multicentric Castleman's disease. *Blood* 1999;93:3643–3653.

108. Zumo L, Grewal RP. Castleman's disease-associated neuropathy: no evidence of human herpesvirus type 8 infection. *J Neurol Sci* 2002;195: 47–150.

109. Philips ED, el-Mahdi AM, Humphrey RL, et al. The effect of the radiation treatment on the polyneuropathy of multiple myeloma. *J Can Assoc Radiol* 1972;23:103–106.

110. Benito-Leon J, Lopez-Rios F, Rodriguez-Martin FJ, et al. Rapidly deteriorating polyneuropathy associated with osteosclerotic myeloma responsive to intravenous immunoglobulin and radiotherapy. *J Neurol Sci* 1998;158:113–117.

111. Rotta FT, Bradley WG. Marked improvement of severe polyneuropathy associated with multifocal osteosclerotic myeloma following surgery, radiation, and chemotherapy. *Muscle Nerve* 1997;20:1035–1037.

112. Parra R, Fernandez JM, Garcia-Bragado F, et al. Successful treatment of peripheral neuropathy with chemotherapy in osteosclerotic myeloma. *J Neurol* 1987;234:261–263.

113. Kuwabara S, Hattori T, Shimoe Y, et al. Long term melphalan-prednisolone chemotherapy for POEMS syndrome. *J Neurol Neurosurg Psychiatry* 1997;63:385–387.

114. Rovira M, Carreras E, Blade J, et al. Dramatic improvement of POEMS syndrome following autologous haematopoietic cell transplantation. *Br J Haematol* 2001;115:373–375.

115. Hogan WJ, Lacy MQ, Wiseman GA, et al. Successful treatment of POEMS syndrome with autologous hematopoietic progenitor cell transplantation. *Bone Marrow Transplant* 2001;28:305–309.

116. Kikuchi M. Lymphadenitis showing focal reticulum cell hyperplasia with nuclear debris and phagocytes: a clinicopathologic study (in Japanese). *Nippon Ketsucki Gakkai Zasshi* 1972;35:379–382.

117. Fujimoto Y, Kozima Y, Yamaguchi K. Cervical subacute necrotizing lymphadenitis. A new clinicopathologic entity. *Naika* 1972;20:920–927.

118. Dorfman RF, Berry GJ. Kikuchi's histiocytic necrotizing lymphadenitis: an analysis of 108 cases with emphasis on differential diagnosis. *Semin Diagn Pathol* 1988;5:329–345.

119. Kikuchi M. Histiocytic necrotizing lymphadenitis (Kikuchi-Fujimoto disease) in Japan. *Am J Surg Pathol* 1991;15:197–198.

120. Kuo TT. Kikuchi's disease (histiocytic necrotizing lymphadenitis): a clinicopathologic study of 79 cases with an analysis of histologic subtypes, immunohistology, and DNA ploidy. *Am J Surg Pathol* 1995; 19:798–809.

121. Kosch M, Schmid KW, Hausberg M, et al. [Kikuchi-Fujimoto disease: the differential diagnosis of cervical lymphadenitis with recurrent attacks of fever]. *Dtsch Med Wochenschr* 1999;124:213–216.

122. Yabe H, Sinzato I, Hashimoto K. [Necrotizing lymphadenitis presenting as mesenteric lymphadenopathy]. *Rinsho Ketsueki* 1999;40:658–662.

123. Miller WT Jr, Perez-Jaffe LA. Cross-sectional imaging of Kikuchi disease. *J Comput Assist Tomogr* 1999;23:548–551.

124. Spies J, Foucar K, Thompson CT, LeBoit PE. The histopathology of cutaneous lesions of Kikuchi's disease (necrotizing lymphadenitis): a report of five cases. *Am J Surg Pathol* 1999;23:1040–1047.

125. Imai K, Yokozeki H, Nishioka K. Kikuchi's disease (histiocytic necrotizing lymphadenitis) with cutaneous involvement. *J Dermatol* 2002;29:587–592.

126. Sato Y, Kuno H, Oizumi K. Histiocytic necrotizing lymphadenitis (Kikuchi's disease) with aseptic meningitis. *J Neurol Sci* 1999;163:187–191.

127. Wilkinson CE, Nichol F. Kikuchi-Fujimoto disease associated with polymyositis. *Rheumatology (Oxford)* 2000;39:1302–1304.

128. Sugiyama A, Araki E, Arakawa K, et al. [A case of subacute necrotizing lymphadenitis complicated with brachial plexus neuritis]. *Rinsho Shinkeigaku* 1998;38:941–944.

129. Keogh MA, Williamson RA, Denaro CP. Kikuchi's disease associated with parotidomegaly, thyroiditis and a rash in a young man. *Aust N Z J Med* 2000;30:633–634.

130. Taguri AH, McIlwaine GG. Bilateral panuveitis: a possible association with Kikuchi-Fujimoto disease. *Am J Ophthalmol* 2001;132:419–421.

131. Blewitt RW, Kumar SN, Abraham JS. Recurrence of Kikuchi's lymphadenitis after 12 years. *J Clin Pathol* 2000;53:157–158.

132. Sierra ML, Vegas E, Blanco-Gonzalez JE, et al. Kikuchi's disease with multisystemic involvement and adverse reaction to drugs. *Pediatrics* 1999;104:e24.

133. Tsai MK, Huang HF, Hu RH, et al. Fatal Kikuchi-Fujimoto disease in transplant recipients: a case report. *Transplant Proc* 1998;30:3137–3138.

134. Tanaka T, Ohmori M, Yasunaga S, et al. DNA typing of HLA class II genes (HLA-DR, -DQ and -DP) in Japanese patients with histiocytic necrotizing lymphadenitis (Kikuchi's disease). *Tissue Antigens* 1999; 54:246–253.

135. Amir AR, Amr SS, Sheikh SS. Kikuchi-Fujimoto disease: report of familial occurrence in two human leukocyte antigen-identical non-twin sisters. *J Int Med* 2002;252:79–83.

136. Dalkilic E, Karakoc Y, Tolunay S, Yurtkuran M. Systemic lupus erythematosus presenting as Kikuchi-Fujimoto disease. *Clin Exp Rheumatol* 2001;19:226.

137. Chen YH, Lan JL. Kikuchi disease in systemic lupus erythematosus: clinical features and literature review. *J Microbiol Immunol Infect* 1998;31:187–192.

138. Cousin F, Grezard P, Roth B, et al. Kikuchi disease associated with Still disease. *Int J Dermatol* 1999;38:464–467.

139. Laeng RH, Stamm B. Kikuchi's histiocytic necrotizing lymphadenitis driven by activated cytolytic T-cells: an example associated with systemic scleroderma. *Histopathology* 1999;34:373–374.

140. Meyer O, Kahn MF, Grossin M, et al. Parvovirus B19 infection can induce histiocytic necrotizing lymphadenitis (Kikuchi's disease) associated with systemic lupus erythematosus. *Lupus* 1991;1:37–41.

141. Huh J, Chi HS, Kim SS, et al. A study of the viral etiology of histiocytic necrotizing lymphadenitis (Kikuchi-Fujimoto disease). *J Korean Med Sci* 1998;13:27–30.

142. Chiu CF, Chow KC, Lin TY, et al. Virus infection in patients with histiocytic necrotizing lymphadenitis in Taiwan. Detection of Epstein-Barr virus, type I human T-cell lymphotropic virus, and parvovirus B19. *Am J Clin Pathol* 2000;113:774–781.

143. Krueger GR, Huetter ML, Rojo J, et al. Human herpesvirus HHV-4 (EBV) and HHV-6 in Hodgkin's and Kikuchi's diseases and their relation to proliferation and apoptosis. *Anticancer Res* 2001;21:2155–2161.

144. Stéphan JL, Jeannoël P, Chanoz J, et al. Epstein-Barr virus-associated Kikuchi disease in two children. *J Pediatr Hematol Oncol* 2001;23:240–243.

145. Martinez-Vazquez C, Potel C, Angulo M, et al. Nosocomial Kikuchi's disease—a search for herpesvirus sequences in lymph node tissues using PCR. *Infection* 2001;29:143–147.

146. Huh J, Kang GH, Gong G, et al. Kaposi's sarcoma-associated herpesvirus in Kikuchi's disease. *Hum Pathol* 1998;29:1091–1096.

147. Ereno C. Kikuchi lymphadenitis and AIDS [Letter]. *Histopathology* 1999;34:273.

148. Bataille V, Harland CC, Behrens J, et al. Kikuchi disease (histiocytic necrotizing lymphadenitis) in association with HTLV1. *Br J Dermatol* 1997;136:610–612.

149. Feller AC, Lennert K, Stain H, et al. Immunohistology and aetiology of histiocytic necrotizing lymphadenitis. Report of three instructive cases. *Histopathology* 1983;7:825–839.

150. Rodriguez Martorell J, Martin MV, Baez JM, et al. [Kikuchi-Fujimoto necrotizing lymphadenitis associated with brucellosis]. *Sangre (Barc)* 1992;37:201–204.

151. Felgar RE, Furth EE, Wasik MA, et al. Histiocytic necrotizing lymphadenitis (Kikuchi's disease): in situ end-labeling, immunohistochemical, and serologic evidence supporting cytotoxic lymphocyte-mediated apoptotic cell death. *Mod Pathol* 1997;10:231–241.

152. Ura H, Yamada N, Torii H, et al. Histiocytic necrotizing lymphadenitis (Kikuchi's disease): the necrotic appearance of the lymph node cells is caused by apoptosis. *J Dermatol* 1999;26:385–389.

153. Chamulak GA, Brynes RK, Nathwani BN. Kikuchi-Fujimoto disease mimicking malignant lymphoma. *Am J Surg Pathol* 1990;14:514–518.

154. el Mezni F, Mrad K, el Mezni-Benzarti A, et al. Kikuchi-Fujimoto subacute necrotizing lymphadenitis: two histologic forms observed in one patient. *Ann Pathol* 1998;18:422–424.

155. Sumiyoshi Y, Kikuchi M, Ohshima K, et al. A case of histiocytic necrotizing lymphadenitis with bone marrow and skin involvement. *Virchows Arch A Pathol Anat Histol* 1992;420:275–279.

156. Tsai MK, Huang HF, Hu RH, et al. Fatal Kikuchi-Fujimoto disease in transplant recipients: a case report. *Transplant Proc* 1998;30:3137–3138.

157. O'Neill D, O'Grady J, Variend S. Child fatality with pathological features of histiocytic necrotizing lymphadenitis (Kikuchi-Fujimoto disease). *Pediatr Pathol Lab Med* 1998;18:79–88.

158. Facchetti F, de Wolf-Peeters C, van den Oord JJ, et al. Plasmacytoid monocytes (so-called plasmacytoid T-cells) in Kikuchi's lymphadenitis: an immunohistologic study. *Am J Clin Pathol* 1989;92:42–50.

159. Rivano MT, Falini B, Stein H, et al. Histiocytic necrotizing lymphadenitis without granulocytic infiltration (Kikuchi's lymphadenitis). Morphological and immunohistochemical study of eight cases. *Histopathology* 1987;11:1013–1027.

160. Pileri SA, Facchetti F, Ascani S, et al. Myeloperoxidase expression by histiocytes in Kikuchi's and Kikuchi-like lymphadenopathy. *Am J Pathol* 2001;159:915–924.

161. Medeiros LJ, Kaynor B, Harris NL. Lupus lymphadenitis: report of a case with immunohistologic studies on frozen sections. *Hum Pathol* 1989;20:295–299.

162. Schnitzer B. Reactive lymphoid hyperplasias. In: Jaffe ES, ed. *Surgical pathology of the lymph nodes and related organs*. Philadelphia: WB Saunders, 1995:98–132.

163. Schapers RF, Reif R, Lennert K, Knapp W. Mesenteric lymphadenitis due to *Yersinia enterocolitica*. *Virchows Arch A Pathol Anat Histol* 1981;390:127–138.

164. Margileth AM, Wear DJ, English CK. Systemic cat scratch disease: report of 23 patients with prolonged or recurrent severe bacterial infection. *J Infect Dis* 1987;155:390–402.

165. Zangwill KM, Hamilton DH, Perkins BA, et al. Cat scratch disease in Connecticut. Epidemiology, risk factors, and evaluation of a new diagnostic test. *N Engl J Med* 1993;329:8–13.

166. Niedobitek G, Herbst H, Young LS, et al. Patterns of Epstein-Barr virus infection in non-neoplastic lymphoid tissue. *Blood* 1992;79:2520–2526.

167. Norton AJ, Ramsay AD, Isaacson PG. Antigen preservation in infarcted lymphoid tissue. A novel approach to the infarcted lymph node using monoclonal antibodies effective in routinely processed tissues. *Am J Surg Pathol* 1988;12:759–767.

168. Cho KJ, Lee SS, Khang SK. Histiocytic necrotizing lymphadenitis. A clinicopathologic study of 45 cases with in situ hybridization for Epstein-Barr virus and hepatitis B virus. *J Korean Med Sci* 1996;11:409–414.

169. Mahadeva U, Allport T, Bain B, et al. Haemophagocytic syndrome and histiocytic necrotizing lymphadenitis (Kikuchi's disease). *J Clin Pathol* 2000;53:636–638.

170. Wong CY, Law GT, Shum TT, et al. Pulmonary haemorrhage in a patient with Kikuchi disease. *Monaldi Arch Chest Dis* 2001;56:118–120.

171. Yoshino T, Mannami T, Ichimura K, et al. Two cases of histiocytic necrotizing lymphadenitis (Kikuchi-Fujimoto's disease) following diffuse large B-cell lymphoma. *Hum Pathol* 2000;31:1328–1331.

172. Hochberg MC. Updating the American College of Rheumatology revised criteria for the classification of systemic lupus erythematosus. *Arthritis Rheum* 1997;40:1725.

173. Hochberg MC. Systemic lupus erythematosus. *Rheum Dis Clin North Am* 1990;16:617–639.

174. Fox RA, Rosahn PD. The lymph nodes in disseminated lupus erythematosus. *Am J Pathol* 1943;19:73–79.

175. Navratil JS, Ahearn JM. Apoptosis, clearance mechanisms, and the development of systemic lupus erythematosus. *Curr Rheumatol Rep* 2001;3:191–198.

176. Tsao BP. An update on genetic studies of systemic lupus erythematosus. *Curr Rheumatol Rep* 2002;4:359–367.

177. Klemperer P, Pollack AD, Baehr C. Pathology of disseminated lupus erythematosus. *Arch Pathol Lab Med* 1941;32:569–631.

178. Moore RD, Weisberger AS, Bowerfind ES. Histochemical studies of lymph nodes in disseminated lupus erythematosus. *Arch Pathol Lab Med* 1956;62:472–478.

179. Eisner MD, Amory J, Mullaney B, et al. Necrotizing lymphadenitis associated with systemic erythematosus. *Semin Arthritis Rheum* 1996;26:477–482.

180. Kojima M, Nakamura S, Morishita Y, et al. Reactive follicular hyperplasia in the lymph node lesions from systemic lupus erythematosus patients: a clinicopathological and immunohistological study of 21 cases. *Pathol Int* 2000;50:304–312.

181. Godman GD, Deitch AD, Klemperer P. The composition of the LE and hematoxylin bodies of systemic lupus erythematosus. *Am J Pathol* 1958;34:1–23.

182. Komocsi A, Tovari E, Pajor L, et al. Histiocytic necrotizing lymphadenitis preceding systemic lupus erythematosus. *J Eur Acad Dermatol Venereol* 2001;15:476–480.

183. Blornadal L, Lofstrom B, Yin L, et al. Increased cancer incidence in a Swedish cohort of patients with systemic lupus erythematosus. *Scand J Rheumatol* 2002;31:66–71.

184. Green JA, Dawson AA, Walker W. Systemic lupus erythematosus and lymphoma. *Lancet* 1978;2:753–756.

185. Upchurch KS, Medeiros LJ. Case records of the Massachusetts General Hospital. Weekly clinicopathological exercises. Case 38-1988. A 58-year-old woman with fever, sweats, congestive heart failure, and lymphadenopathy after treatment of diagnosis of systemic lupus erythematosus. *N Engl J Med* 1988;319:768–781.

186. Rosai J, Dorfman RF. Sinus histiocytosis with massive lymphadenopathy. A newly recognized benign clinicopathological entity. *Arch Pathol* 1969;87:63–70.

187. Rosai J, Dorfman RF. Sinus histiocytosis with massive lymphadenopathy: a pseudolymphomatous benign disorder. Analysis of 34 cases. *Cancer* 1972;30:1174–1188.

188. Foucar E, Rosai J, Dorfman R. Sinus histiocytosis with massive lymphadenopathy (Rosai-Dorfman disease): review of the entity. *Semin Diagn Pathol* 1990;7:19–73.

189. Welbeck JE. Sinus histiocytosis and massive lymphadenopathy in two Ghanaian brothers. *Trop Doct* 2000;30:182–183.

190. Bankaci M, Morris RF, Stool SE, et al. Sinus histiocytosis with massive lymphadenopathy. Report of its occurrence in two siblings with retropharyngeal involvement in both. *Ann Otol Rhinol Laryngol* 1978;87:327–331.

191. Marsh WL Jr, McCarrick JP, Harlan DM. Sinus histiocytosis with massive lymphadenopathy. Occurrence in identical twins with retroperitoneal disease. *Arch Pathol Lab Med* 1988;112:298–301.

192. Chu P, LeBoit PE. Histologic features of cutaneous sinus histiocytosis (Rosai-Dorfman disease): study of cases both with and without systemic involvement. *J Cutan Pathol* 1992;19:201–206.

193. Levine EA, Landry MM. Rosai-Dorfman disease of soft tissue. *Surgery* 1994;115:650–652.

194. Wenig BM, Abbondanzo SL, Childers EL, et al. Extranodal sinus histiocytosis with massive lymphadenopathy (Rosai-Dorfman disease) of the head and neck. *Hum Pathol* 1993;24:483–492.

195. Zimmerman LE, Hidayat AA, Grantham RL, et al. Atypical cases of sinus histiocytosis (Rosai-Dorfman disease) with ophthalmological manifestations. *Trans Am Ophthalmol Soc* 1988;86:113–135.

196. Lauwers GY, Perez-Atayde A, Dorfman RF, et al. The digestive system manifestations of Rosai-Dorfman disease (sinus histiocytosis with massive lymphadenopathy): review of 11 cases. *Hum Pathol* 2000;31:380–385.

197. Grote HJ, Moesenthin M, Foss HD, et al. Osseous manifestation of Rosai-Dorfman disease (sinus histiocytosis with massive lymphadenopathy). A case report and review of the literature. *Gen Diagn Pathol* 1998;143:341–345.

198. Carpenter RJ 3rd, Banks PM, McDonald TJ, et al. Sinus histiocytosis with massive lymphadenopathy (Rosai-Dorfman disease): report of a case with respiratory tract involvement. *Laryngoscope* 1978;88:1963–1969.

199. Green I, Dorfman RF, Rosai J. Breast involvement by extranodal Rosai-Dorfman disease: report of seven cases. *Am J Surg Pathol* 1997;21:664–668.

200. Andriko JA, Morrison A, Colegial CH, et al. Rosai-Dorfman disease isolated to the central nervous system: a report of 11 cases. *Mod Pathol* 2001;14:172–178.

201. Deodhare SS, Ang LC, Bilbao JM. Isolated intracranial involvement in Rosai-Dorfman disease: a report of two cases and review of the literature. *Arch Pathol Lab Med* 1998;122:161–165.

202. Levine PH, Jahan N, Murari P, et al. Detection of human herpesvirus 6 in tissues involved by sinus histiocytosis with massive lymphadenopathy (Rosai-Dorfman disease). *J Infect Dis* 1992;166:291–295.

203. Luppi M, Barozzi P, Garber R, et al. Expression of human herpes virus-6 antigens in benign and malignant lymphoproliferative diseases. *Am J Pathol* 1998;153:815–823.

204. Foucar E, Rosai J, Dorfman RF, et al. Immunologic abnormalities and their significance in sinus histiocytosis with massive lymphadenopathy. *Am J Clin Pathol* 1984;82:515–525.

205. Jadus MR, Sekhon S, Barton BE, et al. Macrophage colony stimulatory factor-activated bone marrow macrophages suppress lymphocytic responses through phagocytosis: a tentative *in vitro* model of Rosai-Dorfman disease. *J Leukoc Biol* 1995;57:936–942.

206. Paulli M, Bergamaschi G, Tonon L, et al. Evidence for a polyclonal nature of the cell infiltrate in sinus histiocytosis with massive lymphadenopathy (Rosai-Dorfman disease). *Br J Haematol* 1995;91:415–418.

207. Eisen RN, Buckley PJ, Rosai J. Immunophenotypic characterization of sinus histiocytosis with massive lymphadenopathy (Rosai-Dorfman disease). *Semin Diagn Pathol* 1990;7:74–82.

208. Herzog KM, Tubbs RR. Langerhans cell histiocytosis. *Adv Anat Pathol* 1998;5:347–358.

209. Lieberman PH, Jones CR, Steinman RM, et al. Langerhans cell (eosinophilic) granulomatosis. A clinicopathologic study encompassing 50 years. *Am J Surg Pathol* 1996;20:519–552.

210. Lu D, Estalilla OC, Manning JT Jr, et al. Sinus histiocytosis with massive lymphadenopathy and malignant lymphoma involving the same lymph node: a report of four cases and review of the literature. *Mod Pathol* 2000;13:414–419.

211. Foucar E, Rosai J, Dorfman RF. Sinus histiocytosis with massive lymphadenopathy. An analysis of 14 deaths occurring in a patient registry. *Cancer* 1984;54:1834–1840.

212. Pulsoni A, Anghel G, Falcucci P, et al. Treatment of sinus histiocytosis with massive lymphadenopathy (Rosai-Dorfman disease): report of a case and literature review. *Am J Hematol* 2002;69:67–71.

213. Colleoni M, Gaion F, Perasole A, et al. Evidence of responsiveness to chemotherapy in aggressive Rosai-Dorfman disease. *Eur J Cancer* 1995;3:424.

214. Palomera L, Domingo JM, Olave T, et al. Sinus histiocytosis with massive lymphadenopathy: complete response to low-dose interferon-alpha. *J Clin Oncol* 1997;15:2176.

215. Antonius JI, Farid SM, Baez-Giangreco A. Steroid-responsive Rosai-Dorfman disease. *Pediatr Hematol Oncol* 1996;13:563–570.

216. Lennert K. *Malignant lymphomas other than Hodgkin's disease*. New York: Springer Verlag, 1978.

217. Hansmann ML, Fellbaum C, Hui PK, Moubayed P. Progressive transformation of germinal centers with and without association to Hodgkin's disease. *Am J Clin Pathol* 1990;93:219–226.

218. Osborne BM, Butler JJ. Clinical implications of progressive transformation of germinal centers. *Am J Surg Pathol* 1984;8:725–733.

219. Osborne BM, Butler JJ, Gresik MV. Progressive transformation of germinal centers: comparison of 23 pediatric patients to the adult population. *Mod Pathol* 1992;5:135–140.

220. Hicks J, Flaitz C. Progressive transformation of germinal centers: review of histopathologic and clinical features. *Int J Pediatr Otorhinolaryngol* 2002;65:195–202.

221. Ferry JA, Zukerberg LR, Harris NL. Florid progressive transformation of germinal centers. A syndrome affecting young men, without early progression to nodular lymphocyte predominance Hodgkin's disease. *Am J Surg Pathol* 1992;16:252–258.

222. Lennert K, Hansmann M. Progressive transformation of germinal centers: clinical significance and lymphocytic predominance Hodgkin's disease: the Kiel experience. *Am J Surg Pathol* 1987;11:149–150.

223. Dorfman R. Progressive transformation of germinal centers and lymphocyte predominant Hodgkin's disease: the Stanford experience. *Am J Surg Pathol* 1987;11:150–151.

224. Bräuninger A, Yang W, Wacker H-H, et al. B-cell development in progressively transformed germinal centers: similarities and differences with classical germinal centers and lymphocyte-predominant Hodgkin disease. *Blood* 2001;97:714–719.

225. Sneller MC, Wang J, Dale JK, et al. Clinical, immunologic, and genetic features of an autoimmune lymphoproliferative syndrome associated with abnormal lymphocyte apoptosis. *Blood* 1997;89:1341–1348.

226. Nguyen PL, Ferry JA, Harris NL. Progressive transformation of germinal centers and nodular lymphocyte predominance Hodgkin's disease: a comparative immunohistochemical study. *Am J Surg Pathol* 1999;23:27–33.

227. Osborne BM, Butler JJ. Follicular lymphoma mimicking progressive transformation of germinal centers. *Am J Clin Pathol* 1987;88:264–269.

228. Saltzstein S, Ackerman LV. Lymphadenopathy induced by anticonvulsant drugs and mimicking clinically and pathologically malignant lymphomas. *Cancer* 1959;12:164–170.

229. Abbondanzo SL, Irey NS, Frizzera G. Dilantin-associated lymphadenopathy. Spectrum of histopathologic patterns. *Am J Surg Pathol* 1995;19:675–686.

230. De Vriese AS, Philippe J, Van Renterghem DM, et al. Carbamazepine hypersensitivity syndrome: report of 4 cases and review of the literature. *Medicine (Baltimore)* 1995;74:144–151.

231. Katzin WE, Julius CJ, Tubbs RR, et al. Lymphoproliferative disorders associated with carbamazepine. *Arch Pathol Lab Med* 1990;114:1244–1248.

232. Kruger G, Harris D, Sussman E. Effect of dilantin in mice. II. Lymphoreticular tissue atypia and neoplasia after chronic exposure. *Z Krebsforsch Klin Onkol Cancer Res Clin Oncol* 1972;78:290–302.

233. Sinnige HA, Boender CA, Kuypers EW, et al. Carbamazepine-induced pseudolymphoma and immune dysregulation. *J Intern Med* 1990;227:355–358.

234. Dosch HM, Jason J, Gelfand EW. Transient antibody deficiency and abnormal T-suppressor cells induced by phenytoin. *N Engl J Med* 1982;306:406–409.

235. Gennis MA, Vemuri R, Burns EA, et al. Familial occurrence of hypersensitivity to phenytoin. *Am J Med* 1991;91:631–634.

236. Rosenthal CJ, Noguera CA, Coppola A, et al. Pseudolymphoma with mycosis fungoides manifestations, hyperresponsiveness to diphenylhydantoin, and lymphocyte disregulation. *Cancer* 1982;49:2305–2314.

237. Di Lernia V, Viglio A, Cattania M, et al. Carbamazepine-induced, CD30+, primary, cutaneous, anaplastic large-cell lymphoma. *Arch Dermatol* 2001;137:675–676.

238. Jeng YM, Tien HF, Su IJ. Phenytoin-induced pseudolymphoma: reevaluation using modern molecular biology techniques. *Epilepsia* 1996;37:104–107.

CHAPTER 43

Unique Aspects of Primary Extranodal Lymphomas

Mary K. Gospodarowicz, Judith A. Ferry, and Franco Cavalli

Approximately 53,900 new cases of lymphoma and 24,400 deaths occurred in the United States in 2002 (1). Non-Hodgkin's lymphoma is the fifth to sixth most common cause of cancer, after prostate, lung, breast, colorectal, uterine, ovarian, and bladder tumors, or 4% to 5% of new cases. The incidence of non-Hodgkin's lymphoma in western countries has increased substantially in the last 20 years, with the Surveillance, Epidemiology, and End Results (SEER) age-adjusted incidence rates increasing by approximately 80% between 1973 and 1997 (2,3). More than one third of new lymphomas arise from sites other than lymph nodes, even those with no native lymphoid tissue. Extranodal presentations of lymphoma account for between 24% and 48% of new lymphoma cases and often present as localized disease. The outcomes of extranodal lymphomas are difficult to ascertain. Most reported data are limited to single-institution retrospective reviews. In prospective trials, extranodal lymphomas are included together with nodal lymphomas. Recently, the International Extranodal Lymphoma Study Group has originated a number of retrospective and prospective trials to clarify the management issues distinct to extranodal presentations (3a).

The etiology of extranodal lymphomas is multifactorial and includes congenital, acquired, and iatrogenic immune suppression; autoimmune disease; infections, both viral and bacterial; and exposure to pesticides and other environmental agents (see Chapter 44). Although considerable progress has been made in the understanding of gastric lymphoma and its relationship to *Helicobacter pylori*, the precise cause of most lymphomas remains to be elucidated.

The exact definition of extranodal lymphoma remains controversial. The first area of controversy relates to the definition of extranodal lymphomas. Criteria for the diagnosis of primary extranodal lymphoma have been proposed by Dawson for gastrointestinal lymphomas and further refined by Lewin and Herrmann (4–6). The original Dawson criteria stipulated that for a

designation of primary extranodal lymphoma, patients had to present with their main disease manifestation in an extranodal site and have no more than regional lymph node involvement, with no peripheral lymph node involvement and no liver or spleen involvement. Later, these criteria were relaxed to allow for contiguous involvement of other organs (e.g., liver, spleen) and for distant nodal disease, providing that the extranodal lesion was the presenting site and constituted the predominant disease bulk. The designation of stage III and IV lymphomas as primary extranodal lymphomas is debatable. Variable reporting criteria make it difficult to establish the true incidence of primary or localized extranodal lymphomas. Extranodal involvement occurring in the presence of predominantly nodal or disseminated disease may represent secondary extranodal disease spread. Some authors deal with this by discussing stage I and II presentation only as primary extranodal lymphomas, whereas others include as extranodal lymphomas those presentations with a "dominant" extranodal component with only a minor nodal component (7). The second area of controversy is designation of extranodal versus extralymphatic site. The taxonomy in extranodal lymphomas deserves comment insofar as the Ann Arbor Classification recognizes Waldeyer's ring, thymus, spleen, appendix, and Peyer's patches of the small intestine as lymphatic tissues and does not consider them as extranodal lesions. However, most clinicians separate nodal from extranodal presenting sites rather than lymphatic and extralymphatic sites, and for purposes of this review, we use the extranodal definition as indicating presentation outside lymph node areas.

PATHOLOGY

The histologic spectrum of extranodal lymphoma differs from that of nodal lymphoma, with a predominance of frequently localized diffuse large-cell lymphomas, the occurrence of extranodal marginal zone B-cell lymphoma of mucosa-associated lymphoid tissue (MALT) type as a distinct group of lymphomas with homing properties of lymphoma cells, and a paucity of follicular lymphomas. Homing of lymphocytes refers to a controlled pattern of traffic that directs specific lymphocytes to a specific lymphoid tissue in the body. The trafficking of lymphocytes plays a major role in the physiology of the immune system and the implementation of the immune mechanisms (8). The mature lymphocytes have the ability to recirculate continuously between the blood and the lymph. Lymphocyte recirculation is an essential component of the functional immune system. Adhesive interactions between recirculating lymphocytes and the high endothelial venules are mediated by lymphocyte homing receptors (integrins) that recognize tissue-specific molecules expressed on the endothelium (addressins). Homing mechanisms have been implicated in the biology of primary extranodal lymphomas of the skin and gastrointestinal tract, which have several characteristic features that might relate to their trafficking properties (8). Most significant is a marked inclination to spread or recur in the skin or at mucosal gastrointestinal sites, respectively, which is best explained by tissue-specific homing. The identification of the mucosal homing receptor $\alpha_4\beta_7$ integrin that binds to mucosal addressin cellular adhesion molecule MAdCAM-1, a vascular recognition addressin selectively expressed on mucosal endothelium, supports the unique character of gastrointestinal and other MALT lymphomas (8,9). In skin lymphomas, the dissemination is presumably mediated by cutaneous lymphocyte antigen, a skin homing receptor, which is selectively expressed on cutaneous T-cell lymphomas and interacts with E-selectin on skin endothelium. L-selectin mediates the tissue-specific positioning of lymphocytes in peripheral lymph nodes (8). Although in some sites almost all lymphomas are of the same type with identical histology, such as diffuse large B-cell lymphoma in testis, in other sites, a broad spectrum of types of lymphoma is seen. For example, in intestine, in addition to diffuse large B-cell lymphoma; enteropathy-associated T-cell lymphoma; marginal zone B-cell lymphoma, including the distinctive subtype known as *immunoproliferative small intestinal disease*; mantle cell lymphoma; and follicular lymphoma occur. Another site with a spectrum of histologic types of lymphoma is the breast. Primary lymphoma of the breast occurring in young women and associated with pregnancy is commonly a high-grade Burkitt-like lymphoma, whereas later in life, marginal zone B-cell lymphomas, follicular lymphomas, and diffuse large B-cell lymphomas occur (10). A broad spectrum of lymphomas also occurs in the skin where mycosis fungoides and other peripheral T-cell lymphomas, including anaplastic (CD30[+]) large-cell lymphomas, low-grade B-cell lymphomas, and large B-cell lymphomas, are all seen. Although histology is diverse, many primary skin lymphomas exhibit homing properties to the skin, regardless of histologic type. Histologic type is the main determinant of prognosis in both nodal and extranodal lymphomas. However, the specific presenting site is also of importance in extranodal lymphomas. For example, in spite of the other factors being equal, the behavior and prognosis of diffuse large B-cell lymphoma of the brain, the testis, and the bone are all different from one another. The types of lymphomas most commonly encountered in different extranodal sites are shown in Table 43.1. The pathologic features of spe-

TABLE 43.1. *Extranodal lymphoma types most often encountered in different extranodal sites*

Site	Type of lymphoma	Associations
Head and neck		
Waldeyer's ring	Diffuse large B-cell lymphoma	GI involvement
	Follicular lymphoma	—
	Burkitt's lymphoma	—
	Mantle cell lymphoma	—
Paranasal sinuses	Diffuse large B-cell lymphoma	—
Nasal cavity	Extranodal natural killer/T-cell lymphoma	EBV[+]
	Diffuse large B-cell lymphoma	—
Salivary gland	Marginal zone B-cell lymphoma	Sjögren's syndrome
	Follicular lymphoma	—
	Diffuse large B-cell lymphoma	—
Thyroid	Diffuse large B-cell lymphoma	Hashimoto's disease
	Marginal zone B-cell lymphoma	Hashimoto's disease
Ocular adnexa	Marginal zone B-cell lymphoma	—
	Follicular lymphoma	—
Larynx	Diffuse large B-cell lymphoma	—
	Marginal zone B-cell lymphoma	—

(continued)

TABLE 43.1. *Continued*

Site	Type of lymphoma	Associations
Thoracic cavity		
Lung	Marginal zone B-cell lymphoma	Subset: autoimmune disease
	Diffuse large B-cell lymphoma (subtype: lymphomatoid granulomatosis)	Immunocompromise, EBV+
Pleura	Primary effusion lymphoma	HIV+, Kaposi's–sarcoma-associated herpesvirus positive, EBV+
	Pyothorax-associated lymphoma	Tuberculosis positive, EBV+
Heart	Diffuse large B-cell lymphoma	Subset: immunosuppressed
GI and hepatobiliary tract		
Stomach	Diffuse large B-cell lymphoma	—
	Marginal zone B-cell lymphoma	*Helicobacter pylori*
Intestine	Diffuse large B-cell lymphoma	—
	Marginal zone B-cell lymphoma (subtype: immunoproliferative small intestinal disease)	—
	Burkitt's lymphoma	—
	Enteropathy-type intestinal T-cell lymphoma	Celiac disease
	Mantle cell lymphoma	Lymphomatous polyposis
	Follicular lymphoma	Duodenal, most cases
Liver	Diffuse large B-cell lymphoma	—
	Burkitt's lymphoma	—
	Marginal zone B-cell lymphoma	—
Pancreas	Diffuse large B-cell lymphoma	—
Genitourinary tract		
Testis	Diffuse large B-cell lymphoma	—
Ovary	Diffuse large B-cell lymphoma	—
	Burkitt's lymphoma	—
	Follicular lymphoma	—
Uterus, cervix, vagina	Diffuse large B-cell lymphoma	—
	Follicular lymphoma	—
Kidney	Diffuse large B-cell lymphoma	—
	Follicular lymphoma	—
Urinary bladder	Marginal zone B-cell lymphoma	Cystitis
	Diffuse large B-cell lymphoma	—
Urethra	Diffuse large B-cell lymphoma	—
	Marginal zone B-cell lymphoma	—
Miscellaneous		
Breast	Diffuse large B-cell lymphoma	—
	Marginal zone B-cell lymphoma	—
	Follicular lymphoma	—
	Burkitt's lymphoma	Pregnancy, lactation
Bone	Diffuse large B-cell lymphoma	—
	Lymphoblastic lymphoma	Children
Adrenal	Diffuse large B-cell lymphoma	—

EBV, Epstein-Barr virus; GI, gastrointestinal; HIV, human immunodeficiency virus.

TABLE 43.2. *Lymphomas found in extranodal sites*[a]

Type of lymphoma	Extranodal sites	Composition	Usual immunophenotype	Genotype
B-cell lymphomas				
Marginal zone B-cell lymphoma, mucosa-associated lymphoid tissue type	Stomach, intestines, parotid, ocular adnexa, lungs, thyroid, many others	Small lymphocytes, marginal zone B cells, plasma cells, reactive follicles, lymphoepithelial lesions	Monotypic sIg–/+, cIg+/–, CD20+, CD5–, CD10–, CD43+/–	IgH clonally rearranged; no t(11;14); no t(14;18)
Diffuse large B-cell lymphoma	GI tract, Waldeyer's ring, bone, testis, many others	Large centrocytes, centroblasts, immunoblastic, anaplastic large B cells	Monotypic sIg+, CD20+, bcl-2+/–, bcl-6+/–, CD10–/+, CD5–/+, CD43+/–	IgH clonally rearranged; t(14;18), t(8;14), or bcl-6 abnormalities are sometimes found
Burkitt's lymphoma	Ileocecal area, ovary, bones of jaw, Waldeyer's ring	Medium-sized atypical lymphoid cells with round nuclei, basophilic cytoplasm, tingible body macrophages	Monotypic sIgM+, CD20+, CD10+, bcl-6+, bcl-2–, Ki67 ~100%	IgH clonally rearranged; t(8;14), t(2;8) or (8;22) (c-myc)
Mantle cell lymphoma	GI tract (multiple lymphomatous polyposis), Waldeyer's ring	Small to medium-sized, slightly irregular cells with scant cytoplasm	Monotypic sIgMD+, CD20+, CD5+, CD10–, CD43+, cyclin D1+	IgH clonally rearranged; t(11;14)
Follicular lymphoma	Parotid, ocular adnexa, GI tract, breast, others	Mixture of centrocytes and centroblasts, follicular dendritic cells	Monotypic sIg+, CD20+, CD10+, bcl-6+, bcl-2+, CD5–, CD43–	IgH clonally rearranged; t(14;18) usually found
NK/T-cell lymphomas				
Extranodal NK/T-cell lymphoma, nasal type	Nasal cavity, GI tract, testis	Small, medium-sized, or large atypical lymphoid cells, necrosis, vascular damage	cCD3+, CD56+	T-cell receptor genes germline in almost all cases; Epstein-Barr virus positive
Enteropathy-type intestinal T-cell lymphoma	GI tract, especially jejunum	Small to medium-sized cells or large bizarre cells, many admixed reactive cells	CD3+, CD4–/CD8– >CD8+	T-cell receptor genes clonally rearranged

GI, gastrointestinal; Ig, immunoglobulin; NK, natural killer.
[a]Excludes bone marrow, spleen, and skin.

cific types of lymphoma are similar in different extranodal sites; pathologic features are summarized in Table 43.2.

PRESENTING SITES

The spectrum of presenting sites is vast, but in most comprehensive reports, primary lymphomas affecting the stomach and Waldeyer's ring are the most common. In the classic report by Freeman et al. of the SEER experience from 1950 to 1964, stomach lymphoma was most common, followed by intestine, tonsil, and skin (11). Waldeyer's ring lymphomas are frequently considered to be nodal presentations and, therefore, are not included in all extranodal lymphoma statistics. The recent SEER report found stomach, skin, intestine, and brain to be the most common sites of extranodal lymphoma (12). In a population-based study from Denmark, d'Amore found stomach, intestine, skin, and bone to be the most common sites of presentation. Referral patterns may affect institutional experience with primary extranodal lymphoma (13). In the Princess Margaret Hospital experience (see below),

Waldeyer's ring lymphoma (mostly tonsil) and stomach lymphoma were consistently the most common extranodal sites over the last 30 years (14). However, in the last 10 years at the Princess Margaret Hospital, fewer stomach and intestinal lymphomas were referred, whereas there were proportionately more primary bone and extradural lymphomas (Table 43.2). Less common but distinct primary extranodal sites for the development of lymphoma include other head and neck sites (salivary gland, paranasal sinus, gingiva, nasal cavity), orbit, thyroid, breast, lung, male and female genital tract (testis, prostate, ovary, cervix, uterine corpus), urinary bladder, and soft-tissue lymphomas. The least common sites of primary extranodal lymphoma include heart, muscle, kidney, pleura, adrenal gland, liver, and dura mater.

PATIENT CHARACTERISTICS AND PRESENTATION

The characteristics of patients with nodal and extranodal lymphomas are similar, although patients with primary extranodal lymphomas tend to be older and have a lower male to female ratio. In both localized nodal and extranodal lymphomas, stage I disease is seen in two thirds of patients. B symptoms at presentation are uncommon. Presenting symptoms depend on the site of origin and do not differ significantly from symptoms of other malignancies affecting that specific organ. Gastric lymphomas present typically with symptoms of peptic ulcer, and bowel lymphomas present with obstruction, blood loss, or diarrhea, whereas bone lymphoma and some other primary extranodal lymphomas usually present with pain. Tumor bulk at presentation is also closely related to primary site. Characteristically, cutaneous and orbital lymphomas are visible and, therefore, diagnosed early; extradural lymphomas present early but with symptoms and with small bulk disease, whereas gastrointestinal lymphomas or, not infrequently, thyroid lymphomas (especially if associated with preexisting goiter), present with bulk disease. In the absence of nodal involvement, primary extranodal lymphoma is often not suspected, thereby making the histologic diagnosis particularly important. One cannot distinguish clinically lymphoma from carcinoma. Immunophenotypic and histochemical analysis may be required to make this distinction.

APPROACH TO MANAGEMENT

Patient Assessment

The assessment of anatomic extent is similar to that for nodal lymphoma. All patients should be assessed using the template applicable to all lymphoma patients. This includes history with the documentation of B symptoms; complete physical examination; complete blood cell count and lactate dehydrogenase; imaging with computed tomography of neck, chest, abdomen, and pelvis; and bone marrow biopsy. In some centers, gallium scans or positron emission tomography scans are performed routinely. In addition to the routine lymphoma work-up, specific tests to define local disease extent in presenting extranodal sites and potential high-risk areas for occult disease are investigated. Specifically, it is very important to image the head and neck region with computed tomography or magnetic resonance imaging to define disease extent in extranodal lymphomas presenting in the head and neck region and with magnetic resonance imaging for primary bone lymphoma or extranodal lymphomas involving soft tissues (15). Endoscopy should be used as appropriate to define local disease extent in airways, gastrointestinal tract, and urinary tract. In *H. pylori*–related gastric lymphoma, a C14 breath test is useful to ascertain eradication of infection. Cerebrospinal fluid cytology is an essential part of the assessment of primary central nervous system lymphomas, and also of lymphomas involving parameningeal sites, such as extradural or paranasal sinus lymphomas, and primary testis lymphoma because of their pattern of relapse.

Principles of Treatment

In most situations, patients' lymphomas are treated with curative intent. A palliative approach is used in situations in which, due to the condition of the patient or the extent or location of the disease, a radical treatment carries no chance of cure. The principles of the management of extranodal lymphoma follow those of their nodal counterparts with several exceptions. Specific histologic type, tumor bulk, and stage are the main factors in selecting therapy. However, tumor location and pattern of disease should also be considered. Primary extranodal lymphomas may be locally invasive and extensive, and it is very important to document the extent of the initial involvement. Computed tomography of the head and neck and magnetic resonance imaging of spine or bone, although not usually part of routine staging procedures for lymphoma, may be extremely useful. The exact disease extent has to be established before starting chemotherapy, as it is very difficult to plan involved-field radiation therapy in the absence of this information.

The principles of management of patients with extranodal lymphomas are in general analogous to those of the nodal lymphomas. They are based primarily on anatomic disease extent that is documented using the Ann Arbor staging system. The currently accepted histologic classification, the World Health Organization Classification, is based on the lineage (B cell, T cell, or natural killer cell), stage of differentiation (precursor or mature), and clinical presentation of lymphoma in nodal or extranodal site (16). Specific lymphoma entities exhibit a range of morphologic grade and clinical aggressiveness, but grade is treated as a variable within the entity rather than as a basis for classification. In addition to histology and stage, factors known to influence the outcome in patients with extranodal lymphomas include local tumor bulk, number of extranodal sites, lactate dehydrogenase, and performance status (17,18). The latter three and stage are attributes comprising the International Prognostic Index (19). Extranodal lymphomas may involve paired organs such as bilateral parotid glands and bilateral orbital involvement. The Ann Arbor Classification does not directly address the issue of stage designation in such situations. However, the prognosis of such presentations is usually that of stage I disease rather than stage IV disease; therefore, we discuss these presentations in the context of localized disease. The presenting extranodal site may by itself carry an adverse prognosis, as seen in central nervous system lymphoma and testis lymphoma (20,21). In stage I and II disease, local therapy is routinely used, both for cure and local control. However, the recognition of occult distant disease mandates the use of chemotherapy in patients with large-cell or mantle cell lymphomas. In stage III and IV disease, the mainstay of treatment is chemotherapy, and local treatment is not routinely used, although it may still have a role for sites of bulky disease or incomplete response, particularly in a location where local control is desired (e.g., extradural space). The addition of rituximab to CHOP [cyclophosphamide, hydroxydaunomycin, Oncovin (vincristine), and prednisone] chemotherapy has been shown to be of benefit for patients 60 years of age or older and is being explored in other groups of patients (22). Chemotherapy alone is used in lymphoblastic and Burkitt's lymphoma. All of these principles are based on clinical observations and past experience rather than knowledge of basic genetic or biologic factors.

Surgery

The role of surgery in the management of extranodal lymphoma is poorly defined. Stage I primary extranodal lymphoma may be cured with surgery alone, but in general, surgical cure is infrequent. However, resection of the primary tumor may be helpful in obtaining local control of tumor such as in gastrointestinal lymphoma, especially localized intestinal disease, and testis lymphoma (23–25). However, because radiation therapy and chemotherapy are also used, aggressive surgical approaches with compromise of cosmesis or function are not indicated. Specifically, there is no need for amputation in bone lymphoma, mastectomy in breast lymphoma, cystectomy in bladder lymphoma, or abdominoperineal resection for rectal lymphoma. Accordingly, an accurate preoperative or intraoperative diagnosis is essential. For example, in the approach to treatment of parotid tumors, in which radical surgical resection carries a risk of nerve injury, early histologic identification of lymphoma prevents unnecessary damage to the facial nerve.

Radiation Therapy

Local disease control is an important consideration in extranodal lymphoma, as presentation with bulk disease is common, organ function may be at risk and tumor may compress vital structures, such as spinal cord or airway. These factors and the fact that lymphomas in sanctuary sites (brain, testis) are not easily controlled with chemotherapy alone make radiation therapy a more important tool in the management of extranodal lymphomas than their nodal counterparts. The principle of radiation therapy is to deliver an adequate radiation dose to the target volume, including the full extent of disease with appropriate margins. The proper design of radiation therapy plans takes into consideration all staging data, awareness of normal anatomy, familiarity with common routes of lymphatic spread, and appreciation of the radiation tolerance of normal organs and tissues. The correct application of dose and fractionation schedule should assure local control with minimization of acute and late complications. The technique should guarantee reproducibility of treatment on a daily basis. Current radiation therapy techniques include the use of custom-designed fields that conform to an individual patient's anatomy and tumor location. The commonly used radiation therapy plans use involved-field radiation therapy. Involved-field radiation therapy implies treatment to the extranodal site and its immediate lymph node drainage area. The dose of radiation therapy required to achieve local control varies depending on histologic type and tumor bulk (26). There are no prospective, randomized trials designed to determine the optimal radiation therapy dose in the combined modality therapy setting, and a survey of expert radiation oncologists showed significant variation (27) within a range of 30 to 45 Gy. In the setting of combined modality therapy, excellent local control has been obtained with doses of 30 to 35 Gy delivered in 1.75 to 3.00 Gy fractions (28,29). Although the local control in most lymphomas treated with radiation therapy is excellent, a subset of patients in whom local control is much lower has been identified. Local control in lymphomas resistant to CHOP chemotherapy has been achieved in less than 50% of patients (30). There is a suggestion that higher doses are required in chemoresistant disease. However, even with a radiation therapy dose in excess of 40 Gy, local failures have been observed in patients who do not respond or who develop local recurrence after chemotherapy.

Chemotherapy and Combined Modality Therapy

Distant failure has been well documented in localized disease treated with radiation therapy alone (26,31–34). Chemotherapy has been documented to cure patients with diffuse large-cell lymphoma. Such an approach has been shown to improve local control over that obtained with radiation therapy alone and to reduce distant relapse rates. It is important to note that in cases in which no response or only partial response to chemotherapy is observed the dose of radiation therapy has to be increased (30). In patients with localized MALT, follicular, and other small-cell lymphomas, although distant failure is common, there is no evidence that addition of chemotherapy improves survival.

Assessment of Response and Follow-Up

The key determinant of cure is the ability to attain a complete remission. In patients treated with radiation therapy alone, response is usually assessed 4 to 5 weeks after the completion of therapy. The assessment of response includes examination of the organ of presentation and follow-up general examination to rule out disease progression. In patients treated with chemotherapy or combined modality therapy in which chemotherapy is used first, the response is assessed after one or two courses of chemotherapy and every 1 to 2 months thereafter. Remission assessment comprises the demonstration of disease-free status on general assessment and also at an organ-specific level with well-defined criteria (35). Issues that require special consideration include

- Knowledge of the pattern of relapse is helpful in planning follow-up procedures. In situations in which local relapse is uncommon, as in orbital lymphoma, completely resected gastric lymphoma, or small-bulk Waldeyer's ring lymphoma, long-term repeated imaging or endoscopic examination of the presenting site is not routinely indicated. However, follow-up should include a complete physical examination with particular attention to any new adenopathy or unusual symptoms. Although most recurrences in patients with aggressive lymphoma occur within 2 to 3 years after the diagnosis, late relapse occurs. Accordingly, prolonged follow-up is indicated in all patients.

- Evaluation of an organ or tissue that is anatomically or architecturally abnormal as a result of prior involvement by lymphoma such as central nervous system lymphoma.
- Primary bone lymphoma presents persisting radiologic and magnetic resonance imaging abnormalities posttreatment, and bone scan almost certainly identifies changes that cannot distinguish active disease from bone healing and remodeling. Resolution of gallium or positron emission tomography activity may be helpful in such cases.
- The evaluation of paired organs/sites, such as testis, kidney, salivary and lacrimal glands, eye and orbit, lung, breast, and ovary, particularly when one organ has been the primary site of disease and may have been removed as part of initial therapy. The increased risk of disease recurrence or progression in the paired "normal" organ is well established.

After establishment of complete remission, the schedule of follow-up assessment reflects the expectation of events and their time course. Consideration must be directed to

Histology: Late recurrence risk is seen in patients with marginal zone or follicular lymphoma, whereas it is less common in diffuse large B-cell lymphoma or T-cell lymphoma.

Organ of presentation: Certain primary extranodal lymphomas, such as primary central nervous system lymphoma, recur locally or within the tissues of origin with a much higher probability than at remote sites.

Bulk of disease at presentation site and the use of locoregional irradiation in the treatment plan: Tumor bulk in an unresected organ predicts for both local and distant relapse. Local disease control in a site that received a tumoricidal dose of radiation therapy is expected unless substantial tumor bulk was present at the time of radiation therapy.

Management of relapse usually involves chemotherapy. However, in patients who relapse with localized disease, retreatment with chemotherapy and radiation may offer a higher chance of prolonged disease control. In selected circumstances of follicular lymphoma or MALT lymphoma with localized small-bulk recurrence, radiation therapy alone may offer prolonged disease control.

SPECIFIC EXTRANODAL PRESENTATIONS

Lymphomas Presenting in the Head and Neck Region

It is evident that considering all the lymphomas arising in the head and neck region as a single group is simply the heritage of a historical topographic distinction, related to the fact that this anatomic region is the second most common site of localized extranodal presentation of non-Hodgkin's lymphoma. However, it is clear that different lymphoma entities can arise within the head and neck area. The localization of tumor presentation by site reveals tonsil to be the most common, followed by nasopharynx, oral cavity, salivary glands, paranasal sinuses, and base of tongue. The signs and symptoms of a non-Hodgkin's lymphoma may be similar to those of a head and neck squamous cancer, and only by biopsy can the distinction be made. Long-term results in patients presenting with extranodal lymphomas in the head and neck area vary greatly, depending not only on histology but also on sites of presentation. In a series of 156 patients with head and neck lymphomas, the 5-year survival according to site was as follows: salivary gland (61%), oral cavity (57%), tonsil (49%), base of tongue (47%), nasopharynx (36%), and paranasal sinuses (12%) (36).

Waldeyer's Ring Lymphoma

There is controversy as to whether tonsils and Waldeyer's ring in general should be considered as nodal or extranodal sites. Although different biologic and histologic characteristics would instead argue for having these lymphomas considered among the neoplasms of peripheral lymph nodes, most authors include them among extranodal sites. Full staging procedures are mandatory because approximately one of three patients has disseminated disease. An important aspect of the natural history of Waldeyer's ring lymphoma is its relationship to gastrointestinal tract involvement. Therefore, gastrointestinal tract investigations belong among the recommended staging procedures. Patients may present with dysphagia, airway obstruction, or a mass lesion in the throat.

Tonsillar lymphoma is the most common site of involvement in Waldeyer's ring; the other sites include nasopharynx and base of the tongue. The most common histologic type is diffuse large B-cell lymphoma, accounting for at least 60% of cases. Other types include follicular lymphoma, Burkitt's lymphoma, mantle cell lymphoma, marginal zone B-cell lymphoma, and peripheral T-cell lymphoma (37–39). Among children, Burkitt's lymphoma is much more common than it is among adults (40). In the past, published results reflected the use of radiation therapy alone, using involved-field techniques and moderate radiation doses (35 to 50 Gy). High local control rates with overall survival rates of 50% to 60% for stage IE lesions and 25% to 50% for IIE lesions were recorded (41–43). After radiation therapy, the majority of failures occurred distant to the radiation field, indicating a high risk of occult systemic disease with apparently localized Waldeyer's ring presentations. In the past two decades, combined modality therapy with anthracy-cline-based chemotherapy and involved-field radiation became a standard approach. Aviles et al. validated this approach in a prospective randomized trial (44), demonstrating the superiority of combined modality therapy in this disease. The 5-year failure-free survival was 48% for radiation therapy, 45% for chemotherapy alone, and 83% for the combined modality arm ($p < .001$) (44). Others have shown local control rates in excess of 80% and overall survival rates of 60% to 75% (45,46). Combined modality therapy is now a standard approach to the management of localized Waldeyer's ring diffuse large-cell lymphoma.

Paranasal Sinuses and Nasal Cavity Lymphoma

In the Western world most series show a low incidence of sinonasal lymphoma. A University of Virginia series showed only 1.5% of all non-Hodgkin's lymphoma occurring in the nasal cavity and paranasal sinuses. The Kiel registry of 33,402 cases showed only 0.14% of lymphomas occurred in the nasal cavity. In both of these western series, B-cell lineage predominated with 74% to 85% of cases. Clinically, nasal lymphomas present with symptoms of nasal obstruction and epistaxis. Signs of more advanced disease include facial swelling, proptosis, hard-palate perforation, and cranial-nerve palsies (47). When locally advanced, these tumors may invade the adjacent nasopharynx, paranasal sinuses, oropharynx, and palate. Sinonasal lymphomas are relatively rare in the Western world, but in Asian countries, they are the second most frequent lymphoma after lymphomas of the gastrointestinal tract (48). Two main types of lymphoma are found in the sinonasal area: diffuse large B-cell lymphoma and extranodal natural killer/T-cell lymphoma (49). Paranasal sinus lymphomas are almost all diffuse large B-cell lymphoma, whereas most lymphomas arising in the nasal cavity are extranodal natural killer/T-cell lymphoma followed by diffuse large B-cell lymphoma (50–52). In Western populations, paranasal diffuse large B-cell lymphoma is more common, whereas natural killer/T-cell lymphoma is more common in Asian and South American populations. Natural killer/T-cell lymphomas are more commonly associated with angioinvasion, necrosis, and bone erosion, occurring in the sixth and eighth decade of life. Because of these destructive features, sinonasal lymphomas were often designated with the descriptive yet nonspecific name of *lethal midline granuloma*. However, now the extranodal natural killer/T-cell lymphoma is recognized as a distinct clinico-pathologic entity. The lymphomas are composed of small, medium-sized, or large atypical lymphoid cells or a mixture of different-sized cells associated with vascular damage, necrosis, and, sometimes, pseudoepitheliomatous hyperplasia (Fig. 43.1 and Color Plate 71). Immunophenotyping usually shows cytoplasmic CD3$^+$ and CD56$^+$ cells with T-cell receptor genes in a germline configuration, consistent with natural killer cell lymphoma. In a small minority, tumor cells express surface CD3 and show clonal rearrangement of the T-cell receptor genes consistent with true T-cell lymphoma. In virtually all

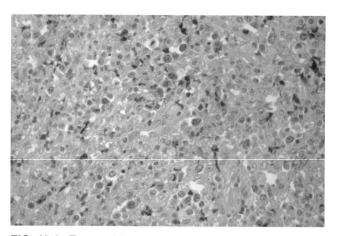

FIG. 43.1. Extranodal natural killer/T-cell lymphoma, nasal cavity. Scattered atypical cells are present in a background of necrotic debris.

cases, Epstein-Barr virus can be detected in neoplastic cells by *in situ* hybridization techniques (53). Tumors with an identical phenotype and genotype may occur in other extranodal sites, most commonly in the skin, subcutis, and gastrointestinal tract, although referred to as *extranodal natural killer/T-cell lymphomas, nasal-type*. In a Chinese study of 175 patients, an overall 5-year survival of 65% and disease-free survival of 57% were noted. Stage IE lesions were most common, with more than one half being limited to the nasal cavity with others demonstrating extension beyond the nasal cavity. The vast majority were natural killer/T-cell lymphomas. The overall survival at 5 years for limited IE lesions was 90%, compared with 57% for extensive IE lesions. The addition of chemotherapy to radiation produced no benefit, although local failure with radiation therapy was substantial (47,54,55). A Stanford report detailed 16 cases (ten B cell, four T cell, and two natural killer cell) treated with combined modality therapy and central nervous system prophylaxis. The overall survival at 5 years was 29%, with a median survival of 18 months. All T- and natural killer–cell patients were dead of disease by 6 months. The report concluded that paranasal sinus/nasal cavity disease is aggressive, requiring combined modality therapy and central nervous system prophylaxis, with a recommendation that natural killer/T-cell disease may require early intensification of therapy to improve progression-free control rates (56). The M.D. Anderson group reported 70 patients with paranasal/nasal cavity disease (57). The M.D. Anderson series, as well as the Massachusetts General Hospital experience, showed that principal factors influencing outcome were stage IE disease and low T category (T1-3 lesions vs. T4), low International Prognostic Index score (0 vs. 1 to 3 vs. 4 or 5), and combined modality therapy (49,57). Only one case of central nervous system progression was identified, suggesting that the risk of central nervous system involvement is low other than in cases with erosion of the base of the skull (57). Historically, treatment has varied among different series and has included radiation alone, chemotherapy alone, or combined modality therapy. Combined modality therapy was not always associated with an improved outcome; however, it is important to note that these series included patients not treated with anthracycline-based regimens and included mixtures of B- and T-cell lymphomas. Presently, for patients presenting with B-cell lymphomas and localized disease, CHOP-type chemotherapy followed by radiation therapy is appropriate. For natural killer/T-cell lymphoma of nasal type, early treatment intensification with high-dose chemotherapy and stem cell support is being tested in prospective clinical trials.

Salivary Gland Lymphoma

Most of the knowledge acquired concerns lymphomas of salivary glands, the vast majority of which are located in the parotid. Salivary gland lymphomas account for 5% to 10% of all salivary gland tumors and somewhat less than 5% of lymphomas at all sites. Three main types of lymphoma occur in salivary glands: marginal zone B-cell lymphoma, follicular lymphoma, and diffuse large B-cell lymphoma, with roughly equal numbers of each type. Other types are rare. The follicular lymphomas tend to arise in intraparotid lymph nodes rather than in the salivary gland parenchyma. They have pathologic features similar to those of follicular lymphoma, arising in nodes away from the parotid. The diffuse large B-cell lymphomas may arise *de novo* or via transformation of a low-grade lymphoma. A recent International Extranodal Lymphoma Study Group study showed that salivary glands are the most common localization among extragastric marginal zone lymphomas (58). Patients usually present with a painless mass, most often in the parotid, followed by the submandibular gland—only occasionally in the sublingual gland or minor salivary glands. Bilateral presentations are frequent. Marginal zone lymphomas of the salivary gland are frequently associated with Sjögren's syndrome. Lymphoepithelial sialoadenitis is characteristic of Sjögren's syndrome and not infrequently represents a precursor lesion for the development of marginal zone lymphoma. Marginal zone B-cell lymphomas generally follow an indolent course and tend to remain localized for prolonged periods of time and are associated with excellent prognosis (59). A recent study of marginal zone B-cell lymphoma of the parotid glands showed a 90% 5-year overall survival and a 100% complete-response rate. No advantage in complete-response rate or time to treatment failure was seen for combined modality therapy over radiation therapy alone (44). Disfiguring surgery should be avoided because radiation therapy, chemotherapy, or the combination of chemotherapy and radiotherapy are all very effective in achieving local control. The role of surgery should be limited to excisional biopsy, whereas further therapy has to be tailored to stage and especially the histologic subtype; radiotherapy is used for localized low-grade lymphomas and combined modality approaches using doxorubicin-containing regimens for aggressive histologies. As is the case for all other MALT sites, salivary gland lymphomas presenting with these histologic types are very sensitive to the monoclonal antibody rituxan; however, the

relative merit and the final role of this new modality in the treatment plan of MALT lymphomas have still to be ascertained (58). Radiation offers excellent local control for limited-stage salivary gland lymphoma but may aggravate xerostomia already produced by Sjögren's. The overall survival at 5 years approaches 70% to 80%, but there is a continuing distant-relapse risk, characteristic of the natural history of these lymphomas. No proven benefit has been documented for chemotherapy in the management of MALT tumors, although the combined modality approach using anthracycline-based chemotherapy is standard treatment for those transformed to large-cell lymphoma.

Thyroid Lymphoma

Primary thyroid lymphoma occurs most frequently in older female patients with a history of Hashimoto's thyroiditis. Marginal zone lymphomas and stage I lymphomas carry a better prognosis than other histologic types (60). Patients usually present with painless unilateral or bilateral enlargement of the thyroid gland. Occasionally, very rapid enlargement of the thyroid may cause obstruction of the trachea with respiratory compromise. The majority of lymphomas are diffuse large B-cell type, and almost all of the remainder are marginal zone lymphomas (Fig. 43.2 and Color Plate 72). Many of the diffuse large B-cell lymphomas have a component of marginal zone lymphoma consistent with large-cell transformation of the underlying low-grade lymphoma. Rare cases of other types, including follicular lymphoma, Burkitt's lymphoma, and peripheral T-cell lymphoma, have been reported (1,61). Surgery is a diagnostic procedure and is not considered a definitive intervention for thyroid lymphoma, and an occasional patient may require tracheotomy to relieve airway obstruction at diagnosis. With locoregional radiation therapy to a moderate dose of 35 to 45 Gy, local control is achieved in more than 75% of patients and is greater than 95% in patients with MALT histology. Overall, survival rates at 5 years range from 40% to 75%, with relapse-free rates of 38% to 64%, depending on prognostic attributes (62–64). For MALT histology, radiation therapy alone is recommended. For diffuse large B-cell lymphoma, with or without a MALT component, given the high distant relapse rates with radiation therapy alone, chemotherapy alone or, more commonly, chemotherapy and radiation therapy has become the standard treatment approach. Systemic progression is noted commonly in the gastrointestinal tract, liver, and spleen. A link among the gastrointestinal tract, Waldeyer's ring, and thyroid lymphoma has been observed. Central nervous system involvement is rare. Localized thyroid lymphoma of large B-cell type is treated with combined modality therapy. With chemotherapy and radiation, local control, survival, and relapse-free survival exceed 70% to 80% (63).

Lymphoma of Ocular Adnexa

Lymphomas of ocular adnexa are lymphomas arising in the tissues and structures that surround the eye: the conjunctiva,

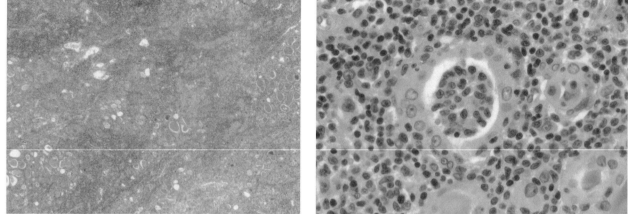

FIG. 43.2. Thyroid gland, marginal zone lymphoma, arising in association with Hashimoto's thyroiditis. **A:** Hashimoto's thyroiditis with patchy lymphocytic infiltrate and oxyphil change of thyroid follicles. **B:** Marginal zone lymphoma with a lymphoepithelial lesion composed of an aggregate of neoplastic cells within the lumen of a thyroid follicle with oxyphil change.

lacrimal gland, orbital soft tissues, and eyelids. Ocular adnexal lymphoma is considerably more common than intraocular lymphoma (lymphoma of the eye). Lymphomas arising in these two sites should be clearly distinguished because of their different natural histories; intraocular lymphoma is a subset of primary central nervous system lymphoma and is associated with a much worse prognosis than ocular adnexal lymphoma. The lymphomas of the ocular adnexa presenting anteriorly as conjunctival lesions are usually small, characteristically salmon pink, nodular, or plaque-like lesions in the conjunctiva, with symptoms of blurred vision, chemosis, and epiphora. The posteriorly located lesions present with swelling, palpable or visible mass, and proptosis. Pain and systemic symptoms are uncommon, but with increasing bulk of the lesion, pressure and double vision may occur. Sixty percent to 75% of cases are extranodal marginal zone B-cell lymphomas. The next most common type is follicular lymphoma, followed by diffuse large B-cell lymphoma. Other types of B-cell lymphoma may present occasionally with ocular adnexal involvement. T-cell lymphoma is very uncommon. Primary Hodgkin's disease has not been documented in this site (65–67). Thus, in the ocular adnexa, there is a marked predominance of low-grade B-cell lymphomas. Histologic features are similar to those seen in other sites. The marginal zone lymphomas are composed of small lymphocytes and marginal zone cells, often with admixed reactive follicles. There may be a component of neoplastic plasma cells, sometimes forming aggregates, or, in cases involving the conjunctiva, a prominent subepithelial layer. Marginal zone cells often invade the overlying conjunctival epithelium, but surprisingly, well-formed lymphoepithelial lesions are only rarely found when marginal zone lymphoma involves the lacrimal gland. The immunophenotypic and genotypic features of ocular adnexal lymphoma are similar to those of the same type of lymphoma occurring in other sites (68). Treatment is directed at cure while preserving vision and the

integrity of the orbit. Extensive surgery should be avoided, as it is entirely unnecessary. Most orbital lesions are easily controlled with low to moderate doses of radiation therapy. Conjunctiva lesions may be treated with direct photon beams. Treatment with an anterior field or electron beam provides satisfactory therapy for anterior lesions limited to the eyelid or bulbar conjunctiva, with the advantage of sparing orbital structures, compared with the use of a megavoltage photon beam. Radiation therapy to 20 to 30 Gy in 10 to 20 daily fractions for small B-cell lymphomas results in a local control rate in excess of 95% (69–74). Higher doses are not required, and their use results in higher acute and long-term morbidity. Fewer data are available for large B-cell lymphomas; however, the dose-control data suggest that for patients with small tumors, a dose of 35 Gy in 1.75 to 2.00 Gy fractions provides excellent local control. For patients with bigger large B-cell tumors, short duration anthracycline-based chemotherapy (e.g., CHOP for three courses) followed by radiation therapy to a dose of 30 to 35 Gy in 1.50 to 1.75 Gy daily fractions is recommended. The complications of radiation therapy, commonly seen when doses of 40 Gy or more are used, include cataract formation, keratitis, and dry eye. The tolerance dose of the lacrimal gland is 40 Gy in 20 daily fractions (73). Damage to the optic nerve and retina should not be seen with a radiation therapy dose of 40 Gy or less.

The overall actuarial 10-year survival rates for orbital lymphomas reported in the literature are 75% to 80%. These excellent survival rates are likely due to a preponderance of indolent B-cell lymphomas. After a complete response, the risk of locoregional failure is extremely low (74). The most common site of relapse is the contralateral orbit, but generalized disease is occasionally seen. Distant failure rates vary from 20% to 50%, but as in other cases of low-grade lymphoma, failures can be successfully managed, and prolonged survival is common. In patients presenting with diffuse large B-cell lymphoma, particularly with bulky orbital lesions, the risk of distant failure is 30% to 60%. Occasionally, for a patient with bulky tumor, whose cornea cannot be protected, the use of radiation therapy alone to high doses may result in severe radiation complications. In such cases, the use of chemotherapy alone or combined modality is preferable.

Lymphomas Presenting in the Gastrointestinal Tract

Gastric Lymphoma

Diffuse large B-cell lymphoma is the most common type of gastric lymphoma (see Color Plate 73A), followed closely by marginal zone lymphoma. An uncertain proportion of the large B-cell lymphomas represent large-cell transformation of marginal zone lymphomas. Other lymphomas are much less common. A major change in the management of gastric lymphoma occurred after the identification of *H. pylori* as the etiologic agent for many cases of gastric marginal zone lymphoma.

Gastric MALT lymphoma typically occurs in patients older than 40 years of age but can occur at any age. The sex incidence is equal. The presenting symptoms are usually those of nonspecific dyspepsia and are more suggestive of gastritis or peptic ulcer than a neoplastic lesion. Likewise, endoscopy more often shows inflamed, sometimes eroded mucosa rather than a tumor mass. Patients with marginal zone lymphoma are more likely to present with mild to moderate symptoms, whereas those with diffuse large-cell lymphoma are more likely to have symptoms of bleeding and perforation.

Historically, the therapeutic strategies in gastric lymphoma were based on surgical approaches. Surgical resection with postoperative radiation therapy or postoperative chemotherapy was standard. In the past decade, approaches without surgery using primary chemotherapy followed by radiation therapy have been shown to produce equivalent results (75,76). Nonsurgical approaches have not been directly compared to outcomes incorporating partial gastrectomy. Surgery alone using partial or total gastrectomy has been reported to cure a proportion of patients, mostly those with low-grade lymphomas (25,77). Surgery alone, especially partial gastrectomy, requires careful follow-up because marginal zone lymphoma is a multifocal disease, and stump recurrences have been reported. Studies with long-term follow-up report relapse-free rates and survival inferior to those of studies in which adjuvant therapy has been used. d'Amore, in a retrospective review of the Danish Lymphoma Study Group experience, found that patients with gastric lymphoma who received radiation therapy as part of their therapy had a reduced relative risk of relapse (78). In previous Princess Margaret Hospital experience, patients with stage IA and IIA gastric lymphoma treated with complete gross surgical resection and low-dose (20 to 25 Gy) postoperative radiation therapy had an 86% 10-year relapse-free survival (79–81). In this favorable group of patients, the depth of stomach-wall invasion did not affect the outcome. Others have shown good results in patients with complete resection of tumor followed by chemotherapy alone or combined modality therapy (82). It

is uncertain whether the favorable outcome in these reports was the effect of surgery or low tumor bulk allowing complete surgical resection. Surgical resection is associated with a significant morbidity and mortality, and its use in an unselected patient population may have an adverse effect on outcome.

Chemotherapy alone or chemotherapy followed by radiation therapy may produce similar results. Maor and colleagues reported a series of 34 patients treated with chemotherapy and radiation therapy without gastrectomy; 24 did not require gastrectomy (83). Taal and colleagues reported a 64% disease-free survival at 4 years in patients treated with radiation therapy alone without prior tumor resection (84). The updated Amsterdam experience treating gastric lymphoma with chemotherapy and radiation therapy or radiation therapy alone without an attempt at surgical resection revealed a 5-year relapse-free survival of 85% in stage I and 58% in stage II patients (84,85). The modern approach to the management of gastric lymphoma is based on histology and is outlined below.

Diffuse Large B-Cell Lymphoma of the Stomach

The modern approach to the management of diffuse large B-cell lymphoma of the stomach follows the principles for treatment of nodal lymphoma. Patients are staged clinically with computed tomography of the abdomen, gastroscopy, and endoscopic ultrasound. The combined modality approach with CHOP chemotherapy followed by involved-field radiation therapy is the standard management for stage I and II disease. Toxicity of radiation therapy can be reduced using three-dimensional conformal techniques and minimizing the radiation therapy dose to the kidneys and the liver (86). Studies of the reproducibility of three-dimensional gastric radiation therapy are ongoing. In cases in which tumor regression is observed after CHOP chemotherapy, excellent permanent local control and survival are observed. However, in chemoresistant cases, surgical resection may be considered, as local control with radiation therapy for large-bulk chemorefractory disease is less than optimal.

The approach to treatment of gastric lymphoma has radically changed in the past decade. With conservative approaches having proved successful, the need for routine gastrectomy has been eliminated. However, the approach to this disease is not consistent. Gastric lymphoma is at the crossroads of the expertise of gastroenterologists, oncologists, and hematologists. Gastroenterologists are more likely to use endoscopic ultrasound to stage these patients and are far more inclined to recommend surgery, whereas hematologists and oncologists are more likely to stage the patients with the emphasis on systemic disease and use chemotherapy with or without radiation therapy.

Intestinal Lymphoma

In this category, small bowel lymphoma is by far the most common presentation, with large bowel or rectal lymphoma being less frequent. Presenting symptoms vary from feeling of abdominal fullness, nausea, diarrhea, and abdominal pain to bowel obstruction and perforation. Because of these nonspecific presenting symptoms, many patients require laparotomy for diagnosis and have resection of bowel lesions at diagnosis.

Distinct clinicopathologic entities include intestinal marginal zone lymphoma, some of which are immunoproliferative small intestinal disease (or α-chain disease), diffuse large B-cell lymphoma, enteropathy-associated T-cell lymphoma, Burkitt's lymphoma, mantle cell lymphoma, and follicular lymphoma (87). The majority of primary intestinal lymphomas are large-cell tumors of B-cell lineage, although considerable diversity exists in histologic subtypes, with distinct clinicopathologic features underscoring the importance of lymphoma typing (88).

The management of diffuse large B-cell lymphoma is usually with surgery followed by chemotherapy. In patients in whom complete tumor resection is not feasible, chemotherapy followed by radiation therapy is standard (79,80). The outcome reported in the literature varies, depending on the extent of disease and histology. In a large series of intestinal lymphomas, Domizio documented a 75% 5-year survival for patients with B-cell lymphomas and only a 25% 5-year survival for those with T-cell tumors (89). The poor outcome of patients with intestinal T-cell lymphoma has also been documented in the British National Lymphoma Investigation group experience (90) and in Danish experience (13). Site of involvement was also of prognostic significance, with lesions in the terminal ileum having the best survival, but this is likely due to association between site and histology, with terminal ileum lymphomas being usually of B-cell type. Other prognostic factors in primary intestinal lymphoma include age, performance status, B symptoms, and mesenteric lymph node involvement (stage II disease) (13,90).

Immunoproliferative intestinal disease, alpha heavy chain disease, and *Mediterranean lymphoma* all refer to various manifestations of an unusual subtype of marginal zone lymphoma affecting the small intestine (87,91). Patients are mostly young adults from the Middle East who present with severe malabsorption, diarrhea, and weight loss. Approximately one half of them have free alpha heavy chains, without associated light chain, in the serum (alpha heavy-chain disease). The lymphoma typically shows diffuse thickening of a long segment of the small intestine. Microscopic examination shows a broad layer of plasma cells beneath which is a variably prominent layer of marginal zone B cells. The plasma cells express alpha heavy chain, usually without light chain. Patients are often malnourished and have a poor performance status and frequently cannot tolerate standard therapy. Overall survival has been poor, probably partly due to late diagnosis. Several authors have reported that treatment with the tetracycline group of antibiotics can produce clinical, histologic, and immunologic remissions. Remissions have also been described after chemotherapy, and more recently, a report of regression of duodenal immunoproliferative intestinal disease after treatment of *H. pylori* was described (92). The role of radiation therapy and surgical resection remains to be defined. Despite several available treatments, immunoproliferative intestinal disease may be a highly lethal disease with reported survival rates as low as 23% at 5 years

(93). Patients with resectable stage I or II$_1$ disease have a 5-year survival of 40% to 47%, compared with 0% to 25% for unresectable or stage II$_2$ disease. After a prolonged time, often many years, immunoproliferative intestinal disease may transform into an aggressive immunoglobulin A–positive diffuse large B-cell lymphoma (94).

Enteropathy-type intestinal T-cell lymphoma is a rare lymphoma usually affecting older adults with a history of celiac disease. Patients present with severe abdominal pain due to obstruction or perforation. This lymphoma preferentially involves the jejunum, producing circumferentially oriented linear ulcers, typically unassociated with prominent bowel-wall thickening or a large mass. The adjacent mucosa usually shows villous atrophy. The lymphomas may be composed of small- to medium-sized atypical lymphoid cells or of large, atypical, sometimes anaplastic large cells, with an abnormal T-cell immunophenotype (Fig. 43.3). Admixed reactive cells may be abundant, sometimes obscuring the neoplastic population. Patients are often severely malnourished and frequently cannot tolerate aggressive therapy. This, combined with the aggressive nature of the lymphoma, leads to a very poor prognosis for this disease (68,95).

Mantle cell lymphoma of the small intestine most often takes the form of innumerable small, superficially located polypoid lesions referred to as *multiple lymphomatous polyposis*. The histologic and immunophenotypic features are similar to mantle cell lymphoma in other sites (96). The prognosis for mantle cell lymphoma is poor in spite of aggressive chemotherapy, similar to its nodal equivalent.

Follicular lymphoma arising in the gastrointestinal tract has an unexplained predilection to involve the duodenum. The follicular lymphoma may take the form of mucosal nodularity or larger, deeply invasive masses. The lymphomas are usually low grade and show histologic, immunophenotypic, and genotypic features that are similar to those of primary nodal follicular lymphomas. The prognosis is good (97,98).

Rectal presentations are less common than other sites in the lower intestinal tract. Diffuse small non–cleaved-cell lymphoma is the most common, although diffuse large-cell lymphomas also occur (99). Treatment usually includes chemotherapy and radiation therapy (30 to 40 Gy in 1.5 to 2.0 Gy daily fractions) for patients presenting with bulky lesions or intermediate-grade lymphoma. Involved-field radiation therapy alone (30 to 35 Gy in 1.50 to 1.75 Gy daily fractions) has been successful in providing long-term disease control for MALT lymphoma of the rectum. Abdominoperineal resection should be discouraged, as there is no evidence that it improves local control or survival.

Lymphomas Presenting in the Genitourinary System

Testicular Lymphoma

Malignant lymphoma of the testis is a rare disease representing 5% of all testicular tumors and only 1% of all lymphomas, with an incidence of 0.26 per 100,000 men (100,101).

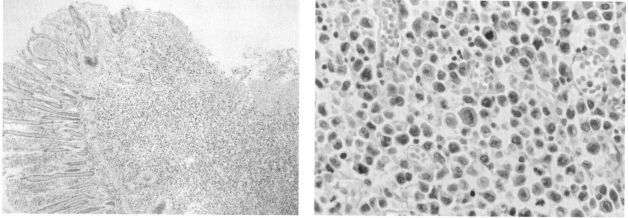

FIG. 43.3. Enteropathy-type intestinal T-cell lymphoma. **A:** Low power shows small intestine with a dense, atypical cellular infiltrate associated with ulceration. Intact mucosa is present focally. **B:** High power shows large, bizarre lymphoid cells that proved to be T cells on immunophenotyping.

Lymphoma, however, is still the most common testicular tumor in men older than 60 years of age (7,101,102), and approximately 85% of patients with testicular lymphoma are older than 60 years of age. Bilateral testicular tumors may be found at diagnosis, or contralateral involvement may develop years later and has been observed in up to 35% of cases (100,103,104). The demonstration of monoclonality in metachronous contralateral testis lymphoma suggests that bilateral involvement is a manifestation of the same disease (105). Most testicular lymphomas are diffuse large B-cell lymphomas. Isolated cases of natural killer/T-cell lymphomas, nasal type; T-cell lymphomas; and follicular lymphomas have been reported (106,107). The molecular or genetic features of diffuse large-cell lymphomas presenting in testis versus other organs have not been studied widely. More than 50% of patients present with stage I disease limited to testis, and approximately 20% present with stage II disease. Presentation with stage III disease is uncommon. The assessment of the patient with testis lymphoma is similar to other lymphomas. However, in addition to the routine tests, staging investigations should include cerebrospinal fluid cytology, and in some centers, brain imaging is recommended. Orchiectomy is both diagnostic and therapeutic, providing local tumor control. Rarely, orchiectomy has been curative, attesting that primary testis lymphoma can present as truly localized disease (104). However, in most cases, occult distant disease is present. Primary testicular lymphoma has been recognized as a highly lethal disease, with overall 5-year survival rates ranging from 16% to 50% with a median survival of 12 to 24 months. The characteristic pattern of failure is mostly distant, with a high proportion of relapses in extranodal sites, including skin, lung, pleura, soft tissue, and Waldeyer's ring. Central nervous system relapse, both meningeal as well as in brain parenchyma, is frequent, as is recurrence in the contralateral testis (21,103,108). Retroperitoneal radiation therapy in stage I disease is no longer used; however, patients with stage II disease receive radiation therapy as part of the combined modality approach recommended for stage II diffuse large-cell lymphoma presenting in other sites.

The introduction of adjuvant chemotherapy resulted in an improved relapse-free rate and survival (109,110). Connors et al. treated patients with a 6-week course of MACOP-B [methotrexate, Adriamycin (doxorubicin), cyclophosphamide, Oncovin (vincristine), prednisone, bleomycin] or three cycles of CHOP and observed survival of 93% with a median follow-up of 44 months (109). However, other authors did not observe these excellent survival results, although chemotherapy appears to have improved the short-term survival (108,111,112). The pattern of failure in the central nervous system has led to a recommendation for routine central nervous system prophylaxis with, at least, intrathecal chemotherapy (21,111). Its value, however, is controversial because central nervous system failures have been observed in patients who received intrathecal chemotherapy. Many central nervous system failures occur in brain parenchyma rather than meninges, and some also occur several years after the initial presentation.

Failure in the contralateral testis is well documented and occurs in 5% to 35% of patients. Low-dose radiation therapy (25 to 30 Gy in 10 to 15 daily fractions) to the contralateral testis eliminates the risk of failure at this site, carries little morbidity in this elderly patient population, and is recommended for all patients with primary testicular lymphoma (21). In the Princess Margaret Hospital experience, 26 patients treated with prophylactic scrotal radiation therapy had no failure in the contralateral testis, compared with a 12.5% recurrence in patients without scrotal radiation therapy. This is consistent with the Manchester experience that scrotal irradiation prevents a relapse in the contralateral testicle in 100% of patients (113). The International Extranodal Lymphoma Study Group conducted a retrospective study of 373 patients with a diagnosis of primary testicular diffuse large-cell lymphoma (102). The majority of patients (75%) received chemotherapy; combined modality therapy was used in 39% of patients. In addition, 34% of patients received prophylactic scrotal radiation therapy, but only 18% had prophylactic intrathecal chemotherapy. The 5-year survival was 48%, and the 10-year survival was 27%. The outcome of patients who received anthracycline-based chemotherapy was better than that of those who did not receive it. Central nervous system failures occurred up to 10 years after initial presentation and were observed in 54 patients. The actuarial 5- and 10-year risks of central nervous system relapse were 20% and 35%, respectively. Prophylactic intrathecal chemotherapy was associated with an improved progression-free survival. A continuous risk of recurrence in the contralateral testis (15% at 3 years, 40% at 15 years) was observed in patients who had not received prophylactic scrotal radiation therapy. The International Extranodal Lymphoma Study Group study represents the largest body of information on outcomes of patients with testis lymphoma to date (102). The disease is rare, making randomized trials virtually impossible to mount. These data suggest that the use of chemotherapy, prophylactic intrathecal chemotherapy, and prophylactic scrotal radiation therapy is associated with an improved outcome. Furthermore, the recent report of improved response to treatment and improved survival in elderly patients by the addition of rituximab to CHOP chemotherapy is promising (22). The International Extranodal Lymphoma Study Group data suggest that intrathecal chemotherapy may indeed control microscopic meningeal disease. Intrathecal chemotherapy may decrease the risk of meningeal failure but is unlikely to affect the risk of failure in brain parenchyma. Prevention of parenchymal brain relapse can be addressed with the use of methotrexate chemotherapy or prophylactic cranial radiation therapy. In small-cell lung cancer, prophylactic cranial radiation therapy is used in patients with limited disease who achieve complete remission. It has been shown to reduce the rate of central nervous system metastasis and improve the progression-free and overall survival (114,115). Noting the frequency of central nervous system relapse in testicular lymphoma, control of occult central nervous system disease may well increase the overall survival in these patients. There are few published data regarding the benefit of prophylactic cranial radiation therapy in testis lymphoma.

Bladder Lymphoma

Primary lymphoma of the urinary bladder is very rare, but a number of case reports and small series of patients have been documented. Patients commonly present with frequency, dysuria, and occasionally hematuria. Cystoscopic examination shows a submucosal mass with an edematous and friable mucosa. Biopsy usually reveals marginal zone B-cell lymphoma, frequently arising on a background of chronic cystitis. Marginal zone lymphomas of the bladder are usually localized and are associated with a particularly good prognosis (116). The next most common type is diffuse large B-cell lymphomas, some of which arise through large-cell transformation of marginal zone lymphoma. Other types are rare (117,118).

Treatment has traditionally involved partial cystectomy or radiotherapy to the pelvis. The prognosis is related to histologic type and extent of tumor (119). As for other extranodal lymphomas, indolent lymphomas may be managed with radiation therapy alone, but large-cell lymphomas should be treated with anthracycline-based chemotherapy followed by local radiation therapy. There are limited data regarding the optimal dose and technique of radiation therapy, but there is no reason to suggest that the sensitivity of the tumor is different from that of other MALT lymphomas. Several reports attest to a favorable prognosis of bladder lymphoma (120,121). Long-term survival has been observed in approximately 40% to 50% of patients, although a small series of four patients with MALT lymphoma was reported by Al-Maghrabi et al., and all patients were controlled by radiotherapy alone, with follow-up ranging between 1 and 13 years (122).

Lymphoma of the Ovary

This is a very rare form of primary extranodal lymphoma. Patients present with abdominal pain or finding of an asymptomatic abdominal mass. Diffuse large B-cell lymphomas are most common, followed by Burkitt's lymphoma and follicular lymphoma. Burkitt's lymphoma is more common among younger patients and patients in areas endemic for Burkitt's lymphoma (123). Treatment with chemotherapy alone may preserve gonadal and hormonal function, but for localized diffuse large B-cell lymphoma, combined modality therapy is recommended. In small series reported over long periods, various forms of treatment have been used singly or in combination. Two- and 5-year overall survival rates of 42% and 24%, respectively, have been cited (124). As lymphomas of the ovary are most commonly of diffuse large B-cell type and clearly are most commonly associated with extensive dissemination, the initial treatment approach should comprise chemotherapy. Radiation therapy may be appropriate in the circumstance of a localized presentation with residual disease postsurgery or after definitive chemotherapy. Local control is, however, a lesser issue, given the usual resection of the presenting lesion and the common pattern of failure being one of systemic disease progression.

Lymphoma of the Uterine Corpus, Uterine Cervix, and Vagina

Lymphomas of uterus, cervix, and vagina usually present in middle-aged women, although presentations at younger ages occur. Cervical lymphomas are much more common than those arising in the uterine corpus or vagina. Abnormal vaginal bleeding is the most common symptom. These lymphomas are often bulky and deeply invasive. By far, the most common type is diffuse large B-cell lymphoma, followed by follicular lymphoma and rare cases of Burkitt's lymphoma, marginal zone B-cell lymphoma, and others (117,125). The diffuse large B-cell lymphomas and follicular lymphomas are often associated with sclerosis. The standard therapy for

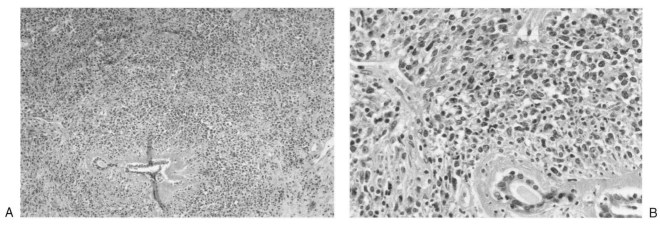

FIG. 43.4. Diffuse large B-cell lymphoma of the breast. **A:** A dense, diffuse infiltrate of lymphoid cells surrounds a small duct in the breast. **B:** High power shows large atypical lymphoid cells adjacent to nonneoplastic mammary epithelium.

patients with stage IE lesions has usually comprised radiation therapy with or without antecedent surgery. There is no evidence that radical surgery is necessary, and, indeed, there is no strong indication for more than a diagnostic biopsy with subsequent detailed staging evaluation. Radiation therapy alone for localized MALT or follicular lymphoma offers a very high probability of local control. Combined chemotherapy and radiation therapy for diffuse large B-cell tumors are appropriate, and, given the impact of radiation therapy on ovarian function in those in the reproductive age range, the use of chemotherapy alone has been recommended with some clinical justification. A 5-year overall survival rate of 73% is quoted by Harris and Scully (126), with an 89% 5-year rate for patients with stage IE disease. Important prognostic factors include stage and histology. Local failure is very uncommon after surgery and radiation therapy for endometrial, cervical, or vaginal lymphoma (127). Progression of primary vaginal lymphoma in the subcutaneous tissues of the abdominal wall, intraabdominal lymph nodes, lung, and inguinal lymph nodes has been noted (128).

Breast Lymphoma

Primary lymphoma of the breast is a rare disease that accounts for less than 0.05% of all breast malignancies and less that 1% of all non-Hodgkin's lymphomas. It comprises only 2% of localized extranodal lymphomas. Almost all tumors are of B-cell lineage, with diffuse large B-cell type predominant (Fig. 43.4), although follicular and marginal zone lymphomas (Fig. 43.5) are also described. The usual presentation is with a discrete painless mass, although aggressive presentations with rapid painful enlargement of one or both breasts also occur. The latter presentation may be associated with pregnancy and is characteristic of a Burkitt's or other aggressive lymphoma. A spectrum of histologic types is seen in primary breast lymphoma, from marginal zone lymphoma to diffuse large B-cell to Burkitt's lymphoma (129–131). The largest individual series with clinical follow-up has been reported by Giardini et

al. (132). Thirty-five patients presenting with stage I or II disease were identified over a 30-year period. The most common histology was diffuse large-cell lymphoma, with only seven patients having indolent histology. With a mean follow-up of 45 months, the overall 5-year survival was 43%. Stage and histology were significant prognostic factors. A number of central nervous system relapses were reported in several series (130). A study of 19 patients by DeBlasio et al. showed a 66% survival at 4 years (133). As for other extranodal lymphomas, diffuse large B-cell lymphomas require combined modality therapy. It is important to note that the completeness of surgical excision does not appear to affect local control. Thus, mastectomy is not recommended, and breast preservation is possible in the majority of cases. Properly planned and delivered radiation therapy results in excellent local control, especially in patients presenting without bulky disease or in those with marginal zone lymphoma. The radiation therapy volume

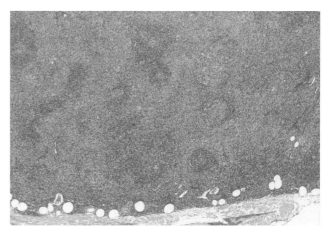

FIG. 43.5. Marginal zone B-cell lymphoma, mucosa-associated lymphoid tissue type of the breast. There is a well-circumscribed but nonencapsulated infiltrate of lymphoid cells within the breast. Follicles are scattered within a diffuse proliferation of marginal zone cells.

should include the whole breast and the ipsilateral axillary lymph nodes. As in other lymphomas, a tumor dose of 35 Gy in 1.75 to 2.00 Gy fractions over 4 weeks achieves excellent local control. The most common sites of failure include lungs, brain, liver, spleen, and distant nodal sites. Isolated central nervous system relapses have been reported. Similarly, late failure in the contralateral breast may occur after therapy of unilateral primary breast lymphoma. Marginal zone lymphoma may be associated with isolated extranodal relapses in other MALT sites. Follicular lymphoma appears to behave in a manner similar to follicular lymphoma arising in lymph nodes (10). The overall survival of patients treated with local treatment methods ranges from 40% to 66% at 5 to 10 years (132,134,135). The local control rates in patients treated with radiation therapy range from 75% to 78% (133,135).

Bone Lymphoma

The clinical presentation of bone lymphoma is variable, with peak incidence in the fifth decade and a slight male preponderance. Symptoms at presentation usually consist of localized bone pain, sometimes accompanied by a soft-tissue mass, although polyostotic presentations are seen. The majority of patients present without systemic symptoms. Open biopsy is often required to make the diagnosis, given the difficulty of performing fine-needle aspiration on a bony lesion. In adults, the lymphoma is virtually always diffuse large B-cell type, with rare cases of Burkitt's lymphoma, CD30+ anaplastic large-cell lymphoma, low-grade lymphoma, and others (136). Among children, half of cases are diffuse large B-cell lymphoma, 40% are precursor B-lymphoblastic lymphoma, and 10% are Burkitt's lymphoma (88,137–139). Cure of lymphoma of bone by surgery alone has been recorded, although this is no longer being considered an appropriate therapy. With radiation therapy, 5- and 10-year overall survival rates of 58% and 53%, respectively, are reported for solitary bone lesions. Key issues relating to local control are the intramedullary and soft-tissue extent of disease in relation to radiation therapy volume. Magnetic resonance imaging has been particularly important in revealing extension of disease not visualized before by routine x-rays or bone scan. Treatment approaches using radiation therapy alone have indicated high levels of local control, approximately 85%, but unacceptable rates of local or marginal failure (20%) probably related to underestimation of tumor extent and bulk, and a systemic failure rate approaching 50%. Patients with localized diffuse large B-cell lymphoma of bone should be treated with combined modality therapy, comprising initial anthracycline-based chemotherapy and subsequent radiation therapy to a dose of 35 Gy. There is no indication for central nervous system prophylaxis. With chemotherapy followed by radiotherapy, the overall survival and relapse-free rates should exceed 70% at 5 years (140–143). Children are usually treated with chemotherapy alone to avoid development of radiation-induced sarcoma; outcome is favorable (139). Bone lymphoma carries with it the special complication of risk of fracture, caused by the tumor or by the treatment. Chemotherapy may induce avascular necrosis, and radiotherapy may induce fractures. Radiation therapy–induced fracture seems related to radiation therapy dose, with doses in excess of 50 Gy increasing the risk (144).

Extradural Lymphoma

Primary extradural lymphoma presents with pain or progressive neurologic deficit. When present, spinal cord compression constitutes a medical emergency. Histologic diagnosis is imperative, and surgical biopsy, with or without decompression, is the first step in management. Complete tumor removal is unnecessary because further therapy is always required. The main objectives of surgery in the setting of spinal cord compression include adequate decompression of the spinal cord and removal of tissue appropriate for histologic diagnosis. Postoperative therapy has historically involved radiation therapy to the affected area of the spine. Radiation therapy is delivered using megavoltage photon therapy, with dose to the tumor limited to 35 to 40 Gy in 1.75 to 2.00 Gy fractions. Doses in excess of 45 to 50 Gy are excessive and carry a risk of radiation myelitis. The radiation therapy volume should take into account the presence of any paraspinal mass or regional lymph node involvement. Radiation therapy results in good local disease control but, as with other localized diffuse large-cell lymphomas, is associated with a 40% to 50% distant failure rate. The use of doxorubicin-based chemotherapy after surgery and radiation therapy is associated with a reduced distant failure rate and an improved survival. In the Princess Margaret Hospital experience, the survival of patients treated with radiation therapy alone was 33%, compared with 86% (at a median follow-up of 3 years) for those treated with combined modality therapy (145). Although the traditional approach was to deliver radiation therapy before chemotherapy, this is no longer considered the optimal sequence. Eeles et al. documented that the use of chemotherapy followed by radiation therapy does not compromise neurologic function, as compared with that achieved when radiation therapy is followed by chemotherapy (145,146). A controversial aspect of the management of primary extradural lymphoma relates to the issue of intrathecal central nervous system chemoprophylaxis. Although some have demonstrated extradural involvement as a risk factor for meningeal relapse (147), the Princess Margaret Hospital experience has documented only rare isolated central nervous system relapse in patients treated without central nervous system prophylaxis. The routine use of intrathecal chemotherapy in patients with localized extradural lymphoma and no evidence of dural invasion may be questioned, but careful attention needs to be given to the extent of initial disease and the possibility of dural invasion (145). When dural invasion is suspected, intrathecal therapy is indicated.

Lung Lymphoma

A variety of types of lymphoma arise in the lung, but approximately 70% are marginal zone lymphoma (Fig. 43.6). The next

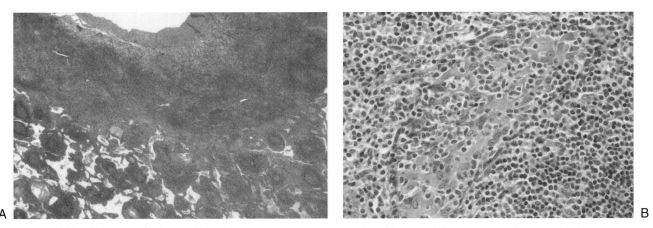

FIG. 43.6. Marginal zone B-cell lymphoma, mucosa-associated lymphoid tissue type of the lung. **A:** A dense cuff of lymphoid cells surrounds a blood vessel (*top*). Away from the vessel, the infiltrate spreads in an interstitial pattern. Reactive follicles punctuate the diffuse infiltrate of marginal zone cells. **B:** Higher power shows marginal zone cells and a lymphoepithelial lesion.

most common (approximately 20%) is diffuse large B-cell lymphoma; at least some of them have transformed from an underlying marginal zone lymphoma. Other uncommon types include follicular lymphoma, Burkitt's lymphoma, CD30+ anaplastic large-cell lymphoma, and others. Some of the marginal zone lymphoma patients have an underlying autoimmune disease, most commonly Sjögren's syndrome (148–152). Pulmonary marginal zone lymphomas are cytologically bland and have indolent behavior, and, as in other sites, they were often formerly believed to be nonneoplastic processes, such as lymphocytic interstitial pneumonia "pseudotumor." Lymphomatoid granulomatosis–type lymphoma is a rare type of Epstein-Barr virus–positive B-cell lymphoma that almost always involves the lungs and that is commonly associated with cutaneous, renal, and central nervous system manifestations. Peripheral T-cell lymphoma rarely involves the lung as a solitary site but may present as multisystem disease (153). Common presentation features include cough, dyspnea, pain, fever, recurrent infections, hemoptysis, or an asymptomatic finding on routine chest radiograph. Radiologic features include pulmonary consolidation, solid pulmonary opacities, hilar adenopathy or pleural effusion. Initial treatment has commonly been surgical resection; however, given current less invasive alternatives to achieve a secure diagnosis, there is no strong indication that resection contributes to outcome. MALT lymphoma is observed or treated with chemotherapy, usually a single alkylating agent. Lesions are commonly responsive to both chemotherapy and radiation therapy, although low tolerance of lung to radiation therapy limits its applicability to treatment of only part of the lung. There is no indication that such treatments are curative, although prolonged survival is common—94% overall survival at 5 years, with a median survival not reached at 10 years and no clear impact of type of therapy on outcome (148). The prognosis is clearly substantially worse for angiocentric and diffuse large-cell lymphomas, even when treated with chemotherapy or combined modality therapy. Systemic progression is common and relapse-free rates of approximately 40% to 50% are expected. T-cell lymphomas have a poor prognosis, with 50% mortality at 2 years even with combined modality therapy.

UNCOMMON SITES OF PRIMARY EXTRANODAL LYMPHOMA

Uncommon Respiratory Tract Lymphomas

Larynx

Primary head and neck lymphomas can infrequently present in the larynx (154,155). Often the presenting symptom is cough. Both marginal zone lymphomas and diffuse large-cell lymphomas (B lineage when immunophenotyped) have been reported. Radiation and combined modality therapy offer excellent local control and cure. Early diagnosis and treatment are important because airway obstruction can occur and result in sudden death.

Trachea

Primary lymphoma of the trachea has been reported, although it is even less common than in the larynx (156). Both MALT lymphomas and large-cell types occur.

Renal Lymphoma

Primary renal lymphoma is very rare. Most reported cases of renal lymphoma have presented with symptoms related to renal involvement, even though staging usually reveals extrarenal spread (117,157–161). In our experience, one patient with stage IE follicular large-cell lymphoma of the kidney was alive without evidence of recurrent disease 15 years after nephrectomy and postoperative radiation to the renal fossa. Similar case reports support primary renal lymphoma as a separate clinical entity (161,162). Patients present with flank pain, anorexia, or hematuria. Those with bilateral disease may have renal insufficiency. More than one-half of cases are diffuse large B-cell lymphoma; the remainder are a variety of high- and low-grade B-cell lymphomas. However, because of the rarity of such cases, no comment can be made regarding the pattern of disease and treatment results; general principles of management should be followed, recognizing important prognostic factors, especially histology.

Prostate Lymphoma

Primary lymphoma of the prostate is extremely rare. There were no cases of localized prostate lymphoma in several large series of patients with localized extranodal lymphoma (13,31,163), although a number of cases, usually in case reports or small series, have been described (117,164). Disease tends to affect older men, although an occasional report includes a younger patient. Patients present with obstructive or irritative urinary symptoms (164,165). The most common type is diffuse large B-cell lymphoma, and the rest are a variety of aggressive and indolent B-cell lymphomas (117,164,166,167). Survival in published cases has been poor, with rapid systemic dissemination of the disease (166), although patients treated more recently with better therapy have had a more favorable outcome (168).

Ureteral Lymphoma

Primary lymphoma of the ureter is rare, probably related to the absence of lymphoid tissue in the ureteral wall. The majority of reported cases are due to extrinsic ureteral compression. Periureteral and peripelvic involvement in the absence of renal involvement is unusual. There are only a few documented cases of primary lymphoma of the ureter (169–171).

Urethral Lymphoma

Primary lymphoma of the urethra is very rare (172–175). Almost all cases of primary urethral lymphoma have been reported in females. The tumor may present on the meatal epithelium and resemble a urethral caruncle or polyp. The pathology usually shows a diffuse large B-cell lymphoma, and some cases may be marginal zone lymphomas (117,176,177). A case of T-cell lymphoma has been reported (173). Long-term disease control in patients managed with radiation therapy alone and in those managed with excision of tumor and radiation therapy or chemotherapy has been reported (172,174,178). As in other cases of large B-cell lymphoma, a short course of Adriamycin (doxorubicin)–based chemotherapy followed by involved-field radiation therapy represents a logical treatment approach.

Pancreas Lymphoma

Primary pancreatic lymphoma accounts for 1% to 3% of all pancreatic malignancies and is rarely considered in the differential diagnosis of pancreatic mass lesions. Patients are usually older than 60 years of age (179). The lesion is defined by computed tomography and is commonly a sizable (3 to 12 cm; median, 8 cm) lesion in the head of the pancreas. Tumors are most commonly of diffuse large-cell type (B lineage when immunophenotyped) (180). Other types are uncommon. There is no indication for radical surgery for primary pancreatic lymphoma. Biliary obstruction is usually managed very effectively with systemic chemotherapy (181). Radiation may have a role for the uncommon indolent lymphoma or for palliation. Combined modality therapy is the appropriate therapy for large B-cell lymphoma, with particular consideration to choice of agents and schedule in patients with obstructive jaundice.

Liver Lymphoma

Primary non-Hodgkin's lymphoma of the liver is exceptionally rare. A recent report cited 68 cases in the literature, including five new cases (182). A relationship of primary lymphoma of the liver to preexisting immunologic disease states, such as systemic lupus erythematosus, acquired immunodeficiency syndrome, cyclosporin/transplantation, and hepatitis B–induced chronic active hepatitis, has been proposed. Fifty percent of patients have B symptoms, most commonly weight loss (183,184). Primary liver lymphoma arises as solitary mass, multiple masses, and rarely as diffuse hepatic enlargement. When recorded, 60% of tumors are of diffuse large B-cell type. Other types include marginal zone lymphoma, Burkitt's lymphoma, and others. The marginal zone lymphomas are centered on portal tracts and form lymphoepithelial lesions with bile duct epithelium (185). T-cell lymphomas are rarely recorded. Chemotherapy, with allowance for any related liver dysfunction particularly if preexistent to lymphoma, appears to be the most appropriate recommendation. Patients with indolent lymphoma have a good prognosis (185,186). Patients with more aggressive lymphomas have a relatively good outcome. In one study, 5-year cause-specific survival was 87% (187).

Lymphoma Affecting Soft Tissues or Muscle

Primary extranodal non-Hodgkin's lymphomas of the soft tissues are extremely rare (188,189). In the Mayo Clinic experience, the primary extranodal soft-tissue lymphoma of the extremities represented 0.11% of all lymphomas (188,189). Patients present with enlarging soft-tissue swelling. Diagnosis is obtained after biopsy or resection of the lesion. In some cases, it may be difficult to distinguish extranodal soft-tissue presentations from the total effacement of an aberrant lymph node by a malignant lymphoma. All histologic types have been reported. Tumors may be confined to the subcutaneous connective tissue or may involve muscle. The principles that apply to the management of other localized lymphomas are appropriate for primary lymphoma of soft tissues. Primary lymphoma arising in the skeletal muscle is even less common (190).

OTHER SITES: HEART, PLEURA, AND ADRENAL

Primary lymphoma of the heart, defined as lymphoma involving only heart and pericardium, is rare. A major subset of patients are immunocompromised because of human immunodeficiency virus infection or iatrogenic immunosuppression for organ transplantation, but cardiac lymphoma also occurs in older patients without immunodeficiency (191–195). In a few reported cases, the diagnosis has been made premortem (196). Presenting symptoms are usually congestive heart failure, pericardial effusion, and occasionally complete heart block. The pathology is usually diffuse large B-cell lymphoma. Prolonged survival has been reported after treatment with chemotherapy (197).

Primary lymphoma of the pleura arising in association with chronic tuberculous pyothorax has been reported in Japan (198). A few cases have been reported in Western countries as a complication of chronic empyema. The majority of cases were Epstein-Barr virus-positive large B-cell lymphomas. The outcome in reported cases treated with chemotherapy was poor.

Few cases of primary adrenal lymphoma have been reported in the literature (199). A number of cases had bilateral involvement of adrenal glands, often associated with adrenal insufficiency. Nearly all cases have been diffuse large B-cell lymphoma, but rare T-cell lymphomas have been reported. Many cases have been managed with surgery and chemotherapy, but survival was poor (199). In recent years, improved diagnostic techniques and therapy have led to a better outcome in the small number of cases reported (200–202).

Primary effusion lymphoma is a large B-cell neoplasm recently included in the World Health Organization Classification of lymphoproliferative disorders. Primary effusion lymphoma usually develops in severely immunocompromised patients, and a strong etiologic relationship is recognized with the human herpesvirus-8/Kaposi's sarcoma-associated herpes virus. Most cases are also Epstein-Barr virus positive (203). The lymphoma develops as a liquid-phase growth in the fluid-filled serous cavities of the body. Its immunophenotype is unusual in that although neoplastic cells express the leukocyte common antigen, they lack pan-B antigen expression; B lineage can be demonstrated with genetic studies. Typically, it displays an aggressive course.

SUMMARY

Extranodal non-Hodgkin's lymphoma encompasses an exceptionally heterogeneous group of diseases that may affect any organ or body part. It is unclear why some sites or organs are affected more than others; however, the role of antigenic stimulation, autoimmunity, and immune dysregulation resulting in genomic instability is an important component of the etiology and pathogenesis of these disorders. This relationship to lymphoma causation is increasingly recognized through observations relating lymphomas to congenital and acquired immunodeficiency states, Hashimoto's and Sjögren's syndrome, Crohn's disease, intestinal immunoproliferative states,

and the role of *H. pylori* in MALT lymphoma of the stomach. Knowledge arising from a more complete understanding of the biology and the genetic basis of lymphoma will undoubtedly lead to improved recognition of distinct clinical entities and refinements in patient management. Treatment results and curability of some tumors may be obscured by the heterogeneity of presentations. Future studies of different treatment strategies recognizing distinct histopathologic entities may help to clarify the outcomes.

REFERENCES

1. Pederson R, Pederson N. Primary non-Hodgkin's lymphoma of the thyroid gland: a population based study. *Histopathology* 1996;28:25–32.
2. Parkin DM, Pisani P, Ferlay J. Global cancer statistics. *CA Cancer J Clin* 1999;49:1, 33–64.
3. Gurney KA, Cartwright RA. Increasing incidence and descriptive epidemiology of extranodal non-Hodgkin lymphoma in parts of England and Wales. *Hematol J* 2002;3:95–104.
3a. International Extranodal Lymphoma Study Group. http://www.ielsg.org/. Accessed 7/15/2003.
4. Lewin K, Ranchod M, Dorfman R. Lymphomas of the gastrointestinal tract: a study of 117 cases presenting with gastrointestinal disease. *Cancer* 1978;42:693–707.
5. Herrmann R, Panahon AM, Barcos MP, et al. Gastrointestinal involvement in non-Hodgkin's lymphoma. *Cancer* 1980;46:215–222.
6. Dawson I, Cornes J, Morson B. Primary malignant lymphoid tumours of the intestinal tract: report of 37 cases with a study of factors influencing prognosis. *Brit J Surg* 1961;49:80–89.
7. Zucca E, Roggero E, Bertoni F, et al. Primary extranodal non-Hodgkin's lymphomas. Part 1: gastrointestinal, cutaneous and genitourinary lymphomas. *Ann Oncol* 1977;8:727–737.
8. Dogan A, Du M, Koulis A, et al. Expression of lymphocyte homing receptors and vascular addressins in low-grade gastric B-cell lymphomas of mucosa-associated lymphoid tissue. *Am J Pathol* 1997;151:1361–1369.
9. Drillenburg P, van der Voort R, Koopman G, et al. Preferential expression of the mucosal homing receptor integrin alpha 4 beta 7 in gastrointestinal non-Hodgkin's lymphomas. *Am J Pathol* 1997;150:919–927.
10. Mattia AR, Ferry JA, Harris NL. Breast lymphoma. A B-cell spectrum including the low grade B-cell lymphoma of mucosa associated lymphoid tissue. *Am J Surg Pathol* 1993;17:574–587.
11. Freeman C, Berg JW, Cutler SJ. Occurrence and prognosis of extranodal lymphomas. *Cancer* 1972;29:252–260.
12. Devesa SS, Fears T. Non-Hodgkin's lymphoma time trends: United States and international data. *Cancer Res* 1992;52:5432–5440.
13. d'Amore F, Christensen BE, Brincker H, et al. Clinicopathological features and prognostic factors in extranodal non-Hodgkin lymphomas. Danish LYFO Study Group. *Eur J Cancer* 1991;27:1201–1208.
14. Sutcliffe SB, Gospodarowicz MK. Localized extranodal lymphomas. In: Keating A, Armitage J, Burnett A, et al., eds. *Hematological oncology*. Cambridge, UK: Cambridge University Press, 1992:189–222.
15. Bangerter M, Griesshammer M, Binder T, et al. New diagnostic imaging procedures in Hodgkin's disease. *Ann Oncol* 1996;4[Suppl 7]:55–59.
16. Harris NL, Jaffe ES, Diebold J, et al. The World Health Organization classification of neoplastic diseases of the haematopoietic and lymphoid tissues: report of the Clinical Advisory Committee Meeting, Airlie House, Virginia, November 1997. *Histopathology* 2000;36:69–86.
17. Shipp M. Prognostic factors in non-Hodgkin's lymphoma [published erratum appears in *Curr Opin Oncol* 1993;5:251]. *Curr Opin Oncol* 1992;4:856–862.
18. Loeffler M, Shipp M, Stein H. 2. Report on the workshop: "Clinical consequences of pathology and prognostic factors in aggressive NHL." *Ann Hematol* 2001;80:B8–B12.
19. The International Non-Hodgkin's Lymphoma Prognostic Factors Project: a predictive model for aggressive non-Hodgkin's lymphoma. *N Engl J Med* 1993;329:987–994.

20. DeAngelis LM. Primary central nervous system lymphoma [Review]. *Recent Results Cancer Res* 1994;135:155–169.
21. Touroutoglou N, Dimopoulos MA, Younes A, et al. Testicular lymphoma: late relapses and poor outcome despite doxorubicin-based therapy. *J Clin Oncol* 1995;13:1361–1367.
22. Coiffier B, Lepage E, Briere J, et al. CHOP chemotherapy plus rituximab compared with CHOP alone in elderly patients with diffuse large-B-cell lymphoma. *N Engl J Med* 2002;346:235–242.
23. Romaguera JE, Velasquez WS, Silvermintz KB, et al. Surgical debulking is associated with improved survival in Stage I-II diffuse large cell lymphoma. *Cancer* 1990;66:267–272.
24. Seifert E, Schulte SE, Stolte M. Long-term results of treatment of malignant non-Hodgkin's lymphoma of the stomach. *Z Gastroenterol* 1992;30:505–508.
25. Thirlby RC. Gastrointestinal lymphoma: a surgical perspective. *Oncology* 1993;7:29–32.
26. Sutcliffe SB, Gospodarowicz MK, Bush RS, et al. Role of radiation therapy in localized non-Hodgkin's lymphoma. *Radiother Oncol* 1985;4:211–223.
27. Tsang RW, Gospodarowicz MK, O'Sullivan B. Staging and management of localized non-Hodgkin's lymphomas: variations among experts in radiation oncology. *Int J Radiat Oncol Biol Phys* 2002;52:643–651.
28. Miller T, Dahlberg S, Cassady J, et al. Three cycles of CHOP plus radiotherapy is superior to eight cycles of CHOP alone for localized intermediate and high grade non-Hodgkin's lymphoma: a Southwest Oncology Group Study, American Society of Clinical Oncology. *J Clin Oncol* 1996:411.
29. Shenkier TN, Voss N, Fairey R, et al. Brief chemotherapy and involved-region irradiation for limited-stage diffuse large-cell lymphoma: an 18-year experience from the British Columbia Cancer Agency. *J Clin Oncol* 2002;20:197–204.
30. Aref A, Narayan S, Tekyi-Mensah S, et al. Value of radiation therapy in the management of chemoresistant intermediate grade non-Hodgkin's lymphoma. *Radiat Oncol Investig* 1999;7:186–191.
31. Gospodarowicz MK, Sutcliffe SB, Brown TC, et al. Patterns of disease in localized extranodal lymphomas. *J Clin Oncol* 1987;5:875–880.
32. Kaminski MS, Coleman CN, Colby TV, et al. Factors predicting survival in adults with stage I and II large-cell lymphoma treated with primary radiation therapy. *Ann Intern Med* 1986;104:747–756.
33. Oguchi M, Ikeda H, Isobe K, et al. Tumor bulk as a prognostic factor for the management of localized aggressive non-Hodgkin's lymphoma: a survey of the Japan Lymphoma Radiation Therapy Group. *Int J Radiat Oncol Biol Phys* 2000;48:161–168.
34. Vaughan Hudson B, Vaughan Hudson G, MacLennan KA, et al. Clinical stage 1 non-Hodgkin's lymphoma: long-term follow-up of patients treated by the British National Lymphoma Investigation with radiotherapy alone as initial therapy. *Br J Cancer* 1994;69:1088–1093.
35. Cheson BD, Horning SJ, Coiffier B, et al. Report of an international workshop to standardize response criteria for non-Hodgkin's lymphomas. *J Clin Oncol* 1999;17:1244.
36. Jacobs C, Hoppe R. Non-Hodgkin's lymphomas of the head and neck: prognosis and patterns of recurrence. *Int J Radiat Oncol Biol Phys* 1985;11:357–364.
37. Harabuchi Y, Tsubota H, Ohguro S, et al. Prognostic factors and treatment outcome in non-Hodgkin's lymphoma of Waldeyer's ring. *Acta Oncol* 1997;36:413–420.
38. Ezzat AA, Ibrahim EM, El Weshi AN, et al. Localized non-Hodgkin's lymphoma of Waldeyer's ring: clinical features, management, and prognosis of 130 adult patients. *Head Neck* 2001;23:547–558.
39. Krol AD, Le Cessie S, Snijder S, et al. Waldeyer's ring lymphomas: a clinical study from the Comprehensive Cancer Center West population based NHL registry. *Leuk Lymphoma* 2001;42:1005–1013.
40. Berkowitz RG, Mahadevan M. Unilateral tonsillar enlargement and tonsillar lymphoma in children. *Ann Otol Rhinol Laryngol* 1999;108:876–879.
41. Conley SF, Staszak C, Clamon GH, et al. Non-Hodgkin's lymphoma of the head and neck: the University of Iowa experience. *Laryngoscope* 1987;97:291–300.
42. Hoppe RT, Burke JS, Glatstein E, et al. Non-Hodgkin's lymphoma, involvement of Waldeyer's ring. *Cancer* 1978;42:1096–1104.
43. Wulfrank D, Speelman T, Pauwels C, et al. Extranodal non-Hodgkin's lymphoma of the head and neck. *Radiother Oncol* 1987;8:199–207.
44. Aviles A, Delgado S, Ruiz H, et al. Treatment of non-Hodgkin's lymphoma of Waldeyer's ring: radiotherapy versus chemotherapy versus combined therapy. *Eur J Cancer B Oral Oncol* 1996;32:19–23.
45. Liang R, Ng RP, Todd D, et al. Management of stage I-II diffuse aggressive non-Hodgkin's lymphoma of the Waldeyer's ring: combined modality therapy versus radiotherapy alone. *Hematol Oncol* 1987;5:223–230.
46. Ossenkoppele GJ, Mol JJ, Snow GB, et al. Radiotherapy versus radiotherapy plus chemotherapy in stages I and II non-Hodgkin's lymphoma of the upper digestive and respiratory tract. *Cancer* 1987;60:1505–1509.
47. Li YX, Coucke PA, Li JY, et al. Primary non-Hodgkin's lymphoma of the nasal cavity: prognostic significance of paranasal extension and the role of radiotherapy and chemotherapy. *Cancer* 1998;83:449–456.
48. Vidal RW, Devaney K, Ferlito A, et al. Sinonasal malignant lymphomas: a distinct clinicopathological category. *Ann Otol Rhinol Laryngol* 1999;108:411–419.
49. Proulx GM, Caudra-Garcia I, Ferry J, et al. Lymphoma of the nasal cavity and paranasal sinuses: treatment and outcome of early-stage disease. *Am J Clin Oncol* 2003;26:6–11.
50. Tomita Y, Ohsawa M, Mishiro Y, et al. The presence and subtype of Epstein-Barr virus in B and T cell lymphomas of the sino-nasal region from the Osaka and Okinawa districts of Japan. *Lab Invest* 1995;73:190–196.
51. Tomita Y, Ohsawa M, Qiu K, et al. Epstein-Barr virus in lymphoproliferative diseases in the sino-nasal region: close association with CD56+ immunophenotype and polymorphic-reticulosis morphology. *Int J Cancer* 1997;70:9–13.
52. Cuadra-Garcia I, Proulx GM, Wu CL, et al. Sinonasal lymphoma: a clinicopathologic analysis of 58 cases from the Massachusetts General Hospital. *Am J Surg Pathol* 1999;23:1356–1369.
53. Jaffe ES, Chan J, Su IJ, et al. Report of the workshop on nasal and related extranodal angiocentric T/natural killer cell lymphomas: definitions, differential diagnosis, and epidemiology. *Am J Surg Pathol* 1996;20:103–111.
54. Liang R, Todd D, Chan TK, et al. Treatment outcome and prognostic factors for primary nasal lymphoma. *J Clin Oncol* 1995;13:666–670.
55. Davison SP, Habermann TM, Strickler JG, et al. Nasal and nasopharyngeal angiocentric T-cell lymphomas. *Laryngoscope* 1996;106:139–143.
56. Hausdorff J, Davis E, Long G, et al. Non-Hodgkin's lymphoma of the paranasal sinuses: clinical and pathological features, and response to combined-modality therapy. *Cancer J Sci Am* 1997;3:303–311.
57. Logston M, Ha C, Kavadi V, et al. Lymphoma of the nasal cavity and paranasal sinuses. *Cancer* 1997;80:477–488.
58. Conconi A. IELSG phase II study of rituximab in MALT lymphoma: final results. Proceedings ASCO, 2002:267, 1067(abst).
59. Wolvius EB, Jiwa NM, van der Valk P, et al. Adenolymphoma and non-Hodgkin's lymphoma of the salivary glands and oral cavity in immunocompetent patients are not associated with latent Epstein-Barr virus. *Oral Oncol* 1997;33:119–123.
60. Laing RW, Hoskin P, Vaughan Hudson B, et al. The significance of MALT histology in thyroid lymphoma: a review of patients from the BNLI and Royal Marsden Hospital. *Clin Oncol* 1994;6:300–304.
61. Derringer GA, Thompson LD, Frommelt RA, et al. Malignant lymphoma of the thyroid gland: a clinicopathologic study of 108 cases. *Am J Surg Pathol* 2000;24:623–639.
62. Blair TJ, Evans RG, Buskirk SJ, et al. Radiotherapeutic management of primary lymphoid lymphoma. *Int J Radiat Oncol Biol Phys* 1985;11:365–370.
63. Tsang R, Gospodarowicz MK, Sutcliffe SB, et al. Non-Hodgkin's lymphoma of the thyroid gland: prognostic factors and treatment outcome. *Int J Radiat Oncol Biol Phys* 1993;27:599–604.
64. Vigliotti A, Kong JS, Fuller LM, et al. Thyroid lymphomas stages IE and IIE: comparative results for radiotherapy only, combination chemotherapy only, and multimodality treatment. *Int J Radiat Oncol Biol Phys* 1986;12:1807–1812.
65. Auw-Haedrich C, Coupland SE, Kapp A, et al. Long term outcome of ocular adnexal lymphoma subtyped according to the REAL classification. Revised European and American Lymphoma. *Br J Ophthalmol* 2001;85:63–69.
66. Coupland SE, Krause L, Delecluse HJ, et al. Lymphoproliferative lesions of the ocular adnexa. Analysis of 112 cases. *Ophthalmology* 1998;105:1430–1441.

67. White WL, Ferry JA, Harris NL, et al. Ocular adnexal lymphoma. A clinicopathologic study with identification of lymphomas of mucosa-associated lymphoid tissue type. *Ophthalmology* 1995;102:1994–2006.

68. Hardman-Lea S, Kerr-Muir M, Wotherspoon AC, et al. Mucosal-associated lymphoid tissue lymphoma of the conjunctiva. *Arch Ophthalmol* 1994;112:1207–1212.

69. Tsang RW, Gospodarowicz MK, Pintilie M, et al. Stage I and II MALT lymphoma: results of treatment with radiotherapy. *Int J Radiat Oncol Biol Phys* 2001;50:1258–1264.

70. Stafford SL, Kozelsky TF, Garrity JA, et al. Orbital lymphoma: radiotherapy outcome and complications. *Radiother Oncol* 2001;59:139–144.

71. Le QT, Eulau SM, George TI, et al. Primary radiotherapy for localized orbital MALT lymphoma. *Int J Radiat Oncol Biol Phys* 2002;52:657–663.

72. Fitzpatrick PJ, Macko SM. Lymphoreticular tumors of the orbit. *Int J Radiat Oncol Biol Phys* 1984;10:333–340.

73. Bessell EM, Henk JM, Wright JE, et al. Orbital and conjunctival lymphoma treatment and prognosis. *Radiother Oncol* 1988;13:237–244.

74. Bhatia S, Paulino AC, Buatti JM, et al. Curative radiotherapy for primary orbital lymphoma. *Int J Radiat Oncol Biol Phys* 2002;54:818–823.

75. Koch P, del Valle F, Berdel WE, et al. Primary gastrointestinal non-Hodgkin's lymphoma: II. Combined surgical and conservative or conservative management only in localized gastric lymphoma—results of the prospective German Multicenter Study GIT NHL 01/92. *J Clin Oncol* 2001;19:3874–3883.

76. Koch P, del Valle F, Berdel WE, et al. Primary gastrointestinal non-Hodgkin's lymphoma: I. Anatomic and histologic distribution, clinical features, and survival data of 371 patients registered in the German Multicenter Study GIT NHL 01/92. *J Clin Oncol* 2001;19:3861–3873.

77. Sano T. Treatment of primary gastric lymphoma: experience in the National Cancer Center Hospital, Tokyo. *Recent Results Cancer Res* 2000;156:104–107.

78. d'Amore F, Brincker M, Gronbaek K, et al. Non-Hodgkin's lymphoma of the gastrointestinal tract: a population-based analysis of incidence, geographic distribution, clinicopathologic presentation features, and prognosis. *J Clin Oncol* 1994;12:1673–1684.

79. Gospodarowicz M, Bush R, Brown T, et al. Curability of gastrointestinal lymphoma with combined surgery and radiation. *Int J Radiat Oncol Biol Phys* 1983;9:3–9.

80. Gospodarowicz MK, Sutcliffe SB, Clark RM, et al. Outcome analysis of localized gastrointestinal lymphoma treated with surgery and postoperative radiation. *Int J Radiat Oncol Biol Phys* 1990;19:1351–1355.

81. Gospodarowicz MK, Pintilie M, Tsang R, et al. Primary gastric lymphoma: brief overview of the recent Princess Margaret Hospital experience. *Recent Results Cancer Res* 2000;156:108–115.

82. Shepherd FA, Evans WK, Kutas G, et al. Chemotherapy following surgery for stages IE and IIE non-Hodgkin's lymphoma of the gastrointestinal tract. *J Clin Oncol* 1988;6:253–260.

83. Maor MH, Velasquez WS, Fuller LM, et al. Stomach conservation in stages IE and IIE gastric non-Hodgkin's lymphoma [see comments]. *J Clin Oncol* 1990;8:266–271.

84. Taal BG, Burgers JM. Primary non-Hodgkin's lymphoma of the stomach: endoscopic diagnosis and the role of surgery. *Scand J Gastroenterol* 1991;188:33–37.

85. Taal BG, Burgers JM, van Heerde P, et al. The clinical spectrum and treatment of primary non-Hodgkin's lymphoma of the stomach [see comments]. *Ann Oncol* 1993;4:839–846.

86. Wirth A, Teo A, Wittwer H, et al. Gastric irradiation for MALT lymphoma: reducing the target volume, fast! *Australas Radiol* 1999;43:87–90.

87. Isaacson PG. Gastrointestinal lymphomas of T- and B-cell types. *Mod Pathol* 1999;12:151–158.

88. Foss HD, Stein H. Pathology of intestinal lymphomas. *Recent Results Cancer Res* 2000;156:33–41.

89. Domizio P, Owen RA, Shepherd NA, et al. Primary lymphoma of the small intestine: a clinicopathological study of 119 cases. *Am J Surg Pathol* 1993;17:429–442.

90. Morton JE, Leyland MJ, Vaughan Hudson G, et al. Primary gastrointestinal non-Hodgkin's lymphoma: a review of 175 British National Lymphoma Investigation cases. *Br J Cancer* 1993;67:776–782.

91. Haber DA, Mayer RJ. Primary gastrointestinal lymphoma. *Semin Oncol* 1988;15:154–169.

92. Fischbach W, Tacke W, Greiner A, et al. Regression of immunoproliferative small intestinal disease after eradication of *Helicobacter pylori*. *Lancet* 1997;349:31–32.

93. Al-Bahrani Z, Al-Mohindry H, Bakir F, et al. Clinical and pathologic subtypes of primary intestinal lymphoma: experience with 132 patients over a 14-year period. *Cancer* 1983;52:1666–1672.

94. Isaacson PG. Gastrointestinal lymphoma. *Hum Pathol* 1994;25:1020–1029.

95. Chott A, Vesely M, Simonitsch I, et al. Classification of intestinal T-cell neoplasms and their differential diagnosis. *Am J Clin Pathol* 1999;111:S68–S74.

96. Hashimoto Y, Nakamura N, Kuze T, et al. Multiple lymphomatous polyposis of the gastrointestinal tract is a heterogenous group that includes mantle cell lymphoma and follicular lymphoma: analysis of somatic mutation of immunoglobulin heavy chain gene variable region. *Hum Pathol* 1999;30:581–587.

97. Bende RJ, Smit LA, Bossenbroek JG, et al. Primary follicular lymphoma of the small intestine: alpha4beta7 expression and immunoglobulin configuration suggest an origin from local antigen-experienced B cells. *Am J Pathol* 2003;162:105–113.

98. Misdraji J, Fernandez del Castillo C, Ferry JA. Follicle center lymphoma of the ampulla of Vater presenting with jaundice: report of a case. *Am J Surg Pathol* 1997;21:484–488.

99. Aosaza K, Ohsawa M, Soma T, et al. Malignant lymphoma of the rectum. *Jpn J Clin Oncol* 1990;20:380–386.

100. Doll DC, Weiss RB. Malignant lymphoma of the testis. *Am J Med* 1986;81:515–524.

101. Moller MB, d'Amore F, Christensen BE. Testicular lymphoma: a population-based study of incidence, clinicopathological correlations and prognosis. The Danish Lymphoma Study Group, LYFO. *Eur J Cancer* 1994;12:1760–1764.

102. Zucca E, Conconi A, Mughal TI, et al. Patterns of outcome and prognostic factors in primary large-cell lymphoma of the testis in a survey by the International Extranodal Lymphoma Study Group. *J Clin Oncol* 2003;21:20–27.

103. Crellin AM, Vaughan Hudson B, Bennett MH, et al. Non-Hodgkin's lymphoma of the testis. *Radiother Oncol* 1993;27:99–106.

104. Sussman EB, Hajdu SI, Lieberman PH, et al. Malignant lymphoma of the testis: a clinicopathologic study of 37 cases. *J Urol* 1977;118:1004–1007.

105. Leite KR, Garicochea B, Srougi M, et al. Monoclonality of asynchronous bilateral lymphoma of the testis. *Eur Urol* 2000;38:774–777.

106. Ferry JA, Harris NL, Young RH, et al. Malignant lymphoma of the testis, epididymis, and spermatic cord. A clinicopathologic study of 69 cases with immunophenotypic analysis. *Am J Surg Pathol* 1994;18:376–390.

107. Chan JKC, Sin VC, Wong KF, et al. Nonnasal lymphoma expressing the natural killer cell marker CD56: a clinicopathologic study of 49 cases of an uncommon aggressive neoplasm. *Blood* 1997;89:4501–4513.

108. Zietman AL, Coen JJ, Ferry JA, et al. The management and outcome of stage IAE non-Hodgkin's lymphoma of the testis [Review]. *J Urol* 1996;155:943–946.

109. Connors JM, Klimo P, Voss N, et al. Testicular lymphoma: improved outcome with early brief chemotherapy. *J Clin Oncol* 1988;6:776–781.

110. Linassier C, Desablens B, Lefrancq T, et al. Stage I-IIE primary non-Hodgkin's lymphoma of the testis: results of a prospective trial by the GOELAMS Study Group. *Clin Lymphoma* 2002;3:167–172.

111. Sasai K, Yamabe H, Tsutsui K, et al. Primary testicular non-Hodgkin's lymphoma: a clinical study and review of the literature. *Am J Clin Oncol* 1997;20:59–62.

112. Tondini C, Ferreri AJ, Siracusano L, et al. Diffuse large-cell lymphoma of the testis. *J Clin Oncol* 1999;17:2854–2858.

113. Read G. Lymphomas of the testis-results of treatment 1960–77. *Clin Radiol* 1982;32:687–692.

114. Auperin A, Arriagada R, Pignon JP, et al. Prophylactic cranial irradiation for patients with small-cell lung cancer in complete remission. Prophylactic Cranial Irradiation Overview Collaborative Group [see comments]. *N Engl J Med* 1999;341:476–484.

115. Arriagada R, Le Chevalier T, Borie F, et al. Prophylactic cranial irradiation for patients with small-cell lung cancer in complete remission [see comments]. *J Natl Cancer Inst* 1995;87:183–190.

116. Yuille FA, Angus B, Roberts JT, et al. Low grade MALT lymphoma of the urinary bladder. *Clin Oncol (R Coll Radiol)* 1998;10:265–266.

117. Ferry JA, Young RH. Malignant lymphoma of the genitourinary tract. *Curr Diagn Pathol* 1997;4:145–169.

118. Kempton CL, Kurtin PJ, Inwards DJ, et al. Malignant lymphoma of the bladder: evidence from 36 cases that low-grade lymphoma of the MALT-type is the most common primary bladder lymphoma. *Am J Surg Pathol* 1997;21:1324–1333.

119. Melekos MD, Matsouka P, Fokaefs E, et al. Primary non-Hodgkin's lymphoma of the urinary bladder. *Eur Urol* 1992;21:85–88.

120. Ohsawa M, Aozasa K, Horiuchi K, et al. Malignant lymphoma of bladder. Report of three cases and review of the literature. [Review]. *Cancer* 1993;72:1969–1974.

121. Heaney JA, Dellellis RA, Rudders RA. Non-Hodgkin's lymphoma arising in the lower urinary tract. *Urology* 1985;25:479–484.

122. Al-Maghrabi J, Kamel-Reid S, Jewett M, et al. Primary low-grade B-cell lymphoma of mucosa-associated lymphoid tissue type arising in the urinary bladder: report of 4 cases with molecular genetic analysis. *Arch Pathol Lab Med* 2001;125:332–336.

123. Dimopoulos MA, Daliani D, Pugh W, et al. Primary ovarian non-Hodgkin's lymphoma: outcome after treatment with combination chemotherapy [Review]. *Gynecol Oncol* 1997;64:446–450.

124. Osborne BM, Robboy SJ. Lymphomas or leukemia presenting as ovaries tumours: an analysis of 42 cases. *Cancer* 1983;52:1933–1943.

125. Vang R, Medeiros LJ, Fuller GN, et al. Non-Hodgkin's lymphoma involving the gynecologic tract: a review of 88 cases. *Adv Anat Pathol* 2001;8:200–217.

126. Harris NL, Scully RE. Malignant lymphoma and granulocytic sarcoma of the uterus and vagina. A clinicopathologic analysis of 27 cases. *Cancer* 1984;53:2530–2545.

127. Stroh EL, Besa PC, Cox JD, et al. Treatment of patients with lymphomas of the uterus or cervix with combination chemotherapy and radiation therapy. *Cancer* 1995;75:2392–2399.

128. Prevot S, Hugol D, Audouin J, et al. Primary non-Hodgkin's malignant lymphoma of the vagina. Report of 3 cases with review of the literature. [Review]. *Pathol Res Pract* 1992;188:78–85.

129. Domchek SM, Hecht JL, Fleming MD, et al. Lymphomas of the breast: primary and secondary involvement. *Cancer* 2002;94:6–13.

130. Ribrag V, Bibeau F, El Weshi A, et al. Primary breast lymphoma: a report of 20 cases. *Br J Haematol* 2001;115:253–256.

131. Thieblemont C, Bastion Y, Berger F, et al. Mucosa-associated lymphoid tissue gastrointestinal and nongastrointestinal lymphoma behavior: analysis of 108 patients. *J Clin Oncol* 1997;15:1624–1630.

132. Giardini R, Piccolo C, Rilke F. Primary non-Hodgkin's lymphomas of the female breast. *Cancer* 1992;69:725–735.

133. DeBlasio D, McCormick B, Straus D, et al. Definitive irradiation for localized non-Hodgkin's lymphoma of breast. *Int J Radiat Oncol Biol Phys* 1989;17:843–846.

134. Jeon HJ, Akagi T, Hoshida Y, et al. Primary non-Hodgkin malignant lymphoma of the breast. An immunohistochemical study of seven patients and literature review of 152 patients with breast lymphoma in Japan [Review]. *Cancer* 1992;70:2451–2459.

135. Liu FF, Clark RM. Primary lymphoma of the breast. *Clin Radiol* 1986;37:567–570.

136. Pettit CK, Zukerberg LR, Gray MH, et al. Primary lymphoma of bone. A B-cell neoplasm with a high frequency of multilobated cells. *Am J Surg Pathol* 1990;14:329–334.

137. Furman WL, Fitch S, Hustu HO, et al. Primary lymphoma of bone in children. *J Clin Oncol* 1989;7:1275–1280.

138. Loeffler JS, Tarbell NJ, Kozakewich H, et al. Primary lymphoma of bone in children: analysis of treatment results with Adriamycin, prednisone, Oncovin (APO), and local radiation therapy. *J Clin Oncol* 1986;4:496–501.

139. Lones MA, Perkins SL, Sposto R, et al. Non-Hodgkin's lymphoma arising in bone in children and adolescents is associated with an excellent outcome: a Children's Cancer Group report. *J Clin Oncol* 2002;20:2293–2301.

140. Christie DR, Barton MB, Bryant G, et al. Osteolymphoma (primary bone lymphoma): an Australian review of 70 cases. Australasian Radiation Oncology Lymphoma Group (AROLG). *Aust N Z J Med* 1999;29:214–219.

141. de Camargo OP, dos Santos Machado TM, Croci AT, et al. Primary bone lymphoma in 24 patients treated between 1955 and 1999. *Clin Orthop* 2002:271–280.

142. Fairbanks RK, Bonner JA, Inwards CY, et al. Treatment of stage IE primary lymphoma of bone. *Int J Radiat Oncol Biol Phys* 1994;28:363–372.

143. Rathmell AJ, Gospodarowicz MK, Sutcliffe SB, et al. Localised lymphoma of bone: prognostic factors and treatment recommendations. The Princess Margaret Hospital Lymphoma Group. *Br J Cancer* 1992;66:603–606.

144. Stokes SH, Walz BJ. Pathologic fracture after radiation therapy for primary non-Hodgkin's malignant lymphoma of bone. *Int J Radiat Oncol Biol Phys* 1983;9:1153–1159.

145. Rathmell AJ, Gospodarowicz MK, Sutcliffe SB, et al. Localized extradural lymphoma: survival, relapse pattern and functional outcome. The Princess Margaret Hospital Lymphoma Group. *Radiother Oncol* 1992;24:14–20.

146. Eeles RA, O'Brien P, Horwich A, et al. Non-Hodgkin's lymphoma presenting with extradural spinal cord compression: functional outcome and survival. *Br J Cancer* 1991;63:126–129.

147. Mackintosh FR, Colby TV, Podolsky WJ, et al. Central nervous system involvement in non-Hodgkin's lymphoma: an analysis of 105 cases. *Cancer* 1982;49:586–595.

148. Cordier JF, Chailleux E, Lauque D, et al. Primary pulmonary lymphomas. A clinical study of 70 cases in nonimmunocompromised patients. *Chest* 1993;103:201–208.

149. Lim JK, Lacy MQ, Kurtin PJ, et al. Pulmonary marginal zone lymphoma of MALT type as a cause of localised pulmonary amyloidosis. *J Clin Pathol* 2001;54:642–646.

150. Li D, Hansmann ML, Zwingers T, et al. Primary lymphomas of the lung: morphological, immunohistochemical and clinical features. *Histopathology* 1990;16:519–531.

151. Kurtin PJ, Myers JL, Adlakha H, et al. Pathologic and clinical features of primary pulmonary extranodal marginal zone B-cell lymphoma of MALT type. *Am J Surg Pathol* 2001;25:997–1008.

152. Rush WL, Andriko JA, Taubenberger JK, et al. Primary anaplastic large cell lymphoma of the lung: a clinicopathologic study of five patients. *Mod Pathol* 2000;13:1285–1292.

153. Montalban C, Obeso G, Gallego A, et al. Peripheral T-cell lymphoma: a clinicopathological study of 41 cases and evaluation of the prognostic significance of the updated Kiel classification. *Histopathology* 1993;22:303–310.

154. Horny HP, Ferlito A, Carbone A. Laryngeal lymphoma derived from mucosa-associated lymphoid tissue. *Ann Otol Rhinol Laryngol* 1996;105:577–583.

155. Kato S, Sakura M, Takooda S, et al. Primary non-Hodgkin's lymphoma of the larynx. *J Laryngol Otol* 1997;111:571–574.

156. Fidias P, Wright C, Harris NL, et al. Primary tracheal non-Hodgkin's lymphoma. A case report and review of the literature. *Cancer* 1996;77:2332–2338.

157. Ferry JA, Harris NL, Papanicolaou N, et al. Lymphoma of the kidney. A report of 11 cases. *Am J Surg Pathol* 1995;19:134–144.

158. Foussard C, Desablens B, Sensebe L, et al. Is the International Prognostic Index for aggressive lymphomas useful for low-grade lymphoma patients? Applicability to stage III-IV patients. The GOELAMS Group, France. *Ann Oncol* 1997;1[Suppl 8]:49–52.

159. Harris GJ, Lager DJ. Primary renal lymphoma [Review]. *J Surg Oncol* 1991;46:273–277.

160. Okuno SH, Hoyer JD, Ristow K, et al. Primary renal non-Hodgkin's lymphoma. An unusual extranodal site [Review]. *Cancer* 1995;75:2258–2261.

161. Poulios C. Primary renal non-Hodgkin lymphoma. *Scand J Urol Nephrol* 1990;24:227–230.

162. Parveen T, Navarro-Roman L, Medeiros LJ, et al. Low-grade B-cell lymphoma of mucosa-associated lymphoid tissue arising in the kidney [see comments]. *Arch Pathol Lab Med* 1993;117:780–783.

163. Tsutsui K, Shibamoto Y, Yamabe H, et al. A radiotherapeutic experience for localized extranodal non-Hodgkin's lymphoma: prognostic factors and re-evaluation of treatment modality. *Radiother Oncol* 1991;21:83–90.

164. Bostwick DG, Iczkowski KA, Amin MB, et al. Malignant lymphoma involving the prostate: report of 62 cases. *Cancer* 1998;83:732–738.

165. Patel DR, Gomez GA, Henderson ES, et al. Primary prostatic involvement in non-Hodgkin lymphoma. *Urology* 1988;32:96–98.

166. Bostwick DG, Mann RB. Malignant lymphomas involving the prostate. A study of 13 cases. *Cancer* 1985;56:2932–2938.

167. Franco V, Florena AM, Quintini G, et al. Monocytoid B-cell lymphoma of the prostate [Review]. *Pathologica* 1992;84:411–417.

168. Sarris A, Dimopoulos M, Pugh W, et al. Primary lymphoma of the prostate: good outcome with doxorubicin-based combination chemotherapy [Review]. *J Urol* 1995;153:1852–1854.

169. Buck DS, Peterson MS, Borochovitz D, et al. Non-Hodgkin lymphoma of the ureter: CT demonstration with pathologic correlation. *Urol Radiol* 1992;14:183–187.

170. Chen HH, Panella JS, Rochester D, et al. Non-Hodgkin lymphoma of ureteral wall: CT findings. *J Comput Assist Tomogr* 1988;12:157–158.

171. Curry NS, Chung CJ, Potts W, et al. Isolated lymphoma of genitourinary tract and adrenals. *Urology* 1993;41:494–498.

172. Nabholtz JM, Friedman S, Tremeaux JC, et al. Non-Hodgkin's lymphoma of the urethra: a rare extranodal entity. *Gynecol Oncol* 1989;35:110–111.

173. Selch MT, Mark RJ, Fu YS, et al. Primary lymphoma of female urethra: long-term control by radiation therapy. *Urology* 1993;42:343–346.

174. Touhami H, Brahimi S, Kubisz P, et al. Non-Hodgkin's lymphoma of the female urethra. *J Urol* 1987;137:991–992.

175. Vogeli T, Engstfeld EJ. Non-Hodgkin lymphoma of the female urethra. *Scand J Urol Nephrol* 1992;26:111–112.

176. Hatcher PA, Wilson DD. Primary lymphoma of the male urethra. *Urology* 1997;49:142–144.

177. Kitamura H, Umehara T, Miyake M, et al. Non-Hodgkin's lymphoma arising in the urethra of a man. *J Urol* 1996;156:175–176.

178. Vapnek JM, Turzan CW. Primary malignant lymphoma of the female urethra: report of a case and review of the literature. *J Urol* 1992;147:701–703.

179. Fischer MA, Kabakow B. Lymphoma of the pancreas. *Mt Sinai J Med* 1987;54:423–426.

180. Nishimura R, Takakuwa T, Hoshida Y, et al. Primary pancreatic lymphoma: clinicopathological analysis of 19 cases from Japan and review of the literature. *Oncology* 2001;60:322–329.

181. Webb TH, Lillemoe KD, Pitt HA, et al. Pancreatic lymphoma. Is surgery mandatory for diagnosis or treatment? *Ann Surg* 1989;209:25–30.

182. Ohsawa M, Aozasa K, Horiuchi K, et al. Malignant lymphoma of the liver. Report of five cases and review of the literature [Review]. *Dig Dis Sci* 1992;37:1105–1109.

183. Anthony PP, Sarsfield P, Clarke T. Primary lymphoma of the liver: clinical and pathologic features of ten patients. *J Clin Pathol* 1990;43:1007–1013.

184. Osborne BM, Butler JJ, Guarda LA. Primary lymphoma of the liver. Ten cases and review of the literature. *Cancer* 1985;56:2902–2910.

185. Isaacson PG, Banks PM, Best PV, et al. Primary low-grade hepatic B-cell lymphoma of mucosa-associated lymphoid tissue (MALT)-type. *Am J Surg Pathol* 1995;19:571–575.

186. Ye MQ, Suriawinata A, Black C, et al. Primary hepatic marginal zone B-cell lymphoma of mucosa-associated lymphoid tissue type in a patient with primary biliary cirrhosis. *Arch Pathol Lab Med* 2000;124:604–608.

187. Page RD, Romaguera JE, Osborne B, et al. Primary hepatic lymphoma: favorable outcome after combination chemotherapy. *Cancer* 2001;92:2023–2029.

188. Scally J, Garrett A. Primary extranodal lymphoma in muscle. *Br J Radiol* 1989;62:81.

189. Travis WD, Banks PM, Reiman HM. Primary extranodal soft tissue lymphoma of the extremities. *Am J Surg Pathol* 1987;11:359–366.

190. Jeffery GM, Golding PF, Mead GM. Non-Hodgkin's lymphoma arising in skeletal muscle. *Ann Oncol* 1991;2:501–504.

191. Chim CS, Chan AC, Kwong YL, et al. Primary cardiac lymphoma. *Am J Hematol* 1997;54:79–83.

192. Rolla G, Bertero MT, Pastena G, et al. Primary lymphoma of the heart. A case report and review of the literature. *Leuk Res* 2002;26:117–120.

193. Saito T, Tamaru J, Kayao J, et al. Cytomorphologic diagnosis of malignant lymphoma arising in the heart: a case report. *Acta Cytol* 2001;45:1043–1048.

194. Zaharia L, Gill PS. Primary cardiac lymphoma. *Am J Clin Oncol* 1991;14:142–145.

195. Kaplan LD, Abrams DI, Feigal E, et al. AIDS-associated non-Hodgkin's lymphoma in San Francisco. *J Am Med Assoc* 1989;261:719–724.

196. Dorsay TA, Ho VB, Rovira MJ, et al. Primary cardiac lymphoma: CT and MR findings. *J Comput Assist Tomogr* 1993;17:978–981.

197. Nand S, Mullen GM, Lonchyna VA, et al. Primary lymphoma of the heart. Prolonged survival with early systemic therapy in a patient. *Cancer* 1991;68:2289–2292.

198. Aozasa K, Ohsawa M, Iuchi K, et al. Prognostic factors for pleural lymphoma patients. *Jpn J Clin Oncol* 1991;21:417–421.

199. Harris GJ, Tio FO, Von Hoff DD. Primary adrenal lymphoma. *Cancer* 1989;63:799–803.

200. Nakatsuka S, Hongyo T, Syaifudin M, et al. Mutations of p53, c-kit, K-ras, and beta-catenin gene in non-Hodgkin's lymphoma of adrenal gland. *Jpn J Cancer Res* 2002;93:267–274.

201. Wu HC, Shih LY, Chen TC, et al. A patient with bilateral primary adrenal lymphoma, presenting with fever of unknown origin and achieving long-term disease-free survival after resection and chemotherapy. *Ann Hematol* 1999;78:289–292.

202. Yamamoto E, Ozaki N, Nakagawa M, et al. Primary bilateral adrenal lymphoma associated with idiopathic thrombocytopenic purpura. *Leuk Lymphoma* 1999;35:403–408.

203. Ascoli V, Lo-Coco F: Body cavity lymphoma. *Curr Opin Pulm Med* 2002;8:317–322.

SECTION VII

Etiology, Epidemiology, and Biology

CHAPTER 44

Overview of the Etiology and Epidemiology of Lymphoma

Patricia Hartge and Sophia S. Wang

Epidemiologists regard non-Hodgkin's lymphoma as a remarkable disease. It exhibits striking patterns of occurrence, which have revealed a large number of causes of specific lymphomas, and yet most of the 56,000 cases of lymphoma that occur yearly in the United States cannot be explained.

Several features of the epidemiology of lymphoma particularly stand out. Cancer registries around the world have reported a steady increase in the occurrence of lymphomas during the second half of the twentieth century. For example, incidence rates in the United States have doubled since the early 1970s. Many analyses conclude that changes in detection of lymphoma do not begin to account for the increase. In many places, human immunodeficiency virus infections have produced a second epidemic superimposed on the unexplained long-term increase of lymphoma. Second, the complexity of lymphoma mirrors the complexity of the immune system. Lymphomas constitute not one but many diseases, and some of the separate entities have distinct etiologies. Third, we can confidently infer that the cause of all lymphomas is immune dysregulation, but we do not understand the specific immune defects at work and the influence of viruses, genes, chemicals, radiation, diet, and aging on the complex natural history of the immune system. In particular, severe immune suppression, whether inborn, medication induced, or viral, dramatically increases lymphoma risk, but the role of mild immune perturbation remains unclear.

These signal features—increasing rates, biologic heterogeneity, and a close tie to severely suppressed immunity—have helped to direct the analytic studies of lymphoma epidemiology. Studies of some rare lymphomas [e.g., Burkitt's lymphoma, mycosis fungoides, mucosa-associated lymphoid tissue (MALT) lymphomas, primary effusion lymphomas, and adult T-cell leukemia/lymphomas] have revealed distinctive and instructive etiology. Lymphomas in childhood may have distinct causes or causes not as easily seen in adult disease; for example, the proportion of disease attribut- able to inherited susceptibility is typically greater at younger ages. Similarly, the lymphomas arising after human immunodeficiency virus infection or after organ transplantation differ in various ways from other lymphomas. Their accelerated development may illuminate the outline of the multistep process of lymphomagenesis.

For exposures to pesticides, organic solvents, and other chemicals on the job and in the general environment, immunologic explanations are speculative at present. If a consistent pattern of lymphoma risk is seen, investigators test various immunologic markers to identify mechanisms. Similarly, dietary and other factors warrant consideration before a specific immune dysregulation is proffered as a biologic rationale. Epidemiologic evaluation of lymphomas attends to the unusual cases with clear immunologic defects as well as to the broad spectrum of lymphomas, taking special note of exposures that have become more common over time.

PATTERNS OF OCCURRENCE

The risk of developing lymphoma or dying from it markedly varies by person, place, and time. The time trend is so dramatic that lymphoma can be described as an epidemic—an epidemic with three distinct phases. The long-term increase in rates began at least as early as 1950. The second phase reflected the addition of the acquired immunodeficiency syndrome (AIDS)–related lymphomas. Most recently, the epidemic growth has subsided, and rates may be reaching a plateau.

The 50-year increase in non-Hodgkin's lymphoma is shown in Figure 44.1 along with the rates for two related cancers, multiple myeloma, and Hodgkin's disease. Mortality from non-Hodgkin's lymphoma increased markedly over the last five decades, from a rate of 3.2 deaths per 100,000 person-years to a rate of 7. Multiple myeloma mortality rates also increased over the half-century, from 1.1 to 3.1. At the same time, Hodgkin's lymphoma mortality rates decreased

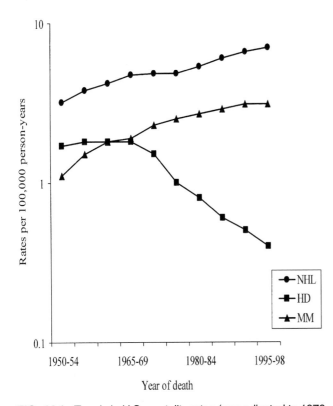

FIG. 44.1. Trends in U.S. mortality rates (age-adjusted to 1970 U.S. standard) for Hodgkin's disease (HD), non-Hodgkin's lymphoma (NHL), and multiple myeloma (MM). (From National Center for Health Statistics, http://www.cdc.gov/nchs. Accessed 07/18/2003.)

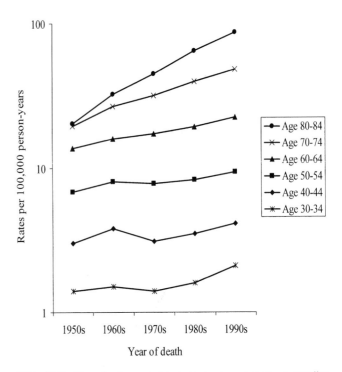

FIG. 44.2. Trends in non-Hodgkin's lymphoma mortality among U.S. white men within selected age groups. (From National Center for Health Statistics, http://www.cdc.gov/nchs. Accessed 07/18/2003.)

from 1.7 to 0.4 deaths per 100,000 person-years. (The effects of the aging of the population have been removed by age adjustment.) Mortality rates are subject to improvements in survival, but they are less sensitive to improvements in diagnostic practices. For that reason, increasing mortality rates provide strong evidence of a real increase in the occurrence of lymphoma. Artifacts of diagnosis explain little of the increase (1).

One intriguing feature of the long-term rise in lymphoma rates is that it has been driven by the very great increases in lymphoma among older people (Fig. 44.2). For example, among white men aged 80 to 84 years, the mortality rate increased from 20 to 86 deaths per 100,000 person-years. By contrast, rates in white men aged 40 to 44 years increased from 3.0 to 4.1. The same fan-shaped pattern of greater rates of increase at older ages appears in incidence, as well as mortality, data and among women as well as men.

The impact of the AIDS epidemic on lymphoma rates appears most starkly in areas with a high prevalence of human immunodeficiency virus infection, such as San Francisco County (Fig. 44.3). When highly active antiretroviral therapy becomes widespread in a particular population, the contribution of human immunodeficiency virus–related lymphoma

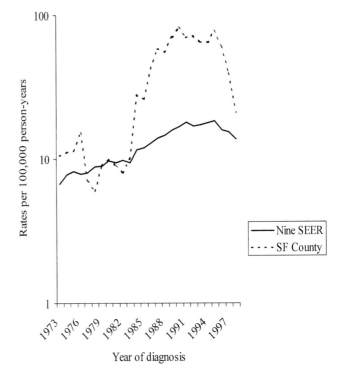

FIG. 44.3. Trends in incidence rates (age-adjusted to 1970 U.S. standard) for non-Hodgkin's lymphoma by year of diagnosis among men aged 20 to 59 years in nine Surveillance, Epidemiology, and End Results (SEER) areas and San Francisco (SF) County.

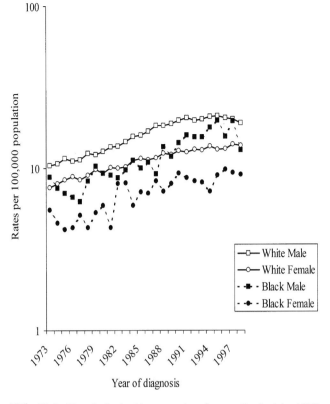

FIG. 44.4. Trends in incidence rates (age-adjusted to 1970 U.S. standard) for non-Hodgkin's lymphoma in nine Surveillance, Epidemiology, and End Results areas.

decreases rapidly (2). The impact on lymphoma rates in a local area can be quite dramatic, yet the overall population rates change much less, depending on the prevalence of human immunodeficiency virus in the population. Since the beginning of the Surveillance, Epidemiology, and End Results program, the yearly incidence rates increased in all sex-race groups and accelerated somewhat during the beginning of the AIDS epidemic (Fig. 44.4). In the most recent years, the rates in white men have not risen at all, but it is too soon to forecast whether the long-term increase will resume.

Gender and ethnicity correlate with non-Hodgkin's lymphoma risk in the United States and elsewhere (3–5). The overall incidence, 16.1 cases diagnosed per 100,000 person-years in the United States, reflects an average of higher rates in white men (20.3) and black men (17.1) and lower rates in white women (13.5) and black women (8.9). The larger size of the elderly female population counterbalances the lower female rates, so approximately 45% of newly diagnosed non-Hodgkin's lymphoma patients are women. Multiple myeloma occurs less often than non-Hodgkin's lymphoma (4.5 vs. 16.1 cases per 100,000 person-years), and Hodgkin's disease occurs much less often (2.7). Men face greater risks than women for both myeloma and Hodgkin's disease. White rates exceed black for Hodgkin's disease, but black rates greatly exceed white for multiple myeloma.

In any time period, advancing age is the overwhelming risk factor for lymphoma, as it is for most cancers. For example, currently among white men in the United States, three cases of lymphoma per 100,000 are diagnosed annually in the age range of 20 to 24 years, but 135 are diagnosed in the age range of 80 to 84 years. Parallel age-specific curves are seen for black and white males and females. (Reported incidence rates appear to decrease after age 85, but these rates are not likely to be accurate.)

Geographic variation in lymphoma rates suggests the importance of environmental effects, some known (human T-cell lymphotrophic virus type I in the Caribbean and Japan or human immunodeficiency virus in San Francisco in the early 1980s) but most unknown. In the United States, deaths per 100,000 person-years among white men vary from approximately four deaths in the south region to approximately eight in the north-central areas (Fig. 44.5). The pattern is very similar in white women (Fig. 44.5), suggesting that the underlying environmental or behavioral factors must be common to men and women. The geography of lymphoma mortality contrasts markedly with the geography of melanoma and nonmelanoma skin cancer (6), an argument against a strong association between ultraviolet radiation and lymphoma risk. Some of the areas with high mortality rates are heavily agricultural, an argument for an effect of pesticides or other farm-related exposures.

International variation in lymphoma risk exceeds the diversity within the United States (Fig. 44.6). In general, rates are lowest in Asia and highest in Western Europe and North America. In areas with lower rates, such as India, Japan, and Colombia, cancer registries recorded substantial increases in lymphoma incidence between approximately 1975 and approximately 1990 (7). (Later data are in press.)

Descriptive local area studies of lymphoma have been conducted to detect clustering that might reveal either an infection or a chemical point source of exposure. An Italian study (8) found slight elevations in an agricultural area and in a heavily industrialized area. A cluster investigation of leukemia and lymphoma in children in northern England found no direct contact among cases, yet closer than expected distance to neighbor cases prompted the authors to suggest transmissible agents in the population of the child's contacts (9). A later study of childhood leukemia and lymphoma near large rural construction sites showed an increase in incidence in the year after construction and the associated influx of population and introduction of new transmissible agents (10).

Because lymphoma comprises a set of diverse pathologic entities, the overall epidemiologic pattern of lymphoma reflects an average of the patterns of the individual entities. Indeed, recent detailed examinations (11,12) reveal that the age effects, the race ratios, and the sex ratios vary among some major histologic subsets of lymphoma in the United States. The age-specific incidence curves for small noncleaved lymphomas, lymphoblastic lymphomas, and immunoblastic lymphomas deviate from the pattern seen overall. Small noncleaved risk increases little with age; lymphoblastic risk decreases to a trough in the 40s and increases again after 50 years of age; and immunoblastic risk increases until 40 years

Males

Mortality rate / 100,000 age-adjusted
1970 US population

- ■ 7.42 to 9.56 (103)
- ▨ 7.07 to 7.42 (101)
- ▦ 6.69 to 7.07 (102)
- ▢ 6.21 to 6.69 (101)
- □ 3.83 to 6.21 (101)
- ▨ Sparse Data (0)

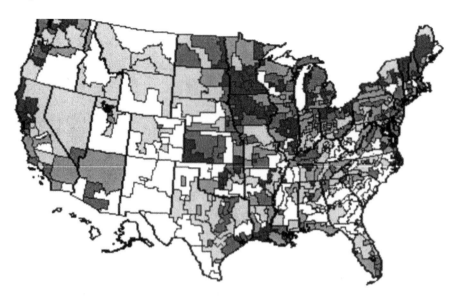

Females

Mortality rate / 100,000 age-adjusted
1970 US population

- ■ 5.14 to 6.44 (103)
- ▨ 4.83 to 5.14 (101)
- ▦ 4.56 to 4.83 (102)
- ▢ 4.22 to 4.56 (101)
- □ 2.69 to 4.22 (101)
- ▨ Sparse Data (0)

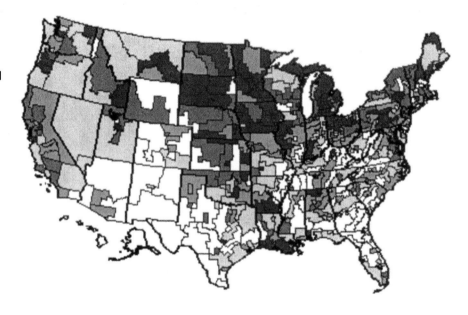

FIG. 44.5. Non-Hodgkin's lymphoma mortality rates among white males and females from 1970 to 1994 by state economic area. (From National Cancer Institute. Cancer Mortality Maps & Graphs. http://www3.cancer.gov/atlasplus/. Accessed 07/18/2003.)

of age, plateaus until 60 years of age, and increases again. The overall sex ratio for lymphoma incidence is approximately three males to two females, but it is closer to 1:1 for follicular and greater than 2:1 for immunoblastic, lymphoblastic, and small noncleaved, the high-grade histologies. The ratio of white to black incidence is highest (3:1) for follicular tumors and much lower (3:5) for peripheral T-cell tumors.

It is difficult to dissect the long-term time trends in lymphoma according to histologic subset because of changes in classification in lymphoma, but certain features are evident. The incidence of non-Hodgkin's lymphoma diagnosed in extranodal sites, approximately 27% of all cases from 1978 to 1995 in the United States, has risen faster than the inci-

dence of nodal lymphomas. High-grade non-Hodgkin's lymphoma incidence has increased the most, and incidence of both follicular small cell and diffuse small cell have been decreasing since the mid-1970s (11).

RISK FACTORS FOR LYMPHOMAS

Epidemiologists have examined a wide range of potential risk factors as they relate to the broad spectrum of lymphomas. Family and personal histories of cancer and of immune-related and other diseases have been studied extensively. Medical conditions and viral infections characterized by marked or moderate immune suppression have been explored

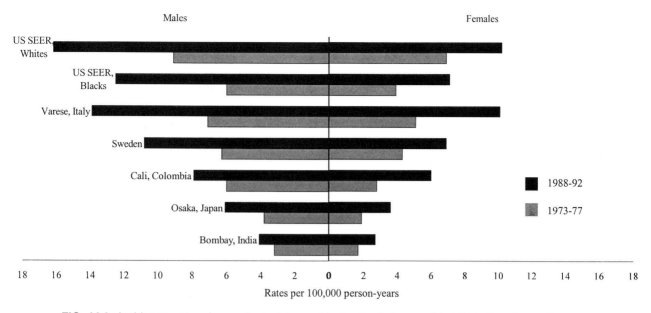

FIG. 44.6. Incidence rates (age-adjusted to world standard) for non-Hodgkin's lymphoma by sex. SEER, Surveillance, Epidemiology, and End Results. (From *Cancer incidence in five continents*, vols. IV and VII. Lyon, France: International Agency for Research on Cancer; and nine SEER registries.)

in detail, with increasing attention to biologic markers of immune function. A somewhat distinct line of epidemiologic research has focused on factors that are not definitely linked to an immune mechanism but that nonetheless appear to influence lymphoma risk. Occupational and environmental exposures to radiation (ionizing, ultraviolet, and electric and magnetic fields) and chemicals (especially pesticides and organic solvents) have all been examined. Finally, factors related to other cancers have been studied simply to detect whether they could also alter lymphoma risk. Dietary and reproductive patterns have been explored, along with personal exposures, such as hair coloring.

Personal and Family History of Cancers

People with one or more first-degree relatives who had non-Hodgkin's lymphoma face approximately twice the average risk of developing non-Hodgkin's lymphoma, according to the most accurate studies, which are based on registries that capture all confirmed cancers in a population over several generations, such as in Utah (13) and Sweden (14). Additional information comes from the numerous case-control studies of non-Hodgkin's lymphoma. Although the relative risk estimates in case-control studies tend to be slightly inflated by under-reporting in controls and over-reporting in cases, the magnitude of the distortion is modest, and the patterns of risk parallel those seen in registry studies. Several other cancers consistently appear in excess in families of non-Hodgkin's lymphoma patients: leukemia, Hodgkin's disease, and multiple myeloma (15,16). The fraction of all lymphomas attributable to family history is probably less than 3%.

Siblings of lymphoma patients may have higher risk than children of lymphoma patients (14), suggesting the possibility of X-linked or recessive inheritance. One large case-control analysis suggested that environmental risks may vary according to family history or that familial risk might vary according to histologic subtypes (17,18). Likely mode of inheritance, interaction of the familial risk with other factors, and histologic specificity all require more investigation with larger data sets with reasonably accurate family history data.

People who have survived certain other cancers are at increased risk of developing non-Hodgkin's lymphoma. Some result from therapy for the first cancer, but some reflect common etiology, including the other lymphoproliferative and the hematopoietic malignancies. Survivors of childhood Hodgkin's disease apparently have seven times the ordinary risk of non-Hodgkin's lymphoma (19). In a large Swedish series, Hodgkin's survivors diagnosed in middle and late adulthood also had greatly increased non-Hodgkin's lymphoma risk; survivors of lymphoid leukemias had four times the usual non-Hodgkin's lymphoma risk, and survivors of myeloma had two times the risk (20).

The development of skin cancers after lymphoma has received special attention because of the sunlight hypothesis; slightly increased risks have been reported from many series and registries. People diagnosed with basal cell or squamous cell skin cancers had twice the risk of lymphoma in a Swiss registry study (21). In U.S. registry data on 55,000 melanoma survivors, lymphoma risk was increased 40% after skin melanoma, especially in the first few years after melanoma (22). It may be relevant that skin cancers and lymphomas are the most common cancers to arise from post-transplant immunosuppression.

A complementary observation arises from the studies of second primary cancers: People who survive non-Hodgkin's lymphoma are at increased risk of particular malignancies, including the same blood, lymph, and skin cancers that are seen in excess preceding non-Hodgkin's lymphoma, but also some other cancers. In an analysis of 6,000 non-Hodgkin's lymphoma survivors, risks were at least doubled for Hodgkin's disease, leukemias, melanoma, and brain cancers. In a recent cancer registry study of 62,000 U.S. non-Hodgkin's lymphoma survivors, skin melanoma risk increased 75% (22). Epidemiologic investigations of second cancers, discussed in greater detail elsewhere in this volume, typically study either a moderately large series of patients who have been followed after treatment and whose treatment data are recorded in some detail or a population-based registry of patients with less information on treatment but with much larger numbers. For non-Hodgkin's lymphoma, the approaches have produced complementary and mutually consistent findings on which cancers cluster with non-Hodgkin's lymphoma, but observers debate the relative importance of effects of therapy versus common etiology.

Primary Immunosuppression

Children and adults with primary or acquired immune deficiencies face enormous and well-documented increases in risk for lymphoproliferative diseases, including lymphomas (23). Immune deficiencies associated with lymphoma risk include congenital immune deficiency diseases; immunosuppression after organ transplant; autoimmune disorders; and immunosuppression by infectious agents, such as human immunodeficiency virus (24,25). In general, the strength of association between immune deficiencies and lymphoma risk mirrors the degree of immune deficiency.

Congenital or primary immune deficiencies consist of genetically determined diseases that affect host immune function, including ataxia-telangiectasia, Wiskott-Aldrich syndrome, and common variable immunodeficiency (23,26). Other primary immune deficiencies leading to increased lymphoma risk include X-linked lymphoproliferative disease and severe combined immunodeficiency (23). These diseases are associated with lymphoma independent of other risk factors. The differences in their mechanisms for immune modulations and in their lymphoma risks provide clues regarding pathogenesis. As many as one fourth of all patients with congenital immune deficiencies develop cancers during their lifetime (one half of them lymphomas) (27). Consistent with the large degree of immune deficiency in these disorders, the associated lymphomas tend to be clinically aggressive, high-grade malignancies.

Individuals with ataxia-telangiectasia have a 50-fold to 150-fold excess risk of cancer in general; approximately 10% of children with ataxia-telangiectasia develop lymphoma (24). This autosomal-recessive disorder is caused by mutations of both alleles in the ataxia-telangiectasia gene (ataxia-telangiectasia mutated) on the long arm of chromosome 11 (11q22.3). The ataxia-telangiectasia–mutated gene encodes for an enzyme that regulates cell division after DNA damage. *Ataxia-telangiectasia* is a genetic neurodegenerative disorder with early onset, characterized by cerebellar ataxia in which coordination of voluntary movements is progressively impaired, oculocutaneous telangiectasia, and cellular and humoral immunodeficiency. The frequency of ataxia-telangiectasia ranges from 1 per 40,000 to 1 per 300,000 births (28). Lymphomas developing in individuals with ataxia-telangiectasia are largely B cell in type, and contrary to most primary immune deficiency–related lymphomas, Epstein-Barr virus is not usually present (24).

Wiskott-Aldrich syndrome, an X-linked recessive disorder caused by mutations in the long arm of the Wiskott-Aldrich syndrome protein gene (Xp11.23-p11.22), encompasses immunodeficiency, eczema, thrombocytopenia, and recurrent infections. Wiskott-Aldrich syndrome occurs in four per million live male births in the United States. Fourteen percent of boys with Wiskott-Aldrich syndrome develop lymphomas, nearly all of them with Epstein-Barr virus in the tumors (24). Wiskott-Aldrich syndrome–related lymphomas are primarily large-cell immunoblastic lymphomas, B cell in type, and extranodal, with central nervous system involvement in one fourth of the lymphomas (24).

Common variable immunodeficiency, a heterogeneous collection of rare genetic immunodeficiency disorders characterized by abnormalities in immune maturation, leads to antibody deficiency, hypogammaglobulinemia (e.g., reduction in immunoglobulins in serum), and recurrent bacterial infections. Probably an autosomal-recessive disorder, common variable immunodeficiency affects approximately 1 in 10,000 to 100,000 men and women. Approximately 1.4% to 7.0% of people with common variable immunodeficiency develop lymphoproliferative disease and lymphoma (29). Common variable immunodeficiency–associated lymphomas are primarily extranodal and B cell in type (27).

X-linked lymphoproliferative disease is caused by mutations in the SAP/SH2D1A gene. The Epstein-Barr virus genome is present in virtually all tissue samples from X-linked lymphoproliferative disease lymphomas (24), and the syndrome itself includes defective immune response to Epstein-Barr virus infection. It is estimated that 20% to 35% of boys with X-linked lymphoproliferative disease develop lymphoma (24,30). X-linked lymphoproliferative disease–associated lymphomas are usually extranodal and B cell in type, including small cleaved and immunoblastic lymphomas (24). Other congenital immunodeficiencies associated with higher frequency of lymphomas include severe combined immunodeficiency, hyperimmunoglobulin M syndrome, Chédiak-Higashi syndrome, B-cell proliferative syndrome, and Bruton's agammaglobulinemia.

Autoimmune Disorders

There is mounting evidence that lymphomas also occur in higher frequencies in some autoimmune disorders, notably rheumatoid arthritis, systemic lupus erythematosus, Sjögren's syndrome, and celiac disease (31). Rheumatoid arthritis, a common inflammatory connective-tissue disease, has been linked to both B- and T-cell lymphomas in several cohort studies. Finnish investigators have demonstrated a twofold increase in risk for lymphoma in a registry-based study (32,33). Swedish and Danish investigators have also reported similar excess risk (34,35). For Felty's syndrome, a rare complication affecting 1% of rheumatoid arthritis patients, a higher eightfold increase in risk for lymphoma has been reported based on a retrospective cohort study of U.S. men (36).

The association among autoimmune diseases, such as rheumatoid arthritis, however, needs to be dissected from effects of simultaneous medication usage. A Finnish study using registry data demonstrated excess risk of lymphoma for rheumatoid arthritis patients receiving cyclophosphamide (32). In a review of autoimmune rheumatic diseases (37), rheumatoid arthritis patients who were on immunosuppressive therapies (e.g., azathioprine, cyclophosphamide, and chlorambucil) had ten times the risk for lymphoma, with longer use and higher doses correlating with level of risk. Although case reports of lymphomas in arthritis patients implicate methotrexate, these associations are not yet definitive (37).

Sjögren's syndrome affects 2 to 4 million individuals in the United States, predominantly women. It is characterized by the progressive destruction of salivary and lacrimal glands and an increased risk for developing lymphoproliferative diseases, mainly B-cell lymphoma. This long-recognized association (38) has been demonstrated with very high risk estimates in case series (39–41). Recent data from the Finnish Cancer Registry, in which 676 patients with primary Sjögren's syndrome and 709 with secondary Sjögren's syndrome were followed for malignancies, show that lymphoma risk increases fourfold with secondary Sjögren's syndrome and ninefold with primary Sjögren's syndrome (42).

Systemic lupus erythematosus patients have a substantially increased risk for B-cell lymphoma (43,44). Animal models provide additional evidence of a causal association (45). Although the early risk estimates, such as a 44-fold increase, were too high (46), subsequent studies of various designs confirm the association. A fivefold increase in risk of lymphomas appeared in Danish Cancer Registry data (43). A population-based case-control study in Italy estimated an eightfold increase in lymphoma risk for systemic lupus erythematosus patients (47); lymphoma risk increased sevenfold in a Canadian cohort of 297 systemic lupus erythematosus patients followed for 12 years (48).

Celiac disease patients also exhibit elevated rates of lymphoma, for example, as recently reported from an Italian cohort (49). Although both B- and T-cell lymphomas have been reported in celiac disease patients, there appears to be a predominance for extranodal T-cell lymphomas. In the primary immune syndromes, very high lymphoma risk accompanies the high degree of immune deficiency. Further evidence comes from examining lymphoma risk in the setting of acquired immunosuppression. Transplant recipients

and other patients undergoing immunosuppressive therapies and individuals immunosuppressed by infectious agents, such as human immunodeficiency virus, suffer excess risk of lymphoma, often evident almost immediately after suppression occurs.

Organ Transplant

Lymphoma arising in organ transplant recipients on immunosuppressive therapy has long been recognized (23,50,51). These posttransplant lymphomas tend to be high-grade, extranodal B-cell lymphomas (24). This association is correlated to the type of transplantation, the size of the organ transplanted, and the degree of immunosuppression needed to forestall rejection (23). Data from a large multicenter study in Europe and North America show lymphomas occurring in 0.2% of kidney transplant recipients and in 1.2% of heart transplant recipients during the first year, rates which are 20 and 120 times higher, respectively, than those seen in the general population (52,53).

Similarly, the use of specific medications (e.g., cyclosporin A, monoclonal antibodies for T-cell depletion, prednisone, and azathioprine) correlates with the risk of developing posttransplant lymphoma. In the Collaborative Transplant Study, higher doses of cyclosporin and azathioprine were used in heart transplant recipients, compared with kidney transplant recipients (54); lymphoma incidence in heart transplant patients was threefold greater than in kidney transplant patients. Furthermore, individuals needing cyclosporin A, azathioprine, and steroids simultaneously showed the highest lymphoma incidence (53).

Two other features of transplantation lymphomas warrant comment. Cessation of immunosuppressive therapies appears to lead to regression of lymphomas (55). Second, Epstein-Barr virus DNA occurs in virtually all tumors from transplantation (56).

Common Medical Conditions, Medications, and Procedures

In blood transfusion recipients, elevated risk of developing lymphomas has also been reported (57). Early initial studies reported a twofold increase in risk (58,59), but subsequent studies have been less consistent, as summarized in a recent review of the literature (57). Most studies specifically assessed allogeneic blood transfusions, prevalent since 1987. In a cohort study of Iowa women, those who reported having received blood transfusion showed a 60% increased risk for subsequent lymphomas. The excess risk was most evident for low-grade nodal lymphoma, specifically follicular and small lymphocytic lymphoma, although the histology-specific estimates were imprecise because of small numbers.

Finally, various common diseases and medications have been associated with lymphomas in one or two studies but not established as risk factors. People with asthma, allergies, and eczema have been inconsistently reported as showing decreased risk of developing lymphomas (60–63). Vaccinations (63) and injection drug use (64) may alter risk. One study found increased risk with use of amphetamines (65), another with endometriosis (28), and another with adult-onset diabetes (66). Perhaps consideration of distinct lymphomas or of biomarkers of immunity will clarify this area. For now, epidemiologic studies investigate leads on this wide range of medical conditions and medications but continue to focus mostly on medical factors with moderately large immune modulating potential.

Viruses and Other Infectious Agents

Viruses and other infectious agents play a critical role in the etiology of lymphomas. They may operate by depressing immune function (e.g., human immunodeficiency virus), by influencing inflammation, or by other mechanisms. The link between specific infectious agents and lymphoma risk varies by preexisting immunosuppressive conditions, by the nature of the infectious agents, and by lymphoma subtype. Well-established associations include those between human immunodeficiency virus and aggressive B-cell lymphomas, human T-cell lymphotrophic virus type I and adult T-cell leukemia/lymphomas, Epstein-Barr virus and Burkitt's lymphoma, and human herpesvirus-8/Kaposi's sarcoma–associated herpesvirus and primary effusion lymphoma. It also appears likely that *Helicobacter pylori* infection plays a crucial role in the development of MALT lymphomas in the gastrointestinal tract. Associations with lymphomas have also been suggested but not established for hepatitis C virus and simian virus 40. Epidemiologic studies of infectious agents and lymphomas include both examination of tumor tissue to identify DNA sequences of these agents and serologic measurements of host immune response to exposure from these agents.

Retroviruses

Human T-cell lymphotrophic virus type I was the first retrovirus established as a cause of lymphoma, specifically of adult T-cell leukemia/lymphomas (25,67). Human T-cell lymphotrophic virus type I infection, endemic in southern Japan and the Caribbean, is rare elsewhere. Human T-cell lymphotrophic virus type I can be transmitted in early life and by sexual activity, injection drug use, and blood transfusion. Because of the 20- to 40-year incubation period for adult T-cell leukemia/lymphomas, even in populations in which human T-cell lymphotrophic virus type I infection is endemic, less than 5% of individuals infected with human T-cell lymphotrophic virus type I live long enough to develop adult T-cell leukemia/lymphomas (68).

Human immunodeficiency virus stands as the major known cause of lymphoma. Indeed, non-Hodgkin's lymphoma is a defining event in the diagnosis of AIDS in a patient who has the human immunodeficiency virus (69), following early observation of aggressive lymphoma cases

among young gay men in California cancer registries (41,70). A recent review of AIDS and lymphoma (71) identifies lymphoma as the second most frequent cancer occurring in human immunodeficiency virus patients; among specific AIDS populations, such as intravenous drug abusers and hemophiliacs, lymphoma is the most frequent cancer (23). Individuals with AIDS face a 60-fold increase in risk for lymphomas, primarily extranodal B-cell lymphomas (72,73). Although the risk is well established, the etiologic sequence of events from human immunodeficiency virus to lymphoma remains to be completely delineated. Notably, human immunodeficiency virus infects T cells, yet most AIDS–related lymphomas are B-cell lymphomas, and lymphoma risk varies with the duration and degree of immunosuppression. Apparently, immunosuppression rather than human immunodeficiency virus infection itself plays the critical role in lymphomagenesis (41).

With the introduction and widespread use of highly active antiretroviral therapy, lymphoma incidence rates have begun to decrease. A metaanalysis of 20 studies on AIDS–related lymphomas examining the effect of widespread highly active antiretroviral therapy usage was recently conducted (74). Results from the metaanalysis show that incidence of lymphomas declined 40%, from 6.2 per 1,000 person-years in 1992 to 1996 to 3.6 in 1997 to 1999. Several large cohort studies do not yet reflect this decline (75,76), and the effects of highly active antiretroviral therapy on lymphoma incidence worldwide remain uncertain at this writing (71).

Herpesviruses

Among the herpesviruses, both Epstein-Barr virus and human herpesvirus-8 can cause particular lymphomas (Burkitt's and primary effusion lymphoma, respectively), and Epstein-Barr virus plays a role, not yet fully understood despite intensive investigation, in many other lymphomas. Human herpesvirus-8, a rare herpesvirus, shows a tight relationship to one particular lymphoma. First identified as the cause of Kaposi's sarcoma, human herpesvirus-8 was linked to lymphoma in 1995 (77). Specific lymphoma subtypes associated with human herpesvirus-8 include multicentric Castleman's disease and body cavity–based lymphoma, also known as *primary effusion lymphoma* (41). These lymphoma subtypes appear to develop in settings of profound immunosuppression, particularly for primary effusion lymphoma (78). Human herpesvirus-8 has been reported in all primary effusion lymphoma tumors, many of which are also coinfected with human immunodeficiency virus (77,79). In addition, 90% of primary effusion lymphomas contain both human herpesvirus-8 and Epstein-Barr virus (80). Although the numbers of lymphomas resulting from human herpesvirus-8 infection account for only a small fraction of all lymphomas, a clear understanding of this remarkable association may elucidate the mechanisms of lymphoma pathogenesis (41).

Epstein-Barr virus presents a more complex picture. The International Agency for Research on Cancer classifies Epstein-Barr virus as a proven human carcinogen (81). Epstein-Barr virus was first identified in Burkitt's lymphoma in Africa, where it is endemic. Ubiquitous Epstein-Barr virus infection occurs early in life in many regions of Africa and in Papua New Guinea (82). Nearly all Burkitt's lymphomas arising in endemic regions are associated with Epstein-Barr virus infection, but only a minority (20% to 34%) of sporadic Burkitt's lymphomas arising in Western countries harbor Epstein-Barr virus (83,84).

Epstein-Barr virus occurs in lymphomas other than Burkitt's but presumably as a passenger rather than a cause in many of them. The strength of association between Epstein-Barr virus and lymphomas differs among subtypes and correlates closely with degree of immunosuppression. Virologists detect Epstein-Barr virus in 33% to 67% of AIDS–related lymphomas, depending on the method (41), but in few of the high-grade lymphomas of human immunodeficiency virus type 1–negative patients. On the other hand, Epstein-Barr virus appears in all lymphomas arising posttransplantation and in lymphomas of the central nervous system. In Wiskott-Aldrich syndrome and X-linked lymphoproliferative disease, all lymphomas contain Epstein-Barr virus, but this is not so for other hereditary immune disorders (24,25).

How does Epstein-Barr virus infection lead to lymphoma development? Serum bank studies shed light on the sequence of events. A cohort study of 240,000 people in Norway and the United States reported two- to threefold increases in risk for lymphoma associated with Epstein-Barr virus antibody titers (85). Similarly, a Finnish cohort followed for 12 years reported a threefold increase in risk for lymphoma in people with elevated Epstein-Barr virus antibodies (86,87). The modest serology effects, the variation in viral detection in tumors, and the studies of immunocompromised cohorts implicate Epstein-Barr virus as a cofactor but not the major agent in many forms of lymphoma. Epstein-Barr virus can produce lymphoma in an immunodeficient host, but immunosuppression seems to be required (80).

Other members of the herpesvirus family, including human T-cell lymphotrophic virus type II, human herpesvirus-6, and cytomegalovirus, do not appear to predispose to lymphoma (23).

Other Viruses

Although many epidemiologic studies in Italy, Japan, the United States, and Europe have examined whether chronic infection by hepatitis C virus alters the risk of developing lymphoma, the issue remains unresolved. Hepatitis C virus is lymphotrophic and associated with mixed cryoglobulinemia, a B-lymphocyte proliferative disorder (88). The first report on lymphomas and hepatitis C virus, from Italy in 1994, found seroprevalence of 34% in 50 patients (89). Subsequent Italian studies have reported similar high hepatitis C virus seroprevalence in lymphoma patients, but U.S. studies have not, with hepatitis C virus prevalence rates ranging from 1.4% to 22% (90,91). Studies elsewhere show no association. A recent comprehensive review found the current evidence unconvincing (92). If hepatitis C virus infection does elevate risk, investigators need to identify specific lymphomas and account for coinfections, such as those from hepatitis B virus, particularly because hepatitis B virus is also prevalent in populations in which hepatitis C virus–lymphoma association has been reported (92).

Recently, two laboratories reported detecting simian virus 40 DNA sequences in a large proportion of lymphomas (93,94). Early experimental studies in laboratory animals suggested the link (95). Controversial simian virus 40 associations have been reported but not confirmed for mesothelioma and other tumors (96–98). Further epidemiologic studies probably will test the simian virus 40–lymphoma hypothesis by examining DNA in tumors and measuring serum antibody levels.

Nonviral Infections

Infection with *H. pylori* greatly increases the risk of developing gastric B-cell lymphoma, according to a small number of relatively consistent epidemiologic studies. Because gastric B-cell lymphoma accounts for 10% of all lymphomas, the *H. pylori*–lymphoma relation potentially affects many cases. In a prospective study of populations in the United States and Norway, individuals with detectable *H. pylori* immunoglobulin G antibodies suffered a sixfold increase in risk for gastric lymphomas (99). Investigators examining a series of Japanese gastric lymphoma patients (100) pinpointed MALT lymphoma as most strongly linked. This observation fits with the epidemiologic studies of peptic ulcer and gastric lymphoma, which demonstrate a stronger association for MALT (101). Further, low-grade gastric B-cell MALT lymphoma regresses after antibiotic treatment eradicates the *H. pylori* infection (102). Because lymphocytes are not present normally at sites in which MALT develops, investigators infer that *H. pylori* attracts and activates the lymphocytes that develop into lymphoma at those sites (103). Meanwhile, the etiology of *H. pylori*–negative gastric MALT lymphomas remains unclear (104).

Radiation

Ionizing radiation, the prototypic cause of many forms of malignancy, plays a minor role in lymphomagenesis (105). This lack of radiosensitivity stands out in comparison to leukemia. Atomic bomb survivors had no increased risk of death from lymphomas (106). Most studies of workers exposed to ionizing radiation find no excess risk of lymphomas. For example, Chinese medical x-ray workers had substantially elevated risk of leukemia but not lymphoma (107). Similarly, large case-control studies of lymphoma comparing job histories typically found no association with ionizing radiation (108). Diagnostic x-rays do not appear to increase risk. For example, twins exposed *in utero* had increased risk of leukemia but not lymphoma (109). Ionizing radiation apparently does increase lymphoma risk in one setting, namely when medical treatments involve very high-dose radiation (110,111).

Nonionizing radiation in the form of electric and magnetic fields around power lines has been investigated as a potential cause of lymphomas in childhood or adulthood. Early case-control studies of childhood cancer and electric and magnetic fields reported some evidence of an association with lymphomas, often with a very few lymphoma cases combined with leukemias, but subsequent studies have had widely varying results. In adults, various occupational studies have been conducted. For example, investigators studying 51 lymphomas within a cohort of Canadian electric utility workers interpreted their results as favoring an association, but the risk estimates were very imprecise because of the small sample size and did not show dose response (112). A study of 154 lymphomas in a U.S. cohort of such workers showed a weakly positive association (113). A recent critical review of the entire electric and magnetic fields' literature found little evidence supporting such a childhood lymphoma association and a few inconclusive studies pertinent to adult disease (114).

Lymphoma researchers hypothesized that ultraviolet radiation might increase risk, based on the association between skin cancers and lymphomas as second primary tumors, the parallel increase in skin cancer and lymphoma incidence over the last half of the twentieth century, and the effect of sunlight on various markers of immunity. Several other lines of evidence bear on the issue: risk of lymphomas according to residential latitude or solar radiation measures, risk in workers with occupational exposures to sunlight, and strength of the associations between biologic markers of immune response or of lymphocyte damage and ultraviolet radiation.

Lymphoma diagnoses do not exhibit seasonality (115). Does residential exposure to sunlight correlate with lymphoma? Consistently negative patterns appear in the United States, both for lymphomas overall (116,117) and cutaneous lymphoma (118), even though melanoma and other skin cancers unambiguously follow latitude. Positive correlations appear in Sweden (119) and in England and Wales (120).

Workers with outdoor jobs get considerable sunlight exposure compared with office workers and, therefore, ought to be at higher lymphoma risk, according to the hypothesis. Among electric utility workers (121), 188 lymphoma patients had similar exposure to sunlight on the job as the total cohort. A comparison of 33,000 cancer deaths from lymphomas in 24 states and twice as many control deaths (117) found no difference in occupational sunlight exposures. Among Swedish construction workers (122), the incidence of lymphomas was similar in those with medium or low ultraviolet exposure and nonsignificantly elevated in those with high.

Mechanistic studies that could explain a putative sunlight effect include a recent report that levels of HPRT-mutations and BCL2 translocations monitored in the population rise and fall with ultraviolet levels (123). Another group reported that differences in DNA damage in mononuclear cells correlate with environmental ultraviolet and also with sun behaviors. Such reports, although intriguing models, do not provide strong evidence for the hypothesis because the link between the biomarker and lymphoma risk is quite unclear. With some current evidence for and some against, epidemiologic studies are pursuing the sunlight-lymphoma hypothesis.

Occupational Exposures

Several occupations have been associated with increased lymphoma risk in multiple studies, notably farming, forestry, paper and pulp, rubber manufacture, woodworking, dry cleaning, and metal work (87). In several studies, workers with exposure to herbicides, particularly phenoxyacetic acids, show a roughly twofold risk of developing lymphomas, but the association is not fully established (124). Herbicide and other pesticides first were linked to increased lymphoma risk in several case-control and cohort studies conducted in the 1980s (125–128). In addition, some studies have linked lymphoma risk to chlorophenols, which are used in the production of chlorinated organic chemicals, including phenoxy herbicides, and also as fungicides and wood preservatives (129). Additional investigation (130) suggests increased risk for herbicides and fungicides but not for insecticide. One recent case-control study found only a very weak association for chlorophenol (131), and another found associations for pesticides and herbicides, but specific compounds were unknown (132).

Some organic solvents that are used in an enormous variety of jobs have been associated with lymphoma risk in several studies. Despite considerable inconsistency in the literature, partly resulting from varying amounts and quality of exposure information, it seems likely that several organic solvents can lead to increased lymphoma risk. Trichloroethylene and tetrachloroethylene ("perchlorethylene"), degreasing agents used in dry cleaning and other industries, have been associated with lymphomas; in a 1995 review, the International Agency for Research on Cancer found "limited evidence for the carcinogenicity of trichloroethylene" and noted the studies of lymphomas. They concluded that tetrachloroethylene is probably carcinogenic to humans and noted the studies of lymphomas (133). One study of aircraft maintenance workers employed several decades ago found increased risk of developing lymphomas in workers exposed to solvents (134); a more recently employed cohort of manufacturers had little or no increased risk (135). A recent study of Danish workers exposed to trichloroethylene found lymphoma risk more than tripled (136); another study of aerospace workers with trichloroethylene exposure saw no excess risk (137). In a pooled case-control analysis, workers who handled white spirits, paint thinner and other solvents, and gasoline faced excess risk (138). A recent Canadian case-control study reported increased risk to workers exposed to benzidine (132).

Benzene exposure, a risk factor for leukemia, probably does not play a large role in lymphoma (139). One metaanalysis of multiple cohorts comprising more than 300,000 petroleum workers concluded that there was no increased lymphoma risk (140), but the lack of information on which workers were exposed could easily obscure a risk. Based on a few positive studies, other commentators believe better measures of exposure may reveal lymphoma risk (141).

Barbers and hairdressers have increased lymphoma risk in some studies (142,143), as do chemists and lab technicians (144,145). (This association has been noted in support of the hypothesis that personal use of hair dyes increases risk.) Asbestos exposure was linked to lymphomas in an early report, but subsequent studies have found no association (146). A study linking Swedish census data to death records for nearly 3 million people found a disproportionate lymphoma risk in several white collar jobs and in rail and road transport workers, telecommunications workers, and telegraph and radio operators (147).

Pursuing the occupational exposures that may cause lymphomas requires accurate and detailed exposure data, information on factors that could confound, and adequate expected numbers of lymphomas (particularly subtypes) in specific jobs. In many cohort studies, details of occupational exposures are measured, but other possible lymphoma risk factors are unknown, leading to possible confounding. Many modern case-control interview studies have industrial hygienists review the occupational histories and assess likely exposures. In these studies, confounders usually are measured, but the number of subjects in any particular job is small, leading to imprecise results and chance associations. Studies created by linking population registries gain statistical power but generally lack confounder data and detailed exposure data, which tends to obscure any real risks. Occupational epidemiologists use a mixture of these approaches to balance strengths and weaknesses of the evidence.

Water, Air, and General Environment

Apart from workers, many members of the general population are exposed to low levels of organochlorines, pesticides, solvents, and other compounds potentially related to lymphomas. The effects of these environmental exposures are largely unstudied. Diet can be a source of exposure, although usually at low concentration, to polychlorinated biphenyls and other organic compounds that have been associated with lymphoma risk when they occur in higher concentration in occupational studies. Drinking water can be a source of exposure to many organic compounds. A New Jersey ecologic study found slightly elevated rates of lymphomas in municipalities with high levels of trichloroethylene and tetrachloroethylene (148). In a case-control study in Nebraska, measured nitrate levels in drinking water were

associated with moderately increased risk (149). A cohort study of Iowa women did not find an association. However, numbers were small, and the analysis was limited to those on public water supplies (150). Further studies should resolve this issue.

Blood and tissue levels of organic compounds reflect an integration of dietary, environmental, occupational, or personal exposures and may be more likely than questionnaire data or environmental measures to reveal any excess risk that exists. In sera collected in 1974 in the United States, levels of polychlorinated biphenyls correlated with a fourfold gradient in risk of subsequent lymphomas, and levels of DDT (dichlorodiphenyltrichloroethane) correlated with a slight increase (151). A correlation study in 22 states in the United States found no correlation between population levels of the DDT derivative dichlorodiphenyldichloroethane in adipose tissue and rate of lymphoma (152). A case-control study found an association of blood levels of both polychlorinated biphenyls and chlordane with lymphoma risk (153). These preliminary reports need to be confirmed in larger studies.

Dietary Patterns

Diet could affect lymphoma risk, quite apart from any contamination by toxic compounds, perhaps by influencing immune function or DNA damage repair pathways. More than a dozen studies have analyzed usual diet in some detail in relation to lymphoma risk. No dietary risk factor is clearly established to date, but several studies have implicated diets high in fat, meat, or animal protein and diets low in vegetables or fruits. Relative risks in the range of 1.5 to 2.0 are reported, high enough to be of scientific and clinical interest but low enough to make accurate determination of risks challenging.

In a cohort of 88,000 nurses, those with high consumption of fat, especially of transunsaturated fat, had approximately twice the risk of developing lymphoma as did those with low consumption (154); those with high intake of vegetables, and fruits to a lesser extent, had a 40% to 50% reduced risk of lymphoma (155), with each effect measured holding the other one constant. In a cohort of 35,000 Iowa women (156), risk was greater in those who consumed more animal fat and lower in those consuming more fruits. Case-control studies in Italy (157) and Nebraska (158) found somewhat similar patterns.

Milk has been inconsistently reported and now appears unlikely to matter. Alcohol has no apparent effect on overall lymphoma risk (159); neither does coffee or tea consumption (160,161). Physical activity on the job appears unrelated to risk (162). Exercise influences some measures of immune function, so this hypothesis may still be examined in studies measuring recreational and total exercise.

Reproductive and Hormonal

Pregnancy produces transient changes in immunity, and several studies have assessed whether number or timing of pregnancies or births affects the risk of developing lymphomas. Despite a few early reports of an association (163,164), a thorough examination of a large cohort of Swedish women (165) convincingly demonstrated that pregnancy history does not alter risk of adult lymphoma. Less information exists on childhood lymphomas, but one study suggested increased risk to children delivered by Cesarean section (166).

Miscellaneous Chemical Exposures

Several studies have examined whether people who use hair dyes face increased risk of lymphoma, recently reviewed in relation to similar data on myeloma and leukemia (167). Several case-control studies suggested a doubling of risk in some groups of users, especially of darker colors or permanent dye, for example (168), but two cohort studies found no effect overall or among permanent users (169,170). The cohort studies had the advantage of collecting data before the lymphomas occurred but the disadvantage of less detail on the type and timing of exposure. The issue is not fully resolved, but the data available at this writing suggest no increased lymphoma risk to the large majority of hair color users.

Tobacco use leads to many forms of cancer and, therefore, warrants examination in relation to lymphoma. One recent cohort study in women found that smokers had a moderately increased risk of follicular lymphoma but not of diffuse, small lymphocytic, or other types (171). A large combined case-control study (172) reported no association in men and a slightly increased risk in women, especially for diffuse or small lymphocytic lymphoma. Many large, well-designed studies have shown no smoking effect (173–175). It is possible that genetically susceptible subpopulations or particular histologic types could eventually be linked to tobacco, but the positive findings in some studies and some subgroups do not yet form a consistent pattern. In most people, it seems likely that smoking produces little or no change in risk of developing most forms of lymphoma.

EPIDEMIOLOGY AND NON-HODGKIN'S LYMPHOMA GENETICS

Chromosomal Abnormalities

Chromosomal abnormalities are a hallmark of lymphoma, and specific chromosomal translocations are known to be associated with specific histologic subtypes of lymphoma (176). One of the initial chromosomal translocations identified was t(8;14)(q24;q32) in Burkitt's lymphoma (177). Other well-characterized translocations include t(14;18) in follicular lymphoma, t(11;14) in mantle cell lymphoma, t(9;14) in lymphoplasmacytoid lymphoma, and t(3;22) in diffuse large B-cell lymphoma (30,176). In addition to chromosomal translocations, chromosomal gains, losses, and specific somatic mutations also lead to activation of proto-oncogenes; more recently, tumor suppressor gene inactivation has also been observed in lymphomas (176,178). One

recent case-control study separated cases with a t(14;18) translocation and found a stronger link to pesticide use (179). Future epidemiologic analyses will pursue the idea of etiologies linked to chromosomal abnormalities.

Genetic Susceptibility

Epidemiologists have begun to pursue genetic susceptibility factors related to many exposures, endogenous and exogenous, in relation to risks of various malignancies. For lymphomas, the role of genetic polymorphisms remains relatively unexplored. In particular, identifying susceptibility genes that play a role in the immune pathways or in metabolic pathways of environmental risk factors for various lymphomas is a promising area of research.

The primary pathways involved in lymphoma etiology are those that play a role in the regulation of immune function. The four key classes of genes involved in regulating immune function are: (a) inflammatory and regulatory cytokines; (b) Th1/Th2 cytokines, which regulate cell-mediated immunity and antibody response; (c) genes involved in innate immunity, which play a key role in bacterial and viral infection; and (d) chemokines, which play a major role in acute and chronic inflammation. Current disease models provide additional clues regarding the involvement of these classes of genes. In individuals with primary immune diseases, one major biologic factor contributing to lymphoma development is an imbalance in cytokine production [e.g., reduced production of interferons and interleukin (IL)-2] (27). In allogeneic transfusions, there exists evidence suggesting that the immune response is shifted to a Th2 type, resulting in secretion of the IL-4, IL-5, IL-6, and IL-10 cytokines, and away from a Th1 response in which IL-2, interferon-γ, and lymphotoxin are secreted (57). Whereas AIDS–related lymphomas also appear to be associated with high levels of IL-10, IL-6, and tumor necrosis factor-α, Epstein-Barr virus appears to inhibit interferon-γ and IL-2 production (41). Given the lymphocytic origin of lymphoma, the role of cytokines in lymphocyte proliferation, and the consistent association between chronic antigenic stimulation and lymphoma, a comprehensive assessment of genetic polymorphisms in these immunologic genes is invaluable in the understanding of lymphoma etiology.

In addition, factors that regulate the metabolism of environmental and occupational chemical exposures may also be important in modifying lymphoma risk. Many solvents, pesticides (organophosphate and organochlorine insecticides), and dioxins are biotransformed by enzymes that are subject to genetic modification. For example, phase I enzymes are responsible for activation of many of these chemicals and are coded by a variety of genes, including the cytochrome P450s, CYP1A1, CYP1A2, and CYP2E1. Genes, such as the glutathione-S-transferases, are responsible for steps leading to detoxification and excretion and possess polymorphisms manifesting decreased or lack of enzyme activity (180). Understanding the role of genetic polymorphisms in the context of environmental exposures provides the potential to elucidate mechanistic pathways involved in lymphoma as well as elucidate the role of these unclear risk factors.

Gene Expression in Tumors

Finally, microarray technology used to distinguish among lymphoma subtypes offers great promise not only for understanding progression and tailoring therapy but also for unlocking etiology. A recent study of diffuse large B-cell lymphomas used microarray analysis to identify molecular profiles within this lymphoma subtype (181,182). By comparing malignant and normal lymphoid cells on the "Lymphochip," a microarray chip consisting of immune genes, cancer genes, and genes expressed in lymphoid cells (183), two molecularly distinct profiles were uncovered for diffuse large B-cell lymphoma. These two molecular profiles indicated diffuse large B-cell lymphomas were derived from different stages of B-cell differentiation. One molecular profile expressed genes characteristic of germinal center B cells (germinal center B–like diffuse large B-cell lymphoma), and the other expressed genes characteristic of genes normally inducted during *in vitro* activation of peripheral blood B cells (activated B–like diffuse large B-cell lymphoma). Patients with germinal center B–like disease survived longer (182). Now limited to small numbers of clinical specimens, the technology is rapidly evolving and may soon be useful in etiologic studies.

FUTURE EPIDEMIOLOGIC RESEARCH ON NON-HODGKIN'S LYMPHOMAS

Table 44.1 briefly summarizes the major risk factors for developing non-Hodgkin's lymphomas. Except as noted, the effect refers to risk of non-Hodgkin's lymphomas as a whole. We now know that particular infectious agents often produce lymphomas that are clinically or immunohistochemically distinctive. We will come to understand the etiology of lymphomas, in part, by chipping away at the problem one small, homogeneous subset at a time. On the other hand, the majority of follicular and diffuse B-cell lymphomas remain unexplained. Many epidemiologists believe that either dividing the common lymphomas according to molecular or genetic profile or dividing the population according to genetic susceptibility or better biologic exposure measure will uncover more etiologically distinctive subsets. It can be hoped that such biologically driven schemes also will illuminate the causal pathways in general.

Striking individual case reports will continue to yield new clues. Epidemiologists also will continue to follow AIDS patients, agricultural workers, populations exposed to particular viruses, and other especially informative groups to measure their risks of developing lymphoma. Increasingly, these studies will include biologic measures of immune status, environmental samples of exposure levels, and detailed evaluation of tumor histology. Advances in multiple myeloma, chronic lymphocytic and other leukemias, and nonmalignant immune

TABLE 44.1. *Overview of risk factors for developing non-Hodgkin's lymphomas*

Risk	Factor
↑↑↑	Age
↑	Male gender
↑↑	Non-Hodgkin's lymphomas in family
↑	Hodgkin's disease or multiple myeloma in family
↑	History of Hodgkin's disease
↑↑↑	Inherited immunodeficiency
↑↑↑	Acquired immunodeficiency syndrome
↑↑↑	Immunosuppression posttransplant
↑↑	Human immunodeficiency virus infection
↑↑↑	Human T-cell lymphotrophic virus type I → adult T-cell leukemia/lymphoma
↑↑	*Helicobacter pylori* → mucosa-associated lymphoid tissue
↑↑↑	Epstein-Barr virus → Burkitt's lymphoma
↑↑↑	Human herpesvirus-8 → primary effusion lymphoma
?↑	Hepatitis C virus
?↑	Simian virus 40
↑	Severe arthritis
?↑	Infectious mononucleosis
?↑	Blood transfusions
?↓	Asthma
?↓	Allergies
↑	Occupational pesticides (farmers, grain handlers, applicators)
↑	Occupational solvent exposures
?↑	Serum dioxin level
?↑	Serum polychlorinated biphenyl level
—	Ionizing radiation
—	Smoking
?↑↓	Hair dyes
?↑	Nitrates, nitrosamines
?↑	Diet: meat, protein
?↓	Diet: vegetables, fruits
?↑↓	Sunlight

↑↑↑, relative risk, 5+; ↑↑, relative risk, 3–4; ↑, relative risk, 2; ↓, decreased risk; ↑↓, conflicting data; ?, uncertain; —, no association.

conditions will also be examined for possible relevance to lymphoma. Increasingly sophisticated models of the immune system and its controlling genetic pathways, in addition to advancing technology, will present an enormous array of options for analyzing data gathered in epidemiologic lymphoma studies. Surveillance of trends in the population will focus on the impact of highly active antiretroviral therapy on the occurrence of lymphomas around the world. Descriptive studies will pursue histology-specific patterns increasingly as the use of the World Health Organization Revised European-

American Lymphoma Classification scheme extends to more cases and more years.

If analytic investigations in the general population (case-control, cohort, and cross-sectional studies) need to subdivide lymphomas into various subsets to discover etiology, they need very large case groups. Metaanalyses, cooperative parallel studies, and consortia will arise to meet this need. Biospecimens collected before diagnosis offer special opportunities to assess pathogenesis. Because of the relative rarity of lymphomas in the general population, even the largest cohorts with stored blood samples typically yield a few hundred lymphoma cases at most. Studies with these precious prediagnosis biologic specimens will be used primarily to confirm and clarify risks already seen elsewhere. At the same time that etiologic studies exploit the heterogeneity of lymphomas, an integrated picture of the causal pathways should emerge.

ACKNOWLEDGMENTS

We thank Dr. Susan Devesa for expert guidance on descriptive statistics. We thank Katrina Wahl for editorial assistance and graphic presentation.

REFERENCES

1. Hartge P, Devesa SS. Quantification of the impact of known risk factors on time trends in non-Hodgkin's lymphoma incidence. *Cancer Res* 1992;52:5566s–5569s.
2. Clarke CA, Glaser SL. Epidemiologic trends in HIV-associated lymphomas. *Curr Opin Oncol* 2001;13:354–359.
3. National Cancer Institute. Surveillance, Epidemiology, and End Results. http://www.seer.cancer.gov/. Accessed 07/17/2003..
4. *Cancer incidence in five continents*. Lyon, France: International Agency for Research on Cancer, 1982.
5. *Cancer incidence in five continents*. Lyon, France: International Agency for Research on Cancer, 1997.
6. Petralia SA, Dosemeci M, Adams EE, et al. Cancer mortality among women employed in health care occupations in 24 US states, 1984–1993. *Am J Ind Med* 1999;36:159–165.
7. Hartge P, Devesa SS, Fraumeni JF Jr. Hodgkin's and non-Hodgkin's lymphomas. *Cancer Surv* 1994;19–20:423–453.
8. Masala G, DiLollo S, Picoco C, et al. Incidence rates of leukemias, lymphomas and myelomas in Italy: geographic distribution and NHL histotypes. *Int J Cancer* 1996;68:156–159.
9. Alexander FE, McKinney PA, Moncrieff KC, et al. Residential proximity of children with leukaemia and non-Hodgkin's lymphoma in three areas of northern England. *Br J Cancer* 1992;65:583–588.
10. Kinlen LJ, Dickson M, Stiller CA. Childhood leukaemia and non-Hodgkin's lymphoma near large rural construction sites, with a comparison with Sellafield nuclear site. *BMJ* 1995;310:763–768.
11. Groves FD, Linet MS, Travis LB, et al. Cancer surveillance series: non-Hodgkin's lymphoma incidence by histologic subtype in the United States from 1978 through 1995. *J Natl Cancer Inst* 2000;92:1240–1251.
12. Herrinton LJ. Epidemiology of the revised European-American Lymphoma Classification subtypes. *Epidemiol Rev* 1998;20:187–203.
13. Goldgar DE, Easton DF, Cannon-Albright LA, et al. Systematic population-based assessment of cancer risk in first-degree relatives of cancer probands. *J Natl Cancer Inst* 1994;86:1600–1608.
14. Dong C, Hemminki K. Modification of cancer risks in offspring by sibling and parental cancers from 2,112,616 nuclear families. *Int J Cancer* 2001;92:144–150.
15. Holly EA, Lele C, Bracci PM, et al. Case-control study of non-Hodgkin's lymphoma among women and heterosexual men in the San Francisco Bay Area, California. *Am J Epidemiol* 1999;150:375–389.
16. Zhu K, Levine RS, Gu Y, et al. Non-Hodgkin's lymphoma and family history of malignant tumors in a case-control study (United States). *Cancer Causes Control* 1998;9:77–82.
17. Zhu K, Levine RS, Brann EA, et al. Risk factors for non-Hodgkin's lymphoma according to family history of haematolymphoproliferative malignancies. *Int J Epidemiol* 2001;30:818–824.
18. Pottern LM, Linet M, Blair A, et al. Familial cancers associated with subtypes of leukemia and non-Hodgkin's lymphoma. *Leuk Res* 1991;15:305–314.
19. Metayer C, Lynch CF, Clarke EA, et al. Second cancers among long-term survivors of Hodgkin's disease diagnosed in childhood and adolescence. *J Clin Oncol* 2000;18:2435–2443.
20. Dong C, Hemminki K. Second primary neoplasms among 53 159 haematolymphoproliferative malignancy patients in Sweden, 1958–1996: a search for common mechanisms. *Br J Cancer* 2001;85:997–1005.
21. Levi F, Randimbison L, Te VC, et al. Non-Hodgkin's lymphomas, chronic lymphocytic leukaemias and skin cancers. *Br J Cancer* 1996;74:1847–1850.
22. Goggins WB, Finkelstein DM, Tsao H. Evidence for an association between cutaneous melanoma and non-Hodgkin lymphoma. *Cancer* 2001;91:874–880.
23. Knowles DM. Immunodeficiency-associated lymphoproliferative disorders. *Mod Pathol* 1999;12:200–217.
24. Levine AM. Lymphoma complicating immunodeficiency disorders. *Ann Oncol* 1994;5[Suppl 2]:29–35.
25. Mueller N. Overview of the epidemiology of malignancy in immune deficiency. *J Acquir Immune Defic Syndr* 1999;21:S5–S10.
26. Filipovich AH, Mathur A, Kamat D, et al. Lymphoproliferative disorders and other tumors complicating immunodeficiencies. *Immunodeficiency* 1994;5:91–112.
27. Filipovich AH, Mathur A, Kamat D, et al. Primary immunodeficiencies: genetic risk factors for lymphoma. *Cancer Res* 1992;52:5465s–5467s.
28. Olsen JH, Hahnemann JM, Borresen-Dale AL, et al. Cancer in patients with ataxia-telangiectasia and in their relatives in the nordic countries. *J Natl Cancer Inst* 2001;93:121–127.
29. Elenitoba-Johnson KS, Jaffe ES. Lymphoproliferative disorders associated with congenital immunodeficiencies. *Semin Diagn Pathol* 1997;14:35–47.
30. Morra E. The biological markers of non-Hodgkin's lymphomas: their role in diagnosis, prognostic assessment and therapeutic strategy. *Int J Biol Markers* 1999;14:149–153.
31. Ehrenfeld M, Abu-Shakra M, Buskila D, et al. The dual association between lymphoma and autoimmunity. *Blood Cells Mol Dis* 2001;27:750–756.
32. Hakulinen T, Isomaki H, Knekt P. Rheumatoid arthritis and cancer studies based on linking nationwide registries in Finland. *Am J Med* 1985;78:29–32.
33. Kauppi M, Hakala M. Prevalence of cervical spine subluxations and dislocations in a community-based rheumatoid arthritis population. *Scand J Rheumatol* 1994;23:133–136.
34. Gridley G, McLaughlin JK, Ekbom A, et al. Incidence of cancer among patients with rheumatoid arthritis. *J Natl Cancer Inst* 1993;85:307–311.
35. Mellemkjaer L, Linet MS, Gridley G, et al. Rheumatoid arthritis and cancer risk. *Eur J Cancer* 1996;32A:1753–1757.
36. Gridley G, Klippel JH, Hoover RN, et al. Incidence of cancer among men with the Felty syndrome. *Ann Intern Med* 1994;120:3539.
37. Leandro MJ, Isenberg DA. Rheumatic diseases and malignancy—is there an association? *Scand J Rheumatol* 2001;30:185–188.
38. Bloch KJ, Buchanan WW, Wohl MJ, et al. Sjögren's syndrome. A clinical, pathological, and serological study of sixty-two cases. 1965. *Medicine (Baltimore)* 1992;71:386–401.
39. Kassan SS, Thomas TL, Moutsopoulos HM, et al. Increased risk of lymphoma in sicca syndrome. *Ann Intern Med* 1978;89:888–892.
40. Valesini G, Priori R, Bavoillot D, et al. Differential risk of non-Hodgkin's lymphoma in Italian patients with primary Sjögren's syndrome. *J Rheumatol* 1997;24:2376–2380.
41. Cohen K, Scadden DT. Non-Hodgkin's lymphoma: pathogenesis, clinical presentation, and treatment. *Cancer Treat Res* 2001;104:201–230.

42. Kauppi M, Pukkala E, Isomaki H. Elevated incidence of hematologic malignancies in patients with Sjögren's syndrome compared with patients with rheumatoid arthritis (Finland). *Cancer Causes Control* 1997;8:201–204.

43. Mellemkjaer L, Andersen V, Linet MS, et al. Non-Hodgkin's lymphoma and other cancers among a cohort of patients with systemic lupus erythematosus. *Arthritis Rheum* 1997;40:761–768.

44. Pettersson T, Rosenlof, K, Friman C, et al. Successful treatment of the anemia of rheumatoid arthritis with subcutaneously administered recombinant human erythropoietin. Slower response in patients with more severe inflammation. *Scand J Rheumatol* 1993;22:188–193.

45. Mellors RC. Autoimmune and immunoproliferative diseases of NZB/Bl mice and hybrids. *Int Rev Exp Pathol* 1966;5:217–252.

46. Pettersson T, Pukkala E, Teppo L, et al. Increased risk of cancer in patients with systemic lupus erythematosus. *Ann Rheum Dis* 1992;51:437–439.

47. Vineis P, Crosignani P, Sacerdote C, et al. Haematopoietic cancer and medical history: a multicentre case control study. *J Epidemiol Community Health* 2000;54:431–436.

48. Cibere J, Sibley J, Haga M. Systemic lupus erythematosus and the risk of malignancy. *Lupus* 2001;10:394–400.

49. Corrao G, Corraza GR, Bagnardi V, et al. Mortality in patients with coeliac disease and their relatives: a cohort study. *Lancet* 2001;358:356–361.

50. Penn I, Hammond W, Brettschneider L, et al. Malignant lymphomas in transplantation patients. *Transplant Proc* 1969;1:106–112.

51. Hoover R, Fraumeni JF Jr. Risk of cancer in renal-transplant recipients. *Lancet* 1973;2:55–57.

52. Opelz G, Henderson R. Incidence of non-Hodgkin lymphoma in kidney and heart transplant recipients. *Lancet* 1993;342:1514–1516.

53. Opelz G, Schwarz V, Henderson R, et al. Non-Hodgkin's lymphoma after kidney or heart transplantation: frequency of occurrence during the first posttransplant year. *Transpl Int* 1994;7[Suppl 1]:S353–S356.

54. Swinnen LJ, Costanzo-Nordin MR, Fisher SG, et al. Increased incidence of lymphoproliferative disorder after immunosuppression with the monoclonal antibody OKT3 in cardiac-transplant recipients. *N Engl J Med* 1990;323:1723–1728.

55. Bayerdorffer E, Neubauer A, Rudolph B, et al. Regression of primary gastric lymphoma of mucosa-associated lymphoid tissue type after cure of Helicobacter pylori infection. MALT Lymphoma Study Group. *Lancet* 1995;345:1591–1594.

56. Swinnen LJ. Transplantation-related lymphoproliferative disorder: a model for human immunodeficiency virus-related lymphomas. *Semin Oncol* 2000;27:402–408.

57. Cerhan JR, Wallace RB, Dick F, et al. Blood transfusions and risk of non-Hodgkin's lymphoma subtypes and chronic lymphocytic leukemia. *Cancer Epidemiol Biomarkers Prev* 2001;10:361–368.

58. Cerhan JR, Wallace RB, Folsom AR, et al. Transfusion history and cancer risk in older women. *Ann Intern Med* 1993;119:8–15.

59. Blomberg J, Moller T, Olsson H, et al. Cancer morbidity in blood recipients—results of a cohort study. *Eur J Cancer* 1993;29A:2101–2105.

60. Doody MM, Linet MS, Glass AG, et al. Leukemia, lymphoma, and multiple myeloma following selected medical conditions. *Cancer Causes Control* 1992;3:449–456.

61. Mills PK, Beeson WL, Fraser GE, et al. Allergy and cancer: organ site-specific results from the Adventist Health Study. *Am J Epidemiol* 1992;136:287–295.

62. Eriksson NE, Holmen A, Hogstedt B, et al. A prospective study of cancer incidence in a cohort examined for allergy. *Allergy* 1995;50:718–722.

63. Holly EA, Lele C. Non-Hodgkin's lymphoma in HIV-positive and HIV-negative homosexual men in the San Francisco Bay Area: allergies, prior medication use, and sexual practices. *J Acquir Immune Defic Syndr Hum Retrovirol* 1997;15:211–222.

64. Bernstein L, Ross RK. Prior medication use and health history as risk factors for non-Hodgkin's lymphoma: preliminary results from a case-control study in Los Angeles County. *Cancer Res* 1992;52:5510s–5515s.

65. Doody MM, Linet MS, Glass AG, et al. Risks of non-Hodgkin's lymphoma, multiple myeloma, and leukemia associated with common medication. *Epidemiology* 1996;7:131–139.

66. Cerhan JR, Wallace RB, Folsom AR, et al. Medical history risk factors for non-Hodgkin's lymphoma in older women. *J Natl Cancer Inst* 1997;89:314–318.

67. Manns A, Cleghorn FR, Falk RT, et al. Role of HTLV-I in development of non-Hodgkin lymphoma in Jamaica and Trinidad and Tobago. The HTLV Lymphoma Study Group. *Lancet* 1993;342:1447–1450.

68. Siegel R, Gartenhaus R, Kuzel T. HTLV-I associated leukemia/lymphoma: epidemiology, biology, and treatment. *Cancer Treat Res* 2001;104:75–88.

69. Centers for Disease Control. Revision of the CDC surveillance case definition for acquired immunodeficiency syndrome. *MMWR Morb Mortal Wkly Rep* 1987;36[Suppl]:1s–5s.

70. Ziegler JL, Bragg K, Abrams D, et al. High-grade non-Hodgkin's lymphoma in patients with AIDS. *Ann N Y Acad Sci* 1984;437:412–419.

71. Bower M. Acquired immunodeficiency syndrome-related systemic non-Hodgkin's lymphoma. *Br J Haematol* 2001;112:863–873.

72. Beral V, Peterman T, Berkelman R, et al. AIDS-associated non-Hodgkin lymphoma. *Lancet* 1991;337:805–809.

73. Beral V, Bull D, Darby S, et al. Risk of Kaposi's sarcoma and sexual practices associated with faecal contact in homosexual or bisexual men with AIDS. *Lancet* 1992;339:632–635.

74. Beral V, Newton R, Sitas F. Human herpesvirus 8 and cancer. *J Natl Cancer Inst* 1999;91:1440–1441.

75. Jacobson LP, Yamashita TE, Detels R, et al. Impact of potent antiretroviral therapy on the incidence of Kaposi's sarcoma and non-Hodgkin's lymphomas among HIV-1-infected individuals. Multicenter AIDS Cohort Study. *J Acquir Immune Defic Syndr* 1999;21[Suppl 1]:S34–S41.

76. Matthews GV, Bower M, Mandalia S, et al. Changes in acquired immunodeficiency syndrome-related lymphoma since the introduction of highly active antiretroviral therapy. *Blood* 2000;96:2730–2734.

77. Cesarman E, Chang Y, Moore PS, et al. Kaposi's sarcoma-associated herpesvirus-like DNA sequences in AIDS-related body-cavity-based lymphomas. *N Engl J Med* 1995;332:1186–1191.

78. Cesarman E, Knowles DM. Kaposi's sarcoma-associated herpesvirus: a lymphotropic human herpesvirus associated with Kaposi's sarcoma, primary effusion lymphoma, and multicentric Castleman's disease. *Semin Diagn Pathol* 1997;14:54–66.

79. Karcher DS, Alkan S. Human herpesvirus-8-associated body cavity-based lymphoma in human immunodeficiency virus-infected patients: a unique B-cell neoplasm. *Hum Pathol* 1997;28:801–808.

80. IARC monographs. *Epstein-Barr virus and Kaposi's sarcoma herpes virus/human herpes virus 8.* Lyon, France: International Agency for Research on Cancer, 1997.

81. *IARC monographs on the evaluation of carcinogenic risks to humans, schistosomes, liver flukes and* Helicobacter pylori. Lyon, France: International Agency for Research on Cancer, 1994.

82. Niedobitek G, Meru N, Delecluse HJ. Epstein-Barr virus infection and human malignancies. *Int J Exp Pathol* 2001;82:149–170.

83. zur HH, Schulte-Holthausen H, Klein G, et al. EBV DNA in biopsies of Burkitt tumours and anaplastic carcinomas of the nasopharynx. *Nature* 1970;228:1056–1058.

84. Hummel M, Anagnostopoulos I, Korbjuhn P, et al. Epstein-Barr virus in B-cell non-Hodgkin's lymphomas: unexpected infection patterns and different infection incidence in low- and high-grade types. *J Pathol* 1995;175:263–271.

85. Mueller N, Mohar A, Evans A, et al. Epstein-Barr virus antibody patterns preceding the diagnosis of non-Hodgkin's lymphoma. *Int J Cancer* 1991;49:387–393.

86. Lehtinen T, Lumio J, Dillner J, et al. Increased risk of malignant lymphoma indicated by elevated Epstein-Barr virus antibodies—a prospective study. *Cancer Causes Control* 1993;4:187–193.

87. Scherr PA, Mueller NE. Non-Hodgkin's lymphoma. In: Schottenfeld D, Fraumeni JF, eds. *Cancer epidemiology and prevention.* New York: Oxford University Press, 1996.

88. Cacoub P, Fabiani FL, Musset L, et al. Mixed cryoglobulinemia and hepatitis C virus. *Am J Med* 1994;96:124–132.

89. Ferri C, Caracciolo F, Zignego AL, et al. Hepatitis C virus infection in patients with non-Hodgkin's lymphoma. *Br J Haematol* 1994;88:392–394.

90. King PD, Wilkes JD, Diaz-Arias AA. Hepatitis C virus infection in non-Hodgkin's lymphoma. *Clin Lab Haematol* 1998;20:107–110.

91. Zuckerman E, Zuckerman T, Levine AM, et al. Hepatitis C virus infection in patients with B-cell non-Hodgkin lymphoma. *Ann Intern Med* 1997;127:423–428.

92. Hausfater P, Rosenthal E, Cacoub P. Lymphoproliferative diseases and hepatitis C virus infection. *Ann Med Interne (Paris)* 2000;151:53–57.

93. Shivapurkar N, Harada K, Reddy J, et al. Presence of simian virus 40 DNA sequences in human lymphomas. *Lancet* 2002;359:851–852.

94. Vilchez RA, Madden CR, Kozinetz CA, et al. Association between simian virus 40 and non-Hodgkin lymphoma. *Lancet* 2002;359:817–823.

95. Diamandopoulos GT. Leukemia, lymphoma, and osteosarcoma induced in the Syrian golden hamster by simian virus 40. *Science* 1972;176:173–175.

96. Carbone M, Pass HI, Rizzo P, et al. Simian virus 40-like DNA sequences in human pleural mesothelioma. *Oncogene* 1994;9:1781–1790.

97. Strickler HD, Rosenberg PS, Devesa SS, et al. Contamination of poliovirus vaccines with simian virus 40 (1955–1963) and subsequent cancer rates. *JAMA* 1998;279:292–295.

98. Strickler HD. A multicenter evaluation of assays for detection of SV40 DNA and results in masked mesothelioma specimens. *Cancer Epidemiol Biomarkers Prev* 2001;10:523–532.

99. Parsonnet J, Friedman GD, Vandersteen DP, et al. *Helicobacter pylori* infection and the risk of gastric carcinoma. *N Engl J Med* 1991;325:1127–1131.

100. Nakamura S, Yao T, Aoyagi K, et al. *Helicobacter pylori* and primary gastric lymphoma. A histopathologic and immunohistochemical analysis of 237 patients. *Cancer* 1997;79:3–11.

101. Vineis P, Crosignani P, Sacerdote C, et al. Hematopoietic cancer and peptic ulcer: a multicentre case-control study. *Carcinogenesis* 1999;20:1459–1463.

102. Wotherspoon AC, Doglioni C, Diss TC, et al. Regression of primary low-grade B-cell gastric lymphoma of mucosa-associated lymphoid tissue type after eradication of *Helicobacter pylori*. *Lancet* 1993;342:575–577.

103. Beales IL, Calam J. Pathogenic mechanisms in *Helicobacter pylori* infection. *Hosp Med* 1998;59:186–190.

104. Wotherspoon AC, Dogan A, Du MQ. Mucosa-associated lymphoid tissue lymphoma. *Curr Opin Hematol* 2002;9:50–55.

105. Boice JD Jr. Radiation and non-Hodgkin's lymphoma. *Cancer Res* 1992;52:5489s–5491s.

106. Shimizu Y, Kato H, Schull WJ. Studies of the mortality of A-bomb survivors. 9. Mortality, 1950–1985: part 2. Cancer mortality based on the recently revised doses (DS86). *Radiat Res* 1990;121:120–141.

107. Wang JX, Inskip PD, Boice JD Jr, et al. Cancer incidence among medical diagnostic x-ray workers in China, 1950 to 1985. *Int J Cancer* 1990;45:889–895.

108. Eheman CR, Tolbert PE, Coates RJ, et al. Case-control assessment of the association between non-Hodgkin's lymphoma and occupational radiation with doses assessed using a job exposure matrix. *Am J Ind Med* 2000;38:19–27.

109. Inskip PD, Harvey EB, Boice JD Jr, et al. Incidence of childhood cancer in twins. *Cancer Causes Control* 1991;2:315–324.

110. Ron E, Boice JD Jr, Hamburger S, et al. Mortality following radiation treatment for infertility of hormonal origin or amenorrhoea. *Int J Epidemiol* 1994;23:1165–1173.

111. Weiss HA, Darby SC, Doll R. Cancer mortality following x-ray treatment for ankylosing spondylitis. *Int J Cancer* 1994;59:327–338.

112. Villeneuve PJ, Agnew DA, Miller AB, et al. Non-Hodgkin's lymphoma among electric utility workers in Ontario: the evaluation of alternate indices of exposure to 60 Hz electric and magnetic fields. *Occup Environ Med* 2000;57:249–257.

113. Schroeder JC, Savitz DA. Lymphoma and multiple myeloma mortality in relation to magnetic field exposure among electric utility workers. *Am J Ind Med* 1997;32:392–402.

114. Ahlbom IC, Cardis E, Green A, et al. Review of the epidemiologic literature on EMF and Health. *Environ Health Perspect* 2001;109[Suppl 6]:911–933.

115. Douglas S, Cortina-Borja M, Cartwright R. A quest for seasonality in presentation of leukaemia and non-Hodgkin's lymphoma. *Leuk Lymphoma* 1999;32:523–532.

116. Hartge P, Devesa SS, Grauman D, et al. Non-Hodgkin's lymphoma and sunlight. *J Natl Cancer Inst* 1996;88:298–300.

117. Freedman DM, Zahm SH, Dosemeci M. Residential and occupational exposure to sunlight and mortality from non-Hodgkin's lymphoma: composite (threefold) case-control study. *BMJ* 1997;314:1451–1455.

118. Newton R. Solar ultraviolet radiation is not a major cause of primary cutaneous non-Hodgkin's lymphoma. *BMJ* 1997;314:1483–1484.

119. Adami J, Gridley G, Nyren O, et al. Sunlight and non-Hodgkin's lymphoma: a population-based cohort study in Sweden. *Int J Cancer* 1999;80:641–645.

120. Bentham G. Association between incidence of non-Hodgkin's lymphoma and solar ultraviolet radiation in England and Wales. *BMJ* 1996;312:1128–1131.

121. van Wijngaarden E, Savitz DA. Occupational sunlight exposure and mortality from non-Hodgkin lymphoma among electric utility workers. *J Occup Environ Med* 2001;43:548–553.

122. Hakansson N, Floderus B, Gustavsson P, et al. Occupational sunlight exposure and cancer incidence among Swedish construction workers. *Epidemiology* 2001;12:552–557.

123. Bentham G, Wolfreys AM, Liu Y, et al. Frequencies of hprt(-) mutations and bcl-2 translocations in circulating human lymphocytes are correlated with United Kingdom sunlight records. *Mutagenesis* 1999;14:527–532.

124. Zahm SH. Mortality study of pesticide applicators and other employees of a lawn care service company. *J Occup Environ Med* 1997;39:1055–1067.

125. Hoar SK, Blair A, Holmes FF, et al. Agricultural herbicide use and risk of lymphoma and soft-tissue sarcoma. *JAMA* 1986;256:1141–1147.

126. Hardell L, Eriksson M, Lenner P, et al. Malignant lymphoma and exposure to chemicals, especially organic solvents, chlorophenols and phenoxy acids: a case-control study. *Br J Cancer* 1981;43:169–176.

127. Wingle DT, Semenciw RM, Wilkins K, et al. Mortality study of Canadian male farm operators: non-Hodgkin's lymphoma mortality and agricultural practices in Saskatchewan. *J Natl Cancer Inst* 1990;82:575–582.

128. Zahm SH, Weisenburger DD, Babbitt PA, et al. A case-control study of non-Hodgkin's lymphoma and the herbicide 2,4-dichlorophenoxyacetic acid (2,4-D) in eastern Nebraska. *Epidemiology* 1990;1:349–356.

129. Hardell L, Eriksson M, Degerman A. Exposure to phenoxyacetic acids, chlorophenols, or organic solvents in relation to histopathology, stage, and anatomical localization of non-Hodgkin's lymphoma. *Cancer Res* 1994;54:2386–2389.

130. Hardell L, Eriksson M. A case-control study of non-Hodgkin lymphoma and exposure to pesticides. *Cancer* 1999;85:1353–1360.

131. Garabedian MJ, Hoppin JA, Tolbert PE, et al. Occupational chlorophenol exposure and non-Hodgkin's lymphoma. *J Occup Environ Med* 1999;41:267–272.

132. Mao Y, Hu J, Ugnat AM, et al. Non-Hodgkin's lymphoma and occupational exposure to chemicals in Canada. Canadian Cancer Registries Epidemiology Research Group. *Ann Oncol* 2000;11[Suppl 1]:69–73.

133. McGregor DB, Heseltine E, Moller H. Dry cleaning, some solvents used in dry cleaning and other industrial chemicals. IARC meeting, Lyon, 7–14 February 1995. *Scand J Work Environ Health* 1995;21:310–312.

134. Blair A, Hartge P, Stewart PA, et al. Mortality and cancer incidence of aircraft maintenance workers exposed to trichloroethylene and other organic solvents and chemicals: extended follow up. *Occup Environ Med* 1998;55:161–171.

135. Boice JD Jr, Marano DE, Fryzek JP, et al. Mortality among aircraft manufacturing workers. *Occup Environ Med* 1999;56:581–597.

136. Hansen J, Raaschou-Nielson O, Christensen JM, et al. Cancer incidence among Danish workers exposed to trichloroethylene. *J Occup Environ Med* 2001;43:133–139.

137. Morgan RW, Kelsh MA, Zhao K, et al. Mortality of aerospace workers exposed to trichloroethylene. *Epidemiology* 1998;9:424–431.

138. Persson B, Fredrikson M. Some risk factors for non-Hodgkin's lymphoma. *Int J Occup Med Environ Health* 1999;12:135–142.

139. Savitz DA, Andrews KW. Review of epidemiologic evidence on benzene and lymphatic and hematopoietic cancers. *Am J Ind Med* 1997;31:287–295.

140. Wong O, Raabe GK. Non-Hodgkin's lymphoma and exposure to benzene in a multinational cohort of more than 308,000 petroleum workers, 1937 to 1996. *J Occup Environ Med* 2000;42:554–568.

141. O'Connor SR, Farmer PB, Lauder I. Benzene and non-Hodgkin's lymphoma. *J Pathol* 1999;189:448–453.

142. Boffetta P, Andersen A, Lynge E, et al. Employment as hairdresser and risk of ovarian cancer and non-Hodgkin's lymphomas among women. *J Occup Med* 1994;36:61–65.

143. Lamba AB, Ward MH, Weeks JL, et al. Cancer mortality patterns among hairdressers and barbers in 24 US states, 1984 to 1995. *J Occup Environ Med* 2001;43:250–258.

144. Burnett C, Robinson C, Walker J. Cancer mortality in health and science technicians. *Am J Ind Med* 1999;36:155–158.

145. Hoar SK, Pell S. A retrospective cohort study of mortality and cancer incidence among chemists. *J Occup Med* 1981;23:485–494.

146. Becker N, Berger J, Bolm-Audorff U. Asbestos exposure and malignant lymphomas—a review of the epidemiological literature. *Int Arch Occup Environ Health* 2001;74:459–469.

147. Cano MI, Pollan M. Non-Hodgkin's lymphomas and occupation in Sweden. *Int Arch Occup Environ Health* 2001;74:443–449.

148. Cohn P, Klotz J, Bove F, et al. Drinking water contamination and the incidence of leukemia and non-Hodgkin's lymphoma. *Environ Health Perspect* 1994;102:556–561.

149. Ward MH, Mark SD, Cantor KP, et al. Drinking water nitrate and the risk of non-Hodgkin's lymphoma. *Epidemiology* 1996;7:465–471.

150. Weyer PJ, Cerhan JR, Kross BC, et al. Municipal drinking water nitrate level and cancer risk in older women: the Iowa Women's Health Study. *Epidemiology* 2001;12:327–338.

151. Rothman N, Cantor KP, Blair A, et al. A nested case-control study of non-Hodgkin lymphoma and serum organochlorine residues. *Lancet* 1997;350:240–244.

152. Cocco P, Kazerouni N, Zahm SH. Cancer mortality and environmental exposure to DDE in the United States. *Environ Health Perspect* 2000;108:1–4.

153. Hardell L, Lindstrom G, van Bavel B, et al. Adipose tissue concentrations of dioxins and dibenzofurans, titers of antibodies to Epstein-Barr virus early antigen and the risk for non-Hodgkin lymphoma. *Environ Res* 2001;87:99–107.

154. Zhang S, Hunter DJ, Rosner BA, et al. Dietary fat and protein in relation to risk of non-Hodgkin's lymphoma among women. *J Natl Cancer Inst* 1999;91:1751–1758.

155. Zhang SM, Hunter DJ, Rosner BA, et al. Intakes of fruits, vegetables, and related nutrients and the risk of non-Hodgkin's lymphoma among women. *Cancer Epidemiol Biomarkers Prev* 2000;9:477–485.

156. Chiu BC, Cerhan JR, Folsom AR, et al. Diet and risk of non-Hodgkin lymphoma in older women. *JAMA* 1996;275:1315–1321.

157. Tavani A, Pregnolato A, La Vecchia C, et al. A case-control study of reproductive factors and risk of lymphomas and myelomas. *Leuk Res* 1997;21:885–888.

158. Ward MH, Zahm SH, Weisenburger DD, et al. Dietary factors and non-Hodgkin's lymphoma in Nebraska (United States). *Cancer Causes Control* 1994;5:422–432.

159. Brown LM, Gibson R, Burmeister LF, et al. Alcohol consumption and risk of leukemia, non-Hodgkin's lymphoma, and multiple myeloma. *Leuk Res* 1992;16:979–984.

160. Tavani A, Negri E, Franceschi S, et al. Coffee consumption and risk of non-Hodgkin's lymphoma. *Eur J Cancer Prev* 1994;3:351–356.

161. Zheng W, Doyle TJ, Kushi LH, et al. Tea consumption and cancer incidence in a prospective cohort study of postmenopausal women. *Am J Epidemiol* 1996;144:175–182.

162. Zahm SH, Hoffman-Goetz L, Dosemici M, et al. Occupational physical activity and non-Hodgkin's lymphoma. *Med Sci Sports Exerc* 1999;31:566–571.

163. Miller AB, Barclay TH, Choi NW, et al. A study of cancer, parity and age at first pregnancy. *J Chronic Dis* 1980;33:595–605.

164. Olsson H, Olsson ML, Ranstam J. Late age at first full-term pregnancy as a risk factor for women with malignant lymphoma. *Neoplasma* 1990;37:185–190.

165. Adami HO, Tsaih S, Lambe M, et al. Pregnancy and risk of non-Hodgkin's lymphoma: a prospective study. *Int J Cancer* 1997;70:155–158.

166. Adami J, Glimelius B, Cnattingius S, et al. Maternal and perinatal factors associated with non-Hodgkin's lymphoma among children. *Int J Cancer* 1996;65:774–777.

167. Correa A, Jackson L, Mohan A, et al. Use of hair dyes, hematopoietic neoplasms, and lymphomas: a literature review. II. Lymphomas and multiple myeloma. *Cancer Invest* 2000;18:467–479.

168. Zahm SH, Weisenburger DD, Babbitt PA, et al. Use of hair coloring products and the risk of lymphoma, multiple myeloma, and chronic lymphocytic leukemia. *Am J Public Health* 1992;82:990–997.

169. Grodstein F, Hennekens CH, Colditz GA, et al. A prospective study of permanent hair dye use and hematopoietic cancer. *J Natl Cancer Inst* 1994;86:1466–1470.

170. Altekruse SF, Henley SJ, Thun MJ. Deaths from hematopoietic and other cancers in relation to permanent hair dye use in a large prospective study (United States). *Cancer Causes Control* 1999;10: 617–625.

171. Parker AS, Cerhan JR, Dick F, et al. Smoking and risk of non-Hodgkin lymphoma subtypes in a cohort of older women. *Leuk Lymphoma* 2000;37:341–349.

172. Zahm SH, Weisenburger DD, Holmes FF, et al. Tobacco and non-Hodgkin's lymphoma: combined analysis of three case-control studies (United States). *Cancer Causes Control* 1997;8:159–166.

173. McLaughlin JK, Hrubec Z, Blot WJ, et al. Smoking and cancer mortality among U.S. veterans: a 26-year follow-up. *Int J Cancer* 1995;60:190–193.

174. Adami J, Nyren O, Bergstrom R, et al. Smoking and the risk of leukemia, lymphoma, and multiple myeloma (Sweden). *Cancer Causes Control* 1998;9:49–56.

175. Tavani A, Negri E, Franceschi S, et al. Smoking habits and non-Hodgkin's lymphoma: a case-control study in northern Italy. *Prev Med* 1994;23:447–452.

176. Chaganti RS, Nanjangud G, Schmidt H, et al. Recurring chromosomal abnormalities in non-Hodgkin's lymphoma: biologic and clinical significance. *Semin Hematol* 2000;37:396–411.

177. Dalla-Favera R, Lombardi L, Pelicci PG, et al. Mechanism of activation and biological role of the c-myc oncogene in B-cell lymphomagenesis. *Ann N Y Acad Sci* 1987;511:207–218.

178. Misra RR, Pinsky PF, Srivastava S. Prognostic factors for hematologic cancers. *Hematol Oncol Clin North Am* 2000;14:907.

179. Schroeder JC, Olshan AF, Baric R, et al. Agricultural risk factors for t(14;18) subtypes of non-Hodgkin's lymphoma. *Epidemiology* 2001; 12:701–709.

180. Strange RC, Fryer AA. Chapter 19. The glutathione S-transferases: influence of polymorphism on cancer susceptibility. *IARC Sci Publ* 1999;231–249.

181. Staudt LM. Gene expression profiling of lymphoid malignancies. *Ann Rev Med* 2002;53:303–318.

182. Alizadeh AA, Eisen MB, Davis RE, et al. Distinct types of diffuse large B-cell lymphoma identified by gene expression profiling. *Nature* 2000;403:503–511.

183. Alizadeh A, Eisen M, Davis RE, et al. The lymphochip: a specialized cDNA microarray for the genomic-scale analysis of gene expression in normal and malignant lymphocytes. *Cold Spring Harb Symp Quant Biol* 1999;64:71–78.

CHAPTER 45

Lymphoma and Abnormalities of the Immune System

J. Patrick Whelan and David T. Scadden

Immune abnormalities have long been associated with neoplastic risk, particularly with an increased risk of lymphoma. The nature of the immune defects enhancing lymphomagenesis may be quite broad in range, from the severe immunodeficiency states of acquired immunodeficiency syndrome (AIDS), organ transplant, or congenital immune dysfunction to the aberrantly active autoimmune disorders of Sjögren's syndrome or autoimmune thyroiditis. The predisposition to malignant transformation has, in both settings, been attributed to an imbalanced response to immune stimuli. In the context of immunodeficiency, this imbalance may be manifest as an inability to constrain viruses with a direct transforming capability, such as Epstein-Barr virus, or may be due to the persistent immune stimulation of uncontrolled viral or other microbial infection. The autoimmune syndromes are believed to result from an ongoing stimulation, either directly by self-antigen or by exogenous antigens that cross-react with self and lead to autostimulation.

In a similar fashion, the antigenic drive of persistent infection with *Helicobacter pylori* or hepatitis C virus is believed to provide the background proliferation necessary for lymphomatous outgrowth. Control of these two infections has been associated with regression of the related lymphomas [1,2], but control of antigenic stimulation in these and other settings is often not sufficient to eliminate the tumor, largely because of secondary genetic events. For example, those *H. pylori*–associated tumors that fail to regress appear to have undergone a secondary transforming mutation, such as t(11;18) (q21;q21), causing a fusion between an apoptosis inhibiting gene (AP12) and an NF-κB activator (MALT-1). Another example is t(1;14)(p22;q32), which enhances Bcl-10 expression and NF-κB activation [2,3].

Using the AIDS as a model, one begins to see the important role that chronic opportunistic infection can play in the genesis of a variety of different cancers (Table 45.1). Perhaps equally compelling is the fact that most common cancers are not increased in incidence among AIDS patients, including several with a known infectious etiology (Table 45.2). This highlights the generally accepted notion that the genesis of cancers in general, and lymphoma in particular, is a complex and evolving interplay of genetic, infectious, and immunologic phenomena. All three may participate in the transformation process in lymphomas that develop in the context of autoimmune disease or states of immunodeficiency. This chapter focuses specifically on the tumors seen in individuals with inadequate host defense, but lessons learned may be more applicable to immune dysregulation in other settings and perhaps to lymphoid malignancies more broadly.

ACQUIRED IMMUNODEFICIENCY SYNDROME–RELATED LYMPHOMA

It is now estimated that 40 million individuals are infected with human immunodeficiency virus type 1. The most lethal complication of this disease is non-Hodgkin's lymphoma [4]. The relative risk of death from opportunistic infection has changed for many infectious complications but has remained stubbornly persistent for AIDS-related lymphoma. The characteristic features of this opportunistic neoplasm, however, have changed markedly in the context of antiretroviral therapy.

Epidemiology

Risk for developing AIDS-related lymphoma is dependent on a number of factors, including genetic background; the use of combination, highly active antiretroviral therapy; and, perhaps, human immunodeficiency virus risk group. Overall, the risk of developing lymphoma for human immunodeficiency virus–positive patients is estimated to be 60- to 110-fold greater than that of the general population. Among human immunodeficiency virus infected individuals, there also appears to be a varying prevalence of lymphoma, with the

TABLE 45.1. *Cancers associated with human immunodeficiency virus infection*[a]

Tumor type	Viral cofactor	Relative risk	Reference
Kaposi's sarcoma and angiosarcoma	Kaposi's sarcoma–associated herpesvirus	310–83,000	223, 226
Non-Hodgkin's lymphoma	EBV	113–165	223, 227, 231
Anal carcinoma[b]	HPV	31.7	226, 228
Hodgkin's lymphoma	EBV	7.6	223, 229, 231
Leiomyosarcoma (pediatric)	EBV	7.2	230, 231
Multiple myeloma[c]	?	4.5–5.8	223, 232, 233
Seminoma[d]	Cytomegalovirus, herpes simplex virus?	2.9	224, 234
Conjunctival squamous cell carcinoma	HPV	Not available	235, 236

EBV, Epstein-Barr virus; HPV, human papilloma virus.
[a]Not including lung cancer and basal cell carcinoma, which have high incidence in the human immunodeficiency virus (HIV) population but not independently of other risk factors.
[b]Grulich et al. have shown that there is no clear association between degree of immune deficiency and risk for anal carcinoma, and that anal carcinoma in this setting has a different natural history from that seen in transplant-related disease. Increased relative risk independent of other risk factors, such as that for cervical cancer, may be difficult to ascertain.
[c]Another study found no increased risk for multiple myeloma in Italian patients (225).
[d]Based on three testicular tumors among a cohort of 430 HIV-seropositive individuals.

diagnosis being approximately twice as common among whites, compared with those of African descent, and among men, compared with women (5). The estimated incidence of lymphoma among those with advanced immunodeficiency overall is 1.6% per year (6).

Genetic associations with AIDS-related lymphoma include polymorphism in a chemokine-encoding, gene affecting B-cell proliferation. Chemokines are known to influence immune cell proliferation and to be critical in modulating the immune response to pathogenic infections. The prototypic chemokine is stroma-derived growth factor-1 (SDF-1), which was first identified based on its ability to alter B-cell proliferative responses. Assessing chemokine or chemokine receptor polymorphisms in populations infected with human immunodeficiency virus, Rabkin and colleagues found that variant 3' regions of the SDF-1 gene were associated with a higher risk of AIDS-related lymphoma (7). Heterozygotes were noted to have a twofold increase in risk, whereas homozygotes had a fourfold increased risk of lymphoma. Because this polymorphism is found in 37% of whites but only 11% of blacks, it is believed to contribute to the racial disparity in AIDS-related lymphoma. Other chemokine alterations may also affect lymphoma incidence. The same authors have studied lymphoma incidence among people with a deletion within the CCR5 chemokine receptor gene (CCR5-delta32) that has been shown to be protective against human immunodeficiency

TABLE 45.2. *Infection-related cancers not increased in acquired immunodeficiency syndrome patients*

Tumor type	Viral cofactor	Relative risk	Reference
Hepatocellular carcinoma	Hepatitis C virus and hepatitis B virus	0.8	237,238
Nasopharyngeal carcinoma	EBV	0.8	239
Endemic Burkitt's lymphoma	EBV	1.0[a]	240
Cervical carcinoma	HPV	0.8	238,241
Maltoma[b]	*Helicobacter pylori*[c]	NA	242,243
Acute T-cell leukemia	Human T-cell leukemia virus type 1	NA	244,245

EBV, Epstein-Barr virus; HPV, human papilloma virus; NA, not available.
[a]Odds ratio, based on 3 of 54 cases of endemic Burkitt's lymphoma occurring in human immunodeficiency virus (HIV)–positive children, compared with 5% of Ugandan child controls; possibly related to poor survival of infected children by vertical transmission.
[b]Specific risk not rigorously studied but not reported in any large series.
[c]References refer to studies showing HIV population is not at increased risk for *H. pylori* infection.

TABLE 45.3. *Expression of Epstein-Barr virus latent genes in disease*

Pattern of latency	EBER	EBNA-1	EBNA-2	EBNA-3	LMP-1	LMP-2	Disease
Latency I	+	+	−	−	−	−	Burkitt's lymphoma, gastric carcinoma
Latency II	+	+	−	−	+	+	Nasopharyngeal carcinoma, Hodgkin's disease
Latency III	+	+	+	+	+	+	Infectious mononucleosis, B-cell lymphoproliferative disorder, X-linked lymphoproliferative disorder, pyothorax-associated lymphoma
Healthy carrier	+	±	−	−	−	+	Not applicable

EBER, Epstein-Barr virus–encoded RNA; EBNA, Epstein-Barr virus nuclear antigen; LMP, latent membrane protein.
Adapted from Hiraki A, et al. Genetics of Epstein-Barr virus infection. *Biomed Pharmacother* 2001;55:369–372 (246).

virus 1 infection in homozygotes and to retard the progression of human immunodeficiency virus disease in heterozygotes. They found that this CCR5 deletion also decreases the risk of lymphoma among human immunodeficiency virus–infected individuals by approximately threefold. CCR5-delta32 may decrease the sensitivity of target cells to the RANTES chemokine, for which CCR5 is a physiologic receptor. Decreased responsiveness to RANTES may result in altered B-cell function, either directly or through T-cell–mediated events (8). Therefore, regulatory genes of the immune system may enhance or decrease an individual's likelihood of developing a lymphoproliferative disease.

In addition to genetic background, the state of decline in immune function is highly relevant for developing malignant complications of human immunodeficiency virus. This is perhaps most evident in the case of Kaposi's sarcoma in which the natural history has most clearly been altered because potent treatment for human immunodeficiency virus has entered clinical practice. Kaposi's sarcoma is believed to be caused by a herpesvirus distantly related to Epstein-Barr virus (9), described in some detail below. Although the incidence of this infection-related neoplasm was already declining before the availability of human immunodeficiency virus protease inhibitor therapy, the impact of human immunodeficiency virus control on this tumor is such that it is now a relative rarity among human immunodeficiency virus–infected individuals (10–12). The use of effective antiretroviral therapy and the resultant improvement in immune function have been associated both with regression of Kaposi's sarcoma in individual patients and with a marked decrease in Kaposi's sarcoma incidence at a population level, with estimates of decline as high as 80-fold (11–15).

Primary central nervous system lymphoma, a subset of non-Hodgkin's lymphomas seen in AIDS, has undergone changes in incidence as dramatic as Kaposi's sarcoma. This is a lymphoma virtually uniformly associated with Epstein-Barr virus present in the tumor tissue. Although this complication of far-advanced human immunodeficiency virus disease was much less common than Kaposi's sarcoma (and thus its decline less well documented), centers in the United

States that previously saw cases on a monthly basis are now seeing them perhaps only once a year. This is an agonal manifestation of AIDS that is now seen predominantly among those who have either failed antiretroviral therapy or for whom it is not available.

The relationship of primary central nervous system lymphoma in AIDS to human immunodeficiency virus therapy and thereby immune status is highly analogous to another setting for lymphoma and immunodeficiency. Like AIDS-related primary central nervous system lymphoma, cases of posttransplant lymphoproliferative disorder uniformly demonstrate Epstein-Barr virus infection in the tumor tissue. Both tumors manifest a profile of Epstein-Barr virus latent gene expression [Epstein-Barr nuclear antigen (EBNA) 1-6 and latent membrane protein (LMP)–1-2, a type III pattern as noted in Table 45.3] seen when Epstein-Barr virus is used to transform B cells *in vitro* (16,17). Among these gene products are those readily targeted by cytotoxic T lymphocytes. Indeed, lymphocytes recognizing these gene products have been shown to enable regression of posttransplant lymphoproliferative disease. Although increased lymphocytes of this specificity in the peripheral blood after antiretroviral therapy have not specifically been shown, the association of reduced incidence of primary central nervous system lymphoma with immune reconstitution after antiretroviral therapy may well be a result of improving cytotoxic T lymphocyte immunity. It should be noted, however, that numbers of cells alone may not define the ability of the host immune system to respond. Even among human immunodeficiency virus–infected individuals with detectable Epstein-Barr virus–specific cytotoxic T lymphocytes, there are abnormalities in cell function that have been linked to Epstein-Barr virus–associated lymphoproliferation (18).

In contrast to the primary central nervous system lymphoma subset of AIDS-related lymphomas, the risk of systemic lymphomas is less dramatically reduced by highly active antiretroviral therapy (12,19). The systemic lymphomas of AIDS are known to have a more complex pathophysiology (discussed below) that likely accounts for this difference in the impact of highly active antiretroviral therapy. Overall, the estimated decline in systemic lymphomas is approximately two- to sevenfold since the introduction of potent antiretroviral therapy (10,20–22). The largest study to date was an observational cohort analysis of 8,500 human immunodeficiency virus–positive individuals across Europe (EuroSIDA) (21). The incidence of all subtypes of lymphoma was significantly reduced after 1999 when the use of combination antiretroviral therapy was commonplace, compared with the period before highly active antiretroviral therapy (marked in this study as September 1995). Similarly, an international multicohort study found a reduction of approximately twofold after the introduction of highly active antiretroviral therapy (20). Of note, this latter series assessed subtypes of lymphomas and observed the greatest difference in immunoblastic and primary central nervous system lymphoma—those lymphomas most associated with Epstein-Barr virus, although presence of the Epstein-Barr virus genome in the tumor specimens was not specifically evaluated. It is interesting to note that Burkitt's lymphoma and Hodgkin's disease appeared to be largely unaffected (20). Therefore, the effect of antiretroviral therapy and, by extension, immune function appears to be nonhomogeneous. The association with Epstein-Barr virus may be part of the explanation, but a complex interplay of immunity and lymphocyte growth control are likely involved.

Pathophysiology

There are a number of different participating factors that may alter the ability of lymphocytes to proliferate and ultimately transform. Perhaps the simplest scenario is that in which an infectious agent alters the growth regulatory machinery of an infected cell directly. Human immunodeficiency virus itself has been implicated in rare instances of this growth dysregulation. Within the lymphocyte pool, the strict T-cell tropism of human immunodeficiency virus appears capable of inducing the extremely rare T-cell non-Hodgkin's lymphomas that have been occasionally reported (23,24). At least some of these tumors have been assessed in detail and found to have an insertion site for human immunodeficiency virus 1 in the host genome that may relate to the transformation of the clone. For example, integration of human immunodeficiency virus 1 into the *fur* locus, just upstream of the *c-fes/fps* protooncogene, has been documented and may account for the ability of these cells to proliferate rather than apoptose (25).

A far more common scenario in which a virus may directly participate involves gamma herpesviruses. Among the members of the gamma herpesvirus family, two have been implicated in AIDS-related lymphomas and in immunodeficiency-related lymphomas generally: Epstein-Barr virus and Kaposi's sarcoma–associated herpesvirus. Two subsets of AIDS-related lymphoma are distinctly characterized by the presence of these two viruses as primary contributing factors; primary central nervous system lym-

phomas (as noted above) are infected with Epstein-Barr virus, and primary effusion lymphomas almost universally demonstrate infection with Kaposi's sarcoma–associated herpesvirus. The molecular basis for the contribution of these viruses to dysregulated growth of lymphocytes is described elsewhere in this book (Chapter 39). In brief, the Epstein-Barr virus gene most directly associated with transforming capability, and which is widely expressed in primary central nervous system lymphomas, is LMP-1 (26,27). LMP-1 mimics the activation of tumor necrosis factor receptor family members such as CD40, a known receptor for T-cell–generated B regulatory signals. LMP-1 codons 185-211 interact directly with members of the tumor necrosis receptor–associated factor family and activate the signaling pathway (28). This results in enhanced expression of the transcription factor NF-κB and results in transformation of B lymphocytes.

Kaposi's sarcoma–associated herpesvirus (also known as *human herpesvirus-8* or *HHV-8*) shares only limited homology with Epstein-Barr virus and specifically does not have an LMP-1 homolog. Its mechanism of transformation remains controversial, although a number of viral gene products have the capability of transforming immortalized cell lines when ectopically expressed. These include a constitutively activated member of the chemokine receptor family [vGPCR, also known as *open reading frame (ORF) 74*], a Bcl-2 homolog affecting apoptosis (KSbcl-2 or ORF16), a cyclin D homolog altering cell proliferative kinetics (K cyclin or ORF 72), and a viral interleukin (IL)-6 with potent biologic activity (vIL-6 or K2) (29–33). Expression of vGPCR alters other regulatory genes, including vIL-6 and vascular endothelial growth factor in lymphoid cells (34). The viral IL-6 is capable of not only inducing IL-6 effects on cells at a distance but having the ability to undermine host cell antiviral mechanisms, specifically inhibiting the effects of interferon-α. Indeed, the virus has co-opted the interferon-α response and produces increased vIL-6 in response to it, enabling an autocrine drive of infected cell proliferation. In addition, Kaposi's sarcoma–associated herpesvirus encodes an interferon regulatory factor homolog (vIRF1 or K9) that is capable of repressing interferon-induced host genes and inhibiting pathways of apoptosis normally enhanced by interferon, thereby further impairing a critical host antiviral defense mechanism (35,36).

Beyond the effects on cell growth and interferon action, a number of other viral-induced means of avoiding host immune response are encoded by Kaposi's sarcoma–associated herpesvirus (37). Kaposi's sarcoma–associated herpesvirus may be capable of altering immune recognition of virus-infected cells through inhibition of the MHC class I–dependent pathway of antigen presentation. Kaposi's sarcoma–associated herpesvirus infection has been associated with decreased transport associated protein 1 (TAP-1) expression, leading to class I–restricted insensitivity to cytotoxic T lymphocyte cytotoxicity (38). The virus has also been reported to downregulate class I MHC expression on infected host cells through targeting of MHC-I to endocytic degradation (39). Expression of Kaposi's sarcoma–associated herpesvirus gene products K3 and K5 has been shown to specifically decrease MHC expression on the cell surface, thereby preventing cells from presenting antigen critical for cytotoxic T lymphocyte recognition and targeting (40). Loss of class I may make a cell more susceptible to natural killer cell killing; however, K5 also downregulates two ligands critical for cell attachment to natural killer cells: ICAM-1 and B7-2. Therefore, K5 expression can markedly inhibit not just cytotoxic T lymphocyte targeting but also natural killer cell–mediated cytotoxicity toward Kaposi's sarcoma–associated herpesvirus–infected cells (41).

Other immune-modulating effects may also impair the host response to Kaposi's sarcoma–associated herpesvirus–infected cells. Specifically, the Kaposi's sarcoma–associated herpesvirus genome encodes a chemokine analog of macrophage inflammatory protein-II (vMIP-II) that may alter the nature of the cellular response to infected cells. This chemokine selectively attracts T-helper 2 (Th2) cells and monocytes but has no effect on Th1 cells, dendritic cells, or natural killer cells (42). This may tip the balance of the immune response toward the Th2 end of the spectrum, a response not generally associated with an effective antiviral defense. Therefore, Kaposi's sarcoma–associated herpesvirus has used multiple modalities to subvert immune targeting, with a resultant augmentation of the virus's ability to persist and perhaps transform infected cells in the host.

The role of herpesviruses is clearest in the relatively small number of AIDS patients who develop primary effusion lymphoma (very rare Kaposi's sarcoma–associated herpesvirus–infected tumors with or without Epstein-Barr virus coinfection) or primary central nervous system lymphoma (Epstein-Barr virus alone). Although these relatively direct viral-based methods of altering target cell growth play a role in these specific subsets, other mechanisms are clearly at work in the majority of AIDS-related lymphomas. Aside from these two minor subsets, other lymphomas in AIDS patients are often negative for Epstein-Barr virus, which, for example, infects only approximately 30% of AIDS-related Burkitt's (also referred to as *small noncleaved cell*) lymphomas (43). Of those tumors that are Epstein-Barr virus infected, the type III latent gene pattern—characteristic of other B-cell lymphoproliferative disorders—is not consistently observed (44–46). Some of these lymphomas appear to express a profile of Epstein-Barr virus genes more consistent with that seen in Hodgkin's disease (type II pattern), and the large proportion of those without Epstein-Barr virus has a range of other genetic abnormalities. Among AIDS-related large-cell lymphomas, approximately 80% are Epstein-Barr virus infected, and genetic abnormalities identified have included mutually exclusive subsets with rearrangements of the Bcl-6 (21%) and c-myc (21%) transcription factor genes; mutations in the p53 tumor suppressor gene were not observed (47). The pattern is somewhat different in AIDS-related lymphoma of Burkitt's histology, with c-myc rearrangements being almost universal (as in non–human immunodeficiency virus–associated forms of Burkitt's lymphoma), p53 mutations seen in 61%, and Bcl-6 rearrangements very uncommon (48–51). There is no clear link between Epstein-Barr virus and any specific genetic mutation other than those more classically noted for each histologic subtype (48–51).

Both endemic and human immunodeficiency virus–associated Burkitt's tumors have been generally lumped together as being derived from the germinal center because both express the BCL6 gene that is characteristic of germinal center cells but not of more differentiated progeny (as discussed below) (52). Curiously, one early study found that although both endemic and AIDS-associated Burkitt's lymphomas display activating c-myc translocations into either the heavy- or light-chain immunoglobulin gene loci, the translocation of the AIDS-associated Burkitt's tumors is unique. In the human immunodeficiency virus patient, the c-myc translocates primarily to the immunoglobulin heavy-chain gene switch region rather than disrupting the more proximal joining region (characteristic of the endemic tumors) (53). This strongly suggests that the rearrangement in the HIV-associated tumors occurs at the time of class switching in the secondary lymphoid organs rather than during early B-cell differentiation in the bone marrow when recombination of the variable, diversity, and joining segments of the immunoglobulin genes is taking place. Because class switching in each B cell occurs later than the recombination of the variable, diversity and joining segments in the cells immunoglobulin locus, the cell of origin in the AIDS-related Burkitt's lymphomas may be a germinal-center or post–germinal-center B cell. Considered in the context of their expression of Bcl-6, however, the data suggest that the cell of origin is from the germinal-center.

Even among the lymphomas in which Epstein-Barr virus or Kaposi's sarcoma–associated herpesvirus is found, other independent genetic abnormalities may cooperatively contribute to lymphomagenesis. For example, the cyclin D homolog of Kaposi's sarcoma–associated herpesvirus induces cytokinesis defects and polyploidy, which normally induces p53-mediated apoptosis. However, in the absence of p53, aneuploid cells may persist and can contribute to malignant potential (54). In addition, activated c-myc may enhance the tumorigenicity of cells infected with Epstein-Barr virus (55). Among AIDS-associated large-cell lymphomas, a curious reciprocal relationship has been found between expression of Bcl-6 (in approximately 50% of these tumors) and LMP-1, which appear to mutually repress the expression of the other (56). Because Bcl-6 is not expressed in the post–germinal center–derived immunoblastic form of large-cell lymphoma (57), many of these tumors strongly express LMP-1 when Epstein-Barr virus infected. In contrast, Epstein-Barr virus infection of the large noncleaved cell variety of large-cell lymphoma (germinal center derived and expressing Bcl-6) apparently results in transformation without expression of the LMP-1 Epstein-Barr virus oncogene. Clearly, the interactions between host and viral gene products are complex and yet to be fully elucidated.

Although direct effects of herpesviruses may be relevant for transformation, and the interaction with other somatic mutations in host cells may enhance tumorigenicity, these events alone are unlikely to account for the high incidence of lymphoma in AIDS patients. Human immunodeficiency virus–induced impairment of the immune system is likely to provide the critical context in which lymphoma can emerge. In the absence of adequate immune reactivity, proliferation of Epstein-Barr virus– or Kaposi's sarcoma–associated herpesvirus–infected cells can occur and may facilitate secondary transforming events. Furthermore, B-cell growth kinetics independent of secondary herpesvirus infection appear to be altered in the presence of human immunodeficiency virus infection. This is clinically manifest as the frequent lymphadenopathy and hypergammaglobulinemia seen in human immunodeficiency virus–infected individuals. Human immunodeficiency virus may directly contribute to the process through antigenic drive, and there are reports that human immunodeficiency virus envelope glycoprotein (gp) may directly enhance B-cell activation (58,59). Human immunodeficiency virus gp120 envelope gene products capable of interacting with the CXCR-4 chemokine receptor, in particular, may affect changes in B-cell proliferation because this receptor is known to provide a growth-promoting signal to B-cell subsets and is the receptor for SDF-1 noted above (60–64). Perturbation of the T-cell compartment with enhancement of Th2 subpopulations and release of B-cell–stimulatory IL-10 and IL-4 likely further augment proliferation (65,66). With control of human immunodeficiency virus replication, B-cell stimulation through these direct and indirect mechanisms may be reduced, resulting in decreased hypergammaglobulinemia after successful highly active antiretroviral therapy.

Clinical Biology

The histology of AIDS-related lymphoma can be large-cell anaplastic or small cell (Burkitt's). As noted above, the origin of the malignant cells has been frequently characterized as being germinal-center or post–germinal-center B cell. Subsets of tumors may derive from distinct stages of B-cell differentiation. For example, Carbone and colleagues have characterized specific subtypes of B cells based on their staining with antibodies against Bcl-6 (associated with germinal-center cells), MUM1/IRF4 (associated with late or post–germinal-center cells), and CD138/syndican-1 (associated with post–germinal-center cells) (67). They noted that germinal-center cell staining was seen in the majority of large-cell or Burkitt's lymphomas; late germinal-center cell staining with large, immunoblastic histology; and post–germinal-center staining

with primary central nervous system, primary effusion, or plasmablastic lymphomas, Hodgkin's lymphoma, and some large immunoblastic systemic lymphomas, all in the setting of human immunodeficiency virus disease.

Systemic AIDS-related lymphomas frequently involve tissues outside the confines of lymph nodes and therefore have a wide array of possible clinical presentations. Extranodal sites that are particularly favored include gastrointestinal tract, bone marrow, and central nervous system, although virtually any tissue may be involved (44,68–85). Histologic subsets do have some discriminating patterns of involvement. For example, large-cell tumors preferentially involve the gastrointestinal tract, whereas Burkitt's tumors can reach the bone marrow and meninges (75,86). The presenting symptoms of lymphoma do not appear to be appreciably affected by highly active antiretroviral therapy (87,88).

Histologic subtypes of systemic AIDS-related lymphoma may have significant differences beyond mode of presentation. Patients with Burkitt's lymphoma and human immunodeficiency virus tend to have a less severe degree of immunosuppression than other histologic subtypes (89). In those cases of Burkitt's that are Epstein-Barr virus infected, the viral gene expression pattern is unusual in that two Epstein-Barr virus–encoded RNAs and only a single protein-encoding gene (EBNA-1) are expressed (the type I program of latent gene expression) (90). Cytotoxic T lymphocyte recognition of Epstein-Barr virus–infected cells typically does not target EBNA-1, a result of an inability of infected cells to process this protein for class I MHC-dependent antigen presentation (91). The basis for the approximately 1,000-fold increase in risk for Burkitt's lymphoma among human immunodeficiency virus–infected individuals is unknown, and whether these patients should be treated differently than those with other histologic subtypes is unclear.

Due to the high incidence of central nervous system involvement noted early in the human immunodeficiency virus epidemic [20% in one study (73)], it has become commonplace to more aggressively evaluate the central nervous system in patients with systemic AIDS-related lymphoma. This has generally included imaging and cerebrospinal fluid sampling studies, and many centers prophylactically treat all patients with intrathecal therapy. Particular attention should be paid to those in whom Epstein-Barr virus is documented in the primary tumor, as this has been shown to be of strong predictive value for patients with increased risk for central nervous system relapse (p = .003) (92). The same study also defined extranodal involvement as a strong predictive factor (p = .006). Whether such criteria can be used to subselect those in whom central nervous system prophylaxis may be restricted has not been tested formally. The data do support targeting intrathecal chemotherapy to patients with Epstein-Barr virus in the tumor tissue and those with extranodal involvement of high-risk sites such as marrow, testis, or paranasal sinus (93).

As noted above, the prognosis for patients with AIDS-related lymphoma before highly active antiretroviral therapy was poor but appears to be changing with the overall improvement in health status and tolerance of chemotherapy afforded by control of human immunodeficiency virus. Prognostic factors have mostly been defined before the advent of highly active antiretroviral therapy and may need to be revised with broader, more current experience. However, the largest multivariate analysis to date indicated that CD4 count less than 100 cells per mm^3, age older than 35 years, intravenous drug use, and stage III/IV disease were negative prognostic factors (94). When only one or none of these factors was present, the overall survival was 46 weeks; when two factors were present, 44 weeks; and when three or four factors were present, 18 weeks.

The International Prognostic Index (95) has been validated as a useful means of stratifying risk in aggressive lymphomas outside the context of AIDS but has not been broadly applied to date in AIDS-related lymphoma. A study of 46 patients did indicate that a high International Prognostic Index score was predictive of poor outcome (96), and other reports have indicated that factors used in the International Prognostic Index, such as elevated lactate dehydrogenase (97) or age older than 40 years, do provide independent prognostic information in AIDS-related lymphoma. In the context of highly active antiretroviral therapy, it is likely that the International Prognostic Index can be used to define risk in AIDS-related lymphoma and will be tested in current trials. Of note, Burkitt's histology has not been consistently found to be of prognostic significance. Treatment protocols so far have generally included this subset of patients with other histologic groups and not detected a distinct outcome. However, as more information is gained in the era of highly active antiretroviral therapy, in which other human immunodeficiency virus complications may play less of a role in outcome, it is believed likely that this histologic subset may distinguish itself as more problematic. Whether more aggressive treatment programs should be applied to this group in the setting of human immunodeficiency virus disease remains undefined.

Primary effusion lymphoma is a rare and unique form of systemic lymphoma associated with AIDS. It is a liquid phase hematologic malignancy that rarely involves the blood or lymph nodes and generally does not present with a tumor mass. Rather, body cavity effusion (98–100) laden with large anaplastic or immunoblastic–appearing cells is the presenting hallmark. The cells immunophenotypically bear surface CD45 (common leukocyte antigen) but do not stain with antibodies specific for B-cell (CD20 or CD19) or T-cell (CD3) antigens. Molecular analysis of tumor cells does demonstrate rearrangement of the variable, diversity and joining segments of the immunoglobulin locus, defining the cells as being of B-cell origin. Unique among the AIDS-related lymphomas, these cells also are uniformly found to contain the Kaposi's sarcoma–associated herpesvirus genome and, as noted above, frequently demonstrate coinfection with Epstein-

Barr virus. These tumors are not restricted to human immunodeficiency virus–related immunodeficiency and may be found in other immunodeficient states. They provide a unique and intriguing paradigm for virus-induced human malignancy.

Another rare form of systemic AIDS-related lymphoma is that of plasmablastic lymphoma of the oral cavity (101). This is an aggressive B-cell lymphoma that is distinct from other human immunodeficiency virus–related large-cell lymphomas in its presentation, histology, and immunohistochemistry (CD20 is not expressed). Epstein-Barr virus is often, but not uniformly, present in these tumors.

POSTTRANSPLANT LYMPHOPROLIFERATIVE DISEASE

Epidemiology

Posttransplant lymphoproliferative disease is a severe complication of organ transplantation resulting from iatrogenic immunosuppression. Posttransplant lymphoproliferative disease is the most common malignancy in the posttransplantation population; the other major complicating neoplasms are Kaposi's sarcoma, basal cell carcinoma, and cutaneous squamous cell carcinomas, which are generally less frequent or severe. Posttransplant lymphoproliferative disease is seen both early and late after transplantation, with distinct pathophysiologic factors distinguishing these two settings. In the immediate posttransplant setting, posttransplant lymphoproliferative disease is uniformly Epstein-Barr virus related. The median time to onset of posttransplant lymphoproliferative disorder has been variably reported but was 10 months after surgery in a series of 4,000 consecutive liver transplants in one retrospective series (122). The frequency of posttransplant lymphoproliferative disorder, and perhaps its timing, is related to the magnitude of immunosuppression (123). For this reason, lung and multiorgan transplants are generally associated with a higher incidence and more rapid onset of disease than kidney transplants. European centers using regimens that are less immunosuppressive generally see less posttransplant lymphoproliferative disease than centers in the United States. In one multicenter study of more than 50,000 patients, the incidence of posttransplant lymphoproliferative disease during the first posttransplant year was 1.2%, with subsequent years estimated at 0.3% per year in cardiac transplant recipients, but these rates vary considerably depending on the center (124).

A number of features factor into the risk of developing posttransplant lymphoproliferative disease. Perhaps most important is whether the organ recipient is Epstein-Barr virus seropositive before transplant and whether the recipient is a child or an adult. The incidence of posttransplant lymphoproliferative disease is significantly greater (approximately threefold) in children, probably due to the lower incidence of preceding Epstein-Barr virus infection, and is approximately

24-fold higher in Epstein-Barr virus–seronegative versus Epstein-Barr virus–seropositive recipients (122,125,126). In those not previously exposed to Epstein-Barr virus, primary Epstein-Barr virus infection via the graft or from transfusions during surgery can result in florid lymphoproliferative disease that is generally polymorphic and polyclonal and responds to reduction in immunosuppression (127). Although often mentioned in conjunction with posttransplant lymphoproliferative disease in previously Epstein-Barr virus–infected adults or children, the pathophysiology of disease in patients with perioperatively acquired Epstein-Barr virus is distinct, as discussed below.

The extent of immunosuppression is one of several reported risk factors, and studies have indicated that the therapeutic use of antibodies directed against T cells (for graft rejection) provides a particular enhancement of risk (128). Alcoholic cirrhosis, and notably the presence of hepatitis C, as a cause of liver failure in liver transplants also appears to increase the risk of posttransplant lymphoproliferative disease for reasons that are not clear (129).

When assessing patients in the posttransplant setting, it has been reported that elevated titers of Epstein-Barr virus viral load in the blood (greater than 25,000 copies/µg DNA) are associated with the development of posttransplant lymphoproliferative disease and have been correlated with a suppression of Epstein-Barr virus–reactive T cells (126,130). Inversion of these parameters has been associated with improvement in posttransplant lymphoproliferative disorder, usually seen in conjunction with a decrease in therapeutic immunosuppression.

The late-occurring lymphoproliferative disorders seen in the posttransplant patient are not Epstein-Barr virus associated, may be B or T cell in origin, and are generally similar to lymphoma in the immunocompetent population.

Pathophysiology

Posttransplantation lymphoproliferative disorders often have a polymorphic histologic appearance that may complicate diagnosis and likely reflect some of the underlying pathophysiologic differences within this group. Knowles has advocated dividing posttransplant lymphoproliferative disease into plasmacytic hyperplasias, polymorphic lymphoproliferative disorders, and malignant lymphomas/multiple myeloma (131). The plasmacytic hyperplasias are polyclonal and generally regress spontaneously after withdrawal of immunosuppression. The malignant lymphomas are monoclonal, possess a variety of genetic alterations, and generally progress despite aggressive therapy. The polymorphic lymphoproliferative disorders are also monoclonal but display variable clinical behavior, their progression and response to chemotherapy apparently correlating with BCL6 gene mutation (131–133). These correlations between clonality and mutation, with responsiveness to alteration of immune suppression, support the following model: In the posttransplant setting, Epstein-Barr virus reactivation induces a reactive lymphoid hyperplasia. The lifting of phar-

macologic suppression results in restoration of the ability to control the consequences of Epstein-Barr virus lytic replication through rejuvenated cytotoxic T-lymphocyte responsiveness. The recalcitrance of some more blastoid posttransplant lymphoproliferative disease tumor types to the lifting of immune suppression supports the notion that these tumors represent a fundamentally different disease process. Epstein-Barr virus may serve as an initiation factor in this subset, but progression may be secondary to genomic mutation and resultant dysregulation of the cell cycle; thus, restoration of an anti–Epstein-Barr virus cytotoxic T-lymphocyte response may no longer be sufficient to control a rapidly progressive tumor.

Overall, posttransplant lymphoproliferative disease may be regarded as a relatively straightforward failure of immune control of Epstein-Barr virus. Pharmacologically induced immune suppression is clearly the central factor in the susceptibility and may serve as a model for the genesis of similar lymphomas in the broader context of autoimmune disease and congenital immunodeficiency. Other genetic traits (e.g., a polymorphism in the hMSH2 DNA mismatch repair gene) (134) and environmental factors (e.g., alcohol use) (135) likely also contribute to lymphomagenesis in these patients, but any discussion of causation must begin with a focus on the host interaction with chronic Epstein-Barr virus infection.

Despite its ubiquity as a chronic infecting agent in more than 90% of adults worldwide, Epstein-Barr virus was first identified in 1964 by a British team (136) that found viral particles in tumor biopsies from patients with the endemic non-Hodgkin's lymphoma subtype first identified in African children by Burkitt in 1958 (137). B lymphocytes appear to be the most important targets of primary infection through exposure to oral secretions. Patients with the infectious mononucleosis symptom complex demonstrate activated B-cell blasts in the paracortical region of the tonsils (138). Epstein-Barr virus–infected T cells and oropharyngeal epithelial cells are only rarely identified during acute mononucleosis (139). Viral particles release their double-stranded linear DNA in the B-cell cytoplasm, subsequently circularizing and surreptitiously assuming control of cellular replication. This viral episome is transcriptionally active in as few as three of the more than 90 viral genes (140). As many as ten latency genes are active in in vitro–transformed B cells, which are sufficient to cause a relative immortalization of the host cell. This parsimony of viral gene expression is believed to contribute significantly to the ability of the virus to hide from immune recognition in the normal host.

Independent of the immune suppression factor, the specific steps leading to transformation of infected B lymphocytes are still poorly understood. Three different latency gene expression patterns (Table 45.3) have been described in most Epstein-Barr virus–related lymphomas, constituted by different combinations of the ten genes expressed in B-cell lines transformed in vitro. All three patterns are represented among posttransplant lymphoproliferative disease patients, with the full complement expressed in polymorphic lymphoproliferative disease and a more restricted expression profile in monoclonal lymphomas (139). Mice expressing a transgene for one of the latency membrane proteins (LMP-1) develop B-cell lymphomas (141). LMP-1 appears to function through constitutive activation of certain elements in the CD40 pathway (142), which normally acts as an essential mediator of T-cell help for B-lymphocyte proliferation and differentiation. Like CD40, LMP-1 engages at least four of the tumor necrosis factor receptor–associated signal transduction factors (TRAF 1, 2, 3, and 5) and the JAK3 kinase, leading in part to the constitutive activation of the NF-κB and AP-1 transcription factors and the resultant obstruction of the cell's apoptotic program.

Successful suppression of viral replication is maintained in large part by the generation of cytotoxic T cells directed against several splice products of the EBNA genes. The ability of renal transplant patients who develop posttransplant lymphoproliferative disease to respond to therapy (acyclovir treatment and a decrease in immunosuppression) has been shown to correlate with the recovery of the CD8+ cytotoxic T-lymphocyte population (143). This suggests that the mechanism behind regression of posttransplant lymphoproliferative disease in the setting of the withdrawal of immune suppression is the release of pharmacologic impairment of cytotoxic T-lymphocyte function. Because of the ubiquity of Epstein-Barr virus infection in posttransplant lymphoproliferative disease, it is tempting to speculate that the invigoration of cytotoxic T-lymphocyte function restores a previously suppressed ability to control Epstein-Barr virus in these patients. Indeed, administration of autologous Epstein-Barr virus–specific cytotoxic T lymphocytes has also been shown to induce regression of posttransplant lymphoproliferative disorder in both renal transplant patients (144) and after allogeneic bone marrow transplantation (145). One of these studies (144) found that in three patients with Epstein-Barr virus reactivation in association with lymphoproliferation, serum Epstein-Barr virus DNA concentrations dropped as much as three logs, back to the control range, within 1 month after cytotoxic T-lymphocyte infusion.

While posttransplant lymphoproliferative disease is generally due to Epstein-Barr virus if seen in the first 2 years posttransplant, there can be rare cases of Epstein-Barr virus–negative tumors, including Kaposi's sarcoma–associated herpesvirus–related primary effusion lymphomas. Primary effusion lymphoma associated with Kaposi's sarcoma–associated herpesvirus in the tumor has been reported in a patient post-heart allograft who had a prior history of Kaposi's sarcoma (146).

Clinical Biology

Posttransplant lymphoproliferative disease after solid-organ transplantation often presents as lymphadenopathy or a mass. Like AIDS–related lymphomas, extranodal involvement is common. Sites of particular proclivity are the central nervous system and the gastrointestinal tract. A site not uncommonly involved is that of the allograft itself, in which presumably the antigenic stimulation is greatest in magnitude and perturbations in immune regulation may be most dramatic. The transplanted organ has been estimated to be involved in approximately 20% of cases involving heart, lung, or liver transplants. Depending on the nature of the lymphomatous infiltration, distinguishing between posttransplant lymphoproliferative disease and graft rejection may be difficult and may require biopsy and supportive clinical information such as Epstein-Barr virus viral load.

The clinical approach to patients with posttransplant lymphoproliferative disease is generally multistep. It involves reduction in immunosuppression, as tolerated. Anti-herpesvirus agents are often given, although their use outside the context of primary Epstein-Barr virus infection is highly controversial. These antiviral medications generally target the viral thymidine kinase, a gene only expressed during the lytic replication phase of the viral life cycle. Consequently, use of these drugs is appropriate in posttransplant lymphoproliferative disease resulting from primary Epstein-Barr virus infection in recipients who were Epstein-Barr virus seronegative at the time of transplant. In contrast, these antivirals are unlikely to impact the predominantly latent viral expression seen in posttransplant lymphoproliferative disease of the polymorphic or monoclonal type. In patients who do not respond to reduction in immunosuppressive drugs or are critically ill at presentation, treatment with the anti-CD20 monoclonal antibody rituximab may be highly successful (147–149). The use of rituximab has been reported in only limited studies to date, but the results are highly encouraging. The apparent toxicities are relatively few, although hypogammaglobulinemia is an expected and potentially important clinical outcome. Interestingly, rituximab induces a reduction in Epstein-Barr virus viral load, but this reduction does not exactly correlate with antitumor effect; quite probably, different populations of B cells are producing Epstein-Barr virus versus those that are malignant (150). For those patients who are refractory to anti-CD20, other antibody therapies may be useful, but no published results are available. Cytotoxic chemotherapy is another alternative, although the sensitivity of patients to the toxic side effects of these agents is increased (151).

AUTOIMMUNE DISEASE

Immune dysregulation is evident in all the rheumatic diseases. A selective susceptibility to lymphomagenesis in a subset of these conditions (Table 45.4) offers a novel avenue toward identifying those elements of the immune response that normally protect against lymphoma.

People with an established diagnosis of diffuse connective tissue disease are at increased risk for a subsequent diagnosis of lymphoma. Many of these individuals appear to have abnormalities in the way their immune system controls infection with Epstein-Barr virus, which commonly infects

TABLE 45.4. *Lymphoma in patients with inflammatory disease*

Condition	Major clinical manifestation	Pathology	Relative risk of NHL	Reference
Rheumatoid arthritis	Polyarthritis, morning stiffness, erosions, anemia, cutaneous nodules, interstitial lung disease	HD, acute nonlymphoblastic leukemia, chronic myelogenous leukemia, NHL	31.8 (men) 18.8 (women)	159 —
Sjögren's syndrome	Sicca complex, dry skin, dry cough, arthritis, maltoma, neuropathy	Lymphoplasmacytic	44	177
Systemic lupus	Rash, serositis, arthritis, neuropsychiatric problems	NHL	5.2–44.0	173–175
Autoimmune thyroiditis	Goiter, metabolic abnormalities, hoarseness, stridor	High-grade B-cell maltoma	40–80	184
Henoch-Schönlein purpura	Purpura, nephritis, arthritis, abdominal angina	NHL, HD	—	247
Lymphomatoid granulomatosis	Pulmonary, skin, renal and central nervous system nodules	High-grade B-cell lymphoma	—	248
Celiac disease	Malabsorption, osteomalacia, anemia, ataxia	Intraepithelial lymphocyte–derived smal-bowel T-cell	43	249
Crohn's disease	Diarrhea, abdominal pain, fever, weight loss, fatigue	B- and T-cell lymphoma	3.96 (men)[a]	191

HD, Hodgkin's disease; NHL, non-Hodgkin's lymphoma.
[a]Incidence rate ratio representing incidence rate standardized to age and gender distribution (191).

patients with rheumatic disease as it does the general population. Because Epstein-Barr virus has a well-established role in the genesis of a variety of malignancies, this new research offers some potential insight into the possible contributions of disordered immunity, opportunistic viral infection, and incompletely controlled inflammation in the genesis of lymphoma and related conditions in individuals suffering from autoimmune disease.

Rheumatoid Arthritis

For many years, comparisons have been drawn between the destructive process evident in the joints of patients with rheumatoid arthritis and the process of oncogenesis (152,153). Hyperplasia, neovascularization, and invasion are three of the cardinal characteristics of the inflamed rheumatoid synovium. At a genetic level, numerous studies have demonstrated that, like many varied tumor types, rheumatoid synovial tissue both overexpresses proto-oncogenes (e.g., *ras* and *rac*) and develops selective mutations in them (e.g., *p53*) (154). Synovial neoplasia do occur, with three different solid tumors of synovium generally recognized: synovial sarcoma, synovial chondrosarcoma, and pigmented villonodular synovitis.

Uncontrolled inflammation has been shown to contribute to the development of certain malignancies such as gastric maltomas arising more often in the context of *H. pylori* infection of the stomach and cholangiocarcinoma being vastly increased in people with sclerosing cholangitis. If the simple fact of uncontrolled inflammation was responsible for excess cancer morbidity in rheumatoid arthritis patients, one might expect the three synovial solid-tumor types to be more prevalent in rheumatoid arthritis patients than in the general population. But curiously, none of these three rare tumors is seen more frequently in rheumatoid arthritis patients. Furthermore, the rheumatoid synovium itself has a distinct pathology from all three, lacking the hyperchromatic DNA, atypical mitotic figures, and large nucleoli seen in many anaplastic processes.

Because rheumatoid arthritis is a systemic disease, one might expect these patients to be at increased risk for a variety of more common solid tumors. But just as they have no increased risk for synovial cancers, rheumatoid arthritis patients appear not to be at increased and independent risk for extraarticular solid tumors. One study of 20,700 Danish patients followed over a 10-year period was the first to break down different tumor types among individuals with rheumatoid arthritis (155). The relative risk of all solid tumors was 1.08 (95% confidence interval, 1.03 to 1.13), compared with age-matched controls. The only individual solid tumor with an increased standardized incidence ratio was lung cancer. But because smoking is a significant risk factor for the development of rheumatoid arthritis (156), an independent increased susceptibility to lung cancer has not been established.

In contrast, both Hodgkin's disease and non-Hodgkin's lymphoma have been demonstrated in multiple studies to occur at a higher age-adjusted incidence among rheumatoid arthritis patients, compared with the general population

(155,157,158). Increased prevalence of myeloma and leukemia may also occur (157,158). The first large cohort analysis of cancer morbidity was carried out on a consecutive series of 489 patients with rheumatoid arthritis in Birmingham, England, over a 14-year period and followed for an additional 5 years (159). Hematopoietic malignancies showed a relative risk of 8.7, independent of rheumatoid arthritis duration or the use of cytotoxic or other immunosuppressive drugs. Perhaps most interesting was the gender analysis, which showed an increased relative risk in men of 31.8, compared with 18.8 in women. Even more dramatically, men showed an increased relative risk of 28.6 for Hodgkin's disease, which was not observed with any greater frequency among women followed in the study, compared with controls. This gender disparity with regard to Hodgkin's disease susceptibility was similarly observed in another study (158) in which an apparently decreased incidence of leukemia among women with rheumatoid arthritis led to an overall absence of increased risk for lymphoproliferative disorders in women altogether.

Gender disparities in susceptibility to lymphoma are particularly intriguing among rheumatoid arthritis patients because of the different epidemiology and disease manifestations between men and women with rheumatoid arthritis. Women are affected by rheumatoid arthritis approximately three times more often than men. But women tend to get the disease earlier, with increased incidence in the postpartum period and an overall population peak incidence between the ages 50 and 52 years (159a). In contrast, men have a rising incidence of rheumatoid arthritis throughout life that continues to increase past 70 years of age and may be related to the decline in endogenous androgens (160). Furthermore, men who contract rheumatoid arthritis tend to have more severe disease, compared with women (161,162), with higher likelihood of associated lung disease and systemic vasculitis. One conclusion may be that men who do develop rheumatoid arthritis have a loss of those genetically based mechanisms that normally protect men from developing rheumatoid arthritis and most other autoimmune diseases. Factors such as these that serve to maintain immune system homeostasis in the postinfectious period may also be operative in protecting against lymphoproliferative disorders, and their dysfunction may consequently predispose both to systemic connective tissue disease and to lymphoma.

The relationship between treatment for rheumatoid arthritis and the development of lymphoproliferative disorders is controversial, with numerous suggestive case reports (163) but no validation in large series (164). Early studies had shown an increased risk in patients receiving cyclophosphamide (165) or chlorambucil (166), but neither of these drugs has been widely used in rheumatoid arthritis since the advent of methotrexate therapy in the 1980s and the very effective biologic agents in the late 1990s.

Of greater interest is a new literature on methotrexate-associated lymphoma (167). Most intriguing is the apparent frequency with which these tumors regress after cessation of therapy. One analysis of nine new cases and review of 28 published cases (168) found that 10 of 16 patients who were diagnosed with lymphoma at the time of methotrexate discontinuation subsequently experienced a complete or partial spontaneous remission with no other therapy. Of these responders, eight of the nine that were studied showed evidence of Epstein-Barr virus infection in the tumor. Only one of six without evidence of Epstein-Barr virus responded to methotrexate withdrawal. A more recent prospective study was performed, seeking to identify all rheumatoid arthritis patients in France over a 3-year period who developed lymphoma while on methotrexate (169,170). The estimated annual incidence of lymphoma was 33.3 per 100,000 population for male rheumatoid arthritis patients treated with methotrexate and 16.7 per 100,000 for women. The standardized mortality ratio was 1.07, based on the observed lymphoma incidence in the general French population when adjusted for age and gender, suggesting no increased risk of lymphoma for these rheumatoid arthritis patients. In contrast, the standardized mortality ratio for Hodgkin's disease was 7.4, with 27.8 cases per 100,000 treated male patients (2.8/100,000 women), with the number of cases also much higher than those expected based on U.S. population incidence of Hodgkin's disease. This association had not been previously reported.

One is tempted to speculate that the success of methotrexate in treating the systemic inflammation in rheumatoid arthritis patients could decrease the established risk of lymphoma generally, although causing a small increase in the risk for both Hodgkin's disease and non-Hodgkin's lymphoma associated with dysregulation of anti–Epstein-Barr virus immunity. The overall result might be neutral with regard to the lymphoma incidence in methotrexate-treated patients, at least with regards to lymphoma. An important new study has suggested that all-cause mortality is strongly decreased in rheumatoid arthritis patients who are treated with methotrexate, particularly cardiac-related death (171). All in all, cytotoxic treatments for rheumatoid arthritis are unlikely to play a significant role in the genesis of the increased susceptibility to non-Hodgkin's lymphoma, and the balance of benefit for disease activity and overall mortality strongly favor the use of drugs such as methotrexate.

Systemic Lupus Erythematosus

Systemic lupus has a societal prevalence approximately tenfold lower than rheumatoid arthritis and affects women approximately nine times more often than men. Excess activation of both B and T cells contributes to the pathophysiologic hallmark of lupus, namely the production of diverse autoreactive antibodies. Several mouse models of lupus have demonstrated a propensity to development of lymphoproliferative phenomena with evolution to lymphoma (172). Furthermore, diffuse lymphadenopathy is an almost universal feature of lupus at the time of diagnosis, with pathology generally demonstrating a reactive hyperplasia or occasionally a necrotizing histiocytic adenitis.

So perhaps it is not surprising that lupus patients also demonstrate an increased risk for lymphoma in the Danish hospital registry in which the rheumatoid arthritis association was originally established (173), with a relative risk of 5.2 (95% confidence interval, 2.2 to 10.3), compared with the general population. This finding validated an earlier study in a smaller cohort (174) that found a relative risk of 44 based on identification of four cases among 182 women with lupus. Closer analysis of the larger cohort with coexistent lupus and lymphoma (173) showed a somewhat higher risk in men, who represented 37% of the cases (compared with approximately 11% of the overall lupus population). Also of interest was the absence of any other hematologic malignancies besides lymphoma, suggesting some specificity for this susceptibility.

Lupus is a highly heterogeneous disorder, with various combinations of only four criteria out of 11 necessary to meet consensus study criteria for the American College of Rheumatology. No association with a particular disease type or severity has been identified (175), with reported cases occurring across the age spectrum (12 to 83 years) and independent of lupus duration (1 to 30 years). Abu-Shakra et al. note that none of the studies on cancer incidence in lupus patients has identified an increased risk of Hodgkin's disease and that the epidemiology of those lupus patients who did develop Hodgkin's disease matched closely those in the general population (175).

Sjögren's Syndrome

Henrik Sjögren, the eponymous Swedish ophthalmologist, originally described keratoconjunctivitis sicca in a group of patients who also had rheumatoid arthritis. Although common in the rheumatoid arthritis population, keratoconjunctivitis sicca can occur as an isolated symptom complex without another underlying connective tissue disease and is referred to in these patients with primary keratoconjunctivitis sicca as *primary Sjögren's syndrome* or *Sjögren's disease*. Primary Sjögren's was the first connective tissue disease in which an increased susceptibility to lymphoma was demonstrated (176,177), and this association is the best studied among all the rheumatic diseases.

Compared with prevailing gender-matched cancer rates, the relative risk of lymphoma in Sjögren's patients has been estimated to be 43.8 among 136 women with sicca syndrome cared for at the National Institutes of Health (177). A more recent retrospective study of 765 Sjögren's patients found malignant lymphoma in 4.3% (178). Eighty-eight percent of the 33 cases identified were women, the median age was 58 years (range, 33 to 82), the median time from Sjögren's diagnosis to identification of lymphoma was 7.5 years, and only two patients had lymphoma at the time of presentation for sicca symptoms. A true incidence in this population is difficult to estimate, in part because many of these patients experience a relatively long latency period of symptoms before Sjögren's diagnosis, typically measured in years.

Like lupus patients, primary Sjögren's patients frequently demonstrate dysregulation of humoral immunity with the expression of autoantibodies directed against nuclear antigens. A particular association is known with more specific antibodies against the Ro and La ribonucleoprotein antigens. B cells grown from isolated salivary gland biopsies in these patients are oligoclonal in nature and demonstrate selective expression of certain immunoglobulin heavy-chain variable region genes (179). These abnormalities may contribute to the genesis of lymphoma in these patients, and anatomic localization is typically in the cervical lymph nodes or salivary glands. Ironically, dysfunction of B lymphocytes and humoral immunity have not yet been shown to play a significant role in the pathogenesis of Sjögren's itself. Immunohistology of the salivary and lacrimal glands that are primarily affected in the disease shows a vast predominance of CD4+ T lymphocytes, many of which are reactive with Ro antigen-derived peptides (180).

A review of 15 epidemiologic studies (181) describes more than one half showing that between 6% and 10% of all Sjögren's patients eventually develop lymphoma. Two of these studies (182,183), with a total of 362 Sjögren's patients, showed no lymphoma development in those with either isolated sicca symptoms or secondary Sjögren's syndrome; only those with primary Sjögren's appeared to be at increased risk. The only *prospective* study looking for lymphoma in Sjögren's patients generated data suggesting that people with onset before 45 years of age had a 60-fold increased risk over the general population (177).

Thyroid Disease

Hashimoto's thyroiditis is commonly found in middle-aged women with rheumatoid arthritis, lupus, or Sjögren's syndrome. This lymphoid infiltrative disease of the thyroid gland also appears to be associated with local lymphoma. One large population-based study found these lymphomas to be almost exclusively B lymphoid in origin, with 83% considered high grade (184).

The incidence of lymphoma in the thyroid gland has been estimated in a Danish population-based study as two cases per million population per year (184), with at least 66% of patients having had preexisting thyroiditis. An older clinicopathologic study of British patients with the disease suggested that "most, if not all, cases of thyroid gland lymphoma arise in a setting of Hashimoto's thyroiditis" (185). The condition is significantly more likely among patients with Hashimoto's than in those with nodular goiter, so there appears to be a relationship between lymphomagenesis and the inflammatory process. Even so, the prevalence of thyroid lymphoma among Hashimoto's patients is probably less than 1% (186). Thus, coincidental genetic or environmental factors may be contributing to the genesis of both inflammatory thyroiditis and thyroid lymphoma, and the former is not necessarily causative of the latter. Nevertheless, a pathophysiologic progression has been proposed that begins with inflammation of the foregut-derived thyroid epithelium, causing transformation of infiltrating parafollicular B cells to a low-grade lymphoma and finally converting to a mucosa-associated lymphoid tissue–like high-grade lymphoma (185).

Lymphomatoid Granulomatosis

This condition was described in 1972 (187) as a multisystem disease with a focal and transmural angiocentric pleomorphic cell infiltrate. Lymphomatoid granulomatosis is classified as an angiocentric immunoproliferative lesion, along with angiocentric lymphoma. Both have mostly pulmonary symptoms, presenting with lower lobe nodules that can progress to cavitation. Lymphomatoid granulomatosis is male predominant (2:1) and affects primarily whites. Reported in a patient as young as 7 years of age, with mean age of diagnosis at 47 years (188), pediatric lymphomatoid granulomatosis frequently involves upper airways and sinuses and most commonly affects children with leukemia or leukemia in remission.

Henoch-Schönlein Purpura

A more recently described association between hematologic malignancy and rheumatic disease was suggested for adults diagnosed after 40 years of age with Henoch-Schönlein purpura (189). Whereas only 10% of 19 cases reviewed involved lymphoma, more than one third had hematologic malignancies of some type. Compared with a control population of 158 adults with Henoch-Schönlein purpura but no subsequent diagnosis of neoplasia, people with Henoch-Schönlein purpura were predominantly men (8.5 times more than women) with arthritis who were older and who had suffered no obvious precedent respiratory or gastrointestinal illness (a common forerunner of Henoch-Schönlein purpura onset).

Inflammatory Disease of the Small Bowel

Inflammatory disease of the small bowel has an important association with local lymphoma. In general, most intestinal lymphomas are high-grade tumors of the Burkitt's or diffuse large B-cell type, but low-grade marginal zone and follicular center cell lymphomas occur. Infrequently, distal small-bowel high-grade B- or T-cell lymphoma arises in Crohn's disease patients, whose cancer risk is primarily for adenocarcinoma.

In contrast to most primary small-bowel lymphoma, which has a B-cell phenotype, people with gluten-sensitive enteropathy have a distinct susceptibility to lymphoma derived from intraepithelial T lymphocytes. Also known as *celiac disease* or *nontropical sprue*, this condition is a widely prevalent autoimmune disease directed against tissue transglutaminase and other bowel antigens. One half of all malignancies in these patients are lymphomas, and 80% of these arise in the small bowel (190). A large prospective study published in 2001 found that lymphoma was the leading cause of death among 1,072 adult patients, and most excess mortality occurred within 3 years of diagnosis (191). One large retrospective series of 30 cases found that two thirds of patients presented with nonspecific gastrointestinal symptoms and the other one third with an acute abdomen. All cases were localized to the jejunum or proximal ileum, and 5-year survival was only 11% (192). Because celiac disease can be asymptomatic, one may wonder if occult disease is a risk factor for the insidious development of lymphoma more generally. A large survey of 653 Italian patients diagnosed with lymphoma found that only approximately 1% subsequently tested positive for celiac disease serology, suggesting that mostly patients with significant gastrointestinal symptomatology were the ones likely to develop lymphoma subsequently (193).

CONGENITAL IMMUNODEFICIENCY

International attention to the link between congenital immune dysfunction and lymphoma was raised when a boy with X-linked severe combined immune deficiency, maintained for 12 years within a sterile "bubble" created by the National Aeronautic and Space Administration, died of lymphoma shortly after putatively life-saving bone marrow transplantation. This highly publicized event occurred after he received a bone marrow transplant from his Epstein-Barr virus–positive sister, experienced Epstein-Barr virus transformation, and succumbed to the resultant aggressive lymphoma (194). Although Epstein-Barr virus plays a role in lymphoma development among the many different forms of congenital immune deficiency, each manifests a different frequency and form of hematologic and other malignancy (Table 45.5). Nevertheless, this case illustrates the role that the immune system plays in protecting otherwise susceptible individuals from hematologic malignancy in general and transformation by ubiquitous herpesviruses in particular.

With some exceptions, congenital immunodeficiency-associated lymphoproliferative disorders of diverse origins share several features that distinguish them from spontaneous lymphoma and other lymphoproliferative disease (195). First, lymphoma occurs significantly more often in children with congenital immunodeficiency as a percent of all cancers (one half to two thirds) than does lymphoma in the general pediatric population (approximately 12%) or in posttransplant immune deficient children (approximately 30%). Second, congenital immunodeficiency-associated lymphoproliferative disorder has a different anatomic localization; with the exception of ataxia-telangiectasia, most congenital immunodeficiency-associated lymphoproliferative disorders occur at extranodal sites. In particular, the central nervous system and gastrointestinal tract appear uniquely susceptible to local infiltrative disease. Third, impaired immune defenses against Epstein-Barr virus result in a high rate of B-cell transformation; excepting again ataxia-telangiectasia, congenital immunodeficiency-associated lymphoproliferative disorder patients frequently develop Epstein-Barr virus–expressing lymphoproliferation

TABLE 45.5. *Distribution of neoplasms in immunodeficient children with cancer*

Cohort at risk	Non-Hodgkin's lymphoma	Hodgkin's disease (%)	Leukemia (%)	Other tumors
General pediatric population	6.7	5.6	30	Brain tumors, 11.7%
Wiskott-Aldrich syndrome	59–75	4	9	—
Ataxia-telangiectasia	41–66	7–10	17–27	Adenocarcinoma, 9.4%
Common variable immuno-deficiency	45–62	4–8	7–19	Adenocarcinoma, 16.4%
Severe combined immuno-deficiency	31–76	7–20	12–20	Adenocarcinoma, 2.4%
Other primary immunodefi-ciencies	16–33	8–14	7–33	Cervical carcinoma, myeloma, Bowen's intraepidermal carcinoma

Adapted from Mueller BU, Pizzo PA. Cancer in children with primary or secondary immunodeficiencies. *J Pediatr* 1995;126: 1–10.

secondary both to natural infection and to posttransplant transformation, as in the case described above. Finally, the histology of these lymphomas is typically of the diffuse large-cell type and is associated with rapid clinical progression in untreated patients.

In a national registry of cancer among patients with immunodeficiency, the largest group of congenital immunodeficiency-associated lymphoproliferative disorders was attributable to ataxia-telangiectasia. Common variable immunodeficiency constitutes an idiopathic acquired condition with a susceptibility to almost as many malignancies. After infection, lymphoproliferative disease is the next leading cause of death for patients with congenital immunodeficiency, whose risk may approach 10,000-fold, compared with the general pediatric population (196).

Ataxia-Telangiectasia

Mutations spread throughout the 66 exons of the large ATM gene on chromosome 11q22-23, when inherited from both parents, are capable of compromising DNA repair and leading to dramatic defects in cell-mediated and natural killer cell immunity (197). Approximately 10% of children who are ATM homozygotes are believed to develop cancer, primarily in the lymphocytic lineages. The ATM gene product appears to function both in the initiation of double-stranded DNA break repair and in triggering a pause in cell-cycle progression to facilitate this repair. Inactivation of the gene has also been identified in cases of spontaneous mantle cell lymphoma and in both B- and T-cell leukemias.

At least five different functional domains have been identified in addition to the critical kinase domain in the ATM gene (198). This multifunctionality and the identification of more than 100 distinct ATM mutations scattered throughout the gene may explain the considerable phenotypic heterogeneity among affected homozygotes, although few missense mutations have been found. As suggested above, the biology of ATM-associated lymphoma differs from other immuno-

deficiencies. Most of these lymphomas are not Epstein-Barr virus infected and do not have characteristic *c-myc* translocations. T-cell lymphomas predominate by more than 5:1 over B-cell lymphomas, and there is no increased incidence of myeloid malignancy. The reason for this distinction may lie in a preferential disruption of the T-cell receptor gene rearrangement process in T lymphocytes, compared with recombination of the immunoglobulin loci of B cells, although functional ATM is required for both (199).

Clinically, blacks with ataxia-telangiectasia appear disproportionately affected by lymphoma. One widely cited retrospective study of 263 homozygous patients found a 750-fold increased risk for blacks and a 252-fold increase in risk for white individuals, compared with the general population (200).

X-Linked Immunodeficiency

Bruton's agammaglobulinemia patients suffer onset of lymphoma in the late infancy period (201). Most affected individuals have a mutation in the BTK gene, which is critical for early B-cell development and for signaling through surface immunoglobulin. For instance, btk has been shown to be essential for the generation of the critical transcriptional factor NF-κB in response to immunoglobulin ligation by antigen (202,203). Consequently, these children are unable to form germinal centers, have markedly decreased levels of serum immunoglobulin, and are significantly impaired in mounting T-cell–dependent humoral immune responses (204). Their state of immune compromise results in susceptibility to infection with the common encapsulated bacterial pathogens of infancy (e.g., *Haemophilus influenzae* and *Streptococcus pneumoniae)*, mycoplasma pneumonia, and common enteroviruses.

Little is known about the molecular pathogenesis of lymphoma in these patients. Healthy older X-linked agammaglobulinemia patients apparently lack evidence for infection with Epstein-Barr virus (205). With no detectable B cells in their peripheral circulation, these people may escape

Epstein-Barr virus infection by virtue of a poverty of susceptible pharyngeal B cells available to the virus. Alternately, btk may itself play some role in Epstein-Barr virus infection. The Epstein-Barr virus status of lymphomas in Bruton's patients is unclear. Perhaps Epstein-Barr virus infection in early infancy is possible and contributes to high-grade lymphomagenesis during that early window. With regard to lymphomagenesis, the absence of significant humoral immunity in these patients could predispose them to an unusual susceptibility to early Epstein-Barr virus or other environmental factors contributing to lymphoma development.

Another possibility is a role for btk as a tumor suppressor gene. Although mutated btk proteins have not been shown to act directly in lymphomagenesis, several potential mechanisms could be envisioned. The btk protein functions both as an upregulator of apoptosis in response to ionizing radiation (206) and as an inhibitor of apoptosis through the Fas cell-surface apoptosis apparatus (207). Additionally, btk has been shown to translocate to the B-cell nucleus when activated (208). The absence of btk in cell lines from affected patients results in the upregulation of a variety of important signaling genes in the cell, suggesting the possibility of btk being a transcriptional regulator (209). By playing a role in both regulation of apoptosis and transcriptional activation or suppression, btk loss may result directly in an increased susceptibility to lymphoma.

A distinct entity called *X-linked lymphoproliferative disease* is associated with mutation in the SLAM-associated protein (*SAP*, also known as *SH2D1A*, which associates with the signaling lymphocytic activation molecule) gene on chromosome Xq25 and results in profound susceptibility to Epstein-Barr virus infection (210). This protein is expressed only in activated T cells and natural killer cells and in selected Burkitt's lymphoma lines, but not in activated B cells (211). Nonetheless, the lymphoma observed in X-linked lymphoproliferative patients is primarily of the B-cell phenotype. The small noncleaved type (Burkitt) predominates, but multiple other types have been described. Anatomically, these lymphomas predominantly occur in the ileocecal area of the small bowel and have been reported infiltrating the liver, kidney, and central nervous system (212). Even in those individuals not infected with Epstein-Barr virus, lymphoma appears to develop eventually in approximately one half of affected men (210). Because the disease gene is not expressed in B cells and because affected children are comparatively resistant to lymphoma development after bone marrow transplant, B-cell transformation may be a result of broadly impaired immunity that includes (but is not limited to) the inability to control Epstein-Barr virus infection.

Wiskott-Aldrich Syndrome

Central nervous system disease appears to predominate among the diffuse, high-grade lymphomas that constitute one half of all malignancies in Wiskott-Aldrich patients. The tumors are almost exclusively extranodal with a large-cell immunoblastic phenotype and are distinctly lacking in Burkitt's or lymphoblastic histology (213). These patients share a mutation in the Wiskott-Aldrich–associated protein, which interacts downstream of the BTK (Bruton's) gene in the immunoglobulin-signaling pathway (214). Seventy-five percent of all cancers in these patients are lymphomas, and one survey found them to be universally infected with Epstein-Barr virus (215).

Common Variable Immunodeficiency

Individuals who contract common variable immunodeficiency, the most common prevalent acquired deficiency of immune function not related to the human immunodeficiency virus, have low immunoglobulin levels and develop an inability to respond humorally to vaccination or other antigen exposure. Patients present with encapsulated bacterial infections, such as those seen in children with Bruton's hypogammaglobulinemia, with prominent susceptibility to otitis and sinusitis (216). Some patients initially diagnosed with irritable bowel syndrome have turned out to have common variable immunodeficiency, which is also frequently accompanied by symptoms of diarrhea and crampy abdominal pain. A high incidence of atrophic gastritis, possibly related to *H. pylori* infection, appears to put these patients at risk for developing gastric carcinomas (217). But common variable immunodeficiency patients in general are at increased risk for gastrointestinal and central nervous system lymphomas. The likelihood of lymphoma increases with age at onset of disease, with one estimate of 8.5% in those diagnosed with common variable immunodeficiency after 16 years of age (218). Clinical presentation crosses a spectrum from atypical or reactive lymphoid hyperplasia to malignancy, with a predominance of benign disease (219). Most patients have no identifiable genetic defect, but mutations have been found in the CD40 ligand, BTK (Bruton's), and SAP (X-linked lymphoproliferative) genes (220).

Severe Combined Immunodeficiency

Multiple genetic defects have been identified in different severe combined immunodeficiency patients that simultaneously impair both cellular and humoral immunity, manifested by severe infections from the time that maternal antibodies disappear from an infant's circulation (221). These children fall prey to infection in most cases unless immune reconstitution takes place. Among those who receive identical or haploidentical bone marrow, a susceptibility subsequently emerges to posttransplant lymphoproliferative disease. Often this is related to naturally acquired or transplant-transmitted Epstein-Barr virus infection, as in the case noted above of the 12-year-old boy who ultimately succumbed to monoclonal transformation of his own B cells (194). As in Wiskott-Aldrich syndrome, lymphoma represents 75% of all malignancies in severe combined immunodeficiency patients and is almost exclusively Epstein-Barr virus related (201).

REFERENCES

1. Wotherspoon AC, et al. *Helicobacter pylori*-associated gastritis and primary B-cell gastric lymphoma. *Lancet* 1991;338:1175–1176.
2. Willis TG, et al. Bcl10 is involved in t(1;14)(p22;q32) of MALT B cell lymphoma and mutated in multiple tumor types. *Cell* 1999;96:35–45.
3. Du MQ, et al. BCL10 gene mutation in lymphoma. *Blood* 2000;95:3885–3890.
4. Chaisson RE. HIV becomes world's leading infectious cause of death. *Hopkins HIV Rep* 1999;11:1.
5. Beral V, et al. AIDS-associated non-Hodgkin lymphoma [see comments]. *Lancet* 1991;337:805–809.
6. Moore RD, Chaisson RE. Natural history of HIV infection in the era of combination antiretroviral therapy. *AIDS* 1999;13:1933–1942.
7. Rabkin CS, et al. Chemokine and chemokine receptor gene variants and risk of non-Hodgkin's lymphoma in human immunodeficiency virus-1-infected individuals. *Blood* 1999;93:1838–1842.
8. Dean M, et al. Reduced risk of AIDS lymphoma in individuals heterozygous for the CCR5-delta32 mutation. *Cancer Res* 1999;59:3561–3564.
9. Chang Y, et al. Identification of herpesvirus-like DNA sequences in AIDS-associated Kaposi's sarcoma [see comments]. *Science* 1994;266:865–869.
10. Grulich AE, et al. Decreasing rates of Kaposi's sarcoma and non-Hodgkin's lymphoma in the era of potent combination anti-retroviral therapy. *AIDS* 2001;15:629–633.
11. Rabkin C, et al. Kaposi's sarcoma and non-Hodgkin's lymphoma incidence trends in AIDS Clinical Trial Group study participants. *J Acquir Immune Defic Syndr* 1999;21[Suppl 1]:S31–S33.
12. Biggar RJ. AIDS-related cancers in the era of highly active antiretroviral therapy. *Oncology (Huntingt)* 2001;15:439–448; discussion, 448–449.
13. Jacobson LP, et al. Impact of potent antiretroviral therapy on the incidence of Kaposi's sarcoma and non-Hodgkin's lymphomas among HIV-1-infected individuals. Multicenter AIDS Cohort Study. *J Acquir Immune Defic Syndr* 1999;21[Suppl 1]:S34–S41.
14. Buchbinder SP, et al. Combination antiretroviral therapy and incidence of AIDS-related malignancies. *J Acquir Immune Defic Syndr* 1999;21[Suppl 1]:S23–S26.
15. Rabkin CS, et al. Declining incidence of Kaposi's sarcoma in ACTG trials. *J Acquir Immune Defic Syndr Hum Retrovirol* 1998;17.
16. Young L, et al. Expression of Epstein-Barr virus transformation-associated genes in tissues of patients with EBV lymphoproliferative disease. *N Engl J Med* 1989;321:1080–1085.
17. Sample J, Kieff E. Transcription of the Epstein-Barr virus genome during latency in growth-transformed lymphocytes. *J Virol* 1990;64:1667–1674.
18. van Baarle D, et al. Dysfunctional Epstein-Barr virus (EBV)-specific CD8(+) T lymphocytes and increased EBV load in HIV-1 infected individuals progressing to AIDS-related non-Hodgkin lymphoma. *Blood* 2001;98:146–155.
19. Grulich AE. AIDS-associated non-Hodgkin's lymphoma in the era of highly active antiretroviral therapy. *J Acquir Immune Defic Syndr* 1999;21[Suppl 1]:S27–S30.
20. Highly active antiretroviral therapy and incidence of cancer in human immunodeficiency virus-infected adults. *J Natl Cancer Inst* 2000;92(22):1823–1830.
21. Kirk O, et al. Non-Hodgkin lymphoma in HIV-infected patients in the era of highly active antiretroviral therapy. *Blood* 2001;98:3406–412.
22. Besson C, et al. Changes in AIDS-related lymphoma since the era of highly active antiretroviral therapy. *Blood* 2001;98:2339–2344.
23. Herndier BG, et al. Acquired immunodeficiency syndrome-associated T-cell lymphoma: evidence for human immunodeficiency virus type 1-associated T-cell transformation. *Blood* 1992;79:1768–1774.
24. Lust JA, et al. T-cell non-Hodgkin lymphoma in human immunodeficiency virus-1-infected individuals. *Am J Hematol* 1989;31:181–187.
25. Shiramizu B, Herndier BG, McGrath MS. Identification of a common clonal human immunodeficiency virus integration site in human immunodeficiency virus-associated lymphomas. *Cancer Res* 1994;54:2069–2072.
26. Liebowitz D. Epstein-Barr virus and a cellular signaling pathway in lymphomas from immunosuppressed patients [see comments]. *N Engl J Med* 1998;338:1413–1421.
27. Camilleri-Broet S, et al. Overexpression of BCL-2, BCL-X, and BAX in primary central nervous system lymphomas that occur in immunosuppressed patients. *Mod Pathol* 2000;13:158–165.
28. Izumi KM, Kieff ED. The Epstein-Barr virus oncogene product latent membrane protein 1 engages the tumor necrosis factor receptor-associated death domain protein to mediate B lymphocyte growth transformation and activate NF-kappaB. *Proc Natl Acad Sci U S A* 1997;94:12592–12597.
29. Moore PS, et al. Molecular mimicry of human cytokine and cytokine response pathway genes by KSHV. *Science* 1996;274:1739–1744.
30. Arvanitakis L, et al. Human herpesvirus KSHV encodes a constitutively active G-protein-coupled receptor linked to cell proliferation [see comments]. *Nature* 1997;385:347–350.
31. Cheng EH, et al. A Bcl-2 homolog encoded by Kaposi sarcoma-associated virus, human herpesvirus 8, inhibits apoptosis but does not heterodimerize with Bax or Bak. *Proc Natl Acad Sci U S A* 1997;94:690–694.
32. Cesarman E, et al. Kaposi's sarcoma-associated herpesvirus contains G protein-coupled receptor and cyclin D homologs which are expressed in Kaposi's sarcoma and malignant lymphoma. *J Virol* 1996;70:8218–8223.
33. Chatterjee M, et al. Viral IL-6-induced cell proliferation and immune evasion of interferon activity. *Science* 2002;298:1432–1435.
34. Cannon M, Philpott NJ, Cesarman E. The Kaposi's sarcoma-associated herpesvirus G protein-coupled receptor has broad signaling effects in primary effusion lymphoma cells. *J Virol* 2003;77:57–67.
35. Li M, et al. Kaposi's sarcoma-associated herpesvirus viral interferon regulatory factor. *J Virol* 1998;72:5433–5440.
36. Seo T, et al. Viral interferon regulatory factor 1 of Kaposi's sarcoma-associated herpesvirus interacts with a cell death regulator, GRIM19, and inhibits interferon/retinoic acid-induced cell death. *J Virol* 2002;76:8797–8807.
37. Means RE, et al. Immune evasion strategies of Kaposi's sarcoma-associated herpesvirus. *Curr Top Microbiol Immunol* 2002;269:187–201.
38. Brander C, et al. Impaired CTL recognition of cells latently infected with Kaposi's sarcoma-associated herpes virus. *J Immunol* 2000;165:2077–2083.
39. Coscoy L, Ganem D. A viral protein that selectively downregulates ICAM-1 and B7-2 and modulates T cell costimulation. *J Clin Invest* 2001;107:1599–1606.
40. Ishido S, et al. Downregulation of major histocompatibility complex class I molecules by Kaposi's sarcoma-associated herpesvirus K3 and K5 proteins. *J Virol* 2000;74:5300–5309.
41. Ishido S, et al. Inhibition of natural killer cell-mediated cytotoxicity by Kaposi's sarcoma-associated herpesvirus K5 protein. *Immunity* 2000;13(3):365–374.
42. Sozzani S, et al. The viral chemokine macrophage inflammatory protein-II is a selective Th2 chemoattractant. *Blood* 1998;92:4036–4039.
43. Neri A, et al. Epstein-Barr virus infection precedes clonal expansion in Burkitt's and acquired immunodeficiency syndrome-associated lymphoma. *Blood* 1991;77:1092–1095.
44. Levine AM. Acquired immunodeficiency syndrome-related lymphoma. *Blood* 1992;80:8.
45. Hamilton-Dutoit SJ, et al. AIDS-related lymphoma. Histopathology, immunophenotype, and association with Epstein-Barr virus as demonstrated by in situ nucleic acid hybridization. *Am J Pathol* 1991;138:149–163.
46. Hamilton-Dutoit SJ, et al. Identification of EBV-DNA in tumour cells of AIDS-related lymphomas by in-situ hybridisation [Letter]. *Lancet* 1989;1:554–552.
47. Gaidano G, et al. Rearrangements of the BCL-6 gene in acquired immunodeficiency syndrome-associated non-Hodgkin's lymphoma: association with diffuse large-cell subtype. *Blood* 1994;84:397–402.
48. Shiramizu B, et al. Molecular and immunophenotypic characterization of AIDS-associated, Epstein-Barr virus-negative, polyclonal lymphoma. *J Clin Oncol* 1992;10:383–389.
49. Pelicci PG, et al. Multiple monoclonal B cell expansions and c-myc oncogene rearrangements in acquired immune deficiency syndrome-related lymphoproliferative disorders. Implications for lymphomagenesis. *J Exp Med*, 1986;164:2049–2060.
50. Ballerini P, et al. Multiple genetic lesions in acquired immunodeficiency syndrome-related non-Hodgkin's lymphoma. *Blood* 1993;81:166–176.

51. Levine AM, Shibata D, Sullivan-Halley J, et al. Epidemiological and biological study of aquired immunodeficiency syndrome–related lymphoma in the country of Los Angeles: preliminary results. *Cancer Res* 1992;52[19 Suppl]:5482s–5484s.

52. Gaidano G, Carbone A, Dalla-Favera R. Genetic basis of acquired immunodeficiency syndrome-related lymphomagenesis. *J Natl Cancer Inst Monogr* 1998;23:95–100.

53. Neri A, et al. Different regions of the immunoglobulin heavy-chain locus are involved in chromosomal translocations in distinct pathogenetic forms of Burkitt lymphoma. *Proc Natl Acad Sci U S A* 1988; 85:2748–2752.

54. Verschuren EW, et al. The oncogenic potential of Kaposi's sarcoma-associated herpesvirus cyclin is exposed by p53 loss in vitro and in vivo. *Cancer Cell* 2002;2:229–241.

55. Lombardi L, Newcomb EW, Dalla-Favera R. Pathogenesis of Burkitt lymphoma: expression of an activated c-myc oncogene causes the tumorigenic conversion of EBV-infected human B lymphoblasts. *Cell* 1987;49:161–170.

56. Carbone A, et al. BCL-6 protein expression in AIDS-related non-Hodgkin's lymphomas: inverse relationship with Epstein-Barr virus-encoded latent membrane protein-1 expression. *Am J Pathol* 1997;150: 155–165.

57. Agarwal B, et al. Lymphoid neoplasms in HIV-positive individuals in India. *J Acquir Immune Defic Syndr* 2002;29:181–183.

58. Kehrl JH, et al. Lymphokine production by B cells from normal and HIV-infected individuals. *Ann N Y Acad Sci* 1992;651:220–227.

59. Yarchoan R, Redfield RR, Broder S. Mechanisms of B cell activation in patients with acquired immunodeficiency syndrome and related disorders. Contribution of antibody-producing B cells, of Epstein-Barr virus-infected B cells, and of immunoglobulin production induced by human T cell lymphotropic virus, type III/lymphadenopathy-associated virus. *J Clin Invest* 1986;78:439–447.

60. Davis CB, et al. Signal transduction due to HIV-1 envelope interactions with chemokine receptors CXCR4 or CCR5. *J Exp Med* 1997;186:1793–1798.

61. Madani N, et al. gp120 envelope glycoproteins of human immunodeficiency viruses competitively antagonize signaling by coreceptors CXCR4 and CCR5. *Proc Natl Acad Sci U S A* 1998;95:8005–8010.

62. Popik W, Pitha PM. Early activation of mitogen-activated protein kinase kinase, extracellular signal-regulated kinase, p38 mitogen-activated protein kinase, and c-Jun N-terminal kinase in response to binding of simian immunodeficiency virus to Jurkat T cells expressing CCR5 receptor. *Virology* 1998;252:210–217.

63. Popik W, Hesselgesser JE, Pitha PE. Binding of human immunodeficiency virus type 1 to CD4 and CXCR4 receptors differentially regulates expression of inflammatory genes and activates the MEK/ERK signaling pathway. *J Virol* 1998;72:6406–6413.

64. Su SB, et al. Inhibition of tyrosine kinase activation blocks the down-regulation of CXC chemokine receptor 4 by HIV-1 gp 120 in CD4+ T cells. *J Immunol* 1999;162:7128–7132.

65. Clerici M, et al. Role of interleukin-10 in T helper cell dysfunction in asymptomatic individuals infected with the human immunodeficiency virus. *J Clin Invest* 1994;93:768–775.

66. Muller F, et al. Possible role of interleukin-10 (IL-10) and CD40 ligand expression in the pathogenesis of hypergammaglobulinemia in human immunodeficiency virus infection: modulation of IL-10 and Ig production after intravenous Ig infusion. *Blood* 1998;92:3721–3729.

67. Carbone A, et al. Expression profile of MUM1/IRF4, BCL-6, and CD138/syndecan-1 defines novel histogenetic subsets of human immunodeficiency virus-related lymphomas. *Blood* 2001;97:744–751.

68. Katler SP, Riggs SA, Cabanillas F. Aggressive non-Hodgkin's lymphoma in immunocompromised homosexual males. *Blood* 1985;66.

69. Ioachim HL, et al. Acquired immunodeficiency syndrome-associated lymphomas: clinical, pathologic, immunologic, and viral characteristics of 111 cases. *Hum Pathol* 1991;22: 659–673.

70. Ziegler JL, et al. Acquired immunodeficiency syndrome-associated lymphomas: clinical, pathologic, immunologic, and viral characteristics of 111 cases. *N Engl J Med* 1984;311:565–570.

71. Lowenthal DA, et al. AIDS-related lymphoid neoplasia. The Memorial Hospital experience. *Cancer* 1988;61:2325–2337.

72. National Cancer Institute sponsored study of classifications of non-Hodgkin's lymphomas: summary and description of a working formulation for clinical usage. The Non-Hodgkin's Lymphoma Pathologic Classification Project. *Cancer* 1982;49:2112–2135.

73. Levine AM, Wernz JC, Kaplan L. Low-dose chemotherapy with central nervous system prophylaxis and zidovudine maintenance in AIDS-related lymphoma. *JAMA* 1991;266:84–88.

74. Gill PS, et al. Primary central nervous system lymphoma in homosexual men. Clinical, immunologic, and pathologic features. *Am J Med* 1985;78:742–748.

75. Gill PS, Levine AM, Krailo M. AIDS-related malignant lymphoma: results of prospective treatment trials. *J Clin Oncol* 1987;5:1322–1328.

76. Knowles DM, Chamulak GA, Subar M. Lymphoid neoplasia associated with the acquired immunodeficiency syndrome (AIDS): the New York University Medical Center experience with 105 patients. *Ann Intern Med* 1988;108:744–753.

77. Bermudez MA, et al. Non-Hodgkin's lymphoma in a population with or at risk for acquired immunodeficiency syndrome: indications for intensive chemotherapy. *Am J Med* 1989;86:71.

78. Kaplan LD, Abrams DI, Feigal E. AIDS-associated non-Hodgkin's lymphoma in San Francisco. *JAMA* 1989;261:719–724.

79. Kaplan MH, et al. Neoplastic complications of HTLV-III infection. Lymphomas and solid tumors. *Am J Med*, 1987;82:389–396.

80. Kaplan LD, et al. Clinical and virologic effects of recombinant human granulocyte-macrophage colony-stimulating factor in patients receiving chemotherapy for human immunodeficiency virus-associated non-Hodgkin's lymphoma: results of a randomized trial. *J Clin Oncol* 1991;9:929–940.

81. Remick SC, McSharry JJ, Wolf BC. Novel oral combination chemotherapy in the treatment of intermediate-grade and high-grade AIDS-related non-Hodgkin's lymphoma. *J Clin Oncol* 1993;11:1691–1702.

82. Freter CE. Acquired immunodeficiency syndrome-associated lymphomas. *J Natl Cancer Inst Monogr* 1990;10:45–54.

83. von Gunten CF, Von Roenn JH. Clinical aspects of human immunodeficiency virus-related lymphoma. *Curr Opin Oncol* 1992;4:894–899.

84. Raphael M, et al. Histopathologic features of high-grade non-Hodgkin's lymphomas in acquired immunodeficiency syndrome. The French Study Group of Pathology for Human Immunodeficiency Virus-Associated Tumors. *Arch Pathol Lab Med* 1991;115:15–20.

85. Burkes RL, et al. Rectal lymphoma in homosexual men. *Arch Intern Med* 1986;146:913–915.

86. Ziegler JL, et al. Non-Hodgkin's lymphoma in 90 homosexual men. Relation to generalized lymphadenopathy and the acquired immunodeficiency syndrome. *N Engl J Med* 1984;311:565–570.

87. Levine AM, et al. Evolving characteristics of AIDS-related lymphoma. *Blood* 2000;96:4084–4090.

88. Matthews GV, et al. Changes in acquired immunodeficiency syndrome-related lymphoma since the introduction of highly active antiretroviral therapy. *Blood* 2000;96:2730–2734.

89. Gabarre J, et al. Human immunodeficiency virus-related lymphoma: relation between clinical features and histologic subtypes. *Am J Med* 2001;111:704–711.

90. Rowe M, et al. Differences in B cell growth phenotype reflect novel patterns of Epstein-Barr virus latent gene expression in Burkitt's lymphoma cells. *EMBO J* 1987;6:2743–2751.

91. Levitskaya J, et al. Inhibition of ubiquitin/proteasome-dependent protein degradation by the Gly-Ala repeat domain of the Epstein-Barr virus nuclear antigen 1. *Proc Natl Acad Sci U S A* 1997;94:12616–12621.

92. Cingolani A, et al. Epstein-Barr virus infection is predictive of CNS involvement in systemic AIDS-related non-Hodgkin's lymphomas [in process citation]. *J Clin Oncol* 2000;18:3325–3330.

93. Scadden DT. Epstein-Barr virus, the CNS, and AIDS-related lymphomas: as close as flame to smoke. *J Clin Oncol* 2000;18:3323–3324.

94. Straus DJ, et al. Prognostic factors in the treatment of human immunodeficiency virus-associated non-Hodgkin's lymphoma: analysis of AIDS Clinical Trials Group protocol 142—low-dose versus standard-dose m-BACOD plus granulocyte-macrophage colony-stimulating factor. National Institute of Allergy and Infectious Diseases. *J Clin Oncol* 1998;16:3601–3606.

95. Shipp MA, et al. Identification of major prognostic subgroups of patients with large-cell lymphoma treated with m-BACOD or M-BACOD. *Ann Intern Med* 1986;104:757–765.

96. Navarro JT, et al. International Prognostic Index is the best prognostic factor for survival in patients with AIDS-related non-Hodgkin's lymphoma treated with CHOP. A multivariate study of 46 patients. *Haematologica* 1998;83:508–513.

97. Vaccher E, et al. Age and serum lactate dehydrogenase level are independent prognostic factors in human immunodeficiency virus-related non-Hodgkin's lymphomas: a single-institute study of 96 patients. *J Clin Oncol* 1996;14:2217–2223.

98. Cesarman E, et al. Kaposi's sarcoma-associated herpesvirus-like DNA sequences in AIDS-related body-cavity-based lymphomas [see comments]. *N Engl J Med* 1995;332:1186–1191.

99. Nador RG, et al. Primary effusion lymphoma: a distinct clinicopathologic entity associated with the Kaposi's sarcoma-associated herpes virus. *Blood* 1996;88:645–656.

100. Karcher DS, Alkan S. Human herpesvirus-8-associated body cavity-based lymphoma in human immunodeficiency virus-infected patients: a unique B-cell neoplasm. *Hum Pathol* 1997;28:801–808.

101. Delecluse HJ, et al. Plasmablastic lymphomas of the oral cavity: a new entity associated with the human immunodeficiency virus infection. *Blood* 1997;89:1413–1420.

102. Reference deleted.

103. Reference deleted.

104. Reference deleted.

105. Reference deleted.

106. Reference deleted.

107. Reference deleted.

108. Reference deleted.

109. Reference deleted.

110. Reference deleted.

111. Reference deleted.

112. Reference deleted.

113. Reference deleted.

114. Reference deleted.

115. Reference deleted.

116. Reference deleted.

117. Reference deleted.

118. Reference deleted.

119. Reference deleted.

120. Reference deleted.

121. Reference deleted.

122. Jain A, et al. Posttransplant lymphoproliferative disorders in liver transplantation: a 20-year experience. *Ann Surg* 2002;236:429-36; discussion, 436–437.

123. Ramalingam P, et al. Posttransplant lymphoproliferative disorders in lung transplant patients: the Cleveland Clinic experience. *Mod Pathol* 2002;15:647–656.

124. Opelz G, Henderson R. Incidence of non-Hodgkin lymphoma in kidney and heart transplant recipients. *Lancet* 1993;342:1514–1516.

125. Allen U, et al. Epstein-Barr virus-related post-transplant lymphoproliferative disease in solid organ transplant recipients, 1988–97: a Canadian multi-centre experience. *Pediatr Transplant* 2001;5:198–203.

126. Smets F, Sokal EM. Epstein-Barr virus-related lymphoproliferation in children after liver transplant: role of immunity, diagnosis, and management. *Pediatr Transplant* 2002;6:280–287.

127. Hayashi RJ, et al. Posttransplant lymphoproliferative disorder in children: correlation of histology to clinical behavior. *J Pediatr Hematol Oncol* 2001;23:14–18.

128. Duvoux C, et al. Risk factors for lymphoproliferative disorders after liver transplantation in adults: an analysis of 480 patients. *Transplantation* 2002;74:1103–1109.

129. McLaughlin K, et al. Increased risk for posttransplant lymphoproliferative disorder in recipients of liver transplants with hepatitis C. *Liver Transpl* 2000;6:570–574.

130. Stevens SJ, et al. Role of Epstein-Barr virus DNA load monitoring in prevention and early detection of post-transplant lymphoproliferative disease. *Leuk Lymphoma* 2002;43:831–840.

131. Knowles DM. Immunodeficiency-associated lymphoproliferative disorders. *Mod Pathol* 1999;12:200–217.

132. Chadburn A, et al. The morphologic and molecular genetic categories of posttransplantation lymphoproliferative disorders are clinically relevant. *Cancer* 1998;82:1978–1987.

133. Cesarman E, et al. BCL-6 gene mutations in posttransplantation lymphoproliferative disorders predict response to therapy and clinical outcome. *Blood* 1998;92:2294–2302.

134. Paz-y-Mino C, et al. A polymorphism in the hMSH2 gene (gIVS12-6T>C) associated with non-Hodgkin lymphomas. *Cancer Genet Cytogenet* 2002;133:29–33.

135. Chiu BC, et al. Alcohol consumption, family history of hematolymphoproliferative cancer, and the risk of non-Hodgkin's lymphoma in men. *Ann Epidemiol* 2002;12:309–315.

136. Epstein MA, Achong BG, Barr YM. Virus particles in cultured lymphoblasts from Burkitt's lymphoma. *Lancet* 1964;1:702–703.

137. Burkitt DA. Sarcoma involving the jaws in African children. *Br J Surg* 1958;45:218–223.

138. Niedobitek G, et al. Identification of Epstein-Barr virus-infected cells in tonsils of acute infectious mononucleosis by in situ hybridization. *Hum Pathol* 1989;20:796–799.

139. Niedobitek G, Meru N, Delecluse H. Epstein-Barr virus infection and human malignancies. *Int J Exp Pathol* 2001;82:149–170.

140. Tierney RJ, et al. Epstein-Barr virus latency in blood mononuclear cells: analysis of viral gene transcription during primary infection and in the carrier state. *J Virol* 1994;68:7374–7385.

141. Kulwichit W, et al. Expression of the Epstein-Barr virus latent membrane protein 1 induces B cell lymphoma in transgenic mice. *Proc Natl Acad Sci U S A* 1998;95:11963–11968.

142. Uchida J, et al. Mimicry of CD40 signals by EBV LMP1 in B lymphocyte responses. *Science* 1999;286:300–303.

143. Porcu P, et al. Successful treatment of posttransplantation lymphoproliferative disorder (PTLD) following renal allografting is associated with sustained CD8$^+$ T-cell restoration. *Blood* 2002;100:2341–2348.

144. Rooney CM, et al. Use of gene-modified virus-specific T lymphocytes to control Epstein-Barr-virus-related lymphoproliferation. *Lancet* 1995;345:9–13.

145. Rooney CM, et al. Infusion of cytotoxic T cells for the prevention and treatment of Epstein-Barr virus-induced lymphoma in allogeneic transplant recipients. *Blood* 1998;92:1549–1555.

146. Jones D, et al. Primary-effusion lymphoma and Kaposi's sarcoma in a cardiac-transplant recipient [see comments]. *N Engl J Med* 1998;339:444–449.

147. Faye A, et al. Chimaeric anti-CD20 monoclonal antibody (rituximab) in post-transplant B-lymphoproliferative disorder following stem cell transplantation in children. *Br J Haematol* 2001;115:112–118.

148. Milpied N, et al. Humanized anti-CD20 monoclonal antibody (Rituximab) in post transplant B-lymphoproliferative disorder: a retrospective analysis on 32 patients. *Ann Oncol* 2000;11[Suppl 1]:113–116.

149. Berney T, et al. Successful treatment of posttransplant lymphoproliferative disorder with prolonged rituximab treatment in intestinal transplant recipients. *Transplantation* 2002;74:1000–1006.

150. Yang J, et al. Characterization of Epstein-Barr virus-infected B cells in patients with posttransplantation lymphoproliferative disease: disappearance after rituximab therapy does not predict clinical response. *Blood* 2000;96:4055–4063.

151. Swinnen LJ, et al. Aggressive treatment for postcardiac transplant lymphoproliferation. *Blood* 1995;86:3333–3340.

152. Sporn MB, Harris ED Jr. Proliferative diseases. *Am J Med* 1981;70:1231–1235.

153. Fassbender HG, Gay S. Synovial processes in rheumatoid arthritis. *Scand J Rheumatol* 1988;76:1–7.

154. Firestein GS. The immunopathogenesis of rheumatoid arthritis. *Curr Opin Rheumatol* 1991;3:398–406.

155. Mellemkjaer L, et al. Rheumatoid arthritis and cancer risk. *Eur J Cancer* 1996;7:1753–1757.

156. Karlson EW, et al. A retrospective cohort study of cigarette smoking and risk of rheumatoid arthritis in female health professionals. *Arthritis Rheum* 1999;42:910–917.

157. Isomaki HA, Hakulinen T, Joutsenlahti U. Excess risk of lymphomas, leukemia and myeloma in patients with rheumatoid arthritis. *J Chronic Dis* 1978;31:691–696.

158. Gridley G, et al. Incidence of cancer among patients with rheumatoid arthritis. *J Natl Cancer Inst* 1993;17:307–311.

159. Prior P. Cancer and rheumatoid arthritis: epidemiologic considerations. *Am J Med* 1985;78:15–21.

159a. Karlson E, *personal communication.*

160. Tengstrand B, Carlstrom K, Hafstrom I. Bioavailable testosterone in men with rheumatoid arthritis: high frequency of hypogonadism. *Rheumatology* 2002;41:285–289.

161. Bajocchi G, et al. Elderly onset rheumatoid arthritis: clinical aspects. *Clin Exp Rheumatol* 2000;18[4 Suppl 20]:S49–S50.

162. Furst DE. Predictors of worsening clinical variables and outcomes in rheumatoid arthritis. *Rheum Dis Clin North Am* 1994; 20:309–319.

163. Abu-Shakra M, Buskila D, Shoenfeld Y. Rheumatoid arthritis and cancer. In: Shoenfeld Y, Gershwin ME, eds. *Cancer and autoimmunity.* Amsterdam: Elsevier, 2000:19–30.
164. Kinlen LJ. Malignancy in autoimmune diseases. *J Autoimmun* 1992;5:363–371.
165. Baker GL, et al. Malignancy following treatment of rheumatoid arthritis with cyclophosphamide. *Am J Med* 1987;83:1–9.
166. Patapanian H, et al. The oncogenicity of chlorambucil in rheumatoid arthritis. *Br J Rheumatol* 1988;27:44–47.
167. Kremer JM. Is methotrexate oncogenic in patients with rheumatoid arthritis? *Semin Arthritis Rheum* 1997:785–787.
168. Salloum E, et al. Spontaneous regression of lymphoproliferative disorders in patients treated with methotrexate for rheumatoid arthritis and other rheumatic diseases. *J Clin Oncol* 1996;14:1943–1949.
169. Sibilia J, Mariette X. Methotrexate treatment and mortality in rheumatoid arthritis. *Lancet* 2002;360:1096–1097.
170. Mariette X, et al. Lymphomas in rheumatoid arthritis patients treated with methotrexate: a 3-year prospective study in France. *Blood* 2002;99:3909–3915.
171. Choi HK, et al. Methotrexate and mortality in patients with rheumatoid arthritis: a prospective study. *Lancet* 2002;359:1173–1177.
172. Theofilopoulos AN. Murine models of lupus. In: Lahita RG, ed. *Systemic lupus erythematosus.* New York: Churchill Livingstone, 1992.
173. Mellemkjaer L, et al. Non-Hodgkin's lymphoma and other cancers among a cohort of patients with systemic lupus erythematosus. *Arthritis Rheum* 1997;40:761–768.
174. Pettersson T, et al. Increased risk of cancer in patients with systemic lupus erythematosus. *Ann Rheum Dis* 1992;51:437–439.
175. Abu-Shakr, M, Buskila D, Shoenfeld Y. Systemic lupus erythematosus and cancer. In: Shoenfeld Y, Gershwin ME, eds. *Cancer and autoimmunity.* Amsterdam: Elsevier, 2000:31.
176. Tala, N, Bunim JJ. Development of malignant lymphoma in the course of Sjögren's syndrome. *Am J Med* 1964;37:529–540.
177. Kassan SS, et al. Increased risk of lymphoma in sicca syndrome. *Ann Int Med* 1978;89:888–892.
178. Voulgarelis M, et al. Malignant lymphoma in primary Sjögren's syndrome: a multi-center, retrospective, clinical study by the European Concerted Action on Sjögren's Syndrome. *Arthritis Rheum* 1999;42:1765–1772.
179. Fox RI, et al. Expression of a cross-reactive idiotype on rheumatoid factor in patients with Sjögren's syndrome. *J Immunol* 1986;136:477–483.
180. Namekawa T, et al. Identification of SSA reactive T cells in labial salivary glands form patients with Sjögren's syndrome. *J Rheumatol* 1995;20:92–99.
181. Ramos-Casals M, Garcia-Carrasco M, Font J, Cervera R. Sjögren's syndrome and lymphoproliferative diseases. In: Shoenfeld Y, Gershwin ME, eds. *Cancer and autoimmunity.* Amsterdam: Elsevier Science, 2000:55.
182. Kruize AA, et al. Long-term follow-up of patients with Sjögren's syndrome. *Arthritis Rheum* 1996;39:297–303.
183. Valesini G, et al. Differential risk of non-Hodgkin's lymphoma in Italian patient with primary Sjögren's syndrome. *J Rheumatol* 1997;24:2376–2380.
184. Pedersen RK, Pedersen NT. Primary non-Hodgkin's lymphoma of the thyroid gland: a population based study. *Histopathology* 1996;28:25–32.
185. Hyjek E, Isaacson PG. Primary B cell lymphoma of the thyroid and its relationship to Hashimoto's thyroiditis. *Hum Pathol* 1988;19:1315–1326.
186. Holm LE, Blomgren H, Lowhagen T. Cancer risks in patients with chronic lymphocytic thyroiditis. *N Engl J Med* 1985;312:601–604.
187. Liebow AA, Carrington CR, Friedman PJ. Lymphomatoid granulomatosis. *Hum Pathol* 1972;3:457–558.
188. Katzenstein AL, Carrington CB, Liebow AA. Lymphomatoid granulomatosis: a clinicopathologic study of 152 cases. *Cancer* 1979;43:360–373.
189. Pertuiset E, et al. Adult HSP associated with malignancy. *Semin Arthritis Rheum* 2000;29:360–367.
190. Swinson CM, et al. Coeliac disease and malignancy. *Lancet* 1983;1:111–115.
191. Corrao G, et al. Mortality in patients with coeliac disease and their relatives: a cohort study. *Lancet* 2001;358:356–361.
192. Egan LJ, et al. Celiac-associated lymphoma. A single institution experience of 30 cases in the combination chemotherapy era. *J Clin Gastroenterol* 1995;21:123–129.
193. Catassi C, et al. Risk of non-Hodgkin lymphoma in celiac disease. *JAMA* 2002;287:1413–1419.
194. Shearer WT, et al. Epstein-Barr virus-associated B-cell proliferations of diverse clonal origins after bone marrow transplantation in a 12-year-old patient with severe combined immunodeficiency. *N Engl J Med* 1985;312:1151–1159.
195. Oertel SH, Riess H. Immunosurveillance, immunodeficiency and lymphoproliferations. *Recent Results Cancer Res* 2002;159:1–8.
196. Mueller BU, Pizzo PA. Cancer in children with primary or secondary immunodeficiencies. *J Pediatr* 1995;126:1–10.
197. Boultwood J. Ataxia telangiectasia gene mutations in leukaemia and lymphoma. *J Clin Pathol* 2001;54:512–516.
198. Gronbaek K, et al. ATM mutations are associated with inactivation of the ARF-TP53 tumor suppressor pathway in diffuse large B-cell lymphoma. *Blood* 2002;100:1430–1437.
199. Taylor AM, et al. Leukemia and lymphoma in ataxia telangiectasia. *Blood* 1996;87:423–438.
200. Morrell D, Cromartie E, Swift M. Mortality and cancer incidence in 263 patients with ataxia-telangiectasia. *J Natl Cancer Inst* 1986;77:89–92.
201. Filipovich A, et al. Immune-mediated hematologic oncologic disorders, including Epstein-Barr virus infection. In: Stiehm E, ed. *Immunologic disorders in infants & children.* Philadelphia: WB Saunders, 1996:855–889.
202. Petro JB, et al. Bruton's tyrosine kinase is required for activation of IκB kinase and nuclear factor κB in response to B cell receptor engagement. *J Exp Med* 2000;191:1745–1754.
203. Bajpai UD, et al. Bruton's tyrosine kinase links the B cell receptor to nuclear factor κB activation. *J Exp Med* 2000;191:1735–1744.
204. Maas A, Hendriks RW. Role of Bruton's tyrosine kinase in B cell development. *Dev Immunol* 2001;8:171–181.
205. Faulkner GC, et al. X-linked agammaglobulinemia patients are not infected with Epstein-Barr virus: implications for the biology of the virus. *J Virol* 1999;73:1555–1564.
206. Uckun FM, et al. BTK as a mediator of radiation-induced apoptosis in DT-40 lymphoma B cells. *Science* 1996;273:1096–1100.
207. Vassilev A, et al. Bruton's tyrosine kinase as an inhibitor of the Fas/CD95 death-inducing signaling complex. *J Biol Chem* 1999;274:1646–1656.
208. Mohamed AJ, et al. Nucleocytoplasmic shuttling of Bruton's tyrosine kinase. *J Biol Chem* 2000;275:40614–40619.
209. Islam TC, et al. Expression profiling in transformed human B cells: influence of btk mutations and comparison to B cell lymphomas using filter and oligonucleotide arrays. *Eur J Immunol* 2002;32:982–993.
210. Schuster V, Kreth HW. X-linked lymphoproliferative disease is caused by deficiency of a novel SH2 domain-containing signal transduction adaptor protein. *Immunol Rev* 2000;178:21–28.
211. Nagy N, et al. The X-linked lymphoproliferative disease gene product SAP is expressed in activated T and NK cells. *Immunol Lett* 2002;82:141–147.
212. MacGinnitie AJ, Geha R. X-linked lymphoproliferative disease: genetic lesions and clinical consequences. *Curr Allergy Asthma Rep* 2002;2:361–367.
213. Cotelingam JD, et al. Malignant lymphoma in patients with the Wiskott-Aldrich syndrome. *Cancer Invest* 1985;3:515–522.
214. Baba Y, et al. Involvement of Wiskott-Aldrich syndrome protein in B-cell cytoplasmic tyrosine kinase pathway. *Blood* 1999;93:2003–2012.
215. Filipovich AH, et al. Primary immunodeficiencies: genetic risk factors for lymphoma. *Cancer Res* 1992;52[19 Suppl]:5465s–5467s.
216. Van der Hilst JC, Smits BW, van der Meer JW. Hypogammaglobulinaemia: cumulative experience in 49 patients in a tertiary care institution. *Neth J Med* 2002;60:140–147.
217. Zullo A, et al. Gastric pathology in patients with common variable immunodeficiency. *Gut* 1999;45:77–81.
218. Groopman JE, Broder S. Cancers in AIDS and other immunodeficiency states. In DeVita VT, Hellman S, Rosenberg SA, eds. *Cancer: principles and practice of oncology.* Philadelphia: JB Lippincott Co, 1989:1958–1959.
219. Sander CA, et al. Lymphoproliferative lesions in patients with common variable immunodeficiency syndrome. *Am J Surg Pathol* 1992;16:1170–1182.

220. Morra M, et al. Alterations of the X-linked lymphoproliferative disease gene SH2D1A in common variable immunodeficiency syndrome. *Blood* 2001;98:1321–1325.
221. Buckley RH. Advances in the understanding and treatment of human severe combined immunodeficiency. *Immunol Res* 2000;22:237–251.
222. Reference deleted.
223. Goedert JJ, et al. Spectrum of AIDS-associated malignant disorders [see comments]. *Lancet* 1998;351:1833–1839.
224. Lyter DW, et al. Incidence of human immunodeficiency virus-related and nonrelated malignancies in a large cohort of homosexual men. *J Clin Oncol* 1995;13:2540–2546.
225. Franceschi S, et al. Risk of cancer other than Kaposi's sarcoma and non-Hodgkin's lymphoma in persons with AIDS in Italy. Cancer and AIDS Registry Linkage Study. *Br J Cancer* 1998;78:966–970.
226. Biggar RJ, Rabkin CS. The epidemiology of AIDS-related neoplasms. *Hematol Oncol Clin North Am* 1996;10(5):997–1010.
227. Cote TR, et al. Non-Hodgkin's lymphoma among people with AIDS: incidence, presentation and public health burden. AIDS/Cancer Study Group. *Int J Cancer* 1997;73(5):645–650.
228. Melbye M, et al. High incidence of anal cancer among AIDS patients. The AIDS/Cancer Working Group. *Lancet* 1994;343(8898):636–639.
229. Franceschi S, et al. Risk of cancer other than Kaposi's sarcoma and non-Hodgkin's lymphoma in persons with AIDS in Italy. Cancer and AIDS Registry Linkage Study. *Br J Cancer* 1998;78(7):966–970.
230. McClain KL, et al. Association of Epstein-Barr virus with leiomyosarcomas in children with AIDS [see comments]. *N Engl J Med* 1995;332(1):12–18.
231. Biggar RJ, Frisch M, Goedert JJ. Risk of cancer in children with AIDS. AIDS-Cancer Match Registry Study Group. *JAMA* 2000;284(2):205–209.
232. Biggar RJ, et al. Risk of other cancers following Kaposi's sarcoma: relation to acquired immunodeficiency syndrome. *Am J Epidemiol* 1994;139(4):362–368.
233. Grulich AE, et al. Rates of non-AIDS-defining cancers in people with HIV infection before and after AIDS diagnosis. *AIDS* 2002;16(8):1155–1161.
234. Remick SC. Non-AIDS-defining cancers. *Hematol Oncol Clin North Am* 1996;10(5):1203–13.
235. Ateenyi-Agaba C. Conjunctival squamous-cell carcinoma associated with HIV infection in Kampala, Uganda. *Lancet* 1995;345(8951):695–696.
236. Goedert JJ, Cote TR. Conjunctival malignant disease with AIDS in USA. *Lancet* 1995;346(8969):257–258.
237. Darby SC, et al. Mortality from liver cancer and liver disease in haemophilic men and boys in UK given blood products contaminated with hepatitis C. UK Haemophilia Centre Directors' Organisation. *Lancet* 1997;350(9089):1425–1431.
238. Beral V, Newton R. Overview of the epidemiology of immunodeficiency-associated cancers. *J Natl Cancer Inst Monogr* 1998(23):1–6.
239. Melbye M, et al. Nasopharyngeal carcinoma: an EBV-associated tumour not significantly influenced by HIV-induced immunosuppression. The AIDS/Cancer Working Group. *Br J Cancer* 1996;73(8):995–997.
240. Parkin DM, et al. Non-Hodgkin lymphoma in Uganda: a case-control study. *AIDS* 2000;14(18):2929–2936.
241. Rabkin CS, et al. Incidence of lymphomas and other cancers in HIV-infected and HIV-uninfected patients with hemophilia. *JAMA* 1992;267(8):1090–1094.
242. Battan R, et al. Helicobacter pylori infection in patients with acquired immune deficiency syndrome. *Am J Gastroenterol* 1990;85(12):1576–1579.
243. Crump M, Gospodarowicz M, Shepherd FA. Lymphoma of the gastrointestinal tract. *Semin Oncol* 1999;26(3):324–337.
244. Hishida O, et al. Serological survey of HIV-1, HIV-2 and human T-cell leukemia virus type 1 for suspected AIDS cases in Ghana. *AIDS* 1994;8(9):1257–1261.
245. Giacomo M, et al. Human T-cell leukemia virus type II infection among high risk groups and its influence on HIV-1 disease progression. *Eur J Epidemiol* 1995;11(5):527–533.
246. Hiraki A, et al. Genetics of Epstein-Barr virus infection. *Biomed Pharmacother* 2001;55(7):369–372.
247. Pertuiset E, et al. Adult Henoch-Schönlein purpura associated with malignancy. *Semin Arthritis Rheum* 2000;29(6):360–367.
248. Fauci AS, et al. Lymphomatoid Granulomatosis. Prospective clinical and therapeutic experience over 10 years. *N Engl J Med* 1982;306(2):68–74.
249. Ferguson A, Kingstone K. Coeliac disease and malignancies. *Acta Paediatr Suppl* 1996;412:78–81.

CHAPTER 46

Infectious Agents and Lymphoma

Richard Frederick Ambinder

Several infectious agents have been implicated in the pathogenesis of lymphoma. Infectious agents have been associated with only a small fraction of lymphoma worldwide. Furthermore, among those infected by these agents, lymphoma remains a relatively uncommon outcome. Some, such as Epstein-Barr virus and *Helicobacter pylori*, are ubiquitous, whereas others, such as human adult T-cell leukemia/lymphoma virus 1, are highly restricted in geographic distribution. But in each case, the infectious agent is considerably more widespread than the associated malignancy or malignancies. Although several viruses are classified as "tumor" viruses, tumorigenesis is not a part of the normal life cycle but always results from a combination of rare circumstances. Among the infectious agents themselves, there is great diversity: viral and bacterial, genomes that are single stranded or double stranded, and genomes that are composed of DNA or RNA. The diversity of the infectious agents, in terms of mechanisms of pathogenesis, is illustrated by consideration of the very different associations of the pathogens and their genomes with the tumor cell and maintenance of the malignant phenotype (Table 46.1). Thus, Epstein-Barr virus and Kaposi's sarcoma-associated herpesvirus (human herpesvirus-8) DNAs are maintained as episomes in tumor cells and are actively transcribed. Present evidence suggests that their presence is necessary to maintain the malignant character of the cells that harbor them. Human adult T-cell leukemia/lymphoma virus 1 proviral DNA is found integrated into the tumor cell genome, but the contribution of ongoing transcription to maintenance of the transformed state in established tumors is unknown. The proviral DNA may have been important only early in the pathogenesis of the tumors. Human immunodeficiency virus, hepatitis C virus, and *H. pylori* genomes are not found in lymphoma cells. However, there is evidence that, at least in some instances, the presence of each of these latter pathogens contributes to the maintenance of malignancy.

Broadly speaking, there are two pathways through which infectious agents lead to lymphoma. The first pathway involves infection of cells that will become malignant or whose progeny will become malignant. The second pathway does not involve the infection of target cells. Rather, lymphocytes, responding to the stimulus supplied by the infectious agent, become malignant. At least some members of the class of agents that directly infect the cells that will become malignant have infection of lymphocytes and proliferation of infected cells as a required part of the agent's life cycle. These agents have evolved means to persist in replicating cells either by episomal replication in tandem with replication of host cell DNA or by integration into the host cell DNA. This class includes Epstein-Barr virus and human adult T-cell leukemia/lymphoma virus 1. Members of the class of agents that does not infect cells destined to become malignant spread through rounds of replication of the infectious agent that are independent of host cell replication. This class includes human immunodeficiency virus, *H. pylori*, and possibly hepatitis C.

GAMMAHERPESVIRUSES

The recognition of a high incidence zone of Burkitt's lymphoma in equatorial Africa and the discovery of a herpesvirus in the tumor provided the first evidence that some human tumors might be viral in origin (1). Although greeted with considerable skepticism, the notion was made biologically plausible by the discovery that Epstein-Barr virus immortalized B cells *in vitro*. However, the discovery that the virus was not confined to equatorial Africa, but was ubiquitous, dashed any hopes that the relationship between virus and tumor might be simple and straightforward. The observation that the virus produced lymphomas after experimental infection in cotton-top marmosets and owl monkeys and that viral DNA was present in several different types of lymphomas, as well as a range of other malignancies, suggested that, although complex, the presence of viral DNA in tumor tissue was likely to be more than an epiphenomenon. Decades later, the link between Kaposi's sarcoma-associated herpesvirus and lymphoma was much more rapidly accepted (2,3).

Epstein-Barr virus and Kaposi's sarcoma-associated herpesvirus are gammaherpesviruses and, like other herpesviruses, have a life cycle that involves two alternative states of infection (4–6). *Lytic infection* is synonymous with productive infection

TABLE 46.1. *Infectious agents associated with lymphoma*

Pathogen	Infectious agent genome in tumor cell	Productive replication of infectious agent required for maintenance of the transformed state	Tumor cell antigen receptors specific for infectious agent
Epstein-Barr virus	Yes	No	No
Kaposi's sarcoma–associated herpesvirus	Yes	?	No
Human adult T-cell leukemia/lymphoma virus 1	Yes	No	No
Human immunodeficiency virus type 1	No	No	No
Hepatitis C	No	Probably, in at least some cases	Probably, in at least some cases
Helicobacter pylori	No	Probably, in at least some cases	?

and is associated with expression of the viral enzymes involved in replicating viral DNA and proteins that are incorporated into new virions. *Latent infection* is associated with persistence of the viral genome but not the production of new virions. As with other herpesviruses, although infection is generally controlled in the immunocompetent host, latent infection persists indefinitely with periodic reactivation of lytic infection.

Viral genomes of each virus are packaged as double-stranded linear DNA molecules in enveloped icosahedral capsids. In latently infected cells, viral genomes are maintained as multicopy circular DNA episomes. These episomes replicate once per cell cycle using cellular proteins and replication machinery (7–9). Only one viral protein is required for replication in latency. The Epstein-Barr virus protein required is the Epstein-Barr nuclear antigen 1 (EBNA1). The Kaposi's sarcoma-associated herpesvirus protein required is the latency nuclear antigen (LANA). Both viral proteins seem to tether viral episomes to chromatin. Latency in viral infection should not be regarded as synonymous with "inactive." During latent infection, viral gene expression profoundly affects cellular function. Several different patterns of latency viral gene expression are recognized for Epstein-Barr virus. It is predominantly in states of latency that Epstein-Barr virus and Kaposi's sarcoma–associated herpesvirus are found in tumor tissue.

Aspects of Epstein-Barr Virus Infection

Epstein-Barr virus is a ubiquitous virus found in all adult populations throughout the world (10). The virus is transmitted in saliva. Primary infection is usually asymptomatic and occurs in childhood. However, when delayed until adolescence or adulthood, infection is commonly associated with the syndrome of infectious mononucleosis, characterized by cervical lymphadenopathy, pharyngitis, hepatosplenomegaly, atypical lymphocytosis, and the appearance of heterophile antibodies.

Epstein-Barr virus has a tropism for B lymphocytes, although a variety of other cell types, including T cells, monocytes, and epithelial cells, are infected *in vitro* and *in vivo* (11). Virion attachment and virion entry are distinct processes. B-cell attachment involves an interaction between CD21, a component of the complement receptor, and the

viral envelope glycoprotein gp350/220; entry requires a complex of three additional viral glycoproteins, gH, gL, and gp42, and an interaction with HLA class II acting as a coreceptor. Attachment to epithelial cells involves gH; entry does not involve gp42 or HLA class II and requires complexes of viral glycoproteins that lack gp42.

In contrast to infection of other cell types, infection of resting B cells leads to cell proliferation (Fig. 46.1). This proliferation leads to the spread of virus-infected cells throughout the B-cell compartment. In acute infectious mononucleosis, as many as several percent of B cells may be Epstein-Barr virus infected (12). Viral antigen expression in proliferating cells leads to a massive T-cell response characterized in part by expansion of activated CD45RO+CD8+ T cells (13). Tetramer staining shows that much of this response targets immunodominant epitopes from immediate early and early proteins of the lytic cycle. Subsequently, latent epitopes are targeted, particularly from members of the EBNA3 family of nuclear antigens (EBNA3A, 3B, and 3C). As the cellular immune response is established, expression of viral antigens serves to target proliferating B cells for immune destruction. Ultimately, Epstein-Barr virus persists in resting B lymphocytes with very limited viral gene expression (14–17). As detailed below, very different patterns of viral latency gene expression are associated with virus-driven proliferation of lymphocytes shortly after primary infection or *in vitro* versus the resting B lymphocytes that harbor infection in most seropositive individuals (15–18). Observations of patients treated with acyclovir suggest that chronic maintenance of the infected B-cell reservoir does not require lytic infection because the number of latently infected B cells in the blood is unaffected. Virus is periodically shed in the saliva of seropositive individuals. Whether this virus is derived from B cells in the mucosa or epithelial cells is unknown. Acyclovir treatment eliminates lytic viral replication, as evidenced by the inability to detect Epstein-Barr virus in throat washings (19).

B-Lymphocyte Immortalization and the Epstein-Barr Virus Genes Required

One of the properties of the virus of most interest with regard to lymphomagenesis is the ability to mediate growth trans-

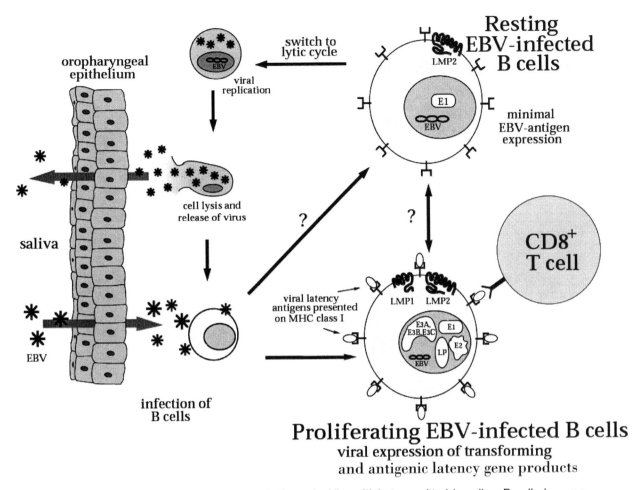

oropharyngeal epithelium

switch to lytic cycle

viral replication

Resting EBV-infected B cells

LMP2

minimal EBV-antigen expression

cell lysis and release of virus

saliva

?

?

CD8⁺ T cell

viral latency antigens presented on MHC class I

LMP1 LMP2

E3A, E3B,E3C   E1

EBV

LP   E2

EBV

infection of B cells

Proliferating EBV-infected B cells
viral expression of transforming
and antigenic latency gene products

FIG. 46.1. The Epstein-Barr virus (EBV) life cycle. Virus (*) is transmitted in saliva. B cells become infected. Viral protein expression leads to proliferation, with expansion of the infected B-cell pool. Viral DNA is in episomal form (∞). Proliferating cells express Epstein-Barr nuclear antigen (EBNA) 1, 2, 3A, 3B, 3C, LP, latent membrane protein (LMP)-1, and LMP2. Expression of these antigens, particularly the immunodominant EBNA3A, 3B, and 3C render infected cells susceptible to killing by CD8⁺ cytotoxic T cells. Some infected cells with limited antigen expression elude this surveillance. The viral proteins that drive proliferation are not expressed in these cells, and the cells are not cycling. These infected cells constitute the major latency reservoir of infection. Intermittently, lytic cycle yields new virions that are released into saliva. MHC, major histocompatibility complex. (Artwork courtesy of M. Victor Lemas.)

formation of primary B cells into long-term proliferating lymphoblastoid cell lines. Such cell lines are tumorigenic in severe combined immunodeficiency mice (20). Recombinant genetic analysis has identified the viral genes required for immortalization (Fig. 46.2) (5). These include EBNA1, EBNA2, and latent membrane protein-1 (LMP1).

EBNA1 is required for the maintenance of the viral genome. It binds to the viral origin of replication used in latency replication and interacts with chromatin, tethering viral episomes to chromatin and acting as a transcriptional transactivator (21). There is a report that EBNA1 expression driven by an immunoglobulin (Ig) heavy chain promoter/enhancer in a transgenic model is associated with an increased incidence of B-cell lymphoma (22,23). However, other evidence has been presented that EBNA1 does not directly impact on cellular transcription in lymphoblasts and

that its only contribution to lymphocyte immortalization may be in episomal maintenance (24).

EBNA2 is a transcriptional transactivator that regulates viral and cellular gene expression, stimulating G0 to G1 cell-cycle progression (25). In these effects, EBNA2 mimics activated NOTCH, an evolutionarily conserved surface receptor that mediates cell–cell signaling and influences cell fate and tissue development. Both activated NOTCH and EBNA2 target promoters through the cellular DNA-binding protein CBF1/RBP-Jk. Bound to DNA, CBF1/RBP-Jk acts as a transcriptional repressor, bringing to target promoters a histone deacetylase complex (26). EBNA2 and NOTCH compete away the core-pressor complex and interact with coactivator proteins, including pCAF, CBP, and p300. Viral promoters driving EBNA2 itself and other EBNAs are activated as well as the LMP1 promoter and the promoters of particular cellular genes, including

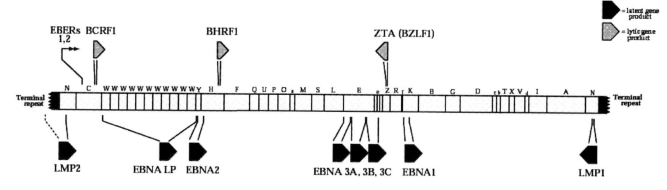

FIG. 46.2. Map of the viral genome. Viral genes discussed in the text are indicated. BamHI restriction fragments are designated by letters and associated vertical bars. A variable number of terminal repeats are present at the ends of the genome. EBER, Epstein-Barr–encoded RNAs; EBNA, Epstein-Barr nuclear antigen; LMP, latent membrane protein. (Artwork courtesy of M. Victor Lemas.)

CD23. Members of the EBNA3 family (EBNA3A, 3B, 3C) have a common structure, origin, and function, in part by modulating the NOTCH signaling pathway. EBNA3A and 3C are required for immortalization, whereas EBNA3B is dispensable.

LMP1 is a member of the tumor necrosis factor receptor superfamily, most closely resembling CD40, an important B-cell activation receptor (27). LMP1 is an integral membrane protein with cytoplasmic amino terminus, cytoplasmic carboxyl terminus, and six hydrophobic transmembrane domains that spontaneously oligomerize, leading to constitutive aggregation and constitutive signaling in the absence of ligand (Fig. 46.3). *In vitro* expression is associated with transformation of immortalized rodent fibroblast cell lines, as marked by loss of contact inhibition, anchorage independent growth, and tumorigenesis in nude mice (28). In transgenic mice, expression under the control of an Ig heavy-chain regulatory locus leads to B-cell lymphomagenesis (29). Expression leads to rapid activation of stress-activated protein kinases; activation of NF-κB; induction of activation markers, including CD23, CD30, and CD40; induction of cell adhesion molecules, including ICAM-1 and LFA-3; induction of antiapoptotic genes, including BCL2; and induction of interleukin (IL) 6. LMP1 also recruits signaling adapter molecules that associate with specific regions (C-terminal activation regions, CTAR1 and CTAR2), including tumor necrosis factor receptor–associated factors (TRAF) 1, 2, and 3 and tumor necrosis factor receptor–associated death domain (TRADD) (30). In all of these regards, LMP1 resembles activated CD40. However, whereas activated CD40 also mediates TRAF degradation, LMP1 does not (31). AP-1 and Stats 1 and 3 are also activated. Strain variation, particularly in the carboxyl terminus, is well recognized, with some variants activating NF-κB more efficiently, whereas others activate AP-1 more efficiently.

Other Epstein-Barr Virus Latency Genes

Other Epstein-Barr virus genes are not required for lymphocyte immortalization but are expressed in immortalized lym-

phocytes and may play important roles in the viral life cycle and in tumorigenesis. LMP2A modulates the signaling pathways associated with the B-cell receptor complex such that neither B-cell receptor engagement by antigen nor the absence of such engagement is fatal to the virus-harboring B cell. B-cell receptor engagement normally leads to Ca_2^+ flux and would precipitate lytic replication (Ca_2^+ flux being a potent lytic cycle activator) and B-cell death. However, in the presence of LMP2A, B-cell receptor engagement does not lead to Ca_2^+ flux. Conversely, LMP2A also substitutes for a B-cell receptor–mediated survival signal such that, in a transgenic mouse model, expression of LMP2A prevents death of B cells lacking membrane Ig (31,32). Both properties may contribute to the survival of Epstein-Barr virus–infected B cells *in vivo* and to the survival of tumor cells expressing the protein. The Epstein-Barr–encoded RNAs 1 and 2 (EBERs) are the most abundant viral transcripts in Epstein-Barr virus–infected lymphocytes (33). These RNA polymerase III transcripts do not code for protein, and their function remains uncertain. In Burkitt's cells that have lost their viral episomes and associated malignant characteristics, reintroduction of the EBERs confers clonability in soft agarose, tumorigenicity in immunodeficient mice, resistance to apoptosis, and other growth properties (33,34). Other RNAs collectively referred to as the *BARTs* (*BamHI A right*-ward *t*ranscripts) are expressed in latently infected lymphocytes and in tumors (35,36). Transcription start sites and splicing patterns in this region are complex, and the proteins encoded and their functions remain poorly understood.

Epstein-Barr Virus Lytic Cycle Viral Genes

The lytic cycle is initiated by expression of the viral ZTA protein (Fig. 46.2) (37,38). This is a DNA-binding bZIP transcription factor whose expression initiates a cascade of events that leads to expression of delayed early genes and late genes and ultimately packaging and release of infectious virus. ZTA mediates viral DNA replication at the lytic origin

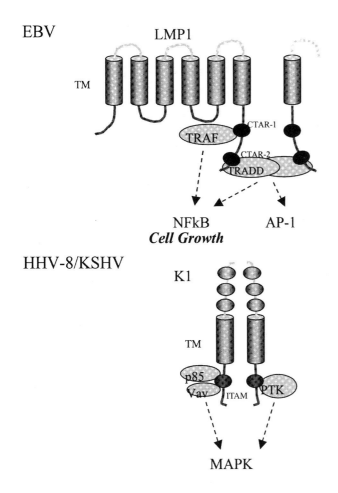

FIG. 46.3. Two gammaherpesvirus membrane proteins: latent membrane protein (LMP)-1 and K1. LMP1, an Epstein-Barr virus (EBV) protein, mediates intracellular signaling through interactions with signaling proteins TRAF (tumor necrosis factor receptor–associated factors) and TRADD (tumor necrosis factor receptor–associated death domain). NF-κB and AP-1 are activated. LMP1 is expressed in a variety of EBV-associated lymphomas, including a subset of posttransplant lymphomas, primary central nervous system lymphoma in acquired immunodeficiency syndrome patients, and Hodgkin's lymphoma. In a transgenic mouse model and in rodent cell lines, it is transforming. K1, a human herpesvirus-8/Kaposi's sarcoma–associated herpesvirus (HHV-8/KSHV) protein, also mediates intracellular signaling through immunoreceptor tyrosine-based activation motif (ITAM) that can bind signaling kinases (Vav, p85, and Syk) and protein tyrosine kinases (PTK) to mediate calcium mobilization and tyrosine phosphorylation. It is not known to be expressed in lymphomas or other malignancies. (Artwork courtesy of John Nicholas.)

of replication and induces cell-cycle arrest. Among the lytic genes encoded by the virus are three with homology to cellular genes implicated in tumorigenesis. These are viral BCL2 family members, BHRF1 and BALF1, and a viral

IL10 homolog BCRF1. BHRF1 shares functional properties with BCL2, whereas BALF1 appears to serve as an inhibitor of BHRF1 antiapoptotic activity (39). Insofar as the expression of the BCL2 family members is limited to lytically infected cells, any contributions to immortalization or maintenance of the malignant phenotype remain poorly understood. BCRF1 is presumed to modulate immune responses to viral infection. This is a function that presumably might impact on the ability of tumors to escape immune surveillance. However, there is very little evidence to date of expression by tumor cells (40). The synthesis of viral DNA and of the late proteins can be blocked with antiviral agents such as acyclovir and ganciclovir. These agents are phosphorylated by a viral kinase, and their phosphorylated products inhibit the viral DNA polymerase (41,42). However, the growth of the latently infected cells and replication of the episomal genome are not inhibited by these agents.

Epstein-Barr Virus Strain

Two viral strains or biotypes have been recognized. *In vitro* and in murine studies suggest that A strain or type 1 virus is more efficient in immortalization and transformation than the less common B strain (43). The A strain predominates in most studies of tumors. However, B-strain virus is detected in some African Burkitt's lymphoma and in tumors arising in homosexual acquired immunodeficiency syndrome (AIDS) patients (44–46). Whether A strain predominance in tumors reflects increased pathogenicity or just prevalence is not clear. Many variations in viral genes have been described, including variants in EBNA1 and LMP1 (47–49). However, there is little evidence for a high-risk strain.

Immune Response to Epstein-Barr Virus Infection

The humoral response is believed to have little impact on established latent infection, although neutralizing antibodies may play a role in interrupting the spread of infection. CD8+ T-cell responses to lytic antigens appear first; subsequently, responses to latency antigens emerge (13,50,51). Responses to EBNA3A, EBNA3B, and EBNA3C are the immunodominant responses to latency antigens across many HLA types. Transcripts for these antigens disappear from peripheral-blood mononuclear cells with the establishment of chronic infection in healthy seropositive individuals. The only infected cells that persist show limited antigen expression and may thus elude cytotoxic T cells (Fig. 46.1).

Animal Models of Epstein-Barr Virus Lymphomagenesis

A variety of animal models have provided insights into Epstein-Barr virus–associated tumorigenesis (52). Most Old World nonhuman primates harbor Epstein-Barr virus–like herpesviruses. Cross-reactive immunity protects against Epstein-Barr virus infection. However, in the setting of phar-

TABLE 46.2. *Epstein-Barr virus (EBV)–associated lymphoma*

Type of lymphoma	Comment on the association
Burkitt's lymphoma	Marked geographic variation in incidence and EBV association.
Posttransplant B-cell lymphoma	Lymphoma occurring early after transplant is almost always EBV associated.
Posttransplant T-cell lymphoma	Sometimes EBV associated.
Lymphomatoid granulomatosis	Always EBV associated.
Extranodal natural killer/T-cell lymphoma	Nasal type is always EBV associated, others are variably EBV associated.
Acquired immunodeficiency syndrome lymphoma	Approximately 50% EBV associated overall, but some subsets are much more strongly EBV associated such as primary central nervous system lymphomas, plasmablastic oral lymphoma, immunoblastic lymphomas, and primary effusion lymphoma.

macologic or viral immunosuppression, and perhaps other factors, lymphoproliferative disease with Epstein-Barr–like viruses may emerge (53,54). New World primates are naturally infected by more distant gammaherpesviruses (55). Inoculation of some of these primates with Epstein-Barr virus, notably tamarins, leads to B-cell lymphoproliferative disease, and vaccine studies have often focused on these animals (56–58). Mice with severe combined immunodeficiency develop Epstein-Barr virus–associated B-cell tumors after transfer of peripheral blood mononuclear cells from Epstein-Barr virus–seropositive donors or after transfer of peripheral blood mononuclear cells from Epstein-Barr virus–seronegative donors followed by inoculation with Epstein-Barr virus or simply transfer of Epstein-Barr virus–immortalized B-cell lines (20,59). In all of these models, whether primate or human engrafted into mouse, the lymphoproliferative disease is B cell, and patterns of viral gene expression resemble that seen in posttransplant lymphoproliferative disease. An interesting variation has been reported in rabbits in which an Epstein-Barr–like virus isolated from macaques leads to T-cell lymphomas (60). In addition to these models involving virus infection or reactivation, transgenic models of lymphomagenesis involving expression of viral genes (LMP1 and EBNA1) in B cells have been alluded to above (23,29).

Epstein-Barr Virus–Associated Lymphoma

Tumors of B-, T-, and natural killer–cell origin may all be Epstein-Barr virus associated (Table 46.2). Three characteristic patterns of viral gene expression in tumors have been recognized (Fig. 46.4). Burkitt's lymphoma shows the most restricted pattern, with only a single viral antigen expressed in most tumor cells (114,115). Hodgkin's lymphoma, some of the diffuse large B-cell lymphomas in immunodeficient patients, and extranodal natural killer/T-cell lymphomas express EBNA1 and the latency membrane antigens (LMP1 and 2) (112,116). Some posttransplant lymphomas and Epstein-Barr virus–associated AIDS lymphomas express the complete spectrum of latency antigens (56,61–64). Definitive determination of the presence of Epstein-Barr virus in tumor tissue requires *in situ* hybrid-

ization for the EBER transcripts or detection of viral antigens by immunohistochemistry. Because of variability of antigen expression in Epstein-Barr virus–associated lymphomas, the inability to detect particular viral antigens, such as LMP1 or EBNA2, should not be regarded as evidence that the lesion is not virus associated (65,66). Some Epstein-Barr virus–associated tumors, such as Burkitt's lymphoma, do not express any viral antigens other than EBNA1, and reagents to detect EBNA1 are not widely used because of lack of commercial availability and issues related to cross-reactivity. Specific lymphomas and their associations are discussed below.

Epstein-Barr virus association may be useful in facilitating diagnosis and guiding therapy. There is general agreement that the number of Epstein-Barr virus genomes in peripheral blood mononuclear cells is increased in association with posttransplant lymphoproliferative disease, although there is striking variability in absolute values in healthy seropositives across studies (5,79–83). Monitoring viral genome copy number has also been believed to be useful in monitoring response to therapy (83,84). However, for rituximab therapy at least, there is a very consistent decrease in viral copy number in cells even in patients whose tumors are progressing (5). Virus load has also been measured in whole blood, serum, or plasma (85–93). Cell-free DNA (plasma or serum) may reflect either the presence of infectious virus or the presence of DNA released by dying cells. Monitoring viral DNA in serum has been shown to be an important prognosticator in natural killer/T-cell lymphoma of the nasal type as well as in nasopharyngeal carcinoma (67,94,95).

Burkitt's Lymphoma

The frequency of the Epstein-Barr virus association is highest in equatorial Africa. Chromosome translocations involving the C-MYC locus on chromosome 8 and an Ig locus, most commonly the heavy-chain locus on chromosome 14, are found in both endemic and sporadic Burkitt's lymphoma. However, characteristic break points differ between endemic and sporadic tumors and perhaps between Epstein-Barr virus–positive and Epstein-Barr virus–negative tumors (68).

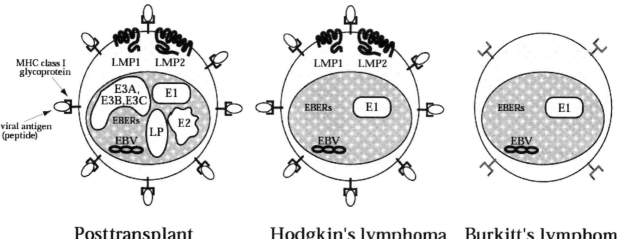

FIG. 46.4. Viral gene expression in three types of lymphoma. Posttransplant lymphoproliferative disease is often associated with expression of the full range of viral latency antigens expressed in immortalized B cells. Hodgkin's lymphoma is associated with a more restricted pattern. Burkitt's lymphoma is associated with the most restricted pattern. In Burkitt's lymphoma, major histocompatibility complex (MHC) class I molecules are often downregulated, and antigens are not processed for presentation. EBER, Epstein-Barr–encoded RNAs; EBV, Epstein-Barr virus; LMP, latent membrane protein. (Artwork courtesy of M. Victor Lemas.)

The role of Epstein-Barr virus in these tumors remains uncertain (69). EBNA1 is the only viral protein consistently expressed in these tumors, although rare cells expressing other latency antigens or lytic antigens have been described (70). In addition, LMP2 RNA is detected (71). Experiments with a Burkitt's cell line (Akata) suggest that loss of the episome is associated with loss of the malignant phenotype (72,73). When recombinant viral genes were engineered into the cells that have lost their viral episomes and their tumorigenicity, the EBERs and EBNA1 restored tumorigenicity, whereas EBNA1 alone did not (34,72,73). The genesis of the very restricted viral gene expression phenotype in Burkitt's lymphoma has been the source of much speculation. Does the restricted pattern of viral gene expression reflect viral gene regulation in germinal-center cells or does the tumor arise from lymphoblastoid B cells expressing the full spectrum of latency antigens after some sort of selection process? Recently, a subset of Burkitt's tumors have been described in which a deletion of the EBNA2 gene has occurred consistent with a selection process (74). Antagonism between the effects of high-level C-MYC expression and EBNA2 expression has been noted; thus, silencing of EBNA2 may be critical to the pathogenesis of the tumor (75).

Although the tumor harbors viral genomes, it is remarkably impervious to CD8+ T-cell immune surveillance. This resistance is a consequence of several factors, including lack of expression of immunodominant viral proteins and lack of antigen-processing machinery (76). Downregulation of antigen-processing machinery is a consequence of high-level c-myc expression even in the absence of any immune selection (77).

Burkitt's lymphomas occurring outside the endemic region of Africa are only variably (25% to 80%) associated with virus (78,79). The determinants of virus association remain essentially unknown but must not be simply immunodeficiency insofar as only a minority of human immunodeficiency virus–associated Burkitt's lymphomas are Epstein-Barr virus associated (80). Strain differences have been recognized, but present evidence suggests that many of these reflect the predominant viral subtype in a given population. The possibility has been considered that Epstein-Barr virus may contribute to the pathogenesis of sporadic tumors but be lost from the malignant clone (81). Fragments of the viral genome have been reported in Burkitt's from nonendemic regions in tumors that, by standard pathologic screens (e.g., EBER *in situ* hybridization), would have been missed (82).

Natural Killer/T-Cell Lymphoma and Leukemia

Extranodal natural killer/T-cell tumors have been classified into nasal, intestinal, and subcutaneous panniculitis-like (83). Each may be Epstein-Barr virus associated, with anatomic site and geography both affecting the degree of association. Natural killer/T-cell lymphomas of the nasal type are a group of aggressive malignancies that express CD56. Most common in Asia, nasal tumors are almost always associated with Epstein-Barr virus (84–89). The pattern of viral gene expression is similar to that in Epstein-Barr virus–associated Hodgkin's disease (i.e., EBNA1, LMP1, and LMP2 are expressed but not EBNA2, 3A, 3B, or 3C) (90). Epstein-Barr virus is also present in most cases of natural killer–cell leukemia, and the presence of virus is one of the features that distinguishes it from a more indolent natural killer–cell lymphoproliferative disorder (91–93).

Lymphoma Arising in the Setting of Immunodeficiency

Congenital immunodeficiencies associated with lymphoproliferative diseases include severe combined immunodeficiency, ataxia-telangiectasia, Wiskott-Aldrich syndrome, hyper IgM syndrome, and X-linked lymphoproliferative disease (94–98). Epstein-Barr virus infection in such patients may manifest as fatal infectious mononucleosis, dysgammaglobulinemia, and lymphoma. Types of Epstein-Barr–associated lymphoma associated with congenital immunodeficiency include diffuse large B-cell lymphoma, including primary central nervous system lymphoma; Burkitt's lymphoma; polymorphic lymphoproliferations resembling those seen in the posttransplant setting; and Epstein-Barr virus–associated Hodgkin's lymphoma. Some lymphomas in congenital immunodeficiency syndromes, notably ataxia-telangiectasia but even in X-linked lymphoproliferative disease, are not Epstein-Barr virus associated.

Organ and marrow transplantations are also associated with lymphoproliferative disease (99–107). Depending on the organ transplanted, the immunosuppressive regimen, and patient characteristics (age, whether the recipient has previously been exposed to Epstein-Barr virus), approximately 0.5% to 10% of organ transplant recipients develop posttransplantation lymphoproliferative disorders. Categories of lymphoproliferative disease include plasmacytic hyperplasia (often a manifestation of primary Epstein-Barr virus infection in the posttransplant period), polymorphic B-cell posttransplant lymphoproliferative disease, and monomorphic posttransplant lymphoproliferative disease (108–111). The latter includes diffuse large B-cell lymphoma, Burkitt's or Burkitt-like lymphoma, plasma-cell myeloma, plasmacytoma, and some peripheral T-cell lymphomas. Epstein-Barr virus is associated with B-cell lymphoproliferative disease in this setting, with the exception of lesions that occur very late after transplantation. A subset of the T-cell lymphomas is also Epstein-Barr virus associated. Hodgkin's lymphoma is also increased in transplant recipients and is consistently Epstein-Barr virus associated. The observation that some cases of posttransplant proliferation regress if immunosuppression is withdrawn or reduced and that others regress with adoptive cellular therapy suggests that lack of immune surveillance plays a critical role in the pathogenesis of these lesions (112–114). When immune approaches fail, this may reflect resistance to cytotoxic T cells, which may result from downregulation or deletion of immunodominant Epstein-Barr virus genes commonly targeted by cytotoxic T cells, acquisition of new genetic lesions, or both (108,115).

Human immunodeficiency virus infection is associated with lymphomagenesis, and this is often Epstein-Barr virus associated. Particular anatomic sites and particular histologies show especially strong Epstein-Barr virus associations. Thus, primary central nervous system lymphomas in AIDS patients are virtually always Epstein-Barr virus associated

(116,117). Similarly, lymphomas that involve the central nervous system in AIDS patients are usually Epstein-Barr virus associated (118). Diffuse large B-cell lymphomas with immunoblastic features, primary effusion lymphomas, plasmablastic oral lymphomas, and Hodgkin's lymphomas also are usually Epstein-Barr virus associated (119–124). Epstein-Barr virus–associated diffuse large B-cell lymphomas with immunoblastic features in AIDS patients often express the full spectrum of Epstein-Barr virus latency genes and are similar to posttransplant lymphoma in this regard. In contrast, primary effusion lymphomas show a highly restricted pattern of Epstein-Barr virus gene expression, most closely resembling the pattern of expression seen in Burkitt's lymphoma.

A variety of other lymphomas have Epstein-Barr virus associations, perhaps reflecting immune dysfunction. These include lymphomas arising in association with the use of methotrexate, lymphomas arising in association with chronic suppuration, and lymphomatoid granulomatosis (125–127).

Aspects of Kaposi's Sarcoma–Associated Herpesvirus Infection

Human herpesvirus-8/Kaposi's sarcoma–associated herpesvirus was discovered in association with Kaposi's sarcoma. Serologic evidence of viral infection is most common in homosexual men and in certain southern European, Mediterranean, and African populations (128). The mode of transmission is poorly understood. *In vivo*, the virus is found in B cells, endothelial cells, epithelial cells, and macrophages.

The latency genes of the virus include LANA, vIRF3, v-cyclin, K15, and the T0.7 transcript (129–137). Several of these have properties that suggest they might contribute to tumorigenesis. LANA, in addition to tethering the viral episome to chromatin, interacts with cellular transcriptional regulatory proteins, including p53, Rb, and components of the SAP30 corepressor complex, to bring about alterations in increased cell survival and proliferation. LANA also sequesters glycogen synthase kinase 3 in the nucleus, resulting in elevated levels of β catenin, which promotes cell proliferation. K15 is a transmembrane protein predicted to interact with signaling proteins and, like LMP2 of Epstein-Barr virus, to interrupt B-cell receptor signal transduction. The T0.7 transcripts are incompletely understood but code for kaposin A, a protein that leads to focus formation, anchorage-independent growth, and tumorigenicity in immortalized murine cell lines (138). Some of its effects are mediated through its association with cytohesin-1, a guanine nucleotide exchange factor, which regulates integrin activity. In fact, a dominant-negative cytohesin-1 inhibited kaposin A–induced focus formation and restored normal actin organization. vIRF3 is expressed only in B cells and binds to and inhibits the apoptotic activity of p53 and interferes with cellular IRFs (139,140).

An IL6 homolog, vIL6, is encoded by the virus (141). The viral cytokine is similar in its actions to IL6 but differs in the details. For example, cells that express only gp130 (one of two subunits that bind human IL6) respond to vIL6. Expression is increased after lytic cycle induction. The viral genome encodes a multitude of other proteins that are expressed in productive lytic infection that have properties that suggest a possible role in transformation. Among these are K1, a transmembrane protein with a functional immunoreceptor tyrosine-based activation motif that can bind several signaling kinases to mediate calcium mobilization and tyrosine phosphorylation. The gene substitutes for a herpesvirus saimirii–transforming gene in a marmoset lymphoma model, transforms murine fibroblast lines *in vitro*, and leads to tumorigenesis in transgenic mice (142,143). However, there is no evidence that it is actually expressed in lymphoma, so any contribution to transformation remains highly speculative.

Kaposi's Sarcoma–Associated Herpesvirus–Associated Lymphoma

Primary effusion lymphoma occurs mainly, but not exclusively, in patients with human immunodeficiency virus infection and involves body cavities and extranodal sites. These cells are typically dually infected with human herpesvirus-8/Kaposi's sarcoma–associated herpesvirus and with Epstein-Barr virus, but only infected cells of human herpesvirus-8/Kaposi's sarcoma–associated herpesvirus have been described (144). The cells are monoclonal with Ig gene rearrangement but express few of the usual markers of B-cell differentiation. No consistent cytogenetic abnormality is identified. The full spectrum of viral latency proteins noted above is expressed, including vIRF3. Lytic gene expression is present in a small population of cells (145,146). vIL6 is detected in a higher fraction of tumor cells than other lytic gene products, and the possibility has been raised that vIL6 can be expressed without lytic induction (147,148). vIL6 can be detected by enzyme-linked immunosorbent assay in some malignant effusions at levels believed to be of biologic significance (149).

Multicentric Castleman's disease is often associated with human herpesvirus-8/Kaposi's sarcoma–associated herpesvirus, particularly in patients with human immunodeficiency virus infection and in transplant patients (150,151). Immunohistochemistry and *in situ* hybridization show the presence of virus in the B cells of the follicular mantle. These cells express LANA, vIRF3, vIL6, vIRF1, and vGCR (147,152). This pattern of gene expression is less restrictive than that seen in primary effusion lymphoma or in Kaposi's sarcoma.

HUMAN RETROVIRUSES

The discovery of the two human retroviruses implicated in human malignancy, human adult T-cell leukemia/lymphoma virus 1 and human immunodeficiency virus type 1, followed clinical characterization of associated disease. Thus, the description of the syndrome of adult T-cell leukemia/lymphoma and its peculiar geographic clustering in 1977 led to the study of T-cell lymphoblastoid cell lines and peripheral T cells harboring human adult T-cell leukemia/lymphoma virus 1 (153–156). Similarly, recognition of the syndrome of acquired immunodeficiency, including the increased incidence of high-grade B-cell lymphomas in homosexual men, led to culture and characterization of human immunodeficiency virus type 1.

Since the early 1900s, retroviruses have been known to be associated with malignancies in animals. Acutely transforming retroviruses induce tumors within days of infection. These viruses carry *onc* genes derived from cellular genes often in place of the viral genes. Expression of the *onc* genes leads to transformation of infected cells, whereas the loss of required viral genes renders them replication defective, except in the presence of a helper virus, which supplies required functions. Although these viruses integrate as part of their life cycle, the site of integration is not important to their ability to transform. Chronically transforming retroviruses produce tumors slowly. They lack an *onc* gene but transform by integration of the viral genome near key cellular genes (insertional mutagenesis). Thus, the site of integration is central to their role in transformation. The study of acute and chronic transforming retroviruses has led to many insights into the molecular biology of tumorigenesis, but neither of these general mechanisms of transformation appear to be involved with human retroviruses and their associated tumors.

Thus human adult T-cell leukemia/lymphoma virus 1 leads to the development of malignancy only after a latency period of decades and in less than 5% of infected individuals (157). There is no targeted integration site or sites that are crucial to tumorigenesis, although a preference for A/T-rich sequences has been suggested (158). Malignant cells carry the human adult T-cell leukemia/lymphoma virus 1 genome, but it is largely silent. Human immunodeficiency virus type 1 also leads to malignancy only in a minority of infected individuals and typically after years of infection. Even more distant from the established animal models of acute and chronic transforming retroviruses than human adult T-cell leukemia/lymphoma virus 1, human immunodeficiency virus is generally not even present in the tumors it engenders. For both viruses, malignancy is a complex multistep process.

Retroviruses consist of two identical, plus-sense single-stranded RNA molecules that are noncovalently linked. Viral proteins include coat proteins encoded by the ENV gene, nonglycosylated core proteins encoded by the GAG gene, and nonstructural proteins encoded by the POL gene. The latter include the reverse transcriptase and Rnase H, which together generate double-stranded circular proviral DNA from single-stranded viral RNA, the viral integrase that mediates integration of the proviral DNA into the host genome, and the protease, which processes large precursor polyproteins.

Human retroviruses include both endogenous and exogenous viruses. There are 100 to 1,000 copies of endogenous human retroviruses in the genome. These persist as genetic elements in chromosomal DNA. Most have defects or have become pseudogenes. However, some are complete viruses.

None of the endogenous human retroviruses is known to be associated with malignancy. The exogenous retroviruses, in contrast, are horizontally transmitted and include both of the human retroviruses associated with malignancy.

In addition to the core proteins, envelope proteins, and reverse transcriptase encoded by other retroviruses, these retroviruses encode other proteins. Human adult T-cell leukemia/lymphoma virus 1 belongs to a group of retroviruses that includes human adult T-cell leukemia/lymphoma virus 2, simian T-cell lymphotropic viruses, and bovine leukemia virus (159). These viruses encode regulatory proteins tax and rex. Human immunodeficiency virus type 1 and human immunodeficiency virus type 2 are lentiviruses. These viruses encode additional open reading frames involved in regulatory functions, particularly related to protein synthesis.

After cell entry, reverse transcriptase within the viral capsid initiates synthesis of DNA from plus-sense RNA. The RNA is displaced, and the DNA is used as a template to generate a complementary DNA strand. The double-stranded proviral DNA is ultimately transported into the nucleus. Then the viral integrase (also carried within the virion) mediates integration into the host genome. This process is not site specific. Both viruses establish lifelong infection.

Aspects of Human Adult T-Cell Leukemia/Lymphoma Virus 1 Infection

Human adult T-cell leukemia/lymphoma virus 1 is endemic in parts of southwestern Japan, the Caribbean basin, sub-Saharan Africa, South America, and the southeastern United States. Worldwide, an estimated 10 to 20 million people are infected. In the highest prevalence endemic areas, up to 15% of normal blood donors are infected, whereas in nonendemic areas, less than 1% are positive. Transmission is believed to require infected cells, as little, if any, cell-free virus is found in plasma (160). Virus-infected cells may be transmitted in breast milk or in semen. Sexual transmission rarely occurs from female to male. The virus is associated with human adult T-cell leukemia/lymphoma virus 1–associated myelopathy and tropical spastic paraparesis as well as other inflammatory illnesses in addition to adult T-cell leukemia/lymphoma (161–163).

Human adult T-cell leukemia/lymphoma virus 1 infection is believed to require infected allogeneic cells, insofar as there is no evidence of cell-free virus in vivo (164). Similarly, in vitro viral-cell entry usually requires direct cell-to-cell interactions such as cocultivation of irradiated virus-producing cells with target cells. Free virus has very little infectivity. Evidence has been presented that a protein encoded by chromosome 17 functions as a viral receptor (165). A wide variety of cell types may be infected, but most proviral DNA in peripheral blood mononuclear cells is found in CD4+ T cells. Little or no cell-free virus is present in plasma.

Infected CD4+ T cells typically contain a single integrated provirus (166). Proliferation of these cells is driven by the tax protein. The genetic stability of the viral genome (in contrast to human immunodeficiency virus type 1) is one piece of evidence in favor of the interpretation that expansion of proviral DNA is mainly mediated by cellular proliferation rather than viral replication. Cellular replication of integrated proviral DNA involves proofreading, whereas the viral reverse transcriptase lacks proofreading and is highly error prone. Clonal expansion of infected T cells results in an increase in proviral DNA load.

These infected cells engender a very active cytotoxic T-cell response against targeting the tax protein, and up to 10% of CD8+ T cells may target a single tax epitope (167,168). Tax-expressing cells are efficiently killed (169). Ultimately, this includes CD8+ T cells specific for human adult T-cell leukemia/lymphoma virus 1 targets. Activation of CD8+ T cells specific for human adult T-cell leukemia/lymphoma virus 1 by human adult T-cell leukemia/lymphoma virus 1–infected CD4+ T cells or dendritic cells enhances their susceptibility to human adult T-cell leukemia/lymphoma virus 1 infection. Human adult T-cell leukemia/lymphoma virus 1–specific CD8+ T cells thus become infected, making them targets for a fratricidal immune response (169). Resulting specific immune impairment may contribute to viral persistence.

Viral messenger RNA is detectable only at low levels in peripheral blood mononuclear cells, probably reflecting the powerful cytotoxic T-cell response and resultant short half-life of tax-expressing cells (170,171).

Tax

The Px region at the 3' end of the genome encodes tax, rex, and other regulatory proteins. Both tax and rex regulate expression of viral genes. Tax transactivates the viral long terminal repeat. Rex permits the accumulation of unspliced gag messenger RNA and efficient expression of GAG gene products. Tax also transactivates cellular genes, including transcription factors, lymphokines, and their receptors (166,172). Among genes and pathways affected are many involved in T-cell differentiation, proliferation, and cell-cycle regulation. These include the NF-κB pathway and serum response factor (SRF)- and activating transcription factor/cyclic AMP responsive element binding protein (ATF/CREB)-responsive genes. Tax also interacts with CDK4, leading to the phosphorylation of the Rb protein (173).

In parallel with its effects on cell cycling, tax also interferes with cellular DNA repair pathways. It inhibits the human mitotic checkpoint protein (MAD1) and competes with p53 for p300/CBP binding, interfering with the DNA-damage sentinel checkpoint at the G1 to S junction (173–175).

Animal Models

Human adult T-cell leukemia/lymphoma virus 1 infection has been studied in rabbit, rat, and nonhuman primate (marmoset, cynomolgus, and squirrel monkey) models (164,176–180). These models have been used to study transmission, viral replication and persistence, and protection conferred by vaccines.

Tax has been studied in several murine transgenic models (181–183). When expressed from the human granzyme B promoter, tax protein leads to peripheral lymphomas consisting of CD8⁺ T cells and natural killer cells. These tumors express high levels of NF-κB, and their proliferation is blocked by sodium salicylate and cyclopentenone prostaglandins.

Human Adult T-Cell Leukemia/Lymphoma Virus 1 and Lymphoma

Only human adult T-cell leukemia/lymphoma virus 1 infection at birth or in infancy is associated with adult T-cell leukemia/lymphoma (184). Acquisition in adulthood is not by blood transfusion, injection drug use, or sexual contact. Present evidence suggests a multistage process requiring decades.

The process likely begins with oligoclonal expansions of virus-infected cells. As suggested above, the tax protein must play a critical role in driving these expansions, which can be readily demonstrated by virtue of unique proviral integration sites in peripheral blood mononuclear cells of infected patients (166). The frequency of abundant circulating clones varies among patient populations, with the highest frequency in adult T-cell leukemia/lymphoma patients, an intermediate frequency in human adult T-cell leukemia/lymphoma virus 1–associated myelopathy and tropical spastic paraparesis patients, and the lowest frequency in asymptomatic carriers.

The determinants of progression are largely unknown, but a variety of cellular genetic lesions, including inactivation of tumor-suppressor genes and aneuploidy, have been identified in adult T-cell leukemia/lymphoma (185,186). These may in part reflect viral interference with cellular pathways involved in DNA repair and chromosomal segregation during clonal expansion (174,185,187). A defect in the mitotic spindle assembly checkpoint may not only explain progression to malignancy but also poor responses to chemotherapy with microtubule inhibitors (185).

Immune escape for tumor clones also seems likely to be important. Four mechanisms have been discussed: downregulation of viral gene expression, downregulation of MHC class I molecules, mutations or deletions in the tax protein eliminating targeted epitopes, and T-cell deficiency possibly reflecting T-cell fratricide (169,188–190).

The possibility has also been raised that strongyloidiasis is a cofactor in the development of adult T-cell leukemia/lymphoma (166). Both *Strongyloides stercoralis* and human adult T-cell leukemia/lymphoma virus 1 are endemic in the same regions. Proviral load is higher in peripheral blood mononuclear cells from patients with dual infection than in those with human adult T-cell leukemia/lymphoma virus 1 alone. The incidence of strongyloidiasis in Martinique in the French West Indies is greater in adult T-cell leukemia/lymphoma patients than in asymptomatic human adult T-cell leukemia/lymphoma virus 1 carriers, and the incubation period for adult T-cell leukemia/lymphoma may be shortened in patients with *S. stercoralis* infection.

Aspects of Human Immunodeficiency Virus Type 1 Infection

Human immunodeficiency virus type 1 infection is worldwide but is endemic in central Africa. Human immunodeficiency virus type 2 is a related virus that is most closely akin to simian immunodeficiency virus and is found in West Africa. Both cause AIDS. In nonendemic regions, human immunodeficiency virus is found mainly in homosexual and bisexual men, injection drug users, transfusion recipients, sexual partners of infected people, and infants born to infected mothers. Sexual contact, blood exposure, and perinatal exposure are all modes of transmission. After infection, there is a slow progressive depletion of CD4⁺ T cells. Progressive immunodeficiency is associated with opportunistic infections and malignancies.

The human immunodeficiency virus genome is similar to the human adult T-cell leukemia/lymphoma virus in that it encodes regulatory tat and rev proteins analogous to tax and rex. In addition, it encodes at least four regulatory proteins: nef, vif, vpu, and vpr. Human immunodeficiency virus infects CD4⁺ T cells, monocytes, macrophages, follicular dendritic cells, and a variety of neural, glial, and intestinal cells. CD4 and a chemokine receptor, CCR5 or CXCR4, are required for cellular entry. CCR5 mutations are rare but when homozygous are protective from human immunodeficiency virus infection.

In contrast to human adult T-cell leukemia/lymphoma virus 1, viral infection typically results in cell lysis, with budding of huge numbers of virions from the cell surface, releasing free virus. Infected CD4⁺ T cells die rather than proliferate. Thus, replication of the viral genome is solely via the reverse transcriptase, and host cell polymerases play no role. As a consequence, there is considerable genomic variation and antigenic heterogeneity, even in isolates obtained from individuals over the course of their infection. Human immunodeficiency virus infection is associated with polyclonal B-cell activation and hypergammaglobulinemia (191). The role of human immunodeficiency virus infection of B cells in mediating these phenomena remains poorly understood (192). However, B-cell stimulatory activity has been attributed to the nef protein and to gp41 (193,194).

Human Immunodeficiency Virus and Lymphoma

Human immunodeficiency virus–associated lymphoma is seen in all populations of human immunodeficiency virus–infected people worldwide (195–197). Predominantly aggressive B-cell lymphomas, their occurrence has been incorporated into the definition of clinical AIDS and accounts for approximately 3% of clinical AIDS cases in the United States (198). The incidence of lymphoma is increased approximately 1% annually in human immunodeficiency virus–infected individuals in recent data (199,200).

The lymphomas that are seen in association with human immunodeficiency virus infection are heterogeneous. They include Burkitt's lymphoma, diffuse large B-cell lymphoma, primary effusion lymphoma, plasmablastic lymphoma of the oral cavity, and Hodgkin's lymphoma. In the era before highly active antiretroviral therapy, primary central nervous system lymphoma occurred with a 3,600-fold greater incidence among people with a diagnosis of AIDS than in the general population (201). With the advent of highly active antiretroviral therapy, the incidence of primary central nervous system lymphoma and perhaps some other lymphomas in AIDS patients appears to have decreased (199,200,202,203).

Lymphomagenesis, in the setting of human immunodeficiency virus infection, is complex and multifactorial. Although most tumors are monoclonal, oligoclonal and polyclonal tumors have been reported, highlighting the complexity of the pathogenesis (204,205). Viral cofactors must contribute to pathogenesis insofar as approximately 50% of these tumors are Epstein-Barr virus associated. Still other lymphomas, the primary effusion lymphomas, are associated with both Epstein-Barr virus and Kaposi's sarcoma–associated herpesvirus/human herpesvirus-8 or the latter alone (3). And others, notably Burkitt's lymphoma, are not generally Epstein-Barr virus associated (80). Immunocompromise must be an important contributing factor, and it is worth noting that in patients with marked CD4$^+$ T-cell lymphopenia, lymphomas resemble posttransplant lymphoproliferative disease in that they are usually extranodal and Epstein-Barr virus associated, with broad expression of Epstein-Barr virus latency genes (206). However, other AIDS–associated lymphomas are not associated with marked CD4$^+$ T-cell lymphopenia (207,208).

Little evidence suggests that human immunodeficiency virus directly infects malignant clones of B cells and human immunodeficiency virus proviral DNA is rarely found in tumors. The precise role that human immunodeficiency virus type 1 plays, particularly in the lymphomas that do not carry Epstein-Barr virus, is not well characterized. Chronic antigenic stimulation is often presumed to be a contributing factor. Evidence in support of the idea comes from the observation that B-cell activation, hypergammaglobulinemia, and generalized lymphadenopathy commonly precede lymphoma development (209). In patients with paraproteins, monoclonal IgG κ paraproteins that specifically recognize the human immunodeficiency virus type 1 p24 gag antigen have been identified. However, in a recent study, lymphoma-derived Ig genes from AIDS-related lymphomas were assayed for AIDS reactivity, and none of the tumor-related Igs bound to human immunodeficiency virus proteins. (210).

HEPATITIS C VIRUS

Studies of transmission of parenterally acquired hepatitis to chimpanzees led to the identification of the hepatitis C virus, an enveloped single-stranded positive-sense RNA of approximately 10 kb (211,212). Infection is usually asymptomatic or mild, but up to 70% of infected individuals show chronic active hepatitis, cirrhosis, or both, and approxi-

mately 20% progress to chronic liver disease. Hepatitis C infection has emerged as the leading cause of liver transplantation in the United States and as an important cause of hepatoma worldwide. Recognition of an impact of hepatitis C on B-cell proliferative disease began with the observation that hepatitis C is also the leading cause of mixed cryoglobulinemia (213,214). Mixed cryoglobulinemia was known to evolve to B-cell lymphoma on occasion, and evidence for an association with B-cell lymphomas, even in patients without mixed cryoglobulinemia, followed (215,216).

Aspects of Hepatitis C Infection

Hepatitis C is similar in many regards to members of the *Flavivirus* genus of arthropod-borne viruses. However, there is no evidence of arthropod-borne transmission. Indeed, natural routes of transmission remain unknown. Seropositives usually have a history of intravenous drug use, transfusion, or other parenteral exposure. Neither sexual nor perinatal transmission appears to be common. The overall prevalence worldwide is approximately 3% and appears to variously reflect unsafe injections, unsafe uses of medical equipment, and injection drug use (217).

Hepatitis C virus is a single-stranded RNA virus that encodes no DNA intermediate and is not capable of integrating into host cell DNA (Fig. 46.5). Because the intact virus does not replicate efficiently in any tissue culture system, aspects of its molecular biology have often been inferred but not demonstrated directly. A single open reading frame is translated to yield a polyprotein of approximately 3,000 amino acids. This is processed to yield a nucleocapsid protein, two envelope glycoproteins (E1 and E2), and nonstructural proteins that include a helicase/protease and a replicase (RNA-dependent RNA polymerase). Both glycoproteins include hypervariable regions. Viral entry is poorly understood, but low density lipoprotein receptors and CD81 are candidate viral receptors (218,219). Recently, evidence has emerged that hepatitis C can infect B cells *in vivo* and *in vitro* (220). Six genotypes have been identified worldwide based on nucleic acid sequence variation throughout the viral genome (221). Within isolates, quasispecies emerge, reflecting accumulation of mutations during viral replication in a host.

Humoral immune responses in hepatitis C–infected patients predominantly target the E2 protein, with antibodies against this protein being detected in 88% of the chronically infected. The hypervariable region of E2 has been compared to the V3 loop of the human immunodeficiency virus because of the rapid mutation in this region, suggesting immune selection. One manifestation of the humoral response in some individuals is type II mixed cryoglobulinemia, a systemic vasculitis characterized by deposition of immune complexes in blood vessel walls (213,222). The complexes consist of a monoclonal IgM (typically κ) with specificity for IgG, polyclonal IgG with specificity for hepatitis C antigens, and hepatitis C antigens themselves.

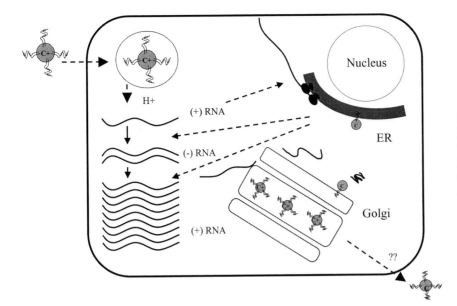

FIG. 46.5. Hepatitis C life cycle. Hepatitis C binds to receptors and is endocytosed. The viral RNA is translated to synthesize a viral polyprotein that is cleaved to yield the nucleocapsid protein, glycoproteins, and nonstructural replication proteins, including an RNA-dependent RNA polymerase. Many copies of the original positive strand RNA are made. Messenger RNA is transported into the proteins of the viral envelope. The capsid assembles around the viral RNA and the virus buds from the host membrane. ER, endoplasmic reticulum.

Hepatitis C and Lymphoma

Splenic and nodal marginal zone lymphomas have been most commonly linked to hepatitis C (216,223–225). Epidemiologic evidence in favor of the association comes from Italy, Southern California, and Japan, where the prevalence of hepatitis C infection among patients with B-cell lymphoma is 9% to 32%. Although the epidemiologic evidence is clearest for low-grade lymphomas, higher grade lymphomas may also be hepatitis C associated.

One explanation for the association of hepatitis C with lymphoma relates to chronic antigenic stimulation. Evidence in support of this idea comes from the observations suggesting that lymphoma cell proliferation is antigen driven. A restricted V gene repertoire (VH1-69 and Vκ3-A27) is common to human monoclonal antibodies established from hepatitis C carriers, mixed cryoglobulinemia, and hepatitis C–associated lymphoma (226,227). The restricted Ig gene usage is all the more striking, given that it differentiates hepatitis C–associated marginal zone lymphomas from other marginal zone lymphomas (228). In hepatitis C–associated lymphomas, there is homology in the CDR3 regions consistent with response to a common epitope, and, in at least one case, Ig rescued from hepatitis C–associated lymphoma was shown to bind a conserved epitope of the E2 glycoprotein (229). Further evidence comes from studies of patients with hepatitis C treated with antiviral therapy. Patients without clinically evident lymphoma but with clonally expanded B cells, as detected by polymerase chain reaction analysis, were treated with interferon-α alone or in combination with ribavirin. In 77% of patients with monoclonal IgH rearrangement and 86% of patients with t(14;18), these polymerase chain reaction markers of clonality disappeared, an effect that was closely associated with hepatitis C virus clearance (230). In a series of patients with splenic lymphoma with villous lymphocytes, tumor regression followed the disappear-

ance of viral RNA in 10 of 11 patients treated with interferon or interferon and ribavirin (231,232). However, polymerase chain reaction assays showed persistence of clonal B cells.

Whether antigen and antigen variation are sufficient for lymphomagenesis or whether there must be another sort of interaction between virus and B cells is not clear. The possibility has been raised that hepatitis C might engage the CD19/CD21/CD81 complex as well as the B-cell receptor. Dual engagement might reduce the threshold for B-cell activation and proliferation (229,233). Alternatively, hepatitis C may directly infect B cells and modulate relevant pathways (220). The hepatitis C core protein and the nonstructural protein NS3 have been reported to transform cells in tissue culture, cooperate with other genes in transforming cells, or lead to malignancy when expressed as transgenes in mice (234–236).

SV40 AND POLYOMAVIRUSES

Other DNA viruses have well-documented transforming properties and may play a role in lymphomagenesis. Possible links with polyomaviruses and particularly SV40 with human lymphoma have recently attracted attention (237–240). Polyomaviruses are commonly transforming in animals that are not their natural hosts. Viral proteins (tumor or "T" antigens) lead to an alteration in cell cycle. In cells from species that are not permissive for viral replication, progeny virus are not produced, and the cells that harbor these cell-cycle perturbing viral genes are not killed by viral lysis, resulting in transformation. A similar circumstance is created when T antigens are expressed in transgenic mice. The antigens are transforming, with the affected cell type being largely dependent on the promoter used to express them. Investigation of the mechanisms involved has provided important insights into processes of tumorigenesis and cell-cycle control, particularly with regard to tumor-suppressor genes. Viral DNA in tumors may persist in episomes or may integrate (241). Integration is nonspecific and does not involve a viral integrase. SV40 is transforming for lymphocytes *in vitro* and is associated with lymphoma among other tumors in rodents. In this setting, the viral genome is present in all tumor cells (241).

Possible mass cross-species infection might have been a consequence of the poliovirus vaccination program. Before 1963, SV40-contaminated tissue cultures were used to grow the poliovirus used in vaccines. A direct link has been reported in two recent polymerase chain reaction–based studies that identified SV40 T antigen sequences in 43% and 42% of lymphomas (238,239). However, a study of lymphoma specimens from Italy and Spain using polymerase chain reaction with the sensitivity to detect ten copies of the viral genome in 200,000 genome equivalents detected SV40 sequences much less commonly and never detected both right and left ends of the genome in lymphoma (240). The discrepancies are not readily attributed to geographic differences because contaminated polio vaccines were distributed in the United States and southern Europe over similar periods. Thus, at present, the role that SV40 plays in lymphomagenesis remains uncertain.

HELICOBACTER AND OTHER BACTERIAL INFECTION

The discovery of the association between *H. pylori* and peptic ulcer disease was initially greeted with skepticism but ultimately led to a profound change in thinking about the etiology of peptic ulcer disease and its treatment. Before the contribution of *H. pylori* was recognized, chemical neutralization of acidity was the major therapeutic objective. Afterward, eradication of infection was the therapeutic objective. Similarly, in gastric lymphoma, standard cytotoxic chemotherapy or radiation therapy approaches have given way to antibiotics. The success of antibiotics in treating malignancy has reinvigorated efforts to identify infectious agents associated with other lymphomas and has broadened the spectrum of infectious agents under consideration beyond viral agents.

Helicobacter were linked with gastric lymphoma by a series of observations. It was noted that mucosa-associated lymphoid tissue (MALT) was seen in the stomachs of patients with *Helicobacter* infection but not in the stomachs of uninfected individuals (242,243). In a nested case-control study, patients with gastric lymphoma were significantly more likely than matched controls to have evidence of previous *H. pylori* infection, as assessed by serology (244). The importance of the association was reinforced by the observation that the organism was present in most gastric lymphomas, with the association being strongest in early lesions and the observation that treatment with antibiotics to eradicate *Helicobacter* resulted in regression of a majority of such tumors (245). As with each of the other infectious agents linked to lymphoma, only a small fraction of those infected

progress to lymphoma, underscoring that this evolution is a complex multistep process.

Aspects of *Helicobacter* Infection

Helicobacter are microaerophilic, nonsporulating, gram-negative, curved or spiral rods distinguished by multiple sheathed flagellae (246). *H. pylori* may adhere to gastric epithelium or reside in the mucous layer of the stomach, but the organism does not invade tissues. Adherence to gastric epithelium is facilitated by the appearance of adherence pedestals on epithelial cells (247,248). The process is orchestrated by the bacteria through secretion of the CagA protein, CagA insertion into mucosal cells, CagA phosphorylation by a tyrosine kinase, and resultant actin polymerization. Urease production from ammonia neutralizes gastric acid, making these organisms uniquely adapted to colonization of the stomach. Transmission is believed to be person to person (fecal–oral, oral–oral), and the major reservoir is human, but waterborne transmission may also be important in some regions (249). The prevalence of infection varies widely among populations, but approximately one half of the world's population is infected (249). The lifetime risk of infection is greatest in developing countries, where more than one half of the population is infected by the age of 10 years. In developed countries, only 5% to 10% of children are seropositive by this age. 13_C breath tests that detect the presence of the bacterial urease by the release of labeled CO_2 show that children may acquire and clear the infection several times in succession. Infection rates increase with age. In adults in developed countries, the annual incidence of infection is approximately 1%. Both environmental and host genetic factors have been implicated in explaining infection rates among different groups. High titers of serum IgA and IgG antibodies develop in infected people. Whether they are protective is unknown. They reside in the mucous layer of the stomach. Some adhere to the epithelium. Urease production allows these microorganisms to degrade host urea into ammonia and thus neutralize gastric acid, making them uniquely adapted to colonize the human stomach. The organism does not invade tissues. The CagA protein is secreted and inserted into cells of the gastric mucosa, where it is phosphorylated by a tyrosine kinase, leading to actin polymerization and the appearance of adherence pedestals (247,248).

H. pylori is linked to gastritis, peptic ulcer disease, and gastric malignancy. Infection is usually associated with a superficial gastritis characterized by a mononuclear infiltrate, disruption of the epithelial gland structure, and decrease in overlying mucous (246). Inflammation has been attributed to production of urease, a vacuolating cytotoxin, and the CagA protein. Duodenal ulcer disease seems to follow antral gastritis and to be associated with excessive acid production. Progressive gastric atrophy and, less commonly, gastric cancer follow gastritis involving the acid-secreting corpus region and are associated with hypochlorhydria.

Duodenal ulceration and gastric cancer appear to be mutually exclusive consequences of infection. Outcomes are not simply explained by bacterial strain differences, and evidence has been marshaled to suggest that host genetic polymorphisms may play a determining role (250,251).

Helicobacter, Other Bacterial Infections, and Lymphoma

The observation of MALT in the stomachs of patients with *Helicobacter* infection, but not in others, provided one of the initial clues to the link between *Helicobacter* and lymphoma (242,243). Serologic study showed that patients with gastric lymphoma were significantly more likely than matched controls to have antibody titers to *H. pylori* (244). The association was reinforced by the observation that the organism itself is present in most gastric lymphomas, with the association being strongest in early lesions (245). Finally, the demonstration that treatment with antibiotics results in regression of such tumors confirmed the importance of the association. As with each of the other infectious agents linked to lymphoma, only a small fraction of those infected progress to lymphoma, underscoring that this evolution is a complex multistep process.

H. pylori, more clearly than any other infectious agent, seems to be linked to lymphoma through the immune response it elicits. MALT lymphomas are hypermutated post–germinal center cells that have undergone antigen selection (252). *In vitro* low-grade gastric lymphoma cells proliferate only in the combined presence of *H. pylori* and T lymphocytes but not in their absence (253). Finally, with antibiotic treatment, gastric MALT regresses, and a substantial fraction of gastric MALT lymphomas regress (254).

Animal models (e.g., ferrets, mice, cats, dogs) have provided some insights (255). None mimic the full spectrum of human *Helicobacter*–associated disease, particularly ulceration or gastric carcinoma. However, lymphocytic infiltrates are common consequences of accompanying infection in several. *Helicobacter felis*, *Helicobacter heilmannii*, and *H. pylori* all colonize the mouse stomach indefinitely. Each produces MALT-like lesions that, in some instances, evolve into low-grade and even high-grade lymphomas in murine and other animal models (255–257). Antibiotic treatment results in regression of the lymphomas in some instances.

Other bacterial infections have also been implicated in lymphomagenesis. *Borrelia burgdorferi*, the spirochete that causes Lyme disease, has been associated with cutaneous B-cell lymphoma (258). Evidence of the association comes from polymerase chain reaction detection studies, culture, or serology. In some cases, tumors have regressed after antibiotic treatment. Evidence for the association has mainly been reported from Europe. Studies in the United States have not confirmed the association (259,260). At present, it is unclear whether these different findings reflect strain variation or other factors.

CONCLUSION

Lymphoma is the exceptional outcome of infection with each of the agents discussed. In some instances, such as with human adult T-cell leukemia/lymphoma virus 1 and *H. pylori* infection, decades elapse between primary infection and the development of lymphoma, giving testimony to the multistep character of the process required to generate malignancy. Among the agents whose genetic material is incorporated into the genetic material of lymphoma, two (human adult T-cell leukemia/lymphoma virus 1 and Epstein-Barr virus) have in common that their life cycle involves expansion of the infected cell population in the lymphoid compartment by induction of the proliferation of infected lymphocytes and replication of viral DNA in these lymphocytes by cellular polymerases. Perturbation of NF-κB pathways is also a common feature. Agents whose genetic material is not incorporated into the genetic material of the lymphoma (hepatitis C, *H. pylori*) have in common extreme variability in antigens with generation of quasispecies. These agents generate lymphocyte proliferation through antigen receptors or other signal transduction pathways that involve cell-surface molecules. Consideration of these divisions may not only be important for understanding pathogenesis but perhaps for therapy as well. When the infectious agent is incorporated into the lymphoma genome, present evidence suggests little benefit to intervention with drugs that inhibit viral enzymes involved in replication. However, when the role the infectious agent plays is exogenous and involves antigen receptors, then removal of antigen load with antiinfective agents may be therapeutic with regard to the lymphoma. An emerging area of research with regard to both sorts of infectious agents and lymphoma is the role that host genetic factors play.

REFERENCES

1. Epstein MA. Reflections on Epstein-Barr virus: some recently resolved old uncertainties. *J Infect* 2001;43:111–115.
2. Cesarman E, Chang Y, Moore PS, et al. Kaposi's sarcoma-associated herpesvirus-like DNA sequences in AIDS-related body-cavity-based lymphomas. *N Engl J Med* 1995;332:1186–1191.
3. Cesarman E, Knowles DM. The role of Kaposi's sarcoma-associated herpesvirus (KSHV/HHV-8) in lymphoproliferative diseases. *Semin Cancer Biol* 1999;9:165–174.
4. Rickinson AB. Epstein-Barr virus. In: Fields BN, Knipe DM, Howley PM, et al., eds. *Fields virology*, 4th ed. Philadelphia: Lippincott Williams & Wilkins, 2001:2575–2627.
5. Kieff E. Epstein-Barr virus and its replication. In: Fields BN, Knipe DM, Howley PM, et al., eds. *Fields virology*, 4th ed. Philadelphia: Lippincott Williams & Wilkins, 2001:2511–2573.
6. Moore PS, Chang Y. Molecular virology of Kaposi's sarcoma-associated herpesvirus. *Philos Trans R Soc Lond B Biol Sci* 2001;356:499–516.
7. Hung SC, Kang MS, Kieff E. Maintenance of Epstein-Barr virus (EBV) oriP-based episomes requires EBV-encoded nuclear antigen-1 chromosome-binding domains, which can be replaced by high-mobility group-I or histone H1. *Proc Natl Acad Sci U S A* 2001;98:1865–1870.
8. Garber AC, Shu MA, Hu J, et al. DNA binding and modulation of gene expression by the latency-associated nuclear antigen of Kaposi's sarcoma-associated herpesvirus. *J Virol* 2001;75:7882–7892.
9. Krithivas A, Fujimuro M, Weidner M, et al. Protein interactions targeting the latency-associated nuclear antigen of Kaposi's sarcoma-associated herpesvirus to cell chromosomes. *J Virol* 2002;76:11596–11604.

10. Cohen JI. Epstein-Barr virus infection. *N Engl J Med* 2000;343:481–492.
11. Li L, Liu D, Hutt-Fletcher L, et al. Epstein-Barr virus inhibits the development of dendritic cells by promoting apoptosis of their monocyte precursors in the presence of granulocyte macrophage-colony-stimulating factor and interleukin-4. *Blood* 2002;99:3725–3734.
12. Ryon JJ, Hayward SD, MacMahon EM, et al. In situ detection of lytic Epstein-Barr virus infection: expression of the NotI early gene and viral interleukin-10 late gene in clinical specimens. *J Infect Dis* 1993; 168:345–351.
13. Hislop AD, Annels NE, Gudgeon NH, et al. Epitope-specific evolution of human CD8(+) T cell responses from primary to persistent phases of Epstein-Barr virus infection. *J Exp Med* 2002;195:893–905.
14. Miyashita EM, Yang B, Babcock GJ, et al. Identification of the site of Epstein-Barr virus persistence *in vivo* as a resting B cell. *J Virol* 1997;71:4882–4891.
15. Tierney RJ, Steven N, Young LS, et al. Epstein-Barr virus latency in blood mononuclear cells: analysis of viral gene transcription during primary infection and in the carrier state. *J Virol* 1994;68:7374–7385.
16. Yang J, Tao Q, Flinn IW, et al. Characterization of Epstein-Barr virus-infected B cells in patients with posttransplantation lymphoproliferative disease: disappearance after rituximab therapy does not predict clinical response. *Blood* 2000;96:4055–4063.
17. Thorley-Lawson DA. Epstein-Barr virus: exploiting the immune system. *Nature Rev Immunol* 2001;1:75–82.
18. Qu L, Rowe DT. Epstein-Barr virus latent gene expression in uncultured peripheral blood lymphocytes. *J Virol* 1992;66:3715–3724.
19. Yao QY, Ogan P, Rowe M, et al. Epstein-Barr virus-infected B cells persist in the circulation of acyclovir-treated virus carriers. *Int J Cancer* 1989;43:67–71.
20. Mosier DE. Viral pathogenesis in hu-PBL-SCID mice. *Semin Immunol* 1996;8:255–262.
21. Wu H, Kapoor P, Frappier L. Separation of the DNA replication, segregation, and transcriptional activation functions of Epstein-Barr nuclear antigen 1. *J Virol* 2002;76:2480–2490.
22. Tsimbouri P, Drotar ME, Coy JL, et al. bcl-xL and RAG genes are induced and the response to IL-2 enhanced in EmuEBNA-1 transgenic mouse lymphocytes. *Oncogene* 2002;21:5182–5187.
23. Wilson JB, Bell JL, Levine AJ. Expression of Epstein-Barr virus nuclear antigen-1 induces B cell neoplasia in transgenic mice. *EMBO J* 1996;15:3117–3126.
24. Kang MS, Hung SC, Kieff E. Epstein-Barr virus nuclear antigen 1 activates transcription from episomal but not integrated DNA and does not alter lymphocyte growth. *Proc Natl Acad Sci U S A* 2001;98:15233–15238.
25. Lee JM, Lee KH, Weidner M, et al. Epstein-Barr virus EBNA2 blocks Nur77-mediated apoptosis. *Proc Natl Acad Sci U S A* 2002;99:11878–11883.
26. Hsieh JJ, Zhou S, Chen L, et al. CIR, a corepressor linking the DNA binding factor CBF1 to the histone deacetylase complex. *Proc Natl Acad Sci U S A* 1999;96:23–28.
27. Uchida J, Yasui T, Takaoka-Shichijo Y, et al. Mimicry of CD40 signals by Epstein-Barr virus LMP1 in B lymphocyte responses. *Science* 1999;286:300–303.
28. Wang D, Liebowitz D, Kieff E. An EBV membrane protein expressed in immortalized lymphocytes transforms established rodent cells. *Cell* 1985;43:831–840.
29. Kulwichit W, Edwards RH, Davenport EM, et al. Expression of the Epstein-Barr virus latent membrane protein 1 induces B cell lymphoma in transgenic mice. *Proc Natl Acad Sci U S A* 1998;95:11963–11968.
30. Lam N, Sugden B. CD40 and its viral mimic, LMP1: similar means to different ends. *Cell Signal* 2003;15:9–16.
31. Bishop GA, Busch LK. Molecular mechanisms of B-lymphocyte transformation by Epstein-Barr virus. *Microbes Infect* 2002;4:853–857.
32. Caldwell RG, Wilson JB, Anderson SJ, et al. Epstein-Barr virus LMP2A drives B cell development and survival in the absence of normal B cell receptor signals. *Immunity* 1998;9:405–411.
33. Nanbo A, Takada K. The role of Epstein-Barr virus-encoded small RNAs (EBERs) in oncogenesis. *Rev Med Virol* 2002;12:321–326.
34. Ruf IK, Rhyne PW, Yang H, et al. Epstein-Barr virus small RNAs potentiate tumorigenicity of Burkitt lymphoma cells independently of an effect on apoptosis. *J Virol* 2000;74:10223–10228.
35. Chen H, Smith P, Ambinder RF, et al. Expression of Epstein-Barr virus BamHI-A rightward transcripts in latently infected B cells from peripheral blood. *Blood* 1999;93:3026–3032.
36. Raab-Traub N. Epstein-Barr virus in the pathogenesis of NPC. *Semin Cancer Biol* 2002;12:431–441.
37. Wu FY, Chen H, Wang SE, et al. CCAAT/enhancer binding protein alpha interacts with ZTA and mediates ZTA-induced p21(CIP-1) accumulation and G(1) cell cycle arrest during the Epstein-Barr virus lytic cycle. *J Virol* 2003;77:1481–1500.
38. Deng Z, Chen CJ, Zerby D, et al. Identification of acidic and aromatic residues in the Zta activation domain essential for Epstein-Barr virus reactivation. *J Virol* 2001;75:10334–10347.
39. Bellows DS, Howell M, Pearson C, et al. Epstein-Barr virus BALF1 is a BCL-2-like antagonist of the herpesvirus antiapoptotic BCL-2 proteins. *J Virol* 2002;76:2469–2479.
40. Boulland ML, Meignin V, Leroy-Viard K, et al. Human interleukin-10 expression in T/natural killer-cell lymphomas: association with anaplastic large cell lymphomas and nasal natural killer-cell lymphomas. *Am J Pathol* 1998;153:1229–1237.
41. Moore SM, Cannon JS, Tanhehco YC, et al. Induction of Epstein-Barr virus kinases to sensitize tumor cells to nucleoside analogues. *Antimicrob Agents Chemother* 2001;45:2082–2091.
42. Feng WH, Israel B, Raab-Traub N, et al. Chemotherapy induces lytic EBV replication and confers ganciclovir susceptibility to EBV-positive epithelial cell tumors. *Cancer Res* 2002;62:1920–1926.
43. Cohen JI, Picchio GR, Mosier DE. Epstein-Barr virus nuclear protein 2 is a critical determinant for tumor growth in SCID mice and for transformation *in vitro*. *J Virol* 1992;66:7555–7559.
44. Frank D, Cesarman E, Liu YF, et al. Posttransplantation lymphoproliferative disorders frequently contain type A and not type B Epstein-Barr virus. *Blood* 1995;85:1396–1403.
45. Tao Q, Yang J, Huang H, et al. Conservation of Epstein-Barr virus cytotoxic T-cell epitopes in posttransplant lymphomas: implications for immune therapy. *Am J Pathol* 2002;160:1839–1845.
46. Yao QY, Croom-Carter DS, Tierney RJ, et al. Epidemiology of infection with Epstein-Barr virus types 1 and 2: lessons from the study of a T-cell-immunocompromised hemophilic cohort. *J Virol* 1998;72:4352–4363.
47. Fassone L, Cingolani A, Martini M, et al. Characterization of Epstein-Barr virus genotype in AIDS-related non-Hodgkin's lymphoma. *AIDS Res Hum Retroviruses* 2002;18:19–26.
48. Schafer H, Berger C, Aepinus C, et al. Molecular pathogenesis of Epstein-Barr virus associated posttransplant lymphomas: new insights through latent membrane protein 1 fingerprinting. *Transplantation* 2001; 72:492–496.
49. Gutierrez MI, Kingma DW, Sorbara L, et al. Association of EBV strains, defined by multiple loci analyses, in non-Hodgkin lymphomas and reactive tissues from HIV positive and HIV negative patients. *Leuk Lymphoma* 2000;37:425–429.
50. Redchenko IV, Rickinson AB. Accessing Epstein-Barr virus-specific T-cell memory with peptide-loaded dendritic cells. *J Virol* 1999;73:334–342.
51. Yang J, Lemas VM, Flinn IW, et al. Application of the ELISPOT assay to the characterization of CD8(+) responses to Epstein-Barr virus antigens. *Blood* 2000;95:241–248.
52. Johannessen I, Crawford DH. In vivo models for Epstein-Barr virus (EBV)-associated B cell lymphoproliferative disease (BLPD). *Rev Med Virol* 1999;9:263–277.
53. Castanos-Velez E, Heiden T, Ekman M, et al. Proliferation and apoptosis-related gene expression in experimental acquired immunodeficiency syndrome-related simian lymphoma. *Blood* 1999;93:1364–1371.
54. Schmidtko J, Wang R, Wu CL, et al. Posttransplant lymphoproliferative disorder associated with an Epstein-Barr-related virus in cynomolgus monkeys. *Transplantation* 2002;73:1431–1439.
55. Cho Y, Ramer J, Rivailler P, et al. An Epstein-Barr-related herpesvirus from marmoset lymphomas. *Proc Natl Acad Sci U S A* 2001;98:1224–1229.
56. Young LS, Finerty S, Brooks L, et al. Epstein-Barr virus gene expression in malignant lymphomas induced by experimental virus infection of cottontop tamarins. *J Virol* 1989;63:1967–1974.
57. Wilson AD, Lovgren-Bengtsson K, Villacres-Ericsson M, et al. The major Epstein-Barr virus (EBV) envelope glycoprotein gp340 when incorporated into Iscoms primes cytotoxic T-cell responses directed against EBV lymphoblastoid cell lines. *Vaccine* 1999;17:1282–1290.
58. Morgan AJ. Epstein-Barr virus vaccines. *Vaccine* 1992;10:563–571.
59. Rowe M, Young LS, Crocker J, et al. Epstein-Barr virus (EBV)-associated lymphoproliferative disease in the SCID mouse model: impli-

cations for the pathogenesis of EBV-positive lymphomas in man. *J Exp Med* 1991;173:147–158.

60. Ferrari MG, Rivadeneira ED, Jarrett R, et al. HV(MNE), a novel lymphocryptovirus related to Epstein-Barr virus, induces lymphoma in New Zealand white rabbits. *Blood* 2001;98:2193–2199.

61. Hamilton-Dutoit SJ, Pallesen G. A survey of Epstein-Barr virus gene expression in sporadic non-Hodgkin's lymphomas. Detection of Epstein-Barr virus in a subset of peripheral T-cell lymphomas. *Am J Pathol* 1992;140:1315–1325.

62. Hamilton-Dutoit SJ, Rea D, Raphael M, et al. Epstein-Barr virus-latent gene expression and tumor cell phenotype in acquired immunodeficiency syndrome-related non-Hodgkin's lymphoma. Correlation of lymphoma phenotype with three distinct patterns of viral latency. *Am J Pathol* 1993;143:1072–1085.

63. Gratama JW, Zutter MM, Minarovits J, et al. Expression of Epstein-Barr virus-encoded growth-transformation-associated proteins in lymphoproliferations of bone-marrow transplant recipients. *Int J Cancer* 1991;47:188–192.

64. Murray PG, Swinnen LJ, Constandinou CM, et al. BCL-2 but not its Epstein-Barr virus-encoded homologue, BHRF1, is commonly expressed in posttransplantation lymphoproliferative disorders. *Blood* 1996;87:706–711.

65. Ambinder RF, Mann RB. Detection and characterization of Epstein-Barr virus in clinical specimens. *Am J Pathol* 1994;145:239–252.

66. Ambinder RF, Mann RB. Epstein-Barr-encoded RNA in situ hybridization: diagnostic applications. *Hum Pathol* 1994;25:602–605.

67. Lei KI, Chan LY, Chan WY, et al. Diagnostic and prognostic implications of circulating cell-free Epstein-Barr virus DNA in natural killer/T-cell lymphoma. *Clin Cancer Res* 2002;8:29–34.

68. Shiramizu B, Barriga F, Neequaye J, et al. Patterns of chromosomal breakpoint locations in Burkitt's lymphoma: relevance to geography and Epstein-Barr virus association. *Blood* 1991;77:1516–1526.

69. Takada K. Role of Epstein-Barr virus in Burkitt's lymphoma. *Curr Top Microbiol Immunol* 2001;258:141–151.

70. Niedobitek G, Agathanggelou A, Rowe M, et al. Heterogeneous expression of Epstein-Barr virus latent proteins in endemic Burkitt's lymphoma. *Blood* 1995;86:659–665.

71. Tao Q, Robertson KD, Manns A, et al. Epstein-Barr virus (EBV) in endemic Burkitt's lymphoma: molecular analysis of primary tumor tissue. *Blood* 1998;91:1373–1381.

72. Komano J, Maruo S, Kurozumi K, et al. Oncogenic role of Epstein-Barr virus-encoded RNAs in Burkitt's lymphoma cell line Akata. *J Virol* 1999;73:9827–9831.

73. Komano J, Sugiura M, Takada K. Epstein-Barr virus contributes to the malignant phenotype and to apoptosis resistance in Burkitt's lymphoma cell line Akata. *J Virol* 1998;72:9150–9156.

74. Kelly G, Bell A, Rickinson A. Epstein-Barr virus-associated Burkitt lymphomagenesis selects for downregulation of the nuclear antigen EBNA2. *Nat Med* 2002;8:1098–1104.

75. Pajic A, Staege MS, Dudziak D, et al. Antagonistic effects of c-myc and Epstein-Barr virus latent genes on the phenotype of human B cells. *Int J Cancer* 2001;93:810–816.

76. Khanna R, Burrows SR, Suhrbier A, et al. EBV peptide epitope sensitization restores human cytotoxic T cell recognition of Burkitt's lymphoma cells. Evidence for a critical role for ICAM-2. *J Immunol* 1993;150:5154–5162.

77. Staege MS, Lee SP, Frisan T, et al. MYC overexpression imposes a nonimmunogenic phenotype on Epstein-Barr virus-infected B cells. *Proc Natl Acad Sci U S A* 2002;99:4550–4555.

78. Rao CR, Gutierrez MI, Bhatia K, et al. Association of Burkitt's lymphoma with the Epstein-Barr virus in two developing countries. *Leuk Lymphoma* 2000;39:329–337.

79. Sandlund JT, Gorban ZI, Berard CW, et al. Large proportion of Epstein-Barr virus-associated small noncleaved cell lymphomas among children with non-Hodgkin's lymphoma at a single institution in Moscow, Russia. *Am J Clin Oncol* 1999;22:523–525.

80. Subar M, Neri A, Inghirami G, et al. Frequent c-myc oncogene activation and infrequent presence of Epstein-Barr virus genome in AIDS-associated lymphoma. *Blood* 1988;72:667–671.

81. Srinivas SK, Sample JT, Sixbey JW. Spontaneous loss of viral episomes accompanying Epstein-Barr virus reactivation in a Burkitt's lymphoma cell line. *J Infect Dis* 1998;177:1705–1709.

82. Razzouk BI, Srinivas S, Sample CE, et al. Epstein-Barr Virus DNA recombination and loss in sporadic Burkitt's lymphoma. *J Infect Dis* 1996;173:529–535.

83. Jaffe ES, Krenacs L, Kumar S, et al. Extranodal peripheral T-cell and NK-cell neoplasms. *Am J Clin Pathol* 1999;111:S46–S55.

84. Chan JK, Yip TT, Tsang WY, et al. Detection of Epstein-Barr viral RNA in malignant lymphomas of the upper aerodigestive tract. *Am J Surg Pathol* 1994;18:938–946.

85. Chan JK, Sin VC, Wong KF, et al. Nonnasal lymphoma expressing the natural killer cell marker CD56: a clinicopathologic study of 49 cases of an uncommon aggressive neoplasm. *Blood* 1997;89:4501–4513.

86. Arber DA, Weiss LM, Albujar PF, et al. Nasal lymphomas in Peru. High incidence of T-cell immunophenotype and Epstein-Barr virus infection. *Am J Surg Pathol* 1993;17:392–399.

87. Elenitoba-Johnson KS, Zarate-Osorno A, Meneses A, et al. Cytotoxic granular protein expression, Epstein-Barr virus strain type, and latent membrane protein-1 oncogene deletions in nasal T-lymphocyte/natural killer cell lymphomas from Mexico. *Mod Pathol* 1998;11:754–761.

88. Gutierrez MI, Spangler G, Kingma D, et al. Epstein-Barr virus in nasal lymphomas contains multiple ongoing mutations in the EBNA-1 gene. *Blood* 1998;92:600–606.

89. Quintanilla-Martinez L, Franklin JL, Guerrero I, et al. Histological and immunophenotypic profile of nasal NK/T cell lymphomas from Peru: high prevalence of p53 overexpression. *Hum Pathol* 1999;30:849–855.

90. Chiang AK, Tao Q, Srivastava G, et al. Nasal NK- and T-cell lymphomas share the same type of Epstein-Barr virus latency as nasopharyngeal carcinoma and Hodgkin's disease. *Int J Cancer* 1996;68:285–290.

91. Gelb AB, van de Rijn M, Regula DP Jr, et al. Epstein-Barr virus-associated natural killer-large granular lymphocyte leukemia. *Hum Pathol* 1994;25:953–960.

92. Kawa-Ha K, Ishihara S, Ninomiya T, et al. CD3-negative lymphoproliferative disease of granular lymphocytes containing Epstein-Barr viral DNA. *J Clin Invest* 1989;84:51–55.

93. Hart DN, Baker BW, Inglis MJ, et al. Epstein-Barr viral DNA in acute large granular lymphocyte (natural killer) leukemic cells. *Blood* 1992;79:2116–2123.

94. Filipovich AH MA, Robison L, et al. Lymphoproliferative disorders associated with primary immunodeficiencies. In: Margath I, ed. *The non-Hodgkin's lymphomas*, 2nd ed. London: Oxford University Press, 1995:459–471.

95. Morra M, Howie D, Grande MS, et al. X-linked lymphoproliferative disease: a progressive immunodeficiency. *Annu Rev Immunol* 2001;19:657–682.

96. Harrington DS, Weisenburger DD, Purtilo DT. Malignant lymphoma in the X-linked lymphoproliferative syndrome. *Cancer* 1987;59:1419–1429.

97. Williams LL, Rooney CM, Conley ME, et al. Correction of Duncan's syndrome by allogeneic bone marrow transplantation. *Lancet* 1993;342:587–588.

98. Strahm B, Rittweiler K, Duffner U, et al. Recurrent B-cell non-Hodgkin's lymphoma in two brothers with X-linked lymphoproliferative disease without evidence for Epstein-Barr virus infection. *Br J Haematol* 2000;108:377–382.

99. Swinnen LJ. Organ transplant-related lymphoma. *Curr Treat Options Oncol* 2001;2:301–308.

100. Zutter MM, Martin PJ, Sale GE, et al. Epstein-Barr virus lymphoproliferation after bone marrow transplantation. *Blood* 1988;72:520–529.

101. Martin PJ, Shulman HM, Schubach WH, et al. Fatal Epstein-Barr-virus-associated proliferation of donor B cells after treatment of acute graft-versus-host disease with a murine anti-T-cell antibody. *Ann Intern Med* 1984;101:310–315.

102. Antin JH, Bierer BE, Smith BR, et al. Selective depletion of bone marrow T lymphocytes with anti-CD5 monoclonal antibodies: effective prophylaxis for graft-versus-host disease in patients with hematologic malignancies. *Blood* 1991;78:2139–2149.

103. Gerritsen EJ, Stam ED, Hermans J, et al. Risk factors for developing EBV-related B cell lymphoproliferative disorders (BLPD) after non-HLA-identical BMT in children. *Bone Marrow Transplant* 1996;18:377–382.

104. Jabado N, Le Deist F, Cant A, et al. Bone marrow transplantation from genetically HLA-nonidentical donors in children with fatal inherited disorders excluding severe combined immunodeficiencies: use of two monoclonal antibodies to prevent graft rejection. *Pediatrics* 1996;98:420–428.

105. Shapiro RS, McClain K, Frizzera G, et al. Epstein-Barr virus associ-

ated B cell lymphoproliferative disorders following bone marrow transplantation. *Blood* 1988;71:1234–1243.

106. Witherspoon RP, Fisher LD, Schoch G, et al. Secondary cancers after bone marrow transplantation for leukemia or aplastic anemia. *N Engl J Med* 1989;321:784–789.

107. Bhatia S, Ramsay NK, Steinbuch M, et al. Malignant neoplasms following bone marrow transplantation. *Blood* 1996;87:3633–3639.

108. Cesarman E, Chadburn A, Liu YF, et al. BCL-6 gene mutations in posttransplantation lymphoproliferative disorders predict response to therapy and clinical outcome. *Blood* 1998;92:2294–2302.

109. Knowles DM, Cesarman E, Chadburn A, et al. Correlative morphologic and molecular genetic analysis demonstrates three distinct categories of posttransplantation lymphoproliferative disorders. *Blood* 1995;85:552–565.

110. Harris NL, Ferry JA, Swerdlow SH. Posttransplant lymphoproliferative disorders: summary of Society for Hematopathology Workshop. *Semin Diagn Pathol* 1997;14:8–14.

111. Swerdlow SH. Classification of the posttransplant lymphoproliferative disorders: from the past to the present. *Semin Diagn Pathol* 1997;14:2–7.

112. Porcu P, Eisenbeis CF, Pelletier RP, et al. Successful treatment of posttransplantation lymphoproliferative disorder (PTLD) following renal allografting is associated with sustained CD8(+) T-cell restoration. *Blood* 2002;100:2341–2348.

113. Rooney CM, Smith CA, Ng CY, et al. Use of gene-modified virus-specific T lymphocytes to control Epstein-Barr-virus-related lymphoproliferation. *Lancet* 1995;345:9–13.

114. Papadopoulos EB, Ladanyi M, Emanuel D, et al. Infusions of donor leukocytes to treat Epstein-Barr virus-associated lymphoproliferative disorders after allogeneic bone marrow transplantation. *N Engl J Med* 1994;330:1185–1191.

115. Gottschalk S, Ng CY, Perez M, et al. An Epstein-Barr virus deletion mutant associated with fatal lymphoproliferative disease unresponsive to therapy with virus-specific CTLs. *Blood* 2001;97:835–843.

116. MacMahon EM, Glass JD, Hayward SD, et al. Epstein-Barr virus in AIDS-related primary central nervous system lymphoma. *Lancet* 1991;338:969–973.

117. Camilleri-Broet S, Davi F, Feuillard J, et al. AIDS-related primary brain lymphomas: histopathologic and immunohistochemical study of 51 cases. The French Study Group for HIV-Associated Tumors. *Hum Pathol* 1997;28:367–374.

118. Cingolani A, Gastaldi R, Fassone L, et al. Epstein-Barr virus infection is predictive of CNS involvement in systemic AIDS-related non-Hodgkin's lymphomas. *J Clin Oncol* 2000;18:3325–3330.

119. Knowles DM. Molecular pathology of acquired immunodeficiency syndrome-related non-Hodgkin's lymphoma. *Semin Diagn Pathol* 1997;14:67–82.

120. Delecluse HJ, Anagnostopoulos I, Dallenbach F, et al. Plasmablastic lymphomas of the oral cavity: a new entity associated with the human immunodeficiency virus infection. *Blood* 1997;89:1413–1420.

121. Audouin J, Diebold J, Pallesen G. Frequent expression of Epstein-Barr virus latent membrane protein-1 in tumour cells of Hodgkin's disease in HIV-positive patients. *J Pathol* 1992;167:381–384.

122. Siebert JD, Ambinder RF, Napoli VM, et al. Human immunodeficiency virus-associated Hodgkin's disease contains latent, not replicative, Epstein-Barr virus. *Hum Pathol* 1995;26:1191–1195.

123. Tirelli U, Serraino D, Spina M, et al. Epstein-Barr virus-encoded latent membrane protein-1 expression as prognostic factor in AIDS-related non-Hodgkin's lymphoma. *AIDS* 1995;9:99–100.

124. Horenstein MG, Nador RG, Chadburn A, et al. Epstein-Barr virus latent gene expression in primary effusion lymphomas containing Kaposi's sarcoma-associated herpesvirus/human herpesvirus-8. *Blood* 1997;90:1186–1191.

125. Mariette X, Cazals-Hatem D, Warszawki J, et al. Lymphomas in rheumatoid arthritis patients treated with methotrexate: a 3-year prospective study in France. *Blood* 2002;99:3909–3915.

126. Copie-Bergman C, Niedobitek G, Mangham DC, et al. Epstein-Barr virus in B-cell lymphomas associated with chronic suppurative inflammation. *J Pathol* 1997;183:287–292.

127. Wilson WH, Kingma DW, Raffeld M, et al. Association of lymphomatoid granulomatosis with Epstein-Barr viral infection of B lymphocytes and response to interferon-alpha 2b. *Blood* 1996;87:4531–4537.

128. Boshoff C, Weiss R. AIDS-related malignancies. *Nat Rev Cancer* 2002;2:373–382.

129. Kedes DH, Lagunoff M, Renne R, et al. Identification of the gene encoding the major latency-associated nuclear antigen of the Kaposi's sarcoma-associated herpesvirus. *J Clin Invest* 1997;100:2606–2610.

130. Kellam P, Boshoff C, Whitby D, et al. Identification of a major latent nuclear antigen, LNA-1, in the human herpesvirus 8 genome. *J Hum Virol* 1997;1:19–29.

131. Rainbow L, Platt GM, Simpson GR, et al. The 222- to 234-kilodalton latent nuclear protein (LNA) of Kaposi's sarcoma-associated herpesvirus (human herpesvirus 8) is encoded by orf73 and is a component of the latency-associated nuclear antigen. *J Virol* 1997;71:5915–5921.

132. Cesarman E, Nador RG, Bai F, et al. Kaposi's sarcoma-associated herpesvirus contains G protein-coupled receptor and cyclin D homologs which are expressed in Kaposi's sarcoma and malignant lymphoma. *J Virol* 1996;70:8218–8223.

133. Chang Y, Moore PS, Talbot SJ, et al. Cyclin encoded by KS herpesvirus. *Nature* 1996;382:410.

134. Thome M, Schneider P, Hofmann K, et al. Viral FLICE-inhibitory proteins (FLIPs) prevent apoptosis induced by death receptors. *Nature* 1997;386:517–521.

135. Choi JK, Lee BS, Shim SN, et al. Identification of the novel K15 gene at the rightmost end of the Kaposi's sarcoma-associated herpesvirus genome. *J Virol* 2000;74:436–446.

136. Poole LJ, Zong JC, Ciufo DM, et al. Comparison of genetic variability at multiple loci across the genomes of the major subtypes of Kaposi's sarcoma-associated herpesvirus reveals evidence for recombination and for two distinct types of open reading frame K15 alleles at the right-hand end. *J Virol* 1999;73:6646–6660.

137. Sadler R, Wu L, Forghani B, et al. A complex translational program generates multiple novel proteins from the latently expressed kaposin (K12) locus of Kaposi's sarcoma-associated herpesvirus. *J Virol* 1999;73:5722–5730.

138. Li H, Komatsu T, Dezube BJ, et al. The Kaposi's sarcoma-associated herpesvirus K12 transcript from a primary effusion lymphoma contains complex repeat elements, is spliced, and initiates from a novel promoter. *J Virol* 2002;76:11880–11888.

139. Burysek L, Pitha PM. Latently expressed human herpesvirus 8-encoded interferon regulatory factor 2 inhibits double-stranded RNA-activated protein kinase. *J Virol* 2001;75:2345–2352.

140. Rivas C, Thlick AE, Parravicini C, et al. Kaposi's sarcoma-associated herpesvirus LANA2 is a B-cell-specific latent viral protein that inhibits p53. *J Virol* 2001;75:429–438.

141. Nicholas J, Ruvolo VR, Burns WH, et al. Kaposi's sarcoma-associated human herpesvirus-8 encodes homologues of macrophage inflammatory protein-1 and interleukin-6. *Nat Med* 1997;3:287–292.

142. Lee H, Veazey R, Williams K, et al. Deregulation of cell growth by the K1 gene of Kaposi's sarcoma-associated herpesvirus. *Nat Med* 1998;4:435–440.

143. Prakash O, Tang ZY, Peng X, et al. Tumorigenesis and aberrant signaling in transgenic mice expressing the human herpesvirus-8 K1 gene. *J Natl Cancer Inst* 2002;94:926–935.

144. Carbone A, Cilia AM, Gloghini A, et al. Establishment and characterization of EBV-positive and EBV-negative primary effusion lymphoma cell lines harbouring human herpesvirus type-8. *Br J Haematol* 1998;102:1081–1089.

145. Parravicini C, Chandran B, Corbellino M, et al. Differential viral protein expression in Kaposi's sarcoma-associated herpesvirus-infected diseases: Kaposi's sarcoma, primary effusion lymphoma, and multicentric Castleman's disease. *Am J Pathol* 2000;156:743–749.

146. Katano H, Sato Y, Kurata T, et al. Expression and localization of human herpesvirus 8-encoded proteins in primary effusion lymphoma, Kaposi's sarcoma, and multicentric Castleman's disease. *Virology* 2000;269:335–344.

147. Cannon JS, Nicholas J, Orenstein JM, et al. Heterogeneity of viral IL-6 expression in HHV-8-associated diseases. *J Infect Dis* 1999;180:824–828.

148. Staskus KA, Sun R, Miller G, et al. Cellular tropism and viral interleukin-6 expression distinguish human herpesvirus 8 involvement in Kaposi's sarcoma, primary effusion lymphoma, and multicentric Castleman's disease. *J Virol* 1999;73:4181–4187.

149. Aoki Y, Yarchoan R, Wyvill K, et al. Detection of viral interleukin-6 in Kaposi sarcoma-associated herpesvirus-linked disorders. *Blood* 2001;97:2173–2176.

150. Soulier J, Grollet L, Oksenhendler E, et al. Kaposi's sarcoma-associated herpesvirus-like DNA sequences in multicentric Castleman's disease. *Blood* 1995;86:1276–1280.

151. Dupin N, Diss TL, Kellam P, et al. HHV-8 is associated with a plasmablastic variant of Castleman disease that is linked to HHV-8-positive plasmablastic lymphoma. *Blood* 2000;95:1406–1412.

152. Chiou CJ, Poole LJ, Kim PS, et al. Patterns of gene expression and a transactivation function exhibited by the vGCR (ORF74) chemokine receptor protein of Kaposi's sarcoma-associated herpesvirus. *J Virol* 2002;76:3421–3439.

153. Uchiyama T, Yodoi J, Sagawa K, et al. Adult T-cell leukemia: clinical and hematologic features of 16 cases. *Blood* 1977;50:481–492.

154. Morgan DA, Ruscetti FW, Gallo R. Selective in vitro growth of T lymphocytes from normal human bone marrows. *Science* 1976;193:1007–1008.

155. Hinuma Y, Nagata K, Hanaoka M, et al. Adult T-cell leukemia: antigen in an ATL cell line and detection of antibodies to the antigen in human sera. *Proc Natl Acad Sci U S A* 1981;78:6476–6480.

156. Yoshida M, Miyoshi I, Hinuma Y. Isolation and characterization of retrovirus from cell lines of human adult T-cell leukemia and its implication in the disease. *Proc Natl Acad Sci U S A* 1982;79:2031–2035.

157. Hollsberg P, Hafler DA. Seminars in medicine of the Beth Israel Hospital, Boston. Pathogenesis of diseases induced by human lymphotropic virus type I infection. *N Engl J Med* 1993;328:1173–1182.

158. Leclercq I, Mortreux F, Cavrois M, et al. Host sequences flanking the human T-cell leukemia virus type 1 provirus in vivo. *J Virol* 2000;74:2305–2312.

159. Slattery JP, Franchini G, Gessain A. Genomic evolution, patterns of global dissemination, and interspecies transmission of human and simian T-cell leukemia/lymphotropic viruses. *Genome Res* 1999;9:525–540.

160. Wodarz D, Nowak MA, Bangham CR. The dynamics of HTLV-I and the CTL response. *Immunol Today* 1999;20:220–227.

161. Gessain A, Barin F, Vernant JC, et al. Antibodies to human T-lymphotropic virus type-I in patients with tropical spastic paraparesis. *Lancet* 1985;2:407–410.

162. McKown K, Trigg L, Cremer M. Human T lymphotropic virus I, myelopathy, polymyositis and synovitis. *J Rheumatol* 1993;20:594–595.

163. Nelson PN, Lever AM, Bruckner FE, et al. Polymerase chain reaction fails to incriminate exogenous retroviruses HTLV-I and HIV-1 in rheumatological diseases although a minority of sera cross react with retroviral antigens. *Ann Rheum Dis* 1994;53:749–754.

164. Mortreux F, Kazanji M, Gabet AS, et al. Two-step nature of human T-cell leukemia virus type 1 replication in experimentally infected squirrel monkeys (*Saimiri sciureus*). *J Virol* 2001;75:1083–1089.

165. Tajima Y, Tashiro K, Camerini D. Assignment of the possible HTLV receptor gene to chromosome 17q21-q23. *Somat Cell Mol Genet* 1997;23:225–227.

166. Mortreux F, Gabet AS, Wattel E. Molecular and cellular aspects of HTLV-1 associated leukemogenesis in vivo. *Leukemia* 2003;17:26–38.

167. Bieganowska K, Hollsberg P, Buckle GJ, et al. Direct analysis of viral-specific CD8+ T cells with soluble HLA-A2/Tax11-19 tetramer complexes in patients with human T cell lymphotropic virus-associated myelopathy. *J Immunol* 1999;162:1765–1771.

168. Jeffery KJ, Usuku K, Hall SE, et al. HLA alleles determine human T-lymphotropic virus-I (HTLV-I) proviral load and the risk of HTLV-I-associated myelopathy. *Proc Natl Acad Sci U S A* 1999;96:3848–3853.

169. Hanon E, Stinchcombe JC, Saito M, et al. Fratricide among CD8(+) T lymphocytes naturally infected with human T cell lymphotropic virus type I. *Immunity* 2000;13:657–664.

170. Asquith B, Hanon E, Taylor GP, et al. Is human T-cell lymphotropic virus type I really silent? *Philos Trans R Soc Lond B Biol Sci* 2000;355:1013–1019.

171. Richardson JH, Hollsberg P, Windhagen A, et al. Variable immortalizing potential and frequent virus latency in blood-derived T-cell clones infected with human T-cell leukemia virus type I. *Blood* 1997;89:3303–3314.

172. Yoshida M. Multiple viral strategies of HTLV-1 for dysregulation of cell growth control. *Annu Rev Immunol* 2001;19:475–496.

173. Haller K, Wu Y, Derow E, et al. Physical interaction of human T-cell leukemia virus type 1 Tax with cyclin-dependent kinase 4 stimulates the phosphorylation of retinoblastoma protein. *Mol Cell Biol* 2002;22:3327–3338.

174. Jin DY, Spencer F, Jeang KT. Human T cell leukemia virus type 1 oncoprotein Tax targets the human mitotic checkpoint protein MAD1. *Cell* 1998;93:81–91.

175. Van PL, Yim KW, Jin DY, et al. Genetic evidence of a role for ATM in functional interaction between human T-cell leukemia virus type 1 Tax and p53. *J Virol* 2001;75:396–407.

176. Taguchi H, Sawada T, Fukushima A, et al. Bilateral uveitis in a rabbit experimentally infected with human T-lymphotropic virus type I. *Lab Invest* 1993;69:336–339.

177. Miyoshi I, Yoshimoto S, Kubonishi I, et al. Infectious transmission of human T-cell leukemia virus to rabbits. *Int J Cancer* 1985;35:81–85.

178. Ishiguro N, Abe M, Seto K, et al. A rat model of human T lymphocyte virus type I (HTLV-I) infection. 1. Humoral antibody response, provirus integration, and HTLV-I-associated myelopathy/tropical spastic paraparesis-like myelopathy in seronegative HTLV-I carrier rats. *J Exp Med* 1992;176:981–989.

179. Yamanouchi K, Kinoshita K, Moriuchi R, et al. Oral transmission of human T-cell leukemia virus type-I into a common marmoset (*Callithrix jacchus*) as an experimental model for milk-borne transmission. *Jpn J Cancer Res* 1985;76:481–487.

180. Ibuki K, Funahashi SI, Yamamoto H, et al. Long-term persistence of protective immunity in cynomolgus monkeys immunized with a recombinant vaccinia virus expressing the human T cell leukaemia virus type I envelope gene. *J Gen Virol* 1997;78:147–152.

181. Grassmann R, Berchtold S, Radant I, et al. Role of human T-cell leukemia virus type 1 X region proteins in immortalization of primary human lymphocytes in culture. *J Virol* 1992;66:4570–4575.

182. Portis T, Grossman WJ, Harding JC, et al. Analysis of p53 inactivation in a human T-cell leukemia virus type 1 Tax transgenic mouse model. *J Virol* 2001;75:2185–2193.

183. Portis T, Harding JC, Ratner L. The contribution of NF-kappa B activity to spontaneous proliferation and resistance to apoptosis in human T-cell leukemia virus type 1 Tax-induced tumors. *Blood* 2001;98:1200–1208.

184. Blattner WA. Human T-lymphotrophic viruses and diseases of long latency. *Ann Intern Med* 1989;111:4–6.

185. Kasai T, Iwanaga Y, Iha H, et al. Prevalent loss of mitotic spindle checkpoint in adult T-cell leukemia confers resistance to microtubule inhibitors. *J Biol Chem* 2002;277:5187–5193.

186. Yamada Y, Hatta Y, Murata K, et al. Deletions of p15 and/or p16 genes as a poor-prognosis factor in adult T-cell leukemia. *J Clin Oncol* 1997;15:1778–1785.

187. Marriott SJ, Lemoine FJ, Jeang KT. Damaged DNA and miscounted chromosomes: human T cell leukemia virus type I tax oncoprotein and genetic lesions in transformed cells. *J Biomed Sci* 2002;9:292–298.

188. Kannagi M, Matsushita S, Harada S. Expression of the target antigen for cytotoxic T lymphocytes on adult T-cell-leukemia cells. *Int J Cancer* 1993;54:582–588.

189. Ohashi T, Hanabuchi S, Suzuki R, et al. Correlation of major histocompatibility complex class I downregulation with resistance of human T-cell leukemia virus type 1-infected T cells to cytotoxic T-lymphocyte killing in a rat model. *J Virol* 2002;76:7010–7019.

190. Furukawa Y, Kubota R, Tara M, et al. Existence of escape mutant in HTLV-I tax during the development of adult T-cell leukemia. *Blood* 2001;97:987–993.

191. Rosenberg ZF, Fauci AS. Immunopathogenesis of HIV infection. *Faseb J* 1991;5:2382–2390.

192. De Silva FS, Venturini DS, Wagner E, et al. CD4-independent infection of human B cells with HIV type 1: detection of unintegrated viral DNA. *AIDS Res Hum Retroviruses* 2001;17:1585–1598.

193. Chirmule N, Kalyanaraman VS, Saxinger C, et al. Localization of B-cell stimulatory activity of HIV-1 to the carboxyl terminus of gp41. *AIDS Res Hum Retroviruses* 1990;6:299–305.

194. Chirmule N, Oyaizu N, Saxinger C, et al. Nef protein of HIV-1 has B-cell stimulatory activity. *AIDS* 1994;8:733–734.

195. Ziegler JL, Beckstead JA, Volberding PA, et al. Non-Hodgkin's lymphoma in 90 homosexual men. Relation to generalized lymphadenopathy and the acquired immunodeficiency syndrome. *N Engl J Med* 1984;311:565–570.

196. Franceschi S, Dal Maso L, La Vecchia C. Advances in the epidemiology of HIV-associated non-Hodgkin's lymphoma and other lymphoid neoplasms. *Int J Cancer* 1999;83:481–485.

197. Goedert JJ, Cote TR, Virgo P, et al. Spectrum of AIDS-associated malignant disorders. *Lancet* 1998;351:1833–1839.

198. Levine AM. AIDS-related malignancies: the emerging epidemic. *J Natl Cancer Inst* 1993;85:1382–1397.

199. Jones JL, Hanson DL, Dworkin MS, et al. Effect of antiretroviral therapy on recent trends in selected cancers among HIV-infected persons. Adult/Adolescent Spectrum of HIV Disease Project Group. *J Acquir Immune Defic Syndr* 1999;21[Suppl 1]:S11–S17.

200. Jacobson LP, Yamashita TE, Detels R, et al. Impact of potent antiretroviral therapy on the incidence of Kaposi's sarcoma and non-Hodgkin's lymphomas among HIV-1-infected individuals. Multicenter AIDS Cohort Study. *J Acquir Immune Defic Syndr* 1999;21[Suppl 1]:S34–S41.

201. Cote TR, Manns A, Hardy CR, et al. Epidemiology of brain lymphoma among people with or without acquired immunodeficiency syndrome. AIDS/Cancer Study Group. *J Natl Cancer Inst* 1996;88:675–679.

202. Rabkin CS. AIDS and cancer in the era of highly active antiretroviral therapy (HAART). *Eur J Cancer* 2001;37:1316–1319.

203. Grulich AE, Li Y, McDonald AM, et al. Decreasing rates of Kaposi's sarcoma and non-Hodgkin's lymphoma in the era of potent combination anti-retroviral therapy. *AIDS* 2001;15:629–633.

204. Pelicci PG, Knowles DM 2nd, Arlin ZA, et al. Multiple monoclonal B cell expansions and c-myc oncogene rearrangements in acquired immune deficiency syndrome-related lymphoproliferative disorders. Implications for lymphomagenesis. *J Exp Med* 1986;164:2049–2060.

205. Herndier BG, Kaplan LD, McGrath MS. Pathogenesis of AIDS lymphomas. *AIDS* 1994;8:1025–1049.

206. Pedersen C, Gerstoft J, Lundgren JD, et al. HIV-associated lymphoma: histopathology and association with Epstein-Barr virus genome related to clinical, immunological and prognostic features. *Eur J Cancer* 1991;27:1416–1423.

207. Gabarre J, Raphael M, Lepage E, et al. Human immunodeficiency virus-related lymphoma: relation between clinical features and histologic subtypes. *Am J Med* 2001;111:704–711.

208. Davi F, Delecluse HJ, Guiet P, et al. Burkitt-like lymphomas in AIDS patients: characterization within a series of 103 human immunodeficiency virus-associated non-Hodgkin's lymphomas. Burkitt's Lymphoma Study Group. *J Clin Oncol* 1998;16:3788–3795.

209. Grulich AE, Wan X, Law MG, et al. B-cell stimulation and prolonged immune deficiency are risk factors for non-Hodgkin's lymphoma in people with AIDS. *AIDS* 2000;14:133–140.

210. Cunto-Amesty G, Przybylski G, Honczarenko M, et al. Evidence that immunoglobulin specificities of AIDS-related lymphoma are not directed to HIV-related antigens. *Blood* 2000;95:1393–1399.

211. Choo QL, Kuo G, Weiner AJ, et al. Isolation of a cDNA clone derived from a blood-borne non-A, non-B viral hepatitis genome. *Science* 1989;244:359–362.

212. Liang TJ, Rehermann B, Seeff LB, et al. Pathogenesis, natural history, treatment, and prevention of hepatitis C. *Ann Intern Med* 2000;132:296–305.

213. Agnello V, Chung RT, Kaplan LM. A role for hepatitis C virus infection in type II cryoglobulinemia. *N Engl J Med* 1992;327:1490–1495.

214. Misiani R, Bellavita P, Fenili D, et al. Hepatitis C virus infection in patients with essential mixed cryoglobulinemia. *Ann Intern Med* 1992;117:573–577.

215. Ferri C, La Civita L, Caracciolo F, et al. Non-Hodgkin's lymphoma: possible role of hepatitis C virus. *JAMA* 1994;272:355–356.

216. Silvestri F, Pipan C, Barillari G, et al. Prevalence of hepatitis C virus infection in patients with lymphoproliferative disorders. *Blood* 1996;87:4296–4301.

217. Wasley A, Alter MJ. Epidemiology of hepatitis C: geographic differences and temporal trends. *Semin Liver Dis* 2000;20:1–16.

218. Agnello V, Abel G, Elfahal M, et al. Hepatitis C virus and other *Flaviviridae* viruses enter cells via low density lipoprotein receptor. *Proc Natl Acad Sci U S A* 1999;96:12766–12771.

219. Pileri P, Uematsu Y, Campagnoli S, et al. Binding of hepatitis C virus to CD81. *Science* 1998;282:938–941.

220. Sung VM, Shimodaira S, Doughty AL, et al. Establishment of B-cell lymphoma cell lines persistently infected with hepatitis C virus in vivo and in vitro: the apoptotic effects of virus infection. *J Virol* 2003;77:2134–2146.

221. Zein NN. Clinical significance of hepatitis C virus genotypes. *Clin Microbiol Rev* 2000;13:223–235.

222. De Vita S, De Re V, Gasparotto D, et al. Oligoclonal non-neoplastic B cell expansion is the key feature of type II mixed cryoglobulinemia: clinical and molecular findings do not support a bone marrow pathologic diagnosis of indolent B cell lymphoma. *Arthritis Rheum* 2000;43:94–102.

223. Izumi KM, Kaye KM, Kieff ED. The Epstein-Barr virus LMP1 amino acid sequence that engages tumor necrosis factor receptor associated factors is critical for primary B lymphocyte growth transformation. *Proc Natl Acad Sci U S A* 1997;94:1447–1452.

224. Izumi T, Sasaki R, Shimizu R, et al. Hepatitis C virus infection in Waldenström's macroglobulinemia. *Am J Hematol* 1996;52:238–239.

225. Zuckerman E, Zuckerman T, Levine AM, et al. Hepatitis C virus infection in patients with B-cell non-Hodgkin lymphoma. *Ann Intern Med* 1997;127:423–428.

226. Arima N, Tei C. HTLV-I Tax related dysfunction of cell cycle regulators and oncogenesis of adult T cell leukemia. *Leuk Lymphoma* 2001;40:267–278.

227. Ivanovski M, Silvestri F, Pozzato G, et al. Somatic hypermutation, clonal diversity, and preferential expression of the VH 51p1/VL kv325 immunoglobulin gene combination in hepatitis C virus-associated immunocytomas. *Blood* 1998;91:2433–2442.

228. Marasca R, Vaccari P, Luppi M, et al. Immunoglobulin gene mutations and frequent use of VH1-69 and VH4-34 segments in hepatitis C virus-positive and hepatitis C virus-negative nodal marginal zone B-cell lymphoma. *Am J Pathol* 2001;159:253–261.

229. Quinn ER, Chan CH, Hadlock KG, et al. The B-cell receptor of a hepatitis C virus (HCV)-associated non-Hodgkin lymphoma binds the viral E2 envelope protein, implicating HCV in lymphomagenesis. *Blood* 2001;98:3745–3749.

230. Zuckerman E, Zuckerman T, Sahar D, et al. The effect of antiviral therapy on t(14;18) translocation and immunoglobulin gene rearrangement in patients with chronic hepatitis C virus infection. *Blood* 2001;97:1555–1559.

231. El-Sabban ME, Merhi RA, Haidar HA, et al. Human T-cell lymphotropic virus type 1-transformed cells induce angiogenesis and establish functional gap junctions with endothelial cells. *Blood* 2002;99:3383–3389.

232. Hermine O, Lefrere F, Bronowicki JP, et al. Regression of splenic lymphoma with villous lymphocytes after treatment of hepatitis C virus infection. *N Engl J Med* 2002;347:89–94.

233. Fearon DT, Carroll MC. Regulation of B lymphocyte responses to foreign and self-antigens by the CD19/CD21 complex. *Annu Rev Immunol* 2000;18:393–422.

234. Sakamuro D, Furukawa T, Takegami T. Hepatitis C virus nonstructural protein NS3 transforms NIH 3T3 cells. *J Virol* 1995;69:3893–3896.

235. Ray RB, Meyer K, Ray R. Hepatitis C virus core protein promotes immortalization of primary human hepatocytes. *Virology* 2000;271:197–204.

236. Moriya K, Fujie H, Shintani Y, et al. The core protein of hepatitis C virus induces hepatocellular carcinoma in transgenic mice. *Nat Med* 1998;4:1065–1067.

237. Malkin D. Simian virus 40 and non-Hodgkin lymphoma. *Lancet* 2002;359:812–813.

238. Shivapurkar N, Harada K, Reddy J, et al. Presence of simian virus 40 DNA sequences in human lymphomas. *Lancet* 2002;359:851–852.

239. Vilchez RA, Madden CR, Kozinetz CA, et al. Association between simian virus 40 and non-Hodgkin lymphoma. *Lancet* 2002;359:817–823.

240. Capello D, Rossi D, Gaudino G, et al. Simian virus 40 infection in lymphoproliferative disorders. *Lancet* 2003;361:88–89.

241. Butel JS, Lednicky JA. Cell and molecular biology of simian virus 40: implications for human infections and disease. *J Natl Cancer Inst* 1999;91:119–134.

242. Stolte M, Eidt S. Lymphoid follicles in antral mucosa: immune response to *Campylobacter pylori*? *J Clin Pathol* 1989;42:1269–1271.

243. Wyatt JI, Rathbone BJ. Immune response of the gastric mucosa to *Campylobacter pylori*. *Scand J Gastroenterol Suppl* 1988;142:44–49.

244. Parsonnet J, Hansen S, Rodriguez L, et al. *Helicobacter pylori* infection and gastric lymphoma. *N Engl J Med* 1994;330:1267–1271.

245. Nakamura S, Yao T, Aoyagi K, et al. *Helicobacter pylori* and primary gastric lymphoma. A histopathologic and immunohistochemical analysis of 237 patients. *Cancer* 1997;79:3–11.

246. Passaro DJ, Chosy EJ, Parsonnet J. *Helicobacter pylori*: consensus and controversy. *Clin Infect Dis* 2002;35:298–304.

247. Odenbreit S, Puls J, Sedlmaier B, et al. Translocation of *Helicobacter pylori* CagA into gastric epithelial cells by type IV secretion. *Science* 2000;287:1497–1500.

248. Segal ED, Cha J, Lo J, et al. Altered states: involvement of phosphorylated CagA in the induction of host cellular growth changes by *Helicobacter pylori*. *Proc Natl Acad Sci U S A* 1999;96:14559–14564.

249. Parsonnet J, Shmuely H, Haggerty T. Fecal and oral shedding of *Helicobacter pylori* from healthy infected adults. *JAMA* 1999;282:2240–2245.

250. El-Omar EM, Carrington M, Chow WH, et al. Interleukin-1 polymorphisms associated with increased risk of gastric cancer. *Nature* 2000;404:398–402.

251. El-Omar EM, Carrington M, Chow WH, et al. The role of interleukin-1 polymorphisms in the pathogenesis of gastric cancer. *Nature* 2001;412:99.

252. Qin Y, Greiner A, Trunk MJ, et al. Somatic hypermutation in low-grade mucosa-associated lymphoid tissue-type B-cell lymphoma. *Blood* 1995;86:3528–3534.

253. Hussell T, Isaacson PG, Crabtree JE, et al. The response of cells from low-grade B-cell gastric lymphomas of mucosa-associated lymphoid tissue to *Helicobacter pylori*. *Lancet* 1993;342:571–574.

254. Wotherspoon AC, Doglioni C, Diss TC, et al. Regression of primary low-grade B-cell gastric lymphoma of mucosa-associated lymphoid tissue type after eradication of *Helicobacter pylori*. *Lancet* 1993; 342:575–577.

255. Chiang KY, Hazlett LJ, Godder KT, et al. Epstein-Barr virus-associated B cell lymphoproliferative disorder following mismatched related T cell-depleted bone marrow transplantation. *Bone Marrow Transplant* 2001;28:1117–1123.

256. Brander C, Suscovich T, Lee Y, et al. Impaired CTL recognition of cells latently infected with Kaposi's sarcoma-associated herpes virus. *J Immunol* 2000;165:2077–2083.

257. Enno A, O'Rourke J, Braye S, et al. Antigen-dependent progression of mucosa-associated lymphoid tissue (MALT)-type lymphoma in the stomach. Effects of antimicrobial therapy on gastric MALT lymphoma in mice. *Am J Pathol* 1998;152:1625–1632.

258. Hofbauer GF, Kessler B, Kempf W, et al. Multilesional primary cutaneous diffuse large B-cell lymphoma responsive to antibiotic treatment. *Dermatology* 2001;203:168–170.

259. Brander C, O'Connor P, Suscovich T, et al. Definition of an optimal cytotoxic T lymphocyte epitope in the latently expressed Kaposi's sarcoma-associated herpesvirus kaposin protein. *J Infect Dis* 2001; 184:119–126.

260. Munksgaard L, Frisch M, Melbye M, et al. Incidence patterns of Lyme disease and cutaneous B-cell non-Hodgkin's lymphoma in the United States. *Dermatology* 2000;201:351–352.

CHAPTER 47

Developmental and Functional Biology of B Lymphocytes

Ralf Küppers and Klaus Rajewsky

B lymphocytes are important components of the adaptive immune response. Their important role in the control of infections becomes evident from the fact that humans with deficiencies in the generation of functional B cells suffer from severe diseases (1). The main task of B cells is to search for foreign antigens, such as infectious agents, and to produce large amounts of specific antibody once activated by such antigens to mediate their elimination from the body. To combat an extremely diverse variety of foreign antigens, each newly generated B cell in the body is equipped with a distinct antigen receptor. This formidable task is accomplished by the structure of the gene segments coding for the variable part of the antibody molecule. Antibodies are composed of heavy and light chains, and the variable regions of both are encoded by distinct gene segments (called *V*, *D*, and *J* for the heavy chain and *V* and *J* for the two types of light chain genes, kappa and lambda) that need to be somatically rearranged to give rise to functional V region genes (Fig. 47.1). This modal structure of the immunoglobulin (Ig) loci allows an essentially limitless diversity to be generated. Even further diversity of antibody molecules is accomplished in later stages of B-cell development, when antigen-activated B lymphocytes undergo the process of somatic hypermutation. As the production of antigen-specific antibodies is the main role of B cells in the immune response, it is perhaps not surprising that the life of these cells is dominated from the beginning to the end by selection of the appropriate cell surface receptor in the various stages of development (2).

GENERATION OF B LYMPHOCYTES

Development of B-Cell Precursors

B lymphocytes are generated in the bone marrow from hematopoietic stem cells. The development of B cells is regulated by an ordered rearrangement of the antigen receptor genes and selection of the cells at successive stages of development for appropriate receptor molecules (2). The first B-lineage cells are called *pro B cells*. In these cells, D_H to J_H gene rearrangements occur often but not always on both IgH alleles, which are located on chromosome 14. In humans, there are 27 D_H and six J_H gene segments available for this process (3,4). In the next step, one of approximately 50 functional V_H gene segments is rearranged to a $D_H J_H$ joint (Fig. 47.1) (5). As the joining sites of the V_H, D_H, and J_H gene segments are variable and often modified by the addition of non–germline-encoded nucleotides, the V_H to $D_H J_H$ rearrangement can be either productive or nonproductive (discussed in more detail below). Only productive IgH gene rearrangements can give rise to a heavy chain protein. If the first $V_H D_H J_H$ rearrangement is nonproductive, the B-cell precursor has a second chance to generate a productive IgH gene rearrangement by using the second IgH allele. Productively rearranged IgH genes are expressed together with a surrogate light chain that is comprised of two proteins, λ5 and VpreB, and the signal transducing molecules Igα and Igβ (CD79a and CD79b); this structure is called the *pre B-cell receptor*. Cells are then selected for expression of the pre B-cell receptor (it is, however, not yet clarified whether expression on the cell surface is needed or whether assembly of this complex in the endoplasmic reticulum is sufficient; it is also not known whether the receptor needs to bind to some ligand for signaling). Expression of this receptor has several consequences: The cells, which are now called *pre B cells*, discontinue further IgH gene rearrangements, divide several times, and then initiate light chain gene rearrangements (2). As further IgH gene rearrangements are prevented once a pre B cell carries a productive V_H gene rearrangement, B cells usually express only one IgH allele, a phenomenon called *allelic exclusion*.

There are two light chain loci in the human, the Igκ locus on chromosome 2 and the Igλ locus on chromosome 22. In the κ locus, there are, depending on the haplotype, 30 to 35

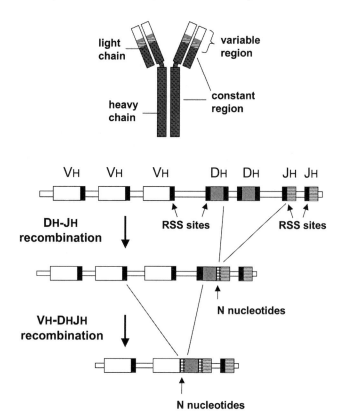

FIG. 47.1. Structure of the antibody and outline of V(D)J recombination. The upper part depicts the structure of the antibody molecule, which is comprised of two identical heavy and two identical light chains. Heavy, as well as light, chains consist of a variable and a constant part. The variable regions mediate antigen binding, whereas the constant region of the heavy chain determines the effector functions of the antibody. The lower part depicts the principle of V(D)J recombination at the heavy chain locus. During heavy chain gene rearrangements, first 1 of 27 D_H gene segments is joined to one of six J_H gene segments. The intervening DNA is deleted from the chromosome as a circle and later lost from the cell. The recombination is mediated by cutting the DNA at the recombination signal sequence (RSS) sites. In the second step, one of approximately 50 functional V_H genes is recombined to a $D_H J_H$ joint. At the V-D and D-J joining sites, additional diversity is generated by the removal of nucleotides from the ends of the gene segments and the addition of non–germline-encoded N nucleotides.

functional Vκ gene segments and five Jκ segments, whereas in the λ locus there are 30 to 37 functional Vλ gene segments and four functional Jλ gene segments available for recombination (6–10). Pre B cells usually first perform light chain gene rearrangements on κ loci, and only if these fail to give rise to a productive light chain gene, the Igλ locus is rearranged. This is suggested by the fact the normal and malignant human κ-expressing B cells in most cases have the λ locus in germline configuration, whereas λ-expressing B cells carry rearranged κ loci (11–13). A productive light chain gene rearrangement is then expressed. If the corresponding light chain cannot pair with the heavy chain of the cell, further light chain gene rearrangements can be performed (see below). If the light chain can pair with the heavy chain and be expressed on the cell surface, the cells are now called *immature B cells*. These cells undergo a further selection process before they can become mature B cells. The immature B cells are tested for binding of the B-cell receptor to autoantigens. Cells that show strong binding to such antigens are either removed by apoptosis or they reinitiate light chain gene rearrangements to replace the originally expressed light chain by a novel one (receptor editing), so that the cells may now express a B-cell receptor without autoreactivity (14). If the immature B cells also pass this last selection process, they become mature B cells and are allowed to leave the bone marrow microenvironment to enter the peripheral immune system. Mature B cells express, with rare exceptions, only one light chain gene, either of the κ or λ isotype (allelic and isotype exclusion). Whereas immature B cells carry only IgM on their surface, mature B cells coexpress IgM and IgD. Approximately 60% of mature human B cells express κ light chains; 40% express λ light chains.

V Gene Recombination and Antibody Diversity

V gene recombination is guided by specific sequences flanking the V, D, and J gene segments, the recombination signal sequences. These sites are composed of a conserved heptamer, a spacer of either 12 or 23 base pairs' length, and a conserved nonamer (15). The sites are present at the 3' end of V gene segments, at the 5' ends of J gene segments, and at both ends of D_H gene segments (Fig. 47.1). Rearrangement takes place only between gene segments with different spacer lengths (12/23 base pair rule). For example, in the human IgH locus, V and J gene segments have recombination signal sequences with 23 base pair spacers, whereas the recombination signal sequences of D_H gene segments contain 12 base pair spacers. This ensures that rearrangement cannot happen between two V gene segments and that a V_H gene is not directly joined to a J_H gene.

The enzymatic machinery that controls V gene recombination is largely known [reviewed in (15)]. Only two of the enzymes involved in the process are lymphocyte specific, namely the recombination-activating genes RAG-1 and RAG-2. These enzymes recognize the recombination signal sequences and introduce DNA double-strand breaks precisely between the heptamer of the recombination signal sequences and the respective gene segment (16). This happens in a complex in which the ends of the two rearranging gene segments are brought close to each other. The ends of the gene segments (coding ends) are closed by the generation of hairpin loops, whereas the ends of the recombination signal sequences (signal ends) have a blunt end structure. In the next step, the coding ends are opened at a variable position along the hairpin. This may create short palindromic sequences (P nucleotides) that contribute to the diversity of the joining sites. The coding ends are usually further modified, either by the exonucleolytic loss of some base pairs or by the introduction of additional, non–germline-encoded bases (N nucleotides). The latter is mediated by the enzyme terminal deoxynucleotidyl transferase. After these modifications, the coding ends are joined. These modifications of the joining sites vastly increase the diversity of the antigen-binding sites, thereby significantly contributing to the essentially limitless diversity of antibody molecules. The signal ends of the intervening DNA are usually closed to a circle, which is released from the complex and later lost from the cell. However, when the rearranging gene segments are not in the same transcriptional orientation, as it is the case for approximately one-half of the human Vκ gene segments in relation to the Jκ genes (8), V gene recombination does not result in the deletion of the intervening DNA but in an inversion, without loss of DNA from the chromosome.

Besides the lymphocyte-specific RAG proteins (and optionally terminal deoxynucleotidyl transferase), the enzymatic recombination machinery is composed of ubiquitously expressed enzymes involved in double-stranded DNA repair, that is DNA-PKcs, the Ku70 and Ku80 proteins, XRCC4, DNA ligase IV, and the Artemis protein (15). Artemis was only recently identified as a component of the recombination complex and in a complex with DNA-PKcs plays an important role in the opening of the hairpin and the trimming of the overhangs (17,18). If any of the components of the V gene recombination machinery are lacking, V gene recombination is blocked, and no or only few mature lymphocytes develop.

Due to the modifications introduced at the ends of the rearranging gene segments, the correct reading frame of the Ig gene, defined by the start codon in the leader peptide of the V gene segment, can be retained or lost in the V(D)J joining reaction. In in-frame rearrangements, the J gene segment and the following C gene to which the V region gene is precisely spliced are read in the correct reading frame and can thus be translated into protein (note that many D elements of heavy chain rearrangements can be read in all three possible reading frames). However, if the reading frame is lost, the C gene is not read in the correct reading frame, and the rearrangement is out-of-frame (Fig. 47.2). Often, premature stop codons are encountered in the incorrectly translated C genes. As the codons are nucleotide triplets, only one-third of the rearrangements are in-frame. Moreover, some in-frame rearrangements are nonproductive because a stop codon can be generated at the breakpoints of recombination.

The high frequency of nonproductive V gene rearrangements potentially results in a massive wastage of B-cell precursors that did not succeed in generating productive heavy and light chain gene rearrangements. However, the loss of cells is reduced, as on the heavy chain locus, a second recombination attempt can be made on the second IgH allele. For the light chains, there are even four loci available (two κ and two λ). Moreover, the structure of the light chain loci allows for repeated V-J rearrangements on a given allele: If a first rearrangement is nonproductive, a second attempt can be made if upstream unrearranged V and downstream germline J seg-

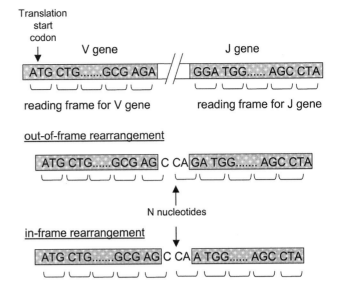

FIG. 47.2. V gene rearrangements can be in-frame or out-of-frame. Shown are two possible outcomes of a V_L to J_L joining. The reading frame of the V gene segment is defined by the start codon of the leader exon (leader exon and V segment are not distinguished here). There is also only one functional reading frame for the J gene segment, as this is directly spliced to the constant region gene, which codes for an immunoglobulin (Ig) light chain protein only in one reading frame. If the removal of nucleotides from the ends of the V and J segments and the addition of N nucleotides results in a reading frame in which the J gene segment (and consequently the C gene) are read in the correct frame, the rearrangement is in-frame (note that in-frame rearrangements can be nonfunctional if a stop codon is generated at the V-J joint). In out-of-frame rearrangements, the number of nucleotides between the last complete V codon and the first complete J codon is not a multiple of three, so that the J segment and, consequently, the C segment are not translated in the correct reading frame. Such rearrangements are nonfunctional, as they do not code for an Ig light chain protein. Note that out-of-frame rearrangements do not necessarily generate stop codons at the joining site or in the J gene. Usually, stop codons are encountered in the C gene segments if they are translated in the wrong reading frame, resulting in premature translation stop. The correct codons defined in the germline and the codons used after rearrangement are indicated below the sequences.

ments are still present. For the heavy chain locus, this kind of additional rearrangement is not possible, as all germline D_H gene segments are deleted in the first $V_HD_HJ_H$ recombination, and a direct V_H to J_H joining is not allowed, as discussed above. However, most human V_H gene segments contain an internal heptamer sequence close to the 3' end of the coding sequence, and the analysis of pre B-cell leukemias indicates that this internal heptamer can be used to perform a V_H gene replacement in which an upstream V_H germline gene replaces a V_H gene segment in a $V_HD_HJ_H$ joint (19). However, it is not known whether V_H gene replacement is used at a significant frequency in the development of normal B cells.

B CELLS IN T-CELL–DEPENDENT IMMUNE RESPONSES

Initiating T-Cell–Dependent Immune Responses

If foreign antigens cross the epithelial layers of the body and enter human tissues, they are taken up by resident dendritic cells. These dendritic cells then migrate to the T-cell zone of local lymph nodes where they present antigenic peptides on MHC class II molecules. This results in the specific recruitment and activation of antigen-specific T helper cells. B cells that enter lymph nodes through high endothelial venules also migrate through the T-cell zones on their way to the B-cell follicles. If a B cell encounters cognate antigen in the T-cell zone, it is retained in this area and becomes activated (20). Antigen-specific T and B cells can now interact and stimulate each other. As a consequence, B cells start to proliferate, and clusters of proliferating B cells, called *primary foci*, become visible a few days after initiation of the immune response (20). A fraction of these B cells differentiates into short-lived plasma cells and produces a first wave of antibody (21). Other antigen-specific B cells of the foci migrate

into primary B-cell follicles where they then initiate the germinal center reaction (Fig. 47.3) (21). Experiments in the mouse indicate that the primary foci usually involute after a few days (22).

Germinal Center Reaction

Antigen-activated B cells that migrate from the T-cell zone into primary B-cell follicles start to vigorously proliferate and differentiate into centroblasts (23). The resident resting B cells of the primary follicle are moved away from the follicle center and build a corona of resting cells around the germinal center, the mantle zone. After some days, two distinct compartments of the germinal center can be histologically recognized, the dark zone and the light zone (Fig. 47.4). The dark zone is dominated by proliferating centroblasts and harbors a loose network of follicular dendritic cells, whereas the light zone is mainly composed of non–cycling centrocytes, a dense network of follicular dendritic cells and T helper cells (23). In the course of their clonal expansion, centroblasts activate the process of somatic hypermutation, which intro-

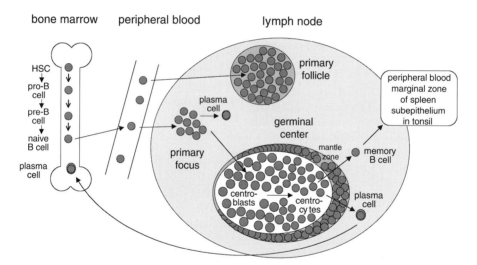

FIG. 47.3. B-cell developmental pathways. B cells are generated in the bone marrow (or during fetal development in the liver) from hematopoietic stem cells. B-cell precursors that performed D_H-J_H rearrangements at their immunoglobulin (Ig) H loci are called *pro B cells*. D_H-J_H rearrangements are usually followed by V_H to $D_H J_H$ rearrangements, and the cells expressing a functional heavy chain rearrangement are termed *pre B cells*. The cells then perform rearrangements at their light chain loci. Cells expressing a functional (and nonautoreactive) B-cell receptor are allowed to mature and leave the bone marrow as naïve B cells. Naïve B cells are found in the peripheral blood; in secondary lymphoid organs, they constitute primary B-cell follicles and the mantle zone of secondary B-cell follicles. Early steps in adaptive immune responses usually take place in the T-cell area of lymphoid organs, where antigen-activated B cells are in contact with T cells and dendritic cells. The interaction of these cells stimulates B-cell proliferation, leading to the generation of primary B-cell foci in the T-cell area. Some of the B cells differentiate into (presumably short-lived) plasma cells. Other activated B cells migrate into B-cell follicles, where they undergo massive clonal expansion and establish germinal centers (see Fig. 47.4 details of the germinal center reaction). Positively selected germinal center B cells differentiate to memory B cells or plasmablasts and leave the germinal center. Many plasma cell precursors home to the bone marrow, where these long-lived cells can secrete large amounts of antibody. Memory B cells are found in the peripheral blood and also in lymphoid organs. In tonsils, they are mainly located in the subepithelial region; in the spleen, they are a major constituent of the marginal zone.

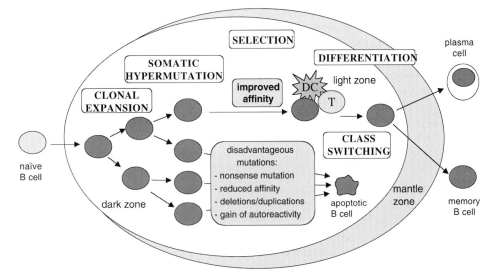

FIG. 47.4. The germinal center (GC) reaction. Antigen-activated B cells that receive appropriate T-cell help are driven into primary B-cell follicles where they establish GCs. In the GC, a dark zone and a light zone can be distinguished. The dark zone mainly consists of proliferating GC B cells, the centroblasts, whereas the GC B cells in the light zone, the centrocytes, are resting B cells. The GC is surrounded by a mantle of resting, naïve B cells, which constitute the primary follicle. In proliferating GC B cells, the process of somatic hypermutation is activated, which leads to the introduction of mutations at a high rate specifically into the immunoglobulin V region genes of the proliferating B cells. Most mutations are disadvantageous for the cells such as when they result in reduced affinity of the B-cell receptor to the respective antigen. B cells acquiring such mutations undergo apoptosis. Only a few GC B cells acquire affinity-increasing mutations, and these cells are positively selected. The selection process presumably takes place mainly in the light zone, where the centrocytes are in close contact with CD4 T cells and follicular dendritic cells. A fraction of the centrocytes undergo class-switch recombination. Finally, antigen-selected GC B cells differentiate to memory B cells or plasma cells and leave the GC microenvironment.

duces mutations at a high rate into the V region genes of the antigen receptor (24–26) (see below). Thereby, antibody variants are generated. The centroblasts then move to the light zone where they are selected based on the affinity of their B-cell receptor to the respective antigen (Fig. 47.4). Germinal center B cells expressing a B-cell receptor with increased affinity are able to appropriately interact with germinal center T cells and follicular dendritic cells and be positively selected (27,28). Likely, the vast majority of germinal center B cells acquire disadvantageous mutations and undergo apoptosis. These cells are taken up by macrophages, which are also present in the germinal center (29). Selected germinal center B cells likely undergo repeated rounds of proliferation, mutation, and selection, resulting in a very efficient selection of germinal center B cells with high-affinity B-cell receptors (30).

In many germinal center B cells, the Ig genes are not only modified at the level of the V region genes by somatic hypermutation but also by altering the isotype of the IgH constant region genes. This change from IgM and IgD expression to IgG, IgA, or IgE is performed by a somatic recombination process termed *class-switch recombination* (see below).

Based on the detection of RAG transcripts or protein in germinal center B cells and V gene recombination intermediates in both human and mouse, it has been suggested that V gene recombination may be reinitiated in germinal center B cells (31–34). This would enable these cells to revise their antigen receptors, such as by replacing the originally expressed light chain gene by a novel one, and would represent a further means of antibody diversification in germinal center B cells besides somatic hypermutation. However, more recent studies question the original reports. For example, monitoring RAG expression with a reporter gene in mice showed that RAG2 expression is not reinitiated in germinal center B cells and in the periphery restricted to immature B cells presumably recently immigrated from the bone marrow (35). In the human, there is now indication that RAG- and terminal deoxynucleotidyl transferase–expressing tonsillar B cells are mostly found outside germinal centers, perhaps also representing immature B cells (36). Hence, although there are some examples of normal or disease-associated human B cells that show indication for receptor revision, the contribution of receptor revision to shaping the memory B-cell compartment in the human seems to be modest at most (37).

Finally, the selected germinal center B cells differentiate into memory B cells or plasma cell precursors and leave the germinal center microenvironment. The signals that regulate these different developmental pathways are not yet fully understood. However, *in vitro* experiments suggest that incubation of germinal center B cells with interleukin (IL)-2 and IL-10 and cross-linking of CD40 or cross-linking of the B-cell receptor together with IL-4 stimulation induces differentiation of the cells to a resting B-cell population resembling memory B cells (38,39). Treatment of germinal center B cells with recombinant CD23 and IL-1α results in the development of cells sharing features with plasma cells (40). It is intriguing that the CD40 ligand is expressed by germinal center T cells (41), and CD23 is highly expressed by follicular dendritic cells (42). Studies in the mouse indicate that plasma cells generated in the germinal center are very long-lived, so that they are able to sustain high serum antibody levels (43,44).

Somatic Hypermutation

Somatic hypermutation is a process by which point mutations are introduced into productively or nonproductively rearranged V region genes at a high rate (10^{-3} to 10^{-4}/bp/cell division) (45). The mutations are introduced into the DNA over a distance of 1.5 to 2.0 kilobases, beginning downstream of the V gene promoter and extending into the intron between variable and constant region genes. The constant region genes themselves are not targeted by somatic hypermutation. Most of the mutations are single nucleotide exchanges, but deletions and duplications of various length can also be found, accounting for approximately 4% to 5% of the mutation events in human B cells (46). The pattern of somatic mutations is not random. There is an intrinsic preference for transitions (replacement of a purine by a purine base or a pyrimidine by a pyrimidine base) over transversions (replacement of a purine by a pyrimidine base or vice versa), and several hot spot motifs of somatic hypermutation have been identified (47). The most prominent hot spot is the RGYW motif (with R representing A or G, Y representing C or T, and W defining A or T) (48,49).

Studies in the mouse revealed that somatic hypermutation depends on transcription of the target sequence, although the V gene promoter can be replaced by other promoters (50,51). Likewise, the target sequence does not have to be a (rearranged) V gene but can be any sequence downstream of the promoter (52). In contrast, the Ig enhancers represent indispensable elements for somatic hypermutation, as their deletion severely impairs somatic hypermutation (50). Hence, the target for hypermutation of Ig V genes is defined by an active promoter in close association with the Ig-specific enhancers.

In the human, somatic hypermutation appears to be not absolutely specific for rearranged Ig genes. So far, two genes have been identified that acquire mutations in germinal center B cells at a significant frequency and with a mutation pattern consistent with somatic hypermutation. The bcl-6 gene

is found mutated in its 5' region in approximately one-third of human germinal center and memory B cells (53,54). Also, the CD95 gene carries mutations in its 5' region in a small fraction of germinal center B cells (55). The molecular features of these genes causing them to be targeted by the hypermutation machinery are still unclear.

Recent studies in the mouse showed that somatic hypermutation is accompanied by DNA strand breaks in the V region genes, but it is debated whether these are single- or double-strand breaks and whether they occur mainly in the G1 or the G2/M phase of the cell cycle (46,56–59). The detection of strand breaks in V region genes of germinal center B cells supports a model in which such breaks are first introduced into the DNA, followed by an error-prone DNA repair. A number of DNA repair enzymes were tested for their involvement in somatic hypermutation, but they showed little if any direct effect on the generation of somatic mutations. More recently, a potential role of error-prone DNA polymerases in the somatic hypermutation process was analyzed. The error-prone DNA polymerases ζ and ι represent attractive candidates for such polymerases (60,61).

The most dramatic recent advance in the field was the discovery of the essential role of activation-induced cytidine deaminase (AID) in both somatic hypermutation and class-switch recombination (62,63). The role of AID as a master regulator of these processes is suggested by the fact that AID deficiency in humans results in the autosomal-recessive form of the hyper-IgM syndrome, which is characterized by the absence of class-switch recombination and a lack of somatic hypermutation (63), and that ectopic AID expression is sufficient to cause somatic hypermutation and class switching of transgenic constructs in non-B cells (64,65). AID may function in somatic hypermutation by deaminating cytosine bases in the DNA, resulting in the generation of uracil, which is not a normal base in DNA, and this may induce an error-prone DNA repair (66,67).

Although it is clear that somatic hypermutation is a hallmark of germinal center B cells and that at least the vast majority of B cells with mutated Ig genes are derived from germinal center B cells, it is an intriguing question whether hypermutation may occur in human B cells also outside of the germinal center microenvironment. Several observations are in favor of this idea: (a) In lymphotoxin α-deficient mice that lack germinal centers, somatically mutated V genes have been identified after immunization (68); (b) in a CD95-deficient transgenic mouse strain in which the B cells produce an autoreactive antibody, somatic hypermutation occurs in B cells proliferating outside B-cell follicles (69); (c) hyper-IgM patients who appear to lack germinal centers due to a deficiency in the CD40 ligand gene lack classical memory B cells but have an IgM+IgD+CD27+ B-cell population with somatically mutated Ig genes (70). This raises the interesting possibility that the mutated IgD+ B cells are generated in a germinal center–independent way (70). However, it may well be that CD40L-independent germinal center or germinal center–like structures supporting somatic hypermutation but not class-switching exist in some lymphoid organs of hyper-IgM patients. This is reminiscent of the situation in CD19-deficient mice, which do not develop germinal centers in spleen and lymph nodes on immunization but have these structures in Peyer's patches (71). It is also noteworthy that hyper-IgM patients with a deficiency in the CD40 gene apparently lack a population of somatically mutated IgD⁺CD27⁺ B cells (72). Regarding the mouse models indicating germinal center–independent hypermutation, it should be noted that hypermutation is observed only under unphysiologic conditions such as the need for CD95 gene deficiency in the Ig receptor transgenic strain and the need for repeated and adjuvant-enhanced immunization of lymphotoxin α mice. The latter mice do not generate high-affinity (somatically mutated) B cells under "normal" immunization conditions (73). Taken together, some human B cells may acquire somatic mutations in a germinal center–independent manner, but direct evidence for this is still weak.

Class-Switch Recombination

Class-switch recombination is—besides somatic hypermutation—the second B-cell–specific process that modifies the Ig genes. By class-switching, the Ig heavy chain constant region gene expressed by a B cell is changed. Naïve B cells express IgM and IgD on their surface as a result of differential splicing of the corresponding messenger RNA transcripts, but after antigen activation, the IgH class of the B-cell receptor is often changed to IgG, IgA, or IgE. This alters the effector functions of the antibody molecule. For example, IgA dimers can cross epithelial layers and can be secreted into the gut lumen, and IgG can bind to specific receptors on phagocytic cells (Fcγ receptors), thereby improving pathogen recognition and binding by those cells.

In the human, there are nine IgH constant (C_H) region genes, one Cμ, one Cδ, four Cγ, two Cα, and one Cε genes (74). These gene segments are located downstream of the V, D, and J gene segments on chromosome 14. Class switching is mediated by a somatic recombination process that results in deletion of the originally expressed IgH genes (usually IgM and IgD) and their replacement by one of the further downstream-located IgH genes.

The class-switch recombination process is initiated by transcription from promoters upstream of the C_H genes (75). These transcripts contain a first exon (I exon) located upstream of repetitive elements, the switch regions, that is spliced to the C_H exons. The generation of these germline transcripts and their splicing is mandatory for the class-switch recombination process, but it is not yet clarified whether the role of this transcription is mainly in regulating the accessibility of the IgH locus for the recombination machinery or whether the germline transcripts are directly involved in the recombination process (76,77).

In the next step, DNA breaks (either double-strand breaks or staggered single-strand breaks) are introduced into the repetitive switch regions of the two C_H genes involved in the class-switching process (Fig. 47.5). The intervening DNA is excised

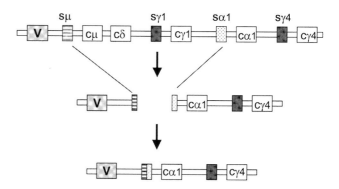

FIG. 47.5. Class-switch recombination. Class switching is initiated by transcription through the repetitive switch regions and the C_H genes involved in the recombination process, followed by splicing of the transcripts (not shown). In the next step, DNA strand breaks are introduced in the switch regions. The DNA between the two switch sites is deleted as a circle (not shown) and later lost from the cell. As a result of the class-switch recombination process, a downstream C_H gene is now juxtaposed to the V region gene, so that this C_H gene is now expressed instead of the original one.

as a circle (switch circle) that is later lost from the cell, and the two switch regions are joined. Class switching usually results in replacement of the originally expressed Cμ (and Cδ) gene by a downstream C_H gene, but there is also indication that sequential class-switching processes can take place (78).

The enzymes involved in the regulation of class-switch recombination are only partly known. The later steps of the process appear to be mediated by the components of nonhomologous end-joining DNA repair. A master regulator and perhaps the only B-cell–specific component of class switching is the AID protein, as its ectopic expression is sufficient to induce class switching of an extrachromosomal construct even in fibroblasts, as discussed above (64).

Most class switching takes place in the germinal center microenvironment, which is evident from the fact that nearly all class-switched B cells and plasma cells in the human carry somatically mutated V region genes and, hence, the hallmark of a germinal center passage. However, class-switch recombination—mostly to Cγ2—can also take place in T-cell–independent immune responses (79,80).

B CELLS IN T-CELL–INDEPENDENT IMMUNE RESPONSES

Although humoral immune responses against most protein antigens are dependent on T helper cells, antibodies against many bacterial antigens can also be produced in humans or mice lacking a thymus or with other T-cell deficiencies. Such thymus-independent (TI) antigens fall into two classes, TI-1 and TI-2 antigens. TI-1 antigens result in a polyclonal B-cell activation and can thus also be considered as B-cell mitogens. TI-2 antigens are characterized by highly repetitive structures (81). This allows for a strong cross-linking of the B-cell receptor on the surface of the B cells. TI-2 antigens are typically bacterial capsular polysaccharides. Immune responses of the TI-II type are, however, not completely T-cell independent because mouse strains lacking all T cells are impaired in immune responses against TI-2 antigens (81). The exact role of T cells in these responses is not yet understood. There are indications that specific subsets of B cells are mainly involved in T-cell–independent immune responses, namely CD5+ B cells and a fraction of marginal zone B cells (see below).

REGULATION OF B-CELL DEVELOPMENT AND DIFFERENTIATION BY TRANSCRIPTION FACTORS

The appropriate expression of genes needed for the generation of B cells and the execution of specific functions at distinct stages of differentiation is regulated by the coordinated activity of a series of transcription factors (Fig. 47.6). One of the factors needed for the earliest stages of B-cell development is PU.1, which is expressed exclusively in hematopoietic cells (82). PU.1 plays a role not only for the development of B cells but also of macrophages. Although very high expression of this ets-type transcription factor favors the development of macrophages, moderate expression results in a preferential generation of B cells (83). Among the target genes of PU.1 in early B-cell development is the IL-7 receptor, which is essential for B-cell development in the bone marrow.

The E12 and E47 gene products of the E2A gene are members of the basic helix-loop-helix family of transcription factors. They are widely expressed, but homodimeric complexes appear to be restricted to B-lineage cells (84). The E2A proteins are involved in the expression and rearrangement of Ig genes (84). Hence, E2A is essential for the development of pro B cells from a common lymphoid precursor. Another transcription factor needed for the development of pro B cells is the early B-cell factor, which is expressed at all stages of B-cell differentiation, excluding plasma cells (85). Genes activated by the early B-cell factor include the transcription factor Pax-5 (see below); the B-cell receptor–associated signal-transducing molecule CD79b; λ5, a component of the pre B-cell receptor; and kappa light chains.

The key molecule for the commitment of cells to the B lineage is the transcription factor B-cell–specific activating protein, the product of the Pax-5 gene. Mouse models revealed that in the absence of Pax-5 B-cell development is arrested at the pro B-cell stage and that these cells that carry $D_H J_H$ joints have retained the capacity to give rise to other lineages, such as T cells and monocytes (86,87). Thus, one of the main functions of Pax-5 appears to be the suppression of alternative developmental pathways in B-lineage precursors and the commitment of these cells to the B-lymphoid lineage. Critical B-cell–specific genes are positively controlled by B-cell–specific activating protein, including CD19 and CD79a. The Pax-5 gene

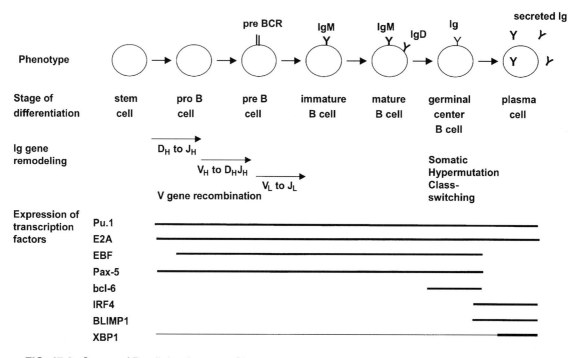

FIG. 47.6. Stages of B-cell development. Given are the main stages of B-cell development in the human. It is indicated at which stages immunoglobulin (Ig) genes are remodeled by V gene recombination, somatic hypermutation, or class-switch recombination. The expression pattern of several key transcription factors for B-cell development is shown. Note that this list does not include all known transcription factors involved in B-cell development. IRF4 and Blimp1 are starting to be expressed in a small subset of germinal center B cells in the light zone with plasmacytoid features. These cells are already Bcl-6−.

is also expressed in mature B cells and appears to play a role in these cells to maintain their B-cell identity (88,89).

For the differentiation of activated B cells to germinal center B cells, the transcriptional repressor bcl-6 is critical, as bcl-6–deficient mice are unable to generate germinal centers (90,91). bcl-6 is upregulated in B cells before they enter the germinal center, highly expressed in germinal center B cells, and downregulated before the cells differentiate to memory or plasma cells (92,93). bcl-6 regulates a large number of genes in germinal center B cells (94). For example, expression of early activation markers is downregulated. Rapid proliferation of germinal center B cells is mediated by bcl-6 through repression of the cell-cycle inhibitor p27kip1 and by activating c-myc, which is essential for cell proliferation, through repression of a c-myc repressor. Moreover, bcl-6 represses transcription factors important for plasma cell differentiation (see below), thereby arresting cells at the germinal center B-cell stage of development as long as bcl-6 is expressed.

When germinal center B cells differentiate into plasma cells, major changes in gene expression happen. This is accompanied by downregulation of several transcription factors that are expressed during early B-cell development and in mature B cells, such as early B-cell factor and Pax-5. Moreover, as already discussed, downregulation of bcl-6 is needed to allow germinal center B cells to terminally differentiate. However, several transcription factors are upregulated in plasma cells, namely the B-lymphocyte–induced maturation protein-1 (Blimp-1), the interferon regulatory factor-4 (IRF-4, also called *MUM-1*), and the X-box–binding protein-1 (XBP-1). Expression of Blimp-1 and IRF-4 is already detectable in a small subset of germinal center B cells that are located in the light zone and resemble early plasma cells, suggesting that the differentiation of germinal center B cells toward plasma cells is initiated in the germinal center microenvironment (95,96).

Blimp-1 is a transcriptional repressor that is involved in the repression of many genes, including BCL-6, Pax-5, C-MYC, CD19, CD20, and MHC class II [summarized in (97)]. Thus, Blimp-1 downregulates many germinal center B-cell functions and activates plasma cell functions. Blimp-1 is repressed by bcl-6 (94); hence, the balance between bcl-6 and Blimp-1 is a key determinant for the switch from a germinal center B cell to a plasma cell fate. IRF-4 can associate with several other transcription factors, such as PU.1 and SpiB, and the lack of plasma cells in IRF-4–deficient mice suggests an important role in plasma cell development (98). So far, little is known about the genes regulated by this factor besides a potential involvement in the regulation of Ig transcription. XBP-1 is an activating, ubiquitously expressed transcription factor that is highly upregulated in plasma cells (99). The critical target genes of XBP-1 are still unknown, but like in the case of IRF-4, no plasma cells develop in mice in the absence of XBP-1 (99). This transcription factor is repressed by the Pax-5 gene product (100), which is likely one of the reasons why downregulation of Pax-5 is a prerequisite for the development of plasma cells.

PERIPHERAL B-CELL COMPARTMENT

B Cells in the Peripheral Blood

In the fetus and in the first years after birth, most B cells in the peripheral blood express the CD5 antigen (101). This antigen was originally identified as a T-cell marker but was later also found on a subset of B cells. Studies in the mouse suggested that CD5 B cells are mainly involved in T-cell–independent immune responses (type II) and are responsible for production of a large fraction of "natural" serum antibodies (102). As these cells also show a restricted V gene usage and appear to be self-replenishing, it has been speculated that they represent a separate, perhaps evolutionary old, B-cell lineage important as a first line of defense against common infectious agents. However, more recent experiments suggest that B-cell receptor engagement is critical for the development of CD5 B cells, leading to the "induced-differentiation" model for the generation of these cells (102). Whether human CD5 B cells are equivalent to murine CD5 B cells is debatable. Human CD5 B cells share with murine CD5 B cells in that they are the predominant B-cell population early in life and that they only very rarely have participated in germinal center reactions, as they mostly carry unmutated V region genes (103–105). Moreover, murine CD5 B cells regularly become an oligoclonal population in old animals, and a development of clonal expansions among CD5 B cells was recently also observed in a few percent of elderly humans (106). However, there are also differences. For example, the restricted V_H gene repertoire that is characteristic for murine CD5 B cells is observed only among human fetal CD5 B cells but not in adults (103,107). In adult humans, CD5 B cells account for approximately 15% of the peripheral blood B-cell pool.

The largest distinct population of B cells in the peripheral blood are conventional (i.e., CD5⁻) naïve B cells (Table 47.1). These cells usually account for 45% of the B-cell pool in adults (108). Naïve B cells coexpress IgM and IgD on their surface and are characterized by unmutated V region genes.

Class-switched B cells, expressing IgG, IgA, or IgE, were classically considered to represent the population of memory B cells that were generated in germinal center reactions. Most, if not all, of these cells, which represent approximately 10% to 15% of B cells in the peripheral blood (Table 47.1), indeed carry somatically mutated V region genes. However, class-switched cells appear to be not the only memory B cells in the human. Somatically mutated Ig genes are also a hallmark of cells expressing IgM without significant levels of IgD (IgM-only B cells) (109). These cells share several other features with class-switched cells, supporting their close relationship: Both B-cell subsets can under similar stimulation conditions differentiate into plasma cells, whereas naïve B cells are resistant to these stimuli (110). Both subsets are lacking in hyper-IgM patients who apparently lack germinal centers due to a defect in the CD40 ligand gene (70). Moreover, IgM-only and class-switched B cells share expression of the CD27 surface molecule, a member of the tumor necrosis factor receptor family that plays an

TABLE 47.1. *Cellular composition of the peripheral blood B-cell compartment[a]*

B-cell subset	Phenotype				Average frequency (%)	Average mutation frequency of V_H genes (%)
	sIg	CD27	CD5	CD20		
Pre–germinal center						
Naïve conventional	IgM+IgD+	−	+	+	45	0
CD5+	IgM+IgD+	−	+	+	15	0[b]
Post–germinal center						
IgM+IgD+ memory	IgM+IgD+	+	−	+	15	5
IgM-only	IgM+IgD$^{low/−}$	+	−	+	10	6
Class switched	IgG+ or IgA+	+	−	+	15	6
IgD-only	IgM−IgD+	+	−	+	<1	12
Plasmablasts	sIg$^{low/−}$	+	−	−	<2	7[c]

sIg, surface immunoglobulin.

[a]The average frequency of the various B-cell subsets in the peripheral blood of healthy adults and their Ig gene mutation loads can vary among individuals. Whether IgM+IgD+CD27+ B cells are a post–germinal center B-cell subset is debated (70). A further small B-cell subset, not shown in the table, accounts for 0.5% to 1.0% of peripheral blood B cells and is characterized by coexpression of light chains and surrogate light chains (112). This population consists of pre– as well as post–germinal center B cells.

[b]A small fraction of CD5-expressing B cells carries mutated V genes (103–105).

[c]So far, mutation frequency only determined for plasmablasts from a patient affected by systemic lupus erythematosus (114).

important role in B-cell differentiation toward plasma cells (108). Naïve B cells with unmutated Ig genes lack CD27 expression (108).

It is interesting that a subset of IgM+IgD+ B cells also expresses CD27 (110). These B cells, which represent up to 20% of IgD+ B cells and approximately 10% to 15% of all B cells in the peripheral blood, also carry somatically mutated V region genes, suggesting that they also represent a subset of memory B cells and that CD27 thus likely represents a marker for memory B cells in the human (108). Consequently, naïve, pre–germinal center B cells in humans have the phenotype IgM+IgD+CD27−. That IgM+IgD+CD27+ B cells belong to the memory B-cell compartment is also supported by phenotypic and functional similarities to IgM-only and class-switched memory B cells (108,110). However, the presence of IgM+IgD+CD27+ B cells with mutated Ig genes in CD40 ligand–deficient hyper-IgM patients may indicate that these cells derive from a separate developmental pathway independent of germinal centers, as discussed above (70).

A peculiar and rare peripheral blood B-cell subset is the population of B cells expressing IgD without IgM (IgD-only B cells), which are also found in tonsillar tissues (108,111). These cells performed an unusual class-switch recombination, resulting in the deletion of the Cμ gene, although retaining the Cδ gene, so that they express IgD in the complete absence of IgM. These cells carry the highest Ig V gene mutation load of all human B-cell subsets (average of 12% to 14%). The frequency of IgD-only B cells among all B cells in the peripheral blood is usually less than 1% (108). A further peculiarity of these cells is their predominant expression of lambda light chains. The role of these cells in humoral immunity is presently unclear.

Another peculiar peripheral blood B-cell subset is defined by coexpression of kappa or lambda light chains and surrogate light chains (112). These cells account for 0.5% to 1.0% of the B cells in peripheral blood. Based on the V gene mutation status and CD27 expression pattern, this population includes both pre– as well as post–germinal center B cells (112). As the light chain and surrogate light chain coexpressing B cells express low levels of RAG messenger RNA and show a significantly biased antibody repertoire, it has been suggested that they may represent cells expressing autoreactive and edited B-cell receptors. Indeed, these cells have been found enriched in the joints of patients with rheumatoid arthritis (112).

Plasma cells are mainly found in lymphoid tissues (see below), and they are rare in the peripheral blood. The frequency of CD38^{high}CD20^{low} cells, which include plasma cells and their immediate precursors, plasmablasts, usually is in the range of 1% to 2% among all B-lineage cells (113,114).

B-Cell Subsets in Tissues

In secondary lymphoid tissues [i.e., lymph nodes, spleen, and Peyer's patches of the mucosa-associated lymphoid tissue (MALT)], mature B cells of distinct differentiation stages can be found in distinct histologic structures (Fig.47.7). Naïve B cells populate primary follicles in lymph nodes and spleen. As discussed earlier, when a germinal center develops in a primary follicle, these cells are pushed aside and constitute the mantle zone of the germinal center in the secondary follicle.

In the white pulp of the spleen, a distinct B-cell compartment is located around the mantle zone of germinal centers, the marginal zone. Many of the B cells in this area are IgM+IgD$^{−/low}$, and most of the cells carry somatically mutated

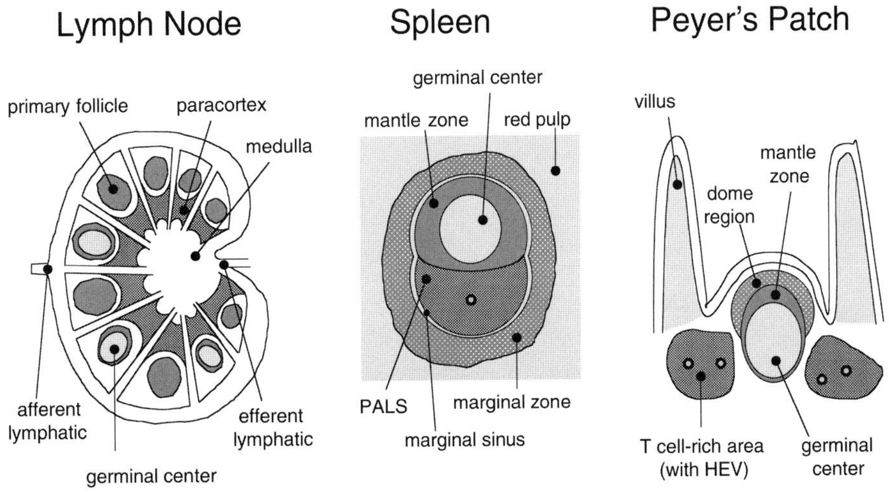

Lymph Node   Spleen   Peyer's Patch

FIG. 47.7. Schematic structures of secondary lymphoid organs. Lymph node: The cortex of lymph nodes consists mainly of primary B-cell follicles or germinal centers. The paracortex is an area rich in T lymphocytes. In the medulla, macrophages and plasma cells are found. The lymph enters the lymph node through afferent lymphatics and leaves the lymph node through efferent lymphatics. The structure of blood vessels is not shown. Spleen: A detailed view of a white pulp area surrounded by red pulp is shown. The white pulp is composed of a germinal center surrounded by a mantle zone and the T-cell–rich periarteriolar lymphoid sheath. A high endothelial venule is shown in the center of the T-cell zone. The white pulp is surrounded by the marginal zone. The space between the marginal zone and the central parts of the white pulp is called the *marginal sinus*. The mantle zone is mainly composed of immunoglobulin D+ (IgD+) naïve B cells, whereas many marginal zone B cells show features of IgD–memory B cells. Many plasma cells migrate to the red pulp. Peyer's patch: A Peyer's patch lymph node and two villi are shown. In the villi, many plasma cells are found. In the lymph node area, one can distinguish a T-cell–rich area with high endothelial venules and a B-cell area. In the B-cell area, a germinal center, surrounded by a mantle zone, is shown. Adjacent to the mantle zone, a dome region is found. Whereas the mantle zone is populated mainly by naïve B cells, the dome region consists mainly of memory B cells. HEV, high endothelial venules; PALS, periarteriolar lymphoid sheaths.

V region genes (115–117). Hence, the marginal zone is a reservoir of (IgM only) memory B cells. However, a subset of marginal zone B cells is responsive to T-cell–independent type II antigens, suggesting that naïve B cells, albeit at a low frequency, are also present in the marginal zone (118). In Peyer's patches, a structure corresponding to the marginal zone of the spleen is seen around the mantle zones of germinal centers. Like in the spleen, these cells mostly represent memory B cells, as they harbor mutated Ig genes and lack IgD expression (119). In human tonsils, which are also components of the MALT, a distinct marginal zone is missing. Here, memory B cells are located mainly in the subepithelial region (120). A clear marginal zone is also lacking in lymph nodes. However, in several types of infections, a population of B cells can be discerned near sinus structures of the lymph node. These B cells have a more pronounced cytoplasm than naïve B cells, similar to memory B cells in the spleen and tonsil. Because of morphologic similarities to monocytes, these cells are designated *monocytoid B cells*. The monocytoid B-cell population appears to be a mixture of pre–germinal center and memory B cells (117,121).

Also, terminally differentiated B-lineage cells (i.e., plasma cells) show a typical distribution in lymphoid tissues. In the spleen, plasma cells are mainly found in the red pulp, although their numbers are relatively low in lymph nodes. Many plasma cells generated in germinal centers migrate to the bone marrow, which is, therefore, an important microenvironment for serum antibody production. However, approximately 80% of human plasma cells are found in extrafollicular areas of Peyer's patches along the intestine (122). Most of these plasma cells carry mutated Ig V genes, suggesting that they developed in germinal centers (123,124).

RELATIONSHIP OF NORMAL B CELLS TO B-CELL NEOPLASMS

Typing B-Cell Tumors to Their Normal Counterparts

As outlined in more detail in other chapters of this book, considerable efforts have been made to identify the cellular origin of the various types of lymphomas. Often, the immunophenotype of the tumor cells or the histology was suggestive for the normal counterpart of the lymphoma cells. For example, the derivation of follicular lymphoma cells from transformed germinal center B cells is suggested by the observations that the tumor cells share several surface markers with normal germinal center B cells (e.g., bcl-6) and morphologically resemble these cells by the follicular growth pattern of the lymphoma and the associa-

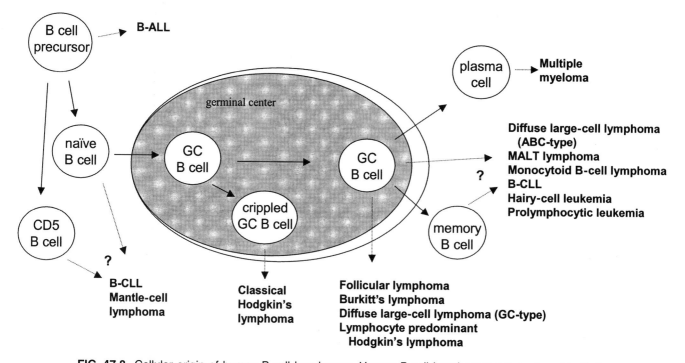

FIG. 47.8. Cellular origin of human B-cell lymphomas. Human B-cell lymphomas are assigned to their putative normal counterparts. Mantle zone lymphomas are assigned to naïve or CD5 B cells, as they carry unmutated immunoglobulin (Ig) genes in most cases. However, a few cases with mutated Ig genes have been described. In B-cell chronic lymphocytic leukemia (B-CLL) , approximately one half of the cases carries unmutated Ig genes, whereas the other half is characterized by mutated Ig genes. In mantle cell lymphoma and B-CLL, the expression of CD5 by the leukemic cells indicates a derivation from CD5 B cells. However, a derivation from conventional naïve B cells that upregulated CD5 expression after transformation can not be excluded. As somatic hypermutation is considered a germinal center (GC) B cell-specific process, the detection of ongoing mutation (at least during early phases of tumor clone expansion) is an indication for a GC B-cell origin of the tumor clone. Intraclonal V gene diversity is typical for follicular lymphoma and lymphocyte predominant Hodgkin's lymphoma. Moreover, a fraction of Burkitt's lymphomas and mucosa-associated lymphoid tissue (MALT) lymphomas and approximately one-half of diffuse large-cell lymphomas show ongoing V gene mutation. A derivation of these diffuse large-cell lymphomas from GC B cells is also supported by their gene expression profile, which closely resembles normal GC B cells (GC-type diffuse large-cell lymphomas) (148). For a number of lymphomas, it is not clear whether the tumor precursors are GC or post-GC B cells, including diffuse large-cell lymphomas with a gene expression profile resembling *in vitro*–activated B cells (ABC-type diffuse large-cell lymphomas). However, it is likely that also in most of these instances, important steps in the transformation process take place in the GC. ABC, activated B cell; B-ALL, B-cell acute lymphoblastic leukemia.

tion of the tumor B cells with follicular dendritic cells and CD4 T cells. However, for other B-cell lymphomas, the origin of the lymphoma cells was less evident. When V gene mutation patterns turned out to identify distinct stages of B-cell development, Ig gene sequence analyses were performed by many groups to gain insight into the cellular origin of B-cell lymphomas [reviewed in (125–127)]. These studies revealed that a surprisingly large number of mature B-cell lymphomas are derived from germinal center or post–germinal center B cells, as they carry somatically mutated Ig genes (Fig. 47.8). Among B-cell non-Hodgkin's lymphomas, somatically mutated Ig V genes were found in diffuse large-cell lymphomas, follicular lymphomas, Burkitt's lymphomas, MALT lymphomas, hairy-cell leukemia, prolymphocytic leukemia, lymphoplasmacytoid lymphomas, and monocytoid B-cell lymphoma (126,127).

Also, the Hodgkin's and Reed-Sternberg cells of classical and lymphocyte predominant Hodgkin's lymphoma and multiple myelomas are characterized by somatically mutated Ig genes (128–133). Unmutated V region genes are typical for mantle cell lymphomas, although a small fraction of cases carry mutated V region genes (134,135). The situation is also diverse in B-cell chronic lymphocytic leukemia. Here, approximately one-half of the cases harbor unmutated Ig genes, whereas the other one-half is characterized by mutated Ig genes (136,137). It is interesting that the lack of somatic mutations in B-cell chronic lymphocytic leukemia is associated with a poorer prognosis for the patients (136,137).

As the somatic hypermutation process is active in germinal center B cells but silenced when the cells further differentiate into memory B or plasma cells, the detection of intraclonal sequence diversity in the rearranged V genes of a lymphoma B-cell clone indicates that somatic hypermutation is still active (at least during the early phase of tumor clone expansion) in the lymphoma and, hence, that the tumor derives from malignant transformation of germinal center B cells. Such intraclonal V gene diversity is typical for follicular lymphoma, Burkitt's lymphoma, many MALT lymphomas, a subset of diffuse large-cell lymphomas, and lymphocyte-predominant Hodgkin's lymphoma (126,127). The Reed-Sternberg cells in classical Hodgkin's lymphoma carry mutated Ig genes but lack ongoing mutation (131,133,138). Nevertheless, there is strong indication that these cells also represent transformed germinal center B cells: In approximately one-fourth of cases, somatic mutations were detected in originally productive V gene rearrangements that rendered these rearrangements nonfunctional (131,139). As such mutations usually result in a very efficient elimination of the cells in the germinal center, the Reed-Sternberg cells likely derive from pre–apoptotic germinal center B cells that were rescued by some transforming event(s) (131,139).

Role of the Germinal Center Reaction and Immunoglobulin Gene Remodeling Processes in Lymphomagenesis

The cellular origin of most human B-cell lymphomas from germinal center or post–germinal center B cells suggests that the development of these lymphomas occurs or is at least initiated in the germinal center microenvironment. One important feature of germinal center B cells in this regard is likely the vigorous proliferation of these cells, which may by itself represent a risk for malignant transformation. Moreover, reciprocal chromosomal translocations involving Ig loci and resulting in the dysregulated expression of oncogenes are a hallmark of many B-cell lymphomas (140–142). The molecular structure of the translocations suggests that many of them are generated as byproducts of class-switch recombination or somatic hypermutation (143). Hence, occasional failures in the control of these molecular processes likely play a decisive role in the generation of chromosomal translocations and, consequently, the pathogenesis of B-cell lymphomas. Somatic hypermutation may be involved in lymphomagenesis not only by causing chromosomal translocations but also by targeting non-Ig genes. The bcl-6 gene is mutated in many B-cell lymphomas, and some of these mutations may well cause deregulated expression of the protein. The CD95 gene is mutated in a small fraction of germinal center B cells and a considerable fraction of germinal center B-cell–derived lymphomas, in particular those associated with autoimmune phenomena (55,144,145). Destructive CD95 gene mutations may rescue germinal center B cells from apoptosis mediated via the CD95 pathway and may enable lymphoma cells to avoid elimination by CD95 ligand–expressing T cells.

Somatic hypermutation may play a particularly important role in the pathogenesis of diffuse large-cell lymphomas. In these lymphomas, targeting of multiple proto-oncogenes (c-myc, Pax-5, Rho/TTF, Pim-1) by somatic hypermutation

was observed (146). These genes were found mutated only in diffuse large-cell lymphomas but not at significant frequency in other B-cell lymphomas or normal germinal center B cells, pointing to a diffuse large-cell lymphoma–specific process. The aberrant hypermutation activity in these lymphoma cells (or their precursors) may cause lymphomagenesis not only by changing gene regulation or the coding sequence but also by mediating chromosomal translocations involving these proto-oncogenes. Indeed, each of these genes is involved in chromosomal translocations, and the translocation breakpoints in these genes overlap with the regions that are targeted by hypermutation (146).

Besides somatic hypermutation and class switching, V gene recombination is likely involved in the generation of chromosomal translocations such as bcl-1/IgH translocations in mantle cell lymphoma and bcl-2/IgH translocations in follicular lymphomas (143). As V gene recombination predominantly, if not exclusively, takes place in the bone marrow and likely only rarely, if at all, in the germinal center, V gene recombination–associated chromosomal translocations presumably happen in the bone marrow during early B-cell development. Notably, in the case of follicular lymphoma, the bcl-2 translocation—although likely acquired already during development of the respective cell in the bone marrow—may become effective only when a cell with such a translocation becomes a germinal center B cell. These cells normally downregulate bcl-2 expression and become sensitive to apoptosis (147), which is prevented in cells with bcl-2 translocation.

Taking these aspects together, it becomes evident that the germinal center plays a decisive role not only for normal B-cell differentiation and effective immune responses but also for the development of most mature B-cell lymphomas in the human.

ACKNOWLEDGMENTS

Ralf Küppers is supported by the Deutsche Forschungsgemeinschaft through SFB502 and a Heisenberg Award of the Deutsche Forschungsgemeinschaft. Klaus Rajewsky is supported by SFB502.

REFERENCES

1. Buckley RH. Primary immunodeficiency diseases due to defects in lymphocytes. *N Engl J Med* 2000;343:1313–1324.
2. Rajewsky K. Clonal selection and learning in the antibody system. *Nature* 1996;381:751–758.
3. Corbett SJ, Tomlinson IM, Sonnhammer EL, et al. Sequence of the human immunoglobulin diversity (D) segment locus: a systematic analysis provides no evidence for the use of DIR segments, inverted D segments, "minor" D segments or D-D recombination. *J Mol Biol* 1997;270:587–597.
4. Ravetch JV, Siebenlist U, Korsmeyer S, et al. Structure of the human immunoglobulin mu locus: characterization of embryonic and rearranged J and D genes. *Cell* 1981;27:583–591.
5. Cook GP, Tomlinson IM. The human immunoglobulin VH repertoire. *Immunol Today* 1995;16:237–242.
6. Hieter PA, Maizel JV, Leder P. Evolution of human immunoglobulin kappa J region genes. *J Biol Chem* 1982;257:1516–1522.
7. Kawasaki K, Minoshima S, Nakato E, et al. One-megabase sequence analysis of the human immunoglobulin lambda gene locus. *Genome Res* 1997;7:250–261.

8. Schäble KF, Zachau HG. The variable genes of the human immunoglobulin kappa locus. *Biol Chem Hoppe Seyler* 1993;374:1001–1022.

9. Vasicek TJ, Leder P. Structure and expression of the human immunoglobulin lambda genes. *J Exp Med* 1990;172:609–620.

10. Williams SC, Frippiat JP, Tomlinson IM, et al. Sequence and evolution of the human germline V lambda repertoire. *J Mol Biol* 1996;264:220–232.

11. Bräuninger A, Goossens T, Rajewsky K, et al. Regulation of immunoglobulin light chain gene rearrangements during early B cell development in the human. *Eur J Immunol* 2001;31:3631–3637.

12. Hieter PA, Korsmeyer SJ, Waldmann TA, et al. Human immunoglobulin kappa light-chain genes are deleted or rearranged in lambda-producing B cells. *Nature* 1981;290:36–372.

13. Korsmeyer SJ, Hieter PA, Sharrow SO, et al. Normal human B cells display ordered light chain gene rearrangements and deletions. *J Exp Med* 1982;156:975–985.

14. Nemazee D. Receptor editing in B cells. *Adv Immunol* 2000;74:89–126.

15. Fugmann SD, Lee AI, Shockett PE, et al. The RAG proteins and V(D)J recombination: complexes, ends, and transposition. *Annu Rev Immunol* 2000;18:495–527.

16. McBlane JF, van Gent DC, Ramsden DA, et al. Cleavage at a V(D)J recombination signal requires only RAG1 and RAG2 proteins and occurs in two steps. *Cell* 1995;83:387–395.

17. Ma Y, Pannicke U, Schwarz K, et al. Hairpin opening and overhang processing by an Artemis/DNA-dependent protein kinase complex in nonhomologous end joining and V(D)J recombination. *Cell* 2002;108:781–794.

18. Moshous D, Callebaut I, de Chasseval R, et al. Artemis, a novel DNA double-strand break repair/V(D)J recombination protein, is mutated in human severe combined immune deficiency. *Cell* 2001;105:177–186.

19. Wasserman R, Yamada M, Ito Y, et al. VH gene rearrangement events can modify the immunoglobulin heavy chain during progression of B-lineage acute lymphoblastic leukemia. *Blood* 1992;79:223–228.

20. MacLennan IC, Gulbranson-Judge A, Toellner KM, et al. The changing preference of T and B cells for partners as T-dependent antibody responses develop. *Immunol Rev* 1997;156:53–66.

21. Jacob J, Kelsoe G. In situ studies of the primary immune response to (4-hydroxy-3-nitrophenyl)acetyl. II. A common clonal origin for periarteriolar lymphoid sheath-associated foci and germinal centers. *J Exp Med* 1992;176:679–687.

22. Jacob J, Kassir R, Kelsoe G. In situ studies of the primary immune response to (4-hydroxy-3-nitrophenyl)acetyl. I. The architecture and dynamics of responding cell populations. *J Exp Med* 1991;173:1165–1175.

23. MacLennan IC. Germinal centers. *Annu Rev Immunol* 1994;12:117–139.

24. Berek C, Berger A, Apel M. Maturation of the immune response in germinal centers. *Cell* 1991;67:1121–1129.

25. Jacob J, Kelsoe G, Rajewsky K, et al. Intraclonal generation of antibody mutants in germinal centres. *Nature* 1991;354:389–392.

26. Küppers R, Zhao M, Hansmann ML, et al. Tracing B cell development in human germinal centres by molecular analysis of single cells picked from histological sections. *EMBO J* 1993;12:4955–4967.

27. Jacob J, Przylepa J, Miller C, et al. In situ studies of the primary immune response to (4-hydroxy-3-nitrophenyl)acetyl. III. The kinetics of V region mutation and selection in germinal center B cells. *J Exp Med* 1993;178:1293–1307.

28. Weiss U, Zoebelein R, Rajewsky K. Accumulation of somatic mutants in the B cell compartment after primary immunization with a T cell-dependent antigen. *Eur J Immunol* 1992;22:511–517.

29. Nakamura M, Yagi H, Kayaba S, et al. Death of germinal center B cells without DNA fragmentation. *Eur J Immunol* 1996;26:1211–1216.

30. Kepler TB, Perelson AS. Cyclic reentry of germinal center B cells and the efficiency of affinity maturation. *Immunol Today* 1993;14:412–415.

31. Han S, Zheng B, Schatz DG, et al. Neoteny in lymphocytes: Rag1 and Rag2 expression in germinal center B cells. *Science* 1996;274:2094–2097.

32. Han S, Dillon SR, Zheng B, et al. V(D)J recombinase activity in a subset of germinal center B lymphocytes. *Science* 1997;278:301–305.

33. Meffre E, Papavasiliou F, Cohen P, et al. Antigen receptor engagement turns off the V(D)J recombination machinery in human tonsil B cells. *J Exp Med* 1998;188:765–772.

34. Papavasiliou F, Casellas R, Suh H, et al. V(D)J recombination in mature B cells: a mechanism for altering antibody responses. *Science* 1997;278:298–301.

35. Monroe RJ, Seidl KJ, Gaertner F, et al. RAG2:GFP knockin mice reveal novel aspects of RAG2 expression in primary and peripheral lymphoid tissues. *Immunity* 1999;11:201–212.

36. Meru N, Jung A, Baumann I, et al. Expression of the recombination-activating genes in extrafollicular lymphocytes but no apparent reinduction in germinal center reactions in human tonsils. *Blood* 2002;99:531–537.

37. Goossens T, Bräuninger A, Klein U, et al. Receptor revision plays no major role in shaping the receptor repertoire of human memory B cells after the onset of somatic hypermutation. *Eur J Immunol* 2001;31:3638–3648.

38. Arpin C, Dechanet J, Van Kooten C, et al. Generation of memory B cells and plasma cells in vitro. *Science* 1995;268:720–722.

39. Choe J, Kim HS, Armitage RJ, et al. The functional role of B cell antigen receptor stimulation and IL-4 in the generation of human memory B cells from germinal center B cells. *J Immunol* 1997;159:3757–3766.

40. Liu YJ, Cairns JA, Holder MJ, et al. Recombinant 25-kDa CD23 and interleukin 1 alpha promote the survival of germinal center B cells: evidence for bifurcation in the development of centrocytes rescued from apoptosis. *Eur J Immunol* 1991;21:1107–1114.

41. Vyth-Dreese FA, Dellemijn TA, Majoor D, et al. Localization in situ of the co-stimulatory molecules B7.1, B7.2, CD40 and their ligands in normal human lymphoid tissue. *Eur J Immunol* 1995;25:3023–3029.

42. Johnson GD, Hardie DL, Ling NR, et al. Human follicular dendritic cells (FDC): a study with monoclonal antibodies (MoAb). *Clin Exp Immunol* 1986;64:205–213.

43. Slifka MK, Antia R, Whitmire JK, et al. Humoral immunity due to long-lived plasma cells. *Immunity* 1998;8:363–372.

44. Manz RA, Thiel A, Radbruch A. Lifetime of plasma cells in the bone marrow. *Nature* 1997;388:133–134.

45. Kocks C, Rajewsky K. Stable expression and somatic hypermutation of antibody V regions in B-cell developmental pathways. *Annu Rev Immunol* 1989;7:537–559.

46. Goossens T, Klein U, Küppers R. Frequent occurrence of deletions and duplications during somatic hypermutation: implications for oncogene translocations and heavy chain disease. *Proc Natl Acad Sci U S A* 1998;95:2463–2468.

47. Wagner SD, Neuberger MS. Somatic hypermutation of immunoglobulin genes. *Annu Rev Immunol* 1996;14:441–457.

48. Neuberger MS, Milstein C. Somatic hypermutation. *Curr Opin Immunol* 1995;7:248–254.

49. Rogozin IB, Kolchanov NA. Somatic hypermutagenesis in immunoglobulin genes. II. Influence of neighbouring base sequence on mutagenesis. *Biochimica Biophysica Acta* 1992;1171:11–18.

50. Betz AG, Milstein C, Gonzalez-Fernandez A, et al. Elements regulating somatic hypermutation of an immunoglobulin kappa gene: critical role for the intron enhancer/matrix attachment region. *Cell* 1994;77:239–248.

51. Fukita Y, Jacobs H, Rajewsky K. Somatic hypermutation in the heavy chain locus correlates with transcription. *Immunity* 1998;9:105–114.

52. Yelamos J, Klix N, Goyenechea B, et al. Targeting of non-Ig sequences in place of the V segment by somatic hypermutation. *Nature* 1995;376:225–229.

53. Pasqualucci L, Migliazza A, Fracchiolla N, et al. BCL-6 mutations in normal germinal center B cells: evidence of somatic hypermutation acting outside Ig loci. *Proc Natl Acad Sci U S A* 1998;95:11816–11821.

54. Shen HM, Peters A, Baron B, et al. Mutation of BCL-6 gene in normal B cells by the process of somatic hypermutation of Ig genes. *Science* 1998;280:1750–1752.

55. Müschen M, Re D, Jungnickel B, et al. Somatic mutation of the CD95 gene in human B cells as a side-effect of the germinal center reaction. *J Exp Med* 2000;192:1833–1840.

56. Bross L, Fukita Y, McBlane F, et al. DNA double-strand breaks in immunoglobulin genes undergoing somatic hypermutation. *Immunity* 2000;13:589–597.

57. Faili A, Aoufouchi S, Gueranger Q, et al. AID-dependent somatic hypermutation occurs as a DNA single-strand event in the BL2 cell line. *Nat Immunol* 2002;3:815–821.

58. Papavasiliou FN, Schatz DG. Cell-cycle-regulated DNA double-stranded breaks in somatic hypermutation of immunoglobulin genes. *Nature* 2000;408:216–221.

59. Sale JE, Neuberger MS. TdT-accessible breaks are scattered over the immunoglobulin V domain in a constitutively hypermutating B cell line. *Immunity* 1998;9:859–869.

60. Faili A, Aoufouchi S, Flatter E, et al. Induction of somatic hypermutation in immunoglobulin genes is dependent on DNA polymerase iota. *Nature* 2002;419:944–947.

61. Zan H, Komori A, Li Z, et al. The translesion DNA polymerase zeta plays a major role in Ig and bcl-6 somatic hypermutation. *Immunity* 2001;14:643–653.

62. Muramatsu M, Kinoshita K, Fagarasan S, et al. Class switch recombination and hypermutation require activation-induced cytidine deaminase (AID), a potential RNA editing enzyme. *Cell* 2000;102:553–563.

63. Revy P, Muto T, Levy Y, et al. Activation-induced cytidine deaminase (AID) deficiency causes the autosomal recessive form of the hyper-IgM syndrome (HIGM2). *Cell* 2000;102:565–575.

64. Okazaki IM, Kinoshita K, Muramatsu M, et al. The AID enzyme induces class switch recombination in fibroblasts. *Nature* 2002;416:340–345.

65. Yoshikawa K, Okazaki IM, Eto T, et al. AID enzyme-induced hypermutation in an actively transcribed gene in fibroblasts. *Science* 2002;296:2033–2036.

66. Di Noia J, Neuberger MS. Altering the pathway of immunoglobulin hypermutation by inhibiting uracil-DNA glycosylase. *Nature* 2002;419:43–48.

67. Petersen-Mahrt SK, Harris RS, Neuberger MS. AID mutates *E. coli* suggesting a DNA deamination mechanism for antibody diversification. *Nature* 2002;418:99–103.

68. Matsumoto M, Lo SF, Carruthers CJ, et al. Affinity maturation without germinal centres in lymphotoxin-alpha-deficient mice. *Nature* 1996;382:462–466.

69. William J, Euler C, Christensen S, et al. Evolution of autoantibody responses via somatic hypermutation outside of germinal centers. *Science* 2002;297:2066–2070.

70. Weller S, Faili A, Garcia C, et al. CD40-CD40L independent Ig gene hypermutation suggests a second B cell diversification pathway in humans. *Proc Natl Acad Sci U S A* 2001;98:1166–1170.

71. Gardby E, Lycke NY. CD19-deficient mice exhibit poor responsiveness to oral immunization despite evidence of unaltered total IgA levels, germinal centers and IgA-isotype switching in Peyer's patches. *Eur J Immunol* 2000;30:1861–1871.

72. Ferrari S, Giliani S, Insalaco A, et al. Mutations of CD40 gene cause an autosomal recessive form of immunodeficiency with hyper IgM. *Proc Natl Acad Sci U S A* 2001;98:12614–12619.

73. Wang Y, Huang G, Wang J, et al. Antigen persistence is required for somatic mutation and affinity maturation of immunoglobulin. *Eur J Immunol* 2000;30:2226–2234.

74. Hofker MH, Walter MA, Cox DW. Complete physical map of the human immunoglobulin heavy chain constant region gene complex. *Proc Natl Acad Sci U S A* 1989;86:5567–5571.

75. Honjo T, Kinoshita K, Muramatsu M. Molecular mechanism of class switch recombination: linkage with somatic hypermutation. *Annu Rev Immunol* 2002;20:165–196.

76. Hein K, Lorenz MG, Siebenkotten G, et al. Processing of switch transcripts is required for targeting of antibody class switch recombination. *J Exp Med* 1998;188:2369–2374.

77. Lorenz M, Jung S, Radbruch A. Switch transcripts in immunoglobulin class switching. *Science* 1995;267:1825–1828.

78. Zhang K, Mills FC, Saxon A. Switch circles from IL-4-directed epsilon class switching from human B lymphocytes. Evidence for direct, sequential, and multiple step sequential switch from mu to epsilon Ig heavy chain gene. *J Immunol* 1994;152:3427–3435.

79. Barrett DJ, Ayoub EM. IgG2 subclass restriction of antibody to pneumococcal polysaccharides. *Clin Exp Immunol* 1986;63:127–134.

80. Shackelford PG, Granoff DM. IgG subclass composition of the antibody response of healthy adults, and normal or IgG2-deficient children to immunization with *H. influenzae* type b polysaccharide vaccine or Hib PS-protein conjugate vaccines. *Monogr Allergy* 1988;23:269–281.

81. Mond JJ, Lees A, Snapper CM. T cell-independent antigens type 2. *Annu Rev Immunol* 1995;13:655–692.

82. Scott EW, Simon MC, Anastasi J, et al. Requirement of transcription factor PU.1 in the development of multiple hematopoietic lineages. *Science* 1994;265:1573–1577.

83. DeKoter RP, Singh H. Regulation of B lymphocyte and macrophage development by graded expression of PU.1. *Science* 2000;288:1439–1441.

84. Kee BL, Quong MW, Murre C. E2A proteins: essential regulators at multiple stages of B-cell development. *Immunol Rev* 2000;175:138–149.

85. Reya T, Grosschedl R. Transcriptional regulation of B-cell differentiation. *Curr Opin Immunol* 1998;10:158–165.

86. Nutt SL, Heavey B, Rolink A, et al. Commitment to the B-lymphoid lineage depends on the transcription factor Pax5. *Nature* 1999;401:556–562.

87. Rolink AG, Nutt SL, Melchers F, et al. Long-term *in vivo* reconstitution of T-cell development by Pax5-deficient B-cell progenitors. *Nature* 1999;401:603–606.

88. Horcher M, Souabni A, Busslinger M. Pax5/BSAP maintains the identity of B cells in late B lymphopoiesis. *Immunity* 2001;14:779–790.

89. Nutt SL, Eberhard D, Horcher M, et al. Pax5 determines the identity of B cells from the beginning to the end of B-lymphopoiesis. *Int Rev Immunol* 2001;20:65–82.

90. Dent AL, Shaffer AL, Yu X, et al. Control of inflammation, cytokine expression, and germinal center formation by BCL-6. *Science* 1997;276:589–592.

91. Ye BH, Cattoretti G, Shen Q, et al. The BCL-6 proto-oncogene controls germinal-centre formation and Th2- type inflammation. *Nat Genet* 1997;16:161–170.

92. Cattoretti G, Chang CC, Cechova K, et al. BCL-6 protein is expressed in germinal-center B cells. *Blood* 1995;86:45–53.

93. Onizuka T, Moriyama M, Yamochi T, et al. BCL-6 gene product, a 92- to 98-kD nuclear phosphoprotein, is highly expressed in germinal center B cells and their neoplastic counterparts. *Blood* 1995;86:28–37.

94. Shaffer AL, Yu X, He Y, et al. BCL-6 represses genes that function in lymphocyte differentiation, inflammation, and cell cycle control. *Immunity* 2000;13:199–212.

95. Angelin-Duclos C, Cattoretti G, Lin KI, et al. Commitment of B lymphocytes to a plasma cell fate is associated with Blimp-1 expression *in vivo*. *J Immunol* 2000;165:5462–5471.

96. Falini B, Fizzotti M, Pucciarini A, et al. A monoclonal antibody (MUM1p) detects expression of the MUM1/IRF4 protein in a subset of germinal center B cells, plasma cells, and activated T cells. *Blood* 2000;95:2084–2092.

97. Calame KL. Plasma cells: finding new light at the end of B cell development. *Nat Immunol* 2001;2:1103–1108.

98. Mittrucker HW, Matsuyama T, Grossman A, et al. Requirement for the transcription factor LSIRF/IRF4 for mature B and T lymphocyte function. *Science* 1997;275:540–543.

99. Reimold AM, Iwakoshi NN, Manis J, et al. Plasma cell differentiation requires the transcription factor XBP-1. *Nature* 2001;412:300–307.

100. Reimold AM, Ponath PD, Li YS, et al. Transcription factor B cell lineage-specific activator protein regulates the gene for human X-box binding protein 1. *J Exp Med* 1996;183:393–401.

101. Bhat NM, Kantor AB, Bieber MM, et al. The ontogeny and functional characteristics of human B-1 (CD5+ B) cells. *Int Immunol* 1992;4:243–252.

102. Berland R, Wortis HH. Origins and functions of B-1 cells with notes on the role of CD5. *Annu Rev Immunol* 2002;20:253–300.

103. Brezinschek HP, Foster SJ, Brezinschek RI, et al. Analysis of the human VH gene repertoire. Differential effects of selection and somatic hypermutation on human peripheral CD5(+)/IgM+ and CD5(−)/IgM+ B cells. *J Clin Invest* 1997;99:2488–2501.

104. Fischer M, Klein U, Küppers R. Molecular single-cell analysis reveals that CD5-positive peripheral blood B cells in healthy humans are characterized by rearranged V kappa genes lacking somatic mutation. *J Clin Invest* 1997;100:1667–1676.

105. Geiger KD, Klein U, Bräuninger A, et al. CD5-positive B cells in healthy elderly humans are a polyclonal B cell population. *Eur J Immunol* 2000;30:2918–2923.

106. Rawstron AC, Green MJ, Kuzmicki A, et al. Monoclonal B lymphocytes with the characteristics of "indolent" chronic lymphocytic leukemia are present in 3.5% of adults with normal blood counts. *Blood* 2002;100:635–639.

107. Schroeder HW Jr, Wang JY. Preferential utilization of conserved immunoglobulin heavy chain variable gene segments during human fetal life. *Proc Natl Acad Sci U S A* 1990;87:6146–6150.

108. Klein U, Rajewsky K, Küppers R. Human immunoglobulin (Ig)M⁺IgD⁺ peripheral blood B cells expressing the CD27 cell surface antigen carry somatically mutated variable region genes: CD27 as a general marker for somatically mutated (memory) B cells. *J Exp Med* 1998;188:1679–1689.

109. Klein U, Küppers R, Rajewsky K. Evidence for a large compartment of IgM-expressing memory B cells in humans. *Blood* 1997;89:1288–1298.

110. Agematsu K, Nagumo H, Yang FC, et al. B cell subpopulations separated by CD27 and crucial collaboration of CD27⁺ B cells and helper T cells in immunoglobulin production. *Eur J Immunol* 1997;27:2073–2079.

111. Liu YJ, de Bouteiller O, Arpin C, et al. Normal human IgD⁺IgM⁻ germinal center B cells can express up to 80 mutations in the variable region of their IgD transcripts. *Immunity* 1996;4:603–613.

112. Meffre E, Davis E, Schiff C, et al. Circulating human B cells that express surrogate light chains and edited receptors. *Nat Immunol* 2000;1:207–213.

113. Arce E, Jackson DG, Gill MA, et al. Increased frequency of pre-germinal center B cells and plasma cell precursors in the blood of children with systemic lupus erythematosus. *J Immunol* 2001;167:2361–2369.

114. Odendahl M, Jacobi A, Hansen A, et al. Disturbed peripheral B lymphocyte homeostasis in systemic lupus erythematosus. *J Immunol* 2000;165:5970–5979.

115. Dunn-Walters DK, Isaacson PG, Spencer J. Analysis of mutations in immunoglobulin heavy chain variable region genes of microdissected marginal zone (MGZ) B cells suggests that the MGZ of human spleen is a reservoir of memory B cells. *J Exp Med* 1995;182:559–566.

116. Tangye SG, Liu YJ, Aversa G, et al. Identification of functional human splenic memory B cells by expression of CD148 and CD27. *J Exp Med* 1998;188:1691–1703.

117. Tierens A, Delabie J, Michiels L, et al. Marginal-zone B cells in the human lymph node and spleen show somatic hypermutations and display clonal expansion. *Blood* 1999;93:226–234.

118. Martin F, Kearney JF. Marginal-zone B cells. *Nat Rev Immunol* 2002;2:323–335.

119. Dunn-Walters DK, Isaacson PG, Spencer J. Sequence analysis of rearranged IgVH genes from microdissected human Peyer's patch marginal zone B cells. *Immunology* 1996;88:618–624.

120. Liu YJ, Barthelemy C, de Bouteiller O, et al. Memory B cells from human tonsils colonize mucosal epithelium and directly present antigen to T cells by rapid up-regulation of B7-1 and B7-2. *Immunity* 1995;2:239–248.

121. Stein K, Hummel M, Korbjuhn P, et al. Monocytoid B cells are distinct from splenic marginal zone cells and commonly derive from unmutated naive B cells and less frequently from postgerminal center B cells by polyclonal transformation. *Blood* 1999;94:2800–2808.

122. Brandtzaeg P, Halstensen TS, Kett K, et al. Immunobiology and immunopathology of human gut mucosa: humoral immunity and intraepithelial lymphocytes. *Gastroenerology* 1989;97:1562–1584.

123. Dunn-Walters DK, Isaacson PG, Spencer J. Sequence analysis of human IgVH genes indicates that ileal lamina propria plasma cells are derived from Peyer's patches. *Eur J Immunol* 1997;27:463–467.

124. Fischer M, Küppers R. Human IgA- and IgM-secreting intestinal plasma cells carry heavily mutated VH region genes. *Eur J Immunol* 1998;28:2971–2977.

125. Klein U, Goossens T, Fischer M, et al. Somatic hypermutation in normal and transformed human B cells. *Immunol Rev* 1998;162:261–280.

126. Küppers R, Klein U, Hansmann M-L, et al. Cellular origin of human B-cell lymphomas. *N Engl J Med* 1999;341:1520–1529.

127. Stevenson FK, Sahota SS, Ottensmeier CH, et al. The occurrence and significance of V gene mutations in B cell-derived human malignancy. *Adv Cancer Res* 2001;83:81–116.

128. Baker BW, Deane M, Gilleece MH, et al. Distinctive features of immunoglobulin heavy chain variable region gene rearrangement in multiple myeloma. *Leuk Lymphoma* 1994;14:291–301.

129. Bakkus MH, Heirman C, Van Riet I, et al. Evidence that multiple myeloma Ig heavy chain VDJ genes contain somatic mutations but show no intraclonal variation. *Blood* 1992;80:2326–2335.

130. Braeuninger A, Küppers R, Strickler JG, et al. Hodgkin and Reed-Sternberg cells in lymphocyte predominant Hodgkin disease represent clonal populations of germinal center-derived tumor B cells. *Proc Natl Acad Sci U S A* 1997;94:9337–9342.

131. Kanzler H, Küppers R, Hansmann ML, et al. Hodgkin and Reed-Sternberg cells in Hodgkin's disease represent the outgrowth of a dominant tumor clone derived from (crippled) germinal center B cells. *J Exp Med* 1996;184:1495–1505.

132. Marafioti T, Hummel M, Anagnostopoulos I, et al. Origin of nodular lymphocyte-predominant Hodgkin's disease from a clonal expansion of highly mutated germinal-center B cells. *N Engl J Med* 1997;337:453–458.

133. Marafioti T, Hummel M, Foss H-D, et al. Hodgkin and Reed-Sternberg cells represent an expansion of a single clone originating from a germinal center B-cell with functional immunoglobulin gene rearrangements but defective immunoglobulin transcription. *Blood* 2000;95:1443–1450.

134. Hummel M, Tamaru J, Kalvelage B, et al. Mantle cell (previously centrocytic) lymphomas express VH genes with no or very little somatic mutations like the physiologic cells of the follicle mantle. *Blood* 1994;84:403–407.

135. Thorselius M, Walsh S, Eriksson I, et al. Somatic hypermutation and V(H) gene usage in mantle cell lymphoma. *Eur J Haematol* 2002;68:217–224.

136. Damle RN, Wasil T, Fais F, et al. Ig V gene mutation status and CD38 expression as novel prognostic indicators in chronic lymphocytic leukemia. *Blood* 1999;94:1840–1847.

137. Hamblin TJ, Davis Z, Gardiner A, et al. Unmutated Ig V(H) genes are associated with a more aggressive form of chronic lymphocytic leukemia. *Blood* 1999;94:1848–1854.

138. Bräuninger A, Hansmann ML, Strickler JG, et al. Identification of common germinal-center B-cell precursors in two patients with both Hodgkin's disease and non-Hodgkin's lymphoma. *N Engl J Med* 1999;340:1239–1247.

139. Küppers R. Molecular biology of Hodgkin's lymphoma. *Adv Cancer Res* 2002;44:277–312.

140. Dalla-Favera R, Gaidano G. Molecular biology of lymphomas. In: De Vita VT, Hellman S, Rosenberg SA, eds. *Cancer: principles and practice of oncology*, 6th ed. Philadelphia: Lippincott Williams & Wilkins, 2001:2215–2235.

141. Siebert R, Rosenwald A, Staudt LM, et al. Molecular features of B-cell lymphoma. *Curr Opin Oncol* 2001;13:316–324.

142. Willis TG, Dyer MJ. The role of immunoglobulin translocations in the pathogenesis of B-cell malignancies. *Blood* 2000;96:808–822.

143. Küppers R, Dalla-Favera R. Mechanisms of chromosomal translocations in B cell lymphomas. *Oncogene* 2001;20:5580–5594.

144. Gronbaek K, Straten PT, Ralfkiaer E, et al. Somatic Fas mutations in non-Hodgkin's lymphoma: association with extranodal disease and autoimmunity. *Blood* 1998;92:3018–3024.

145. Müschen M, Rajewsky K, Krönke M, et al. The origin of CD95 gene mutations in B cell lymphoma. *Trends Immunol* 2002;23:75–80.

146. Pasqualucci L, Neumeister P, Goossens T, et al. Hypermutation of multiple proto-oncogenes in B-cell diffuse large-cell lymphomas. *Nature* 2001;412:341–346.

147. Liu YJ, Mason DY, Johnson GD, et al. Germinal center cells express bcl-2 protein after activation by signals which prevent their entry into apoptosis. *Eur J Immunol* 1991;21:1905–1910.

148. Alizadeh AA, Eisen MB, Davis RE, et al. Distinct types of diffuse large B-cell lymphoma identified by gene expression profiling. *Nature* 2000;403:503–511.

CHAPTER 48

Developmental and Functional Biology of T Lymphocytes

Jacques J. M. van Dongen, Frank J. T. Staal, and Anton W. Langerak

The development of T lymphocytes in the thymus and their regulatory and cytotoxic cellular functions in peripheral lymphoid organs play a central role in the antigen-specific immune response. The tightly regulated process of T-cell differentiation with the stepwise rearrangements in the T-cell receptor (TCR) genes and selection processes are essential to mediate T-cell responses with well-suited antigen-specific receptors.

Multistep deregulation and malignant transformation can occur at multiple stages of T-cell differentiation and T-cell–mediated immune responses, resulting in immature (thymocytic) or mature (postthymic) T-cell malignancies. This chapter summarizes the molecular background of the TCR repertoire, the stepwise T-cell differentiation processes, the T-cell effector functions, and the immunophenotypic and genotypic characteristics of normal, as compared with malignant, T cells.

T-CELL RECEPTOR MOLECULES AND T-CELL RECEPTOR REPERTOIRE

T-Cell Receptor Molecules and Their Encoding Genes

The ability of human T lymphocytes to specifically recognize millions of different antigens and antigenic epitopes is based on the enormous diversity (at least 10^{10}) of their antigen-specific receptors, better known as *TCR molecules* (1–3). Being distinct per T lymphocyte, each single T lymphocyte expresses approximately 10^5 TCR molecules with identical antigen specificity. TCR molecules consist of two generally disulfide-linked chains. Two different types of TCR are known: the "classical" TCRαβ receptor, consisting of a TCRα and a TCRβ chain, and the "alternative" TCRγδ receptor, comprised of a TCRγ and a TCRδ chain (2,4). The majority of mature T lymphocytes (85% to 98%) in peripheral blood and in most lymphoid tissues are TCRαβ+, whereas only a minority (2% to 15%) express TCRγδ (4). Both types of TCR molecules are closely associated with

CD3 protein chains, required for transmembrane signal transduction of the TCR-CD3 complex (Fig. 48.1) (3).

Each TCR chain consists of two domains: one variable domain involved in actual recognition of antigens and one constant domain that mediates the effector function resulting in signaling through CD3. To recognize all antigenic epitopes, an extensive repertoire of variable domains of TCR molecules is needed. If this entire repertoire is encoded by separate genes, these would occupy a major part of the human genome. However, because the variable domains are encoded by a single exon that is formed through distinct combinations of gene segments, only a limited set of gene segments are able to encode the required diversity of TCR molecules (2,5). In the case of the *TCRB* and *TCRD* loci, this concerns the combination of variable (V), diversity (D), and joining (J) gene segments, whereas the *TCRA* and *TCRG* gene complexes only contain V and J gene segments (Fig. 48.2) (2,4).

The human *TCRA* and *TCRB* loci contain large sets of Vα and Vβ gene segments (60-65), which can be further subdivided into families based on homology at the DNA level (Table 48.1). The nine V gene segments of the human *TCRG* gene complex are generally subdivided into four families, three of which are single-member families; the human *TCRD* locus consists of six V segments. Human J gene segments are generally more sparse than V gene segments, ranging from four for *TCRD*, five for *TCRG*, to 13 for *TCRB*; the 61 different J segments of the *TCRA* locus are exceptional. Finally, two Dβ and three Dδ gene segments exist (Table 48.1). The constant domains of the TCR chains are encoded by C gene segments; *TCRA* and *TCRD* loci each contain a single C gene segment, whereas *TCRB* and *TCRG* loci comprise two C gene segments (Fig. 48.2) (6–14).

Gene Rearrangement or V(D)J Recombination

During early T-cell differentiation, V, (D), and J gene segments from the germline repertoire of the various TCR gene

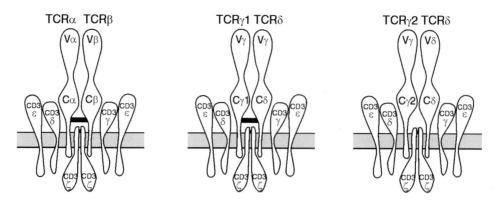

FIG. 48.1. Schematic diagram of human T-cell receptor (TCR) αβ and TCRγδ molecules. Both types of TCR molecules are associated with CD3 protein chains, which are involved in signal transduction. The proteins of TCRγδ receptor that are derived from Cγ1 sequences are disulfide linked, whereas this interchain disulfide bond is lacking if the TCRγ chain is derived from Cγ2 sequences. Most TCRγδ⁺ T lymphocytes in peripheral blood use disulfide-linked TCR chains because of selection for Vδ2-Jδ1/Vγ9-Jγ1.2 receptors. Vα, Vβ, Vγ, and Vδ are variable domains of TCR chains; Cα, Cβ, Cγ, and Cδ are constant domains of TCR chains.

complexes are coupled via a tightly regulated process (see later); this process is called *gene rearrangement* or *V(D)J recombination*. The resulting specific combination of V, (D), and J segments in each T lymphocyte is also known as *V(D)J*

exon (1,2,5,15). V(D)J recombination is a complex process involving several proteins, which together form the recombinase enzyme system. Next to regulatory DNA binding proteins, the products of the lymphoid-specific recombinase

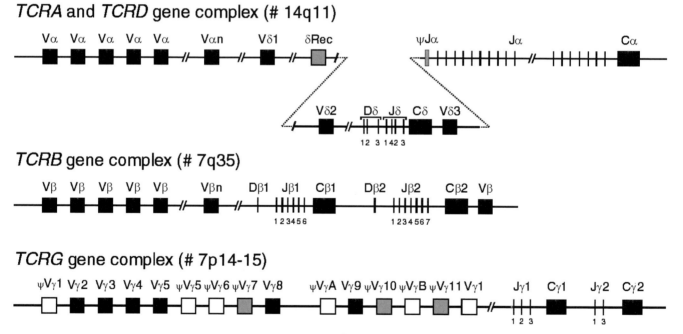

FIG. 48.2. Schematic diagram of the human T-cell receptor gene complexes. The *TCRA* gene complex consists of approximately 60 V gene segments, a stretch of 61 J gene segments, and one C gene segment. The *TCRB* gene complex contains approximately 65 V gene segments and two C gene segments, both of which are preceded by a D gene segment and six or seven J gene segments. The *TCRG* gene complex consists of a restricted number of V gene segments (six functional segments and nine pseudosegments) and two C gene segments, each preceded by two to three J gene segments. The *TCRD* gene complex comprises several V (three true Vδ segments and several Vα/Vδ segments), three D, four J, and one C gene segment. The major part of the *TCRD* gene complex is located between the Vα and Jα gene segments and is flanked by the δREC and ψJα gene segments, which are involved in *TCRD* gene deletions that occur before *TCRA* gene rearrangements. Pseudogenes (ψ) are indicated as open symbols.

TABLE 48.1. *Estimated number of human V, D, and J gene segments that can potentially be involved in T-cell receptor (TCR) gene rearrangements*[a]

Gene segment	TCRA	TCRB	TCRG	TCRD
V (family)	~60 (32)	~65 (30)	9 (4)	7[b]
D	—	2	—	3
J (family)	61[b]	13	5 (3)	4

[a]Numbers are based on the international ImMunoGeneTics database (126). Numbers in parentheses reflect families.
[b]These numbers include the nonfunctional ψJα gene segment (*TCRA* locus) and the δREC gene segment (*TCRD* locus).

activating genes 1 and 2 (RAG1 and RAG2 proteins) are the main constituents of the recombinase complex (16–18). RAG 1 and RAG 2 specifically bind to the recombination signal sequences (RSS), which flank the 3' side of V gene segments, both sides of D gene segments, and the 5' side of J gene segments (19–21). These RSS elements consist of conserved palindromic heptamer (CACAGTG) and nonamer (ACAAAAACC) sequences, separated by either 12 or 23 base pair spacer regions (19–21). After the introduction of double-strand breaks between the RSS and the rearranging gene segment, a hairpin structure is formed at the coding end of the break (Fig. 48.3). This hairpin has to be opened before religation to another gene segment via several enzymes known to be involved in double-strand break repair; this results in the so-called coding joint (Fig. 48.3). During the coding joint formation, deletion and random insertion of

nucleotides can occur, leading to imprecise coupling of gene segments. The RSS ends of the breaks fuse head to tail to form the so-called signal joint, which is generally removed from the genomic DNA in the form of an excision circle (Fig. 48.3) (2,19,20). Such TCR excision circles (TRECs) are relatively stable molecules, which do not replicate on cell division; consequently, they are diluted out on proliferation of the developing T cells. This characteristic has prompted the development of quantitative assays for analysis of TREC levels as measure for thymic output of recent thymic emigrants (22,23). TREC analysis has been used to study thymic output in different age groups and different pathophysiologic conditions (e.g., during human immunodeficiency virus type 1 infection) (22,24).

In Figure 48.4, an example of a *TCRB* gene rearrangement is illustrated. Initially, a coding joint is formed between a Jβ gene segment and one of the Dβ gene segments, whereas the 3' Dβ RSS and the Jβ RSS form a signal joint in the excision circle or TREC. In a second step rearrangement, coupling of one of many Vβ gene segments results in a complete V(D)J exon as well as another TREC with the signal joint of the Vβ RSS and the 5' Dβ RSS. The rearranged gene is subsequently transcribed into a precursor messenger RNA, which is further processed into mature mRNA by splicing out all intronic, noncoding sequences and coupling of the V(D)J exon and the C exons (Fig. 48.4) (2). Similar rearrangement and transcription processes occur in all other TCR loci as well. Although the signal joints that are formed during TCR gene recombination are generally present on TRECs, this is not the case for one exceptional type of rearrangement. On inversional rearrangement, which occurs in the case of V

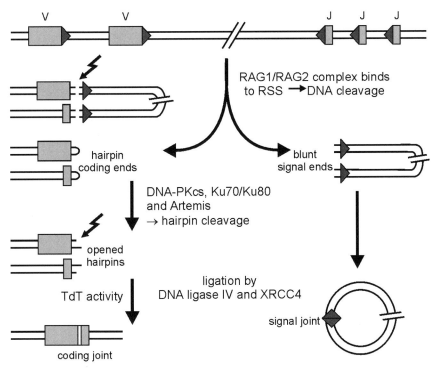

FIG. 48.3. Scheme of the V(D)J recombination mechanism. RAG1 and RAG2 bind to recombination signal sequences (RSS), resulting in double-strand breaks. After cleavage, hairpin structures are formed at the coding ends, whereas the RSS blunt ends fuse to form a signal joint. Further processing results in opening of the hairpins via several enzymes known to be involved in double strand break repair (DNA-PK$_{CS}$, Ku70/Ku80, and Artemis). Finally, opened hairpins are religated (involving DNA ligase IV and XRCC4) to a coding joint and are further diversified by the action of terminal deoxynucleotidyl transferase (TdT), which introduces nucleotides in a template-independent way.

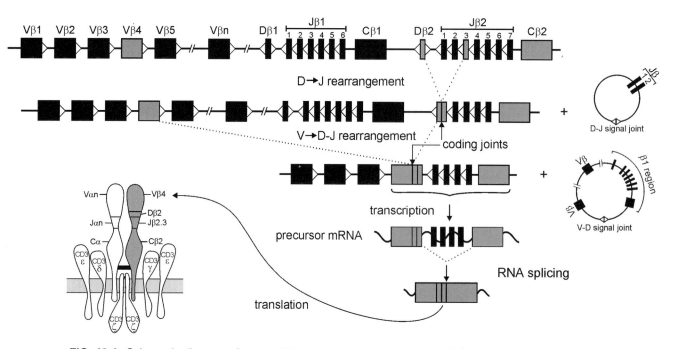

FIG. 48.4. Schematic diagram of sequential rearrangement steps, transcription, and translation of the *TCRB* gene during T-cell differentiation. In this example, first a Dβ2 to Jβ2.3 rearrangement occurs, followed by Vβ4 to Dβ2-Jβ2.3 rearrangement, resulting in the formation of a Vβ4Dβ2Jβ2.3 coding joint. The rearranged *TCRB* gene is transcribed into precursor messenger RNA (mRNA), spliced into mature mRNA, and finally translated into a TCRβ protein. The two extrachromosomal TCR excision circles (TRECs) that are formed during this recombination process are indicated as well; they contain the D-J signal joint and V-D signal joint, respectively.

gene segments in inverted orientation (e.g., the Vβ20 or Vδ3 gene segments) (13), the signal joint and other intervening sequences between the two coding elements are not removed as TREC but are preserved on the genome.

As TCR recombinations are complex processes with imprecise joining of gene segments, approximately two out of three joinings are out-of-frame (1). This high frequency of out-of-frame rearrangements may explain why most T cells have biallelic *TCRB* and *TCRG* gene rearrangements (5,25). In addition, replacement gene rearrangements appear to occur that are assumed to rescue precursor T cells with nonproductive TCR genes. In *TCRB* and *TCRD* loci, this concerns D-J replacements, whereas V-J replacements replace preexisting V-J joinings in *TCRA* and *TCRG* loci (26–28). Both types of replacements can occur repeatedly in the same TCR gene complex as long as germline V, (D), and J gene segments are available. Another type of secondary rearrangement concerns V gene segment replacement in a complete V(D)J exon by an upstream V gene segment. This process is mediated via an internal heptamer RSS in the 3' part of the V gene segments (29,30).

T-Cell Receptor Repertoire

The complete repertoire of TCR molecules of T lymphocytes is shaped by V(D)J recombination mechanisms in the TCR gene loci. The extent of this potential primary repertoire is determined by two levels of diversity: combinatorial diversity [different V(D)J combinations] and junctional diversity (due to imprecise joining of V, D, and J gene segments) (1).

Combinatorial diversity results from all possible combinations of available functional V, D, and J gene segments per TCR locus and the pairing of two different functional protein chains per TCR molecule (TCRα with TCRβ and TCRγ with TCRδ) (1). As the *TCRB* gene complex probably contains at least approximately 45 functional Vβ gene segments, 2 Dβ gene segments, and 13 functional Jβ gene segments, coupling results in many possible Vβ-Dβ-Jβ combinations (more than 1,000). Together with the many combinations of the approximately 45 functional Vα and 50 functional Jα gene segments, a potential combinatorial diversity of more than 2×10^6 can be obtained (Table 48.2).

The combinatorial diversity of TCRγδ molecules is less extensive due to the limited number of functional V, D, and J gene segments in the encoding gene complexes. Still, because of multiple Dδ gene segment usage, a potential combinatorial repertoire of more than 5,000 TCRγδ molecules can be produced. The numbers of different TCRαβ and TCRγδ molecules are based on the assumption of random usage of available functional V, D, and J gene segments. However, there are indications for preferential gene segment usage. TCRαβ+ cells tend to use Jβ2 gene segments more frequently than Jβ1 gene segments (31), whereas peripheral TCRγδ+ T lymphocytes exhibit preferential usage of Vγ9-Jγ1.2 and Vδ2-Jδ1 gene segments (32,33). Alternatively, gene segment usage

TABLE 48.2. *Estimation of potential primary repertoire of human T-cell receptor (TCR) molecules*

Repertoire	TCRαβ molecules		TCRγδ molecules	
	TCRα	TCRβ	TCRγ	TCRδ
Number of functional gene segments[a]				
V gene segments	45	44–47	6	6
D gene segments	—	2[b]	—	3[b]
J gene segments	50	13	5	4
Combinatorial diversity	>2 × 10^6		>5000	
Junctional diversity	+	++	+	+++
Estimation of total repertoire	>10^12		>10^12	

+, limited (range 0–20 nt); ++, extensive (range 0–35 nt); +++, very extensive (range 7–55 nt).
[a]Numbers are based on the international ImMunoGeneTics database (126).
[b]In *TCRD* gene rearrangements, multiple D segments might be used; this implies that the number of junctions can vary from one to four. In *TCRB* gene rearrangements, generally only one D gene segment is used.

might be random, but overrepresentation of certain receptor types would be explained by clonal selection and expansion of particular receptor specificities in peripheral tissues (34).

The other type of diversity, *junctional diversity*, is based on deletion of nucleotides at the ends of the rearranging gene segments as well as random insertion of nucleotides (N region nucleotides) between the coupled gene segments (junctional region). Insertion of N region nucleotides at the 3' ends of DNA breakpoints is mediated by terminal deoxynucleotidyl transferase (TdT) and occurs in a template-independent way (35). Absence or decreased TdT activity, as in early fetal thymocytes, leads to the virtual absence of N region insertion in TCR gene rearrangement, but the junctional regions of rearranged TCR genes in late fetal and postnatal thymocytes do contain N regions (36,37). The junctional regions of TCR genes encode the so-called complementarity determining regions 3 (CDR3), which are involved in antigen recognition and which function as unique lymphocyte-specific ("fingerprint-like") sequences. N region insertion thus drastically increases diversity of antigen recognition by TCR chains and TCR molecules. This especially holds true for *TCRB* and *TCRD* gene rearrangements in which multiple couplings (V-D, D-J, and even D-D) can be present within a junctional region. The enormous junctional diversity of TCRδ chains thereby compensates for the relatively low number of different V, D, and J combinations (Table 48.2).

STAGES OF T-CELL DIFFERENTIATION

Immunophenotype of Thymocyte Subsets

T cells develop from common lymphoid progenitor cells that seed the thymus from the fetal liver or bone marrow (38). In

most differentiation schemes, thymocyte subsets are phenotypically distinguished by the expression of CD4 and CD8 coreceptors: Thymocytes are either double negative (DN), double positive (DP), or single positive (SP) for these two cell surface antigens (Fig. 48.5). During the DN stage, thymocytes can be subdivided into subpopulations based on the expression of the CD34 stem cell marker and CD1a (for a recent review, see reference 39). The earliest cells in the human thymus phenotypically resemble hematopoietic stem cells and are CD34+CD38−CD1a− (40). CD38 expression is rapidly acquired, and the CD34+CD38+CD1a− cells represent cells that behave as multipotent progenitor cells having the capacity to develop not only into the T-cell lineage but also into natural killer cells, dendritic cells, and B cells. The thymus is an important site for the development of natural killer cells and probably dendritic cells but a very minor site for B-cell development (41). After acquisition of CD1a expression on the progenitor cells (CD34+CD1a+), T-cell commitment is established (Fig. 48.5). This is because the first TCR gene rearrangements occur at this transition, concomitant with increased expression of the pre-Tα gene.

During transition to the next stage of T-cell maturation, the pre–T-cell stage (DN3 in the mouse), the cells shut down proliferation (42), and *TCRB* genes start to rearrange. During the immature single positive stage, the TCRβ protein chain is expressed at the cell surface, complexed to pre-Tα as the pre–TCR complex. In the mouse, these immature single positive cells express CD8, whereas in humans, they express CD4 (Fig. 48.5). In both species, the immature single positive cells represent a stage of rapid proliferation, driven by signals via the pre–TCR complex (TCRβ selection). This process generates DP cells, which comprise 85% to 90% of thymocytes. As soon as the DP thymocytes express CD3/TCRαβ, they undergo positive selection (for self-MHC) and negative selection (against autoreactivity) (43). The selected cells develop into CD4 or CD8 SP cells with high CD3/TCRαβ expression, which exit the thymus and become circulating T cells that reside in blood and peripheral lymphoid organs (Fig. 48.5).

Rearrangement Processes during T-Cell Differentiation

Antigen recognition by T lymphocytes is dependent on successful rearrangement of TCR genes through the process of V(D)J recombination. During early T-cell differentiation, *TCRD* genes rearrange first, followed by *TCRG* gene rearrangements (44). This might result in TCRγδ+ T lymphocytes, provided that these rearrangements are functional. TCRαβ+ T lymphocytes most probably develop via a separate differentiation lineage, with *TCRB* gene rearrangements taking place before *TCRA* gene rearrangements (Fig. 48.6). *TCRA* gene rearrangements are preceded by deletion of the *TCRD* gene, which is for the major part located between the Vα and Jα gene segments (Fig. 48.2). This *TCRD* gene deletion process is primarily mediated via rearrangement of the flanking δREC and ΨJα gene segments. These rearrangement and deletion processes in the *TCRA/TCRD* locus prob-

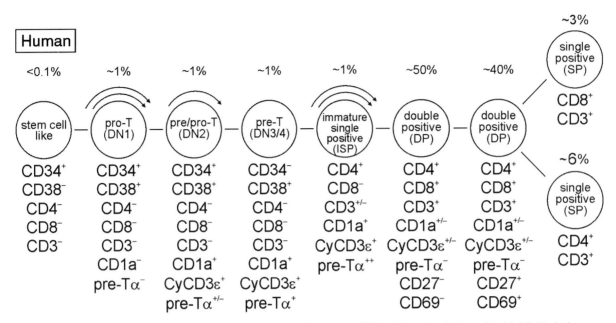

FIG. 48.5. Stages of human T-cell development in the thymus. This scheme is designed to highlight similarities with mouse T-cell development. Cells that are not yet T-cell committed seed the thymus. These first two stages represent a minute fraction (less than 1%) of all thymocytes. The most common cell type in the thymus is the DP thymocyte (85% to 90%), which gives rise to both CD4 (4% to 9%) and CD8 (2% to 5%) single-positive (SP) cells. DN, double negative; DP, double positive; ISP, immature single positive; SP, single positive.

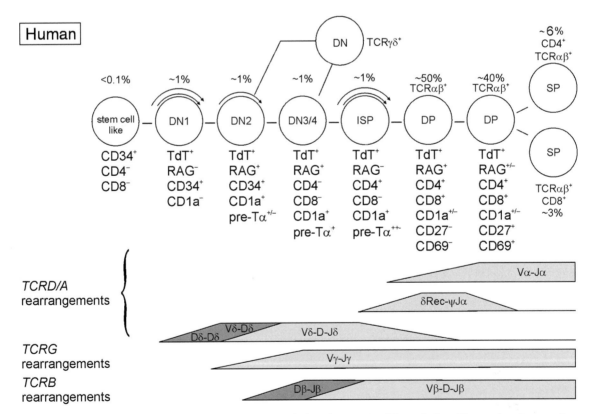

FIG. 48.6. T-cell receptor (TCR) rearrangements during thymocyte differentiation. The major stages of T-cell development are depicted with the corresponding start of rearrangements of the TCR loci. The δREC-ψJα elements are involved in deletion of the *TCRD* locus, which is necessary for efficient rearrangement of the *TCRA* locus (Fig. 48.2). DN, double negative; DP, double positive; ISP, immature single positive; SP, single positive; TdT, terminal deoxynucleotidyl transferase.

ably play a crucial role in the divergence of the TCRγδ and TCRαβ differentiation pathways, although it is still unclear in which differentiation stage this divergence occurs. The fact that virtually all TCRαβ⁺ T lymphocytes have rearranged *TCRG* genes and that a large part of the TCRγδ⁺ T lymphocytes have rearranged *TCRB* genes is remarkable and suggests that both differentiation lineages might share a common origin (Fig. 48.6).

In the earliest human thymocyte subset (CD34⁺CD1a⁻), recombination is initiated in the *TCRD* locus, with incomplete Dδ2-Dδ3 and Vδ2-Dδ3 couplings as the most early rearrangements. *TCRG* recombinations start in the next stage (CD34⁺CD1a⁺), in which *TCRD* rearrangements are further completed, and incomplete *TCRB* (Dβ-Jβ) rearrangements start (45). During transition to the next stage (pre–T-cell stage), the thymocytes stop proliferating, and the *TCRB* genes further rearrange into complete Vβ-Jβ joints. During the immature single positive stage in humans, the protein product of the *TCRB* gene is expressed at the cell surface together with the pre-Tα chain, forming the pre-TCR complex, leading to expansion of cells expressing a functional TCRβ chain (45). Finally, after rearranging their *TCRA* gene, the DP cells express TCRαβ and undergo (positive and negative) selection, followed by maturation into CD4⁺ or CD8⁺ SP cells with high TCRαβ expression (Fig. 48.6).

Positive and Negative Selection during T-Cell Differentiation

The rescue of DP thymocytes from programmed cell death via interaction of their TCR with peptide/self-MHC complexes is called *positive selection*. When a DP thymocyte recognizes no MHC molecules with appreciable affinity, neither a positive nor a negative signal is given, and the thymocyte dies "by neglect." Positive selection ensures that mature T cells can recognize foreign antigens preferentially in the context of self-MHC molecules (46,47) (Fig. 48.7). DP thymocytes also undergo *negative selection*, which refers to the process of eliminating potentially self-reactive cells via apoptosis. In general, these cells bear TCR molecules with high affinity for self-peptide/self-MHC complexes and are likely to be autoreactive (Fig. 48.7). Selection for low-affinity interaction with peptide/MHC determines that CD4⁺ T cells become helper T cells, and CD8⁺ T cells become cytotoxic T cells (Fig. 48.7). That is, almost all CD4⁺ T cells have TCR molecules that recognize peptides bound to self-MHC class II and are programmed to become cytokine-secreting helper T cells, whereas most of the CD8⁺ T cells have receptors recognizing self-MHC class I molecules and are determined to become cytotoxic effector cells (48).

Specialized cells in the thymic cortex mediate positive and negative selection. Positive selection involves interaction of DP thymocytes with cortical epithelial cells, whereas negative selection is driven by a variety of antigen-presenting cells in the thymic stroma that are bone-marrow derived such as dendritic cells and macrophages (Fig. 48.7) (49).

Signal Transduction via the Pre–T-Cell Receptor and T-Cell Receptor Molecules

Signaling via the pre-TCR complex and mature TCR molecules provides important signals during T-cell differentiation (proliferation, positive selection, apoptosis). The events from triggering of a receptor and transmission of this signal inside the cell via signaling molecules to activation of transcription factors leading to specific changes in gene expression is referred to as *signal transduction*. Because of its relevance to both thymocyte differentiation and activation of mature T lymphocytes, we briefly discuss signaling via TCR molecules (50,51).

The complete TCR complex consists of a highly diverse TCR chain, complexed to nonvariant CD3 molecules (one CD3γ, one CD3δ, two CD3ε and two CD3ζ molecules), which are responsible for transduction of the signals via the TCR complex. The TCR molecules themselves have very short intracellular domains incapable of signaling. Signaling from the TCR complex is dependent on the presence of so-called immunoreceptor tyrosine-based activation motif in the CD3 chains. immunoreceptor tyrosine-based activation motifs are composed of two tyrosine residues separated by 13 amino acids. The pre-TCR complex has a similar make-up, except that the TCRβ chain is not associated with a TCRα chain but with the invariant pre-Tα protein.

When antigen binds the TCR molecule, the tyrosines of the immunoreceptor tyrosine-based activation motifs become phosphorylated by the protein tyrosine kinases Lck and Fyn. Lck is constitutively associated with CD4 and CD8; Fyn associates with CD3ζ and ε on receptor clustering. Lck is activated when CD4 or CD8 are clustered with the TCR when it binds its peptide/MHC ligand. Both Lck and Fyn phosphorylate the immunoreceptor tyrosine-based activation motifs in the CD3 complex (Fig. 48.8). This then recruits another tyrosine kinase, ZAP-70, to bind to the immunoreceptor tyrosine-based activation motifs of the CD3ζ chains. Lck subsequently activates ZAP-70, which then phosphorylates the linker proteins LAT (linker of activation in T cells) and SLP-76. Several signaling routes are subsequently activated, one via the small G protein Ras, which via the Raf kinase activates the so-called MAP kinase pathway, which consists of several serine/threonine protein kinases that are activated by subsequent phosphorylation steps (Ras, Raf, MEK, ERK). Ultimately, the MAP kinase pathway activates transcription factors important for cell proliferation (Fig. 48.8), such as NF-κB, NFAT, and Elk.

ZAP-70 also activates PLC-γ1, which cleaves phosphatidylinositol bisphosphate (PIP$_2$) into diacylglycerol (DAG) and inositol trisphosphate (IP$_3$). IP$_3$ is responsible for increasing intracellular levels of free calcium, which is an important signal for various calcium-binding proteins and kinases involved in cell proliferation and apoptosis. DAG together with calcium can activate protein kinase C (PKC). PKC activates the important NF-κB transcription factor by phosphorylation and activation of a series of kinases that phosphorylate an inhibitor molecule, IκB, that traps the NF-κB transcription factor in the cytoplasm. Phosphorylation of IκB leads to its

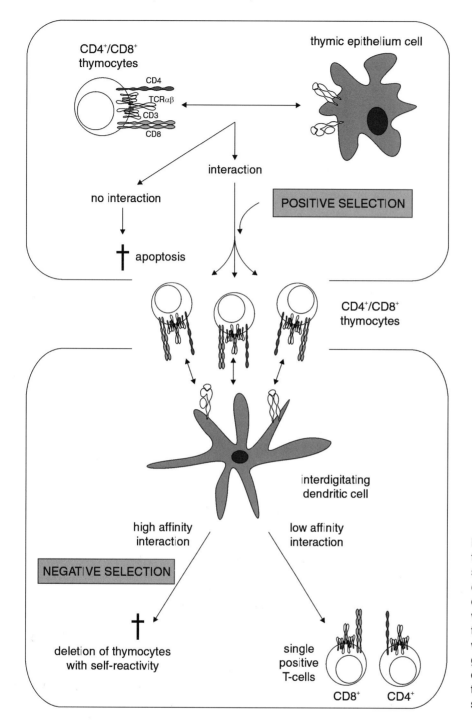

FIG. 48.7. Positive and negative selection in the thymus. The thymic stroma selects for those T-cell receptor (TCR) αβ+ T cells that have useful TCRs by contact of the TCR and its coreceptor with self-MHC on thymic cortical epithelial cells (positive selection). Also within the thymus, professional antigen-presenting cells of bone marrow origin delete potentially harmful cells that recognize self-antigens (negative selection).

breakdown and release of NF-κB from its inhibition in the cytoplasm. NF-κB then migrates to the nucleus to activate its target genes (Fig. 48.8). The calcium signal also is important to activate the calcineurin phosphatase. This phosphatase dephosphorylates NF-AT, thereby activating nuclear import of this transcription factor.

Transcriptional Regulation of T-Cell Differentiation

Regulation of gene expression, resulting in cell-specific or differentiation stage–specific gene expression profiles,

can occur at multiple levels, such as induction of locus accessibility, transcription initiation, RNA splicing, mRNA stability, translation, and posttranslational modification (52). Transcription initiation is probably the most critical regulatory step in control of gene expression. Several different (types of) transcription factors have been shown to be essential for T-cell differentiation. Evidence for this has for a large part come from studies on mice with targeted disruptions in the genes encoding these transcription factors, leading to characteristic blocks in thymocyte differentiation. The most important transcrip-

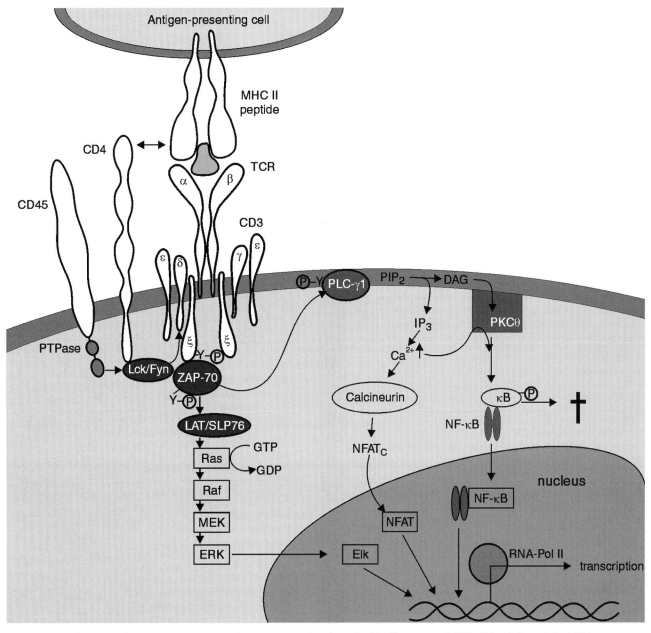

FIG. 48.8. Signal transduction pathways emanating from the T-cell receptor (TCR). Stimulation of the TCR via antigen/MHC and the CD4 or CD8 coreceptor leads to activation of the Lck and Fyn tyrosine kinases (PTK). These kinases phosphorylate the immunoreceptor tyrosine-based activation motif in the CD3 chains. CD3ζ now recruits the ZAP-70 PTK, which then activates SOS adapter molecule and the phospholipase PLCγ1. The latter cleaves phosphatidylinositol bisphosphate (PIP_2) into inositol trisphosphate (IP_3) and diacylglycerol (DAG), leading to increases in intracellular free calcium and activation of protein kinase C (PKC) Θ. PKC and other kinases can phosphorylate IκB, which is subsequently degraded, releasing the NF-κB transcription factor from cytoplasmic retention to activate target genes in the nucleus. The NFAT transcription factor is activated via the phosphatase calcineurin. The Ras/Raf/MAP kinase pathway activates the Elk transcription factor. Ultimately, target genes involved in proliferation, apoptosis, and differentiation are activated. GDP, guanosine diphosphate; GTP, guanosine triphosphate; PTPase, protein tyrosine phosphatase.

tion factors known to date to be involved in T-cell differentiation are summarized here: ikaros, GATA-3, E2A, and Tcf-1 (Fig. 48.9). These factors may become important markers for staging of malignant counterparts of immature thymocytes in the future. For instance, the transcription factor Tcf-1 is already in use to distinguish immature myeloid leukemias from immature T-cell leukemias (53). *Ikaros* is a lymphoid-restricted, zinc-finger transcription factor (54,55) related to Helios and Aiolos. Mice expressing a stable dominant-negative form of

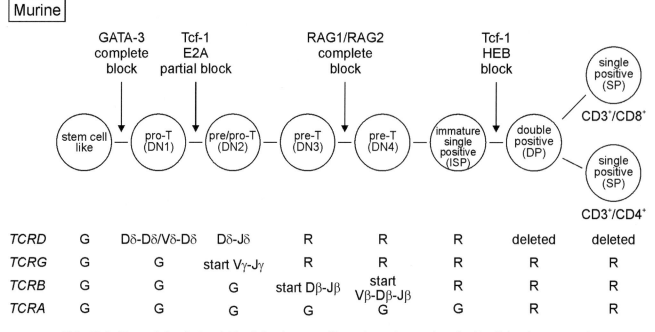

FIG. 48.9. Transcription factors in T-cell development. Shown is a scheme of murine T-cell development and those stages of differentiation in which development is blocked in mice with specific targeted mutations in the transcription factor indicated. The basic mechanisms governing murine and human T-cell development are conserved, as evidenced from blocks at similar stages in *in vitro* experiments with human thymocytes. DN, double negative; DP, double positive; ISP, immature single position; SP, single positive.

Ikaros lacked all T, B, and natural killer cells and their precursors.

GATA-3 expression is confined to stem cells, common lymphoid precursors, and pro-T and pre-T cells but not to precursors of other hematopoietic lineages. Data from several different experimental approaches demonstrate an essential role for GATA-3 in T-cell commitment, probably already at the stage of development of T-lineage precursors in fetal liver and bone marrow.

Basic helix-loop-helix (bHLH) transcription factors consist of a basic (DNA binding) domain and a helix-loop-helix (dimerization) region and have been implicated in gene regulation and differentiation of many cell types, including lymphoid cells. Class I bHLH proteins comprise E2A, HEB, and E2-2, which are also known as *E proteins* for their capacity to bind to E-box sequences (CANNTG) within regulatory elements. During lymphoid differentiation, E protein dimers are the major players. In addition to their B-cell deficiency (56), E2A$^{-/-}$ mice exhibit a defect in T-cell differentiation (56). HEB$^{-/-}$ mice display a partial block in T-cell differentiation at the transition from DN to DP cells, which is later than in E2A$^{-/-}$ mice. E-box binding sites have been recognized in enhancers of the *TCRD/TCRA* locus as well as the *TCRB* locus, suggesting a role for E proteins in regulation of TCR recombination (57).

Tcf-1 is a highly T-cell–specific transcription factor in mice and humans. Complete disruption of Tcf-1 results in a partial block of T-cell differentiation at the DN 1 to DN 2 and immature single positive to DP transitions. Tcf-1 is not an active transcription factor by itself but requires the interaction with the Wnt effector β-catenin (58).

Interaction between membrane-bound *Notch* and one of its ligands results in proteolytic cleavage of Notch (59). On cleavage, the intracellular Notch domain is released and translocates to the nucleus to interact with *CBF-1/RBP-Jκ*, thereby converting it from a repressor to an activator of gene transcription (59). Recent data from reconstitution experiments suggest that Notch signaling may play a critical role in promoting progression through several major checkpoints during T-cell differentiation, including the choice of T-lineage or B-lineage commitment; the choice between TCRαβ and TCRγδ lineages; and, in the case of TCRαβ T cells, between CD4$^+$ and CD8$^+$ lineages (60).

POSTTHYMIC T-CELL MATURATION AND EFFECTOR FUNCTION

Once T cells have completed their development in the thymus, they enter the bloodstream. The relative frequency and the absolute numbers of T lymphocytes and their subsets in peripheral blood are age dependent, with high numbers in younger age groups (particularly younger than 2 years of age) (Table 48.3). These higher numbers are probably directly related to the encountering of many new antigens and the subsequent immune responses during the first 2 years of life.

The blood T lymphocytes migrate to peripheral lymphoid organs (Peyer's patches, tonsil, lymph nodes) where they encounter antigen and where immune responses are initiated. The naïve T lymphocytes mature into effector T lympho-

TABLE 48.3. *Absolute counts of blood T lymphocytes and their subsets[a]*

Age group	TCRαβ+	CD4+CD3+	CD8+CD3	TCRγδ+	Natural killer cells
Neonatal cord blood (n = 35)	1.5–3.5	1.0–2.5	0.4–1.5	0.05–0.20	0.5–1.5
Children <9 mo (n = 164)	2.5–6.0	1.7–4.0	0.7–1.8	0.05–0.30	0.3–0.8
Children 9–24 mo (n = 103)	2.0–5.0	1.2–3.8	0.5–1.5	0.10–0.40	0.2–0.8
Children 2–15 yr (n = 91)	1.0–3.0	0.5–1.8	0.4–1.2	0.10–0.40	0.1–0.6
Adults (n = 51)	0.8–1.7	0.4–1.2	0.2–0.7	0.05–0.20	0.1–0.4

TCR, T-cell receptor.
[a]The indicated values concern the 25–75 percentiles in 10^9/L.

cytes after interaction with antigen/MHC complexes on antigen-presenting cells. The initial activation of naïve T lymphocytes requires a costimulatory signal in addition to the signal via the TCR. Costimulatory signals are given via CD28, but other molecules, including adhesion molecules (LFA-1, ICAM-3), can serve this function as well (61,62).

Naïve CD8+ T lymphocytes emerging from the thymus are already predestined to become cytotoxic cells, even though they do not yet express high levels of cytotoxic molecules. Virus-infected cells present viral antigens via their MHC class I molecules to the CD8+ T lymphocytes, which subsequently

are activated. The activated CD8+ T lymphocytes can kill the target cells that display the viral antigens (Fig. 48.10A). This killing is done via specialized molecules such as perforin, which makes holes in the cell membrane of the target cell, proteases called *granzymes*, and cytokines, such as tumor necrosis factor-α. Also, cell–cell mediated apoptotic signals are given via interaction of Fas ligand on the cytotoxic T cells, with Fas on the virus-infected target cell (Fig. 48.10A).

Naïve CD4 T lymphocytes can differentiate on activation in either T helper 1 (T_H1) or T helper 2 (T_H2) cells, which differ in the cytokines they produce and their effector func-

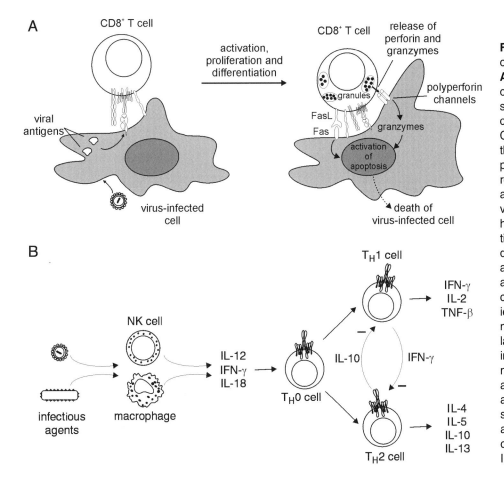

FIG. 48.10. Effector cell functions of mature CD4+ and CD8+ T cells. **A:** After encounter of viral antigens on infected cells, antigens are presented via MHC class I to CD8+ cytotoxic T cells. The activated CD8+ T cells kill then target cells that display fragments of cytosolic pathogens (mostly viruses). Via release of perforin and granzymes and interaction of Fas-FasL, the virally infected cell is killed. **B:** CD4+ helper T cells differentiate on activation in either T_H1 or T_H2 cells, which differ in the cytokines they produce and their effector function. T_H1 cells activate macrophages and induce B cells to produce opsonizing antibodies. They are mostly involved in cell-mediated immunity and produce large amounts of interferon (IFN)-γ, interleukin (IL)-12, IL-3, and tumor necrosis factor(TNF)-β. T_H2 cells activate B cells to make neutralizing antibodies; they help induce class switching in B cells and have variable effects on macrophages. Typical T_H2 cytokines are IL-4, IL-5, IL-6, and IL-10. NK, natural killer.

tion (63). The fate of naïve T lymphocytes is determined during the first encounter with antigen. T_H1 cells activate macrophages and induce B lymphocytes to produce opsonizing antibodies. They are mostly involved in cell-mediated immunity (e.g., for the response against intracellular pathogens) and produce large amounts of interferon-γ, interleukin (IL)-12, and tumor necrosis factor-β. T_H2 cells activate B cells to make neutralizing antibodies; they help induce class switching in B cells and have variable effects on macrophages. Typical T_H2 cytokines are IL-4, IL-5, IL-6, IL-10, and IL-13 (Fig. 48.10B).

The term *natural killer cells* was originally assigned on a merely functional basis to lymphoid cells capable of lysing certain tumor cells in the absence of prior stimulation (for review see reference 64). Regarding their origin, clear evidence has now been provided both in mice and humans that natural killer cells and T lymphocytes may derive from a common precursor. That is, mature natural killer cells can be obtained *in vitro* from CD34$^+$ cells isolated from umbilical cord blood, bone marrow, and even human thymus when cultured in the presence of appropriate feeder cells or IL-15.

The molecular mechanism allowing natural killer cells to discriminate between normal cells and tumor cells, predicted by the "missing self hypothesis," has been clarified only in recent years. Thus, natural killer cells recognize MHC class I molecules through surface receptors delivering signals that inhibit, rather than activate, natural killer cells. As a consequence, natural killer cells lyse target cells that have lost expression of MHC class I molecules, as frequently occurs in tumors and in cells infected by certain viruses.

Several mechanisms control discrimination between self and non-self, including the thymic deletion of autoreactive T cells and the induction of anergy in the periphery. In addition to these passive mechanisms, evidence has accumulated for the active suppression of autoreactivity by a population of regulatory or suppressor T cells that coexpress CD4 and CD25 (the IL-2 receptor α-chain) (65). CD4$^+$ CD25$^+$ regulatory T cells are powerful inhibitors of T-cell activation both *in vivo* and *in vitro*. These cells have received a lot of interest lately from basic researchers as well as clinicians. Obviously, they could play a critical regulatory role in many pathologic conditions.

NORMAL T LYMPHOCYTES AND THEIR RELATIONSHIP TO T-CELL NEOPLASIA

Immunophenotype

The various types of acute and chronic T-cell leukemias and T-cell lymphomas can be regarded as the malignant counterparts of immature (thymic) or more mature (postthymic) T lymphoid cells (Fig. 48.11). Apart from morphologic and cytochemical features, the normal (precursor) T cells and their malignant counterparts can be characterized by immunophenotyping, using antibodies directed against (membrane bound or intracellular) leukocyte antigens (Fig. 48.11).

Immunophenotype of Thymic-Derived T-Cell Neoplasms

Approximately 15% to 20% of childhood acute lymphoblastic leukemias and 20% to 25% of adult acute lymphoblastic leukemias belong to the T lineage. Virtually all T-cell acute lymphoblastic leukemias are positive for TdT, CD2, CD7, and CyCD3; further discrimination of subtypes is possible on the basis of CD1, CD3, CD4, CD5, and CD8 reactivity (Table 48.4) (66–70). T-cell acute lymphoblastic leukemias are often classified in three main subtypes using CD1 and CD3: immature T-cell acute lymphoblastic leukemia (CD1$^-$/CD3$^-$), common (cortical) thymocytic T-cell acute lymphoblastic leukemia (CD1$^+$/CD3$^{+ \text{ or } -}$), and mature T-cell acute lymphoblastic leukemia (CD1$^-$/CD3$^+$) (Table 48.4). Immature T-cell lymphoblastic leukemias can be further subdivided into the rare CD5$^-$ prothymocytic T-cell lymphoblastic leukemia (pro–T-cell acute lymphoblastic leukemia) and the CD5$^+$ immature thymocytic T-cell lymphoblastic leukemia (pre–T-cell acute lymphoblastic leukemia). These immature T-cell lymphoblastic leukemias have a poor prognosis, whereas the CD1$^+$ common thymocytic T-cell lymphoblastic leukemia is characterized by a much better outcome under intensive treatment. This difference in outcome probably reflects the apoptosis sensitivity of the normal thymocytic counterparts of these T-cell lymphoblastic leukemias (68,69,71,72). Membrane CD3$^+$ T-cell lymphoblastic leukemias, which constitute approximately 35% of all T-cell lymphoblastic leukemias, are further subdivided in TCRαβ$^+$ (20% of T-cell lymphoblastic leukemia) and TCRγδ$^+$ (15% of T-cell lymphoblastic leukemia) subgroups (4); event free survival is better in TCRγδ$^+$ T-cell lymphoblastic leukemias. The various types of T-cell lymphoblastic leukemias and the T-cell lymphoblastic lymphomas form a continuous spectrum of lymphoblastic T-cell malignancies. CD3$^+$ T-cell lymphoblastic leukemias and T-cell lymphoblastic lymphomas seem to be highly comparable in many features, despite a single report claiming a difference in the type of TCR molecule (TCRαβ vs. TCRγδ) that is expressed (73).

Immunophenotype of Postthymic T-Cell Neoplasms

Mature T/natural killer–cell neoplasms are also called *postthymic T-cell neoplasms* because they do not express TdT or CD1 antigen. This group consists of several types of chronic T/natural killer–cell leukemias and mature T/natural killer–cell lymphomas (74–77). They comprise approximately 5% to 10% of all mature lymphoid neoplasms. Immunophenotypic analysis helps to identify these subtypes as separate entities that show their characteristic disease course, prognosis, and treatment possibilities. Consequently, in the recent World Health Organization classification of hematopoietic tumors, immunologic marker analysis plays a major role next to morphology (reviewed in references 78 and 79). One of the most important antibodies is CD3, which enables discrimination between CD3$^+$ T-cell neoplasms and CD3$^-$ natural killer–cell neoplasms, such as the aggressive natural killer–cell leukemia and the mostly natural killer–type extranodal/nasal lymphoma (Table 48.5). Most postthymic CD3$^+$ T-cell neoplasms express TCRαβ, with

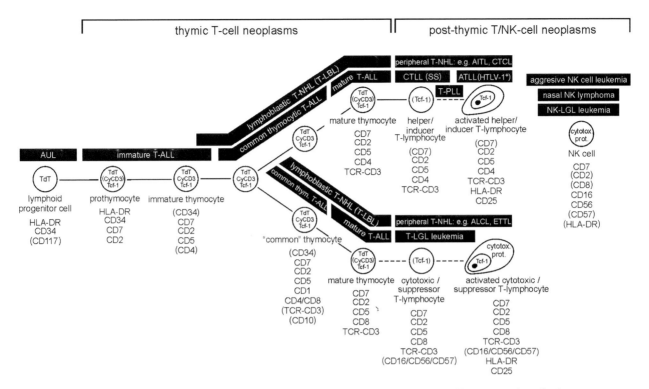

FIG. 48.11. Hypothetic scheme of T/natural killer (NK) lymphoid differentiation. The expression of relevant immunologic markers is indicated for each differentiation stage; markers in parentheses are not always expressed. The bars represent the various types of leukemias and non-Hodgkin's lymphomas (NHL) as presumed malignant counterparts of lymphoid T cells on maturational arrest. AITL, angioimmunoblastic T-cell lymphoma; ALCL, anaplastic large-cell lymphoma; ALL, acute lymphoblastic leukemia; ATLL, adult T-cell leukemia lymphoma; AUL, acute undifferentiated leukemia; CTCL, cutaneous T-cell lymphoma; CTLL (SS), cutaneous T-cell leukemia lymphoma (mycosis fungoides/Sézary syndrome); ETTL, enteropathy-type T-cell lymphoma; HTLV-1, human T-cell leukemia virus type I; LBL, lymphoblastic lymphoma; LGL, large granular lymphocyte; PLL, prolymphocytic leukemia; TCR, T-cell receptor; TdT, terminal deoxynucleotidyl transferase.

TABLE 48.4. *Immunophenotypic characteristics of T-cell acute lymphoblastic leukemia (T-ALL)*

| Marker | Immature T-ALL | | Common thymocytic T-ALL | | |
	Prothymocytic (pro T-ALL)	Immature thymocytic (pre T-ALL)	SmCD3⁻	SmCD3⁺	Mature T-ALL
TdT	++	++	++	++	++
CD1	−	−	++	++	−
CD2	+	++	++	++	++
CyCD3	++	++	++	++	++
CD3	−	−	−	++	++
CD4⁻/CD8⁻	++	+	−	−	−
CD4⁺/CD8⁻	−	±	±	±	+
CD4⁻/CD8⁺	−	±	±	±	±
CD4⁺/CD8⁺	−	−	+	+	±
CD5	−	++	++	++	++
CD7	++	++	++	++	++
TCRαβ	−	−	−	60–70%	60–70%
TCRγδ	−	−	−	30–40%	30–40%

−, <10% of T-ALL positive; ±, 10–25% of T-ALL positive; +, 25–75% of T-ALL positive; ++, >75% of T-ALL positive; TCR, T-cell receptor; TdT, terminal deoxynucleotidyl transferase.

TABLE 48.5. *Major immunophenotypic characteristics of postthymic T/natural killer (NK)–cell neoplasms*

Postthymic T/NK-cell neoplasms[a]	TCRαβ phenotype		TCRγδ phenotype	NK phenotype	Cytotoxic granule proteins
	CD4	CD8			
T-cell prolymphocytic leukemia	+	±	−	−	−
T-cell large granular lymphocytic leukemia	Rare	~70%	~10%	~15%	+
Aggressive NK-cell leukemia	−	−	−	+	+
Adult T-cell leukemia/lymphoma	+	Rare	−	−	−
Extranodal/nasal T/NK lymphoma	−	−	−	+	+
Enteropathy-type T-cell lymphoma	−	±	−	−	−
Hepatosplenic T-cell lymphoma	−	−	+	−	+
Subcutaneous panniculitis-like T-cell lymphoma	−	75%	25%	−	+
Mycosis fungoides/Sézary syndrome	+	Rare	Rare	−	−
Primary cutaneous anaplastic large-cell lymphoma	+	−	−	−	+
Peripheral T-cell lymphoma, unspecified	+	−	−	−	Rare
Angioimmunoblastic T-cell lymphoma	+	±	−	−	−
Anaplastic large-cell lymphoma	±	Rare	−	−	+

−, negative; ±, occasionally positive; +, positive; TCR, T-cell receptor.
[a]Postthymic T/NK-cell neoplasms as defined according to the World Health Organization Classification of tumors of hematopoietic and lymphoid tissues.

only a minority expressing TCRγδ. Nevertheless, in some entities, such as T-cell large granular lymphocytic leukemia or hepatosplenic T-cell lymphoma, TCRγδ cases are more abundant than in others (80,81). However, generally TCRγδ⁺ mature T-cell neoplasms are more rare than TCRγδ⁺ T-cell lymphoblastic leukemias. A major subdivision within the group of postthymic TCRαβ⁺ T-cell neoplasms concerns CD4 or CD8 positivity, largely reflecting the helper or cytotoxic origin of their normal counterparts, respectively. Most chronic T-cell leukemias, including T-cell prolymphocytic leukemia and adult T-cell leukemia/lymphoma, are largely of CD4 phenotype, except for T-cell large granular lymphocytic leukemia, which generally show a CD8⁺/CD57⁺ cytotoxic origin (Table 48.5). T-cell prolymphocytic leukemia and adult T-cell leukemia/lymphoma typically express CD7 and CD25 antigens, respectively. Also, the various T-cell lymphomas are generally characterized as CD4⁺ or CD8⁺: Angioimmunoblastic lymphoma, peripheral T-cell lymphoma unspecified, and various types of cutaneous T-cell lymphoma (including mycosis fungoides and its leukemic variant Sézary syndrome) are mostly CD4⁺, whereas others are CD8⁺, such as the enteropathy-type and subcutaneous panniculitis-like T-cell lymphoma (Table 48.5). In many of the CD8⁺ postthymic neoplasms as well as in TCRγδ⁺ and natural killer–cell types, cytotoxic granule proteins can be detected; this also holds for anaplastic large cell lymphomas and their cutaneous variants, which are both often CD4⁺ (Table 48.5).

Immunogenotype

Given the observation that the various types of T-cell lymphomas and leukemias strongly resemble normal lymphoid (precursor) cells (67), the vast majority also contain rear-

ranged TCR genes. However, neoplasms might exhibit curious types of rearrangements, which are rare or absent in normal T lymphocytes. One example concerns the so-called cross-lineage *IGH* gene rearrangements, which are found in 10% to 15% of T-cell lymphoblastic leukemias (25,82–85) and which are probably due to the continuous activity of the recombinase enzyme system after malignant transformation in these precursor T-cell leukemias.

T-Cell Receptor Gene Recombination Patterns in Thymic-Derived T-Cell Neoplasms

CD3⁻, TCRαβ⁺, and TCRγδ⁺ T-cell lymphoblastic leukemias/T-cell lymphoblastic lymphomas show major differences in TCR gene rearrangement patterns (Table 48.6) (4,25). Although the frequency of TCR gene rearrangements in T-cell lymphoblastic leukemias in general is very high, approximately 10% of CD3⁻ T-cell lymphoblastic leukemias still have all TCR genes in germline configuration (4,25); this mainly concerns immature CD1⁻/CD3⁻ T-cell lymphoblastic leukemia of the prothymocytic/pro–T-cell lymphoblastic leukemia type (Table 48.6). The *TCRD* genes in CD3⁻ T-cell lymphoblastic leukemias are rearranged in most cases (approximately 80%) and contain biallelic deletions in approximately 10% of cases (4,13). As expected, all TCRγδ⁺ T-cell lymphoblastic leukemias have *TCRG* and *TCRD* gene rearrangements, and the vast majority (approximately 95%) also contain *TCRB* gene rearrangements (Table 48.6) (13,86). All TCRαβ⁺ T-cell lymphoblastic leukemias contain *TCRB* and *TCRG* gene rearrangements and have at least one deleted *TCRD* allele (equals *TCRA* rearrangement); the second *TCRD* allele is also deleted in two-thirds of cases (Table 48.6)

TABLE 48.6. *Frequencies of T-cell receptor (TCR) gene rearrangements and deletions in human T/natural killer (NK)–cell neoplasms*

T/NK-cell neoplasm	TCRB R (%)	TCRG R (%)	TCRD R (%)	TCRD D (%)
Thymic derived				
CD3⁻ T-ALL (T-LBL)	85	90	80	10
TCRγδ⁺ T-ALL (T-LBL)	95	100	100	0
TCRαβ⁺ T-ALL (T-LBL)	100	100	35	65
Postthymic				
ATLL, CTLL, T-PLL[a]	100	100	10–25	75–90
TCRαβ⁺ T-LGL[b]	100	100	<25	>75
TCRγδ⁺ T-LGL[b]	~50	100	100	0
NK-LGL[b]	0	0	0	0
T-NHL[c]	80	60–100	<35?	>60?

ATLL, adult T-cell leukemia/lymphoma; CTLL, cutaneous T-cell leukemia/lymphoma; D, both alleles deleted; R, at least one allele rearranged; T-ALL, T-cell acute lymphoblastic leukemia; T-LBL, T-cell lymphoblastic lymphoma; T-LGL, T-cell large granular lymphocytic leukemia; T-NHL, T-cell non-Hodgkin's lymphoma; T-PLL, T-cell prolymphocytic leukemia.
[a]The majority of ATLL, CTLL, and T-PLL are of TCRαβ⁺ type.
[b]Most LGL proliferations are TCRαβ⁺ (70–80%), and minorities are TCRγδ⁺ (10–15%) or belong to the NK lineage (10–15%).
[c]Except for γδ hepatosplenic lymphoma and some cases of TCR⁻ anaplastic large-cell lymphoma, many postthymic T-NHLs are TCRαβ⁺.

(13,25). Despite persistent V(D)J recombinase activity in the T-cell lymphoblastic leukemia blasts, a comparative diagnosis-relapse study in 26 T-cell lymphoblastic leukemia patients revealed a high stability of clonal TCR rearrangements; continuing and secondary rearrangements were apparent in 0%, 14%, and 20% of *TCRD*, *TCRG*, and *TCRB* gene rearrangements, respectively (86a). Oligoclonality at diagnosis is rarely seen in T-cell lymphoblastic leukemias (25,86a), except for a few CD3⁻ T-cell lymphoblastic leukemias showing polyclonal δREC-ψJα rearrangements that can be interpreted as continuing rearrangements aiming at TCRαβ expression (87). *TCRA* rearrangements have not been studied in detail so far.

T-Cell Receptor Gene Recombination Patterns in Postthymic T-Cell Neoplasms

As the vast majority of chronic T-cell leukemias (T-cell prolymphocytic leukemia, adult T-cell leukemia/lymphoma, T-cell large granular lymphocytic leukemia) concern TCRαβ⁺ T-cell malignancies, *TCRB* rearrangements are found in virtually all samples (95% to 100%) (Table 48.6). Only the small subgroup of TCRγδ⁺ T-cell large granular

lymphocytic leukemia lacks *TCRB* recombinations in approximately 50% of cases. *TCRG* rearrangements are very frequent in both TCRγδ⁺ and TCRαβ⁺ chronic leukemias. In contrast, most TCRαβ⁺ T-cell leukemias show monoallelic or biallelic deletions of their *TCRD* loci, which correlates with their expression of TCRα chains. Only a minority of cases, including all TCRγδ⁺ T-cell large granular lymphocytic leukemias, have rearranged *TCRD* genes (Table 48.6). Natural killer–large granular lymphocytic leukemias completely lack TCR rearrangements.

The membrane TCR expression of postthymic T-cell non-Hodgkin's lymphoma also largely reflects its TCR gene recombination patterns. Because most T-cell non-Hodgkin's lymphoma types are TCRαβ⁺, except for (TCRγδ⁺) hepatosplenic T-cell lymphomas and some TCR⁻ anaplastic large-cell lymphomas, *TCRB* and *TCRG* rearrangements are very frequent but (slightly) less than those found in chronic T-cell leukemias (Table 48.6). The frequency of *TCRD* rearrangements is not exactly known but is estimated to be less than 35%, whereas *TCRD* deletions are probably found in more than 60% of cases (Table 48.6).

T-Cell Receptor Clonality Detection in T-Cell Neoplasms

Because T-cell leukemias are clonal cell proliferations, the TCR gene rearrangements are assumed to be identical in all cells of the leukemic clone (25,88–91). This is the basis of clonality assessment in lymphoproliferations (25). Detection of clonal TCR gene rearrangements is possible via polymerase chain reaction methods. As *TCRG* and *TCRD* loci contain a limited number of V and J gene segments (Table 48.1 and Fig. 48.2) (10,13), only a restricted number of polymerase chain reaction primers is sufficient to analyze the various *TCRG* and *TCRD* gene rearrangements. In contrast, polymerase chain reaction analysis of *TCRA* and *TCRB* gene rearrangements requires many more (family) primers, especially for the many different V and J gene segments in *TCRA* and *TCRB* genes (Table 48.1 and Fig. 48.2) (7,8,92–95). Reverse transcriptase polymerase chain reaction analysis of *TCRA* and *TCRB* V(D)J-C transcripts still requires many different V (family) primers but in combination with only a single C primer (92–94,96). False-negative results, due to primer sets that do not recognize all involved TCR gene segments, might be overcome by using specific primers for every individual V and J gene segment in multiplex polymerase chain reactions.

Polymerase chain reaction–based detection of clonal TCR gene rearrangements is relatively easy if the percentage of leukemic cells is high (e.g., greater than 90%). In such cell samples, the background of TCR gene rearrangements of normal, polyclonal cells generally does not hamper proper interpretation. However, if a sample contains substantial numbers of polyclonal T cells, many polyclonal TCR polymerase chain reaction products are present as well, stressing the need to discriminate between clonal (leukemia derived) and polyclonal (reactive) polymerase chain reaction prod-

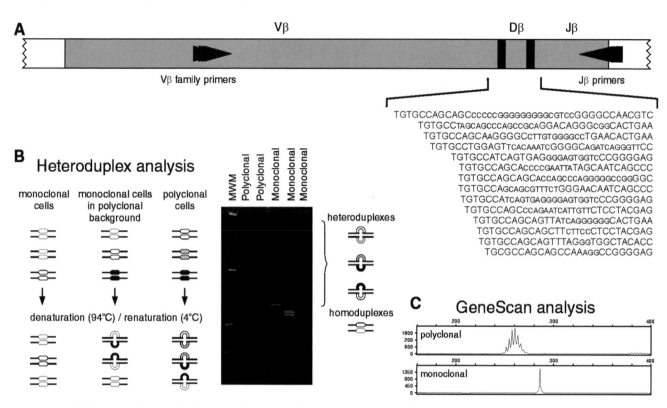

FIG. 48.12. Schematic diagram of the heteroduplex analysis and GeneScan analysis techniques. Rearranged T-cell receptor (TCR) genes (*TCRB* in the example) show heterogeneity (in size and nucleotide composition) in their junctional regions. This heterogeneity of rearranged TCR polymerase chain reaction (PCR) products is used in heteroduplex analysis (size and composition) and GeneScan analysis (size) to discern between products derived from monoclonal and polyclonal lymphoid cell populations. In heteroduplex analysis, PCR products are heat-denatured (5 minutes, 94°C) and subsequently rapidly cooled (1 hour, 4°C) to induce duplex (homo- or heteroduplex) formation. In cell samples consisting of clonal lymphoid cells, the PCR products of rearranged TCR genes give rise to homoduplexes after denaturation and renaturation, whereas in samples that contain polyclonal lymphoid cell populations, the single-strand PCR fragments mainly form heteroduplexes, which result in a background smear of slowly migrating fragments on electrophoresis. In GeneScan analysis, fluorochrome-labeled rearranged TCR products are first denatured before high resolution fragment analysis of the resulting single-strand fragments. Monoclonal cell samples give rise to PCR products of identical size, whereas in polyclonal samples, many different TCR PCR products are formed, which show a characteristic Gaussian size distribution.

ucts. Methods exploiting the junctional diversity of rearranged TCR genes to discriminate between identical (clonal) and heterogeneous (polyclonal) polymerase chain reaction products include a.o. heteroduplex analysis (97,98) and GeneScan/fragment analysis (Fig. 48.12) (99,100).

T-Cell Receptor Vβ Detection via Monoclonal Antibodies

Molecular methods for clonality detection and repertoire analysis of (aberrant) T-cell populations can be time-consuming and labor intensive, and, most important, do not allow precise quantitative evaluation. However, the recent availability of a set of well-defined Vβ antibodies enables flow cytometric analysis of the TCR Vβ repertoire. Using normal values in healthy controls of different age groups as a reference (Fig. 48.13), clonal T-cell populations can be identified in a quantitative manner (101,102). In a comparative study

using 28 thymic-derived T-cell neoplasms and 47 postthymic mature T-cell neoplasms, Vβ flow cytometric results appeared to correlate completely with *TCRB* polymerase chain reaction results. As the complete set of antibodies covers 65% to 70% of all TCR Vβ domains, flow cytometric assays served to identify restricted Vβ usage in two-thirds of the monoclonal T-cell neoplasms (Fig. 48.14); in the other cases, a major T-cell population did not stain with any of the antibodies, which is indirect evidence for the homogenous character of these samples in line with the molecular data (96,103). In the future, quantitative flow cytometric Vβ analyses might, thus, (partly) replace the more expensive and cumbersome molecular TCR repertoire studies. Likewise, Vγ and Vδ analysis in the case of TCRγδ T-cell proliferations might also (partly) be performed by flow cytometry using Vγ and Vδ antibodies, although the small Vγ/Vδ repertoire makes this more difficult than Vβ analysis.

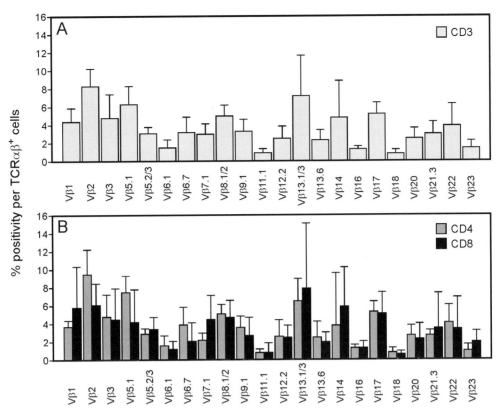

FIG. 48.13. Flow cytometric Vβ analysis in healthy individuals. Schematic overview of mean values and standard deviations for Vβ positivity within T-cell receptor (TCR) αβ⁺/CD3⁺ T lymphocytes **(A)** and within TCRαβ⁺/CD4⁺ and TCRαβ⁺/CD8⁺ T lymphocytes **(B)**.

Deregulated Differentiation Leading to T-Cell Neoplasia

Illegitimate V(D)J Recombination Leading to Chromosome Aberrations in Thymocytes

T-cell neoplasms harbor characteristic TCR gene recombination patterns (13,86,104–106), and also nonphysiologic rearrangements between TCR loci and proto-oncogenes can occur (107). This is particularly the case in T-cell lymphoblastic leukemias, in which several types of chromosome aberrations involving the *TCRD* (chromosome region 14q11) and *TCRB* (7q34-35) loci have been described (Table 48.7). Such translocations are most likely mediated

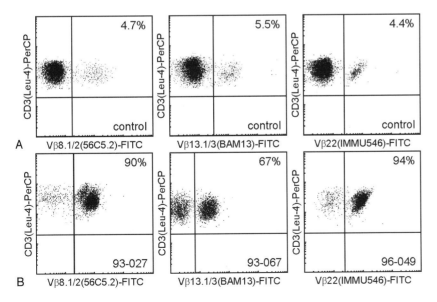

FIG. 48.14. Flow cytometric Vβ analysis in patients with mature T-cell proliferations. Examples of Vβ8.1/2, Vβ13.1/3, and Vβ22 reactivity within CD3⁺ T lymphocytes of healthy controls **(A)** and three different monoclonal T-cell neoplasms **(B)**.

TABLE 48.7. *Nonrandom chromosome aberrations in T-cell acute lymphoblastic leukemia (T-ALL)*

Chromosome aberration	Relative frequency of T-ALL (%)	Involved gene	Involved T-cell receptor gene
1p32 aberrations	20–25	*TAL1*	*TCRD/TCRB*
t(11;14)(p13;q11)/t(7;11)(q35;p13)	7	*LMO2*	*TCRD/TCRB*
t(11;14)(p15;q11)	1	*LMO1*	*TCRD*
t(10;14)(q24;q11)/t(7;10)(q35;q24)	4	*HOX11*	*TCRD/TCRB*
t(8;14)(q24;q11)	2	*MYC*	*TCRD*
t(7;9)(q34;q32)	2	*TAL2*	*TCRB*
t(7;9)(q34;q34)	2	*TAN1*	*TCRB*
t(1;7)(p32;q34)	1	*LCK*	*TCRB*
t(7;19)(q34;p13)	1	*LYL1*	*TCRB*
t(5;14)(q35;q11)/t(5;14)(q35;q32)	15–20	*HOX11L2/(RANBp17)*	*TCRD/CTIP2[a]*

[a]CTIP2 is also known as BCL11B.

via mechanisms closely resembling physiologic V(D)J gene rearrangements. This is supported by the presence of RSS or RSS-like elements in the breakpoint regions of several of these genes. As a result of these illegitimate V(D)J recombinations, proto-oncogenes on the partner chromosomes are activated through regulatory elements of the translocated TCR gene. The best known example concerns ectopic expression of the transcription factor TAL1 on t(1;14)(p32;q11) and t(1;7)(p32;q35) (Table 48.7). Together, with microdeletions of chromosome region 1p32 that also give rise to TAL1 overexpression, these aberrations are found in a considerable subgroup of 20% to 25% of all T-cell lymphoblastic leukemias (108–110). In addition to TAL1, other transcription factors can be activated inappropriately by translocation of TCR genes. This concerns other bHLH transcription factors, such as MYC, TAL2, and LYL1, and also LIM domain factors LMO1 and LMO2 (Table 48.7) (111,112). Recently, the cryptic translocation t(5;14)(q35;q32), resulting in HOX11L2 overexpression, has been described and was found to be related to poor outcome (113,114).

So far, illegitimate V(D)J recombination involving TCR loci has not been described in more mature T-cell neoplasms. One exceptional type of TCR rearrangement is found in these patients as well as T-cell neoplasms that develop in ataxia-telangiectasia and Nijmegen breakage syndrome patients. This concerns the so-called trans-rearrangements between the *TCRB* and *TCRG* loci through t(7;7) or inversion 7 (115–118). However, although described in a T-cell lymphoblastic leukemia case as well (119), these trans-rearrangements are not believed to play a direct role in oncogenesis; they are rather considered to be a general indicator of the risk of lymphoma development through genomic instability in such patients.

Inappropriate Transcriptional Activation in Thymocytes

As a general result of translocations in human T-cell lymphoblastic leukemia, transcription factors are inappropriately activated, leading to deregulated thymocyte differentiation. In the case of tissue-specific bHLH factors, it has been hypothesized that their ectopic expression in T-lymphocyte precursors causes heterodimerization with class I bHLH factors (e.g., E2A and HEB) that are normally expressed in these cells. As a result, key regulator functions of these E proteins in thymocyte differentiation are blocked, which contributes to malignant transformation and subsequently T-cell lymphoblastic leukemia development (120,121). In addition, the presumed tumor suppressor function of E2A might be blocked. Consistent with the E protein inactivation hypothesis is the rapid development of immature T-cell lymphomas in E2A$^{-/-}$ mice (56).

Another family of regulatory factors known to be involved in human T-cell lymphoblastic leukemia is the Notch receptor family, which normally controls cell fate decisions (122,123). Notch1, truncated by a chromosomal translocation leading to a constitutively active intracellular domain (TAN-1), plays a role in T-cell lymphoblastic leukemia leukemogenesis (124).

Recent gene profiling studies have revealed that even though only 30% of human T-cell lymphoblastic leukemias have chromosomal translocations, T-cell lymphoblastic leukemias can be organized into clusters with common gene expression signatures (125). This is due to the fact that the *LYL1*, *HOX11*, and *TAL1* oncogenes that define these groups can also be overexpressed via other mechanisms than translocations. It is interesting that the three gene expression–based groups appeared to correspond to different thymic subsets that are blocked in differentiation by transcription factor overexpression (125). Moreover, they represented distinct clinical subtypes with different prognosis. HOX11+ T-cell lymphoblastic leukemias (derived from early cortical thymocytes) are associated with a relatively favorable prognosis, whereas LYL1+ (prothymocyte-derived cases) and TAL1+ (late cortical thymocyte-derived cases) show a less favorable outcome.

Although inappropriate transcriptional activation, either due to translocation or other mechanisms responsible for increased expression of several classes of transcription factors, seems to be a general principle contributing to aberrant thymocyte development and subsequent malignant transformation, much less is known yet about similar mechanisms in more mature T-cell neoplasias. Many of the molecular genetic events involved in lymphomagenesis and leukemogenesis of postthymic T lymphocytes, therefore, still remain to be identified.

CONCLUSION

Insight into normal T-cell differentiation and T-cell function is essential to understand the origin and characteristics of T-cell malignancies. Although malignantly transformed cells differ in some aspects from their normal counterparts, most phenotypic and genotypic characteristics are identical.

Transformation of T-cells might be mediated via several different events, such as aberrant TCR gene rearrangements leading to oncogene activation, inappropriate apoptosis leading to proliferation instead of cell death, or unwanted activation and subsequent proliferation. This implies that malignant transformation might be caused by seemingly minor defects in several molecular steps during normal T-cell differentiation, TCR gene rearrangement processes, positive and negative selection processes, activation and TCR molecule signaling processes, and T helper and cytotoxic functions. Understanding the regulation of these processes supports the understanding of malignant transformation.

Over the last decade, progress in the immunodiagnosis of T-cell malignancies was based on

1. Advances in immunophenotyping of normal and malignant T cells, particularly by use of multiparameter flow cytometry with quadruple labelings. This progress allowed more detailed characterization and classification of T-cell malignancies (Fig. 48.11 and Table 48.5).

2. Novel developments in clonality diagnostics, particularly based on the polymerase chain reaction–mediated detection of clonal TCR gene rearrangements (Fig. 48.12 and Table 48.6) and TCR gene–related chromosome aberrations (Table 48.7). Clonality assessment appeared to be highly valuable in the diagnosis of mature T-cell malignancies, particularly in patients who have many reactive T lymphocytes in suspect lesions.

3. New possibilities for evaluation of treatment effectiveness by detection of minimal residual disease in blood and bone marrow during and after treatment. Minimal residual disease detection in T-cell malignancies is possible by use of Vβ antibodies in part of the patients. However, in virtually all patients, polymerase chain reaction–based techniques can be applied for minimal residual disease detection, using the junctional regions of rearranged TCR genes as leukemia-specific polymerase chain reaction targets.

It can be foreseen that current developments in genomics and proteomics (including gene expression profiling and antibody or tissue arrays) will further contribute to the insight in normal and malignant T-cell development. Subsequent multidisciplinary translational research will play a key role in the further improvement of diagnostics and treatment of patients with T-cell malignancies.

REFERENCES

1. Davis MM, Bjorkman PJ. T-cell antigen receptor genes and T-cell recognition. *Nature* 1988;334:395–402.
2. Owen MJ, Lamb JR. *Immune recognition*. Oxford, UK: IRL Press, 1988.
3. Borst J, Brouns GS, de Vries E, et al. Antigen receptors on T and B lymphocytes: parallels in organization and function. *Immunol Rev* 1993;132:49–84.
4. van Dongen JJ, Comans-Bitter WM, Wolvers-Tettero IL, Borst J. Development of human T lymphocytes and their thymus-dependency. *Thymus* 1990;16:207–234.
5. van Dongen JJ, Wolvers-Tettero IL. Analysis of immunoglobulin and T cell receptor genes. Part I: basic and technical aspects. *Clin Chim Acta* 1991;198:1–91.
6. Yoshikai Y, Clark SP, Taylor S, et al. Organization and sequences of the variable, joining and constant region genes of the human T-cell receptor alpha-chain. *Nature* 1985;316:837–840.
7. Griesser H, Champagne E, Tkachuk D, et al. The human T cell receptor alpha-delta locus: a physical map of the variable, joining and constant region genes. *Eur J Immunol* 1988; 8:641–644.
8. Toyonaga B, Yoshikai Y, Vadasz V, et al. Organization and sequences of the diversity, joining, and constant region genes of the human T-cell receptor beta chain. *Proc Natl Acad Sci U S A* 1985;82:8624–8628.
9. Quertermous T, Strauss WM, Van Dongen JJ, Seidman JG. Human T cell gamma chain joining regions and T cell development. *J Immunol* 1987;138:2687–2690.
10. Lefranc MP, Rabbitts TH. The human T-cell receptor gamma (TRG) genes. *Trends Biochem Sci* 1989;14:214–218.
11. Zhang XM, Tonnelle C, Lefranc MP, Huck S. T cell receptor gamma cDNA in human fetal liver and thymus: variable regions of gamma chains are restricted to V gamma I or V9, due to the absence of splicing of the V10 and V11 leader intron. *Eur J Immunol* 1994;24:571–578.
12. Takihara Y, Tkachuk D, Michalopoulos E, et al. Sequence and organization of the diversity, joining, and constant region genes of the human T-cell delta-chain locus. *Proc Natl Acad Sci U S A* 1988;85:6097–6101.
13. Breit TM, Wolvers-Tettero IL, Beishuizen A, et al. Southern blot patterns, frequencies, and junctional diversity of T-cell receptor-delta gene rearrangements in acute lymphoblastic leukemia. *Blood* 1993;82:3063–3074.
14. Davodeau F, Peyrat MA, Hallet MM, et al. Characterization of a new functional TCR J delta segment in humans. Evidence for a marked conservation of J delta sequences between humans, mice, and sheep. *J Immunol* 1994;153:137–142.
15. Tonegawa S. Somatic generation of antibody diversity. *Nature* 1983; 302:575–581.
16. Schatz DG, Oettinger MA, Baltimore D. The V(D)J recombination activating gene, RAG-1. *Cell* 1989;59:1035–1048.
17. Oettinger MA, Schatz DG, Gorka C, Baltimore D. RAG-1 and RAG-2, adjacent genes that synergistically activate V(D)J recombination. *Science* 1990;248:1517–1523.
18. McBlane JF, van Gent DC, Ramsden DA, et al. Cleavage at a V(D)J recombination signal requires only RAG1 and RAG2 proteins and occurs in two steps. *Cell* 1995;83:387–395.
19. Lieber MR. The mechanism of V(D)J recombination: a balance of diversity, specificity, and stability. *Cell* 1992;70:873–876.
20. Lieber MR. The role of site-directed recombinases in physiologic and pathologic chromosomal rearrangements. In: Kirsch IR, ed. *The causes and consequences of chromosomal aberrations*. Boca Raton, FL: CRC Press, 1993:239–275.
21. van Gent DC, Ramsden DA, Gellert M. The RAG1 and RAG2 proteins establish the 12/23 rule in V(D)J recombination. *Cell* 1996;85:107–113.
22. Hazenberg MD, Verschuren MC, Hamann D, et al. T cell receptor excision circles as markers for recent thymic emigrants: basic

aspects, technical approach, and guidelines for interpretation. *J Mol Med* 2001;79:631–640.

23. Ye P, Kirschner DE. Reevaluation of T cell receptor excision circles as a measure of human recent thymic emigrants. *J Immunol* 2002;168:4968–4979.

24. Hazenberg MD, Otto SA, Cohen Stuart JW, et al. Increased cell division but not thymic dysfunction rapidly affects the T-cell receptor excision circle content of the naive T cell population in HIV-1 infection. *Nat Med* 2000;6:1036–1042.

25. van Dongen JJ, Wolvers-Tettero IL. Analysis of immunoglobulin and T cell receptor genes. Part II: possibilities and limitations in the diagnosis and management of lymphoproliferative diseases and related disorders. *Clin Chim Acta* 1991;198:93–174.

26. Marolleau JP, Fondell JD, Malissen M, et al. The joining of germ-line V alpha to J alpha genes replaces the preexisting V alpha-J alpha complexes in a T cell receptor alpha, beta positive T cell line. *Cell* 1988;55:291–300.

27. McCormack WT, Liu M, Postema C, et al. Excision products of TCR V alpha recombination contain in-frame rearrangements: evidence for continued V(D)J recombination in TCR+ thymocytes. *Int Immunol* 1993;5:801–804.

28. Huang C, Kanagawa O. Ordered and coordinated rearrangement of the TCR alpha locus: role of secondary rearrangement in thymic selection. *J Immunol* 2001;166:2597–2601.

29. Golub R, Huang CY, Kanagawa O, Wu GE. Valpha gene replacement in a TCRalpha knock-in mouse. *Eur J Immunol* 2001;31:2919–2925.

30. Golub R. V gene replacement in T and B lymphocytes: illicit or regimented rearrangement? *Arch Immunol Ther Exp (Warsz)* 2002;50:255–262.

31. Leiden JM, Dialynas DP, Duby AD, et al. Rearrangement and expression of T-cell antigen receptor genes in human T-lymphocyte tumor lines and normal human T-cell clones: evidence for allelic exclusion of Ti beta gene expression and preferential use of a J beta 2 gene segment. *Mol Cell Biol* 1986; 6:3207–3214.

32. Triebel F, Hercend T. Subpopulations of human peripheral T gamma delta lymphocytes. *Immunol Today* 1989;10:186–188.

33. Borst J, Wicherink A, Van Dongen JJ, et al. Non-random expression of T cell receptor gamma and delta variable gene segments in functional T lymphocyte clones from human peripheral blood. *Eur J Immunol* 1989;19:1559–1568.

34. Breit TM, Wolvers-Tettero IL, van Dongen JJ. Unique selection determinant in polyclonal V delta 2-J delta 1 junctional regions of human peripheral gamma delta T lymphocytes. *J Immunol* 1994;152: 2860–2864.

35. Desiderio SV, Yancopoulos GD, Paskind M, et al. Insertion of N regions into heavy-chain genes is correlated with expression of terminal deoxytransferase in B cells. *Nature* 1984;311:752–755.

36. Elliott JF, Rock EP, Patten PA, et al. The adult T-cell receptor delta-chain is diverse and distinct from that of fetal thymocytes. *Nature* 1988;331:627–631.

37. Breit TM, Wolvers-Tettero IL, Bogers AJ, et al. Rearrangements of the human TCRD-deleting elements. *Immunogenetics* 1994;40:70–75.

38. Kondo M, Weissman IL, Akashi K. Identification of clonogenic common lymphoid progenitors in mouse bone marrow. *Cell* 1997;91:661–672.

39. Spits H. Development of alphabeta t cells in the human thymus. *Nat Rev Immunol* 2002;2:760–772.

40. Peault B. Human T-cell lineage development in foetal thymus-engrafted SCID mice. *Res Immunol* 1994;145:124–128; discussion, 155–158.

41. Spits H, Blom B, Jaleco AC, et al. Early stages in the development of human T, natural killer and thymic dendritic cells. *Immunol Rev* 1998;165:75–86.

42. Shortman K, Wu L. Early T lymphocyte progenitors. *Annu Rev Immunol* 1996;14:29–47.

43. Hogquist KA, Jameson SC, Bevan MJ. The ligand for positive selection of T lymphocytes in the thymus. *Curr Opin Immunol* 1994;6:273–278.

44. McVay LD, Carding SR. Generation of human gammadelta T-cell repertoires. *Crit Rev Immunol* 1999;19:431–460.

45. Blom B, Verschuren MC, Heemskerk MH, et al. TCR gene rearrangements and expression of the pre-T cell receptor complex during human T-cell differentiation. *Blood* 1999;93:3033–3043.

46. Pawlowski TJ, Staerz UD. How are alpha beta T cells positively selected in the thymus? *Behring Inst Mitt* 1994:94–103.

47. Hogquist KA. Signal strength in thymic selection and lineage commitment. *Curr Opin Immunol* 2001;13:225–231.

48. Germain RN. T-cell development and the CD4-CD8 lineage decision. *Nat Rev Immunol* 2002;2:309–322.

49. Anderson G, Harman BC, Hare KJ, Jenkinson EJ. Microenvironmental regulation of T cell development in the thymus. *Semin Immunol* 2000;12:457–464.

50. Sen J. Signal transduction in thymus development. *Cell Mol Biol (Noisy-le-grand)* 2001;47:197–215.

51. Rothenberg EV. Signaling mechanisms in thymocyte selection. *Curr Opin Immunol* 1994;6:257–265.

52. Ernst P, Smale ST. Combinatorial regulation of transcription. I: general aspects of transcriptional control. *Immunity* 1995;2:311–319.

53. Castrop J, van Wichen D, Koomans-Bitter M, et al. The human TCF-1 gene encodes a nuclear DNA-binding protein uniquely expressed in normal and neoplastic T-lineage lymphocytes. *Blood* 1995;86:3050–3059.

54. Georgopoulos K, Moore DD, Derfler B. Ikaros, an early lymphoid-specific transcription factor and a putative mediator for T cell commitment. *Science* 1992;258:808–812.

55. Georgopoulos K, Bigby M, Wang JH, et al. The Ikaros gene is required for the development of all lymphoid lineages. *Cell* 1994;79:143–156.

56. Bain G, Engel I, Robanus Maandag EC, et al. E2A deficiency leads to abnormalities in alphabeta T-cell development and to rapid development of T-cell lymphomas. *Mol Cell Biol* 1997;17:4782–4791.

57. Bain G, Murre C. The role of E-proteins in B- and T-lymphocyte development. *Semin Immunol* 1998;10:143–153.

58. van de Wetering M, Cavallo R, Dooijes D, et al. Armadillo coactivates transcription driven by the product of the *Drosophila* segment polarity gene dTCF. *Cell* 1997;88:789–799.

59. Struhl G, Adachi A. Nuclear access and action of notch in vivo. *Cell* 1998;93:649–660.

60. Pui JC, Allman D, Xu L, et al. Notch1 expression in early lymphopoiesis influences B versus T lineage determination. *Immunity* 1999;11:299–308.

61. Schwartz JC, Zhang X, Nathenson SG, Almo SC. Structural mechanisms of costimulation. *Nat Immunol* 2002;3:427–434.

62. Bour-Jordan H, Blueston JA. CD28 function: a balance of costimulatory and regulatory signals. *J Clin Immunol* 2002;22:1–7.

63. Reiner SL. Helper T cell differentiation, inside and out. *Curr Opin Immunol* 2001;13:351–355.

64. Colucci F, Di Santo JP, Leibson PJ. Natural killer cell activation in mice and men: different triggers for similar weapons? *Nat Immunol* 2002;3:807–813.

65. Shevach EM. CD4+ CD25+ suppressor T cells: more questions than answers. *Nat Rev Immunol* 2002;2:389–400.

66. Foon KA, Todd RF 3rd. Immunologic classification of leukemia and lymphoma. *Blood* 1986;68:1–31.

67. van Dongen JJ, Adriaansen HJ, Hooijkaas H. Immunophenotyping of leukaemias and non-Hodgkin's lymphomas. Immunological markers and their CD codes. *Neth J Med* 1988;33:298–314.

68. Pui CH, Behm FG, Crist WM. Clinical and biologic relevance of immunologic marker studies in childhood acute lymphoblastic leukemia. *Blood* 1993;82:343–362.

69. Ludwig WD, Raghavachar A, Thiel E. Immunophenotypic classification of acute lymphoblastic leukaemia. *Baillieres Clin Haematol* 1994;7:235–262.

70. Bene MC, Castoldi G, Knapp W, et al. Proposals for the immunological classification of acute leukemias. European Group for the Immunological Characterization of Leukemias. *Leukemia* 1995;9.

71. Niehues T, Kapaun P, Harms DO, et al. A classification based on T cell selection-related phenotypes identifies a subgroup of childhood T-ALL with favorable outcome in the COALL studies. *Leukemia* 1999:13.

72. Pullen J, Shuster JJ, Link M, et al. Significance of commonly used prognostic factors differs for children with T cell acute lymphocytic leukemia (ALL), as compared to those with B-precursor ALL. A Pediatric Oncology Group (POG) study. *Leukemia* 1999;13:1696–1707.

73. Gouttefangeas C, Bensussan A, Boumsell L. Study of the CD3-associated T-cell receptors reveals further differences between T-cell acute lymphoblastic lymphoma and leukemia. *Blood* 1990;75:931–934.

74. Bain B. *Leukemia diagnosis: a guide to the FAB classification*. Philadelphia: JB Lippincott Co, 1990.

75. Bennett JM, Catovsky D, Daniel MT, et al. Proposals for the classification of chronic (mature) B and T lymphoid leukaemias. French-American-British (FAB) Cooperative Group. *J Clin Pathol* 1989;42: 567–584.

76. Catovsky D, Matutes E. Leukemias of mature T cells. In: Knowles DM, ed. *Neoplastic hematopathology*. Baltimore: Williams & Wilkins, 1992:1267.

77. Matutes E, Brito-Babapulle V, Swansbury J, et al. Clinical and laboratory features of 78 cases of T-prolymphocytic leukemia. *Blood* 1991;78:3269–3274.

78. Harris NL, Jaffe ES, Diebold J, et al. World Health Organization classification of neoplastic diseases of the hematopoietic and lymphoid tissues: report of the Clinical Advisory Committee meeting-Airlie House, Virginia, November 1997. *J Clin Oncol* 1999;17:3835–3849.

79. Jaffe ES, Harris NL, Stein H, Vardiman J. *WHO classification of tumours: pathology and genetics of tumours of the haematopoietic and lymphoid tissues*. Lyon, France: IARC Press, 2001.

80. Loughran TP Jr. Clonal diseases of large granular lymphocytes. *Blood* 1993;82:1–14.

81. Semenzato G, Zambello R, Starkebaum G, et al. The lymphoproliferative disease of granular lymphocytes: updated criteria for diagnosis. *Blood* 1997;89:256–260.

82. Greaves MF, Chan LC, Furley AJ, et al. Lineage promiscuity in hemopoietic differentiation and leukemia. *Blood* 1986;67:1–11.

83. Adriaansen HJ, Soeting PW, Wolvers-Tettero IL, van Dongen JJ. Immunoglobulin and T-cell receptor gene rearrangements in acute non-lymphocytic leukemias. Analysis of 54 cases and a review of the literature. *Leukemia* 1991;5:744–751.

84. Beishuizen A, Verhoeven MA, van Wering ER, et al. Analysis of Ig and T-cell receptor genes in 40 childhood acute lymphoblastic leukemias at diagnosis and subsequent relapse: implications for the detection of minimal residual disease by polymerase chain reaction analysis. *Blood* 1994;83:2238–2247.

85. Szczepanski T, Pongers-Willemse MJ, Langerak AW, et al. Ig heavy chain gene rearrangements in T-cell acute lymphoblastic leukemia exhibit predominant DH6-19 and DH7-27 gene usage, can result in complete V-D-J rearrangements, and are rare in T-cell receptor alpha beta. *Blood* 1999;93.

86. Langerak AW, Wolvers-Tettero IL, van den Beemd MW, et al. Immunophenotypic and immunogenotypic characteristics of TCRgammadelta+ T cell acute lymphoblastic leukemia. *Leukemia* 1999;13:206–214.

86a. Sczepanski T, Van der Velden VHJ, Ratt T, Jacobs DCH, et al. Comparative analysis of T-cell receptor gene rearrangements at diagnosis and relapse of T-cell acute lymphoblastic leukemia (T-ALL) shows high stability of clinical markers for monitoring of minimal residual disease and reveals the occurrence of secondary T-ALL. *Leukemia* 2003 (*in press*).

87. Breit TM, Verschuren MC, Wolvers-Tettero IL, et al. Human T cell leukemias with continuous V(D)J recombinase activity for TCR-delta gene deletion. *J Immunol* 1997;159:4341–4349.

88. Felix CA, Wright JJ, Poplack DG, et al. T cell receptor alpha-, beta-, and gamma-genes in T cell and pre-B cell acute lymphoblastic leukemia. *J Clin Invest* 1987;80:545–556.

89. Furley AJ, Mizutani S, Weilbaecher K, et al. Developmentally regulated rearrangement and expression of genes encoding the T cell receptor-T3 complex. *Cell* 1986;46:75–87.

90. Williams ME, Innes DJ Jr, Borowitz MJ, et al. Immunoglobulin and T cell receptor gene rearrangements in human lymphoma and leukemia. *Blood* 1987;69:79–86.

91. van Dongen JJ, Quertermous T, Bartram CR, et al. T cell receptor-CD3 complex during early T cell differentiation. Analysis of immature T cell acute lymphoblastic leukemias (T-ALL) at DNA, RNA, and cell membrane level. *J Immunol* 1987;138:1260–1269.

92. Oksenberg JR, Stuart S, Begovich AB, et al. Limited heterogeneity of rearranged T-cell receptor V alpha transcripts in brains of multiple sclerosis patients. *Nature* 1991;353:94.

93. Broeren CP, Verjans GM, Van Eden W, et al. Conserved nucleotide sequences at the 5' end of T cell receptor variable genes facilitate polymerase chain reaction amplification. *Eur J Immunol* 1991;21:569–575.

94. Doherty PJ, Roifman CM, Pan SH, et al. Expression of the human T cell receptor V beta repertoire. *Mol Immunol* 1991;28:607–612.

95. Wei S, Charmley P, Robinson MA, Concannon P. The extent of the human germline T-cell receptor V beta gene segment repertoire. *Immunogenetics* 1994;40:27–36.

96. Langerak AW, van Den Beemd R, Wolvers-Tettero IL, et al. Molecular and flow cytometric analysis of the Vbeta repertoire for clonality assessment in mature TCRalphabeta T-cell proliferations. *Blood* 2001;98:165–173.

97. Bottaro M, Berti E, Biondi A, et al. Heteroduplex analysis of T-cell receptor gamma gene rearrangements for diagnosis and monitoring of cutaneous T-cell lymphomas. *Blood* 1994;83:3271–3278.

98. Langerak AW, Szczepanski T, van der Burg M, et al. Heteroduplex PCR analysis of rearranged T cell receptor genes for clonality assessment in suspect T cell proliferations. *Leukemia* 1997;11:2192–2199.

99. Kneba M, Bolz I, Linke B, Hiddemann W. Analysis of rearranged T-cell receptor beta-chain genes by polymerase chain reaction (PCR) DNA sequencing and automated high resolution PCR fragment analysis. *Blood* 1995;86:3930–3937.

100. Linke B, Bolz I, Pott C, et al. Use of UITma DNA polymerase improves the PCR detection of rearranged immunoglobulin heavy chain CDR3 junctions. *Leukemia* 1995;9:2133–2137.

101. McCoy JP Jr, Overton WR, Schroeder K, et al. Immunophenotypic analysis of the T cell receptor V beta repertoire in CD4+ and CD8+ lymphocytes from normal peripheral blood. *Cytometry* 1996;26:148–153.

102. van den Beemd R, Boor PP, van Lochem EG, et al. Flow cytometric analysis of the Vbeta repertoire in healthy controls. *Cytometry* 2000;40:336–345.

103. Lima M, Almeida J, Santos AH, et al. Immunophenotypic analysis of the TCR-Vbeta repertoire in 98 persistent expansions of CD3(+)/TCR-alpha-beta(+) large granular lymphocytes: utility in assessing clonality and insights into the pathogenesis of the disease. *Am J Pathol* 2001;159.

104. Langerak AW, Wolvers-Tettero IL, van Dongen JJ. Detection of T cell receptor beta (TCRB) gene rearrangement patterns in T cell malignancies by Southern blot analysis. *Leukemia* 1999;13:965–974.

105. Moreau EJ, Langerak AW, van Gastel-Mol EJ, et al. Easy detection of all T cell receptor gamma (TCRG) gene rearrangements by Southern blot analysis: recommendations for optimal results. *Leukemia* 1999;13:1620–1626.

106. Szczepanski T, Langerak AW, Willemse MJ, et al. T cell receptor gamma (TCRG) gene rearrangements in T cell acute lymphoblastic leukemia reflect "end-stage" recombinations: implications for minimal residual disease monitoring. *Leukemia* 2000;14:1208–1214.

107. Hwang LY, Baer RJ. The role of chromosome translocations in T cell acute leukemia. *Curr Opin Immunol* 1995;7:659–664.

108. Begley CG, Aplan PD, Denning SM, et al. The gene SCL is expressed during early hematopoiesis and encodes a differentiation-related DNA-binding motif. *Proc Natl Acad Sci U S A* 1989;86:10128–10132.

109. Breit TM, Mol EJ, Wolvers-Tettero IL, et al. Site-specific deletions involving the tal-1 and sil genes are restricted to cells of the T cell receptor alpha/beta lineage: T cell receptor delta gene deletion mechanism affects multiple genes. *J Exp Med* 1993;177:965–977.

110. Fitzgerald TJ, Neale GA, Raimondi SC, Goorha RM. c-tal, a helix-loop-helix protein, is juxtaposed to the T-cell receptor-beta chain gene by a reciprocal chromosomal translocation: t(1;7)(p32;q35). *Blood* 1991;78:2686–2695.

111. Xia Y, Brown L, Yang CY, et al. TAL2, a helix-loop-helix gene activated by the (7;9)(q34;q32) translocation in human T-cell leukemia. *Proc Natl Acad Sci U S A* 1991;88:11416–11420.

112. Mellentin JD, Smith SD, Cleary ML. lyl-1, a novel gene altered by chromosomal translocation in T cell leukemia, codes for a protein with a helix-loop-helix DNA binding motif. *Cell* 1989;58:77–83.

113. Bernard OA, Busson-LeConiat M, Ballerini P, et al. A new recurrent and specific cryptic translocation, t(5;14)(q35;q32), is associated with expression of the Hox11L2 gene in T acute lymphoblastic leukemia. *Leukemia* 2001;15:1495–1504.

114. Mauvieux L, Leymarie V, Helias C, et al. High incidence of Hox11L2 expression in children with T-ALL. *Leukemia* 2002;16:2417–2422.

115. Stern MH, Lipkowitz S, Aurias A, et al. Inversion of chromosome 7 in ataxia telangiectasia is generated by a rearrangement between T-cell receptor beta and T-cell receptor gamma genes. *Blood* 1989;74:2076–2080.

116. Kobayashi Y, Tycko B, Soreng AL, Sklar J. Transrearrangements between antigen receptor genes in normal human lymphoid tissues and in ataxia telangiectasia. *J Immunol* 1991;147:3201–3209.

117. Retiere C, Halary F, Peyrat MA, et al. The mechanism of chromosome 7 inversion in human lymphocytes expressing chimeric gamma beta TCR. *J Immunol* 1999;162:903–910.

118. Hinz T, Allam A, Wesch D, et al. Cell-surface expression of transrearranged Vgamma-cbeta T-cell receptor chains in healthy donors and in ataxia telangiectasia patients. *Br J Haematol* 2000;109.

119. Bernard O, Groettrup M, Mugneret F, et al. Molecular analysis of T-cell receptor transcripts in a human T-cell leukemia bearing a t(1;14) and an inv(7); cell surface expression of a TCR-beta chain in the absence of alpha chain. *Leukemia* 1993;7:1645–1653.

120. Murre C. Intertwining proteins in thymocyte development and cancer. *Nat Immunol* 2000;1:97–98.

121. Herblot S, Steff AM, Hugo P, et al. SCL and LMO1 alter thymocyte differentiation: inhibition of E2A-HEB function and pre-T alpha chain expression. *Nat Immunol* 2000;1:138–144.

122. Osborne B, Miele L. Notch and the immune system. *Immunity* 1999; 11:653–663.

123. Screpanti I, Bellavia D, Campese AF, et al. Notch, a unifying target in T-cell acute lymphoblastic leukemia? *Trends Mol Med* 2003;9: 30–35.

124. Ellisen LW, Bird J, West DC, et al. TAN-1, the human homolog of the *Drosophila* notch gene, is broken by chromosomal translocations in T lymphoblastic neoplasms. *Cell* 1991;66:649–661.

125. Ferrando AA, Neuberg DS, Staunton J, et al. Gene expression signatures define novel oncogenic pathways in T cell acute lymphoblastic leukemia. *Cancer Cell* 2002;1:75–87.

126. Lefranc MP. IMGT, the international ImMunoGeneTics database. *Nucleic Acids Res* 2001;29:207–209.

CHAPTER 49

Cytogenetics of Lymphoma

R. S. K. Chaganti and Gouri Nanjangud

Over the past three decades, chromosome analysis has provided crucial insights into neoplastic transformation of the cell, tumorigenesis, and clinical behavior of tumors. Because of the ease with which chromosome preparations can be obtained, leukemias, especially acute leukemias, lead the way, with lymphomas and solid tumors following behind. Cytogenetic analysis of hematopoietic tumors has been instrumental in the identification of recurring translocations and in the establishment of the principle that such translocations cause deregulation of genes at the breakpoints by a variety of molecular mechanisms, leading to derailment of the cell's normal functional or developmental fate and initiating aberrant proliferation. They also have shown, especially in acute leukemias, that certain chromosome changes are associated with good outcome and others with poor outcome, thereby enabling therapeutic decisions based on the results of chromosome analysis. In contrast to leukemias, until recently, detailed cytogenetic information on non-Hodgkin's lymphomas was unavailable for most lymphoma subsets, which made the understanding of the genetic basis of the morphologic and biologic complexity and clinical behavior of these tumors difficult. Lymphomas arise in cells undergoing B- and T-lineage differentiation and present complex histologic and immunologic phenotypes and clinical behavior. As a result, their biology has been difficult to understand and their classification into biologically or clinically meaningful subsets has been difficult to accomplish. Over the past two decades, several systems of lymphoma classification have been devised, the most recent being the one proposed by the World Health Organization (1). This classification recognizes three main groups and multiple subsets within each group: lymphomas of B cells, T cell/natural killer cell, and Hodgkin's disease. The emphasis of these classification efforts has been to relate the morphologic and immunologic phenotypes of tumors to the stage in lineage development of the putative precursor cell, on the one hand, and to clinical endpoints, such as response to treatment and patient survival, on the other. Over the past decade, there has been a sustained increase in the cytogenetic data on lymphomas that is beginning to allow a new view of the role of chromosome changes in lymphoma biology and clinical behavior. The more recent studies have included conventional cytogenetic methods, such as Q-banding and G-banding, as well as the more recent molecularly based techniques, such as fluorescence *in situ* hybridization, spectral karyotyping, multicolor fluorescent *in situ* hybridization, and chromosome-based and array-based comparative genomic hybridization. This combination of the conventional and the new methods of cytogenetic analysis has enabled the identification of a bewildering array of novel, recurring chromosome abnormalities, some of which are of clinical relevance. In this review, the methodologies used in modern cytogenetic analysis are first discussed, followed by a review of association of recurring chromosome abnormalities with biologic and clinical features of lymphomas.

CYTOGENETIC METHODS

Since the discovery by Levan and Tjio and Ford and Hamerton in 1956 (2,3) that human cells possess 46 chromosomes (23 pairs of autosomes and the X and Y sex chromosomes), the history of human cytogenetics has been one of continuous discovery, aided by impressive advances in methodology. The first of these, perhaps the most important, was the observation by Hsu that hyposmotic treatment swells cells and leads to dispersion of chromatin and chromosomes. Hyposmotic treatment in combination with treatment with the metaphase-arresting drug colchicine scatters chromosomes, thereby enabling their ready counting and identification (4). This was followed by the discovery by Nowell and Hungerford that treatment of peripheral blood lymphocytes with phytohemagglutinin leads to their stimulation to undergo mitosis, thus providing a ready source of dividing cells from the body for chromosome analysis (5). These initial discoveries led to a rapid demonstration that constitutional chromosome abnormalities contribute significantly to the etiology of infertility, reproductive loss, birth defects, and mental retardation. The first successful application of cytogenetics to neoplastic disease was the discovery by Nowell and Hungerford that in chronic myelogenous leukemia one of the small acrocentric ("G-group") chromosomes was replaced by a much smaller acrocentric chromosome that appeared to be diagnostic of this disorder and was termed the *Philadelphia (Ph) chromosome*, after the city of its discovery (5). During the 1970s, experimenters tried special stains or chemical treatments to expose structural variation along the length of the chromosome to aid in the further identification of individual chromosomes and their regions. This effort was remarkably successful and led to the development of several so-called banding methods that provided the basis for detailed subregional mapping of the human chromosomal complement as well as the development of a system of nomenclature for description of the normal and abnormal chromosome complements. This nomenclature, designated the *International System for Human Chromosome Nomenclature* (6), is updated from time to time based on new information and continues to be the currently accepted tool for chromosome description (7). The development of the banding techniques also had a significant effect on the efforts, then underway, in unraveling the molecular organization of the chromatin and the chromosomes.

The banding techniques that have had the most impact on cytogenetic analysis were the so-called quinacrine (Q-), Giemsa (G-), centromeric (C-), and reverse (R-) banding methods. In Q-banding, the chromosomes on a metaphase preparation stained with quinacrine dihydrochloride exhibit brighter fluorescence of A-T rich regions, compared with G-C rich regions. The pattern of this bright and dull fluorescence is consistent and yields a reproducible "banding" pattern (8). In G-banding, the chromosome preparation is subjected to treatment with sodium salt citrate at a warm temperature or a mild and brief treatment with an enzyme, such as trypsin, followed by staining with a weak solution of Giemsa. This procedure also leads to a linear differentiation of the chromosome into darkly stained and lightly stained regions or bands that correspond to the brightly fluorescent and dully fluorescent regions revealed by Q-banding (9,10). Currently, G-banding is the method of choice for most cytogenetic analysis (Fig. 49.1). R-banding is produced by incubation of the chromosome preparation in very hot phosphate buffer, followed by staining with Giemsa (11). R-banding yields a banding pattern that is the reverse of G-banding; thus, bands staining dark with G-banding stain light and vice versa. C-banding involves treating the chromosomes on a metaphase preparation with a weak solution of alkali, such as barium hydroxide, for a few seconds, followed by staining with Giemsa, as in the case of G-banding (12). C-banding suppresses staining all along the chromosome, except at the centromeric heterochromatic regions. Application of C-banding was instrumental in discovering constitutional polymorphisms in the heterochromatin segments around the centromeric regions of human chromosomes (13). Together, these banding techniques are collectively referred to as *con-*

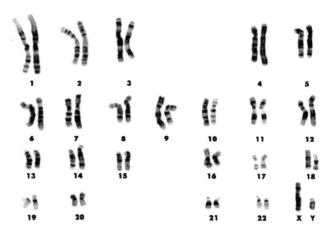

FIG. 49.1. G-banded karyotype of a normal male (46, XY).

ventional cytogenetic or *banding methods*. These techniques have been responsible for the delineation of a large number of dysmorphic syndromes and are routinely used in the pre- and postnatal diagnosis of birth defects and infertility.

The first major discovery in neoplastic disease using conventional cytogenetic methods was the discovery by Rowley that the Ph chromosome is the result of a reciprocal translocation between chromosomes 9 and 22, with breaks at 9q34 and 22q11 (14). Conventional cytogenetics techniques have been applied to characterize the karyotypes of thousands of tumors, especially of the hematopoietic lineage. They are routinely used in the diagnostic, follow-up, and prognostic evaluation of leukemias. With regard to lymphomas, more than 8,000 tumors have been karyotyped and, as discussed in the subsequent sections of this review, have had identified aberrations associated with specific histologic subtypes as well as some that are associated with clinical outcome.

The major technical development during the 1980s was the linking of the methods of cytogenetics with those of molecular genetics. Following molecular techniques, such as Southern blotting (15), in which specific genomic sequences labeled with radioactive nucleotides (probe) are hybridized to total genomic DNA immobilized on nitrocellulose or nylon membranes to ascertain the status of the genomic DNA relevant to the probe, investigators began to hybridize probes *in situ* on to metaphase chromosomes to identify and map the positions of the probes on the chromosomes. Initially, the probes were tagged by radiolabeled nucleotides (3H) (16) and soon after by fluorescently labeled nucleotides. The latter method of labeling and hybridization, called *fluorescence* in situ *hybridization*, developed into a powerful methodology to map genes and to seek the status of a variety of chromosomal lesions in the genomes of cancer cells such as gain, loss, and rearrangement at metaphase as well as at interphase (17). Among the most impressive of these in B-cell lymphomas is the detection at interphase of the common recurring translocations such as t(14;18)(q32;q21) and t(11;14)(q13;q32) (Color Plate 74). A variation of fluorescent *in situ* hybridization is whole chromosome painting, in which the probe comprises fluorescently labeled DNA of an entire chromosome obtained usually by flow sorting of individual chromosomes, followed by DNA amplification by polymerase chain reaction and labeling (18,19). Fluorescent *in situ* hybridization and whole chromosome painting are extremely powerful techniques and have the ability of resolving complex aberrations (Color Plate 75). In the case of lymphomas, fluorescent *in situ* hybridization and whole chromosome painting have been applied numerous times to resolve complex translocations and other rearrangements. Because the probes are fluorescently labeled, appropriate absorption and emission wavelengths need to be used to visualize or capture the images of the fluorescent patterns generated. In the case of fluorescent *in situ* hybridization and whole chromosome painting, generally no more than two colors are used, and signal detection is achieved by use of appropriate filters. More recently, these two techniques have been further enhanced by developing a technology that enables simultaneous hybridization of DNA from all 23 chromosomes with a set number of labels in a combinatorial fashion to a metaphase cell. In this system, discrimination of 23 different colors at the same time is achieved, but the available filter systems are inadequate to discriminate the emission spectra. This is accomplished by the use of spectral separation methods, which lead to the term *spectral karyotyping* for this type of analysis (Color Plate 76) (20). Spectral karyotyping is a powerful technique and is increasingly being used to interrogate tumor karyotypes to define changes. Lymphomas are beginning to be analyzed by spectral karyotyping; currently, the most comprehensive data come from two large ascertainments, one of diffuse large B-cell lymphoma and the other of follicular lymphoma (21,22).

The molecular cytogenetic methods discussed above are designed to interrogate cell preparations containing metaphase or interphase chromosomes using specific DNA probes from the genome, ranging in size from 1 Kbp to a whole chromosome. Whereas fluorescent *in situ* hybridization and whole chromosome painting are not suited for high throughput analysis of the genome, spectral karyotyping is suited for such an analysis. However, spectral karyotyping most effectively detects rearrangements, less so gains and losses, and not at all high copy number changes such as amplifications.

During the past decade, methods to scan the entire genome for gains, losses, and amplification solely based on analysis of DNA have been developed, which truly integrate cytogenetics with molecular genetics. The first of these is comparative genomic hybridization, a method in which target (tumor) and control (normal, e.g., as placenta) DNAs are differentially labeled (typically, green and red for tumor and control) and cohybridized under appropriate conditions to a standard metaphase preparation from normal cells (23). The images are captured using a charge coupled device camera and analyzed by a software. Increase (gain or amplification) in the number of copies of DNA regions within the tumor chromosomes is reflected as excess hybridization on the normal metaphase chromosome (excess green color from tumor), and deficiency (loss) in the number of copies of DNA regions within the tumor chromosomes is reflected as deficient hybridization (excess red color from normal) (Color Plate 77). The one caveat about this assay is the fact that altered regions need to be at least 10 Mbp in extent to be reliably detected by comparative genomic hybridization. This method also cannot identify rearrangements. Nevertheless, large numbers of tumors of different histologies have been screened by comparative genomic hybridization and have provided valuable information, especially in regard to gains and amplifications (24). In the case of lymphomas, a large number of tumors of different histologies have been screened by comparative genomic hybridization, although diffuse large B-cell lymphoma received the most attention. In this review, these data are discussed along with the discussion of cytogenetic changes in the different histologic subsets. The major contribution of comparative genomic hybridization analysis to lymphoma cytogenetics so far is the discovery that chromosomal (and hence gene) amplification is a frequent event, possibly associating with advanced stage (25).

An extension of chromosomal comparative genomic hybridization is array-based comparative genomic hybridization in which the normal metaphase chromosome preparation as the hybridization substrate for the differentially labeled tumor and normal DNAs is replaced by an "array," comprising a variety of DNA targets such as expressed sequence tags (cDNA), PI artificial chromosome, or bacterial artificial chromosome elements printed on a glass slide (Color Plate 78) (26,27). Signals from cohybridization of differentially labeled tumor and normal DNA are read by a laser and generate large volumes of data that require special biostatistical analysis tools to define presence or absence of loss, gain, and amplification and the copy DNA number in gains and amplifications. In principle, arrays representing the entire genome in any chosen configuration can be constructed. In practice, however, the currently used expressed sequence tag arrays contain 10,000 to 12,000 elements. The currently used bacterial artificial chromosome arrays generally represent a 1 to 4 Mbp resolution of the genome. Because expressed sequence tag arrays mainly represent expressed genes, they provide the opportunity to not only identify the amplified genes in the target amplicon but also to assess the expression status of the individual amplified genes within an amplicon (28). Bacterial artificial chromosome arrays, on the other hand, are well suited for the precise delineation of the limits of the amplicons. However, amplicon-specific expressed sequence tag arrays or other methods need to be used to identify overexpressed targets in a given amplicon. Nevertheless, array-based comparative genomic hybridization promises to be an exciting new approach to rapidly identify amplified and overexpressed genes in tumors that may have biologic and clinical significance. Array-based comparative genomic hybridization analysis of lymphomas is in very early stages.

CHROMOSOME ABNORMALITIES IN LYMPHOMA: AN OVERVIEW

Conventional cytogenetics identify chromosome abnormalities in cancer cells as gains and losses of entire chromosomes and breaks and rearrangements leading to a variety of abnormalities, such as translocations, inversions, deletions, and partial gains and losses of chromosomes. Fluorescent *in situ* hybridization and spectral karyotyping, as discussed above, enhance the resolution of conventional banding. Comparative genomic hybridization technologies, on the other hand, enhance the resolution of detection of gains and losses and, in addition, identify high copy number changes of DNA sequences resulting from amplification of chromosome regions.

Chromosome Breakage

Recent banding and spectral karyotyping analysis of large series of follicular lymphomas and diffuse large B-cell lymphomas have defined the extent and pattern of chromosome breakage that occurs in these two subsets of lymphoma. The most informative of these studies were the detailed analyses of large, consecutively ascertained series of follicular lymphoma (294 cases) and diffuse large B-cell lymphoma (215 cases) using conventional cytogenetic and spectral karyotyping methods from a single institution that identified more than 1,000 breakpoints in each of these subsets (Color Plate 79) (21,22,29). The same analyses identified recurring (greater than 10%) breakpoints that included 1p36, 1q11-21, 3q27, 6q15, 6q21, 6q25, 10q22, 10q24, 12q13, 14q32, and 18q21 in follicular lymphoma and 1p22, 1p36, 1q21, 3p21, 3q27, 6q21, 8q24, 14q32, and 18q21 in diffuse large B-cell lymphoma. The incidence of these breakpoints differed not only among follicular lymphoma and diffuse large B-cell lymphoma but also among the t(14;18)(q32;q21) positive and negative subsets of follicular lymphoma (Color Plate 79). A greater number of breakpoints and structural abnormalities were identified by spectral karyotyping analysis, compared with banding analysis (21,22). In addition to redefining many of the breakpoints and abnormalities identified by G-banding (Color Plate 80A), the spectral karyotyping analysis also identified 13 new breakpoints in diffuse large B-cell lymphoma (Color Plate 80B).

Chromosome Translocation

Nonrandom chromosome translocations that involve IG and TCR genes with a variety of other genes are the hallmark of lymphoid neoplasms. These translocations are considered to arise as errors during intragenic physiologic rearrangements that assemble productive copies of IG and TCR genes during normal B- and T-cell development (30). Overall, individual translocations tend to be specific for breakpoints and show a high degree of association with histologic subsets (Table 49.1). The first translocation to be so analyzed was t(8;14)(q24;q32) in Burkitt's lymphoma, in which the MYC proto-oncogene mapped at 8q24 was shown to rearrange with the IGH gene mapped at 14q32 (31). The expression of the rearranged MYC gene is deregulated, being brought under the transcriptional regulation of the IG gene promoter/enhancer machinery by replacement of MYC regulatory sequences with those of the IG genes. The MYC coding sequences are not affected by the translocation that results in abnormal expression of a normal

protein. In virtually all cases of such IG gene–associated translocations molecularly analyzed so far, the target gene is deregulated in its expression without altering the protein encoded by it. A related mechanism of activation of oncogenes recently identified in lymphoma and multiple myeloma is insertion of IG gene sequences in the vicinity of target genes (32,33). The genes involved in these translocations and insertions participate in diverse cellular functions such as cell-cycle control, apoptosis, regulation of cell growth and differentiation, and tumor metastasis. However, the predominant class of genes affected are transcription regulators, several of which play important roles in normal lymphoid cell development (Table 49.1). It is also noteworthy that a second type of gene deregulation by translocation has also been recognized in lymphoma, namely, generation of fusion transcripts and proteins, a phenomenon more commonly encountered in leukemias and sarcomas (Table 49.1).

More recent studies of follicular lymphoma and diffuse large B-cell lymphoma by G-banding and spectral karyotyping have shown that recurring translocations, in addition to those involving IG and TCR genes, are prevalent (Table 49.2). The biologic or clinical significance of these translocations has not yet been investigated, although they appear to associate, to some extent, with tumor progression, at least in follicular lymphoma (21,29). The functional consequence of gene deregulation in lymphoid lineage development and lymphomagenesis is not discussed here; these data can be found in Chapter 50 in this book.

Chromosome Gain, Loss, and Amplification

Whole chromosome, as well as partial chromosome, gains and losses are a consistent feature of lymphomas (34), although the biologic or clinical significance of most of them is yet to be delineated. Recent G-banding and spectral karyotyping studies of follicular lymphoma and diffuse large B-cell lymphoma have permitted mapping of minimal regions of gain and loss in these subsets.

Genomic amplification leading to overexpression of genes associated with cell proliferation or resistance to drug treatment has been shown to be an important pathway to tumor progression and adverse clinical outcome in a number of solid tumor types (35). Gene amplification as a significant factor in the biology and clinical behavior of lymphoma has, however, not been recognized until recently. Cytogenetic lesions indicative of gene amplification, such as double minute chromosomes and homogeneously staining regions, have been noted in occasional B-cell lymphomas, but their significance remains undetermined (36).

Recent comparative genomic hybridization analysis of B-cell lymphoma subsets identified gain, loss, and amplification of multiple chromosomal regions in chronic lymphocytic leukemia, splenic marginal zone lymphoma, multiple myeloma, extranodal marginal zone lymphoma of mucosa-associated lymphoid tissue type, follicular lymphoma, and diffuse large B-cell lymphoma. These data are summarized in

TABLE 49.1. *Genes deregulated in non-Hodgkin's lymphoma and their normal cellular function*

Lymphoma subset	Translocation	Gene	Normal function
Chronic lymphocytic leukemia/small lympho-cytic leukemia	t(11;14)(q13;q32)	BCL1	Cell-cycle regulation
	t(14;19)(q32;q13)	BCL3	Transcription regulation
	t(2;14)(p13;q32)	BCL11A	Transcription regulation
Lymphoplasmacytic lymphoma	t(9;14)(p13;q32)	PAX5	Transcription regulation
Plasma cell myeloma (multiple myeloma)	t(11;14)(q13;q32)	BCL1	Cell-cycle regulation
	t(4;14)(p16.3;q32)	FGFR3 and MMSET	Growth regulation
	t(6;14)(p16;q32)	MUM1	Transcription regulation
	t(6;14)(p21;q32)	CCND3	Cell cycle regulation
	t(14;16)(q32;q23)	CMAF	Transcription regulation
	t(1;14)(q21;q32)	IRTA1 and IRTA2	Immune response
Splenic marginal zone lymphoma/splenic lym-phoma with villous lymphocytes	t(2;7)(p12;q22)	CDK6	Cell-cycle regulation
Extranodal marginal zone lymphoma of mucosa-associated lymphoid tissue type	t(1;14)(p21;q32)	BCL10	Apoptosis regulation
	t(11;18)(q21;q21)	CIAP2/MLT	Apoptosis regulation
	t(14;18)(q32;q21)	MALT1	?
	t(6;14)(p21;q32)	CCND3	Cell-cycle regulation
Mantle cell lymphoma	t(11;14)(q13;q32)	BCL1	Cell-cycle regulation
Follicular lymphoma or diffuse large B-cell lym-phoma	t(14;18)(q32;q21)	BCL2	Apoptosis regulation
	t(3;14)(q27;q32)	BCL6	Transcription regulation
	t(8;14)(q24;q32)	MYC	Transcription regulation
	t(8;12;14)(q24;q24;q32)	BCL7A	?
	t(10;14)(q24;q32)	NFKB2	Transcription regulation
	t(14;15)(q32;q11-13)	BCL8	?
	t(1;14)(q21;q32)	MUC1	Signal transduction
	t(1;22)(q21;q11)	FCGR2B	Immune response
	t(1;14)(q21;q32)	FCGR2B	Immune response
	t(1;14)(q21;q32)	BCL9	?
	t(3;3)(q27;q29)	BCL6/TFRR	Iron metabolism
	t(3;4)(q27;p13)	BCL6/TTF	Signal transduction
	t(3;6)(q27;p21)	BCL6/PIM1	Signal transduction
	t(3;7)(q27;q32)	BCL6/H4	Cell-cycle regulation
	t(3;7)(q27;p12)	BCL6/IKAROS	Lymphoid differentiation
	t(3;11)(q27;q23)	BCL6/BOB1	Transcription regulation
	t(3;13)(q27;q14)	BCL6/LCP1	Cell adhesion
	t(3;14)(q27;q32)	BCL6/HSP89a	Cell metabolism
	t(3;16)(q27;p11)	BCL6/IL21	Growth regulation
	t(3;16)(q27;p13))	BCL6/CIITA	MHC regulation
	t(3;18)(q27;p11)	BCL6/EIF4A2	Transcription regulation
Burkitt's lymphoma	t(8;14)(q24;q32)	MYC	Transcription regulation
Anaplastic large-cell lymphoma	t(2;5)(p23;q25)	ALK/NPM	?/Internuclear transport
T-cell/null-cell lymphoma	t(1;2)(q25;p23)	TPM3/ALK	Muscle development/?
	t(2;3)(p23;q21)	TFGL/ALK	?
	t(2;3)(p23;q21)	TFGS/ALK	?
	t(2;17)(p23;q23)	CLTC/ALK	Organelle biogenesis/?
	inv(2)(p23q35)	ATIC/ALK	Purine biosynthesis/?

TABLE 49.2. *Secondary recurring translocations in follicular lymphoma and diffuse large B-cell lymphoma*

Breakpoint	Translocation	Breakpoint	Translocation
1p11	der(1)t(1;1)(p11;q21)^{SKY}	1q25	der(4)t(1;4)(q25;q35)
1p22	t(1;14)(p22;q23)	3q27	t(2;3)(q21-23;q27)
1p32	t(1;13)(p32;q14)^{SKY}		t(3;12)(q27;p11)
	der(1)t(1;1)(p32;q12-21)		t(3;12)(q27;q22)
1p36	t(1;17)(p32;q21)		t(3;16)(q21;p13)
	t(1;6)(p36;p22)		t(3;4)(p21;q21)
	t(1;7)(p36;q22)		t(3;5)(p25;p13)
	t(1;7)(p36;q22)		t(3;5)(q27;q13)
	t(1;9)(p36;q13)		t(3;5)(q27;q15)
	der(1)t(1;1)(p36;q12-21)		t(3;8)(q27;q13)
	der(1)t(1;1)(p36;q25)		t(3;9)(q27;p13)
	der(1)(1;2)(p36;p11)	8q11	der(6)t(6;8)(q11;q11)^{SKY}
	der(1)t(1;2)(p36;q21)		t(7;8)(q22;q11)^{SKY}
	der(1)t(1;2)(p36;q31)	8q22	t(8;22)(q22;q13)
	der(1)t(1;3)(p36;p21)	8q24	t(8;9)(q24;p13)
	der(1)t(Y;1)(q12;p36)	9p13	t(6;9)(p25;p13)
1q12	der(18)(t(1;18)(q12;p11)		t(9;9)(q13;p13)
	der(3)t(1;3)(q12; p26)	9p22	t(9;19)(p22;q13)
1q21	t(1;7)(q21;q22)^{SKY}	9q13	der(13)t(9;13)(q13;q34)
	t(1;8)(q21; q24)	10q24	t(10;12)(q24;q22)
	der(4)t(1;4)(q21;q35)	11q13	der(5)t(5;11)(q15;q13)
	der(6)t(1;6)(q21;q21)		t(11;17)(q13;p13)
	der(9)t(1;9)(q21;p24)	12q24	t(12;15)(q24;q15)
	der(12)t(1;12)(q21;q13)	13q10	t(13;14)(q10;q10)
	der(12)t(1;12)(q21;q24),	13q14	t(13;22)(q14;q13)
	der(13)t(1;13)(q21;q34)	14q32	der(14)t(3;14)(q21;q32)^{SKY}
	der(17)t(1;17)(q21;q11)		t(6;14)((p21;q32)
	der(19)t(1;19)(q21;q13)		der(14)t(12;14)(q13;q32)
	der(22)t(1;22)(q21;q13)		t(12;14)(p11;q32)
	der(X)t(X;1)(q28;q21)		t(14;22)(q32;q11)

SKY, identified by spectral karyotyping alone.

Table 49.3 and in the relevant sections that discuss the cytogenetics of the various subsets. The most important result emerging from these studies is the discovery that chromosomal amplification occurs at more than a dozen sites in B-cell lymphoma. Such amplification predicts gene amplification. Previous to the application of the comparative genomic hybridization method, chromosomal amplification has not been documented as a consistent feature of lymphoma.

Combined use of comparative genomic hybridization and Southern blotting has led to the identification of amplification of MYC, BCL2, and REL genes in small numbers of cases of lymphoma (25,37–39). One study screened a panel of tumors by Southern blotting and demonstrated that REL was amplified in more than 20% of diffuse large B-cell lymphomas (40). Using a combination of comparative genomic hybridization and candidate gene approach, a recent study sought to map amplified chromosomal regions and identify amplified genes within them

in a large panel of diffuse large B-cell lymphoma biopsies obtained at diagnosis. This study identified nine sites of chromosomal amplification (1q21-23, 2p12-16, 8q24, 9q34, 12q12-14, 13q32, 16p12, 18q21-22, and 22q12) and amplification of target genes within these sites (more than four copies) of REL (2p12), MYC (8q24), BCL2 (18q21), and CDK4, MDM2, and GLI (12q13-14). In the tumor panel assayed, there was no overlap between amplification and translocation affecting REL, MYC, and BCL2 genes, suggesting that translocation and amplification represent independent pathways to deregulated expression of these genes in B-cell lymphoma (25). Further candidate gene, positional cloning, or microarray-based approaches can be expected to identify additional amplified genes mapping in the amplified chromosomal regions, with the potential to provide new clues to the genetic basis of progression and clinical behavior of diffuse large B-cell lymphoma and other subsets of B-cell lymphoma.

TABLE 49.3. *Recurring clonal chromosomal abnormalities in non-Hodgkin's lymphomas and their diagnostic and prognostic significance*

Lymphoma subset	Diagnostic	Progression/transformation	Poor outcome	Good outcome
		Clinical markers		
B-cell chronic lymphocytic leukemia/small lympho-cytic leukemia	—	+12, del(11q), del(6q), del(17p), t/der(14)(q32)	+12, del(11q), del(17p)	del(13q)
Lymphoplasmacytic lymphoma	t(9;14)(p13;q32)	—	—	—
Plasma cell myeloma (multi-ple myeloma)	—	—	−13/del(13q)	—
Extranodal marginal zone lym-phoma of mucosa-associ-ated lymphoid tissue type	t(11;18)(q21;q21)– low grade	—	—	—
Follicular lymphoma	t(14;18)(q32;q21)	t/der(1q), +7, del(6q), del(17p), t(8;14)(q24;q32)	del(17p), t(8;14)(q24;q32)	—
Mantle cell lymphoma	t(11;14)(q13;q32)	—	del(17p)	—
Diffuse large B-cell lymphoma	—	der(1)(q21), +7, del(6q), del(17p)	der(1q21), del(6q)	—
Burkitt's lymphoma	t(8;14)(q24;q32)	dup(1q)	—	—
Anaplastic large-cell T/null-cell lymphoma	—	—	—	t(2;5)(p23;q25)

More recently, an effort has been made to apply array-based comparative genomic hybridization methodology to the analysis gene amplification in lymphoma. In one study, genomic aberrations were measured in a series of paired biopsy samples from patients who presented initially with follicular lymphoma and subsequently transformed to diffuse large B-cell lymphoma using a bacterial artificial chromosome array with clone elements selected at a resolution of 1 megabase of the genome (41). Associated with transformation, a heterogenous pattern of acquired genomic abnormalities was noted that included loss, gain, and amplification. Some of the regions identified were previously reported to associate with transformation by comparative genomic hybridization and other methods. However, because the targets on the array comprised large regions of the genome (± 1 Mbp), they did not yield information on specific genes whose genomic status in the tumors has altered. Nevertheless, screening the same tumors using a whole genome complementary DNA array, differential expression of some targets mapping to the regions of gain/loss was identified. These early studies point to the feasibility and promise of this technology in identifying functionally relevant candidates in altered chromosomal regions.

RELEVANCE OF CHROMOSOME ABNORMALITIES IN LYMPHOMA: HISTOLOGIC AND CLINICAL CORRELATIONS

Several nonrandom chromosome abnormalities are now associated with morphologic and clinical features of lymphoma subsets, although the available data are by no means as precise and useful as those in the case of acute leukemias. These data

are discussed below, and the clinical associations are summarized in Table 49.4.

B-Cell Neoplasms

Much of the currently available information on the cytogenetics of lymphomas comes from B-cell neoplasms. The subsets, such as follicular lymphoma and diffuse large B-cell lymphoma, have been extensively studied due to their clinical significance and presence of IG gene–associated translocations.

B-Cell Chronic Lymphocytic Leukemia/ Small Lymphocytic Lymphoma

Clonal chromosome abnormalities have been noted in 50% to 60% of chronic lymphocytic leukemia cases by conventional cytogenetics and in more than 80% of the cases by fluorescent *in situ* hybridization. The most frequent abnormality is del(13)(q14), followed by del(11q), +12, del(6q), del(17p), +8q, and +3q (42). Recurring translocations affecting the *IG* gene sites, although rare in chronic lymphocytic leukemia (more than 2%), include t(14;19)(q32;q13), t(14;18)(q32;q21), and t(11;14)(q13;q32) (42–45). These translocations are often found in atypical chronic lymphocytic leukemia in association with +12. Familial cases of chronic lymphocytic leukemia show an increased incidence of loss of Xp11-p21, 2p12-p14, and 4q11-q21 and gain of Xp21 and Xq22-qter, compared with sporadic chronic lymphocytic leukemia cases (46).

Karyotypic evolution has been noted in approximately 16% of the cases. Del(6q), del(11q), and del(17p) are the most frequently acquired changes. Del(11q) and del(17p) have been suggested to

TABLE 49.4. *Recurring minimal regions of gain and loss and high level amplification in non-Hodgkin's lymphoma*

Lymphoma subset	Minimal region of gain	Minimal region of loss	High level amplification
Mature peripheral B-cell neoplasms			
B-cell chronic lymphocytic leukemia/small lymphocytic leukemia	12q13-15	6q15, 6q21-23, 6q27, 11q22-23, 13q14, 17p13	—
Lymphoplasmacytic lymphoma with Waldenström's macroglobulinemia	—	6q21	—
Splenic marginal zone lymphoma/splenic lymphoma with villous lymphocytes	1q21-25, 3q23, 3q25-29, 4q25-28, 5q13-15, 9q32, 12q15-21, 20q	7q31-32, 17p13	3q26-29, 2p13-15,18q21-22
Hairy-cell leukemia	5q13-q31	—	—
Plasma cell myeloma (multiple myeloma)	1q12-41, 2q25-27, 7q22, 8q24, 9q34, 11q13-22, 15q24, 19q13	13q14, 16q, 17p13	—
Extranodal marginal zone lymphoma of mucosa-associated lymphoid tissue type	1q25-31, 3q21-23, 3q25-29, 18q21-23, Xp22	—	3q26-29
Nodal marginal zone lymphoma	3q21-23, 3q25-29, 18q21-23	—	—
Follicular lymphoma	7p11-p22, 7q22-q36, 8q24, 12p11-13, 12q11-15, 12q22-24, 18q21, Xp11-23, Xq22-28	6q15, 6q21-25	2p12-16, 6p21, 8q24, 12q13
Mantle cell lymphoma	3q26-29, 7p13-22, 8q24, 12q13-15	1p22, 6q15, 6q25, 9p21, 11q22-23, 13q14, 17p13	2p24-25, 3q26-29, 7p22, 8q24, 13q32, 10p12, 18q21 (*BCL2*), Xq27-28
Diffuse large B-cell lymphoma	1q21, 1q25-32, 3q26-29, 7q32-34, 12p11-13, 12q11-15, 12q22-24, 13q22, 18q21,Xp11-23, Xq25-26	1p34-36, 8p21-23, 9p21-23, 6q21 6q23-25, 17p13	1q21-23, 2p12-16, 6p21, 8q24, 12q12-14, 18q21
Primary mediastinal large B-cell lymphoma	2p13-15, 2p24-25, 9p22-24, Xp11, Xq23-28	—	2p14-15, 9p23-24, Xp11-21, Xq22-28
Mature peripheral T-cell neoplasms			
T-cell prolymphocytic lymphoma	8q11-24	—	—
Extranodal T/natural killer–cell lymphoma, nasal type	17q11-21	6q16-27, 13q14-34, 11q22-25, 17p13	—
Adult T-cell lymphoma/leukemia (human T-cell leukemia virus type 1 positive)	7q21-35, 14q32, 3q21-26	6q14-16, 6q21-22, 6q27, 10p11-13, 13q32-34	—
Hepatosplenic γ/δ T-cell lymphoma	7q11-q36	—	—
Mycosis fungoides/Sézary syndrome	17q11-21, 18q11-23	1p33-36, 6q15-23, 9p11-21, 9q34, 10q11-25, 17p13, 19p11-13	—

be important independent prognostic factors that identify subgroups of patients with rapid disease progression and short survival in multivariate analyses (42,47–52). The prognostic impact of del(6q) and +12 is controversial (42,48,50,53,54). Del(13q) as the sole aberration suggests a favorable prognosis (50).

B-Cell Prolymphocytic Leukemia

B-cell prolymphocytic leukemia may present *de novo* or evolve from B-cell chronic lymphocytic leukemia and is characterized by complex hyperdiploid karyotypes. The t(11;14)(q13;q32) has been frequently noted. Other recurring chromosome changes include +12, rearrangements of 1p/q, del(6q), del(11)(q23), and del(13)(q14) (55–57).

Lymphoplasmacytic Lymphoma

Approximately 50% of cases exhibit a t(9;14)(p13;q32) translocation. Posttreatment tumors show increased karyotypic complexity, characterized by abnormalities affecting chromosomes 1 and 7 and dup(17q) (58).

Splenic Marginal Zone Lymphoma (± Villous Lymphocytes)

The most common recurring abnormality identified in this subset is del(7)(q23), which has been noted as the sole abnormality in some cases. In addition, +3q, +5q, +9q, +12q, +18, and +20q and rearrangement of 1p34, 1q21, and 8q have been frequently noted. High level amplification has been noted at 3q26-29, 5p11-15, and 17q22-25 (59–63). Coexistence of +3q and del(7q) is rare (62). In splenic lymphoma with villous lymphocytes, the leukemic counterpart of splenic marginal zone lymphoma, t(11;14)(q13;q32) is common, while +3 is less frequent than in splenic marginal zone lymphoma (64,65). Other frequent changes in splenic lymphoma with villous lymphocytes include rearrangements of 2p11, del(7q), +12, and del(13q) (65–68). Chromosome loss identified by comparative genomic hybridization has been associated with a poor clinical outcome (60).

Hairy-Cell Leukemia

Approximately two-thirds of the patients with hairy-cell leukemia are characterized by multiple unrelated or partially related cytogenetically abnormal clones. Pericentric inversions and interstitial deletions of 5q13, +5q, inv/del(2)(q11), and inv/del(19q) are common. The t(11;14)(q13;q32) translocation has been observed sporadically. The variant form of hairy-cell leukemia often exhibits +12 and rearrangements of 7q32-34 (69–72).

Plasma Cell Myeloma (Multiple Myeloma)/Plasmacytoma

Clonal chromosome abnormalities have been detected only in 30% to 50% of cases by G-banding, whereas deletions have been noted in virtually all cases by fluorescent *in situ* hybridization (73,74). Translocations affecting band 14q32, noted in more than 60% of cases, are the most frequent aberrations. They identify molecular subtypes and possibly comprise the earliest genetic events in the pathogenesis of multiple myeloma (75). Using cytogenetic and molecular methods, more than 20 different translocation partners of 14q32 have been identified, although only a few of them are recurring. The t(11;14)(q13;q21), t(4;14)(p16;q32), and t(14;16)(q32;q23) translocations account for the majority of *IGH*-associated translocations. Other recurring partner sites include 1q10-12, 1q21-25, 2p23, 3q21, 4q22-33, 6p21, 6p25, 8q24, 9p13, 11q23, 20q12, 21q22, and 22q12 (74–77). Rearrangements of chromosomes 1, 3p, 11q, 19q, and 6q are also common. Numeric abnormalities have been noted in virtually all cases, with -13 as the most common. Other frequent changes include +1, +3, +5, +7, +9, +11, +15, and +19 (78,79). In addition to these abnormalities identified by conventional banding methods, spectral karyotyping and comparative genomic hybridization studies have revealed increased rearrangements of 3q27, 17q24-25, and 20q11; gain of 5p, 6p, 8q, 11q, 12q, 17q, and 22q; and loss of 1p, 6q, 8p, 16q, and X. High level copy number increase was noted affecting 1q, 5, 7, 8q, 9q, 11q, 14q, 15, and 19 (80–84). The incidence of 19q gain has been noted at a much higher rate in comparative genomic hybridization analysis, compared with banding analysis, and was also seen as a unique change in two cases (83). A comparatively higher incidence of -2q, -6p, -13, +1, +18, and +X and absence of

+ 3, +6, +9, +11, and +15 have been noted in primary plasma cell leukemia (82,85).

The extent of karyotypic abnormality in multiple myeloma correlates with clinical stage. Approximately 20% of stage I, 60% of stage III, and more than 80% of extramedullary plasmacytomas exhibit aberrant karyotypes (78,79). Monosomy 13 is associated with transition or progression of monoclonal gammopathies of undetermined significance to multiple myeloma (86–88). Hypodiploidy, t/del(11q), -13/del(3q), and rearrangements of 17p have been suggested to carry an adverse prognosis (78,79,89–93).

Extranodal Marginal Zone Lymphoma of Mucosa-Associated Lymphoid Tissue Type

In the low-grade tumors, clonal chromosomal abnormalities are seen in 65% of cases, and the karyotypes tend to be simple. Approximately 20% to 60% of the cases exhibit a t(11;18)(q21;q21), usually as a unique abnormality (94,95). The t(14;18)(q32;q21) and t(1;14)(p22;q32) translocations have been documented in 18% and less than 5% of cases, respectively, and have often been found in high-grade tumors in association with additional genetic abnormalities (96,97). The translocation t(8;14)(q24;q32) has been documented in some high-grade tumors (98). Other abnormalities found in both low- and high-grade tumors, but at a greater incidence in high-grade tumors, include +3/3q+, rearrangements of 1p/q and 14q32, +7, +12, +18, +X, +8q, +11q, del(6q), and -17/del(17p) (98–102).

Nodal Marginal Zone B-Cell Lymphoma (± Monocytoid B Cells)

Cytogenetic data on this subgroup are limited. Rearrangements of 1p/q, +3/+3q, +12, and +18 have been noted to be frequent (59,103). No clinical associations have been identified.

Follicular Lymphoma

The hallmark of follicular lymphoma is the t(14;18)(q32;21) translocation, which is seen in more than 75% of cases. The t(3;14)(q27;q32) and t(8;14)(q24;q32) translocations have been noted in more than 25% and more than 5% of the cases, respectively (34,104). Follicular lymphomas are also characterized by a large number of additional recurring translocations that do not involve the IG gene sites (22). Breakpoints (10% or more) in follicular lymphoma, as shown by conventional cytogenetic methods and spectral karyotyping, cluster at 1p11-13, 1p36, 1q11-21, 2p11-13, 3q27, 6q11-15, 6q21, 6q25-27, 8q24, 9p13, 10q22, 10q24, 12q11-13, 14q32, 17q11-21, and 18q21 (22,105–107). More than 75% of follicular lymphomas show gains and losses of chromosomes. Gains of chromosomes X, 1, 2, 3, 8, 9, 6, 7, 11, 12, 17, and 18 and loss of chromosomes 6, 10, and 17 are common. Regions of common cytogenetic gains have been mapped at 1q21-44, 11q13-q23, 12q13-22, and 18p11.3-q21, and regions of common cytogenetic deletions have been mapped at 6q13, 6q15, 6q21-25, 6q27, 10q22-24, and 17p11-13 (22,105–107).

The cytogenetic features of the t(14;18)(q32;q21) positive and negative subsets of follicular lymphoma differ significantly (22). The latter are karyotypically complex, present with higher histologic grade (grade 2-3b), and associate significantly with t(3;14)(q27;q32)/t(3q27) and t(8;14)(q24;q32), +1/1q, +3p/q, and +9q. Several additional breaks (at 12q11-13 and 17q11-21) and gains (+X, +2p/q, +16, +17q, and +21) have also been noted at a greater frequency in the t(14;18)(q32;q21) negative follicular lymphomas, compared with t(14;18)(q32;q21) positive subset, as revealed by spectral karyotyping. The t(3;14)(q27;q32)/t(3q27) and t(8;14)(q24;q32) translocations are mutually exclusive, indicating that the t(14;18)(q32;q21) negative subset is cytogenetically heterogenous and possibly comprises subgroups characterized by t(3q27), t(8;14)(q24;q32), and other nonrandom abnormalities (22). It has been previously shown that the t(8;14)(q24;q32) in follicular lymphoma in the absence of t(14;18)(q32;q21) is cytogenetically and molecularly distinct from the t(8;14)(q24;q32) seen in high-grade lymphoma and does not involve the MYC gene (108). Among the t(14;18)(q32;q21) negative subgroup, cases with t(3q27) tend to have a greater degree of karyotypic instability (22). The t(14;18)(q32;q21) positive follicular lymphomas, on the other hand, usually present with grade 1 histology and associate with +7 and rearrangements of 1p36 (105,107,109).

Karyotypic complexity has been shown to increase with histologic grade. Although the cytogenetic differences between the histologic grades are significantly different, their overall pattern is consistent with an evolution from low to high grade, rather than comprising distinct entities (22,67,106,107,110,111). Observed associations with other morphologic features include MZD with t(8;14)(q24;q32) as well as with t(8q24), sclerosis with presence of t(14;18)(q32;q21), and prominent FDC component with absence of t(3q27) and t(8q24). A high reactive T-cell component appears to be less common among cases with t(14;18)(q32;q21) (22).

Most follicular lymphomas eventually progress clinically, and in 40% to 70% of the cases, this progression is associated with histologic transformation to diffuse large B-cell lymphoma (112). Abnormalities reported to associate with histologic progression and transformation include del(1)(p26) and rearrangements of 1q21-32, +1, +2, +3, +7, del(6q), +7, +8/8q, +9/9q, del(10)(q22-q24), +12/12q, del(13q), +17/17q, del(17p), +18/18q, and +X (105,107,109,113–115). Among these, del(1)(p36), +1q, +7/7q, +9q, del(10)(q22-23), and +12/12q tend to associate with progression in the t(14;18)(q32;q21) positive subset, and breaks at 1q11-21, +3/3p, +6/6p, and +18/18q tend to associate with progression in the t(14;18)(q32;q21) negative subset (22). In contrast to the other lymphoma subsets, deregulation of genes via chromosome translocations is also common in the progression/transformation of follicular lymphoma, particularly the t(14;18)(q32;q21) positive subset (Table 49.2) (22).

The t(14;18)(q32;q21) translocation is not believed to be of prognostic significance by itself. Presence of t(8;14)(q32;q21) involving MYC in association with t(14;18)(q32;q21) marks an aggressive clinical course, whereas the clinical course of follicular lymphoma with t(8;14)(q24;q32) (without involvement of MYC) alone appears to be similar to that of other follicular lymphoma (116). In some studies, a poor clinical outcome has been noted in patients with deletions of 6q (113,117).

Mantle Cell Lymphoma

The cytogenetic hallmark of mantle cell lymphoma is the t(11;14)(q13;q32) translocation (118). Translocations involving chromosomes 3, 8, 10, 13, and 17 are frequently encountered in addition to t(11;14)(q13;q32). More than 50% of cases with t(11;14)(q13;q32) show additional multiple karyotypic abnormalities, including rearrangements of 3q, +1q, and +12 and deletions of 1p, 6q, 9p, 10q, 11q, 13q, 14q, 17p, and -Y (119–122). The breakpoints cluster at 1p21-22, 1p31-32, 1q21, 6q11-15, 6q23-25, 8q24, 9p21-24, 11q13-23, 13q12-14, and 17p12-13. Comparative genomic hybridization studies have identified frequent gains of 3q, 6p, 7q, 8q, 12p, 12q, 15q, and 17q and losses of 1p, 5p, 6q, 8p, 11q, and 13q. Among these, gain of 3q26.1-29 and loss of 11q22-23 are the most common. High level amplification has been identified at several regions, predominantly at 3q27-29, 18q23, and Xq28 (123–125). The blastoid variant of mantle cell lymphoma is characterized by polyploid karyotypes and increased gain/amplification of the sites mentioned above (124,126). Leukemic and nodal mantle cell lymphoma showed a similar genomic pattern; however, abnormalities affecting chromosomes 8q24, 9p22-24, 16q24, 17, 21, and 22 and del(8p) appeared to be more common in leukemic mantle cell lymphoma (127,128). Patients with an increased number of abnormalities -17p and +Xq tend to have a poorer outcome (119,124,125).

Diffuse Large B-Cell Lymphoma

The majority of diffuse large B-cell lymphomas are characterized by complex hyperdiploid karyotypes. The most frequent recurring translocations in this histology are t(14;18)(q21;q32), followed by t(3q27) and t(8;14)(q24;q32). The band 3q27 manifests promiscuity in rearrangement, and a number of recurring (Table 49.2) as well as nonrecurring partner chromosomal sites have been documented (29,105,129). Several additional recurring translocation breakpoints have been identified (1p22, 1q21, 1p36, 3p21, 6q21, 8q24, and 22q11), including 13 new breakpoints detected by spectral karyotyping (Xp11, 4p11, 4p14, 5q11, 11p11, 12p11, 16p11, 16q11-13, 17q11, 17q23, 18p11, 18q11, and 20q11-13) (Color Plate 80B). As a group, diffuse large B-cell lymphoma cases lacking 14q32 rearrangements show a higher degree of chromosome instability and a tendency to gain additional chromosome changes other than translocations (29). Frequent numerical abnormalities noted (more than 10%) in diffuse large B-cell lymphoma include +3, +7, +12, +X, +11, +18, -X, and -Y. Chromosomes 1, 3, 6, 7, 9, and 17 frequently display RCDs (29,129). Gains and losses have been detected at a much higher frequency by spectral karyotyping and comparative genomic hybridization analysis, comprising gains at 1q21-23, 2p13-22, 2q21, 3q27-29, 8q24, 9p11-24, 9q34, 12q12-14, 13q32, 16p12, 17q11-21, 18q21-22, 19q11-13, 22q12, and Xq25-26 and losses at 8p, 6q11-13, 13q22-32, 18p11-13, and 22q (25,39,130,131). Chromosomal amplification as a frequent phenomenon in diffuse large B-cell lymphoma has been recognized only through comparative genomic hybridization studies. These studies so far identified 16 sites of amplification (1q21, 2p13-15, 3q21-22, 6p21, 8q12, 8q24, 9p12-13, 9q34, 10p11-12, 11q23-24, 12q13, 12q15, 13q33-34, 15q22-24, 16p12, and 18q21) of which six were recurring (1q21, 2p13-15, 8q24, 12q13, 13q33-34, and 18q21) (130). In several tumor types, gene amplification has been shown to correlate with progression and clinical outcome (35), indicating that gene amplification may play a significant role in lymphoma progression and clinical outcome. The functionally amplified target genes in these chromosomal amplicons are yet to be identified.

A number of studies have suggested that patterns of chromosomal abnormalities between nodal and extranodal diffuse large B-cell lymphoma may be distinct; however, these data have generally not been confirmed by study of large cohorts. In one large prospectively ascertained cohort, amplification of REL, initially identified by amplification of 2p13-15 in comparative genomic hybridization studies, was suggested to be associated with extranodal presentation of diffuse large B-cell lymphoma (40). Most primary mediastinal diffuse large B-cell lymphomas show gain of chromosome 9p and the X chromosome. Up to 30% of cases also exhibit gains of 2p and 12q (38,130,132–134). Gains of 18q21, seen in more than one-third of the cases, represent the most frequent imbalance in primary diffuse large B-cell lymphoma of the central nervous system (135–137). The most common abnormalities in primary gastric diffuse B-cell lymphomas include del(6q) gain/amplification of 3q and +12 (138–140).

Several studies have attempted to correlate cytogenetic findings with clinical features or patient outcome of diffuse large B-cell lymphoma, and the results have been contradictory. Most studies have failed to show a consistent association between the recurring translocations t(3q27), t(14;18)(q32;q21), and t(8;14)(q24;q32) and clinical outcome (141–144). In some G-banding studies, changes, such as +2/2p, +3/3p, +5, +6, or +18, -7, del(6q), abnormalities of 17 [-17,del(17p) and i(17q)], and breaks or duplications of 1q have been suggested to correlate with advanced stage disease and poor prognosis (129,145,146). In the spectral karyotyping analysis, rearrangements affecting 3q27, 2q31, and 7q22 significantly associated with advanced stage disease or poor treatment response in one study (21).

Burkitt's Lymphoma

A t(8;14)(q24;q32) or its variants t(8;22)(q24;q11) and t(2;8)(p12;q24) are seen in virtually every case and are the hallmark of Burkitt's lymphoma (146). Duplication or structural alterations of 1q leading to partial trisomy are the most

frequent additional changes. The involved regions are heterogeneous but always include 1q21-32. Other chromosomal changes detected include del(6q), del(9p), del(13q), +7, and, +12 (146,147).

T-Cell and Natural Killer–Cell Neoplasms

Due to their rarity and histologic overlap, many of the T-cell lymphoma subtypes remain cytogenetically ill-defined, with the exception of anaplastic large-cell lymphoma.

T-Cell Prolymphocytic Leukemia

T-cell prolymphocytic leukemia is generally characterized by complex karyotypes. Abnormalities of chromosome 8, including i(8)(q10), t(8;8)(p13;q11), and +8 and del(8p), inv(14)(q11q32), or t(14;14)(q11;q32), are the most frequent cytogenetic abnormalities reported. Less frequent abnormalities include del(6q), del(11q), del(12p), and -14, del(17p) (49,148–150). Patients with the inherited disorder ataxia-telangiectasia are prone to develop T-cell prolymphocytic leukemia with a t(X;14)(q28;q11), which is often noted in association with T-cell proliferation before the onset of leukemia (151).

Natural Killer–Cell Lymphoma/Leukemia

Little is known about the cytogenetics of this disorder, due to its rarity and difficulty in obtaining adequate tumor samples. Karyotypes are usually hyperdiploid and more complex in the nasal-type lymphomas, compared with the aggressive natural killer–cell lymphoma/leukemia. The most common abnormalities include del(6q) or i(6p) and +7. Other nonrandom abnormalities reported include +X, i(1q), +8, and rearrangements involving 17p/q, 1q, 13q, and 11q (152,153). Comparative genomic hybridization studies have shown frequent gains at 1p32-pter, 6p, 11q, 12q, 17q, 19p, 20q, and Xp and losses at 6q16-q27, 13q14-q34, 11q22-q25 , 17p13, and X (153,154).

Adult T-Cell Lymphoma/Leukemia (Human T-Cell Leukemia Virus Type 1 Positive)

Clonal chromosomal abnormalities have been detected in virtually every case. Translocations and inversions involving 14q32 or 14q11 and del(6)(q15-21) are the most frequent abnormalities in this subset. Other cytogenetic changes include -X,-Y,+3,+7, and +21 and deletions of 10p, 3q, 5q, 9q, 1p, and 7p. Among these, +3, +7, -X, and del(6q) are found predominantly in acute adult T-cell lymphoma/leukemia and may be associated with progression (155–157). The karyotypes tend to be hyperdiploid and more complex in the acute stage than in the chronic or smoldering stages. Abnormalities affecting 1q, 10p, 12q, and 14q have been shown to correlate with one or more of the following clinical features: hepatosplenomegaly, elevated lactate dehydrogenase, hypercalcemia, and unusual immunophenotype—all indicators of clinical severity of adult T-cell lymphoma/leukemia. Six or more breaks and abnormalities affecting chromosomes 1, 2q, 3q, 9p, 14q, and 17q have been shown to correlate with shorter survival (156).

Hepatosplenic γ/δ T-Cell Lymphoma

The most frequently reported cytogenetic abnormalities in this subset are i(7q), +8, and -Y. I(7q) has been observed as the sole abnormality in some cases, although in sequential studies it has been shown to evolve during the course of the disease (158,159).

Mycosis Fungoides/Sézary Syndrome

Mycosis fungoides is characterized by multiple nonclonal chromosome abnormalities, whereas Sézary syndrome usually presents clonal hyperdiploid/near-tetraploid chromosome complements. The most common abnormality is -10. Chromosomes frequently involved in translocations are 1p, 1q, 11q, 14q, 2p, 10q, 7q, 9q, 12q, 7p, 8q, and 13q, with breakpoints clustering at bands 1p11, 1p36, 2p11-24, 13q11-14, 14q11, and 14q32. Deletions commonly affect 6q, 1q, 3p, 7, 1p, and 2p. (160,161). The presence of clonal abnormalities correlates with advanced stage disease and decreased survival (161).

Peripheral T-Cell Lymphoma, Not Otherwise Characterized

Clonal chromosome abnormalities are more frequent and complex in high-grade lesions, compared with low-grade lesions. Translocations involving 14q11, 14q32, 7q34, 7p15, 5q23-32, dup(5)(q23-32), +5, +7/+7q, del(1p), -13/del(13q), and del(6q) are frequent (162,163). T-zone lymphoma and lymphoepithelioid lesions frequently display +3 (163).

Angioimmunoblastic T-Cell Lymphoma

Angioimmunoblastic T-cell lymphoma is characterized by karyotypically unrelated abnormal clones. Such clones can be found in up to 90% of the cases. Nonrandom chromosomal changes include +3, +5, and +X, with the combinations +3 and +X and +3 and +5 as the most frequent. Other recurring changes include del(1)(p31-32), dup(6p), t/del(6q), -7/+7q, and -13/del(13q). Sites frequently involved in structural rearrangements include 3p24-25, 4p13, 6q21-25, 9q2, 12q13, 14q11, and 14q32 (163–165). In the only published study, presence of cytogenetically abnormal clones correlated with a significantly lower incidence of therapy-induced remission and shortened survival (166).

Anaplastic Large-Cell Lymphoma, T Cell/Null Cell

Anaplastic large-cell lymphoma is characterized by the presence of t(2;5)(p23;q35) (95,167). Molecular genetic and immunohistochemical studies have shown that this translocation is predominant in children and young adults with primary nodal CD30+ anaplastic large-cell lymphoma of T-cell/

null-cell lineage (168,169). The karyotypes of cases with anaplastic morphology are usually more complex than those with nonanaplastic morphology (168).

Cytogenetic, molecular, and immunohistochemical studies have also identified several variant translocations/rearrangements that activate ALK at 2p23 (Table 49.3) (169). Additional chromosome changes are frequently encountered and include +7, +X, -Y, +9, del (6q), and del (17p) (147,168). Clinically, t(2;5)(p23;q25) and ALK+ patients carry a better prognosis, compared with ALK− patients (147,170).

CHROMOSOME CHANGES THAT ASSOCIATE WITH CLINICAL BEHAVIOR IN MULTIPLE HISTOLOGIC SUBSETS

Abnormalities of chromosomes 1, 6, and 17 have been noted in virtually all lineages of cancer (hematopoietic, epithelial, mesenchymal, neuronal, and germ cell). Several studies also have shown that abnormalities involving these chromosomes are associated with a poor clinical outcome of patients. These descriptive cytogenetic data strongly indicate involvement of multiple genes located on these chromosomes in tumorigenesis per se.

Chromosomes 1 and 6

Abnormalities of both chromosomes 1 and 6, mostly translocations or deletions, have been reported in at least 15% of low- and high-grade lymphomas. The breakpoints mainly cluster in 1p32-36, 1q21-23, and 6q13-27 regions (171,172). They may be found in association with or independent of t(14;18)(q32;q21) or other IG gene–associated translocations (29,146,147). In general, these abnormalities have been uniformly associated with overall poor prognosis in all histologic types of lymphoma, especially diffuse large B-cell lymphoma (146). Molecular breaks at 1q21-22 have been found to be heterogeneous (172). So far, three breakpoint clusters have been identified by molecular genetic analysis, associated with BCL9 (97), FCGR2B (173,174), and MUC1 (175) genes. Among these, MUC1 deregulation resulting from a t(1;14)(q21;q32) best fits the model for a progression-associated genetic change (175).

Chromosome 17

Structural abnormalities of chromosome 17 also are a frequent finding in many malignancies and have been reported in up to 20% of lymphomas, involving both the long and short arms as well as formation of i(17q) (147). The TP 53 gene mapped at 17p13 plays a pathogenetic role in at least some of these cases. Although no specific recurring breakpoint has been identified, 17p- or all alterations of chromosome 17, either at initial diagnosis or as part of clonal evolution, have been significantly associated with a higher risk of transformation of low-grade lymphoma to high-grade lymphoma to diffuse large B-cell lymphoma and adverse prognosis in follicular lymphoma and other histologic subtypes of lymphoma (142,176–179).

CONCLUSION

In this review, we have attempted to provide a summary of the current state of lymphoma cytogenetics. In the first section, the technical developments that led to the development of this field were discussed in the historical context, and accomplishments of the classical techniques and the promise of the new techniques have been highlighted. This was followed by an overall critique of the types of chromosome changes seen in lymphomas and their possible biologic significance. The third section comprises a detailed description of nonrandom chromosomal changes in the various lymphoma subsets recognized by the World Health Organization Classification (1) and their possible clinical relevance. Overall, although lymphoma cytogenetics has been slow in developing, the work of several groups over the past decade provided new information and opened new avenues of investigation in regard to understanding the biology of this disease and its clinical behavior. This new information, together with the new molecularly based cytogenetic technologies that have become available, augers a productive future ahead. Lymphomas represent an exciting model not only because they are tumors that arise in a complex developmental lineage but also because they occupy a position in between leukemias and solid tumors in terms of biologic evolution of tumors, hence serving as models for both types of malignancies.

REFERENCES

1. Harris NL, Jaffe ES, Diebold J, et al. World Health Organization classification of neoplastic diseases of the hematopoietic and lymphoid tissues: report of the Clinical Advisory Committee meeting-Airlie House, Virginia, November 1997. *J Clin Oncol* 1999;17:3835–3849.
2. Tjio JH, Levan A. The chromosome number of man. *Hereditas* 1956;42:1–6.
3. Ford CE, Hamerton JL. The chromosomes of man. *Nature* 1956;178:1020.
4. Hsu T. Mammalian chromosomes *in vitro*. I. The karyotype of man. *J Hered* 1952;43:172.
5. Nowell PC, Hungerford DA. A minute chromosome in human chronic granulocytic leukemia. *Science* 1960;132:1197.
6. ISCN. Harnden DG, Klinger HP, eds. *An international system for human cytogenetic nomenclature*. Basel: S. Karger, 1985.
7. ISCN. Mitleman F, ed. *An international system for human cytogenetic nomenclature*. Basel: S. Karger, 1995.
8. Caspersson T, Zech L, Johansson C. Differential banding of alkylating fluorochromes in human chromosomes. *Exp Cell Res* 1970;60:315–319.
9. Sumner A, Evans HJ, Buckland RA. A new technique for distinguishing between human chromosomes. *Nature New Biol* 1971;232:31–32.
10. Seabright M. A rapid banding technique for human chromosomes. *Lancet* 1971;2:971–972.
11. Dutrillaux B, Lejeune J. Sur une novelle technique d'analyse du caryotype human. *C R Acad Sci Paris* 1971;272:2638–2640.
12. Sumner AT. A simple technique for demonstrating centromeric heterochromatin. *Exp Cell Res* 1972;75:304–306.
13. Chen TR. Karyotype analysis utilizing differentially stained constitutive heterochromatin of human and murine chromosomes. *Chromosoma* 1971;34:51–72.
14. Rowley JD. A new consistent chromosomal abnormality chronic myelogenous leukemia identified by quinacrine fluorescence and Giemsa staining. *Nature* 1973;243:290–292.
15. Southern EM. Detection of specific sequences among DNA fragments separated by gel electrophoresis. *J Mol Biol* 1975;98:503–517.
16. Neel BG, Jhanwar SC, Chaganti RS, et al. Two human c-onc genes are located on the long arm of chromosome 8. *Proc Natl Acad Sci U S A* 1982;79:7842–7846.
17. Tonnies H. Modern molecular cytogenetic techniques in genetic diagnostics. *Trends Mol Med* 2002;8:246–250.
18. Meltzer PS, Guan XY, Burgess A, et al. Rapid generation of region specific probes by chromosome microdissection and their application. *Nat Genet* 1992;1:24–28.
19. Pinkel D, Straume T, Gray JW. Cytogenetic analysis using quantitative, high-sensitivity, fluorescence hybridization. *Proc Natl Acad Sci U S A* 1986;83:2934–2938.
20. Schrock E, du Manoir S, Veldman T, et al. Multicolor spectral karyotyping of human chromosomes. *Science* 1996;273:494–497.
21. Nanjangud G, Rao PH, Hegde A, et al. Spectral karyotyping identifies new rearrangements, translocations, and clinical associations in diffuse large B-cell lymphoma. *Blood* 2002;99:2554–2561.
22. Nanjangud G, Naresh KN, Teruya-Feldstein J, et al. Cytogenetic analysis of follicular lymphoma: chromosome instability associated with t(14;18)(q32;q21) positive and negative subsets, histologic grade, progression, and transformation (*submitted*).
23. Kallioniemi A, Kallioniemi OP, Sudar D, et al. Comparative genomic hybridization for molecular cytogenetic analysis of solid tumors. *Science* 1992;258:818–821.
24. Struski S, Doco-Fenzy M, Cornillet-Lefebvre P. Compilation of published comparative genomic hybridization studies. *Cancer Genet Cytogenet* 2002;135:63–90.
25. Rao PH, Houldsworth J, Dyomina K, et al. Chromosomal and gene amplification in diffuse large B-cell lymphoma. *Blood* 1998;92:234–240.
26. Pollack JR, Perou CM, Alizadeh AA, et al. Genome-wide analysis of DNA copy-number changes using cDNA microarrays. *Nat Genet* 1999;23:41–46.
27. Pinkel D, Segraves R, Sudar D, et al. High resolution analysis of DNA copy number variation using comparative genomic hybridization to microarrays. *Nat Genet* 1998;20:207–211.
28. Bourdon V, Naef F, Rao PH, et al. Genomic and expression analysis of the 12p11-p12 amplicon using EST arrays identifies two novel amplified and overexpressed genes. *Cancer Res* 2002;62:6218–6223.
29. Cigudosa JC, Parsa NZ, Louie DC, et al. Cytogenetic analysis of 363 consecutively ascertained diffuse large B-cell lymphomas. *Genes Chromosomes Cancer* 1999;25:123–133.
30. Haluska FG, Croce CM. Molecular mechanisms of chromosome translocation in human B- and T-cell neoplasia. *Ann N Y Acad Sci* 1987;511:196–206.
31. Dalla-Favera R, Lombardi L, Pelicci PG, et al. Mechanism of activation and biological role of the c-myc oncogene in B-cell lymphomagenesis. *Ann N Y Acad Sci* 1987;511:207–218.
32. Chaganti SR, Rao PH, Chen W, et al. Deregulation of BCL6 in non-Hodgkin lymphoma by insertion of IGH sequences in complex translocations involving band 3q27. *Genes Chromosomes Cancer* 1998;23:328–336.
33. Gabrea A, Bergsagel PL, Chesi M, et al. Insertion of excised IgH switch sequences causes overexpression of cyclin D1 in a myeloma tumor cell. *Mol Cell* 1999;3:119–123.
34. Chaganti RS, Nanjangud G, Schmidt H, et al. Recurring chromosomal abnormalities in non-Hodgkin's lymphoma: biologic and clinical significance. *Semin Hematol* 2000;37:396–411.
35. Schwab M. Oncogene amplification in solid tumors. *Semin Cancer Biol* 1999;9:319–325.
36. Ben-Yehuda D, Houldsworth J, Parsa NZ, et al. Gene amplification in non-Hodgkin's lymphoma. *Br J Haematol* 1994;86:792–797.
37. Bentz M, Werner CA, Dohner H, et al. High incidence of chromosomal imbalances and gene amplifications in the classical follicular variant of follicle center lymphoma. *Blood* 1996;88:1437–1444.
38. Joos S, Otano-Joos MI, Ziegler S, et al. Primary mediastinal (thymic) B-cell lymphoma is characterized by gains of chromosomal material including 9p and amplification of the REL gene. *Blood* 1996;87:1571–1578.
39. Monni O, Joensuu H, Franssila K, et al. DNA copy number changes in diffuse large B-cell lymphoma—comparative genomic hybridization study. *Blood* 1996;87:5269–5278.

40. Houldsworth J, Mathew S, Rao PH, et al. REL proto-oncogene is frequently amplified in extranodal diffuse large cell lymphoma. *Blood* 1996;87:25–29.

41. Martinez-Climent JA, Alizadeh AA, Segraves R, et al. Transformation of follicular lymphoma to diffuse large cell lymphoma is associated with a heterogeneous set of DNA copy number and gene expression alterations. *Blood* 2002 (*in press*).

42. Crossen PE. Genes and chromosomes in chronic B-cell leukemia. *Cancer Genet Cytogenet* 1997;94:44–51.

43. Michaux L, Dierlamm J, Wlodarska I, et al. t(14;19)/BCL3 rearrangements in lymphoproliferative disorders: a review of 23 cases. *Cancer Genet Cytogenet* 1997;94:36–43.

44. Nanjangud G, Naresh KN, Nair CN, et al. Translocation (11;14)(q13;q32) and overexpression of cyclin D1 protein in a CD23-positive low-grade B-cell neoplasm. *Cancer Genet Cytogenet* 1998;106:37–43.

45. Cuneo A, Balboni M, Piva N, et al. Atypical chronic lymphocytic leukaemia with t(11;14)(q13;q32): karyotype evolution and prolymphocytic transformation. *Br J Haematol* 1995;90:409–416.

46. Summersgill B, Thornton P, Atkinson S, et al. Chromosomal imbalances in familial chronic lymphocytic leukaemia: a comparative genomic hybridisation analysis. *Leukemia* 2002;16:1229–1232.

47. Chevallier P, Penther D, Avet-Loiseau H, et al. CD38 expression and secondary 17p deletion are important prognostic factors in chronic lymphocytic leukaemia. *Br J Haematol* 2002;116:142–150.

48. Shaw GR, Kronberger DL. TP53 deletions but not trisomy 12 are adverse in B-cell lymphoproliferative disorders. *Cancer Genet Cytogenet* 2000;119:146–154.

49. Juliusson G, Gahrton G. Cytogenetics in CLL and related disorders. *Baillieres Clin Haematol* 1993;6:821–848.

50. Dohner H, Stilgenbauer S, Benner A, et al. Genomic aberrations and survival in chronic lymphocytic leukemia. *N Engl J Med* 2000;343:1910–1916.

51. Dohner H, Stilgenbauer S, James MR, et al. 11q deletions identify a new subset of B-cell chronic lymphocytic leukemia characterized by extensive nodal involvement and inferior prognosis. *Blood* 1997;89:2516–2522.

52. Stilgenbauer S, Lichter P and Dohner H. Genetic features of B-cell chronic lymphocytic leukemia. *Rev Clin Exp Hematol* 2000;4:48–72.

53. Stilgenbauer S, Bullinger L, Lichter P, et al. Genetics of chronic lymphocytic leukemia: genomic aberrations and V(H) gene mutation status in pathogenesis and clinical course. *Leukemia* 2002;16:993–1007.

54. Stilgenbauer S, Bullinger L, Benner A, et al. Incidence and clinical significance of 6q deletions in B cell chronic lymphocytic leukemia. *Leukemia* 1999;13:1331–1334.

55. Brito-Babapulle V, Pittman S, Melo JV, et al. Cytogenetic studies on prolymphocytic leukemia. 1. B-cell prolymphocytic leukemia. *Hematol Pathol* 1987;1:27–33.

56. Lens D, Matutes E, Catovsky D, et al. Frequent deletions at 11q23 and 13q14 in B cell prolymphocytic leukemia (B-PLL). *Leukemia* 2000;14:427–430.

57. Schlette E, Bueso-Ramos C, Giles F, et al. Mature B-cell leukemias with more than 55% prolymphocytes. A heterogeneous group that includes an unusual variant of mantle cell lymphoma. *Am J Clin Pathol* 2001;115:571–581.

58. Offit K, Parsa NZ, Filippa D, et al. t(9;14)(p13;q32) denotes a subset of low-grade non-Hodgkin's lymphoma with plasmacytoid differentiation. *Blood* 1992;80:2594–2599.

59. Dierlamm J, Pittaluga S, Wlodarska I, et al. Marginal zone B-cell lymphomas of different sites share similar cytogenetic and morphologic features. *Blood* 1996;87:299–307.

60. Hernandez JM, Garcia JL, Gutierrez NC, et al. Novel genomic imbalances in B-cell splenic marginal zone lymphomas revealed by comparative genomic hybridization and cytogenetics. *Am J Pathol* 2001;158:1843–1850.

61. Mateo M, Mollejo M, Villuendas R, et al. 7q31-32 allelic loss is a frequent finding in splenic marginal zone lymphoma. *Am J Pathol* 1999;154:1583–1589.

62. Sole F, Salido M, Espinet B, et al. Splenic marginal zone B-cell lymphomas: two cytogenetic subtypes, one with gain of 3q and the other with loss of 7q. *Haematologica* 2001;86:71–77.

63. Sole F, Woessner S, Florensa L, et al. Frequent involvement of chromosomes 1, 3, 7 and 8 in splenic marginal zone B-cell lymphoma. *Br J Haematol* 1997;98:446–449.

64. Gruszka-Westwood AM, Matutes E, Coignet LJ, et al. The incidence of trisomy 3 in splenic lymphoma with villous lymphocytes: a study by FISH. *Br J Haematol* 1999;104:600–604.

65. Troussard X, Mauvieux L, Radford-Weiss I, et al. Genetic analysis of splenic lymphoma with villous lymphocytes: a Groupe Francais d'Hematologie Cellulaire (GFHC) study. *Br J Haematol* 1998;101:712–721.

66. Garcia-Marco JA, Nouel A, Navarro B, et al. Molecular cytogenetic analysis in splenic lymphoma with villous lymphocytes: frequent allelic imbalance of the RB1 gene but not the D13S25 locus on chromosome 13q14. *Cancer Res* 1998;58:1736–1740.

67. Gruszka-Westwood AM, Hamoudi R, Osborne L, et al. Deletion mapping on the long arm of chromosome 7 in splenic lymphoma with villous lymphocytes. *Genes Chromosomes Cancer* 2003;36:57–69.

68. Oscier DG, Matutes E, Gardiner A, et al. Cytogenetic studies in splenic lymphoma with villous lymphocytes. *Br J Haematol* 1993;85:487–491.

69. Dierlamm J, Stefanova M, Wlodarska I, et al. Chromosomal gains and losses are uncommon in hairy cell leukemia: a study based on comparative genomic hybridization and interphase fluorescence in situ hybridization. *Cancer Genet Cytogenet* 2001;128:164–167.

70. Vallianatou K, Brito-Babapulle V, Matutes E, et al. p53 gene deletion and trisomy 12 in hairy cell leukemia and its variant. *Leuk Res* 1999;23:1041–1045.

71. Brito-Babapulle V, Matutes E, Oscier D, et al. Chromosome abnormalities in hairy cell leukaemia variant. *Genes Chromosomes Cancer* 1994;10:197–202.

72. Haglund U, Juliusson G, Stellan B, et al. Hairy cell leukemia is characterized by clonal chromosome abnormalities clustered to specific regions. *Blood* 1994;83:2637–2645.

73. Drach J, Kaufmann H. New developments and treatment in multiple myeloma: new insights on molecular biology. *Ann Oncol* 2002;13[Suppl 4]:43–47.

74. Kuehl WM, Bergsagel PL. Multiple myeloma: evolving genetic events and host interactions. *Nat Rev Cancer* 2002;2:175–187.

75. Chesi M, Kuehl WM, Bergsagel PL. Recurrent immunoglobulin gene translocations identify distinct molecular subtypes of myeloma. *Ann Oncol* 2000;11[Suppl 1]:131–135.

76. Bergsagel PL, Nardini E, Brents L, et al. IgH translocations in multiple myeloma: a nearly universal event that rarely involves c-myc. *Curr Top Microbiol Immunol* 1997;224:283–287.

77. Avet-Loiseau H, Gerson F, Magrangeas F, et al. Rearrangements of the c-myc oncogene are present in 15% of primary human multiple myeloma tumors. *Blood* 2001;98:3082–3086.

78. Calasanz MJ, Cigudosa JC, Odero MD, et al. Cytogenetic analysis of 280 patients with multiple myeloma and related disorders: primary breakpoints and clinical correlations. *Genes Chromosomes Cancer* 1997;18:84–93.

79. Feinman R, Sawyer J, Hardin J, et al. Cytogenetics and molecular genetics in multiple myeloma. *Hematol Oncol Clin North Am* 1997;11:1–25.

80. Sawyer JR, Lukacs JL, Munshi N, et al. Identification of new nonrandom translocations in multiple myeloma with multicolor spectral karyotyping. *Blood* 1998;92:4269–4278.

81. Rao PH, Cigudosa JC, Ning Y, et al. Multicolor spectral karyotyping identifies new recurring breakpoints and translocations in multiple myeloma. *Blood* 1998;92:1743–1748.

82. Gutierrez NC, Hernandez JM, Garcia JL, et al. Differences in genetic changes between multiple myeloma and plasma cell leukemia demonstrated by comparative genomic hybridization. *Leukemia* 2001;15:840–845.

83. Cigudosa JC, Rao PH, Calasanz MJ, et al. Characterization of nonrandom chromosomal gains and losses in multiple myeloma by comparative genomic hybridization. *Blood* 1998;91:3007–3010.

84. Avet-Loiseau H, Andree-Ashley LE, et al. Molecular cytogenetic abnormalities in multiple myeloma and plasma cell leukemia measured using comparative genomic hybridization. *Genes Chromosomes Cancer* 1997;19:124–133.

85. Garcia-Sanz R, Orfao A, Gonzalez M, et al. Primary plasma cell leukemia: clinical, immunophenotypic, DNA ploidy, and cytogenetic characteristics. *Blood* 1999;93:1032–1037.

86. Lloveras E, Sole F, Florensa L, et al. Contribution of cytogenetics and in situ hybridization to the study of monoclonal gammopathies of undetermined significance. *Cancer Genet Cytogenet* 2002;132:25–29.

87. Fonseca R, Bailey RJ, Ahmann GJ, et al. Genomic abnormalities in monoclonal gammopathy of undetermined significance. *Blood* 2002;100:1417–1424.

88. Avet-Loiseau H, Li JY, Morineau N, et al. Monosomy 13 is associated with the transition of monoclonal gammopathy of undetermined significance to multiple myeloma. Intergroupe Francophone du Myelome. *Blood* 1999;94:2583–2589.

89. Fassas AB, Spencer T, Sawyer J, et al. Both hypodiploidy and deletion of chromosome 13 independently confer poor prognosis in multiple myeloma. *Br J Haematol* 2002;118:1041–1047.

90. Fonseca R, Harrington D, Oken MM, et al. Biological and prognostic significance of interphase fluorescence in situ hybridization detection of chromosome 13 abnormalities (delta13) in multiple myeloma: an eastern cooperative oncology group study. *Cancer Res* 2002;62:715–720.

91. Smadja NV, Bastard C, Brigaudeau C, et al. Hypodiploidy is a major prognostic factor in multiple myeloma. *Blood* 2001;98:2229–2238.

92. Perez-Simon JA, Garcia-Sanz R, Tabernero MD, et al. Prognostic value of numerical chromosome aberrations in multiple myeloma: a FISH analysis of 15 different chromosomes. *Blood* 1998;91:3366–3371.

93. Calasanz MJ, Cigudosa JC, Odero MD, et al. Hypodiploidy and 22q11 rearrangements at diagnosis are associated with poor prognosis in patients with multiple myeloma. *Br J Haematol* 1997;98:418–425.

94. Ott G, Katzenberger T, Greiner A, et al. The t(11;18)(q21;q21) chromosome translocation is a frequent and specific aberration in low-grade but not high-grade malignant non-Hodgkin's lymphomas of the mucosa-associated lymphoid tissue (MALT-) type. *Cancer Res* 1997;57:3944–3948.

95. Rosenwald A, Ott G, Stilgenbauer S, et al. Exclusive detection of the t(11;18)(q21;q21) in extranodal marginal zone B cell lymphomas (MZBL) of MALT type in contrast to other MZBL and extranodal large B cell lymphomas. *Am J Pathol* 1999;155:1817–1821.

96. Streubel B, Lamprecht A, Dierlamm J, et al. T(14;18)(q32;q21) involving IGH and MALT1 is a frequent chromosomal aberration in MALT lymphoma. *Blood* 2003;101:2335–2339.

97. Willis TG, Jadayel DM, Du MQ, et al. Bcl10 is involved in t(1;14)(p22;q32) of MALT B cell lymphoma and mutated in multiple tumor types. *Cell* 1999;96:35–45.

98. Ott MM, Rosenwald A, Katzenberger T, et al. Marginal zone B-cell lymphomas (MZBL) arising at different sites represent different biological entities. *Genes Chromosomes Cancer* 2000;28:380–386.

99. Watanobe I, Takamori S, Kojima K, et al. Numerical chromosomal abnormality in gastric MALT lymphoma and diffuse large B-cell lymphoma. *J Gastroenterol* 2002;37:691–696.

100. Barth TF, Bentz M, Leithauser F, et al. Molecular-cytogenetic comparison of mucosa-associated marginal zone B-cell lymphoma and large B-cell lymphoma arising in the gastrointestinal tract. *Genes Chromosomes Cancer* 2001;31:316–325.

101. Wotherspoon AC, Finn TM, Isaacson PG. Trisomy 3 in low-grade B-cell lymphomas of mucosa-associated lymphoid tissue. *Blood* 1995;85:2000–2004.

102. Starostik P, Patzner J, Greiner A, et al. Gastric marginal zone B-cell lymphomas of MALT type develop along 2 distinct pathogenetic pathways. *Blood* 2002;99:3–9.

103. Dierlamm J, Wlodarska I, Michaux L, et al. Genetic abnormalities in marginal zone B-cell lymphoma. *Hematol Oncol* 2000;18:1–13.

104. Knutsen T. Cytogenetic mechanisms in the pathogenesis and progression of follicular lymphoma. *Cancer Surv* 1997;30:163–192.

105. Offit K, Jhanwar SC, Ladanyi M, et al. Cytogenetic analysis of 434 consecutively ascertained specimens of non-Hodgkin's lymphoma: correlations between recurrent aberrations, histology, and exposure to cytotoxic treatment. *Genes Chromosomes Cancer* 1991;3:189–201.

106. Horsman DE, Connors JM, Pantzar T, et al. Analysis of secondary chromosomal alterations in 165 cases of follicular lymphoma with t(14;18). *Genes Chromosomes Cancer* 2001;30:375–382.

107. Knutsen T. Cytogenetic changes in the progression of lymphoma. *Leuk Lymphoma* 1998;31:1–19.

108. Ladanyi M, Offit K, Chaganti RS. Variant t(8;14) translocations in non-Burkitt's non-Hodgkin's lymphomas. *Blood* 1992;79:1377–1379.

109. Whang-Peng J, Knutsen T, Jaffe ES, et al. Sequential analysis of 43 patients with non-Hodgkin's lymphoma: clinical correlations with cytogenetic, histologic, immunophenotyping, and molecular studies. *Blood* 1995;85:203–216.

110. Ott G, Katzenberger T, Lohr A, et al. Cytomorphologic, immunohistochemical, and cytogenetic profiles of follicular lymphoma: 2 types of follicular lymphoma grade 3. *Blood* 2002;99:3806–3812.

111. Bosga-Bouwer AG, Van Imhoff GW, Boonstra R, et al. Follicular lymphoma grade 3B includes 3 cytogenetically defined subgroups

112. Bastion Y, Sebban C, Berger F, et al. Incidence, predictive factors, and outcome of lymphoma transformation in follicular lymphoma patients. *J Clin Oncol* 1997;15:1587–1594.

113. Tilly H, Rossi A, Stamatoullas A, et al. Prognostic value of chromosomal abnormalities in follicular lymphoma. *Blood* 1994;84:1043–1049.

114. Juneja S, Matthews J, Lukeis R, et al. Prognostic value of cytogenetic abnormalities in previously untreated patients with non-Hodgkin's lymphoma. *Leuk Lymphoma* 1997;25:493–501.

115. Bernell P, Arvidsson I, Jacobsson B. Gain of chromosome 7, which marks the progression from indolent to aggressive follicle centre lymphomas, is restricted to the B-lymphoid cell lineage: a study by FISH in combination with morphology and immunocytochemistry. *Br J Haematol* 1999;105:1140–1144.

116. Ladanyi M, Offit K, Parsa NZ, et al. Follicular lymphoma with t(8;14)(q24;q32): a distinct clinical and molecular subset of t(8;14)-bearing lymphomas. *Blood* 1992;79:2124–2130.

117. Viardot A, Moller P, Hogel J, et al. Clinicopathologic correlations of genomic gains and losses in follicular lymphoma. *J Clin Oncol* 2002;20:4523–4530.

118. Weisenburger DD, Armitage JO. Mantle cell lymphoma—an entity comes of age. *Blood* 1996;87:4483–4494.

119. Cuneo A, Bigoni R, Rigolin GM, et al. Cytogenetic profile of lymphoma of follicle mantle lineage: correlation with clinicobiologic features. *Blood* 1999;93:1372–1380.

120. de Boer CJ, van Krieken JH, Schuuring E, et al. Bcl-1/cyclin D1 in malignant lymphoma. *Ann Oncol* 1997;8[Suppl 2]:109–117.

121. Wlodarska I, Pittaluga S, Hagemeijer A, et al. Secondary chromosome changes in mantle cell lymphoma. *Haematologica* 1999;84:594–599.

122. Au WY, Gascoyne RD, Viswanatha DS, et al. Cytogenetic analysis in mantle cell lymphoma: a review of 214 cases. *Leuk Lymphoma* 2002;43:783–791.

123. Monni O, Oinonen R, Elonen E, et al. Gain of 3q and deletion of 11q22 are frequent aberrations in mantle cell lymphoma. *Genes Chromosomes Cancer* 1998;21:298–307.

124. Bea S, Ribas M, Hernandez JM, et al. Increased number of chromosomal imbalances and high-level DNA amplifications in mantle cell lymphoma are associated with blastoid variants. *Blood* 1999;93:4365–4374.

125. Allen JE, Hough RE, Goepel JR, et al. Identification of novel regions of amplification and deletion within mantle cell lymphoma DNA by comparative genomic hybridization. *Br J Haematol* 2002;116:291–298.

126. Ott G, Kalla J, Ott MM, et al. Blastoid variants of mantle cell lymphoma: frequent bcl-1 rearrangements at the major translocation cluster region and tetraploid chromosome clones. *Blood* 1997;89:1421–1429.

127. Onciu M, Schlette E, Medeiros LJ, et al. Cytogenetic findings in mantle cell lymphoma cases with a high level of peripheral blood involvement have a distinct pattern of abnormalities. *Am J Clin Pathol* 2001;116:886–892.

128. Martinez-Climent JA, Vizcarra E, Sanchez D, et al. Loss of a novel tumor suppressor gene locus at chromosome 8p is associated with leukemic mantle cell lymphoma. *Blood* 2001;98:3479–3482.

129. Jerkeman M, Johansson B, Akerman M, et al. Prognostic implications of cytogenetic aberrations in diffuse large B-cell lymphomas. *Eur J Haematol* 1999;62:184–190.

130. Palanisamy N, Abou-Elella AA, Chaganti SR, et al. Similar patterns of genomic alterations characterize primary mediastinal large-B-cell lymphoma and diffuse large-B-cell lymphoma. *Genes Chromosomes Cancer* 2002;33:114–122.

131. Berglund M, Enblad G, Flordal E, et al. Chromosomal imbalances in diffuse large B-cell lymphoma detected by comparative genomic hybridization. *Mod Pathol* 2002;15:807–816.

132. Barth TF, Leithauser F, Moller P. Mediastinal B-cell lymphoma, a lymphoma type with several characteristics unique among diffuse large B-cell lymphomas. *Ann Hematol* 2001;80[Suppl 3]:B49–B53.

133. Scarpa A, Moore PS, Rigaud G, et al. Genetic alterations in primary mediastinal B-cell lymphoma: an update. *Leuk Lymphoma* 2001;41:47–53.

134. Bentz M, Barth TF, Bruderlein S, et al. Gain of chromosome arm 9p is characteristic of primary mediastinal B-cell lymphoma (MBL): comprehensive molecular cytogenetic analysis and presentation of a novel MBL cell line. *Genes Chromosomes Cancer* 2001;30:393–401.

135. Montesinos-Rongen M, Zuhlke-Jenisch R, Gesk S, et al. Interphase cytogenetic analysis of lymphoma-associated chromosomal break-

points in primary diffuse large B-cell lymphomas of the central nervous system. *J Neuropathol Exp Neurol* 2002;61:926–933.

136. Weber T, Weber RG, Kaulich K, et al. Characteristic chromosomal imbalances in primary central nervous system lymphomas of the diffuse large B-cell type. *Brain Pathol* 2000;10:73–84.

137. Rickert CH, Dockhorn-Dworniczak B, Simon R, et al. Chromosomal imbalances in primary lymphomas of the central nervous system. *Am J Pathol* 1999;155:1445–1451.

138. Peters K, Zettl A, Starostik P, et al. Genetic imbalances in primary gastric diffuse large B-cell lymphomas: comparison of comparative genomic hybridization, microsatellite, and cytogenetic analysis. *Diagn Mol Pathol* 2000;9:58–65.

139. Starostik P, Greiner A, Schultz A, et al. Genetic aberrations common in gastric high-grade large B-cell lymphoma. *Blood* 2000;95:1180–1187.

140. Chan WY, Wong N, Chan AB, et al. Consistent copy number gain in chromosome 12 in primary diffuse large cell lymphomas of the stomach. *Am J Pathol* 1998;152:11–16.

141. Romaguera JE, Pugh W, Luthra R, et al. The clinical relevance of t(14;18)/BCL-2 rearrangement and DEL 6q in diffuse large cell lymphoma and immunoblastic lymphoma. *Ann Oncol* 1993;4:51–54.

142. Bastard C, Deweindt C, Kerckaert JP, et al. LAZ3 rearrangements in non-Hodgkin's lymphoma: correlation with histology, immunophenotype, karyotype, and clinical outcome in 217 patients. *Blood* 1994;83:2423–2427.

143. Kramer MH, Hermans J, Wijburg E, et al. Clinical relevance of BCL2, BCL6, and MYC rearrangements in diffuse large B-cell lymphoma. *Blood* 1998;92:3152–3162.

144. Vitolo U, Gaidano G, Botto B, et al. Rearrangements of bcl-6, bcl-2, c-myc and 6q deletion in B-diffuse large-cell lymphoma: clinical relevance in 71 patients. *Ann Oncol* 1998;9:55–61.

145. Offit K, Wong G, Filippa DA, et al. Cytogenetic analysis of 434 consecutively ascertained specimens of non-Hodgkin's lymphoma: clinical correlations. *Blood* 1991;77:1508–1515.

146. Offit K, Chaganti RS. Chromosomal aberrations in non-Hodgkin's lymphoma. Biologic and clinical correlations. *Hematol Oncol Clin North Am* 1991;5:853–869.

147. Johansson B, Mertens F, Mitelman F. Cytogenetic evolution patterns in non-Hodgkin's lymphoma. *Blood* 1995;86:3905–3914.

148. Maljaei SH, Brito-Babapulle V, Hiorns LR, et al. Abnormalities of chromosomes 8, 11, 14, and X in T-prolymphocytic leukemia studied by fluorescence in situ hybridization. *Cancer Genet Cytogenet* 1998;103:110–116.

149. Schlegelberger B, Himmler A, Bartles H, et al. Recurrent chromosome abnormalities in peripheral T-cell lymphomas. *Cancer Genet Cytogenet* 1994;78:15–22.

150. Soulier J, Pierron G, Vecchione D, et al. A complex pattern of recurrent chromosomal losses and gains in T-cell prolymphocytic leukemia. *Genes Chromosomes Cancer* 2001;31:248–254.

151. Madani A, Choukroun V, Soulier J, et al. Expression of p13MTCP1 is restricted to mature T-cell proliferations with t(X;14) translocations. *Blood* 1996;87:1923–1927.

152. Ohshima K, Haraokaa S, Ishihara S, et al. Analysis of chromosome 6q deletion in EBV-associated NK cell leukaemia/lymphoma. *Leuk Lymphoma* 2002;43:293–300.

153. Wong KF. Genetic changes in natural killer cell neoplasms. *Leuk Res* 2002;26:977–978.

154. Siu LL, Wong KF, Chan JK, et al. Comparative genomic hybridization analysis of natural killer cell lymphoma/leukemia. Recognition of consistent patterns of genetic alterations. *Am J Pathol* 1999;155:1419–1425.

155. Kamada N, Sakurai M, Miyamoto K, et al. Chromosome abnormalities in adult T-cell leukemia/lymphoma: a karyotype review committee report. *Cancer Res* 1992;52:1481–1493.

156. Itoyama T, Chaganti RS, Yamada Y, et al. Cytogenetic analysis and clinical significance in adult T-cell leukemia/lymphoma: a study of 50 cases from the human T-cell leukemia virus type-1 endemic area, Nagasaki. *Blood* 2001;97:3612–3620.

157. Tsukasaki K, Krebs J, Nagai K, et al. Comparative genomic hybridization analysis in adult T-cell leukemia/lymphoma: correlation with clinical course. *Blood* 2001;97:3875–3881.

158. Jonveaux P, Daniel MT, Martel V, et al. Isochromosome 7q and trisomy 8 are consistent primary, non-random chromosomal abnormalities associated with hepatosplenic T gamma/delta lymphoma. *Leukemia* 1996;10:1453–1455.

159. Alonsozana EL, Stamberg J, Kumar D, et al. Isochromosome 7q: the primary cytogenetic abnormality in hepatosplenic gammadelta T cell lymphoma. *Leukemia* 1997;11:1367–1372.

160. Mao X, Lillington D, Scarisbrick JJ, et al. Molecular cytogenetic analysis of cutaneous T-cell lymphomas: identification of common genetic alterations in Sézary syndrome and mycosis fungoides. *Br J Dermatol* 2002;147:464–475.

161. Thangavelu M, Finn WG, Yelavarthi KK, et al. Recurring structural chromosome abnormalities in peripheral blood lymphocytes of patients with mycosis fungoides/Sézary syndrome. *Blood* 1997;89:3371–3377.

162. Lepretre S, Buchonnet G, Stamatoullas A, et al. Chromosome abnormalities in peripheral T-cell lymphoma. *Cancer Genet Cytogenet* 2000;117:71–79.

163. Schlegelberger B, Feller AC. Classification of peripheral T-cell lymphomas: cytogenetic findings support the updated Kiel classification. *Leuk Lymphoma* 1996;20:411–416.

164. Schlegelberger B, Feller A, Godde E, et al. Stepwise development of chromosomal abnormalities in angioimmunoblastic lymphadenopathy. *Cancer Genet Cytogenet* 1990;50:15–29.

165. Kaneko Y, Maseki N, Sakurai M, et al. Characteristic karyotypic pattern in T-cell lymphoproliferative disorders with reactive "angioimmunoblastic lymphadenopathy with dysproteinemia-type" features. *Blood* 1988:;72:413–421.

166. Schlegelberger B, Zwingers T, Hohenadel K, et al. Significance of cytogenetic findings for the clinical outcome in patients with T-cell lymphoma of angioimmunoblastic lymphadenopathy type. *J Clin Oncol* 1996;14:593–599.

167. Mason DY, Bastard C, Rimokh R, et al. CD30-positive large cell lymphomas ("Ki-1 lymphoma") are associated with a chromosomal translocation involving 5q35. *Br J Haematol* 1990;74:161–168.

168. Weisenburger DD, Gordon BG, Vose JM, et al. Occurrence of the t(2;5)(p23;q35) in non-Hodgkin's lymphoma. *Blood* 1996;87:3860–3868.

169. Falini B. Anaplastic large cell lymphoma: pathological, molecular and clinical features. *Br J Haematol* 2001;114:741–760.

170. Morris SW, Xue L, Ma Z, et al. Alk+ CD30+ lymphomas: a distinct molecular genetic subtype of non-Hodgkin's lymphoma. *Br J Haematol* 2001;113:275–295.

171. Gaidano G, Hauptschein RS, Parsa NZ, et al. Deletions involving two distinct regions of 6q in B-cell non-Hodgkin lymphoma. *Blood* 1992;80:1781–1787.

172. Itoyama T, Nanjungud G, Chen W, et al. Molecular cytogenetic analysis of genomic instability at the 1q12-22 chromosomal site in B-cell non-Hodgkin lymphoma. *Genes Chromosomes Cancer* 2002;35:318–328.

173. Callanan MB, Le Baccon P, Mossuz P, et al. The IgG Fc receptor, FcgammaRIIB, is a target for deregulation by chromosomal translocation in malignant lymphoma. *Proc Natl Acad Sci U S A* 2000;97:309–314.

174. Chen W, Palanisamy N, Schmidt H, et al. Deregulation of FCGR2B expression by 1q21 rearrangements in follicular lymphomas. *Oncogene* 2001;20:7686–7693.

175. Dyomin VG, Palanisamy N, Lloyd KO, et al. MUC1 is activated in a B-cell lymphoma by the t(1;14)(q21;q32) translocation and is rearranged and amplified in B-cell lymphoma subsets. *Blood* 2000;95:2666–2671.

176. Levine EG, Bloomfield CD. Cytogenetics of non-Hodgkin's lymphoma. *J Natl Cancer Inst Monogr* 1990:7–12.

177. Schouten HC, Sanger WG, Weisenburger DD, et al. Chromosomal abnormalities in untreated patients with non-Hodgkin's lymphoma: associations with histology, clinical characteristics, and treatment outcome. The Nebraska Lymphoma Study Group. *Blood* 1990;75:1841–1847.

178. Rodriguez MA, Ford RJ, Goodacre A, et al. Chromosome 17- and p53 changes in lymphoma. *Br J Haematol* 1991;79:575–582.

179. Schoch C, Rieder H, Stollmann-Gibbels B, et al. 17p anomalies in lymphoid malignancies: diagnostic and prognostic implications. *Leuk Lymphoma* 1995;17:271–279.

CHAPTER 50

Molecular Genetics of Lymphoma

Riccardo Dalla-Favera and Laura Pasqualucci

Many advances have been made in the understanding of the pathogenesis of non-Hodgkin's lymphoma derived from B cells (B-cell non-Hodgkin's lymphoma), whereas with few exceptions, the molecular basis of T-cell–derived non-Hodgkin's lymphoma remains relatively undefined. This chapter focuses on: (a) the putative cellular derivation of the various subtypes of non-Hodgkin's lymphoma, (b) the mechanisms of genetic alteration that are associated with the development of non-Hodgkin's lymphoma, and (c) the description of the most frequent and biologically important genetic lesions associated with the major subtypes of non-Hodgkin's lymphoma. Additional details can be found in the chapters describing each non-Hodgkin's lymphoma subtype.

CELLULAR DERIVATION OF LYMPHOMA

The cellular derivation of non-Hodgkin's lymphomas can be identified by comparing the lineage and the differentiation stage of a given type of lymphoma with the features proper for the different maturation stages of normal lymphocytes. To date, the cellular derivation of lymphomas arising from B cells (approximately 85% of the cases) has been sufficiently clarified, whereas it is still relatively undefined in the case of lymphomas originating from T cells (approximately 15% of the cases).

B lymphocytes are generated in the bone marrow as precursor B cells, which first undergo immunoglobulin (Ig) gene rearrangements of the heavy chain locus, followed by rearrangements of the light chain loci (1,2). Immature B cells, which express a functional surface antibody acting as an antigen receptor, are positively selected into the peripheral B-cell pool, whereas cells failing to express a functional antigen receptor are eliminated within the bone marrow (1). For many B cells, the subsequent maturation steps are linked to the encounter with the antigen and to the formation of germinal centers, the sites where B cells are selected based on their affinity to T-cell–dependent antigens (3). The germinal center is constituted by a dark zone, characterized by rapidly proliferating B cells called *centro-blasts*, and by a light zone, in which B cells cease to proliferate and mature to centrocytes, which are induced to differentiate

through interactions with follicular dendritic cells and T helper cells (Fig. 50.1) (4). Within the germinal center, antigen-activated B cells accumulate somatic point mutations in their rearranged heavy and light chain genes, a phenomenon known as *somatic hypermutation*, which modifies the affinity of their surface antibody to the antigen (3,5). Only B cells that have acquired mutations leading to high-affinity binding are positively selected and differentiate into memory B cells or plasma cells, whereas the majority of B cells are eliminated by apoptosis within the germinal center (6). Thus, the presence of somatic mutations in the variable (V) region of Ig genes can be used as a marker of germinal center transit, allowing the definition of two categories of B-cell lymphoma (7):

(a) Non-Hodgkin's lymphoma lacking IgV mutations. This category includes pre–germinal center–derived non-Hodgkin's lymphomas such as most cases of mantle cell lymphoma. In addition, this category includes tumors deriving from B cells that did not undergo a germinal center reaction, such as approximately one-third of B-cell chronic lymphocytic leukemia/small lymphocytic lymphoma cases (7).

(b) Non-Hodgkin's lymphoma with IgV mutations. These tumors are derived from germinal center or post–germinal center B cells. Among all non-Hodgkin's lymphomas, subtypes associated with IgV somatic hypermutation include Burkitt's lymphoma, follicular lymphoma, lymphoplasmacytic lymphoma, mucosa-associated lymphoid tissue (MALT) lymphoma, and diffuse large B-cell lymphoma (7–15). In addition, the majority of B-cell chronic lymphocytic leukemias/small lymphocytic lymphomas are believed to originate from post–germinal center memory B cells (15).

MECHANISMS OF GENETIC LESION IN LYMPHOMA

Similar to most types of cancer, the pathogenesis of lymphoma represents a multistep process that involves the clonal accumulation of multiple genetic lesions affecting proto-oncogenes and tumor suppressor genes. Nonetheless, several features distinguish the mechanism and type of genetic

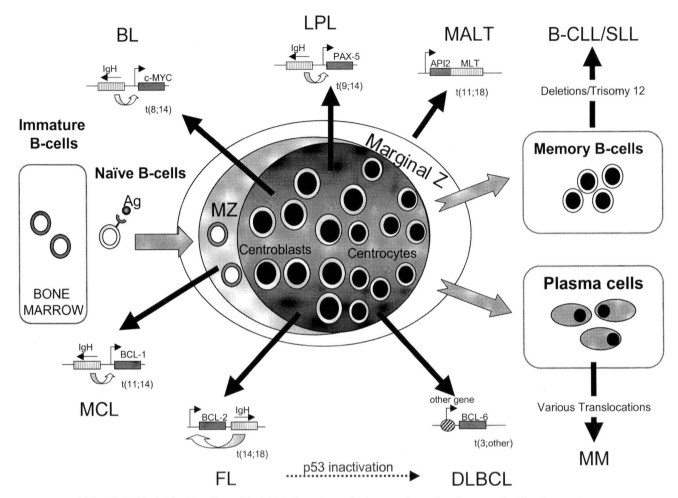

FIG. 50.1. Model for B-cell non-Hodgkin's lymphoma histogenesis and pathogenesis. The figure shows a schematic representation of a lymphoid follicle, constituted by the germinal center (GC) and the mantle zone (MZ) along with the surrounding marginal zone (Marginal Z). B cells that have successfully rearranged their V(D)J genes in the bone marrow move to peripheral lymphoid organs as naïve B cells. On encounter with a T-cell–dependent antigen (Ag), B cells become proliferating centroblasts in the GC and eventually mature into centrocytes. These events are associated with the activation of somatic hypermutation and immunoglobulin (Ig) isotype switch. Only GC B cells with high affinity for the antigen are positively selected to exit the GC and further differentiate into plasma cells or memory B cells, whereas low-affinity clones are eliminated by apoptosis. Based on the absence or presence of somatically mutated IgV genes, B-cell non-Hodgkin's lymphoma may be distinguished into two broad histogenetic categories: (a) B-cell non-Hodgkin's lymphoma derived from pre-GC B cells and devoid of Ig mutations, exemplified in the figure by mantle cell lymphoma (MCL); and (b) B-cell non-Hodgkin's lymphoma derived from B cells that have transited through the GC and harbor Ig mutations, exemplified in the figure by follicular lymphoma (FL), lymphoplasmacytoid lymphoma (LPL), mucosa-associated lymphoid tissue (MALT) lymphoma, diffuse large B-cell lymphoma (DLBCL), and Burkitt's lymphoma (BL). In B-cell chronic lymphocytic leukemia/small lymphocytic lymphoma (B-CLL/SLL), more than 50% of the cases carry mutated Ig genes, suggesting a derivation from a GC-experienced B cell, possibly a memory B cell. The genetic lesion most commonly associated to the various lymphoma subtypes is schematically shown for each tumor type. In the case of B-CLL/SLL, as well as in a subset of DLBCL, the relevant cancer-related gene has not been identified. MM, multiple myeloma.

lesions associated with lymphoma from those associated with solid tumors, especially the ones deriving from epithelial tissues. Cytogenetic studies have shown that the genome of lymphoma cells is relatively stable and is not affected by the massive instability typical of many solid tumors, particularly carcinomas (16). Lymphoma, with the possible exception of MALT lymphoma, appears also devoid of defects in DNA mismatch repair genes observed in some hereditary cancer predisposition syndromes as well as, more rarely, in most types of sporadic tumors (17–20). Conversely, the

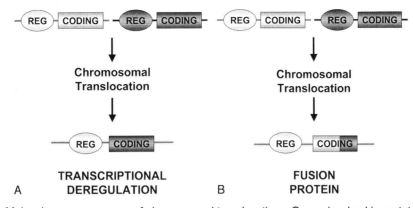

FIG. 50.2. Molecular consequences of chromosomal translocations. Genes involved in prototypic chromosomal translocations are shown schematically, with their regulatory (REG) and coding sequences. Only one side of the balanced, reciprocal translocations is indicated. Chromosomal translocations may lead to two different outcomes. In the case of transcriptional deregulation **(A)**, the normal REG sequences of the proto-oncogene are removed and substituted with REG sequences derived from the partner chromosome. The proto-oncogene coding sequences become, therefore, juxtaposed to heterologous REG sequences, resulting in dysregulated expression of the proto-oncogene. The novel REG regions can derive from the immunoglobulin loci or from other loci. In the case of fusion proteins **(B)**, the coding sequences of the two involved genes are joined in-frame into a chimeric transcriptional unit encoding for a novel fusion protein whose biochemical properties are distinct from those of the native proteins.

genome of lymphoma cells is characterized by few, sometimes single, nonrandom chromosomal abnormalities, commonly represented by chromosomal translocations (21).

At the molecular level, the genetic lesions identified so far in lymphomas include activation of oncogenes—either by chromosomal translocations or by mutations introduced by the aberrant activity of the somatic hypermutation mechanism—and inactivation of tumor suppressor loci, which can occur by chromosomal deletion and mutation. In addition, the genome of certain lymphoma subtypes can be altered via the introduction of exogenous genes by various types of oncogenic viruses.

Chromosomal Translocations

Chromosomal translocations are found in malignancies derived from the hematopoietic system, including the lymphoid system, and in sarcomas. As in other types of tumors, chromosomal translocations associated with non-Hodgkin's lymphoma represent reciprocal and balanced recombination events between two specific chromosomes, which are recurrently associated with a given tumor type and clonally represented in each tumor case.

The mechanisms responsible for chromosomal translocations are not clearly understood. Several observations suggest that the translocation process occurs most likely during Ig and TCR gene rearrangements in B and T cells, respectively, as a consequence of errors in the mechanisms that mediate the remodeling of these genes during lymphoid cell development. In particular, chromosomal translocations may derive from errors of: (a) the variable diversity joining (VDJ) recombination machinery, which functions in immature B

cells; (b) the class-switch recombination mechanism, which functions in mature B cells both within and outside the germinal centers; and (c) the somatic hypermutation mechanism, which operates in germinal center B cells (22,23). Because VDJ recombination, class-switch recombination, and, possibly, somatic hypermutation involve double-strand DNA breaks (24–26), translocations may represent the outcome of illegitimate recombinations that occur between antigen receptor loci (Ig and TCR) and other loci or between non-Ig loci.

The common feature of all chromosomal translocations associated with non-Hodgkin's lymphoma is the presence of a proto-oncogene in the proximity of the chromosomal recombination sites. In most cases, the structure of the proto-oncogene and, in particular, its coding domain are not affected by the translocation, but the pattern of expression of the involved gene is altered as a consequence of the juxtaposition of heterologous regulatory sequences derived from the partner chromosome (proto-oncogene deregulation) (Fig. 50.2). Two distinct types of proto-oncogene deregulation may be distinguished, including homotopic and heterotopic deregulation. Homotopic deregulation occurs when a proto-oncogene, whose expression is tightly regulated in normal lymphoid cells, becomes constitutively expressed in the lymphoma. Conversely, heterotopic deregulation occurs when the proto-oncogene, which is normally not expressed in lymphoid cells, undergoes ectopic expression in the tumor cells.

An alternative mechanism of oncogene activation by chromosomal translocation is represented by the juxtaposition of coding sequences derived from the two involved genes, which result in gene fusions coding for a novel chimeric protein (Fig. 50.2). This mechanism, which is common in chro-

TABLE 50.1. *Chromosomal translocations associated with non-Hodgkin's lymphoma (NHL)*

NHL histologic subtype	Translocation	Proto-oncogene involved	Mechanism of proto-oncogene activation	Proto-oncogene function
Mantle cell lymphoma	t(11;14)(q13;q32)	*BCL1* (cyclinD1)	Transcriptional deregulation	Cell-cycle regulator
Burkitt's lymphoma	t(8;14)(q24;q32), t(2;8)(p11;q24), t(8;22)(q24;q11)	*cMYC*	Transcriptional deregulation	Transcription factor regulating cell proliferation and growth
Follicular lymphoma	t(14;18)(q32;q21), t(2;18)(p11;q21), t(18;22)(q21;q11)	*BCL2*	Transcriptional deregulation	Negative regulator of apoptosis
Mucosa-associated lymphoid tissue lymphoma	t(11;18)(q21;q21)	API2/MLT	Fusion protein	API2 has antiapoptotic activity
	t(1;14)(p22;q32)	BCL10	Transcriptional deregulation	Antiapoptosis (?)
Diffuse large B-cell lymphoma	der(3)(q27)	BCL6	Transcriptional deregulation	Transcriptional repressor required for germinal center formation
Lymphoplasmacytic lymphoma	t(9;14)(p13;q32)	PAX5	Transcriptional deregulation	Transcription factor regulating B-cell proliferation and differentiation
T-cell anaplastic large-cell lymphoma	t(2;5)(p23;q35)	*NPM-ALK*	Fusion protein	*ALK* is a tyrosine kinase

mosomal translocations associated with acute leukemias, is rarely associated with non-Hodgkin's lymphoma. Examples are represented by the t(11;18) of MALT lymphoma and the t(2;5) of T-cell anaplastic lymphoma.

The molecular cloning of the genetic loci involved in the translocations most frequently associated with various non-Hodgkin's lymphoma subtypes has led to the identification of a number of proto-oncogenes implicated in lymphomagenesis (Table 50.1). The structural and functional consequences of each chromosomal translocation associated with non-Hodgkin's lymphoma are described in the sections Molecular Pathogenesis of B-Cell Non-Hodgkin's Lymphoma and Molecular Pathogenesis of T-Cell Non-Hodgkin's Lymphoma.

Aberrant Somatic Hypermutation

Recently, it has been shown that the process of somatic hypermutation can malfunction and target non-Ig genes in a large fraction of diffuse large B-cell lymphoma cases (27). In normal germinal center B cells, the somatic hypermutation process targets the V region of the Ig genes as well as the 5' region of other genes, including the *BCL6* proto-oncogene, the genes encoding the Fas/CD95 apoptosis receptor, and the CD79 component of the B-cell receptor (28–33). Whereas hypermutation of IgV sequences allows the selection of B cells with increased affinity for the antigen, the role of mutations found in these other genes remains obscure. In more than 50% of diffuse large B-cell lymphoma cases, the somatic hypermutation mechanism appears to misfire and target the 5' sequences of a number of additional genes, including several proto-oncogenes, such as *PIM1*, which encodes a signal transduction molecule with proven oncogenic

potential; *cMYC*, which encodes a transcription factor involved in the control of cell proliferation and differentiation and is one of the most frequently altered human oncogenes; *PAX5*, which encodes a transcription factor necessary for B-cell proliferation and whose expression is deregulated by chromosomal translocations in lymphoplasmacytic lymphoma; and *RhoH/TTF*, which encodes for a small G protein belonging to the RAS superfamily (27). In the case of *PIM1* and *cMYC*, the mutations affect nontranslated as well as coding regions, leading to amino acid changes with potential functional consequences. This abnormal activity may represent a powerful mechanism of malignant transformation because it may have an effect on a multitude of genes, only part of which may have been identified so far. However, a comprehensive characterization of the potentially extensive genetic damage caused by aberrant somatic hypermutation is still lacking.

Other Mechanisms of Proto-Oncogene Alteration

Additional mechanisms can alter the structure or the pattern of expression of proto-oncogenes in non-Hodgkin's lymphoma. Proto-oncogene amplification is substantially less common than in epithelial cancers, yet it can be observed in some high-grade non-Hodgkin's lymphomas, as exemplified by the case of *REL* amplifications in diffuse large B cell lymphoma (34). Gene amplification may involve many other unknown chromosomal sites, which are likely to be revealed by the extensive use of advanced cytogenetic techniques such as comparative genomic hybridization (35). Point mutations, presumably independent of the somatic hypermutation mechanism, rarely target the *RAS* proto-oncogenes in non-Hodgkin's lymphoma, despite the fact that these genes are among the most frequently mutated ones in other types of human cancer (36).

Inactivation of Tumor Suppressor Genes

Although deletions and mutations of the *p53* tumor suppressor gene represent the most common genetic alteration in human cancer (37), these lesions are relatively rare in non-Hodgkin's lymphoma and are restricted to the late stages of follicular lymphoma and Burkitt's lymphoma (38–40). The mechanism of *p53* inactivation in non-Hodgkin's lymphoma is similar to that detected in other types of tumor and occurs through point mutation of one allele and chromosomal deletion of the second allele (37).

Non-Hodgkin's lymphomas are also associated with specific chromosomal deletions, suggesting the loss of still unidentified tumor suppressor genes. The most frequent of these deletions involves the long arm of chromosome 6 (6q) (16,41). The observation that 6q deletions may occur as the sole cytogenetic abnormality in some non-Hodgkin's lymphoma cases (16) and are associated with poor prognosis (21) strongly supports a pathogenetic role for these alterations. Deletions of chromosome 13q14 represent the most frequent lesion in B-cell chronic lymphocytic leukemia/small lymphocytic lymphoma, occurring in more than 50% of cases (16). Mapping studies have ruled out the involvement of the *RB1* tumor suppressor gene, which is also located on chromosome 13q14, and have suggested the presence of a distinct tumor suppressor gene in the same region (42–48).

Finally, tumor suppressor inactivation can occur via epigenetic mechanisms such as transcriptional inactivation by hypermethylation of the promoter region. This mechanism is responsible for the lack of expression of the *p16* tumor suppressor gene in a variety of non-Hodgkin's lymphoma subtypes (49–53).

Oncogenic Viruses

Oncogenic viruses introduce foreign genes into their target cells or alter cellular genes by inserting their genome. Three distinct viruses are associated with the pathogenesis of specific non-Hodgkin's lymphoma subtypes: the human T-cell leukemia virus type I, the Epstein-Barr virus, and the human herpesvirus-8.

Human T-Cell Leukemia Virus Type I

Human T-cell leukemia virus type I, the first human pathogenic retrovirus isolated, is the etiologic agent of the malignant CD4+ adult T-cell leukemia/lymphoma (54–56). Unlike acutely transforming retroviruses, the human T-cell leukemia virus type I genome does not encode a viral oncogene (54–56). In addition, this retrovirus does not transform T cells by *cis*-activation of an adjacent cellular proto-oncogene

because the provirus appears to integrate randomly within the host genome. Rather, the pathogenetic effect of human T-cell leukemia virus type I seems to be due to viral production of a *trans*-regulatory protein (human T-cell leukemia virus type I tax) that markedly increases expression of all viral gene products and transcriptionally activates the expression of certain host genes, including interleukin *(IL)*-2, the α-chain of the IL-2 receptor (CD25), *c-SIS*, *c-FOS*, and granulocyte-macrophage colony-stimulating factor (54–61). The central role of these genes in normal T-cell activation and growth, coupled to direct experimental evidence, supports the notion that tax-mediated activation of these host genes represents an important mechanism by which human T-cell leukemia virus type I initiates T-cell transformation (62). In addition, there are suggestions that tax may mediate DNA damage as a consequence of either inactivation of the *p53* checkpoint or a repression of DNA repair functions (63,64). Recently, it has been shown that tax may abrogate a mitotic checkpoint by targeting the TXBP181 cellular gene, a homolog of the yeast mitotic checkpoint MAD1 protein (65). These features of tax are consistent with the fact that adult T-cell leukemia/lymphoma cells are karyotypically abnormal and frequently present as pleomorphic multinucleated giant cells (66,67).

Epstein-Barr Virus

Epstein-Barr virus was initially identified in cases of endemic Burkitt's lymphoma from Africa; subsequently, Epstein-Barr virus was also detected in a fraction of sporadic forms of Burkitt's lymphomas, acquired immunodeficiency syndrome–associated lymphomas, and primary effusion lymphomas (39,68–77). On infection of a B lymphocyte, the Epstein-Barr virus genome is transported into the nucleus where it exists predominantly as an extrachromosomal circular molecule (episome) (68). The formation of circular episomes is mediated by the cohesive terminal repeats, which are represented by a variable number of tandem repeats sequence (68,78). Because of this termini heterogeneity, the number of tandem repeats sequences enclosed in newly formed episomes may differ considerably, thus representing a constant clonal marker of the episome and, consequently, of a single infected cell (68,78). Evidence for a pathogenetic role of the virus in Epstein-Barr virus–infected non-Hodgkin's lymphomas is at least twofold: (a) It is well recognized that Epstein-Barr virus is able to significantly alter the growth of B cells (68), and (b) Epstein-Barr virus–infected lymphomas usually display a single form of fused Epstein-Barr virus termini, suggesting that Epstein-Barr virus was present in the single cell from which the clonal expansion of the tumor originated (39,70).

Human Herpesvirus-8

Human herpesvirus-8 is a gammaherpesvirus that was initially identified in tissues of acquired immunodeficiency syndrome–related Kaposi's sarcoma and subsequently found to infect a peculiar type of lymphoma, known as *primary effusion lymphoma* (79–84), as well as a substantial fraction of multicentric Castleman's disease (85). Phylogenetic analysis has shown that the closest relative of human herpesvirus-8 is herpesvirus saimiri, a gamma-2 herpesvirus of primates associated with T-cell lymphoproliferative disorders (85–87). As with other gammaherpesviruses, human herpesvirus-8 is also lymphotropic because it can be found in lymphocytes both *in vitro* and *in vivo* (79–84). Lymphoma cells naturally infected by human herpesvirus-8 harbor the viral genome in its episomal configuration and display a marked restriction of viral gene expression, suggesting a pattern of latent infection (87). Human herpesvirus-8 carries several genes that may behave as oncogenes, including a gene homologous to the cellular D-type cyclins, a G protein coupled receptor displaying constitutive activation, and several genes encoding for molecules that share high homology with cellular cytokines (viral IL-6) and chemokines (viral MIP-1α, MIP-II) (88–90). However, because primary effusion lymphoma cells carry latent human herpesvirus-8 infection, only a restricted subset of viral genes is expressed *in vivo*, including viral cyclin D and viral IL-6 (88–91).

MOLECULAR PATHOGENESIS OF B-CELL NON-HODGKIN'S LYMPHOMA

Specific genetic lesions have been found associated with distinct B-cell non-Hodgkin's lymphoma subtypes classified according to the World Health Organization Classification of lymphoid neoplasia (92,93). The following section focuses on well-characterized lesions associated with major B-cell non-Hodgkin's lymphoma subtypes, including mantle cell lymphoma, diffuse large B-cell lymphoma, follicular lymphoma, Burkitt's lymphoma, MALT lymphoma, B-cell chronic lymphocytic leukemia/small lymphocytic lymphoma, and lymphoplasmacytic lymphoma. The molecular pathogenesis of other B-cell non-Hodgkin's lymphoma types is far less understood.

Mantle Cell Lymphoma

Chromosomal Translocations Involving BCL1

Mantle cell lymphoma is typically associated with t(11;14) (q13;q32), which can be detected in up to 70% of cases (Fig. 50.1 and Table 50.1) (93–99). The t(11;14)(q13;q32) translocation juxtaposes the BCL1 locus at 11q13 to the IgH locus, leading to homotopic deregulation of BCL1 (also known as *CCND1* or *PRAD1*) (100–102). The BCL1 gene encodes for cyclin D1, a member of the D-type G1 cyclins that regulate the early phases of cell cycle (97,103–106). The consistent and selective clustering of BCL1 expression with non-Hodgkin's lymphoma carrying t(11;14) strongly suggests that this gene is indeed the critical target of the t(11;14)(q13;q32) (97,103–106). By deregulating cyclin D1, t(11;14) is believed to deregulate cell-cycle control because this molecule acts primarily as a growth factor

sensor, integrating extracellular signals with the cell-cycle clock (107). The pathogenetic role of BCL1 deregulation in human neoplasia is suggested by the ability of cyclin D1 overexpression to transform cells *in vitro* and to contribute to B cell lymphomagenesis in transgenic mice (108–110).

Other Genetic Alterations

Less common genetic lesions, observed in aggressive variants of mantle cell lymphoma, include inactivation of the tumor suppressor genes p53 and p16 and mutations of the ATM gene. Mutations of p53 and deletions of the short arm of chromosome 17, frequently associated with p53 overexpression, occur in up to 15% of the cases and represent a marker of poor prognosis (111,112). Inactivation of p16 by deletion, mutation, or hypermethylation can be detected in approximately one-half of the cases belonging to the aggressive variant of mantle cell lymphoma, which is characterized by a blastoid cell morphology (50). Finally, ATM mutations, mainly associated with 11q22-23 deletions, have been identified more recently in this lymphoma subtype (113,114).

Burkitt's Lymphoma

Chromosomal Translocations Involving the cMYC Proto-Oncogene

Burkitt's lymphoma includes several variants (i.e., sporadic Burkitt's lymphoma, endemic Burkitt's lymphoma, and acquired immunodeficiency syndrome–associated Burkitt's lymphoma) (92,93). All Burkitt's lymphoma cases, including the leukemic variants, are associated with chromosomal translocations involving the cMYC locus on chromosome 8q24 and three alternative chromosomal regions, each one containing an Ig locus: IgH, Igκ, or Igλ (Table 50.1 and Fig. 50.3) (115–120). The IgH locus is involved in 80% of the cases, leading to t(8;14)(q24;q32). The remaining cases are characterized by t(2;8)(p11;q24), involving the Igκ locus (15% of cases), and t(8;22)(q24;q11), involving Igλ (5% of cases) (Table 50.1).

Although relatively homogeneous at the microscopic level, these translocations are very heterogeneous at the molecular level. The t(8;14) breakpoints are located 5' and centromeric to *cMYC*, whereas in t(2;8) and t(8;22), they map 3' to *cMYC* (115–120). Further molecular heterogeneity derives from the exact breakpoint sites on chromosomes 8 and 14 of t(8;14) (Fig. 50.3). In endemic Burkitt's lymphoma, the translocation generally involves sequences on chromosome 8, which are located at undefined distance [more than 100 kilobase (kb)] 5' to *cMYC*, and sequences on chromosome 14 within or in proximity of the Ig J_H region (121,122). In sporadic Burkitt's lymphoma, t(8;14) preferentially involves sequences located within or immediately 5' (less than 3 kb) to *cMYC* on chromosome 8 and sequences on chromosome 14 mapping within the Ig switch regions (121,122).

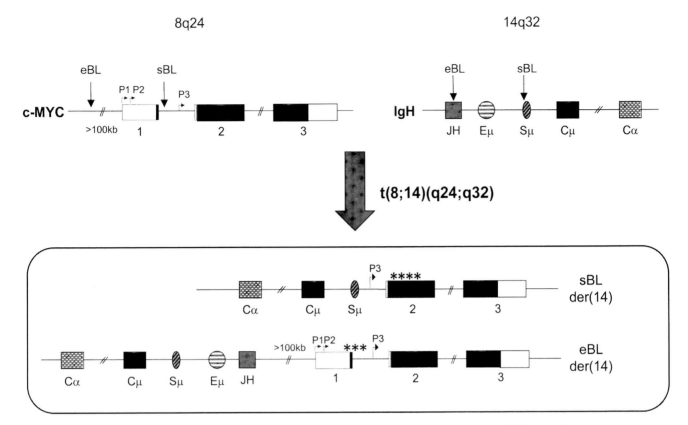

FIG. 50.3. Schematic representation of chromosomal translocations involving the *cMYC* locus. The germline configuration of the *cMYC* gene on chromosome 8q24 and the IgH locus on chromosome 14q32 are schematically shown (*top*). In its germline configuration, *cMYC* is comprised of three exons. Coding regions are indicated by black boxes, whereas noncoding regions are indicated by white boxes. The two major *cMYC* promoters within exon 1 (P1 and P2) and the minor P3 promoter, located 5' to exon 2, are shown by arrows. In the IgH locus, symbols represent the joining (J), switch (S), and constant (C) regions as well as the Ig enhancer (E). The breakpoint clusters associated with sporadic Burkitt's lymphoma (sBL) and endemic Burkitt's lymphoma (eBL) are indicated for both the 8q24 and the 14q32 chromosomal regions. Two distinct types of translocations can be recognized that preferentially associate with either sBL or eBL. In the case of t(8;14) of sBL, the breakpoints involve sequences within the intron 1 of the cMYC locus and sequences in the proximity of the Sμ region on the IgH locus. As a consequence, the cMYC gene is decapitated of its first exon. Because the physiologically active promoters of *cMYC* are removed, a novel transcriptional initiation site (P3), located within *cMYC* intron 1, is activated in *cMYC* alleles affected by this translocation. Notably, although the coding region of the translocated *cMYC* alleles is left intact, at the nucleotide level, these alleles frequently harbor point mutations (schematically represented by asterisks) within their exon 2 sequences, which lead to amino acid changes in the cMYC protein. The RNA transcribed from t(8;14) of sBL is comprised of *cMYC* exons 2 and 3, preceded by an abnormally transcribed sequence of intron 1 that starts from the novel transcriptional initiation site. Because the *cMYC* coding region remains intact, a normally sized cMYC protein is produced. In the case of t(8;14) of eBL, the *cMYC* breakpoint involves sequences on chromosome 8 located more than 100 kilobase (kb) 5' to the gene and sequences on chromosome 14 within or in proximity to the Ig JH region. The genomic configuration of the translocated *cMYC* allele is thus apparently preserved. However, *cMYC* alleles involved by t(8;14) of eBL consistently harbor point mutations clustering around the exon 1/intron 1 border, where *cMYC* regulatory regions are located (see asterisks). In addition and in common with t(8;14) of sBL, mutations within the cMYC exon 2 coding sequence are frequently detected in *cMYC* alleles affected by t(8;14) of eBL. The transcript from t(8;14) of eBL includes *cMYC* exons 1 through 3 and encodes for a normally sized cMYC protein. The functional consequences of t(8;14) on the expression of translocated *cMYC* alleles in both sBL and eBL are described in detail in the text. Only one side of the balanced, reciprocal t(8;14)(q24;q32) is shown. Variant translocations involving the *cMYC* locus and the Ig light chain genes are not shown.

The common effect of t(8;14), t(2;8), and t(8;22) is the ectopic activation (heterotopic deregulation) of *cMYC* expression in germinal center B cells, which normally do not express *cMYC* (123,124). Two distinct mechanisms may be responsible for *cMYC* deregulation: (a) juxtaposition of *cMYC* to heterologous enhancers derived from the Ig loci; and (b) structural alterations in the 5' regulatory sequences of the gene, which putatively alter the responsiveness to cell factors regulating its expression. In fact, the *cMYC* exon 1/ intron 1 boundary, where *cMYC* regulatory sequences are located, is either decapitated by the translocation or mutated in the translocated alleles (Fig. 50.3) (115–120,125). In addition to heterotopic deregulation, oncogenic conversion of *cMYC* may also be due to amino acid substitutions in the gene exon 2, which encodes the transactivation domain of the cMYC protein (126,127). These mutations are believed to affect various aspects of cMYC function, including the stability of the protein and its response to p107, a nuclear protein related to *RB1* (128,129).

The product of *cMYC* is a ubiquitously expressed nuclear phosphoprotein that functions as a transcriptional regulator, controlling cell proliferation, differentiation, and apoptosis (130–132). *In vivo*, cMYC is found mainly in heterodimeric complexes with the related protein MAX, and such interaction is required for cMYC-induced stimulation of transcription and cell proliferation (133–138). Conversely, MAX can form heterodimers with MAD and MXI1, two basic helix-loop-helix/leucine zipper proteins that act as negative regulators of transcription (139,140). In non-Hodgkin's lymphoma carrying *cMYC* translocations, it is conceivable that constitutive expression of cMYC leads to the prevalence of cMYC/ MAX complexes over MAD/MAX and MXI1/MAX heterodimers, thus inducing positive growth regulation. In fact, expression of cMYC regulates transcription of a subset of target genes involved in cell metabolism, protein synthesis, and telomere maintenance (131,141). Substantial experimental evidence documents that the constitutive expression of cMYC can influence the growth of B cells *in vitro* and *in vivo*, consistent with a role in B-cell lymphomagenesis. *In vitro*, the expression of *cMYC* oncogenes transfected into Epstein-Barr virus–immortalized human B cells, a potential natural target for *cMYC* activation in Epstein-Barr virus–positive Burkitt's lymphoma, leads to their malignant transformation (142). *In vivo*, the targeted expression of *cMYC* oncogenes in the B-cell lineage of transgenic mice leads to the development of B-cell malignancy (143,144).

Other Genetic Alterations

Additional genetic lesions associated with Burkitt's lymphoma include p53 deletion/mutation, which is found in 30% of cases (Table 50.2) (38), and deletions of 6q, which are detected in approximately 30% of cases (41). Inactivation of p16 has also been reported in a fraction of cases (145). Another lesion that may contribute to the development of this malignancy is monoclonal Epstein-Barr virus infection, present in virtually all cases of endemic Burkitt's lymphoma and in approximately 30% of sporadic Burkitt's lymphoma (Table 50.2) (69–73). Because Epstein-Barr virus infection in Burkitt's lymphoma displays a latent infection phenotype characterized by the lack of expression of both Epstein-Barr virus–transforming antigens latent membrane protein-1 and Epstein Barr nuclear antigen 2, the precise pathogenetic role of the virus in these tumors remains controversial.

Follicular Lymphoma

Chromosomal Translocations Involving the BCL2 Proto-Oncogene

The most common chromosomal translocation associated with follicular lymphoma is represented by t(14;18)(q32;q21), which can be detected in 80% to 90% of the cases independent of the

---

TABLE 50.2. *Frequency of genetic lesions associated with B-cell non-Hodgkin's lymphoma*

Non-Hodgkin's lymphoma subtype	BCL1	BCL2	BCL6	cMYC	PAX5	API2/MLT	BCL10	p53	p16	EBV
B-cell chronic lymphocytic leukemia/small lymphocytic lymphoma	–	–	–	–	–	–	–	10%	–	–
Mantle cell lymphoma	70%	–	–	–	–	–	–	20%[a]	50%[a]	–
Burkitt's lymphoma	–	–	–	100%	–	–	–	30%	30%	30–100%[b]
Follicular lymphoma	–	90%	Rare	–	–	–	–	–	–	–
Mucosa-associated lymphoid tissue lymphoma	–	–	–	–	–	60%	Rare	–		
Diffuse large B-cell lymphoma	–	30%	35%	20%	–	–	–	30%	30%	–
Lymphoplasmacytic lymphoma	–	–	–	–	50%	–	–	–	–	–

–, molecular lesion or viral infection not involved; where positive, the percentage of affected cases is indicated.
[a]Fifty percent of the aggressive mantle cell lymphoma variant.
[b]Thirty percent in sporadic Burkitt's lymphoma; 100% in endemic Burkitt's lymphoma.

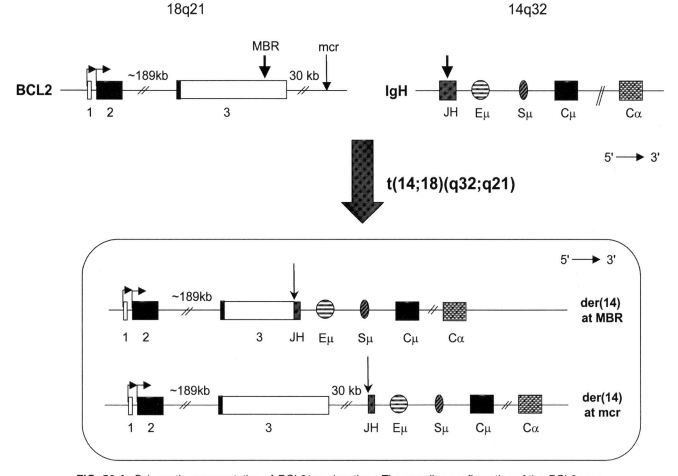

FIG. 50.4. Schematic representation of *BCL2* translocations. The germline configuration of the *BCL2* gene on chromosome 18q21 and part of the immunoglobulin H (IgH) locus on chromosome 14q32 are shown in the figure (*top*, not in scale). In its germline configuration, the *BCL2* gene is comprised of three exons separated by a large intron between exon 2 and exon 3. Black boxes represent coding regions, whereas white boxes represent noncoding regions. Only part of the IgH locus [from the switch (S) region to the constant (C) α region] is schematically shown. Color-coded symbols represent the joining (J), S, and C regions of IgH as well as the Ig enhancer (E). Alternative transcription initiation sites are indicated by arrows. In the majority of cases, t(14;18) breaks cluster within two regions: a major breakpoint region (MBR) in the 3' untranslated sequences and a minor cluster region (mcr) located approximately 20 kilobase (kb) downstream of the gene. The 14q32 breakpoint (indicated by a vertical arrow) maps within the JH segment. The molecular consequences of t(14;18)(q32;q21), including both the MBR and mcr types of translocations, are depicted in the bottom panel of the figure, only one side of the reciprocal, balanced translocation being shown. The translocation causes the juxtaposition of an intact *BCL2* coding domain telomeric and in the same transcriptional orientation to the IgH locus. Because the *BCL2* coding region is preserved, the chimeric *BCL2*/IgH transcript gives rise to a wild-type BCL2 protein, whose expression is dysregulated (see Chromosomal Translocations Involving the BCL2 Proto-Oncogene for a description of the functional consequences of BCL2 translocations on the transcriptional regulation of BCL2).

cytologic subtype (Table 50.1 and Fig. 50.1) (92,93). In this translocation, the rearrangement joins the BCL2 gene at its 3' untranslated region to an Ig J$_H$ segment (Fig. 50.4), resulting in homotopic deregulation of BCL2 expression (146–150). Approximately 70% of the breakpoints on chromosome 18 cluster within the major breakpoint region, whereas the remaining 5% to 25% usually map to the more distant minor cluster region (146–150). Rearrangements involving the 5' flanking region of BCL2 have also been reported in a minority of cases

(151). The consequence of the translocation is the presence within the cells of constitutively high levels of BCL2 protein, resulting from both enhanced transcription and, possibly, more efficient RNA processing (152,153).

BCL2 is a 26-kD integral membrane protein that has been localized to mitochondria, endoplasmic reticulum, and perinuclear membrane (154–158). The main function of the BCL2 protein is to control the cell threshold to enter apoptosis or programmed cell death. In the B-cell compartment, BCL2 appears to be important for the emergence of long-living memory cells by promoting survival of antigen-selected germinal center cells (159). Deregulation of BCL2 expression may contribute to the pathogenesis of follicular lymphoma by preventing apoptosis in germinal center cells that are normally destined to die (160). Indeed, *BCL2*-Ig transgenic mice develop a pattern of polyclonal hyperplasia characterized by mature, long-lived B cells resting in G0 (161,162). Despite the morphologic similarities, this pattern contrasts with the consistent monoclonality of human follicular lymphoma, indicating that *BCL2* activation is not sufficient for lymphoma development and that other genetic lesions or host factors are required. In fact, with time and analogous to the human disease, a fraction of the indolent follicular hyperplasia observed in *BCL2*-Ig transgenic mice progresses to aggressive, clonal diffuse large-cell lymphomas that have acquired additional genetic lesions (see below) (163).

Other Genetic Alterations

Deletions of chromosome 6 are found in approximately 20% of cases (41), whereas other genes commonly involved in lymphomagenesis, such as *cMYC* and *p53*, do not appear to be altered during the development of follicular lymphoma. Over time, follicular lymphoma tends to convert into an aggressive lymphoma with a diffuse large-cell architecture (Fig. 50.1) (92,93). This histologic transformation is generally accompanied by the accumulation of *p53* mutations and, in approximately 40% of cases, by inactivation of *p16* (Fig. 50.1) (40,50,164). In rare cases, rearrangements of *cMYC* may also occur during transformation of follicular lymphoma in diffuse large B-cell lymphoma (165).

Diffuse Large B-Cell Lymphoma

In contrast with other non-Hodgkin's lymphoma subtypes, diffuse large B-cell lymphoma is characterized by a marked biologic, phenotypic, and clinical heterogeneity. Based on the identification of different gene expression profiles and on their highly variable clinical course, it is believed that diffuse large B-cell lymphoma comprises multiple, presently unrecognized disease entities (166–168). This marked heterogeneity reflects in part the complex molecular pathogenesis of this disease, which includes specific lesions (i.e., rearrangements of the *BCL6* gene) as well as alterations common to other non-Hodgkin's lymphoma subtypes.

Alterations Affecting the BCL6 Locus

Chromosomal translocations affecting band 3q27 represent the most common and specific genetic abnormality associated with *de novo* diffuse large B-cell lymphoma (21,169). These alterations were shown to be "promiscuous" in that they involved balanced, reciprocal recombinations between the 3q27 region, containing the *BCL6* locus, and various alternative chromosomal partners in different diffuse large

B-cell lymphoma cases (170–174). The partner sites include, but are not limited to, those harboring the Ig heavy (14q32) or light (2p11, 22q11) chain genes.

The *BCL6* gene encodes for a 95-kD nuclear phosphoprotein belonging to the POZ/zinc-finger family of transcription factors (175). The BCL6 protein acts as a potent transcriptional repressor of promoter sequences containing its specific DNA recognition motif (176,177). In the B-cell lineage, expression of the BCL6 protein is restricted to germinal center cells, whereas it is absent in pre–germinal center B cells or in their differentiated progenies such as memory B cells and plasma cells (178,179). Mice deficient for BCL6 are not able to form germinal centers in response to T-cell–dependent antigens and, consequently, completely lack affinity maturation (180,181). Therefore, BCL6 appears to be a master regulator of germinal center development in which it represses the transcription of genes involved in activation, differentiation, apoptosis, and cell-cycle arrest, thereby favoring proliferation and survival (182–184).

Chromosomal translocations cause rearrangements of the *BCL6* gene in approximately 35% of diffuse large B-cell lymphoma cases and in a minority (5% to 10%) of follicular lymphoma cases (185). These rearrangements juxtapose the intact coding domain of *BCL6* downstream and in the same transcriptional orientation to heterologous sequences derived from the partner chromosome, including IgH (14q23), Igκ (2p11), Igλ (22q11), and at least twenty other chromosomal sites unrelated to the Ig loci (Fig. 50.5) (79,186,187). Among the genes identified so far in the partner chromosomal site are: *RhoH/TTF* (small guanosine triphosphatase of the RAS superfamily associated with cytoskeleton) (188), *BOB1* (B-cell coactivator) (189), L-*plastin* (actin-binding protein) (190), *H4* (histone) (191,192), *IKAROS* (193), *HSP89A* (heat shock protein) (194), MHC class II transactivator (*CIITA*), *PIM1* (serine threonine kinase), eukaryotic initiation factor 4AII (translation factor), and the transferrin receptor (195,196). The majority of these translocations result in a fusion transcript in which the promoter region and the exon 1 of Bcl6 are replaced by sequences derived from the partner gene (Fig. 50.5) (79,186,187). The common denominator of these promoters, when compared with BCL6, is a broader spectrum of activity throughout B-cell development, including expression in the post–germinal center differentiation stage such as immunoblasts and plasma cells (186). Consequently, the translocation is believed to prevent the downregulation of BCL6 expression that is normally associated with differentiation into post–germinal center cells. It is hypothesized that deregulated expression of a normal *BCL6* gene product may play a critical role by enforcing the proliferative phenotype typical of germinal center cells. However, a transgenic mouse model supporting this hypothesis has not been obtained yet.

In addition to chromosomal translocations, the 5' regulatory sequences of *BCL6* can be altered by multiple somatic mutations in up to 75% of diffuse large B cell lymphoma cases (29,164,197). These mutations, however, are introduced in normal germinal center B cells and are believed to be generated by

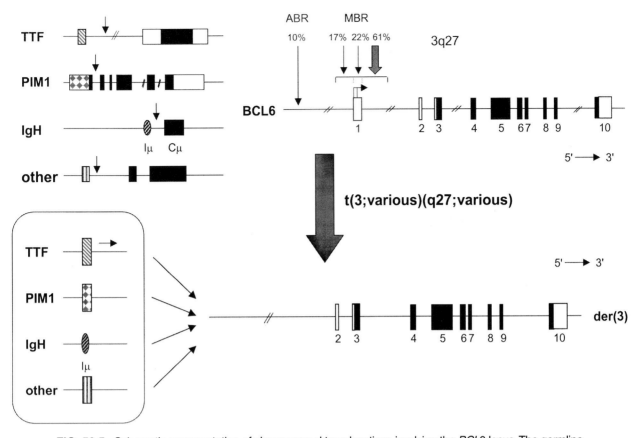

FIG. 50.5. Schematic representation of chromosomal translocations involving the *BCL6* locus. The germline configuration of the *BCL6* gene on chromosome 3q27 is shown in the upper-right panel of the figure, whereas representative *BCL6* translocation partners, including *TTF*, *PIM1*, immunoglobulin H (IgH), and other hypothetic genes (other), are shown on the upper-left panel. *BCL6* is comprised of ten exons, represented by empty (noncoding) and solid (coding) boxes. Arrows indicate the major and minor *BCL6* promoters in exon 1. The distribution and frequency of *BCL6* breaks within the major breakpoint cluster (MBR) and the alternative breakpoint cluster (ABR) are also shown (*vertical arrows*). The bottom panel shows the schematic representation of several derivatives on chromosome 3 after t(3q27) chromosomal translocations. Independent of the partner chromosome involved, the translocation decapitates the *BCL6* alleles of variable portions of their 5' noncoding domain. Novel sequences derived from the partner chromosomes are juxtaposed 5' to the *BCL6* coding sequences, providing heterologous regulatory sequences with distinct expression patterns such as the IgH germline transcript promoter Iμ (or Iγ) in the case of t(3;14), the *RhoH/TTF* promoter in the case of t(3;4), and the *PIM1* promoter in the case of t(3;6). Because the genomic configuration of the *BCL6* coding domain downstream to the breakpoint site is preserved, the translocation leads to deregulated expression of a normal BCL6 protein. Only one side of the balanced, reciprocal translocation is shown.

the same somatic hypermutation mechanism that targets Ig genes (29,30,33,197). Consistent with their association with the physiologic germinal center reaction, *BCL6* mutations are found in a fraction of all B-cell tumors carrying mutated IgV sequences and displaying a germinal center or post–germinal center phenotype, including B-cell chronic lymphocytic leukemia, Burkitt's lymphoma, follicular lymphoma, MALT lymphoma, and multiple myeloma as well as diffuse large B-cell lymphoma (29,33,164,197–199). Functional analysis of a number of mutated *BCL6* alleles has shown that some mutations are specifically associated with diffuse large B-cell lymphoma because they are not found in normal germinal center cells or in other B-cell malignancies (200). These mutations deregulate BCL6 transcription by disrupting an autoregulatory circuit in

which the BCL6 protein controls its own level of expression by binding to the promoter region of the gene (200,201). The full extent of *BCL6* mutations deregulating gene expression has not been characterized, indicating that the fraction of diffuse large B-cell lymphoma carrying abnormal BCL6 expression cannot be determined.

Aberrant Somatic Hypermutation

Approximately 50% of diffuse large B-cell lymphomas are associated with an aberrant activity of the somatic hypermutation mechanism (27). This aberrant activity targets several proto-oncogenes, including *cMYC*, *PIM1*, *PAX5*, and *RhoH/TTF* (see Mechanisms of Genetic Lesion in Lymphoma:

Aberrant Somatic Hypermutation). The number and identity of the genes targeted by the aberrant hypermutation mechanism vary in different cases and are still largely undefined. This mechanism may be responsible for the heterogeneity of diffuse large B-cell lymphoma via the alteration of different cellular pathways in different cases.

Other Genetic Lesions

Diffuse large B-cell lymphoma can be found associated with mutations and deletions of the *p53* tumor suppressor gene—mostly detectable in cases originating from the transformation of follicular lymphoma and therefore associated with chromosomal translocations involving *BCL2* (40). In addition, diffuse large B-cell lymphomas are associated with a variety of chromosomal translocations, including those involving the *cMYC* and *BCL2* loci, which, however, appear to be mutually exclusive with those involving BCL6 (21). In addition, a few sites of amplification have been identified, including those containing known proto-oncogenes as *REL*, *cMYC*, and *BCL2* (34,202). Finally, deletion or lack of expression of the *p16* tumor suppressor gene and mutations of the *ATM* gene have been reported in a minority of cases (203,204). Overall, the relative distribution of all these lesions has not been comprehensively assessed in large panels of diffuse large B-cell lymphoma cases.

Mucosa-Associated Lymphoid Tissue Lymphomas

Most cases of gastric MALT lymphomas are associated with *Helicobacter pylori* infection (205). It has been suggested that gastric MALT lymphomas may be dependent on antigen stimulation by *H. pylori* because the malignant lymphoid cells respond to *H. pylori* antigens and because the lymphoma may regress, at least partially, on eradication of infection (206). The potential role of antigen in MALT lymphoma pathogenesis is further supported by the observation that MALT lymphoma cells harbor the genotypic hallmark of antigen-experienced B cells (i.e., somatic hypermutation of Ig genes) (207–209).

Cytogenetic studies have pointed to several abnormalities specifically associated with these tumors. The most frequent of these abnormalities is t(11;18) (q21; q21) (16), which is observed in approximately 50% of MALT lymphomas independent of the site of origin (210,211). The genes involved in the t(11;18) are *API2* on 11q21 and *MLT* (*MALT-lymphoma translocation*) on 18q21. *API2* belongs to the family of *inhibitor of apoptosis proteins* (IAP), which plays an evolutionary conserved role in regulating programmed cell death in diverse species. The function of *MLT* appears to be to induce the activation of the NF-κB transcription complex (212). The *API2/MLT* fusion protein resulting from t(11;18)(q21;q21) appears also to activate the NF-κB complex, with antiapoptotic effects that may contribute to the pathogenesis of MALT lymphomas (210–212).

The second chromosomal abnormality associated with MALT lymphomas is t(1;14)(p22;q32), which occurs in a small fraction of cases and causes alterations of the *BCL10* gene (213,214). *BCL10* encodes an aminoterminal caspase recruitment domain homologous to that found in several apoptotic molecules (213,214). The wild type *BCL10* gene activates the NF-κB signaling cascade and is able to induce apoptosis in different cell types. It is interesting that the BCL10 protein forms a complex and synergizes with the MALT1 protein to activate the NF-κB transcription complex and inhibits apoptosis in normal cells (212). Thus, it is possible that both translocations associated with MALT lymphomas act on the same antiapoptotic pathway, with analogous biologic consequences in lymphomagenesis (212).

Finally, MALT lymphomas are associated with trisomy of chromosome 3, for which no molecular characterization is available (215), and with genetic alterations commonly detected in other lymphoma types, including *BCL6* rearrangements or mutations and *p53* mutations (33,164,216–218).

Small Lymphocytic Lymphoma/B-Cell Chronic Lymphocytic Leukemia

Different from other types of malignancies derived from mature B cells, the pathogenesis of B-cell chronic lymphocytic leukemia/small lymphocytic lymphoma is much less understood (Fig. 50.1). Despite initial suggestions, it is now well established that "true" cases of B-cell chronic lymphocytic leukemia/small lymphocytic lymphoma [i.e., CD5+ and CD23+ according to the World Health Organization and the Revised European-American Lymphoma classifications (1,2)] are unique among lymphoid neoplasia in that they lack chromosomal translocations (Table 50.2) (219,220). This important difference may be due to the distinct cell of origin of these tumors. Although B-cell chronic lymphocytic leukemia/small lymphocytic lymphoma has been traditionally viewed as a tumor of naïve, pre–germinal center B cells, approximately 50% of the cases have been shown to harbor mutations of Ig or *BCL6* genes (15,199,219,221–223), which are well-established markers of germinal center transit. Furthermore, gene expression profile analysis of B-cell chronic lymphocytic leukemia has suggested that the cases with mutated and germline Ig genes both derive from memory B cells (224,225). Because the mechanisms that generate chromosomal translocations (Ig gene rearrangements and hypermutation) are no longer active in memory cells, these observations may explain the fact that the genome of B-cell chronic lymphocytic leukemia/small lymphocytic lymphoma is characterized by other types of genetic alterations, including chromosomal deletions, trisomies, and point mutations.

Trisomy 12 is found in approximately 35% of B-cell chronic lymphocytic leukemia/small lymphocytic lymphoma cases evaluated by interphase fluorescent *in situ* hybridization and correlates with a poor survival (220,226). Based on karyotypic and deletion mapping studies, it is likely that the 13q14 chromosomal region harbors a novel tumor suppressor gene that is involved at high frequency in B-cell chronic lymphocytic leukemia/small lymphocytic lymphoma. In fact, deletions of 13q14 occur in approximately 60% of cases when analyzed by sensitive molecular tools, but the relevant gene has not been identified (46,47,220). Deletions of 6q define a subset of B-cell chronic lymphocytic leukemia/small lymphocytic lymphoma cases displaying prolymphocytic features (41,220). Mutations of the *p53* gene and loss of heterozygosity in 17p, the *p53* site, are found in a small fraction (10% to 15%) of cases (38,220). A higher frequency of *p53* alterations is observed after transformation of B-cell chronic lymphocytic leukemia/small lymphocytic lymphoma to Richter's syndrome, a highly aggressive lymphoma with a poor clinical outcome (38), suggesting that *p53* may be involved in the genetic mechanisms underlying B-cell chronic lymphocytic leukemia/small lymphocytic lymphoma progression. Finally, a small fraction of B-cell chronic lymphocytic leukemia/small lymphocytic lymphoma harbors mutations of the *ataxia-telangiectasia mutated* (*ATM*) gene (198,227–229). Because these mutations may occur in the patient germline, *ATM* mutations may account, at least in part, for the familial cases of the disease.

Lymphoplasmacytic Lymphoma

More than one-half of the cases of lymphoplasmacytic lymphoma are associated with the t(9;14)(p13;q32) translocation, a recurrent chromosomal abnormality in B cell non-Hodgkin's lymphoma (Fig. 50.1 and Table 50.1) (230). The chromosomal breakpoints of t(9;14)(p13;q32) involve the IgH locus on chromosome 14q32 and, on chromosome 9p13, a genomic region containing the *PAX5* (paired homeobox-5) gene (231–233). *PAX5* encodes a B-cell specific transcription factor involved in the control of B-cell proliferation and differentiation (234). Presumably, the juxtaposition of *PAX5* to the IgH locus in non-Hodgkin's lymphoma carrying t(9;14)(p13;q32) causes the deregulated expression of the gene, thus contributing to tumor development (231–233). No other genetic lesions have been detected at significant frequency in lymphoplasmacytic lymphoma (Table 50.2).

MOLECULAR PATHOGENESIS OF T-CELL NON-HODGKIN'S LYMPHOMA

Only a few categories of mature T-cell lymphoid malignancies have been investigated in detail at the molecular level. These include Ki-1[+]/CD30[+] anaplastic large-cell lymphoma, adult T-cell leukemia/lymphoma, T-cell prolymphocytic leukemia, and, to a lesser extent, cutaneous T-cell lymphoma (92,93).

T-Cell Anaplastic Large-Cell Lymphoma

Conventional karyotyping analysis of anaplastic large-cell lymphoma cases has shown a unique translocation involving bands 2p23 and 5q35 in a substantial fraction of cases (16). Molecular characterization of the breakpoints revealed that the t(2;5)(p23;q35) translocation causes the fusion of two genes, the nucleophosmin (NPM) gene encoding for a nucle-

olar phosphoprotein on chromosome 5 and the anaplastic lymphoma kinase (ALK) gene encoding for a novel orphan receptor tyrosine kinase on chromosome 2 (235). This fusion generates an 80-kD fusion protein in which the aminoterminal portion of NPM is joined to the entire cytoplasmic catalytic portion of ALK (235). NPM-ALK has been shown to have transforming ability *in vitro* (236,237) and *in vivo* using retroviral mediated gene transfer (238,239). Most recently, targeted expression of NPM-ALK in T lymphocytes induced lymphoid malignancies in mice, demonstrating a direct causative role for NPM-ALK in human lymphoma (240). The fusion of NPM to ALK has two distinct consequences, both of which are important in the oncogenic properties of the fusion protein. First, it leads to the ectopic expression of NPM-ALK in T cells (236). Second, it results in the constitutive activation of ALK activity due to oligomerization mediated by the NPM segment. This activated kinase function, in turn, activates the mitogenic signal transduction pathway through phospholipase Cγ (236,237).

Ten to 20% of ALK[+] anaplastic large-cell lymphomas express ALK fusion proteins other than NPM-ALK (239, 241,242). In these other translocations involving tyrosine kinases, the ALK breakpoints are the same as in the classic (2;5) translocation. Like NPM-ALK, the alternative ALK fusion proteins have functional tyrosine kinase activity (242).

Adult T-Cell Leukemia/Lymphoma

The malignant cells of adult T-cell leukemia/lymphoma are infected by the human T-cell leukemia virus type I retrovirus in 100% of cases (243). The retroviral gene Tax has been shown to have a critical role for the pathogenesis of adult T-cell leukemia/lymphoma. Tax can transform T cells both *in vitro* and in transgenic animals by regulating the expression of cellular genes, including those encoding IL-2 and the IL-2 receptor (243,244). However, based on the observation of the low incidence of adult T-cell leukemia/lymphoma in human T-cell leukemia virus type I–infected patients and the long latency (10 to 30 years) of the disease, it is clear that Tax alone is not sufficient for full-blown malignancy, and additional genetic lesions are required (243). The hypothesis is supported by the observation that p53 is inactivated in 40% of adult T-cell leukemia/lymphoma cases (245).

T-Cell Prolymphocytic Leukemia

T-cell prolymphocytic leukemia is frequently associated with abnormalities of chromosome 11, the most common ones being represented by monosomy 11, partial or terminal deletions of 11q, and unbalanced translocations involving the 11q arm (16). The target gene of these abnormalities has been recently identified as the *ATM* gene, which is also responsible for the hereditary disorder ataxia-telangiectasia (246,247). Although *ATM* is mutated in the germline of ataxia-telangiectasia patients, in cases of T-cell prolymphocytic leukemia, the mutations are of somatic origin (246,247). Mutations of *ATM* in T-cell prolymphocytic leukemia associate with deletion of the second allele and lead to the absence, premature truncation, or alteration of the *ATM* gene product, consistent with the inactivation model of tumor suppressor genes (246,247). The *ATM* gene is involved in cell-cycle regulation and DNA repair, which, in fact, have been shown to be defective in T-cell prolymphocytic leukemia cells (248).

Cutaneous T-Cell Lymphoma

The most frequent known genetic lesion associated with cutaneous T-cell lymphoma is the rearrangement of the NF-κB-2/Lyt-10 gene, which is present in approximately 15% of cases (249,250). The NF-κB-2 gene encodes a component of the NF-κB transcription factor complex, which is involved in regulating cell proliferation, differentiation, activation, and apoptosis in response to a variety of extracellular signals (251,252). In non-Hodgkin's lymphoma, rearrangements cluster within the 3' terminal ankyrin-coding domain of the NF-κB-2 gene, resulting in the generation of a protein truncated at its C terminal, which occasionally is fused to heterologous proteins (249). These alterations convert NF-κB-2 from a repressor to a constitutive transcriptional activator, possibly leading to abnormal expression of genes that enforce proliferation and survival (253).

REFERENCES

1. Burrows PD, Cooper MD. B cell development and differentiation. *Curr Opin Immunol* 1997;9:239–244.
2. Willerford DM, Swat W, Alt FW. Developmental regulation of V(D)J recombination and lymphocyte differentiation. *Curr Opin Genet Dev* 1996;6:603–609.
3. Rajewsky K. Clonal selection and learning in the antibody system. *Nature* 1996;381:751–758.
4. MacLennan IC. Germinal centers. *Annu Rev Immunol* 1994;12:117–139.
5. Wagner SD, Neuberger MS. Somatic hypermutation of immunoglobulin genes. *Annu Rev Immunol* 1996;14:441–457.
6. McHeyzer-Williams LJ, Driver DJ, McHeyzer-Williams MG. Germinal center reaction. *Curr Opin Hematol* 2001;8:52–59.
7. Küppers R, Klein U, Hansmann ML, Rajewsky K. Cellular origin of human B-cell lymphomas. *N Engl J Med* 1999;341:1520–1529.
8. Muller-Hermelink HK, Greiner A. Molecular analysis of human immunoglobulin heavy chain variable genes (IgVH) in normal and malignant B cells. *Am J Pathol* 1998;153:1341–1346.
9. Bahler DW, Levy R. Clonal evolution of a follicular lymphoma: evidence for antigen selection. *Proc Natl Acad Sci U S A* 1992;89:6770–6774.
10. Tamaru J, Hummel M, Marafioti T, et al. Burkitt's lymphomas express VH genes with a moderate number of antigen-selected somatic mutations. *Am J Pathol* 1995;147:1398–1407.
11. Bertoni F, Cazzaniga G, Bosshard G, et al. Immunoglobulin heavy chain diversity genes rearrangement pattern indicates that MALT-type gastric lymphoma B cells have undergone an antigen selection process. *Br J Haematol* 1997;97:830–836.
12. Küppers R, Rajewsky K, Hansmann ML. Diffuse large cell lymphomas are derived from mature B cells carrying V region genes with a high load of somatic mutation and evidence of selection for antibody expression. *Eur J Immunol* 1997;27:1398–1405.
13. Sahota SS, Garand R, Bataille R, et al. VH gene analysis of clonally related IgM and IgG from human lymphoplasmacytoid B-cell tumors with chronic lymphocytic leukemia features and high serum monoclonal IgG. *Blood* 1998;91:238–243.
14. Fais F, Gaidano G, Capello D, et al. Immunoglobulin V region gene use and structure suggest antigen selection in AIDS-related primary effusion lymphomas. *Leukemia* 1999;13:1093–1099.
15. Fais F, Ghiotto F, Hashimoto S, et al. Chronic lymphocytic leukemia B cells express restricted sets of mutated and unmutated antigen receptors. *J Clin Invest* 1998;102:1515–1525.
16. Mitelman F, Mertens F, Johansson B. A breakpoint map of recurrent chromosomal rearrangements in human neoplasia. *Nat Genet* 1997;15:417–474.
17. Bedi GC, Westra WH, Farzadegan H, et al. Microsatellite instability in primary neoplasms from HIV+ patients. *Nat Med* 1995;1:65–68.
18. Eshleman JR, Markowitz SD. Microsatellite instability in inherited and sporadic neoplasms. *Curr Opin Oncol* 1995;7:83–89.
19. Gamberi B, Gaidano G, Parsa N, et al. Lack of microsatellite instability is rare in B-cell non-Hodgkin's lymphomas. *Blood* 1997;89:975–979.
20. Furlan D, Bertoni F, Cerutti R, et al. Microsatellite instability in gastric MALT lymphomas and other associated neoplasms. *Ann Oncol* 1999;10:783–788.
21. Offit K, Wong G, Filippa DA, et al. Cytogenetic analysis of 434 consecutively ascertained specimens of non-Hodgkin's lymphoma: clinical correlations. *Blood* 1991;77:1508–1515.
22. Goossens T, Klein U, Küppers R. Frequent occurrence of deletions and duplications during somatic hypermutation: implications for oncogene translocations and heavy chain disease. *Proc Natl Acad Sci U S A* 1998;95:2463–2468.
23. Küppers R, Dalla-Favera R. Mechanisms of chromosomal translocation in B-cell lymphoma. *Oncogene* 2001.
24. Papavasiliou FN, Schatz DG. Cell-cycle-regulated DNA double-stranded breaks in somatic hypermutation of immunoglobulin genes. *Nature* 2000;408:216–221.
25. Bross L, Fukita Y, McBlane F, et al. DNA double-strand breaks in immunoglobulin genes undergoing somatic hypermutation. *Immunity* 2000;13:589–597.
26. Bross L, Muramatsu M, Kinoshita K, et al. DNA double-strand breaks: prior to but not sufficient in targeting hypermutation. *J Exp Med* 2002;195:1187–1192.
27. Pasqualucci L, Neumeister P, Goossens T, et al. Hypermutation of multiple proto-oncogenes in B-cell diffuse large-cell lymphomas. *Nature* 2001;412:341–346.
28. Klein U, Goossens T, Fischer M, et al. Somatic hypermutation in normal and transformed human B cells. *Immunol Rev* 1998;162:261–280.
29. Pasqualucci L, Migliazza A, Fracchiolla N, et al. BCL-6 mutations in normal germinal center B cells: evidence of somatic hypermutation acting outside Ig loci. *Proc Natl Acad Sci U S A* 1998;95:11816–11821.
30. Shen HM, Peters A, Baron B, et al. Mutation of BCL-6 gene in normal B cells by the process of somatic hypermutation of Ig genes. *Science* 1998;280:1750–1752.
31. Müschen M, Re D, Jungnickel B, et al. Somatic mutation of the CD95 gene in human B cells as a side-effect of the germinal center reaction. *J Exp Med* 2000;192:1833–1840.
32. Gordon MS, Kanegai CM, Doerr JR, Wall R. Somatic hypermutation of the B cell receptor genes B29 (Igbeta, CD79b) and mb1 (Igalpha, CD79a). *Proc Natl Acad Sci U S A* 2003;100:4126–4131.
33. Peng HZ, Du MQ, Koulis A, et al. Nonimmunoglobulin gene hypermutation in germinal center B cells. *Blood* 1999;93:2167–2172.
34. Houldsworth J, Mathew S, Rao PH, et al. REL proto-oncogene is frequently amplified in extranodal diffuse large cell lymphoma. *Blood* 1996;87:25–29.
35. Chaganti RS, Nanjangud G, Schmidt H, Teruya-Feldstein J. Recurring chromosomal abnormalities in non-Hodgkin's lymphoma: biologic and clinical significance. *Semin Hematol* 2000;37:396–411.
36. Neri A, Knowles DM, Greco A, et al. Analysis of RAS oncogene mutations in human lymphoid malignancies. *Proc Natl Acad Sci U S A* 1988;85:9268–9272.
37. Hollstein M, Sidransky D, Vogelstein B, Harris CC. p53 mutations in human cancers. *Science* 1991;253:49–53.
38. Gaidano G, Ballerini P, Gong JZ, et al. p53 mutations in human lymphoid malignancies: association with Burkitt lymphoma and chronic lymphocytic leukemia. *Proc Natl Acad Sci U S A* 1991;88:5413–5417.
39. Ballerini P, Gaidano G, Gong JZ, et al. Multiple genetic lesions in acquired immunodeficiency syndrome-related non-Hodgkin's lymphoma. *Blood* 1993;81:166–176.
40. Lo Coco F, Gaidano G, Louie DC, et al. p53 mutations are associated with histologic transformation of follicular lymphoma. *Blood* 1993;82:2289–2295.

41. Gaidano G, Hauptschein RS, Parsa NZ, et al. Deletions involving two distinct regions of 6q in B-cell non-Hodgkin lymphoma. *Blood* 1992;80:1781–1787.

42. Brown AG, Ross FM, Dunne EM, et al. Evidence for a new tumour suppressor locus (DBM) in human B-cell neoplasia telomeric to the retinoblastoma gene. *Nat Genet* 1993;3:67–72.

43. Devilder MC, Francois S, Bosic C, et al. Deletion cartography around the D13S25 locus in B cell chronic lymphocytic leukemia and accurate mapping of the involved tumor suppressor gene. *Cancer Res* 1995;55:1355–1357.

44. Liu Y, Hermanson M, Grander D, et al. 13q deletions in lymphoid malignancies. *Blood* 1995;86:1911–1915.

45. Garcia-Marco JA, Caldas C, Price CM, et al. Frequent somatic deletion of the 13q12.3 locus encompassing BRCA2 in chronic lymphocytic leukemia. *Blood* 1996;88:1568–1575.

46. Kalachikov S, Migliazza A, Cayanis E, et al. Cloning and gene mapping of the chromosome 13q14 region deleted in chronic lymphocytic leukemia. *Genomics* 1997;42:369–377.

47. Migliazza A, Bosch F, Komatsu H, et al. Nucleotide sequence, transcription map, and mutation analysis of the 13q14 chromosomal region deleted in B-cell chronic lymphocytic leukemia. *Blood* 2001;97:2098–2104.

48. Bullrich F, Veronese ML, Kitada S, et al. Minimal region of loss at 13q14 in B-cell chronic lymphocytic leukemia. *Blood* 1996;88:3109–3115.

49. Drexler HG. Review of alterations of the cyclin-dependent kinase inhibitor INK4 family genes p15, p16, p18 and p19 in human leukemia-lymphoma cells. *Leukemia* 1998;12:845–859.

50. Pinyol M, Cobo F, Bea S, et al. p16(INK4a) gene inactivation by deletions, mutations, and hypermethylation is associated with transformed and aggressive variants of non-Hodgkin's lymphomas. *Blood* 1998;91:2977–2984.

51. Herman JG, Civin CI, Issa JP, et al. Distinct patterns of inactivation of p15INK4B and p16INK4A characterize the major types of hematological malignancies. *Cancer Res* 1997;57:837–841.

52. Martinez-Delgado B, Richart A, Garcia MJ, et al. Hypermethylation of P16ink4a and P15ink4b genes as a marker of disease in the follow-up of non-Hodgkin's lymphomas. *Br J Haematol* 2000;109:97–103.

53. Martinez-Delgado B, Robledo M, Arranz E, et al. Hypermethylation of p15/ink4b/MTS2 gene is differentially implicated among non-Hodgkin's lymphomas. *Leukemia*. 1998;12:937–941.

54. Ferreira OC Jr, Planelles V, Rosenblatt JD. Human T-cell leukemia viruses: epidemiology, biology, and pathogenesis. *Blood Rev* 1997;11:91–104.

55. Uchiyama T. Human T cell leukemia virus type I (HTLV-I) and human diseases. *Annu Rev Immunol* 1997;15:15–37.

56. Yoshida M. Howard Temin Memorial Lectureship. Molecular biology of HTLV-1: deregulation of host cell gene expression and cell cycle. *Leukemia* 1997;11[Suppl 3]:1–2.

57. Inoue J, Seiki M, Taniguchi T, et al. Induction of interleukin 2 receptor gene expression by p40x encoded by human T-cell leukemia virus type 1. *EMBO J* 1986;5:2883–2888.

58. Cross SL, Feinberg MB, Wolf JB, et al. Regulation of the human interleukin-2 receptor alpha chain promoter: activation of a nonfunctional promoter by the transactivator gene of HTLV-I. *Cell* 1987;49:47–56.

59. Fujii M, Sassone-Corsi P, Verma IM. c-fos promoter trans-activation by the tax1 protein of human T-cell leukemia virus type I. *Proc Natl Acad Sci U S A* 1988;85:8526–8530.

60. Wano Y, Feinberg M, Hosking JB, et al. Stable expression of the tax gene of type I human T-cell leukemia virus in human T cells activates specific cellular genes involved in growth. *Proc Natl Acad Sci U S A* 1988;85:9733–9737.

61. Nimer SD, Gasson JC, Hu K, et al. Activation of the GM-CSF promoter by HTLV-I and -II tax proteins. *Oncogene* 1989;4:671–676.

62. Arima N. Autonomous and interleukin-2-responsive growth of leukemic cells in adult T-cell leukemia (ATL): a review of the clinical significance and molecular basis of ATL cell growth. *Leuk Lymphoma* 1997;26:479–487.

63. Uittenbogaard MN, Giebler HA, Reisman D, Nyborg JK. Transcriptional repression of p53 by human T-cell leukemia virus type I Tax protein. *J Biol Chem* 1995;270:28503–28506.

64. Jeang KT, Widen SG, Semmes OJ, Wilson SH. HTLV-I trans-activator protein, tax, is a trans-repressor of the human beta-polymerase gene. *Science* 1990;247:1082–1084.

65. Jin DY, Spencer F, Jeang KT. Human T cell leukemia virus type 1 oncoprotein Tax targets the human mitotic checkpoint protein MAD1. *Cell* 1998;93:81–91.

66. Poiesz BJ, Ruscetti FW, Gazdar AF, et al. Detection and isolation of type C retrovirus particles from fresh and cultured lymphocytes of a patient with cutaneous T-cell lymphoma. *Proc Natl Acad Sci U S A* 1980;77:7415–7419.

67. Kikuchi M, Mitsui T, Takeshita M, et al. Virus associated adult T-cell leukemia (ATL) in Japan: clinical, histological and immunological studies. *Hematol Oncol* 1986;4:67–81.

68. Kieff E, Leibowitz D. Oncogenesis by herpesvirus. In: Weinberg RA, ed. *Oncogenes and the molecular origin of cancer*. Cold Spring Harbor, NY: Cold Spring Harbor Laboratory Press, 1989:259.

69. zur Hausen H, Schulte-Holthausen H, Klein G, et al. EBV DNA in biopsies of Burkitt tumours and anaplastic carcinomas of the nasopharynx. *Nature* 1970;228:1056–1058.

70. Neri A, Barriga F, Inghirami G, et al. Epstein-Barr virus infection precedes clonal expansion in Burkitt's and acquired immunodeficiency syndrome-associated lymphoma. *Blood* 1991;77:1092–1095.

71. Pelicci PG, Knowles DM 2nd, Arlin ZA, et al. Multiple monoclonal B cell expansions and c-myc oncogene rearrangements in acquired immune deficiency syndrome-related lymphoproliferative disorders. Implications for lymphomagenesis. *J Exp Med* 1986;164:2049–2060.

72. Hamilton-Dutoit SJ, Pallesen G. A survey of Epstein-Barr virus gene expression in sporadic non-Hodgkin's lymphomas. Detection of Epstein-Barr virus in a subset of peripheral T-cell lymphomas. *Am J Pathol* 1992;140:1315–1325.

73. Carbone A, Gaidano G, Gloghini A, et al. Differential expression of BCL-6, CD138/syndecan-1, and Epstein-Barr virus-encoded latent membrane protein-1 identifies distinct histogenetic subsets of acquired immunodeficiency syndrome-related non-Hodgkin's lymphomas. *Blood* 1998;91:747–755.

74. Horenstein MG, Nador RG, Chadburn A, et al. Epstein-Barr virus latent gene expression in primary effusion lymphomas containing Kaposi's sarcoma-associated herpesvirus/human herpesvirus-8. *Blood* 1997;90:1186–1191.

75. Larocca LM, Capello D, Rinelli A, et al. The molecular and phenotypic profile of primary central nervous system lymphoma identifies distinct categories of the disease and is consistent with histogenetic derivation from germinal center-related B cells. *Blood* 1998;92:1011–1019.

76. Fassone L, Bhatia K, Gutierrez M, et al. Molecular profile of Epstein-Barr virus infection in HHV-8-positive primary effusion lymphoma. *Leukemia* 2000;14:271–277.

77. Cingolani A, Gastaldi R, Fassone L, et al. Epstein-Barr virus infection is predictive of CNS involvement in systemic AIDS-related non-Hodgkin's lymphomas. *J Clin Oncol* 2000;18:3325–3330.

78. Raab-Traub N, Flynn K. The structure of the termini of the Epstein-Barr virus as a marker of clonal cellular proliferation. *Cell* 1986;47:883–889.

79. Chang Y, Cesarman E, Pessin MS, et al. Identification of herpesvirus-like DNA sequences in AIDS-associated Kaposi's sarcoma. *Science* 1994;266:1865–1869.

80. Cesarman E, Chang Y, Moore PS, et al. Kaposi's sarcoma-associated herpesvirus-like DNA sequences in AIDS-related body-cavity-based lymphomas. *N Engl J Med* 1995;332:1186–1191.

81. Carbone A, Gloghini A, Vaccher E, et al. Kaposi's sarcoma-associated herpesvirus DNA sequences in AIDS-related and AIDS-unrelated lymphomatous effusions. *Br J Haematol* 1996;94:533–543.

82. Gaidano G, Pastore C, Gloghini A, et al. Distribution of human herpesvirus-8 sequences throughout the spectrum of AIDS-related neoplasia. *AIDS* 1996;10:941–949.

83. Carbone A, Gaidano G. HHV-8-positive body-cavity-based lymphoma: a novel lymphoma entity. *Br J Haematol* 1997;97:515–522.

84. Gaidano G, Carbone A. Primary effusion lymphoma: a liquid phase lymphoma of fluid-filled body cavities. *Adv Cancer Res* 2001;80:115–146.

85. Soulier J, Grollet L, Oksenhendler E, et al. Kaposi's sarcoma-associated herpesvirus-like DNA sequences in multicentric Castleman's disease. *Blood* 1995;86:1276–1280.

86. Roizmann B, Desrosiers RC, Fleckenstein B, et al. The family Herpesviridae: an update. The Herpesvirus Study Group of the International Committee on Taxonomy of Viruses. *Arch Virol* 1992;123:425–449.

87. Moore PS, Gao SJ, Dominguez G, et al. Primary characterization of a herpesvirus agent associated with Kaposi's sarcomae. *J Virol* 1996;70:549–558.

88. Chang Y, Moore PS, Talbot SJ, et al. Cyclin encoded by KS herpesvirus. *Nature* 1996;382:410.

89. Moore PS, Boshoff C, Weiss RA, Chang Y. Molecular mimicry of human cytokine and cytokine response pathway genes by KSHV. *Science* 1996;274:1739–1744.

90. Arvanitakis L, Geras-Raaka E, Varma A, et al. Human herpesvirus KSHV encodes a constitutively active G-protein-coupled receptor linked to cell proliferation. *Nature* 1997;385:347–350.

91. Carbone A, Gloghini A, Bontempo D, et al. Proliferation in HHV-8-positive primary effusion lymphomas is associated with expression of HHV-8 cyclin but independent of p27(kip1). *Am J Pathol* 2000;156:1209–1215.

92. Jaffe ES, Harris NL, Stein H, Vardiman JW, eds. *World Health Organization classification of tumors, pathology and genetics of tumors of hematopoietic and lymphoid tissues.* Lyon: IARC Press, 2001.

93. Harris NL, Jaffe ES, Stein H, et al. A revised European-American classification of lymphoid neoplasms: a proposal from the International Lymphoma Study Group. *Blood* 1994;84:1361–1392.

94. Berger F, Felman P, Sonet A, et al. Nonfollicular small B-cell lymphomas: a heterogeneous group of patients with distinct clinical features and outcome. *Blood* 1994;83:2829–2835.

95. Fisher RI, Dahlberg S, Nathwani BN, et al. A clinical analysis of two indolent lymphoma entities: mantle cell lymphoma and marginal zone lymphoma (including the mucosa-associated lymphoid tissue and monocytoid B-cell subcategories): a Southwest Oncology Group study. *Blood* 1995;85:1075–1082.

96. Raffeld M, Jaffe ES. bcl-1, t(11;14), and mantle cell-derived lymphomas. *Blood* 1991;78:259–263.

97. Rimokh R, Berger F, Delsol G, et al. Rearrangement and overexpression of the BCL-1/PRAD-1 gene in intermediate lymphocytic lymphomas and in t(11q13)-bearing leukemias. *Blood* 1993;81:3063–3067.

98. Callanan M, Leroux D, Magaud JP, Rimokh R. Implication of cyclin D1 in malignant lymphoma. *Crit Rev Oncog* 1996;7:191–203.

99. Campo E, Raffeld M, Jaffe ES. Mantle cell lymphoma. *Semin Hematol* 1999;36:115–127.

100. Tsujimoto Y, Yunis J, Onorato-Showe L, et al. Molecular cloning of the chromosomal breakpoint of B-cell lymphomas and leukemias with the t(11;14) chromosome translocation. *Science* 1984;224:1403–1406.

101. Tsujimoto Y, Jaffe E, Cossman J, et al. Clustering of breakpoints on chromosome 11 in human B-cell neoplasms with the t(11;14) chromosome translocation. *Nature* 1985;315:340–343.

102. Erikson J, Finan J, Tsujimoto Y, et al. The chromosome 14 breakpoint in neoplastic B cells with the t(11;14) translocation involves the immunoglobulin heavy chain locus. *Proc Natl Acad Sci U S A* 1984;81:4144–4148.

103. Withers DA, Harvey RC, Faust JB, et al. Characterization of a candidate bcl-1 gene. *Mol Cell Biol* 1991;11:4846–4853.

104. Motokura T, Bloom T, Kim HG, et al. A novel cyclin encoded by a bcl1-linked candidate oncogene. *Nature* 1991;350:512–515.

105. Rosenberg CL, Wong E, Petty EM, et al. PRAD1, a candidate BCL1 oncogene: mapping and expression in centrocytic lymphoma. *Proc Natl Acad Sci U S A* 1991;88:9638–9642.

106. Seto M, Yamamoto K, Iida S, et al. Gene rearrangement and overexpression of PRAD1 in lymphoid malignancy with t(11;14)(q13;q32) translocation. *Oncogene* 1992;7:1401–1406.

107. Murakami MS, Strobel MJ, Vande Woude JF. Cell cycle regulation, oncogenes, and antineoplastic drugs. In: Mendelsohn J, Howley PM, Israel MA, Liotta LA, eds. *The molecular basis of cancer. Vol. 3.* Philadelphia: WB Saunders, 1995.

108. Jiang W, Kahn SM, Zhou P, et al. Overexpression of cyclin D1 in rat fibroblasts causes abnormalities in growth control, cell cycle progression and gene expression. *Oncogene* 1993;8:3447–3457.

109. Bodrug SE, Warner BJ, Bath ML, et al. Cyclin D1 transgene impedes lymphocyte maturation and collaborates in lymphomagenesis with the myc gene. *EMBO J* 1994;13:2124–2130.

110. Lovec H, Grzeschiczek A, Kowalski MB, Moroy T. Cyclin D1/bcl-1 cooperates with myc genes in the generation of B-cell lymphoma in transgenic mice. *EMBO J* 1994;13:3487–3495.

111. Greiner TC, Moynihan MJ, Chan WC, et al. p53 mutations in mantle cell lymphoma are associated with variant cytology and predict a poor prognosis. *Blood* 1996;87:4302–4310.

112. Louie DC, Offit K, Jaslow R, et al. p53 overexpression as a marker of poor prognosis in mantle cell lymphomas with t(11;14)(q13;q32). *Blood* 1995;86:2892–2899.

113. Camacho E, Hernandez L, Hernandez S, et al. ATM gene inactivation in mantle cell lymphoma mainly occurs by truncating mutations and missense mutations involving the phosphatidylinositol-3 kinase domain and is associated with increasing numbers of chromosomal imbalances. *Blood* 2002;99:238–244.

114. Schaffner C, Idler I, Stilgenbauer S, et al. Mantle cell lymphoma is characterized by inactivation of the ATM gene. *Proc Natl Acad Sci U S A* 2000;97:2773–2778.

115. Dalla-Favera R. Chromosomal translocations involving the c-myc oncogene in lymphoid neoplasia. In: Kirsch IR, ed. *The causes and consequences of chromosomal aberrations.* Boca Raton, FL: CRC Press, 1993:312.

116. Dalla-Favera R, Bregni M, Erikson J, et al. Human c-myc onc gene is located on the region of chromosome 8 that is translocated in Burkitt lymphoma cells. *Proc Natl Acad Sci U S A* 1982;79:7824–7827.

117. Dalla-Favera R, Martinotti S, Gallo RC, et al. Translocation and rearrangements of the c-myc oncogene locus in human undifferentiated B-cell lymphomas. *Science* 1983;219:963–967.

118. Taub R, Kirsch I, Morton C, et al. Translocation of the c-myc gene into the immunoglobulin heavy chain locus in human Burkitt lymphoma and murine plasmacytoma cells. *Proc Natl Acad Sci U S A* 1982;79:7837–7841.

119. Davis M, Malcolm S, Rabbitts TH. Chromosome translocation can occur on either side of the c-myc oncogene in Burkitt lymphoma cells. *Nature* 1984;308:286–288.

120. Hollis GF, Mitchell KF, Battey J, et al. A variant translocation places the lambda immunoglobulin genes 3' to the c-myc oncogene in Burkitt's lymphoma. *Nature* 1984;307:752–755.

121. Neri A, Barriga F, Knowles DM, et al. Different regions of the immunoglobulin heavy-chain locus are involved in chromosomal translocations in distinct pathogenetic forms of Burkitt lymphoma. *Proc Natl Acad Sci U S A* 1988;85:2748–2752.

122. Pelicci PG, Knowles DM 2nd, Magrath I, Dalla-Favera R. Chromosomal breakpoints and structural alterations of the c-myc locus differ in endemic and sporadic forms of Burkitt lymphoma. *Proc Natl Acad Sci U S A* 1986;83:2984–2988.

123. Klein U, Tu Y, Stolovitzky GA, et al. Transcriptional analysis of the B cell germinal center reaction. *Proc Natl Acad Sci U S A* 2003;100:2639–2644.

124. Cattoretti G, Mattioli M, Shaknovich R, et al. Lack of c-Myc expression in germinal center B cells: implications for the pathogenesis of GC-derived lymphomas. *Blood.* 2003;100(13)[Supp1]: abstract 567.

125. Cesarman E, Dalla-Favera R, Bentley D, Groudine M. Mutations in the first exon are associated with altered transcription of c-myc in Burkitt lymphoma. *Science* 1987;238:1272–1275.

126. Bhatia K, Huppi K, Spangler G, et al. Point mutations in the c-Myc transactivation domain are common in Burkitt's lymphoma and mouse plasmacytomas. *Nat Genet* 1993;5:56–61.

127. Bhatia K, Spangler G, Gaidano G, et al. Mutations in the coding region of c-myc occur frequently in acquired immunodeficiency syndrome-associated lymphomas. *Blood* 1994;84:883–888.

128. Gu W, Bhatia K, Magrath IT, et al. Binding and suppression of the Myc transcriptional activation domain by p107. *Science* 1994;264:251–254.

129. Gregory MA, Hann SR. c-Myc proteolysis by the ubiquitin-proteasome pathway: stabilization of c-Myc in Burkitt's lymphoma cells. *Mol Cell Biol* 2000;20:2423–2435.

130. Eisenman RN. Deconstructing myc. *Genes Dev* 2001;15:2023–2030.

131. Dang CV. c-Myc target genes involved in cell growth, apoptosis, and metabolism. *Mol Cell Biol* 1999;19:1–11.

132. Lutz W, Leon J, Eilers M. Contributions of Myc to tumorigenesis. *Biochim Biophys Acta* 2002;1602:61–71.

133. Amati B, Dalton S, Brooks MW, et al. Transcriptional activation by the human c-Myc oncoprotein in yeast requires interaction with Max. *Nature* 1992;359:423–426.

134. Amati B, Brooks MW, Levy N, et al. Oncogenic activity of the c-Myc protein requires dimerization with Max. *Cell* 1993;72:233–245.

135. Blackwood EM, Eisenman RN. Max: a helix-loop-helix zipper protein that forms a sequence-specific DNA-binding complex with Myc. *Science* 1991;251:1211–1217.

136. Blackwood EM, Luscher B, Eisenman RN. Myc and Max associate in vivo. *Genes Dev* 1992;6:71–80.

137. Kretzner L, Blackwood EM, Eisenman RN. Myc and Max proteins possess distinct transcriptional activities. *Nature* 1992;359:426–429.

138. Gu W, Cechova K, Tassi V, Dalla-Favera R. Opposite regulation of

gene transcription and cell proliferation by c-Myc and Max. *Proc Natl Acad Sci U S A* 1993;90:2935–2939.

139. Ayer DE, Kretzner L, Eisenman RN. Mad: a heterodimeric partner for Max that antagonizes Myc transcriptional activity. *Cell* 1993;72:211–222.

140. Zervos AS, Gyuris J, Brent R. Mxi1, a protein that specifically interacts with Max to bind Myc-Max recognition sites. *Cell* 1993;72:223–232.

141. Coller HA, Grandori C, Tamayo P, et al. Expression analysis with oligonucleotide microarrays reveals that MYC regulates genes involved in growth, cell cycle, signaling, and adhesion. *Proc Natl Acad Sci U S A* 2000;97:3260–3265.

142. Lombardi L, Newcomb EW, Dalla-Favera R. Pathogenesis of Burkitt lymphoma: expression of an activated c-myc oncogene causes the tumorigenic conversion of EBV-infected human B lymphoblasts. *Cell* 1987;49:161–170.

143. Kovalchuk AL, Qi CF, Torrey TA, et al. Burkitt lymphoma in the mouse. *J Exp Med* 2000;192:1183–1190.

144. Adams JM, Harris AW, Pinkert CA, et al. The c-myc oncogene driven by immunoglobulin enhancers induces lymphoid malignancy in transgenic mice. *Nature* 1985;318:533–538.

145. Klangby U, Okan I, Magnusson KP, et al. p16/INK4a and p15/INK4b gene methylation and absence of p16/INK4a mRNA and protein expression in Burkitt's lymphoma. *Blood* 1998;91:1680–1687.

146. Bakhshi A, Jensen JP, Goldman P, et al. Cloning the chromosomal breakpoint of t(14;18) human lymphomas: clustering around JH on chromosome 14 and near a transcriptional unit on 18. *Cell* 1985;41:899–906.

147. Tsujimoto Y, Finger LR, Yunis J, et al. Cloning of the chromosome breakpoint of neoplastic B cells with the t(14;18) chromosome translocation. *Science* 1984;226:1097–1099.

148. Cleary ML, Galili N, Sklar J. Detection of a second t(14;18) breakpoint cluster region in human follicular lymphomas. *J Exp Med* 1986;164:315–320.

149. Cleary ML, Sklar J. Nucleotide sequence of a t(14;18) chromosomal breakpoint in follicular lymphoma and demonstration of a breakpoint-cluster region near a transcriptionally active locus on chromosome 18. *Proc Natl Acad Sci U S A* 1985;82:7439–7443.

150. Cleary ML, Smith SD, Sklar J. Cloning and structural analysis of cDNAs for bcl-2 and a hybrid bcl-2/immunoglobulin transcript resulting from the t(14;18) translocation. *Cell* 1986;47:19–28.

151. Buchonnet G, Jardin F, Jean N, et al. Distribution of BCL2 breakpoints in follicular lymphoma and correlation with clinical features: specific subtypes or same disease? *Leukemia* 2002;16: 1852–1856.

152. Ngan BY, Chen-Levy Z, Weiss LM, et al. Expression in non-Hodgkin's lymphoma of the bcl-2 protein associated with the t(14;18) chromosomal translocation. *N Engl J Med* 1988;318:1638–1644.

153. Graninger WB, Seto M, Boutain B, et al. Expression of Bcl-2 and Bcl-2-Ig fusion transcripts in normal and neoplastic cells. *J Clin Invest* 1987;80:1512–1515.

154. Hockenbery D, Nunez G, Milliman C, et al. Bcl-2 is an inner mitochondrial membrane protein that blocks programmed cell death. *Nature* 1990;348:334–336.

155. Korsmeyer SJ. Bcl-2 initiates a new category of oncogenes: regulators of cell death. *Blood* 1992;80:879–886.

156. Nunez G, Seto M, Seremetis S, et al. Growth- and tumor-promoting effects of deregulated BCL2 in human B-lymphoblastoid cells. *Proc Natl Acad Sci U S A* 1989;86:4589–4593.

157. Chao DT, Korsmeyer SJ. BCL-2 family: regulators of cell death. *Annu Rev Immunol* 1998;16:395–419.

158. Vaux DL, Cory S, Adams JM. Bcl-2 gene promotes haemopoietic cell survival and cooperates with c-myc to immortalize pre-B cells. *Nature* 1988;335:440–442.

159. Nunez G, Hockenbery D, McDonnell TJ, et al. Bcl-2 maintains B cell memory. *Nature* 1991;353:71–73.

160. Smith KG, Light A, O'Reilly LA, et al. bcl-2 transgene expression inhibits apoptosis in the germinal center and reveals differences in the selection of memory B cells and bone marrow antibody-forming cells. *J Exp Med* 2000;191:475–484.

161. McDonnell TJ, Deane N, Platt FM, et al. bcl-2-immunoglobulin transgenic mice demonstrate extended B cell survival and follicular lymphoproliferation. *Cell* 1989;57:79–88.

162. McDonnel TJ, Nunez G, Platt FM, et al. Deregulated Bcl-2-immunoglobulin transgene expands a resting but responsive immunoglobulin M and D-expressing B-cell population. *Mol Cell Biol* 1990;5:1901–1907.

163. McDonnell TJ, Korsmeyer SJ. Progression from lymphoid hyperpla-

sia to high-grade malignant lymphoma in mice transgenic for the t(14; 18). *Nature* 1991;349:254–256.

164. Capello D, Vitolo U, Pasqualucci L, et al. Distribution and pattern of BCL-6 mutations throughout the spectrum of B-cell neoplasia. *Blood* 2000;95:651–659.

165. Yano T, Jaffe ES, Longo DL, Raffeld M. MYC rearrangements in histologically progressed follicular lymphomas. *Blood* 1992;80:758–767.

166. Dalla-Favera R, Gaidano G. Molecular biology of lymphomas. In: DeVita VT, Hellman S, Rosenberg SA, eds. *Cancer. Principles and practice of oncology*. Philadelphia: Lippincott Williams & Wilkins, 2001:2215–2235.

167. Alizadeh AA, Eisen MB, Davis RE, et al. Distinct types of diffuse large B-cell lymphoma identified by gene expression profiling. *Nature* 2000;403:503–511.

168. Shipp MA, Ross KN, Tamayo P, et al. Diffuse large B-cell lymphoma outcome prediction by gene-expression profiling and supervised machine learning. *Nat Med* 2002;8:68–74.

169. Offit K, Jhanwar S, Ebrahim SA, et al. t(3;22)(q27;q11): a novel translocation associated with diffuse non-Hodgkin's lymphoma. *Blood* 1989;74:1876–1879.

170. Baron BW, Nucifora G, McCabe N, et al. Identification of the gene associated with the recurring chromosomal translocations t(3;14)(q27;q32) and t(3;22)(q27;q11) in B-cell lymphomas. *Proc Natl Acad Sci U S A* 1993;90:5262–5266.

171. Kerckaert JP, Deweindt C, Tilly H, et al. LAZ3, a novel zinc-finger encoding gene, is disrupted by recurring chromosome 3q27 translocations in human lymphomas. *Nat Genet* 1993;5:66–70.

172. Ye BH, Lista F, Lo Coco F, et al. Alterations of a zinc finger-encoding gene, BCL-6, in diffuse large-cell lymphoma. *Science* 1993;262:747–750.

173. Ye BH, Rao PH, Chaganti RS, Dalla-Favera R. Cloning of bcl-6, the locus involved in chromosome translocations affecting band 3q27 in B-cell lymphoma. *Cancer Res* 1993;53:2732–2735.

174. Miki T, Kawamata N, Arai A, et al. Molecular cloning of the breakpoint for 3q27 translocation in B-cell lymphomas and leukemias. *Blood* 1994;83:217–222.

175. Zollman S, Godt D, Prive GG, et al. The BTB domain, found primarily in zinc finger proteins, defines an evolutionarily conserved family that includes several developmentally regulated genes in *Drosophila*. *Proc Natl Acad Sci U S A* 1994;91:10717–10721.

176. Chang CC, Ye BH, Chaganti RS, Dalla-Favera R. BCL-6, a POZ/zinc-finger protein, is a sequence-specific transcriptional repressor. *Proc Natl Acad Sci U S A* 1996;93:6947–6952.

177. Dalla-Favera R, Migliazza A, Chang CC, et al. Molecular pathogenesis of B cell malignancy: the role of BCL-6. *Curr Top Microbiol Immunol* 1999;246:257–263.

178. Cattoretti G, Chang CC, Cechova K, et al. BCL-6 protein is expressed in germinal-center B cells. *Blood* 1995;86:45–53.

179. Allman D, Jain A, Dent A, et al. BCL-6 expression during B-cell activation. *Blood* 1996;87:5257–5268.

180. Ye BH, Cattoretti G, Shen Q, et al. The BCL-6 proto-oncogene controls germinal-centre formation and Th2-type inflammation. *Nat Genet* 1997;16:161–170.

181. Dent AL, Shaffer AL, Yu X, et al. Control of inflammation, cytokine expression, and germinal center formation by BCL-6. *Science* 1997; 276:589–592.

182. Shaffer AL, Yu X, He Y, et al. BCL-6 represses genes that function in lymphocyte differentiation, inflammation, and cell cycle control. *Immunity* 2000;13:199–212.

183. Baron BW, Anastasi J, Thirman MJ, et al. The human programmed cell death-2 (PDCD2) gene is a target of BCL6 repression: implications for a role of BCL6 in the down-regulation of apoptosis. *Proc Natl Acad Sci U S A* 2002;99:2860–2865.

184. Niu H, Cattoretti G, Dalla-Favera R. BCL6 controls the expression of the B7-1/CD80 costimulatory receptor in germinal center B cells. *J Exp Med*. 2003;198:211.

185. Lo Coco F, Ye BH, Lista F, et al. Rearrangements of the BCL6 gene in diffuse large cell non-Hodgkin's lymphoma. *Blood* 1994;83:1757–1759.

186. Yoshida S, Kaneita Y, Aoki Y, et al. Identification of heterologous translocation partner genes fused to the BCL6 gene in diffuse large B-cell lymphomas: 5'-RACE and LA-PCR analyses of biopsy samples. *Oncogene* 1999;18:7994–7999.

187. Akasaka T, Ohno H, Mori T, Okuma M. Long distance polymerase chain reaction for detection of chromosome translocations in B-cell lymphoma/leukemia. *Leukemia* 1997;11[Suppl 3]:316–317.

188. Dallery E, Galiegue-Zouitina S, Collyn-d'Hooghe M, et al. TTF, a gene encoding a novel small G protein, fuses to the lymphoma-associated LAZ3 gene by t(3;4) chromosomal translocation. *Oncogene* 1995;10:2171–2178.

189. Galieque Zouitina S, Quief S, Hildebrand MP. The B cell transcriptional coactivator BOB1/OBF1 gene fuses to the LAZ3/BCL6 gene by t(3;11)(q27;q23.1) chromosomal translocation in a B cell leukemia line (Karpas 231). *Leukemia* 1996;10:579–587.

190. Galiegue-Zouitina S, Quief S, Hildebrand MP, et al. Nonrandom fusion of L-plastin(LCP1) and LAZ3(BCL6) genes by t(3;13)(q27;q14) chromosome translocation in two cases of B-cell non-Hodgkin lymphoma. *Genes Chromosomes Cancer* 1999;26:97–105.

191. Kurata M, Maesako Y, Ueda C, et al. Characterization of t(3;6)(q27;p21) breakpoints in B-cell non-Hodgkin's lymphoma and construction of the histone H4/BCL6 fusion gene, leading to altered expression of Bcl-6. *Cancer Res* 2002;62:6224–6230.

192. Akasaka T, Miura I, Takahashi N, et al. A recurring translocation, t(3;6)(q27;p21), in non-Hodgkin's lymphoma results in replacement of the 5' regulatory region of BCL6 with a novel H4 histone gene. *Cancer Res* 1997;57:7–12.

193. Hosokawa Y, Maeda Y, Ichinohasama R, et al. The Ikaros gene, a central regulator of lymphoid differentiation, fuses to the BCL6 gene as a result of t(3;7)(q27;p12) translocation in a patient with diffuse large B-cell lymphoma. *Blood* 2000;95:2719–2721.

194. Xu WS, Liang RH, Srivastava G. Identification and characterization of BCL6 translocation partner genes in primary gastric high-grade B-cell lymphoma: heat shock protein 89 alpha is a novel fusion partner gene of BCL6. *Genes Chromosomes Cancer* 2000;27:69–75.

195. Chen W, Iida S, Louie DC, et al. Heterologous promoters fused to BCL6 by chromosomal translocations affecting band 3q27 cause its deregulated expression during B-cell differentiation. *Blood* 1998;91:603–607.

196. Ye BH, Chaganti S, Chang CC, et al. Chromosomal translocations cause deregulated BCL6 expression by promoter substitution in B cell lymphoma. *EMBO J* 1995;14:6209–6217.

197. Migliazza A, Martinotti S, Chen W, et al. Frequent somatic hypermutation of the 5' noncoding region of the BCL6 gene in B-cell lymphoma. *Proc Natl Acad Sci U S A* 1995;92:12520–12524.

198. Capello D, Carbone A, Pastore C, et al. Point mutations of the BCL-6 gene in Burkitt's lymphoma. *Br J Haematol* 1997;99:168–170.

199. Pasqualucci L, Neri A, Baldini L, et al. BCL-6 mutations are associated with immunoglobulin variable heavy chain mutations in B-cell chronic lymphocytic leukemia. *Cancer Res* 2000;60:5644–5648.

200. Pasqualucci L, Migliazza A, Basso K, et al. Mutations of the BCL6 proto-oncogene disrupt its negative autoregulation in diffuse large B-cell lymphoma. *Blood* 2003;101:2914–2923.

201. Wang X, Li Z, Naganuma A, Ye BH. Negative autoregulation of BCL-6 is bypassed by genetic alterations in diffuse large B cell lymphomas. *Proc Natl Acad Sci U S A* 2002;99:15018–15023.

202. Rao PH, Houldsworth J, Dyomina K, et al. Chromosomal and gene amplification in diffuse large B-cell lymphoma. *Blood* 1998;92:234–240.

203. Gronbaek K, Worm J, Ralfkiaer E, et al. ATM mutations are associated with inactivation of the ARF-TP53 tumor suppressor pathway in diffuse large B-cell lymphoma. *Blood* 2002;100:1430–1437.

204. Bai M, Vlachonikolis J, Agnantis NJ, et al. Low expression of p27 protein combined with altered p53 and Rb/p16 expression status is associated with increased expression of cyclin A and cyclin B1 in diffuse large B-cell lymphomas. *Mod Pathol* 2001;14:1105–1113.

205. Parsonnet J, Hansen S, Rodriguez L, et al. *Helicobacter pylori* infection and gastric lymphoma. *N Engl J Med* 1994;330:1267–1271.

206. Wotherspoon AC, Doglioni C, Diss TC, et al. Regression of primary low-grade B-cell gastric lymphoma of mucosa-associated lymphoid tissue type after eradication of Helicobacter pylori. *Lancet* 1993;342:575–577.

207. Qin Y, Greiner A, Trunk MJ, et al. Somatic hypermutation in low-grade mucosa-associated lymphoid tissue-type B-cell lymphoma. *Blood* 1995;86:3528–3534.

208. Thiede C, Alpen B, Morgner A, et al. Ongoing somatic mutations and clonal expansions after cure of *Helicobacter pylori* infection in gastric mucosa-associated lymphoid tissue B-cell lymphoma. *J Clin Oncol* 1998;16:3822–3831.

209. Hallas C, Greiner A, Peters K, Muller-Hermelink HK. Immunoglobulin VH genes of high-grade mucosa-associated lymphoid tissue lymphomas show a high load of somatic mutations and evidence of antigen-dependent affinity maturation. *Lab Invest* 1998;78:277–287.

210. Lucas PC, Yonezumi M, Inohara N, et al. Bcl10 and MALT1, independent targets of chromosomal translocation in malt lymphoma, cooperate in a novel NF-kappa B signaling pathway. *J Biol Chem* 2001;276:19012–19019.

211. Dierlamm J, Baens M, Wlodarska I, et al. The apoptosis inhibitor gene API2 and a novel 18q gene, MLT, are recurrently rearranged in the t(11;18)(q21;q21)p6 associated with mucosa-associated lymphoid tissue lymphomas. *Blood* 1999;93:3601–3609.

212. Akagi T, Motegi M, Tamura A, et al. A novel gene, MALT1 at 18q21, is involved in t(11;18) (q21;q21) found in low-grade B-cell lymphoma of mucosa-associated lymphoid tissue. *Oncogene* 1999;18:5785–5794.

213. Willis TG, Jadayel DM, Du MQ, et al. Bcl10 is involved in t(1;14)(p22;q32) of MALT B cell lymphoma and mutated in multiple tumor types. *Cell* 1999;96:35–45.

214. Zhang Q, Siebert R, Yan M, et al. Inactivating mutations and overexpression of BCL10, a caspase recruitment domain-containing gene, in MALT lymphoma with t(1;14)(p22;q32). *Nat Genet* 1999;22:63–68.

215. Ott G, Kalla J, Steinhoff A, et al. Trisomy 3 is not a common feature in malignant lymphomas of mucosa-associated lymphoid tissue type. *Am J Pathol* 1998;153:689–694.

216. Du M, Peng H, Singh N, et al. The accumulation of p53 abnormalities is associated with progression of mucosa-associated lymphoid tissue lymphoma. *Blood* 1995;86:4587–4593.

217. Gaidano G, Volpe G, Pastore C, et al. Detection of BCL-6 rearrangements and p53 mutations in MALT-lymphomas. *Am J Hematol* 1997;56:206–213.

218. Gaidano G, Carbone A, Pastore C, et al. Frequent mutation of the 5' noncoding region of the BCL-6 gene in acquired immunodeficiency syndrome-related non-Hodgkin's lymphomas. *Blood* 1997;89:3755–3762.

219. Dohner H, Stilgenbauer S, Dohner K, et al. Chromosome aberrations in B-cell chronic lymphocytic leukemia: reassessment based on molecular cytogenetic analysis. *J Mol Med* 1999;77:266–281.

220. Stilgenbauer S, Bullinger L, Lichter P, Dohner H. Genetics of chronic lymphocytic leukemia: genomic aberrations and V(H) gene mutation status in pathogenesis and clinical course. *Leukemia* 2002;16:993–1007.

221. Oscier DG, Thompsett A, Zhu D, Stevenson FK. Differential rates of somatic hypermutation in V(H) genes among subsets of chronic lymphocytic leukemia defined by chromosomal abnormalities. *Blood* 1997;89:4153–4160.

222. Schroeder HW Jr, Dighiero G. The pathogenesis of chronic lymphocytic leukemia: analysis of the antibody repertoire. *Immunol Today* 1994;15:288–294.

223. Stevenson F, Sahota S, Zhu D, et al. Insight into the origin and clonal history of B-cell tumors as revealed by analysis of immunoglobulin variable region genes. *Immunol Rev* 1998;162:247–259.

224. Rosenwald A, Alizadeh AA, Widhopf G, et al. Relation of gene expression phenotype to immunoglobulin mutation genotype in B cell chronic lymphocytic leukemia. *J Exp Med* 2001;194:1639–1647.

225. Klein U, Tu Y, Stolovitzky GA, et al. Gene expression profiling of B cell chronic lymphocytic leukemia reveals a homogeneous phenotype related to memory B cells. *J Exp Med* 2001;194:1625–1638.

226. Navarro B, Garcia-Marco JA, Jones D, et al. Association and clonal distribution of trisomy 12 and 13q14 deletions in chronic lymphocytic leukaemia. *Br J Haematol* 1998;102:1330–1334.

227. Bullrich F, Rasio D, Kitada S, et al. ATM mutations in B-cell chronic lymphocytic leukemia. *Cancer Res* 1999;59:24–27.

228. Stankovic T, Weber P, Stewart G, et al. Inactivation of ataxia telangiectasia mutated gene in B-cell chronic lymphocytic leukaemia. *Lancet* 1999;353:26–29.

229. Starostik P, Manshouri T, O'Brien S, et al. Deficiency of the ATM protein expression defines an aggressive subgroup of B-cell chronic lymphocytic leukemia. *Cancer Res* 1998;58:4552–4557.

230. Offit K, Parsa NZ, Filippa D, et al. t(9;14)(p13;q32) denotes a subset of low-grade non-Hodgkin's lymphoma with plasmacytoid differentiation. *Blood* 1992;80:2594–2599.

231. Busslinger M, Klix N, Pfeffer P, et al. Deregulation of PAX-5 by translocation of the Emu enhancer of the IgH locus adjacent to two alternative PAX-5 promoters in a diffuse large-cell lymphoma. *Proc Natl Acad Sci U S A* 1996;93:6129–6134.

232. Iida S, Rao PH, Ueda R, et al. Chromosomal rearrangement of the

PAX-5 locus in lymphoplasmacytic lymphoma with t(9;14)(p13;q32). *Leuk Lymphoma* 1999;34:25–33.

233. Iida S, Rao PH, Nallasivam P, et al. The t(9;14)(p13;q32) chromosomal translocation associated with lymphoplasmacytoid lymphoma involves the PAX-5 gene. *Blood* 1996;88:4110–4117.

234. Morrison AM, Nutt SL, Thevenin C, et al. Loss- and gain-of-function mutations reveal an important role of BSAP (Pax-5) at the start and end of B cell differentiation. *Semin Immunol* 1998;10:133–142.

235. Morris SW, Kirstein MN, Valentine MB, et al. Fusion of a kinase gene, ALK, to a nucleolar protein gene, NPM, in non-Hodgkin's lymphoma. *Science* 1994;263:1281–1284.

236. Bischof D, Pulford K, Mason DY, Morris SW. Role of the nucleophosmin (NPM) portion of the non-Hodgkin's lymphoma-associated NPM-anaplastic lymphoma kinase fusion protein in oncogenesis. *Mol Cell Biol* 1997;17:2312–2325.

237. Bai RY, Dieter P, Peschel C, et al. Nucleophosmin-anaplastic lymphoma kinase of large-cell anaplastic lymphoma is a constitutively active tyrosine kinase that utilizes phospholipase C-gamma to mediate its mitogenicity. *Mol Cell Biol* 1998;18:6951–6961.

238. Lange K, Uckert W, Blankenstein T, et al. Overexpression of NPM-ALK induces different types of malignant lymphomas in IL-9 transgenic mice. *Oncogene* 2003;22:517–527.

239. Kuefer MU, Look AT, Pulford K, et al. Retrovirus-mediated gene transfer of NPM-ALK causes lymphoid malignancy in mice. *Blood* 1997;90:2901–2910.

240. Chiarle R, Gong JZ, Guasparri I, et al. NPM-ALK transgenic mice spontaneously develop T-cell lymphomas and plasma cell tumors. *Blood* 2003;101:1919–1927.

241. Falini B, Pulford K, Pucciarini A, et al. Lymphomas expressing ALK fusion protein(s) other than NPM-ALK. *Blood* 1999;94:3509–3515.

242. Hernandez L, Pinyol M, Hernandez S, et al. TRK-fused gene (TFG) is a new partner of ALK in anaplastic large cell lymphoma producing two structurally different TFG-ALK translocations. *Blood* 1999;94:3265–3268.

243. Smith MR, Greene WC. Molecular biology of the type I human T-cell leukemia virus (HTLV-I) and adult T-cell leukemia. *J Clin Invest* 1991;87:761–766.

244. Bex F, Gaynor RB. Regulation of gene expression by HTLV-I Tax protein. *Methods* 1998;16:83–94.

245. Cesarman E, Chadburn A, Inghirami G, et al. Structural and functional analysis of oncogenes and tumor suppressor genes in adult T-cell leukemia/lymphoma shows frequent p53 mutations. *Blood* 1992;80:3205–3216.

246. Vorechovsky I, Luo L, Dyer MJ, et al. Clustering of missense mutations in the ataxia-telangiectasia gene in a sporadic T-cell leukaemia. *Nat Genet* 1997;17:96–99.

247. Stilgenbauer S, Schaffner C, Litterst A, et al. Biallelic mutations in the ATM gene in T-prolymphocytic leukemia. *Nat Med* 1997;3:1155–1159.

248. Westphal CH. Cell-cycle signaling: Atm displays its many talents. *Curr Biol* 1997;7:R789–R792.

249. Neri A, Chang CC, Lombardi L, et al. B cell lymphoma-associated chromosomal translocation involves candidate oncogene lyt-10, homologous to NF-kappa B p50. *Cell* 1991;67:1075–1087.

250. Neri A, Fracchiolla NS, Roscetti E, et al. Molecular analysis of cutaneous B- and T-cell lymphomas. *Blood* 1995;86:3160–3172.

251. Siebenlist U, Franzoso G, Brown K. Structure, regulation and function of NF-kappa B. *Annu Rev Cell Biol* 1994;10:405–455.

252. de Martin R, Schmid JA, Hofer-Warbinek R. The NF-kappaB/Rel family of transcription factors in oncogenic transformation and apoptosis. *Mutat Res* 1999;437:231–243.

253. Chang CC, Zhang J, Lombardi L, et al. Rearranged NFKB-2 genes in lymphoid neoplasms code for constitutively active nuclear transactivators. *Mol Cell Biol* 1995;15:5180–5187.

Index

Page numbers followed by *f* indicate figures; numbers followed by *t* indicate tables.

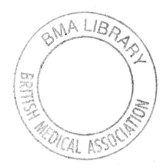